PATHOLOGY OF THE FEMALE REPRODUCTIVE TRACT

Content Strategist: Michael Houston
Content Development Specialist: Martin Mellor Publishing Services Ltd
Project Manager: Lucía Pérez
Design: Ellen Zanolle
Illustration Manager: Jennifer Rose
Illustrator: Richard Tibbitts, Antbits Ltd

PATHOLOGY OF THE FEMALE REPRODUCTIVE TRACT

George L. Mutter MD
Professor of Pathology
Harvard Medical School
Division of Women's and Perinatal Pathology
Brigham and Women's Hospital
Boston, MA, USA

Jaime Prat MD, PhD, FRCPath
Professor and Chairman of Pathology
Hospital de la Santa Creu i Sant Pau
Autonomous University of Barcelona
Barcelona, Spain

For additional online content visit expertconsult.com

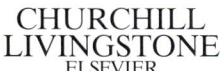

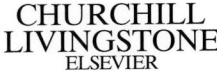

© 2014, Elsevier Limited. All rights reserved.

First edition 2002
Second edition 2009

The right of George L. Mutter and Jaime Prat to be identified as author of this work has been asserted by them in accordance with the Copyright, Designs and Patents Act 1988.

No part of this publication may be reproduced or transmitted in any form or by any means, electronic or mechanical, including photocopying, recording, or any information storage and retrieval system, without permission in writing from the publisher. Details on how to seek permission, further information about the Publisher's permissions policies and our arrangements with organizations such as the Copyright Clearance Center and the Copyright Licensing Agency, can be found at our website: www.elsevier.com/permissions.

This book and the individual contributions contained in it are protected under copyright by the Publisher (other than as may be noted herein).

Notices
Knowledge and best practice in this field are constantly changing. As new research and experience broaden our understanding, changes in research methods, professional practices, or medical treatment may become necessary.

Practitioners and researchers must always rely on their own experience and knowledge in evaluating and using any information, methods, compounds, or experiments described herein. In using such information or methods they should be mindful of their own safety and the safety of others, including parties for whom they have a professional responsibility.

With respect to any drug or pharmaceutical products identified, readers are advised to check the most current information provided (i) on procedures featured or (ii) by the manufacturer of each product to be administered, to verify the recommended dose or formula, the method and duration of administration, and contraindications. It is the responsibility of practitioners, relying on their own experience and knowledge of their patients, to make diagnoses, to determine dosages and the best treatment for each individual patient, and to take all appropriate safety precautions.

To the fullest extent of the law, neither the Publisher nor the authors, contributors, or editors, assume any liability for any injury and/or damage to persons or property as a matter of products liability, negligence or otherwise, or from any use or operation of any methods, products, instructions, or ideas contained in the material herein.

ISBN: 9780702044977
e-book ISBN: 9780702055447

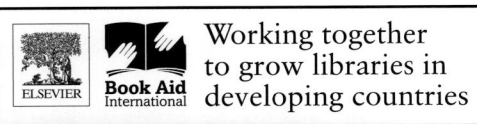

Printed in China

Contents

Extended Table of Contents   vii
Preface   xxiii
List of Contributors   xxv
Acknowledgements   xxix

1. Embryology   1
   George L. Mutter, Stanley J. Robboy

2. Disorders of Sexual Development   18
   Stanley J. Robboy, George L. Mutter

3. Vulvar Dermatoses and Infections   48
   M. Angelica Selim, Mai P. Hoang, Bruce R. Smoller, Christopher R. Shea

4. Vulvar Squamous Lesions   79
   Demaretta S. Rush, Edward J. Wilkinson

5. Vulvar Cysts, Adenocarcinoma, Melanocytic, and Miscellaneous Lesions   95
   Victor G. Prieto, M. Angelica Selim

6. Vulvar Mesenchymal Neoplasms and Tumor-Like Conditions   116
   Marisa R. Nucci, Cristopher D.M. Fletcher

7. Vagina   132
   Sarah Bean, Jaime Prat, Stanley J. Robboy

8. Cervical Benign and Non-Neoplastic Conditions   160
   Anais Malpica

9. Biology of Cervical Squamous Neoplasia   188
   Cornelia L. Trimble, Rachel Katzenellenbogen

10. Cervical Squamous Intraepithelial Lesions   200
    C. Simon Herrington, Jan P.A. Baak, George L. Mutter

11. Cervical Squamous Cell Carcinoma   232
    Thomas C. Wright, Jr.

12. Cervical Glandular Neoplasia   251
    Emanuela D'Angelo, Jaime Prat

13. Miscellaneous Cervical Neoplasms   275
    Anais Malpica

14. The Normal Endometrium   290
    Rex C. Bentley, George L. Mutter, Stanley J. Robboy

15. Exogenous Hormones and their Effects on the Endometrium   310
    Rex C. Bentley

16. Endometritis, Metaplasias, Polyps, and Miscellaneous Changes   326
    George L. Mutter, Joseph W. Carlson

17. Endometrial Hyperplasia without Atypia and EIN   349
    George L. Mutter

18. Endometrial Adenocarcinoma   370
    George L. Mutter, Jaime Prat

19. Uterine Smooth Muscle Tumors   402
    Emanuela D'Angelo, Bradley J. Quade, Jaime Prat

20. Endometrial Stromal Tumors, Mixed Müllerian Tumors, Adenomyosis, Adenomyomas and Rare Sarcomas   425
    Esther Oliva

21. Fallopian Tube   459
    Elke A. Jarboe

22. Endometriosis   487
    George L. Mutter

23. Normal Ovaries, Inflammatory and Non-Neoplastic Conditions   509
    Ruthy Shaco-Levy, Stanley J. Robboy

24. Non-Neoplastic and Tumor-Like Conditions of the Ovary   535
    Emanuela F. Veras, Jennifer H. Crow, Stanley J. Robboy

25. Ovarian Epithelial-Stromal Tumors. Serous Tumors   564
    Jaime Prat, Elke Jarboe

26. Ovarian Mucinous Tumors   591
    Jaime Prat

27. Ovarian Endometrioid, Clear Cell, Transitional, and Mixed Epithelial–Stromal Tumors   608
    Jaime Prat

#	Chapter	Page
28	Ovarian Sex Cord–Stromal and Steroid Cell Tumors *Jaime Prat*	642
29	Ovarian Germ Cell Tumors *Jaime Prat*	670
30	Metastatic Tumors of the Ovary *Emanuela D'Angelo, Jaime Prat*	694
31	The Peritoneum *Emanuela D'Angelo, Jaime Prat*	716
32	Implantation and Placenta *Eoghan E. Mooney*	741
33	Non-Neoplastic Maternal Gestational Diseases *Eoghan E. Mooney, Emma M. Doyle*	769
34	Gestational Trophoblastic Disease *Kyu-Rae Kim*	784
35	Gross Description and Processing of Specimens *Brooke Howitt, George L. Mutter*	812
36	Practical Biomarkers for Female Genital Tract Lesions *W. Glenn McCluggage*	828
APPENDIX A	FIGO Staging of Cancers of the Female Genital Tract *George L. Mutter, Jaime Prat*	846
APPENDIX B	Online Resources *George L. Mutter*	850
Index		855

Extended Table of Contents

1 EMBRYOLOGY
GEORGE L. MUTTER, STANLEY J. ROBBOY

Introduction	1
Gonadal Development	1
Role of Germ Cells	11
Müllerian and Wolffian Duct Development	11
The Müllerian Duct to Week 8	11
External Influence on the Developing Embryonic Genital Tract Ducts	12
The Müllerian Duct after Week 8	14
The Müllerian Duct during the Second Trimester	14
External Genitalia	15

2 DISORDERS OF SEXUAL DEVELOPMENT
STANLEY J. ROBBOY, GEORGE L. MUTTER

Disorders of Genital Differentiation (Disorders Generally Associated with a Normal Chromosome Constitution and Normal Gonad)	18
Female Pseudohermaphroditism (Female Intersex)	18
Fetal Defects	18
Maternal Influence	22
Male Pseudohermaphroditism (Male Intersex)	22
Primary Gonadal Defects	22
End-Organ Defects	25
Disorders of Sex Determination (Disorders Associated with Abnormal Sex Chromosomes and Abnormal Gonadal Formation)	30
Sexual Ambiguity Infrequent	31
Klinefelter Syndrome	31
Turner Syndrome	32
XX Male (Sex Reversal)	35
Pure Gonadal Dysgenesis	35
Defect in the Wilms' Tumor Suppressor (*WT1*) Gene	36
Sexual Ambiguity Frequent	36
46,XY Disorders of Sex Development (Mixed Gonadal Dysgenesis)	36
Gonadoblastoma	40
XY Female (Sex Reversal)	42
True Hermaphroditism	43

3 VULVAR DERMATOSES AND INFECTIONS
M. ANGELICA SELIM, MAI P. HOANG, BRUCE R. SMOLLER, CHRISTOPHER R. SHEA

Introduction	48
Common Dermatoses Affecting the Vulva	49
Spongiotic Dermatitis (Eczemas)	49
General Clinical and Pathologic Features of Spongiotic Dermatitis	49
Clinical Patterns of Vulvar Spongiotic Dermatitis	49
Hints on Histopathologic Interpretation of Vulvar Spongiotic Dermatitis	54
Chronic Dermatitides	54
Lichen Simplex Chronicus (Formerly Squamous Cell Hyperplasia or Hyperplastic Dystrophy)	54
Psoriasis	54
Less Common Dermatoses that Frequently Involve the Vulva	55
Lichenoid Dermatoses	55
Lichen Sclerosus	55
Lichen Planus	57
Bullous Disorders	58
Pemphigus Vulgaris	58
Pemphigus Vegetans	60
Bullous Pemphigoid and Cicatricial Pemphigoid	61
Chronic Bullous Dermatosis of Childhood and Adult Linear IgA Bullous Dermatosis	61
Inherited Dermatoses	61
Hailey–Hailey Disease	61
Epidermolysis Bullosa	62
Darier Disease (Keratosis Follicularis)	62
Warty Dyskeratoma	62
Other Inflammatory Diseases Affecting the Vulva	63
Plasma Cell Vulvitis (Vulvitis of Zoon)	63
Erythema Multiforme and Stevens–Johnson Syndrome	63
Behçet Disease	63
Crohn Disease	64
Hidradenitis Suppurativa	64
Vulvar Pain Syndromes	65
Vulvar Vestibulitis	65
Dysesthetic Vulvodynia	65

Pigmentary Alterations	65
Hyperpigmentation	65
Hyperpigmentation Due to Melanin in Vulvar Skin	65
Hyperpigmentation Due to Increased Keratin in Stratum Corneum	65
Hypopigmentation	66
Postinflammatory Hypopigmentation (Leukoderma)	66
Vitiligo	66
Drugs	66
Fixed Drug Eruptions (Dermatitis Medicamentosa)	66
Vulvar Infections and Infestations	67
Bacterial Infections	67
Staphylococcal Infections	67
Streptococcal Infections (Necrotizing Fasciitis)	67
Syphilis	67
Gonorrhea	68
Chancroid	69
Chlamydial Infection (Lymphogranuloma Venereum)	69
Granuloma Inguinale (Donovanosis)	69
Fungal Infections	69
Candidiasis	69
Pityriasis Versicolor	69
Tinea Cruris	70
Viral Infections	70
Herpes Virus Infection	70
Varicella Zoster Virus Infection (Vulvar Shingles)	71
Other Virus Infections	71
Molluscum Contagiosum	71
Human Papillomavirus Infections	72
Protozoal Infections	73
Trichomoniasis	73
Infestations	73
Scabies	73
Pubic (Crab) Lice (*Phthirus pubis*)	74
Glossary of Common Clinical Dermatologic Terms	74
Glossary of Common Dermatopathologic Terms	75
Terms Applied to the Surface Keratin Layer	75
Terms Applied to the Epidermis	75
Terms Applied to the Dermis	76

4 VULVAR SQUAMOUS LESIONS

DEMARETTA S. RUSH, EDWARD J. WILKINSON

Benign Squamous Neoplasms	79
Condyloma Acuminatum	79
Seborrheic Keratosis	79
Keratoacanthoma	80
Squamous Intraepithelial Lesions of the Vulva (VIN)	81
HPV-Related Low- and High-Grade Squamous Intraepithelial Lesions (VIN 1–3)	81
High-Grade VIN, Differentiated or Simplex Type	86
Squamous Cell Carcinoma	87
Uncommon Subtypes of Squamous Cell Carcinoma	91
Verrucous Carcinoma	91
Basal Cell Carcinoma	92
Sebaceous Carcinoma	93

5 VULVAR CYSTS, ADENOCARCINOMA, MELANOCYTIC, AND MISCELLANEOUS LESIONS

VICTOR G. PRIETO, M. ANGELICA SELIM

Cysts	95
Follicular ('Epidermoid') Cyst	95
Steatocystoma Multiplex	96
Bartholin Cyst	96
Mucinous Cyst	97
Ciliated Cyst (Paramesonephric Cyst)	97
Paraurethral (Skene) Gland Cyst	97
Mesonephric-Like Cyst	97
Cyst of the Canal of Nuck	98
Extramammary Paget Disease	98
Melanocytic Lesions	101
Lentigo	101
Common Acquired Melanocytic Nevus	101
Melanocytic Nevus of the Genital Type	102
Blue Nevus (Dermal Melanocytoma)	102
Atypical (Dysplastic, Clark) Nevus	102
Melanoma	103
Skin Appendage Neoplasms and Lesions of the Anogenital Mammary-Like Glands	106
Hidradenoma Papilliferum (Papillary Hidradenoma or Mammary-Like Gland Adenoma of the Vulva)	106
Syringoma	106
Trichoepithelioma	107
Vascular Lesions	108
Infantile Hemangioma ('Strawberry' Hemangioma)	108
Venous Malformation (Cavernous Hemangioma)	108
Deep Lymphatic Malformation (Cavernous Lymphangioma)	108
Miscellaneous Lesions	109
Acrochordon (Fibroepithelial Polyp, Skin Tag, Squamous Papilloma)	109
Endometriosis	109
Heterotopic Breast	109

Rare Tumors and Tumor-Like Conditions	110
Langerhans Cell Histiocytosis (Histiocytosis X)	110
Merkel Cell Carcinoma (Trabecular Carcinoma, Small Cell Carcinoma of the Skin, Primary Cutaneous Neuroendocrine Carcinoma)	110
Metastatic Tumors	112
Tumors of the Bartholin Gland	112
Urethra	113
Urethral Caruncle	113
Urethral Carcinoma	113

6 VULVAR MESENCHYMAL NEOPLASMS AND TUMOR-LIKE CONDITIONS

MARISA R. NUCCI, CHRISTOPHER D.M. FLETCHER

Tumor-Like Conditions	116
Fibroepithelial–Stromal Polyp (Pseudosarcoma Botryoides)	116
Nodular Fasciitis	117
Benign Neoplasms	118
Angiomyofibroblastoma	118
Cellular Angiofibroma	119
Prepubertal Vulvar Fibroma	120
Dermatofibroma (Fibrous Histiocytoma)	121
Granular Cell Tumor	122
Leiomyoma	122
Lymphangioma Circumscriptum	123
Angiokeratoma	124
Other Rare Tumors	124
Locally Recurrent Neoplasms	125
Deep Angiomyxoma (Deep 'Aggressive' Angiomyxoma)	125
Superficial Angiomyxoma (Cutaneous Myxoma)	126
Dermatofibrosarcoma Protuberans	127
Malignant Neoplasms	128
Leiomyosarcoma	128
So-Called Proximal-Type Epithelioid Sarcoma	128
Liposarcoma	129
Other Rare Sarcomas	129

7 VAGINA

SARAH BEAN, JAIME PRAT, STANLEY J. ROBBOY

Development	132
Anatomy	133
Histology and Physiology	133
Mesonephric Ducts	135
Developmental Disorders	136
Benign Effects of Diethylstilbestrol on the Vagina	136
Gross Structural Changes of the Vagina and Cervix	136
Vaginal Adenosis	136
Imperforate Hymen	139
Vaginal Agenesis	139
Transverse Vaginal Septum	139
Miscellaneous Congenital Disorders	139
Inflammatory Disorders	139
Vaginitis	139
Malakoplakia	140
Tampon-Related Lesions and Toxic Shock Syndrome	141
Noninfectious Inflammatory Diseases	141
Ligneous Vaginitis	141
Vaginal Cysts	141
Cysts of the Introitus	142
Tumor-Like Conditions	142
Fibroepithelial Polyps	142
Prolapsed Fallopian Tube	143
Granulation Tissue Nodule	143
Postoperative Spindle Cell Nodule	143
Microglandular Hyperplasia	143
Endometriosis	144
Benign Tumors	144
Benign Mixed Tumor	144
Müllerian Papilloma	144
Leiomyoma	145
Rhabdomyoma	145
Angiomyofibroblastoma	145
Miscellaneous Benign Tumors	146
Squamous Neoplasia	146
HPV Infection	146
Squamous Intraepithelial Lesion (VaIN)	146
Invasive Squamous Cell Carcinoma	148
Verrucous Carcinoma	149
Warty Carcinoma	150
Papillary Squamotransitional Cell Carcinoma	150
Small Cell Carcinoma	150
Clear Cell Adenocarcinoma	150
Adenocarcinoma, Non-Clear Cell Types	153
Other Primary Malignant Tumors of the Vagina	153
Malignant Melanoma	153
Leiomyosarcoma	154
Miscellaneous Tumors	154
Malignant Vaginal Tumors in Childhood	154
Embryonal Rhabdomyosarcoma	154
Yolk Sac Tumor	156
Lymphoma	156
Secondary Tumors of the Vagina	157

8 CERVICAL BENIGN AND NON-NEOPLASTIC CONDITIONS

ANAIS MALPICA

Normal Structure	160
Anatomy	160
Native (Original) Squamous Epithelium	160
Hormonal Influences on Squamous Epithelium	162
Basal Cell Hyperplasia	163
Squamous Cell Hyperplasia	164
Native (Original) Cervical Glandular Epithelium	164
Physiologic Changes in the Cervix and the Formation of the Transformation Zone	165
Squamous Metaplasia	166
The Congenital Transformation Zone (CTZ)	169
Histogenesis of the Congenital Transformation Zone	169
Inflammatory Cervicitis and Reactive Changes	170
Infective Cervicitis	170
C. Trachomatis	171
Tuberculosis	172
Syphilis	172
HSV	173
Cytomegalovirus (CMV)	173
Human Papilloma Virus (HPV)	174
Schistosomiasis	174
Epithelial Inflammatory Changes	175
Healing/Regenerating Epithelium	175
Metaplasias	176
Tubal, Endometrioid, and Tuboendometrioid Metaplasia	176
Intestinal Metaplasia	177
Lesions of the Endocervical Glandular Epithelium	177
Endocervical Tunnel Clusters	177
Deep Nabothian Cysts	179
Lobular Endocervical Glandular Hyperplasia	179
Diffuse Laminar Endocervical Glandular Hyperplasia	180
Lesions Related to Exogenous Stimuli	180
Microglandular Hyperplasia	180
Arias-Stella Reaction	181
Decidual Change	182
Radiation Changes	182
Other Non-Neoplastic Conditions	183
Endometriosis	183
Mesonephric Remnants and Hyperplasia	183
Mesonephric Duct Remnants	183
Mesonephric Duct Hyperplasia	184
Cervical Polyp	185
Ectopic Tissue	186
Prostatic Tissue	186
Glial Tissue	186
Sebaceous Glands	186

9 BIOLOGY OF CERVICAL SQUAMOUS NEOPLASIA

CORNELIA L. TRIMBLE, RACHEL KATZENELLENBOGEN

Introduction	188
HPV Infection	188
Low-Grade Squamous Intraepithelial Lesions (CIN1)	191
High-Grade Squamous Intraepithelial Lesions (CIN 2/3)	191
Mechanisms of Oncogenesis	192
The HPV E6 and E7 Oncoproteins	192
Naturally Occurring Immune Responses to HPV Antigens	193
Tissue-Resident Immune Cells	194
Hpv Vaccines	194
Primary Prevention: Early Detection and Prophylactic Vaccines	194
Secondary Prevention: Immune-Based Therapies	195
Vaccine Immunogenicity	195
Future Directions	196

10 CERVICAL SQUAMOUS INTRAEPITHELIAL LESIONS

C. SIMON HERRINGTON, JAN P.A. BAAK, GEORGE L. MUTTER

Introduction	200
Squamous Intraepithelial Lesions (SILs)	202
Nomenclature	202
Features	203
Changes of HPV Infection	203
Nuclear Abnormalities	205
Mitotic Activity	205
Differentiation, Maturation, and Stratification	206
Disease States: Types of SIL	207
LSIL (Condyloma/CIN 1)	208
High-Grade Squamous Intraepithelial Lesions (CIN 2–3)	212
Areas of Diagnostic Difficulty	214
The Scant Endocervical Curettage	214
Lesions Suspicious for, but Subdiagnostic of, SIL	215
Basal Cell Hyperplasia	215
Immature Squamous Metaplasia and Atypical Squamous Metaplasia	215
Repair (Reactive Epithelial Changes)	216

Low Estrogen States and Atrophy	216
Thin Epithelium	216
Invasive Squamous Cell Carcinoma	217
Artifact	217
Stratified Mucin-Producing Intraepithelial Lesion	217
Congenital Transformation Zone (See also Chapter 8)	218
Miscellaneous Conditions	218
Biomarkers	218
p16	218
Ki-67	218
ProExC	218
HPV Typing	219
Histologic Features of SIL (CIN) Affecting Management and Prognosis	219
Involvement of Endocervical Gland Crypts	219
Resection Margins	220
Invasive Disease	221
Regression and Progression to Invasive Carcinoma	221
Regression	221
Progression	222
Correlation between Cytology and Histology	**223**
Distribution and Site of Origin of SIL	**224**
Colposcopy	**224**
Normal Colposcopic Findings	225
Original Squamous Epithelium	225
Columnar Epithelium	225
Squamous Metaplasia	225
Abnormal Colposcopic Findings	226
Mosaic and Punctation	226
Acetowhite Epithelium	227
Leukoplakia	228
Atypical Vessels	228
Suspect Frank Invasive Carcinoma	228
Congenital Transformation Zone	228
Other Colposcopic Findings	228

11 CERVICAL SQUAMOUS CELL CARCINOMA

THOMAS C. WRIGHT, JR.

Epidemiology and Staging	**232**
Types of Cervical Malignancies	**233**
Superficially Invasive Squamous Cell Carcinoma	**233**
Depth of Invasion	234
Tumor Volume and Lateral Extent of Spread	234
Lymphovascular Invasion	234
Morphologic Features	235
Stromal Invasion	235
Measuring Depth of Invasion and Lateral Extent of Spread	236
Assessing Presence of LVI	237
Assessing Surgical Margins	237
Squamous Cell Carcinoma	**238**
Microscopic Features Used in Classification	239
Microscopic Grading	241
Additional Microscopic Features	241
Clinicopathologic Correlation	242
Prognostic Features	243
Histopathologic Prognostic Features	243
Tumor Size	244
Peritumoral Lymphatic Vessel Density	244
Biomarkers	244
Differential Diagnosis	244
Special Considerations	**245**
Cervical Stump Carcinoma	245
Effects of Radiotherapy on Cervical Carcinoma	245
Micrometastasis	246
'Mucin-Secreting' Carcinoma	246
Histologic Variants	**246**
Verrucous Squamous Cell Carcinoma	246
Warty Squamous Cell Carcinoma	247
Papillary Squamous Cell Carcinoma	247
Lymphoepithelioma-Like Squamous Cell Carcinoma	247
Papillary Squamotransitional Cell Carcinoma	248

12 CERVICAL GLANDULAR NEOPLASIA

EMANUELA D'ANGELO, JAIME PRAT

Preinvasive Glandular Lesions	**251**
Adenocarcinoma In Situ	**251**
Adenocarcinoma	**257**
Microinvasive (Early Invasive) Adenocarcinoma	257
Invasive Adenocarcinoma	259
Adenocarcinoma, Usual-Type	259
Mucinous Adenocarcinoma, Intestinal-Type	262
Mucinous Adenocarcinoma, Signet-Ring Cell-Type	262
Mucinous Adenocarcinoma Gastric-Type (Minimal Deviation Adenocarcinoma)	263
Villoglandular Adenocarcinoma	265
Endometrioid Adenocarcinoma	267
Minimal Deviation Adenocarcinoma, Endometrioid Type	267
Clear Cell Adenocarcinoma	267
Serous Adenocarcinoma	268
Mesonephric Adenocarcinoma	269

Adenosquamous Carcinoma	270
Glassy Cell Carcinoma	271

13 MISCELLANEOUS CERVICAL NEOPLASMS

ANAIS MALPICA

Epithelial Tumors	275
Adenoid Basal Carcinoma (Adenoid Basal Epithelioma)	275
Adenoid Cystic Carcinoma	277
Neuroendocrine Tumors	277
Typical (Classic) Carcinoid Tumor	277
Atypical Carcinoid Tumor	277
Small Cell Neuroendocrine Carcinoma	278
Large Cell Neuroendocrine Carcinoma	280
Biphasic Tumors	281
Adenofibroma	281
Adenomyoma	281
Adenosarcoma	281
Carcinosarcoma (Malignant Mixed Müllerian Tumor)	282
Rhabdomyosarcoma	283
Smooth Muscle Tumors (Leiomyoma and Leiomyosarcoma)	283
Malignant Peripheral Nerve Sheath Tumor	283
Primitive Neuroectodermal Tumor/ Ewing Sarcoma	284
Alveolar Soft Part Sarcoma	284
Blue Nevus	284
Malignant Melanoma	284
Lymphoma and Leukemia	285
Metastatic Tumors to the Cervix	286
Other Types of Cervical Neoplasms	287

14 THE NORMAL ENDOMETRIUM

REX C. BENTLEY, GEORGE L. MUTTER, STANLEY J. ROBBOY

Components of the Normal Endometrium	290
Surface Epithelium	292
Glandular Cells	292
Stromal Cells	293
Endometrial Lymphocytes	294
Blood Vessels	295
Endometrium during the 28 Day Idealized Normal Menstrual Cycle	295
Menstrual Endometrium (Days 1–3 of 28)	297
Proliferative Phase (Days 4–15 of 28)	298
Interval Endometrium (Day 16 of 28)	299
Secretory Endometrium (Days 17–28 of 28)	299
Early Secretory Phase, Days 16–18: Changing Vacuolar Patterns	299
Mid-Secretory Phase, Days 19–21: Increasing Stromal Edema	300
Late Secretory Phase, Days 22–28: Predecidual Change	301
Endometrium after Menopause	303
Methods of Endometrial Sampling	304
Dilatation and Curettage	304
Vabra Aspirator	304
Pipelle Biopsy	305
Cytologic Evaluation of the Endometrium	305
Direct Endometrial Cytologic Sampling	305
Hysteroscopy	305
Endometrial Resection and Ablation	305
Problems in Interpretation of Endometrial Specimens	307
Adequacy	307
Dissociation Artifact	307
Telescoping Artifact	308
Fixation Artifact	308
Legitimate Tissue Contaminants	308

15 EXOGENOUS HORMONES AND THEIR EFFECTS ON THE ENDOMETRIUM

REX C. BENTLEY

Introduction	310
Estrogens	310
Progestins	312
Oral Contraceptives	313
Combined OCs	314
Pure Progestin OCs ('Mini-Pill')	315
Long-Term, Progestin-Only OCs	315
Hormone Replacement Therapy	315
Unopposed Estrogen HRT	316
Cyclic Estrogen–Progesterone HRT	316
Combined Estrogen–Progesterone HRT	317
Other Hormonal Agents	318
Tamoxifen	318
Other Selective Estrogen Receptor Modulators	319
Aromatase Inhibitors	319
Phytoestrogens and Other Dietary Agents	319
Clomiphene/Ovulation Induction Therapy	320
Progesterone Receptor Modulators	320
GnRH Agonists and Antagonists	321
Gonadotropins	321

Corticosteroids	321
Danazol	321
Treatment of Endometrial Lesions with Progestins	321
Progestin Therapy of Persistent Estrogen States (Hyperplasia)	322
Progestin Therapy of Neoplastic Lesions: EIN and Carcinoma	322

16 ENDOMETRITIS, METAPLASIAS, POLYPS, AND MISCELLANEOUS CHANGES

GEORGE L. MUTTER, JOSEPH W. CARLSON

Inflammatory and Infectious Processes	326
Endometritis	326
Nonspecific Endometritis	327
Specific Forms of Endometritis	328
Chlamydia Trachomatis and *Neisseria Gonorrhoeae*	328
Mycoplasma	328
Cytomegalovirus	328
Herpes Simplex Virus	329
Tuberculous Endometritis	329
Actinomyces Israeilii	330
Other Forms of Endometritis	330
Granulomatous Endometritis	330
Histiocytic Endometritis	330
Postpartum and Postabortal Endometritis	330
Pyometra	331
Endometrial Metaplasias	331
Epithelial Metaplasias	332
Tubal Metaplasias	332
Squamous Metaplasia	333
Ichthyosis Uteri	334
EIN with Squamous Morules	334
Isolated Squamous Morules	335
Mucinous Metaplasia	336
Benign Mucinous Changes	337
EIN and Adenocarcinoma with Mucinous Differentiation	338
Secretory Metaplasia	339
Metaplasias to Nonspecific Cell Types	340
Eosinophilic Metaplasia	340
Micropapillary Metaplasia	340
Papillary Syncytial Metaplasia	341
Micropapillary 'Hobnail' Metaplasia	341
Mesenchymal Metaplasias	342
Osseous Metaplasia	342
Endometrial Extramedullary Hemopoiesis	342
Endometrial Polyps	342
Atypical Polypoid Adenomyoma	345
Miscellaneous Conditions	345
Asherman's Syndrome	345
Radiation Effect	346
The Effects of the IUD on the Endometrium	346
Endometrial Ablation	347

17 ENDOMETRIAL HYPERPLASIA WITHOUT ATYPIA AND EIN

GEORGE L. MUTTER

Introduction and Terminology	349
Two Diseases	350
The Spectrum of Non-Atypical Endometrial Hyperplasias	350
Disordered Proliferative Endometrium: a Prelude to Non-Atypical Hyperplasia	352
Non-Atypical Hyperplasia	353
Non-Atypical Hyperplasia with Superimposed Progestin Effect	355
Withdrawal Shedding Following Non-Atypical Hyperplasia	355
Normal Endometrium	356
Endometrial Polyps	356
Postmenopausal Cystic Atrophy	356
Exclusion of EIN	357
EIN, Atypical Hyperplasia	357
Cancer Outcomes in Women with EIN	358
Molecular Etiology and Natural History	358
Mutation and Clonal Growth in EIN	358
Latent Precancers—a Preclinical Phase Within Normal Tissues	359
Specific EIN Diagnostic Criteria	360
Exclusion of Benign Mimics	362
Exclusion of Carcinoma	363
Common EIN Diagnostic Problems	364
Non-Localizing (Widespread) EIN	364
EIN Within an Endometrial Polyp	365
Localizing Lesions Subdiagnostic for EIN	365
Excessively Fragmented Tissue	365
Non-Endometrioid EIN	366
Hormonally Treated EIN	366
Special Studies for EIN Diagnosis	367
Biomarkers: *PAX2* and *PTEN*	367
Quantitative Histomorphometry	367
Management of EIN	368
Hysterectomy	368
Hormonal Therapy	368

18 ENDOMETRIAL ADENOCARCINOMA

GEORGE L. MUTTER, JAIME PRAT

Introduction	370
An Oversimplified View of Endometrial Adenocarcinoma: Types 1 and 2	370
Molecular Pathology of Type 1 and 2 Cancers	372
Classification of Endometrial Adenocarcinoma	372
Risk Factors in Endometrial Carcinoma	373
Estrogens and Estrogen-Associated Conditions	373
Obesity	373
Diabetes	373
Polycystic Ovary Syndrome	373
Ovarian Sex Cord–Stromal Tumors	373
Other Risk Factors	373
Heritable Risk	373
Tamoxifen	374
Reproductive Factors	374
Cigarette Smoking	374
Endometrioid Adenocarcinoma and Its Variants	374
Precursor Lesions: Endometrial Intraepithelial Neoplasia/Atypical Hyperplasia	381
Variants of Endometrioid Carcinoma	382
Serous carcinoma	387
Serous Endometrial Intraepithelial Carcinoma (EIC)	389
Clear Cell Adenocarcinoma	391
Mixed Types of Carcinoma	393
Carcinosarcoma	393
Other Types of Endometrial Carcinoma	394
Undifferentiated Carcinoma	394
Squamous Cell Carcinoma	394
Synchronous Endometrial and Ovarian Carcinoma	395
Tumors Metastatic to the Endometrium	395
Prognostic Factors in Endometrial Carcinoma	396
Histologic Type	396
Histologic Grade	396
Stage and Depth of Myometrial Invasion	396
Lymphovascular Invasion	397
Age	397
Steroid Hormone Receptors	397
The Spread of Endometrial Carcinoma	398

19 UTERINE SMOOTH MUSCLE TUMORS

EMANUELA D'ANGELO, BRADLEY J. QUADE, JAIME PRAT

Introduction	402
Leiomyoma	402
Variants of Leiomyoma	405
Mitotically Active Leiomyoma	405
Cellular Leiomyoma	405
Hemorrhagic Cellular Leiomyoma and Hormone-Induced Changes	406
Degenerated Leiomyoma	406
Leiomyoma Treated by Interventional Radiology	407
Leiomyoma with Bizarre Nuclei (So-Called 'Atypical' Leiomyoma)	408
Epithelioid Leiomyoma	409
Myxoid Leiomyoma	410
Leiomyomas with Heterologous Elements	411
Unusual Growth Patterns of Leiomyomas	411
Diffuse Leiomyomatosis and Myometrial Hypertrophy	411
Intravenous Leiomyomatosis	411
Benign Metastasizing Leiomyoma	412
Disseminated Peritoneal Leiomyomatosis	413
Leiomyosarcoma	414
Histologic Diagnosis of Leiomyosarcoma	416
Diagnostic Criteria	417
Molecular Genetics	418
Prognosis and Treatment	419
Atypical Smooth Muscle Tumors (So-Called Smooth Muscle Tumors of Uncertain Malignant Potential)	420

20 ENDOMETRIAL STROMAL TUMORS, MIXED MÜLLERIAN TUMORS, ADENOMYOSIS, ADENOMYOMAS AND RARE SARCOMAS

ESTHER OLIVA

Endometrial Stromal Tumors	425
Introduction	425
Endometrial Stromal Nodule	425
Low-Grade Endometrial Stromal Sarcoma	427
Endometrial Stromal Variants	428
High-Grade Endometrial Stromal Sarcoma	435
Undifferentiated Endometrial Sarcoma	435
Uterine Tumors Resembling Ovarian Sex Cord Tumors	436
Mixed Müllerian Tumors	438
Introduction	438
Müllerian Adenofibroma	438
Müllerian Adenosarcoma	439
Malignant Mixed Müllerian Tumor (Carcinosarcoma)	443
Adenomyosis	446
Adenomyomas	447
Endocervical- and Endometrioid-Type Adenomyomas	447
Atypical Polypoid Adenomyoma	449
PEComa	450

Other Rare Sarcomas	452	Adenofibroma	478
Rhabdomyosarcoma	452	Leiomyomas	479
Primitive Neuroectodermal Tumor (Ewing/Peripheral or Central Types)	453	Other Benign Tumors	479
		Borderline Tumors	479
Alveolar Soft Part Sarcoma	453	Malignant Tumors	479
		Primary Carcinoma of the Fallopian Tube	479
		Carcinosarcoma	483
		Other Malignant Tumors	483
		Tumors Metastatic to the Fallopian Tube	483
		Female Adnexal Tumor of Wolffian Origin	484

21 FALLOPIAN TUBE

ELKE A. JARBOE

Introduction	459
Anatomy, Histology, and Function of the Fallopian Tube	459
Anatomy	459
Histology	460
Mucosal Epithelial Alterations	461
Secretory Cell Outgrowths and p53 Signatures	461
Other Mucosal Epithelial Proliferations	462
Function	462
Sperm Transport	462
Ovum Transport	462
Approach to Examining Tubal Specimens	462
Bilateral Tubal Ligation for Sterilization	462
Salpingectomy for Tubal Ectopic Gestation	463
Salpingectomy (with or Without Oophorectomy And/or Hysterectomy)	463
The SEE-FIM Protocol	463
Non-Neoplastic Lesions	463
Inflammation of the Fallopian Tubes	463
Infectious Salpingitis	464
Non-Granulomatous Salpingitis	464
Granulomatous Salpingitis	467
Salpingitis Isthmica Nodosa	469
Tubal Pregnancy	470
Cysts	472
Paramesonephric Cysts	473
Mesonephric Cysts	473
Mesothelial Inclusion Cysts	473
Metaplasias and Rests	474
Mucinous Metaplasia	474
Endometriosis and Endosalpingiosis	474
Transitional Metaplasia	474
Adrenal Rest	475
Pseudodecidual Change (Ectopic Decidua)	475
Torsion of the Fallopian Tube	475
Prolapse of the Fallopian Tube	476
Epithelial Proliferation Associated with Salpingitis	476
Tumors of the Fallopian Tube	477
Benign Tumors	477
Adenomatoid Tumor	477
Serous Cystadenoma	478

22 ENDOMETRIOSIS

GEORGE L. MUTTER

Introduction	487
Clinical Features of Endometriosis	487
Distribution of Endometriosis	488
Epidemiology of Endometriosis	488
Pathogenesis of Endometriosis	489
Transplantation	489
Metaplastic Theory	490
Intrinsic Abnormalities of Endometriotic Tissue	490
Local Feedback between Estrogen Production and Inflammation	490
Altered Stromal–Epithelial Interaction	490
Etiologic Factors in Endometriosis	490
Genetic Factors	490
Congenital Anatomic Abnormalities	491
Systemic Hormonal Factors	491
Peritoneal Environment	491
Angiogenesis	491
Morphologic Features of Endometriosis	491
Considerations at Specific Anatomic Locations	498
Ovary	498
Peritoneal Surfaces	499
Fallopian Tube	499
Cervix	499
Gastrointestinal Tract	500
Urinary Tract	500
Abdominal Wall	500
Lymph Nodes	500
Clinical Classification of Endometriosis	501
Infertility in Endometriosis	501
Endometriosis Presenting as a Benign Solid Tumor	501
Florid Endometriosis	501
Polypoid Endometriosis	502
Malignancy in Endometriosis	502
Frequency and Types of Malignancies	503
Atypical Endometriosis and the Pathogenesis of Malignancy	504

23 NORMAL OVARIES, INFLAMMATORY AND NON-NEOPLASTIC CONDITIONS

RUTHY SHACO-LEVY, STANLEY J. ROBBOY

Anatomy, Histology, and Function	509
Anatomy	509
Histology	509
Physiology	510
Ovarian Development	510
Folliculogenesis	510
Follicular Maturation	511
Formation of the Corpus Luteum	512
Involution of the Corpus Luteum	513
Follicular Atresia	514
The Hormonal Background of the Ovarian Cycle	515
The Ovarian Hilum and Its Vicinity	516
Follicular Failure	517
Follicular Dysgenesis (Dysplasia)	517
Ovarian Failure	517
Afollicular Ovarian Failure (Primary Ovarian Insufficiency, Premature Follicular Depletion)	518
Follicular Ovarian Failure. Resistant Ovary Syndrome (Savage Syndrome, Gonadotropin-Insensitivity Syndrome)	520
Autoimmune Oophoritis	520
Hypogonadotropic Hypogonadism	522
Anomalies of Ovarian Development and Descent	523
Ectopic Ovarian Tissue	523
Dystopic Ovaries	523
Ovarian Agenesis	523
Splenogonadal Fusion	523
'Uterus-Like Mass' Replacing Ovary	523
Infectious Inflammatory Diseases	524
Bacterial Oophoritis	524
Pelvic Inflammatory Disease	524
Xanthogranulomatous Oophoritis	524
Malacoplakia	525
Actinomycosis	525
Tuberculosis	526
Viral Oophoritis	526
Mumps	526
Cytomegalovirus	527
Parasitic Oophoritis	527
Schistosomiasis (Bilharziasis)	527
Enterobiasis	528
Echinococcosis	529
Fungal Oophoritis	529
Coccidioidomycosis	529
Blastomycosis	529
Noninfectious Inflammatory Diseases	529
Sarcoidosis	529
Crohn Disease	529
Cortical Granulomas	530
Isolated Noninfectious Granulomas	530
Autoimmune Oophoritis	530
Necrotizing Arteritis	530
Giant Cell Arteritis	531
Polyarteritis Nodosa	531
Postpartum Ovarian Vein Thrombophlebitis	531

24 NON-NEOPLASTIC AND TUMOR-LIKE CONDITIONS OF THE OVARY

EMANUELA F. VERAS, JENNIFER H. CROW, STANLEY J. ROBBOY

Dysfunctional Cysts	535
Cysts Derived From Preovulatory Follicles (Follicular Cysts)	536
Corpus Luteum Cysts	538
Corpus Albicans Cysts	539
Simple (Unclassified) Cysts	540
Tumor-Like Lesions Associated with Pregnancy	540
Luteomas of Pregnancy (Nodular Theca–Lutein Hyperplasia of Pregnancy)	540
Multiple Theca–Lutein Cysts (Hyperreactio Luteinalis)	542
Solitary Luteinized Follicular Cysts of Pregnancy and Puerperium	542
Leydig (Hilus) Cell Hyperplasia	543
Deciduosis (Ectopic Decidua)	543
Ovarian Granulosa Cell Proliferations of Pregnancy	544
Ovarian Pregnancy	544
Primary Ovarian Trophoblastic Disease	545
Other Ovarian Lesions	546
Torsion	546
Disseminated Peritoneal Leiomyomatosis	546
Ovarian Neoplasms	546
Reactive Stromal Tumor-Like Lesions	546
Polycystic Ovary Syndrome	546
Stromal Hyperplasia and Hyperthecosis	548
Leydig (Hilus) Cell Hyperplasia	551
Massive Ovarian Edema and Fibromatosis	552
Massive Ovarian Edema	552
Fibromatosis	554

EXTENDED TABLE OF CONTENTS xvii

Sequelae of Surgery or Trauma	556
Ovarian Remnant Syndrome (Residual or Remnant Ovary Syndrome)	556
Ovarian 'Drilling' for Polycystic Ovary Syndrome	557
Splenosis (Autotransplantantion of Splenic Tissue)	557
Iatrogenic Disorders of the Ovaries	558
Radiotherapy Damage	558
Chemotherapeutic and Immunosuppressive Drugs	558
Oral Contraceptives	558
Progesterone	559
Danazol	559
(GnRH) Analogs	559
Ovulation-Induction Agents	559
Tamoxifen	560
Ovarian Hemorrhage and Adnexal Torsion	560
Ovarian Hemorrhage	560
Adnexal Torsion	560
Müllerianosis and Reactive Mesothelial Lesions	561

25 OVARIAN EPITHELIAL-STROMAL TUMORS. SEROUS TUMORS

JAIME PRAT, ELKE JARBOE

Epithelial/Stromal Tumors	564
Borderline Tumors	565
Carcinomas	565
Benign and Borderline Serous Tumors	565
Benign Serous Tumors	565
Serous Borderline Tumors	567
Pseudoinvasion, Autoimplants, and Mesothelial Cell Hyperplasia	569
Micropapillary Pattern	569
Microinvasion	571
Peritoneal Implants	572
Serous Borderline Tumors in Lymph Nodes	578
Serous Borderline Tumors of the Peritoneum	579
Serous Carcinomas	580
Low-Grade Serous Carcinomas	580
High-grade Serous Carcinomas	582

26 OVARIAN MUCINOUS TUMORS

JAIME PRAT

General Features	591
Benign Mucinous Tumors	592
Mucinous Borderline Tumors	593
Mucinous Borderline Tumors, Endocervical-Like	593
Mucinous Borderline Tumors, Gastrointestinal Type	595
Mucinous Cystic Tumors Associated with Pseudomyxoma Peritonei	598
Mucinous Adenocarcinomas	600
Mural Nodules	604

27 OVARIAN ENDOMETRIOID, CLEAR CELL, TRANSITIONAL, AND MIXED EPITHELIAL-STROMAL TUMORS

JAIME PRAT

Endometrioid Tumors	608
Epithelial Tumors	609
Benign Endometrioid Tumors	609
Borderline Endometrioid Tumors	610
Endometrioid Carcinomas	611
Simultaneous Endometrioid Carcinomas of the Ovary and Endometrium	618
Mixed Tumors (Tumors with a Sarcomatous Component)	618
Malignant Mesodermal Mixed Tumors (Carcinosarcomas)	618
Müllerian Adenosarcomas	620
Endometrioid Stromal Sarcomas	621
Tumors of Smooth Muscle	623
Leiomyomas	623
Leiomyosarcomas	623
Myxoid Leiomyosarcoma	624
Clear Cell Tumors	624
Benign Clear Cell Tumors	625
Borderline Clear Cell Tumors	625
Clear Cell Adenocarcinomas	626
Transitional Cell Tumors	629
Benign Brenner Tumor	629
Borderline and Malignant Brenner Tumors	630
Squamous Cell Lesions	633
Epidermoid (Squamous Cell) Cysts	633
Squamous Cell Carcinomas	633
Mixed Epithelial Tumors	633
Undifferentiated Carcinomas	634
Miscellaneous and Unclassified Tumors	635
Small Cell Undifferentiated Carcinoma, Hypercalcemic Type	635
Small Cell Carcinoma, Pulmonary Type	636
Undifferentiated Carcinoma of Non-Small Cell (Neuroendocrine) Type	636
Cysts and Adenomas of the Rete Ovarii	636
Adenomatoid Tumors	636
Hepatoid Carcinomas	637
Female Adnexal Tumors of Wolffian Origin	637

28 OVARIAN SEX CORD–STROMAL AND STEROID CELL TUMORS

JAIME PRAT

General Features	642
Granulosa Cell Tumors	643
Adult Granulosa Cell Tumor	643
Juvenile Granulosa Cell Tumor	647
Thecoma	650
Typical Form	650
Luteinized Thecoma	651
Fibroma	652
Cellular Fibroma	653
Fibrosarcoma	654
Sclerosing Stromal Tumor	654
Signet-Ring Stromal Tumor	655
Microcystic Stromal Tumor	655
Sertoli–Stromal Cell Tumors	656
Sertoli Cell Tumors	656
Sertoli-Leydig Cell Tumors	656
Sex Cord Tumor with Annular Tubules	661
Gynandroblastoma	661
Steroid Cell Tumors	662
Stromal Luteoma	662
Leydig Cell Tumor	663
Steroid Cell Tumor, Adrenal Cortical Type	664
Steroid Cell Tumor (NOS)	664
Endocrine Syndromes Associated with Ovarian Tumors	665
Ovarian Tumors with Functioning Stroma	665
Hypercalcemia	666
Hyperthyroidism	666
Carcinoid Syndrome	666
Zollinger–Ellison Syndrome	666
Hyperprolactinemia	667
Cushing Syndrome	667
Hypoglycemia	667
Hyperaldosteronism	667

29 OVARIAN GERM CELL TUMORS

JAIME PRAT

General Features	670
Dysgerminoma	671
Yolk Sac Tumor (Primitive Endodermal Tumor)	674
Embryonal Carcinoma	678
Polyembryoma	678
Nongestational Choriocarcinoma	679
Teratomas	679
Mature Teratomas	679
Immature Teratomas	681
Monodermal Teratomas	683
Struma Ovarii	683
Carcinoids	684
Neuroectodermal-Type Tumors	686
Carcinoma in Dermoid Cysts	688
Squamous Cell Carcinoma	688
Adenocarcinoma	688
Mixed Malignant Germ Cell Tumors	688
Mixed Germ Cell Sex Cord–Stromal Tumor	688
Gonadoblastoma	688

30 METASTATIC TUMORS OF THE OVARY

EMANUELA D'ANGELO, JAIME PRAT

General Features	694
Mode of Spread	694
Site of Origin	696
Intestinal Carcinomas	696
Krukenberg Tumor	699
Carcinoid Tumors	701
Breast Carcinoma	702
Tumors of the Pancreas, Biliary Tract, and Liver	703
Tumors of the Appendix	704
Renal Tumors	705
Tumors of the Urinary Tract	706
Adrenal Gland Tumors	707
Malignant Melanoma	707
Pulmonary and Mediastinal Tumors	707
Uterine Tumors	707
Lymphoma and Leukemia	709
Peritoneal Tumors	710
Extragenital Sarcomas	711
Summary	712

31 THE PERITONEUM

EMANUELA D'ANGELO, JAIME PRAT

Normal Peritoneum	716
Inflammatory and Reactive Lesions	716
Granulomatous Peritonitis	717
Tuberculosis	717
Suture Materials	717
Surgical Glove Powder	717
Contrast Media	717
Intestinal Contents	717
Cystic Teratoma (Dermoid Cyst) Rupture	717
Keratin	717

Cauterized Tissue	718
Cesarean Delivery	718
Non-Granulomatous Histiocytic Lesions	718
Fibrosing Lesions	718
Tumor-Like Lesions	719
Mesothelial Hyperplasia	719
Peritoneal Inclusion Cysts	720
Ovarian Remnant Syndrome	721
Supernumerary or Accessory Ovaries	721
Splenosis	721
Trophoblastic Implants	723
Infarcted Appendix Epiploica	723
Mesothelial Neoplasms	**723**
Adenomatoid Tumor	723
Well-Differentiated Papillary Mesothelioma	723
Diffuse Malignant Mesothelioma	724
Miscellaneous Primary Tumors	**727**
Intra-Abdominal Desmoplastic, Small Round Cell Tumor	727
Solitary Fibrous Tumor of Peritoneum ('Fibrous Mesothelioma')	728
Inflammatory Myofibroblastic Tumor	729
Other Tumors	729
Metastatic Tumors	**729**
Pseudomyxoma Peritonei	729
Gliomatosis Peritonei	732
Strumosis Peritonei	732
Lesions of the Secondary Müllerian System	**733**
Endometriosis	733
Peritoneal Serous Lesions	733
Endosalpingiosis	733
Intranodal Glands of Müllerian Type (Müllerian Inclusion Cysts)	734
Serous Tumors (Primary and Metastatic)	735
Serous Borderline Tumor	735
Serous Carcinoma (of Peritoneal Origin)	735
Psammocarcinoma	735
Endocervicosis	735
Peritoneal Endometrioid, Clear Cell, and Transitional Cell Lesions	735
Deciduosis	735
Disseminated Peritoneal Leiomyomatosis	735

Examination of the Placenta	745
Umbilical Cord	745
Membranes	748
Meconium on Cord and Membranes	749
Architectural and Developmental Abnormalities	750
Placental Weight	751
Fetal Surface of Placenta	751
Maternal Surface of the Placenta	752
Cut Surface	752
Infarction	752
Perivillous Fibrin Deposition and Maternal Floor 'Infarction'	753
Hematoma	754
Subchorial Thrombosis (Breus Mole)	755
Intervillous Thrombosis	755
Other Conditions	755
Multiple Gestation	755
Microscopic Lesions of the Placenta	**757**
Placental Inflammation and Infection	757
Chronic Chorioamnionitis and Deciduitis	758
Membrane and Decidual Hypoxic Lesions	758
Eosinophilic/T-Cell Vasculitis	758
Villitis	758
Chronic Histiocytic Intervillositis	759
Vascular Lesions	759
Fetal Vessel Thrombi	759
Maternal Vessel Pathology	761
Fetal and Maternal Vascular Disease and Thrombophilia	761
Chorangiosis	762
Chorangiomatosis	762
Villous Maturity	762
Villous Edema	763
Persistant Fetal Normoblastemia	764
Miscellaneous Villous Changes	764
Non-Trophoblastic Tumors of the Placenta	764
Chorangioma	764
Chorangiocarcinoma (Chorangiomas with Trophoblastic Proliferation)	764
Intraplacental Choriocarcinoma	764
Teratomas	765
Metastatic Tumor	766

32 IMPLANTATION AND PLACENTA

EOGHAN E. MOONEY

Introduction	741
Anatomy and Embryology	741
Implantation and Early Pregnancy	741
Functional Unit of the Placenta	745

33 NON-NEOPLASTIC MATERNAL GESTATIONAL DISEASES

EOGHAN E. MOONEY, EMMA M. DOYLE

Early Pregnancy Loss (Spontaneous Miscarriage)	769
Mid to Late Pregnancy Loss	771
Abruption	771

Hypertensive Disorders	772
Pre-Eclampsia	772
Intrauterine Growth Restriction	773
Confined Placental Mosaicism	774
Adverse Neurologic Outcome: Neonatal Encephalopathy and Cerebral Palsy	774
Diabetes Mellitus	775
Hydrops Fetalis (Maternal Rhesus Isoimmunization)	775
Placenta Creta	775
Postpartum Hemorrhage and Subinvolution	776
Maternal Sickle Cell Trait and Disease	776
Twin Pregnancy	777
Prolonged Pregnancy	777
Maternal Infections and the Placenta	777
Cytomegalovirus	777
Parvovirus B19	778
Rubella	779
Varicella Zoster	779
Herpes Simplex	779
HIV	780
Human Papillomavirus	780
Toxoplasmosis	780
Malaria	781
Syphilis	781
Listeriosis	781
Other Organisms	781

34 GESTATIONAL TROPHOBLASTIC DISEASE

KYU-RAE KIM

Introduction	784
Overview of Early Placental Development	784
Villous Trophoblast	784
Extravillous (Intermediate) Trophoblast	785
Trophoblast Immunohistochemical Markers	787
Molar Gestational Trophoblastic Disease	788
Complete Hydatidiform Mole	788
Early (First Trimester) Complete Hydatidiform Moles	791
Advanced (Second Trimester) Complete Hydatidiform Moles	791
Partial Hydatidiform Mole	795
Adverse Clinical Outcomes in Molar Disease	798
Persistent Trophoblastic Disease	798
Recurrent Hydatidiform Mole	799
Invasive Mole	799
Trophoblastic Neoplasia	800
Choriocarcinoma	800
Choriocarcinoma Associated with Full-Term Pregnancy and Intraplacental Choriocarcinoma	802
Placental Site Trophoblastic Tumor	803
Epithelioid Trophoblastic Tumor	805
Non-Neoplastic Trophoblastic Lesions	807
Placental Site Nodule or Plaque	807
Exaggerated Placental Site (Reaction)	809

35 GROSS DESCRIPTION AND PROCESSING OF SPECIMENS

BROOKE HOWITT, GEORGE L. MUTTER

Introduction	812
Section Codes and the Report	813
Section Codes	813
Location of Section Codes in the Report	813
Specimen and Site Identification	814
General Aspects of Gross Decription and Cutting in of Specimens	814
Gross Description	814
Inking	815
Drawings and Photographs	815
Fixatives	815
Number of Sections Required	815
Synoptic Checklists	815
Vulva	815
Excisional Biopsies	815
Wide Local Excision	815
Skinning Vulvectomy	816
Simple (or Total) Vulvectomy	816
Radical Vulvectomy	816
Cervix	817
Punch Biopsies	817
Endocervical Curettage	817
Cervical Cone Biopsy/Excision and Trachelectomy	817
Hysterectomy for Malignant Cervical Disease	818
Uterine Corpus	818
Endometrial Biopsies and Curettings	818
Uterus Removed for Benign or Functional Disease	818
Supracervical Hysterectomy	820
Malignant Uterine Disease	820
Endometrial Sampling for Products of Conception	821
Uterus Removed during Obstetric Procedures	821
Fallopian Tube	821
Sterilization	822
Tubal Ectopic Pregnancy	822
Prophylactic Salpingectomy (with or without Oophorectomy)	822
Tubal Neoplasm	822

Ovary	822
General Rules	822
Large Cystic or Neoplastic Ovaries	823
Microscopic Sections	823
Staging Operations	824
Fetus and Placenta	824
Second Trimester Fetus	824
Placenta	825
Twin Placenta	826

36 PRACTICAL BIOMARKERS FOR FEMALE GENITAL TRACT LESIONS

W. GLENN MCCLUGGAGE

Introduction	828
Broad Spectrum Differentiation Markers	828
Epithelial Markers	828
Cytokeratins	828
Broad Spectrum Cytokeratins	829
CAM 5.2	829
CK7 and 20	829
CK5/6	830
Other Cytokeratins	830
Epithelial Membrane Antigen and Ber-EP4	831
Mesenchymal Cell Markers	831
Vimentin	831
Smooth Muscle Markers	831
Skeletal Muscle Markers	832
Endometrial Stromal Markers	832
CD10	832
Mesothelial Markers	832
Calretinin	832
Blood Vessel Markers	832
CD34	832
Narrow Spectrum Differentiation Markers	832
Trophoblastic Markers	833
β-hCG	833
Placental Alkaline Phosphatase	833
Human Placental Lactogen	833
Mel-CAM (CD146)	833
HLA-G	833
Melanocytic Markers	833
HMB45	833
Melan-A (MART-1)	833
S-100	833
Neuroendocrine Markers	833
Lymphoid Markers	834

Markers of Altered Function in Disease States	834
Tumor Markers	834
CA19.9	834
Carcinoembryonic Antigen	834
CA125 (OC125)	834
Inhibin	834
OCT3/4	835
HIK1083	835
CDX-2	835
Alpha-Fetoprotein	835
Hep-PAR1	835
Muc Antibodies	835
CD99	835
Thyroid Transcription Factor 1	836
Prostatic-Specific Antigen and Prostatic Acid Phosphatase	836
Glypican 3	836
SALL 4	836
Steroidogenic Factor 1	836
ALK1	836
HER-2/NEU	836
Tumor Suppressor Genes	836
WT1	836
DPC4	837
p53	837
p63	837
PTEN	837
Proto-Oncogenes	838
Bcl-2	838
CD117 (C-Kit)	838
Cell Cycle and Nuclear Proliferation	838
Ki-67 (MIB1) and Proliferating Cell Nuclear Antigen	838
p16	838
p57	839
Cyclin D1	839
Cyclin E	839
ProExC	839
Hormone Receptors	839
Estrogen Receptor and Progesterone Receptor	839
Androgen Receptor	840
Oxytocin Receptor	840
Cell Adhesion Markers	840
β-Catenin	840
E-Cadherin	840
Other Markers	840
PAX8	840
PAX2	841
HMGA2	841
Hepatocyte Nuclear Factor 1-β	841
FOXL2	841
IMP-3 and IMP-2	841
DOG1	841

Preface

In this third edition of *Pathology of the Female Reproductive Tract*, the new editorial team seeks to present new concepts and findings as a background to furthering patient management. By so doing, we hope to improve communication between the pathologist and the clinician, which is essential for optimal patient care. Balancing the broad range of contents has not been an easy task. We have deleted sections deemed no longer relevant, while retaining classic material still pertinent for today's practice. For example, we kept and even expanded the clinical discussions because pathologists should be aware of the therapeutic implications of their diagnosis, and clinicians should be able to understand the meaning of a pathology report. Only in this way we can promote optimal patient care

The most significant changes made with respect to the previous edition include the following:

The diseases of the lower genital tract related to HPV are comprehensively presented in six separate chapters including one (Chapter 9) exclusively devoted to the molecular biology of cervical squamous neoplasia, early detection, and prophylactic vaccines. Even if it has been unilaterally proposed by the Lower Anogenital Tract Squamous Terminology (LAST) group, the unified nomenclature with two-tier (LSIL and HSIL) system for all HPV-related preinvasive squamous lesions of the lower anogenital tract has been adhered to throughout.

Endometrial carcinomas and their precursors are presented in two chapters (Chapters 17 and 18). Besides an in-depth discussion of prototypic endometrioid and nonendometrioid (serous) carcinomas which includes clinicopathologic features, differential diagnosis and treatment, the clinical and molecular characteristics of some unique tumor histotypes (such as clear cell carcinomas and carcinosarcomas that do not fit into either of the two main types) are also analyzed. Uterine sarcomas are also presented in two chapters (Chapters 19 and 20) dominated by the clinicopathologic features of leiomyosarcomas and endometrial stromal sarcomas respectively. Among the latter tumors, the prematurely eliminated high-grade endometrial stromal sarcoma has been resurrected, based upon its distinctive histologic and molecular characteristics.

Recent advances in epidemiology, molecular genetics and therapy, have confirmed the older 1960s idea that ovarian epithelial cancer is not one, but many diseases not only exhibiting different morphology, but also different genetic risk factors, precursor lesions, patterns of spread, molecular events during oncogenesis, response to chemotherapy, and prognosis. Accordingly, the five main types of ovarian carcinoma, accounting for 98% of the total, are presented in three separate chapters (Chapters 25–27) emphasizing conventional histopathology and differential diagnosis, as well as immunohistochemistry and molecular genetic analysis.

The increasing demonstration of both intraepithelial high-grade serous carcinoma and putative precursor epithelial lesions in the distal fallopian tube, particularly in women carrying BRCA1 mutations, are discussed in detail on the chapters dealing with diseases of the fallopian tube (Chapter 21) and serous tumors of the ovary (Chapter 25). The relative importance of the fallopian tube mucosa compared with the ovarian surface epithelium (mesothelium) in the genesis of high-grade serous ovarian cancers is still a subject of debate. Similarly, the increasing evidence that both endometrioid and clear cell carcinomas of the ovary originate from ovarian endometriosis and the role of AT-rich interactive domain 1A gene (ARID1A) mutations in endometrioid and clear cell carcinogenesis are presented on Chapter 27. The diagnostic value of FOXL2 and pluripotency stem cell markers is discussed in the chapters dealing with ovarian sex cord–stromal and germ cell tumors (Chapters 28 and 29), respectively.

Regarding molecular diagnosis and biomarkers, we have been pragmatic in keeping those which have already demonstrated added value in clinical practice, or might become so in the foreseeable future. Furthermore, the range of histopathologic variants of the main gynecological and obstetrical tumors and tumor-like conditions can be quite broad. It would be impossible to rigidly consider all morphologic variants as separate entities, much less illustrate them well. Rather, aggregation by disease mechanism, clinical outcome, and available therapies has guided us throughout. In this regard, we admit a tendency to 'lump' diagnoses along clinicopathologic lines, rather than 'splitting' them according to morphologic variations.

We are strongly aware that, in today's wired society, the latest information can outdate any published text. Nevertheless, the essence of this work is to give the most accurate review of what is currently available.

George L. Mutter
Jaime Prat

List of Contributors

Jan P.A. Baak MD, PhD
Professor of Pathology, Department of Pathology, Stavanger University Hospital, Stavanger, Norway

Sarah Bean MD
Assistant Professor, Department of Pathology, Duke University Medical Center, Durham, NC, USA

Rex C. Bentley MD
Professor of Pathology, Duke University Medical Center, Durham, NC, USA

Joseph W. Carlson MD, PhD
Specialist Physician, Department of Pathology and Cytology, Karolinska University Hospital, Stockholm, Sweden

Jennifer H. Crow MD
Assistant Professor, Department of Pathology, Duke University, Durham, NC, USA

Emanuela D'Angelo MD, PhD
Associate Professor of Pathology, Autonomous University of Barcelona, Hospital de la Santa Creu i Sant Pau, Barcelona, Spain

Emma M. Doyle MB, MRCOG
Lecturer in Pathology, School of Medicine and Medical Science, University College Dublin, Dublin, Ireland

Christopher D.M. Fletcher MD, FRCPath
Vice Chair, Anatomic Pathology, Brigham & Women's Hospital; Chief of Onco-Pathology, Dana-Farber Cancer Institute; Professor of Pathology, Harvard Medical School, Boston, MA, USA

C. Simon Herrington MA, MB BS, DPhil, FRCP, FRCPath
Professor of Pathology, Division of Cancer Research, Medical Research Institute, University of Dundee, Dundee, UK

Mai P. Hoang MD
Associate Professor of Pathology, Department of Pathology, Harvard Medical School, Massachusetts General Hospital, Boston, MA, USA

Brooke Howitt MD
Soft Tissue Pathology Fellow, Department of Pathology, Women's and Perinatal Division, Brigham and Women's Hospital, Boston, MA, USA

Elke A. Jarboe MD
Assistant Professor, Department of Pathology, University of Utah Health Sciences Center, Salt Lake City, UT, USA

Rachel Katzenellenbogen MD
Assistant Professor, Pediatrics, University of Washington; Adjunct Assistant Professor, Global Health, University of Washington, Seattle, WA, USA

Kyu-Rae Kim MD, PhD
Professor, Department of Pathology, University of Ulsan College of Medicine, ASAN Medical Center, Seoul, Korea

Anais Malpica MD
Professor of Pathology and Gynecologic Oncology, Department of Pathology, MD Anderson Cancer Center, The University of Texas, Houston, TX, USA

W. Glenn McCluggage MD
Professor of Gynecological Pathology, Department of Pathology, Belfast Health and Social Care Trust, Belfast, Northern Ireland, UK

Eoghan E. Mooney MB, BCh, BAO
Consultant Histopathologist, Department of Pathology and Laboratory Medicine, National Maternity Hospital, Dublin, Ireland

George L. Mutter MD
Professor of Pathology, Harvard Medical School, Division of Women's and Perinatal Pathology, Brigham and Women's Hospital, Boston, MA, USA

Marisa R. Nucci MD
Associate Professor of Pathology, Harvard Medical School; Associate Pathologist, Department of Pathology, Division of Women's and Perinatal Pathology, Brigham and Women's Hospital, Department of Pathology, Boston, MA, USA

Esther Oliva MD
Professor of Pathology, Harvard Medical School; Pathologist, Massachusetts General Hospital, Boston, MA, USA

Jaime Prat MD, PhD, FRCPath
Professor and Chairman, Department of Pathology, Hospital de la Santa Creu i Sant Pau, Autonomous University of Barcelona, Barcelona, Spain

Victor G. Prieto MD, PhD
Professor of Pathology and Dermatology; Section Chief, Dermatopathology, Department of Pathology, University of Texas; Director of Dermatopathology, Department of Pathology, MD Anderson Cancer Center, Houston, TX, USA

Bradley J. Quade MD
Associate Professor of Pathology, Harvard Medical School; Division of Women's and Perinatal Pathology, Brigham and Women's Hospital, Boston, MA, USA

Stanley J. Robboy MD
Professor of Pathology; Professor of Obstetrics and Gynecology, Department of Pathology, Duke University Medical Center, Durham, NC, USA

Demaretta S. Rush MD
Assistant Professor, Department of Pathology, Immunology and Laboratory Medicine, University of Florida College of Medicine, Gainesville, FL, USA

M. Angelica Selim MD
Professor of Pathology and Dermatology; Director of Dermatopathology, Department of Pathology, Duke University Medical Center, Durham, NC, USA

Ruthy Shaco-Levy MD
Senior Gynecological Pathologist, Department of Pathology, Soroka University Medical Center, Beer-Sheva, Israel

Christopher R. Shea MD
Eugene J. Van Scott Professor in Dermatology, The University of Chicago Medicine, Chicago, IL, USA

Bruce R. Smoller MD
Executive Vice President, United States and Canadian Academy of Pathology, Augusta, GA, USA

Cornelia L. Trimble MD
Associate Professor, Gynecology/Obstetrics, Oncology, Pathology, Johns Hopkins University School of Medicine, Baltimore, MD, USA

Emanuela F. Veras MD
Private Practice, East Georgia Diagnostic Services, Inc., Statesboro, GA, USA

Edward J. Wilkinson MD
Professor and Vice Chairman, Department of Pathology, Immunology and Laboratory Medicine, University of Florida College of Medicine, Gainesville, FL, USA

Thomas C. Wright, Jr. MD
Professor Emeritus and Special Lecturer of Pathology and Cell Biology, Columbia University, New York, NY, USA

To Robert E. Scully MD (1921–2012)
Pioneering pathologist, educator, and gentleman

Acknowledgements

This book began with Malcolm Anderson's 1991 *Female Reproductive System* in the Symmers Systemic Pathology Series, becoming a standalone first edition text in 2002 with Stanley Robboy, Malcolm Anderson, and Peter Russell as editors, and an expanded second edition with additional co-editors (George Mutter, Jaime Prat, Rex Bentley). Although an international project from its inception, these editors greatly increased the roster of authors through targeted recruitment, and created a truly collaborative international environment. These works always kept the reader in mind: presenting expertly curated content in a cleanly written and clinically relevant style.

Dr. Robboy facilitated the transition to this third edition as he turned his attention to another phase of a storied career. He is extraordinarily prescient in anticipating how the practice of pathology might best serve our patients in the context of a complex healthcare system. Soon after the second edition of this book was published, he decided he could best implement many of his goals by running for the Presidency of the College of American Pathologists, a successful endeavor which led to his inauguration in 2011. It was in anticipation of his duties with the CAP, that a period of smooth transition to the current editors followed.

All of the current authors have taken valuable time from their professional, and all too often personal, schedules to contribute their expertise. This is a precious gift in an increasingly busy and overcommitted world. We are most grateful to have the opportunity to work with such a world-class team of experts who have enlightened us all in the process. We would also like to recognize the contributions of authors from prior editions, as we have built upon their solid foundation.

The gracious support of our families and colleagues is what made it possible to engage the many distractions and long hours of extra work necessary for this book. We have succeeded only because of their understanding, and we should acknowledge that it is them who make it all worthwhile.

Lastly, the staff at Elsevier has been outstanding, especially Michael Houston who originally commissioned this book and has now seen it through every edition. A special thanks to the efforts of Martin Mellor and Lucía Pérez throughout the long editorial process.

George L. Mutter and Jaime Prat

Embryology

George L. Mutter, Stanley J. Robboy

CHAPTER OUTLINE

Introduction	1	External Influence on the Developing Embryonic Genital Tract Ducts	12
Gonadal Development	1	The Müllerian Duct after Week 8	14
Role of Germ Cells	11	The Müllerian Duct during the Second Trimester	14
Müllerian and Wolffian Duct Development	11	External Genitalia	15
The Müllerian Duct to Week 8	11		

INTRODUCTION

Understanding normal development of the embryonic genital tract gives insight into many disorders encountered in the female. These can range from relatively simple arrests of development or malformation (described by organ) to more complex abnormalities of sexual development that result from dysembryogenesis (see Chapter 2), and, in some cases, to help understand the origin of some tumors, particularly sex cord–stromal and germ cell tumors of the ovary. Most early insights have come from understanding human mutations. During more recent years, targeted mutations using mouse models have disclosed key roles for genes that had not been anticipated previously. Many regulators of gonadal development are receptors, signal transduction elements, transcription factors, extracellular ligands, and even intracellular signaling pathways mediating downstream transcriptional responses. Recently published references[1-7] provide extensive reviews and, to some degree, competing theories.

Most of the female genital tract is of mesodermal origin. Germ cells are of endodermal origin. The vulva and the epithelial lining of the vagina are ectoderm. The chronology and sequence of events that underlie the development of the female genital tract are summarized in Figures 1.1 and 1.2, and in Table 1.1. Table 1.2 lists specific genes involved in the initial steps of sexual development.

In the broadest view, sex determination takes place in three sequential steps.[8] The first is chromosomal sex determination, which occurs as a result of fertilization. Gonadal sex determination, the second critical event, results when the potential gonads actually transform into ovaries or testes in accord with the available chromosomal information. Third, the secondary sex characteristics develop along female or male lines as determined by the preponderant estrogenic or androgenic hormonal milieu present systemically. Sexual identity, not to be discussed here, includes a person's sense of self (gender identity) and his/her attraction to others.

GONADAL DEVELOPMENT

Prior to the period when sex determination begins, the indifferent gonad arises from the gonadal ridge that, with the mesonephros, lies longitudinally on the dorsal aspect of the celomic cavity. At this time, the indifferent gonad is 'unisex' or, more properly, 'bipotential' due to its ability to develop into a testis or an ovary depending upon the embryo's genetic makeup.

In humans and other mammals, the karyotype 'XY' genetically defines the sex as male, whereas 'XX' defines the female sex. Sex is determined by the presence or absence of a signal from the substance initially called the testis determining factor and now recognized as the gene called *SRY* (*S*ex determining *R*egion *Y*) in the human and *SRY* in the mouse. The gene is found on the Y chromosome. Testes are formed if this gene is expressed by the embryo before the urogenital ridge differentiates. Further male development occurs under the influence of hormones secreted later by the testes. Without *SRY*, the gonads differentiate as ovaries and the embryo develops as a female. The timely expression of *SRY* is critical to the development of male sex. In its absence, the embryo develops a female phenotype, regardless of genetic sex. Although for years believed to occur by default, a gene has been identified in women (R-spondin1, RSPO1)[9] critical for development of the ovary through signaling pathways.[10]

The *SRY* gene is located in the region just central to the pseudoautosomal pairing region at the distal end of the short arm of the Y chromosome.[11] The pseudoautosomal pairing region is named for the two limited regions at the distal ends of the short and long arms of the Y chromosome where sequence identity with the X chromosome permits pairing and recombination during male meiosis.[12] The

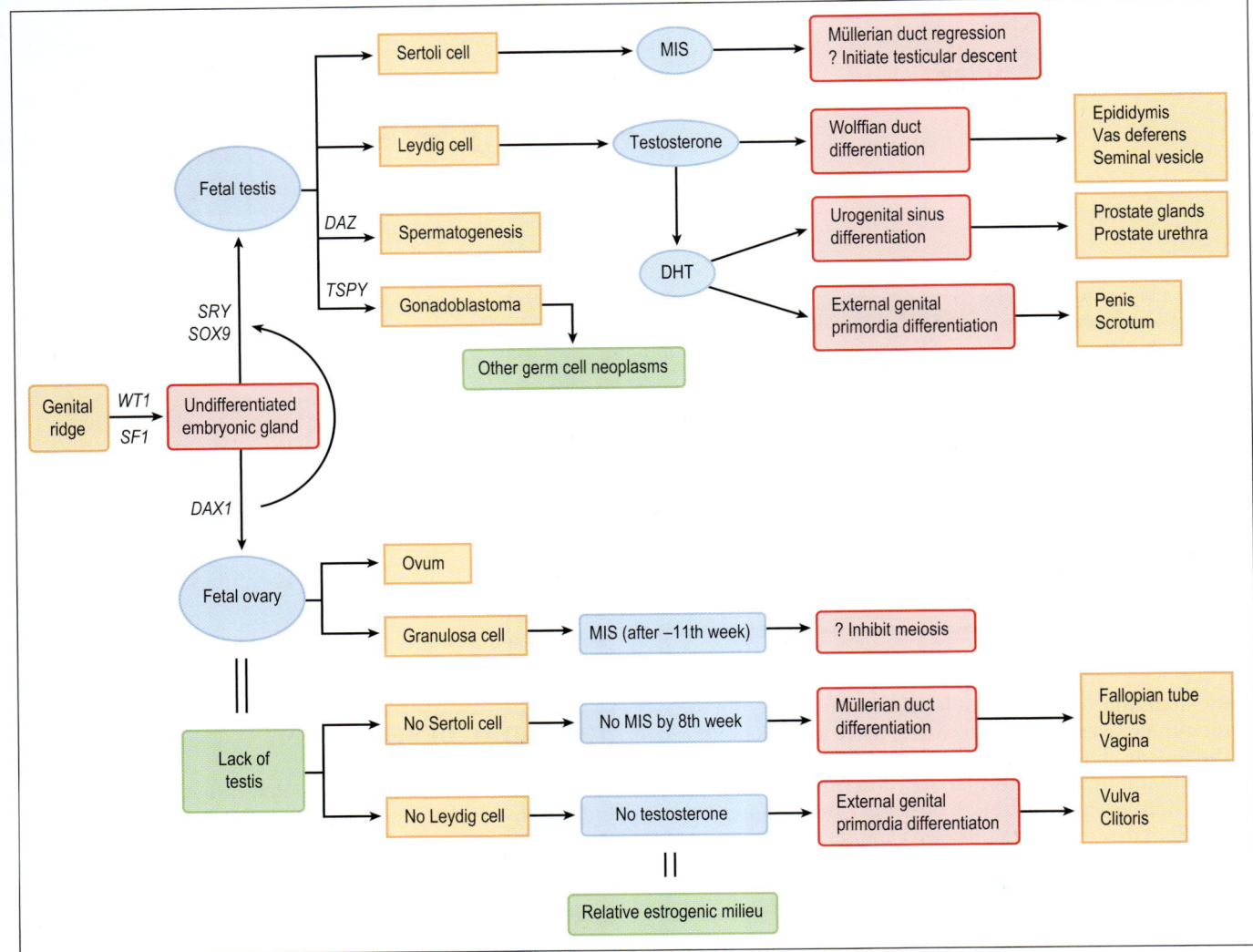

Figure 1.1 Pathophysiology of genital tract development.

gene, which has a strongly conserved motif,[13] encodes for a DNA binding protein, which is the binding activity product (transcriptional switch) that orchestrates the action of other genes. It does so by initiating a cascade of gene expression that regulates the development of the testis, not all of which are known or understood.

Several lines of evidence support this thesis. These include that the:

- *SRY* gene is absent from the normal X chromosome and somatic chromosomes
- *SRY* gene is present on the X chromosome of 'sex-reversed' XX human males
- Homologous gene in the mouse is initially expressed just before sexual differentiation begins
- *SRY* gene acts in the absence of germ cells
- *SRY* gene in the chromosomally female embryo causes it to develop as a male.[14]

Rare examples have also been identified where single base pair point mutations in the *SRY* gene or in promoter regions essential for gene expression render an XY patient as a phenotypic female with a streak gonad.[15]

Early on, *SRY* initiates induction of somatic cell migration from the mesonephros into the gonad[16] and induces indifferent cells in the genital ridge to differentiate into Sertoli cells. This is the first type of cell required to form in the embryonic testis.[17] With monoclonal antibodies, an *SRY* protein has been found in the nuclei of Sertoli cells and germ cells.[18] Several other genes are thought to be important in Sertoli cell function. *SOX9*, which is named for it being an *SRY*-related high motility gene box group, in the mouse is active in pre-Sertoli cells[19] and results in XY human females when mutations inactivate the gene. *SF1*, which *SOX9* helps regulate, is another important gene that is an orphan nuclear receptor expressed in the gonadal ridge in precursor cells of Sertoli and stromal cells. It appears as a master regulator of the reproductive system because it regulates the expression of numerous genes required for gland development and hormone synthesis.[20–22] Mutations in this gene in humans have been responsible for adrenal

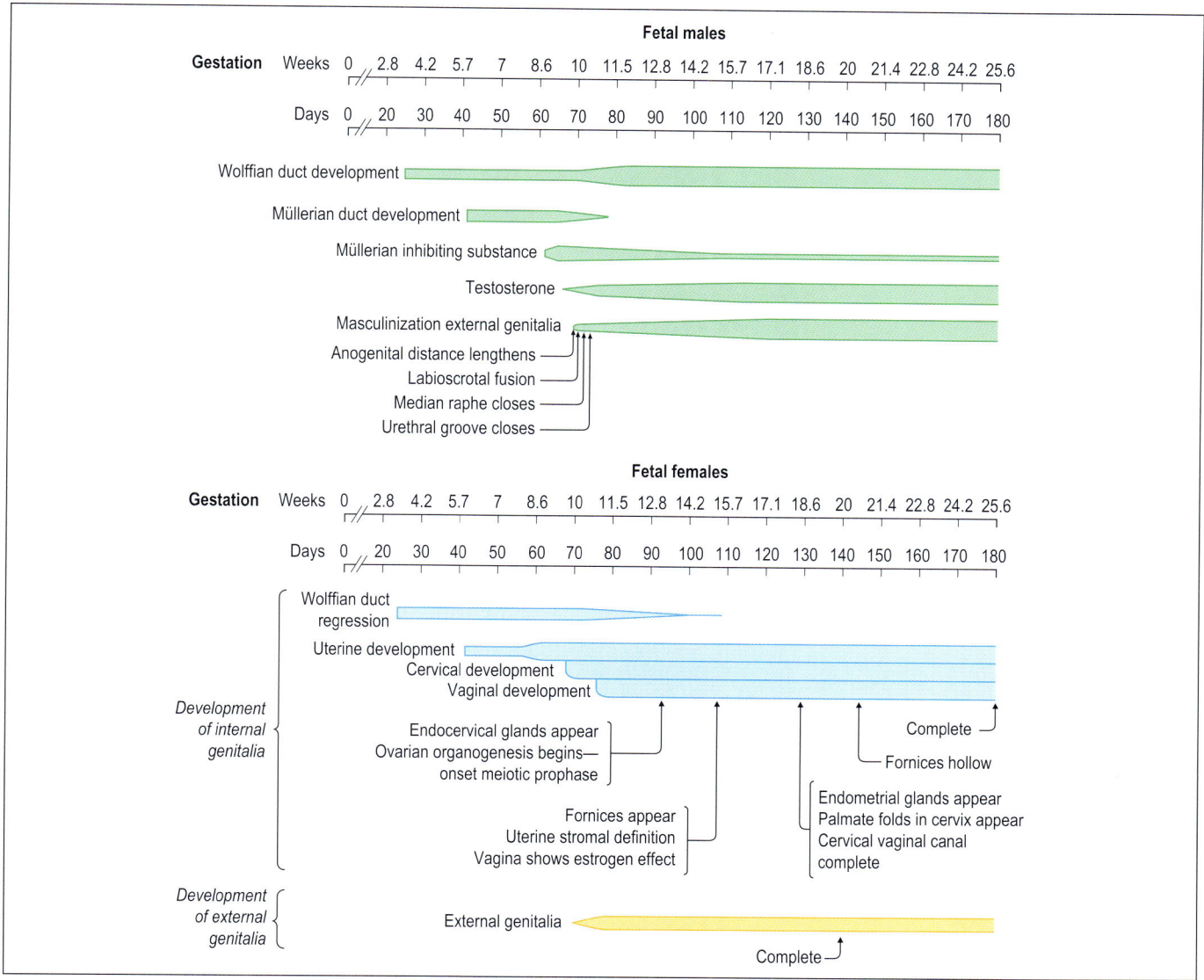

Figure 1.2 Normal sexual development. Embryologic development is determined by several factors, all of which are time specific during embryogenesis.

insufficiency associated with gonadal dysgenesis.[23] The gene *DAX1*, which is required at several points in embryonic testis development,[24] also plays a key role in sex determination. Overexpression causes varying degrees of gonadal dysgenesis, and at high doses in the mouse, male-to-female sex reversal occurs. Additional references[8,12,22,25] describe in greater detail the genes involved in the rapidly evolving science of male sex determination.

In the event that the embryo does not express *SRY* on a time-sensitive basis as a transcription factor, and therefore does not develop a testis, then other genes that are responsible for the development of the ovary activate later. In the goat, studies on XX sex reversal in polled (horned) goats have led to the discovery of a female-specific locus critical for ovarian differentiation (see later discussion about *FOXL2*).

During the development of both male and female human embryos, but before the gonads develop, the primordial germ cells migrate from the yolk sac to the urogenital ridges via the caudal part of the hindgut approximately 3 weeks after fertilization (Figure 1.3). The yolk sac, which is of considerable size (Figure 1.4), is easily recognized by its reactivity to α-fetoprotein. This migratory event is independent of eventual sex. The germ cells are large and prominent, and have clear cytoplasm and vesicular nuclei. Once they synthesize glycogen and alkaline phosphatase, they are easily identified histochemically by their demonstration of placental-like alkaline phosphatase (PLAP) and CD117 (c-kit).

At about this time, the mesothelium on the medial surface of the urogenital ridge, which itself is located ventral to the mesonephric rudiments, begins to proliferate. By the fifth week, while still in the indifferent stage, the parenchyma is a thin wisp, measuring less than 1 mm in thickness and several millimeters in width (Figures 1.5 and 1.6). Several transcription factors, including Wilms' tumor 1 (*WT1*) and steroidogenic factor 1 (*SF1*), are involved in the

Table 1.1 Synopsis of Stages of Normal Embryologic Development

Postovulatory Week	Crown–Rump at Beginning of Week	Sequence of Events (Top to Bottom) Within Stated Week
1 week	0.2 mm	Uterine implantation (0.2 mm).
2 weeks	1.5 mm	Primitive pit forms. No somites yet.
3 weeks	2.0 mm	1–3 somites. Pronephric tubules form; pronephric (mesonephric) duct arises and grows caudad as solid cord (2.5 mm). Primordial germ cells first discernible in yolk sac near caudal part of embryo (2–3 mm). Pronephros degenerated, but mesonephric duct reaches cloaca (3–5 mm). Primordial germ cells discernible in hindgut (3–5 mm). Primordial germ cells discernible in mesonephric ridges (5 mm).
4 weeks	7 mm	Primordial germ cells discernible in gonadal ridge, which itself at this time is a thin mesodermal proliferation (7 mm). Cloaca divides into rectum and urogenital sinus. Müllerian ducts appear as funnel-shaped opening of celomic epithelium.
5 weeks	12 mm	Indifferent gonad bulges into celom (12 mm). Primitive sex cords appear (16–17 mm).
6 weeks	18 mm	Müllerian ducts about half distance to urogenital sinus. Testis anatomically distinct with seminiferous tubules and capsule (tunica albuginea).
7 weeks	23 mm	Ovaries initially identified by absence of distinct seminiferous tubules (23 mm). Müllerian ducts elongate and near urogenital sinus (23 mm). Müllerian ducts in apposition; sinusal tubercle appears (23–28 mm). Müllerian ducts lose sensitivity to MIS at 25 mm, but regression effect not observed until 31–35 mm.
8 weeks	29 mm	Müllerian ducts fuse and in contact with urogenital sinus (29 mm).
9 weeks	43 mm	Müllerian duct regression in response to MIS completed by 43–55 mm. Testes and ovaries acquire capacity to secrete characteristic hormones at same stage of development; testosterone coincides with histologic development of Leydig cells and immediately precedes virilization of genital tract; ovary not yet differentiated; rate-limiting step is appearance of 3-α-hydroxysteroid dehydrogenase, which is 50-fold more abundant in testis than in ovary; ovary converts testosterone to estradiol, which testis cannot do; later regulation shifted to pituitary–placenta gonadotropins where testosterone → estradiol controlled by conversion of cholesterol to pregnenolone. Müllerian ducts completely fused (entire septum gone); caudal aspect proliferates; epithelium lining canal stratifies (2–3 cells layers thick).
10 weeks	60 mm	Anogenital distance lengthens. Testosterone synthesis sufficient to induce development of mesonephric duct into definitive structures (epididymis, vas deferens, and seminal vesicle). Subsequently, testosterone converted peripherally into 5-α-dihydrotestosterone, which causes the following transformations: Urogenital sinus → prostate Genital tubercle → glans penis Genital folds → penis (only 3.5 mm long) Genital swelling → scrotum Fusion of labioscrotal folds. Closure of median raphe. Closure of urethral groove. Phallus in both sexes 3 mm long; thereafter grows in males 0.72 mm/week and females 0.20 mm/week. Mesonephric ducts regress if not stimulated by testosterone. Vaginal plate first seen distinctly (complete at 140 mm; week 17). Initially, upper uterovaginal canal is large and oval in cross section, mostly lined by pseudostratified columnar epithelium. Extensive growth begins caudally; cells stratify. Uterovaginal canal occluded caudally, progresses cranially.
11 weeks	71 mm	Primordial follicles appear. Seminal vesicles develop. Testis at inguinal ring. Extensive uterovaginal growth continues caudally.
12 weeks	93 mm	Cervical glands appear; wavy, but undifferentiated. Vaginal rudiment approaches vestibule. True ovarian organogenesis begins with onset of meiotic prophase.
13 weeks	105 mm	Male urethral organogenesis complete.

Table 1.1 Continued

Postovulatory Week	Crown–Rump at Beginning of Week	Sequence of Events (Top to Bottom) Within Stated Week
14 weeks	116 mm	Primary folds of mucosa give uterine lumen W-shaped appearance on cross section. Vaginal rudiment reaches level of vestibular glands; uterovaginal canal (15 mm total length) divisible into vagina (one-half), cervix (one-third), and corpus (one-sixth); boundaries ill-defined. Isthmus readily distinguishable. Stromal layers of uterus begin definition. Solid epithelial anlage of anterior and posterior fornices appear. Vagina begins to show slight estrogen effect.
15 weeks	130 mm	Fallopian tube begins active growth phase, begins to coil. Vaginal plate completed; lower end reaches vestibule; upper end extends into endocervical canal. Female urogenital sinus becomes shallow vestibule. Primary follicles of ovary appear.
16 weeks	142 mm	Vaginal plate longest and begins to canalize. Corpus glands appear as slight outpouchings.
17 weeks	153 mm	Palmate folds of cervix appear (forerunner adult cervix). Mucoid development of cervix begins. Smooth muscle of uterus appears. Estrogen effect apparent throughout vagina. Cavitation of vaginal canal completed.
18 weeks	164 mm	Fornices hollow.
19 weeks	177 mm	
20 weeks	186 mm	Dramatic increase in growth and coiling of fallopian tube (about 3 mm/week to week 34).
21 weeks	197 mm	
22 weeks	208 mm	Differentiation of muscular layer of uterus complete. Fundus well marked; uterus assumes adult form. Graafian follicles appear.
24 weeks	230 mm	
26 weeks	250 mm	
28 weeks	270 mm	
30 weeks	290 mm	
34 weeks	328 mm	
38 weeks	362 mm	Birth.

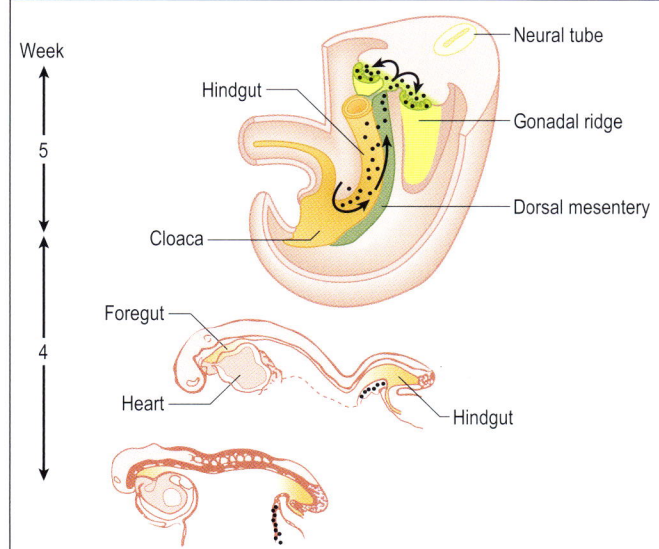

Figure 1.3 Migration of germ cells in the human embryo. At the end of the third week, epiblast-derived cells present in the yolk sac near the allantoic base have differentiated into primordial germ cells, the latter having migrated by the fifth week along the dorsal mesentery of the hindgut to the gonadal ridges.

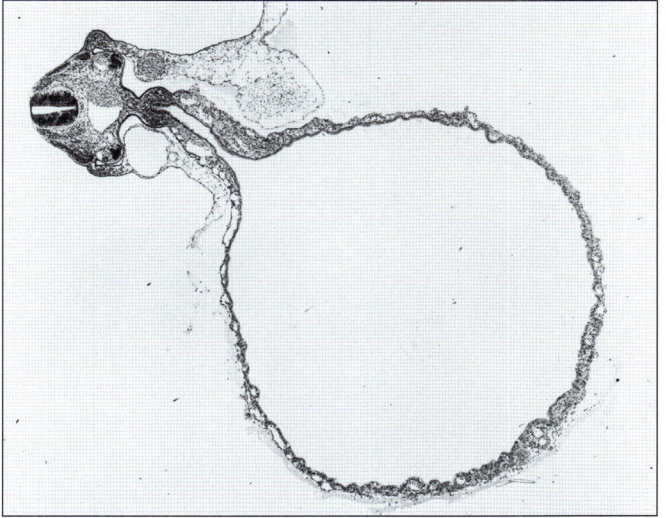

Figure 1.4 The yolk sac connects to the hindgut, along which germ cells migrate, day 28.

Table 1.2 Genes Involved in Sex Determination

Gene	Origin of Name	Localization	Expressed by	Function	Phenotype if Abnormal
Testis determining					
SRY = NR5A1	Sex determining region Y (nuclear receptor subfamily 5, group A, member 1)	Yp11	Genital ridge and Sertoli cells	Transcription factor	XY gonadal dysgenesis
SOX9	Srybox	17q24	Sertoli cells	Transcription factor	Campomelic dysplasia with XY gonadal dysgenesis
SF1	Steroidogenic factor-1	9q33	Ovary, adrenal gland and Sertoli cells	Transcription factor	Gonadal and adrenal agenesis in mouse
WT1	Wilms' tumor suppressor gene	11p13	Primordial gonad and kidney	Transcription factor	Denys–Drash and Frasier syndromes
DAX1 = NR0B1	DAX1, DSS-AHC on the X chromosome, where DSS is dosage sensitive sex reversal gene AHC is adrenal hypoplasia congenital gene (nuclear receptor subfamily 0, group B, member 1)	Xp21.3	Genital ridge	Transcription factor	XY gonadal dysgenesis
DMRT1, DMRT2	Double sex and mab-3 related transcription factor 1	9p24.3	Testis	High and low expression, respectively, required for testis and ovarian differentiation	XY sex reversal
Ovary determining					
FOXL2	Forkhead box L2	3q23	Genital ridge, ovarian follicular cells	Forkhead transcription factor	Premature ovarian failure
WNT4	Wingless-related integration site 4 (wingless-type MMTV integration site family, member 4)	1p35	Leydig cells	Signaling molecule for pattern formation	Rokitansky–Kuster–Hauser syndrome
Phenotype determining					
AMH (MIS)	Anti-müllerian hormone (müllerian inhibiting substance, type 1)	19q13	Sertoli cells and in secondary follicle granulosa cells	Causes regression of fetal müllerian ducts, inhibits Leydig cells	Persistent müllerian duct syndrome
AMHR2 MISR II	Anti-müllerian hormone type 2 receptor Müllerian inhibiting substance II	12q12–13	Primary sex cords; and müllerian duct	Serine threonine kinase receptor	Persistent müllerian duct syndrome

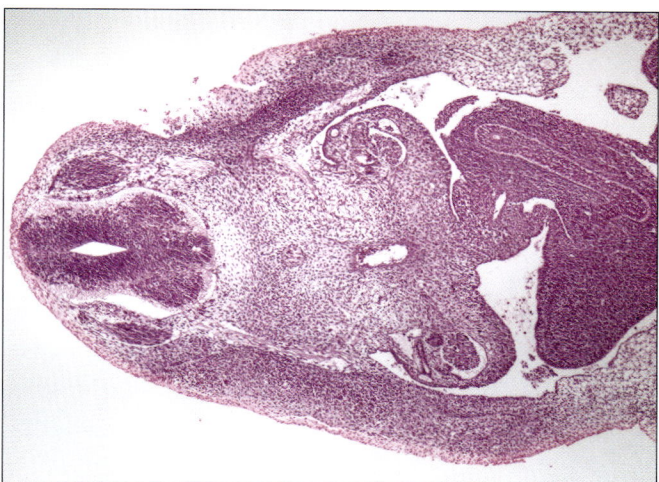

Figure 1.5 The gonadal ridge in the 7 mm embryo (5 weeks) is much thinner than the width of the mesonephros.

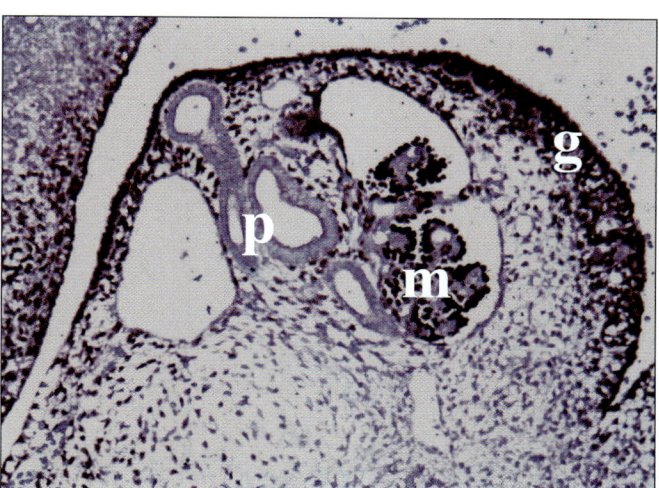

Figure 1.7 *WT1* is expressed in the mesonephros (m) and the genital ridge (g) (about day 33). The residual pronephric ducts (p) do not react.

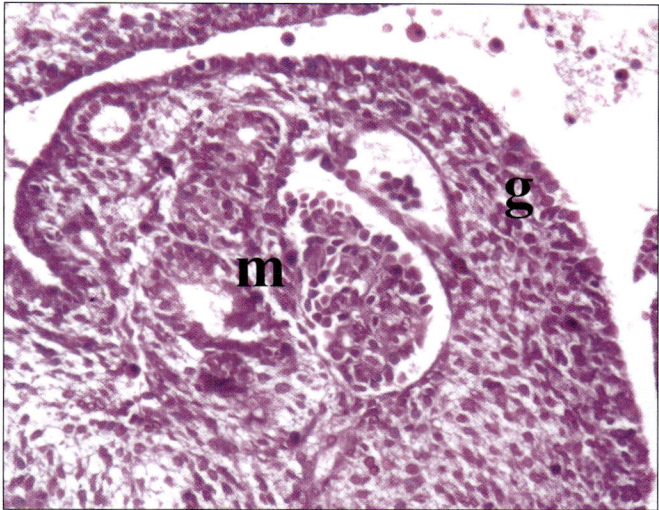

Figure 1.6 Detail of mesonephros (m) and gonadal ridge (g), 7 mm embryo.

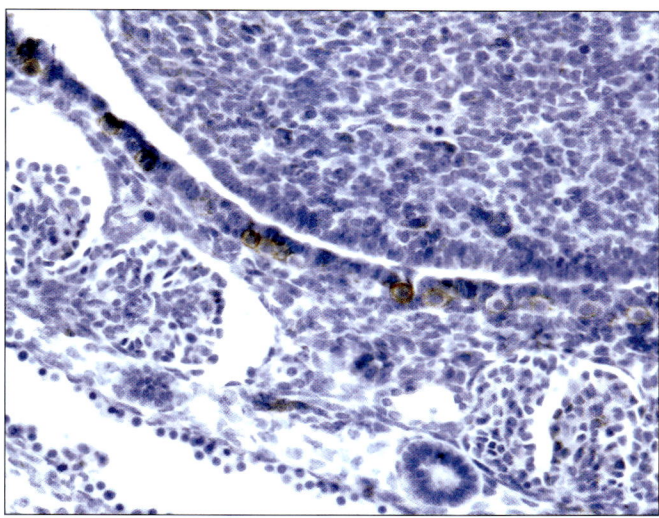

Figure 1.8 C-kit reactive germ cells (brown) in the genital ridge (about 33 days).

earliest processes of gonad formation, regardless of the direction to which the gonad differentiates (Figure 1.7). These transcription factors act on the somatic cells in the gonadal primordia, but do not affect the germ cells themselves, which are still easily identifiable by their reactivity for PLAP and c-kit (Figure 1.8). Over the next several weeks the ridge develops into a recognizable, but undifferentiated, gonad (Figures 1.9 and 1.10).

During the initial stages of both testicular and ovarian development, the gonads develop independent of whether the primordial germ cells are present or absent or have proliferated abnormally. An early manifestation of the normally developing gonad is the appearance in the gonad of primary sex cords, which are temporary branched structures containing the proliferating germ cells and support cells (Figures 1.11 and 1.12). This process begins during the fifth week. The sex cords, the exact embryologic derivation of which is uncertain but seemingly dependent on the migration of mesonephric interstitial cells, lack a basement membrane and basal myoid cells. In a manner not yet understood, in the presence of *SRY* and with the participation of the rete and mesonephric apparatus, the sex cords transform into the tubules, which become cords of epithelial-like cells that extend from the rete in the hilus of the gonad into the medulla. The level of the connection is less important than the field effect of induction of epithelial–mesenchymal differentiation (Figure 1.13).

In females, germ cells continue to increase in number (Figures 1.14 and 1.15) until ovarian differentiation is apparent at approximately 15 weeks, as shown by the emergence of primordial follicles. In many other respects, until this time the ovarian tissue continues to resemble the indifferent gonad, unlike the testis, which becomes anatomically distinct with early tubular formation and immature Sertoli

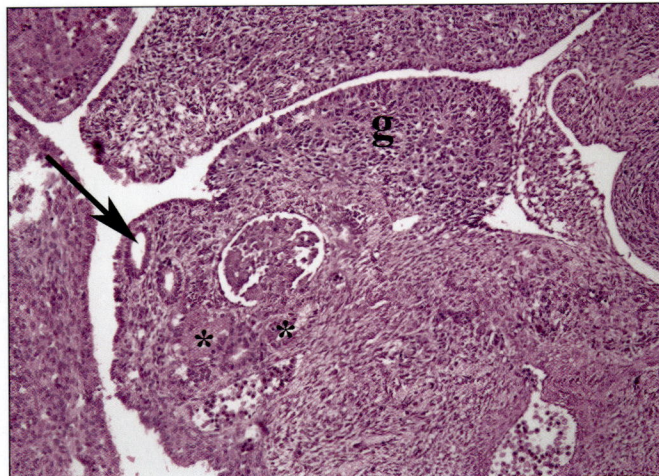

Figure 1.9 Undifferentiated gonad (g) with wolffian (asterisks) and müllerian (arrow) ducts and adjacent mesonephros containing glomerular structures (about 42 days).

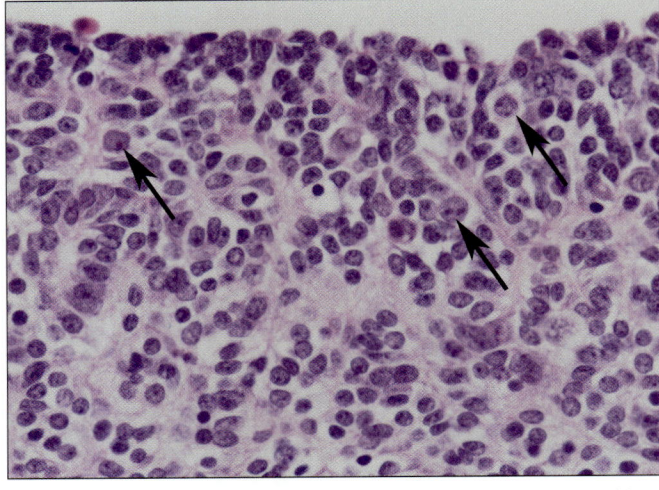

Figure 1.12 Germ cells with enlarged nuclei (arrows) are evident within the poorly formed sex cords in this 56 day gonad.

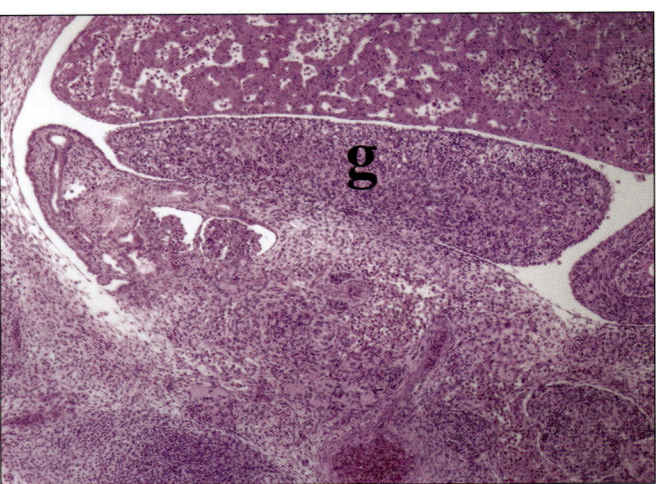

Figure 1.10 Undifferentiated gonad (g) showing enlargement and development of characteristic gonadal shape (about 45 days).

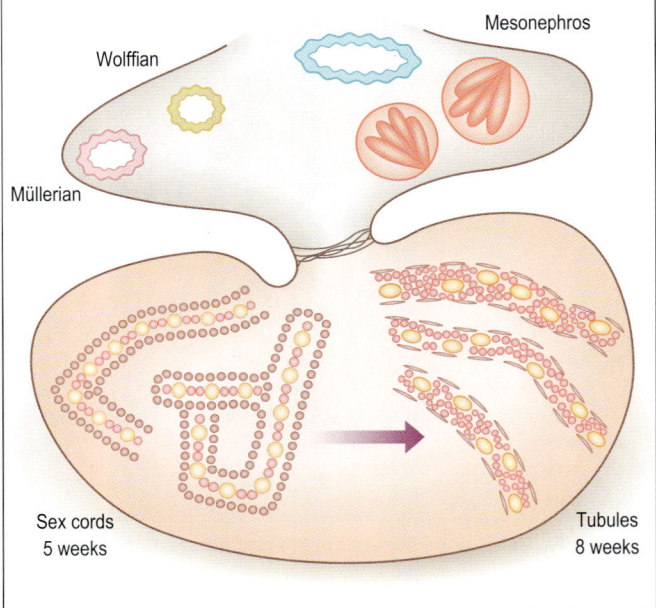

Figure 1.13 Testicular development in male embryo from 5–8 weeks of gestation. Within the bean-like gonad the primary sex cords develop under the influence of migrating mesonephric cells, which induce a mesenchymal to epithelial switch of differentiation similar to that happening in the metanephros under the action of *WT1*. The conversion of the sex cords to tubules is induced by the rete, which is under *SRY* control, and connected to the tubules. The primary sex cords (left) are composed of primary germ cells (yellow) and stromal cells that have acquired epithelial features. Tubular differentiation (right) features acquisition of myoid cells and a peripheral basement membrane and more centrally located Sertoli (pink) and germ cells (yellow).

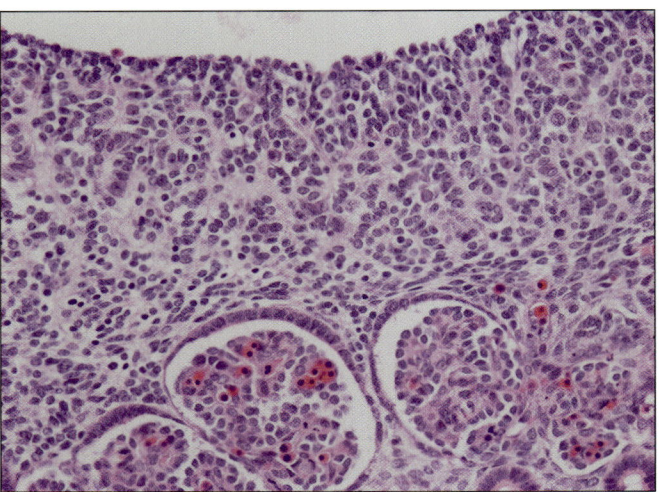

Figure 1.11 Sex cords become more prominent in this still indifferent gonad. Mesonephric glomeruli present underneath (about 56 days).

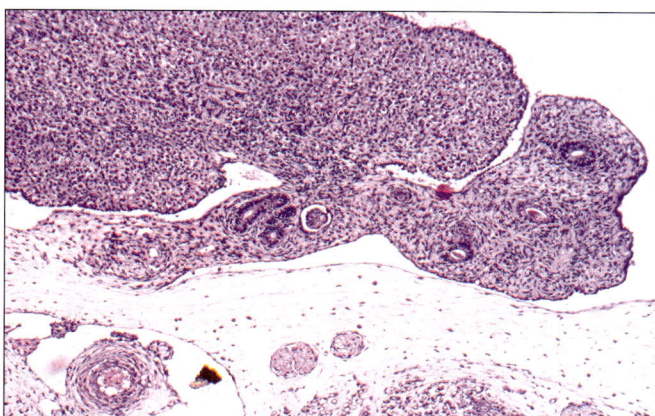

Figure 1.14 Ovarian volume is greater than in prior weeks, 10 week fetus.

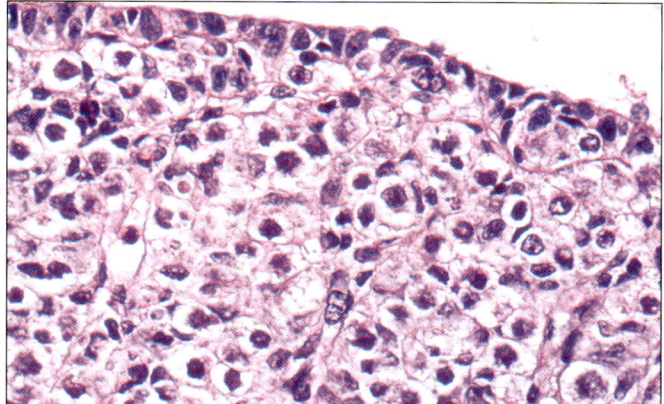

Figure 1.15 Ovary with numerous oogonia before primordial follicles develop, 10 week fetus.

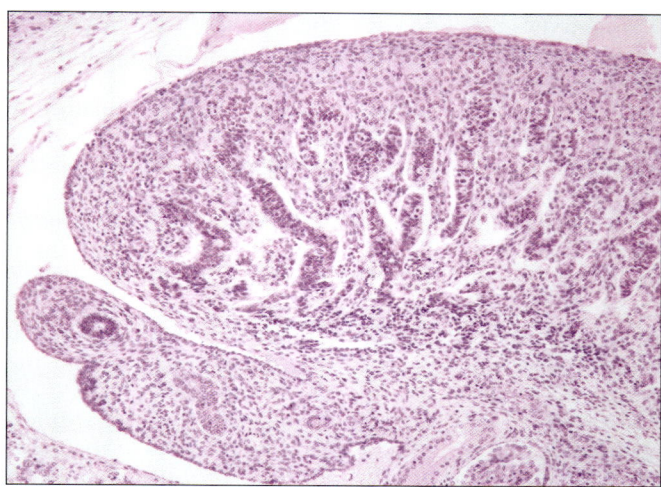

Figure 1.16 The testis capsule (tunica albuginea) separates early seminiferous tubules from the surface, approximately 10 weeks (70 days).

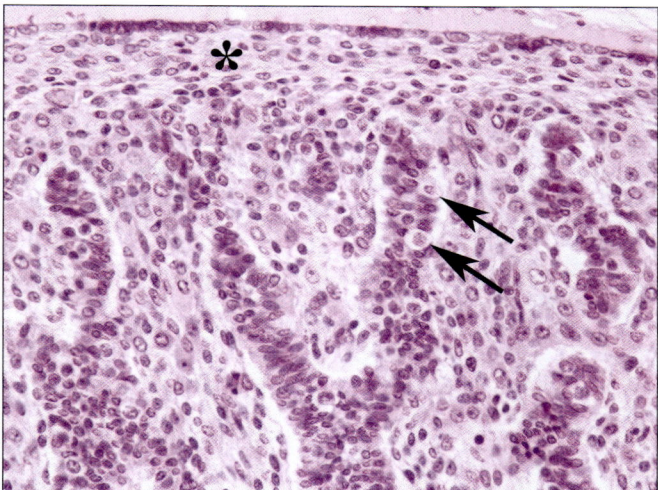

Figure 1.17 Testis with seminiferous tubules, intratubal germ cells (arrows), and overlying tunica (asterisk), 10 week fetus.

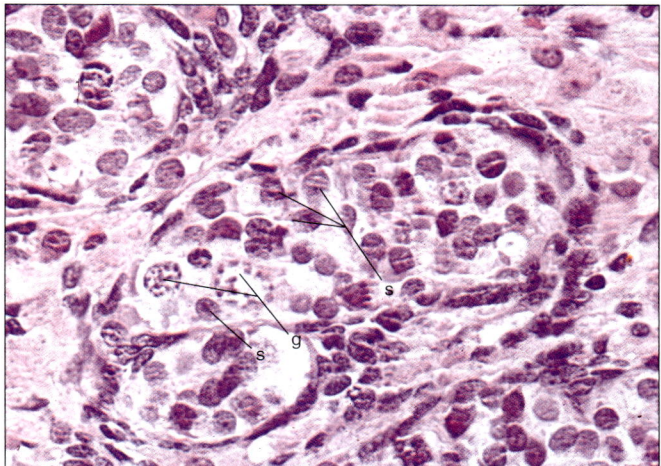

Figure 1.18 Testis with seminiferous tubules and intratubal germ cells, 19 week fetus. g, germ cell; s, Sertoli cell.

cells by postovulation day 44. (In this chapter, all dates given are postovulation.)

In the male, one of the first easily recognized testis-specific structures that can be identified is its capsule, or tunica albuginea (Figures 1.16 and 1.17), which is first evident at approximately 50 days. The tunica is a zone of spindle cells that develops and separates the epithelial cords from the surface. The cords become the testicular tubules as the epithelial cells differentiate into the tall, clear, flask-shaped Sertoli cells of the testis and myoid (peritubular contractile) cells appear just outside the basement membrane. The gonadal stromal cells become the interstitial or Leydig cells. In normal development, the germ cells are initially located in the lumen and move eventually between the Sertoli cells to lie on the basement membrane at the base of the tubules (Figure 1.18). The primordial germ cells preferentially colonize the medullary region of the presumptive gonads.[14] Even in the absence of germ cells, the somatic tissues of the undifferentiated embryonic gonad are capable of developing into a testis, albeit lacking spermatogonia and spermatogenesis.[26]

At some later time, another gene of the Y chromosome comes into play and activates the process for the development of normal spermatogenesis. The gene, called *DAZ* (*D*eleted in *AZ*oospermia), is less well characterized than the *SRY* gene.[27] In the absence of *DAZ*, or at least if not detectable by current methods, sperm will still develop, although defective and few in number, it will still be capable of successful fertility.[28] *DAZ* mutation results in loss of the Y chromosome during mitosis, which leads to the creation of both XO and XY cell lines.

If functional *SRY* is absent (i.e., normal 46,XX females), genes associated with ovarian development activate.[29] *WNT4*, the first signaling molecule identified in the study of sex determination in mice, regulates female sexual development.[13] Part of its function is to repress male sexual differentiation. Patients with defective *WNT4* present with a Mayer–Rokitansky–Hauser-like syndrome with absence of müllerian structures, unilateral renal agenesis, and clinical signs of androgen excess.[30] *FOXL2* is demonstrable in the genital ridge before there is any clear structural organization of the gonads.[31-33] Recent studies in mice have shown a robust female genetic program that activates at the onset of ovarian development.[34]

In the absence of male determining factors, the dividing germ cells are incorporated into a proliferating mass of surface epithelial cells, which results in a thickened cortex that presages the organization of the adult ovary without the development of a separating tunica (Figure 1.19). From the second to the early third trimester, this thickened cortical mass of proliferating epithelial and germ cells divides into small groups demarcated by strands of stromal tissue extending from the medulla to the cortex (Figure 1.20). The small groups of germ cells and epithelial cells further subdivide into primordial follicles composed of single germ cells surrounded by a layer of epithelial cells, the primitive granulosa cells (Figure 1.21). In normal development, each germ cell is characteristically encapsulated in its own (primordial) follicle. Oogonia, not so enveloped, undergo spontaneous apoptosis. This is associated with entry into meiosis and cessation of further proliferation. By puberty, while most of the ovary shows variable concentrations of oocytes (Figure 1.22), some have developed into the antral stage and may become future ovulatory sites (see Chapter 23).

Until about the 15th week, the ovary is an undifferentiated gonad with a streak-like pattern. The primary sex cords begin their development under the influence of mesonephric cells that had migrated earlier and then remained inactive. The mesenchymal to epithelial switch of differentiation starts deeply in the parenchyma as does early primary follicular differentiation, as shown by immunohistochemical demonstration of *FOXL2* nuclear reactivity and the

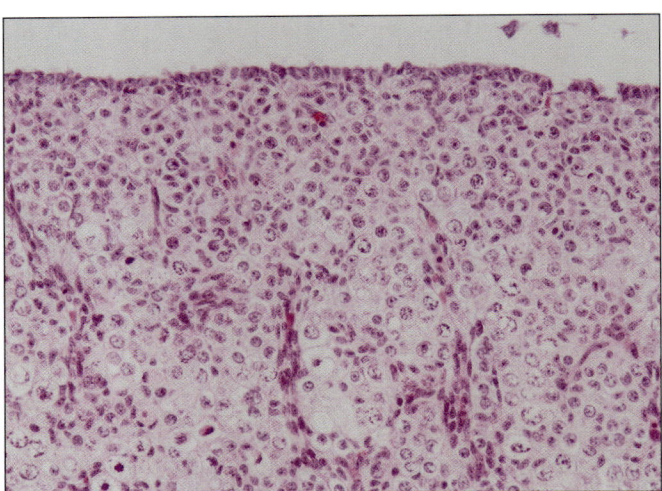

Figure 1.20 Ovary at 15 weeks' gestation showing sheets of germ cells extending to the surface epithelium. Vascular elements divide the oocytes into nests.

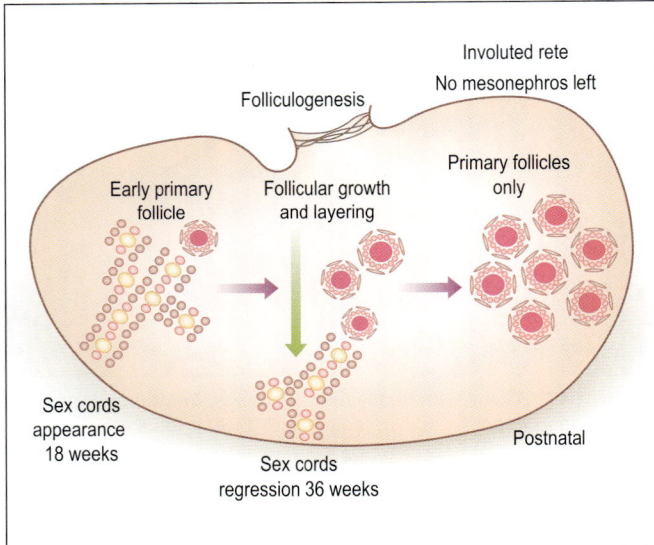

Figure 1.19 Ovarian development from 18 weeks through birth. Until the 18th week of gestation the ovary is an undifferentiated gonad with a streak-like pattern. The primary sex cords begin their development under the influence of mesonephric cells that had migrated earlier and then remained inactive. The mesenchymal to epithelial switch of differentiation starts deeply in the parenchyma as does early primary follicular differentiation, as shown by immunohistochemical demonstration of FOXL2 nuclear reactivity and the appearance of primary follicles of small size. The folliculogenetic process repeats itself in a deeper to more superficial direction with the progressive disappearance of the primary sex cords around 36 weeks' gestation. The growth in follicles occurs under the influence of WT1 like that of metanephric glomeruli in the kidney. Simultaneously, the primary sex cords regress by apoptotic death of the remaining cells. By birth, only primary follicles remain. Primary sex cords (left) are composed of primary germ cells (yellow) and stromal cells acquiring epithelial features. Follicles (left, middle, and right) disclose a central oogonium (large pink) surrounded by follicular (granulosa) cells. A peripheral basement membrane envelops each follicle.

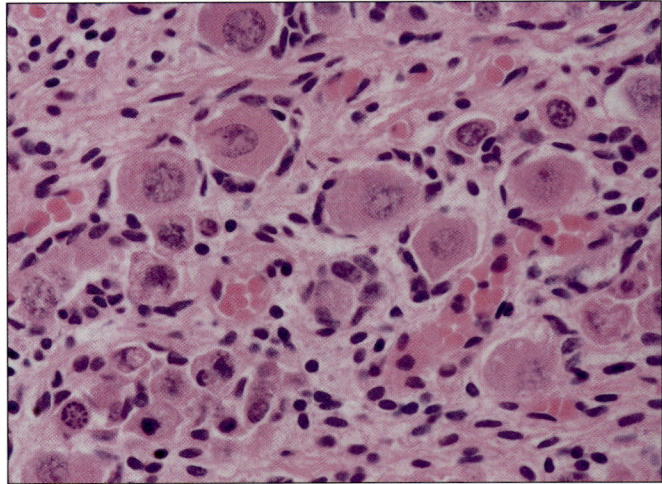

Figure 1.21 Ovary at 36 weeks' gestation showing primordial follicles.

appearance of primary follicles of small size. The folliculogenetic process repeats itself from the deeper to the more superficial with the progressive disappearance of the primary sex cords around 36 weeks' gestation. The growth in follicles occurs under the influence of *WT1*, similar to that for metanephric glomeruli in the kidney. Simultaneously, the primary sex cords regress by apoptotic death of the remaining cells. By birth, only primary follicles remain.

If the normal male genetic constitution (46,XY) is present, some of the early epithelial proliferation contributes to the connection between the sex cords and the mesonephric tubules (rete testis). Where gonads are destined to become ovary, early epithelial proliferation degenerates in the ovarian hilus, leaving a few tubules, the rete ovarii. It is these primordial mesonephric cells that are believed to develop and envelop the individual germ cells and eventually become the follicular granulosa cells. Interstitial (Leydig) cells develop extensively in the stromal tissue of the second trimester female gonad, but degenerate in most cases by term. The few interstitial cells found in the hilus of the adult ovary are called hilus cells (Figure 1.23). Thus, the gonad develops primarily from mesodermal tissues, with the exception of the germ cells, which migrate from the extraembryonic yolk sac to the fetal visceral endoderm.

ROLE OF GERM CELLS

The primordial germ cells, which migrate to the primitive gonad, are not undifferentiated cells. By the time of their migration from the yolk sac to the gonadal ridge, they have attained some developmental potency. Occasionally, germ cells stray during migration and reach ectopic sites. If they do not die, they still may be capable of differentiation, but, remarkably, always differentiate as oocytes regardless of their genetic sex. Even if the cells are in males, they differentiate as XX germ cells would normally in the ovary. It is thought that the absence of Sertoli cell differentiation is important, and the suggestion remains that all germ cells should be viewed potentially as female, regardless of the genetic sex of the patient. Follicular cells also appear important: in their absence, germ cells in ectopic sites usually degenerate and disappear. Thus, the ability of primordial germ cells to develop into oocytes or spermatogenic cells seems to reflect the tissue environment in which they grow rather than their own native chromosomal constitution. The development of the germ cells follows the somatic sex of the gonadal tissue, and not the genetic sex of the germ cells themselves.[35] In the mouse there is evidence that c-kit reactive stem cells present in bone marrow become ovarian-type germ cells.[36]

MÜLLERIAN AND WOLFFIAN DUCT DEVELOPMENT

THE MÜLLERIAN DUCT TO WEEK 8

Regardless of genetic sex, the celomic epithelium in both females and males invaginates at several points on the lateral surface of the paired urogenital ridges beginning at week 5 of embryonic life. They coalesce to form the paired tubes termed the müllerian (paramesonephric) ducts (Figures 1.24 and 1.25). Each of the paired ducts extends caudally in the urogenital ridge immediately lateral to and using the wolffian (mesonephric) duct as a guidewire. For proper müllerian duct migration to occur, the wolffian duct must be present. Spatially lateral to the cephalad aspect of the wolffian ducts, the müllerian ducts then cross over caudally to lie medial to them as they enter the pelvis (Figure 1.26). By the end of week 8 of embryonic life, the müllerian ducts between the two wolffian ducts fuse to form a single structure, which is the anlage of the common uterovaginal canal (Figure 1.27). The tip of the müllerian duct abuts upon the posterior wall of the urogenital sinus immediately between the two orifices of the wolffian ducts (Figure 1.28), approximately at the position of the future cervix.

All of the above occur in both female and male fetuses and are completed before the testis, if the embryo is male, begins to secrete anti-müllerian hormone (AMH), also known as müllerian inhibiting substance (MIS). In the presence of AMH, the müllerian tissues regress, remaining only as rudimentary structures in the maturing male urogenital system.

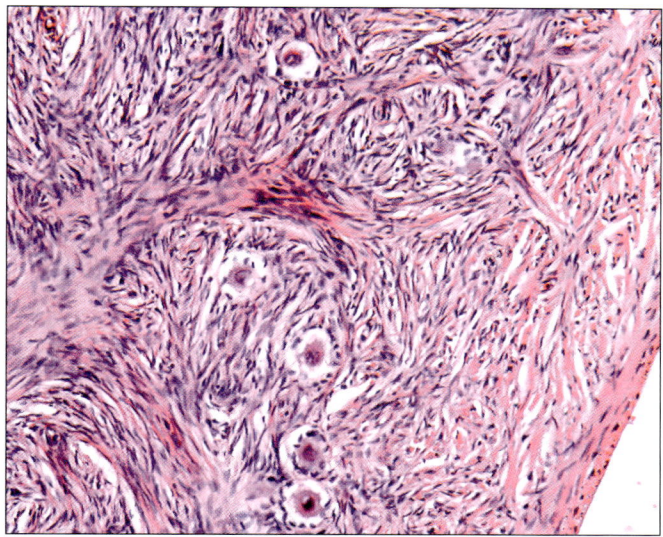

Figure 1.22 Ovary of a 13-year-old child. The primary follicles are widely spaced (H&E).

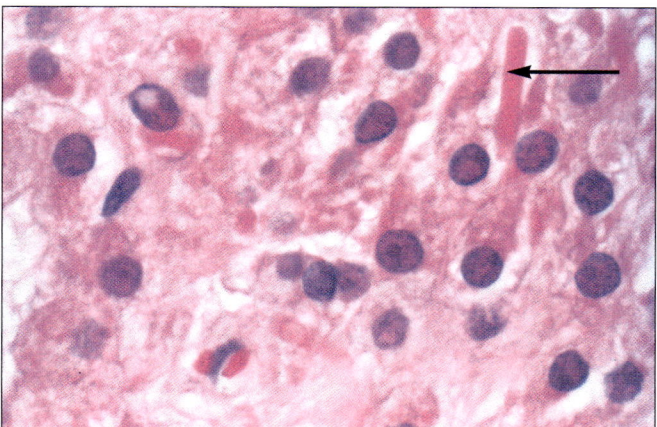

Figure 1.23 Hilus cells with crystalloids of Reinke (arrow) surround a nerve. The crystalloids appear as proteinaceous rods.

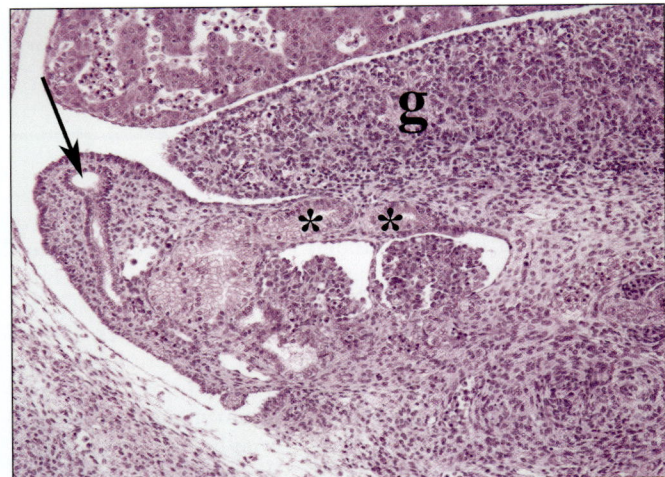

Figure 1.24 The müllerian duct (arrow) formed by invagination of the celomic epithelium adjacent to the mesonephros (paramesonephric) becomes the fallopian tube. Mesonephric tubules in the region of the gonadal hilum (asterisks) remain as the rete ovarii, 6.5 week embryo; g, gonad.

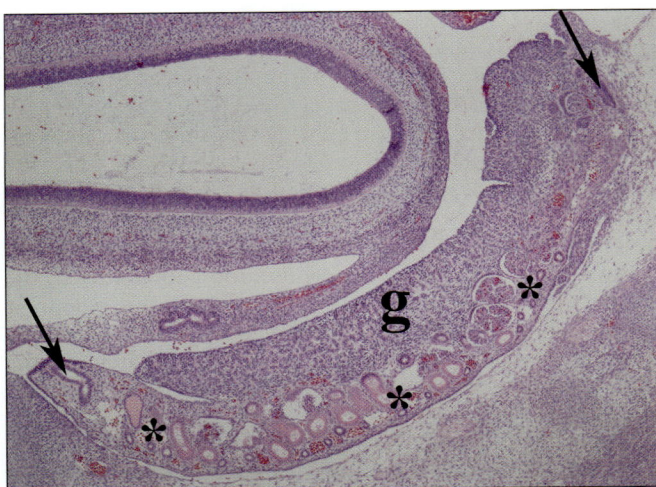

Figure 1.25 Mesonephric (wolffian, asterisks) ducts and mesonephric glomeruli underlie the length of the indifferent gonadal ridge (g). The müllerian duct (paramesonephric duct) forms by invagination at the end of the mesonephros, and courses from a cranial (right arrow) to caudal (left arrow) direction along the gonad as the presumptive fallopian tube. Parasagittal section of 8 week embryo.

EXTERNAL INFLUENCE ON THE DEVELOPING EMBRYONIC GENITAL TRACT DUCTS

Once the male pathway of development has begun, two hormones produced by the fetal testis then control the differentiation of the male phenotype. The first is AMH, which the Sertoli cells produce early during fetal life.[37,38] The primary function of AMH is to cause regression of the müllerian (paramesonephric) ducts in the male fetus, which it does by its effects on the mesenchyme surrounding the duct (Figure 1.29).

AMH is first secreted in effective amounts 56–62 days after fertilization, and the process of müllerian regression is normally completed by about day 77, after which the müllerian tissue is no longer sensitive to AMH. During this critical period, even relatively small amounts of AMH given over a short period of time can cause irreversible damage to the embryonic müllerian tract.[39] In the female, AMH is produced in insignificant amounts during fetal life (as there are no Sertoli cells) and the müllerian ducts develop passively to form the fallopian tubes, uterus, and vaginal wall. Other functions of AMH, secreted later in fetal life, are discussed in the following sections.

AMH has a local action, and inhibits development of the ipsilateral fallopian tube. To prevent development of both the uterus and vagina, both testes must secrete adequate amounts of AMH. Thus, in a patient with a testis and a contralateral streak, the ovary or ovotestis generally has a uterus and vagina and a single fallopian tube on the side with the streak or ovary. AMH immunoreactivity can be observed in Sertoli cell cytoplasm from roughly week 8 of fetal life until puberty. It is detected in the Sertoli cells in the premeiotic seminal pretubules but disappears in older tubules that have shown meiotic development.[38]

Additional functions of AMH have recently been discovered or postulated. In the female, ovarian granulosa cells

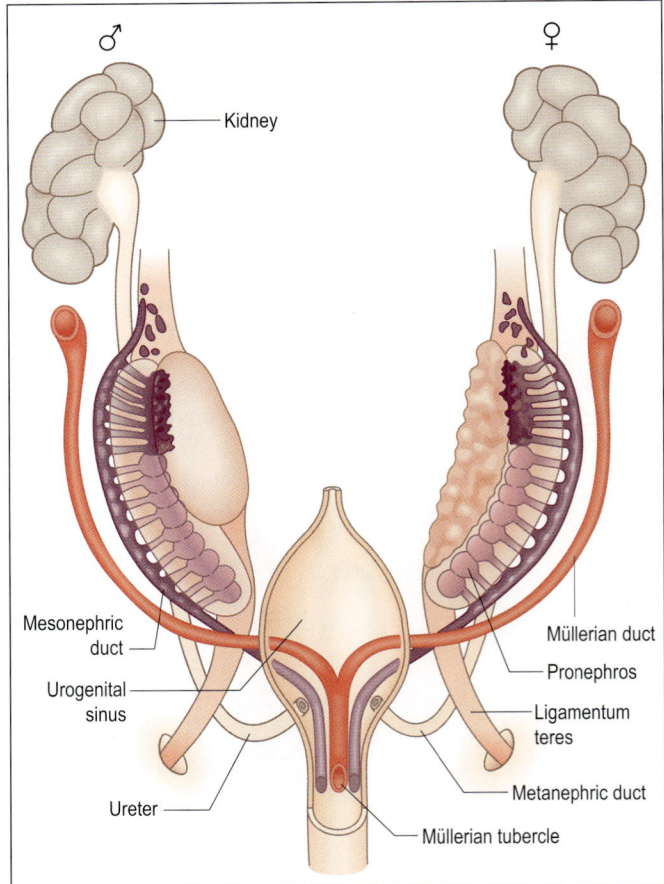

Figure 1.26 The anlage of the genital organs in the indifferent, bisexual stage. The müllerian derivatives are red and the wolffian derivatives are purple.

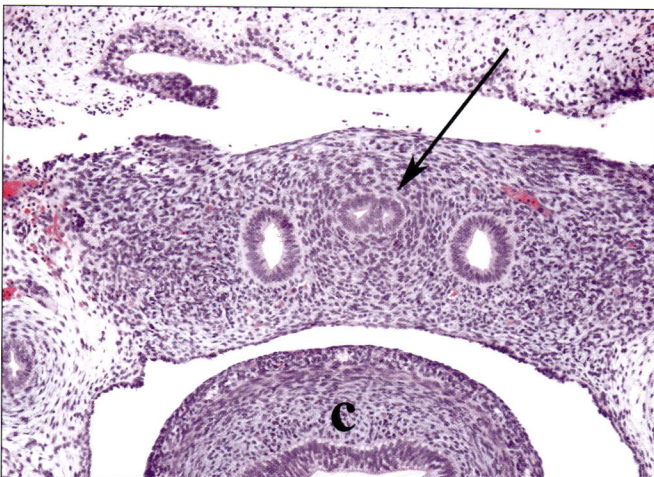

Figure 1.27 The two müllerian ducts fuse (arrow) in the midline within the pelvis, between the two wolffian ducts. The sigmoid colon is adjacent (c). Transverse section of 9.5 week embryo.

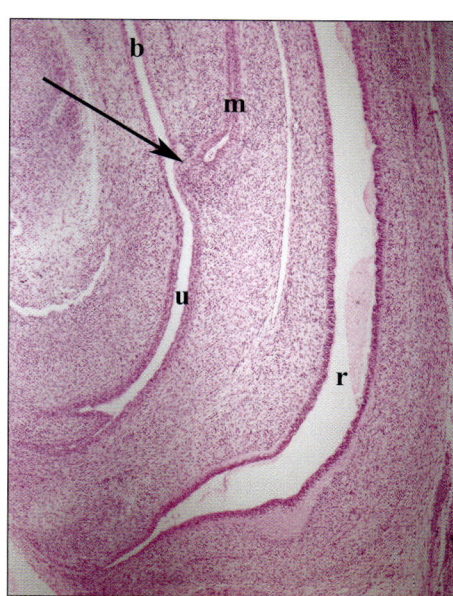

Figure 1.28 Midline sagittal section of female genitalia at 9.5 weeks. The müllerian tubercle (arrow) is the future site of the cervix, located at the juncture of the müllerian duct (m) and urogenital sinus (u). The urogenital sinus in females contributes to the urethra and vaginal wall, with squamous vaginal lining growing upward from the perineum. Rectum (r) and bladder (b) positions are indicated.

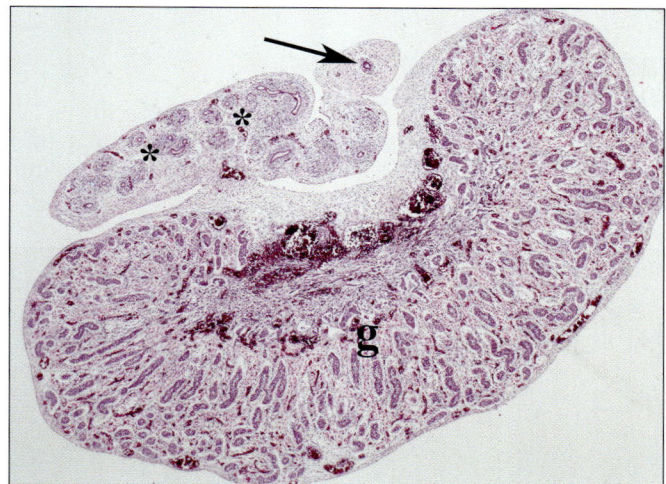

Figure 1.29 AMH secreted by Sertoli cells within the testis (g) leads to involution of the müllerian duct (arrow) until it remains only as a vestigial single duct known as the appendix epididymis. Within the epididymis itself, the wolffian ducts (asterisks) become more prominent, 16 week male fetus.

begin producing AMH only after the müllerian-derived tissues (fallopian tubes, uterus, and vagina) are well developed and no longer susceptible to the regressive effects of AMH. Serum AMH levels in girls rise slowly after birth from nearly undetectable levels until reaching a plateau after 10 years of life. It is then equivalent to the adult male serum concentration. In contrast, the male serum AMH concentration is relatively high at birth, peaks at 4–12 months of age, and then falls progressively to a baseline low adult level by about 10 years of age. A major action of AMH in the young female may be to inhibit oocyte meiosis in the developing follicle. Dramatically high levels of AMH have been found in women with ovarian sex cord tumors, thus serving potentially as a diagnostic marker or method to evaluate the effectiveness of therapy.[40] Another important action of AMH in males may be to initiate testicular descent, principally by its postulated regulatory control over the gubernaculum testis.[41] Anti-AMH is an excellent biomarker for gonadal-stromal tumor in which there is a Sertoli or granulosa cell component.[42]

The second hormone that the fetal testis secretes is testosterone. This androgenic steroid, which is critical for male development, is required for the wolffian (mesonephric) duct to differentiate into the epididymis, vas deferens, and seminal vesicle. Leydig cells appear in the testis around day 54–64 and shortly thereafter begin to produce testosterone (see Huhtaniemi[43] for a fuller analysis of the fetal testis and how it differs significantly from the adult testis). Leydig cell activity is probably stimulated by increased production of chorionic gonadotropin by the placenta at that time. Testosterone acts locally on the ipsilateral wolffian duct by binding to a specific high-affinity intracellular receptor protein. This receptor hormone complex binds DNA to regulate transcription of specific genes that govern further development. In the absence of a testis or inability of a testis to produce testosterone in adequate amounts by 10–12 weeks, or insensitivity of the wolffian duct anlage to testosterone, the epididymis, vas deferens, and seminal vesicle fail to differentiate. Only rarely are abnormally elevated testosterone levels reached sufficiently early during embryogenesis in a female fetus to cause the wolffian duct to differentiate into definitive male organs (androgen administration to the mother during pregnancy, congenital adrenogenital syndrome, and some androgen-secreting ovarian tumors; see Chapter 2).

The development of the stromal component of the genital canal is little studied, but is clearly of major importance.[44] In addition to its role in the development of the walls of the tubular muscular organs (i.e., the vagina, cervix, uterine corpus, and fallopian tubes), there is extensive experimental evidence to indicate that the stroma also directs epithelial development. Thus, the entire structure of the female genital tract is determined by stromal–epithelial interaction.

THE MÜLLERIAN DUCT AFTER WEEK 8

If the embryo is female, or in the case of male intersex in which embryonic müllerian ducts have not been completely inhibited by the AMH that the testis secretes, the ducts continue to grow unimpeded. Cranially, the separate müllerian ducts develop as distinct fallopian tubes (Figure 1.30), and the fused caudal portion as the uterus (Figure 1.31). Caudally, squamous epithelium proliferates from the urogenital sinus, growing up toward the embryonic müllerian ducts to replace the native embryonic glandular epithelium. A column of squamous epithelial cells is formed, termed the 'vaginal plate,' which comes to occupy the entire region of the vagina and exocervix (Figure 1.32). At that time the uterovaginal canal is a straight tube without evidence of a fornix. The vaginal plate is solid. By early in the second trimester, the vaginal plate begins to degenerate, and thus the vagina shows early signs of patency. The epithelium of the vaginal plate gives rise to the epithelium that ultimately lines the vagina and exocervix (Figure 1.33).

THE MÜLLERIAN DUCT DURING THE SECOND TRIMESTER

Smooth muscle appears in the walls of the genital tract between 18 and 20 weeks, although stromal aggregates into circular and longitudinal layers appear earlier. By approximately 24 weeks, the muscular portion is well developed. Vaginal, uterine, and tubal muscular walls develop around the müllerian duct alone, thus excluding the wolffian duct remnants, which are external to the true wall of the canal. Cervical glands appear at about 15 weeks. Rudimentary endometrial glands are present by 19 weeks (Figures 1.34 and 1.35), but the endometrium is poorly developed even at term in most infants.

After about 20 weeks, at the time when estrogen levels have risen in the mother, the squamous epithelium comprising the vaginal plate of the fetus first shows signs of intracytoplasmic glycogen accumulation (Figure 1.33). Eventually,

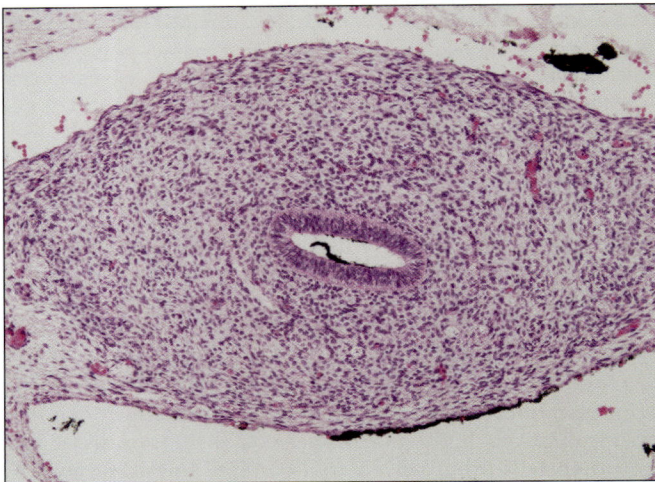

Figure 1.31 The fused müllerian duct develops a thick wall but in the location of the future uterus does not yet have glands or a myometrial layer; 12.5 week female embryo, transverse section.

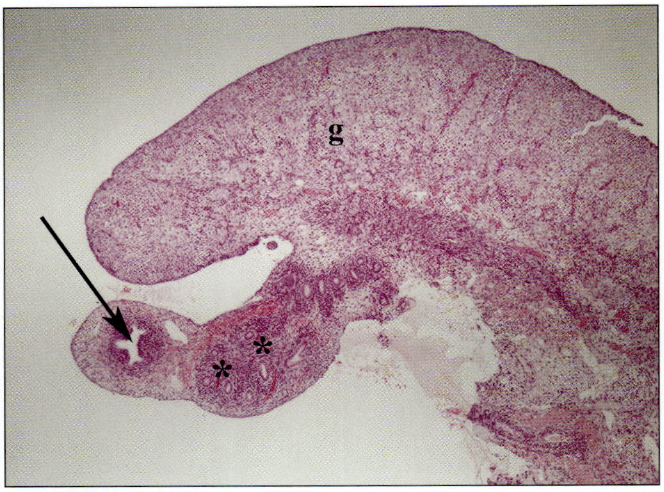

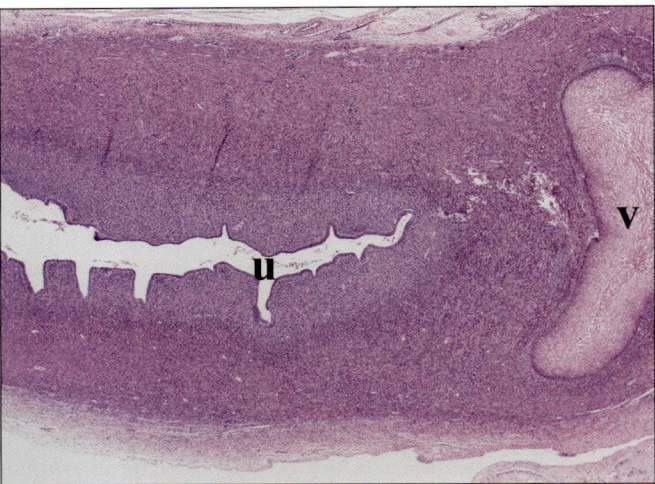

Figure 1.30 In females, the cranial aspect of the müllerian duct (arrow, paramesonephric), near the ovary (g), develops into the fallopian tube during the second trimester. Remnants of the wolffian (asterisks, mesonephric) ducts course alongside, within the mesosalpinx. Relative size of the müllerian and wolffian ducts is reversed in comparable aged male fetuses (see Figure 1.29); 15 week female embryo.

Figure 1.32 The vaginal plate (v) is a mass of squamous cells extending from the vagina in a cranial direction toward the developing uterus (u). They do connect, in this case outside the plane of section. Much of the uterus visible here will become the cervix uteri, as the lumen is further colonized by squamous epithelium; 20 week female embryo, slightly parasagittal section.

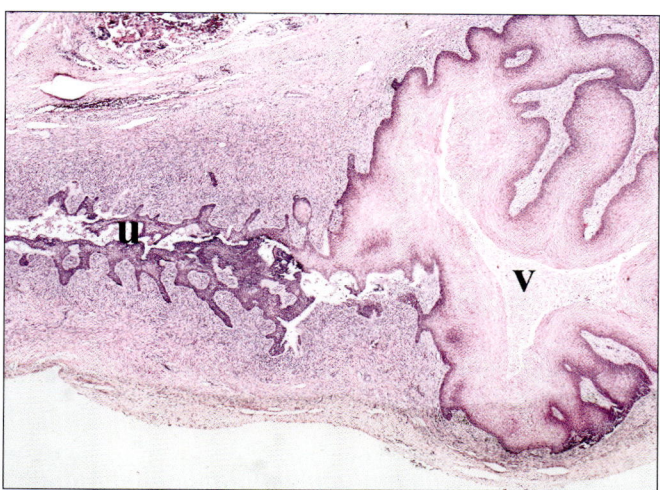

Figure 1.33 Similar perspective to Figure 1.32, only a week or two later, shows further extension of the vaginal squamous epithelium (v) into the fused müllerian duct in the region of the cervix uteri (u). Vaginal squamous epithelium is now highly glycogenated; 21–22 week female embryo.

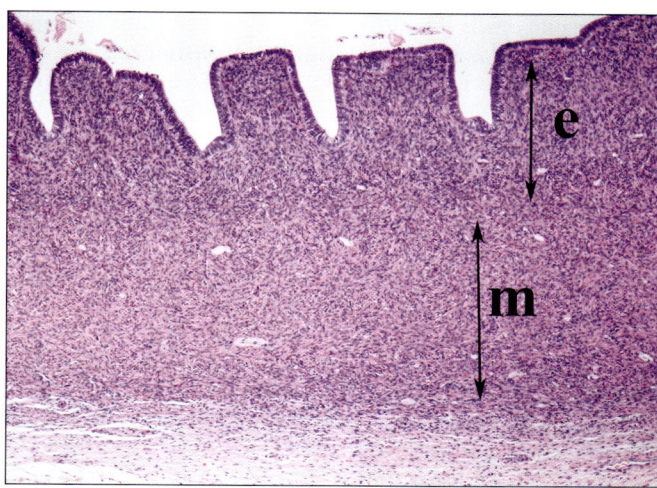

Figure 1.35 Detail of 20 week uterine wall, showing simple endometrial glands, an inner layer of endometrial stroma (e), and outer myometrium (m).

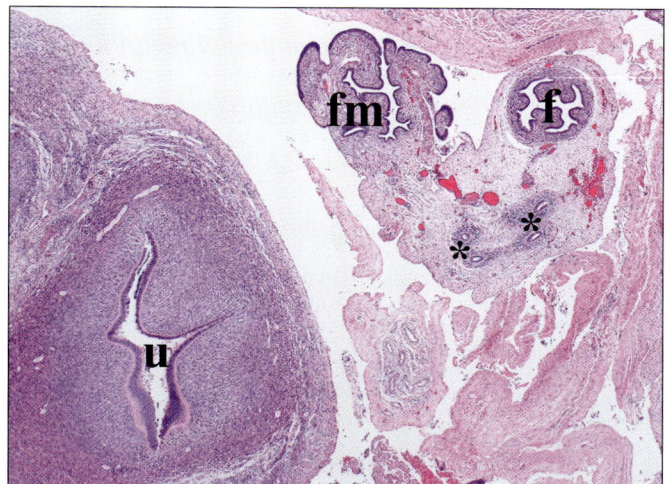

Figure 1.34 The uterus (u), formed by fused müllerian ducts in the midline, develops a thick wall composed of inner endometrial stroma, and outer myometrium. The fallopian tube (f) and fimbria (fm), originally in a cranial location, drop into the pelvis to lie lateral to the uterus. Wolffian duct rests (asterisks) are seen in the mesosalpinx; transverse pelvic section of 20 week female fetus.

there is cellular dissolution and the formation of the fully patent vagina.

EXTERNAL GENITALIA

The appearance of the external genitalia is influenced by the systemic hormonal milieu found in the developing fetus beginning somewhere about week 15. It becomes masculine when exposed to an excess of androgens and female if there is a deficiency of androgens, i.e., a relative excess of estrogens. Androgens have a positive influence on the appearance of the external genitalia. Maternal or inappropriate levels of fetal androgens will virilize a female fetus, while high levels of circulating estrogens in pregnancy have no effect on the male fetus.

Dihydrotestosterone, the active androgen that derives from testosterone, is ultimately responsible for initiating masculinization of the external genitalia and differentiation of the prostate. 5-α reductase, found in the tissues of the external genitalia and urogenital sinus, converts testosterone to dihydrotestosterone, which causes the:

- Genital tubercle to enlarge and form the glans penis
- Genital folds to enlarge and fuse to form the penile shaft with migration of the urethral orifice along the lower border of the shaft to the tip of the glans
- Genital swellings to fuse and form a scrotum
- Urogenital sinus tissues to differentiate into the prostate
- Utricle to regress.

Failure of the external genitalia to develop in males in the presence of testes may be due to a lack of adequate testosterone secretion into the systemic circulation, deficient enzyme (5-α reductase, type II) at the end-organ level to convert testosterone to dihydrotestosterone, or complete end-organ insensitivity (androgen receptor insensitivity). Lesser degrees of deficiency or end-organ insensitivity may result in partial male development characterized by a small penis, hypospadias, deficient formation of the scrotum, or a persistent urogenital sinus (vaginal opening into the urethra). The effects of dihydrotestosterone begin about day 70, with fusion of the labioscrotal folds and closure of the median raphe, and continue at day 74 with closure of the urethral groove. External genital development is complete by day 120–140 (week 18–20).

The urogenital sinus, into which the vagina opens, enlarges as the embryo grows, so that it becomes the vestibule of the adult external genitalia. Consequently, the vestibule is lined, except for a variable portion anterior to the urethral orifice, by the endodermal epithelium of the urogenital sinus. This is clinically important as the endodermal-derived epithelium not only differs morphologically from the mesodermal- and ectodermal-derived epithelium, but also responds differently to a variety of stimuli, notably sex steroids.

The form of the external genitalia results from events that begin during embryonic week 4 in the mesodermal stroma immediately lateral and ventral to the cloacal plate. Just ventral to the plate, the stroma produces paired elevations of the ectoderm, which fuse to form the genital tubercle. Immediately lateral to the cloacal plate on each side, two parallel folds develop by the same mechanism: the more medial urogenital fold is destined to become the labium minor; the more lateral labioscrotal fold becomes the labium major.

The labioscrotal fold extends cranially around the genital tubercle and fuses with its partner on the other side, becoming the mons pubis. At the end of week 6, the urorectal septum fuses with the cloacal plate, thus dividing this structure into the anal membrane posteriorly and the urogenital membrane ventrally. The lateral folds are distributed primarily in relation to the urogenital membrane. In both the male and female, the lateral folds fuse across the midline in front of the anus. In the male, the fusion moves ventrally in zipper-like fashion. The urogenital folds fuse to form a portion of the wall of the penile urethra, and the labioscrotal folds fuse to form the scrotum. As female differentiation reflects the absence of this fusion, it may be difficult to detect, although by the end of the first trimester significant fusion should have occurred in a male fetus.

In summary, female internal organs and external genitalia develop in the absence of hormones secreted by the fetal ovary, and differentiate even when gonads are absent (Figure 1.36). Unless interrupted by the regressive influence of AMH, differentiation of the müllerian ducts proceeds caudally to form fallopian tubes, a uterus, and a vagina. In the absence of the masculinizing effect of dihydrotestosterone, the undifferentiated external genital anlage develops into the vulva. The genital tubercle develops into the clitoris, the genital folds into the labia minora, and the genital swellings into the labia majora. Thus, the infant with ovaries or streak gonads has female internal and external genitalia at birth. Only if the female fetus has systematically elevated levels of androgens before week 10–12 of gestation does any degree of internal male development occur. In such cases, the external genitalia may appear ambiguous or may resemble that of a normal phenotypic male; the vagina in these instances opens into the membranous portion of the urethra. If the androgens are not elevated until after week 20, by which time the external genitalia have fully formed, the only virilizing effect is an enlarged clitoris.

REFERENCES

1. Brennan J, Capel B. One tissue, two fates: molecular genetic events that underlie testis versus ovary development. Nat Rev Genet 2004;5:509–21.
2. Iyer AK, McCabe ER. Molecular mechanisms of DAX1 action. Mol Genet Metab 2004;83:60–73.
3. Kanai Y, Hiramatsu R, Matoba S, Kidokoro T. From SRY to SOX9: mammalian testis differentiation. J Biochem 2005;138:13–9.
4. Mittwoch U. The elusive action of sex-determining genes: mitochondria to the rescue? J Theor Biol 2004;228:359–65.
5. Park SY, Jameson JL. Minireview: transcriptional regulation of gonadal development and differentiation. Endocrinology 2005;146:1035–42.
6. Viger RS, Silversides DW, Tremblay JJ. New insights into the regulation of mammalian sex determination and male sex differentiation. Vitam Horm 2005;70:387–413.
7. Yao HH. The pathway to femaleness: current knowledge on embryonic development of the ovary. Mol Cell Endocrinol 2005;230:87–93.
8. Shimada K. Sex determination and sex differentiation. Avian Poultry Biol Rev 2002;13:1–14.
9. Capel B. R-spondin1 tips the balance in sex determination. Nat Genet 2006;38:1233–4.
10. Chassot AA, Ranc F, Gregoire EP, et al. Activation of beta-catenin signaling by Rspo1 controls differentiation of the mammalian ovary. Hum Mol Genet 2008;7:1264–77.
11. Brennan J, Karl J, Martineau J, et al. SRY and the testis: molecular pathways of organogenesis. J Exp Zool 1998;281:494–500.
12. McElreavey K, Quintana-Murci L. Y chromosome haplogroups: a correlation with testicular dysgenesis syndrome? APMIS 2003;111:106–14.
13. Fleming H. Differentiation in human endometrial cells in monolayer culture: dependence on a factor in fetal bovine serum. J Cell Biochem 1995;57:262–70.
14. Hunter RHF. Mechanisms of sex determination. In: Hunter RHF, editor. Sex determination, differentiation and intersexuality in placental mammals. Cambridge, UK: Cambridge University Press; 1995. p. 22–68.
15. Mendes JR, Strufaldi MW, Delcelo R, et al. Y-chromosome identification by PCR and gonadal histopathology in Turner's syndrome without overt Y-mosaicism. Clin Endocrinol (Oxf) 1999;50:19–26.
16. Tilmann C, Capel B. Mesonephric cell migration induces testis cord formation and Sertoli cell differentiation in the mammalian gonad. Development 1999;126:2883–90.
17. Swain A, Lovell-Badge R. A molecular approach to sex determination in mammals. Acta Paediatr (Suppl) 1997;423:46–9.
18. Salas-Cortes L, Jaubert F, Barbaux S, et al. The human SRY protein is present in fetal and adult Sertoli cells and germ cells. Int J Dev Biol 1999;43:135–40.
19. Moreno-Mendoza N, Harley V, Merchant-Larios H. Cell aggregation precedes the onset of SOX9-expressing preSertoli cells in the genital ridge of mouse. Cytogenet Genome Res 2003;101:219–23.
20. Park SY, Meeks JJ, Raverot G, et al. Nuclear receptors SF1 and DAX1 function cooperatively to mediate somatic cell differentiation during testis development. Development 2005;132:2415–23.
21. Parker KL, Rice DA, Lala DS, et al. Steroidogenic factor 1: an essential mediator of endocrine development. Recent Prog Horm Res 2002;57:19–36.

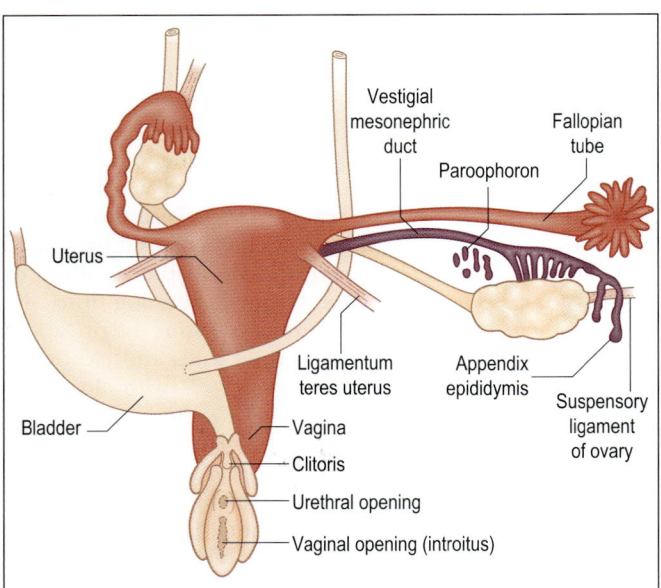

Figure 1.36 Female differentiation of the genital organs.

22. Sekido R, Bar I, Narvaez V, et al. SOX9 is up-regulated by the transient expression of SRY specifically in Sertoli cell precursors. Dev Biol 2004;274:271–9.
23. Mallet D, Bretones P, Michel-Calemard L, et al. Gonadal dysgenesis without adrenal insufficiency in a 46, XY patient heterozygous for the nonsense C16X mutation: a case of SF1 haploinsufficiency. J Clin Endocrinol Metab 2004;89:4829–32.
24. Meeks JJ, Weiss J, Jameson JL. DAX1 is required for testis determination. Nat Genet 2003;34:32–3.
25. Fleming A, Vilain E. The endless quest for sex determination genes. Clin Genet 2005;67:15–25.
26. Short RV. Difference between a testis and an ovary. J Exp Zool 1998;281:359–61.
27. de Kretser DM, Burger HG. The Y chromosome and spermatogenesis. N Engl J Med 1997;336:576–8.
28. Mulhall JP, Reijo R, Alagappan R, et al. Azoospermic men with deletion of the DAZ gene cluster are capable of completing spermatogenesis: fertilization, normal embryonic development and pregnancy occur when retrieved testicular spermatozoa are used for intracytoplasmic sperm injection. Hum Reprod 1997;12:503–8.
29. Choi Y, Rajkovic A. Genetics of early mammalian folliculogenesis. Cell Mol Life Sci 2006;63:579–90.
30. Biason-Lauber A, Konrad D, Navratil F, Schoenle EJ. A WNT4 mutation associated with Müllerian-duct regression and virilization in a 46,XX woman. N Engl J Med 2004;351:792–8.
31. Beysen D, Vandesompele J, Messiaen L, et al. The human FOXL2 mutation database. Hum Mutat 2004;24:189–93.
32. Cocquet J, Pailhoux E, Jaubert F, et al. Evolution and expression of FOXL2. J Med Genet 2002;39:916–21.
33. De Baere E., Copelli S, Caburet S, et al. Premature ovarian failure and forkhead transcription factor FOXL2: blepharophimosis-ptosis-epicanthus inversus syndrome and ovarian dysfunction. Pediatr Endocrinol Rev 2005;2:653–60.
34. Nef S, Schaad O, Stallings NR, et al. Gene expression during sex determination reveals a robust female genetic program at the onset of ovarian development. Dev Biol 2005;287:361–77.
35. Hunter RHF. Differentiation of the gonads. In: Hunter RHF, editor. Sex determination, differentiation and intersexuality in placental mammals. Cambridge, UK: Cambridge University Press; 1995. p. 69–106.
36. Johnson J, Bagley J, Skaznik-Wikiel M, et al. Oocyte generation in adult mammalian ovaries by putative germ cells in bone marrow and peripheral blood. Cell 2005;122:303–15.
37. Josso N, Racine C, di CN, et al. The role of anti-Müllerian hormone in gonadal development. Mol Cell Endocrinol 1998;145:3–7.
38. Rey R, al-Attar L, Louis F, et al. Testicular dysgenesis does not affect expression of anti-müllerian hormone by Sertoli cells in premeiotic seminiferous tubules. Am J Pathol 1996;148:1689–98.
39. Hunter RHF. Differentiation of the genital duct system. In: Hunter RHF, editor. Sex determination, differentiation and intersexuality in placental mammals. Cambridge, UK: Cambridge University Press; 1995. p. 107–38.
40. Lane A, Lee M. Clinical applications of Müllerian inhibiting substance in patients with gonadal disorders. Endocrinologist 1999;9:208–15.
41. Clarnette TD, Sugita Y, Hutson JM. Genital anomalies in human and animal models reveal the mechanisms and hormones governing testicular descent. Br J Urol 1997;79:99–112.
42. Rey R, Sabourin JC, Venara M, et al. Anti-Müllerian hormone is a specific marker of Sertoli- and granulosa-cell origin in gonadal tumors. Hum Pathol 2000;31:1202–8.
43. Huhtaniemi I. Fetal testis—a very special endocrine organ. Eur J Endocrinol 1994;130:25–31.
44. Cunha GR, Boutin EL, Turner T, Donjacour AA. Role of mesenchyme in the development of the urogenital tract. J Clean Technol Environ Toxicol Occ Med 1998;7:179–94.

2 Disorders of Sexual Development

Stanley J. Robboy, George L. Mutter

CHAPTER OUTLINE

Disorders of Genital Differentiation (Disorders Generally Associated with a Normal Chromosome Constitution and Normal Gonad) 18	**Disorders of Sex Determination (Disorders Associated with Abnormal Sex Chromosomes and Abnormal Gonadal Formation)** 30
Female Pseudohermaphroditism (Female Intersex) 18	Sexual Ambiguity Infrequent 31
Male Pseudohermaphroditism (Male Intersex) 22	Sexual Ambiguity Frequent 36

New insights into the biology of sexual development (see Chapter 1) and advances in chromosome analysis are leading to earlier identification and more prompt treatment of the intersexual patient, the results of which facilitate a more normal life for affected individuals.[1,2] It becomes easier to offer more appropriate counseling for gender assignment, hormone treatment, and fertility options and information about the risk of future gonadal malignancy. Based on these various advances, a classification of abnormal sexual development has been developed and refined that correlates gonadal and genital anatomy with chromosomal findings and specific genetic or metabolic defects (Tables 2.1 and 2.2). Thus classification has shifted from one primarily based on genotype (whether a specific gene or whole chromosomal abnormality) to broad phenotypic categories of 'abnormalities of genital differentiation.' These phenotypic abnormalities may be caused by abnormal production or sensitivity of a single hormone, or abnormal gonadal differentiation, usually testicular, with or without chromosomal aberration.[3–5]

The complexity of the subject is evident from studies in which precise assignment of the etiologic cause cannot be determined in nearly half of the cases by a multidisciplinary team of clinicians, biochemists, molecular biologists, and pathologists. The current classification is an integrated approach to this complex group of disorders, organized by clinical presentation and underlying pathophysiology. The classification also groups patients who are at high risk for development of gonadal neoplasia (Table 2.3).

DISORDERS OF GENITAL DIFFERENTIATION (DISORDERS GENERALLY ASSOCIATED WITH A NORMAL CHROMOSOME CONSTITUTION AND NORMAL GONAD)

FEMALE PSEUDOHERMAPHRODITISM (FEMALE INTERSEX)

Female pseudohermaphroditism occurs as a result of relative androgen excess *in utero* in an individual with two ovaries and two X chromosomes (46,XX). The elevated levels of androgen present during embryogenesis usually result in genital ambiguity and may result in a male phenotype.

FETAL DEFECTS

Adrenogenital Syndrome

Congenital adrenal hyperplasia, unlike all other conditions responsible for the appearance of ambiguous genitalia in the newborn, may be life threatening because of a lack of synthesis of specific adrenal steroids. Prompt diagnosis and appropriate therapy are essential. With early treatment, normal external genitalia and fertility can be achieved. The manifestations of the adrenogenital syndrome in the 46,XX individual are most easily understood by examining the simplified biosynthetic pathways of mineralocorticoid, glucocorticoid, and sex steroids (Figure 2.1).[6–8] Two enzymes, 21 hydroxylase and 11β-hydroxylase, participate in the

Table 2.1 Classification of Intersexual Disorders*

Disorders of Genital Differentiation (Disorders Generally Associated with a Normal Chromosome Constitution and Normal Gonad)

FEMALE PSEUDOHERMAPHRODITISM (FEMALE INTERSEX)

Fetal Defect

Adrenogenital syndrome (testosterone overproduction due to adrenocorticoid insufficiency)
  21-Hydroxylase deficiency
  11β-Hydroxylase deficiency
Placental aromatase defect

Maternal Influence

Maternal ingestion of progestins or androgens
Maternal virilizing tumor

MALE PSEUDOHERMAPHRODITISM (MALE INTERSEX)

Gonadal Defects

Testicular regression syndrome (gonadal destruction)
Leydig cell agenesis
  Defective hCG–LH receptor
Defects in testosterone synthesis
  Testosterone and adrenocorticoid insufficiency
    Defect in cholesterol synthesis (Smith–Lemli–Opitz syndrome)
    20,22-Demolase deficiency (STAR deficiency)
    3β-Hydroxylase dehydrogenase deficiency
    17α-Hydroxylase deficiency
  Testosterone insufficiency only
    17,20-Desmolase deficiency
    17β-Hydroxysteroid (17-ketosteroid reductase) dehydrogenase deficiency
  Persistent müllerian duct syndrome (defect in müllerian inhibiting substance system)

End-Organ Defects

Androgen receptor binding deficiency
  Androgen insensitivity syndrome (testicular feminization)
  Incomplete androgen insensitivity syndrome (Reifenstein syndrome)
Peripheral androgen transformation deficiency
  5α-Reductase deficiency

Disorders of Sex Determination (Disorders Generally Associated with an Abnormal Sex Chromosome Constitution Leading to Abnormal Gondal Formation)

SEXUAL AMBIGUITY INFREQUENT

Klinefelter Syndrome (XXY)

Turner Syndrome and Turner-Like (45,X, and X Mosaicism)

XX Male (Sex Reversal)

Pure Gonadal Dysgenesis, Bilateral

Disorders of Wilms' Tumor Gene (WT1)

Denys–Drash syndrome
Frasier syndrome

SEXUAL AMBIGUITY FREQUENT

XY Disorder of Sex Development, Mixed Gonadal Dysgenesis

Turner-like (some forms)
Dysgenetic male pseudohermaphroditism

XY Male to Female Sex Reversal

Steroidogenic Factor 1 (*SF1*) abnormality
Deleted chromosome 9p

True Hermaphroditism

*Idiopathic or unclassified conditions exist within each major category. We assume that each category of male pseudohermaphroditism with defects in specific protein products or receptors has forms where the abnormality is total or partial, or where the defect results from a qualitatively abnormal structure.

---

formation of the glucocorticoids desoxycorticosterone and cortisol and the mineralocorticoid aldosterone, but are unnecessary for synthesis of the sex steroids testosterone, estrone, and estradiol. Deficiency of either enzyme in the 46,XX female leads to elevated adrenocorticotropic hormone (ACTH) products and hence elevated levels of testosterone and other strongly androgenic intermediates, which may result in sexual ambiguity or marked virilization of the newborn's external genitalia (Table 2.4).[9,10]

3β-Hydroxysteroid dehydrogenase is required for testosterone formation. In its absence, the principal androgen to form is the weak androgen dehydroepiandrosterone (DHEA), which has 1/20 the potency of testosterone. Patients with deficiency of this enzyme, therefore, show signs of no more than mild virilization, usually with clitoral hypertrophy but not with labial fusion or anterior displacement of the urethral orifice.[11]

21-Hydroxylase deficiency is inherited as an autosomal recessive trait caused by abnormalities of the *CYP21A2* gene on chromosome 6 (which encodes for cytochrome P450, family 21). It accounts for more than 95% of cases of congenital adrenal hyperplasia, occurring once in 15,000 births, and is especially high in Ashkenazi Jews (1:27 live births). The clinical manifestation of classic congenital adrenogenital syndrome depends upon inactivation of the normally expressed copy of the *CYP21A2* gene. In three-quarters of cases the cause is rearranged inactive elements of a homologous nonexpressed pseudogene, *CYP21A1P*.[6] Deletion of

Table 2.2 Genes Involved in Disorders of Intersex

Gene	Name	Location	Cells Affected	Function	Abnormality
AMH	Anti-Müllerian hormone (MIS type 1)	19p13.3	Sertoli cells	Causes regression of fetal müllerian ducts, inhibits Leydig cells	Persistent müllerian duct syndrome
AMHR2	AMH type 2 receptor	12q13	Primary sex cords	Serine threonine kinase receptor	Persistent müllerian duct syndrome
AR	Androgen receptor	Xq11–12	Target cell depends on cofactor specifics	Androgen receptor, a ligand transcription factor	Male pseudohermaphroditism, complete or partial androgen insensitivity syndrome
CYP11B1	Cytochrome P450, family 11	8q21	Microsome of adrenal, testis, ovary	11β-Hydroxylase	Congenital adrenal hyperplasia
CYP17A1	Cytochrome P450, family 17	10q24–25	Microsome of adrenal, testis, ovary	17-Hydroxylase: 20–22 lyase	Male pseudohermaphroditism
CYP21A2	Cytochrome P450, family 21	6p21.3	Microsome of adrenal, testis, ovary	21-Hydroxylase	Congenital adrenal hyperplasia, female pseudohermaphroditism
DMRT1	Double sex and msb-3 related transcription factor 1	9p24.3	Gonadal ridge	Human testis differentiation	XY male to female sex reversal
HSD17B3	17β-Hydroxysteroid dehydrogenase III	9q22	Microsome of adrenal, testis, ovary	17β-Hydroxysteroid dehydrogenase, 17-ketosteroid reductase 3	Male pseudohermaphroditism
HSD3B2	3β-Hydroxysteroid dehydrogenase type II	1p13.1	Microsome of adrenal, testis, ovary	3β-Hydroxysteroid dehydrogenase type II	Congenital adrenal hyperplasia
NR5A1	Steroidogenic factor-1 (SF1)	9q33	Gonads	Gonadal differentiation and steroidogenesis	XY male to female sex reversal; male pseudohermaphroditism
SRD5A2	Steroid 5α-reductase 2	2p23	Fetal genital skin and male accessory organs	5α-Reductase type 2	Male pseudohermaphroditism
SRY	Sex-determining region Y	Yp11.3	Gonadal ridge	Transcription factor, coordinates testis formation via SOX9	Mutation causes XY gonadal dysgenesis, Translocation causes XX male
STAR	Steroidogenic acute regulatory protein	8p11.2	Mitochondria of adrenal, testis, ovary	Steroidogenic acute regulatory protein	Congenital lipoid adrenal hyperplasia
TSPY1	Testis-specific protein, Y-linked (one component of gonadoblastoma Y gene locus)	Yp11.2	Spermatogonia	Spermatogonial proliferation in a phosphorylation-dependent manner	Gonadoblastoma

Table 2.3 Gonadal Tumors and Abnormal Sexual Development

Tumor	Associated Abnormal Sexual Development
Leydig cell hyperplasia (pseudotumor)	Adrenogenital syndrome
Luteoma of pregnancy	Maternal virilizing tumor
Intratubular germ cell neoplasia	Congenital lipoid adrenal hyperplasia (defect in STAR gene)
Sertoli cell hamartomas; Leydig cell nodules; seminoma	Androgen insensitivity syndrome (testicular feminization)
Mediastinal germ cell tumors	Klinefelter syndrome (XXY)
Rarely, Leydig cell tumors	
Breast cancer; hematologic malignancies	
Non-germ cell (serous carcinoma of ovary; endometrial cancer)	Turner syndrome and Turner-like (X0 and X mosaicism)
Stromal luteoma or hilus cell hyperplasia	
Extragonadal tumor of neurogenic origin	
Wilms' tumor; gonadoblastoma	Denys–Drash syndrome
Gonadoblastoma	Frasier syndrome; 46,XY Disorder of Sex Development
Germinoma; rarely, gonadoblastoma	True hermaphroditism

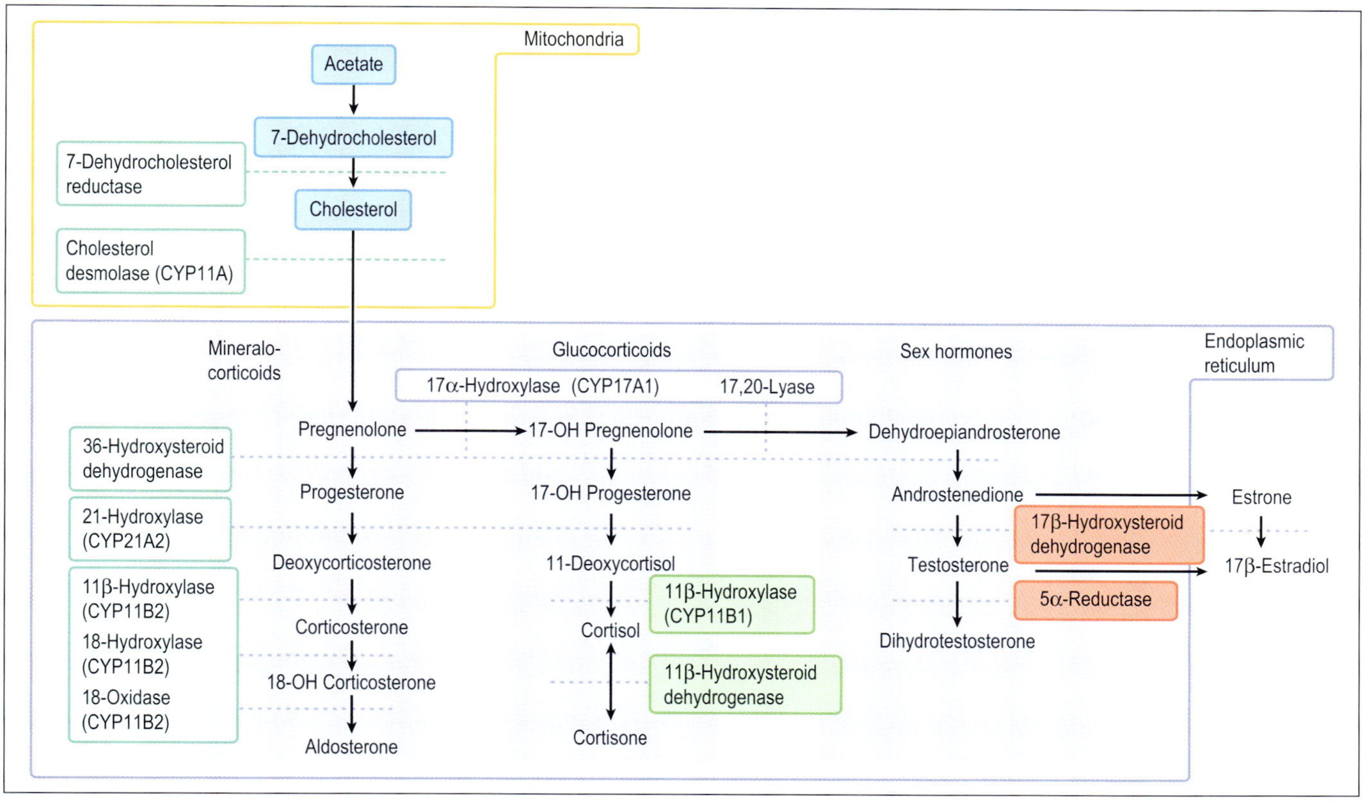

Figure 2.1 Biosynthesis of mineralocorticoids, glucocorticoids, and sex steroids.

Table 2.4 Forms of Adrenal Hyperplasia Affecting the External Genitalia

Deficiency	Syndrome	Ambiguous Genitalia	Postnatal Virilization
STAR protein	—	Males	
3β-Hydroxysteroid dehydrogenase	Classic	Males	Yes
	Non-classic	No	Yes
17α-Hydroxylase	—	Males	No
21-Hydroxylase	Salt wasting	Females	Yes
	Simple virilizing	Females	Yes
	Non-classic	No	Yes
11β-Hydroxylase	Classic	Females	Yes
	Non-classic	No	Yes

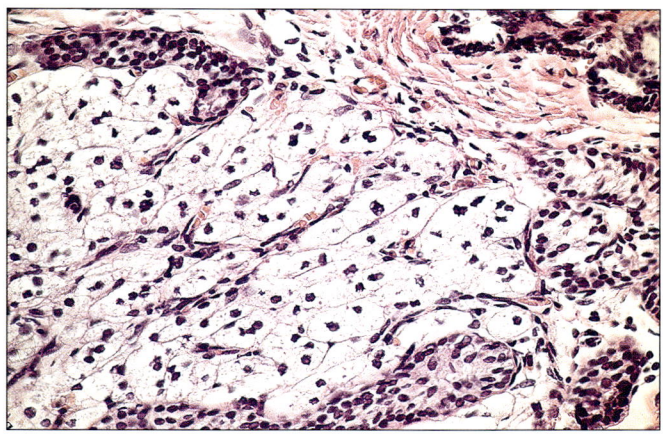

Figure 2.2 Interstitial cell tumor of adrenogenital syndrome. The tumor cells with vacuolated clear cytoplasm, which lie adjacent to immature seminiferous tubules, resemble adrenocortical cells more closely than Leydig cells.

the *CYP21A1* gene itself causes the remaining cases. If the allele carries a defect encoding for a mild defect, then the child will develop a non-classic form of adrenal hyperplasia, which by definition occurs after birth and is never associated with genital ambiguity.[12] This latter syndrome is common, occurring in 1% of all women, and is the major cause of adult-onset virilism.

The extent of virilization in genetic females with adrenogenital syndrome depends upon the timing in fetal life when androgen excess begins. If the onset begins after week 16 of gestation, the clitoris may be enlarged. If earlier, the vagina and urethra may open into a common urogenital sinus. More marked clitoral enlargement and an opening of the urogenital sinus at the clitoral base may mimic penile hypospadias and suggest an even earlier temporal effect. On occasion, the changes have been of such severity that the female infants have been misdiagnosed as cryptorchid males with or without hypospadias. Gonadal tumor development in genetic females with adrenogenital syndrome is rare.

Males who have the adrenogenital syndrome show no evidence of genital ambiguity, but may have an enlarged phallus and a hyperpigmented rugated scrotum. Clinically detectable bilateral testicular nodules occasionally develop during childhood or young adulthood and must be distinguished from true Leydig cell tumors (Figure 2.2).[13] Usually the cells are composed of interstitial cells larger than Leydig cells, secrete cortisol, and respond to treatment with the adrenolytic agent o,p'-DDD (mitotane), indicative that these cells are adrenal or adrenal like in origin. Bilaterality and decreasing tumor size after corticosteroid therapy are features indicative that this testicular 'tumor' of the adrenogenital syndrome is hyperplastic rather than neoplastic.[14]

Placental Aromatase Defect

Placental aromatase deficiency is a rare cause of maternal virilization during pregnancy and pseudohermaphroditism of the female fetus.[15,16] Mutations in the aromatase gene, *CYP19A1*, which causes abnormally low conversion of androstenedione to 17β-estradiol and estrone, result in virilization of the mother and her female fetus because potent androgens that are not converted to estrogens accumulate. The mothers usually show the onset of progressive virilization during the third trimester. The male fetus has normal genitalia.

MATERNAL INFLUENCE

Maternal Ingestion of Progestins or Androgens

Maternal ingestion of synthetic progestins was implicated as a cause of female pseudohermaphroditism in the late 1950s when such treatment was employed for threatened or habitual abortion. Subsequently, progestins have also been implicated in the development of hypospadias in male offspring. Most cases of female pseudohermaphroditism in this category developed after maternal ingestion of Norlutin (17α-ethinyl-19-nortestosterone), less often with ethisterone (17α-ethinyltestosterone), and occasionally after the ingestion of Enovid, diethylstilbestrol, androgens, or the intramuscular administration of progesterone.

Masculinization usually consists of phallic enlargement and variable degrees of labioscrotal fusion, depending on the time during gestation when the therapy was administered. Although the degree of masculinization is usually less than that associated with the adrenogenital syndrome, the sexual ambiguity in female infants has been of such severity in some instances as to result in male sex assignment. The degree of virilization does not progress with age. The gonads and internal genital organs are unaffected, and ovulation, menstruation, and normal secondary female characteristics appear at puberty.

Maternal Virilizing Lesions

A variety of benign and malignant tumors and tumor-like conditions, primary as well as metastatic to the ovary, have been associated with virilization of the mother and/or her female offspring.[17,18] The luteoma of pregnancy and pronounced theca–lutein cysts (hyperreactio luteinalis) are the most common lesions that cause maternal virilization during pregnancy.[19] These are benign hyperplastic lesions of the ovaries encountered most often as an incidental finding at the time of cesarean section or postpartum sterilization, usually in women who are multiparous. Elevated levels of human chorionic gonadotropin (hCG) induce hyperplasia of theca–lutein or stroma–lutein cells, which are responsible for the production of androgen (principally androstenedione). Some female infants become masculinized, with mild enlargement of the clitoris and occasionally minimal degrees of labioscrotal fusion or rugate, hyperpigmented ('scrotal') labia. The nature of these changes indicates that the ovarian nodules do not function until the second half of gestation, which agrees with the occasional onset of masculinization in the mother during the third trimester.

Elevated plasma and tissue levels of testosterone, dihydrotestosterone, androstenedione, and DHEA have been detected in virilized patients. The plasma levels return to normal once the tumor is extirpated. Even without treatment, the nodules regress and disappear soon after delivery. Rarely, a functional luteoma may recur during a subsequent pregnancy.

MALE PSEUDOHERMAPHRODITISM (MALE INTERSEX)

Male pseudohermaphroditism defines a heterogeneous group of intersex conditions where there is an intrauterine state of relative functional androgen deficiency, an apparently normal 46,XY karyotype, and either identifiable testes or evidence that testes were present during fetal development. The external genitalia are usually female or ambiguous, although in certain categories (e.g., testicular regression syndrome) they may appear as phenotypically male. The responsible defect may be in the gonad, leading to deficiency in androgens, deficiency in müllerian inhibiting substance (AMH), or both. Alternatively, end-organ defects in which developing tissues are unresponsive to androgens or müllerian inhibitory substance (MIS) may lead to the abnormal phenotype.

PRIMARY GONADAL DEFECTS

A primary defect of the gonad in an XY karyotype individual may lead to male pseudohermaphroditism by any one of the following mechanisms: regression (destruction) of the gonads or their anlage during intrauterine life; agenesis of the Leydig cells; a specific enzymatic defect in testosterone, dihydrotestosterone synthesis, or receptors to these hormones; or a defect in elaboration or action of AMH.

Testicular Regression Syndrome

Testicular regression syndrome follows the irreparable destruction of both testes at a critical stage of fetal development in an XY individual, with resulting endocrine disturbances. Unilateral testicular destruction does not result in the syndrome.

The phenotype of an affected individual with testicular regression syndrome reflects the specific stage of fetal development during which the testes were damaged. In general, gonadal regression that occurs during embryonic life, before the elaboration of AMH and/or androgenic steroids by the testes, leads to a female phenotype. Regression of the testes during late embryonic through mid-fetal life permits a masculine phenotype (Figure 2.3). Testicular regression has a variety of etiologies, as diverse as inherited genetic defect, intrauterine infection, or infarction. The heterogeneous presentations of this syndrome and its relative rarity have led to numerous and sometimes confusing terms for this disorder, including: true agonadism, testicular dysgenesis, rudimentary testis, vanishing testis, and complete bilateral anorchia. Pure gonadal dysgenesis (Swyer syndrome) has been used to designate some forms of the testicular regression syndrome, but this term is nonspecific and thus best avoided.

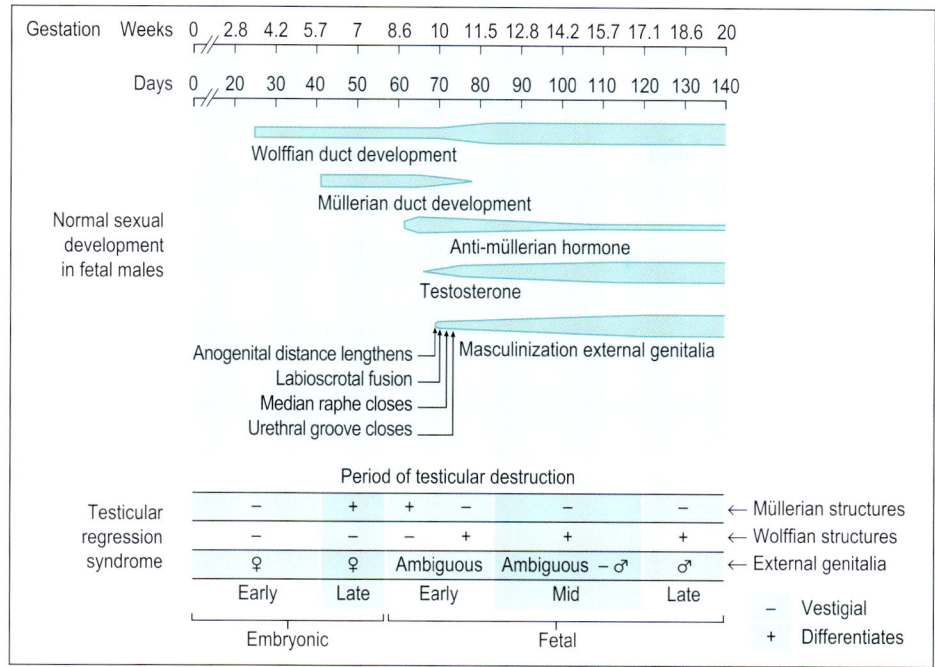

Figure 2.3 Testicular regression syndrome. The phenotypic appearance of the internal genitalia abnormalities relates to the time during embryogenesis when the normal development of the genital tract was damaged.

At one end of the testicular regression syndrome spectrum, the internal genitalia and gonads are absent and the external genitalia are female. Presumably, the urogenital ridge was destroyed in its entirety during early embryonic life, even before the müllerian ducts began to differentiate (prior to day 42). At the other end of the spectrum, which approximates the endpoint of normal genital development, the patients are phenotypic males with infantile to nearly normal male external genitalia, normally differentiated wolffian duct structures, and completely inhibited müllerian duct development. Often in these cases, no gonadal tissue is identified. However, there is sometimes a focus of vascularized fibrosis (85%), hemorrhage or hemosiderin deposition (70%), and calcification (60%) or giant cells at the expected site of the gonad, which is near the residual vas deferens or epididymis (Figure 2.4).[20] Occasionally, atrophic seminiferous tubules may be found amidst the fibrous stroma. Testicular regression presumably develops during the late fetal period (after 120 days) when müllerian structures have already atrophied under the influence of AMH, and testosterone and dihydrotestosterone have exerted a major influence on the normal development of internal and external genitalia, respectively. Torsion and infarction of improperly descended testes have been suggested.[21]

Intermediate in the spectrum of this disorder are patients with ambiguous genitalia and various combinations of wolffian and/or müllerian duct development. Testes that regress during the late embryonic period (days 43–59) usually secrete insufficient testosterone to affect the wolffian duct. The production of AMH is variable, resulting in poorly differentiated or rudimentary müllerian structures (incomplete inhibition). In the absence of systemic androgens, the external genitalia appear female.

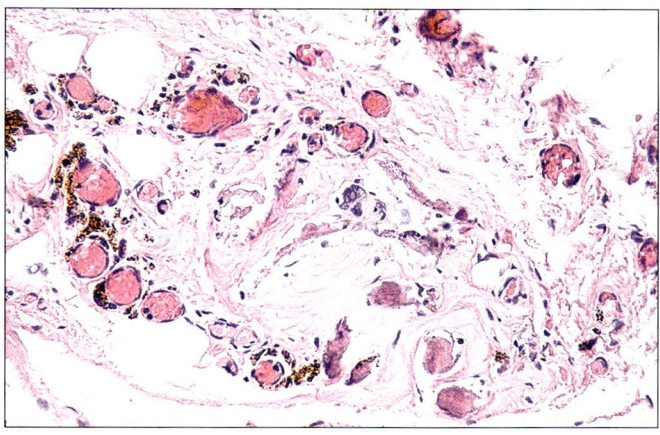

Figure 2.4 Testicular regression syndrome. Vascularized fibrosis, hemosiderin deposition, and calcification are seen at the expected site of both gonads.

Regression of the testes during the early fetal period (days 59–84), which is after Sertoli cell (AMH) and Leydig cell (testosterone) functions have begun or are about to begin, results in an individual with ambiguous external genitalia. Various combinations of wolffian and müllerian structures develop depending on the duration of androgen secretion and müllerian inhibition.

Regression of the testes during the mid-fetal period (days 84–120) results in more advanced masculinization of the external genitalia, although degrees of ambiguity are usually present. Since müllerian duct inhibition is normally completed by day 80, the müllerian structures will have been suppressed and wolffian structures develop.

Leydig Cell Deficiency

Leydig cell deficiency is a rare cause of male pseudohermaphroditism that may have more than one etiology. Some cases may lack Leydig cells altogether, while in others those present are dysfunctional, having an abnormal fibroblast-like morphology.[22] Affected individuals have a 46,XY karyotype and testes with interstitial fibrosis, but lack mature Leydig cells and testosterone production. Tubules with Sertoli cells and, sometimes, immature spermatogonia are found. The müllerian structures are absent, indicating appropriate testicular production of AMH by Sertoli cells during fetal life. The wolffian duct system is developed either partially or fully such that identifiable vasa deferentia and epididymides are present. The phenotype varies and is usually female with unremarkable or ambiguous external genitalia, although unambiguous males with evidence of primary hypogonadism have been reported. The presence of wolffian duct development and the variable degrees of masculinized external genitalia indicate that some Leydig cells must have differentiated and functioned during early fetal life. Luteinizing hormone (LH) levels are elevated in affected individuals. Because this condition is so rare, it is uncertain whether the underlying defect is an absence or a defect of the LH–hCG receptor on the Leydig cell or with some other, unknown, factor arresting Leydig cell development.

Defects in Testosterone Synthesis

Congenital deficiency of any enzyme involved in testosterone production in the testis or adrenal gland results in a state of androgen deficiency (relative estrogen excess). The histologic appearance of the testicular tissue is variable. Although described occasionally as 'normal,' the photomicrographs in some reports have disclosed large clusters of Leydig cells surrounding tubules lined only by Sertoli cells. Spermatogonia are often normal in children, but disappear by puberty.[23] In general, the number of gonads studied for any of the conditions and the ranges of ages studied (infancy, childhood, adulthood) have been limited. Müllerian structures are absent, but wolffian duct structures may be present. The degree to which the external genitalia develop depends upon the type and severity of the defect.

Defect in Cholesterol Synthesis (Smith–Lemli–Opitz Syndrome). Cholesterol synthesis is required for testosterone and all other hormones that the gonads and adrenal glands produce. The Smith–Lemli–Opitz syndrome, inherited as an autosomal recessive trait, results from an enzymatic defect in the last step of cholesterol metabolism (reduction of 7-dehydrocholesterol due to mutations in the *DHCR7* gene).[24] These patients variably show ambiguous genitalia with hypospadias, and more constantly a wide range of other somatic abnormalities including a distinctive facial appearance (microcephaly, ptosis, small upturned nose, micrognathia), cleft palate, and limb anomalies (proximally placed thumbs, polydactyly, and 2–3 toe syndactyly).[25] Several 46,XY infants with female external genitalia and intra-abdominal testes with epididymides and deferent ducts had a normally shaped uterus and vagina.[26,27] The Y chromosome is normal in these cases, with the affected *DHCR7* gene located at 11q13.[27]

Congenital Lipoid Adrenal Hyperplasia. Congenital lipoid adrenal hyperplasia (lipoid CAH), the most severe form of CAH, results from mutations in the steroidogenic acute regulatory (*STAR*) gene as the primary defect (Table 2.2).[28] The *STAR* gene, located on chromosome 8, encodes a protein that helps transport cholesterol into the mitochondria.[29] The principal effect is the absence of cholesterol intermediates capable of converting to pregnenolone. Additional damage occurs from the subsequent steroidogenic loss independent of *STAR*, and results from the effects of the cholesterol esters that accumulate in the adrenal cortex. This leads to cellular damage in the form of salt wasting, hyponatremia, hypovolemia, hyperkalemia, acidosis, and death in infancy. This state of hypergonadotropic hypogonadism shows markedly elevated levels of gonadotropic hormones (LH, follicle-stimulating hormone, ACTH), but markedly impaired synthesis of all gonadal and adrenal cortical steroids, even with trophic stimulation tests.

In the 46,XY male, the external genitalia may be ambiguous to female, but sufficient testosterone must have been secreted during embryogenesis since the internal genitalia are male. Some of these patients may have a palpable gonad in the inguinal canal. These testes disclose immature seminiferous tubules with spermatogonia. Occasional Leydig cells are present. The germ cells may disappear over time, resulting in a Sertoli-only syndrome, although this is not inevitable. Germ cells can persist and rarely develop into intratubular germ cell neoplasia.[30]

CAH. Several inherited enzymatic defects, which cause the syndrome of CAH, involve both the synthesis of adrenal mineralocorticoid and glucocorticoid hormones as well as the adrenal and testicular sex hormones. Because of these genetic defects, one or more adrenal cortical enzymes fail to be synthesized or are defective.

The deficiency of 3β-hydroxylase dehydrogenase, like the 20,22-desmolase deficiency, results in decreased synthesis of mineralocorticoid and glucocorticoid hormones as well as adrenal and testicular sex hormones, and may lead to life-threatening salt wasting in infancy. DHEA, a weak androgen secreted in high amounts, results in slight clitoral enlargement in the female, but rarely completely masculinizes the external genitalia in males. Hence, the male may be born with ambiguous genitalia and may resemble a virilized female. Males in whom the defect is partial may be born with hypospadias, but at puberty develop gynecomastia. Over time, the Sertoli cells, which may initially appear normal, undergo atrophy and the spermatogonia change from abundant to rare to absent. The number of Leydig cells may increase with age, but it is unclear whether the hyperplasia is absolute or relative to the atrophy of other elements.[31]

In contrast to the early age of diagnosis in the above two syndromes, the diagnosis in most patients with 17β-hydroxylase deficiency is not suspected until the anticipated time of puberty or later. Occasionally, detailed steroid analysis of the urine of a newborn male presenting with ambiguous genitalia has been performed, indicating that the correct diagnosis can be made in the young.

Deficiency of two enzymes, 17,20-desmolase and 17-hydroxysteroid dehydrogenase (formerly 17-ketosteroid reductase), results in deficient testosterone synthesis but does not affect the production of either mineralocorticoids or glucocorticoids. The former defect (conversion of 17-hydroxypregnenolone to DHEA) is extremely rare. The patients present with ambiguous external genitalia and inguinal or intra-abdominal testes. Spermatogonia were present in the testes of infants but were absent in the biopsies of their older teenage relatives. All had third-degree hypospadias, but normal male internal ductal differentiation.

Genetic males with 17β-hydroxysteroid dehydrogenase (17β-HSD) deficiency have uniformly been raised as females and have unambiguous female external genitalia. Most are diagnosed at or after puberty when they fail to menstruate and instead show signs of virilization such as clitoromegaly (enlarged phallus) and hirsutism.[32] Breast development may or may not take place. At surgery, müllerian duct derivatives are absent, consistent with normal AMH action. Wolffian duct differentiation, indicative of testosterone secretion during embryogenesis, is normal.[33] The testes present in the inguinal canal or labia majora contain rare to no spermatogonia, and may exhibit numerous Leydig cells. Detailed endocrine studies have shown that testicular 17β-HSD is under a different genetic control from that in extragonadal tissues, and while affected males lack testicular 17β-HSD, the extragonadal activity is normal or enhanced. More than 15 mutations have been identified in the responsible gene.[11,33]

Defect in Müllerian Inhibiting System (AMH and its Receptors)

The persistent müllerian duct syndrome, also known as 'hernia uteri inguinalis,' is a rare form of male pseudohermaphroditism where müllerian duct structures persist in 46,XY phenotypic males (Figure 2.5). Most patients present when young with unilateral or bilateral cryptorchid testes, normal or almost normal male external genitalia, and an inguinal hernia into which prolapses an infantile uterus and fallopian tubes.[34,35] Some patients may be older.[36] The testes are histologically normal, wolffian duct structures are developed, the pubertal development is normal, and a rare patient has been fertile. Treatment is surgical, consisting of orchiopexy and herniorrhaphy with hysterectomy and bilateral salpingectomy.

If at operation any patient has a streak gonad or a tumor rather than bilateral testes, the diagnosis of mixed gonadal dysgenesis should be considered. In most cases of persistent müllerian duct syndrome, the vas deferens is embedded in the wall of the upper vagina and sometimes the müllerian structures must be left intact to preserve the vas deferens. Malignant testicular tumors have been reported in the very rare cases of adult patients with persistent müllerian duct syndrome and uncorrected cryptorchid testes.

Persistent müllerian duct syndrome is a heterogeneous group of disorders caused by at least two different defects in the müllerian inhibiting system. The most common is a defect in the anti-müllerian hormone gene, *AMH* (the protein is also called MIS). The next most common is a defective AMH type II receptor.[37,38] The effect of these abnormalities is that some patients produce no biologically functional AMH, whereas others who produce normal amounts of biologically active AMH have end-organ insensitivity or an abnormality of the timing of AMH secretion. On rare occasion, a germ cell tumor may develop in the gonad, and, exceptionally, a müllerian-type tumor develops in the genital tract.[39]

END-ORGAN DEFECTS

The normal development of the wolffian duct derivatives and the external genitalia requires that these structures be responsive to androgen and that the enzyme 5α-reductase be present in the anlage of the prostate and external genitalia to convert testosterone to dihydrotestosterone. A molecular defect of the androgen receptor system (e.g., unstable androgen receptor or lack of androgen receptor) leads to impaired development of both wolffian duct structures and external genitalia in 46,XY individuals. If only 5α-reductase is absent or defective, the abnormalities in the reproductive tract are confined to the external genitalia and prostate.

Androgen Receptor Disorders (Androgen Insensitivity Syndromes)

Disordered androgen receptor function results in various phenotypes, which range from phenotypic women with intra-abdominal testes, to individuals with ambiguous genitalia, and to phenotypic men with minimal clinical abnormalities. One classification scheme[40] lists four categories, which are in order of increasing virilization (decreasing feminization):

1. Complete testicular feminization
2. Incomplete testicular feminization
3. Reifenstein phenotype: gynecomastia and hypospadias
4. Infertile and/or undervirilized man.

About 70% of cases share an X-linked recessive inheritance through the carrier mothers, the result of mutational defects in the androgen receptor gene, which is in the X chromosome's long arm. In another 30%, the mutation arises *de novo*.[41] Other genetic mutations are known, many of which are limited to individual families.[42,43] These mutations may lead to functional absence of the androgen receptor because the primary sequences of the gene are affected.

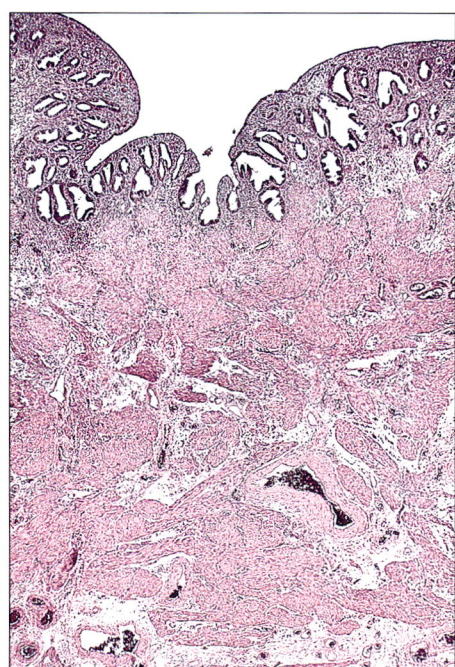

Figure 2.5 Uterus in persistent müllerian duct syndrome.

These patients generally present as complete testicular feminization. The more common defect results from single amino acid substitutions and is associated with the various other forms of the disease as described below. In rare patients the androgen receptor disorder occurs in combination with other unusual karyotypes, e.g., 47,XXY and 47,XYY.

Complete Androgen Receptor Insufficiency (Complete Testicular Feminization). Complete testicular feminization, the most common form of male pseudohermaphroditism, occurs in 1:20,000 newborns. The external genitalia are phenotypically female (Figure 2.6) and, for this reason, the condition is rarely diagnosed before puberty unless an inguinal hernia or labial mass is encountered or unless the disease is known to be familial. Primary amenorrhea is the most common complaint leading to evaluation and subsequent diagnosis. The medical history usually reveals that breast development occurred as expected at puberty, but remains in the pubertal state (Figure 2.7). Pubic and axillary hair is scant (Figure 2.8) and the vagina is shortened. The epididymides are usually cystic and not connected to the testes. The vasa differentia, seminal vesicles, and prostate are absent. As a rule, both the cervix and the uterine corpus are absent. Fallopian tube fragments are found in one-third of cases.[44] The testes are cryptorchid and may be located in the inguinal canal, the pelvis, or rarely the labia.

In the complete or almost complete form of the syndrome, the individual exhibits a female gender identity with normal extragenital erotogenic sensitivity and normal maternal attitude, emphasizing the need to support the patient as a woman, even with reconstructive surgery.[45] This condition should be differentiated from defects in steroidogenic factor-1 mutations (XY, sex reversal with androgen insensitivity-like features) with which it can be confused.

The gonads in infants and young children are relatively normal but, by age 5 years, they show abnormalities. By young adulthood, the gonad is often involved with benign or malignant tumors as described later. If tumors are not present by this age, the gonad is usually small and on section is tan to brown and traversed by thin white bands (Figure 2.9). Microscopic examination of the testicular parenchyma discloses immature seminiferous tubules. At earlier ages, the tubules may be clustered in small aggregates (Figure 2.10), but with time they become more

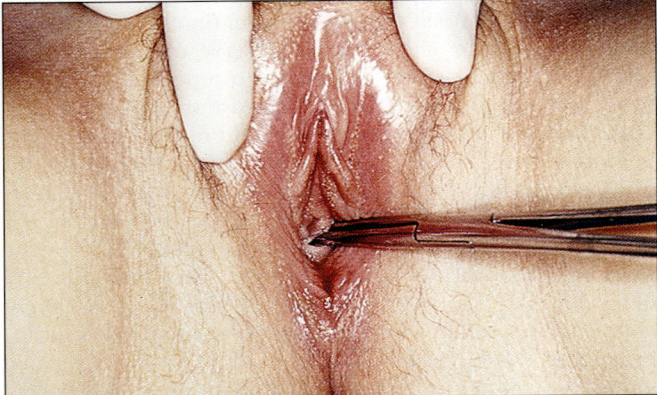

Figure 2.6 'Normal' phenotypic feminine genitalia in androgen insensitivity syndrome.

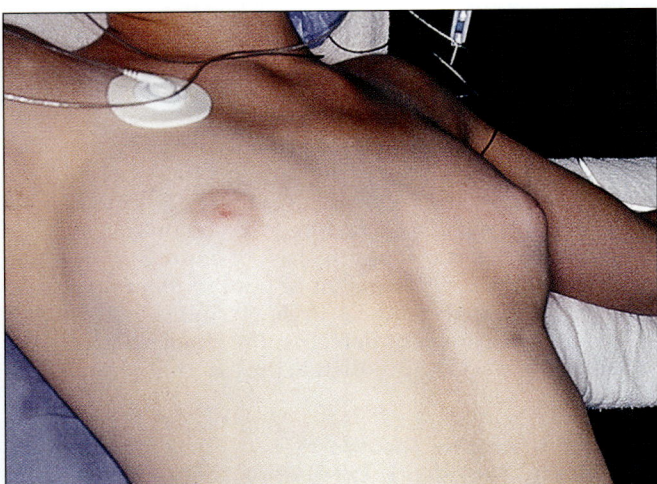

Figure 2.7 Immature breast development and lack of axillary hair in androgen insensitivity syndrome.

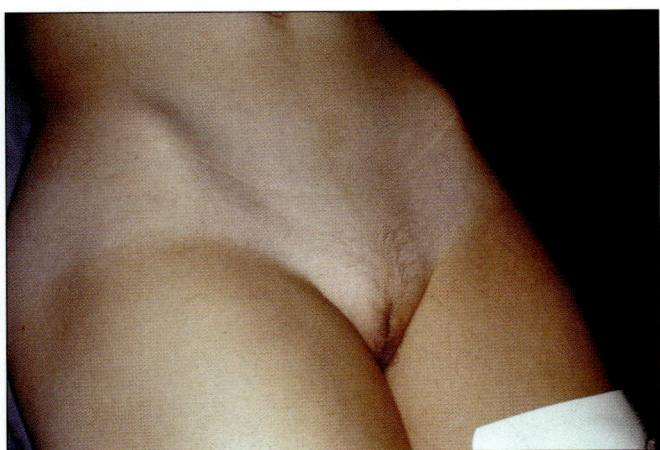

Figure 2.8 Lack of pubic hair in androgen insensitivity syndrome.

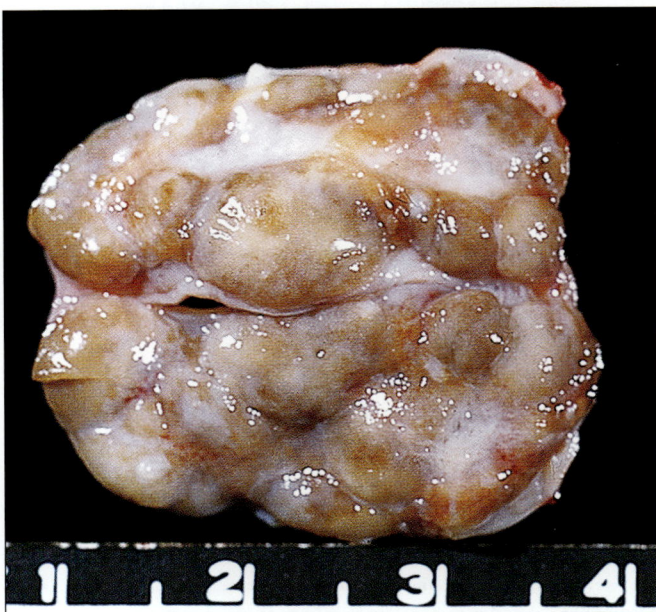

Figure 2.9 Testis in androgen insensitivity syndrome without tumor.

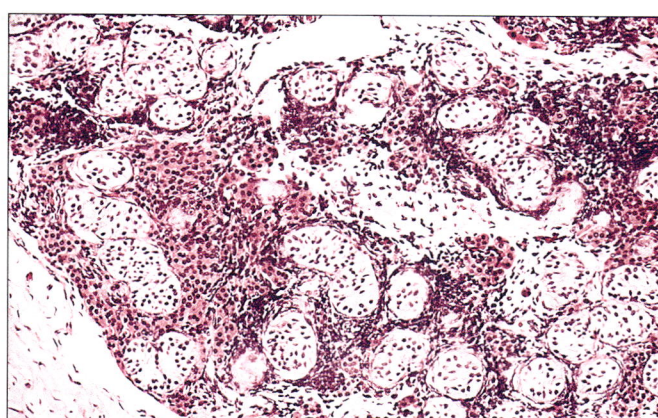

Figure 2.10 Androgen insensitivity syndrome. Immature seminiferous tubules, numerous Leydig cells, and rare foci of immature ovarian-type stroma constitute the testis.

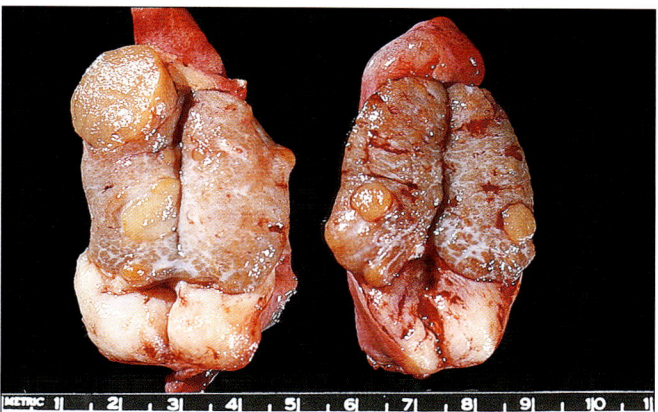

Figure 2.13 Androgen insensitivity syndrome. Several small yellowish Sertoli cell adenomas are present throughout the specimen. The large white mass at the inferior pole may represent a hypertrophied gubernaculum testis or a leiomyoma present since birth.

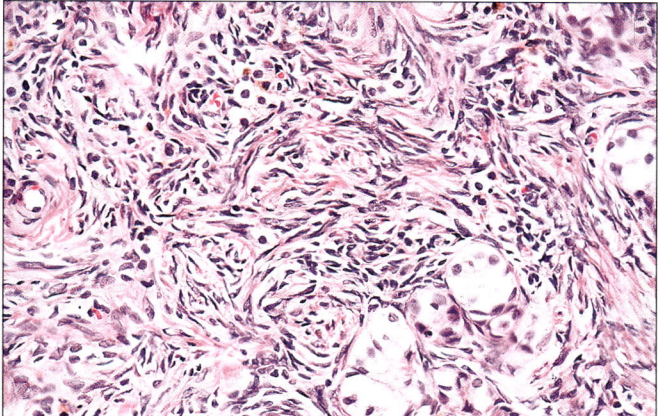

Figure 2.11 Androgen insensitivity syndrome. Scattered immature seminiferous tubules are embedded in the dense ovarian-type cortical stroma present in the testis.

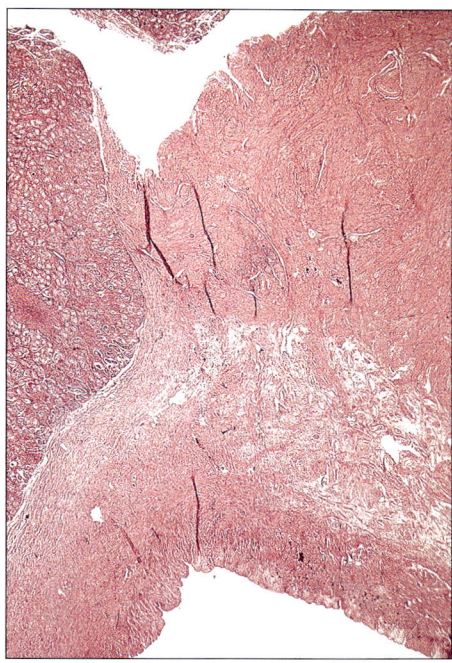

Figure 2.14 Nodule of hypertrophied gubernaculum in androgen insensitivity syndrome.

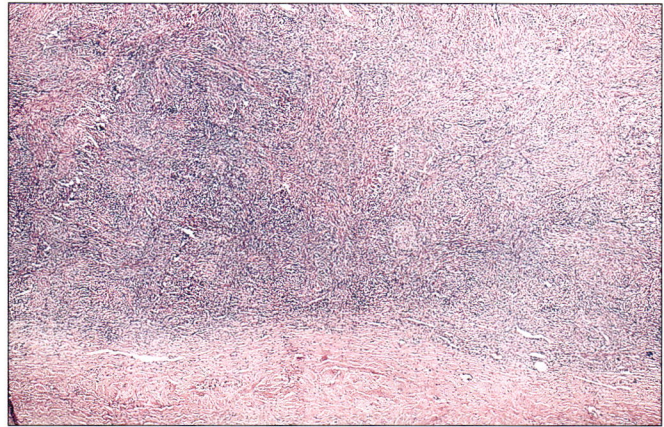

Figure 2.12 Androgen insensitivity syndrome, gonad in an older patient. Dense ovarian-type cortical stroma with extremely rare scattered immature seminiferous tubules constitute the testis.

sparsely distributed (Figure 2.11). Spermatogonia may be present, but spermatogenesis is absent. The number of spermatogonia found is also age dependent, diminishing as the patient ages. The interstitium, which resembles ovarian stroma, is usually abundant at an early age and over time often becomes more fibrous (Figure 2.12). Fetal-type Leydig cells may be abundant. The Leydig cells in individuals with testicular feminization have an ultrastructure typical of cells involved in active hormone synthesis and the systemic androgen levels in these individuals are typically elevated. These findings indicate that the pathologic defect in the testicular feminization syndrome is an end-organ defect and not lack of hormone production by the testes.

Most testes of affected individuals contain multiple benign nodules that are discrete, firm, yellow to brown, and bulge above the sectioned surface (Figure 2.13). These can be hamartomatous (e.g., Sertoli cell adenoma) or neoplastic (e.g., dysgerminoma or gonadoblastoma like). One finding we have seen characteristically is a 1–2 cm firm white nodule of hyalinized smooth muscle leiomyoma-like tissue that is usually present at one pole of the testis (Figure 2.14).

Reactivity for smooth muscle actin confirms its smooth muscle origin (Figure 2.15). Additionally, hamartomatous nodules are present, usually bilaterally, in virtually every case. The typical size varies from 1 mm to 1 cm, but occasionally up to 4 cm.[44] The bulk of the nodule consists of seminiferous tubules lacking lumina (Figure 2.16). Spermatogonia may be present (Figure 2.17). The seminiferous tubules located outside the nodules have a lamina propria that is of normal thickness in prepubertal testes, but thickened and hyalinized in the adult.[46] Sertoli cell adenomas, which average 3 cm in diameter, but range to 25 cm (Figure 2.18), are hamartomas composed predominantly or exclusively of closely packed immature seminiferous tubules lacking lumina and lined by immature, uniform Sertoli cells (Figure 2.19), some with germ cells (Figure 2.20).[44,47] The interstitium in the testes of affected patients often resembles ovarian stroma, and frequently contains Leydig cells (Figure 2.10). On rare occasion, Leydig cell nodules form, and have been considered benign tumors (Figure 2.21). Even though tumors have been reported occasionally as malignant, none has shown evidence of invasion or dissemination grossly or microscopically.[48] In summary, the name applied to each type of nodule is somewhat arbitrary and depends largely upon the types of component present as well as their number and size. Most nodules are classified as hamartomas, Sertoli cell adenomas, or rarely as Leydig cell tumors.

Malignant gonadal tumors develop with increasing frequency with age in patients with testicular feminization. Seminoma is the most commonly encountered gonadal

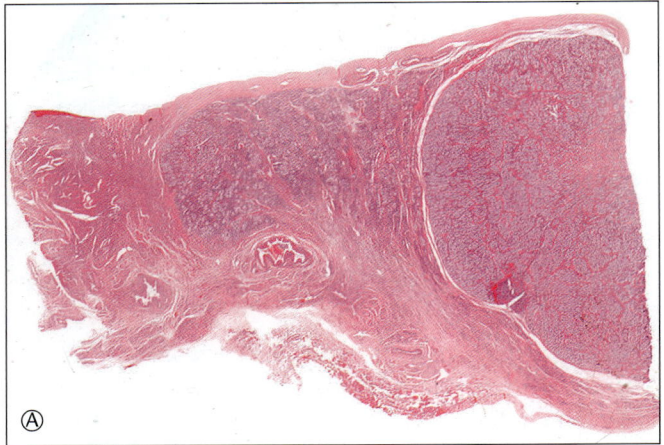
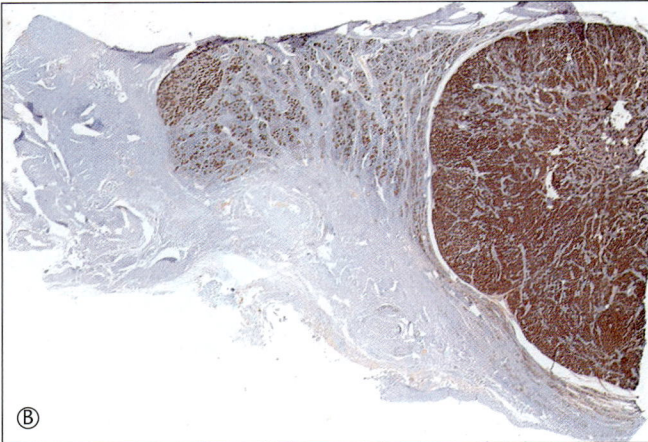
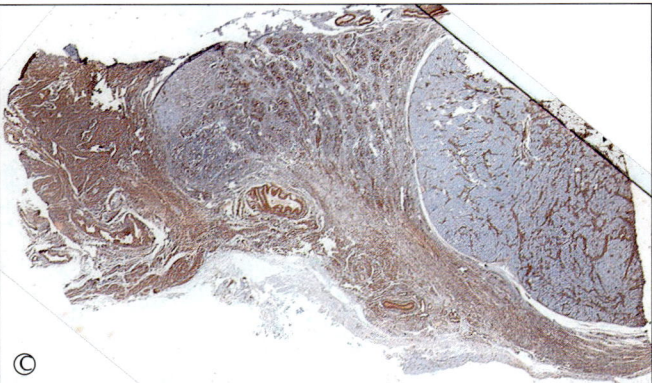

Figure 2.15 **(A)** Androgen insensitivity syndrome with Sertoli adenoma (right) and hypertrophied gubernaculum (left). The adenoma expresses AMH **(B)**, and smooth muscle actin is positive in the gubernaculum **(C)**.

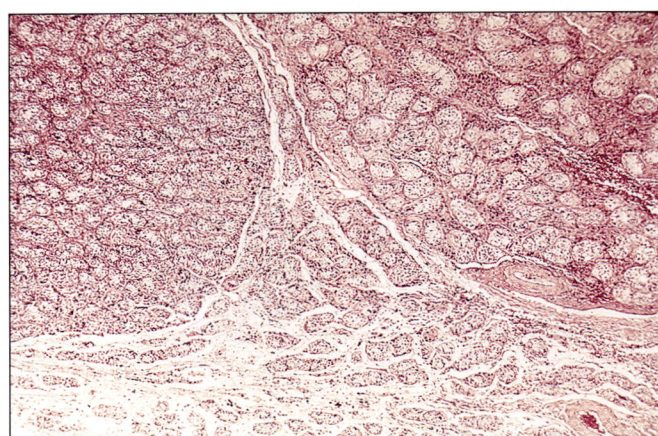

Figure 2.16 Sertoli cell adenoma in androgen insensitivity syndrome. The tubules lack lumens.

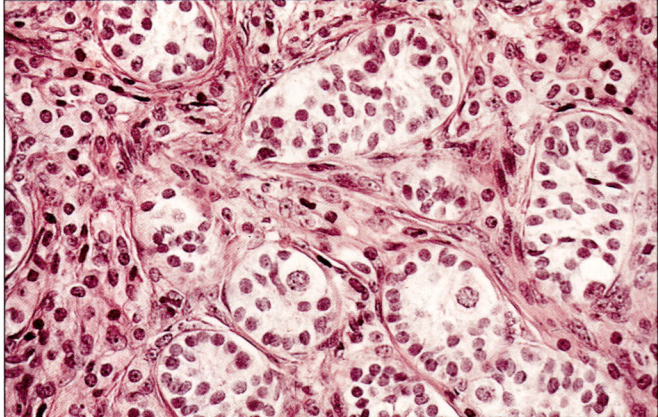

Figure 2.17 Seminiferous tubules with occasional spermatogonia in androgen insensitivity syndrome.

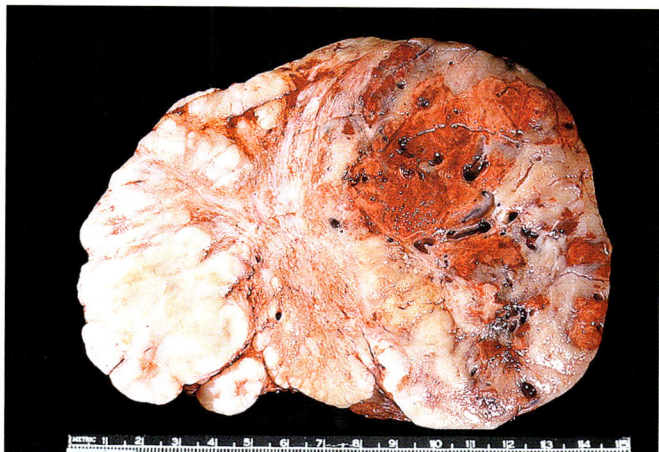

Figure 2.18 Giant Sertoli cell adenoma.

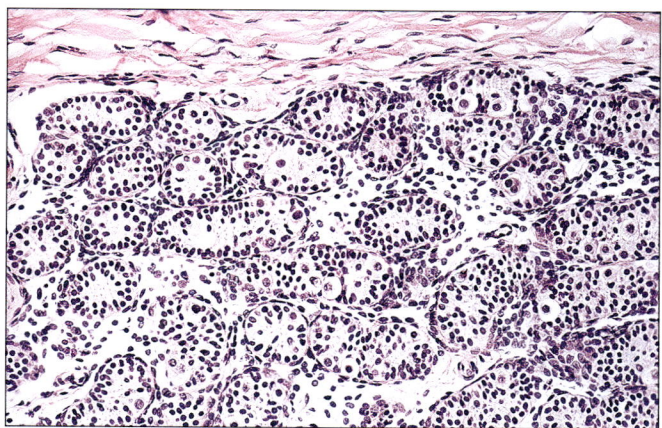

Figure 2.20 Germ cells in Sertoli cell adenoma.

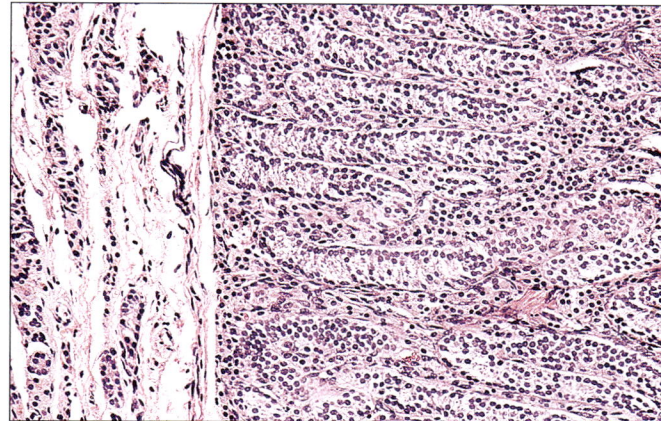

Figure 2.19 Interface of Sertoli cell adenoma (right) and adjacent degenerative seminiferous tubules (left) in androgen insensitivity syndrome.

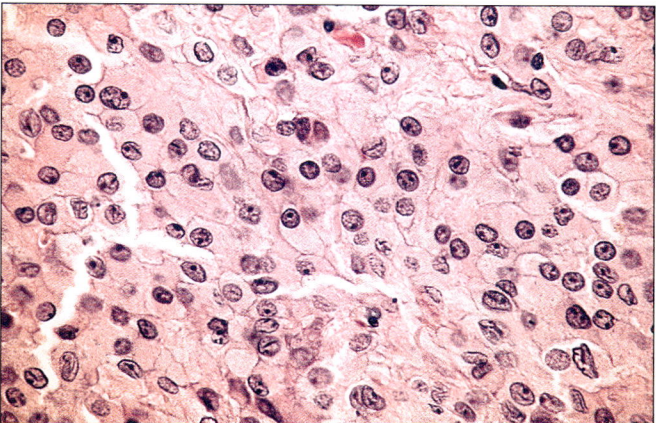

Figure 2.21 Leydig cell tumor in androgen insensitivity syndrome. Detail of a well-circumscribed gross nodule showing sheets of cells with large central nucleus and copious cytoplasm.

malignancy in this syndrome. Intratubular germ cell neoplasia is sometimes seen, either independently or in association with seminoma (Figures 2.22 and 2.23). Other malignant germ cell tumors and malignant sex cord tumors are also encountered rarely. Unlike mixed gonadal dysgenesis in which tumors develop in young individuals, the risk of malignancy in patients with testicular feminization is only 4% by the age of 25 years, but reaches 33% by 50 years.[49] Since malignant tumors rarely develop before completion of puberty, castration can usually be delayed until after adolescence, thus permitting the patient to undergo normal pubertal development with spontaneous female secondary sex characteristics.

Partial Androgen Receptor Insufficiency (Incomplete Testicular Feminization). About 10–50% of patients with the androgen insensitivity syndrome have an incomplete variant.[50,51] The clinical manifestations vary depending on the classification system used. If restricted, it resembles complete testicular feminization except that there is partial fusion of the labioscrotal folds and usually some clitoromegaly at birth. If inclusive of all forms of the androgen insensitivity syndrome that are not considered *complete* testicular feminization, then greater percentages of patients will look and be raised as

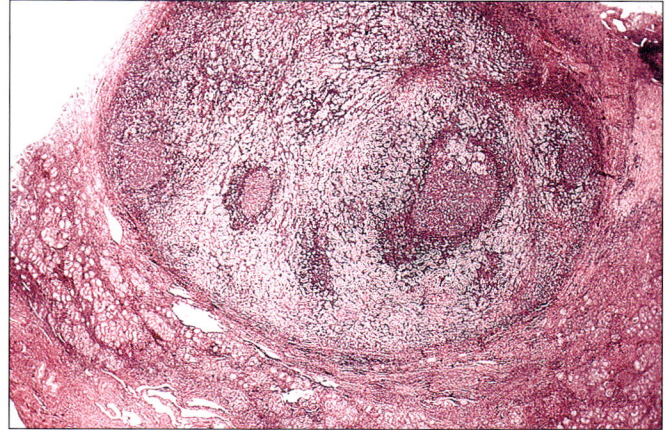

Figure 2.22 Seminoma in androgen insensitivity syndrome.

males.[50,51] Viewed broadly, patients with partial androgen receptor insufficiency form one of the largest groups of intersex patients born with male sex ambiguity.[4] Like the complete form, underdeveloped wolffian duct derivatives are often present. If the diagnosis is established during

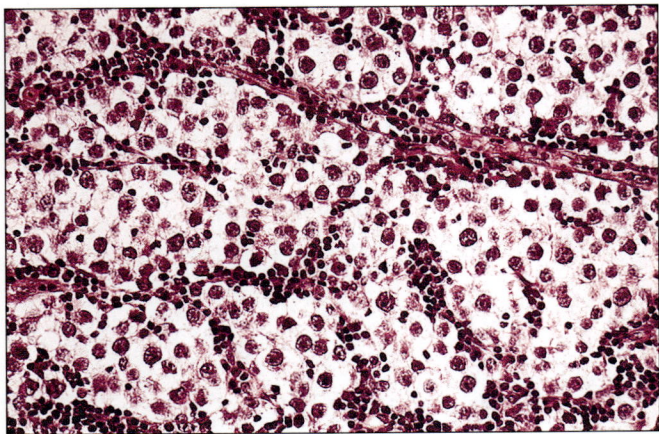

Figure 2.23 Seminoma in androgen insensitivity syndrome. Detail of neoplastic germ cells surrounded by fibrous stroma invested with numerous lymphocytes.

childhood, gonadectomy should be performed before puberty, since disfiguring virilization may accompany breast development at puberty. Estrogen therapy should be given at the appropriate time to initiate feminization. The pathologic findings are those described for the complete form of testicular feminization.[46]

Other Forms. Reifenstein syndrome, infertile male syndrome, and undervirilized male syndrome are other forms of incomplete androgen insensitivity in which the phenotype is male. There are few reports describing the microscopic findings of the gonads.

- Patients with Reifenstein syndrome usually present with gynecomastia and severe hypospadias, like children or teenagers with perineoscrotal hypospadias. However, the phenotypic spectrum is wide, even within the same affected family with a single androgen receptor abnormality in all affected family members. Additional abnormalities include female habitus, azoospermia, cryptorchism, and hypoplasia or absence of wolffian duct structures.
- Infertile male syndrome is a rare androgen receptor defect characterized by a phenotypically normal man with infertility caused by azoospermia.
- In the undervirilized male syndrome, the individual is a male with gynecomastia, a small penis, decreased beard and body hair, a normal male urethra, a normal sperm density, and an identifiable androgen receptor defect. Most affected individuals are infertile.

5α-Reductase Type 2 Deficiency

This is a disorder of testosterone metabolism. Functional deficiency from the mutated enzyme, 5α-reductase 2, impairs the conversion of testosterone to dihydrotestosterone, the hormone that masculinizes the indifferent urogenital sinus and induces development of the prostate.[52] The disorder, formerly known as 'pseudovaginal perineoscrotal hypospadias,' has an autosomal recessive inheritance and is rare. Most reported cases come from family clusters found in a number of relatively isolated geographic locations.[53] Several unrelated patients have had an identical mutation, suggesting a common ancestral founder.[54] The type 2 isoenzyme develops in the fetus and is detectable in the genital skin and the male accessory sex organs. The type 1 isoenzyme is not detectable in the fetus; its activation in skin at the time of puberty is responsible for the clinical virilization these patients later express.

Affected males are usually phenotypically female with female to ambiguous external genitalia at birth.[55] The small clitoris-like phallus lacks a urethral orifice. In most affected individuals the urogenital sinus opens on the perineum and within the sinus an anterior orifice leads to the urethra and a posterior orifice to a blind vaginal pouch. The testes are in the inguinal canals or labia. The müllerian-derived structures are absent whereas wolffian-derived structures (vas deferens, epididymis, and seminal vesicle), the anlagen of which respond to testosterone, are normal.

At puberty, virilization occurs due to type 1 isoenzyme activation, but the breasts fail to develop. The penis lengthens, the bifid scrotum grows and becomes rugated and hyperpigmented, and the testes enlarge and descend. Testicular biopsy specimens reveal spermatogenesis and tubular atrophy in some individuals, complete spermatogenic arrest and Leydig cell hyperplasia in others. The prostate remains rudimentary and the seminal vesicles underdeveloped, which results in affected adults having highly viscous semen and extremely low ejaculate volume. Erection and ejaculation are possible in some affected individuals, but few individuals are fertile.

Neonates with this disorder frequently go unrecognized and are raised as females. After the virilization that accompanies puberty, individuals raised as girls sometimes reverse their sex roles and function as men, often with a stormy period of adjustment. Individuals with a male gender identity benefit from surgical correction of hypospadias and cryptorchism. High doses of testosterone enhance virilization. Persons raised as females who elect to continue to function as females into adulthood benefit from orchiectomy before the onset of puberty to avoid the accompanying virilization. Estrogen therapy is useful to promote feminization. No patients are known to have developed testicular germ cell tumors.

DISORDERS OF SEX DETERMINATION (DISORDERS ASSOCIATED WITH ABNORMAL SEX CHROMOSOMES AND ABNORMAL GONADAL FORMATION)

Additions, deletions, and mosaicism of the sex chromosomes characterize individuals in this category. The gonadal appearance is variable and ranges from a streak gonad to a nearly normal female or male gonad on both gross and microscopic examination. These disorders are subdivided into two broad categories depending on the frequency with which sexual ambiguity occurs.

The pathologist can sometimes suspect that a specimen is from a patient with abnormal sexual development by determining whether a sex chromatin is present. The Barr body, as it is often called, refers to the mass of densely staining chromatin material found at the periphery of the nucleus in patients with more than one X chromosome. The nuclei in smooth muscle cells in arteries are particularly useful for this examination. The number of Barr bodies is one less than the number of 'X' chromosomes present, such that none are evident in an XY male, a single Barr body signifies an XX karyotype, and three Barr bodies an XXXX karyotype (Figures 2.24 and 2.25). Barr bodies are best assessed in cytologic preparations, such as an exfoliative buccal smear or solid tissue touch preparation, but can be seen in a well-stained tissue section. Sex chromosome fluorescent *in situ* hybridization is a more sensitive alternative, and because it is amenable to quantification can be used to assess mosaicism in tissue sections.

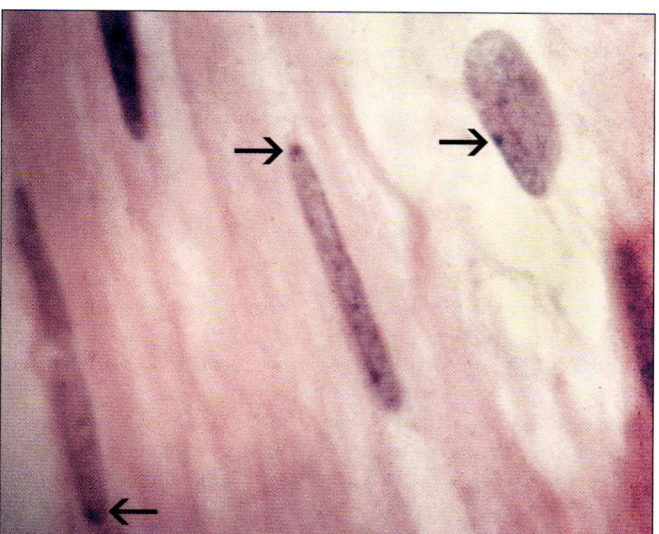

Figure 2.24 Single Barr body, indicating two X chromosomes. The number of sex chromatin masses is one less than the actual number of X chromosomes. A single mass of densely staining chromatin material (arrows) is present at the periphery of the nucleus in this tissue section.

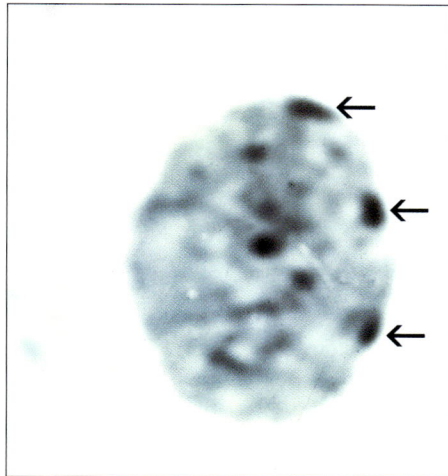

Figure 2.25 Three Barr bodies, indicating four X chromosomes. Three masses of densely staining chromatin material (arrows) are present at the periphery of the nucleus in this cytologic smear. The number of sex chromatin masses is one less than the actual number of X chromosomes.

SEXUAL AMBIGUITY INFREQUENT

KLINEFELTER SYNDROME

Klinefelter syndrome, one of the most common causes of prepubertal delay and primary hypogonadism in males, occurs in about 1 in every 1000 live newborn males and accounts for about 3% of infertile males. The karyotype is usually 47,XXY in four-fifths of cases, which usually results from non-disjunction occurring during meiosis of either paternal or maternal gametes.[56] The remainder have a higher grade chromosomal aneuploidy (48,XXXY, 49,XXXXY, 48,XXYY) or mosaicism (47,XXY/46,XY) caused by non-disjunction during mitosis of the developing zygote. Molecular probe studies have shown that the extra chromosome is equally likely to originate from the mother as the father. In the father they result as an error in the first paternal meiotic division, but in the mother over one-fourth occur (28%) at the second maternal meiotic division.[57] Unlike trisomy 21, which occurs as a failure of the first maternal meiotic division, the likelihood of Klinefelter syndrome is not increased with advancing maternal age.

The clinical picture varies depending on the age at which the diagnosis is first suspected. Some estimate that more than two-thirds of persons with Klinefelter syndrome remain undiagnosed; about 10% are diagnosed prenatally with genetic screening programs, and one-fourth at adolescence or during adult life when the patient presents with gynecomastia, obesity, and signs of infertility, or is evaluated for malignancy.[56] Although infants with Klinefelter syndrome usually have normal external male genitalia at birth, the syndrome is sometimes discovered during evaluations of newborns with hypospadias, micropenis, and small, soft testes or cryptorchism. Before puberty, the only physical signs may be small testes or long-leggedness resulting in a diminished upper to lower body segment ratio. After puberty, signs of androgen deficiency become apparent. The beard and body hairs are frequently sparse. Half of the patients develop gynecomastia (Figures 2.26 and 2.27). By the age of 25 years, two-thirds of patients complain of decreased libido. Frequently associated clinical findings include learning disabilities, behavioral disorders, reduced economic striving, and limited sexual drive. Laboratory tests reveal elevated gonadotropin levels (post puberty), low testosterone levels, and azoospermia.

The Klinefelter testes in adult 47,XXY individuals are small and rarely exceed 2 cm in maximal dimension (Figure 2.28). The seminiferous tubules may show some degenerative changes during fetal life, and by late childhood the primary spermatogonia are already greatly reduced in number. Shortly before the expected time of puberty, the progressive degenerative changes dramatically accelerate.[58] The absence or presence of elastic fibers in the tubular wall indicates whether the process of atrophy began prepubertally or postpubertally (Figure 2.29), respectively. On microscopic examination, the testes in adults are largely atrophic, have hyalinized seminiferous tubules, and have a relative increase in the number of Leydig cells (Figure 2.30). Some tubules may be preserved, but lined only by Sertoli cells. Rarely, an occasional seminiferous tubule of the adult testis contains germ cells in varying stages of maturation. In these cases it is unusual for development to extend beyond the stage of first spermatocyte.[57] If sperm are detected,

32 PATHOLOGY OF THE FEMALE REPRODUCTIVE TRACT

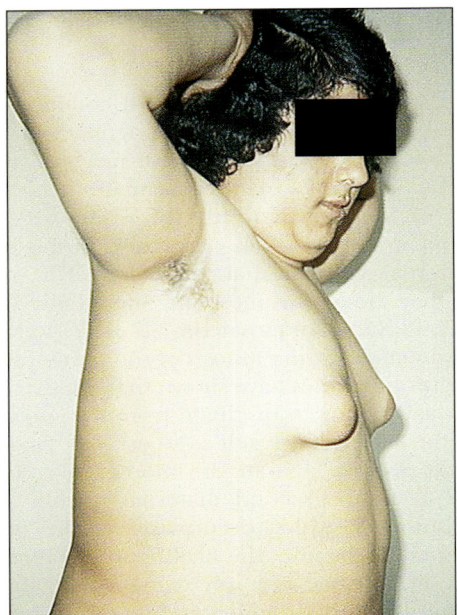

Figure 2.26 Klinefelter syndrome. Gynecomastia is present and axillary hair is absent.

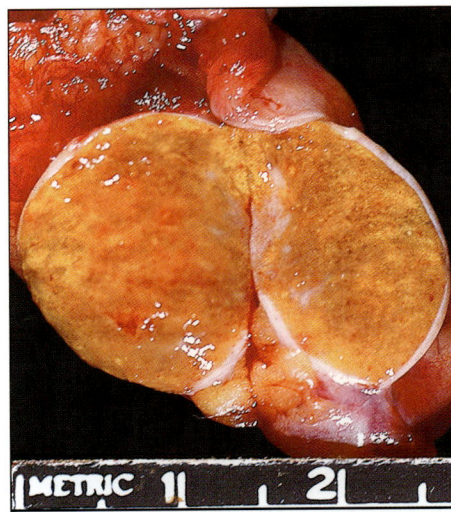

Figure 2.28 Testis in Klinefelter syndrome. The parenchyma is golden-yellow to slightly brown.

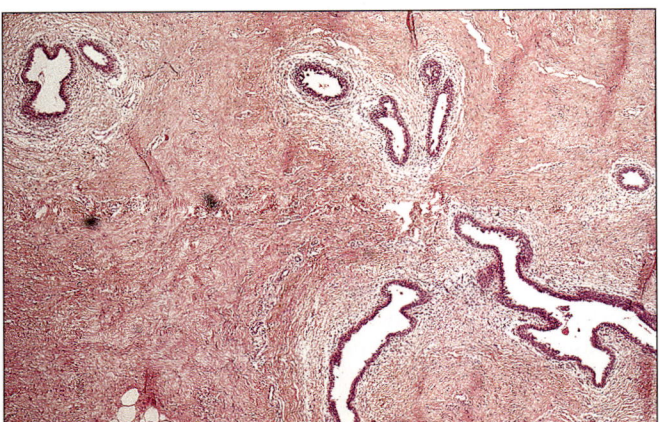

Figure 2.27 Gynecomastia in Klinefelter syndrome. The breast tissue is composed solely of ducts; no lobular tissue is present.

mosaicism, most likely of the 46,XY/47,XXY pattern, should be suspected. Patients with this mosaic karyotype are sometimes fertile.

The Leydig cells become pronounced in number sometime after puberty. Although they appear hyperplastic relative to the atrophic appearance of the other elements, it is uncertain whether the absolute volume is greater than in normal testes. Functionally, the Leydig cells are abnormal, evidenced by the low levels of serum testosterone in the setting of elevated serum LH and follicle-stimulating hormone levels and subnormal increase in response to an hCG challenge.

Various neoplasms have been associated with Klinefelter syndrome. Both gonadal and extragonadal germ cell tumors develop with increased frequency. Most extragonadal tumors occur in the mediastinum as teratoma and embryonal cell carcinoma (teratocarcinoma) or choriocarcinoma.[59,60] In the testis, seminoma, teratoma, and embryonal cell carcinoma have been encountered.[61] Leydig cell tumors are rare (Figure 2.31).[62] The risk of breast carcinoma in men with Klinefelter syndrome may be 20% higher than in normal men. Hematologic malignancies have also been reported, including acute leukemia, Hodgkin disease, malignant lymphoma, and chronic myeloid leukemia.[63]

TURNER SYNDROME

In the classic form, Turner syndrome is a disorder in which sexually immature phenotypic females of short stature have various congenital anomalies and streak gonads. The cytogenetic hallmark is the 45,X karyotype with a sporadic, non-familial pattern of inheritance. Other karyotypes identified less frequently in this syndrome include mosaic 45,X/46,XX and 45,X/47,XXX/46,XX, or additional anomalies of the X chromosome. The X chromosome present is maternal in origin in 71% of cases.[64] Patients with a 45,X/46,XY mosaic karyotype (considered in mixed gonadal dysgenesis) usually present with obvious sexual ambiguity, but sometimes present as phenotypic females with the clinical stigmata of Turner syndrome. Approximately 5% of clinical Turner syndrome patients will have a structurally abnormal Y chromosome at karyotype, and up to 40% have occult Y chromosome sequences by polymerase chain reaction in a mosaic or non-mosaic distribution.[65]

At a molecular level, a specific deficiency has been proposed to help explain the syndrome's development.[66] The gene *RPS4* (ribosomal protein S4) is necessary for ribosomal function. This gene is normally located on the X and Y chromosomes near the pseudoautosomal region and are interchangeable. It is speculated that normal human development requires at least two *RPS4* genes in each cell, and that the Turner phenotype may be due, in part at least, to the presence of only one.

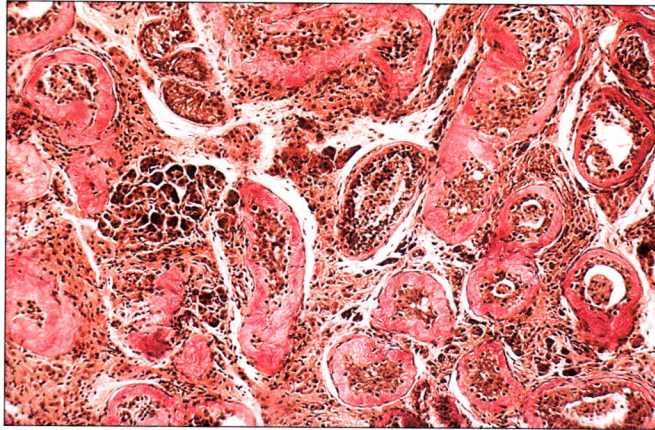
Figure 2.29 Postpubertal end-stage testis in Klinefelter syndrome. Elastic tissue is present in the hyalinized sclerotic wall of seminiferous tubules.

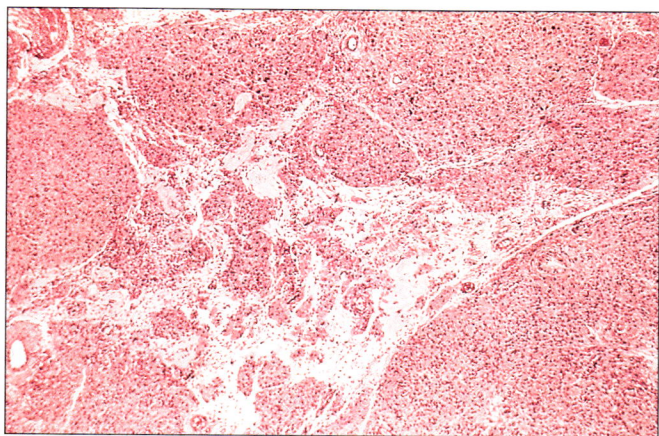
Figure 2.31 Leydig cell neoplasm in Klinefelter syndrome.

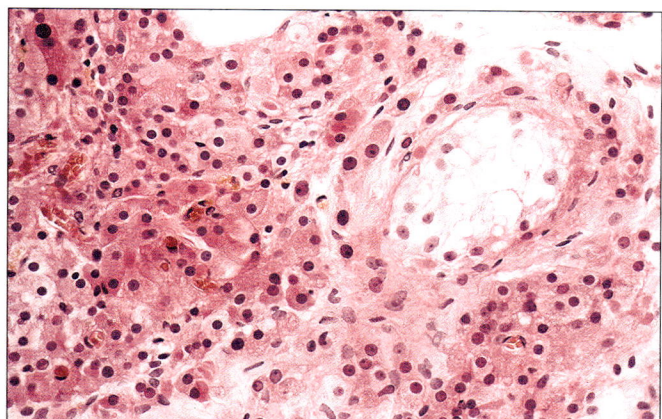
Figure 2.30 Leydig cells surrounding a seminiferous tubule composed only of Sertoli cells in Klinefelter syndrome.

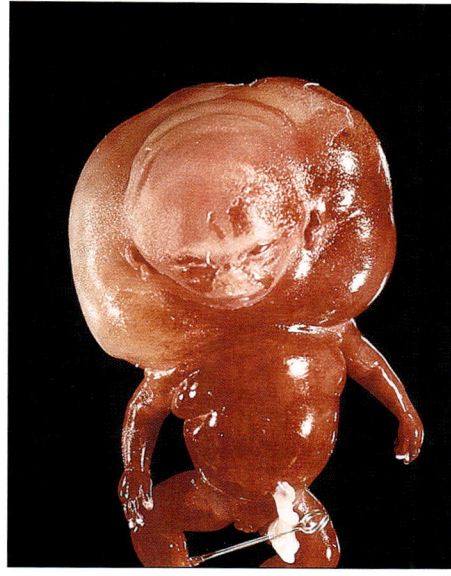
Figure 2.32 Fetus with Turner syndrome. The overt finding related to lymph stasis manifests as swellings of the nape of the neck (cystic hygroma).

About 98% of fetuses with a 45,X karyotype abort. This accounts for the frequency of Turner syndrome being about 1 in 100 conceptions, but only about 1 in 3,000–10,000 liveborn females. In the newborn, the overt findings relate to lymph stasis, which manifests as edema of the dorsum of the hands or feet or, less frequently, as a swelled nape of the neck (cystic hygroma) (Figure 2.32). Later in childhood and in adult life, a webbed neck and elevated distal portion of the nails are residua of more marked swellings present during fetal life and may still provide a clue to the correct diagnosis. A rare, but important, major presentation is hydronephrosis due to ureteropelvic stenosis. All female neonates with a ureteropelvic obstruction should have chromosomal analysis. Congenital anomalies of other organ systems associated with Turner syndrome include a short fourth metacarpal, hypoplastic nails, multiple pigmented nevi, and coarcted aorta. Growth retardation (short stature) is common.[67] More than 40 somatic anomalies are associated with this condition.

Spontaneous puberty occurs in 5–10% of women with Turner syndrome.[68] While most patients will have been diagnosed earlier, those who reach adolescence undiagnosed often present with primary amenorrhea. Examination reveals underdeveloped secondary sex characteristics and a small uterus. Urinary gonadotropins are always elevated and the vaginal smear lacks cornified cells. The buccal smear in a 45,X individual reveals few if any Barr bodies; in those 20% of patients with a mosaic karyotype (usually 45,X/46,XX or 45,X/47,XXX) the smear discloses a subnormal number of chromatin-positive cells (about 5–15% for a female). Only rare patients with Turner syndrome have become pregnant and most of these have been mosaics with a 46,XX cell line. Some of these women have mosaic patterns that are found only after extensive search.[69] Oocyte donation programs have recently proven effective with one center recording 20 clinical pregnancies in 18 women, the majority of whom achieved a liveborn via cesarean section.[70]

At laparotomy, the internal genitalia are female and, although small, are in normal relation to one another. The adult gonads appear as white fibrous streaks, 2–3 cm long and 0.5 cm in diameter, and are located in the position normally occupied by the ovary (Figure 2.33). On microscopic examination a streak consists of an attenuated cortex, a medulla, and a hilus (Figures 2.34 and 2.35). The cortex consists of characteristic ovarian stroma in which the cells are elongated, wavy, and have a conspicuous nucleus with scant cytoplasm. Rete tubules (rete ovarii) and hilar cells are typically present in the hilus region. Oocytes are almost always absent in adults with Turner syndrome. Oocytes are present in normal numbers in 45,X embryos before week 12 of gestation (Figure 2.36), but older fetuses and young children show accelerated rates of oocyte depletion relative to the normal number for the age. Usually before the time of menarche in the normal girl, women with Turner syndrome will have no oocytes, thus leading to primary amenorrhea. These findings are interpreted to suggest that the second X chromosome is necessary for granulosa cell development and primary follicle formation. Without this X chromosome, granulosa cells fail to differentiate and, as a result, the oocytes degenerate.

A significant difference between patients with a 45,X/46,XY mosaic karyotype and those with classic 45,X Turner syndrome is that gonadoblastoma and malignant germ cell tumors are common in patients with the former and rare in the latter. Currently, it is common practice to

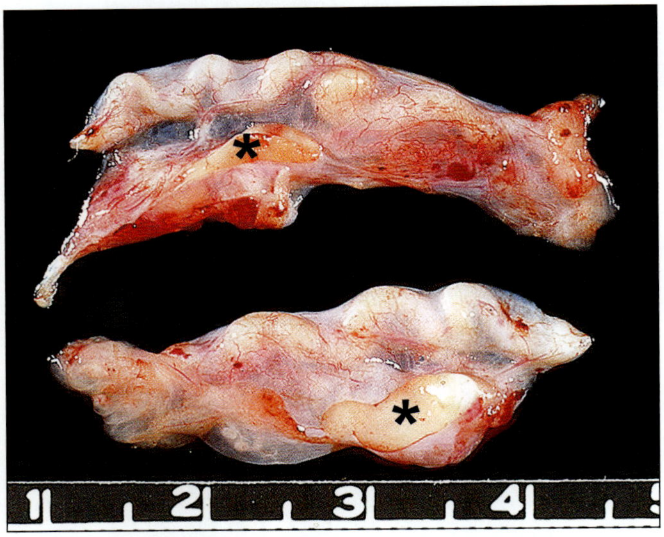

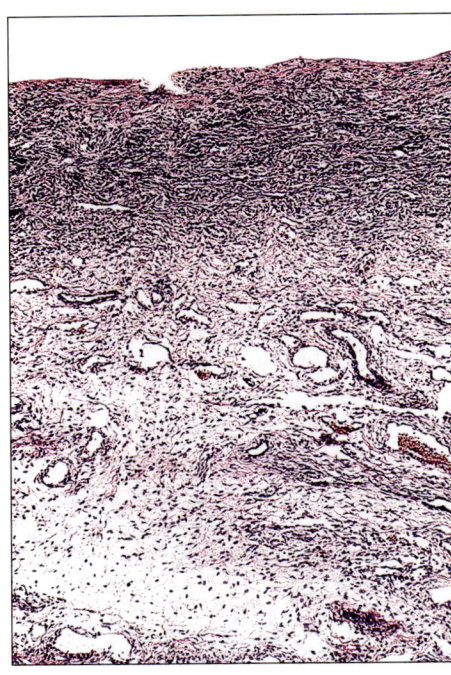

Figure 2.35 Streak ovary in Turner syndrome. The streak consists of an attenuated cortex, a medulla, and a hilus. The cortex consists of characteristic ovarian stroma with cells that have elongated, wavy conspicuous nuclei and scant cytoplasm.

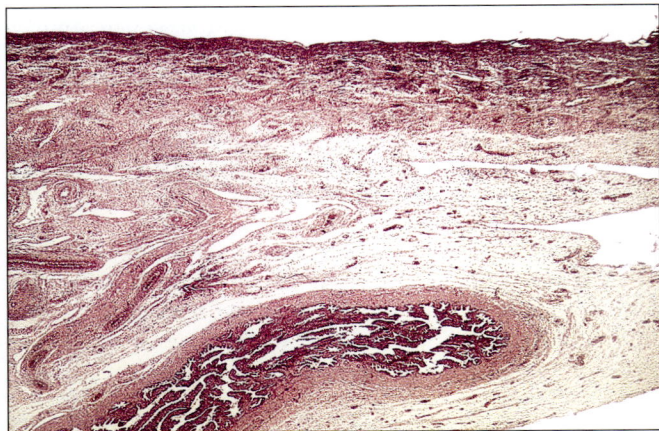

Figure 2.33 Streak ovary in Turner syndrome. The adult gonads appear as white fibrous streaks (asterisks), adjacent to the fallopian tube, located in the position normally occupied by the ovary.

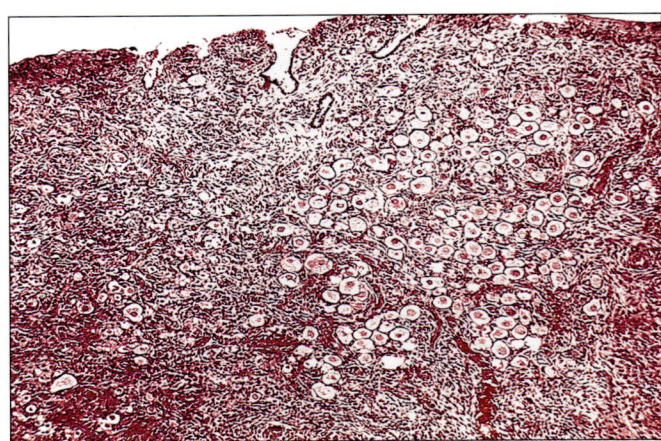

Figure 2.34 Streak ovary in Turner syndrome with adjacent fallopian tube.

Figure 2.36 Embryonic ovary in Turner syndrome. Oocytes are present in normal numbers before week 12 of gestation.

actively exclude Y mosaicism in individuals with Turner syndrome if virilization or a small marker chromosome is seen.[71] Some have recommended that Y chromosomal exclusion should be carried out in all Turner patients.[72] In an occasional instance, microscopic gonadoblastoma or other germ cell tumor has been found in some of these Turner-like patients with a cryptic Y chromosome.[73]

Non-germ cell tumors occur. Some patients also have had virilization with stromal luteoma or hilus cell hyperplasia.[74] Development of neoplasms of the so-called 'surface epithelial type' suggests that the celomic epithelium encapsulating the gonad can undergo malignant change even if the gonad is a streak. Endometrial carcinoma occurred occasionally in those patients who had received long-term, high-dose exogenous estrogen therapy to foster the appearance of the female secondary sex characteristics. Both natural estrogens and synthetic non-steroidal estrogens have been implicated and the duration of usage usually exceeded 3 years. Today, this is so rare that it is not even recognized to occur, although there have been several cases described where the tumor developed even in the absence of hormone replacement therapy.[75] Extragonadal tumors, most often of neurogenic origin, have also been reported in children and young adults.

XX MALE (SEX REVERSAL)

The XX male syndrome is a disorder exhibiting a nearly normal but infertile phenotypic male with a 46,XX karyotype. This syndrome, one of the rarest of all sex chromosome anomalies, occurs in about 1 in 24,000 newborn males.[76] XX males share many characteristics of men with Klinefelter syndrome. Both have a generally masculine appearance, normal or near-normal external genitalia, male psychosexual orientation, normal-to-weak secondary sexual characteristics, normal-to-low androgen levels, and azoospermia. The testes are small with prominent Leydig cells and tubules lined only by Sertoli cells. Like Klinefelter patients, the most common reasons for adult evaluation are infertility and abnormal secondary sexual characteristics. But they also differ. XX males are generally shorter in height, and the frequency of hypospadias and gynecomastia is higher. The frequency of impaired intelligence is not increased in XX males relative to the general population. Increasingly, with ultrasonography and genetic analyses being performed during the gestation, the XX male syndrome is now being discovered prenatally.[77]

The XX male syndrome results from at least three distinctly different mechanisms. About 70% of these patients have a small portion of paternally derived Y chromosome that contains the *SRY* gene present abnormally on the X chromosome. The *SRY* gene is normally found on the short arm of the Y chromosome adjacent to the pseudoautosomal pairing region. During meiosis in the father, an abnormal exchange sometimes leads to the transfer onto the X chromosome of the entire pseudoautosomal region plus the adjacent portion of the Y chromosome with the *SRY* gene. Inheritance of such an X chromosome from the father leads to the Y(+) XX male syndrome. The inheritance pattern of this syndromic form is sporadic. These patients have normal male external genitalia. Apparently, the presence of the *SRY* gene is adequate to lead to normal male phenotype, if its primary downstream target, *SOX9*, is present.[1] Azoospermia in these patients results from the lack of other genes normally found on the Y chromosome necessary for sperm development.

Some patients with the XX male syndrome lack Y-derived DNA. Such Y(−) XX males might occur by two different mechanisms. The first is familial transmission of an autosomal dominant or X-linked inheritance of XX maleness. These patients usually have ambiguous genitalia. This indicates that genes exist that can trigger testis determination when mutated.[78] A second mechanism is chromosomal mosaicism with a prevalent XX lineage. In such patients, the Y-containing cell line might simply be technically too difficult to identify because of the small number of such cells, or selective distribution within gonadal tissues.

PURE GONADAL DYSGENESIS
Usual Form

Pure gonadal dysgenesis and its eponym, Swyer syndrome, historically have encompassed diverse conditions, including testicular regression syndrome at one end of the spectrum and mixed gonadal dysgenesis (now 46,XY disorder of sex development) at the other. As used in this chapter, 'pure gonadal dysgenesis' refers to a phenotypic female where the internal genitalia include müllerian structures (uterus and fallopian tubes) and generally streak gonads, the constellation of which probably still encompasses a multitude of diverse conditions. The patients may appear phenotypically normal or have hypoplastic external genitalia. The pure gonadal dysgenesis syndrome occurs with both 46,XX and 46,XY karyotypes and has both familial and sporadic patterns of inheritance.

The 46,XX type pure gonadal dysgenesis is usually an autosomal recessive disorder, but, less frequently, may be due to an abnormality of the X chromosome, possibly as a mosaic 45,X cell line confined to the gonad.[79] Deletions of the short or long arm of an X chromosome have been identified in some cases. Such patients have greater ovarian development than those with 46,XY pure gonadal dysgenesis or Turner syndrome and present more often with signs of ovarian dysfunction (secondary amenorrhea or infertility) rather than primary gonadal failure (primary amenorrhea). Some patients may also have mosaic cell lines with the *SRY* gene absent in some tissues (peripheral leukocytes), but present in others (testicular tissue).[80]

The 46,XY type pure gonadal dysgenesis is more common than the 46,XX form of the disorder. The syndrome of pure gonadal dysgenesis may be sporadic or familial with either X-linked recessive or autosomal recessive patterns of inheritance.[81,82] Some patients have a mosaic 45,X/46,XY karyotype. The 46,XY type may also involve deletion of the *SRY* gene, a mutated inactive *SRY* gene or a defective promoter cofactor.[83–85] In one series of 14 XY females with pure gonadal dysgenesis, patients who had normal *SRY* had gonads composed of undifferentiated stroma in which there were tubules or a rete structure suggesting some differentiation toward testis. In those cases where there were mutations in *SRY*, no tubules were observed; the gonads were composed exclusively of ovarian-like stroma with sclero-hyaline nodules in some areas. These data also suggested that *SRY* may play a role in rete testis formation.[86]

Patients with 46,XX pure gonadal dysgenesis, as those with Turner syndrome, only rarely have gonadal tumors.

Some have had hilus cell hyperplasia and hilus cell tumors with the usual associated virilizing effects. Epithelial tumors are extremely rare, but of these mucinous tumors occur more frequently than serous.[87] Rare examples of germ cell tumors have been reported,[88] and even though no identifiable Y chromosome component could be detected in some, the possibility of a cryptic Y fragment cannot be excluded. Patients with 46,XY pure gonadal dysgenesis are at high risk for gonadoblastoma and other germ cell tumors, as is true of all patients with streak gonads and a Y chromosome.[85] In one series, 11 of 20 patients had gonadal neoplasms; eight were gonadoblastoma, half of which were bilateral, and eight were dysgerminoma, all unilateral.[89] On this basis, patients with 46,XY pure gonadal dysgenesis might be considered a subset of the broader condition of mixed gonadal dysgenesis.

DEFECT IN THE WILMS' TUMOR SUPPRESSOR (*WT1*) GENE

Denys–Drash Syndrome

Denys–Drash syndrome is a rare disorder that, like Frasier syndrome, results from a mutated Wilms' tumor suppressor (*WT1*) gene, which is located on chromosome band 11p13. The two entities, however, have differing mutations, the heterozygous point mutations altering the zinc finger encoding exons in the former, and mutations in intron 9 of the same gene in the latter.[90] Denys–Drash syndrome consists of congenital nephropathy, Wilms' tumor, and intersex disorders, sometimes with the development of gonadoblastoma. Most children present with renal disease in the form of proteinuria. Most develop Wilms' tumor and nearly all die from renal failure by 3 years of age. Males with ambiguous genitalia are more commonly diagnosed earlier than females in whom the genitalia are normal.[3,91]

Multiple gonadal abnormalities described to date include normal ovaries with signs of early ovarian failures, normal müllerian and wolffian ducts, and normal to dysgenetic testes. Early prophylactic nephrectomy is important to prevent the development of the malignant renal tumors.[92]

Frasier Syndrome

Frasier syndrome, like Denys–Drash syndrome, is rare and results from mutation of intron 9 of the *WT1* gene.[90] The syndrome is defined by male pseudohermaphroditism and progressive glomerulopathy. Patients usually present because of the glomerulopathy, usually with proteinuria as the initial manifestation. During the ensuing work-up, they are found to have normal female external genitalia, streak gonads, XY karyotype, and sometimes gonadoblastoma.[93,94] When raised as a female, a presenting sign may be absence of anticipated pubertal sexual development.[95] The nephropathy is usually focal segmental glomerulosclerosis, which differs from the diffuse mesangial sclerosis seen in Denys–Drash. The renal disease is relentless, but end-stage renal disease may not occur until late childhood.

Abnormal splicing at intron 9 leads to an unbalanced ratio of the WT1 isoforms needed for normal glomerular and gonadal development.[96] Patients with Frasier syndrome have no increased risk for Wilms' tumor because the KTS-negative isoform of the WT1 protein retains its tumor-suppressor function.[97] The elevated risk of gonadoblastoma reflects the overall high risk of tumorigenesis in dysgenetic gonads.

SEXUAL AMBIGUITY FREQUENT

Patients in this category exhibit a wide range of phenotypic appearances and internal genitalia. A Y chromosome, either intact or portions thereof, is often present, usually as part of a mosaic complement. Sexual ambiguity is a common finding. This is an area currently undergoing rapid change as detailed genetic analyses at the molecular level are just beginning to identify an ever-expanding group of conditions that give rise to the phenotype described next. These can be described in a broad sense as 46,XY disorders of sex development, and where a causal genetic locus is known this can be specified along with the designated phenotype. For example, deletion of chromosome 9p can cause deficiency of the linked steroidogenic factor 1, and its attendant clinical abnormalities.

46,XY DISORDERS OF SEX DEVELOPMENT (MIXED GONADAL DYSGENESIS)

Mixed gonadal dysgenesis (MGD) is a heterogeneous syndrome with a 45,X/46,XY or 46,XY karyotype, persistent müllerian duct structures, a dysgenetic testis, and a contralateral streak gonad.[98] It is one of the most frequent causes of male sexual ambiguity.[4] The functional deficit imposed by the abnormal testis is expressed as incomplete inhibition of müllerian development, incomplete differentiation of wolffian duct structures, and incomplete male development of the external genitalia. Often, incomplete mediation of testicular descent occurs, resulting in both internal and external asymmetry of the genitalia and a mixture of male and female features in an individual in whom neither gonad is normal. About two-thirds of affected individuals are raised as females and the remainder as males, in part for psychologic and cultural reasons. Gonadectomy is often part of the intervention, so as to prevent the future development of cancer, which is not uncommon. The subject of gender assignment is multifaceted, and benefits from a multidisciplinary team approach.[99]

Given the overlap, we believe that the syndrome of MGD should be enlarged to incorporate some patients with bilateral streak gonads, streak-like areas but with tubules (described earlier as 46,XY type pure gonadal dysgenesis), or bilateral abnormal testes with a mosaic 45,X/46,XY karyotype (dysgenetic male pseudohermaphroditism) because the clinical, pathologic, and chromosomal features of these syndromes closely resemble each other. In turn, some patients with MGD exhibit the phenotypic features of a Turner-like syndrome.[100,101]

A variety of different genetic abnormalities appear to result in MGD, thus leading to its phenotypic heterogeneity. Partial deletions of both the short and long arms of chromosome Y have been detected in these individuals. Most cases where no detectable Y chromosomal anomaly is observed by conventional chromosome analysis have a Y fragment found when additional testing is performed.[102]

Clinically, MGD is usually detected in the neonate because of ambiguous external genitalia (Figures 2.37 and 2.38). Frequently, a palpable testis bulges through an indirect inguinal hernia or descends completely into the labioscrotal fold, resulting in asymmetry of the genital swellings. This clinical appearance prompted some earlier investigators to name the syndrome 'asymmetric gonadal dysgenesis.' If the

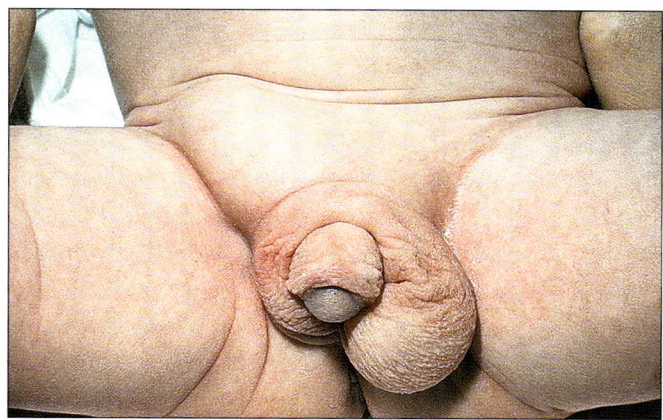

Figure 2.37 External genitalia in mixed gonadal dysgenesis. The left testis had descended into the scrotum; the right streak was in the abdominal cavity. Because of this characteristic appearance, some investigators prefer the name 'asymmetric gonadal dysgenesis' rather than 'mixed gonadal dysgenesis.'

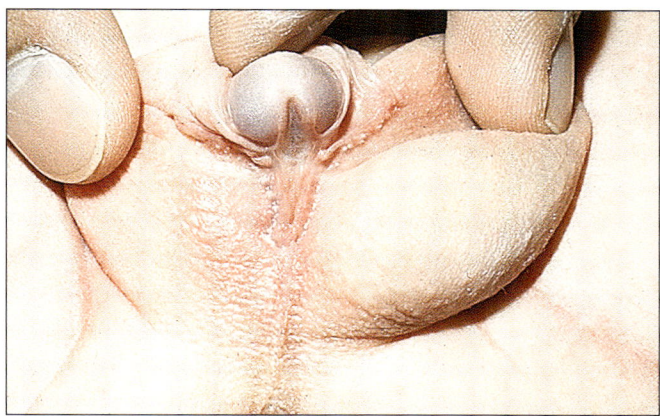

Figure 2.38 External genitalia in mixed gonadal dysgenesis. Only the left testis had descended into the scrotum.

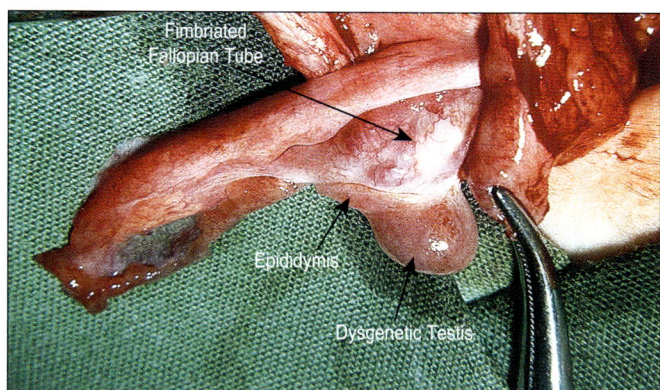

Figure 2.39 Internal genitalia in mixed gonadal dysgenesis.

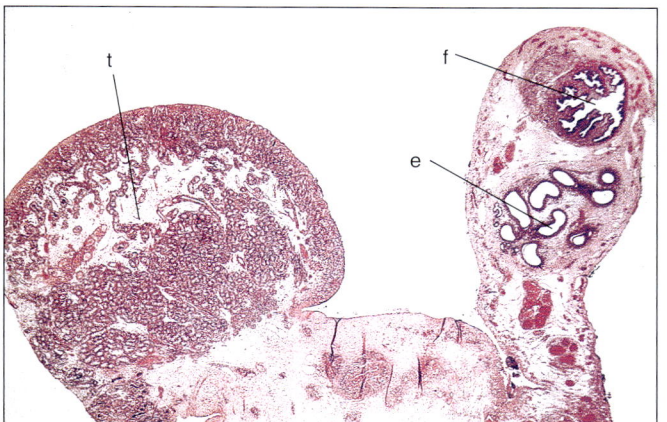

Figure 2.40 Organs in mixed gonadal dysgenesis. Testis (t), fallopian tube (f), and epididymis (e).

gonads are intra-abdominal, the labioscrotal folds may appear as normal labia or as empty scrotal sacs. The condition is likely to go unrecognized unless the clitoris is sufficiently enlarged to mandate investigation, which is common. The gonad that descends is usually a testis, and the streak gonads are always intra-abdominal unless dragged into a 'hernia uteri inguinale.'

Organs derived from the müllerian duct persist in 95% of cases (Figures 2.39 and 2.40).[103,104] The uterus is usually infantile or rudimentary, but occasionally may be normal. The fallopian tubes are frequently bilateral. If a testis is grossly near-normal size and well differentiated, the fimbria of the ipsilateral tube may be absent, but in only one-third of cases is the ipsilateral tube entirely absent. Organs of wolffian duct derivation may also be present, but the frequency is variable. An epididymis is identified in two-thirds of cases and is usually present on the side where there is a testis. The vas deferens is encountered less frequently. The seminal vesicle is identified only rarely, probably because tissue near the bladder/prostate region is not usually removed.

The gonad may be a testis or a streak. Streak gonads may be partially differentiated toward testis, or there may be a suggestion of differentiation toward ovary with gonadal-type stroma and even a very rare primordial follicle, but not ovary, which requires the presence of differentiation with follicles in at least the antral stage. Bilateral gross testes, frequently of an asynchronous degree of maturity, are found in about 15% of cases whereas a unilateral gross testis is found in 60%. The testis is consistently abnormal architecturally, and its organization is divided into three zones, each of which reflects the quantity and type of cellular components present (Figure 2.41). The three zones, which are described below in detail, include: (1) the region of the tunica albuginea or cortex, which exhibits a range of findings from widely spaced seminiferous tubules (Figure 2.42) or differentiation toward streak, usually with ovarian-like stroma, to immature zones indeterminate between female and male structures with primary sex cords (Figure 2.43); (2) the medulla, which is composed of normal or near-normal seminiferous tubules and interstitium (Figure 2.44); and (3) a hilar region with poorly differentiated seminiferous tubules that are only partly differentiated toward testis (Figure 2.41). It is uncertain whether this zone may represent hypertrophied rete testis.

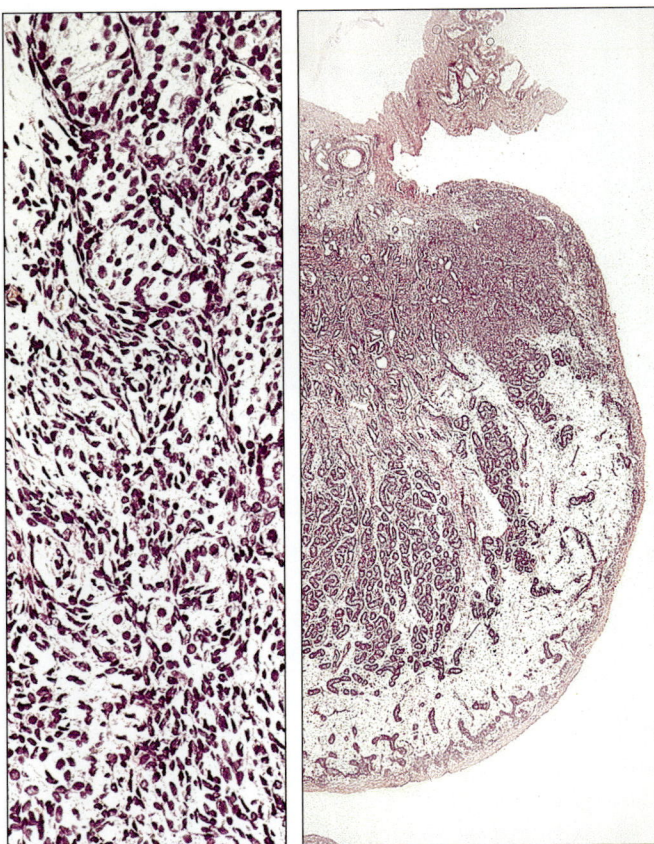

Figure 2.41 Testis in mixed gonadal dysgenesis. The dysgenetic testis has a thin rim of cortex (right bottom), relatively normal medulla (right middle), and hilus (right top), which in detail (left) shows the various tissue components blending together such that they are indistinguishable.

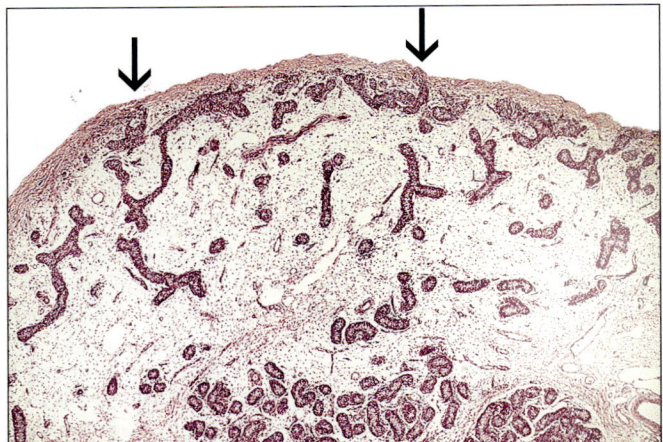

Figure 2.42 Cortex of testis in mixed gonadal dysgenesis. The seminiferous tubules are scattered and penetrate the tunica albuginea to open onto the surface (arrows).

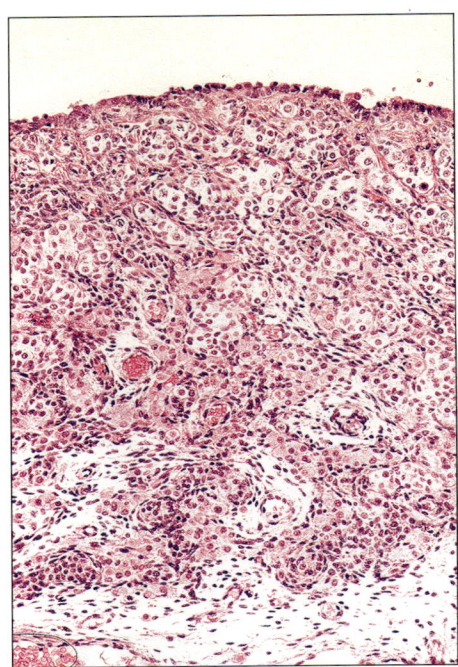

Figure 2.43 Rim of gonadal cortex in mixed gonadal dysgenesis with persistent primary sex cords. It is difficult to determine whether the organ is testis or ovary.

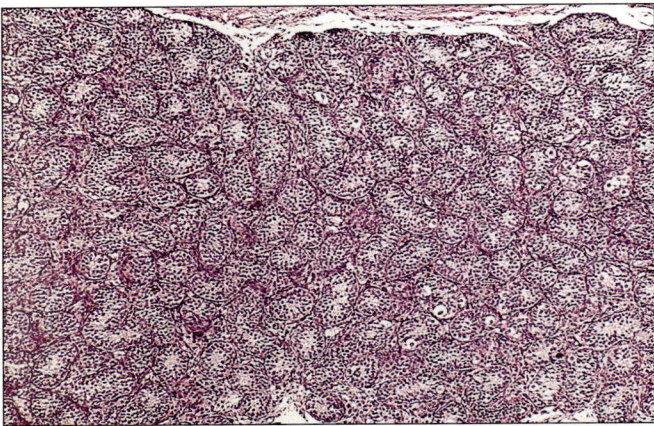

Figure 2.44 Medulla of testis in mixed gonadal dysgenesis. The testicular tissue looks relatively normal.

The superficial cortex may contain seminiferous tubules that are often widely separated by edematous, undifferentiated stroma. Sometimes the tubules penetrate the incompletely formed tunica albuginea and open onto the serosa. Occasionally, broad zones of cortex differentiate slightly toward streak-like ovary, even displaying rare primordial follicles, but, as mentioned above, without more fully developed follicles would still be called a streak (or, as some prefer, a 'streak testis') (Figure 2.45). In some cases it is difficult to distinguish between female and male structures.

The central zone (medulla) of the macroscopic infant testis is usually architecturally and cytologically normal (Figure 2.44). Narrow closed seminiferous tubules are lined by Sertoli cells with abundant cytoplasm. The numbers of spermatogonia vary. Advanced forms of spermatogenic maturation are not observed. Occasionally, the germ cells are seen to lie directly on the basement membrane of the

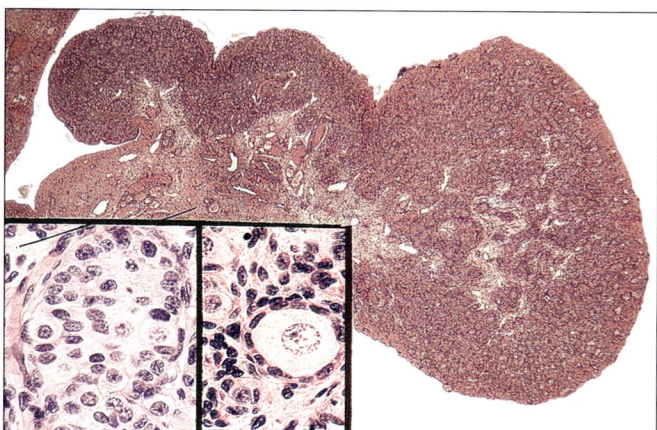

Figure 2.45 Gonad in mixed gonadal dysgenesis. In an unusual finding, some areas show early formation of seminiferous tubules while rare foci disclose primordial follicles, but nothing more advanced in development. Over time, the entire organ will atrophy and appear as a streak gonad.

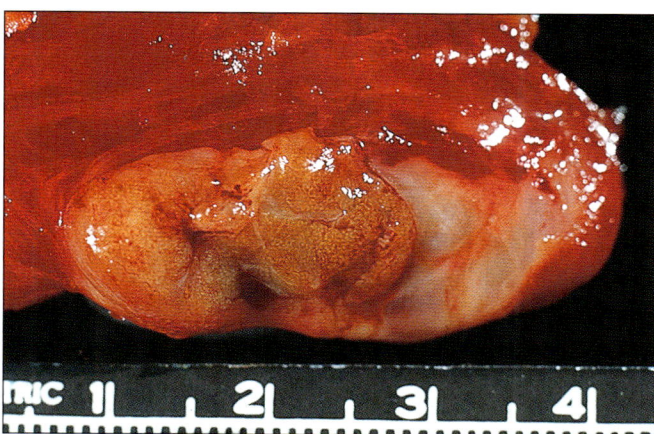

Figure 2.47 Testis in a 35-year-old phenotypic male with mixed gonadal dysgenesis (also Figures 2.48 and 2.49). The tunica albuginea is tan and maximally 1 mm thick. The parenchyma is golden yellow.

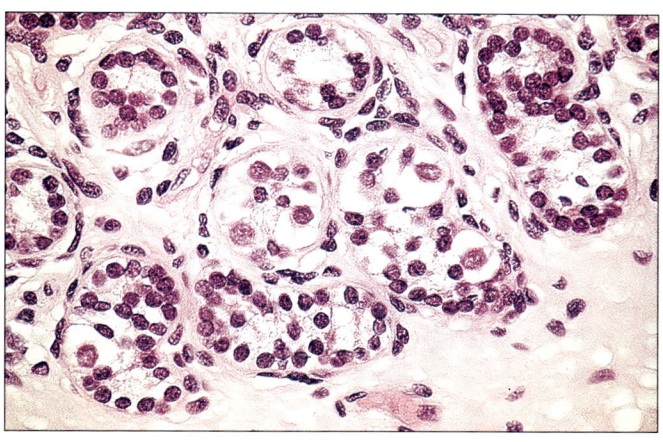

Figure 2.46 Abnormally located germ cells in mixed gonadal dysgenesis. Numerous germ cells lie directly on the basement membrane of the seminiferous tubule rather than being surrounded normally by Sertoli cells.

seminiferous tubule rather than surrounded normally by Sertoli cells (Figure 2.46). Leydig cells are present in small clusters of varying size. The nuclei of the Leydig cells contain finely dispersed chromatin, and the cytoplasm varies from minimal and amphophilic or slightly basophilic to abundant and eosinophilic. In older patients with a small gonad (Figure 2.47), the medulla is atrophic with tubules lined only by Sertoli cells. The tunica albuginea is composed of stroma resembling the stroma of ovarian cortex (Figure 2.48). Seminiferous tubule basement membranes are often thickened (Figure 2.49). Prominent clusters of Leydig cells fill the interstitium.

The architecturally disorganized hilar region discloses seminiferous tubules that are swollen by increased numbers of Sertoli cells and are lined by indistinct basement membranes. These tubules also merge with the surrounding stroma, imparting the appearance of a homogeneous blend of Leydig cells, germ cells, Sertoli cells, and an indeterminate type of interstitial stroma. The region resembles neither fetal ovary nor testis (Figure 2.41). It is uncertain whether some of this region may represent rete testis.

The streak gonads appear similar to those found in Turner syndrome (45,X karyotype). We have not observed a gonad that has been identifiable grossly as an ovary or has been shown microscopically to contain Graafian follicles, corpora lutea, or corpora albicantia. However, the presence of rare primordial follicles or, especially as in the fetal ovary, aggregates of germ cells partially surrounded by immature granulosa cells are evidence that a streak gonad can differentiate toward ovary. Morphologic changes may occur over time in the streak gonads. Myriads of germ cells present in a streak of an infant may degenerate and disappear by puberty (Figure 2.50), resulting in a gonad composed exclusively of fibrous tissue and a few rete tubules.

Tumors develop in about 10% of patients with mixed gonadal dysgenesis.[104] The most common, the gonadoblastoma, is discussed in the following section. Approximately 30% of gonadoblastomas are overgrown by a malignant germ cell tumor, usually germinoma (Figures 2.51 and 2.52); 8% are overgrown by yolk sac tumor, immature teratoma, embryonal carcinoma, or choriocarcinoma. An occasional gonad may also show proliferative sex cord elements and resemble a Sertoli cell tumor[105] or disclose nodules suggestive of a juvenile granulosa cell tumor.[106] Although the gonadoblastoma itself does not metastasize and therefore can be considered as a precancer or an *in situ* malignancy, the typically malignant behavior of the other tumors makes early prophylactic removal of the gonads in all patients advisable. Also, to avoid the consequences of onset of virilization if the patient is to be raised as a female, it is important that gonadectomy be performed before the patient reaches puberty. Patients who have been treated with long-term administration of estrogen may on occasion develop endometrial carcinoma (Figure 2.53). Congenital cardiovascular anomalies have also been reported in patients with MGD.

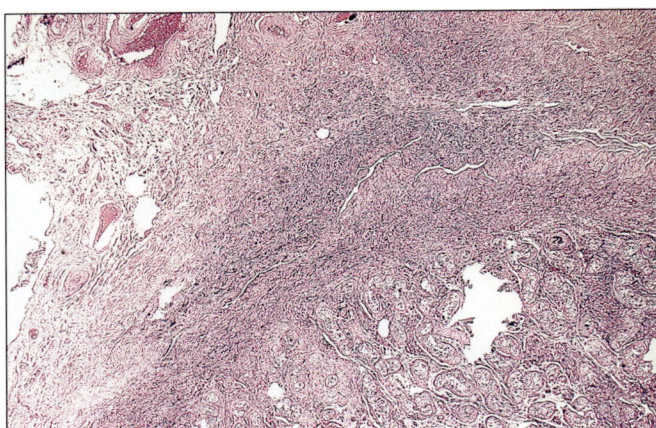

Figure 2.48 Cross section of tunica albuginea in mixed gonadal dysgenesis. The testicular stroma resembles the stroma of ovarian cortex. The medulla contains seminiferous tubules.

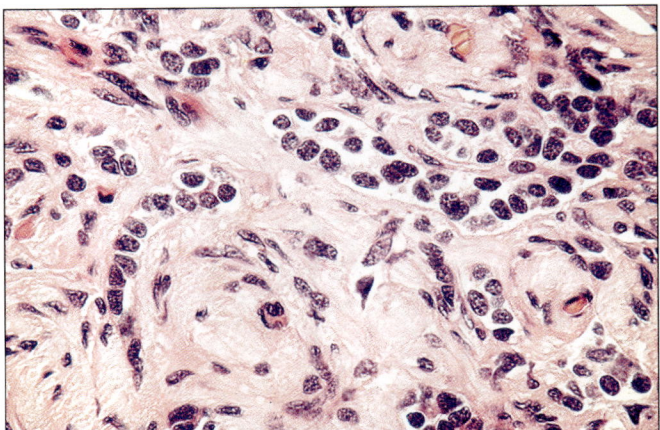

Figure 2.50 Changes over time in mixed gonadal dysgenesis. When the patient was an infant, this streak gonad resembled a fetal ovary with germ cells and immature sex cords or tubules. When the streak gonad was removed in entirety 13 years later, it existed only as several microscopic areas of wispy ovarian-type cortical stroma and rete ovarii.

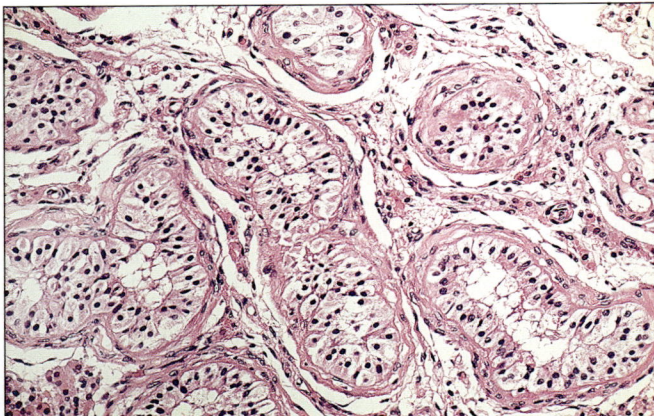

Figure 2.49 Seminiferous tubules lined only by Sertoli cells in mixed gonadal dysgenesis. The interstitium is filled with Leydig cells.

GONADOBLASTOMA

Gonadoblastoma is a precancerous or *in situ* form of germ cell cancer unique to patients with abnormal sexual development. It consists of malignant germ cells that are surrounded individually or in groups or by immature cells that are of sex cord derivation (immature Sertoli/granulosa-like cells). The tumor nearly always occurs in association with a whole or component of a 'Y' chromosome,[107] although cases are known that have arisen in tumors with a 46,XX karyotype and even where the patient has given birth.[108] Although most cases are detected in children or young adults, the tumor may develop prenatally.[109]

Clinical Features

Most gonadoblastomas occur in phenotypic females with abnormal gonads.[107] Some occur in phenotypic males, almost all of whom have cryptorchism or abnormal external or abnormal internal genitalia. Only the rare patient is a normal phenotypic male without apparent abnormal genitals.[110] Nearly all gonadoblastomas occur in patients with MGD. Gonadoblastoma accounts for three-fourths of the

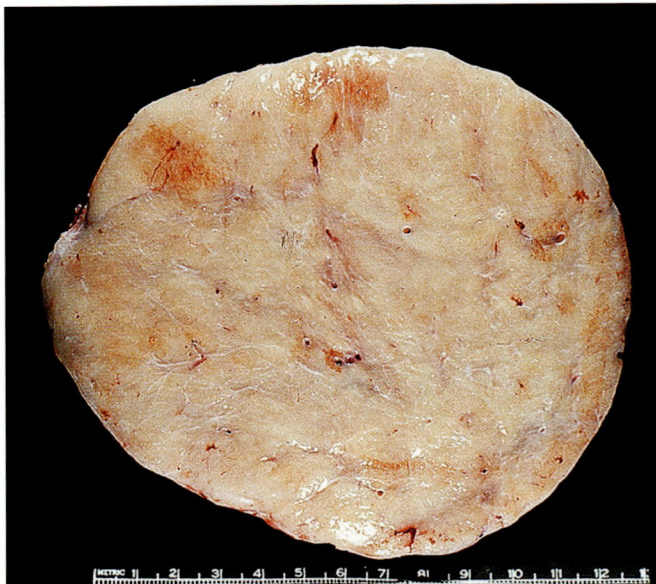

Figure 2.51 A 15 cm dysgerminoma in mixed gonadal dysgenesis arising from gonadoblastoma.

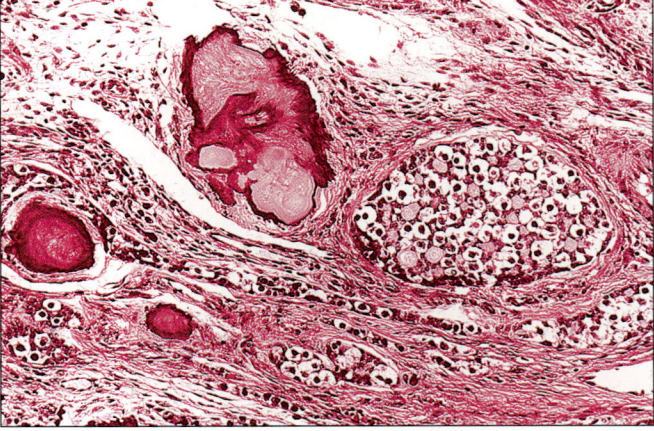

Figure 2.52 Gonadoblastoma with multifocal 'mulberry-like' calcifications.

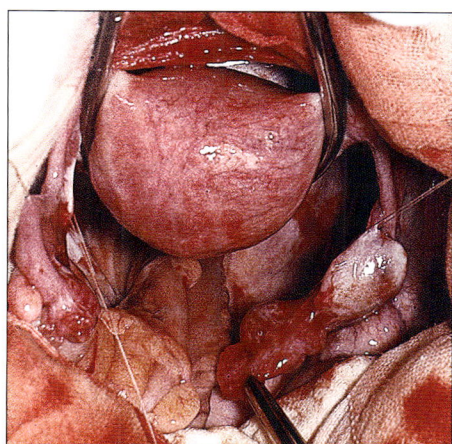

Figure 2.53 Mixed gonadal dysgenesis with ovary, streak gonads, and endometrial adenocarcinoma. The patient had been treated with long-term estrogen therapy.

gonadal tumors arising in dysgenetic gonads and is usually discovered during the first to fourth decades of life. Many of the isolated reports of gonadoblastoma associated with other forms of hermaphroditism described clinically and pathologically may in actuality be examples of MGD.

Genetic Changes

The role of the Y chromosome in the development of cancer is controversial. Since much of the Y chromosome (except for the pseudoautosomal regions at both ends of the chromosomes) neither pairs with nor recombines with the X chromosome during meiosis, it has been difficult to study this chromosome and identify its oncogenic genes and tumor suppressor genes. The gonadoblastoma Y gene locus (*GBY*) appears to be located on the short or long arm of the Y chromosome near the centromere. It may be that more than one gene is involved. Possibly the gonadoblastoma gene functions as an oncogene only in the dysgenetic gonad, and otherwise has a normal function in the normally developing testis. A multicopy gene, called *TSPY1* (testis specific protein Y1), which is an oncogene located in the GBY critical region, has emerged as the most likely GBY candidate.[111] This oncogene is expressed in spermatogonial cells in embryonic and adult testis, where there is some evidence it enhances protein synthesis and participates in control of cell division. Ectopic overexpression in dysgenetic gonads, and its continued overexpression in resultant tumors, is part of the evidence for its oncogenic potential. It has been postulated that inappropriate *TSPY1* expression accelerates cell cycle progression through competition with a related gene product from the X chromosome, *TSPX*.[112]

Pathology

The gross appearance of the gonad with gonadoblastoma (Figure 2.54) varies according to the size of the neoplasm, the presence of calcification (Figure 2.55), and whether the gonadoblastoma has been overgrown by a malignant form of germ cell tumor (usually germinoma). The immunoprofile of the tumor cells shows reactivity with placental alkaline phosphatase (PLAP), c-kit (Figure 2.56A), and FOXL2 (Figure 2.56B).[113] Most gonadoblastomas, if macroscopically

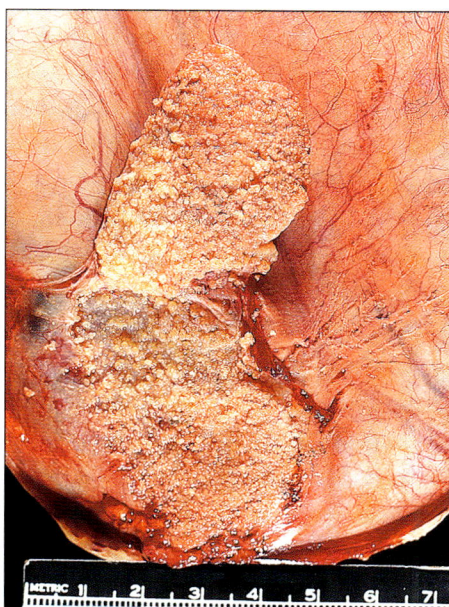

Figure 2.54 Calcified gonadoblastoma. The $5 \times 2 \times 0.5$ cm calcified focus was apparent radiographically.

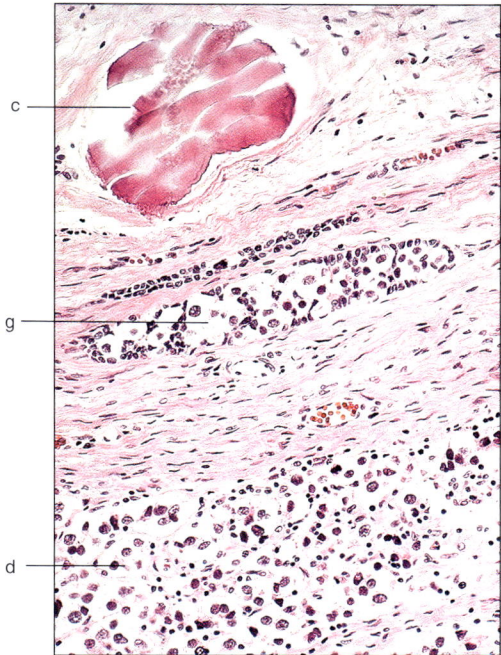

Figure 2.55 Gonadoblastoma with superimposed dysgerminoma. A small focus of calcification (c) lies adjacent to the gonadoblastoma (g) in which malignant germ cells are surrounded by immature granulosa/Sertoli cells. Adjacent is typical dysgerminoma (d), which by definition lacks surrounding sex cord supporting elements.

visible, are small. About 20% of gonadoblastomas arise in a streak gonad and another 20% arise in a dysgenetic testis. A very rare case is found with ovarian tissue or at least dysgenetic gonads with rare primordial follicles. In the remaining cases, the nature of the underlying gonad cannot be determined with certainty because tumor replaces it. About one-fifth of gonadoblastomas are discovered solely because

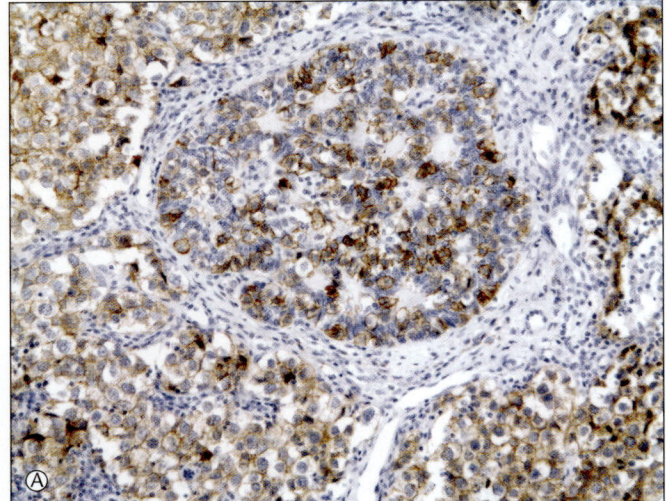

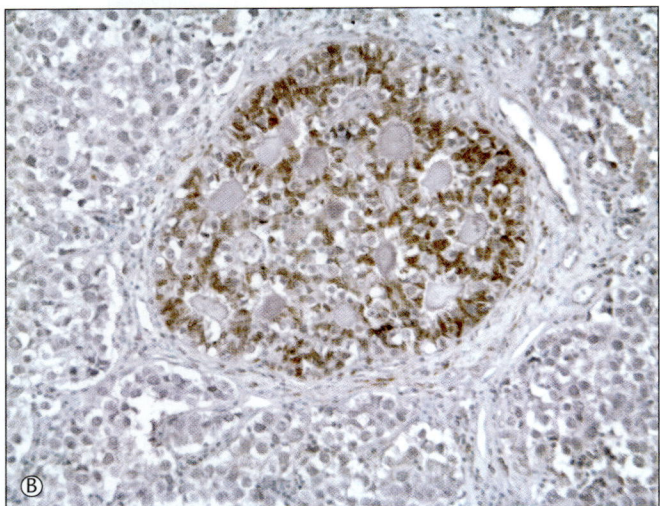

Figure 2.56 Gonadoblastoma showing reactivity with c-kit **(A)** and FOXL2 **(B)**.

a streak gonad was examined microscopically. The contralateral gonad also contains a gonadoblastoma in more than one-third of patients.

On microscopic examination, the gonadoblastoma appears as circumscribed nests of neoplastic germ cells having the cytologic properties of germinoma (dysgerminoma and seminoma) and are encompassed individually or in groups by sex cord derivatives with inconspicuous cytoplasm and small round to oval nuclei resembling immature Sertoli cells (Figures 2.55 and 2.57). The germ cells are of two forms, one of which is an immature small cell form with a high nuclear to cytoplasmic ratio resembling gonocytes/oogonia and believed to be the cell that can progress to dysgerminoma.[114] The small cell also gives rise to the larger and mature form of germ cells, which resemble prespermatogonia/oocytes and have copious amounts of light to clear cytoplasm, usually with a distinct cytoplasmic membrane. The mature large cell is not precancerous. Both types of germ cell have centrally placed nuclei in the cell and obvious macronucleoli that are one to several in number. Histologically, these precancerous germ cells resemble the carcinoma *in situ* germ cells often found in seminiferous tubules that are adjacent to seminomas that develop in genetically normal 46,XY men.

Hyaline, composed of basement membrane material, is found along the margin or as nodules within the nests of gonadoblastoma. In four-fifths of cases, the hyaline material is calcified, initially appearing as small, laminated spheres, which eventually fuse and coalesce into large mulberry-like masses (Figure 2.52). Not infrequently, the only evidence that a dysgerminoma originated in a gonadoblastoma is the presence focally of mulberry-like calcifications. Hormonally active cells that resemble lutein and Leydig cells are found interspersed among the nests of tumor in about two-thirds of cases. These hormonally active cells are found least frequently in non-virilized phenotypic females, more often in virilized females, and most frequently in phenotypic males. To some degree, their appearance may reflect the postpubertal age of the patient when the gonad is examined. Inhibin reactivity and AMH[115] are commonly demonstrable in the surrounding cells, which is in keeping with the sex cord cells (immature Sertoli/granulosa cells) as an integral part of the tumor.

XY FEMALE (SEX REVERSAL)

Steroidogenic factor 1 (*SF1*), coded by the *NR5A1* gene, is an orphan nuclear receptor (i.e., no identified natural ligand) that regulates the transcription of multiple genes implicated in reproduction, steroidogenesis, and male sexual differentiation, including *AMH*, *NR0B1* (*DAX1*), *CYP11A1*, STAR protein, and those encoding steroid hydroxylases, gonadotropins, and aromatase. Some of the heterozygous *SF1* mutations result in a spectrum of end-organ defects similar to that of androgen receptor mutations and were discussed earlier. In rare instances, mutation in *SF1* can lead to a testicular regression-like syndrome with 46,XY sex reversal but without adrenal insufficiency. One patient described had a eunuchoid habitus, no breast development and ambiguous genitalia with an enlarged clitoris, single perineal opening, and without palpable gonads (absence histologically confirmed).[116,117] The rarity of identifying this form of XY sex reversal has suggested that other genes participate in the sex determination cascade.

Deletion of *DMRT1* may cause sex reversal in the genetic XY male.[118] The gene, *DMRT1*, located at 9p24.3 and transcribed only in the embryonic gonads of both sexes and in fetal and adult testis, is required for postnatal differentiation of both somatic and germ cells in the mouse testis. One patient,[118] born with sexually ambiguous genitalia and *DMRT1* deletion, had gonads resembling that of a postnatal testis with normal müllerian regression and wolffian development. One of the two pelvic testes had a poorly developed albuginea. One-third of the gonad at one pole was maldeveloped with ill-defined, large trabeculae rich in abnormal-appearing germ cells. Another patient had no uterus, but a fallopian tube on the right and bilateral ovotestes.[119] The locus on 9p apparently maintains testis differentiation in the male rather than determining the primary sex, since the dysgenetic testes exhibit WT1, SRY, and AMH.

Several 46,XX females, including some of postpubertal age, with deletions at 9p or other abnormalities, showed normal ovarian development, suggesting that the 9p22–p24

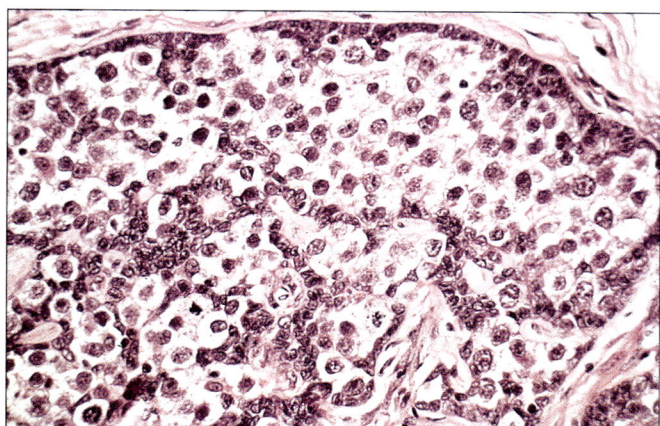

Figure 2.57 Gonadoblastoma with immature granulosa/Sertoli cells surrounding nests of tumor.

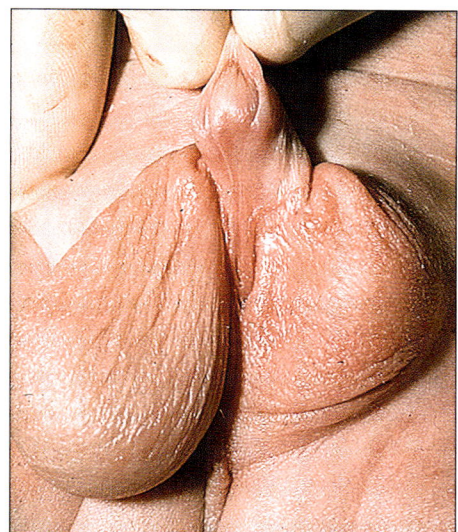

Figure 2.58 True hermaphroditism with bifid scrotum.

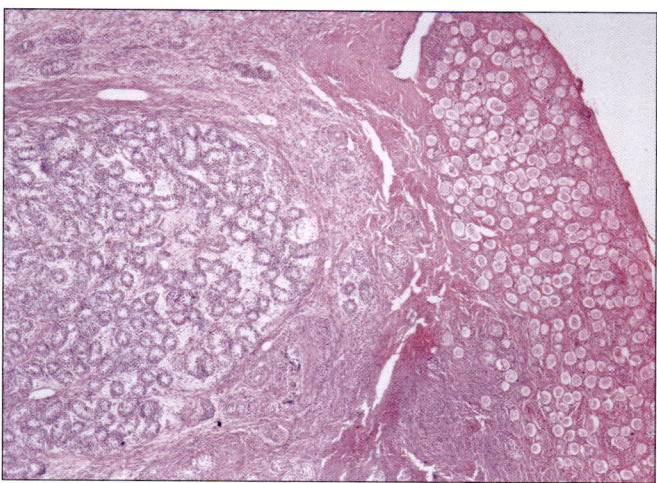

Figure 2.59 Ovotestis in true hermaphrodite. The gonad showed a zone of oocytes indicative of ovary (right), and a separate area of testicular seminiferous tubules (left).

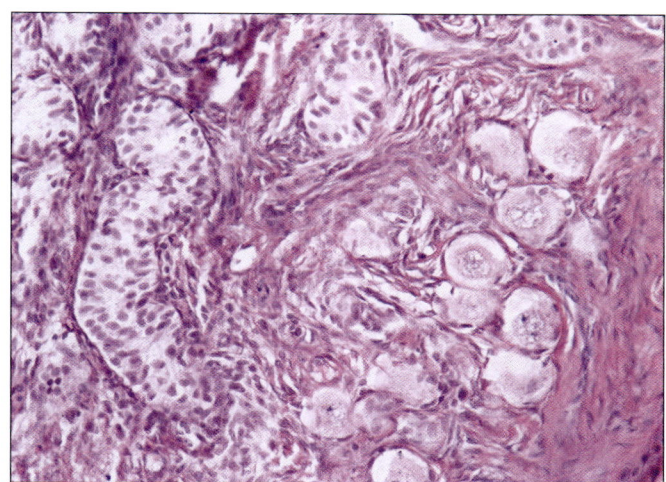

Figure 2.60 Ovotestis in a true hermaphrodite. Detail showing the interface between well-formed oocytes (right) and seminiferous tubules (left).

deletion does not contain a locus required for early ovarian differentiation.[118,119]

TRUE HERMAPHRODITISM

True hermaphroditism is defined as the presence of both testicular and ovarian tissue in a patient. Affected individuals may have either a female or a male phenotype with variable degrees of sexual ambiguity (Figure 2.58). Because the wavy, cortical-type stroma typically seen in the female gonad can be found in both female and male gonads and therefore is nonspecific, follicular structures must be identified to classify gonadal tissue as ovarian and seminiferous tubules to classify the tissue as testicular. In true hermaphrodites, the gonads may be ovary and testis separately or combined in an ovotestis.

True hermaphroditism is a rare condition in both North America and Europe,[120] but one of the more common etiologies of male sexual ambiguity.[4] It is, in contrast, common in Africa, especially in South Africa.[121] Clusters in other geographic locations are known,[122,123] some with data differing from the summary given below.

The ovotestis is the most frequently encountered type of gonad in true hermaphroditism (Figures 2.59 and 2.60).[124] In four-fifths of cases the ovarian and testicular tissues are arranged in an end-to-end fashion. The ovarian portion of an ovotestis has a convoluted surface while the testicular portion is smooth and glistening. Frequently, a distinct line demarcates the two tissues. The firm nature of the palpable ovarian tissue and the soft texture of the testis are valuable clinical signs when evaluating the nature of a gonad in an infant with ambisexual external genitalia. An ovary, which preferentially develops on the left side, is the second most common gonad in true hermaphrodites. Every patient over 15 years of age in one series had either a corpus luteum or a corpus albicans.[121] The testis, which is the gonad least often encountered, develops preferentially on the right.

The location of the gonad is influenced by the type and quantity of gonadal tissue present. Increasing amounts of ovarian tissue increase the probability that the gonad will be in an ovarian position. It is felt that this may be due to deficient or absent AMH, which is needed for the initial descent of the testis to occur. When a gonad with the macroscopic features of an ovary is situated in the inguinal canal or in the labioscrotal fold, the possibility of it being an ovotestis should be seriously considered. The position of the testis is less constant. Most (63%) reside in the scrotum, 14% in the inguinal region, 1% in the internal inguinal ring, and 22% in a normal ovarian position.

The nature of the genital structure adjacent to a gonad in true hermaphroditism depends upon the nature of the gonad, which is in contrast to mixed gonadal dysgenesis in which a fallopian tube is often adjacent to the gonad, regardless of whether it is a testis or a streak. In true hermaphroditism a fallopian tube is adjacent to an ovary and an epididymis or vas deferens is adjacent to a testis. Either a müllerian or wolffian structure, but not both, is adjacent to an ovotestis. AMH appears to be functional. Ninety-five percent of fallopian tubes adjacent to ovotestes have closed ostia. Only 10% of uteri are normal; the other patients have absent uteri (13%), unicornuate uteri (10%), absent cervix (14%), or uterine hypoplasia (46%).

The most common karyotypes in true hermaphroditism are 46,XX (60%), 46,XY (12%), and mosaic (28%), usually 46,XX/46,XY, 46,XY/47,XXY, or least frequently 45,X/46,XY. Patients with a Y chromosome have a two- to threefold increased frequency of having a testis as opposed to an ovotestis. Nearly 75% of true hermaphrodites with an ovary and an ovotestis have a 46,XX karyotype.

As in other disorders of intersex, genetic aberrations appear to play a key role in the development of true hermaphroditism. For example, Y chromosome-specific genes (e.g., *SRY*) have been detected in some 46,XX true hermaphrodites, suggesting one potential mechanism for the development of XX true hermaphroditism, similar to individuals with XX male syndrome.[120] In some series, *SRY* was undetected in the 46,XX patients,[123] indicating that other mechanisms may also be important. But such data must be read with care as other case reports identify examples where the patient may be 46,XX and lack the *SRY* gene in usual cells examined (leukocytes). Yet cells from the gonad itself demonstrate *SRY*.[125] Mutations that mimic the *SRY* gene have been suggested as one possibility where the *SRY* gene was absent.[126] One explanation proposed for patients with an XY chromosome constitution is the possibility that the *SRY* gene, if present, may act at a time too late to stimulate the development of a testis, hence permitting ovarian tissue to develop.

The clinical presentations of true hermaphrodites vary to some extent depending upon their ages at the time of diagnosis. Until recently, the condition often went undetected until adolescence when phenotypic male patients were evaluated for gynecomastia or for cysts in the testis and treated surgically, and phenotypic female patients were evaluated for amenorrhea or failure to develop secondary sex changes. Thus, in one series,[121] three-fourths of patients were raised as males and one-fourth as females. Many patients, however, menstruated and a few became pregnant. Phenotypic males may experience monthly hematuria because of menstruation into a persistent urogenital sinus. With an increased awareness of intersex states, the condition is recognized more often in infants because of ambiguous genitalia, usually in the form of a small phallus (enlarged clitoris).[120,122] Like MGD, the scrotum may be asymmetric, with the larger, more normal-appearing hemiscrotum containing a testis. Among 160 patients the external genitalia were asymmetric in three-fourths (labioscrotal folds in 63% and hemiscrota in 13%).

On microscopic examination, the gonadal tissue often appears normal if the patient is young. In infants, the ovarian tissue contains numerous follicles, whereas the testicular parenchyma discloses normal-appearing seminiferous tubules with spermatogonia. Patients in the reproductive years may have ovarian tissue with structures indicative of ovulation, e.g., follicles, corpora lutea, and corpora albicantia, but spermatogenesis is rare in the testicular portion. The testicular portion of an ovotestis is usually abnormal with incomplete development, loss of germ cells, and tubular sclerosis. Scrotal testes in these patients show less severe changes, sometimes showing faulty spermatogenesis.

At times, distinction between true hermaphroditism and MGD can be difficult, if not impossible. In the newborn, asymmetric ambiguous genitalia may be observed in both conditions. If a streak gonad from a patient with MGD is serially sectioned, a rare primordial follicle may be encountered in what otherwise appears to be a testis with well-developed seminiferous tubules. If the gonad is not removed, over time the gonad will progress to a streak gonad. If the term 'true hermaphroditism' is restricted to those patients in whom the ovarian and testicular tissue are both apparent grossly and the definition of an ovary requires development of at least the antral stage of follicular development, it should usually be possible to segregate more clearly those individuals in whom the ovarian tissue may be functional.

Gonadal tumors occur in less than 3% of affected individuals, and in one large series with long-term follow-up, not at all.[124] Germinoma is the most common type of tumor, but gonadoblastomas and a variety of other tumors have been reported.[127] One case has been reported where the primitive sex cord cellular elements adjacent to seminiferous tubules in a testis gave rise to cancer in the form of a juvenile granulosa cell tumor.[128]

REFERENCES

1. Biason-Lauber A. Control of sex development. Best Pract Res Clin Endocrinol Metab 2010;24:163–86.
2. Hughes IA, Morel Y, McElreavey K, Rogol A. Biological assessment of abnormal genitalia. J Pediatr Urol 2012;8:592–6.
3. Jaubert F, Nihoul-Fekete C, Lortat-Jacob S, et al. [Hermaphroditism pathology]. Ann Pathol 2004;24:499–509.
4. Morel Y, Rey R, Teinturier C, et al. Aetiological diagnosis of male sex ambiguity: a collaborative study. Eur J Pediatr 2002;161:49–59.
5. Robboy SJ, Jaubert F. Neoplasms and pathology of sexual developmental disorders (intersex). Pathology 2007;39:147–63.
6. Carlson AD, Obeid JS, Kanellopoulou N, et al. Congenital adrenal hyperplasia: update on prenatal diagnosis and treatment. J Steroid Biochem Mol Biol 1999;69:19–29.
7. New MI. Diagnosis and management of congenital adrenal hyperplasia. Annu Rev Med 1998;49:311–28.
8. Newfield RS, New MI. 21-hydroxylase deficiency. Ann N Y Acad Sci 1997;816:219–29.
9. Cerame BI, Newfield RS, Pascoe L, et al. Prenatal diagnosis and treatment of 11beta-hydroxylase deficiency congenital adrenal

hyperplasia resulting in normal female genitalia. J Clin Endocrinol Metab 1999;84:3129–34.
10. Ferrari P, Obeyesekere VR, Li K, et al. Point mutations abolish 11 beta-hydroxysteroid dehydrogenase type II activity in three families with the congenital syndrome of apparent mineralocorticoid excess. Mol Cell Endocrinol 1996;119:21–4.
11. Mendonca BB, Arnhold IJ, Bloise W, et al. 17Beta-hydroxysteroid dehydrogenase 3 deficiency in women. J Clin Endocrinol Metab 1999;84:802–4.
12. Moran C, Knochenhauer ES, Azziz R. Non-classic adrenal hyperplasia in hyperandrogenism: a reappraisal. J Endocrinol Invest 1998;21:707–20.
13. Rich MA, Keating MA, Levin HS, Kay R. Tumors of the adrenogenital syndrome: an aggressive conservative approach. J Urol 1998;160:1838–41.
14. Rutgers JL, Young RH, Scully RE. The testicular 'tumor' of the adrenogenital syndrome. A report of six cases and review of the literature on testicular masses in patients with adrenocortical disorders. Am J Surg Pathol 1988;12:503–13.
15. Jones ME, Boon WC, McInnes K, et al. Recognizing rare disorders: aromatase deficiency. Nat Clin Pract Endocrinol Metab 2007;3:414–21.
16. MacGillivray MH, Morishima A, Conte F, et al. Pediatric endocrinology update: an overview. The essential roles of estrogens in pubertal growth, epiphyseal fusion and bone turnover: lessons from mutations in the genes for aromatase and the estrogen receptor. Horm Res 1998;49(Suppl 1):2–8.
17. Fung MF, Vadas G, Lotocki R, et al. Tubular Krukenberg tumor in pregnancy with virilization. Gynecol Oncol 1991;41:81–4.
18. Vauthier-Brouzes D, Vanna Lim-You K, Sebagh E, et al. [Krukenberg tumor during pregnancy with maternal and fetal virilization: a difficult diagnosis. A case report]. J Gynecol Obstet Biol Reprod (Paris) 1997;26:831–3.
19. Vanslooten AJ, Rechner SF, Dodds WG. Recurrent maternal virilization during pregnancy caused by benign androgen-producing ovarian lesions. Am J Obstet Gynecol 1992;167:1342–3.
20. Spires SE, Woolums CS, Pulito AR, Spires SM. Testicular regression syndrome—a clinical and pathologic study of 11 cases. Arch Pathol Lab Med 2000;124:694–8.
21. Smith NM, Byard RW, Bourne AJ. Testicular regression syndrome—a pathological study of 77 cases. Histopathology 1991;19:269–72.
22. Arnhold IJ, Latronico AC, Batista MC, Mendonca BB. Menstrual disorders and infertility caused by inactivating mutations of the luteinizing hormone receptor gene. Fertil Steril 1999;71:597–601.
23. Bale PM, Howard NJ, Wright JE. Male pseudohermaphroditism in XY children with female phenotype. Pediatr Pathol 1992;12:29–49.
24. Opitz JM. RSH (so-called Smith-Lemli-Opitz) syndrome. Curr Opin Pediatr 1999;11:353–62.
25. Porter FD. Human malformation syndromes due to inborn errors of cholesterol synthesis. Curr Opin Pediatr 2003;15:607–13.
26. Bialer MG, Penchaszadeh VB, Kahn E, et al. Female external genitalia and mullerian duct derivatives in a 46,XY infant with the Smith-Lemli-Opitz syndrome. Am J Med Genet 1987;28:723–31.
27. Fukazawa R, Nakahori Y, Kogo T, et al. Normal Y sequences in Smith-Lemli-Opitz syndrome with total failure of masculinization. Acta Paediatr 1992;81:570–2.
28. Khoury K, Ducharme L, Lehoux JG. Family of two patients with congenital lipoid adrenal hyperplasia due to StAR mutation. Endocr Res 2004;30:925–9.
29. Caron KM, Soo SC, Wetsel WC, et al. Targeted disruption of the mouse gene encoding steroidogenic acute regulatory protein provides insights into congenital lipoid adrenal hyperplasia. Proc Natl Acad Sci U S A 1997;94:11540–5.
30. Korsch E, Peter M, Hiort O, et al. Gonadal histology with testicular carcinoma in situ in a 15-year-old 46,XY female patient with a premature termination in the steroidogenic acute regulatory protein causing congenital lipoid adrenal hyperplasia. J Clin Endocrinol Metab 1999;84:1628–32.
31. Mendonca BB, Inacio M, Arnhold IJP, et al. Male pseudohermaphroditism due to 17 beta-hydroxysteroid dehydrogenase 3 deficiency: Diagnosis, psychological evaluation, and management. Medicine 2000;79:299–309.
32. Zhu YS, Katz MD, Imperato-McGinley J. Natural potent androgens: lessons from human genetic models. Baillieres Clin Endocrinol Metab 1998;12:83–113.
33. Andersson S, Moghrabi N. Physiology and molecular genetics of 17 beta-hydroxysteroid dehydrogenases. Steroids 1997;62:143–7.
34. Buchholz NP, Biyabani R, Herzig MJ, et al. Persistent Mullerian duct syndrome. Eur Urol 1998;34:230–2.
35. Rizk DE, Ezimokhai M, Hussein AS, et al. Persistent mullerian duct syndrome. Arch Gynecol Obstet 1998;261:105–7.
36. Erk A, Ozeren S, Ozbay O, et al. Persistent mullerian duct syndrome. A case report. J Reprod Med 1999;44:135–8.
37. Belville C, Josso N, Picard JY. Persistence of Mullerian derivatives in males. Am J Med Genet 1999;89:218–23.
38. Josso N, Belville C, di CN, Picard JY. AMH and AMH receptor defects in persistent Mullerian duct syndrome. Hum Reprod Update 2005;11:351–6.
39. Shinmura Y, Yokoi T, Tsutsui Y. A case of clear cell adenocarcinoma of the mullerian duct in persistent mullerian duct syndrome: the first reported case. Am J Surg Pathol 2002;26:1231–4.
40. McPhaul MJ, Griffin JE. Male pseudohermaphroditism caused by mutations of the human androgen receptor. J Clin Endocrinol Metab 1999;84:3435–41.
41. Kohler B, Lumbroso S, Leger J, et al. Androgen insensitivity syndrome: somatic mosaicism of the androgen receptor in seven families and consequences for sex assignment and genetic counseling. J Clin Endocrinol Metab 2005;90:106–11.
42. Hughes IA, Davies JD, Bunch TI, et al. Androgen insensitivity syndrome. Lancet 2012;380:1419–28.
43. Kanayama H, Naroda T, Inoue Y, et al. A case of complete testicular feminization: laparoscopic orchiectomy and analysis of androgen receptor gene mutation. Int J Urol 1999;6:327–30.
44. Rutgers JL, Scully RE. The androgen insensitivity syndrome (testicular feminization): a clinicopathologic study of 43 cases. Int J Gynecol Pathol 1991;10:126–44.
45. Velidedeoglu HV, Coskunfirat OK, Bozdogan MN, et al. The surgical management of incomplete testicular feminization syndrome in three sisters. Br J Plast Surg 1997;50:212–16.
46. Regadera J, Martinez-Garcia F, Paniagua R, Nistal M. Androgen insensitivity syndrome: an immunohistochemical, ultrastructural, and morphometric study. Arch Pathol Lab Med 1999;123:225–34.
47. Hawkyard S, Poon P, Morgan DR. Sertoli tumour presenting with stress incontinence in a patient with testicular feminization. BJU Int 1999;84:382–3.
48. Iwamoto I, Yanazume S, Fujino T, et al. Leydig cell tumor in an elderly patient with complete androgen insensitivity syndrome. Gynecol Oncol 2005;96:870–2.
49. Manuel M, Katayama K, Jones H. The age of occurrence of gonadal tumors in intersex patients with a Y chromosome. Am J Obstet Gynecol 1976;124:293–300.
50. Hiort O, Sinnecker GH, Holterhus PM, et al. The clinical and molecular spectrum of androgen insensitivity syndromes. Am J Med Genet 1996;63:218–22.
51. Viner RM, Teoh Y, Williams DM, et al. Androgen insensitivity syndrome: a survey of diagnostic procedures and management in the UK. Arch Dis Child 1997;77:305–9.
52. Imperato-McGinley J. 5 alpha-reductase-2 deficiency. Curr Ther Endocrinol Metab 1997;6:384–7.
53. Al-Attia HM. Male pseudohermaphroditism due to 5 alpha-reductase-2 deficiency in an Arab kindred. Postgrad Med J 1997;73:802–7.
54. Skordis N, Patsalis PC, Bacopoulou I, et al. 5alpha-reductase 2 gene mutations in three unrelated patients of Greek Cypriot origin: identification of an ancestral founder effect. J Pediatr Endocrinol Metab 2005;18:241–6.
55. Sinnecker GH, Hiort O, Dibbelt L, et al. Phenotypic classification of male pseudohermaphroditism due to steroid 5 alpha-reductase 2 deficiency. Am J Med Genet 1996;63:223–30.
56. Lanfranco F, Kamischke A, Zitzmann M, Nieschlag E. Klinefelter's syndrome. Lancet 2004;364:273–83.
57. Hunter RHF. Abnormal sexual development in man. In: Hunter RHF, editor. Sex determination, differentiation and intersexuality in placental mammals. Cambridge: Cambridge University Press; 1995. p. 204–38.

58. Aksglaede L, Wikstrom AM, Rajpert-De ME, et al. Natural history of seminiferous tubule degeneration in Klinefelter syndrome. Hum Reprod Update 2006;12:39–48.
59. Aguirre D, Nieto K, Lazos M, et al. Extragonadal germ cell tumors are often associated with Klinefelter syndrome. Hum Pathol 2006;37:477–80.
60. Volkl TM, Langer T, Aigner T, et al. Klinefelter syndrome and mediastinal germ cell tumors. Am J Med Genet A 2006;140:471–81.
61. Matsuki S, Sasagawa I, Kakizaki H, et al. Testicular teratoma in a man with XX/XXY mosaic Klinefelter's syndrome. J Urol 1999;161:1573–4.
62. Okada H, Gotoh A, Takechi Y, Kamidono S. Leydig cell tumour of the testis associated with Klinefelter'tumor's syndrome by molecular analysis of the X chromosome in growth-retarded girls. J Clin Endocrinol Metab 1998;83:1472–6.
63. Keung YK, Buss D, Chauvenet A, Pettenati M. Hematologic malignancies and Klinefelter syndrome. a chance association? Cancer Genet Cytogenet 2002;139:9–13.
64. Devernay M, Bolca D, Kerdjana L, et al. Parental origin of the X-chromosome does not influence growth hormone treatment effect in Turner syndrome. J Clin Endocrinol Metab 2012;97:E1241–8.
65. Oliveira RM, Verreschi IT, Lipay MV, et al. Y chromosome in Turner syndrome: review of the literature. Sao Paulo Med J 2009;127:373–8.
66. Watanabe M, Zinn AR, Page DC, Nishimoto T. Functional equivalence of human X- and Y-encoded isoforms of ribosomal protein S4 consistent with a role in Turner syndrome. Nat Genet 1993;4:268–71.
67. Gicquel C, Gaston V, Cabrol S, Le BY. Assessment of Turner's syndrome by molecular analysis of the X chromosome in growth-retarded girls. J Clin Endocrinol Metab 1998;83:1472–6.
68. Hovatta O. Pregnancies in women with Turner's syndrome. Ann Med 1999;31:106–10.
69. Magee AC, Nevin NC, Armstrong MJ, et al. Ullrich-Turner syndrome: seven pregnancies in an apparent 45,X woman. Am J Med Genet 1998;75:1–3.
70. Foudila T, Soderstrom-Anttila V, Hovatta O. Turner's syndrome and pregnancies after oocyte donation. Hum Reprod 1999;14:532–5.
71. Chu C. Y-chromosome mosaicism in girls with Turner's syndrome. Ann Med 1999;31:106–10.
72. varez-Nava F, Soto M, Sanchez MA, et al. Molecular analysis in Turner syndrome. J Pediatr 2003;142:336–40.
73. Brant WO, Rajimwale A, Lovell MA, et al. Gonadoblastoma and Turner syndrome. J Urol 2006;175:1858–60.
74. Mendes JR, Strufaldi MW, Delcelo R, et al. Y-chromosome identification by PCR and gonadal histopathology in Turner's syndrome without overt Y-mosaicism. Clin Endocrinol (Oxf) 1999;50:19–26.
75. Kocova M, Basheska N, Papazovska A, et al. Girls with Turner's syndrome. Ann Med 1999;31:106–10.
76. Tateno T, Sasagawa I, Ashida J, Nakada T. Deletion of Y chromosome involving the DAZ (deleted in azoospermia) gene in XX males. Arch Androl 1999;42:179–83.
77. Ginsberg NA, Cadkin A, Strom C, et al. Prenatal diagnosis of 46,XX male fetuses. Am J Obstet Gynecol 1999;180:1006–7.
78. Kolon TF, Ferrer FA, McKenna PH. Clinical and molecular analysis of XX sex reversed patients. J Urol 1998;160:1169–72.
79. Meyers CM, Boughman JA, Rivas M, et al. Gonadal (ovarian) dysgenesis in 46,XX individuals: frequency of the autosomal recessive form. Am J Med Genet 1996;63:518–24.
80. Dardis A, Saraco N, Mendilaharzu H, et al. Report of an XX male with hypospadias and pubertal gynecomastia, SRY gene negative in blood leukocytes but SRY gene positive in testicular cells. Horm Res 1997;47:85–8.
81. Bilbao JR, Loridan L, Castano L. A novel postzygotic nonsense mutation in SRY in familial XY gonadal dysgenesis. Hum Genet 1996;97:537–9.
82. Rutgers JL. Advances in the pathology of intersex conditions. Hum Pathol 1991;22:884–91.
83. Scherer G, Held M, Erdel M, et al. Three novel SRY mutations in XY gonadal dysgenesis and the enigma of XY gonadal dysgenesis cases without SRY mutations. Cytogenet Cell Genet 1998;80:188–92.
84. Tsutsumi O, Iida T, Nakahori Y, Taketani Y. Analysis of the testis-determining gene SRY in patients with XY gonadal dysgenesis. Horm Res 1996;46(Suppl 1):6–10.
85. Uehara S, Funato T, Yaegashi N, et al. SRY mutation and tumor formation on the gonads of XP pure gonadal dysgenesis patients. Cancer Genet Cytogenet 1999;113:78–84.
86. Vilain E, Jaubert F, Fellous M, McElreavey K. Pathology of 46,XY pure gonadal dysgenesis: absence of testis differentiation associated with mutations in the testis-determining factor. Differentiation 1993;52:151–9.
87. Lam SK, Yu MY, To KF, et al. Ovarian epithelial tumour in gonadal dysgenesis. A case report and literature review. Aust N Z J Obstet Gynaecol 1996;36:106–9.
88. Morimura Y, Nishiyama H, Yanagida K, Sato A. Dysgerminoma with syncytiotrophoblastic giant cells arising from 46,XX pure gonadal dysgenesis. Obstet Gynecol 1998;92:654–6.
89. Radakovic B, Jukic S, Bukovic D, et al. Morphology of gonads in pure XY gonadal dysgenesis. Coll Antropol 1999;23:203–211.
90. Barbosa AS, Hadjiathanasiou CG, Theodoridis C, et al. The same mutation affecting the splicing of WT1 gene is present on Frasier syndrome patients with or without Wilms' tumor. Hum Mutat 1999;13:146–53.
91. Jaubert F, Vasiliu V, Patey-Mariaud de SN, et al. Gonad development in Drash and Frasier syndromes depends on WT1 mutations. Arkh Patol 2003;65:40–4.
92. Auber F, Lortat-Jacob S, Sarnacki S, et al. Surgical management and genotype/phenotype correlations in WT1 gene-related diseases (Drash, Frasier syndromes). J Pediatr Surg 2003;38:124–9.
93. Saxena AK, van TC, Schultze-Everding A. Frasier syndrome in a pre-menarchal girl: laparoscopic resection of gonadoblastoma. Eur J Pediatr 2006;165:917–19.
94. Wang NJ, Song HR, Schanen NC, et al. Frasier syndrome comes full circle: genetic studies performed in an original patient. J Pediatr 2005;146:843–4.
95. Bonte A, Schroder W, Denamur E, Querfeld U. Absent pubertal development in a child with chronic renal failure: the case of Frasier syndrome. Nephrol Dial Transplant 2000;15:1688–90.
96. de Nanclares GP, Castano L, Bilbao JR, et al. Molecular analysis of Frasier syndrome: mutation in the WT1 gene in a girl with gonadal dysgenesis and nephronophthisis. J Pediatr Endocrinol Metab 2002;15:1047–50.
97. Niaudet P, Gubler MC. WT1 and glomerular diseases. Pediatr Nephrol 2006;21:1653–60.
98. Alvarez-Nava F, Gonzalez S, Soto S, et al. Mixed gonadal dysgenesis: a syndrome of broad clinical, cytogenetic and histopathologic spectrum. Genet Couns 1999;10:233–43.
99. Bidarkar SS, Hutson JM. Evaluation and management of the abnormal gonad. Semin Pediatr Surg 2005;14:118–23.
100. Alvarez-Nava F, Martinez MC, Gonzalez S, et al. FISH and PCR analysis of the presence of Y-chromosome sequences in a patient with Xq-isochromosome and testicular tissue. Clin Genet 1999;55:356–61.
101. Telvi L, Lebbar A, Del PO, et al. 45,X/46,XY mosaicism: report of 27 cases. Pediatrics 1999;104:304–8.
102. Gibbons B, Tan SY, Yu CC, et al. Risk of gonadoblastoma in female patients with Y chromosome abnormalities and dysgenetic gonads. J Paediatr Child Health 1999;35:210–13.
103. Mendez JP, Ulloa-Aguirre A, Kofman-Alfaro S, et al. Mixed gonadal dysgenesis: clinical, cytogenetic, endocrinological, and histopathological findings in 16 patients. Am J Med Genet 1993;46:263–7.
104. Robboy SJ, Miller T, Donahoe PK, et al. Dysgenesis of testicular and streak gonads in the syndrome of mixed gonadal dysgenesis: perspective derived from a clinicopathologic analysis of twenty-one cases. Hum Pathol 1982;13:700–16.
105. Nomura K, Matsui T, Aizawa S. Gonadoblastoma with proliferation resembling Sertoli cell tumor. Int J Gynecol Pathol 1999;18:91–3.
106. Pena-Alonso R, Nieto K, Alvarez R, et al. Distribution of Y-chromosome-bearing cells in gonadoblastoma and dysgenetic testis in 45,X/46,XY infants. Mod Pathol 2005;18:439–45.
107. Scully RE, Young RH, Clement RB. Tumors of the ovary, maldeveloped gonads, fallopian tube, and broad ligament. 3rd ed. Washington, DC: Armed Forces Institute of Pathology; 1998.
108. Zhao S, Kato N, Endoh Y, et al. Ovarian gonadoblastoma with mixed germ cell tumor in a woman with 46, XX karyotype and successful pregnancies. Pathol Int 2000;50:332–5.

109. Jorgensen N, Muller J, Jaubert F, et al. Heterogeneity of gonadoblastoma germ cells: similarities with immature germ cells, spermatogonia and testicular carcinoma in situ cells. Histopathology 1997;30:177–86.
110. Hatano T, Yoshino Y, Kawashima Y, et al. Case of gonadoblastoma in a 9-year-old boy without physical abnormalities. Int J Urol 1999;6:164–6.
111. Lau YF, Li Y, Kido T. Gonadoblastoma locus and the TSPY gene on the human Y chromosome. Birth Defects Res C Embryo Today 2009;87:114–22.
112. Lau YF, Li Y, Kido T. Gonadoblastoma locus and the TSPY gene on the human Y chromosome. Birth Defects Res C Embryo Today 2009;87:114–22.
113. Hersmus R, Kalfa N, de LB, et al. FOXL2 and SOX9 as parameters of female and male gonadal differentiation in patients with various forms of disorders of sex development (DSD). J Pathol 2008;215:31–8.
114. Kersemaekers AM, Honecker F, Stoop H, et al. Identification of germ cells at risk for neoplastic transformation in gonadoblastoma: an immunohistochemical study for OCT3/4 and TSPY. Hum Pathol 2005;36:512–21.
115. Rey R, Sabourin JC, Venara M, et al. Anti-Mullerian hormone is a specific marker of Sertoli- and granulosa-cell origin in gonadal tumors. Hum Pathol 2000;31:1202–8.
116. Correa RV, Domenice S, Bingham NC, et al. A microdeletion in the ligand binding domain of human steroidogenic factor 1 causes XY sex reversal without adrenal insufficiency. J Clin Endocrinol Metab 2004;89:1767–72.
117. Domenice S, Correa RV, Costa EM, et al. Mutations in the SRY, DAX1, SF1 and WNT4 genes in Brazilian sex-reversed patients. Braz J Med Biol Res 2004;37:145–50.
118. Vialard F, Ottolenghi C, Gonzales M, et al. Deletion of 9p associated with gonadal dysfunction in 46,XY but not in 46,XX human fetuses. J Med Genet 2002;39:514–18.
119. Ounap K, Uibo O, Zordania R, et al. Three patients with 9p deletions including DMRT1 and DMRT2: a girl with XY complement, bilateral ovotestes, and extreme growth retardation, and two XX females with normal pubertal development. Am J Med Genet A 2004;130A:415–23.
120. Hadjiathanasiou CG, Brauner R, Lortat-Jacob S, et al. True hermaphroditism: genetic variants and clinical management. J Pediatr 1994;125:738–44.
121. van Niekerk WA, Retief AE. The gonads of human true hermaphrodites. Hum Genet 1981;58:117–22.
122. Damiani D, Fellous M, McElreavey K, et al. True hermaphroditism: clinical aspects and molecular studies in 16 cases. Eur J Endocrinol 1997;136:201–4.
123. Guerra JG, De Mello MP, Assumpcao JG, et al. True hermaphrodites in the southeastern region of Brazil: a different cytogenetic and gonadal profile. J Pediatr Endocrinol Metab 1998;11:519–24.
124. Verkauskas G, Jaubert F, Lortat-Jacob S, et al. The long-term followup of 33 cases of true hermaphroditism: a 40-year experience with conservative gonadal surgery. J Urol 2007;177:726–31.
125. Jimenez AL, Kofman-Alfaro S, Berumen J, et al. Partially deleted SRY gene confined to testicular tissue in a 46,XX true hermaphrodite without SRY in leukocytic DNA. Am J Med Genet 2000;93:417–20.
126. Slaney SF, Chalmers IJ, Affara NA, Chitty LS. An autosomal or X linked mutation results in true hermaphrodites and 46,XX males in the same family. J Med Genet 1998;35:17–22.
127. Talerman A, Verp MS, Senekjian E, et al. True hermaphrodite with bilateral ovotestes, bilateral gonadoblastomas and dysgerminomas, 46,XX/46,XY karyotype, and a successful pregnancy. Cancer 1990;66:2668–72.
128. Tanaka Y, Sasaki Y, Tachibana K, et al. Testicular juvenile granulosa cell tumor in an infant with X/XY mosaicism clinically diagnosed as true hermaphroditism. Am J Surg Pathol 1994;18:316–22.

3 Vulvar Dermatoses and Infections

M. Angelica Selim, Mai P. Hoang, Bruce R. Smoller, Christopher R. Shea

CHAPTER OUTLINE

Introduction	48
Common Dermatoses Affecting the Vulva	49
Spongiotic Dermatitis (Eczemas)	49
Chronic Dermatitides	54
Psoriasis	54
Less Common Dermatoses that Frequently Involve the Vulva	55
Lichenoid Dermatoses	55
Bullous Disorders	58
Inherited Dermatoses	61
Other Inflammatory Diseases Affecting the Vulva	63
Plasma Cell Vulvitis (Vulvitis of Zoon)	63
Erythema Multiforme and Stevens–Johnson Syndrome	63
Behçet Disease	63
Crohn Disease	64
Hidradenitis Suppurativa	64
Vulvar Pain Syndromes	65
Vulvar Vestibulitis	65
Dysesthetic Vulvodynia	65
Pigmentary Alterations	65
Hyperpigmentation	65
Hypopigmentation	66
Drugs	66
Fixed Drug Eruptions (Dermatitis Medicamentosa)	66
Vulvar Infections and Infestations	67
Bacterial Infections	67
Fungal Infections	69
Viral Infections	70
Other Virus Infections	71
Protozoal Infections	73
Infestations	73
Glossary of Common Clinical Dermatologic Terms	74
Glossary of Common Dermatopathologic Terms	75
Terms Applied to the Surface Keratin Layer	75
Terms Applied to the Epidermis	75
Terms Applied to the Dermis	76

INTRODUCTION

The most common diseases affecting the vulva are dermatologic,[1–7] but the clinicians caring for patients with these complaints are usually gynecologists or family practitioners who may lack sophisticated diagnostic and therapeutic skills in skin diseases. Conversely, dermatologists may have interest and expertise in a subset of diseases in this organ. In summary, no single specialist is generally well trained to care for the full spectrum of vulvar diseases. Multidisciplinary clinics, to which different specialists bring their expertise, are often the best forum to efficiently diagnose and treat acute or chronic vulvar diseases.[8,9]

In response to the complexity of vulvar disorders, the International Society for the Study of Vulvovaginal Disease (ISVVD) was founded with one objective: to facilitate clear communication between clinicians and pathologists caring for patients with neoplastic and non-neoplastic vulvar diseases. Accordingly, it discarded its 1987 classification, replacing it in 2006 (Table 3.1) with an entirely different classification based on histopathology.[10,11] And in 2011, a

Table 3.1 2006 ISSVD Classification of Vulvar Dermatoses:[10,11] Pathologic Subsets and Their Clinical Correlates

Spongiotic pattern
    Atopic dermatitis
    Allergic contact dermatitis
    Irritant contact dermatitis
Acanthotic pattern (formerly squamous cell hyperplasia)
    Psoriasis
    Lichen simplex chronicus
    Primary (idiopathic)
    Secondary (superimposed on lichen sclerosus, lichen planus or other vulvar disease)
Lichenoid pattern
    Lichen sclerosus
    Lichen planus
Dermal homogenization/sclerosis pattern
    Lichen sclerosus
Vesiculobullous pattern
    Pemphigoid, cicatricial type
    Linear IgA disease
Acantholytic pattern
    Hailey–Hailey disease
    Darier disease
    Papular genitocrural acantholysis
Granulomatous pattern
    Crohn disease
    Melkersson–Rosenthal syndrome
Vasculopathic pattern
    Aphthous ulcers
    Beçhet disease
    Plasma cell vulvitis

new clinical based classification of inflammatory vulvar diseases was published to assist the clinician to reach a diagnosis based only on clinical findings (see glossaries at the end of this chapter). Currently, the ISSVD considers both classifications as complementary of each other.

This chapter utilizes a multidisciplinary approach. The diseases are organized in order of frequency and classified with a clinical perspective using the type of lesion (patch, papule, nodule, etc.) and the symptoms produced (itch, etc.), combined with the histopathologic pattern of inflammation (Figure 3.1). Both vulvar and extravulvar manifestations are covered. Not uncommonly, the latter features are the key to a correct diagnosis.

The brief glossary of clinical dermatological terms at the end of this chapter defines some of the more commonly used terms in dermatology and dermatopathology. To further enhance this chapter, the common dermatopathologic terms used are also defined in a separate glossary divided into terms that apply to the three main layers: the surface keratin layer, the epidermis, and the dermis.

COMMON DERMATOSES AFFECTING THE VULVA

SPONGIOTIC DERMATITIS (ECZEMAS)

Eczema or spongiotic dermatitis encompasses a variety of diseases with *spongiosis* as a common histologic finding at some stage. The spongiotic tissue reaction shows intracellular and intercellular edema leading to expanded spaces among keratinocytes. Eczema is the leading cause of chronic genital itching. All forms of endogenous and exogenous spongiotic dermatitis can affect the vulva, where they may present acutely or chronically. The location, pattern, and extent of the lesions help to define the different types of eczemas.

GENERAL CLINICAL AND PATHOLOGIC FEATURES OF SPONGIOTIC DERMATITIS

Acute Spongiotic Dermatitis. The term 'eczema' derives from the Greek *ekzein* 'to boil over,' reflecting the clinical appearance of acute lesions. Clinically, it exhibits erythematous macules, papules, and plaques (Figure 3.2). With increasing degrees of spongiosis, lesions become vesicular or bullous and begin to weep or to ooze. The vesicles frequently progress to rupture, and their contents dry to form a surface crust. In the biopsy specimen the epidermis shows a variable amount of spongiosis, hyperkeratosis and parakeratosis, and exocytosis of inflammatory cells. If the spongiosis is considerable, the fluid will collect in intraepidermal vesicles that may contain lymphocytes, neutrophils, eosinophils, and Langerhans cells. Mild papillary dermal edema leading to separation of collagen fibers can be seen in association with telangiectatic vessels. The superficial vascular plexus shows a perivascular mixed inflammatory infiltrate consisting of lymphocytes, neutrophils, and eosinophils. This basic pattern of acute spongiotic dermatitis is altered by scratching or superimposed infections (impetiginization). The former produces excoriations or lichen simplex chronicus (see the following section); the latter is associated with neutrophils in the stratum corneum. Acute inflammation in the stratum corneum should prompt the pathologist to request special stains for bacterial (Brown–Brenn) and fungal (periodic acid–Schiff, PAS, and Gomori methenamine silver, GMS) forms.

Chronic Spongiotic Dermatitis. Clinically the skin exhibits a leathery appearance with accentuation of skin markings (*lichenification*). The skin also changes from red (characteristic of acute spongiotic dermatitis) to brown or hyperpigmented, particularly in racially dark individuals. Scratching from intense pruritus produces excoriations where the surface has been traumatized. Histologically there is variable hyperplasia of the epidermis (acanthosis) with overlying hyperkeratosis and parakeratosis. The elongated rete ridges are separated by a papillary dermis with prominent capillaries and thick collagen fibers arranged perpendicular to the surface. Lymphocytes predominantly are found around upper dermal vessels. In certain biopsy specimens, in the previously described background of chronic dermatitis, there are features associated with acute inflammation, specifically a notable degree of spongiosis. This coexistence of acute and chronic histologic findings is called *subacute spongiotic dermatitis* (Figure 3.3).

CLINICAL PATTERNS OF VULVAR SPONGIOTIC DERMATITIS

Endogenous Vulvar Spongiotic Dermatitis. The two most common endogenous dermatitides are *atopic dermatitis* and

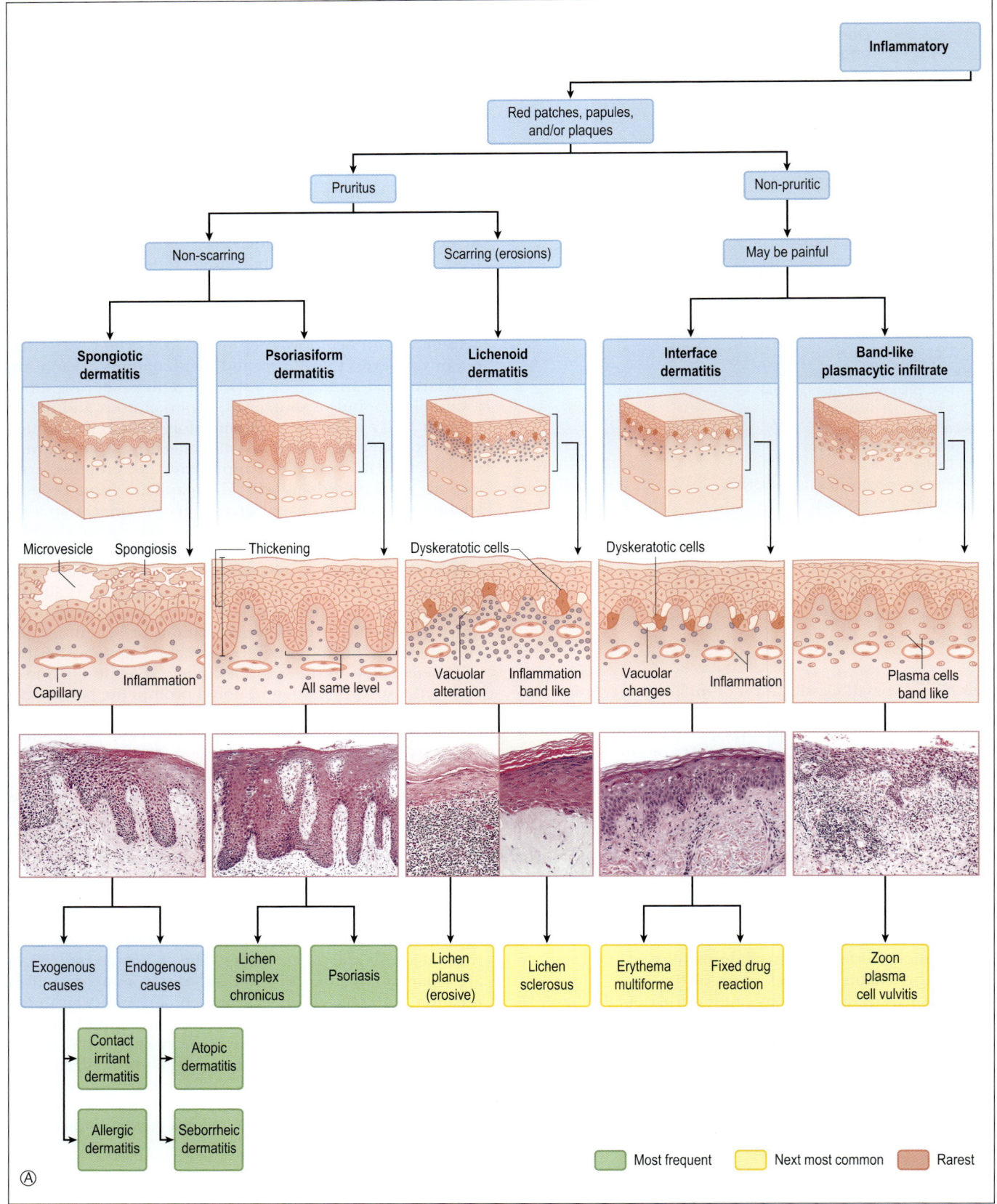

Figure 3.1 Differential diagnoses of vulvar dermatoses. **(A)** Noninfectious inflammatory conditions.

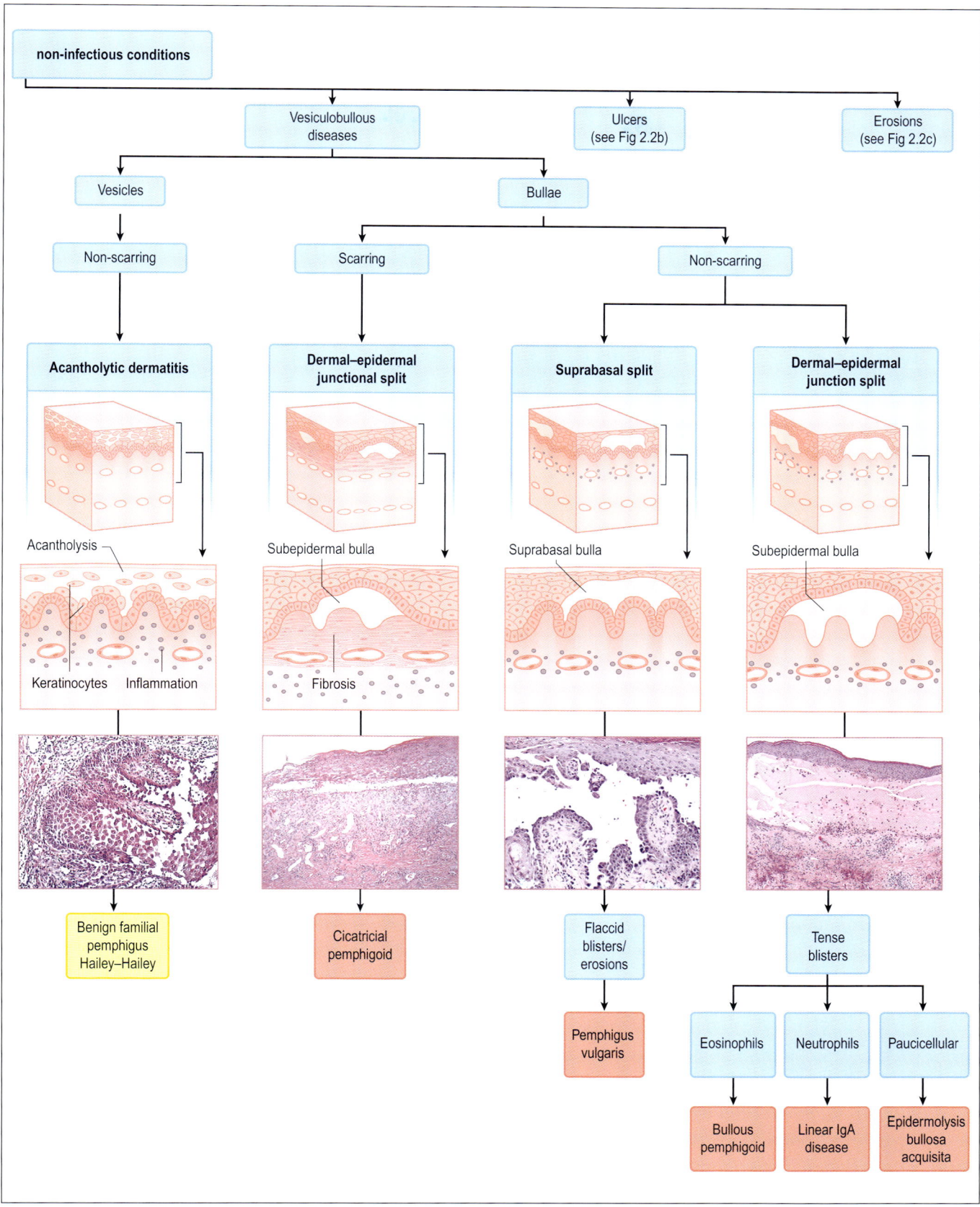

Figure 3.1 Continued.

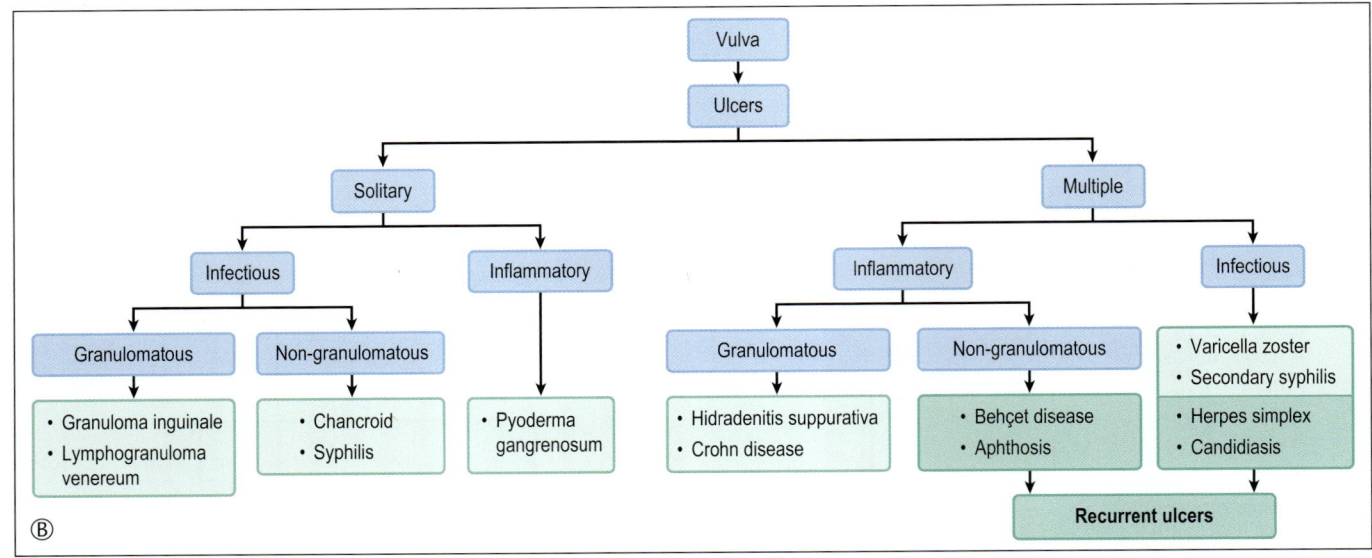

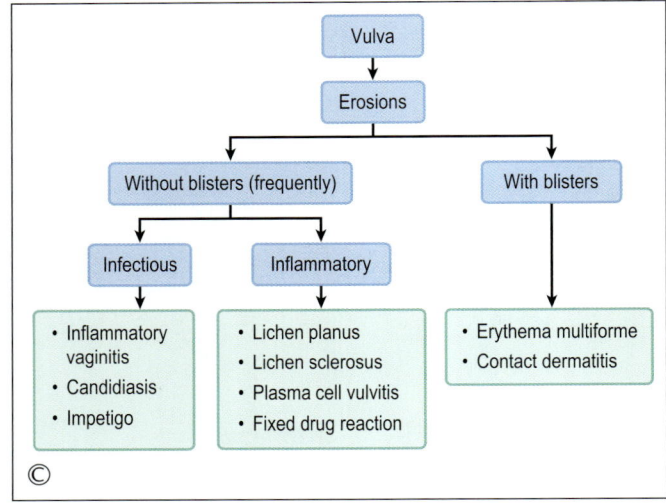

Figure 3.1 Continued. (B) Ulcers. (C) Erosions.

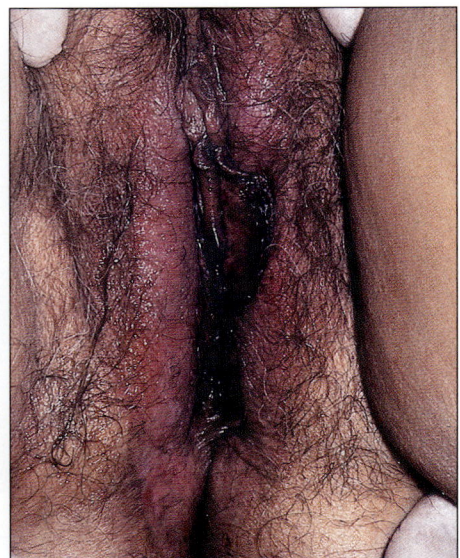

Figure 3.2 Vulvar acute dermatitis (eczema). Erythema and edema are present, with linear excoriations due to scratching.

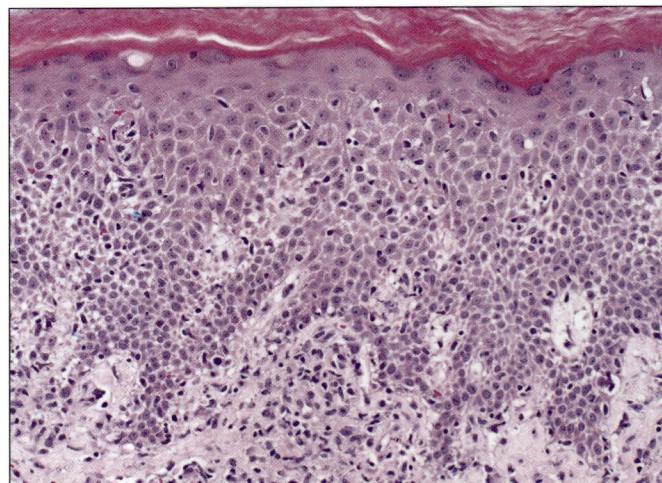

Figure 3.3 Subacute vulvar dermatitis. The epidermis shows both active focal spongiosis (acute dermatitis changs) and rete ridge elongation with collagenization in dermal papillae (chronic dermatitis change).

seborrheic dermatitis. Both diseases can show the entire spectrum of eczematous lesions ranging from erythematous scaly areas to oozing to vesicle formation, ending in lichenification. Few physicians see the acute phase. Most patients seek medical attention only during the subacute to chronic phase. Commonly, the correct diagnosis depends on identifying more distinctive extragenital lesions.

Atopic Dermatitis is a chronic, pruritic inflammation of the skin that affects individuals with personal or family history of atopic diathesis (atopic eczema, asthma, allergic seasonal rhinitis). Among the major diagnostic criteria are the presence of pruritus, chronicity, history of atopy, and lesions with typical morphology such as flexural distribution. Although the etiology and pathogenesis are still unknown, IgE-mediated late phase responses, cytokine imbalances, and cell-mediated reactions may all play important roles. Genetic factors also appear to be involved. One candidate gene is located on chromosome 11q13.5 (note that the gene for the β-subunit of the FCγRI, the high-affinity receptor for IgE, is localized to chromosome 11q12–13). Another gene implicated in the pathogenesis of this disease is on chromosome 16q11–p13 (associated with the *IL4R* gene).

Patients with atopic dermatitis experience pruritus rather than soreness or irritation when suffering from inflamed skin. The rubbing and scratching in turn stimulate and perpetuate the itch in an 'itch–scratch cycle.' Adult women are prone to experience genital eczema in the form of red to hyperpigmented areas, often with subtle changes of excoriation and scale due to the moisture of the area. Biopsies are rarely necessary. The diagnosis is confirmed by the excellent response to therapy, mainly corticosteroid medications.

Seborrheic Dermatitis is a chronic and recurrent dermatitis that manifests as minimally symptomatic, thin, reddish plaques with greasy yellowish scale involving areas of increased sebum production. Genital lesions frequently occur in association with lesions localized in seborrheic areas with skinfold involvement, especially axillae. *Malassezia furfur*, the causative organism of pityriasis versicolor, may play a role in seborrheic dermatitis by inducing an allergic reaction. Seborrheic dermatitis of the external genitalia is prominent in the skinfolds. It affects the hair-bearing skin of the labia majora and perineum. The diagnosis is reached by identifying red scaling plaques on the scalp, central face, and skinfolds, and the absence of *Candida* in cultures of skin scrapings. Similar to atopic dermatitis, the response to therapy confirms the diagnosis.

Exogenous Vulvar Spongiotic Dermatitis. The two most common forms of spongiotic dermatitis with an exogenous cause are irritant contact dermatitis and allergic contact dermatitis.[12–16] The acute clinical presentations of allergic and irritant contact dermatitis have significant overlap and with time both evolve to lichen simplex chronicus.

Irritant Contact Dermatitis occurs when damage to the cutaneous barrier function exceeds the skin's repair mechanisms.[12–14] This dermatitis is an inflammatory reaction to direct toxic effects of a chemical, physical, or mechanical agent. Irritants may remove surface lipids and water-holding substances, damage cell membranes, denature keratins, exert direct cytotoxic effects, liberate cytokines,

Table 3.2 Common Causes of Vulvar Contact Irritant Dermatitis

Water (overwashing)
Soap (overwashing)
Detergents in shower gels and bubble baths
Antiseptic lotions, creams, etc.
Wet-wipes
Deodorant sprays
Cosmetic constituents such as perfumes or preservatives

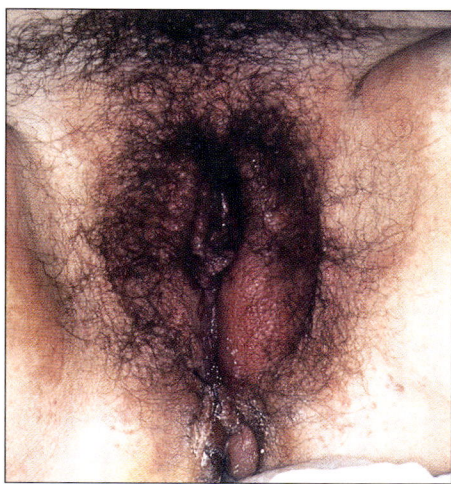

Figure 3.4 Acute contact dermatitis to chlorhexidine. Edema and erythema are present in areas where the antiseptic chlorhexidine solution was applied during an episiotomy.

etc. Vulvar tissue structure, hydration, occlusion, and friction may increase its propensity to inflammation.[17] Irritant contact dermatitis of the vulva occurs most commonly in the form of diaper dermatitis due to urine; this can also occur in adult women experiencing stress incontinence. The most common contact irritants causing vulvar dermatitis are listed in Table 3.2. Contact irritant dermatitis clinically presents with sharply demarcated, erythematous papules and plaques that may be weeping (Figures 3.3 and 3.4) and eroded if acute, or lichenified in chronic cases (see the section Lichen simplex chronicus).[18] The diagnosis is confirmed when the culprit is eliminated and the rash disappears.

Allergic Contact Dermatitis is a cell-mediated type IV delayed hypersensitivity reaction.[12,16] The rash develops 48–72 hours after exposure to the allergen. After sensitization, the patient develops allergic contact dermatitis upon each subsequent exposure. Although one exposure may be sufficient to develop the initial dermatitis, most frequently clinical reactivity becomes manifest only after repetitive exposures. The dermatitis lasts for about 2–3 weeks. As a general rule, infants under five and elderly persons are less liable to develop allergic contact dermatitis as their immune systems tend not to develop type IV hypersensitivity reactions to antigens. If episodes are continuous, a patch test

> **Table 3.3 Common Agents Causing Vulvar Contact Allergic Dermatitis**
>
> Perfumes
> Preservatives in creams
> Topical local anesthetics (such as benzocaine)
> Topical antibiotics and antiseptics
> Nail varnish
> Rubber chemicals in contraceptive devices

may be useful to study the reactants. Table 3.3 lists the common causes of vulvar allergic dermatitis.

HINTS ON HISTOPATHOLOGIC INTERPRETATION OF VULVAR SPONGIOTIC DERMATITIS

Biopsy is rarely obtained on acute lesions of either irritant or allergic contact dermatitis. In such cases, the pathologist's main contribution is to confirm the clinical suspicion of spongiotic dermatitis, and to rule out any other underlying dermatoses such as candidiasis or psoriasis. Performance of fungal stains for vulvar dermatitis can virtually always be justified. Rarely can the histopathologist distinguish the exogenous from the endogenous types with certainty.[15] The cause is more likely to be identified after a detailed clinical history and an expert dermatologic examination. However, certain histologic features may point toward a particular entity such as the following:

- *Keratin changes.* Parakeratosis, particularly when also containing the nuclear remnants of neutrophils, should suggest psoriasis, seborrheic dermatitis, or a fungal infection. The location of parakeratosis around the follicular ostia, and spongiosis accentuated in the epithelium of the follicular infundibula, point toward seborrheic dermatitis.
- *Keratinocytes.* Focal keratinocyte ballooning and apoptosis suggests irritant contact dermatitis. Extensive keratinocyte necrosis, however, suggests erythema multiforme, fixed drug eruption, or dermatitis artefacta.
- *Spongiosis.* Exocytosis of eosinophils into the epidermis suggests fungal infection, allergic contact dermatitis, atopic dermatitis, or drug reaction (or, more rarely, cicatricial pemphigoid or pemphigus vegetans). Neutrophils suggest fungal infection or psoriasis. Increased numbers of Langerhans cells suggest allergic contact dermatitis.
- *Dermal infiltrate.* Eosinophils suggest allergic contact dermatitis. Marked dermal edema and dilatation of lymphatics suggest an urticarial reaction to systemic or topical drugs.

CHRONIC DERMATITIDES

LICHEN SIMPLEX CHRONICUS (FORMERLY SQUAMOUS CELL HYPERPLASIA OR HYPERPLASTIC DYSTROPHY)

Clinical Features

Lichen simplex chronicus is now considered to be equivalent to squamous cell hyperplasia by the ISSVD.[19] Lichen simplex chronicus manifests as thick, scaly plaques arising

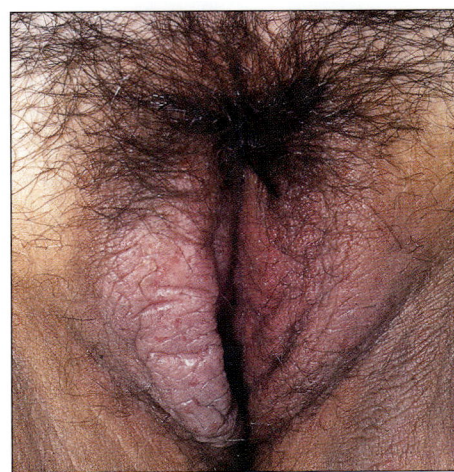

Figure 3.5 Lichen simplex chronicus of the right labium majus. There is thickening and accentuation of skin markings, with surface excoriation due to recent scratching.

after rubbing and scratching in response to pruritus. The areas most frequently affected are the mons pubis and labia majora. These cutaneous changes may be the end point of various types of eczematous dermatitis or be superimposed upon other inflammatory processes (lichen planus, psoriasis, lichen sclerosus, etc.). Sometimes the original process that started the chronic itch/scratch cycle, perpetuating the lichen simplex chronicus changes, may have resolved by the time of the biopsy (i.e., an episode of allergic contact dermatitis, an infection with *Candida*, etc.). Clinically, the presence of thick skin with enhanced cutaneous markings (Figure 3.5) is encompassed by the term 'lichenification,' referring to the rough surface of lichen overgrowing smooth-surfaced rocks. Excoriations and secondary infections may result from the scratching. The pathogenesis of this disorder remains incompletely understood.

Microscopic Features

The histologic features of lichen simplex chronicus are epidermal acanthosis with superficial dermal fibrosis and variable chronic inflammation (Figure 3.6). Hyperkeratosis and parakeratosis may be present. The dermal collagen bundles are thickened and tend to be vertically oriented. There is an inflammatory infiltrate, predominately of lymphocytes in the superficial dermis. The changes are otherwise nonspecific, and the diagnosis is made by exclusion of other dermatoses. When inflammatory exocytosis is marked, special stains for fungal forms (PAS and GMS) or bacteria are particularly recommended.

PSORIASIS

Psoriasis (psoriasis vulgaris) is a chronic, relapsing, inflammatory dermatosis affecting 1–2% of the American population.[20] Psoriasis is inherited as an autosomal dominant trait (diathesis) with incomplete penetrance. Four main genetic loci appear associated with this disease (on chromosomes 17q, 4q, 1q, and 6p).

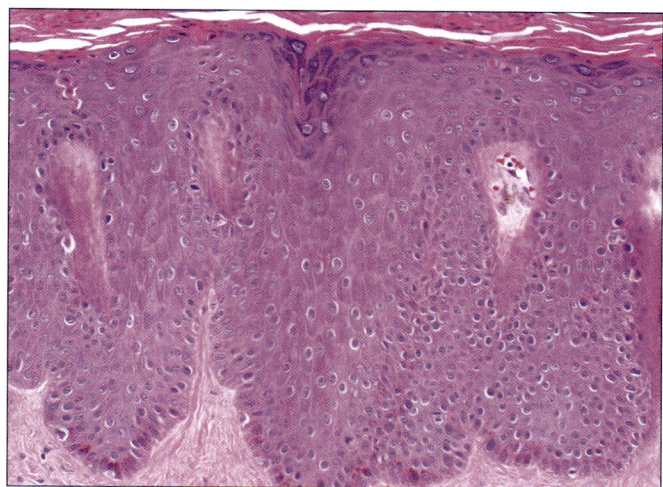

Figure 3.6 Lichen simplex chronicus. The epidermis shows thickening of rete ridges, thickening of the granular layer, and overlying hyperkeratosis.

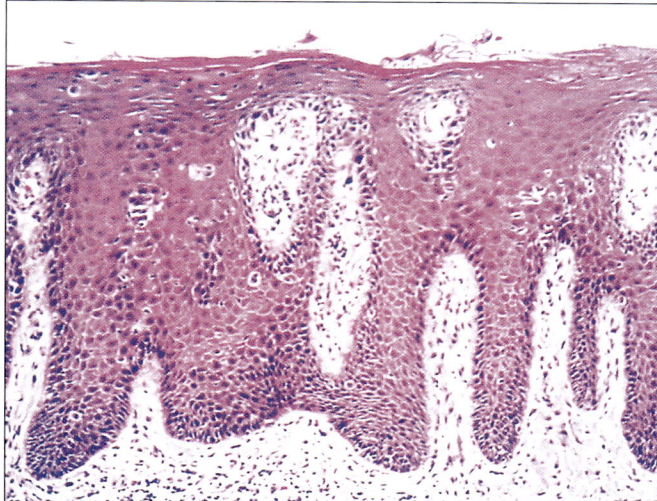

Figure 3.7 Psoriasis. There is psoriasiform hyperplasia of rete ridges with papillary dermal edema and telangiectasia. The parakeratotic scale on the skin surface is not prominent in vulvar psoriasis.

Clinical Features

The most typical clinical presentation is as well-demarcated, red to salmon-colored plaques with loosely adherent, silver scales affecting the extensor surfaces of the extremities (elbows and knees), sacral region, scalp, and nails. The vulva and perineum are involved frequently in combination with typical lesions elsewhere on the body. Psoriasis is infrequently confined solely to the vulva with a reported incidence of 2–5% of psoriatic patients.[20] In the vulva and other intertriginous areas, the silvery scales are lost.[21] The disease affects hair-bearing areas (mons pubis and labia majora), whereas the labia minora are spared. The intense erythema and the well-demarcated borders help to separate psoriasis from eczema. The lesions frequently are symmetric and may persist for years. Persistent, painful intergluteal and perianal fissuring can be a serious complication. Often the diagnosis is established with certainty after typical lesions develop elsewhere on the body.

Microscopic Features

The epidermal changes are hyperkeratosis, parakeratosis, and elongation of the rete ridges to an even length with club-shaped tips of rete ridges, hypogranulosis, and collections of polymorphonuclear leukocytes within the stratum corneum (Munro abscesses) and epidermis (spongiform pustules of Kogoj). Mitotic figures are found at different levels of the epidermis reflecting the significantly increased rate of epithelial turnover. The papillary dermis shows edema with irregularly dilated vessels with a minimal lymphocytic infiltrate and scattered neutrophils (Figure 3.7). Coexistence of staphylococcal infection, repeated scratching, trauma, and chronicity, as well as partial treatment with topical steroids, can affect the histologic features.

Differential Diagnosis

The major differential diagnosis includes chronic spongiotic dermatitis and seborrheic dermatitis. Although both conditions also show psoriasiform hyperplasia, the rete ridges typically are not elongated to an even length as in the psoriasis. In seborrheic dermatitis, the parakeratosis is typically distributed around follicular ostia.

LESS COMMON DERMATOSES THAT FREQUENTLY INVOLVE THE VULVA

LICHENOID DERMATOSES

The two most common conditions in this category are lichen sclerosus and lichen planus.

LICHEN SCLEROSUS

Lichen sclerosus, one of the most common chronic anogenital dermatoses, manifests as thickened and sclerotic dermal collagen.[1] Most patients are middle-aged and elderly women.[22] Sometimes it is familial.[23] Childhood presentation is uncommon, but it is important to remember that it does occur lest it be confused with signs of sexual abuse.[24–26] One-fifth of patients show extragenital involvement as hypopigmented wrinkled patches. Extragenital lesions as a rule do not undergo malignant degeneration. On the other hand, genital lesions may coexist with or subsequently develop squamous cell carcinoma.[27–30] In the vulva the frequency with which squamous cell carcinoma is associated with long-standing lesions of lichen sclerosus is 3–4%,[30] compared with 5.8% in penile lesions (balanitis xerotica obliterans), most of them associated with human papillomavirus (HPV) infection.[31]

Clinical Features

The clinical presentation of lichen sclerosus is protean. The initial lesions consist of flat, ivory to white papules that coalesce to form plaques of varying sizes and shapes. The early erythematous lesions with an edematous center impart a white color, and with time transform to the classic sclerotic lesions. The 'cigarette paper' atrophy in these lesions refers to the progressively wrinkled, flat or slightly depressed surface (Figure 3.8). The symmetrically involved vulva and anus form the classical 'figure-of-eight' or 'hourglass.' In the vulva, lichen sclerosus extends to Hart's line in the vestibule, with

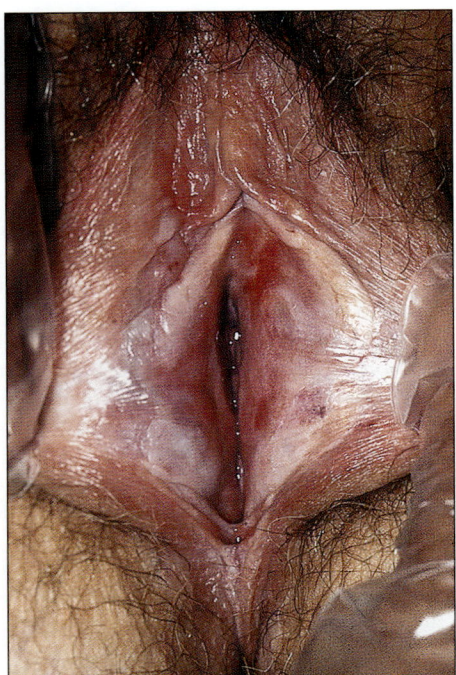

Figure 3.8 Lichen sclerosus. Classic white areas with purpura are present on the labia majora and minora. Partial reabsorption of labia minora is seen.

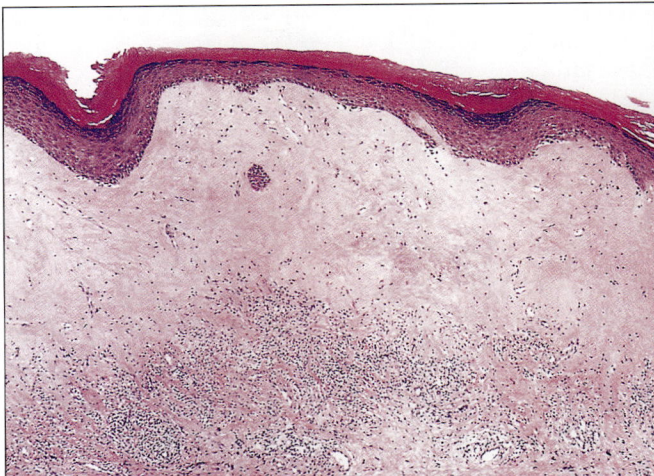

Figure 3.9 Lichen sclerosus. There is a broad band of hyalinized collagen beneath the epidermis, and a band of lymphocytic infiltrate beneath the hyalinization. The characteristic hyalinized band may be very narrow.

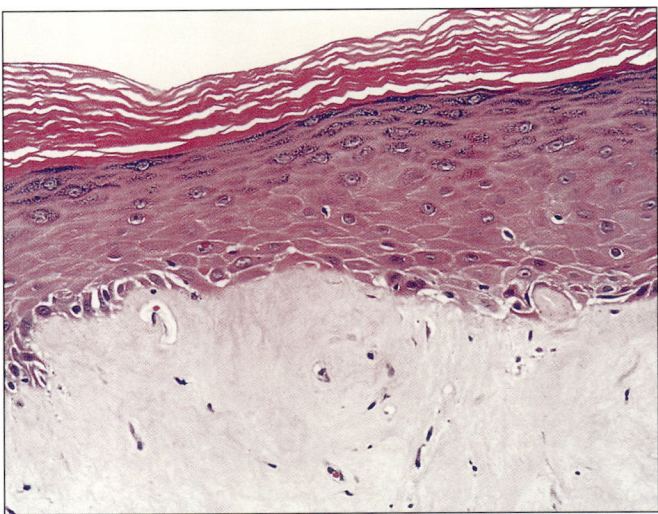

Figure 3.10 Lichen sclerosus. A characteristic feature of lichen sclerosus is irregular damage to the basal layer of the epidermis.

the vaginal mucosa uninvolved. Vulvar lesions may combine atrophic and hypertrophic areas, or may develop lichenification secondary to pruritus-related scratching. Early stage of lichen sclerosus may be difficult to separate from lichen planus and some patients with lichen sclerosus may develop introital lichen planus.[32] This clinical overlap parallels a similar cytokine response between these two diseases.[33]

Lichen sclerosus usually causes severe, intractable itch.[24,25] Occasionally, the condition is asymptomatic and discovered incidentally during a routine pelvic examination. Over time, variable degrees of scarring occur at an unpredictable pace and extent. Often the labia minora partially resorb (Figure 3.8). In severe cases, vulvar stenosis, effaced anatomy, and clitoral phimosis occur. Dyspareunia is common.

Early diagnosis and adequate treatment can prevent the distressing symptoms and severe vulvar deformities. Close surveillance facilitates early detection of squamous cell carcinoma.[34,35] Biopsy has a double role: first to confirm the diagnosis and second to help exclude a malignancy.

Etiology and Pathogenesis

Although the etiology of lichen sclerosus is still unknown, infection may play a potential role, an argument based on the presence of CD8+ and CD57+ lymphocytic infiltrates, a profile usually associated with viral diseases and autoimmune disorders. Direct immunofluorescence studies have shown a deposit of fibrin along the dermoepidermal junction in most of the specimens studied.[36] With an indirect fluorescent technique, IgM and C3 were concentrated along the basal lamina of the epithelium.[36] Studies of the T-cells within lichen sclerosus have identified monoclonal T-cells that are predominantly cytotoxic CD8+ responsible for the destruction of basal keratinocytes.[37] Lichen sclerosus is associated with autoimmune disorders such as vitiligo, pernicious anemia, thyroid disease, etc.[38–41] Individual HLA types (DQ7, DQ8, and DQ9) have been detected more frequently in patients with lichen sclerosus.[38]

Tissue studies of glucose metabolism as well as alkaline phosphatase and adenosine triphosphatase have shown a surprisingly high rate of activity equal to that seen in hyperplastic specimens and greater than that found in normal menopausal skin. The cell cycle protein Ki-67 is present in the basal and many parabasal epithelial cells involved by lichen sclerosus.[42] Collagen metabolism is abnormally active and the number of capillaries is reduced.

Microscopic Features

Lichen sclerosus affects the epidermis and upper dermis. The microscopic findings can vary considerably depending upon the age of the lesion, scratching, excoriation, and treatment. The main features include a thin epidermis with loss of the rete ridges, an underlying zone of homogeneous collagenized edema of variable thickness, and a band of lymphocytic infiltration beneath this zone (Figures 3.9 and 3.10).[43] The squamous epithelium is thinned, but hyperkeratosis may result in some cases from superimposed lichen simplex chronicus. The dermal–epidermal junction may show focal vacuolar change and the basement membrane may fragment, leading to the formation of PAS-positive clumps in the subjacent dermis. Spongiosis may be evident. Mitotic figures are rare or absent. The homogeneous dermal zone usually shows absence of elastic fibers. Both the absence of melanosomes in the keratinocytes and the disappearance of melanocytes contribute to the white clinical appearance.

Clinical Behavior

Lichen sclerosus is a relentless and progressive disease when presenting in most adults, but not uncommonly spontaneously regresses in girls once they reach menarche. Lichen sclerosus sometimes is associated with vulvar squamous carcinoma; however, it is not considered to be a premalignant intraepithelial neoplasm.[27–29] In a report of vulvar squamous cell carcinoma, 61% of the patients had lichen sclerosus.[44] Symptomatic lichen sclerosus is preceded by carcinoma by a mean of 4 years. Among patients with symptomatic vulvar lichen sclerosus, 9% developed vulvar intraepithelial neoplasia (VIN) lesions and 21% invasive squamous cell carcinoma. Differentiated (simplex) type VIN and non-HPV-related squamous cell carcinoma have been associated with vulvar lichen sclerosus.[45] Increased basal expression of Ki-67 appears to identify those cases with high risk of evolving into squamous cell carcinoma.[46,47] Also, aneuploidy has been reported, which correlates with elevated p53 expression.[27] Traditional management has relied on the long-term topical application of testosterone or progesterone. Currently, strong topical corticosteroids produce symptomatic relief and, in some cases, resolution of lichen sclerosus.[48]

LICHEN PLANUS

Lichen planus is a chronic, inflammatory disease of skin and mucous membranes, which occurs most commonly in women older than 40 years of age.[1,15,49] Vulvar pruritus and burning are common symptoms; however, the patient may be asymptomatic.[50,51] White, lace-like plaques (Wickham striae) involving the oral and vaginal mucosa also may be present (Figure 3.11).[52,53] Patients with this condition experience vulvar pain, dyspareunia, and burning. Lichen planus can result in severe introital and vaginal adhesions, scarring, and stenosis.[54–56]

Lichen planus has been associated with immunodeficiency states, internal malignancy, primary biliary cirrhosis, and ulcerative colitis among other conditions. Whereas lichen sclerosus does not affect the vagina, lichen planus can manifest as desquamative vaginitis.

Clinical Features

Half of the women and one-fourth of the men with cutaneous lichen planus have genital involvement. Unfortunately, it is frequently missed, for several reasons. As a mucocutaneous interface, the vulva can be affected by cutaneous, mucosal, or combined patterns. Thus, the clinical appearance may be highly variable ranging from delicate reticulated papules to an erosive desquamative process involving the vagina and vulva (Figure 3.12).[54,55] Within the vulva, the erosive process is typically confined to the vulvar vestibule

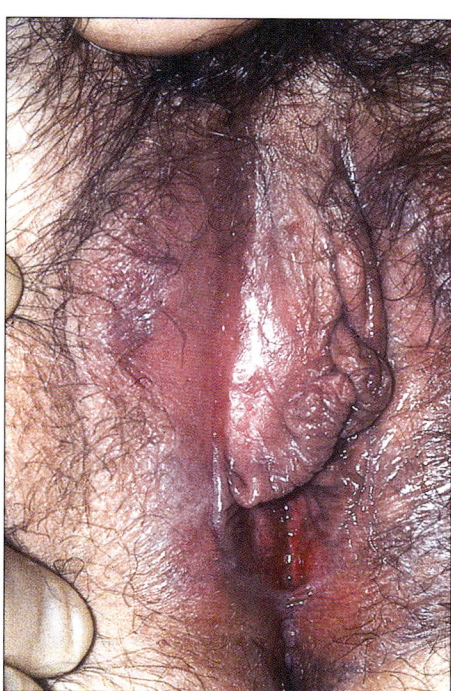

Figure 3.11 Lichen planus in the interlabial creases. Fine white striae and erosions are present.

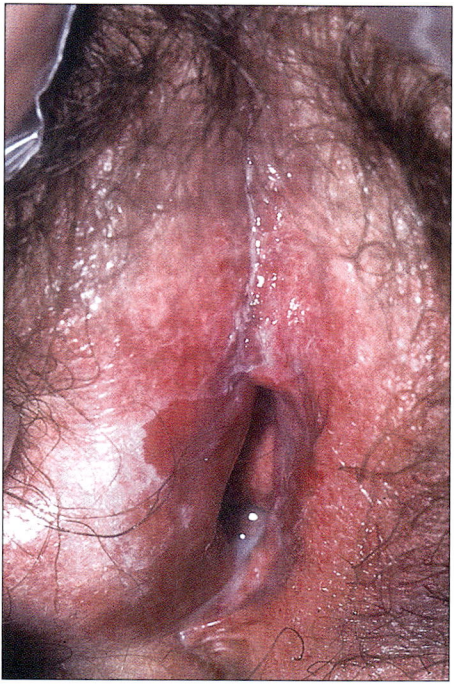

Figure 3.12 Erosive lichen planus. Bright patches of eroded epithelium with a shaggy white edge are present at the vulvar vestibule. Vaginal disease may be present.

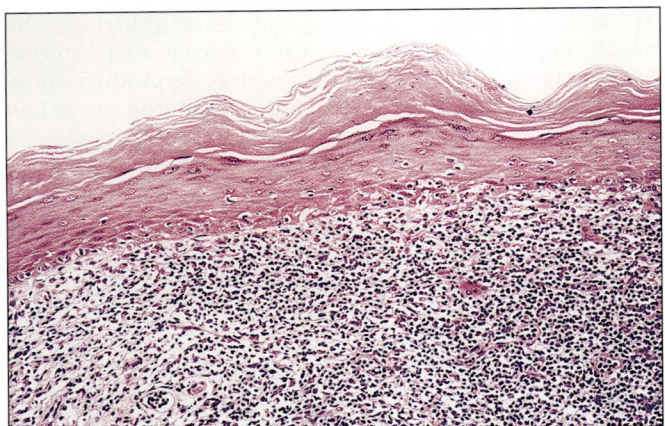

Figure 3.13 Lichen planus. The epidermis shows hyperkeratosis, extensive basal layer destruction, and a dense lichenoid infiltrate at the dermoepidermal junction. In the vulva, the histologic changes are not always as florid and classic as shown here.

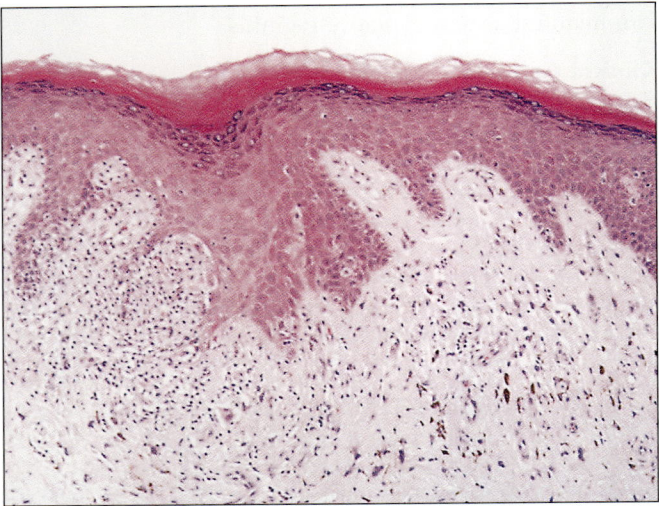

Figure 3.14 Lichen planus. In the vulva, lichen planus changes may be very focal and show superimposed lichen simplex chronicus due to repeated scratching.

and commonly involves the vagina. With advancing disease, there is loss and agglutination of the labia minora and prepuce, associated with thinned epithelium, and shrinkage with stenosis of the vaginal introitus.

Pathology

The histopathologic diagnosis of vulvar lichen planus is often difficult. First, mucous membrane lesions may differ considerably from those occurring on vulvar skin. Second, lichen simplex chronicus frequently coexists, and sometimes there is also associated lichen sclerosus. Finally, the erosive pattern, where the epithelium is lost, may be extremely difficult to diagnose due to sampling problems, secondary infection, and inflammation from topical applications. In the skin, two typical microscopic features help in the histologic diagnosis: a band-like chronic inflammatory infiltrate that is predominantly lymphocytic, with rare plasma cells. The inflammation typically involves the upper dermis and immediate overlying epidermis; and liquefaction necrosis of the basal epithelial cells. These cells appear admixed with chronic inflammatory cells, and degenerated keratinocytes result in the formation of colloid bodies (Civatte bodies) (Figures 3.13 and 3.14).

The fully developed epidermal changes usually seen in classic cutaneous lichen planus (saw-tooth pattern, hypergranulosis, orthokeratosis, etc.) are rarely present in vulvar lesions. Accurate diagnosis is important since the erosive form may require immunosuppressive therapy. Also, the presence of chronic lichen planus in the vulva is a risk factor for squamous cell carcinoma.[35,57,58] The differential diagnosis includes lichenoid drug reactions, which should be suspected if eosinophils are present.

Immunofluorescent studies often reveal fibrin deposition at the dermal–epidermal junction and, occasionally, granular IgM; rarely, C3 and IgG deposits are also present. The clusters of necrotic keratinocytes (colloid bodies) are positive for IgM in up to 87% of cases and, sometimes, C3 and IgG deposits may be helpful for the diagnosis.[59]

The epithelial changes are variable within mucous membranes and include thinning of the epithelium, with ulceration and bullous formation. In contrast to the findings within the skin, plasma cells may be evident with mucosal involvement.

The skin lesions resolve in most cases within 1–2 years, but mucosal lesions may persist longer. Hyperpigmentation is a common sequela after resolution, especially in darker skinned patients.

BULLOUS DISORDERS

The vesiculobullous disorders result from the congenital or acquired formation of antibodies against components involved in the adhesion of keratinocytes.[60] Many of the blistering diseases that affect the skin also involve mucosal sites.[61] In the vulva, friction and trauma foster the development of the blistering disorders, which typically present clinically as soggy, weeping, or erosive to ulcerative lesions. Clinical suspicion needs to be high in patients with erosions. Besides a detailed clinical history and careful physical examination, biopsies of the lesion for light microscopy plus perilesional skin for direct immunofluorescence are important. The most significant primary bullous skin diseases affecting the vulva are the following (Table 3.4):

- Pemphigus vulgaris, and its variant pemphigus vegetans
- Cicatricial pemphigoid
- Linear IgA disease, particularly in children.

PEMPHIGUS VULGARIS

Pemphigus vulgaris is an acquired, autoimmune blistering disease representing 80% of all pemphigus cases.[15] Autoantibodies develop against the desmosomal protein, desmoglein 3, at intercellular sites between keratinocytes, leading to acantholytic blisters that break easily and form erosions.[62,63]

Clinical Features

Most patients have oral blisters that precede cutaneous involvement by weeks to months. The vulvar lesions consist of erythematous, moist, eroded plaques, at the edge of

Table 3.4 Bullous Diseases

Disease	Age	Genital	Mucosal	Separation Plane	Type of Infiltrate	IF site/pattern	Autoantibody Reactant	Location of Antigen	Target
Pemphigus vulgaris	Adults	80%	Most of the cases	Suprabasal	Minimal	ICS/lace-like	IgG	Desmosomes of lower epidermis/mucosa	Desmoglein 3 (mucosal) Desmoglein 3/1 (mucocutaneous)
Pemphigus vegetans	Adults	Intertriginous areas	Frequent	Suprabasal	Neutrophils and eosinophils	ICS/lace-like	IgG	Desmosomes	Desmoglein 3
Bullous pemphigoid	Elderly; rare in childhood	9%	Common	BM: lamina lucida	Eosinophils	BMZ/linear	C3, IgG	Hemidesmosomes	BPA-1 BPA-2
Pemphigoid gestationis	Fertile age	5%	Rare	BM: lamina lucida	Eosinophils	BMZ/linear	C3	Hemidesmosomes	BPA-2
Cicatricial pemphigoid	Middle and old age	55%	Always with major scarring	BM: lamina lucida	Neutrophils and eosinophils	BMZ/linear	C3, IgG	Laminin	BPA-2 and epiligrin
Chronic bullous dermatosis of childhood	Childhood	60%	Common	BM: lamina lucida	Neutrophils	BMZ/linear	IgA	Anchoring filaments	LAD-1-ladinin
Adult linear IgA dermatosis	Adults	Variable	Common	BM: lamina lucida	Neutrophils	BMZ/linear	IgA	Anchoring filaments	LAD-1-ladinin
Epidermolysis bullosa	Babies	Variable	Variable	EB simplex: basal layer EB dystrophica: sublamina densa	Minimal	N/A	N/A	N/A	N/A
Hailey–Hailey disease	Young adult	Common perianal	Very rare	Spinous	N/A	N/A	N/A	N/A	N/A
Darier disease	Young adult		Rare	Suprabasal	N/A	N/A	N/A	N/A	N/A

BM/BMZ, epidermal basement membrane zone; BPA, bullous penphigoid antigen; EB, epidermolysis bullosa; ICS, squamous intercellular substance; IF, immunofluorescence; LAD-1, linear IgA disease antigen homolog; N/A, not applicable.

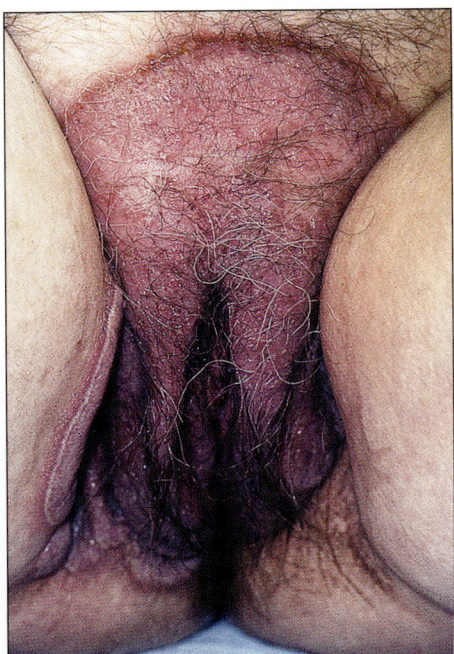

Figure 3.15 Pemphigus vegetans. This disease preferentially involves the genital area and presents with exuberant ('vegetating'), weeping, blistering plaques.

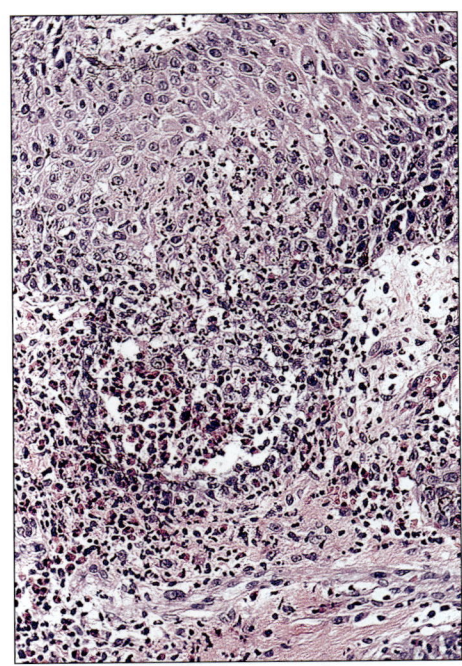

Figure 3.16 Pemphigus vegetans. At an early stage, intraepidermal accumulations of eosinophils are a useful diagnostic picture.

which intact blisters may briefly be seen. The classical skin lesions consist of flaccid blisters on a normal or erythematous base. The blisters break easily leading to eroded and crusted areas. Trunk, groins, axillae, scalp, and face are frequently involved. These lesions extend if pressure is applied to the top of the bullae (positive Asboe-Hansen sign). They heal without scarring. The disease activity can be followed by enzyme linked immunosorbent assay (ELISA) titers of circulating antibody to desmoglein 3. The principal cause of death is infection secondary to corticosteroid treatment. The mortality rate is 5–15%. There are reported cases of cervical and vulvar microinvasive squamous cell carcinoma in association with pemphigus vulgaris.[64]

Microscopic Features

The squamous epithelium shows a suprabasal bulla with scattered neutrophils and eosinophils. Because the disease targets an adhesion protein joining keratinocytes, but not between keratinocytes and basement membrane, the basal keratinocytes remain attached to the dermis, imparting a 'tombstone appearance.' Dermal changes are nonspecific. Unfortunately, the separated upper layers of the epidermis frequently fall off during the biopsy process and all that remains is the dermis with the single layer of intact basal keratinocytes. Thus, a useful histologic clue is the presence of clefts extending deep into adnexal structures. A biopsy that includes the edge of the blister increases the chances of finding some surviving acantholytic keratinocytes. Direct immunofluorescence usually shows IgG, especially IgG_1 and IgG_4, in the intercellular spaces (Table 3.4).[59]

Therapy includes high systemic doses of corticosteroids and cytotoxic agents, plasma pheresis, and supportive measures.

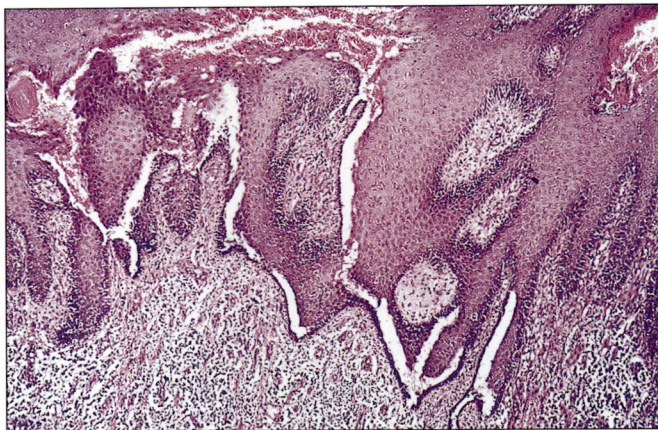

Figure 3.17 Pemphigus vegetans. Acantholytic separation of the hyperplastic epidermis just above the basal layer is characteristic of pemphigus vegetans. There is frequently a chronic inflammatory dermal infiltrate with some inflammatory cells in the epidermis.

PEMPHIGUS VEGETANS

Clinical Features

This rare variant of pemphigus shows well-demarcated, warty erythematous plaques with a moist, ulcerated surface that preferentially involves the pubic, perineal, and perianal areas (Figure 3.15). Rarely, blisters are found at the edges of the plaque. As with pemphigus vulgaris, oral lesions are invariably present, and frequently the presenting feature. 'Vegetans' alludes to the warty appearance of these lesions that may mislead the clinician to diagnose condyloma acuminatum or even squamous cell carcinoma.

Microscopic Features

The microscopic as well as immunofluorescent and immunologic findings are similar to pemphigus vulgaris except for the presence of intraepidermal eosinophilic microabscesses (Figure 3.16) and marked epidermal hyperplasia. The presence of eosinophils and the localized and self-limited character of the disease distinguish it from pemphigus vulgaris. The extreme acanthosis may even suggest squamous cell carcinoma (Figure 3.17). Circulating antibodies of the IgG_2 and IgG_4 subclasses, with strong complement fixation, are commonly present in pemphigus vegetans (Table 3.4).

BULLOUS PEMPHIGOID AND CICATRICIAL PEMPHIGOID

Bullous pemphigoid is a chronic, subepidermal, acquired, autoimmune blistering disease.[65–69] Multiple, tense blisters typically occur on erythematous plaques or normal skin in elderly patients. These patients develop autoantibodies that target basal cells' basement membrane attachment plaque (hemidesmosome).[61] Cicatricial pemphigoid or benign mucous membrane pemphigoid is a chronic bullous disease that affects predominantly oral and ocular membranes and results in scarring and stenosis.[70,71] Anogenital region involvement occurs in 20% of patients. Both bullous and cicatricial pemphigoid can be the result of a drug hypersensitivity reaction. Severe cicatrization with shrinkage may suggest lichen sclerosus or lichen planus;[72] however, in contrast to lichen sclerosus or lichen planus, cicatricial pemphigoid is associated with small blisters and a positive Nikolsky sign, i.e., formation of blisters in unaffected tissue by application of light pressure.[70,71]

Microscopically, there are subepidermal blisters and a mixed inflammatory cell infiltrate within the dermis. Eosinophils are numerous. In cicatricial pemphigoid the lesions evolve to scars. Perilesional direct immunofluorescence usually shows a linear band of IgG with or without C3 at the dermoepidermal junction (Table 3.4). IgA is found in 20% of cases. Systemic corticosteroids and immunosuppressive drugs may be helpful.

CHRONIC BULLOUS DERMATOSIS OF CHILDHOOD AND ADULT LINEAR IgA BULLOUS DERMATOSIS

This is an immunobullous disorder of unknown etiology in which linear deposits of IgA are detected in subepidermal blisters. There are two clinical variants that are commonly regarded as different expressions of the same entity. One is the chronic bullous dermatosis of childhood and the other is the adult linear IgA bullous dermatosis. In the first years of life, chronic bullous dermatosis presents with the abrupt onset of large, tense bullae or 'cluster of jewels' that have a propensity for perioral and perigenital areas, but extend to thighs and lower abdomen. Initially the blisters fill with clear fluid, but secondary infection results in pustules (Figure 3.18). Commonly, this disease resolves in several months. In adults, the clinical presentation is protean and mimics other bullous disorders. Amiodarone, vancomycin, lithium, and nonsteroidal anti-inflammatory drugs (NSAIDs) can induce this immunobullous disorder.

Histologically, there are subepidermal blisters with neutrophilic microabscesses in the papillary dermis, a finding indistinguishable from that seen in dermatitis herpetiformis. Fibrin with leukocytoclasis in the tip of the papilla favors

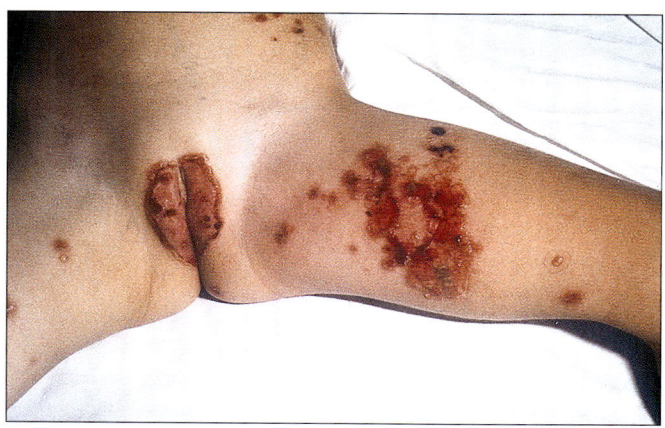

Figure 3.18 Chronic bullous disease of childhood. The disease presents with groups of itchy blisters and erosions. The genital region is often involved.

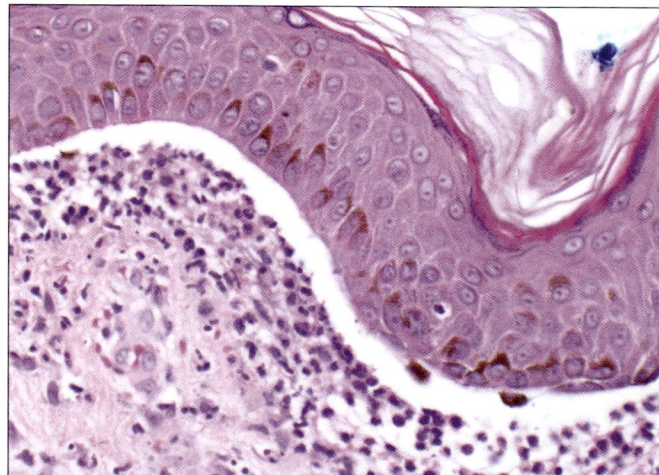

Figure 3.19 Linear IgA disease. The presence of neutrophils parallel to the dermal–epidermal junction points toward linear IgA dermatosis.

dermatitis herpetiformis, while the presence of neutrophils parallel to the dermal–epidermal junction points toward linear IgA dermatosis (Figure 3.19). However, only immunofluorescence definitively separates these two diseases. Bullous pemphigoid is distinguished from IgA dermatosis by the linear IgG basement membrane deposits (Table 3.4).

INHERITED DERMATOSES

HAILEY–HAILEY DISEASE

Hailey–Hailey disease is an acantholytic dermatosis involving flexural areas that usually starts in the late teens.[73,74] It is inherited as an autosomal dominant trait and the responsible gene called *ATP2CL* is mapped to chromosome 3q21–q24. Patients suffer from recurrent clusters of vesicles that evolve into bullae that rupture, leaving crusted, erythematous erosions (Figure 3.20). The disease, when occurring in the perineal region, frequently extends to the vulva. Unusual cases are restricted to the vulva.[75,76] Some may spread to involve the vagina.[77]

Microscopically, early lesions show suprabasal clefting. Acantholytic cells may border the cleft or lie free in the

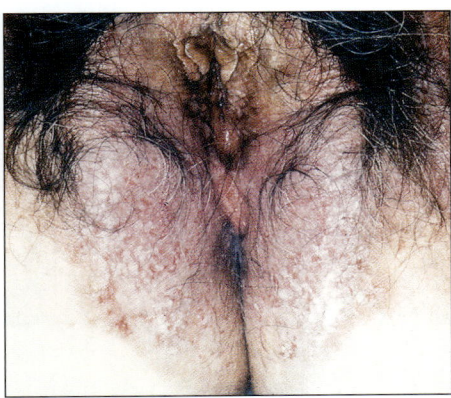

Figure 3.20 Hailey–Hailey disease. This dyskeratotic genodermatosis presented with irritable superficially eroded plaques in flexural sites.

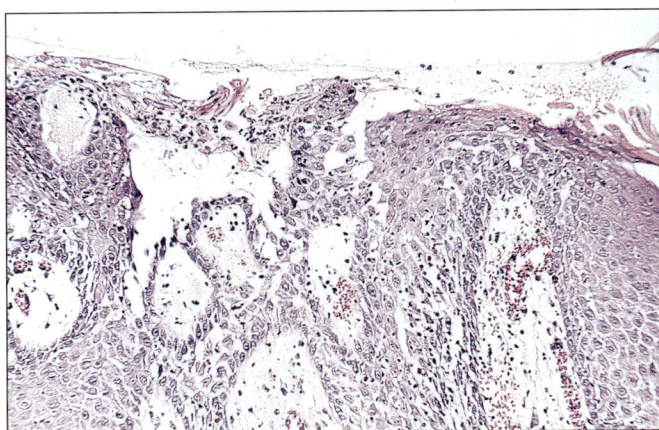

Figure 3.22 Darier disease with suprabasal acantholysis.

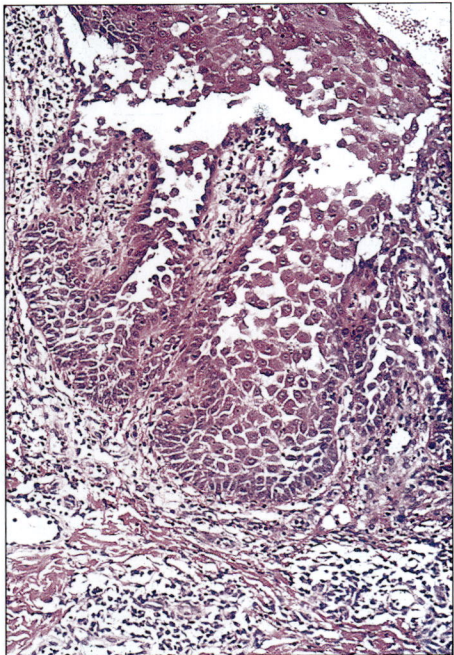

Figure 3.21 Hailey–Hailey disease. The pattern of epidermal acantholysis in Hailey–Hailey disease is characteristic, said to resemble a crumbling brick wall. Compare this pattern of acantholysis with that seen in pemphigus vegetans.

cavity. With time the acantholysis involves the entire epidermis, producing the characteristic image of a 'crumbling, dilapidated brick wall' (Figure 3.21). The acantholysis is more marked than in Darier disease. The broad lesion and degree of inflammation help to distinguish Hailey–Hailey disease from other acantholytic dermatoses. Immunofluorescence tests in difficult cases help separate it from pemphigus vulgaris (Table 3.4). Isolated cases of squamous cell carcinoma have arisen on a background of Hailey–Hailey.[78,79]

EPIDERMOLYSIS BULLOSA

This mechanobullous disease rarely affects the vulva, except in the setting of generalized cutaneous involvement by the severe junctional and dystrophic types.

DARIER DISEASE (KERATOSIS FOLLICULARIS)

Darier disease is a chronic acantholytic dermatosis inherited as an autosomal dominant disorder involving the *ATP2A2* gene located on chromosome 12q23–24.1.[80] It usually appears in adolescence with yellow to brown, crusted papules that affect the seborrheic areas and frequently involves the vulva.[81–83] Darier disease has a predisposition to bacterial, fungal, and viral infections. Follow-up of these patients is recommended due to the rare cases of squamous cell carcinoma associated with this disease.[84]

Microscopically, the keratotic papules disclose acantholysis that involves rete ridges in which a cleft or lacuna forms (Figure 3.22). The papillary dermis typically protrudes into the lacuna, which is lined by a single layer of basal cells (forming so-called 'villi'). Overlying these changes is a thick area of orthokeratosis with focal parakeratosis. Accompanying these features are dyskeratotic cells in the form of 'corp ronds' and 'grains.' Differential diagnosis includes Hailey–Hailey disease, localized acantholytic disease of the vulva, and warty dyskeratoma. Corps ronds are cells located in the upper malpighian layer and stratum corneum with a small pyknotic nucleus, clear perinuclear halo, and bright eosinophilic cytoplasm. The dense and bright peripheral rim of cytoplasm represents aggregates of tonofilaments and keratohyaline granules. Grains are small cells with elongated nuclei and a small amount of cytoplasm; electron microscopy demonstrates premature aggregation of tonofilaments. The synthesis of keratohyaline in association with clumped tonofilaments demonstrated by electron microscopy is distinctive of Darier disease and can separate it from Hailey–Hailey disease (Table 3.4).

WARTY DYSKERATOMA

The histologic features of warty dyskeratoma are essentially similar to those of Darier disease. Unlike Darier disease, which is multifocal, warty dyskeratoma typically involves the head, neck, or vulva as a solitary endophytic lesion. Darier disease usually is congenital, and is carried as an autosomal dominant trait, whereas warty dyskeratoma is not.

OTHER INFLAMMATORY DISEASES AFFECTING THE VULVA

PLASMA CELL VULVITIS (VULVITIS OF ZOON)

A chronic inflammatory disorder of unknown etiology, Zoon vulvitis exhibits extensive plasma cells in the mucosa.[85–88] Patients after middle age present with a solitary, sore, orange-red glistening 1–3 cm lesion on the vestibular mucosa (Figure 3.23).[89,90] On microscopic examination there is a dense and band-like mucosal infiltrate of plasma cells admixed with lymphocytes (Figure 3.24).[91] The epidermis eventually becomes atrophic, with loss of the surface keratin and of the stratum granulosum. The stratum spinosum frequently exhibits flattened, lozenge-shaped keratinocytes separated by mild spongiosis. The basal layer is often irregular and may exhibit exocytosis of lymphocytes. The dermis shows increased numbers of dilated, thin-walled vessels, often with red cell extravasation. Immunohistochemistry for light chain restriction helps exclude plasmacytoma if suspected. The lesions resolve slowly, leaving behind a rusty stain from resolved microhemorrhages. Recurrences are common.

ERYTHEMA MULTIFORME AND STEVENS–JOHNSON SYNDROME

Erythema multiforme is a self-limited cytotoxic reaction triggered by agents such as drugs (antibiotics, oral contraceptives, NSAIDs, etc.) and infections (especially *Mycoplasma* and viral infections, particularly herpes simplex). Stevens-Johnson syndrome, presently been classified with transepidermal necrolysis, presents with painful ulcers of the mouth and genitalia in association with the skin rash.

This disease presents at any age and the skin lesions appear targetoid (central zone of necrosis, blister, or erosion surrounded by erythema and edema) most frequently affecting the extremities in a symmetrical distribution. In the genital region, it usually presents as a bullous eruption.[92] On microscopic examination, scattered apoptotic keratinocytes are present in the epithelium, often associated with intraepithelial vesicle formation, upper dermal edema, and a perivascular lymphocytic infiltrate. Erythema multiforme and Stevens-Johnson syndrome share identical histologic presentation. Erythema multiforme is a clinical diagnosis that usually rests on the clinical history and appearance, and the presence of other lesions outside the vulva. Most episodes are recurrent, lasting on average 2 weeks without sequelae.

BEHÇET DISEASE

Behçet disease is defined by the triad of recurrent oral ulcers, genital ulcers, and ocular inflammation.[93,94] The pathogenesis is unknown. Behçet disease can cause deep ulcerations in the vulva that may lead to labial fenestration and gangrene.[95,96] Aphthous (small ulcers) stomatitis is the initial manifestation in two-thirds of patients.[97] Genital and perianal aphthae are in general larger, deeper, and more painful than oral lesions (Figure 3.25). The histologic features are usually nonspecific, and clinical–pathologic correlation is necessary for diagnosis. Although necrotizing arteritis is frequent and can be considered a cardinal pathologic finding, in the presence of ulceration, it is difficult to determine whether it is primary or secondary. The dermis

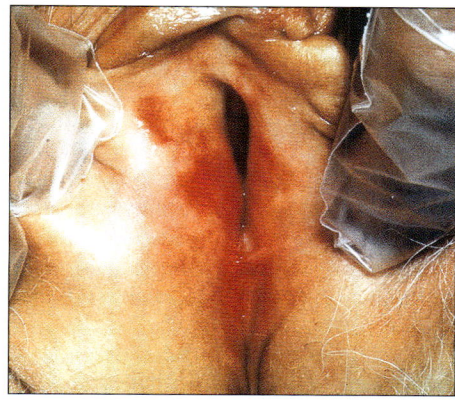

Figure 3.23 Zoon plasma cell vulvitis. Typical orangey-red patches are present on the vestibular mucosa. These are very sore to touch.

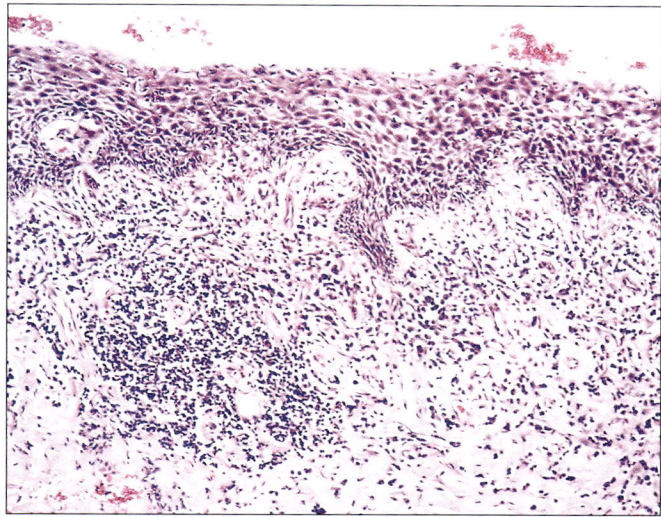

Figure 3.24 Zoon vulvitis. Characteristic histologic features include 'lozenge-shaped' keratinocytes, epidermal atrophy (not seen in this early lesion), and a variable but usually heavy lymphoplasmacytic infiltrate in upper dermis.

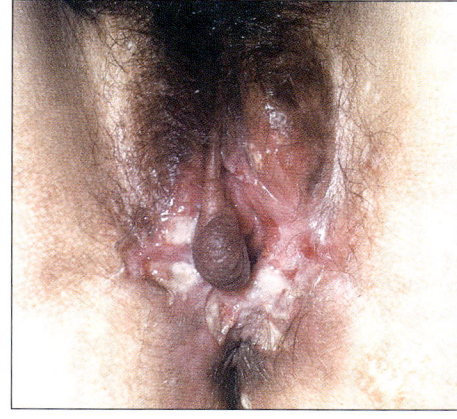

Figure 3.25 Behçet disease. Recurrent deep painful ulcers have developed in the genital epithelium.

often contains a perivascular lymphocytic infiltrate. Endothelial cell swelling also occurs and may result in venous thrombosis. Other manifestations in the skin include erythema nodosum-like lesions. Unlike erythema nodosum, this entity lacks histiocytic granulomas.

CROHN DISEASE

Crohn disease is a granulomatous inflammation, most commonly involving the small bowel, but occasionally the vulva and the perineum in adults and children.[98–101] In fact, genital Crohn disease is more frequent in children than in adults.[102]

The cutaneous changes can both precede the gastrointestinal involvement and lack any correlation in severity between cutaneous and gastrointestinal manifestations. Extraintestinal findings precede the gastrointestinal involvement in one-fourth of cases. The clinical appearance of vulvar Crohn disease is variable. When associated with local colonic disease, perineal ulcers and large, edematous skin tags are characteristic.[100] Sometimes fistulas extend from the affected bowel into perineal and even vulvar skin or Bartholin glands, resulting in indurated, tender, inflamed areas that drain pus. The latter may mimic bartholinitis.[103] Vulvar Crohn disease may occur as erythematous plaques on the labia majora (Figure 3.26) and pubic skin. Occasionally, it may present as chronic sloughing ulcers on the mucosal surfaces of the labia. The pathologic changes include massive dermal and subcutaneous edema, and markedly dilated lymphatics. Noncaseating sarcoidal granulomas are diagnostic (Figure 3.27), but often ill-formed aggregates of histiocytes with variable numbers of lymphocytes are seen instead. Ulcerated or fistulous lesions often show a predominance of secondary features such as fibrosis, chronic inflammation, suppuration, and granulation tissue.

HIDRADENITIS SUPPURATIVA

Hidradenitis suppurativa is chronic folliculitis of apocrine gland-bearing skin, affecting particularly the axilla and vulva. The etiology is unknown. Patients usually present with recurrent painful subcutaneous abscesses, followed by sinuses from which foul pus may drain (Figure 3.28).[104] Suppuration results from secondary infection by a wide range of bacteria, including anaerobes. Squamous cell carcinoma is a rare complication, and has been reported in long-standing lesions.[105]

Hidradenitis suppurativa may be difficult to distinguish from Crohn disease. However, the latter usually does not affect axillae, is not painful, and patients usually have gastrointestinal manifestations. Hidradenitis suppurativa must also be distinguished from Fox–Fordyce disease, with which it sometimes coexists. Fox–Fordyce disease (apocrine miliaria) may present at puberty with pruritic papules of the axillae, vulva, and perianal regions.

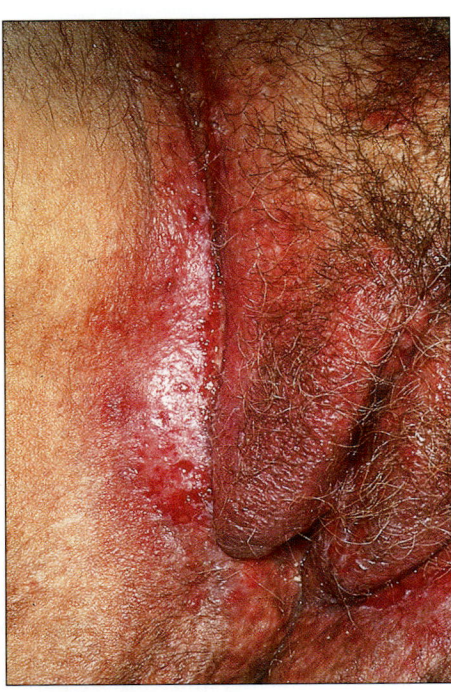

Figure 3.26 Cutaneous Crohn disease of the perineum. The disease has infiltrated eroding plaques of the vulva and perianal skin.

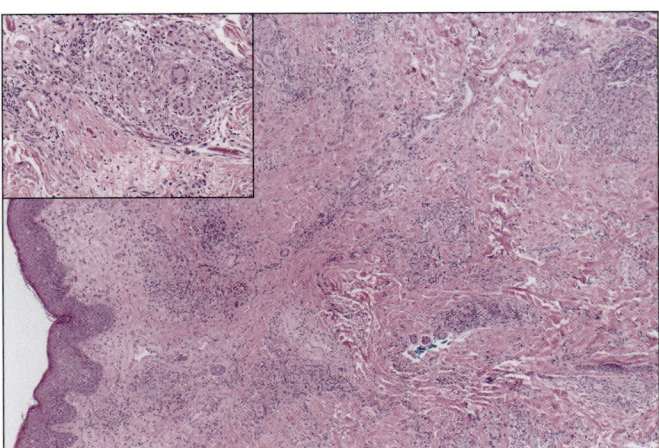

Figure 3.27 Vulvar Crohn disease. The dermis shows a diffuse infiltration of noncaseating granulomas with variable numbers of lymphocytes. Inset: Detail of a noncaseating granuloma.

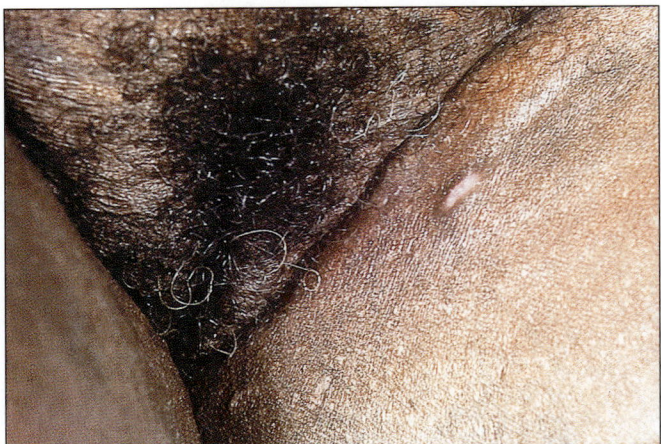

Figure 3.28 Hidradenitis suppurativa. Discharging pustular nodules and sinuses are present in the groin creases.

VULVAR PAIN SYNDROMES

VULVAR VESTIBULITIS

Clinical Features

The vulvar vestibule is the ring of epithelium proximal to Hart's line (see glossaries at the end of this chapter), which is in continuity with the hymen and contains the minor vestibular glands and the openings of the ducts of Bartholin and Skene glands. Vestibulitis is a complex of introital dyspareunia and severe tenderness on light pressure.[106–109] Most women present in their twenties and thirties with dyspareunia. Some patients give a history of severe *Candida* infection or a gynecologic procedure. Examination may show punctate erythema and these areas are likely to be biopsied. The vulva is otherwise normal. Vestibulitis is more common in women with migraine, irritable bowel syndrome, and/or myalgic encephalopathy syndrome.[110] Treatment with low-dose tricyclic antidepressant drugs often brings at least some relief.

Vestibulitis is rarely biopsied, and the histologic changes are nonspecific, subtle, and of dubious significance. Biopsies may show peripheral nerve hyperplasia in the vestibule, without significant inflammation.[111] A sparse lymphocytic infiltrate may surround the necks of the minor vestibular glands.

DYSESTHETIC VULVODYNIA

Clinically, a severe burning sensation affects the entire vulva, often extending onto the perineal skin, upper thighs, and abdominal wall.[113–115] Dysesthetic vulvodynia tends to affect older women with a history of lumbar disc disease, constipation, or previous gynecologic surgery. Physical examination reveals only vulvar atrophic change, without tenderness to palpation. There may be altered sensitivity to light touch over the lower abdomen, pubis, and thighs. A thorough neurologic examination is required to exclude cauda equina lesions or neuralgia of the pudendal nerve. Treatment with low-dose tricyclic antidepressants is often successful.[112]

PIGMENTARY ALTERATIONS

These disorders can be divided by whether the pigmentation is increased (hyperpigmentation) or decreased (hypopigmentation). Before discussing these entities, it is useful to understand physiologic hyperpigmentation. Skin and mucosa in various body sites have different densities of melanocytes. Melanocyte concentration and melanin density are greater in genital skin, particularly in dark-skinned patients. Hormones also affect the level of pigmentation, and pregnancy increases melanogenesis, accentuating physiologic hyperpigmentation.

HYPERPIGMENTATION

Increased pigmentation in the vulvar skin may be due to increased:

- Melanin deposition in the epidermis or dermis
- Thickness of the keratin layer in a verruciform or papillomatous pattern
- Hemosiderin deposition in the upper dermis

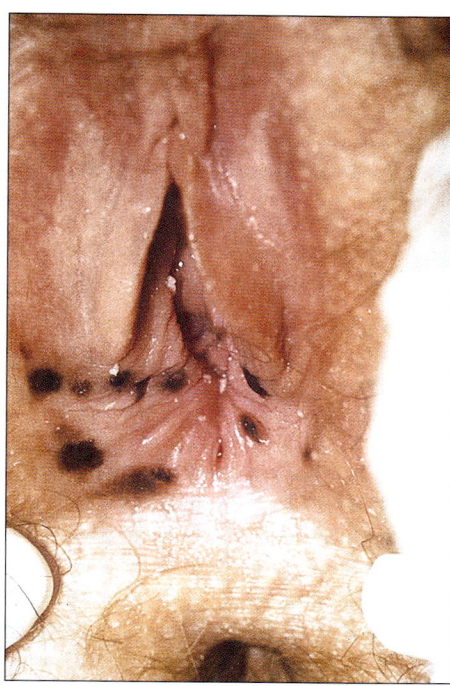

Figure 3.29 Vulvar melanosis (of Laugier). This benign condition of young adults must be distinguished microscopically from pigmented VIN and melanoma.

HYPERPIGMENTATION DUE TO MELANIN IN VULVAR SKIN

The pigmented melanocytic nevi and melanoma are described in Chapter 5.

Idiopathic Acquired Pigmentation (of Laugier)/Vulvar Melanosis. Marked, macular hyperpigmentation appears on the vulva, vagina, and cervix, without a preceding history of trauma or inflammation.[116,117] Lesions can reach several centimeters in diameter. Areas are often multiple (Figure 3.29). The etiology is unknown. Lesions show increased melanin deposition in the basal layer of keratinocytes and dermal melanophages are invariably present.[118] The Masson–Fontana stain serves to emphasize the increased melanin. Immunocytochemical stains show a normal or mildly increased number of melanocytes in the pigmented area. Lesions with melanocytic hyperplasia are best termed *lentigines*.

Postinflammatory Hyperpigmentation. Postinflammatory hyperpigmentation is the most common type of hyperpigmentation and usually results from increased melanin deposition in macrophages in the upper dermis following prolonged damage to epidermal keratinocytes such as in lichen planus, lichenoid drug eruptions, and fixed drug eruptions.

HYPERPIGMENTATION DUE TO INCREASED KERATIN IN STRATUM CORNEUM

Compact orthohyperkeratosis, when arranged flat, gives a pale gross appearance. It appears brown when thrown up into papillary folds. The two most common lesions affecting the vulva are acanthosis nigricans and seborrheic keratoses.

Acanthosis Nigricans. Symmetrical, pigmented, hyperkeratotic plaques in flexural sites, particularly the axillae, neck folds, anogenital region, and groins, characterize this disorder. Mucosal involvement, particularly oral mucosa (lip and tongue), occurs in 25% of cases. Acanthosis nigricans is an abnormal epidermal growth in response to various factors with expression of unusual keratins, such as 18 and 19, in basal keratinocytes. It is important to recognize acanthosis nigricans because of its potential association with underlying disorders, including:

- Multiple *endocrine disorders and congenital syndromes sharing resistance to insulin and hyperinsulinemia.*[119] The effect of high insulin levels on insulin-like growth factor 1 (IGF-1) receptors on keratinocytes is believed to produce the skin changes. Stimulation of the same receptor on ovarian stromal cells can lead to stromal hyperthecosis and hyperandrogenism.
- Rare *familial acanthosis nigricans* is inherited as an autosomal dominant condition and is not linked to insulin resistance. These rare syndromes include: Lelis' syndrome or acanthosis nigricans with ectodermal dysplasia, *s*evere *a*chondroplasia with *d*evelopmental *d*elay and *a*canthosis *n*igricans (SADDAN syndrome), and Crouzon syndrome with acanthosis nigricans.[120,121] The molecular basis of these syndromes is mutations in the fibroblast growth factor receptor 3 (*FGFR3*) gene on chromosome 4p16.3.[122]
- *Drug-induced forms* occasionally occur with various agents including oral contraceptives, nicotinic acid, and the folate acid antagonist triazinate.
- *Paraneoplastic type* or malignancy-associated acanthosis nigricans is a rare disorder usually seen with adenocarcinoma of the stomach or some other part of the gastrointestinal tract.[123] Usually the acanthosis nigricans and the neoplasm are diagnosed simultaneously. Sometimes, the cutaneous manifestation precedes or follows the tumor. Epidermal growth factor and transforming growth factor (TGF-α) are potential factors produced by these tumors and can lead to the abnormal proliferation found in acanthosis nigricans.

Microscopically, the skin lesions show papillomatosis with upwardly projected dermal papillae covered by thinned epidermis. Between the projections, the epidermis shows mild acanthosis with hyperkeratosis. The basal layer is mildly hyperpigmented. Sometimes, mucosal lesions show marked acanthosis and mild chronic inflammation in the submucosa. These lesions can be confused with condyloma acuminatum.

HYPOPIGMENTATION

POSTINFLAMMATORY HYPOPIGMENTATION (LEUKODERMA)

As with hyperpigmentation, hypopigmentation can follow inflammation. A possible mechanism is blockage of the transfer of melanosomes from the melanocytes to the keratinocytes. Destruction of melanocytes is also postulated in lichenoid inflammation. Fungal and yeast infections may cause patchy mild hypopigmentation, particularly in pityriasis versicolor, which appears as pale macules. A PAS stain for fungi may be helpful in evaluating a vulvar biopsy of an irregular hypopigmented area. An important disease showing hypopigmentation is lichen sclerosus. VIN may also present as a white plaque. Histologically, the number of melanocytes is normal, but the melanin content is reduced in the basal layer. Melanin-laden macrophages are occasionally seen in the upper dermis, especially in patients with darker skin. Features of active or resolving inflammatory dermatosis may be noted.

VITILIGO

Vitiligo is an inherited leukoderma in which melanocytes are destroyed in the involved areas. It is usually symmetrical and often involves the perineum. Onset occurs at any age, but half appear before the age of 20 years. The presence of antimelanocyte antibodies supports the immune theory as an effector of melanocytic destruction.[124] Melanocytes sometimes remains in the hair follicles, and it is from the follicular melanocytes that the repigmentation occurs. In cases of depigmentation, it may be difficult to differentiate vitiligo from lichen sclerosus. Both are in the same group of inherited autoimmune disorders and sometimes coexist in the same patient. However, vitiligo is a purely macular lesion, lacking the atrophy or sclerosis of lichen sclerosus. Vulvar skin affected by end-stage vitiligo is completely devoid of melanin within the basal keratinocytes, and melanocytes are entirely absent in the basal layer. The ideal biopsy is taken through the edge of a lesion so that the vitiligo patch can be compared with adjacent normal skin. The edge of the vitiligo lesion may show a narrow zone of degenerating basal melanocytes and a lymphocytic infiltrate in underlying papillary dermis and lower epidermis. The Masson–Fontana stain for melanin and immunohistochemical stains (Melan A and HMB-45) for melanocytes help highlight the differences between the lesion and adjacent normal skin.

DRUGS

Besides topical applications, systemically taken drugs may also elicit various types of skin reactions affecting the vulva. Such reactions are not confined to prescription-only agents. Agents such as aspirin, acetaminophen, alternative or herbal remedies with unknown constituents, and food materials containing dyes or preservatives can also induce skin lesions.

FIXED DRUG ERUPTIONS (DERMATITIS MEDICAMENTOSA)

Fixed drug eruption is an infrequent, but recurrent reaction that occurs each time an individual is exposed to a triggering drug. The classic presentation is that of a single, well-defined, erythematous, round to oval plaque with a dusky center and possible bulla formation leading to erosion. This lesion develops 1–2 weeks after a first exposure. This period is reduced to 24 h in subsequent exposures. More than 100 drugs are known triggering agents, and the most frequent are sulfonamides, tetracyclines, tranquilizers, quinine, phenolphthalein (formerly used in laxatives), and analgesics. The current hypothesis concerning the pathogenesis of fixed drug eruptions is that the eruptions causative drug activates keratinocytes to release cytokines or induces keratinocytes to express surface adhesion molecules, leading to

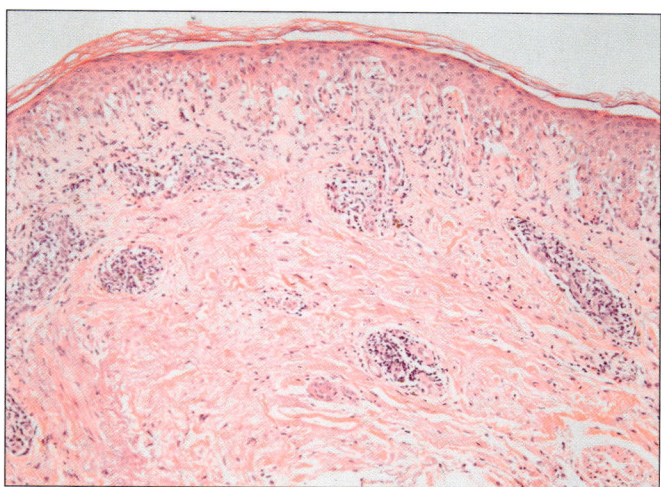

Figure 3.30 Fixed drug eruption. Prominent number of apoptotic keratinocytes is noted at the basal layer. There is underlying patchy and band-like inflammatory infiltrate with pigment incontinence.

activation of epidermal CD8+ T-cells, and subsequent death of keratinocytes by FasL-mediated pathway.[125]

The most common histopathologic findings of fixed drug eruption show a lichenoid inflammatory reaction with basal layer vacuolization and Civatte bodies associated with a heavy, superficial and deep dermal lymphocytic infiltrate (Figure 3.30). The infiltrate sometimes contains a few neutrophils and eosinophils. Damage to the epidermal basal layer leads to release of melanin, which macrophages in the upper dermis capture. While these findings resemble that of erythema multiforme, fixed drug eruption also shows the presence of a mid to deep dermal inflammatory reaction, neutrophils, and prominent melanin incontinence. Histologic findings in drug eruption are usually nonspecific and are only suggestive or supportive of a drug eruption. Patch testing, indirect and direct Coombs tests, other specific laboratory testing, as well as a detailed clinical history, are necessary to precisely diagnose such cases.

VULVAR INFECTIONS AND INFESTATIONS

Vaginal infections may cause vulvar symptoms either by extension or by the irritant effects of vaginal discharge. These disorders will be discussed in Chapter 7.

BACTERIAL INFECTIONS

STAPHYLOCOCCAL INFECTIONS

Similar to any hair-bearing skin, the labia majora or mons pubis may be the sites of a superficial staphylococcal folliculitis and deep folliculitis producing furunculosis (boils). Occlusion, intertrigo, and depilated pubic hair particularly by shaving are important predisposing factors. Other organisms producing similar changes are *Pseudomonas*, *Malassezia furfur*, and dermatophyte fungi. The histologic appearances are identical to superficial and deep folliculitis elsewhere on the body. The exfoliative toxin produced by *Staphylococcus aureus* can induce flaccid blisters or pustules in the genitalia and thighs. Clinical inspection reveals yellow crust and residual superficial erosions immediately after superficial fragile blisters rupture. Diagnosis is made by culture. Focal disease requires only local treatment. Oral antibiotics are the therapy of choice for extensive disease.

STREPTOCOCCAL INFECTIONS (NECROTIZING FASCIITIS)

Streptococcal infection affecting the genital area has a range of clinical presentations varying from superficial cutaneous infection to necrotizing fasciitis, a rapidly progressive necrosis of skin and subcutaneous tissue. The superficial bacterial infection, common in children between 3 and 5 years, has a predominant perianal distribution that can extend to the vulva and vagina. Streptococcal vulvitis and perianal dermatitis can produce tender, well-demarcated red skin with or without scale. Occasionally, anal fistulas with mucoid discharge and vulvar fissures develop. Swabs grow group A or C hemolytic streptococci, and systemic antibiotics are required to clear the infection.

Group A streptococci are among the organisms responsible for *necrotizing fasciitis* together with other anaerobic and aerobic bacteria such as streptococci, *S. aureus*, *Escherichia coli*, *Bacteroides*, and *Clostridium* spp. This rare form of rapidly progressive necrosis of subcutaneous tissue and fascia can be fatal if not recognized early and aggressive therapeutic intervention pursued. The vulva is one of the sites affected, with extension to the perineum and abdominal wall. It usually occurs in diabetics, particularly when complicated by obesity, hypertension, and peripheral vascular disease, or in the immunocompromised host. The infection's origin can be a surgical incision (e.g., episiotomy) or a local abscess of skin or Bartholin gland. At an alarming rate the skin changes from red to dusky gray–blue with bulla formation and necrosis. The soft tissue frequently feels indurated and wooden to palpation. The patient shows signs of toxicity with fever, chills, malaise, shock, and tachycardia. Surgical debridement with extensive reconstructive surgery is the mainstay of treatment. Mortality is high, upward of 40%, especially when diagnosis and debridement have been delayed or invasive group A streptococcus is involved.

Microscopically, extensive necrosis extends from the epidermis, to subcutaneous tissue, to fascia, and sometimes to muscle. Numerous polymorphonuclear leukocytes and mononuclear cells infiltrate the tissue and necrotizing vasculitis with thrombi is apparent. Large numbers of bacterial colonies pervade the upper dermis. Necrotizing fasciitis is often regarded as a form of septic vasculitis.[126]

SYPHILIS

Clinical Features

Syphilis is a chronic, worldwide, sexually transmitted disease caused by the spirochete *Treponema pallidum*. Coinfection with human immunodeficiency virus (HIV) is well recognized. Acquired syphilis is divided into four stages (primary, secondary, latent, and tertiary) with distinct clinical presentations separated by asymptomatic periods. The primary or initial lesion is the chancre, an indurated, painless, shallow ulcer with well-defined borders that appears within 3–4 weeks at the site of inoculation. Multiple lesions occur, especially in immunocompromised patients. The serum exudate from the chancre contains numerous spirochetes, which can be identified by dark-field microscopy, permitting prompt diagnosis. The primary site in women is often on the vulva or perineum; other sites include the cervix, urethra, lip, or tonsillar fossae. The lesion is self-healing within 1–5 weeks leaving a small discrete stellate scar. Regional painless lymphadenopathy presents 3–4 days after the chancre.

Between 4 and 8 weeks after the chancre, untreated patients develop constitutional symptoms and mucocutaneous lesions as part of secondary syphilis. Fever, lymphadenitis, and hepatitis occur in association with an erythematous exanthem of the trunk, genital area, flexor aspect of limbs, and, characteristically, the palms and soles. Atypical presentations may occur in patients with concurrent HIV infection. Pregnant women can infect the fetus via transplacental passage of the spirochete. Some cases of secondary syphilis show large, flat, fleshy, moist papules or *condylomata lata* in the labia and perineum. Condylomata lata are among the most infectious lesions in syphilis; dark-field examination shows numerous treponemes. Such lesions also occur on other mucocutaneous borders. After 3–8 weeks lesions disappear spontaneously. Diagnostic tools in secondary stage include serologic tests that measure antibodies to cardiolipin by rapid plasma reagin (RPR) and venereal disease research laboratory (VDRL) assay. In the setting of HIV infection or immunosuppression, one must be aware of false-negative RPR results or the prozone effect. It occurs when the antibody titers in the infected individual are so high that the visualization of the reaction is impaired.[127] Other methods detect antibodies to surface proteins of *T. pallidum* by *T. pallidum* hemabsorption test (TPHA) or microhemagglutination assay for antibodies to *T. pallidum* (MHA-TP). Latency, the period between healing of the clinical lesions and appearance of late manifestations, can last for many years. The gumma, the classic lesion of tertiary syphilis, is rarely seen on the vulva.

Microscopic Features

If the diagnosis of primary syphilis is suspected clinically, identification of spirochetes by dark-field microscopy is the diagnostic tool *par excellence*. Serologic tests to confirm the diagnosis are essential. A biopsy may be necessary when the chancre has an atypical appearance or it is located in an unusual, nongenital site. Acanthosis of the epidermis is common at the edges of the ulcer, the base of which shows an infiltrate of lymphocytes and plasma cells. Blood vessels show prominent endothelial swelling.

Dieterle, Warthin–Starry, or Steiner stains may demonstrate the spirochetes, but, today, antibodies against *T. pallidum* are available for formalin-fixed paraffin-embedded tissue and represent a more specific and sensitive method (Figure 3.31).[128] In primary syphilis spirochetes are usually identified at the dermal–epidermal junction and within and around superficial dermal blood vessels.

The histologic findings of secondary syphilis vary. The epidermal changes range from normal to hyperplastic with spongiosis. There are variable degrees of plasmacytic infiltrate and vascular endothelial swelling. The perivascular lymphoplasmacytic infiltrate usually involves the superficial and deep vascular plexus. Plasma cells are less prominent in macular lesions (Figure 3.32). The lymphocytic infiltrate can be so exuberant as to simulate lymphoma, but its mixed nature would be rare in such a neoplasm. Early lesions exhibit a neutrophilic vascular reaction with occasional microabscesses. In late syphilitic lesions granulomas of the

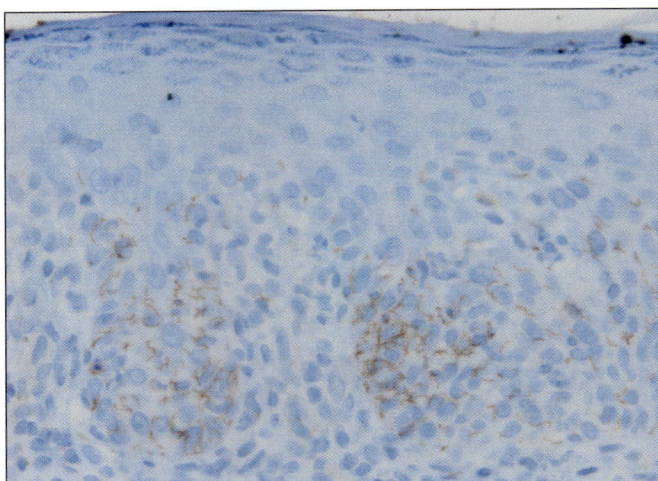

Figure 3.31 *T. pallidum* immunohistochemical stain highlights many spirochetes within the epidermis.

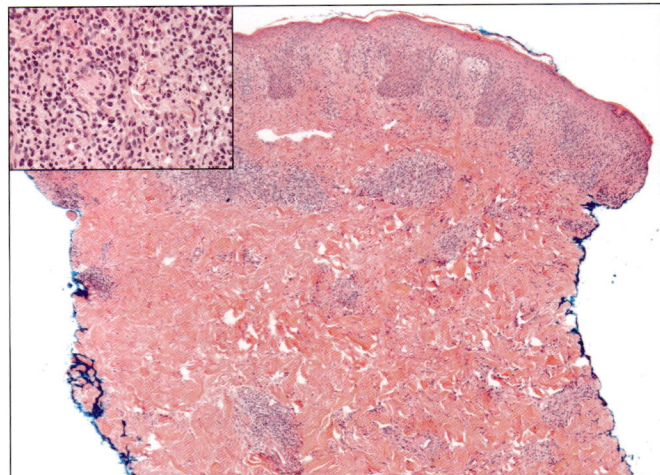

Figure 3.32 Secondary syphilis. An acanthotic epidermis, papillary dermal edema, and superficial as well as deep inflammatory infiltrate are seen. Plasma cells are noted within the dermal infiltrate (inset).

palisading type may simulate granuloma annulare or less frequently sarcoidal type granulomas. Although secondary syphilis occasionally mimics other skin diseases the predominance of plasma cells in the infiltrate is a valuable hint. Condylomata lata have epidermal hyperplasia with hyperkeratosis and patchy parakeratosis. The latter is associated with a superficial and mid-dermal perivascular lymphoplasmacytic infiltrate.

GONORRHEA

Neisseria gonorrhoeae is a Gram-negative diplococcus. Infection primarily affects the urethra but may spread to the vagina and cervix.[129] The paraurethral and Bartholin glands may be infected and, in the latter, an acute abscess may ensue. Gonococcal vulvitis is rare in adult women but is a common feature of infection in prepubertal children. Microbiologic culture is important diagnostically. Primary lesions are often ulcerated with underlying dense dermal neutrophilic infiltrate with abscess formation. Gram-negative intracellular diplococci can be seen.

CHANCROID

This sexually transmitted infection due to the bacterium *Haemophilus ducreyi* is more prevalent in the tropics. Painful ulcers develop on the labia and perineum, and usually are multiple and contiguous, giving the appearance of a large erosion with a granulomatous base. Half of the cases present with enlarged inguinal lymph nodes. If the skin lesion is biopsied, there is usually marked ulceration with an underlying zone of necrosis and inflamed granulation tissue. A Giemsa or Steiner stain shows organisms singly or in short chains, outside or within histiocytes. Smears of the lesions can show the Gram-negative rods in parallel chains ('school of fish'). Selective agars that facilitate the rapid growth of this bacillus, but the low sensitivity of culture, make polymerase chain reaction (PCR) the identification test of choice.

CHLAMYDIAL INFECTION (LYMPHOGRANULOMA VENEREUM)

Chlamydia trachomatis (serotypes L1, L2, and L3) is the obligatory intracellular microorganism responsible for the sexually transmitted lymphogranuloma venereum. This infection is prevalent in tropical climates and women are commonly asymptomatic carriers. The initial lesion is a small, painless papule or vesicle that frequently erodes, healing within several days without residual scar. Subsequently, the infection spreads via the lymphatics and manifests as enlarged painful inguinal and/or femoral lymph nodes. The lymph nodes can evolve to bubo formation leading to spontaneous rupture and sinus tract formation. Without treatment, extensive necrosis and scarring result in lymphedema, which can evolve to elephantiasis of the genitalia. Lymph nodes are occasionally excised for histologic diagnosis and show serpiginous or stellate abscesses with necrotic tissue and neutrophils surrounded by a macrophage and giant-cell granulomatous reaction ('suppurating granulomas'). Only one-third of cases reveal positive cultures. Therefore, the main diagnostic tools are serologic; however, they do not distinguish the different serotypes. A complement fixation titer of more than 1:64 in concert with the clinical findings previously described are diagnostic of lymphogranuloma venereum. A microimmunofluorescence test can detect antichlamydial antibodies to different serologic variants of *C. trachomatis* as well as various PCR-based tests.[130] Treatment is with systemic tetracycline or doxycycline.

GRANULOMA INGUINALE (DONOVANOSIS)

This is a mildly contagious, sexually transmitted disease caused by the bacterium *Klebsiella granulomatis*, which used to be called *Calymmatobacterium granulomatis*, and is endemic in tropical and subtropical areas. The lesions present as small, ulcerated papules on the labia or vaginal introitus, which merge to create hypertrophic, velvety, beefy-red granulation tissue. This is the most frequent, ulcerovegetative form. Papules also can enlarge to become nodules that may become confluent. Extensive matted ulcerations are slow to heal. This slowly progressive, destructive disease leaves disfiguring fibrous scars that, in the absence of treatment, cause extensive genital mutilation. Smears of the lesions show parasitized macrophages, the organisms (Donovan bodies) measure 1–2 μm, with a bipolar staining pattern in silver preparations (Warthin–Starry) giving an appearance of small safety pins.

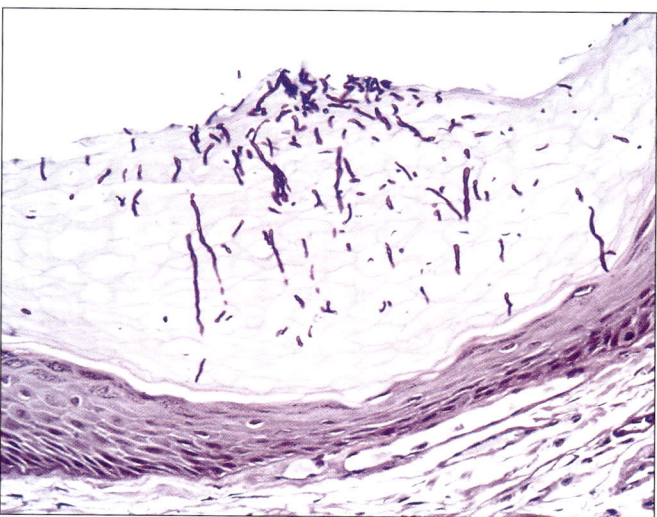

Figure 3.33 *Candida* infection. Candida hyphae and yeasts are present in the thickened keratin layer (D-PAS stain). In this case, there is minimal dermal inflammation.

FUNGAL INFECTIONS

CANDIDIASIS

Clinical Features

Candidiasis is one of the most frequent infections of the genital and anal region.[131,132] *Candida albicans*, the most frequent *Candida* species involved in human infection, is a normal inhabitant of the gastrointestinal tract and is found in the mouth of approximately half of normal individuals. Pregnancy, immunologic and endocrine dysfunction, immunosuppression, high-dose estrogen, antibiotic or systemic corticosteroid therapy, and debilitating states all predispose to clinical infection. Vulvovaginal candidiasis presents with vaginal and vulvar itching and burning, accompanied by vaginal discharge. Women of childbearing years are predominantly affected. A characteristic white curd (*Candida* comes from the Latin *candidus* or dazzling white) appears on the vagina walls. Erythema, edema, and fissuring of the vulva may occur. Diagnosis is confirmed on culture of a high vaginal swab or by finding hyphae and spores on a Gram-stained film from the vaginal discharge. *C. albicans* is the culprit in most cases, but other *Candida* species such as *C. glabrata* and *C. tropicalis* are responsible in a minority and can be more resistant to conventional treatments.

Microscopic Features

The diagnosis of vulvar candidiasis is usually evident once a special stain for fungi is used (Figure 3.33). The presence of parakeratosis with neutrophils that appears disproportionate to the degree of spongiosis should direct the pathologist to request a stain for fungi (PAS or GMS).

PITYRIASIS VERSICOLOR

Pityriasis versicolor or tinea versicolor is a common, noncontagious, superficial fungal infection. *Malassezia globosa* in its mycelial phase is the causative agent. It occasionally involves the labia majora, producing hypopigmented or hyperpigmented patches. Hyperpigmentation may result from large melanosomes, vascular erythema, or orthokeratosis, while hypopigmentation is due to azelaic acid, a tyrosinase inhibitor the organisms produce. Examination with a Wood's lamp accentuates the lesion, producing a dull green fluorescence. These findings differentiate this infection from erythrasma, a *Corynebacterium minutissimum* infection producing a bright, coral-red fluorescence under a Wood's light. The characteristic histologic finding of 'spaghetti and meatballs' is the presence in the stratum corneum of numerous round budding yeasts (blastoconidia) and short septate hyphae (pseudomycelia)

TINEA CRURIS

This superficial dermatophyte infection involves the inner upper thighs and crural folds. *Trichophyton rubrum*, the most frequent causative agent, produces a chronic infection with frequent extension to the buttocks and waist. Characteristic lesions are sharply demarcated, itchy, red patches with erythematous, scaly, advancing borders. The vulva is rarely involved. Heat, sweating, and friction predispose to infection. When topical steroids are inadvertently applied, the appearance can change dramatically and become nondiagnostic; however, the infection ultimately becomes more extensive and inflammatory, with papules and pustules. The annular configuration may be the clue to direct the pathologist to request a PAS stain. Diagnosis rests on cultures of scrapes taken from a scale at the rash's leading edge.

The histologic changes are usually nonspecific. Mild epidermal acanthosis with focal spongiosis and perivascular chronic inflammation is commonly seen. A constant feature is parakeratosis overlying the epidermal changes. The hyphae in the stratum corneum are frequently scanty, but more easily visible with special stains for fungus.

VIRAL INFECTIONS

HERPES VIRUS INFECTION

Clinical Features

Herpes simplex viruses (HSVs), ubiquitous type 1 and type 2 DNA viruses, produce primary infection, latency, and recurrent orolabial and genital disease.[133,134] Genital herpes, the most frequent sexually transmitted disease worldwide, is generally associated with HSV type 2 (70–90%) with a recent increase being noted for type 1 (10–30%).[135,136] In the last two decades, the seroprevalence of HSV type 2 has increased in the United States by 30%, or with one million new primary genital infections yearly. The virus replicates at the site of infection, then travels to the dorsal root ganglia through retrograde axonal flow and remains in a latent phase, with recurrent reactivations occurring spontaneously or following stimuli such as fever, stress, ultraviolet radiation, or immunosuppression.

The first episode of primary infection occurs 3–7 days after exposure, with a prodrome of general malaise associated with nonspecific genital findings. In time, the classic lesions develop, which are vesicles on an erythematous base arranged in clusters that evolve to pustules and/or erosions (Figure 3.34). These lesions are excruciatingly painful. Accompanying regional lymphadenopathy may last for more than a week. The vesicles heal without scarring unless there is secondary infection. Recurrent genital infection is in general milder and even subclinical.

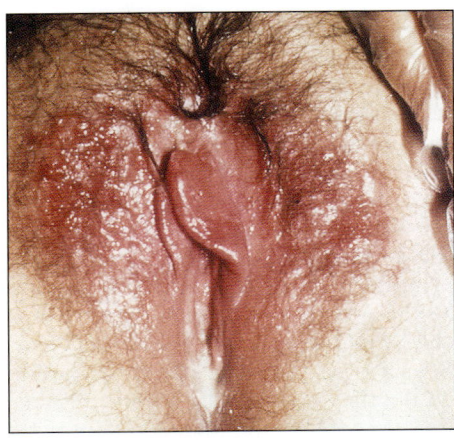

Figure 3.34 Acute herpes simplex infection. The vulva, which shows edema, erythema, and multiple vesicles, is excruciatingly painful.

Genital HSV infection is more severe and protracted in immunosuppressed individuals, who have a tendency to produce pseudoepitheliomatous hyperplasia in chronic clinical cases, simulating verrucous lesions. Recurrence of previous infection is common after transplant surgery. HSV infections in HIV patients can be extensive with severe, nonhealing, painful ulcers. Candidal and bacterial secondary infections are common.

The diagnosis is usually apparent clinically and may be confirmed through serologic tests, tissue culture, direct immunofluorescence, or molecular techniques. Reliable and rapid identification can be made using smears of vesicles (Tzanck preparation) and monoclonal immunofluorescence antibodies. The gold standard is western blot with 99% specificity and sensitivity. PCR is the preferred test to diagnose HSV in cases of systemic spread such as encephalitis.

Microscopic Features

The earliest changes appear in the nucleus of infected keratinocytes, with peripheral clumping of chromatin, homogeneous 'ground-glass' appearance, and ballooning. These early changes start at the basal layer. However, most biopsies include an intraepidermal vesicle resulting from infected cell swelling and losing attachment (ballooning degeneration), and progressive hydropic swelling of cells transforming in large and clear keratinocytes (reticular degeneration) (Figure 3.35). Ballooning changes are specific for viral infection and the cells can be multinucleated, with eosinophilic intranuclear inclusions and/or dense eosinophilic cytoplasm. Ulceration occurs, at the edges of which large, infected keratinocytes with intranuclear inclusions or multinucleated cells are often usually easily identified (Figures 3.36 and 3.37). In the late stages ghost cells remain, which are infected keratinocytes where the intranuclear inclusions have turned from eosinophilic to a slate gray color. Perivascular lymphocytic and neutrophilic inflammation is seen in the upper dermis. Follicles are more often involved in recurrent lesions. If the latter is the predominant finding, the diagnosis of herpes folliculitis can be rendered. Other adnexal structures can be affected, as in herpes syringitis. Eccrine ducts and glands show changes of the viral infection. The nerves in the biopsy specimen can show inflammation, Schwann cell hypertrophy, and viral cytopathic

CHAPTER 3 — VULVAR DERMATOSES AND INFECTIONS

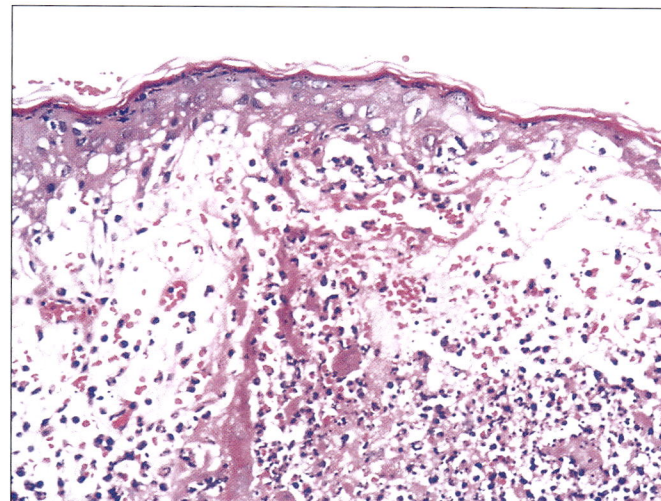

Figure 3.35 Herpes simplex infection. There is extensive destruction of the epidermis at the edge of a blister. The reticular degeneration pattern of epidermal destruction is characteristic of acute herpes/varicella infections of skin but can also be seen in the Stevens–Johnson variant of erythema multiforme.

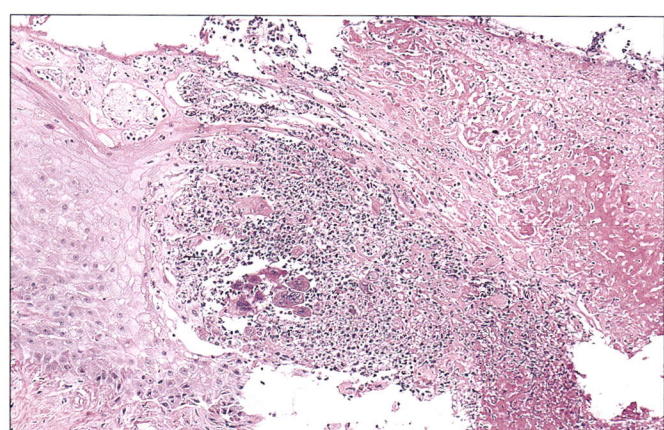

Figure 3.36 Herpes simplex. In herpes simplex there is often severe necrosis of skin appendages and upper dermis. Viral inclusions, while prominent in this slide, may be difficult to see, and immunohistochemical stains may be necessary to identify the viral particles.

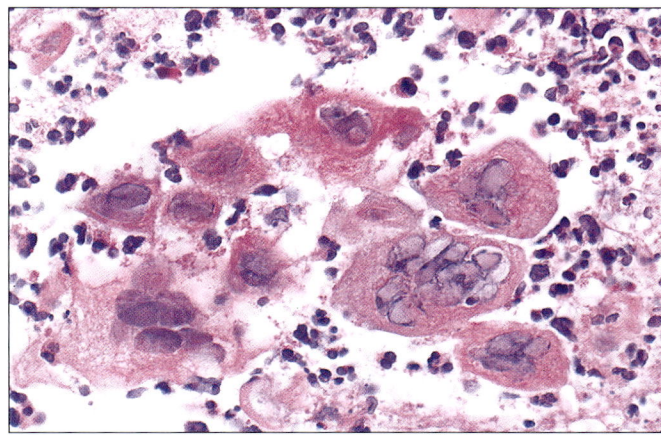

Figure 3.37 Herpes simplex with prominent viral inclusions.

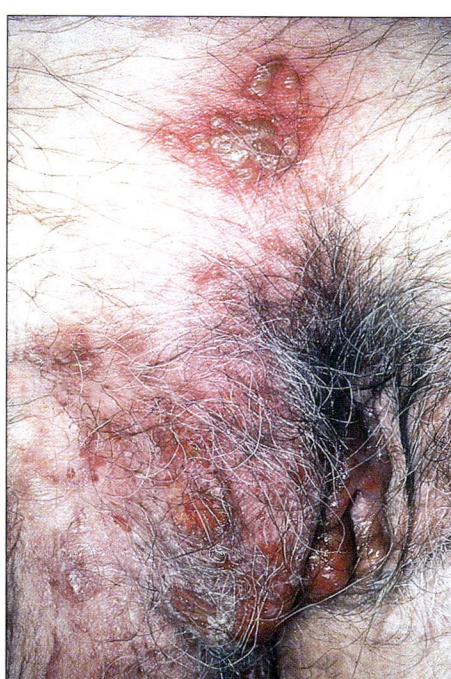

Figure 3.38 Varicella zoster of the vulva and pubis. Unilateral groups of vesicles and pustules have an erythematous base.

changes demonstrating that nerves are not only a conduit for this virus but also a target of infection. Acyclovir may reduce the severity of infection if given early in the course of illness.

VARICELLA ZOSTER VIRUS INFECTION (VULVAR SHINGLES)

Varicella zoster virus is the etiology of both varicella (chicken pox) and herpes zoster (shingles). Ninety percent of children in the United States under the age of 10 years have suffered varicella. Subsequently, the virus can remain latent in nerve ganglia until it is reactivated in 20% of immunocompetent hosts and half of immunosuppressed individuals. Herpes zoster is usually a disease of patients over 50 years. The incidence is increasing in immunocompromised patients, especially those infected with HIV. In most patients herpes zoster starts with a prodrome of pain, pruritus, tingling, or tenderness in a dermatomal distribution. A painful eruption of clustered papules follows, and in a short period of time, the papules transform to vesicles on an erythematous base (Figures 3.38). In the genital area erosions predominate. The distribution of the rash is a strong diagnostic clue. Confirmation comes from direct fluorescence antibodies or PCR viral detection. Microscopically, the changes overlap with those seen in herpes simplex infections (Figure 3.39). Immunoperoxidase stains can be useful in separating herpes simplex from varicella zoster.

OTHER VIRUS INFECTIONS

MOLLUSCUM CONTAGIOSUM

Clinical Features

Molluscum contagiosum is a poxvirus infection exhibiting single or multiple, 2–8 mm dome-shaped papules with a

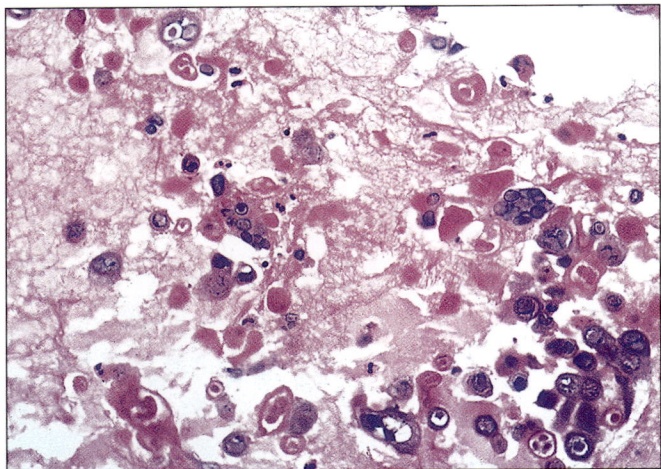

Figure 3.39 Varicella zoster. In an early vesicular lesion the viral inclusion bodies are usually easily seen in the necrotic epithelial cells in blister content.

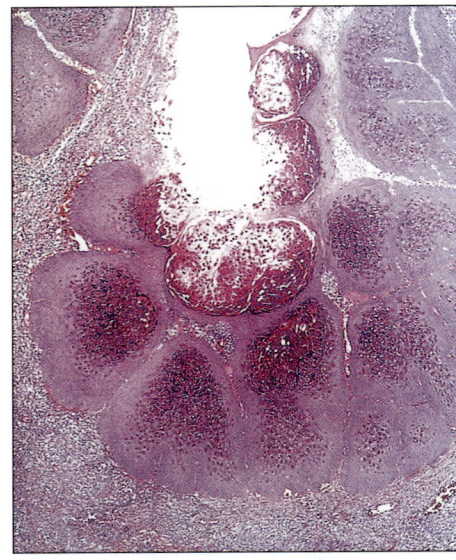

Figure 3.41 Molluscum contagiosum. Each inverted nodule of hyperplastic squamous cells expands into the underlying dermis.

HUMAN PAPILLOMAVIRUS INFECTIONS

Clinical Features

Papillomaviruses are a large group exceeding 100 genotypes of DNA viruses that infect skin and mucosae, producing warts, intraepithelial neoplasia, or invasive squamous cell carcinoma.[137] Genital HPV is a common, sexually transmitted disease affecting predominantly young adults.[138] The vulva, vagina, cervix, and anus are frequent areas of infection. Transmission of this virus can occur from direct contact with individuals who harbor clinical or subclinical HPV lesions. The lesions are in most cases transient, but the virus may recur, persist, or enter a latent phase. Genital warts are by far the most common manifestation and the majority of infections are with HPV types which, in the normal host, carry a low risk of neoplastic change. In immunocompromised patients, HPV infections often persist and increase the risk of developing neoplasms. HPV infections affecting the genital tract can be categorized as follows:

- Those that produce warts on fully keratinized skin, i.e., common and plantar warts.
- Those that cause warts, dysplasia, and squamous cell cancer in the immunosuppressed or in patients with the rare inherited disorder epidermodysplasia verruciformis.
- Those that infect the nasopharyngeal, conjunctival, and anogenital mucosal surfaces. These can be subdivided into low-, intermediate-, and high-risk types for the development of intraepithelial dysplasia and squamous cell cancer.[139] As on the cervix, HPV types 16 and 18 are most definitely linked to vulvar and anal intraepithelial neoplasia and squamous cell carcinoma. However, the risk of cancerous change on the vulva and anal mucosa seems much less than on the cervix.

The clinical presentation will depend on the HPV type, the anatomic location, and the host's immune status. These are the most frequent clinical presentations:

- Condylomata acuminata (singular: condyloma acuminatum) or anogenital warts occur on the nonhair-bearing,

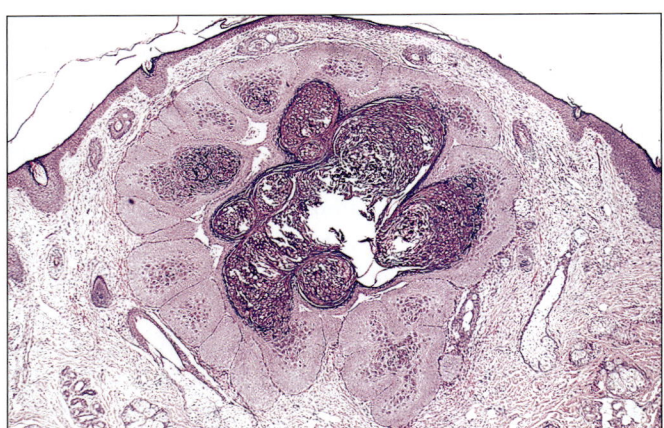

Figure 3.40 Molluscum contagiosum. A well-defined sac encloses the virion colony. The histologic appearances of molluscum contagiosum are pathognomonic and esthetically appealing.

central umbilicated core of white material. This infection predominantly affects children and adolescents. Commonly, spontaneous regression occurs. In adults, molluscum contagiosum occurs principally as a sexually transmitted disease involving the vulvar and perianal regions. Primary or recurrent molluscum contagiosum often complicates HIV disease.

The histologic features of molluscum contagiosum are pathognomonic. An endophytic growth of squamous epithelium arranged as lobules is seen in low power. Eosinophilic inclusion bodies fill the cytoplasm of infected cells above the basal layer. The inclusions can acquire large dimensions and compress the nucleus of the infected keratinocytes to the periphery (Figures 3.40 and 3.41). In a fully evolved lesion, the epidermis ruptures under the pressure of the underlying proliferation almost entirely occupied by viral inclusion, and produces the characteristic small white core. The viral inclusion bodies become more basophilic as they enlarge.

partially keratinized skin of the vulva (labia minora), the perineum, perianal region adjacent to the skin/mucosal interface, or in adjacent areas such as inguinal folds and mons pubis. They are discrete, skin-colored to brown, exophytic papillomas. They acquire a whitish surface when macerated in moist areas. The lesions range from several millimeters to being large and broad based, several centimeters in size, and forming confluent plaques that may extend into the vagina, urethra, or anal canal. One-third of these cases recur. Although malignant transformation is infrequent, the chances are higher than with other types of warts. The most frequent oncogenic HPV types are HPV 16, 18, 31, 33, and 35. The most frequent HPV types associated with the benign lesions are HPV 6 and 11 (see Chapter 9).

- Papular and keratotic warts tend to occur on fully keratinized and hair-bearing skin (e.g., labia majora).
- Flat warts can be found in all situations.

PCR has identified HPV DNA in skin with no clearly defined lesions. Dilute acetic acid will turn these abnormal areas white, albeit the acetowhite coloring only reflects thickening of the squamous epithelium and it is not diagnostic of HPV infection (e.g., acetowhite coloring can be seen in *Candida* infection, psoriasis, lichen planus, or eczema). Detection of this virus has not been only in subclinical lesions but also in normal-appearing skin. Furthermore, the virus is resistant to heat and desiccation. This explains the high recurrence rate of lesions (e.g., 20–50% for genital warts) and supports the consideration that treatment may not prevent transmission of HPV. Genital warts are of concern to the healthcare provider when they occur in prepubertal individuals.

The two major methods for detection of carcinogenic HPV DNA are hybridization with signal amplification and genomic amplification using PCR techniques. Currently, the Food and Drug Administration approved test is the hybridization method, Hybrid Capture 2 (HC2; Qiagen Corporation, Gaithersburg, MD).[140] To date HPV DNA detection by PCR-based methods has been used mainly for research.

Genital warts should be biopsied when there is concern about dysplastic or neoplastic change or when there is diagnostic uncertainty. Presently, no specific antiviral therapy is available. Only therapeutic measurements toward local destruction, removal, or induction of an immunologic response against the lesion are therapeutic considerations. Recently, a recombinant DNA vaccine has been developed that may change how we see HPV infection in the future.

Microscopic Features

The common wart shows papillomatosis with hyperkeratosis and parakeratosis, the latter especially located in the tips of the papillae. The elongated rete ridges often show an inward orientation at the lesion's edge (Figure 3.42). Hypergranulosis with large clumps of basophilic keratohyaline material lie in the valley of the papillomatosis. Koilocytes, which are large vacuolated cells with small pyknotic single or multiple nuclei, are located in the superficial malpighian layer. In flat warts koilocytes present as a more or less continuous line in the upper epidermis. Condylomata acuminata show marked epidermal acanthosis with hyperkeratosis and parakeratosis and a minor component of papillomatosis with only a few vacuolated koilocytes in the upper malpighian layers. Papillomatosis is more rounded at the base than in common warts, and koilocytes are less frequently seen than other variants of warts and are usually present beneath the areas of parakeratosis (Figures 3.43 and 3.44). Coarse keratohyaline granules are commonly present. Changes of lichen simplex chronicus may be superimposed due to trauma to the lesion. The histopathologist needs to know whether the warts have been treated before biopsy. Podophyllin paints and gels are still a common treatment and, if applied within 48 hours of biopsy, the squamous cells may show severe nuclear and cytoplasmic atypia and large numbers of mitotic figures due to metaphase arrest. These changes can persist long after treatment has stopped. These changes may be a pitfall in the diagnosis of intraepidermal malignancy.

PROTOZOAL INFECTIONS

TRICHOMONIASIS

Trichomonas vaginalis, the causative organism, elicits an acute vaginitis, particularly symptomatic when there is a coexisting bacterial vaginitis, as often occurs. The profuse, offensive vaginal discharge is associated with dysuria, dyspareunia, and vulvovaginal soreness. The vulva is acutely inflamed, with marked reddening, and the vaginal wall is similarly reddened, likened to the appearance of a strawberry. Diagnosis is made by demonstrating the presence of the motile, flagellate organisms in a fresh wet saline preparation of the discharge.

INFESTATIONS

SCABIES

Clinical Features

The female mite, *Sarcoptes scabiei* var. *hominis*, infests the epidermis. The primary means of transmission is direct

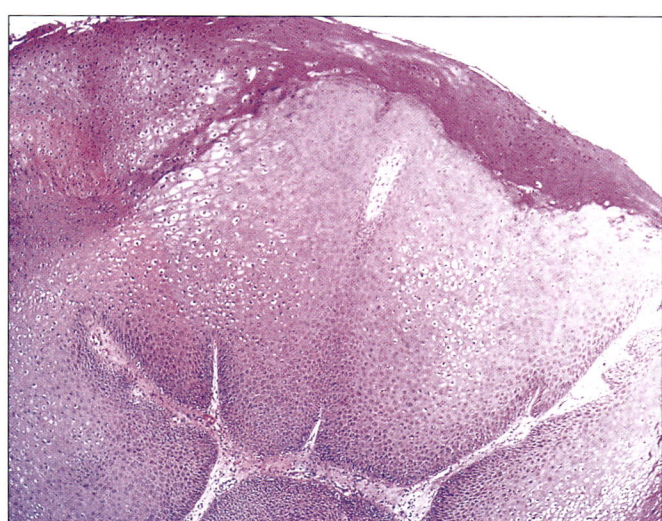

Figure 3.42 Condyloma acuminatum. Hyperplastic thickening of the epidermis with characteristic HPV koilocytosis of many of the epidermal cells.

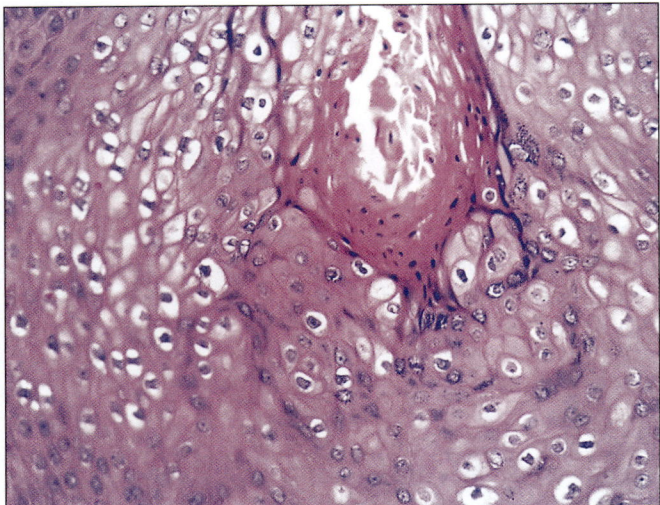

Figure 3.43 Condyloma acuminatum. The koilocytic changes are obvious in most epidermal cells near the surface and are producing parakeratotic keratin.

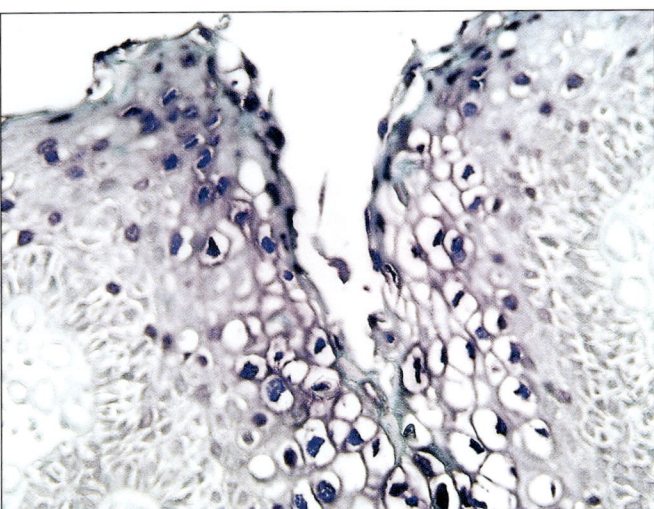

Figure 3.44 Condyloma acuminatum. Positive reaction in the nuclei of koilocytes confirms the presence of HPV (*in situ* hybridization method for HPV).

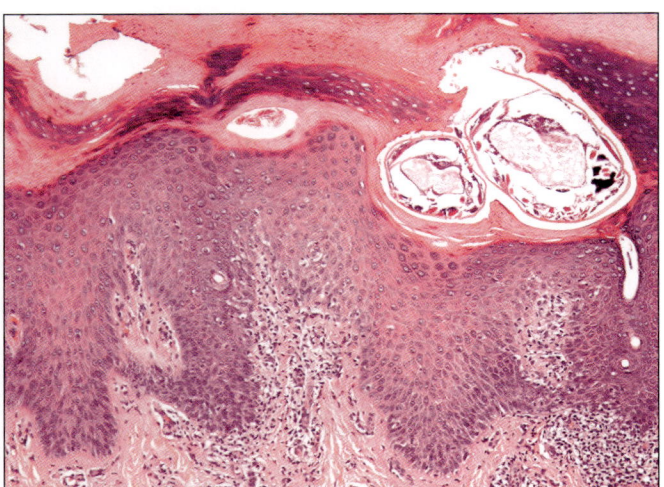

Figure 3.45 Scabies. There is marked hyperkeratosis and epidermal hyperplasia. A mite is seen beneath the stratum corneum.

close contact. The female mite lives out her 30 day life cycle in burrows in the epidermis where she lays her eggs, causing an allergic reaction to the mite protein. The first infestation takes 2–6 weeks before the host is sensitized and develops pruritus. The combination of severe nocturnal itching with the finding of papules/vesicles and visible epidermal burrows in finger webs, nipples, and buttocks are clues to the diagnosis. Secondary bacterial infection is common. In women, the areolae, nipples, and genitals are frequently affected. Persistent nodules affecting the lower trunk, genitalia, and thighs occur in 7% of patients due to a delayed hypersensitivity reaction to the infestation. Crusted scabies, also known as Norwegian scabies, affects immunocompromised patients (elderly individuals, those with HIV, or transplanted patients) or patients suffering from sensory dysfunction (those infected with leprosy or paraplegia). Mites number in the millions in crusted scabies. However, allergic symptoms such as itch are not as pronounced. Clinical confirmation follows by examining skin scrapings with a light microscope and mineral oil to recognize adult mites, eggs, and or fecal pellets. Epiluminescence microscopy is also useful to see mites and eggs.

Microscopic Features

Eggs, larvae, mites, and excreta are located beneath the stratum corneum when the biopsy includes a burrow (Figure 3.45). The epidermis shows spongiosis with exocytosis of eosinophils and occasionally neutrophils. There is a superficial and deep perivascular lymphocytic infiltrate with abundant eosinophils, a reaction similar to that seen with other arthropod infestations or assault. If the eosinophilic infiltrate is exuberant, flame figures (eosinophilic granules lining the collagen fibers) may be seen. Scabetic feces (scybala) or eggs are seen more often than the mite itself in vulvar biopsies. The lesions of persistent nodular scabies have a heavy superficial and deep inflammatory infiltrate including lymphocytes, macrophages, plasma cells, eosinophils, and occasionally atypical mononuclear cells; mites are rarely found. Norwegian scabies shows massive hyperkeratosis and parakeratosis containing numerous mites and psoriasiform epidermal hyperplasia. The dermal changes resemble those of the papulovesicular variant of scabies.

PUBIC (CRAB) LICE (*Phthirus pubis*)

The pubic louse typically affects the axillae and pubis, but any area dense in hair follicles on the trunk or even eyelashes can be colonized. These arthropods feed at night from the patient's blood and cement their eggs to the hair, forming minute gritty projections called nits. The pruritus associated with feeding bites leads to excoriation and secondary bacterial folliculitis. Multiple bluish spots can be seen on the trunk of individuals with pubic lice (maculae ceruleae). The immune status of these patients appears to affect the infestation. Hairs can be extracted and examined under the microscope in the search for eggs. Vulvar biopsy is not required.

GLOSSARY OF COMMON CLINICAL DERMATOLOGIC TERMS[141]

Atopy (adj. atopic): Inherited predisposition to hypersensitivity reactions when exposed to certain allergens. Atopic disorders include asthma, allergic rhinitis, atopic eczema, and urticaria.

Dermatosis (pl. dermatoses): A nonspecific term used to denote a cutaneous eruption, but generally excluding solitary or multiple benign or malignant skin lesions.

Eczematous: A pattern of inflammatory skin changes characterized in the acute stages by erythema and exudation and in the chronic form by dry, scaling, fissured skin.

Erythema: Redness of the skin due to vasodilatation of cutaneous blood vessels. This may result from inflammation or from physiologic or pathologic changes in cutaneous vasculature.

Hart's line: A visible line on the inner surface of the labia minora indicating the change from vestibular epithelium (endoderm derived) to skin (ectodermal derived).

Lichenification: Changes seen in skin after long-standing itching and scratching. The skin becomes thickened with exaggeration of normal skin markings. Hyperpigmentation is often a feature.

Lichenoid: Rashes sharing clinical features (of shiny purple-red papules and plaques) with lichen planus. Examples include certain drug eruptions and photosensitive disorders.

Psoriasiform: A pattern of skin inflammation in which scaling plaques are reminiscent of psoriasis. Certain drug eruptions and forms of cutaneous T-cell lymphoma are examples of psoriasiform rashes.

Vulvar vestibule: That part of the vulva lying between Hart's line and the hymen. Contains the openings of the major and minor vestibular glands.

GLOSSARY OF COMMON DERMATOPATHOLOGIC TERMS

TERMS APPLIED TO THE SURFACE KERATIN LAYER

Hyperkeratosis: Describes thickening of the keratin layer inappropriate to the site. The thickness of the keratin layer varies according to site; for example, it is normally very thin on the trunk, but very thick on the soles and palms. Hyperkeratosis may be **orthokeratotic** (in which the keratin is devoid of nuclear remnants) or **parakeratotic** (in which the keratin layer contains the remnants of nuclei from the underlying epidermis). As a general rule, orthokeratotic hyperkeratosis is associated with a thickening of the granular layer of the epidermis (**hypergranulosis**) and parakeratotic hyperkeratosis is associated with diminution of the granular layer. Parakeratosis is almost always indicative of an active abnormality in the underlying epidermis, which should be sought when parakeratosis is seen. Orthokeratotic hyperkeratosis with hypergranulosis is seen in lichen simplex chronicus (see Figure 3.6). Parakeratosis may be seen in active acute dermatitis (see Figure 3.3) and may be marked in psoriasis (see Figure 3.7).

TERMS APPLIED TO THE EPIDERMIS

Acantholysis: The name given to a process in which there is loss of adhesion and contact between adjacent epidermal keratinocytes such that the cells separate one from the other with breakdown of their linking desmosomal junctions, leading to an increase in the intercellular space. Eventually the intercellular spaces become large and fluid-filled, the separated acantholytic cells tending to become rounded off and floating singly or in small clumps within a variably sized bulla. Acantholysis in the vulva is most commonly seen in Hailey–Hailey disease (see Figure 3.21) and in pemphigus vegetans (see Figure 3.17).

Acanthosis: This term is used to describe inappropriate thickening of the epidermal layer. The thickness of the epidermal layer varies according to site, being thin on the trunk and proximal limbs, and thick in areas such as the palms and soles where the skin is exposed to regular frictional forces. Normally thin epidermis frequently undergoes thickening in response to increased frictional forces; in the vulva this is usually due to repeated scratching (see the section Lichen simplex chronicus). There are particular patterns of acanthosis that may assist in histologic diagnosis.

Basal layer hydropic degeneration: A particular pattern of vacuolation and swelling of the cytoplasm of the basal cells of the epidermis due to the intracellular accumulation of water. This is followed by the death of the affected basal cells, some of which appear as eosinophilic spherical bodies in the basal layer or just beneath, called **colloid** or **Civatte bodies**. In the vulva, the combination of basal layer hydropic degeneration and the presence of colloid/Civatte bodies is most frequently seen in the various patterns of lichen planus (see Figure 3.13), but is also seen elsewhere in the body in systemic lupus erythematosus and dermatomyositis.

Bullae (sing. bulla): A bulla is another form of blister which is larger than a vesicle (a vesicle is less than 5 mm in diameter and a bulla is greater than 5 mm in diameter). Although most vesicles arise within the epidermis, bullae can arise either within the epidermis or beneath the dermoepidermal junction.

Civatte body: See **Basal layer hydropic degeneration**.

Exocytosis: Term used to describe an invasion of the epidermis by inflammatory cells (mainly lymphocytes) in association with spongiosis and vesiculation. It is a common histologic feature of inflammatory skin disease of many types.

Papillomatosis: Term used to describe the histologic appearance of marked exaggeration of the dermal papillae by elongation of rete ridges on the dermoepidermal junction and the throwing up into exaggerated folds of the surface epidermis. In the vulva, papillomatosis of epidermis is most frequently seen in condylomata acuminata and papular and keratotic warts.

Psoriasiform acanthosis: In this pattern, the surface of the epidermis is mainly flat but the thickening is due to marked downward elongation of the rete ridges. The epidermis is therefore not uniformly thickened, the areas between rete ridges often showing marked thinning of the epidermis. This is the pattern of epidermal thickening seen most obviously in active psoriasis, hence its name.

Pustule: A pustule is a vesicle that contains inflammatory cells in large numbers, usually neutrophil polymorphs. The presence of the cells renders the vesicle fluid thick and creamy, and the clinically visible vesicle appears white. Pustules may be seen in the vulva in bacterial infections (particularly staphylococcal and streptococcal) and in some forms of psoriasis.

Spongiosis: The name given to focal intercellular edema of the epidermis leading to partial separation of the epidermal cells by edema fluid, particularly in the prickle cell layer. Accumulation of fluid between epidermal cells causes spaces to appear that may coalesce to form fluid-filled vesicles.

Vesicles: Small discrete accumulations of fluid within the epidermis to form a tiny blister, which may be apparent clinically. Vesicle formation usually follows spongiosis (see above).

TERMS APPLIED TO THE DERMIS

Lichenoid infiltrate: An infiltrate of chronic inflammatory cells (predominantly lymphocytes), which occupies a band-like zone in the upper dermis immediately beneath the dermoepidermal junction. It is a characteristic feature of lichen planus and the very early stages of lichen sclerosus.

Urticaria: Histologically manifested by dermal edema. This may be difficult to detect histologically, but useful clues are the presence in the upper dermis of dilated small lymphatics, and the presence of a distinct pale zone of edema around upper dermal blood vessels. In acute urticaria (rarely biopsied) upper dermal capillaries and venules show margination of neutrophils; in persistent chronic urticaria there is often a scanty perivascular lymphocytic infiltrate in which special stains (e.g., chloroacetate esterase) reveal increased numbers of mast cells. Urticaria of the vulva is an important cause of itchiness, and the histologic diagnosis is frequently missed because the changes are so subtle.

ACKNOWLEDGEMENTS

We would like to thank Dr. Stanley J. Robboy for his contribution to the chapter in the prior edition. We especially thank Dr. Jaime Prat for his insightful editorial comments.

REFERENCES

1. Ball SB, Wojnarowska F. Vulvar dermatoses: lichen sclerosus, lichen planus, and vulval dermatitis/lichen simplex chronicus. Semin Cutan Med Surg 1998;17(3):182–8.
2. Fischer G, Spurrett B, Fischer A. The chronically symptomatic vulva: aetiology and management. Br J Obstet Gynaecol 1995;102(10):773–9.
3. Foster DC. Vulvar disease. Obstet Gynecol 2002;100(1):145–63.
4. Heller DS, Randolph P, Young A, et al. The cutaneous-vulvar clinic revisited: a 5-year experience of the Columbia Presbyterian Medical Center Cutaneous-Vulvar Service. Dermatology 1997;195(1):26–9.
5. Lewis FM. Vulval disease from the 1800s to the new millennium. J Cutan Med Surg 2002;6(4):340–4. [Epub 2002 Apr 15].
6. McKay M. Vulvar dermatoses: common problems in dermatological and gynaecological practice. Br J Clin Pract Suppl 1990;71:5–10.
7. O'Keefe RJ, Scurry JP, Dennerstein G, et al. Audit of 114 non-neoplastic vulvar biopsies. Br J Obstet Gynaecol 1995;102(10):780–6.
8. Sullivan AK, Straughair GJ, Marwood RP, et al. A multidisciplinary vulva clinic: the role of genito-urinary medicine. J Eur Acad Dermatol Venereol 1999;13(1):36–40.
9. Tan AL, Jones R, McPherson G, Rowan D. Audit of a multidisciplinary vulvar clinic in a gynecologic hospital. J Reprod Med 2000;45(8):655–8.
10. Lynch PJ. 2006 International Society for the Study of Vulvovaginal Disease classification of vulvar dermatoses: a synopsis. J Low Genit Tract Dis 2007;11(1):1–2.
11. Lynch PJ, Moyal-Barrocco M, Bogliatto F, et al. 2006 ISSVD classification of vulvar dermatoses: pathologic subsets and their clinical correlates. J Reprod Med 2007;52(1):3–9.
12. Bauer A, Rodiger C, Greif C, et al. Vulvar dermatoses—irritant and allergic contact dermatitis of the vulva. Dermatology 2005;210(2):143–9.
13. Eason EL, Feldman P. Contact dermatitis associated with the use of Always sanitary napkins. CMAJ 1996;154(8):1173–6.
14. Elsner P, Wilhelm D, Maibach HI. Multiple parameter assessment of vulvar irritant contact dermatitis. Contact Dermatitis 1990;23(1):20–6.
15. Hammock LA, Barrett TL. Inflammatory dermatoses of the vulva. J Cutan Pathol 2005;32(9):604–11.
16. Marren P, Wojnarowska F, Powell S. Allergic contact dermatitis and vulvar dermatoses. Br J Dermatol 1992;126(1):52–6.
17. Farage M, Maibach HI. The vulvar epithelium differs from the skin: implications for cutaneous testing to address topical vulvar exposures. Contact Dermatitis 2004;51(4):201–9.
18. Schlosser BJ. Contact dermatitis of the vulva. Dermatol Clin 2010;28(4):697–706. Review.
19. Lynch PJ, Moyal-Barrocco M, Bogliotto F (2007) ISSVD classification of vulvar dermatoses: pathologic subsets and their clinical correlates. J Reprod Med 2007;52:3–9.
20. Meeuwis KA, de Hullu JA, Massuger LF, et al. Genital psoriasis: a systematic literature review on this hidden skin disease. Acta Derm Venereol 2011;91(1):5–11. Review.
21. Wang G, Li C, Gao T, Liu Y. Clinical analysis of 48 cases of inverse psoriasis: a hospital-based study. Eur J Dermatol 2005;15(3):176–8.
22. Carlson JA, Lamb P, Malfetano J, et al. Clinicopathologic comparison of vulvar and extragenital lichen sclerosus: histologic variants, evolving lesions, and etiology of 141 cases. Mod Pathol 1998;11(9):844–54.
23. Friedrich Jr EG, MacLaren NK. Genetic aspects of vulvar lichen sclerosus. Am J Obstet Gynecol 1984;150(2):161–6.
24. Berth-Jones J, Graham-Brown RA, Burns DA. Lichen sclerosus et atrophicus—a review of 15 cases in young girls. Clin Exp Dermatol 1991;16(1):14–7.
25. Loening-Baucke V. Lichen sclerosus et atrophicus in children. Am J Dis Child 1991;145(9):1058–61.
26. Isaac R, Lyn M, Triggs N. Lichen sclerosus in the differential diagnosis of suspected child abuse cases. Pediatr Emerg Care 2007;23(7):482–5.
27. Carlson JA, Ambros R, Malfetano J, et al. Vulvar lichen sclerosus and squamous cell carcinoma: a cohort, case control, and

investigational study with historical perspective; implications for chronic inflammation and sclerosis in the development of neoplasia. Hum Pathol 1998;29(9):932–48.
28. Cattaneo A, Bracco GL, Maestrini G, et al. Lichen sclerosus and squamous hyperplasia of the vulva. A clinical study of medical treatment. J Reprod Med 1991;36(4):301–5.
29. Chiesa-Vottero A, Dvoretsky PM, Hart WR. Histopathologic study of thin vulvar squamous cell carcinomas and associated cutaneous lesions: a correlative study of 48 tumors in 44 patients with analysis of adjacent vulvar intraepithelial neoplasia types and lichen sclerosus. Am J Surg Pathol 2006;30(3):310–8.
30. Hart WR, Norris HJ, Helwig EB. Relation of lichen sclerosus et atrophicus of the vulva to development of carcinoma. Obstet Gynecol 1975;45(4):369–77.
31. Nasca MR, Innocenzi D, Micali G. Penile cancer among patients with genital lichen sclerosus. J Am Acad Dermatol 1999;41(6):911–4.
32. Murphy R. Lichen sclerosus. Dermatol Clin 2010;28(4):707–15.
33. Farrell AM, Dean D, Millard PR, et al. Cytokine alterations in lichen sclerosus: An immunohistochemical study. Br J Dermatol 2006;155(5):931–40.
34. Gomez Rueda N, Garcia A, Vighi S, et al. Epithelial alterations adjacent to invasive squamous carcinoma of the vulva. J Reprod Med 1994;39(7):526–30.
35. Zaki I, Dalziel KL, Solomonsz FA, Stevens A. The under-reporting of skin disease in association with squamous cell carcinoma of the vulva. Clin Exp Dermatol 1996;21(5):334–7.
36. Scrimin F, Rustja S, Radillo O, et al. Vulvar lichen sclerosus: an immunologic study. Obstet Gynecol 2000;95:147–50.
37. Regauer S, Liegl B, Reich O. Early vulvar lichen sclerosus: a histopathological challenge. Histopathology 2005;47:340–7.
38. Marren P, Yell J, Charnock FM, et al. The association between lichen sclerosus and antigens of the HLA system. Br J Dermatol 1995;132(2):197–203.
39. Meyrick Thomas RH, Ridley CM, McGibbon DH, Black MM. Lichen sclerosus et atrophicus and autoimmunity—a study of 350 women. Br J Dermatol 1988;118(1):41–6.
40. Purcell KG, Spencer LV, Simpson PM, et al. HLA antigens in lichen sclerosus et atrophicus. Arch Dermatol 1990;126(8):1043–5.
41. Cooper SM, Ali I, Baldo M, Wojnarowska F. The association of lichen sclerosus and erosive lichen planus of the vulva with autoimmune disease: a case-control study. Arch Dermatol 2008;144(11):1432–5.
42. Scurry J, Beshay V, Cohen C, Allen D. Ki67 expression in lichen sclerosus of vulva in patients with and without associated squamous cell carcinoma. Histopathology 1998; 32:399–404.
43. Hewitt J. Histologic criteria for lichen sclerosus of the vulva. J Reprod Med 1986;31(9):781–7.
44. Leibowitch M. Lichen sclerosus. Semin Dermatol 1996;15(1):42–6.
45. Yang B, Hart WR. Vulvar intraepithelial neoplasia of the simplex (differentiated) type: a clinicopathologic study including analysis of HPV and p53 expression. Am J Surg Pathol 2000; 24:429–41.
46. Raspollini MR, Asirelli G, Moncini D, Taddei GL. A comparative analysis of lichen sclerosus of the vulva and lichen sclerosus that evolves to vulvar squamous cell carcinoma. Am J Obstet Gynecol 2007;197(6):592.e1–5.
47. van der Avoort IA, van der Laak JA, Paffen A, et al. MIB1 expression in basal cell layer: a diagnostic tool to identify premalignancies of the vulva. Mod Pathol 2007;20(7):770–8.
48. Smith YR, Haefner HK. Vulvar lichen sclerosus : pathophysiology and treatment. Am J Clin Dermatol 2004;5(2):105–25.
49. Edwards L. Vulvar lichen planus. Arch Dermatol 1989;125(12):1677–80.
50. Lewis FM. Vulval lichen planus. Br J Dermatol 1998;138(4):569–75.
51. Lewis FM, Shah M, Harrington CI. Vulval involvement in lichen planus: a study of 37 women. Br J Dermatol 1996;135(1):89–91.
52. Eisen D. The vulvovaginal-gingival syndrome of lichen planus. The clinical characteristics of 22 patients. Arch Dermatol 1994;130(11):1379–82.
53. Kirtschig G, Wakelin SH, Wojnarowska F. Mucosal vulval lichen planus: outcome, clinical and laboratory features. J Eur Acad Dermatol Venereol 2005;19(3):301–7.
54. Lotery HE, Galask RP. Erosive lichen planus of the vulva and vagina. Obstet Gynecol 2003;101(5 Pt 2):1121–5.
55. Mann MS, Kaufman RH. Erosive lichen planus of the vulva. Clin Obstet Gynecol 1991;34(3):605–13.
56. Pelisse M. Erosive vulvar lichen planus and desquamative vaginitis. Semin Dermatol 1996;15(1):47–50.
57. Dwyer CM, Kerr RE, Millan DW. Squamous carcinoma following lichen planus of the vulva. Clin Exp Dermatol 1995;20(2):171–2.
58. Franck JM, Young Jr AW. Squamous cell carcinoma in situ arising within lichen planus of the vulva. Dermatol Surg 1995; 21(10):890–4.
59. Helander SD, Rogers 3rd RS. The sensitivity and specificity of direct immunofluorescence testing in disorders of mucous membranes. J Am Acad Dermatol 1994;30(1):65–75.
60. Bernard P, Vaillant L, Labeille B, et al. Incidence and distribution of subepidermal autoimmune bullous skin diseases in three French regions. Bullous Diseases French Study Group. Arch Dermatol 1995;131(1):48–52.
61. Marren P, Wojnarowska F, Venning V, et al. Vulvar involvement in autoimmune bullous diseases. J Reprod Med 1993;38(2):101–7.
62. Malik M, Ahmed AR. Involvement of the female genital tract in pemphigus vulgaris. Obstet Gynecol 2005;106(5 Pt 1):1005–12.
63. Zosmer A, Kogan S, Frumkin A, et al. Unsuspected involvement of the female genitalia in pemphigus vulgaris. Eur J Obstet Gynecol Reprod Biol 1992;47(3):260–3.
64. Bifulco G, Mandato VD, Piccoli R, et al. Early invasive vulvar squamous cell carcinoma arising in a woman with vulvar pemphigus vulgaris and systemic lupus erythematosus. BMC Cancer 2010;10:324.
65. Farrell AM, Kirtschig G, Dalziel KL, et al. Childhood vulval pemphigoid: a clinical and immunopathological study of five patients. Br J Dermatol 1999;140(2):308–12.
66. Goldstein AT, Anhalt GJ, Klingman D, Burrows LJ. Mucous membrane pemphigoid of the vulva. Obstet Gynecol 2005;105(5 Pt 2):1188–90.
67. Guenther LC, Shum D. Localized childhood vulvar pemphigoid. J Am Acad Dermatol 1990;22(5 Pt 1):762–4.
68. Saad RW, Domloge-Hultsch N, Yancey KB, et al. Childhood localized vulvar pemphigoid is a true variant of bullous pemphigoid. Arch Dermatol 1992;128(6):807–10.
69. Urano S. Localized bullous pemphigoid of the vulva. J Dermatol 1996;23(8):580–2.
70. Frith P, Charnock M, Wojnarowska F. Cicatricial pemphigoid diagnosed from ocular features in recurrent severe vulval scarring. Two case reports. Br J Obstet Gynaecol 1991;98(5):482–4.
71. Marren P, Walkden V, Mallon E, Wojnarowska F. Vulval cicatricial pemphigoid may mimic lichen sclerosus. Br J Dermatol 1996;134(3):522–4.
72. Edwards L, Hays S. Vulva r cicatricial pemphigoid as a lichen sclerosus imitator. A case report. J Reprod Med 1992;37(6):561–4.
73. Langenberg A, Berger TG, Cardelli M, et al. Genital benign chronic pemphigus (Hailey–Hailey disease) presenting as condylomas. J Am Acad Dermatol 1992;26(6):951–5.
74. Wieselthier JS, Pincus SH. Hailey–Hailey disease of the vulva. Arch Dermatol 1993;129(10):1344–5.
75. Evron S, Leviatan A, Okon E. Familial benign chronic pemphigus appearing as leukoplakia of the vulva. Int J Dermatol 1984; 23(8):556–7.
76. Hazelrigg DE, Stoller LJ. Isolated familial benign chronic pemphigus. Arch Dermatol 1977;113(9):1302.
77. Vaclavinkova V, Neumann E. Vaginal involvement in familial benign chronic pemphigus (Morbus Hailey–Hailey). Acta Derm Venereol 1982;62(1):80–1.
78. von Felbert V, Hampl M, Talhari C, et al. Squamous cell carcinoma arising from a localized vulval lesion of Hailey–Hailey disease after tacrolimus therapy. Am J Obstet Gynecol 2010;203(3):e5–7.
79. Holst VA, Fair KP, Wilson BB, Patterson JW. Squamous cell carcinoma arising in Hailey–Hailey disease. J Am Acad Dermatol 2000;43(2 Pt 2):368–71.
80. Craddock N, Dawson E, Burge S, et al. The gene for Darier's disease maps to chromosome 12q23–q24.1. Hum Mol Genet 1993;2(11):1941–3.
81. Barrett JF, Murray LA, MacDonald HN. Darier's disease localized to the vulva. Case report. Br J Obstet Gynaecol 1989;96(8):997–9.
82. Ridley CM, Buckley CH. Darier's disease localized to the vulva. Br J Obstet Gynaecol 1991;98(1):112.

83. Salopek TG, Krol A, Jimbow K. Case report of Darier disease localized to the vulva in a 5-year-old girl. Pediatr Dermatol 1993;10(2):146–8.
84. Vázquez J, Morales C, González LO, et al. Vulval squamous cell carcinoma arising in localized Darier's disease. Eur J Obstet Gynecol Reprod Biol 2002;102(2):206–8.
85. Kavanagh GM, Burton PA, Kennedy CT. Vulvitis chronica plasmacellularis (Zoon's vulvitis). Br J Dermatol 1993;129(1):92–3.
86. Salopek TG, Siminoski K. Vulvitis circumscripta plasmacellularis (Zoon's vulvitis) associated with autoimmune polyglandular endocrine failure. Br J Dermatol 1996;135(6):991–4.
87. Scurry J, Dennerstein G, Brenan J, et al. Vulvitis circumscripta plasmacellularis. A clinicopathologic entity? J Reprod Med 1993;38(1):14–8.
88. Yoganathan S, Bohl TG, Mason G. Plasma cell balanitis and vulvitis (of Zoon). A study of 10 cases. J Reprod Med 1994;39(12):939–44.
89. Li Q, Leopold K, Carlson JA. Chronic vulvar purpura: persistent pigmented purpuric dermatitis (lichen aureus) of the vulva or plasma cell (Zoon's) vulvitis? J Cutan Pathol 2003;30(9):572–6.
90. Neri I, Patrizi A, Marzaduri S, et al. Vulvitis plasmacellularis: two new cases. Genitourin Med 1995;71(5):311–3.
91. Brix WK, Nassau SR, Patterson JW, et al. Idiopathic lymphoplasmacellular mucositis-dermatitis. J Cutan Pathol 2010;37(4):426–31.
92. Meneux E, Wolkenstein P, Haddad B, et al. Vulvovaginal involvement in toxic epidermal necrolysis: a retrospective study of 40 cases. Obstet Gynecol 1998;91(2):283–7.
93. Criteria for diagnosis of Behcet's disease. International Study Group for Behcet's Disease. Lancet 1990;335(8697):1078–80.
94. Jorizzo JL, Abernethy JL, White WL, et al. Mucocutaneous criteria for the diagnosis of Behcet's disease: an analysis of clinicopathologic data from multiple international centers. J Am Acad Dermatol 1995;32(6):968–76.
95. Magro CM, Crowson AN. Cutaneous manifestations of Behcet's disease. Int J Dermatol 1995;34(3):159–65.
96. Mangelsdorf HC, White WL, Jorizzo JL. Behcet's disease. Report of twenty-five patients from the United States with prominent mucocutaneous involvement. J Am Acad Dermatol 1996;34(5 Pt 1):745–50.
97. Haidopoulos D, Rodolakis A, Stefanidis K, et al. Behcet's disease: part of the differential diagnosis of the ulcerative vulva. Clin Exp Obstet Gynecol 2002;29(3):219–21.
98. Fenniche S, Mokni M, Haouet S, Ben Osman A. Vulvar Crohn disease: 3 cases. Ann Dermatol Venereol 1997;124(9):629–32.
99. Gunthert AR, Hinney B, Nesselhut K, et al. Vulvitis granulomatosa and unilateral hypertrophy of the vulva related to Crohn's disease: a case report. Am J Obstet Gynecol 2004;191(5):1719–20.
100. Schrodt BJ, Callen JP. Metastatic Crohn's disease presenting as chronic perivulvar and perirectal ulcerations in an adolescent patient. Pediatrics 1999;103(2):500–2.
101. Leu S, Sun PK, Collyer J, et al. Clinical spectrum of vulva metastatic Crohn's disease. Dig Dis Sci 2009;54(7):1565–71.
102. Corbett SL, Walsh CM, Spitzer RF, et al. Vulvar inflammation as the only clinical manifestation of Crohn disease in an 8-year-old girl. Pediatrics 2010;125(6):e1518–22.
103. Fahmy N, Kalidindi M, Khan R. Direct colo-labial Crohn's abscess mimicking bartholinitis. J Obstet Gynaecol 2010;30(7):741–2.
104. Goldberg JM, Buchler DA, Dibbell DG. Advanced hidradenitis suppurativa presenting with bilateral vulvar masses. Gynecol Oncol 1996;60(3):494–7.
105. Short KA, Kalu G, Mortimer PS, Higgins EM. Vulval squamous cell carcinoma arising in chronic hidradenitis suppurativa. Clin Exp Dermatol 2005;30(5):481–3.
106. Furlonge CB, Thin RN, Evans BE, McKee PH. Vulvar vestibulitis syndrome: a clinico-pathological study. Br J Obstet Gynaecol 1991;98(7):703–6.
107. Graziottin A, Brotto LA. Vulvar vestibulitis syndrome: a clinical approach. J Sex Marital Ther 2004;30(3):125–39.
108. Marinoff SC, Turner ML. Vulvar vestibulitis syndrome. Dermatol Clin 1992;10(2):435–44.
109. Gardella C. Vulvar vestibulitis syndrome. Curr Infect Dis Rep 2006;8(6):473–80.
110. Zolnoun D, Hartmann K, Lamvu G, et al. A conceptual model for the pathophysiology of vulvar vestibulitis syndrome. Obstet Gynecol Surv 2006;61(6):395–401; quiz 23.
111. Halperin R, Zehavi S, Vaknin Z, et al. The major histopathologic characteristics in the vulvar vestibulitis syndrome. Gynecol Obstet Invest 2005;59(2):75–9.
112. Davis GD, Hutchison CV. Clinical management of vulvodynia. Clin Obstet Gynecol 1999;42(2):221–33.
113. Edwards L. New concepts in vulvodynia. Am J Obstet Gynecol 2003;189(3 Suppl):S24–30.
114. Haefner HK, Collins ME, Davis GD, et al. The vulvodynia guideline. J Low Genit Tract Dis 2005;9(1):40–51.
115. Sonnendecker EW, Sonnendecker HE, Wright CA, Simon GB. Recalcitrant vulvodynia. A clinicopathological study. S Afr Med J 1993;83(10):730–3.
116. Dupre A, Viraben R. Laugier's disease. Dermatologica 1990;181(3):183–6.
117. Estrada R, Kaufman R. Benign vulvar melanosis. J Reprod Med 1993;38(1):5–8.
118. Barnhill RL, Albert LS, Shama SK, et al. Genital lentiginosis: a clinical and histopathologic study. J Am Acad Dermatol 1990;22(3):453–60.
119. Torley D, Bellus GA, Munro CS. Genes, growth factors and acanthosis nigricans. Br J Dermatol 2002;147(6):1096–101.
120. Samdani AJ. Ectodermal dysplasia with acanthosis nigricans (Lelis' syndrome). J Coll Physicians Surg Pak 2004;14(10):626–7.
121. Arnaud-Lopez L, Fragoso R, Mantilla-Capacho J, Barros-Nunez P. Crouzon with acanthosis nigricans. Further delineation of the syndrome. Clin Genet 2007;72(5):405–10.
122. Leroy JG, Nuytinck L, Lambert J, et al. Acanthosis nigricans in a child with mild osteochondrodysplasia and K650Q mutation in the FGFR3 gene. Am J Med Genet 2007;143A(24):3144–9.
123. Rigel DS, Jacobs MI. Malignant acanthosis nigricans: a review. J Dermatol Surg Oncol 1980;6(11):923–7.
124. Naughton GK, Reggiardo D, Bystryn JC. Correlation between vitiligo antibodies and extent of depigmentation in vitiligo. J Am Acad Dermatol 1986;15(5 Pt 1):978–81.
125. Choi HJ, Ku JK, Kim MY, et al. Possible role of Fas/Fas ligand-mediated apoptosis in the pathogenesis of fixed drug eruptions. Br J Dermatol 2006;154(3):419–25.
126. Hurwitz RM, Leaming RD, Horine RK. Necrotic cellulitis. A localized form of septic vasculitis. Arch Dermatol 1984;120(1):87–92.
127. Smith G, Holman RP. The prozone phenomenon with syphilis and HIV-1 co-infection. South Med J 2004;97(4):379–82.
128. Hoang MP, High WA, Molberg KH. Secondary syphilis: a histologic and immunohistochemical evaluation. J Cutan Pathol 2004;31(9):595–9.
129. Mehrany K, Kist JM, O'Connor WJ, DiCaudo DJ. Disseminated gonococcemia. Int J Dermatol 2003;42(3):208–9.
130. Schachter J, Osoba AO. Lymphogranuloma venereum. Br Med Bull 1983;39(2):151–4.
131. Eckert LO, Hawes SE, Stevens CE, et al. Vulvovaginal candidiasis: clinical manifestations, risk factors, management algorithm. Obstet Gynecol 1998;92(5):757–65.
132. Sobel JD. Candida vulvovaginitis. Semin Dermatol 1996;15(1):17–28.
133. Nader SN, Prober CG. Herpesvirus infections of the vulva. Semin Dermatol 1996;15(1):8–16.
134. Palamaras I, Richardson D, Healy V, et al. An atypical herpetic vulval ulcer in an African woman: an important lesson. Int J STD AIDS 2006;17(6):427–8.
135. Lowhagen GB, Bonde E, Forsgren-Brusk U, et al. The microenvironment of vulvar skin in women with symptomatic and asymptomatic herpes simplex virus type 2 (HSV-2) infection. J Eur Acad Dermatol Venereol 2006;20(9):1086–9.
136. Nahmias AJ, Lee FK, Beckman-Nahmias S. Sero-epidemiological and -sociological patterns of herpes simplex virus infection in the world. Scand J Infect Dis Suppl 1990;69:19–36.
137. Dupin N. Genital warts. Clin Dermatol 2004;22(6):481–6.
138. Beutner KR. Human papilloma virus infection of the vulva. Semin Dermatol 1996;15(1):2–7.
139. Srodon M, Stoler MH, Baber GB, Kurman RJ. The distribution of low and high-risk HPV types in vulvar and vaginal intraepithelial neoplasia (VIN and VaIN). Am J Surg Pathol 2006;30(12):1513–8.
140. Cuzick J, Arbyn M, Sankaranarayanan R, et al. Overview of human papillomavirus-based and other novel options for cervical cancer screening in developed and developing countries. Vaccine 2008;26(Suppl 10):K29–41.
141. Lynch PJ, Moyal-Barracco M, Scurry J, Stockdale C. Terminology and classification of vulvar dermatological disorders: An approach to clinical diagnosis. Low Genit Tract Dis 2012;16(4):339–44.

Vulvar Squamous Lesions

4

Demaretta S. Rush, Edward J. Wilkinson

CHAPTER OUTLINE

Benign Squamous Neoplasms 79	High-grade VIN, Differentiated or Simplex Type 86
Condyloma Acuminatum 79	Squamous Cell Carcinoma 87
Seborrheic Keratosis 79	Uncommon Subtypes of Squamous Cell Carcinoma 91
Keratoacanthoma 80	Verrucous Carcinoma 91
Squamous Intraepithelial Lesions of the Vulva (VIN) 81	Basal Cell Carcinoma 92
HPV-related Low- and High-grade Squamous Intraepithelial Lesions (VIN 1–3) 81	Sebaceous Carcinoma 93

BENIGN SQUAMOUS NEOPLASMS

CONDYLOMA ACUMINATUM

Definition

Condyloma acuminatum is a benign exophytic lesion caused by infection with low-risk human papillomavirus (HPV) subtypes, principally types 6 and 11.

Clinical Features

Condylomata are asymptomatic, usually multiple and often multifocal, presenting as papillary growths varying in size from barely visible on gross examination to several centimeters.

Microscopic Features

On histologic examination, the lesion consists of complex branching fibrovascular cores covered with acanthotic squamous epithelium, frequently with accompanying hyperkeratosis and parakeratosis. Pathognomonic findings include basal and parabasal hyperplasia, with koilocytic atypia, manifested by enlarged, hyperchromatic nuclei with irregular, wrinkled nuclear membranes accompanied by a region of perinuclear clearing or 'halo,' in the upper third of the epithelium (Figures 4.1 and 4.2).

Differential Diagnosis

Immunohistochemical reactivity with Ki-67 in condylomata demonstrates cells active in the cell cycle at all layers of the epithelium, which is helpful to distinguish them from other benign exophytic lesions of the vulva, such as fibroepithelial polyp and seborrheic keratosis. Although warty vulvar intraepithelial neoplasm (VIN) and the warty type of squamous cell carcinoma may show marked koilocytic atypia in the superficial cells, they are distinguished from condyloma by the presence of nuclear atypia and numerous, frequently atypical, mitotic figures in deeper layers of the epithelium. Verrucous carcinoma is grossly similar to condyloma, but is distinguished by its characteristic growth pattern with a pushing invasive border.

Clinical Behavior and Treatment

Condylomata may regress spontaneously, but usually persist and may increase in size or number over time. They are not considered premalignant, and do not progress to high-grade VIN or carcinoma. Small lesions can be treated with topical agents or laser or electro-loop ablation. Extensive lesions may require superficial surgical excision.

SEBORRHEIC KERATOSIS

Definition

Seborrheic keratosis is a benign, frequently pigmented wart-like growth common on the sun-exposed skin of the elderly and less commonly seen on the hair-bearing skin of the vulva.

Clinical Features

The typical appearance is of an elevated, often macular–papular, flesh-toned or hyperpigmented lesion, which is well demarcated from the surrounding skin, giving the impression of being 'stuck-on' to the surface. Because of the superficial, exophytic nature of the lesions, they are prone to irritation and trauma, which may lead to secondary changes of inflammation, erythema, and crusting.

Microscopic Features

The epidermis is thickened by a population of cells with basaloid morphology, without significant nuclear atypia or mitotic activity, and with pronounced surface hyperkeratosis. Pigmentation of the basal and parabasal cells is usually

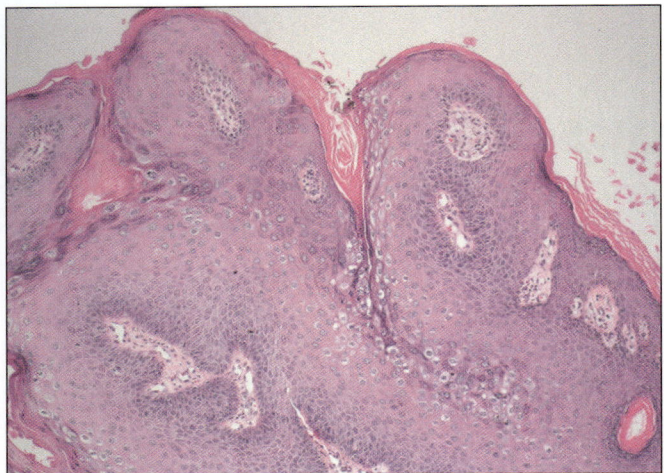

Figure 4.1 Condyloma acuminatum. A complex formation of branching fibrovascular cores is lined by a slightly thickened epithelium with hyperkeratosis apparent on the surface and koilocytic atypia in the superficial third of the epithelium.

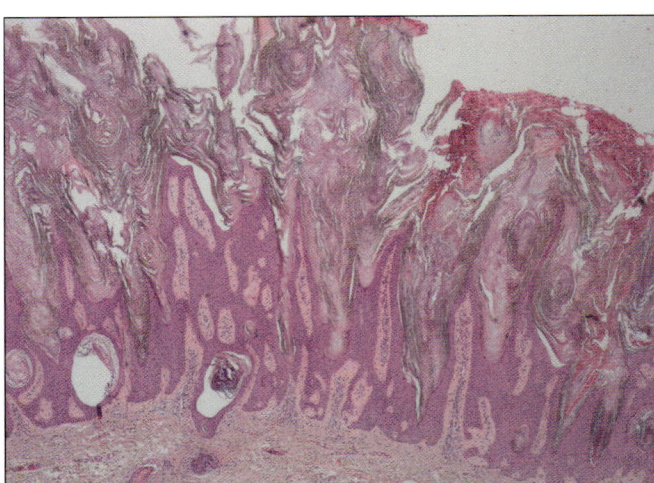

Figure 4.3 Seborrheic keratosis at low power, showing marked hyperkeratosis at the surface and keratin horn cysts toward the base.

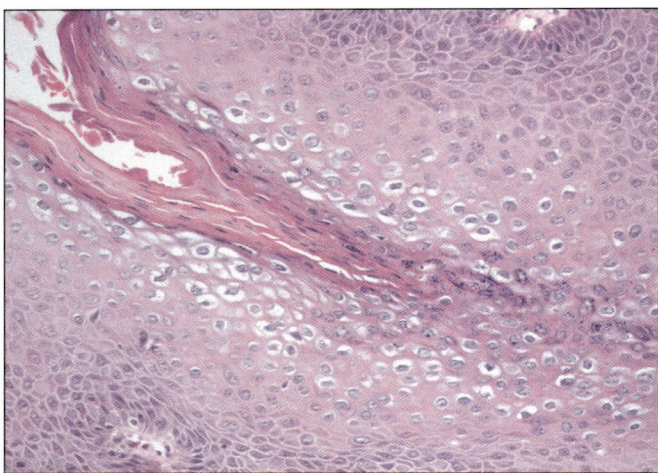

Figure 4.2 Condyloma acuminatum at higher power showing koilocytic atypia and surface parakeratosis.

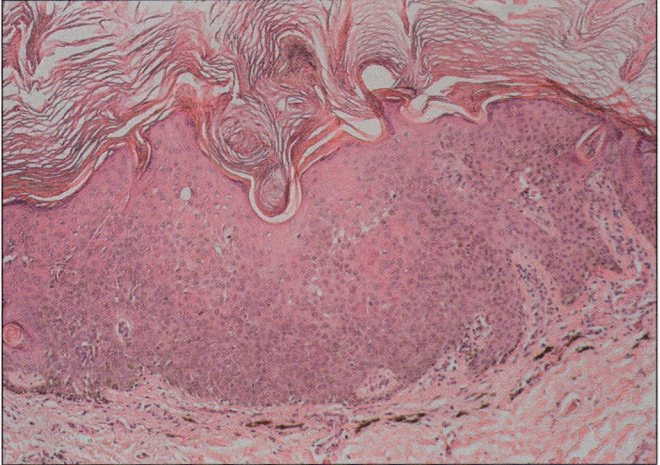

Figure 4.4 Pigmentation of basal cells and numerous squamous eddies in the acanthotic epithelium of seborrheic keratosis.

evident. Invaginations of the surface epithelium result in the accumulation of hyperkeratotic material below the surface of the lesion, in what may appear to be cystic spaces, forming the structures known as 'horn cysts' (Figure 4.3). Follicular plugging with this hyperkeratosis is also typical. 'Squamous eddies,' rounded whorls of squamous cells named for their resemblance to swirling currents in a stream, may be found (Figure 4.4).

Differential Diagnosis

On occasion, reactive changes secondary to trauma or prominence of squamous eddies can be suggestive of squamous cell carcinoma. Key to establishing the correct diagnosis in such cases is the absence of an infiltrative growth pattern. Other entities in the differential diagnosis of seborrheic keratoses on the vulvar skin include condyloma acuminatum, VIN, and melanoma. The papillary architecture and hyperkeratosis of seborrheic keratosis can be suggestive of condyloma, particularly at low power. As seborrheic keratoses are frequently found to contain HPV DNA,[1,2] some authors have maintained that these lesions are, in fact, variants of condyloma,[3] although this remains controversial. The absence of koilocytic atypia in seborrheic keratosis and of keratin horn cysts in condylomata will usually resolve the diagnosis. The lack of significant nuclear atypia or mitotic activity is also of use to differentiate seborrheic keratosis from VIN and melanoma, with immunohistochemistry of further use in distinguishing the latter.

Clinical Behavior and Treatment

Treatment is identical to that of vulvar condylomata; both excisional and topical treatments are available and effective.

KERATOACANTHOMA

Definition

Keratoacanthoma is a distinctive keratinocytic neoplasm characterized by rapid growth and spontaneous regression. Although often considered a low-grade variant of squamous cell carcinoma, this view is not universally accepted,[4-6] and as there have been no reported cases of malignant behavior in cases presenting on the vulva, we present it here as a benign neoplasm.

Clinical Features

Keratoacanthoma characteristically presents as a rapidly growing pink or flesh-colored, firm, well-demarcated dome-shaped lesion with central umbilication. Although common on the sun-exposed skin of the elderly, very few cases occurring on the vulva have been reported.[7-10]

Microscopic Features

The dome-shaped, umbilicated lesion observed on the skin corresponds to an endophytic proliferation of squamous cells forming a keratin-filled crater-like center rimmed by collarette, or 'buttressing lips,' of epidermis. The central squamous cells are well differentiated and tend to become larger toward the center of the proliferation, accumulating abundant glassy, eosinophilic cytoplasm (Figures 4.5 and 4.6). In the early stages of development, mitoses may be numerous and mild to moderate nuclear atypia may be present, but these features regress as the lesion matures, and when well developed only minimal atypia is present. The lesions typically have a rounded, pushing border with a dense inflammatory infiltrate at the base of the lesion.

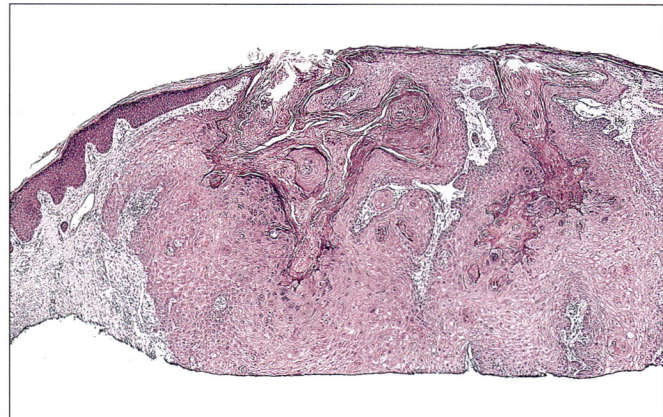

Figure 4.5 Keratoacanthoma at low power, with a 'buttressing lip' of normal epidermis visible on the left side of the lesion.

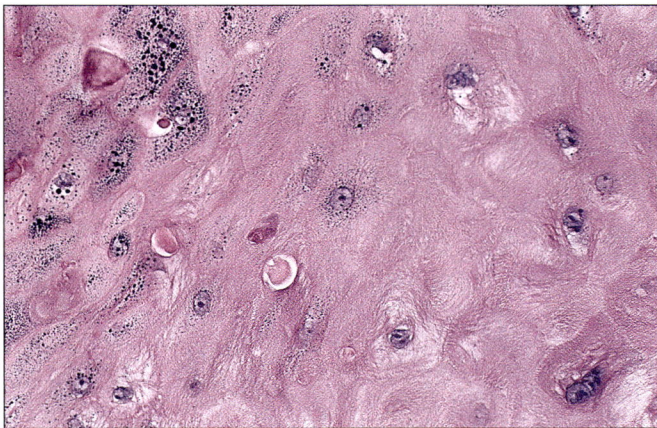

Figure 4.6 Higher magnification of the cells of keratoacanthoma demonstrating the abundant, glassy eosinophilic cytoplasm.

Differential Diagnosis/Clinical Behavior and Treatment

Focal, small, irregular nests of cells, and less commonly perineural or intravascular invasion adjacent to the pushing border of keratoacanthoma may occasionally be seen. Such seemingly infiltrative patterns can be alarming, but in the absence of other features do not warrant a malignant diagnosis.

Untreated, keratoacanthoma typically increases rapidly in size over a period of weeks to months and then may persist for months until finally undergoing spontaneous involution, usually within six months of eruption. Excision is usually curative, with rare recurrences reported.

SQUAMOUS INTRAEPITHELIAL LESIONS OF THE VULVA (VIN)

Definition

About 90% of squamous intraepithelial lesions of the vulva are HPV related, comprising a spectrum of alterations ranging from low-grade squamous intraepithelial lesions VIN (VIN 1), sometimes characterized as 'flat condyloma,' to the severe full-thickness dysplasia of high-grade squamous intraepithelial lesion VIN (VIN 3). Recent proposals from both the International Society for the Study of Vulvovaginal Disease (ISVVD) and the College of Pathologists (CAP)/American Society for Colposcopy and Cervical Pathology (ASCCP) have advocated replacement of the older three-tiered system used to describe these lesions with a two-tiered system (Table 4.1).[11-13]

HPV-RELATED LOW- AND HIGH-GRADE SQUAMOUS INTRAEPITHELIAL LESIONS (VIN 1–3)

Clinical Features

Patients with HPV-related squamous intraepithelial lesions are usually in their thirties or forties, frequently smokers, and frequently have a history of, or concurrent, multifocal

Table 4.1 Commonly Used Classification Schemes for Intraepithelial Disease of the Vulva

1986 VIN Terminology	2009 ISSVD Terminology	2012 CAP/ASCCP Terminology
VIN 1	Condyloma HPV changes	Low grade squamous intraepithelial lesion (VIN 1)
VIN 2	VIN, usual type (uVIN)	High grade squamous intraepithelial lesion (VIN 2–3)
VIN 3	VIN, usual type (uVIN) or VIN, differentiated type (dVIN)	High grade squamous intraepithelial lesion (VIN 2–3) or VIN, differentiated type

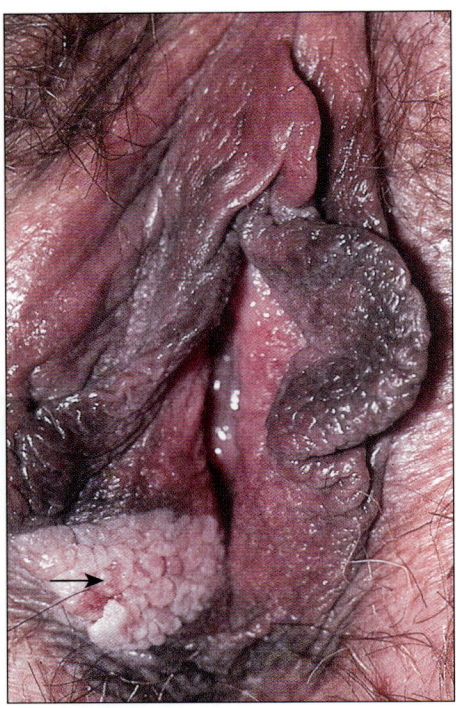

Figure 4.7 Plaque of warty VIN 3 (arrow). The young woman also had cervical dysplasia.

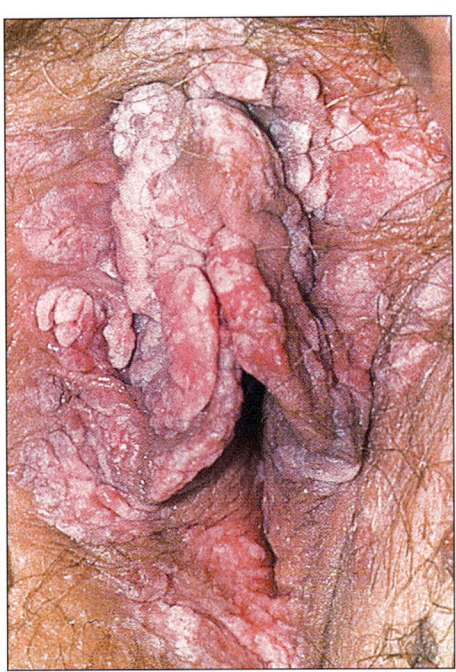

Figure 4.8 Extensive warty VIN 3. This young woman had similar lesions in the perianal skin.

vulvar lesions and/or multicentric oncogenic HPV-related disease, or other sexually transmitted diseases.[14–21] Pruritus is the most common symptom.[20,21] Other symptoms may include pain, ulceration, or dysuria. Approximately 20% of patients are asymptomatic, but may have observed an abnormal area on self-examination.[22,23]

The gross appearance of the lesion is variable. Lesions are usually well demarcated and asymmetric, may appear red, white, pigmented, or mixed, and may be raised, papular, flat, or ulcerated (Figures 4.7 and 4.8).

Pathogenesis/Etiology

The majority of low-grade HPV-related vulvar squamous intraepithelial lesions (LSILs) contain low-risk HPV subtypes, while high-grade lesions (HSILs) typically contain high-risk subtypes, most commonly HPV 16. The estimated time of progression from incident infection to the development of clinical disease has been estimated at 18.5 months.[23]

Microscopic Features

LSIL of the Vulva (VIN 1). Not all authors agree on the value or significance of the category of LSIL (VIN 1), although there is general agreement that it is a rare and poorly reproducible diagnosis.[23–25] The controversy stems from disagreement as to the biologic behavior of these lesions.[12,26–28] Because of its distinctive, albeit uncommon, morphology and its as yet unclear behavior, we prefer to maintain this diagnostic category for flat-macular lesions with epithelial changes resembling those of exophytic condylomata (Figure 4.9).

HSIL of the Vulva (VIN 2–3). For descriptive purposes, high-grade HPV-related lesions of the vulva have been divided into warty and basaloid subtypes. Warty lesions (Figure 4.10A–D) are characterized by a spiky or undulating

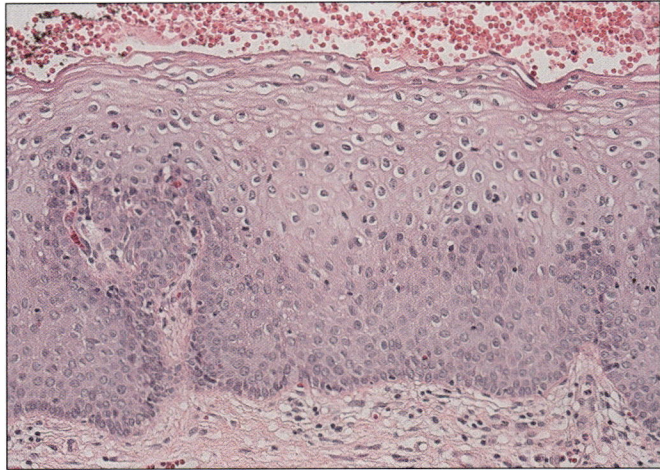

Figure 4.9 VIN 1. Immature cells with architectural disarray are evident in the lower third of the epithelium, and koilocytic atypia is seen in the upper layers of the epithelium without papillary structures.

surface, giving them a condylomatous gross appearance. The markedly thickened epithelium forms wide, deep rete pegs separated by thin dermal papillae that often closely approach the surface. Disorganization and abundant mitotic figures, including abnormal ones, can be seen in all levels of the epithelium, with evidence of maturation and often koilocytic change in the upper layers. Hyperkeratosis is prominent, often with accompanying parakeratosis. Nuclei are enlarged and hyperchromatic, with irregular nuclear membrane contours and prominent pleomorphism. Multinucleated cells, as well as dyskeratotic cells, may be present. An appreciable amount of eosinophilic cytoplasm is present, and the cell borders are easily delineated. Lesions with this morphology were formerly subclassified as VIN 2 or VIN 3, by determination of the proportion of the epithelium populated by

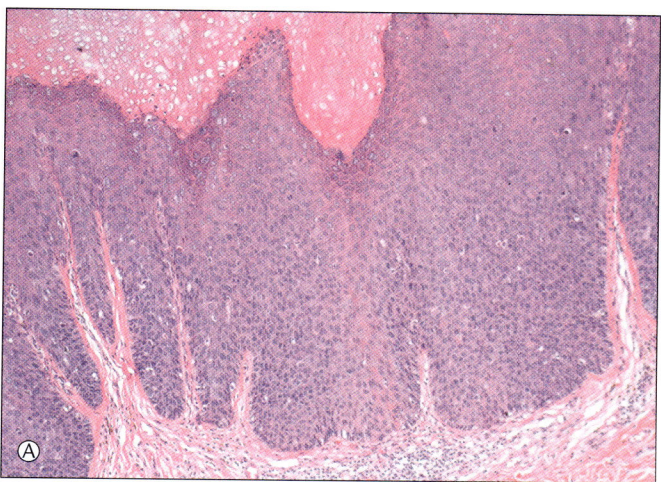
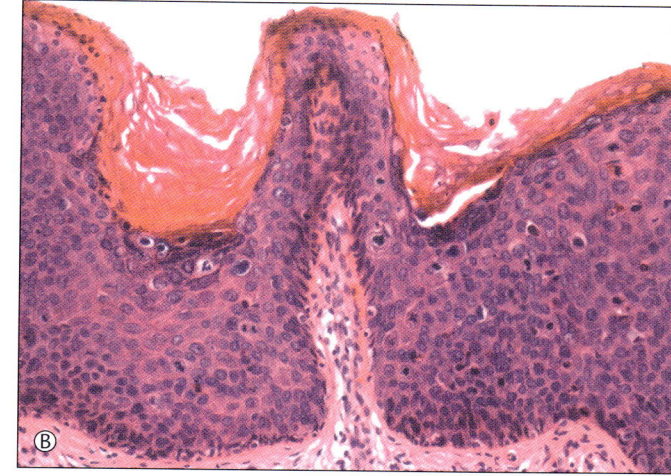
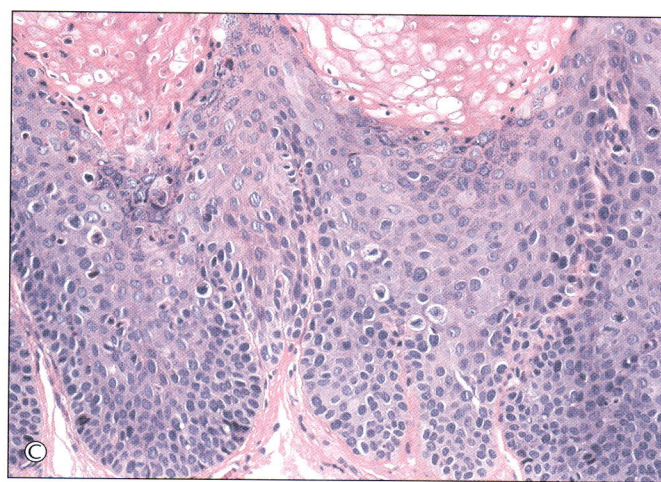
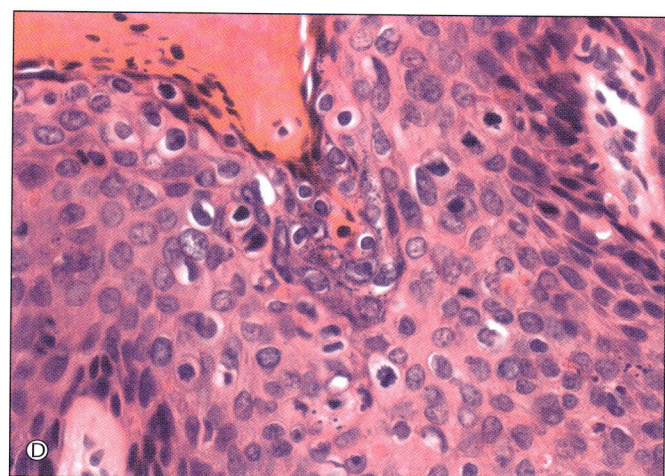

Figure 4.10 **(A)** VIN 3, warty type, showing acanthosis, hyperkeratosis, and widened, deep rete ridges. **(B)** Extension of a long narrow dermal papilla close to the surface is seen in the center of this image. Numerous mitotic figures and dyskeratotic cells can be appreciated throughout all layers of the epithelium. **(C)** Marked nuclear pleomorphism in warty VIN 3, with surface hyperkeratosis and parakeratosis. **(D)** At high power, prominent nuclear atypia, numerous mitotic figures, apoptotic bodies, and dyskeratotic cells are easily identified.

relatively immature cells, with those having immature cells involving no more than two-thirds of the epithelium classified as VIN 2 (Figure 4.11) and those having immature cells involving more than two-thirds of the epithelium as VIN 3.

In contrast to warty lesions, the surface of basaloid lesions is relatively flat. Hyperkeratosis and koilocytosis may be present, but to a lesser degree than is seen in warty lesions. The epithelium is thickened by a relatively uniform population of immature cells with scant cytoplasm, poorly defined cell borders, and enlarged hyperchromatic nuclei (Figure 4.12). As in warty lesions, mitotic activity is readily identified and atypical mitotic figures may be present.

Distinction between warty and basaloid subtypes is not always easy. Mixed forms, containing morphologic features of both types, are not uncommon, and may be designated as such (Figure 4.13), although, as there is no clinical difference between lesions of either morphology, specification is not required for diagnosis.

Routine Biomarkers of Clinical Relevance

Immunohistochemistry for Ki-67 can be useful in identification of LSIL, where it can highlight an abnormal degree of

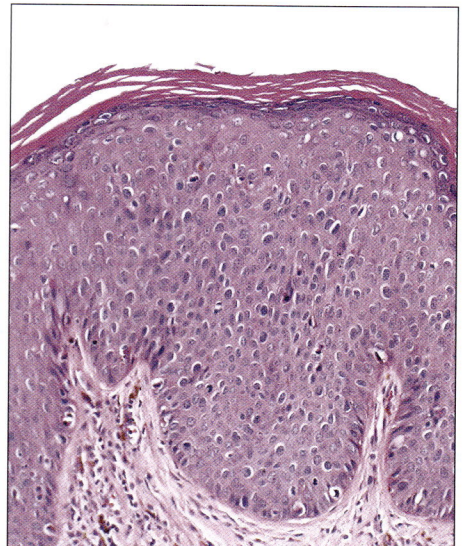

Figure 4.11 VIN 2.

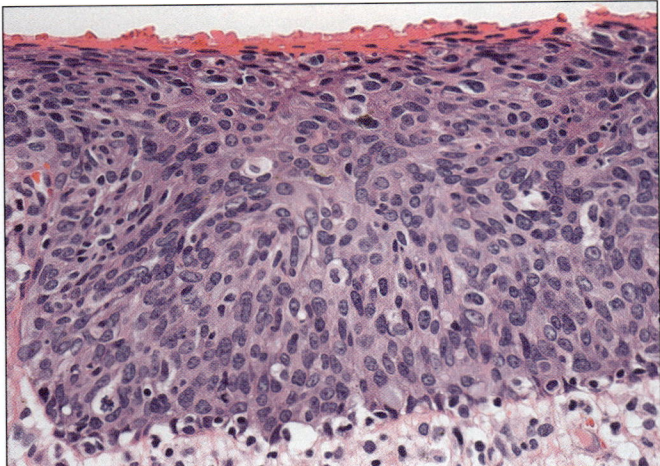

Figure 4.12 VIN 3, basaloid type. A disorganized proliferation of immature cells with nuclear atypia and polymorphism fills the entire thickness of the epithelium.

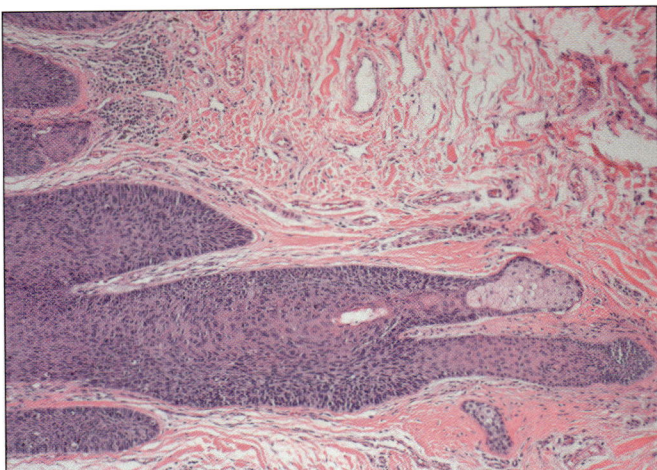

Figure 4.14 VIN 3 with skin appendage involvement. The cells of VIN 3 are palisaded along the periphery of the hair follicle. The involvement does not completely replace the normal epithelium in this case, and the terminal portion of the hair follicle and adjacent sebaceous gland are unaffected. Note how deep the hair follicle extends into the dermis compared with the adjacent epithelium.

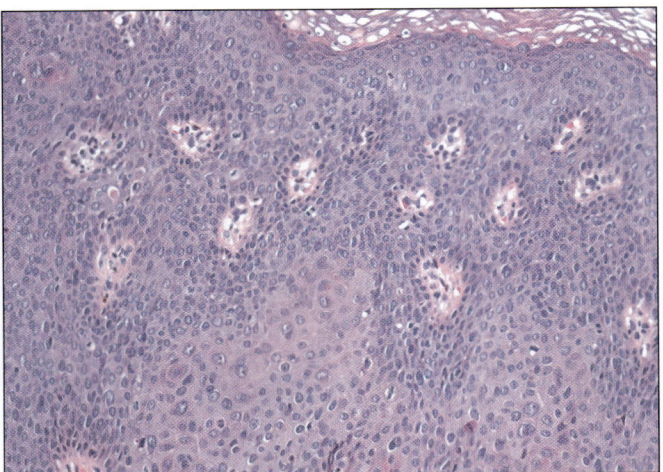

Figure 4.13 Mixed basaloid and warty VIN 3, with evidence of maturation and accumulation of eosinophilic cytoplasm typical of warty lesions in the cells toward the lower right, and more immature basaloid cells along the left edge and middle portion of the image.

proliferation in a cytologically equivocal lesion.[28] Of greater utility in the diagnosis of HSIL is p16^{INK4a}; as a reliable indicator of the presence of high-risk HPV in the vulva,[19,29] it is strongly positive throughout most of the epithelium in HSIL (VIN 3).[19,29,30]

Differential Diagnosis

Although both condyloma acuminatum and warty HSIL (VIN 2–3) may have prominent koilocytic changes, the latter can be distinguished by the presence of atypical, pleomorphic cells in the deeper levels of the epithelium and by the presence of increased mitotic activity, including abnormal mitotic figures, in the upper layers. Seborrheic keratosis and lichen simplex chronicus may have acanthosis and hyperkeratosis, but typically lack the nuclear atypia of HSIL (VIN 2–3). Probably the most common diagnostic dilemma in assessment of HSIL (VIN 2–3) is distinction of truly intraepithelial disease from disease with associated early invasion. This can be complicated by involvement of skin appendages, which may extend quite deeply into the underlying dermis. The distinction rests on the preservation of a distinct epithelial–dermal junction, without an inflammatory response or stromal desmoplasia (Figure 4.14). The border along the basement membrane in intraepithelial lesions should be smooth, while in early invasion irregularly shaped tongues of cells protrude from the basal layer through the basement membrane (Figure 4.15). Often this is accompanied by 'paradoxical maturation' of the cells on the invasive front, with the cells enlarging and accumulating more abundant eosinophilic cytoplasm (Figure 4.16). Early invasive nests of squamous cell carcinoma are small, irregularly shaped, and usually accompanied by a desmoplastic response (Figure 4.17).

Intraoperative Consultation and Sampling/Tissue Issues

Proper attention to specimen orientation and sectioning is critical in processing specimens of HSIL (VIN 2–3), whether for frozen or permanent sections. Resections for this disease can be quite large, and often involve margins in multiple anatomic areas, such as perivaginal, periurethral, and perianal, all on the same specimen. Clear orientation by the surgeon is imperative for optimal pathologic evaluation. Pinning larger specimens to a corkboard prior to fixation will help to prevent tangential sections and curling of the edges of the resected tissue, which can make it difficult or impossible to get properly oriented margin sections. When specimens are submitted for the evaluation of margins, whether by frozen section or permanents, it is advisable to take a perpendicular section from the lesion to the nearest margin so that measurement of the nearest distance from the margin is possible. If no gross lesion is appreciable, it may be preferable to perform en face margins, parallel to the surgical excision margins, to ensure complete assessment.

Clinical Behavior and Treatment

The frequency of recurrence for HSIL (VIN 2–3) is estimated at over 50%,[22] and is said to be more likely in patients who continue to smoke after initial diagnosis,[18] in patients with multifocal disease,[22] and in patients with involved margins on the initial resection, although the last association has not been a uniform finding.[22] Several clinical risk factors for the progression of HSIL (VIN 2–3) to carcinoma have been identified, such as patient age, multicentricity, and multifocality of disease, and immunosuppression, but to date the data remain conflicting on all counts.[14,16,17] Regardless of what the risk factors for progression may be, rates of progression are reported at 5.7–10%,[14,21] and, untreated, HSIL (VIN 2–3) has been found to progress to carcinoma within 8 years.[16] Treatment usually consists of wide local partial superficial vulvectomy or laser ablation.[21,22] Topical treatments are available and currently under investigation, but to date none have been shown to be as effective as surgical treatment.[21]

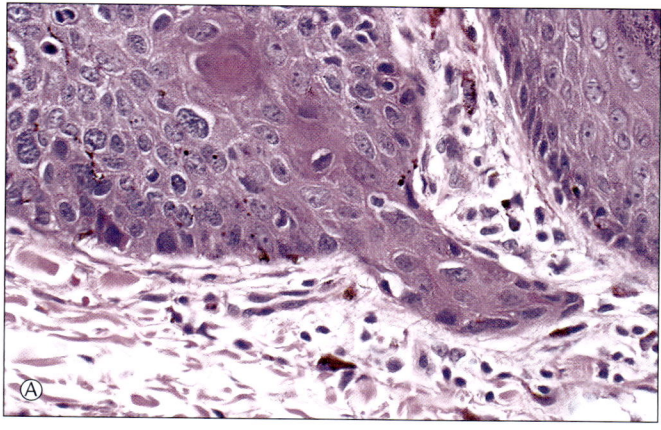

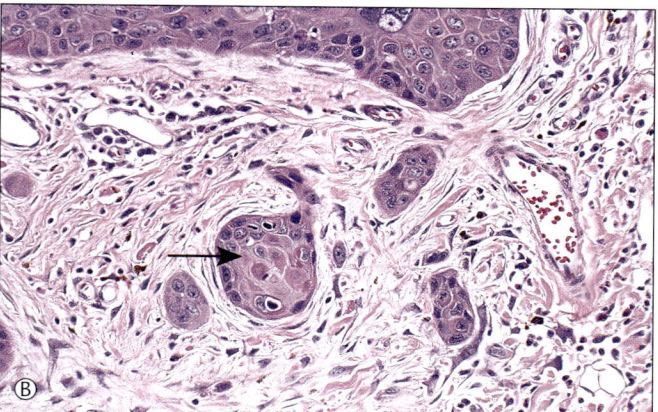

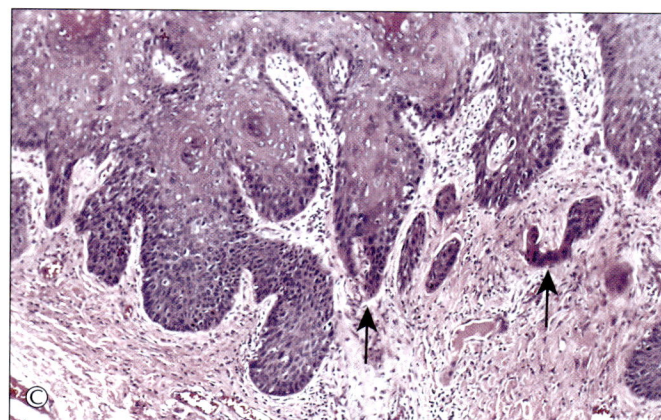

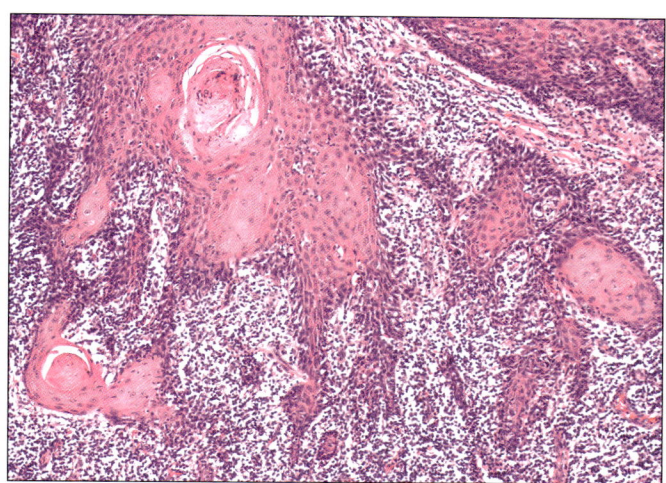

Figure 4.15 Early invasion by squamous cell carcinoma, with irregular fingers and nests protruding into the dermis. Note the 'paradoxical maturation' of the cells toward the center of the larger cell groups.

Figure 4.17 Microinvasive squamous cell cancer. **(A)** Early stromal invasion with a tiny tongue of tumor protruding from the basal most epithelium. **(B)** The small nests of tumor cells are distinctly separate from the overlying epidermis, sometimes have irregular shapes and lie in a desmoplastic stroma, and sometimes exhibit invasive cells with increased and more eosinophilic cytoplasm than neighboring basal cells. The microinvasive component is easy to recognize (arrow). **(C)** Some foci are easily recognized as microinvasive (arrows), whereas the bulbous tips of the overlying epidermis that are composed of small basal cells are considered as VIN 3.

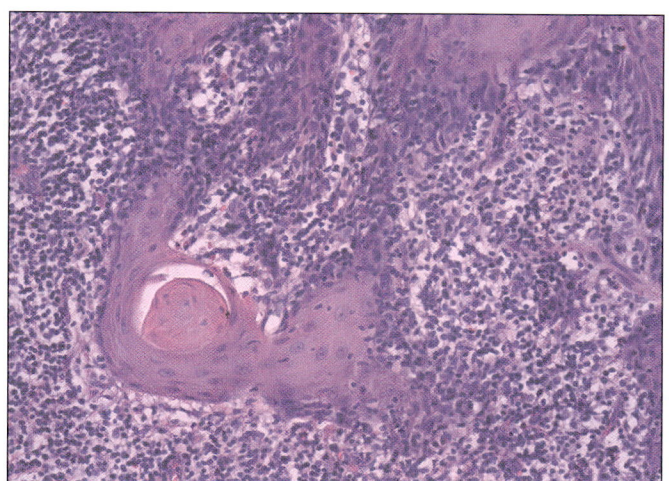

Figure 4.16 'Paradoxical maturation' with formation of a keratin pearl in an irregularly shaped protrusion of early invasion.

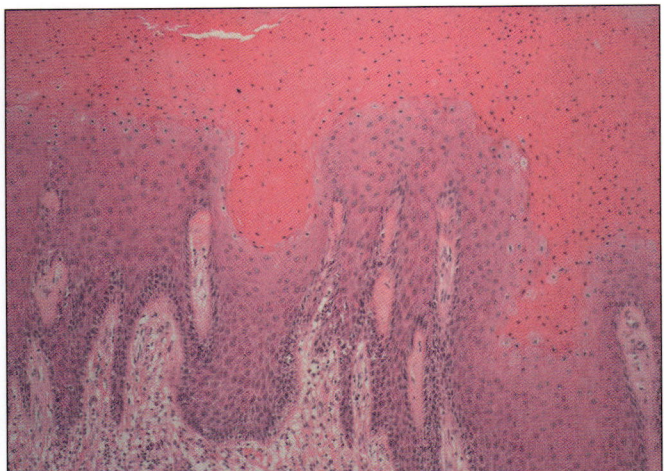

Figure 4.18 VIN 3, differentiated type, with acanthosis, hyperkeratosis, and parakeratosis.

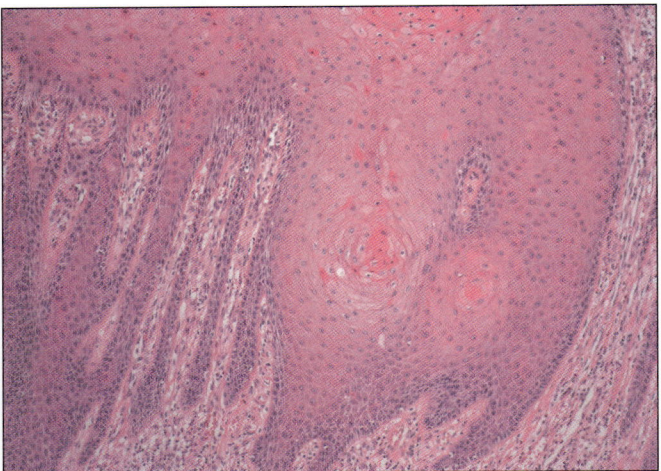

Figure 4.19 Elongated rete ridges of VIN 3, differentiated type, with anastomosis of the rete on the left side of the image and whorls of differentiated squamous cells deep within the rete toward the right side.

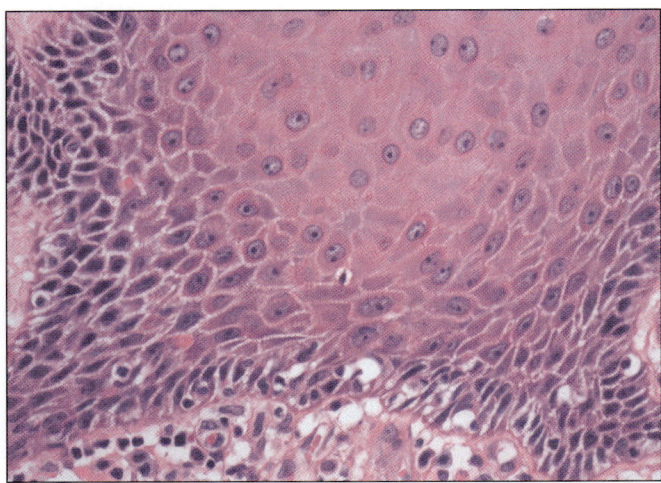

Figure 4.20 Premature maturation of the cells toward the base in VIN 3, differentiated type. The cells contain abundant eosinophilic cytoplasm, clear cell borders with obvious intercellular bridges, and enlarged rounded nuclei with prominent nucleoli.

HIGH-GRADE VIN, DIFFERENTIATED OR SIMPLEX TYPE

Clinical Features

The 'differentiated' or 'simplex' type of VIN does not have an associated low-grade counterpart; all lesions with this morphology qualify as high grade. This type of VIN is not associated with HPV, and consequently the clinical presentation differs from that of HPV-related lesions in that patients are usually older (postmenopausal), are less often smokers, and rarely have multifocal or multicentric intraepithelial disease, but often have an associated benign vulvar condition, typically lichen sclerosus or lichen simplex chronicus.[14,15,17,19–21] The symptoms and gross appearances of these lesions do not differ from those described for HPV-related lesions.

Pathogenesis/Etiology

Because of its frequent association with lichen sclerosus, long-standing lichen sclerosus has been implicated by some authors as a precursor lesion to differentiated VIN and associated carcinoma.[15,17,19,21] Also implicated in the development of differentiated VIN is p53 mutation, and many studies have demonstrated the increased expression of p53 in the basal and suprabasal layers of the epithelium in these lesions.[20,21,26,31–33]

Microscopic Features

In differentiated VIN the most atypical cells are confined to the basal and parabasal layers of the epithelium, while the superficial layers of the epithelium often appear relatively normal, making it easy to overlook. The epithelium may be acanthotic (Figure 4.18), but can also be normal in thickness or even atrophic. An orderly pattern of keratinocyte maturation is present, in contradistinction to the disorder seen in warty and basaloid VIN. The rete pegs are typically elongated, narrow, and branched, and may show an anastomosing pattern (Figure 4.19). The basal cell layer is often expanded by the population of atypical basal and parabasal cells. These cells are characterized by hyperchromatic, irregular, and variably sized nuclei with coarse chromatin and prominent macronucleoli, and a moderate to abundant amount of hypereosinophilic cytoplasm indicative of premature keratinization (Figure 4.20). These cells may form whorled aggregates with or without keratin pearls in the basal portion of the epithelium (Figures 4.21 and 4.22).

Routine Biomarkers of Clinical Relevance

Because differentiated VIN can be so difficult to recognize morphologically, there is great interest in identifying a 'magic marker,' which would distinguish it with greater ease. Hence, much has been made of the use of p53 immunostaining in these lesions, which is reported to show positive reactivity for p53 in the majority of the basal epithelial cells with superficial extension of this reactivity in 66–84% of cases.[17,29,30,32,33] The immunoreactivity, however, is not always consistent throughout the lesion and a similar staining pattern can be seen in several other benign and malignant conditions.[30,32,34] Moreover, p53 staining does not necessarily correlate with gene mutation, raising an additional concern as to the significance and utility of this finding.[33,35] Thus, while p53 immunohistochemical study

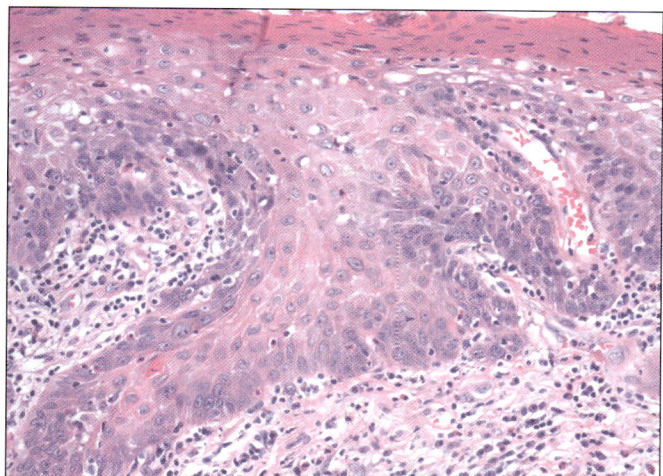

Figure 4.21 Marked cellular atypia in the basal layers of the epithelium in VIN 3, differentiated type. Premature maturation is also evident, as is a dyskeratotic cell adjacent to the basal layers.

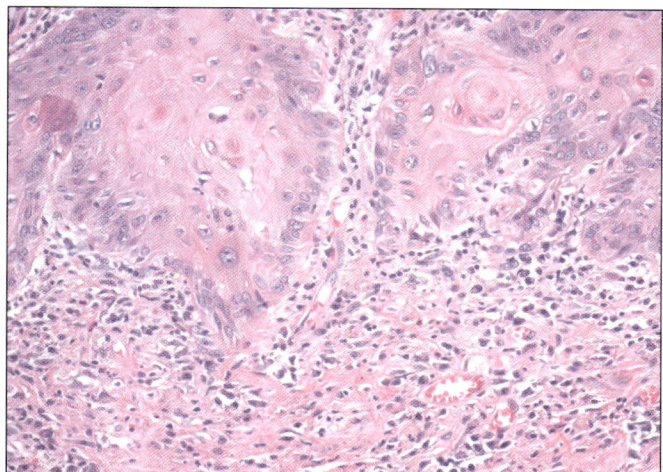

Figure 4.22 At high power, the atypia of the basal cells and premature keratinization with formation of a squamous pearl is more easily appreciated in VIN 3, differentiated type.

may be of value in confirming the diagnosis of differentiated VIN, it appears to be neither sensitive nor specific as a marker, and results must be interpreted with caution.

Differential Diagnosis

Differentiated VIN may be difficult to distinguish from the lichen sclerosus and lichen simplex chronicus that so often accompany it, but these benign conditions do not have keratinocyte atypia of the basal cell layers, disturbance of cell maturation, squamous whorls, or keratin pearls. These latter features may be mimicked by seborrheic keratosis; its lack of significant nuclear atypia should distinguish it from VIN.

Intraoperative Consultation and Sampling/Tissue Issues

Specimens should be handled in the same fashion as HPV-related lesions.

Clinical Behavior and Treatment

There is strong evidence that differentiated VIN is more likely to progress than HPV-related VIN, with reported rates of progression of up to 33%,[14,31] and it appears to do so at a more rapid rate as well.[14,24,32] In one study comparing the association of the two types of VIN with preceding, concurrent, or subsequent invasive carcinoma, the rates were found to be 24.2% for high-grade HPV-related VIN and 83.3% for differentiated VIN.[23] Given this very high association, a diagnosis of differentiated VIN often necessitates a more extensive excision than for HPV-related lesions.[15,21]

SQUAMOUS CELL CARCINOMA

Definition

Squamous cell carcinoma is a malignancy developing from neoplastic cells of squamous epithelium as a progression from high-grade squamous intraepithelial lesions.

Clinical Features

Vulvar carcinoma is relatively uncommon, constituting approximately 4% of all malignancies of the female genital tract, and is most common in women of Caucasian descent.[36] The vast majority of these tumors, estimated at 80–90%, are squamous cell carcinomas.[37]

While the frequency and incidence of HSIL (VIN 2–3) has been found to be increasing over the past 20 years,[14,19,22,38] the incidence of squamous cell carcinoma has remained stable.[21,38] At the same time, there has been a notable trend toward decreasing patient age at diagnosis for both HSIL (VIN 2–3)[16,22] and squamous cell carcinoma.[29] These epidemiologic changes have been attributed to numerous changing clinical factors, including increased prevalence of oncogenic HPV infection; increased awareness of the disease; an increased comfort in the discussion of, and willingness to seek care for, vulvar lesions on the part of younger patients; and an increased clinical knowledge of the disease and the use of biopsy to evaluate suspicious lesions and accomplish earlier diagnosis and treatment.[14,21,22]

Similar to their associated intraepithelial lesions, the clinical presentation of vulvar squamous cell carcinoma varies somewhat with the histologic subtype, as patients with HPV-related tumors tend not only to be younger, and more likely to have a history of other HPV-associated lesions,[32] but also to present with advanced disease.[37] The symptoms of vulvar cancer are similar to those of intraepithelial disease, and may include pruritus, vaginal discharge, dysuria, pain, bleeding, and ulceration. In some cases the patient may palpate or observe a mass. Early tumors may be asymptomatic, and occult carcinoma may be diagnosed on excised lesions clinically judged to be VIN in up to 20% of cases.[12,39–42] Vulvar squamous cell carcinomas are most frequently located on the labia majora or minora and are typically solitary, with about 10% reported to be multifocal (Figures 4.23 and 4.24).[43]

Pathogenesis/Etiology

Increased understanding of the histopathogenesis of this disease has developed along with the changing epidemiology. Beginning in the early 1990s two distinct

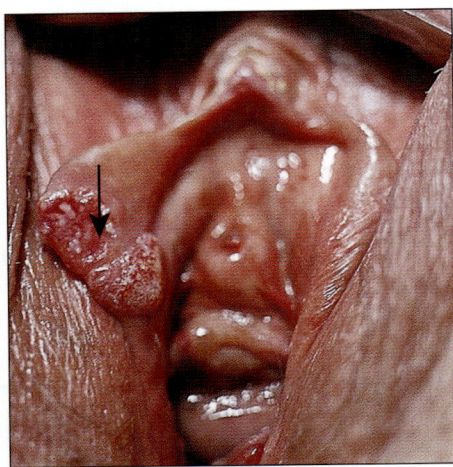

Figure 4.23 Squamous cell carcinoma with ulceration (arrow). This elderly woman had no apparent predisposing disease.

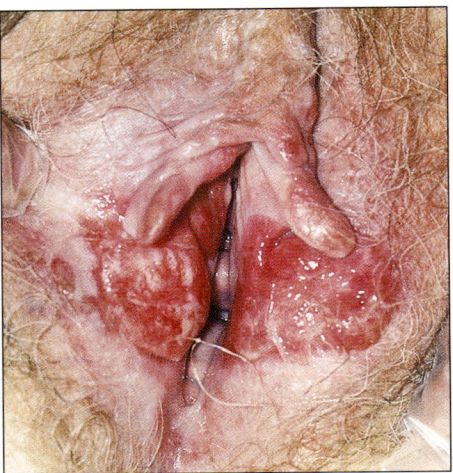

Figure 4.24 Bilateral squamous cell carcinoma ('kissing cancers'). The tumor arose on a background of lichen sclerosus.

clinicopathologic groups of squamous cell carcinoma became distinguishable and it has become clear that two pathogenetic pathways exist for vulvar carcinoma, one HPV related and one not.[44–47] Tumors associated with HPV appear to originate in HPV-positive high-grade VIN of warty and/or basaloid morphology and tend to have similar morphology, while tumors not associated with HPV appear to originate in differentiated VIN, or from some other process, and to have a keratinizing morphology.[17,48,49] Those tumors with warty, basaloid, or mixed morphology, like the associated HSIL, typically occur in younger patients.[20,23,27,50] While HPV-related HSIL is more commonly diagnosed than differentiated VIN, keratinizing carcinoma is the more common type of invasive tumor,[21] indicating that HSIL either less likely to progress than is differentiated VIN or does so at a much slower rate, which explains why the increased diagnosis of intraepithelial disease has not led to a proportionate increase in squamous cell carcinoma.

The details of HPV-driven carcinogenesis have been well characterized in work on cervical cancer, and the mechanisms are presumed to be similar in the vulva and other sites where HPV-associated tumors present. The etiology and mechanisms behind the development of HPV-negative tumors remain somewhat obscure. A large proportion of them demonstrate immunohistochemical reactivity for p53,[35,44] implicating p53 mutation in their pathogenesis. Additional studies have shown other genetic differences between HPV-positive and HPV-negative tumors.[31] Ongoing investigation will undoubtedly provide more detailed understanding of this HPV-independent pathway.

Gross Features

Gross features of vulvar carcinoma are highly variable. The tumor may be unrecognizable grossly, as in cases where occult tumor is found in resections for a diagnosis of VIN, or may be evident as an ulcer, a hyperkeratotic plaque, or an exophytic mass (Figures 4.25 and 4.26).

Microscopic Features

The three principal morphologic patterns seen in squamous cell carcinoma of the vulva are keratinizing, warty, and basaloid types. The majority of squamous cell carcinomas of the vulva are of the well-differentiated, keratinizing variety, and often arise on a background of lichen sclerosus with or without associated differentiated VIN. The morphology of these vulvar tumors is identical to those occurring elsewhere on the skin, and consists of irregularly shaped tongues and nests of squamous cells with abundant eosinophilic cytoplasm frequently showing whorling and forming keratin pearls (Figures 4.27 and 4.28). The cells may invade in broad fronds or in narrow finger-like projections with small clusters and single cells interspersed in irregular patterns. The nuclei show the same atypical features as those of differentiated VIN. Stroma surrounding the invasive tumor shows a desmoplastic response, and a chronic inflammatory response may be seen in the surrounding tissue.

Warty carcinoma is significantly less common, and is distinguished by its exophytic, papillary architecture and koilocytic change toward the epithelial surface. At the base of the lesion, irregularly shaped nests containing dyskeratotic cells and frequently keratin pearls are seen, similar to ordinary squamous cell carcinomas, but usually with a greater degree of nuclear pleomorphism and cytologic atypia (Figure 4.29). It is frequently associated with warty and/or basaloid VIN.

Basaloid carcinoma is an uncommon tumor, consisting of variably sized nests of squamous cells showing little to no maturation. The cells are relatively uniform, with scant cytoplasm and oval nuclei containing evenly distributed, coarsely granular chromatin (Figure 4.30). It is also frequently associated with VIN, usually also of the basaloid type.

Rare cases of squamous cell carcinoma of the vulva, as elsewhere on the skin, have been described with sarcomatoid,[51] plasmacytoid,[52] and pseudoangiosarcomatous[53] differentiation, as well as adenosquamous, giant cell, lymphoepithelioma-like, and papillary squamous cell carcinomas and some tumors that are not otherwise classifiable.[46]

Routine Biomarkers of Clinical Relevance

Similar to their VIN counterparts, warty and basaloid tumors are strongly associated with HPV, particularly type 16, and

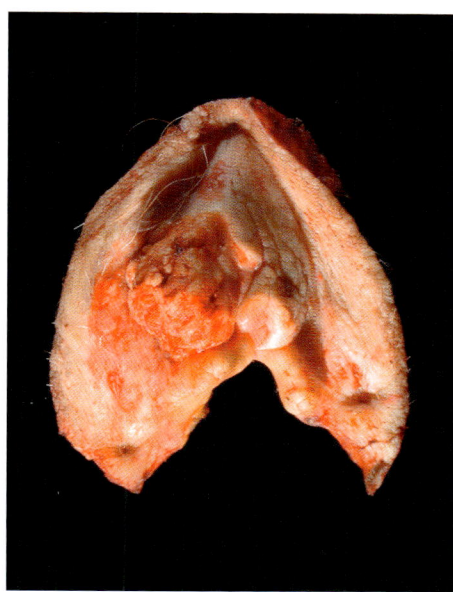

Figure 4.25 Vulvar squamous cell carcinoma forming a large exophytic mass in the clitoral region. (Photo courtesy of Robin Foss, University of Florida College of Medicine, Department of Pathology, Immunology and Laboratory Medicine.)

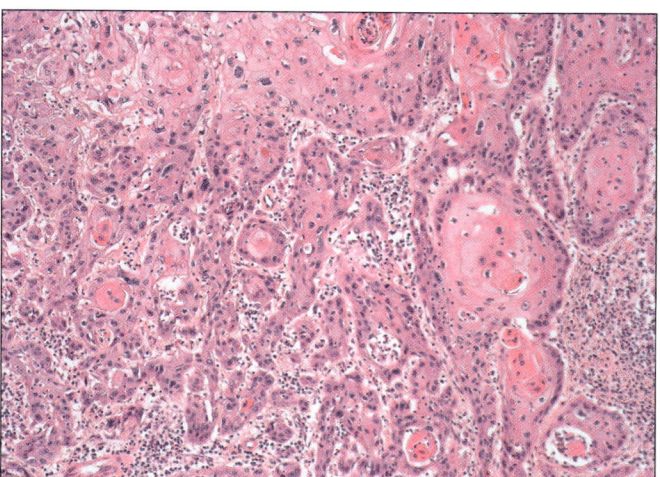

Figure 4.27 Nests and cords of malignant squamous cells permeating the dermis.

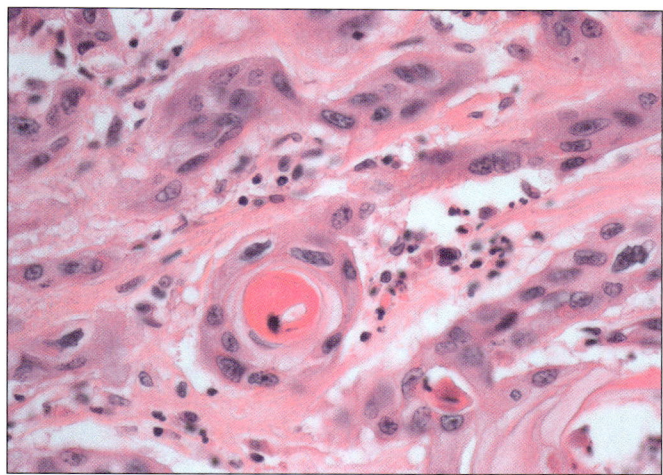

Figure 4.28 Pronounced nuclear atypia and keratin pearl formation, characteristic of invasive squamous cell carcinoma.

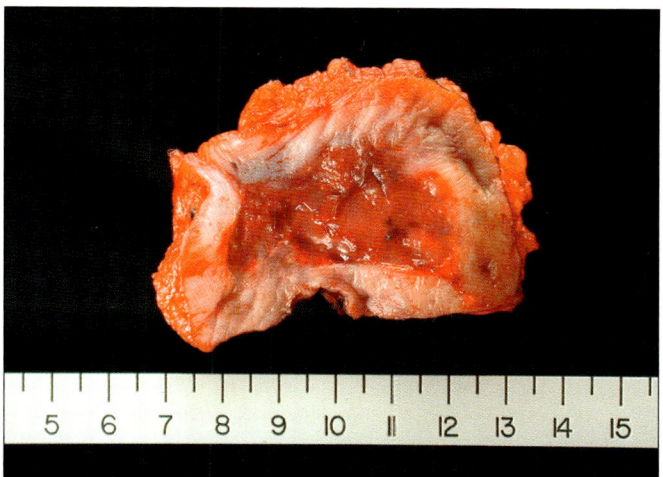

Figure 4.26 Vulvar squamous cell carcinoma forming a large red ulcerated patch. (Photo courtesy of Robin Foss, University of Florida College of Medicine, Department of Pathology, Immunology and Laboratory Medicine.)

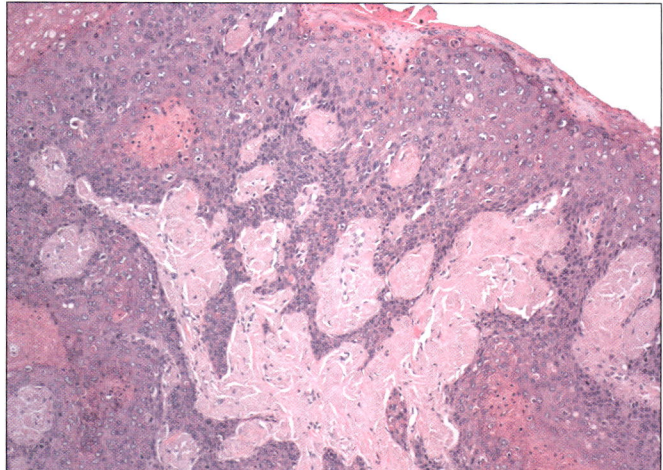

Figure 4.29 Squamous cell carcinoma, warty type. Irregular cords extend from a surface lesion with features typical of warty VIN.

stain for $p16^{INK4a}$.[47–49] Keratinizing squamous cell carcinomas, like their precursor differentiated VIN, are usually HPV negative and negative for $p16^{INK4a}$, but commonly reactive for p53.[48,49]

Differential Diagnosis

The distinction of early invasive carcinoma from VIN has been discussed previously. Other tumors in the differential diagnosis include malignant melanoma, keratoacanthoma, verrucous carcinoma, and basal cell carcinomas. Amelanotic melanomas, in particular, can be difficult to distinguish from squamous cell carcinoma, but can be distinguished by

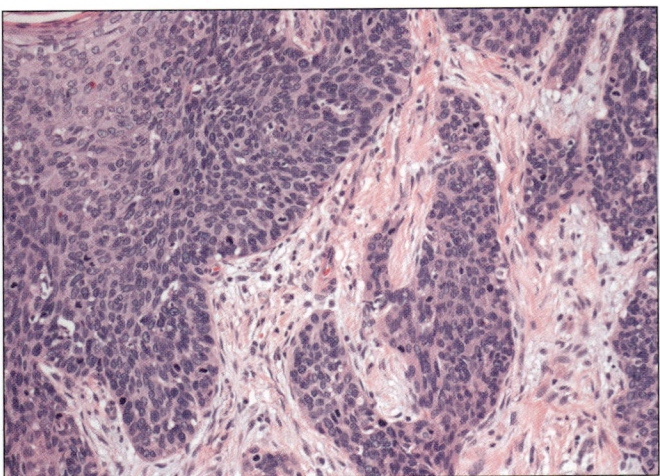

Figure 4.30 Basaloid carcinoma, comprising irregularly shaped nests of immature cells with scant cytoplasm invading the dermis and inducing a desmoplastic response. Associated VIN 3, basaloid type, is present on the left.

positive immunohistochemical stains for S-100, HMB-45, and Melan-A. Differentiation from keratoacanthoma, verrucous carcinoma, and basal cell carcinoma is discussed in the sections of this chapter on those respective lesions.

Intraoperative Consultation and Sampling/Tissue Issues

The majority of squamous cell carcinomas contain adjacent areas of high-grade VIN, with studies reporting the association in 45–100%.[42–44,48] Because concurrent VIN is so often present in these cases, it is important to sample any unusual looking area of the epithelium, even if it is at some distance from the obvious tumor. Likewise, all margins must be sampled even in the absence of gross disease to ensure they are free of intraepithelial disease as well as invasive tumor.

Clinical Behavior and Treatment

The most recent (2009) International Federation of Gynecology and Obstetrics (FIGO) staging system, correlated with the current American Joint Committee on Cancer (AJCC) TNM staging, is shown in Table 4.2, and survival rates by stage are shown in Table 4.3. These data demonstrate the prognostic significance of tumor size, depth of invasion, and extent of local spread, and it is important to include such information in the pathologic report of vulvectomy specimens. A thorough and updated protocol (checklist) for the evaluation of vulvar carcinoma specimens has recently been published by CAP and can be used for further guidance on reporting these cases.

The measurement of the depth of invasion warrants further discussion, as there is often some confusion as to the difference between tumor thickness and tumor depth. In the vulva, measurement of depth of invasion has been standardized as the measurement from the epithelial/dermal junction of the adjacent most superficial dermal papilla to the point of deepest invasion. Proper measurement of this depth is of critical importance, as a depth of 1 mm or less

Table 4.2 Vulvar Tumor Pathologic Staging

Primary Tumor (pT)	FIGO Stage
pTX: Primary tumor cannot be assessed	—
pT0: No evidence of primary tumor	—
pTis: Carcinoma *in situ*	—
pT1a: Lesions 2 cm or less in size, confined to vulva or perineum, and with depth of stromal invasion 1.0 mm or less	IA
pT1b: Lesions more than 2 cm in size or any size with depth of stromal invasion more than 1.0 mm, confined to the vulva or perineum	IB
pT2: Tumor of any size with extension to any adjacent perineal structures including lower/distal one-third urethra, lower/distal one-third vagina, or anal involvement	II
pT3: Tumor of any size with extension to any of the following structures: upper/proximal two-thirds urethra, upper/proximal two-thirds vagina, bladder mucosa, rectal mucosa, or fixed to pelvic bone	IVA
Regional Lymph Nodes (pN)	
pNx: Regional lymph nodes cannot be assessed	
pN0: No regional lymph node metastasis	
pN1:	
N1a: One or two lymph node metastases, each less than 5 mm	IIIA
N1b: One lymph node metastasis 5 mm or greater	IIIA
pN2:	
pN2a: Three or more lymph node metastases each less than 5 mm	IIIB
pN2b: Two or more lymph node metastases each 5 mm or greater	IIIB
pN2c: Lymph node metastasis with extracapsular spread	IIIC
pN3: Fixed or ulcerated regional lymph node metastasis	IVA
Distant Metastasis (pM)	
pM0: No distant metastasis	
pM1: Distant metastasis (including pelvic lymph node metastasis)	IVB

Based on AJCC/UICC TNM, 7th edition (2010) and FIGO 2009 Annual Report and College of American Pathologists, 2010.

in a solitary tumor measuring no more than 2 cm in greatest dimension defines a specific subset of tumors with distinct clinicopathologic features. These tumors, designated as AJCC stage T1a (FIGO IA) or, more recently, by the CAP/ASCCP as 'superficially invasive squamous cell carcinomas (SISCCA),'[16] have a negligible risk of nodal dissemination, and an excellent prognosis.[54,55] There are few data on tumors with a depth of invasion of 1.1–2 mm, but it appears that once the depth of invasion exceeds 2 mm there is clearly a risk of nodal metastases, with recurrences associated with decreased survival. The risks increase with progressive depth of invasion.[56,57] Accordingly, treatment for SISCCA may be limited to partial deep vulvectomy without lymphadenectomy, while tumors with invasion greater than 1 mm require excision of the ipsilateral inguinal nodes as well.[58,59] Bilateral groin dissections are advised if the lesion is in the midline or ipsilateral nodes are positive.[59] There has been a shift in recent years toward increasingly conservative surgery, and total deep vulvectomy with bilateral groin dissection in one large, continuous block, once routine for vulvar carcinomas, is now rarely performed.[58] On the rare occasion when the disease is extremely extensive or advanced at the time of diagnosis, chemotherapy and radiation, rather than surgery, may be the initial treatment of choice, but such nonsurgical treatments have been found to have little value in preventing recurrent disease.[59] Vulvar carcinoma spreads locally into adjacent structures, commonly extending into the vagina and distal urethra, and in advanced cases into the base of the bladder, pelvic bones, rectum, and perirectal tissues. Lymphovascular spread may occur, most commonly involving first the inguinofemoral lymph nodes and then spreading to the deeper pelvic nodes. From there spread may extend to the para-aortic nodes and from there drain into the thoracic duct, from which metastasis to other distant sites may occur by hematogenous dissemination.

Adequate surgical resection is said to achieve local control of disease in 80–90% of cases, even when inguinal lymph nodes are positive.[59] Local recurrence on the vulva is three times more common than recurrence in the groin, pelvis, or distant sites, and carries a better prognosis.[59] Factors associated with an increased risk of local recurrence are margins positive for tumor or VIN, margins less than 8 mm from invasive tumor, the presence of lymphovascular space invasion, greater depth of invasion, and large tumor size.[58,59] The next most frequent site of recurrence is the groin, and when this occurs the prognosis is guarded, with the majority of patients succumbing to disease within 2 years.[57,59] Overall, recurrences most frequently occur in the first 2 years following surgery.[57] Patients with positive inguinal lymph nodes are more likely to have recurrence of tumor, and the risk is increased if the nodal involvement is bilateral.[57,59] Recurrences in the pelvis or distant sites are uncommon, but nearly always fatal.[59] It should be recognized that a fair number of recurrences occur 5 years or later from the initial surgery,[57] and long-term follow-up is imperative.

UNCOMMON SUBTYPES OF SQUAMOUS CELL CARCINOMA

VERRUCOUS CARCINOMA

Verrucous carcinoma is an uncommon subtype of very well-differentiated squamous cell carcinoma with a favorable prognosis. The tumor typically occurs in postmenopausal women, and presents as a papillary, exophytic growth, which in advanced cases may completely obscure the normal vulvar anatomy. It has no consistently documented association with HPV infection.

Microscopic Features

Verrucous carcinoma is characterized by an acanthotic epithelial proliferation of well-differentiated squamous cells with abundant cytoplasm and minimal nuclear atypia or pleomorphism. Abundant hyperkeratosis and parakeratosis is typically present on the surface. The tumor expands and elongates the rete ridges, producing large bulbous nests along the base that advance into the underlying dermis in a pushing, rather than an infiltrative, pattern, which is a distinguishing characteristic of this tumor (Figures 4.31–4.33). A chronic inflammatory infiltrate is commonly found along this advancing border.

Differential Diagnosis

The warty architecture of verrucous carcinoma can suggest a diagnosis of condyloma or warty VIN. The lack of fibrovascular cores within the papillary epithelial formations of verrucous carcinoma as well as the absence of nuclear

Table 4.3 Survival Rates for Squamous Cell Carcinoma by Stage

FIGO Stage	Relative 5 Year Survival Rate	Relative 10 Year Survival Rate
I	93%	87%
II	79%	69%
III	53%	46%
IV	29%	16%

Adapted from www.cancer.org

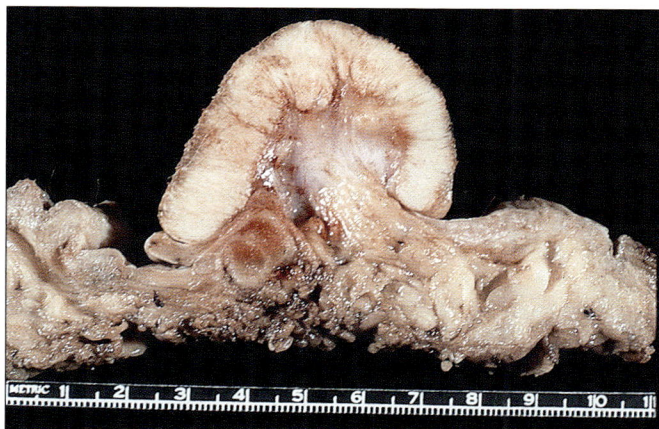

Figure 4.31 Verrucous carcinoma. The mass is large, exophytic, and fungating.

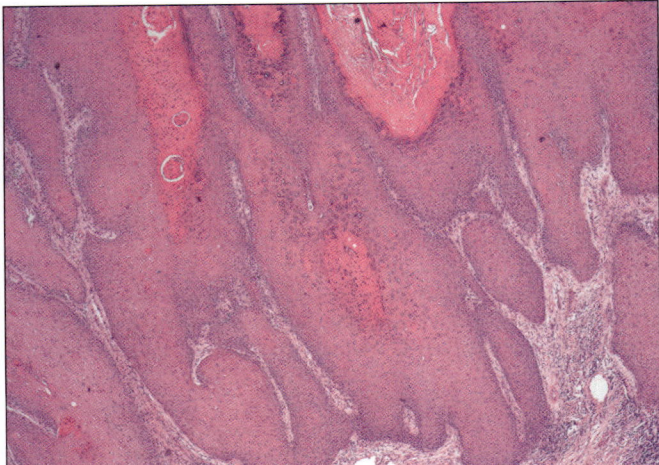

Figure 4.32 Verrucous carcinoma.

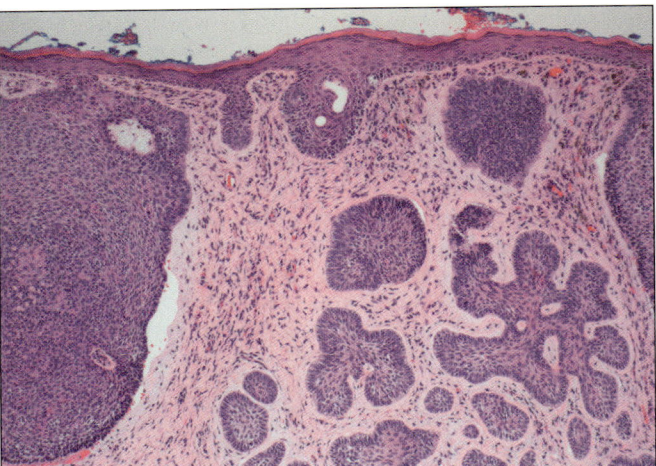

Figure 4.34 Irregular nests with palisading of the cells at the periphery invading the dermis. Notice also the large nest of basal cell carcinoma still in continuity with the basal layer of the epithelium on the left.

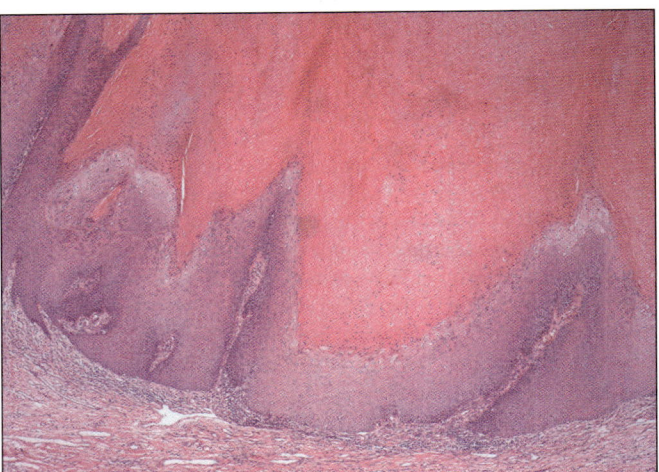

Figure 4.33 Broad, bulbous rete ridges form the invasive front of verrucous carcinoma. Hyperkeratosis is prominent, but the tumor lacks koilocytic atypia.

atypia or koilocytic change will aid in this distinction. It is also important to distinguish verrucous carcinoma from exophytic squamous cell carcinomas of either the warty or keratinizing type, in which cases the characteristic bulbous downgrowths of the rete pegs in verrucous carcinoma, forming a pushing rather than an infiltrative margin, should distinguish it.

Clinical Behavior and Treatment

Although the tumor may be locally aggressive and has a tendency to recur,[60] it very rarely metastasizes, and, in fact, the finding of lymph node metastasis strongly mitigates against the diagnosis and should prompt a thorough re-evaluation of the lesion for areas of typical squamous cell carcinoma. Treatment consists of wide local excision without lymph node dissection.

BASAL CELL CARCINOMA

Basal cell carcinoma is a very common cutaneous tumor, but rare on the vulvar skin, constituting only 1–3% of all vulvar cancers.[61–63] They occur primarily in elderly white women, and the symptoms are similar to those of typical squamous cell carcinoma. The lesions are always solitary and present as firm, well-circumscribed, hypopigmented nodules or plaques, which may ulcerate as the disease progresses. The etiology of this tumor on the sun-exposed skin, where it is a common occurrence, is believed to be exposure to ultraviolet radiation, but the etiology of lesions of the vulva remains obscure. There is no association of basal cell carcinoma with HPV infection.

Microscopic Features

The histologic appearance of basal cell carcinoma of the vulva is no different from that of such tumors elsewhere on the skin. Numerous architectural patterns may occur, alone or in combination, but the features described here are common to most of them. The tumors are composed of small, uniform cells with hyperchromatic, elongated nuclei and scant cytoplasm, and may show abundant mitotic figures and apoptotic bodies. Most tumors maintain a connection with the basal surface of the overlying epithelium, and grow downward in lobules or nests that characteristically show peripheral palisading of the nuclei with haphazard distribution of the cells toward their centers. The tumor nests are embedded in a loose fibrous stroma that may show myxoid change, and frequently a cleft-like retraction space is seen between the tumor cells and this stroma (Figure 4.34).

Differential Diagnosis

The relative uniformity of the cells in basal cell carcinoma aids in distinguishing it from basaloid VIN and squamous cell carcinoma of basaloid type, which are characterized by pronounced nuclear atypia and pleomorphism. Immunostaining for BerEP4 can also be of use in this differential, as its expression is seen in basal cell carcinomas, but not squamous ones. Various trichogenic tumors may also enter the differential, but these tumors do not show the typical clefting or infiltrative pattern typical of basal cell carcinoma and are exceedingly rare in this location.

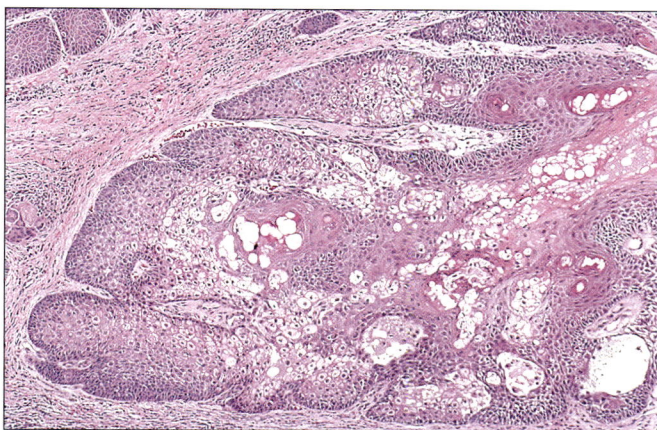

Figure 4.35 Sebaceous carcinoma.

Clinical Behavior and Treatment

As in basal cell carcinoma elsewhere on the skin, basal cell carcinoma of the vulva may be locally invasive and may recur locally, but metastasis is very rare.[61-63] Wide local excision is the treatment of choice, and the prognosis is excellent with the exception of those very rare cases that do metastasize, in which case the disease is rapidly fatal.[61-63]

SEBACEOUS CARCINOMA

Sebaceous carcinoma is a rare, aggressive neoplasm originating from the sebaceous glands of the skin. It is most commonly seen on the eyelid, but rare cases involving the vulva have been reported, a few of which have been associated with VIN.[64-66] It is composed of malignant cells in lobules, tongues, or small clusters in a fibrovascular stroma. The large cells, with large nuclei containing prominent nucleoli and abundant cytoplasm, have a squamoid appearance, particularly at low power. At higher magnification, sebaceous differentiation is manifested by the presence of intracellular lipid producing foaminess or fine vacuolization of the cytoplasm, which may produce scalloping of the edges of the nuclei (Figure 4.35). These sebaceous features are often most prominent toward the center of the cell nests. The tumor may be very deeply invasive, and may metastasize to lymph nodes or distant sites, which must be taken into account when planning for its excision.

REFERENCES

1. Gushi A, Kanekura T, Kanzaki T, Eizuru Y. Detection and sequences of human papillomavirus DNA in nongenital seborrheic keratosis of immunocompetent individuals. J Dermatol Sci 2003;31(2):143–9.
2. Bai H, Cviko A, Granter S, et al. Immunophenotype and viral (human papillomavirus) correlates of vulvar seborrheic keratosis. Hum Pathol 2003;34(6):59–64.
3. Li J, Ackerman AB. 'Seborrheic keratosis' that contain human papillomavirus are condyloma acuminate. Am J Dermatopathol 1994;16(4):398–405.
4. Karaa A, Khachemoune A. Keratoacanthoma: a tumor in search of a classification. Int J Dermatol 2007;46(7):671–8.
5. Schwartz, R. Keratoacanthoma: a clinico-pathologic enigma. Dermatol Surg 2004;30(2 Pt 2):326–33.
6. Weedon D, Malo J, Brooks D, Williamson R. Keratoacanthoma: is it really a variant of squamous carcinoma? ANZ J Surg 2010; 80(3):129–30.
7. Chen W, Koenig C. Vulvar keratoacanthoma: a report of two cases. Int J Gynecol Pathol 2004;23(3):284–6.
8. Gilbey S, Moore D, Look K, Sutton G. Vulvar keratoacanthoma. Obstet Gynecol 1997;89(5 Pt 2):848–50.
9. Ozcan F, Bilgic R, Cesur S. Vulvar keratoacanthoma. APMIS 2006;114(7–8):562–65.
10. Nascimento M, Cominos D, Davies N, Obermair A. Vulval keratoacanthoma. Gynecol Oncol 2005;97(2):674–6.
11. Wilkinson EJ, Kneale B, Lynch PJ. Report of the ISVVD Terminology Committee. J Reprod Med 1986;31:973–4.
12. Heller DS. Report of a new ISSVD classification of VIN. J Low Genit Tract Dis 2007;11(1):46–7.
13. Darragh T, Colgan T, Cox JT, et al. The Lower Anogenital Squamous Terminology Standardization Project for HPV-Associated Lesions: background and consensus recommendations from the College of American Pathologists and the American Society for Colposcopy and Cervical Pathology. J Low Genit Tract Dis 2012;16(3):205–42.
14. Van de Nieuwenhof H, Massurger L, van der Avoort I, et al. Vulvar squamous cell carcinoma development after diagnosis of VIN increases with age. Eur J Cancer 2009;45(5):851–6.
15. Terlou A, Blok L, Helmerhorst T, Beurden M. Premalignant epithelial disorders of the vulva: squamous vulvar intraepithelial neoplasia, vulvar paget's disease and melanoma in situ. Acta Obstet Gynecol Scand 2010;89(6):741–8.
16. Jones R, Rowan D, Stewart A. Vulvar intraepithelial neoplasia: aspects of the natural history and outcome of 405 women. Obstet Gynecol 2005;106(6):1319–26.
17. Hart W. Vulvar intraepithelial neoplasia: historical aspects and current status. Int J Gynecol Pathol 2001;20(1):16–30.
18. Khan AM, Freeman-Wang T, Pisal N, Singer A. Smokers and multicentric vulval intraepithelial neoplasia. J Obstet Gynaecol 2009;29(2):123–5.
19. McCluggage WG. Recent developments in vulvovaginal pathology. Histopathology 2009;54(2):156–73.
20. de Bie RP, van de Nieuwenhoof HP, Bekkers RLM, et al. Patients with usual vulvar intraepithelial neoplasia-related vulvar cancer have an increased risk of cervical abnormalities. Br J Cancer 2009;101(1):27–31.
21. Van de Nieuwenhof HP, van der Avoort IAM, de Hullu JA. Review of squamous premalignant vulvar lesions. Crit Rev Oncol Hematol 2008;68(2):131–56.
22. McNally OM, Mulvany NJ, Pagano R, et al. VIN 3: a clinicopathologic review. Int J Gynecol Cancer 2002;12(5):490–5.
23. Skapa P, Zamecnik J, Hamsikova E, et al. Human papillomavirus (HPV) profiles of vulvar lesions: possible implications for the classification of vulvar squamous cell carcinoma precursors and for the efficacy of prophylactic HPV vaccination. Am J Surg Pathol 2007;31(12):1834–43.
24. Preti M, Mezzetti M, Robertson C, Sideri M. Inter-observer variation in histopathological diagnosis and grading of vulvar intraepithelial neoplasia: results of an European collaborative study. Br J Obstet Gynaecol 2000;107(5):594–9.
25. Garland S, Insinga R, Sings H, et al. Human papilloma virus infections and vulvar disease. Cancer Epidemiol Biomarkers Prev 2009;18(6):1777–84.
26. Srodon M, Stoler M, Baber G, Kurman R. The distribution of low and high risk HPV types in vulvar and vaginal intraepithelial neoplasia. Am J Surg Pathol 2006;30(12):1513–8.
27. Van der Avoort IAM, Shirango H, Hoevanaars BM, et al. Vulvar squamous cell carcinoma as a multifactorial disease following two separate and independent pathways. Int J Gynecol Pathol 2005; 25(1):22–9.
28. Logani S, Lu D, Quint W, et al. Low-grade vulvar and vaginal intraepithelial neoplasia: correlation of histologic features with human papillomavirus DNA detection and MIB-1 immunostaining. Mod Pathol 2003;16(8):735–41.
29. Hoevenaars BM, van der Avoort I, de Wilde P, et al. A panel of p16^{INK4a}, MIB-1 and p53 proteins can distinguish between the 2 pathways leading to vulvar squamous cell carcinoma. Int J Cancer 2008;123(12):2767–73.
30. Santos M, Montagut C, Mellado B, et al. Immunohistochemical staining for p16 and p53 in premalignant and malignant epithelial lesions of the vulva. Int J Gynecol Pathol 2004;23(3):206–14.
31. Yang B, Hart W. Vulvar intraepithelial neoplasia of the simplex (differentiated) type: a clinicopathologic study including analysis

of HPV and p53 expression. Am J Surg Pathol 2000;24(2):429–41.
32. Mulvany N, Allen D. Differentiated intraepithelial neoplasia of the vulva. Int J Gynecol Pathol 2007;27(1):125–35.
33. Pinto A, Miron A, Yassin Y, et al. Differentiated vulvar intraepithelial neoplasia contains Tp53 mutations and is genetically linked to vulvar squamous cell carcinoma. Mod Pathol 2010;23(3):404–12.
34. Medeiros F, Nascimento A, Crum C. Early vulvar squamous neoplasia: advances in classification, diagnosis, and differential diagnosis. Adv Anat Pathol 2005;12(1):20–6.
35. Rolfe KJ, MacLean AB, Crow JC, et al. TP53 mutations in vulval lichen sclerosus adjacent to squamous cell carcinoma of the vulva. Br J Cancer 2003;89(12):2249–53.
36. Saraiya M, Watson M, Wu X, et al. Incidence of in situ and invasive vulvar cancer in the US, 1998–2003. Cancer 2008;113(110 Suppl):2865–72.
37. Tyring S. Vulvar squamous cell carcinoma: guidelines for early diagnosis and treatment. Am J Obstet Gynecol 2003;189(3 Suppl):S17–23.
38. Lanneau G, Argenta P, Lanneau M, et al. Vulvar cancer in young women: demographic features and outcome evaluation. Am J Obstet Gynecol 2009;200(6):645.e1–5.
39. Husseinzadeh N, Recinto C. Frequency of invasive cancer in surgically excised vulvar lesions with intraepithelial neoplasia (VIN 3). Gynecol Oncol 1999;73(1):119–20.
40. Chafe W, Richards A, Morgan L, Wilkinson E. Unrecognized invasive carcinoma in vulvar intraepithelial neoplasia (VIN). Gynecol Oncol 1988;31(1):154–62.
41. Van Seters M, van Beurden M, deCraen A. Is the assumed natural history of vulvar intraepithelial neoplasia III based on enough evidence? A systematic review of 3322 published patients. Gynecol Oncol 2005;97(2):645–51.
42. Poltrerauer S, Dressler A, Grimm C, et al. Accuracy of preoperative vulva biopsy and the outcome of surgery in vulvar intraepithelial neoplasia 2 and 3. Int J Gynecol Pathol 2009;28(6):559–62.
43. Kurman RJ, Ronnett BM, Sherman ME, Wilkinson EJ. Tumors of the cervix, vagina and vulva. 4th series ed. Washington, DC: American Registry of Pathology; 2010.
44. Gargano JW, Wilkinson EJ, Unger ER, et al. Prevalence of human papillomavirus types in invasive vulvar cancers and vulvar intraepithelial neoplasia 3 in the United States before vaccine introduction. J Low Genit Tract Dis 2012;16(4):471–9.
45. Chiesa-Vottero A, Dvoretsky P, Hart WR. Histopathologic study of thin vulvar squamous cell carcinomas and associated cutaneous lesions: a correlative study of 48 tumors in 44 patients with analysis of adjacent vulvar intraepithelial neoplasia types and lichen sclerosus. Am J Surg Pathol 2006;30(3):310–8.
46. Santos M, Landolfi S, Olivella A et al. p16 overexpression identifies HPV-positive vulvar squamous cell carcinomas. Am J Surg Pathol 2006;30(11):1347–56.
47. De Vuyst H, Clifford G, Nascimento M et al. Prevalence and type distribution of human papillomavirus in carcinoma and intraepithelial neoplasia of the vulva, vagina and anus: a meta-analysis. Int J Cancer 2009;124(7):1626–36.
48. Quddus M, Xu C, Steinhoff MM, et al. Simplex (differentiated) type VIN: absence of p16INK4 supports its weak association with HPV and its probable precursor role in non-HPV related vulvar squamous cancers. Histopathology 2005;46(6):709–22.
49. Eva L, Ganesan R, Chan K, et al. Differentiated-type vulval intraepithelial neoplasia has a high-risk association with vulval squamous cell carcinoma. Int J Gynecol Cancer 2009;19(4):741–4.
50. Messing M, Gallup D. Carcinoma of the vulva in young women. Obstet Gynecol 1995;86(1):51–4.
51. Choi D, Lee J, Lee S, et al. Squamous cell carcinoma with sarcomatoid features of the vulva: a case report and review of literature. Gynecol Oncol 2006;103(1):363–7.
52. Tran T, Carlson J. Plasmacytoid squamous cell carcinoma of the vulva. Int J Gynecol Pathol 2008;27(4):601–5.
53. Horn L-C, Liebert U, Edelmann J, et al. Adenoid squamous carcinoma (pseudoangiosarcomatous carcinoma) of the vulva: a rare but highly aggressive variant of squamous cell carcinoma-a report of a case and review of the literature. Int J Gynecol Pathol 2008;27(2):288–91.
54. Yoder B, Rufforny I, Massoll N, Wilkinson E. Stage 1A vulvar squamous carcinoma: an analysis of tumor invasive characteristics and risk. Am J Surg Pathol 2008;32(5):765–72.
55. Herod JJ, Shafi MI, Rollason TP, et al. Vulvar intraepithelial neoplasia with superficially invasive carcinoma of the vulva. Br J Obstet Gynaecol 1996;103(5):453–6.
56. Binder SW, Huang I, Fu YS, et al. Risk factors for the development of lymph node metastasis in vulvar squamous cell carcinoma. Gynecol Oncol 1990;37(1):9–16.
57. Bosquet J, Magrina J, Gaffey T, et al. Long-term survival and disease recurrence in patients with primary squamous cell carcinoma of the vulva. Gynecol Oncol 2005;97(3):828–33.
58. Preti M, Rouzier R, Mariani L, Wilkinson E. Superficially invasive carcinoma of the vulva: diagnosis and treatment. Clin Obstet Gynecol 2005;48(4):862–8.
59. Stehman F, Look K. Carcinoma of the vulva. Obstet Gynecol 2006;107(3):719–33.
60. Gualco M, Bonin S, Foglia G, et al. Morphologic and biologic studies on ten cases of verrucous carcinoma of the vulva supporting the theory of a discrete pathologic entity. Int J Gynecol Cancer 2003;13(3):317–24.
61. Piuria B, Rabinovich A, Dgani R. Basal cell carcinoma of the vulva. J Surg Oncol 1999;70(3):172–6.
62. Mulayim N, Silver D, Ocal I, Babloa E. Vulvar basal cell carcinoma: two unusual presentations and review of the literature. Gynecol Oncol 2001;85(3):532–7.
63. de Giorgi V, Salvini C, Massi D, et al. Vulvar basal cell carcinoma: retrospective study and review of literature. Gynecol Oncol 2005;97(1):192–4.
64. Esconilla P, Grilli R, Canamero M, et al. Sebaceous carcinoma of the vulva. Am J Dermatol 1999;21(15):468–72.
65. Carlson J, McGlennen R, Gomez R, et al. Sebaceous carcinoma of the vulva: a case report and review of the literature. Gynecol Oncol 1996;60(30):489–91.
66. Khan Z, Misra G, Fiander A, Dallimore N. Sebaceous carcinoma of the vulva. Br J Obstet Gynaecol 2003;110(2):227–8.

Vulvar Cysts, Adenocarcinoma, Melanocytic, and Miscellaneous Lesions

5

Victor G. Prieto, M. Angelica Selim

CHAPTER OUTLINE

Cysts	95
Follicular ('Epidermoid') Cyst	95
Steatocystoma Multiplex	96
Bartholin Cyst	96
Mucinous Cyst	97
Ciliated Cyst (Paramesonephric Cyst)	97
Paraurethral (Skene) Gland Cyst	97
Mesonephric-Like Cyst	97
Cyst of the Canal of Nuck	98
Extramammary Paget Disease	98
Melanocytic Lesions	101
Lentigo	101
Common Acquired Melanocytic Nevus	101
Melanocytic Nevus of the Genital Type	102
Blue Nevus (Dermal Melanocytoma)	102
Atypical (Dysplastic, Clark) Nevus	102
Melanoma	103
Skin Appendage Neoplasms and Lesions of the Anogenital Mammary-Like Glands	106
Hidradenoma Papilliferum (Papillary Hidradenoma or Mammary-Like Gland Adenoma of the Vulva)	106
Syringoma	106
Trichoepithelioma	107
Vascular Lesions	108
Infantile Hemangioma ('Strawberry' Hemangioma)	108
Venous Malformation (Cavernous Hemangioma)	108
Deep Lymphatic Malformation (Cavernous Lymphangioma)	108
Miscellaneous Lesions	109
Acrochordon (Fibroepithelial Polyp, Skin Tag, Squamous Papilloma)	109
Endometriosis	109
Heterotopic Breast	109
Rare Tumors and Tumor–Like Conditions	110
Langerhans Cell Histiocytosis (Histiocytosis X)	110
Merkel Cell Carcinoma (Trabecular Carcinoma, Small Cell Carcinoma of the Skin, Primary Cutaneous Neuroendocrine Carcinoma)	110
Metastatic Tumors	112
Tumors of the Bartholin Gland	112
Urethra	113
Urethral Caruncle	113
Urethral Carcinoma	113

CYSTS

FOLLICULAR ('EPIDERMOID') CYST

Definition

Follicular cyst is a cystic dilatation of the hair follicle epithelium.

Clinical Features

Follicular cyst presents as a solitary, creamy-white or yellowish lesion on the labium majus (Figure 5.1). It is generally asymptomatic, but rupture may induce inflammation with enlargement, tenderness, erythema, and induration. Follicular cysts usually occur spontaneously and after age 30. Onset at an early age or occurrence in great numbers should prompt consideration of Gardner syndrome.

Microscopic Features

Most vulvar follicular cysts represent dilatations of the most distal portion of the follicle, the infundibulum, hence they have thin, flat, squamous epithelium lacking rete ridges, contain a granular layer, and are filled with loose-packed

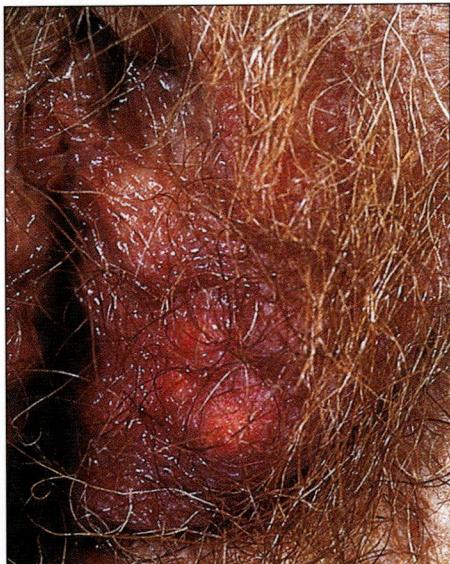

Figure 5.1 Follicular cysts ('epidermal inclusion cysts'). Ruptured cysts become inflamed as a result of foreign body giant cell reaction to keratin leakage.

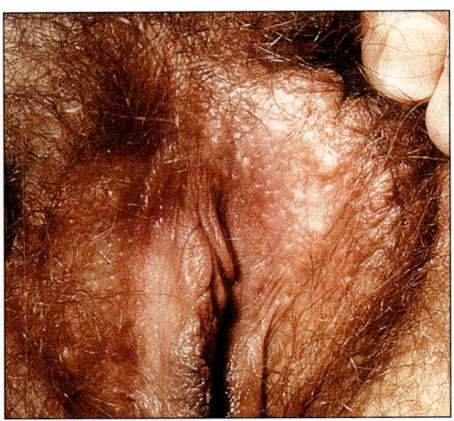

Figure 5.2 Steatocystoma multiplex. This inherited disorder, sometimes involving the genitalia, shows multiple creamy-colored cysts.

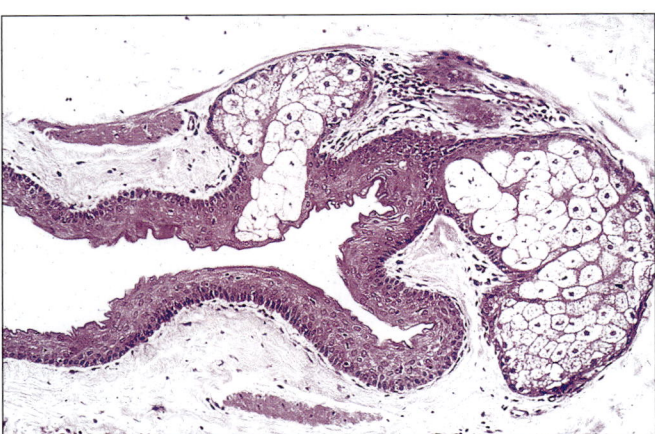

Figure 5.3 Steatocystoma multiplex. Characteristic features include an apparently collapsed cyst with sebaceous units in the wall and a densely eosinophilic thin lining cuticle.

keratin. Its rupture may lead to leakage of keratin, resulting in an acute and chronic inflammatory foreign-body reaction.

STEATOCYSTOMA MULTIPLEX

Definition
Widespread, multiple, thin-walled cysts of the skin, lined by *squamous epithelium*, and including lobules of *sebaceous* cells.

Clinical Features
Steatocystoma multiplex is the dominantly inherited occurrence of numerous small, creamy-colored cysts exhibiting sebaceous ductal differentiation. The lesions usually appear after adolescence and may be solitary. Most common locations are the presternum, axillae, abdomen, and labia majora. Rarely, they first present as multiple vulvar cysts at an older age[1] (Figure 5.2).

Microscopic Features
Steatocystomas are composed of an intricately folded, thin layer of stratified squamous epithelium lined internally by a corrugated, thin, compact, and strongly eosinophilic cuticle, lacking a granular layer. There may be associated small sebaceous glands (Figure 5.3). Although this finding raises the differential diagnosis of dermoid cyst, the latter is extremely rare in the vulva and shows miniaturized hair follicles.

BARTHOLIN CYST

Definition
Bartholin cyst is the cystic dilatation of a major vestibular (Bartholin) gland or its duct.

Clinical Features
Bartholin cyst is the most common form of vulvar cyst, and is the presenting complaint for 2% of women during their annual gynecologic visit.[2] The Bartholin glands (Figure 5.4) are located behind the labia minora and their ducts open into the posterior lateral vestibules, just anterior to the

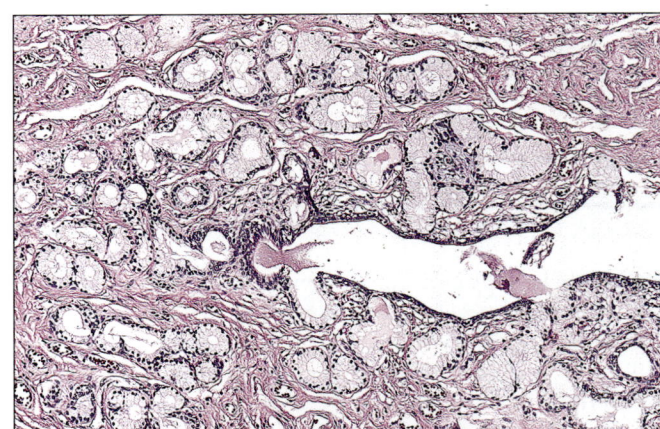

Figure 5.4 Normal Bartholin gland. Simple tubuloalveolar glands with mucin-producing alveoli drain eventually into a central duct lined by transitional epithelium.

hymeneal tegmentum. Bartholin cysts result from blockage of the drainage duct and resultant retention of secretions, perhaps following infection. Bartholin cysts are most common in the reproductive years. If large, they may partially obstruct the introitus. Bartholin cysts usually present as smooth-domed nodules, generally 1–10 cm in diameter. If brown or blue, they may be mistaken clinically for melanocytic nevi. The cysts contain mucoid fluid, which stains with mucicarmine, periodic acid–Schiff (PAS; with and without diastase), and Alcian blue at pH 2.5. They may recur after incision and drainage, and may require surgical excision, particularly in postmenopausal women, to rule out the possibility of associated carcinoma. Bartholin abscess is an acute process usually caused by *Neisseria* gonorrheal infection. Excision, drainage, and antibiotics are the treatments of choice.

Microscopic Features

Bartholin cysts show a lining of transitional epithelium, with frequent focal squamous metaplasia (Figure 5.5). Smaller mucus-filled cysts may show some remnant of the original mucus-secreting glandular epithelium, but it may be flattened or cuboidal. Normal remnants of mucus glands may be presented adjacent to the cyst. Microscopically, the Bartholin duct abscess shows abundant neutrophilic infiltrate within the stroma surrounding the duct.

MUCINOUS CYST

Definition

Mucinous cyst is the cystic dilatation of a minor vestibular gland or its duct.

Clinical Features

True mucinous cysts most commonly occur in the vulvar vestibule, including the medial labium minus and near the Bartholin glands. Onset is typically between puberty and the fourth decade, usually in parous women or those exposed to oral contraceptives. Mucinous cysts are 2 mm to 3 cm in diameter and are usually solitary. They may cause pain or urinary complaints. Excision is curative. They presumably are due to obstruction.

Microscopic Features

These cysts are lined almost entirely by columnar or cuboidal mucus-secreting epithelium like that of endocervical glands without peripheral muscle fibers or myoepithelial cells. Foci of squamous metaplasia are sometimes present; they are considered to be of urogenital sinus origin.[3]

CILIATED CYST (PARAMESONEPHRIC CYST)

An occasional cyst may be lined partially by ciliated columnar epithelium (Figure 5.6). Usually this occurs as a focal change within a mucinous cyst or a Bartholin cyst; it is likely a nonspecific metaplastic change.

PARAURETHRAL (SKENE) GLAND CYST

Definition

Paraurethral gland cyst is the cystic dilatation of the paraurethral (Skene) gland or its duct.

Clinical Features

The paired paraurethral glands (the female homolog of the male prostate gland) are located on either side of the urethral meatus. Ductal occlusion, probably a consequence of infection (e.g., gonococcal), leads to formation of a retention cyst, generally less than 2 cm in size, located in the upper lateral introitus. Paraurethral gland cysts affect from neonates to premenopausal women, with an incidence of 1 per 2000–7000 women.[4] Patients may be asymptomatic or complain of urinary obstruction or dyspareunia. Surgical excision should be done after medical therapy for any underlying infection.[5]

Microscopic Features

Paraurethral gland cysts are probably derived from the duct rather than the acini, and are lined by transitional or stratified squamous epithelium upon a basement membrane, with only rare luminal cells containing intracytoplasmic mucin. Rarely, they contain calculi.

MESONEPHRIC-LIKE CYST

Definition

Mesonephric-like cysts are lined by cuboidal or low columnar epithelium and encased by a small amount of smooth muscle.

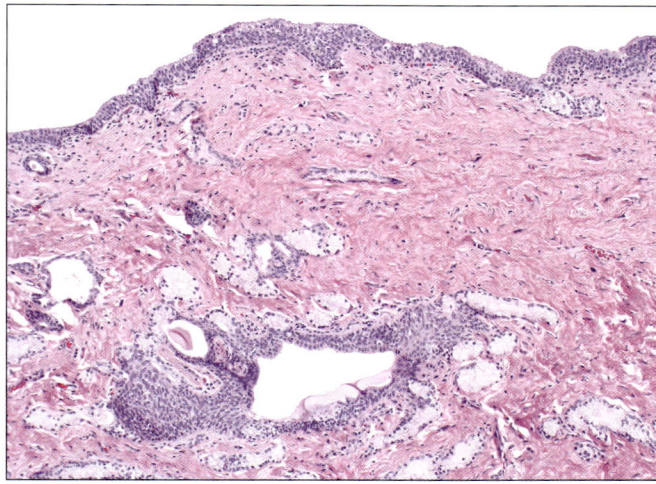

Figure 5.5 Bartholin cyst. The cyst wall (top) is lined by transitional epithelium as it is a duct (center) surrounded by normal mucus glands.

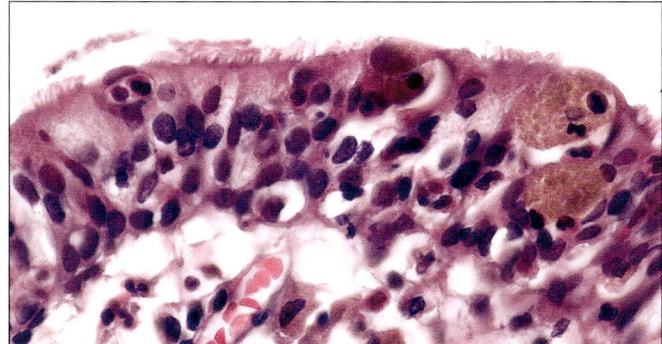

Figure 5.6 Bartholin gland cyst with ciliated cells.

Clinical Features

These cysts occur in the lateral walls of the vulva as superficial, single, domed, blue or red cysts with clear, watery contents. They resemble mesonephric ducts but their embryologic basis is unclear.

CYST OF THE CANAL OF NUCK

Definition

Cyst of the canal of Nuck is a cystic remnant of the processus vaginalis peritonei.

Clinical Features

These cysts are most common in the inguinal canal, where they must be distinguished from hernias. They also occur in the mons pubis and in the superior, outer region of the labium majus. Ultrasonography or magnetic resonance imaging may be helpful for definitive clinical diagnosis. They are homologous to hydroceles in males.[6] The processus vaginalis peritonei (canal of Nuck) is a rudimentary sac of peritoneal mesothelium carried down by the round ligament as it passes through the inguinal canal[7,8] and inserts into the labium majus. Failure of this structure to obliterate normally during fetal development leads to blockage and cystic dilatation. While these cysts are usually solitary, more than one may arise if obstruction occurs at multiple sites. Generally asymptomatic, they may become tender to pressure, and may then require a procedure similar to herniorrhaphy.

Microscopic Features

In their pristine state, these are thin-walled and lined by flattened mesothelium. By the time they present clinically, repeated external trauma has usually induced fibrosis of their walls, reduced or destroyed their mesothelial lining, and caused hemosiderin deposition from old haemorrhage.[9]

EXTRAMAMMARY PAGET DISEASE

Definition

Extramammary Paget disease[10] is a form of *in situ* adenocarcinoma of the squamous mucosa. For a number of these cases, recent evidence suggests an origin from Toker cells, which are found in the breast with clear cytoplasm that reacts for cytokeratin 7 (CK7)[10–13] and are thought to derive from the ostia of the mammary-like glands found in the vulva, perineum, and perianal skin.

Clinical Features

The vulva is the most common site of extramammary Paget disease, accounting for about 5% of all vulvar neoplasms. It usually presents in older women as a moist, red, eroded or eczematous-appearing plaque. One or both sides of the vulva can be involved, often with spread to the perianal skin (Figure 5.7). The plaques are usually irritated and sore, and may be clinically misinterpreted as an inflammatory skin disease (e.g., intertrigo, fungal infections, immunobullous disorders, Hailey–Hailey disease). The diagnosis requires biopsy confirmation.

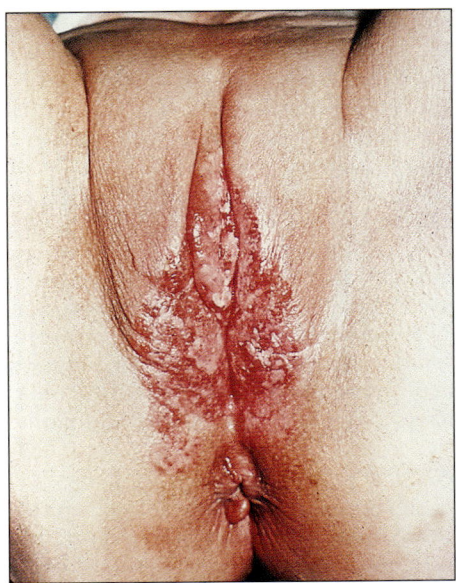

Figure 5.7 Paget disease, which extends to involve the perianal region.

Treatment may be difficult because the disease usually extends well beyond the clinically apparent margins. Moreover, even surgical margin status is not particularly helpful in predicting recurrence, as about a third of patients experience recurrence regardless of whether the margins after initial surgery are positive or negative. The extent of the operation (wide local excision, simple vulvectomy, or modified radical vulvectomy) during the initial treatment also poorly correlates with disease recurrence. Mohs micrographic surgery, topical chemotherapy, and photodynamic therapy may play a role in selected cases. HER-2/neu expression has been demonstrated by some Paget disease of the vulva;[14] thus, some patients may benefit from trastuzumab (Herceptin), a recombinant monoclonal antibody against HER-2/neu.

Microscopic Features

Histologically, the epidermis contains pale-staining cells that are larger than adjacent keratinocytes, arranged singly or in small to large nests (Figure 5.8). When numerous, Paget cells may replace much of the epidermis, which appears swollen and thickened (Figure 5.9). When Paget cells are single or few in number, they appear to be mainly above the basal layer or individually (pagetoid migration) into the upper epidermal layers. Cells appear not to be connected with the basement membrane and thus are different from melanoma *in situ* (see later; Figure 5.10A). Paget cells may even be found growing down hair follicles as well as eccrine glands (Figures 5.11 and 5.12). Occasionally, similar cells may be seen in the underlying dermis (Figure 5.13), indicating invasion. While up to 50% of patients are reported to show invasion in some series,[15] this is a distinctly unusual happening in our experience. Likewise, we find that metastases to lymph nodes are exceedingly rare.

The pale cytoplasm of the Paget cell is usually finely granular, and the nuclei are central and round to oval. Mitotic

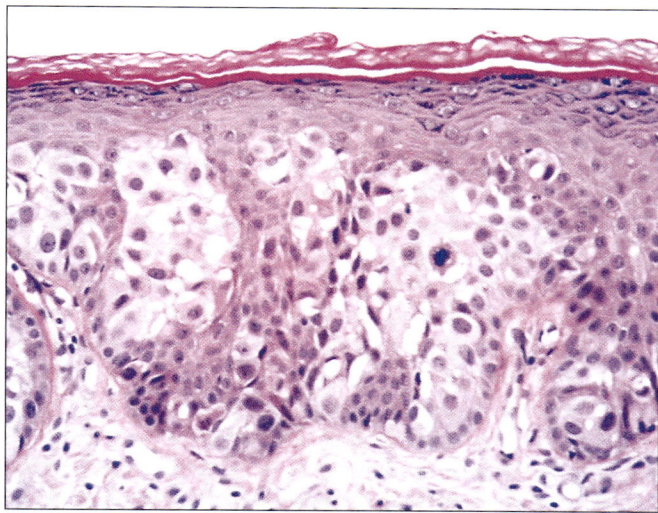

Figure 5.8 Paget disease. Nests of pale-staining tumor cells are located within the epidermis including the upper layers. The nests compress the basal layer of squamous cells.

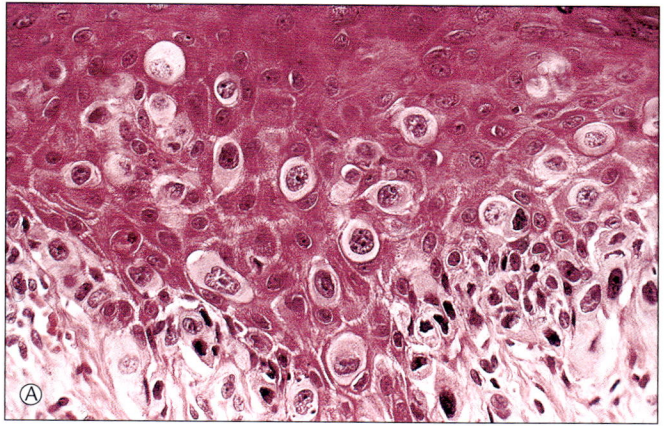

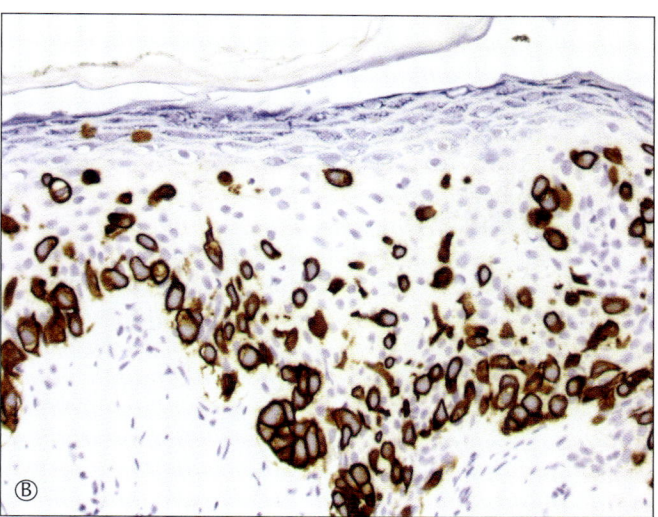

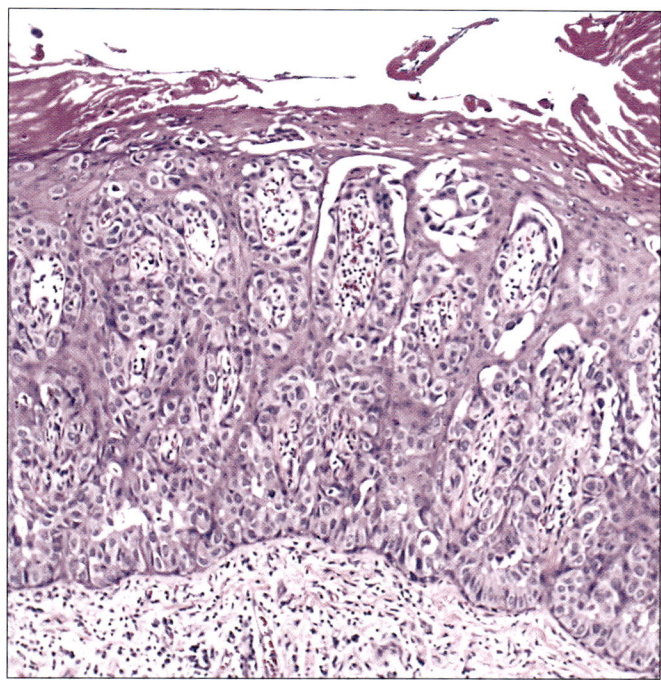

Figure 5.9 Massive Paget disease in which virtually the entire epidermis has been replaced.

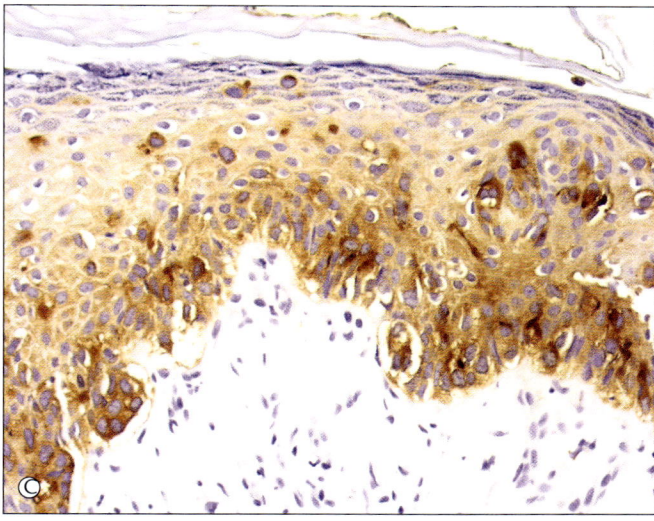

Figure 5.10 Paget disease. **(A)** The tumor cells have abundant pale cytoplasm and are arranged singly or in small clusters within the epidermis. They appear larger than the surrounding keratinocytes. **(B)** Paget cells express CK7 and **(C)** CEA.

figures may be found. On routine staining, Paget disease may be confused with melanoma *in situ*. However, the Paget cells at the basal layer are usually discrete and characteristically compress and displace the normal keratinocytes, whereas melanoma cells generally form a continuous proliferation close to the basement membrane.

Paget cells usually contain intracytoplasmic mucin (neutral and acidic), as highlighted by PAS-diastase, Alcian blue, colloidal iron, and mucicarmine stains. In problematic cases, immunohistochemistry may be useful (Table 5.1),

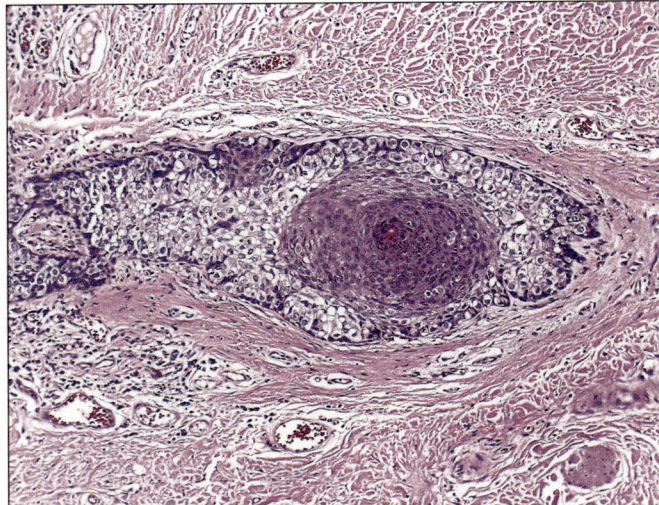

Figure 5.11 Paget disease involving a hair follicle.

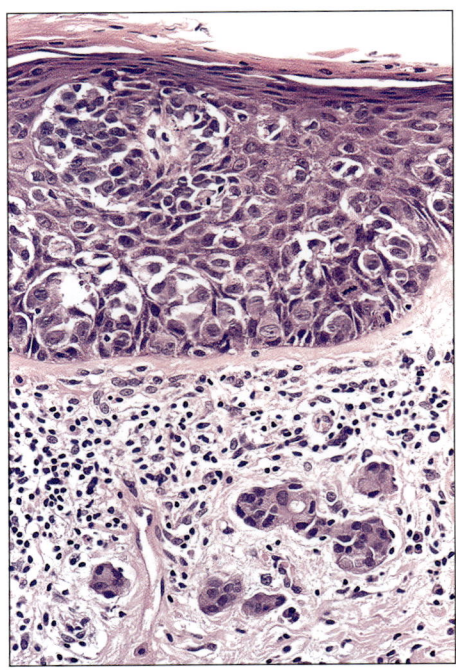

Figure 5.13 Invasive Paget disease.

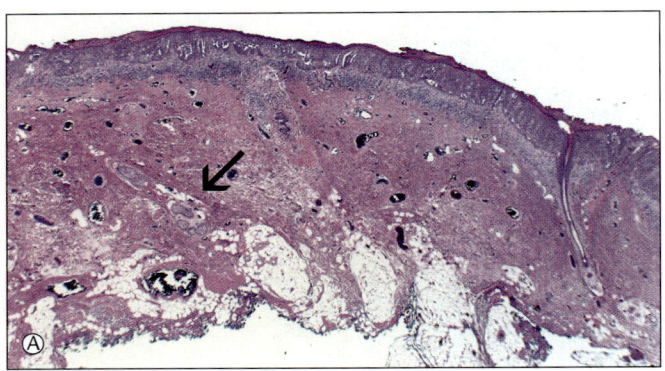

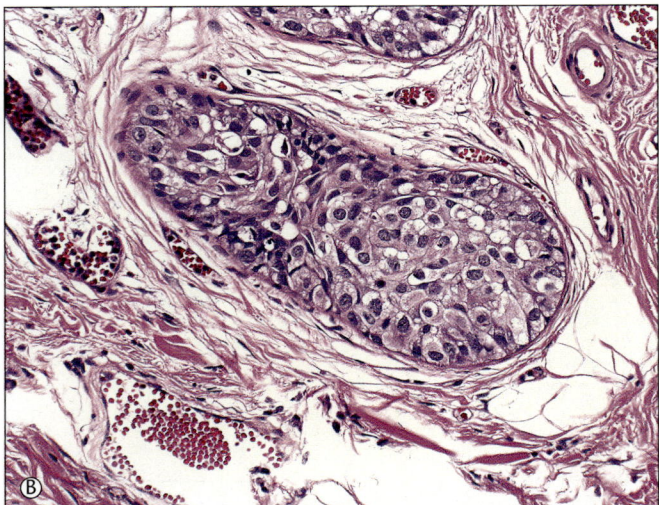

Figure 5.12 Paget disease involving sweat glands. **(A)** Low-power section of skin in which the involved gland (arrow) extends near to the cutaneous fat. **(B)** Detail of gland cut in cross section.

with Paget cells selectively expressing cytokeratins CAM 5.2, CK7 (Figure 5.10B), MUC5AC, carcinoembryonic antigen (CEA) (Figure 5.10C), epithelial membrane antigen (EMA), and gross cystic disease fluid protein-15 (BRST-2). About one-fifth of Paget cases are reactive for CK20.[16] Since S-100 protein is also sometimes expressed, such cases may require study for more specific melanocytic markers (MART-1/Melan-A, HMB45, etc.). A possible pitfall is those cases in which the tumor cells contain melanin pigment since the interspersed melanocytes may show prominent dendrites and thus may be interpreted as melanoma cells.[17] Androgen receptors can be detected in some cases.[18]

The origin of extramammary Paget disease is controversial. Some cases represent epidermotropic adenocarcinomas, but, unlike mammary cases (in which an underlying ductal carcinoma is almost invariably present), an underlying carcinoma is only rarely detected. Other postulated origins include a pluripotential stem cell within the epidermis or *in situ* malignant transformation of cells in the cutaneous sweat ducts as they insert into the epidermis. The most recent works point to the Toker cell[11–13] (Figure 5.14), which in the breast is an intraepidermal clear cell with bland nuclear features that is reactive for CK7 but not CK20.[12] Cytogenetic findings suggest that at least some cases of Paget disease arise multicentrically within the epidermis from pluripotent stem cells,[19] and have a molecular basis differing from other vulvar carcinomas.[20]

Regarding the expression of mucin core proteins, vulvar Paget disease may arise from ectopic MUC5AC-positive cells originating from Bartholin or some other unidentified glands, while the unique expression of MUC2 in perianal Paget disease indicates that its origin from colorectal mucosa differs from that in the vulva.

Table 5.1 Immunohistochemical Panel in the Differential Diagnosis of Extramammary Paget Disease, Squamous Cell Carcinoma, and Melanoma

Diagnosis	Keratin Cocktail	CK7	CK20	S-100	MART-1/HMB45
Paget disease	+	+	–/+*	–**	–
Squamous cell carcinoma	+	+	–	–	–
Melanoma	–	–	–	+	+

*CK20 is usually negative in extramammary Paget disease. However, it is positive in cases of carcinoma of the genitourinary or gastrointestinal tract.
**Rare cases of Paget disease may express S-100.

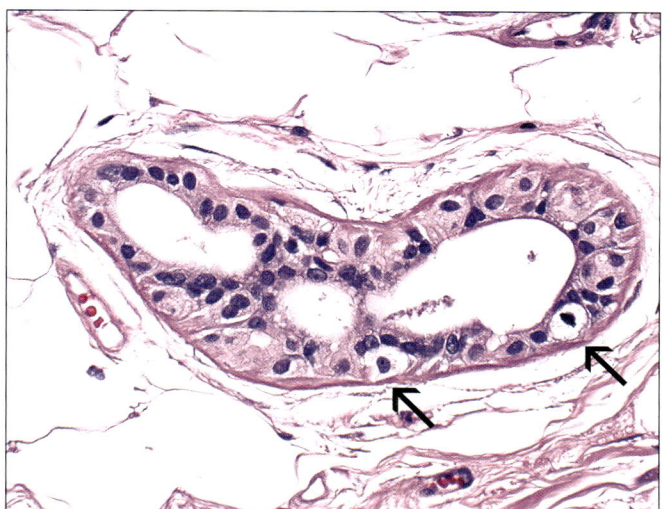

Figure 5.14 Toker cells (arrows) with abundant clear cytoplasm in an isolated anogenital mammary-like gland of the vulva.

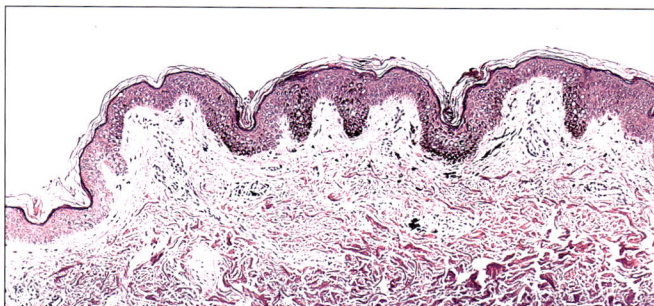

Figure 5.15 Lentigo. Note the hyperpigmentation of basal keratinocytes without apparent increase in the number of melanocytes.

MELANOCYTIC LESIONS

LENTIGO

Definition

A lentigo is a circumscribed macule of increased pigmentation, generally 5 mm or less in diameter, and persisting even in the absence of sun exposure.

Clinical Features

Lentigines are common on the labia majora or minora. They are often deeply pigmented but usually have uniform color, sharp circumscription, and regular borders. Lentigines proper are not precursors of melanoma.[21]

Microscopic Features

The epidermis of a lentigo has elongated rete ridges and increased melanin deposition in the keratinocytes (Figure 5.15). The number of melanocytes should be approximately normal. Furthermore, the melanocytes lack cytologic atypia.

COMMON ACQUIRED MELANOCYTIC NEVUS

Definition

A melanocytic nevus is a benign neoplasm composed of cells exhibiting melanocytic differentiation.

Clinical Features

Melanocytic nevi are the most common neoplasms to occur in humans. An average Caucasian adult has 10 or more. Nevi occur with some frequency on the vulva, usually on the labia majora (Figure 5.16).

Microscopic Features

Intradermal, junctional, and compound nevi resemble those seen elsewhere in the body. A key element in assessing the benignity of a melanocytic lesion is to determine the presence of 'maturation,' i.e., the tendency to undergo a morphologic shift with progressive depth in the dermis as seen on both light microscopy and immunohistochemical expression.[22] Another hallmark of benignity is a tendency for quiescence in the deeper component, with reduced numbers of proliferating cells in the deeper dermis[23] and absence of mitotic figures. In contrast, most melanomas consist of large, pleomorphic cells throughout the entire lesion and exhibit mitotic figures in their deep component. However, an uncommon subset of melanomas exhibits a paradoxical pattern of maturation simulating that of nevi.[24] A possible pitfall is the presence of mitotic figures in otherwise benign nevi from pregnant women.[25]

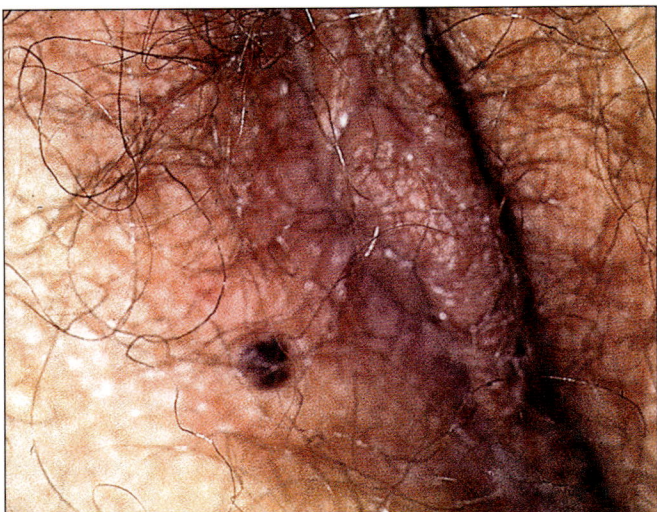

Figure 5.16 Melanocytic nevus. The dark color and slight irregularity of outline and pigmentation intensity in this woman of 52 years is a worrying feature and merits complete excision.

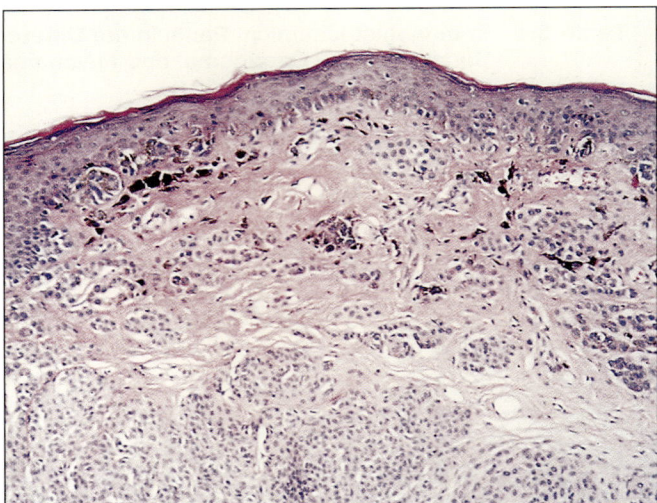

Figure 5.17 Compound nevus of the 'genital' type. Note the focal 'bridging' of the rete ridges and irregular shape and size of junctional nests. There is no evident fibrosis or lymphocytic infiltrate in the subepithelial region.

MELANOCYTIC NEVUS OF THE GENITAL TYPE

Definition
A subset of nevi occurring on the vulva, perineum, or mons pubis exhibits particular stromal changes. It differs from the standard atypical (dysplastic, Clark) nevus, which can be found anywhere, occurs in young individuals, and lacks the characteristic stromal changes seen in the atypical 'dysplastic' nevus.

Clinical Features
Nevi of the genital type are more common on the labia minora or the mucosa of the clitoral region than on the labia majora. They have also been seen in other flexural areas such as the axillae and uncommonly on male genitalia. They occur at a much younger age (median 25 years) than vulvar melanoma.

Microscopic Features
These nevi show confluent and enlarged nests of nevus cells that vary in size, shape, and position at the dermoepidermal junction (Figure 5.17). The nevus cells exhibit reduced cohesion. Finally, the stromal pattern at the dermoepidermal junction is often inconspicuous and nondescript in contrast to the concentric eosinophilic fibroplasia or lamellar fibroplasia seen in the usual atypical (dysplastic) nevus (see later).

BLUE NEVUS (DERMAL MELANOCYTOMA)

Definition
Blue nevus is a benign melanocytic neoplasm consisting almost exclusively of spindle and epithelioid dermal cells associated with prominent melanin pigment.

Clinical Features
Blue nevus is relatively uncommon in the vulva. It is fairly common on the buttock and acral extremities. These nevi are small, blue to black, well-circumscribed lesions, sometimes slightly raised.

Microscopic Features
The dermis has collections of spindle-shaped or dendritic cells containing delicate melanin pigment, intersecting with dense collagen fibers (Figure 5.18). There are also melanophages containing coarse, clumped melanin pigment. In the cellular variant, the nevus cells are packed in dense fascicles, often forming a dumbbell-shaped nodule that may extend into the subcutis. Malignant change in blue nevi is extremely rare.[26] We discourage the use of the term 'malignant blue nevus' and rather recommend 'melanoma blue-nevus type' for such melanoma cases showing spindle cells and pigmented melanocytes/melanophages (i.e., resembling blue nevus). Blue nevi with necrosis or mitotic figures or cytologic atypia are usually described as atypical forms[27] and probably warrant conservative excision.

A related entity is the pigmented epithelioid melanocytoma ('animal-type melanoma').[28] It is unclear whether this lesion is a low-grade melanoma or if it belongs to a spectrum of lesions between blue nevus and melanoma. Most pigmented epithelioid melanocytomas occur in the extremities but some lesions have been described in the vulva. Histologically, they resemble the epithelioid blue nevus seen in patients with the Carney complex. Lymph node metastasis may occur, but visceral metastasis is uncommon.

ATYPICAL (DYSPLASTIC, CLARK) NEVUS

Clinical Features
Both atypical nevi and melanomas customarily are relatively large (>5 mm), poorly circumscribed, and asymmetric, with an irregular border and a range of colors. Atypical nevi represent a strong, independent risk factor for development of melanoma,[29] whether occurring sporadically or in the context of a familial melanoma diathesis. Moreover, there is a strong relationship between melanoma risk and

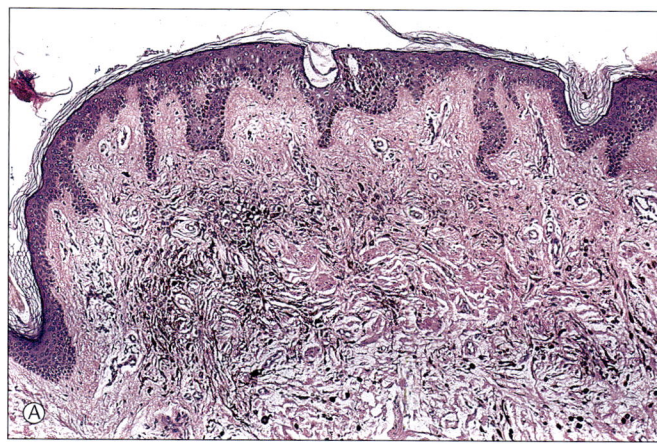

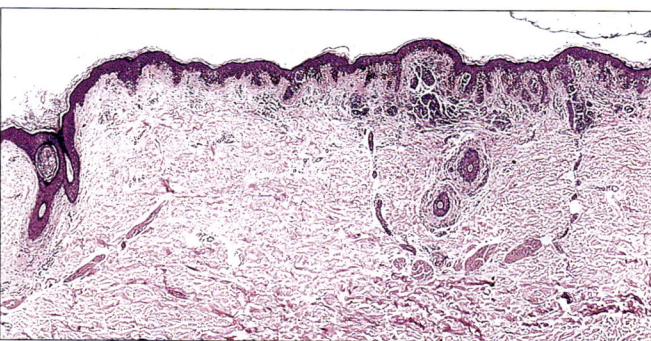

Figure 5.19 Atypical nevus. Features of architectural disorder such as bridging of rete ridges and irregular size and shape of junctional nests. Evidence of a host response with fibrosis, vascular proliferation, and lymphocytic infiltrate with melanophages.

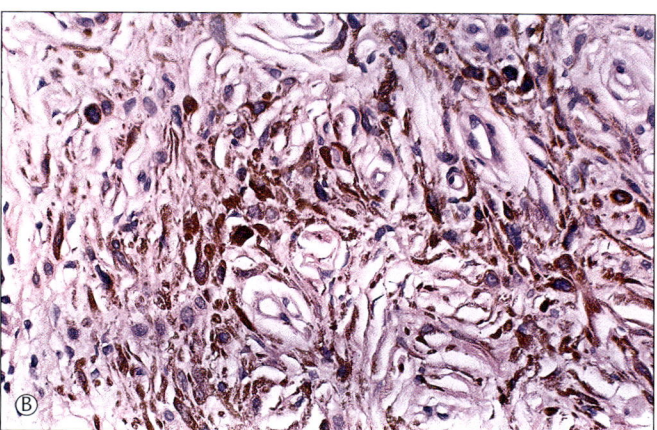

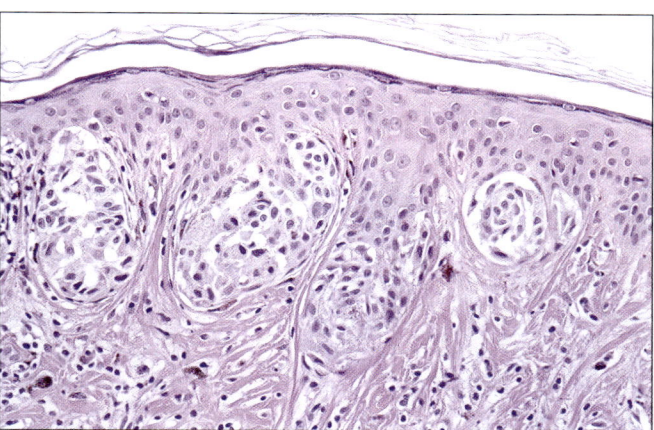

Figure 5.18 **(A)** Blue nevus. **(B)** Dendritic, finely pigmented melanocytes with scattered, coarsely pigmented macrophages.

Figure 5.20 Atypical nevus: detail of nevus cells, dermal fibrosis, and lymphocytic infiltrate.

the number of atypical nevi present. Apart from this role as a simple marker of melanoma risk, atypical nevi themselves may on occasion be precursors to melanoma.

Microscopic Features

The histopathologic features include abnormal architecture, host response, and cytology. In general, there is a high degree of consensus on the defining architectural features of atypical nevi, which include peripheral extension of the junctional component (shoulder) (Figure 5.19), confluence of single melanocytes or via bridging of adjacent rete ridges, and irregular disposition, size, and shape of junctional nests (Figure 5.20).

MELANOMA

Definition

Melanoma is a malignant tumor of melanocytes.

Clinical Features

Vulvar melanoma accounts for 8–10% of all malignant tumors of the vulva.[30–35] It occurs on the clitoris, labia minora, and labia majora with similar frequency, and may develop from a pre-existing pigmented lesion. It affects mainly older women, and only rarely younger women and girls.[36,37] Vulvar bleeding is the most common symptom followed by vulvar mass, vulvar ulcer, and mole.[33]

Except in the rare amelanotic[38] variant, the clinical appearance of melanoma is characteristic. There is usually marked gross asymmetry, border irregularity, and color variegation, sometimes including a play of brown, black, blue, and red (Figures 5.21 and 5.22). A white color suggests regression. Most melanomas have a prominent *in situ* (intraepidermal) component, which presents as a hyperpigmented macule. Elevation to form a plaque or nodule frequently indicates invasion, and is an ominous sign. Development of satellite lesions (approximately in 20% of cases) is a form of local metastasis and is associated with poor prognosis.[33]

Microscopic Features

Historically, melanoma has been classified into four distinct histopathologic subtypes, including superficial spreading melanoma, nodular melanoma, acral–lentiginous (mucosal–lentiginous) melanoma, and lentigo maligna melanoma. Verrucous melanoma has also been described. Acral–lentiginous (mucosal–lentiginous) melanoma is the most common type of vulvar melanoma.

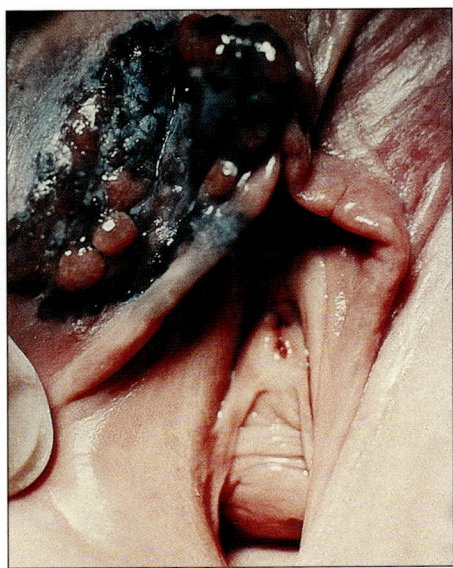

Figure 5.21 Melanoma. The tumor is darkly pigmented, elevated, and nodular.

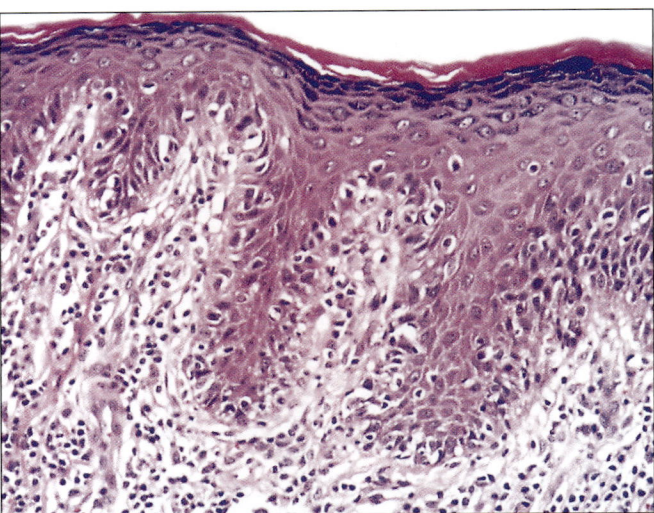

Figure 5.23 Mucosal lentiginous melanoma. The lower levels of the epidermis contain an almost continuous line of atypical melanocytes, somewhat resembling one pattern of Paget disease.

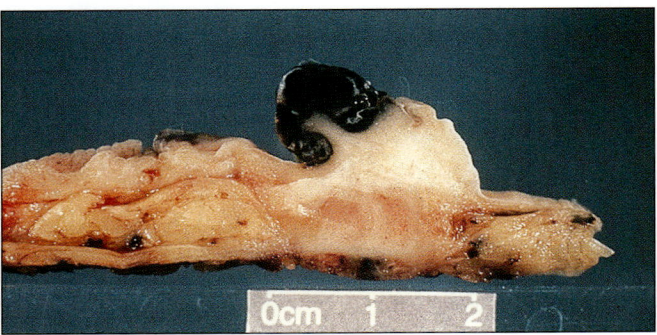

Figure 5.22 Melanoma. Cross section shows the pigmented tumor's invasive nature.

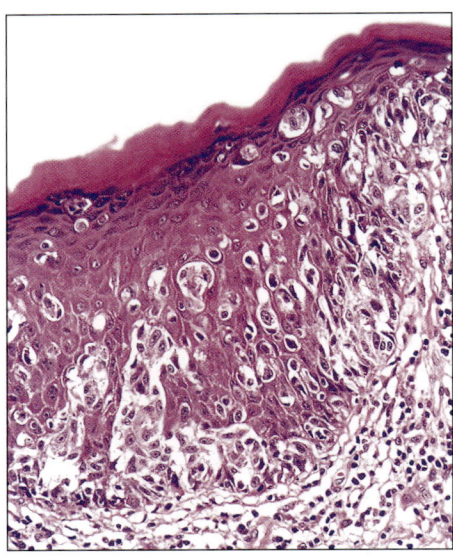

Figure 5.24 Melanoma. Atypical melanocytes, singly and in clumps, migrate into the upper layers of the epidermis ('pagetoid change'), but there is no dermal invasion.

Melanoma *in situ* is composed of atypical melanocytes arranged both singly and in nests within the epithelium (Figure 5.23). Single cells often predominate over nests, and confluence may be extensive. In superficial spreading melanoma, the tumor cells usually exhibit high-grade cytologic atypia (large, pleomorphic nuclei with large nucleoli), as well as marked architectural disorder including pagetoid spread through the upper epidermal layers (Figure 5.24). The radial growth or the atypical melanocytes involves four or more adjacent rete ridges. In nodular melanomas, an intraepithelial component may be seen in continuity with an invasive component, but without a radial growth phase. The so-called acral–lentiginous variants usually show less pagetoid spread and the tumor cells often have less abundant cytoplasm; these melanomas are composed of relatively small but hyperchromatic melanocytes, with a marked tendency to extend along the basal layer of the epidermis and adnexal epithelium. However, the distinctive cellular features of melanoma are seen in the invasive component, which often shows a desmoplastic stromal reaction.

Differential Diagnosis

Vulvar melanoma, particularly of the superficial spreading type, should be distinguished from Paget disease and vulvar intraepithelial neoplasia (VIN). The cells of Paget disease are larger than those of superficial spreading melanoma and, occasionally, form glandular structures. Sarcomatoid squamous cell carcinomas may mimic the invasive component of malignant melanoma of the acral–lentiginous type. However, foci of typical squamous cell carcinoma facilitate the correct diagnosis and are usually encountered in deeper sections. Melanomas are immunoreactive for S-100 protein, HMB45, and Melan-A, whereas the non-melanocytic tumors, (including Paget, VIN, and squamous cell carcinoma) are

Table 5.2 Immunohistochemical Panel Used in the Differential Diagnosis of Squamous Cell Carcinoma, Merkel Cell Carcinoma, Adenocarcinoma, and Melanoma

Diagnosis	Keratin Cocktail	CK7	CK20	CK5/6	CEA	S-100	MART-1/HMB45	Chromogranin Synaptophysin
Squamous cell carcinoma	+	+	−	+	−	−	−	−
Merkel cell carcinoma	+	−*	+	−	−	−	−	+
Adenocarcinoma	−	−	−	−	+	−**	+	−
Melanoma	***	−	−	+	−†	+	+	−

*Some cases of Merkel cell carcinoma may express CK7.
**Rare cases of adenocarcinoma (e.g., Paget disease) may express S-100.
***Up to 10% of melanoma cases may focally express keratins (low molecular weight).
†Rare melanoma cases may focally express CEA.

negative (Table 5.1). Paget disease can be distinguished from melanoma with mucin stains and immunohistochemical reactions for CEA, S-100 protein, HMB45 (or Melan-A), and cytokeratins (Table 5.1). Paget cells typically contain cytoplasmic mucin, as shown with mucicarmine stain, and are immunoreactive for CEA and cytokeratins, whereas melanomas are not. Spindle cell sarcomas and metastatic choriocarcinoma may also enter in the differential diagnosis. Muscle markers for leiomyosarcoma or rhabdomyosarcoma (e.g., desmin, smooth muscle actin) and human chorionic gonadotropin (hCG) for choriocarcinoma may be helpful. Nevertheless, it should be emphasized that the diagnosis of melanoma must be seriously considered when examining any poorly differentiated tumor of the vulva (Table 5.2). To confirm the diagnosis of vulvar melanoma, immunoreactions for epithelial markers (e.g., AE1/3, CK7 and CK20, EMA, CEA, GCDFP-15), neural and neuroendocrine tumor markers (e.g., S-100, chromogranin, synaptophysin, CD56), and melanoma markers may be done (Figure 5.25; Table 5.2).

Clinical Behavior and Treatment

Local recurrences are frequent and the overall 5 year survival rates vary from 37% to 54%, even when the tumor appears localized at initial presentation. Factors that adversely influence survival include ulceration, Clark level IV, tumor thickness (Breslow) exceeding 2 mm, and mitotic count exceeding 10 mitoses per mm^2. Non-diploidy by flow cytometry is also a strong independent risk factor for death.[39]

The Clark level is inapplicable to melanomas arising in vulvar mucosa since it may be difficult to determine the anatomic boundary between the papillary and reticular dermis (distinction between levels III and IV). Thus, it can be applied only to vulvar melanomas arising in keratinized skin. In contrast, the Breslow measurement for thickness is readily applicable in both sites. It measures the distance from the top of the granular layer of the overlying epidermis to the deepest melanoma cells in the dermis. If the tumor is thickest in an area of ulceration (therefore lacking a granular layer), the floor of the ulcer should be used as the starting point for measurement. Periappendageal tumor cells should be measured from the center of that particular appendage and not from the top of the granular layer. For noncutaneous tumors involving the vulvar mucosa, the measurement of the thickness is modified as from the top of the epithelium to the deepest melanoma cell in the mucosa. Lesions measuring <0.76 mm in thickness have little or no metastatic potential. This is also accepted for tumors with a thickness of 1 mm or less. Correlations between the thickness and the level of a vulvar melanoma can be made. Level I (in situ) melanomas have no measurable thickness. Level II melanomas have a thickness of 1 mm or less; level III, from 1 to 2 mm; and level IV melanomas have a thickness exceeding 2 mm without involving the subcutaneous fat.

Mitotic figures are counted as their number per mm^2. This is done in 'hot spots'; i.e., we recommend looking for areas with visible mitotic figures and then counting the number of mitoses in 4½ consecutive high power fields (×40) (his area corresponds to 1 mm^2).[40]

Regression probably represents a negative prognostic factor. The likely explanation is that regressed lesions may previously have attained a greater thickness, and so the measured Breslow thickness may underestimate the tumor's metastatic potential.[41]

Melanomas of the labia minora which involve the urethra and vagina have a particularly poor prognosis, likely related to a delayed diagnosis when compared to melanomas located in more easily accessible areas and because it is difficult to achieve complete surgical excision. Therefore, surveillance and early biopsy are crucial.[42]

As mentioned earlier, the last American Joint Committee on Cancer classification highlights the main histologic features that correlate with worse prognosis and recommends that the pathology reports should include Breslow thickness, ulceration, and number of mitotic figures in the dermis.[43]

Surgical treatment is based on complete local excision, with margins based on the thickness of the tumor. Melanoma *in situ* is usually treated with complete excision of the gross lesion, the full thickness of the underlying dermis, and a 5 mm rim of normal tissue. Invasive melanoma thinner than 1 mm is treated similarly, but with a 1 cm margin. Debate remains about the appropriate margins for deeper melanomas,[44] but some surgeons recommend a 2 or 3 cm margin in thick tumors to decrease the probability of local recurrence. Rarely, radical vulvectomy with lymph node removal

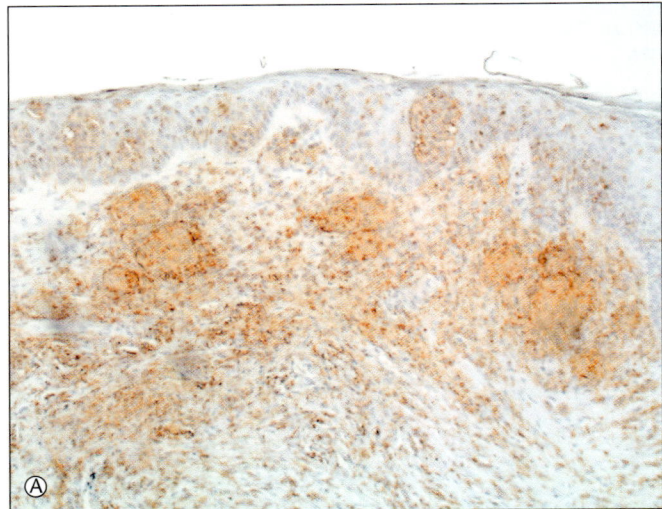
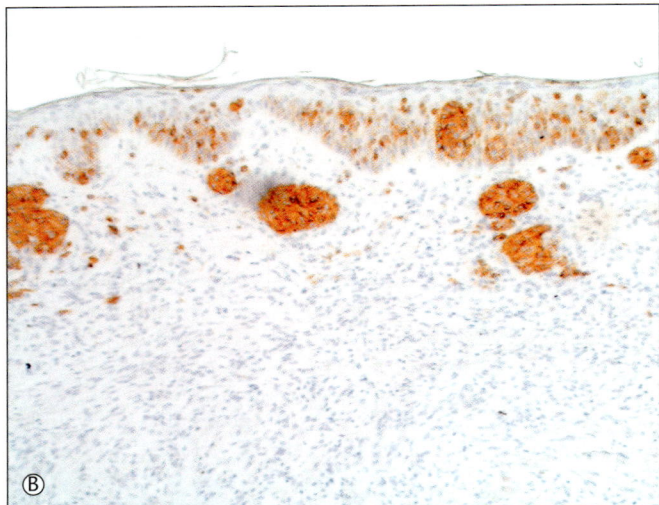
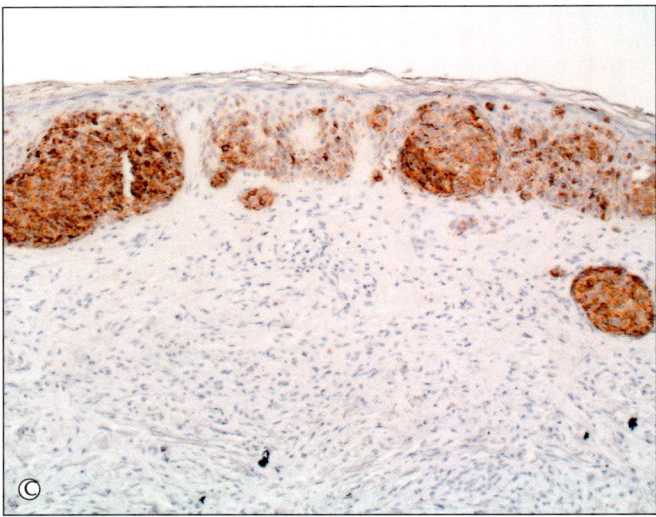

Figure 5.25 Immunohistochemical markers used to confirm the diagnosis of invasive melanoma: **(A)** S-100 protein, **(B)** MART-1, and **(C)** HMB45 antigen. Usually most melanoma cells express S-100 protein but invasive melanoma cells may show only focal expression of MART-1 or HMB45 antigen.

is necessary in large, neglected melanomas or those with urethral, clitoral, or lower vaginal involvement. Complete elective lymphadenectomy is now uncommonly performed for clinically nonpalpable nodes, but sentinel lymph nodes[45] are often removed in tumors 1 mm or greater in thickness, ulcerated tumors, or those with a mitotic index higher than $1/mm^2$. Completion lymphadenectomy may be recommended in cases with positive sentinel node(s).[46]

SKIN APPENDAGE NEOPLASMS AND LESIONS OF THE ANOGENITAL MAMMARY-LIKE GLANDS

The vulvar skin contains hair follicles, eccrine sweat glands, apocrine glands, and sebaceous glands. In the labia majora the sebaceous glands open into the hair follicles (pilosebaceous unit) but in the labia minora they are small and superficial, opening directly onto the mucosal surface.[47] Despite the high concentration of skin appendages in the vulva, tumors derived from them are uncommon.

HIDRADENOMA PAPILLIFERUM (PAPILLARY HIDRADENOMA OR MAMMARY-LIKE GLAND ADENOMA OF THE VULVA)

Definition

Hidradenoma papilliferum is a benign neoplasm with cystic and papillary features, and composed of epithelium exhibiting apocrine differentiation.

Clinical Features

Hidradenoma papilliferum is the only adnexal neoplasm seen frequently on the vulva. It occurs mainly in middle-aged women on the labia majora and the outer lateral surfaces of the labia minora, but may also arise in the perineum. It typically presents as a solitary, round, firm, dome-shaped, occasionally tender nodule, 1–2 cm in diameter (Figure 5.26). Neglected, large lesions may ulcerate and bleed and lead to the formation of Bartholin cyst/abscess by obstruction. Malignant change is very rare. Human papillomavirus infection does not appear to play an etiologic role.[48]

Microscopic Features

These tumors are usually purely intradermal and are roughly spherical. Within a collagenous stroma are epithelial cells in a complex, folded, papillary pattern (Figure 5.27). Each branching papilla has a fibrovascular core and a double-layered epithelium consisting of small, dark-staining myoepithelial cells and an inner layer of columnar or cuboidal cells, some of which are PAS positive. Mitotic count can range from 0 to 5.3 mitoses/mm^2.[49] Oxyphilic metaplasia and areas of solid growth in this lesion are uncommon but may cause a diagnostic challenge.[50] Rarely, mammary-like adenocarcinomas may develop from these adnexal tumors.[51]

SYRINGOMA

Definition

Syringoma is a benign, microcystic neoplasm exhibiting differentiation toward eccrine ducts.

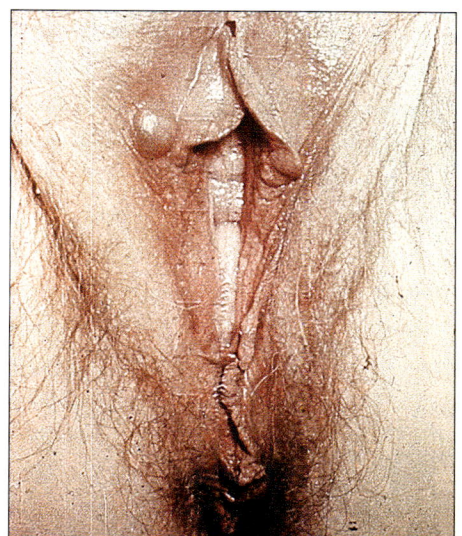

Figure 5.26 Hidradenoma papilliferum involving the right labium.

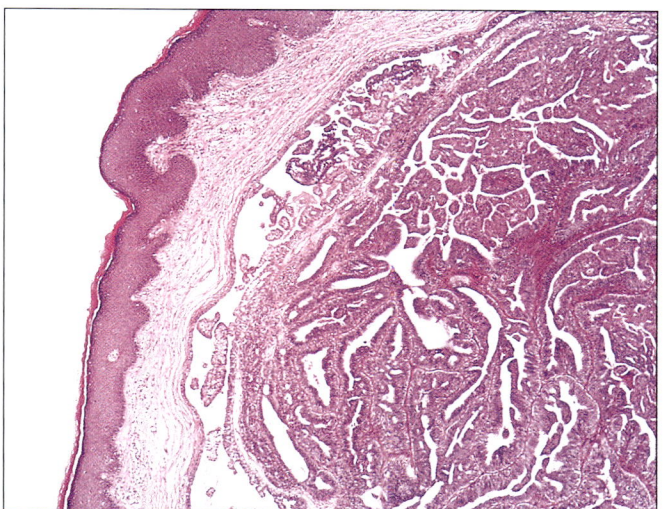

Figure 5.27 Hidradenoma papilliferum. The complex papillary pattern of this dermal sweat gland tumor is characteristic.

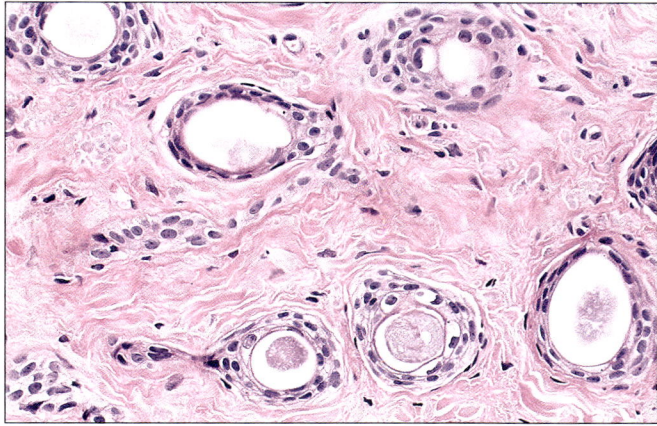

Figure 5.28 Syringoma. Small, benign glands within the subepithelial region.

Clinical Features

Syringoma most often occurs on the eyelid, often as multiple lesions. Labial syringomas may occur in the setting of eruptive syringomatosis. Grossly, the tumors are flesh-colored, dermal papules, less than 3 mm in diameter, most commonly seen in young women. Malignant change is extremely rare.[52] Lesions usually remain small and treatment is rarely necessary. Vulvar pruritus can occur and be aggravated during menses or pregnancy.[53,54]

Microscopic Features

Histologically, syringomas comprise clusters of minute, cystic ductal structures exhibiting a double layer of compressed epithelium, often with curved epithelial extensions attached to some of the microcysts (tadpole or frying-pan appearance) (Figure 5.28). The epithelium may undergo clear-cell change due to abundance of cytoplasmic glycogen. The lumen of the microcysts often contains pink-staining, PAS-positive, proteinaceous material. Usually the stroma surrounding the glandular proliferation is fibrotic. In chondroid syringoma (benign mixed tumor of skin), the stroma is myxocartilaginous. This lesion is histologically identical to the pleomorphic adenoma of the salivary gland.

TRICHOEPITHELIOMA

Definition

Trichoepithelioma is a benign neoplasm exhibiting trichogenic differentiation.

Clinical Features

Trichoepithelioma occurs most often on the head and neck as a flesh-colored papule, 2–8 mm in diameter, but may occur on the vulva. It is usually a solitary, sporadic lesion with onset in childhood or early adulthood.[55] In the less common autosomal dominant form (Brooke–Spiegler syndrome), multiple lesions present in childhood and gradually increase in size; in this setting, trichoepithelioma may be associated with other cutaneous neoplasms such as cylindroma. Either form may be managed by conservative treatment such as shave biopsy or curettage, sometimes combined with electrodesiccation or cryotherapy.

Microscopic Features

Classic trichoepithelioma consists of basaloid cells that closely recapitulate follicular differentiation (Figure 5.29), especially by developing papillary mesenchymal bodies (fibroblastic aggregates resembling abortive follicular papillae) (Figure 5.29, inset) and horn pseudocysts (resembling follicular infundibula). The main histologic differential diagnosis is with basal cell carcinoma. In problematic cases, the presence of mitotic and apoptotic figures, myxoid stroma, and retraction of neoplastic cells from the stroma suggest basal cell carcinoma, whereas well-formed papillary–mesenchymal bodies and a more fibrous stroma suggest trichoepithelioma.[56] In the desmoplastic variant, follicular differentiation is less well developed; aggregates of neoplastic cells, usually including some keratinizing cysts, extend diffusely within a fibrous stroma, and may simulate the morpheiform pattern of basal cell carcinoma or microcystic adnexal carcinoma.

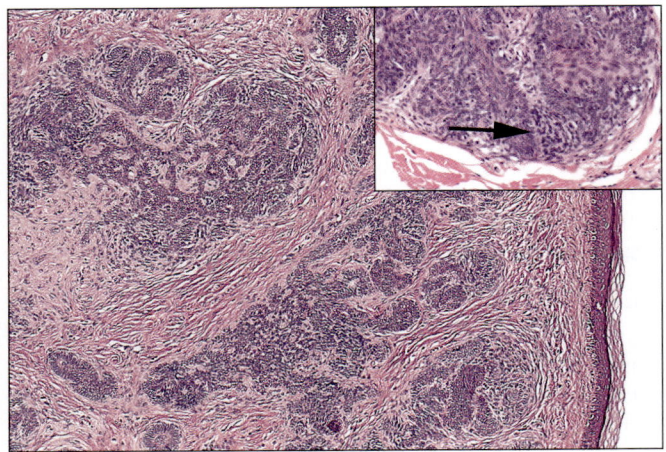

Figure 5.29 Trichoepithelioma. Basaloid cells with an organoid pattern. Inset: condensation of mesenchymal cells immediately adjacent to a cluster of basaloid cells (papillary mesenchymal body) (arrow).

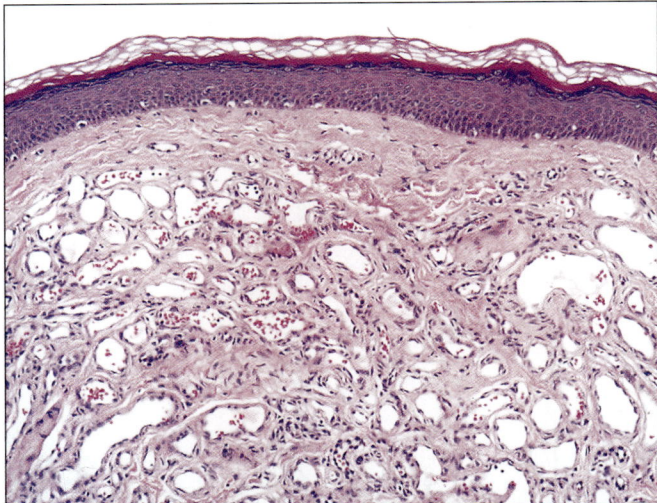

Figure 5.30 Capillary hemangioma. This small dermal angioma is largely composed of capillary-sized channels. It is identical to those seen elsewhere in the skin.

VASCULAR LESIONS

INFANTILE HEMANGIOMA ('STRAWBERRY' HEMANGIOMA)

Definition

Infantile hemangioma is a benign vascular neoplasm with onset in infancy and having a tendency for rapid growth followed by spontaneous regression.

Clinical Features

These lesions have a predilection for the head and neck, but may also occur on the vulva and perianal skin.

In a large revision of gynecologic tumors in childhood and adolescence, hemangiomas of the vulva represent 0.8% of all tumors.[57] They are the most common vascular neoplasm of infancy, affecting 1% of newborns.

Microscopic Features

Lobular collections of small blood vessels are present in the dermis (Figure 5.30). During the early stages of the life cycle, these lesions are hypercellular and composed of numerous capillary-type vessels. In mature lesions, the vessels may become widely dilated. Regressed lesions are fibrotic and usually contain only a few dilated vessels. GLUT-1 is a specific and sensitive marker for infantile hemangiomas, and can aid in their distinction from vascular malformations.[58] Similarly, expression of Wilms' tumor 1 gene (*WT1*) can help distinguish proliferative vascular lesions from malformations.[59]

VENOUS MALFORMATION (CAVERNOUS HEMANGIOMA)

Definition

Venous malformation is a benign vascular lesion representing abnormal structures or widely dilated dermal blood vessels due to aberration in embryologic development. These slow-flow, hemodynamically inactive vessels are present at birth and worsen with time.

Clinical Features

This lesion rarely regresses spontaneously. Use of the term 'cavernous hemangioma' is discouraged as these lesions do not represent a proliferative neoplasm as that name implies. Clinically, most of the time they are asymptomatic lesions with no specific clinical presentation and can range from a small nodule found by routine gynecologic examination to a large unilateral vulvar mass with distortion of labia and perineum.[60]

Microscopic Features

Large blood vessels lined by a thin layer of endothelial cells are present in the dermis and subcutaneous tissue. Fibrin and red cells are numerous, and there may be focal calcification.[61]

DEEP LYMPHATIC MALFORMATION (CAVERNOUS LYMPHANGIOMA)

Definition

Deep lymphatic malformation is a benign lesion presenting as widely dilated, dermal or subcutaneous lymphatic vessels.

Clinical Features

This lesion may involve the whole lower limb and extend onto the vulva. In addition to surface changes similar to those seen in superficial lymphatic malformation, there is often hypertrophy and lymphedema of the affected area.[62] Lymphangiosarcoma is a rare complication with approximately eight cases reported.

Microscopic Features

The dermis or deeper soft tissue contains a mass of anomalous, widely dilated lymphatics, occasionally containing

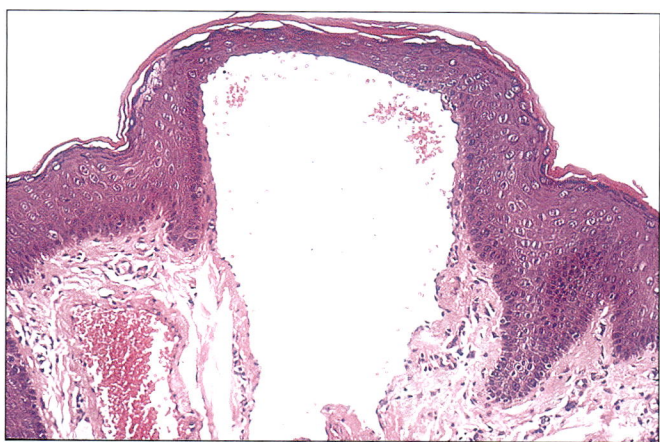

Figure 5.31 Cavernous lymphangioma. Large, dilated vascular spaces with only rare red blood cells.

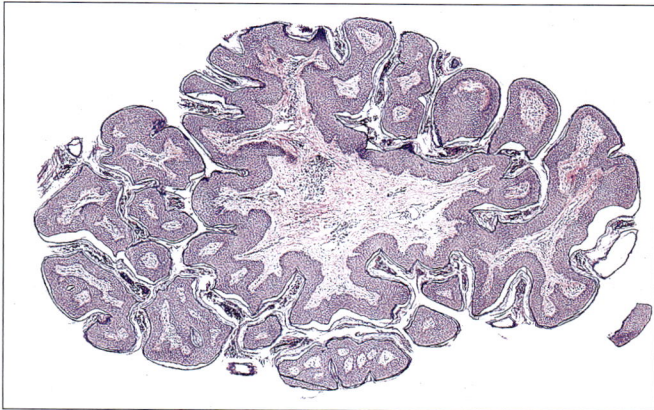

Figure 5.32 Acrochordon/fibroepithelial polyp. Polypoid lesion covered by squamous epithelium and containing a delicate stroma.

scattered red cells and lined by flat endothelium (Figure 5.31). Lymphoid tissue is usually present at the periphery. These lesions express D2-40, a marker commonly associated with lymphatic differentiation.

MISCELLANEOUS LESIONS

ACROCHORDON (FIBROEPITHELIAL POLYP, SKIN TAG, SQUAMOUS PAPILLOMA)

Definition
Acrochordon is a soft, skin-colored or pigmented polyp, ranging from a millimeter to a centimeter in diameter, and arising from a narrow stalk.

Clinical Features
This benign lesion is thought to result from chronic intertriginous rubbing and therefore occurs most commonly in the inguinal folds. Other sites include the mons pubis and labia majora. Acrochordons are more common in obese, middle-aged and elderly women, and are often familial.

Microscopic Features
Acrochordons are composed of a loose fibrovascular stroma covered by epidermis (Figure 5.32). Skin appendages are generally absent. Larger lesions may contain adipose tissue in the stromal core, and are then designated as dermatolipomas (Figure 5.33) or, if occurring in a dermatomal distribution and with a congenital onset, as nevus lipomatosus superficialis. Dermatolipomas may be associated with diabetes mellitus or hyperlipidemia.

ENDOMETRIOSIS

Implants of endometrial tissue into the vulva can occur during uterine curettage, episiotomy, or scar after excision of the Bartholin gland.[63] Areas of endometriosis appear as purplish-blue nodules, and may cause pain or bleeding during menstruation (see Chapter 22).

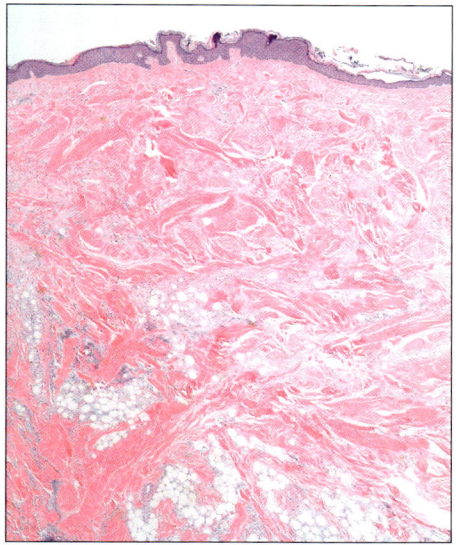

Figure 5.33 Dermatolipoma. Fibroepithelial polyp with superficial adipose tissue next to the epithelium.

HETEROTOPIC BREAST

Clinical Features
A rare finding in the vulva, it most commonly presents as a small, asymptomatic, solitary, mobile nodule not fixed to the overlying skin. It may swell in late pregnancy.

Microscopic Features
There are terminal ducts and lobular units typical of benign breast tissue, with inner columnar epithelium and outer myoepithelial layer. After childbirth it may show changes of lactation. Lesions similar to those found in normal breast may develop. They include sclerosing adenosis, fibroadenoma,[64,65] intraductal papilloma or even carcinoma.[66–70]

RARE TUMORS AND TUMOR-LIKE CONDITIONS

Several tumors and tumor–like conditions encountered rarely in the vulva are described in greater detail in organs where they occur at greater frequencies:

- Juvenile colonic polyp
- Primary yolk sac tumor
- Neurofibromas
- Solitary neurofibroma
- Schwannoma
- Lipoma
- Angiolipoma.

Please also see Chapter 6 for mesenchymal tumors of the vulva.

LANGERHANS CELL HISTIOCYTOSIS (HISTIOCYTOSIS X)

Definition

Langerhans cell histiocytosis (LCH) is a localized or systemic accumulation of neoplastic Langerhans cells.

Clinical Features

LCH is a spectrum of disease characterized by proliferation of specialized Langerhans cells and mature eosinophils. The infiltrate of LCH is sometimes monoclonal, supporting its neoplastic nature.

In the United States the incidence is about 1200 new cases per year. LCH spans a clinical spectrum ranging from an acute, fulminant, disseminated disease of childhood (Letterer–Siwe disease) to solitary or few, indolent, chronic lesions of bone or other organs (eosinophilic granuloma). An intermediate form, showing multifocal, chronic involvement, classically presents as the triad of diabetes insipidus, proptosis, and lytic bone lesions (Hand–Schüller–Christian disease). Approximately one-third of cases of apparently isolated vulvar LCH subsequently evolve to a disseminated form, most commonly involving bones.[71–75]

Eosinophilic granulomas are often asymptomatic, incidental findings discovered during investigation for unrelated disorders, or they may present with bone pain or as a soft-tissue mass. One-third of patients have mucocutaneous lesions, usually infiltrated nodules and ulcerated plaques, in the mouth, axillae, oral, perineal, vulvar, or retroauricular regions.

Microscopic Features

The dermis contains infiltrates of pathologic LCH cells admixed with eosinophils and a lesser number of neutrophils, plasma cells, and lymphocytes (Figure 5.34). The LCH cell is a non-dendritic, ovoid, mononuclear cell, 15–25 mm in diameter, with a folded or reniform nucleus, central nucleolus, and a moderate amount of slightly eosinophilic, homogeneous cytoplasm.

Immunohistochemistry can be helpful for definitive diagnosis. LCH cells strongly express S-100 protein in a cytoplasmic pattern, and also the more specific markers CD1a and langerin (CD207).[76] It should be noted that several cutaneous conditions, e.g., contact dermatitis, mycosis fungoides,

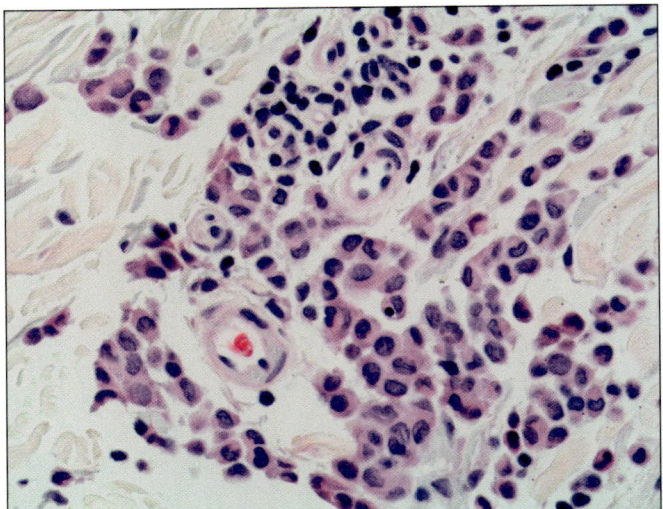

Figure 5.34 Langerhans cell histiocytosis. The tumor infiltrate is composed of pleomorphic Langerhans cells, eosinophils, and lymphocytes. In very young children, the infiltrate is composed almost entirely of Langerhans cells alone ('Letterer–Siwe disease').

and insect bites, show increased numbers of Langerhans cells. However, whereas the cells in LCH appear arranged in clusters and show rounded contours (Figure 5.35A), the reactive Langerhans cells resemble dendritic cells (Figure 5.35B).

MERKEL CELL CARCINOMA (TRABECULAR CARCINOMA, SMALL CELL CARCINOMA OF THE SKIN, PRIMARY CUTANEOUS NEUROENDOCRINE CARCINOMA)

Definition

Merkel cell carcinoma is a malignant primary neoplasm of the skin exhibiting neuroendocrine differentiation. A new polyomavirus, Merkel cell polyomavirus (MCV), was described in 2008 in tumor tissue of patients with Merkel cell carcinoma.[77–78]

Clinical Features

Mean age at diagnosis is about 75 years, and only 5% of cases occur before 50 years. They occur much more commonly in the skin of the head and upper trunk in the elderly, but may originate in the skin of the labia majora. Most present as a solitary, dome-shaped nodule or firm plaque, usually over 2 cm in greatest dimension. They are typically red, violaceous, or purple, with a shiny epidermal surface. Ulceration occurs occasionally.

Microscopic Features

Merkel cell carcinoma is usually located predominantly within the dermis and exhibits neuroendocrine differentiation. An intraepidermal component may be present, but purely intraepidermal cases are rare (Figure 5.36). The tumor may show several architectural patterns. The trabecular pattern consists of interconnecting strands of dermal tumor cells with formation of pseudorosettes and pseudoglands. The intermediate pattern comprises large, solid

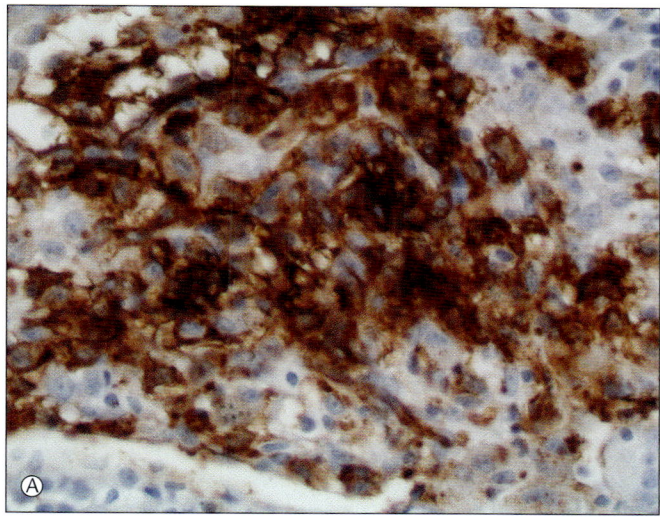

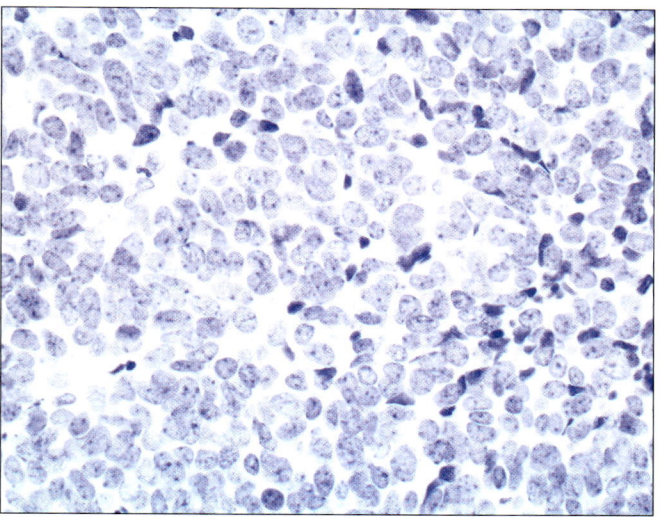

Figure 5.37 Merkel cell carcinoma. Tumor cells show large nuclei with speckled (salt and pepper) chromatin. There are numerous apoptotic bodies and mitotic figures.

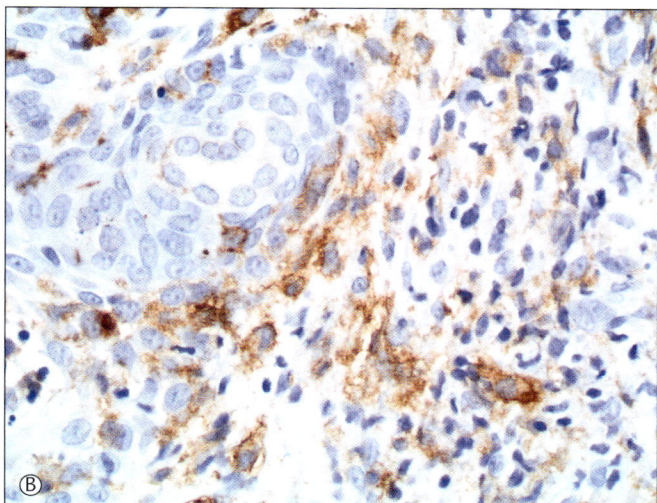

Figure 5.35 In Langerhans cell histiocytosis, Langerhans cells, which are immunoreactive for CD1a, show dense cytoplasm and rounded contour **(A)**; however, in reactive processes Langerhans cells appear as dendritic-shaped cells **(B)**.

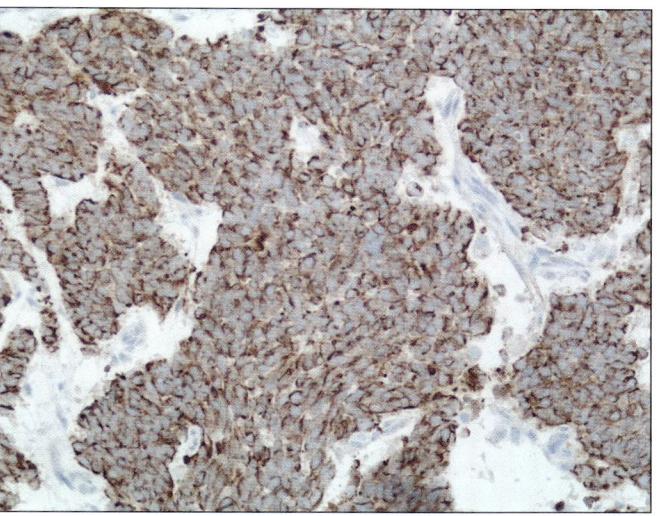

Figure 5.38 Merkel cell carcinoma. CK20 expression shows the characteristic dot-like pattern.

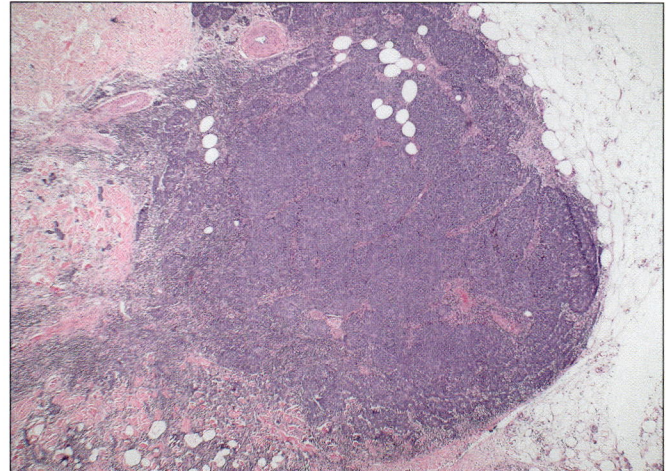

Figure 5.36 Merkel cell carcinoma. The tumor shows large masses of hyperchromatic cells.

nests of neoplastic cells. In the diffuse pattern, tumor cells infiltrate among dermal collagen bundles without forming distinctive organoid aggregates.

The neoplastic cells are round, small, and dark, with inconspicuous nucleoli, central euchromatin, and peripheral heterochromatin (Figure 5.37). Mitotic figures and apoptotic bodies are numerous. Lymphovascular invasion is a sign of adverse prognosis. Tumors exhibiting pagetoid growth may resemble extramammary Paget disease or melanoma,[79] whereas tumors with focal glandular or squamous differentiation mimic adenocarcinoma or squamous cell carcinoma. Immunohistochemistry is helpful for definitive diagnosis. Cytokeratins are expressed in a dot-like paranuclear pattern (Figure 5.38) and serve to distinguish Merkel cell carcinoma from metastatic neuroendocrine carcinoma (e.g., from a pulmonary primary tumor) (Table 5.2).

The tumors metastasize early and extensively via lymphatic vessels and the bloodstream. Overall 2 year survival is 50–70%. Better progression-free survival is seen in patients with high MCV antibody titers.[80] There are rare cases of Merkel cell carcinoma arising from the Bartholin gland. Merkel cell carcinoma has a poor outcome, with dissemination to regional lymph nodes or lung at the time of tumor detection or shortly thereafter.[81]

METASTATIC TUMORS

The most common primary sites of origin for vulvar metastases are the uterine cervix and endometrium, ovary, breast, lung, kidney, and large bowel. About half of the primary tumors are of gynecologic origin.[82] The labium majus is the site most frequently involved.

TUMORS OF THE BARTHOLIN GLAND

Other than cysts, diseases of the Bartholin gland are rare, including hyperplasia, adenoma, and carcinoma.[83–85] The latter are usually adenocarcinomas of various types (40%): papillary (Figure 5.39); mucinous (Figure 5.40); colloid (Figure 5.41); or squamous cell carcinomas (40%), but about 15% are adenoid cystic carcinomas (Figure 5.42),[86] which are histologically similar to those of the salivary glands. The tumors are composed of uniform cells arranged in cords and nests with a cribriform pattern. Cysts filled with eosinophilic basement membrane-like material are also found. Immunoreactivity for cytokeratins and S-100 protein demonstrate a myoepithelial cell component. Carcinoma of Bartholin glands may present as a nodule resembling the

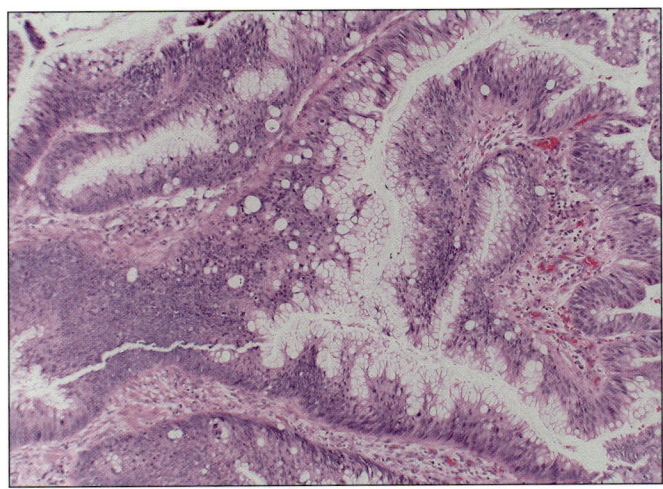

Figure 5.40 Mucinous adenocarcinoma of Bartholin gland.

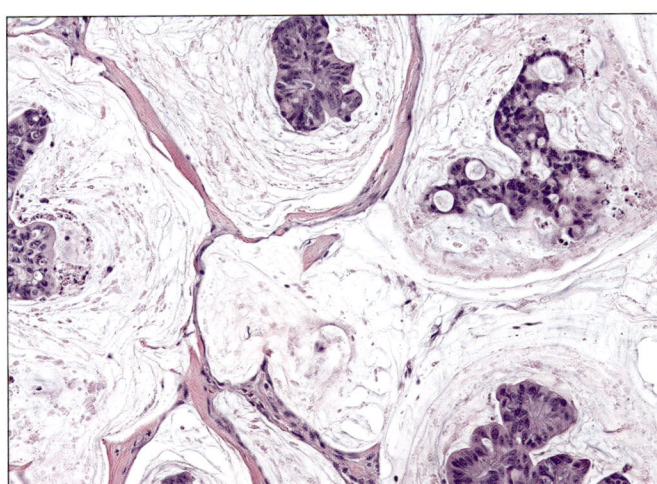

Figure 5.41 Colloid adenocarcinoma of Bartholin gland.

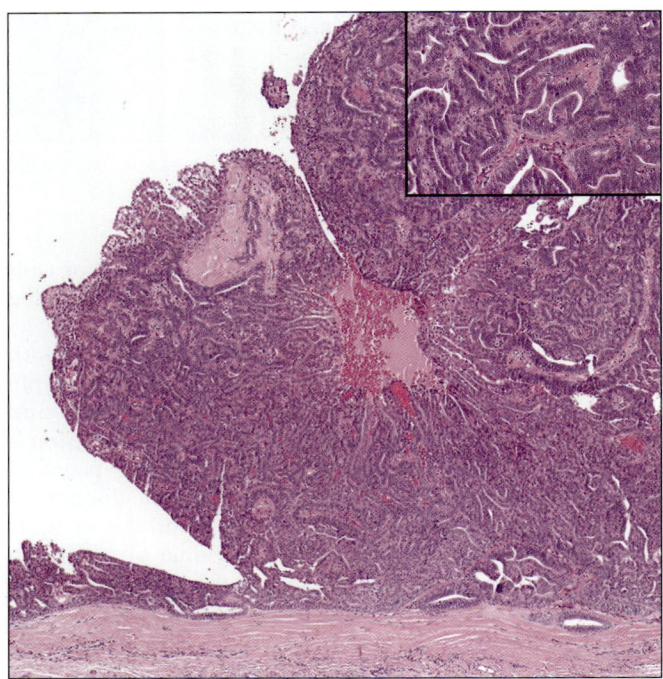

Figure 5.39 Papillary adenocarcinoma of Bartholin gland. Inset: high-power view.

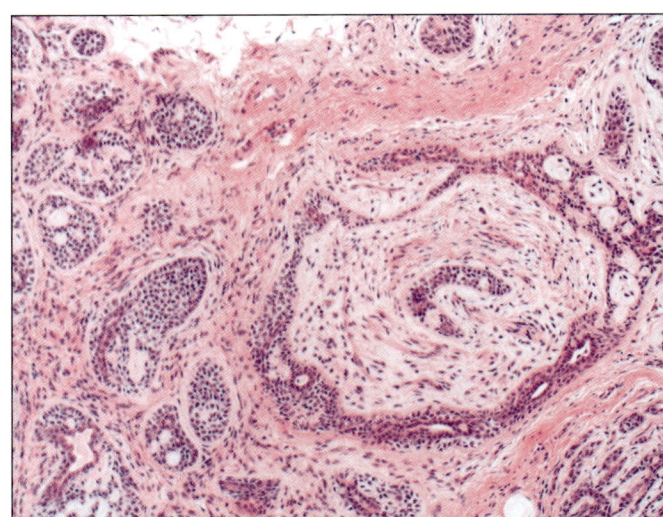

Figure 5.42 Adenoid cystic carcinoma of Bartholin gland.

much more common Bartholin gland cyst. At presentation, about 25% of all Bartholin gland carcinomas have metastasized to the superficial inguinal–femoral nodes. Wide local excision or vulvectomy with excision of inguinal nodes on both sides is the standard treatment. With adenocarcinoma, 5 year survival rates of about 50% can be expected, but this falls to about 20% when nodal metastases exist. Survival rates for squamous cell carcinoma are rather worse, and for adenoid–cystic carcinoma, slightly better.

Adenocarcinomas arising from anogenital mammary-like glands have histopathologic features very similar to those of primary mammary adenocarcinomas, and a few have been associated with breast cancers. Most have a pattern of growth of infiltrating, well-differentiated adenocarcinoma. In some cases, an intraductal carcinoma component has been identified.

URETHRA

URETHRAL CARUNCLE

Definition
The urethral caruncle is a small, fleshy, sometimes painful protrusion of the mucous membrane at the meatus of the female urethra.

Clinical Features
The caruncle may be telangiectatic, papillomatous, or composed of granulation tissue. It is common, usually after menopause, and is often asymptomatic, although it may be painful. Caruncles can be difficult to distinguish clinically from the early stage of the much rarer urethral carcinoma. The cancer, though, tends to bleed readily and is indurated to palpation.

Microscopic Features
Urethral caruncles are protuberant, polypoid masses of urethral stroma containing a dense, lymphohistiocytic infiltrate, admixed with neutrophils if the surface is ulcerated. Sometimes, vascular proliferation is so prominent to resemble a capillary hemangioma or pyogenic granuloma. Islands or cords of urethral epithelium are present, distinguishing the caruncle from urethral prolapse, in which the stroma is edematous, with only a scanty inflammatory infiltrate and no epithelium. Squamous cell carcinoma and amelanotic melanomas have been described arising from caruncles.[87,88]

URETHRAL CARCINOMA

Clinical Features
These rare tumors usually present in elderly women with dysuria, frequency, urgency, and hematuria. They account for <0.02% of malignant neoplasms occurring in women. In the early stages, urethral carcinoma resembles a caruncle or prolapse, but is characteristically firm to palpation, and may be friable and bleed.[89]

Microscopic Features
Almost all primary tumors of the urethra proper are squamous cell carcinomas arising from the squamous epithelium of the anterior third of the urethra. In advanced cases the urethral origin may be hard to identify, and such lesions may resemble an ordinary vulvar squamous cell carcinoma. Small foci of transitional epithelium may be seen, but pure transitional cell carcinoma is extremely rare. Adenocarcinomas of the urethral region are usually derived from the paraurethral glands. The usual squamous or mixed squamous/transitional carcinoma is most often solid, but there may be papillary areas. Spread is by local invasion to the bladder neck, the rest of the vulva, and occasionally the vagina. Lymphatic spread may occur to the superficial inguinal nodes and later the deeper pelvic nodes. The 5 year survival rate is 30–40%, despite surgery and radiotherapy. Large tumors with extensive local involvement and lymph node spread have a much worse prognosis.[90]

ACKNOWLEDGMENT
We would like to thank Drs. Christopher R. Shea and Stanley J. Robboy for their contribution to the chapter in the prior edition. We especially thank Dr. Jaime Prat for his insightful editorial comments.

REFERENCES

1. Rongioletti F, Cattarini G, Romanelli P. Late onset vulvar steatocystoma multiplex. Clin Exp Dermatol 2002;27:445–7.
2. Marzano DA, Haefner HK. The Bartholin gland cyst: past, present, and future. J Low Genit Tract Dis 2004;8:195–204.
3. Robboy SJ, Ross JS, Prat J, et al. Urogenital sinus origin of mucinous and ciliated cysts of the vulva. Obstet Gynecol 1978;51:347–51.
4. Ceylan H, Ozokutan BH, Karakok M, Buyukbese S. Paraurethral cyst: is conservative management always appropriate? Eur J Pediatr Surg 2002;12:212–14.
5. Busto Martín L, Barguti I, Andraca AZ, et al. Cyst of the Skene's gland: report of four cases and bibliographic review. Arch Esp Urol 2010;63:238–42.
6. Caviezel A, Montet X, Schwartz J, et al. Female hydrocele: the cyst of Nuck. Urol Int 2009;82:242–5.
7. Gaeta M, Minutoli F, Mileto A, et al. Nuck canal endometriosis: MR imaging findings and clinical features. Abdom Imaging 2010;35:737–41.
8. Safak AA, Erdogmus B, Yazici B, Gokgoz AT. Hydrocele of the canal of Nuck: sonographic and MRI appearances. J Clin Ultrasound 2007;35:531–2.
9. Ryan JD, Joyce MR, Pierce C, et al. Haematoma in a hydrocele of the canal of Nuck mimicking a Richter's hernia. Hernia 2009;13:643–5.
10. Fanning J, Lambert HC, Hale TM, et al. Paget's disease of the vulva: prevalence of associated vulvar adenocarcinoma, invasive Paget's disease, and recurrence after surgical excision. Am J Obstet Gynecol 1999;180:24–7.
11. Willman JH, Golitz LE, Fitzpatrick JE. Vulvar clear cells of Toker: precursors of extramammary Paget's disease. Am J Dermatopathol 2005;27:185–8.
12. Lundquist K, Kohler S, Rouse RV. Intraepidermal cytokeratin 7 expression is not restricted to Paget cells but is also seen in Toker cells and Merkel cells. Am J Surg Pathol 1999;23:212–19.
13. Belousova IE, Kazakov DV, Michal M, Suster S. Vulvar Toker cells: the long-awaited missing link: a proposal for an origin-based histogenetic classification of extramammary Paget disease. Am J Dermatopathol 2006;28:84–6.
14. Bianco MK, Vasef MA. HER-2 gene amplification in Paget disease of the nipple and extramammary site: a chromogenic in situ hybridization study. Diagn Mol Pathol 2006;15:131–5.
15. Crawford D, Nimmo M, Clement PB, et al. Prognostic factors in Paget's disease of the vulva: a study of 21 cases. Int J Gynecol Pathol 1999;18:351–9.
16. Goldblum JR, Hart WR. Vulvar Paget's disease: a clinicopathologic and immunohistochemical study of 19 cases. Am J Surg Pathol 1997;21:1178–87.

17. Petersson F, Ivan D, Kazakov DV, et al. Pigmented Paget disease—a diagnostic pitfall mimicking melanoma. Am J Dermatopathol 2009;31:223–6.
18. Diaz de Leon E, Carcangiu ML, Prieto VG, et al. Extramammary Paget disease is characterized by the consistent lack of estrogen and progesterone receptors but frequently expresses androgen receptor. Am J Clin Pathol 2000;113:572–5.
19. Teixeira MR, Kristensen GB, Abeler VM, Heim S. Karyotypic findings in tumors of the vulva and vagina. Cancer Genet Cytogenet 1999;111:87–91.
20. Takata M, Hatta N, Takehara K. Tumour cells of extramammary Paget's disease do not show either p53 mutation or allelic loss at several selected loci implicated in other cancers. Br J Cancer 1997;76:904–8.
21. Barnhill RL, Albert LS, Shama SK, et al. Genital lentiginosis: a clinical and histopathologic study. J Am Acad Dermatol 1990;22:453–60.
22. Prieto VG, Shea CR. Use of immunohistochemistry in melanocytic lesions. J Cutan Pathol 2008;35(Suppl 2):1–10.
23. Rudolph P, Schubert C, Schubert B, Parwaresch R. Proliferation marker Ki-S5 as a diagnostic tool in melanocytic lesions. J Am Acad Dermatol 1997;37:169–78.
24. Ruhoy SM, Prieto VG, Eliason SL, et al. Malignant melanoma with paradoxical maturation. Am J Surg Pathol 2000;24:1600–14.
25. Clark Jr WH, Hood AF, Tucker MA, Jampel RM. Atypical melanocytic nevi of the genital type with a discussion of reciprocalparenchymal-stromal interactions in the biology of neoplasia. Hum Pathol 1998;29(Suppl 1):S1–S24.
26. Spatz A, Zimmermann U, Bachollet B, et al. Malignant blue nevus of the vulva with late ovarian metastasis. Am J Dermatopathol 1998;20:408–12.
27. Tran TA, Carlson JA, Basaca PC, Mihm MC. Cellular blue nevus with atypia (atypical cellular blue nevus): a clinicopathologic study of nine cases. J Cutan Pathol 1998;25:252–8.
28. Mandal RV, Murali R, Lundquist KF, et al. Pigmented epithelioid melanocytoma: favorable outcome after 5-year follow-up. Am J Surg Pathol 2009;33:1778–82.
29. Tucker MA, Halpern A, Holly EA, et al. Clinically recognized dysplastic nevi. A central risk factor for cutaneous melanoma. JAMA 1997;277:1439–44.
30. Verschraegen CF, Benjapibal M, Supakarapongkul W, et al. Vulvar melanoma at the M. D. Anderson Cancer Center: 25 years later. Int J Gynecol Cancer 2001;11:359–64.
31. Sugiyama VE, Chan JK, Shin JY, et al. Vulvar melanoma: a multivariable analysis of 644 patients. Obstet Gynecol 2007;110:296–301.
32. Stang A, Streller B, Eisinger B, Jockel KH. Population-based incidence rates of malignant melanoma of the vulva in Germany. Gynecol Oncol 2005;96:216–21.
33. Ragnarsson-Olding BK, Kanter-Lewensohn LR, Lagerlof B, et al. Malignant melanoma of the vulva in a nationwide, 25-year study of 219 Swedish females: clinical observations and histopathologic features. Cancer 1999;86:1273–84.
34. Ragnarsson-Olding BK, Nilsson BR, Kanter-Lewensohn LR, et al. Malignant melanoma of the vulva in a nationwide, 25-year study of 219 Swedish females: predictors of survival. Cancer 1999;86:1285–93.
35. Dunton CJ, Berd D. Vulvar melanoma, biologically different from other cutaneous melanomas. Lancet 1999;354:2013–14.
36. Egan CA, Bradley RR, Logsdon VK, et al. Vulvar melanoma in childhood. Arch Dermatol 1997;133:345–8.
37. Hu DN, Yu GP, McCormick SA. Population-based incidence of vulvar and vaginal melanoma in various races and ethnic groups with comparisons to other site-specific melanomas. Melanoma Res 2010;20:153–8.
38. Ulmer A, Dietl J, Schaumburg-Lever G, Fierlbeck G. Amelanotic malignant melanoma of the vulva. Case report and review of the literature. Arch Gynecol Obstet 1996;259:45–50.
39. Scheistroen M, Trope C, Kaern J, et al. Malignant melanoma of the vulva FIGO stage I: Evaluation of prognostic factors in 43 patients with emphasis on DNA ploidy and surgical treatment. Gynecol Oncol 1996;61:253–8.
40. Frishberg DP, Balch C, Balzer BL, et al. Protocol for the examination of specimens from patients with melanoma of the skin. 2011. Based on AJCC/UICC TNM, 7th edition. College of American Pathologists, http://www.cap.org/apps/docs/committees/cancer/cancer_protocols/2011/SkinMelanoma_11protocol.pdf; 2012.
41. Guitart J, Lowe L, Piepkorn M, et al. Histological characteristics of metastasizing thin melanomas: a case- control study of 43 cases. Arch Dermatol 2002;138:603–8.
42. de Giorgi V, Massi D, Salvini C, et al. Thin melanoma of the vulva: a clinical, dermoscopic-pathologic case study. Arch Dermatol 2005;141:1046–7.
43. Balch CM, Gershenwald JE, Soong SJ, et al. Final version of 2009 AJCC Melanoma staging and classification. J Clin Oncol 2009.
44. Piepkorn M, Barnhill RL. A factual, not arbitrary, basis for choice of resection margins in melanoma. Arch Dermatol 1996;132:811–14.
45. Wechter ME, Gruber SB, Haefner HK, et al. Vulvar melanoma: a report of 20 cases and review of the literature. J Am Acad Dermatol 2004;50:554–62.
46. De Simone P, Silipo V, Buccini P, et al. Vulvar melanoma: a report of 10 cases and review of the literature. Melanoma Res 2008;18:127–33. Review.
47. Woodworth Jr H, Dockerty MB, Wilson RB, Pratt JH. Papillary hidradenoma of the vulva: a clinicopathologic study of 69 cases. Am J Obstet Gynecol 1971;110:501–8.
48. Kazakov DV, Nemcova J, Mikyskova I, et al. Human papillomavirus in lesions of anogenital mammary-like glands. Int J Gynecol Pathol 2007;26:475–80.
49. Sington J, Chandrapala R, Manek S, Hollowood K. Mitotic count is not predictive of clinical behavior in hidradenoma papilliferum of the vulva: a clinicopathologic study of 19 cases. Am J Dermatopathol 2006;28:322–6.
50. Kazakov DV, Mikyskova I, Kutzner H, et al. Hidradenoma papilliferum with oxyphilic metaplasia: a clinicopathological study of 18 cases, including detection of human papillomavirus. Am J Dermatopathol 2005;27:102–10.
51. Shah SS, Adelson M, Mazur MT. Adenocarcinoma in situ arising in vulvar papillary hidradenoma: report of 2 cases. Int J Gynecol Pathol 2008;27:453–6.
52. Gemer O, Piura B, Segal S, Inbar IY. Adenocarcinoma arising in a chondroid syringoma of vulva. Int J Gynecol Pathol 2003;22:398–400.
53. Gerdsen R, Wenzel J, Uerlich M, et al. Periodic genital pruritus caused by syringoma of the vulva. Acta Obstet Gynecol Scand 2002;81:369–70.
54. Huang YH, Chuang YH, Kuo TT, et al. Vulvar syringoma: a clinicopathologic and immunohistologic study of 18 patients and results of treatment. J Am Acad Dermatol 2003;48:735–9.
55. Heller J, Roche N, Hameed M. Trichoepithelioma of the vulva: report of a case and review of the literature. J Low Genit Tract Dis 2009;13:186–7.
56. Bettencourt MS, Prieto VG, Shea CR. Trichoepithelioma: a 19-year clinicopathologic re-evaluation. J Cutan Pathol 1999;26:398–404.
57. Imai A, Furui T, Tamaya T. Gynecologic tumors and symptoms in childhood and adolescence; 10-years' experience. Int J Gynaecol Obstet 1994;45:227–34.
58. Frieden IJ, Rogers M, Garzon MC. Conditions masquerading as infantile haemangioma: Part 1. Australas J Dermatol 2009;50:77–97; quiz 98.
59. Al Dhaybi R, Powell J, McCuaig C, Kokta V. Differentiation of vascular tumors from vascular malformations by expression of Wilms tumor 1 gene: evaluation of 126 cases. J Am Acad Dermatol 2010;63:1052–7.
60. Wang S, Lang JH, Zhou HM. Venous malformations of the female lower genital tract. Eur J Obstet Gynecol Reprod Biol 2009;145:205–8.
61. Coffin CM, Dehner LP. Vascular tumors in children and adolescents: a clinicopathologic study of 228 tumors in 222 patients. Pathol Annu 1993;28(Pt 1):97–120.
62. Watanabe T, Matsubara S, Yamaguchi T, Yamanaka Y. Cavernous lymphangiomas involving bilateral labia minora. Obstet Gynecol 2010;116(Suppl. 2):510–12.
63. Buda A, Ferrari L, Marra C, et al. Vulvar endometriosis in surgical scar after excision of the Bartholin gland: report of a case. Arch Gynecol Obstet 2008;277:255–6.
64. Carter JE, Mizell KN, Tucker JA. Mammary-type fibroepithelial neoplasms of the vulva: a case report and review of the literature. J Cutan Pathol 2008;35:246–9.
65. Kazakov DV, Spagnolo DV, Stewart CJ, et al. Fibroadenoma and phyllodes tumors of anogenital mammary-like glands: a series of 13 neoplasms in 12 cases, including mammary-type juvenile

66. van der Putte SC, van Gorp LH. Adenocarcinoma of the mammary-like glands of the vulva: a concept unifying sweat gland carcinoma of the vulva, carcinoma of supernumerary mammary glands and extramammary Paget's disease. J Cutan Pathol 1994;21:157–63.
67. Abbott JJ, Ahmed I. Adenocarcinoma of mammary-like glands of the vulva: Report of a case and review of the literature. Am J Dermatopathol 2006;28:127–33.
68. Fracchioli S, Puopolo M, De La Longrais IA, et al. Primary "breast-like" cancer of the vulva: a case report and critical review of the literature. Int J Gynecol Cancer 2006;16(Suppl 1):423–8.
69. Lopes G, DeCesare T, Ghurani G, et al. Primary ectopic breast cancer presenting as a vulvar mass. Clin Breast Cancer 2006;7:278–9.
70. Perrone G, Altomare V, Zagami M, et al. Breast-like vulvar lesion with concurrent breast cancer: a case report and critical literature review. In Vivo 2009;23:629–34.
71. Powell JL. Langerhans' cell histiocytosis of the vulva: the Iowa experience. J Reprod Med 2009;54:411.
72. Mottl H, Rob L, Stary J, et al. Langerhans cell histiocytosis of vulva in adolescent. Int J Gynecol Cancer 2007;17:520–4.
73. Ishigaki H, Hatta N, Yamada M, et al. Localised vulva Langerhans cell histiocytosis. Eur J Dermatol 2004;14:412–14.
74. Fernandez Flores A, Mallo S. Langerhans cell histiocytosis of vulva. Dermatol Online J 2006;12:15.
75. Padula A, Medeiros LJ, Silva EG, Deavers MT. Isolated vulvar Langerhans cell histiocytosis: report of two cases. Int J Gynecol Pathol 2004;23:278–83.
76. Chikwava K, Jaffe R. Langerin (CD207) staining in normal pediatric tissues, reactive lymph nodes, and childhood histiocytic disorders. Pediatr Dev Pathol 2004;7:607–14.
77. Hierro I, Blanes A, Matilla A, et al. Merkel cell (neuroendocrine) carcinoma of the vulva. A case report with immunohistochemical and ultrastructural findings and review of the literature. Pathol Res Pract 2000;196:503–9.
78. Foulongne V, Dereure O, Kluger N, et al. Merkel cell polyomavirus DNA detection in lesional and nonlesional skin from patients with Merkel cell carcinoma or other skin diseases. Br J Dermatol 2010;162:59–63.
79. Hashimoto K, Lee MW, D'Annunzio DR, et al. Pagetoid Merkel cell carcinoma: epidermal origin of the tumor. J Cutan Pathol 1998;25:572–9.
80. Touze A, Le Bidre E, Laude H, et al. High levels of antibodies against merkel cell polyomavirus identify a subset of patients with merkel cell carcinoma with better clinical outcome. J Clin Oncol 2011;29:1612–19.
81. Khoury-Collado F, Elliott KS, Lee YC, et al. Merkel cell carcinoma of the Bartholin's gland. Gynecol Oncol 2005;97:928–31.
82. Neto AG, Deavers MT, Silva EG, Malpica A. Metastatic tumors of the vulva: a clinicopathologic study of 66 cases. Am J Surg Pathol 2003;27:799–804.
83. Obermair A, Koller S, Crandon AJ, et al. Primary Bartholin gland carcinoma: a report of seven cases. Aust N Z J Obstet Gynaecol 2001;41:78–81.
84. Kazakov DV, Curik R, Vanecek T, et al. Nodular hyperplasia of the bartholin gland: a clinicopathological study of two cases, including detection of clonality by HUMARA. Am J Dermatopathol 2007;29:385–7.
85. Ben-Harosh S, Cohen I, Bornstein J. Bartholin's gland hyperplasia in a young woman. Gynecol Obstet Invest 2008;65:18–20.
86. Yang SY, Lee JW, Kim WS, et al. Adenoid cystic carcinoma of the Bartholin's gland: report of two cases and review of the literature. Gynecol Oncol 2006;100:422–5.
87. Kaneko G, Nishimoto K, Ogata K, Uchida A. A case of intraepithelial squamous cell carcinoma arising from urethral caruncle. Can Urol Assoc J 2011;5:E14–16.
88. Nakamoto T, Inoue Y, Ueki T, et al. Primary amelanotic malignant melanoma of the female urethra. Int J Urol 2007;14:153–5.
89. Dalbagni G, Zhang ZF, Lacombe L, Herr HW. Female urethral carcinoma: an analysis of treatment outcome and a plea for a standardized management strategy. Br J Urol 1998;82:835–41.
90. Thyavihally YB, Wuntkal R, Bakshi G, et al. Primary carcinoma of the female urethra: single center experience of 18 cases. Jpn J Clin Oncol 2005;35:84–7.

6 Vulvar Mesenchymal Neoplasms and Tumor-Like Conditions

Marisa R. Nucci, Christopher D.M. Fletcher

CHAPTER OUTLINE

Tumor-Like Conditions	116	Angiokeratoma	124
Fibroepithelial–Stromal Polyp (Pseudosarcoma Botryoides)	116	Other Rare Tumors	124
		Locally Recurrent Neoplasms	125
Nodular Fasciitis	117	Deep Angiomyxoma (Deep 'Aggressive' Angiomyxoma)	125
Benign Neoplasms	118		
Angiomyofibroblastoma	118	Superficial Angiomyxoma (Cutaneous Myxoma)	126
Cellular Angiofibroma	119		
Prepubertal Vulvar Fibroma	120	Dermatofibrosarcoma Protuberans	127
Dermatofibroma (Fibrous Histiocytoma)	121	Malignant Neoplasms	128
		Leiomyosarcoma	128
Granular Cell Tumor	122	So-called Proximal-type Epithelioid Sarcoma	128
Leiomyoma	122		
Lymphangioma Circumscriptum	123	Liposarcoma	129
		Other Rare Sarcomas	129

TUMOR-LIKE CONDITIONS

FIBROEPITHELIAL–STROMAL POLYP (PSEUDOSARCOMA BOTRYOIDES)

Definition

A benign polypoid growth that arises from the distinctive subepithelial stroma of the distal female genital tract.

Clinical Features

Fibroepithelial–stromal polyps, which are hormonally sensitive, most commonly occur in the vulvovaginal region of reproductive age women, often during pregnancy. They may, however, also occur in postmenopausal women on hormonal replacement therapy. Often, the polyps are incidental findings discovered during routine gynecologic examination. Symptoms, when present, may include bleeding, discharge, or the sensation of a mass. These lesions are characteristically polypoid or pedunculated, varying in size but usually less than 5 cm, and are typically solitary, although multiple polyps may occur and are usually associated with pregnancy. Evidence supporting that these lesions are hormonally driven, benign, reactive proliferations include: (1) their occurrence during pregnancy, during which they can be multiple and after which they can spontaneously regress; (2) their association with hormonal replacement therapy in postmenopausal women; and (3) expression of estrogen and progesterone receptors by the constituent stromal cells. Incomplete excision or continued hormonal stimulation (e.g., pregnancy) may be associated with recurrence.[1–6]

Pathology

Gross examination typically reveals a polypoid mass with a central fibrovascular core covered by glistening squamous mucosa or skin (Figure 6.1). On occasion, multiple finger-like projections, which may clinically mimic a condyloma, are present. Histologically, these lesions exhibit: (1) a variably cellular spindle cell stroma most often located close to the surface epithelium with scattered stellate and multinucleate stromal cells; (2) a central fibrovascular core; and (3) overlying squamous epithelium or skin, which may exhibit varying degrees of hyperplasia (Figures 6.2 and 6.3).

The stromal component has no clearly defined margin and extends up to the epithelial–submucosal interface. Similar to non-neoplastic vulvar stroma, the stromal cells of these polyps may be reactive for desmin, actin, vimentin, and estrogen and progesterone receptors. The most variable component of these lesions is the stroma, which may exhibit a significant degree of cellularity, nuclear pleomorphism, and mitotic activity, thereby mimicking a malignant

CHAPTER 6 — VULVAR MESENCHYMAL NEOPLASMS AND TUMOR-LIKE CONDITIONS 117

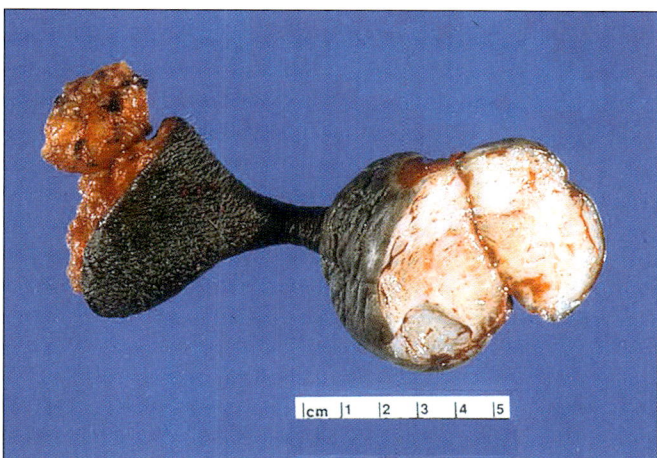

Figure 6.1 Fibroepithelial–stromal polyp. Lesions are typically a polypoid/pedunculated mass. (Courtesy of Dr. J. R. Lewin, Jackson, MS.)

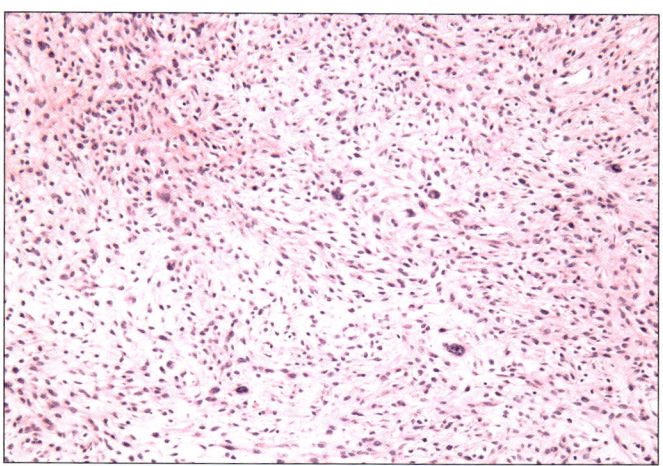

Figure 6.4 Fibroepithelial–stromal polyp, pseudosarcomatous appearance. The stroma is hypercellular and contains cells with enlarged, pleomorphic nuclei.

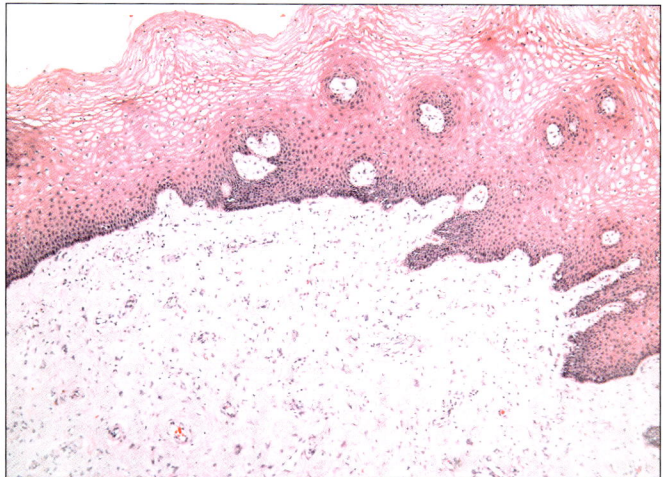

Figure 6.2 Fibroepithelial–stromal polyp. The lesion extends up to the epithelial interface without a clearly definable margin.

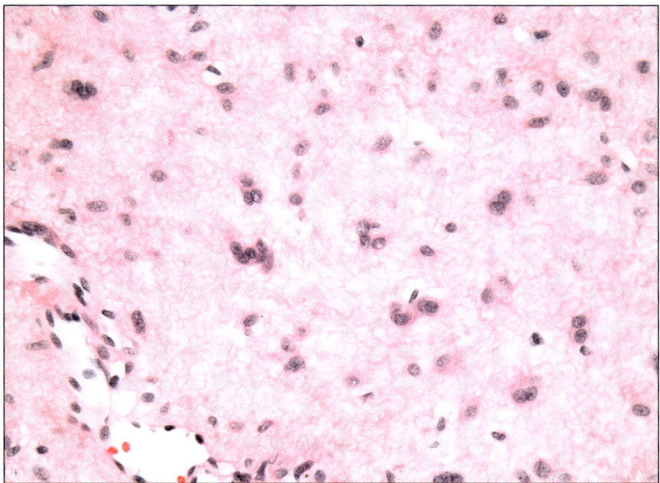

Figure 6.3 Fibroepithelial–stromal polyp. Characteristic appearance of the stellate and multinucleate stromal cells.

process (Figure 6.4).[7–10] These worrisome histologic features are particularly, but not invariably, present in polyps that occur during pregnancy (and account for the historical term 'pseudosarcoma botryoides').[11]

Differential Diagnosis

Pseudosarcomatous stromal polyps can be distinguished from a malignant process by the presence of stellate and multinucleate stromal cells near the epithelial–stromal interface, which are characteristically present in these polyps even in the most floridly pseudosarcomatous examples, and by the lack of an identifiable lesional margin. Fibroepithelial–stromal polyps are also readily distinguished from botryoid embryonal rhabdomyosarcoma as they are rare before puberty and lack both the characteristic hypercellular subepithelial (cambium) layer of sarcoma botryoides and specific markers of skeletal muscle differentiation.[12]

NODULAR FASCIITIS

Definition

A benign, self-limiting myofibroblastic neoplasm characterized by MYH9-USP6 gene fusion that shows rapid growth and spontaneous regression.[13–16]

Clinical Features

Nodular fasciitis typically occurs as a rapidly growing, painful, or tender subcutaneous mass in young adults. It most commonly involves the upper limbs, particularly the forearm; however, it occasionally occurs in the vulva. These lesions are benign and local marginal excision is adequate; if left untreated they will spontaneously regress over a period of months.

Pathology

Similar to its counterparts elsewhere, nodular fasciitis involving the vulva is usually a well-circumscribed, unencapsulated mass that typically measures less than 3 cm in size. Histologically, it is a relatively well-circumscribed cellular proliferation of loosely arranged spindle cells set within a variably edematous or myxoid matrix that may exhibit microcystic change (Figure 6.5). The spindle cells, which are arranged in short interconnecting fascicles, have bipolar eosinophilic cytoplasmic processes with indistinct borders and ovoid nuclei with occasional nucleoli, imparting an overall appearance to the cells that has been likened to tissue culture fibroblasts. Scattered inflammatory cells, particularly lymphocytes, and extravasated red blood cells are commonly present. Osteoclast-like giant cells are also quite common. Immunohistochemically, the spindle cells are typically reactive for smooth muscle actin and negative for desmin. Nodular fasciitis is distinguished from a sarcoma, particularly leiomyosarcoma at this site, by the following: (1) lack of nuclear hyperchromasia or pleomorphism, (2) lack of necrosis, and (3) characteristic reactive 'tissue culture'-like myofibroblastic growth pattern.

BENIGN NEOPLASMS

ANGIOMYOFIBROBLASTOMA

Definition
A benign, nonrecurring tumor composed of myofibroblasts and thin-walled capillaries, which principally occurs in vulvovaginal soft tissue.

Clinical Features
Angiomyofibroblastoma is an uncommon tumor that occurs almost exclusively in the superficial soft tissue of the vulvovaginal region of reproductive age women; however, similar tumors also occur rarely in men in the inguinoscrotal region. Clinically, it is often mistaken for a cyst on examination, in particular a Bartholin gland cyst. Local excision is typically adequate treatment, as these tumors do not recur. Exceptionally, they undergo sarcomatous transformation. Rarely, they may have areas indistinguishable from aggressive angiomyxoma, suggesting that these two tumors may be related. In either of these unusual settings, excision with clear margins is recommended.

Pathology
Tumors are typically small (usually <5 cm), well demarcated, tan/white and may have a rubbery consistency (Figure 6.6). They are composed of plump, round to ovoid or spindle-shaped cells, set within a variably edematous to collagenous matrix with alternating zones of cellularity (Figure 6.7). These cells, which have moderate amounts of eosinophilic cytoplasm and round nuclei with fine chromatin and inconspicuous nucleoli, characteristically cluster around the prominent vascular component, which is composed of numerous delicate, thin-walled capillaries (Figure 6.8). Tumor cells may be binucleate or appear somewhat epithelioid. Mitotic activity is typically sparse and occasional cases may have an adipocytic component. The spindle cells are typically reactive for desmin and negative for actin. In postmenopausal patients, lesional cells may be desmin negative.[17-22]

Differential Diagnosis
Angiomyofibroblastoma is distinguished from aggressive angiomyxoma by its well-circumscribed margin, its prominent vascular component (which is typically composed of

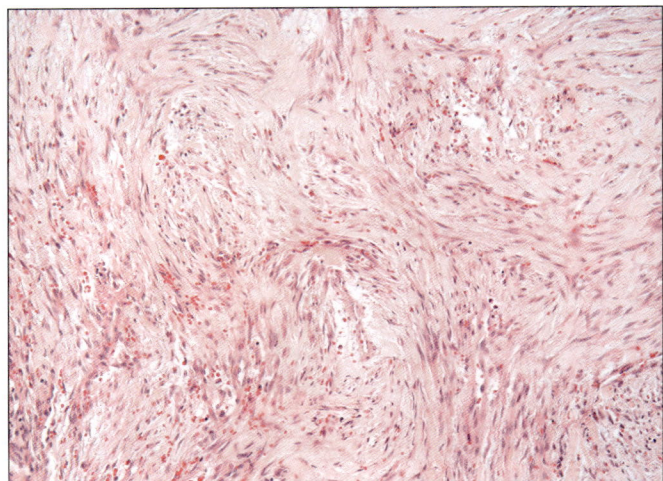

Figure 6.5 Nodular fasciitis. Somewhat fascicular proliferation of spindle cells within an edematous matrix containing extravasated red blood cells.

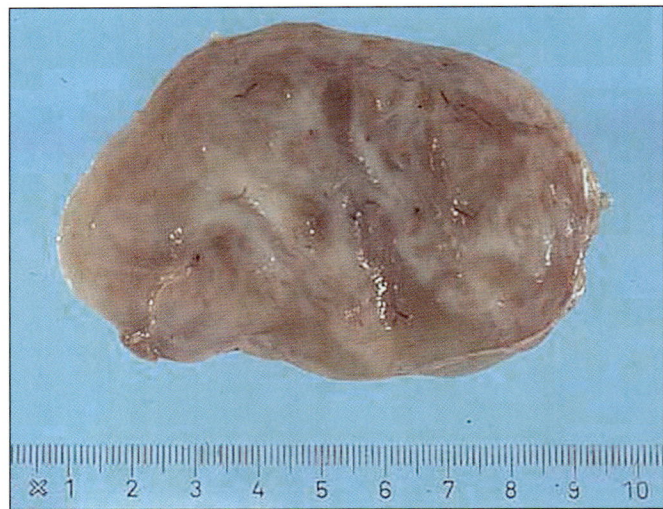

Figure 6.6 Angiomyofibroblastoma. Well-demarcated, tan/white mass. (Courtesy of Professor P. P. Saint-Maur, Paris, France.)

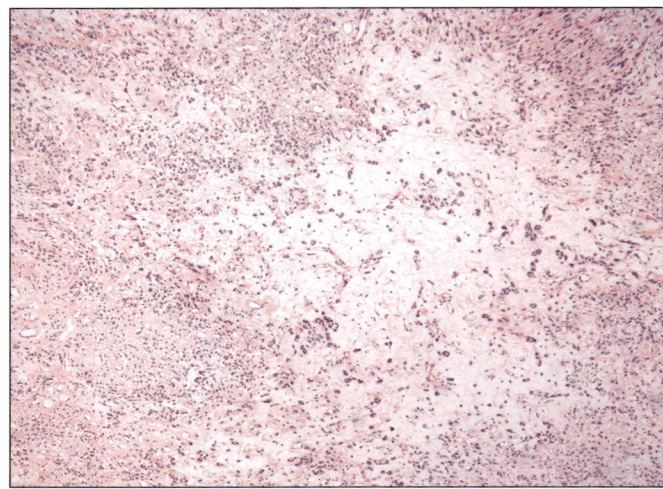

Figure 6.7 Angiomyofibroblastoma. Alternating zones of cellularity are characteristic.

CHAPTER 6 — VULVAR MESENCHYMAL NEOPLASMS AND TUMOR-LIKE CONDITIONS

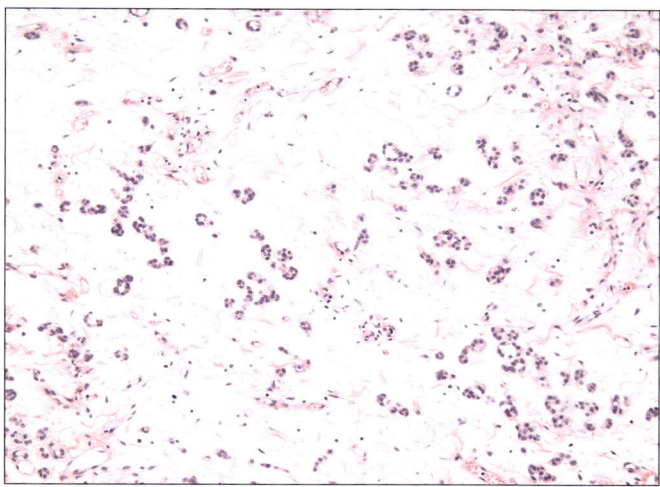

Figure 6.8 Angiomyofibroblastoma. Numerous, thin-walled capillaries are surrounded by clusters of epithelioid and spindle cells.

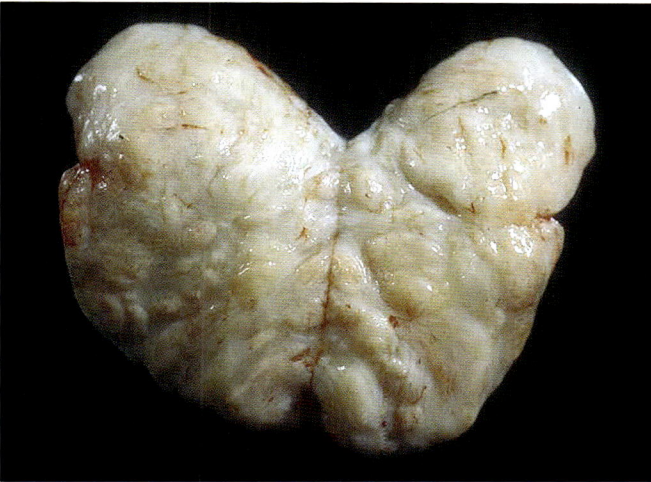

Figure 6.9 Cellular angiofibroma. Bisected solid and well-demarcated, white/tan mass.

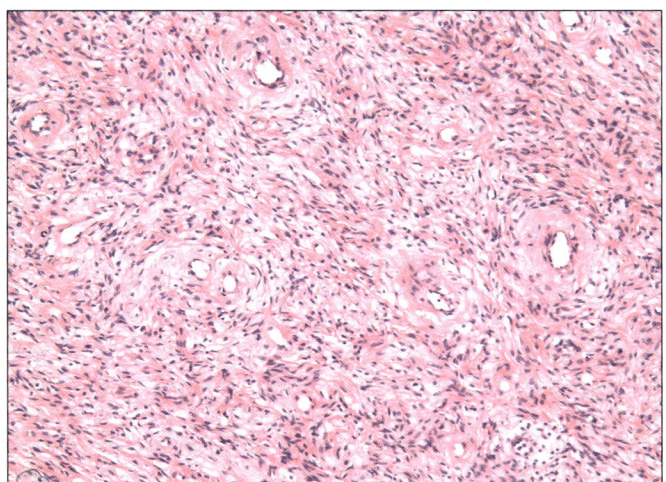

Figure 6.10 Cellular angiofibroma. Numerous medium-sized, thick-walled vessels are surrounded by short intersecting fascicles of bland spindle cells.

smaller caliber vessels), and its alternating zones of cellularity. As both tumors share a similar immunophenotype, distinction is based on morphologic differences (Table 6.1).[23]

CELLULAR ANGIOFIBROMA

Definition

A benign tumor of vulvar mesenchyme composed of a prominent vascular network admixed with bland spindle cells resembling those of spindle cell lipoma.

Clinical Features

Cellular angiofibroma is a rare benign stromal tumor that predominantly occurs in the vulva or perineum of middle-aged women (mean 54 years). Although initially described to occur exclusively at this site, they also occur in the inguinoscrotal region in men (so-called angiomyofibroblastoma-like tumor) and in extragenital sites (e.g., retroperitoneum, skin). In the vulva, they most commonly present as a relatively small (mean 2.7 cm) subcutaneous mass that is well circumscribed and painless. Cellular angiofibroma, if completely excised, behaves in a benign fashion with no recurrent potential. Incomplete excision may lead to regrowth of tumor; therefore, local excision with negative margins is adequate treatment. Very rare cases show sarcomatous transformation.[24–29]

Pathology

On gross examination, cellular angiofibroma typically is gray-white and has a firm, rubbery consistency (Figure 6.9). Histologically, it is usually well circumscribed; however, focal infiltration into surrounding soft tissue may be present. These tumors are characteristically cellular, composed of the following: (1) short, intersecting fascicles of bland, spindle-shaped cells with ovoid nuclei and scant palely eosinophilic cytoplasm; (2) numerous small to medium sized, thick-walled, and often hyalinized blood vessels; and (3) admixed wispy collagen bundles (Figure 6.10). In approximately 25% of cases, a usually minor component of adipose tissue is present. Mitotic activity, although brisk in some cases, is usually infrequent while necrosis and nuclear pleomorphism are typically absent. On occasion, atypia may be present, most commonly in the form of scattered hyperchromatic multinucleated cells (Figure 6.11). Rarely, abrupt transition to a discrete sarcomatous component can occur, which may exhibit features of atypical lipomatous tumor, pleomorphic liposarcoma or pleomorphic sarcoma, not otherwise specified.[29] The spindle cells of cellular angiofibroma are reactive for CD34 in 60% of cases, and less commonly reactive for smooth muscle actin (20%) and desmin (8%). Half of all cases show reactivity for estrogen and progesterone receptors. Keratin, epithelial membrane antigen, and S-100 protein are negative.

Differential Diagnosis

Cellular angiofibroma is distinguished from a smooth muscle tumor by its more prominent vascular component, shorter fascicular growth pattern, and relative lack of eosinophilic cytoplasm. Distinction from angiomyofibroblastoma is based on its uniform cellularity; larger, thick-walled, and hyalinized blood vessels; and spindle cells arranged in

	Fibroepithelial–stromal Polyp	Angiomyofibroblastoma	Cellular Angiofibroma	Superficial Angiomyxoma	Deep Angiomyxoma
Age at presentation	Reproductive age	Reproductive age	Reproductive age	Reproductive age	Reproductive age
Location/configuration	Typically polypoid, pedunculated	Subcutaneous	Subcutaneous	Superficial, subcutaneous, polypoid	Deep seated, not polypoid
Size	Variable	Usually <5 cm	Usually <3 cm	Usually <3 cm	Variable
Margins	Merges with normal	Well circumscribed	Usually well circumscribed; may show focal infiltration	Lobulated, well demarcated	Infiltrative, poorly demarcated
Cellularity	Variable	Alternating hypercellular and hypocellular zones	Uniformly cellular	Hypocellular	Hypocellular
Vessels	Variable, usually large, thick-walled and centrally located	Numerous, capillary sized	Abundant, small to medium sized, often thick walled and hyalinized	Delicate, elongated, thin-walled capillaries	Medium to large, thick-walled; perivascular collagen condensation and myoid bundles
Mitotic index	Variable	Typically low	Variable; may be brisk	Typically low	Rare
Clinical course	Benign, rare recurrences (e.g., during pregnancy)	Benign, no recurrent potential; rare sarcomatous transformation	Benign, no recurrent potential; rare sarcomatous transformation	30% local nondestructive recurrence	30% local, sometimes destructive, recurrence

Table 6.1 Comparison of Common Entities in the Differential Diagnosis of Vulvar Mesenchymal Neoplasms

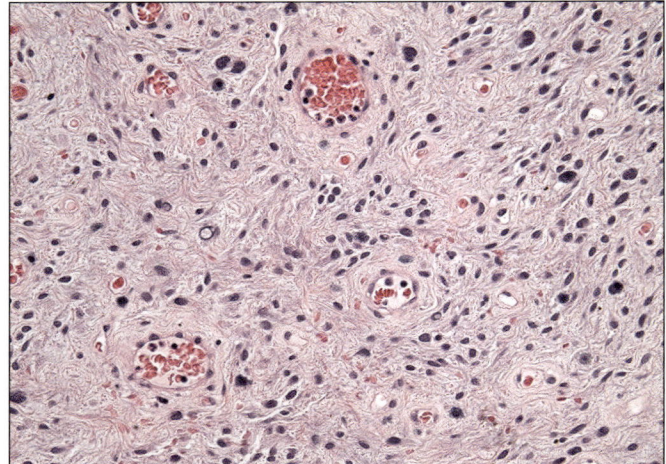

Figure 6.11 Cellular angiofibroma. Stromal cell atypia may occasionally occur.

short intersecting fascicles (Table 6.1).[30] Mammary type myofibroblastoma and cellular angiofibroma are both well-circumscribed tumors composed of short intersecting fascicles of bland, CD34-positive spindle cells within a collagenous stroma; however, the vascular component of the former is typically not as prominent but can show a similar degree of hyalinization. These tumors both have similar genetic changes with loss of 13q14 (*FOXIA1*) and thus likely represent tumors along a spectrum exhibiting varied cellularity and vascularity.

PREPUBERTAL VULVAR FIBROMA

Definition

A poorly circumscribed, hypocellular lesion composed of bland spindle cells within a variably edematous, myxoid, or collagenous matrix that usually occurs in prepubertal girls.[31-32]

Clinical Features

Prepubertal vulvar fibroma most commonly involves the labia majora of girls and usually presents as a painless, gradual vulvar swelling or enlargement. Lesions typically are under 5 cm in size, unilateral, and ill-defined submucosal or subcutaneous masses. While these lesions have been considered neoplastic due to their ability to recur, it has also been proposed that they represent growth of a hormonally responsive vulvar mesenchyme to changes in the hormonal environment at the time of puberty and thus represent a hyperplastic rather than a neoplastic process. Although only a limited number of cases have been studied, the lesions appear to be benign, except for quite frequent local recurrence when incompletely excised.

Pathology

Histologically, these tumors, which are located in submucosal or subcutaneous tissue, are poorly marginated with infiltration into surrounding tissue, including around adnexal structures and nerves, and into adipose tissue (Figure 6.12). In addition, there is no clear interface with the overlying epithelium. The lesion is hypocellular and composed of a patternless proliferation of bland, uniform spindle cells with ovoid nuclei and palely amphophilic cytoplasm set within a variably myxoid, edematous, or collagenous matrix (Figure 6.13). Small to medium sized vessels, some with mural thickening, are present. Mitotic activity is sparse and nuclear pleomorphism is absent. Lesional spindle cells are typically reactive for CD34 but are negative for smooth muscle actin, desmin, and S-100 protein.

DERMATOFIBROMA (FIBROUS HISTIOCYTOMA)

Definition

A benign tumor of dermal connective tissue exhibiting a storiform growth pattern.

Clinical Features

Most commonly occurring on the limbs or trunk of adults, dermatofibroma occasionally involves vulvar skin. Although the clinical appearance is variable, most present as a flesh-colored papule, nodule, or plaque; however, some may be pigmented. The diagnosis may be suspected clinically by the presence of the so-called 'dimpling' sign; pinching of the tumor results in an inward dimpling of the lesion. Complete excision is usually not necessary unless the tumor shows unusual morphologic features (e.g., cellular, aneurysmal, plexiform, deeply infiltrative, or atypical variants) as these subtypes have locally recurrent potential. Following re-excision, very rare cases of these subtypes have been associated with regional lymph node or metastatic deposits in the lung; however, there are no morphologic indicators in the primary that would predict this biologic potential.[33–43]

Pathology

Dermatofibroma exhibits a storiform proliferation of bland spindle cells with varying degrees of hyalinization of the dermal collagen, which is birefringent under polarized light (Figure 6.14). The tumor is relatively well circumscribed; however, entrapment of hyalinized bundles of dermal collagen by the spindle cells at the periphery of the tumor imparts a characteristic pseudoinfiltrative pattern (Figure 6.15). Another characteristic feature is the presence of overlying epidermal hyperplasia, which is common. A number of histologic variants are recognized (although these occur principally outside of the vulva) and include hemosiderotic, lipidized, aneurysmal (angiomatoid), atypical, epithelioid, plexiform, cellular, and deeply penetrating types. The spindle cells are often focally reactive for smooth muscle actin and negative for CD34, although the cellular variant may be reactive for CD34 at the periphery of the tumor. These lesions are often factor XIIIa positive, but most staining is in reactive dermal dendritic cells toward the periphery.[33]

Differential Diagnosis

Dermatofibroma can be distinguished from dermatofibrosarcoma protuberans, its main differential diagnostic

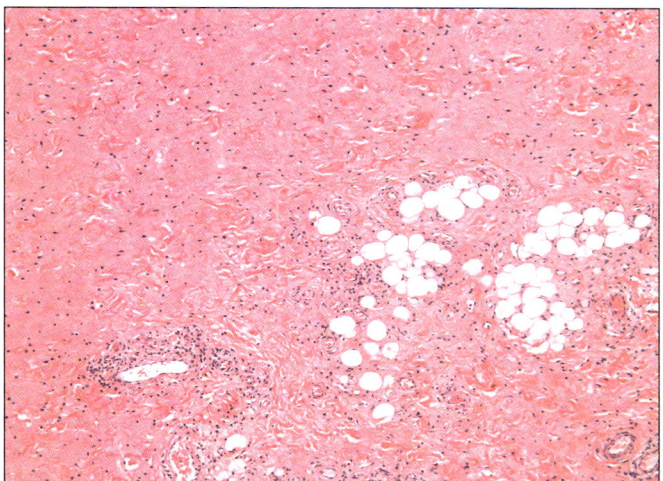

Figure 6.12 Prepubertal fibroma. The lesion is typically poorly marginated with infiltration into adipose tissue.

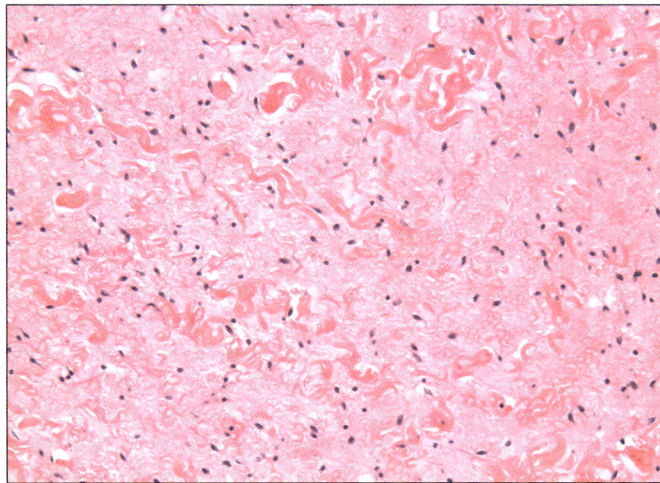

Figure 6.13 Prepubertal fibroma. Hypocellular proliferation of bland spindle cells set within a collagenous matrix.

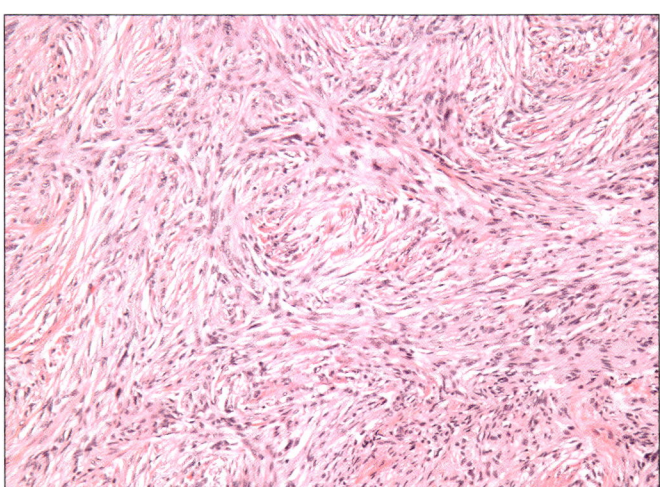

Figure 6.14 Dermatofibroma. Characteristic storiform proliferation of bland spindle cells.

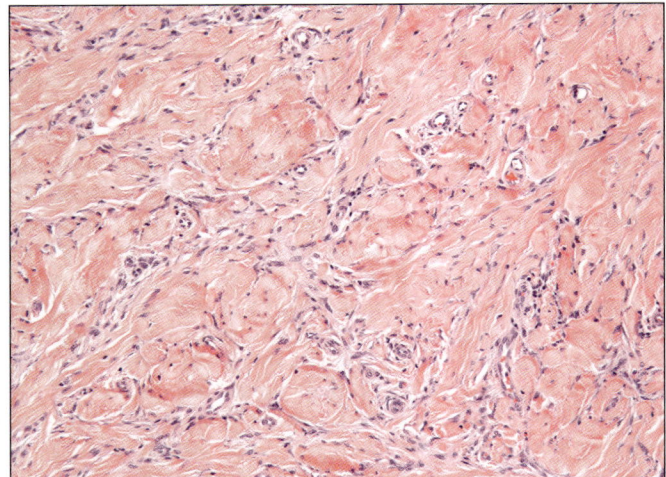

Figure 6.15 Dermatofibroma. At the periphery of the tumor, the neoplastic spindle cells infiltrate around hyalinized collagen bundles in a characteristic pattern.

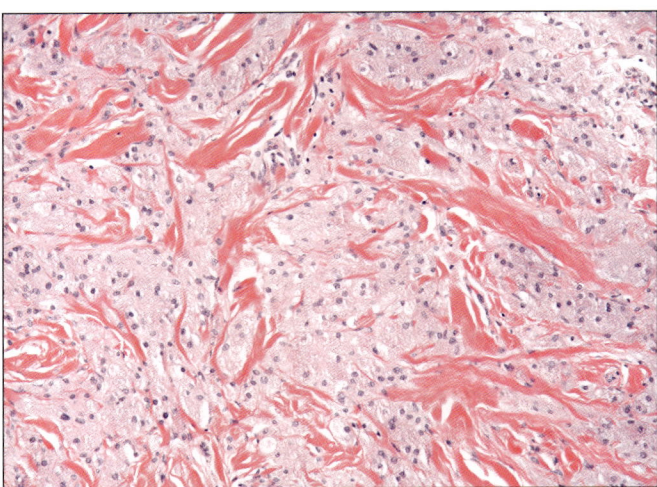

Figure 6.16 Granular cell tumor. Nests and cords of polygonal cells with abundant eosinophilic granular cytoplasm.

consideration, by the following: (1) its lack of infiltration of adipose tissue (although this may be seen in the cellular and deeply penetrating variants), (2) presence of birefringent collagen under polarized light, (3) overlying epidermal hyperplasia, (4) tendency not to infiltrate around adnexal structures, and (5) lack of diffuse reactivity for CD34.[43]

GRANULAR CELL TUMOR

Definition
A tumor of neuroectodermal origin composed of cells that contain distinctive granular cytoplasm due to the accumulation of lysosomes.

Clinical Features
Granular cell tumor is an uncommon neoplasm that typically arises in the skin and subcutaneous tissue of middle-aged adults with a slightly increased frequency in women. Tumors typically involve the head, neck, and trunk region, but may occasionally occur in the vulva, most often the labium majus. Patients usually present with a solitary, slowly growing, asymptomatic nodule that is often discovered incidentally on clinical examination. If present, symptoms may include pain, increased growth, and pruritus. Complete excision with clear margins is standard treatment, although these tumors seldom recur, even if incompletely excised. Malignant examples are rare.[44–49]

Pathology
Granular cell tumors are composed of strands and nests of polygonal cells with abundant eosinophilic granular cytoplasm and small, centrally placed, hyperchromatic nuclei separated by thin fibrous septa (Figure 6.16). Although distinctive, the characteristic granular cytoplasmic change, which is due to the accumulation of lysosomes, is not specific for this tumor type and may be seen in other types of neoplasms, such as smooth muscle tumors. Although many granular cell tumors are relatively well circumscribed, nearly half may show poorly defined or infiltrative margins. Nests of tumor cells adjacent to or surrounding small nerves are common. In addition, the tumor is often associated with overlying pseudoepitheliomatous hyperplasia, which may be mistaken for a squamous neoplasm if the underlying granular cell tumor is overlooked. Granular cell tumors are reactive for S-100 protein, neuron-specific enolase, CD68, and NKI-C3.

Differential Diagnosis
The granular cell tumor is distinctive and few pose diagnostic difficulty. Exclusion of a smooth muscle tumor with granular cell change is the most likely differential diagnostic consideration, which can be accomplished by recognition of areas with typical smooth muscle morphology and architecture as well as coexpression of desmin, caldesmon, and smooth muscle actin.

LEIOMYOMA

Definition
A benign tumor of smooth muscle exhibiting intersecting fascicles of spindle cells with eosinophilic cytoplasm.

Clinical Features
Although genital smooth muscle tumors were initially considered within the category of superficial smooth muscle tumors, which includes pilar leiomyoma and angioleiomyoma, they are now classified separately based upon their differing clinical behavior, histologic features, and criteria for malignancy. Smooth muscle tumors of the distal female genitalia, unlike those of the uterus, are uncommon. They occur over a wide age range but are most common in the fourth and fifth decades and typically present as a painless, well-circumscribed mass usually <3 cm in size. Not uncommonly, the clinical impression is that of a cyst. Local excision

for typical leiomyomas is adequate treatment. For tumors with unusual histologic features associated with recurrent potential (see the following sections), a margin of excision of at least 1 cm is recommended whenever possible, with close, long-term follow-up.[50–55]

Pathology

Similar to uterine smooth muscle tumors, vulvar leiomyomas usually exhibit the characteristic gross appearance of benign smooth muscle tumors of the myometrium but on occasion may have a more homogeneous appearance with less obvious whorling (Figure 6.17). In most instances, they are composed of intersecting fascicles of spindle-shaped cells with moderate amounts of eosinophilic cytoplasm and elongated, blunt-ended nuclei. However, an unusual morphologic pattern, which is commonly present in vulvar smooth muscle tumors, is the variable deposition of myxohyaline matrix, which imparts a plexiform or lacy appearance (Figure 6.18).

Due to the relative infrequency of vulvar smooth muscle tumors in combination with few published series with long-term follow-up, there is continued difficulty in reliably predicting which tumors are benign and which have recurrent potential. While a combination of size, circumscription, nuclear atypia, and mitotic thresholds has been proposed to identify those tumors with recurrent potential, in our experience any mitotic activity, nuclear pleomorphism, or infiltration of surrounding tissue may be associated with local recurrence, sometimes years after the initial excision. These observations suggest that smooth muscle tumors of the vagina and vulva fall along a biologic continuum with regard to their behavior and resist being rigidly classified into benign and malignant categories by currently definable histopathologic criteria.

From a practical standpoint, we advocate use of the term 'atypical smooth muscle tumor' for those cases having any of the following features: (1) mitotic activity, (2) nuclear pleomorphism, or (3) an infiltrative margin. Although published series have not included necrosis as a histologic criterion, leiomyosarcoma should be seriously considered in any smooth muscle neoplasm with coagulative tumor cell necrosis.

There are only case reports regarding the cytogenetic findings of vulvar smooth muscle tumors. In one case, a pericentric inversion (12)(p12q13–14) was described as the sole chromosomal abnormality, which resulted in activation of HMGA2, a gene that appears to be activated in smooth muscle tumors of genital, but not extragenital, origin. A clonal translocation, 46,XX,t(7;8)(p13;q11.2), has also been described in a periurethral smooth muscle tumor, an aberration not previously discovered in smooth muscle tumors from any site.

LYMPHANGIOMA CIRCUMSCRIPTUM

Definition

An abnormality of dermal lymphatic channels exhibiting numerous dilated and cystic lymphatic spaces.[56–60]

Clinical Features

Lymphangioma circumscriptum may be congenital, occurring during infancy and commonly associated with other lymphatic abnormalities such as cystic hygroma or cavernous lymphangioma, or it may be acquired (also termed 'acquired lymphangiectasia'), which most commonly occurs in adults and is associated with secondary lymphatic damage such as that associated with radiotherapy or chronic lymphedema. It most commonly affects the skin and subcutaneous tissue of the trunk, thighs, and buttocks, but occasionally involves the vulva. Clinically, numerous small vesicles filled with clear fluid characterize this lesion. Symptoms typically include swelling, pain, and superimposed infection secondary to excoriation. Management of congenital lesions is local excision, including removal of any large feeding lymphatic channel, which may be deep seated, as incomplete removal is commonly associated with recurrence.

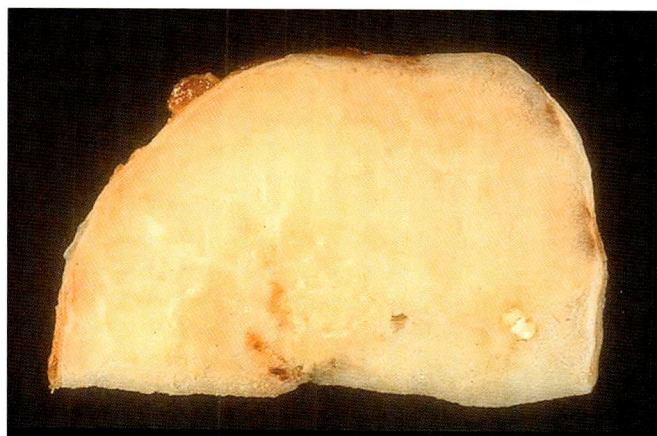

Figure 6.17 Leiomyoma. Well-circumscribed, tan/yellow mass with a homogeneous, glistening cut surface.

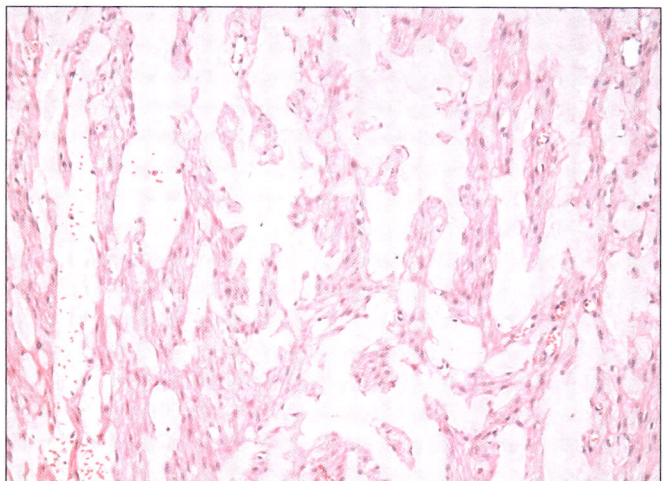

Figure 6.18 Leiomyoma. Abundant myxohyaline matrix deposition is common in benign vulvar smooth muscle tumors.

Pathology

Numerous dilated and cystic lymphatic channels are present, primarily within the papillary dermis, but also within the

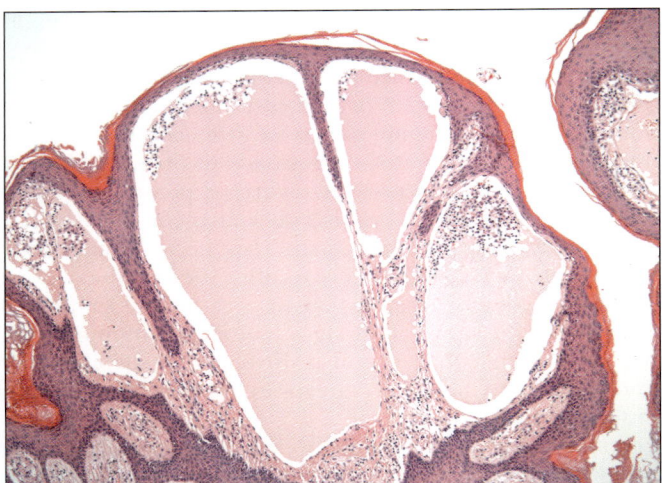

Figure 6.19 Lymphangioma circumscriptum. Numerous dilated lymphatic channels located within the papillary dermis are closely apposed to the overlying epithelium. Note the epidermal hyperplasia and dermal lymphocytic infiltrate.

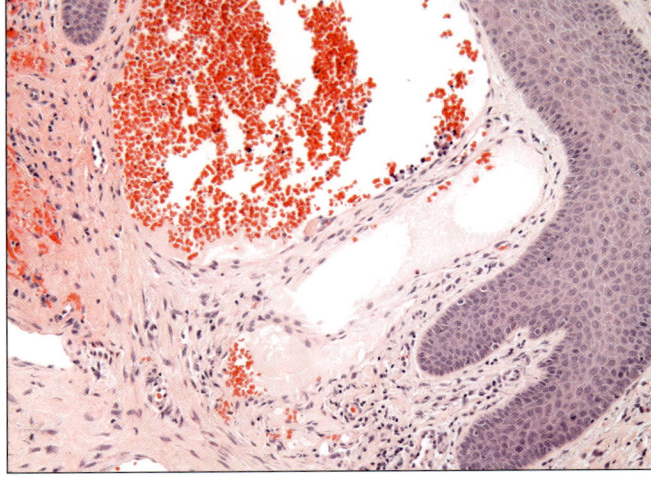

Figure 6.20 Angiokeratoma. Dilated, blood-filled spaces within the papillary dermis are partially surrounded by epithelium.

dermis and subcutaneous tissue. Those located in the papillary dermis are closely apposed to the overlying epithelium, which results in the clinical impression of a vesicle (Figure 6.19). Associated epidermal hyperplasia and a dermal lymphocytic infiltrate are common.

ANGIOKERATOMA

Definition

A lesion composed of superficial ectatic vascular channels associated with epidermal hyperplasia.

Clinical Features

Angiokeratoma involving the vulva occurs over a wide age range, but typically presents before the sixth decade as an asymptomatic, red to purple, papular lesion under 1 cm in size. It often has a warty appearance due to associated epidermal changes. When present, symptoms include bleeding, pain, or pruritus. The lesion may be solitary or multiple, and if multiple should raise the possibility of Fabry disease, a rare X-linked chromosomal disorder of lipid metabolism in which there is a deficiency of lysosomal α-galactosidase.[61–62]

Pathology

Angiokeratoma exhibits closely apposed, dilated, blood-filled vascular spaces within the papillary dermis, partially surrounded by the overlying epithelium (Figure 6.20). The epithelium typically shows acanthosis, hyperkeratosis, and occasionally papillomatosis, resulting in the clinical impression of a warty lesion.

OTHER RARE TUMORS

Vulvar leiomyomatosis[54,63,64] is a rare condition in which patients have numerous, ill-defined, multinodular proliferations of smooth muscle involving the vulvar submucosa.

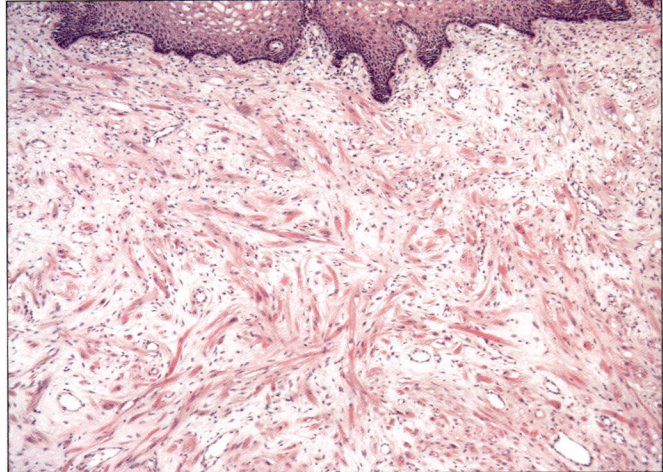

Figure 6.21 Genital rhabdomyoma. Submucosal fascicular proliferation of well-differentiated rhabdomyoblasts.

Genital rhabdomyoma[65–67] most commonly involves the vagina of middle-aged women, but may occasionally occur in the vulva. Lesions are typically polypoid and patients usually present with bleeding or symptoms related to a mass. Histologically, this benign tumor exhibits a somewhat fascicular proliferation of well-differentiated rhabdomyoblasts within the submucosa (Figure 6.21). Cross-striations are usually easily identifiable (Figure 6.22).

Lipoblastoma-like tumor of the vulva[68] is a distinctive benign mesenchymal neoplasm that histologically resembles lipoblastoma in infants. In contrast to the latter, which typically occurs in the trunk and extremities of young boys under 5 years of age, this tumor occurs in young women. Histologically, the tumors are well circumscribed and composed of lobules of immature and mature adipocytes separated by thin fibrous septa resembling myxoid liposarcoma (Figure 6.23).

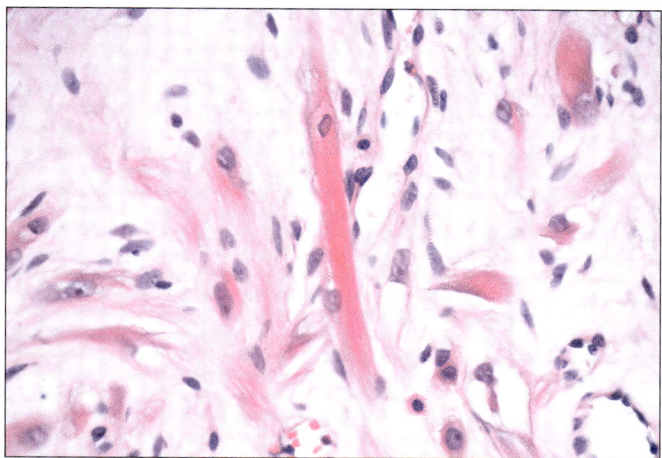

Figure 6.22 Genital rhabdomyoma. Brightly eosinophilic cytoplasmic processes, some of which contain identifiable cross-striations.

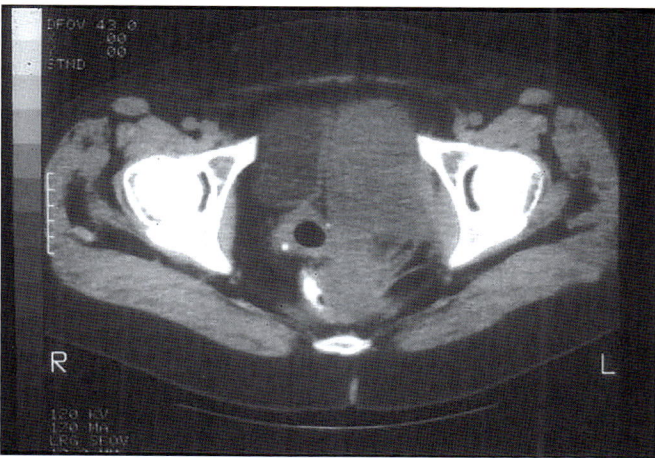

Figure 6.24 Deep angiomyxoma. CT scan showing an infiltrative tumor mass. (Courtesy of Dr. R. W. Fortt, Wales, UK.)

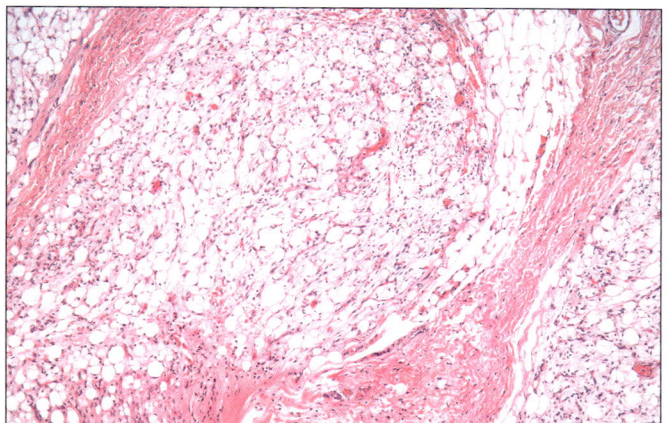

Figure 6.23 Lipoblastoma-like tumor. Lobules of immature adipocytes within a myxoid matrix separated by thin fibrous septa.

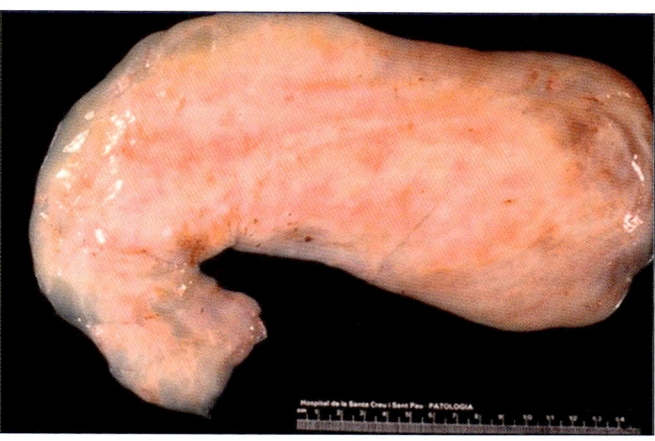

Figure 6.25 Deep angiomyxoma. Tumor appears gelatinous or myxoid.

LOCALLY RECURRENT NEOPLASMS

DEEP ANGIOMYXOMA (DEEP 'AGGRESSIVE' ANGIOMYXOMA)

Definition

A locally infiltrative, non-metastasizing, hypocellular myxoid tumor of the pelvicoperineal region with the potential for local, sometimes destructive, recurrence.

Clinical Features

Deep angiomyxoma occurs principally in the pelvicoperineal region of reproductive age women, with a median incidence in the fourth decade, but rarely also develops in the inguinoscrotal region of men, in whom the median age at presentation is in the sixth to seventh decade. Often the clinical impression is that of a labial cyst, most commonly a Bartholin gland cyst. Tumors vary in size, but are often relatively large (>10 cm) and poorly marginated (Figure 6.24). Although there is a 20–30% risk of local, sometimes destructive recurrence, more than one recurrence is unusual and most are cured by an additional surgical excision with negative margins. Hence the currently preferred terminology is deep angiomyxoma, as these tumors are not as 'aggressive' as originally thought. Besides positive surgical margins, there are no clinical or histopathologic features that predict recurrent potential. Wide local excision with 1 cm margins is considered optimal and adequate treatment.

Pathology

Tumors typically have a gelatinous or myxoid appearance (Figure 6.25), but occasionally may appear more fibrous in a recurrence, presumably due to previous surgical scar tissue. Histologically, deep angiomyxoma is a poorly marginated, paucicellular neoplasm composed of uniformly distributed bland spindle cells with round to ovoid nuclei and moderate amounts of palely eosinophilic cytoplasm, discernible as bipolar or multipolar cell processes (Figure 6.26). The cells are set within a copious myxoid matrix that contains variably sized, but often medium to large, thick-walled, often hyalinized, blood vessels. Condensation of

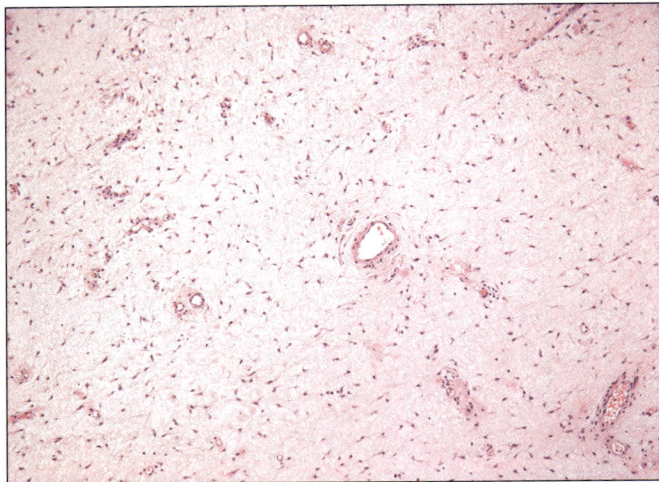

Figure 6.26 Deep angiomyxoma. Paucicellular neoplasm punctuated by medium to large sized blood vessels.

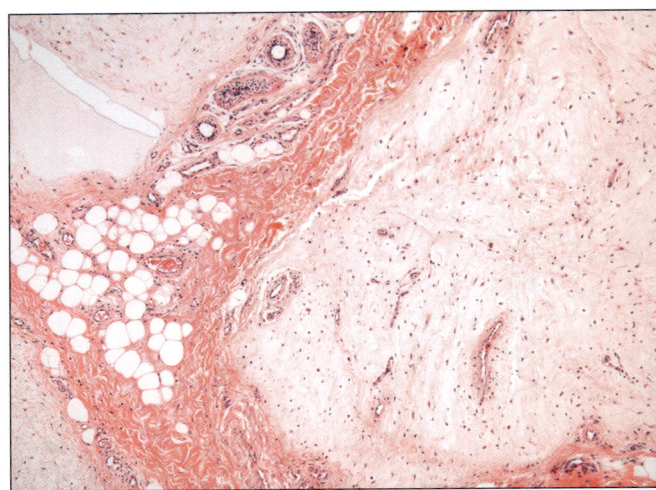

Figure 6.28 Superficial angiomyxoma. Well-demarcated, lobulated growth pattern.

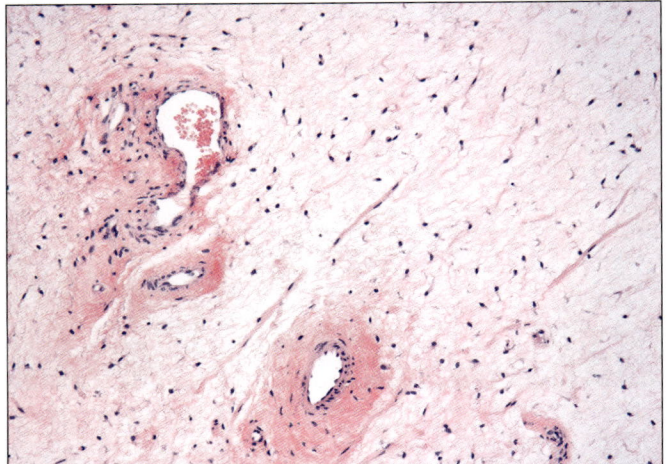

Figure 6.27 Deep angiomyxoma. Bland spindle cells with bipolar processes within a myxoid matrix surround blood vessels with hyalinized walls. Note brightly eosinophilic smooth muscle cells.

delicate fibrillary collagen around the blood vessels is characteristic, as is the presence of bundles of brightly eosinophilic smooth muscle cells (Figure 6.27). The spindle cells are typically reactive for desmin, smooth muscle actin, and estrogen and progesterone receptors, similar to normal vulvar mesenchyme. The spindle cells also can be positive for CD34, HMGA2, and CDK4. The expression of the last two markers is related to the fact that structural rearrangements of 12q15 with involvement of HMGA2, which encodes a factor important in transcriptional regulation, is the most frequent chromosomal aberration observed in deep (aggressive) angiomyxoma. Rearrangements appear to occur in approximately 30% of cases and the 12q15 breakpoint can be either intragenic or extragenic. Consequently, immunohistochemical expression of HMGA2 may only be useful in confirming the diagnosis or assessing margin status in a subset of cases.[69–72]

Differential Diagnosis

The differential diagnosis includes superficial angiomyxoma (see the following section), angiomyofibroblastoma, and an edematous fibroepithelial–stromal polyp (Table 6.1). Deep angiomyxoma is distinguished from angiomyofibroblastoma by its infiltrative margin, its vascular component (which is typically less prominent and composed of larger, thicker walled vessels), and its uniform paucicellularity. Deep angiomyxoma differs from edematous fibroepithelial–stromal polyps by its deep location, its infiltrative margin, its lack of polypoid superficial growth, and its uniformly bland cytomorphology with the lack of the characteristic stellate and multinucleate cells typical of stromal polyps.

SUPERFICIAL ANGIOMYXOMA (CUTANEOUS MYXOMA)

Definition

A superficially located, multilobulated, myxoid neoplasm with a 20–30% risk of local, nondestructive recurrence.

Clinical Features

Superficial angiomyxoma usually involves the head, neck, and trunk region, but does occasionally occur in the vulva. It typically occurs in the fourth decade and patients usually present with a slowly growing, painless, polypoid mass that typically measures less than 5 cm in size. Although usually solitary, multiple lesions may be associated with Carney complex. Approximately one-third of these tumors recur locally if incompletely or marginally excised; therefore, complete excision with clear margins is recommended treatment.[79–81]

Pathology

Histologically, superficial angiomyxoma is a myxoid neoplasm with a distinctive multilobulated growth pattern that is centered in the dermis and superficial subcutaneous tissue (Figure 6.28). The relatively well-demarcated myxoid nodules contain slender spindle and stellate-shaped cells,

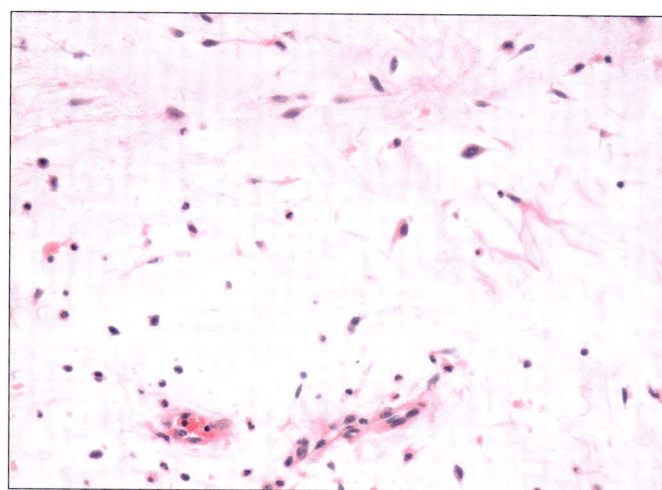

Figure 6.29 Superficial angiomyxoma. Bland spindle- and stellate-shaped cells, delicate capillaries, and a myxoid matrix are characteristic. Note the stromal acute inflammatory cells.

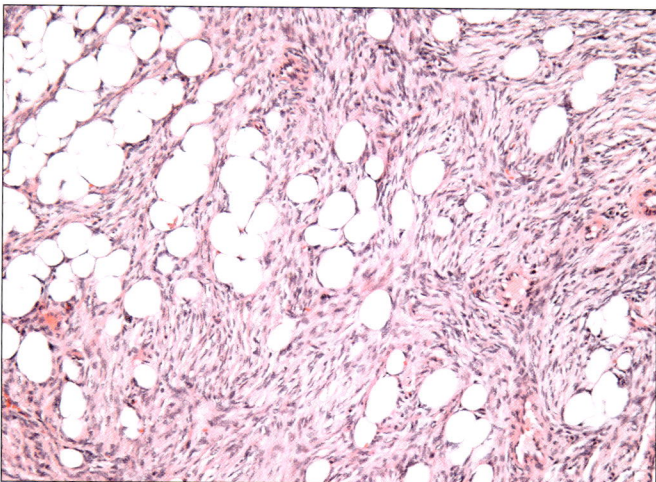

Figure 6.30 Dermatofibrosarcoma protuberans. Storiform proliferation of spindle cells with extension into subcutaneous adipose tissue in a characteristic honeycomb pattern.

delicate thin-walled capillaries, and scattered inflammatory cells, particularly polymorphonuclear leukocytes (Figure 6.29). The presence of acute inflammatory cells is not associated with necrosis or overlying epidermal ulceration and is presumably secondary to the production of a chemotactic factor by the tumor cells. In 10–20% of cases, an epithelial component—usually in the form of a squamous epithelial-lined cyst, buds of basaloid cells, or strands of squamous epithelium—is present, probably as a result of entrapped adnexal structures or stimulation of the overlying epithelium by the tumor. Immunohistochemically, the spindle cells are typically negative for actin, desmin, and S-100 protein.

Differential Diagnosis

Superficial angiomyxoma is distinguished from deep angiomyxoma by the following: (1) its superficial location, (2) well-demarcated margins, (3) lobulated growth pattern, (4) lack of thick-walled blood vessels, and (5) negativity of the lesional cells for desmin (Table 6.1).

DERMATOFIBROSARCOMA PROTUBERANS

Definition

A tumor of dermal connective tissue exhibiting a monomorphic storiform proliferation of fibroblastic spindle cells and infiltration of adipose tissue.

Clinical Features

Dermatofibrosarcoma protuberans most commonly occurs on the trunk, lower extremities, and groin area (although not commonly the vulva proper) of adults, principally between the third and sixth decades. Clinical presentation can vary from a flesh-colored to pigmented papule, plaque, nodule, or exophytic multinodular growth. Wide local excision with clear margins is necessary to prevent recurrence; rare cases (<0.1%) have metastasized, although this figure is higher (~15%) in cases that show higher grade fibrosarcomatous change.

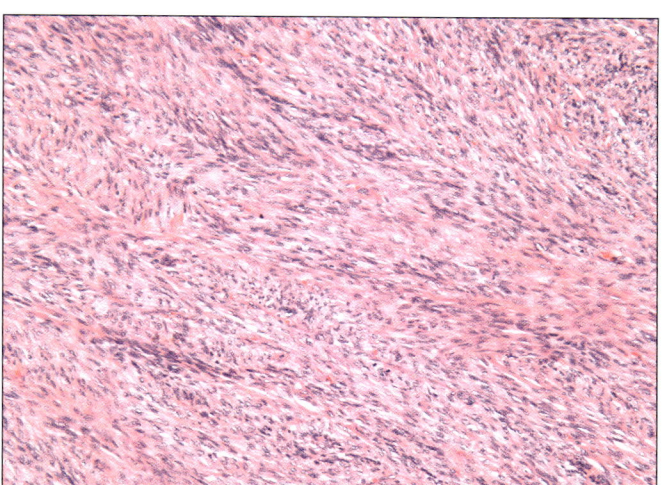

Figure 6.31 Dermatofibrosarcoma protuberans. Fibrosarcomatous change with a fascicular growth pattern.

Pathology

Histologically, the classic appearance of this tumor is that of a poorly circumscribed, storiform proliferation of uniform spindle cells involving the dermis and extending into subcutaneous adipose tissue in a characteristic lace-like or honeycomb pattern (Figure 6.30). A band of uninvolved dermis between the tumor and epidermis, which may be of normal thickness or atrophic, is typically present (Grenz zone). Entrapment of adnexal structures is common. In contrast to benign fibrous histiocytoma, polarizable collagen is typically absent. Some tumors, including those that occur in the vulva, may exhibit fibrosarcomatous change characterized by a herringbone, fascicular growth pattern with increased mitotic activity (Figure 6.31); tumors with this morphologic appearance have metastatic potential. Immunohistochemically, the neoplastic cells are typically diffusely reactive for CD34 and negative for factor XIIIa. Translocation between chromosomes 17 and 22, often in the form of supernumerary ring chromosomes, has been identified by cytogenetic analysis in this tumor type, including cases that have occurred in the vulva. This translocation results in the fusion of two genes, collagen type I α-1 (*COL1A1*) and platelet-derived growth factor β-chain (*PDGFB*).[82–92]

Differential Diagnosis

Dermatofibrosarcoma protuberans differs from dermatofibroma, its main differential diagnostic consideration, by the following: (1) its tendency to infiltrate subcutaneous adipose tissue in a characteristic honeycomb pattern (although extension into adipose tissue may be seen in some cases of fibrous histiocytoma), (2) entrapment of adnexal structures, (3) lack of birefringent collagen under polarized light, (4) lack of overlying epidermal hyperplasia, and (5) diffuse reactivity for CD34.

MALIGNANT NEOPLASMS

LEIOMYOSARCOMA

Definition

A rare sarcoma of vulvar soft tissue showing smooth muscle differentiation.

Clinical Features

Of all sarcomas of the vulva, which as a category are rare, leiomyosarcoma represents the most common subtype. Patients are typically in their fourth or fifth decade and present with symptoms related to a mass. Tumors may be of varying size but are typically under 5 cm. Treatment varies from wide local excision to radical vulvectomy.

Pathology

Histologically, most vulvar leiomyosarcomas have a similar morphologic appearance to those that occur more commonly elsewhere in the female genital tract that are of the spindle cell type (Figure 6.32). Due to the rarity of these lesions, defining criteria to predict those tumors with metastatic potential remains problematic yet of paramount importance due to potential differences in clinical management. Use of the criteria proposed by Tavassoli and Norris[55] is recommended, in which tumors with three or more of the following criteria should be diagnosed as leiomyosarcoma:

- >5 cm in size
- >5 mitoses per 10 HPF
- infiltrative margin
- moderate to severe cytologic atypia.

Although necrosis is excluded in this algorithm, its presence should strongly raise the possibility of malignancy.[52–55,93–95]

SO-CALLED PROXIMAL-TYPE EPITHELIOID SARCOMA

Definition

Large cell variant of epithelioid sarcoma that has a predilection for the genital and perineal regions.

Clinical Features

Patients typically present in the fourth decade with symptoms related to a mass lesion. Tumor size in the genital area is usually under 6 cm but tumor size in general may range up to 20 cm (median, 4 cm). Clinically, the proximal subtype acts more aggressively than the usual (distal) epithelioid sarcoma, with earlier distant metastasis following excision of the primary.

Pathology

Histologically, this tumor exhibits a diffuse and often multinodular proliferation of relatively monomorphic large cells with abundant eosinophilic cytoplasm, imparting an epithelioid appearance. Rhabdoid inclusions are frequent (Figures 6.33 and 6.34). The tumor cells, which contain large vesicular nuclei and prominent nucleoli, commonly invade into subcutaneous or deeper soft tissue. Immunohistochemically, the tumor cells commonly react with keratin and

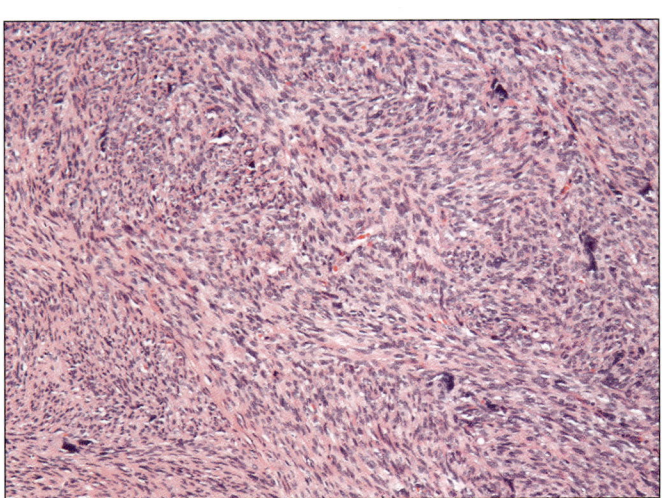

Figure 6.32 Leiomyosarcoma, spindle cell type.

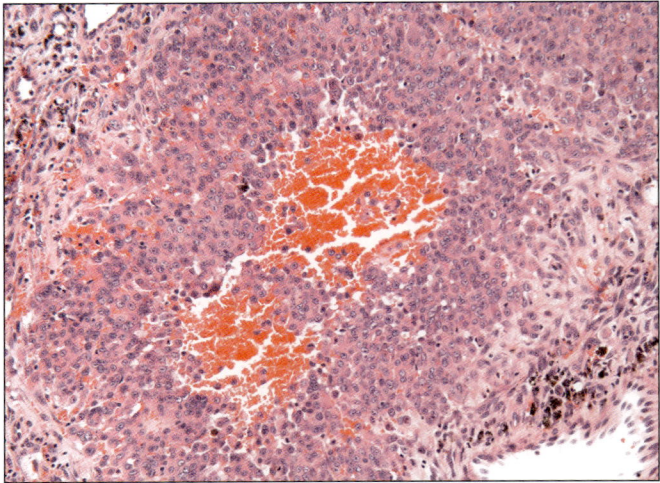

Figure 6.33 Proximal-type epithelioid sarcoma. Multinodular, 'granulomatous' growth pattern.

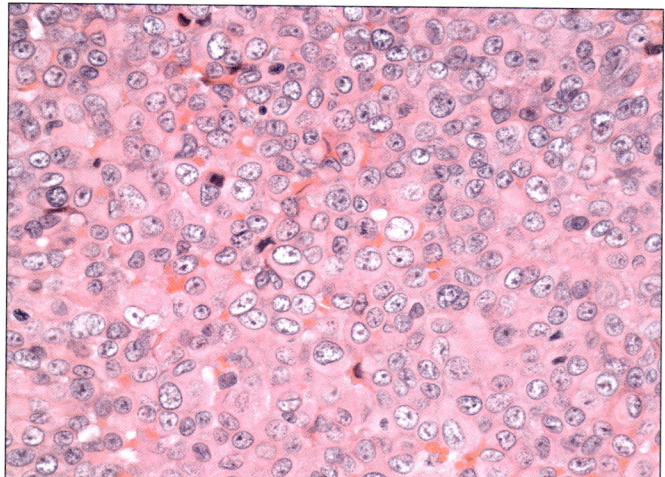

Figure 6.34 Proximal-type epithelioid sarcoma. Tumor cells have abundant eosinophilic cytoplasm and vesicular nuclei. Note the rhabdoid appearance of some cells.

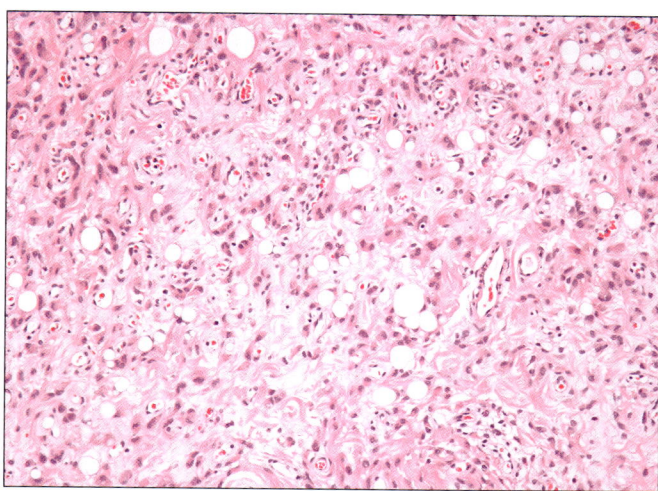

Figure 6.35 Liposarcoma, unusual vulvar variant. Admixture of bland spindle and round cells with numerous bivacuolated lipoblasts.

epithelial membrane antigen. Approximately 50% express CD34 and may occasionally react for desmin and actin. The vast majority show loss of staining for INI1, the product of this ubiquitous chromatin remodeling gene located on chromosome 22q11.2, the expression of which is often lost in these tumors.[96-100]

Differential Diagnosis

In the genital region, the principal differential diagnosis is with carcinoma or melanoma. Proximal-type epithelioid sarcoma is distinguished from poorly differentiated carcinoma by its multinodular growth pattern, coexpression of CD34 and, occasionally, desmin, and lack of an intraepidermal *in situ* component. In addition, it differs from melanoma by the previous features as well as expression of epithelial markers and lack of S-100 protein reactivity.

LIPOSARCOMA

Definition

Malignant mesenchymal neoplasm showing adipocytic differentiation.

Clinical Features

Liposarcoma usually arises in the limbs, trunks, and abdominal cavity, but uncommonly also in the vulva. It occurs predominantly in middle-aged women (median 52 years) on the labia majora and is of varying size but typically is under 8 cm. Many are thought clinically to represent a lipoma. Most are of the well-differentiated subtype and have a similar clinical behavior to those that occur outside the abdominal cavity, that is, complete excision with a clear margin is curative.

Pathology

Histologically, most tumors have the usual morphologic appearance of well-differentiated liposarcoma/atypical lipomatous tumor with variation in adipocyte size, adipocytic nuclear atypia, cellular fibrous septa (often with scattered hyperchromatic stromal cells), and occasional lipoblasts. Some, however, may have an unusual morphology that is unique to tumors that arise at this site. These tumors show an admixture of neoplastic bland spindle and round cells, variably sized adipocytes, and numerous bivacuolated lipoblasts (Figure 6.35). This unusual morphology is not associated with any difference in behavior.[101-104]

OTHER RARE SARCOMAS

Other sarcomas may rarely occur in the vulva and include rhabdomyosarcoma (embryonal, alveolar, and pleomorphic subtypes),[105-107] alveolar soft part sarcoma,[108] Ewing sarcoma,[109,110] angiosarcoma,[93,95] and Kaposi sarcoma,[111,112] among others.

REFERENCES

1. Burt RL, Prichard RW, Kim BS. Fibroepithelial polyp of the vagina. A report of five cases. Obstet Gynecol 1976;47:52S–4S.
2. Chirayil SJ, Tobon H. Polyps of the vagina: a clinicopathologic study of 18 cases. Cancer 1981;47:2904–7.
3. Elliott GB, Reynolds HA, Fidler HK. Pseudo-sarcoma botryoides of cervix and vagina in pregnancy. J Obstet Gynaecol Br Commonw 1967;74:728–33.
4. Hartmann CA, Sperling M, Stein H. So-called fibroepithelial polyps of the vagina exhibiting an unusual but uniform antigen profile characterized by expression of desmin and steroid hormone receptors but no muscle-specific actin or macrophage markers. Am J Clin Pathol 1990;93:604–8.
5. Maenpaa J, Soderstrom KO, Salmi T, Ekblad U. Large atypical polyps of the vagina during pregnancy with concomitant human papilloma virus infection. Eur J Obstet Gynecol Reprod Biol 1988;27:65–9.
6. Miettinen M, Wahlstrom T, Vesterinen E, Saksela E. Vaginal polyps with pseudosarcomatous features. A clinicopathologic study of seven cases. Cancer 1983;51:1148–51.
7. Mucitelli DR, Charles EZ, Kraus FT. Vulvovaginal polyps. Histologic appearance, ultrastructure, immunocytochemical characteristics, and clinicopathologic correlations. Int J Gynecol Pathol 1990;9:20–40.
8. Norris HJ, Taylor HB. Polyps of the vagina. A benign lesion resembling sarcoma botryoides. Cancer 1966;19:227–32.

9. Nucci MR, Fletcher CD. Fibroepithelial stromal polyps of vulvovaginal tissue: from the banal to the bizarre. Pathol Case Rev 1998;3:151–7.
10. Nucci MR, Young RH, Fletcher CD. Cellular pseudosarcomatous fibroepithelial stromal polyps of the lower female genital tract: an underrecognized lesion often misdiagnosed as sarcoma. Am J Surg Pathol 2000;24:231–40.
11. O'Quinn AG, Edwards CL, Gallager HS. Pseudosarcoma botryoides of the vagina in pregnancy. Gynecol Oncol 1982;13: 237–41.
12. Ostor AG, Fortune DW, Riley CB. Fibroepithelial polyps with atypical stromal cells (pseudosarcoma botryoides) of vulva and vagina. A report of 13 cases. Int J Gynecol Pathol 1988;7:351–60.
13. Gaffney EF, Majmudar B, Bryan JA. Nodular fasciitis (pseudosarcomatous fasciitis) of the vulva. Int J Gynecol Pathol 1982;1: 307–12.
14. LiVolsi VA, Brooks JJ. Nodular fasciitis of the vulva: a report of two cases. Obstet Gynecol 1987;69:513–6.
15. Roberts W, Daly JW. Pseudosarcomatous fasciitis of the vulva. Gynecol Oncol 1981;11:383–6.
16. Erickson-Johnson MR, Chou MM, Evers BR, et al. Nodular fasciitis: a novel model of transient neoplasia induced by MYH9-USP6 gene fusion. Lab Invest 2011;91:1427–3.
17. Fletcher CD, Tsang WY, Fisher C, et al. Angiomyofibroblastoma of the vulva. A benign neoplasm distinct from aggressive angiomyxoma. Am J Surg Pathol 1992;16:373–82.
18. Fukunaga M, Nomura K, Matsumoto K, et al. Vulval angiomyofibroblastoma. Clinicopathologic analysis of six cases. Am J Clin Pathol 1997;107:45–51.
19. Hisaoka M, Kouho H, Aoki T, et al. Angiomyofibroblastoma of the vulva: a clinicopathologic study of seven cases. Pathol Int 1995;45:487–92.
20. Laskin WB, Fetsch JF, Tavassoli FA. Angiomyofibroblastoma of the female genital tract: analysis of 17 cases including a lipomatous variant. Hum Pathol 1997;28:1046–55.
21. Nielsen GP, Rosenberg AE, Young RH, et al. Angiomyofibroblastoma of the vulva and vagina. Mod Pathol 1996;9:284–91.
22. Nielsen GP, Young RH, Dickersin GR, Rosenberg AE. Angiomyofibroblastoma of the vulva with sarcomatous transformation ('angiomyofibrosarcoma'). Am J Surg Pathol 1997;21:1104–8.
23. Ockner DM, Sayadi H, Swanson PE, et al. Genital angiomyofibroblastoma. Comparison with aggressive angiomyxoma and other myxoid neoplasms of skin and soft tissue. Am J Clin Pathol 1997;107:36–44.
24. Chen E, Fletcher CD. Cellular angiofibroma with atypia or sarcomatous transformation: clinicopathologic analysis of 13 cases. Am J Surg Pathol, 2010;34:707–14.
25. Flucke U, van Krieken JH, Mentzel T. Cellular angiofibroma: analysis of 25 cases emphasizing its relationship to spindle cell lipoma and mammary-type myofibroblastoma. Mod Pathol 2011;24:82–9.
26. Iwasa Y, Fletcher CD. Cellular angiofibroma: clinicopathologic and immunohistochemical analysis of 51 cases. Am J Surg Pathol 2004;28:1426–35.
27. Laskin WB, Fetsch JF, Mostofi FK. Angiomyofibroblastomalike tumor of the male genital tract: analysis of 11 cases with comparison to female angiomyofibroblastoma and spindle cell lipoma. Am J Surg Pathol 1998;22:6–16.
28. McCluggage WG, Ganesan R, Hirschowitz L, et al. Cellular angiofibroma and related fibromatous lesions of the vulva: report of a series of cases with a morphological spectrum wider than previously described. Histopathology 2004;45:360–8.
29. McCluggage WG, Perenyei M, Irwin ST. Recurrent cellular angiofibroma of the vulva. J Clin Pathol 2002;55:477–9.
30. Nucci MR, Granter SR, Fletcher CD. Cellular angiofibroma: a benign neoplasm distinct from angiomyofibroblastoma and spindle cell lipoma. Am J Surg Pathol 1997;21:636–44.
31. Iwasa Y, Fletcher CD. Distinctive prepubertal vulval fibroma: a hitherto unrecognized mesenchymal tumor of prepubertal girls: analysis of 11 cases. Am J Surg Pathol 2004;28:1601–8.
32. Vargas SO, Kozakewich HP, Boyd TK, et al. Childhood asymmetric labium majus enlargement: mimicking a neoplasm. Am J Surg Pathol 2005;29:1007–16.
33. Abenoza P, Lillemoe T. CD34 and factor XIIIa in the differential diagnosis of dermatofibroma and dermatofibrosarcoma protuberans. Am J Dermatopathol 1993;15:429–34.
34. Calonje E, Fletcher CD. Aneurysmal benign fibrous histiocytoma: clinicopathological analysis of 40 cases of a tumour frequently misdiagnosed as a vascular neoplasm. Histopathology 1995;26: 323–31.
35. Calonje E, Mentzel T, Fletcher CD. Cellular benign fibrous histiocytoma. Clinicopathologic analysis of 74 cases of a distinctive variant of cutaneous fibrous histiocytoma with frequent recurrence. Am J Surg Pathol 1994;18:668–76.
36. Colome-Grimmer MI, Evans HL. Metastasizing cellular dermatofibroma. A report of two cases. Am J Surg Pathol 1996;20:1361–7.
37. Franquemont DW, Cooper PH, Shmookler BM, et al. Benign fibrous histiocytoma of the skin with potential for local recurrence: a tumor to be distinguished from dermatofibroma. Mod Pathol 1990;3:158–63.
38. Gonzalez S, Duarte I. Benign fibrous histiocytoma of the skin. A morphologic study of 290 cases. Pathol Res Pract 1982;174: 379–91.
39. Iwata J, Fletcher CD. Lipidized fibrous histiocytoma: clinicopathologic analysis of 22 cases. Am J Dermatopathol 2000;22:126–34.
40. Kaddu S, McMenamin ME, Fletcher CD. Atypical fibrous histiocytoma of the skin: clinicopathologic analysis of 59 cases with evidence of infrequent metastasis. Am J Surg Pathol 2002;26: 35–46.
41. Requena L, Aguilar A, Lopez Redondo MJ, et al. Multinodular hemosiderotic dermatofibroma. Dermatologica 1990;181:320–3.
42. Singh Gomez C, Calonje E, Fletcher CD. Epithelioid benign fibrous histiocytoma of skin: clinico-pathological analysis of 20 cases of a poorly known variant. Histopathology 1994;24:123–9.
43. Zelger B, Sidoroff A, Stanzl U, et al. Deep penetrating dermatofibroma versus dermatofibrosarcoma protuberans. A clinicopathologic comparison. Am J Surg Pathol 1994;18:677–86.
44. Haley JC, Mirowski GW, Hood AF. Benign vulvar tumors. Semin Cutan Med Surg 1998;17:196–204.
45. Horowitz IR, Copas P, Majmudar B. Granular cell tumors of the vulva. Am J Obstet Gynecol 1995;173:1710–3; discussion 3–4.
46. Kondi-Pafiti A, Kairi-Vassilatou E, Liapis A, et al. Granular cell tumor of the female genital system. Clinical and pathologic characteristics of five cases and literature review. Eur J Gynaecol Oncol 2010;31:222–4.
47. Lack EE, Worsham GF, Callihan MD, et al. Granular cell tumor: a clinicopathologic study of 110 patients. J Surg Oncol 1980;13:301–16.
48. Majmudar B, Castellano PZ, Wilson RW, et al. Granular cell tumors of the vulva. J Reprod Med 1990;35:1008–14.
49. Robertson AJ, McIntosh W, Lamont P, et al. Malignant granular cell tumour (myoblastoma) of the vulva: report of a case and review of the literature. Histopathology 1981;5:69–79.
50. Guardiola MT, Dobin SM, Dal Cin P, et al. Pericentric inversion (12)(p12q13-14) as the sole chromosomal abnormality in a leiomyoma of the vulva. Cancer Genet Cytogenet 2010;199:21–3.
51. Horton E, Dobin SM, Debiec-Rychter M, et al. A clonal translocation (7;8)(p13;q11.2) in a leiomyoma of the vulva. Cancer Genet Cytogenet 2006;170:58–60.
52. Newman PL, Fletcher CD. Smooth muscle tumours of the external genitalia: clinicopathological analysis of a series. Histopathology 1991;18:523–9.
53. Nielsen GP, Rosenberg AE, Koerner FC, et al. Smooth-muscle tumors of the vulva. A clinicopathological study of 25 cases and review of the literature. Am J Surg Pathol 1996;20:779–93.
54. Nucci MR, Fletcher CD. Vulvovaginal soft tissue tumours: update and review. Histopathology 2000;36:97–108.
55. Tavassoli FA, Norris HJ. Smooth muscle tumors of the vulva. Obstet Gynecol 1979;53:213–7.
56. Flanagan BP, Helwig EB. Cutaneous lymphangioma. Arch Dermatol 1977;113:24–30.
57. Peachey RD, Lim CC, Whimster IW. Lymphangioma of skin. A review of 65 cases. Br J Dermatol 1970;83:519–27.
58. Prioleau PG, Santa Cruz DJ. Lymphangioma circumscriptum following radical mastectomy and radiation therapy. Cancer 1978;42:1989–91.
59. Stewart CJ, Chan T, Platten M. Acquired lymphangiectasia ('lymphangioma circumscriptum') of the vulva: a report of eight cases. Pathology 2009;41:448–53.
60. Vlastos AT, Malpica A, Follen M. Lymphangioma circumscriptum of the vulva: a review of the literature. Obstet Gynecol 2003;101:946–54.

61. Cohen PR, Young Jr AW, Tovell HM. Angiokeratoma of the vulva: diagnosis and review of the literature. Obstet Gynecol Surv 1989;44:339–46.
62. Terzakis E, Androutsopoulos G, Zygouris D, et al. Angiokeratoma of the vulva. Eur J Gynaecol Oncol 2011;32:597–8.
63. Faber K, Jones MA, Spratt D, et al. Vulvar leiomyomatosis in a patient with esophagogastric leiomyomatosis: review of the syndrome. Gynecol Oncol 1991;41:92–4.
64. Miner JH. Alport syndrome with diffuse leiomyomatosis. When and when not? Am J Pathol 1999;154:1633–5.
65. Chabrel CM, Beilby JO. Vaginal rhabdomyoma. Histopathology 1980;4:645–51.
66. Hanski W, Hagel-Lewicka E, Daniszewski K. Rhabdomyomas of female genital tract. Report on two cases. Zentralbl Pathol 1991;137:439–42.
67. Iversen UM. Two cases of benign vaginal rhabdomyoma. Case reports. APMIS 1996;104:575–8.
68. Lae ME, Pereira PF, Keeney GL, et al. Lipoblastoma-like tumour of the vulva: report of three cases of a distinctive mesenchymal neoplasm of adipocytic differentiation. Histopathology 2002;40:505–9.
69. Kazmierczak B, Wanschura S, Meyer-Bolte K, et al. Cytogenic and molecular analysis of an aggressive angiomyxoma. Am J Pathol 1995;147:580–5.
70. McCluggage WG, Patterson A, Maxwell P. Aggressive angiomyxoma of pelvic parts exhibits oestrogen and progesterone receptor positivity. J Clin Pathol 2000;53:603–5.
71. Medeiros F, Erickson-Johnson MR, Keeney GL, et al. Frequency and characterization of HMGA2 and HMGA1 rearrangements in mesenchymal tumors of the lower genital tract. Genes Chromosomes Cancer 2007;46:981–90.
72. Micci F, Panagopoulos I, Bjerkehagen B, et al. Deregulation of HMGA2 in an aggressive angiomyxoma with t(11;12)(q23;q15). Virchows Arch 2006;448:838–42.
73. Nucci MR, Weremowicz S, Neskey DM, et al.. Chromosomal translocation t(8;12) induces aberrant HMGIC expression in aggressive angiomyxoma of the vulva. Genes Chromosomes Cancer 2001;32:172–6.
74. Rabban JT, Dal Cin P, Oliva E. HMGA2 rearrangement in a case of vulvar aggressive angiomyxoma. Int J Gynecol Pathol 2006;25:403–7.
75. Rawlinson NJ, West WW, Nelson M, et al. Aggressive angiomyxoma with t(12;21) and HMGA2 rearrangement: report of a case and review of the literature. Cancer Genet Cytogenet 2008;181:119–24.
76. Steeper TA, Rosai J. Aggressive angiomyxoma of the female pelvis and perineum. Report of nine cases of a distinctive type of gynecologic soft-tissue neoplasm. Am J Surg Pathol 1983;7:463–75.
77. Tsang WY, Chan JK, Lee KC, et al. Aggressive angiomyxoma. A report of four cases occurring in men. Am J Surg Pathol 1992;16:1059–65.
78. van Roggen JF, van Unnik JA, Briaire-de Bruijn IH, et al. Aggressive angiomyxoma: a clinicopathological and immunohistochemical study of 11 cases with long-term follow-up. Virchows Arch 2005;446:157–63.
79. Allen PW, Dymock RB, MacCormac LB. Superficial angiomyxomas with and without epithelial components. Report of 30 tumors in 28 patients. Am J Surg Pathol 1988;12:519–30.
80. Calonje E, Guerin D, McCormick D, et al. Superficial angiomyxoma: clinicopathologic analysis of a series of distinctive but poorly recognized cutaneous tumors with tendency for recurrence. Am J Surg Pathol 1999;23:910–7.
81. Fetsch JF, Laskin WB, Tavassoli FA. Superficial angiomyxoma (cutaneous myxoma): a clinicopathologic study of 17 cases arising in the genital region. Int J Gynecol Pathol 1997;16:325–34.
82. Barnhill DR, Boling R, Nobles W, et al. Vulvar dermatofibrosarcoma protuberans. Gynecol Oncol 1988;30:149–52.
83. Bock JE, Andreasson B, Thorn A, et al. Dermatofibrosarcoma protuberans of the vulva. Gynecol Oncol 1985;20:129–35.
84. Davos I, Abell MR. Soft tissue sarcomas of vulva. Gynecol Oncol 1976;4:70–86.
85. Ghorbani RP, Malpica A, Ayala AG. Dermatofibrosarcoma protuberans of the vulva: clinicopathological and immunohistochemical analysis of four cases, one with fibrosarcomatous change, and review of the literature. Int J Gynecol Pathol 1999;18:366–73.
86. Gokden N, Dehner LP, Zhu X, et al. Dermatofibrosarcoma protuberans of the vulva and groin: detection of COL1A1-PDGFB fusion transcripts by RT-PCR. J Cutan Pathol 2003;30:190–5.
87. Leake JF, Buscema J, Cho KR, et al. Dermatofibrosarcoma protuberans of the vulva. Gynecol Oncol 1991;41:245–9.
88. Mentzel T, Beham A, Katenkamp D, et al. Fibrosarcomatous ('high-grade') dermatofibrosarcoma protuberans: clinicopathologic and immunohistochemical study of a series of 41 cases with emphasis on prognostic significance. Am J Surg Pathol 1998;22:576–87.
89. Moodley M, Moodley J. Dermatofibrosarcoma protuberans of the vulva: a case report and review of the literature. Gynecol Oncol 2000;78:74–5.
90. Naeem R, Lux ML, Huang SF, et al. Ring chromosomes in dermatofibrosarcoma protuberans are composed of interspersed sequences from chromosomes 17 and 22. Am J Pathol 1995;147:1553–8.
91. Soergel TM, Doering DL, O'Connor D. Metastatic dermatofibrosarcoma protuberans of the vulva. Gynecol Oncol 1998;71:320–4.
92. Vanni R, Faa G, Dettori T, et al. A case of dermatofibrosarcoma protuberans of the vulva with a COL1A1/PDGFB fusion identical to a case of giant cell fibroblastoma. Virchows Arch 2000;437:95–100.
93. Curtin JP, Saigo P, Slucher B, et al. Soft-tissue sarcoma of the vagina and vulva: a clinicopathologic study. Obstet Gynecol 1995;86:269–72.
94. DiSaia PJ, Rutledge F, Smith JP. Sarcoma of the vulva. Report of 12 patients. Obstet Gynecol 1971;38:180–4.
95. Nirenberg A, Ostor AG, Slavin J, et al. Primary vulvar sarcomas. Int J Gynecol Pathol 1995;14:55–62.
96. Guillou L, Wadden C, Coindre JM, et al. 'Proximal-type' epithelioid sarcoma, a distinctive aggressive neoplasm showing rhabdoid features. Clinicopathologic, immunohistochemical, and ultrastructural study of a series. Am J Surg Pathol 1997;21:130–46.
97. Hollmann TJ, Hornick JL. INI1-deficient tumors: diagnostic features and molecular genetics. Am J Surg Pathol 2011;35:e47–63.
98. Kasamatsu T, Hasegawa T, Tsuda H, et al. Primary epithelioid sarcoma of the vulva. Int J Gynecol Cancer 2001;11:316–20.
99. Kim HJ, Kim MH, Kwon J, et al. Proximal-type epithelioid sarcoma of the vulva with INI1 diagnostic utility. Ann Diagn Pathol 2012;16:411–5.
100. Tholpady A, Lonergan CL, Wick MR. Proximal-type epithelioid sarcoma of the vulva: relationship to malignant extrarenal rhabdoid tumor. Int J Gynecol Pathol 2010;29:600–4.
101. Genton CY, Maroni ES. Vulval liposarcoma. Arch Gynecol 1987;240:63–6.
102. Gondos B, Casey MJ. Liposarcoma of the perineum. Gynecol Oncol 1982;14:133–40.
103. Nucci MR, Fletcher CD. Liposarcoma (atypical lipomatous tumors) of the vulva: a clinicopathologic study of six cases. Int J Gynecol Pathol 1998;17:17–23.
104. Vecchione A, Palazzetti P. [Anatomoclinical considerations on a case of liposarcoma with vulvar localization]. Riv Anat Pathol Oncol 1967;31:177–93.
105. Copeland LJ, Gershenson DM, Saul PB, et al. Sarcoma botryoides of the female genital tract. Obstet Gynecol 1985;66:262–6.
106. Copeland LJ, Sneige N, Stringer CA, et al. Alveolar rhabdomyosarcoma of the female genitalia. Cancer 1985;56:849–55.
107. Imachi M, Tsukamoto N, Kamura T, et al. Alveolar rhabdomyosarcoma of the vulva. Report of two cases. Acta Cytol 1991;35:345–9.
108. Shen JT, D'Ablaing G, Morrow CP. Alveolar soft part sarcoma of the vulva: report of first case and review of literature. Gynecol Oncol 1982;13:120–8.
109. Cetiner H, Kir G, Gelmann EP, et al. Primary vulvar Ewing sarcoma/primitive neuroectodermal tumor: a report of 2 cases and review of the literature. Int J Gynecol Cancer 2009;19:1131–6.
110. McCluggage WG, Sumathi VP, Nucci MR, et al. Ewing family of tumours involving the vulva and vagina: report of a series of four cases. J Clin Pathol 2007;60:674–80.
111. Hall DJ, Burns JC, Goplerud DR. Kaposi's sarcoma of the vulva: a case report and brief review. Obstet Gynecol 1979;54:478–83.
112. Macasaet MA, Duerr A, Thelmo W, et al. Kaposi sarcoma presenting as a vulvar mass. Obstet Gynecol 1995;86:695–7.

7 Vagina

Sarah Bean, Jaime Prat, Stanley J. Robboy

CHAPTER OUTLINE

Development	132	Benign Tumors	144
Anatomy	133	Benign Mixed Tumor	144
Histology and Physiology	133	Müllerian Papilloma	144
Mesonephric Ducts	135	Leiomyoma	145
Developmental Disorders	136	Rhabdomyoma	145
Benign Effects of Diethylstilbestrol on the Vagina	136	Angiomyofibroblastoma	145
		Miscellaneous Benign Tumors	146
Imperforate Hymen	139	Squamous Neoplasia	146
Vaginal Agenesis	139	HPV Infection	146
Transverse Vaginal Septum	139	Squamous Intraepithelial Lesion (VaIN)	146
Miscellaneous Congenital Disorders	139	Invasive Squamous Cell Carcinoma	148
Inflammatory Disorders	139	Verrucous Carcinoma	149
Vaginitis	139	Warty Carcinoma	150
Malakoplakia	140	Papillary Squamotransitional Cell Carcinoma	150
Tampon-related Lesions and Toxic Shock Syndrome	141	Small Cell Carcinoma	150
Noninfectious Inflammatory Diseases	141	Clear Cell Adenocarcinoma	150
Ligneous Vaginitis	141	Adenocarcinoma, Non-clear Cell Types	153
Vaginal Cysts	141	Other Primary Malignant Tumors of the Vagina	153
Cysts of the Introitus	142	Malignant Melanoma	153
Tumor-Like Conditions	142	Leiomyosarcoma	154
Fibroepithelial Polyps	142	Miscellaneous Tumors	154
Prolapsed Fallopian Tube	143	Malignant Vaginal Tumors in Childhood	154
Granulation Tissue Nodule	143	Embryonal Rhabdomyosarcoma	154
Postoperative Spindle Cell Nodule	143	Yolk Sac Tumor	156
Microglandular Hyperplasia	143	Lymphoma	156
Endometriosis	144	Secondary Tumors of the Vagina	157

The vagina acts as a barrier to many potentially invasive microorganisms. Accordingly, it is the site of a variety of infections, both sexually and nonsexually transmitted, and this, in fact, represents the predominant type of pathology of this organ. In contrast, neoplasms are relatively infrequent in this site, which is somewhat unexpected in view of the relationship between infection (e.g., human papillomavirus (HPV) infection) and the development of carcinoma of the vulva and cervix.

DEVELOPMENT

The müllerian ducts first appear as funnel-shaped openings of the celomic mesothelium in the mesonephric ridge at about day 37.[1] They grow caudally as paired tubes, extending to meet the posterior wall of the urogenital sinus. At about day 54, the caudal portions of the müllerian ducts fuse, forming a straight uterovaginal canal lined by simple columnar epithelium. The uterovaginal canal continues to elongate caudally until about day 66. Subsequently, the epithelium from the caudal end of the canal to the external cervical os becomes stratified squamous epithelium due to migration of squamous cells from the urogenital sinus.[2] Stratification of the squamous epithelium progressively occludes the caudal portion of the canal, leading to the development of a solid vaginal plate. In the 16th week, desquamation subsequently results in the canalization of the vaginal plate. Vaginal development is essentially complete by the 18–20th week.

ANATOMY

The vagina, from the Latin *sheath*, extends from the vestibule of the vulva to the uterine cervix, lying posterior (dorsal) to the urinary bladder and anterior (ventral) to the rectum (Figure 7.1). Its axis averages 0° with the vertical and usually more than 90° with the uterus. The ventral wall is shorter than the dorsal wall, but overall the mean vaginal length is 6.2 cm. It surrounds the exocervix and forms vault-like fornices between its cervical attachment and the lateral wall. In the adult, the anterior and posterior walls are slack and remain in contact with each other, whereas the lateral walls remain fairly rigid and separated. This gives an H-shaped appearance to the vaginal canal on cross section. The vagina opens into the vestibule formed from the urogenital sinus. The vestibule lies beneath the urethra and between the inner margins of the labia minora. The vagina, urethra, and ducts of Bartholin glands open into the vestibule.

The vagina is in contact anteriorly with the uterine cervix, the base of the bladder, and the urethra. Posteriorly, the upper fourth of the vaginal wall is bounded by peritoneum and forms the anterior part of the cul-de-sac or pouch of Douglas. The rectovaginal septum connects the adventitia of the middle half of the vagina with the rectum. Laterally, each ureter, crossed by the uterine artery and vein, runs just above the lateral fornix. Caudally (distally), the levator ani and bulbocavernosus muscles partially surround the vagina. Blood is supplied to the vagina primarily by branches of the internal iliac artery, including the uterine, vaginal, middle rectal, and internal pudendal arteries. A complex network of veins surrounds the vagina, forming a plexus that drains into the internal iliac vein. The lymphatics of the proximal anterior vagina and vaginal vault drain primarily into the external iliac lymph nodes. The posterior portion of the vagina drains into the inferior gluteal, sacral, and anorectal lymph nodes, whereas the distal part of the vagina drains into the femoral lymph nodes. As a consequence of extensive anastomotic channels, any pelvic, anorectal, or femoral node may be involved in the lymphatic drainage of any part of the vagina. The innervation of the vagina is principally from the superior hypogastric plexus of the autonomic nervous system.

HISTOLOGY AND PHYSIOLOGY

The vaginal wall consists of three principal layers: mucosa, muscularis, and adventitia (Figure 7.2). The epithelium lining of the mucosa is about 0.4 mm thick and, on gross examination, exhibits a characteristic pattern of folds or rugae separated by furrows of variable depth. The rugal pattern of the vaginal mucosa produces an undulating appearance on microscopic examination in contrast to the flat surface of the cervix. A glycogenated nonkeratinized squamous epithelium, similar to cervical epithelium, lines the luminal surface. The normal vaginal mucosa lacks glands. Its surface is lubricated both by fluids that pass directly through the mucosa and by cervical mucus. The vaginal fluid is acid (pH 4–5) owing to the presence of lactic

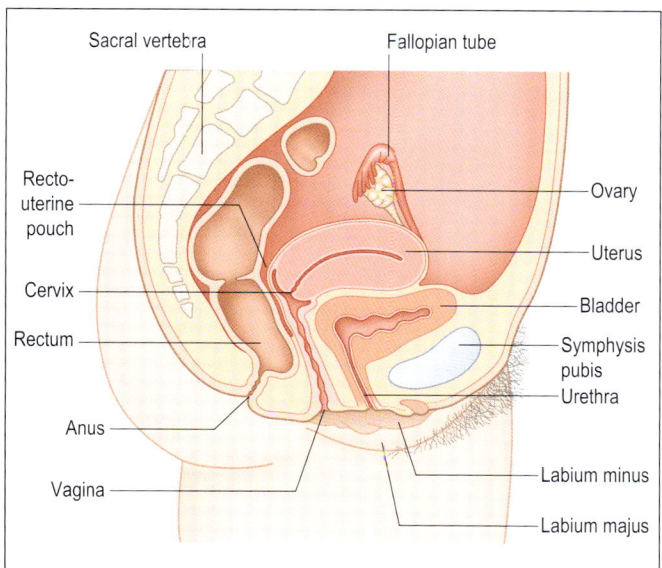

Figure 7.1 Median sagittal section of the female pelvis.

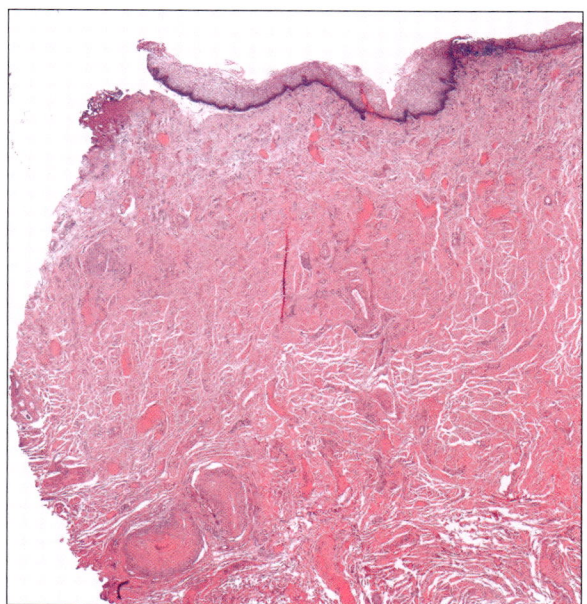

Figure 7.2 Vaginal wall. The vaginal muscularis is composed of intermixed smooth muscle bundles of variable size.

acid produced from the metabolism of epithelial glycogen by *Lactobacillus acidophilus* (bacillus of Döderlein). The fluid's acidity accounts for its considerable bacteriostatic capacity. The degree of acidity is reduced during sexual response and, more significantly, in the presence of pus or menstrual blood, or a paucity of estrogens. Before puberty and, to a lesser extent, after menopause, the vaginal mucosa is thinner and less resistant to infection than during reproductive life.

The mature, stratified squamous epithelium is arbitrarily subdivided into the deep, intermediate, and superficial zones (Figure 7.3). The deep zone contains the basal cell layer and above this the parabasal layer. Both are the active proliferative compartments or germinal beds, as shown by the nuclear proliferation markers (the Ki-67 antigen, which is demonstrable during late G_1, G_2, and M phases of the cell cycle) (Figure 7.4). The basal cell layer consists of a single layer of columnar-like cells, approximately 10 μm thick, the long axis of which is vertically arranged. The cells have a basophilic cytoplasm and relatively large oval nuclei. Mitoses may be present. Occasional melanocytes are also found. The parabasal layer is poorly demarcated from the overlying cell layers and consists usually of about 2–5 layers of small polygonal cells, having a total 14 μm thickness, often with intercellular bridges. The cells have basophilic cytoplasm, relatively large, centrally placed, round nuclei, and occasional mitoses.

The intermediate cell layer is of variable thickness, but generally about 10 rows that are in total about 100 μm thick. The cells have prominent intercellular bridges, a naviculate configuration, and a long cell axis parallel to the surface. The nuclei are round, oval, or irregular, with finely granular chromatin. The cytoplasm is basophilic, although some glycogen may be present. The glycogen accumulates initially in a perinuclear location resulting in a clear zone around the nucleus. This appearance may cause confusion with the perinuclear clearing of koilocytes. However, the presence of nuclear membrane irregularity in koilocytes and the characteristic location of these normal cells in the middle rather than superficial third of the epithelium are helpful distinguishing features.

The superficial layer is also variably thick. The cells are polygonal when viewed from above and flattened when viewed in cross section. The cytoplasm is acidophilic, and the nuclei are centrally located, small, round, and pyknotic. Keratohyalin granules are sometimes seen in the cytoplasm. This layer also contains about 10 rows of squamous cells.

Cyclic changes occur in the vaginal epithelium. Proliferation of the basal layers and general thickening of the epithelium are seen in the first half of the cycle. Estrogens stimulate maturation of the epithelium, as increased numbers of intermediate cells and then superficial cells show (Figure 7.3). A sign of maturation is the significant accumulation of glycogen in the epithelium (Figure 7.5). Although glycogen is found in the intermediate and superficial cells throughout the menstrual cycle, it is particularly abundant during pregnancy. Full maturation to superficial cells does not occur when the estrogenic action is opposed

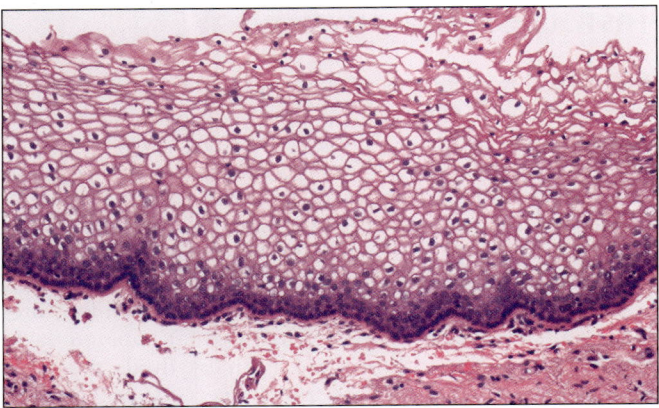

Figure 7.3 Normal vaginal epithelium. The epithelium consists of a single layer of basal cells, several layers of parabasal cells, and thick intermediate and superficial layers of highly glycogenated cells.

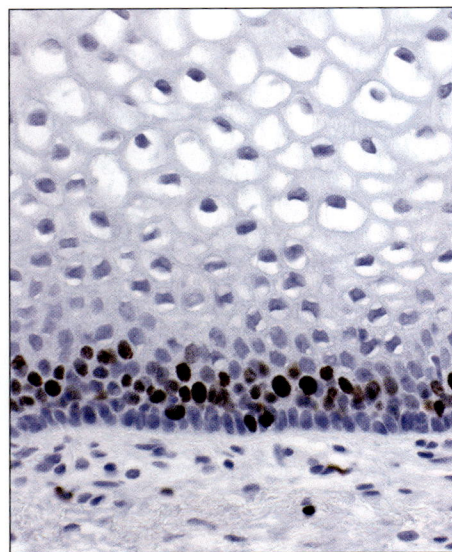

Figure 7.4 Normal vagina. Ki-67 antigen, demonstrable during the late G_1, G_2, and M phases of the cell cycle in the parabasal and basal layer of the normal vaginal mucosa.

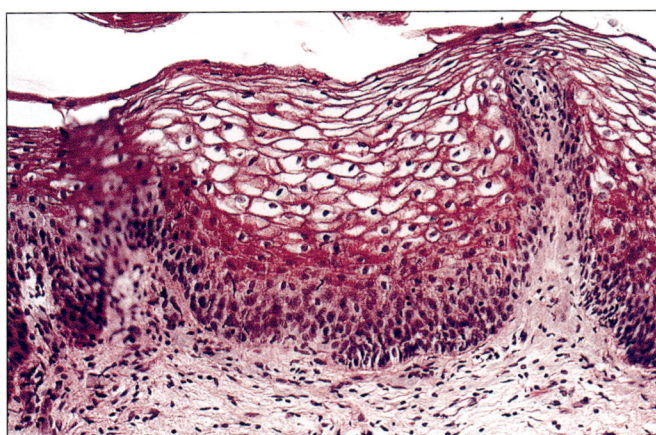

Figure 7.5 Normal vaginal epithelium. Extensive glycogen (red) is present in the thick layers of intermediate and superficial cells (periodic acid–Schiff stain).

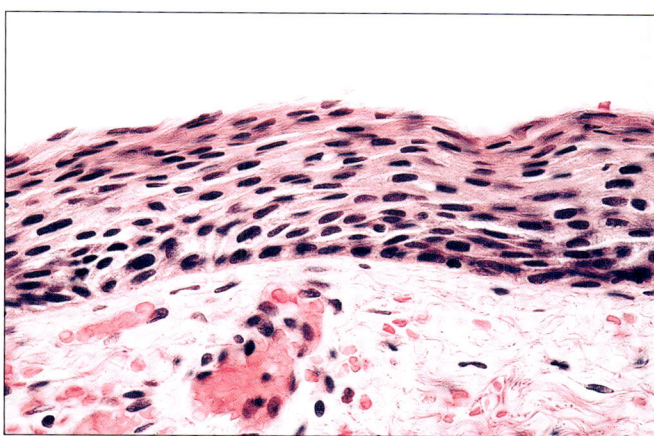

Figure 7.6 Atrophy. In the absence of estrogenic stimulation, the number of cell layers decreases, and virtually all cells are basal and parabasal with minimal cytoplasm.

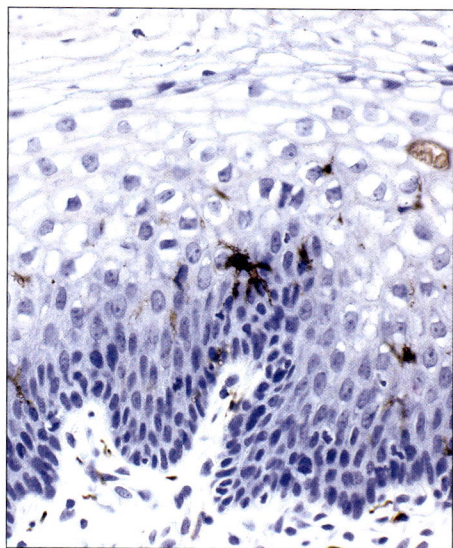

Figure 7.7 Vagina. The dendritic processes of Langerhans cells.

by progesterone. Thus, in the second half of the cycle, after ovulation has taken place, maturation ceases at the level of the intermediate cells. This change is clinically useful; the number of superficial cells in a smear taken from the lateral vaginal wall (and, to a lesser extent, from the ectocervix) compared with the number of intermediate and parabasal cells gives a rough indication of the woman's hormonal status. Variously calculated, although now considered archaic, this relationship gives the maturation index, the cornification index, or the karyopyknotic index (KPI). A high KPI therefore means that unopposed estrogen has stimulated the epithelium. Without hormonal stimulation, the cells atrophy. After menopause, a gradual reduction in the thickness of the epithelium occurs, first with a loss of superficial cells followed by intermediate cells. Thus, the mucosa of late menopausal women may be reduced to only 4–6 layers of parabasal cells (Figure 7.6). Consequently, a normal postmenopausal atrophic epithelium may be erroneously interpreted as a high-grade intraepithelial lesion. Exposure of the postmenopausal vagina to estrogen leads to squamous maturation comparable to that seen in the proliferative phase of reproductive age women.

The lamina propria, which lies beneath the squamous epithelium, consists of a loose fibrovascular stroma containing elastic fibers, nerves, and various mononuclear cells demonstrable by immunocytochemical methods. Dendritic processes of Langerhans cells, about 4 per HPF, are distributed throughout the mucosa.[3] They are found largely in the deeper layers but can extend into the superficial fields (Figure 7.7). CD8 and, to a lesser degree, CD4 T-lymphocytes are also frequently found, whereas macrophages and B-lymphocytes are relatively uncommon.

Sometimes the superficial lamina propria discloses a band-like zone of loose connective tissue that contains atypical polygonal to stellate stromal cells with scant cytoplasm. Many cells are multinucleated or have multilobulated hyperchromatic nuclei. Few are mononucleate. Mitoses are not observed. These atypical stromal cells are thought to give rise to fibroepithelial polyps and have been observed within the cervix, vagina, and vulva. They are myofibroblastic in nature.[4]

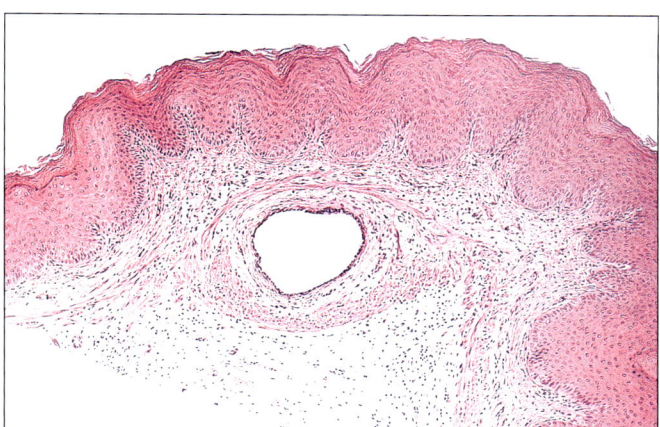

Figure 7.8 Normal mesonephric duct. On cross section it is a single duct in the submucosa surrounded by clusters of smooth muscle bands.

The muscularis is an ill-defined zone of inner circular and outer longitudinal bundles of smooth muscle that is continuous with that of the uterus. Some of the outer longitudinal layers of muscle pass into the lateral pelvic wall to contribute to the cardinal ligaments, while fibers of the bulbocavernosus form a sphincter around the distal vagina. The adventitia is a thin coat of dense connective tissue that contains lymphatics, veins, and nerves and merges with the loose fibrous tissue of the pelvis connecting the vagina to the adjacent structures.

MESONEPHRIC DUCTS

The wolffian ducts, known otherwise as 'mesonephric ducts' or 'Gartner ducts,' are vestigial in the adult female (Figure 7.8). They begin to irreversibly regress if not stimulated by testosterone before week 13 post conception. These paired ducts are most commonly seen in the lateral vaginal walls.

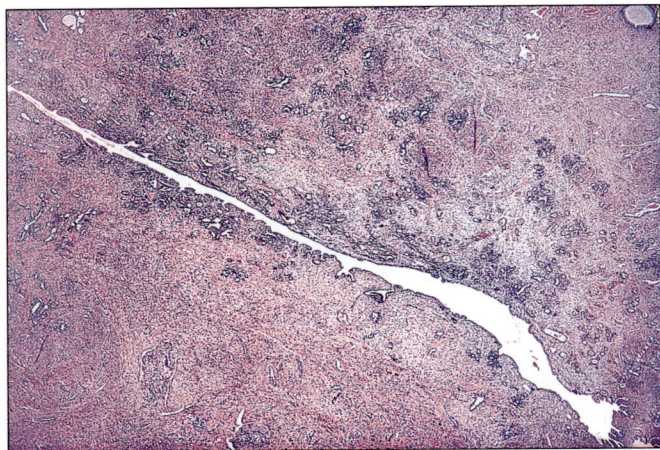

Figure 7.9 Elongated mesonephric duct.

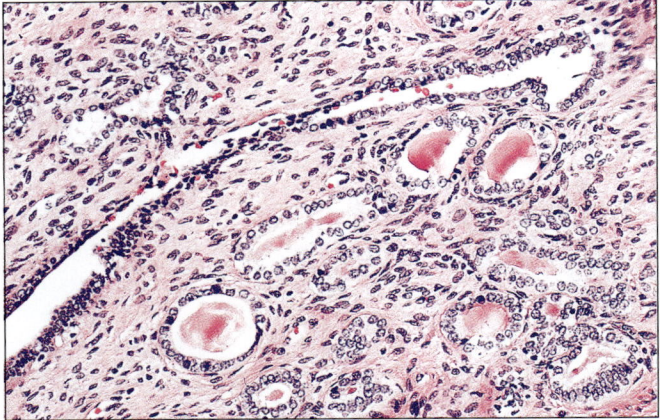

Figure 7.10 Mesonephric duct. Smaller arborized offshoots surround the main duct and show intraluminal eosinophilic secretions.

When encountered by chance in a radical vaginectomy specimen, the ducts are virtually always invisible grossly. Microscopically, the ducts are seen often as central ducts with more peripheral arborized glands. Occasionally, the ducts appear as elongated tubes (Figure 7.9), also with peripheral arborized glands. The lumens are filled frequently with a deeply eosinophilic, hyalinized secretion (Figure 7.10). The single layer of cells lining the ducts is predominantly composed of nuclei. The cytoplasm is scant, relatively translucent, and lacks cilia. The nuclei frequently overlap. The chromatin is strikingly bland. Mitoses are absent. Individual ducts occasionally dilate and become visible cysts. In the cervix, these ducts may appear throughout the wall as mesonephric hyperplasia or even adenoma. Rarely, mesonephric adenocarcinomas arise from these vestigial structures mainly in the cervix or vagina.[5]

DEVELOPMENTAL DISORDERS

Congenital uterine and vaginal malformations result from failure of development, failure of fusion, or septal reabsorption of the müllerian ducts. The spectrum of findings ranges from agenesis to duplications. They are important clinically because of their association with menstrual disorders and impaired fertility. Furthermore, women with müllerian duct anomalies have a significant risk of obstetric complications such as spontaneous abortion, stillbirth, and preterm delivery.

BENIGN EFFECTS OF DIETHYLSTILBESTROL ON THE VAGINA

Diethylstilbestrol (DES), a synthetic, nonsteroidal estrogen promoted for the treatment of habitual abortion and threatened abortion during the mid-1940s and 1950s, profoundly affects the development of the vagina as well as the uterus and fallopian tubes. The pathology associated with *in utero* DES exposure has led to many insights into embryology, anatomy, physiology, and neoplasia of the vagina and their interrelations. In 1971 its use became linked to the rare development of clear cell adenocarcinoma in the vagina and cervix of offspring exposed *in utero*. Upwards of one million daughters may have been so exposed. Subsequently, various non-neoplastic changes were identified in the genital tract of daughters of women receiving DES during pregnancy, such as adenosis, cervical ectropion, various types of cervicovaginal ridges, and structural abnormalities of the uterine corpus and fallopian tube. DES was soon thereafter withdrawn from the market for use during pregnancy

GROSS STRUCTURAL CHANGES OF THE VAGINA AND CERVIX

Various non-neoplastic as well as neoplastic changes occur in DES-exposed offspring. Approximately one-fifth of exposed women demonstrate gross structural changes in the cervix or vagina.[6] The cervix may be hypoplastic and the vaginal fornices may be obliterated. Descriptive designations include coxcomb (hood), collar (rim), pseudopolyp, and ridge. The coxcomb is a protuberant ridge of tissue, usually on the anterior lip of the cervix, which is covered by squamous epithelium and contains cervical stroma. The collar is a low constricting band about a portion of the cervix. The pseudopolyp appears as a polyp due to the presence of a circumferential constricting groove, but in fact is a portion of cervix in which there is a central endocervical canal (Figures 7.11 and 7.12). Gross abnormalities are less common in the vagina than in the cervix. The most common is a transverse partial vaginal septum, which may make examination of the cervix by the naked eye and by colposcopy difficult or impossible. Deformities found in the upper reproductive tract include a T-shaped uterine cavity, constrictions of the uterine cavity, and hypoplasia of the uterine cavity and uterine corpus. These conditions also occur in approximately 2–4% of women who have no prenatal drug history. Over time, many structural changes disappear as the cervix remodels with age. Estimates are that upwards of two-thirds disappear after pregnancy.

VAGINAL ADENOSIS

Most women exposed prenatally to DES have some form of microscopic change in the inner half of the exocervix and many also have vaginal manifestations. The presence of

CHAPTER 7 — VAGINA

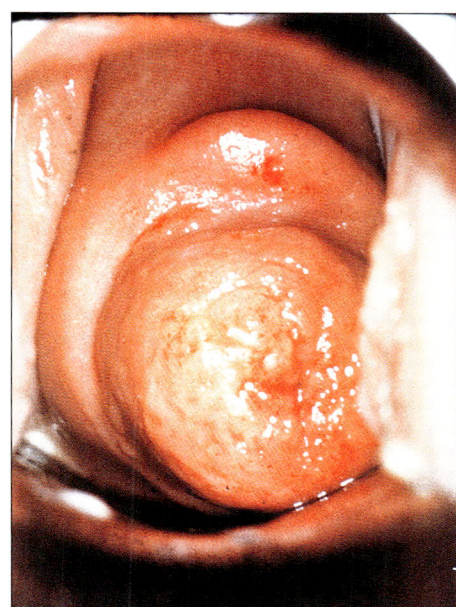

Figure 7.11 DES-associated cervical abnormalities. A coxcomb (upper) and pseudopolyp (middle) are present.

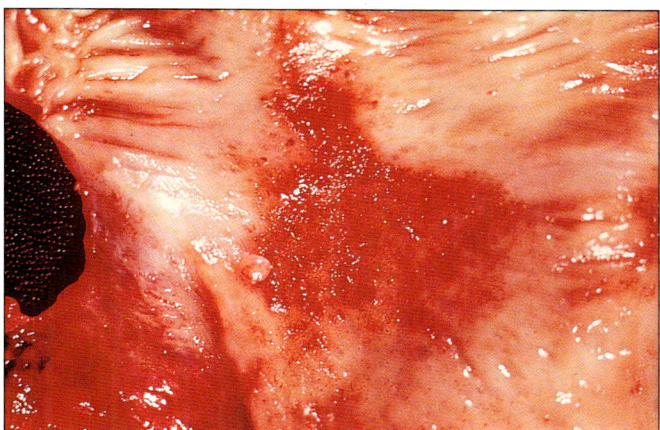

Figure 7.13 Vaginal adenosis.

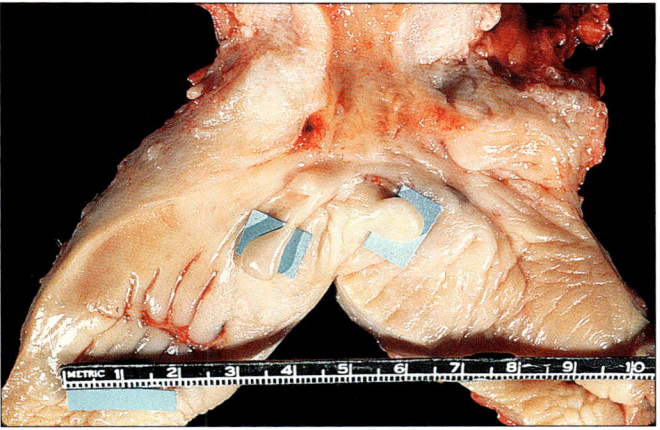

Figure 7.12 DES-associated cervical abnormalities. The entire remains of the upper vagina and exocervix appear as several tiny tags. The cervix is hypoplastic and the fornices are obliterated.

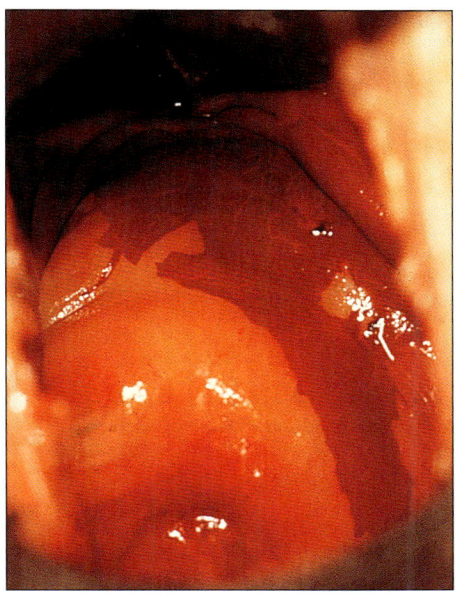

Figure 7.14 Iodine stain of the lower genital tract. Both the cervix and portions of the vagina fail to take up the stain, indicative of a lack of glycogenated squamous epithelium.

glandular tissue in the vagina is called 'adenosis.' Squamous metaplasia represents the normal healing process by which adenosis transforms and heals. Ultimately the vaginal epithelial changes, when completely healed, appear as normal squamous epithelium.

Adenosis should be suspected clinically when the vaginal mucosa discloses red granular spots or patches (Figure 7.13) or fails to stain with an iodine solution (Figure 7.14). On colposcopy, adenosis appears as glandular or metaplastic epithelium that has replaced the squamous epithelium of the vaginal mucosa. It is usually asymptomatic, although some women have vaginal discharge or postcoital bleeding.

Adenosis, with or without squamous metaplasia, involves the upper third of the vagina in 34% of DES-exposed women. The anterior wall is involved more frequently than the posterior wall. These changes extend into the middle third of the vagina in 9% and the lower third in 2% of exposed women. An embryonic form of adenosis is also encountered occasionally.[7] In unexposed women, adenosis of the adult type is rare, but, when present, is identical to that which occurs in exposed women.

There are two adult (or differentiated) forms of adenosis: mucinous and tuboendometrial. Mucinous columnar cells, which by light and electron microscopy resemble those of the normal endocervical mucosa (Figure 7.15), comprise the glandular epithelium most frequently encountered in adenosis (62% of biopsy specimens with vaginal adenosis) and is the type of glandular epithelium most commonly seen by colposcopy. Tuboendometrial glands lined by light and dark cells, which are often ciliated and resemble the cells lining the fallopian tube and endometrium (Figure 7.16), are found in 21% of specimens with adenosis.

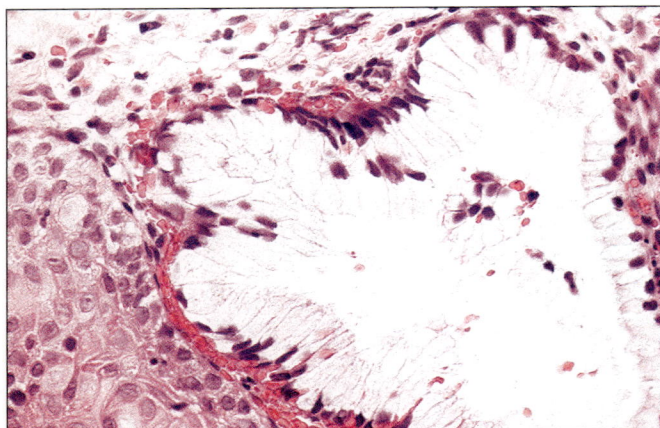

Figure 7.15 Adenosis, mucinous type.

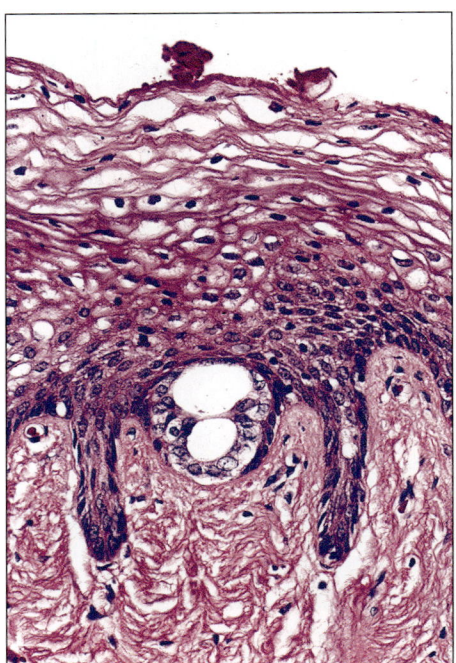

Figure 7.17 Adenosis, fetal (embryonic) type.

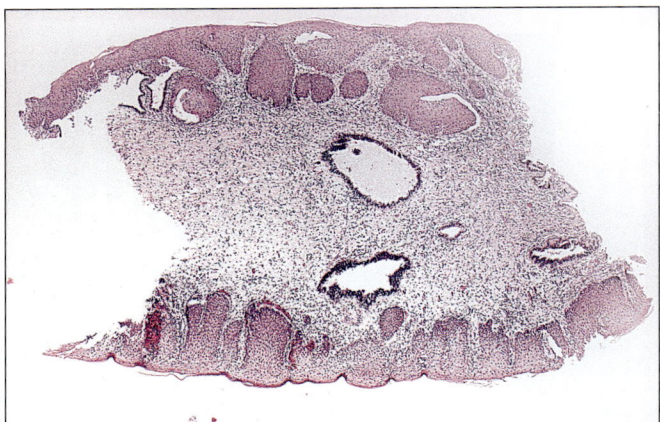

Figure 7.16 Adenosis, tuboendometrial type.

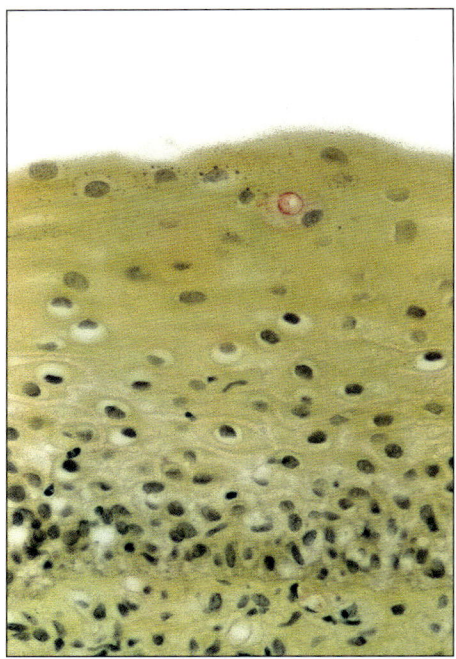

Figure 7.18 Adenosis, intracellular droplet of mucin.

These glands are usually found in the lamina propria and not on the surface of the vagina. The third type of adenosis is embryonic, i.e., a fetal form of adenosis (Figure 7.17). It is the putative precursor from which the adult form of adenosis develops postpubertally. It is this embryonic form that is found in up to 15% of fetuses and stillbirths and occasionally in the vagina of adult women regardless of DES history, and, experimentally, in human embryonic vagina grown in an athymic mouse host in a DES milieu.[2] Remnants of columnar cells, which may be surrounded by metaplastic squamous cells or shown as intracellular droplets of mucin in metaplastic squamous cells, constitute the only evidence for adenosis in 48% of biopsy specimens (Figure 7.18).

DES-exposed women often have abnormal colposcopic findings, i.e., mosaicism and punctation, which are often misinterpreted clinically as dysplasia. The paucity or total lack of glycogen in the early stages of squamous metaplasia accounts for the failure of the epithelium to stain with iodine. The increased vascularity, the slightly tortuous arrangement of the vessels surrounding the pegs in the lamina propria, and the tile-like patterns are responsible for the atypical colposcopic motifs. Hyperkeratosis accounts for the colposcopic findings of leukoplakia. Eventual maturation of the metaplastic squamous epithelium with acquisition of glycogen makes it indistinguishable from the normal (native) squamous epithelium.

Vaginal adenosis must be distinguished in a biopsy from endometriosis, which is also uncommon in the vagina. Apart from the presence of endometrial stroma, which is often not convincingly demonstrable, the glands of endometriosis much more closely resemble those of normal endometrium than do those of adenosis. This difference is at its most obvious during the secretory phase of the cycle. A CD10 immunoreaction may be used to confirm the presence of endometrial stroma. Another useful point in the differential diagnosis is if the glandular epithelium contains any mucinous component. This is virtually never seen in endometriosis.

The changes seen in DES-exposed progeny may be explained in part by the normal embryologic development of the lower genital tract. Both the müllerian ducts and the urogenital sinus are required for the normal vagina to develop. The primitive uterovaginal canal that forms early in embryonic life, initially paired and shortly thereafter merged into a single structure, has a muscular wall lined by columnar (müllerian) epithelium. At about week 10 of gestation, the normal transitional squamous epithelium that lines the urogenital sinus grows upward into the vagina to replace the embryonic columnar (müllerian) epithelium. The squamous epithelium grows to extend as far as what becomes the external cervical os. If the process arrests before the external os is reached, then the area where replacement has not occurred, i.e., usually the upper vagina, retains its original columnar (müllerian) lining. This explains in part what happens as vaginal adenosis develops.

IMPERFORATE HYMEN

Imperforate hymen is the most common congenital anomaly of significance to occur in the vagina, with a frequency of 0.05%. The presence of a thick mucoid secretion that distends the vagina may provide a clue to diagnosis in the neonate, but often an imperforate hymen goes unrecognized until puberty, when there is retention of menstrual detritus.[8,9] If not corrected promptly, infertility may result from endometriosis and pelvic adhesions associated with retrograde menstruation.

VAGINAL AGENESIS

Vaginal agenesis refers to the absence or failure of large portions of the vagina to develop. Complete vaginal agenesis is rare, occurring in about 1 of 6000 live female births.[10] As an isolated defect, it results from incomplete caudal development and fusion of the lower part of the müllerian ducts (müllerian dysgenesis). The external genitalia usually appear normal, except for the introitus, where a short blind pouch may be present. The epithelium is highly glycogenated and normal in all respects since, embryologically, it derives from the urogenital sinus. The defect is often associated with an absent uterus and fallopian tubes (müllerian agenesis or Mayer–Rokitansky–Kuster–Hauser syndrome), and with anomalies of the urinary tract.[11–13] This syndrome provides insight into embryologic development and demonstrates that an intact mesonephric duct is required for the growth and caudal lengthening of the müllerian duct during fetal life. The gonads, not being of müllerian origin, are usually normal. About a fourth of women with vaginal agenesis have a uterus and they may have complications from retrograde menstruation (such as an increased risk of pelvic endometriosis).

TRANSVERSE VAGINAL SEPTUM

A transverse vaginal septum is uncommon,[12] occurring anywhere within the vagina. Some may be related to prenatal DES exposure. A complete septum results in obstructive symptoms similar to an imperforate hymen, whereas a partial septum may allow passage of menstrual flow, but cause dyspareunia or laceration during childbirth. The microscopic appearance of the septum is typically that of a fibrovascular stroma covered on two surfaces by epithelium. The caudal surface is covered by a stratified squamous epithelium of urogenital origin, whereas the cranial aspect shows a glandular müllerian epithelium that has never transformed, as predicted from the arrested embryologic development.

MISCELLANEOUS CONGENITAL DISORDERS

Complete duplication of the vagina with a septum including muscularis extending to the introitus is rare,[14] and typically accompanies cervical and uterine duplication. Longitudinal septa that lack a muscular layer are more common. They often are clinically asymptomatic. Congenital rectovaginal fistulas are often associated with an imperforate anus. Typically, the anus opens into the posterior caudal portion of the vagina, near the fourchette.

INFLAMMATORY DISORDERS

VAGINITIS

'Vaginitis,' a generic term, refers to a vaginal infection from any cause, be it yeast, parasite, or bacterial. Vaginitis, one of the most common maladies in clinical medicine, is the reason cited most often for visits to the gynecologist. The three main categories of vaginitis are related to *Trichomonas vaginalis* infection, *Candida* vaginitis, and bacterial vaginosis.[15]

Bacterial vaginosis is the most common form of vaginitis, accounting for nearly 50% of all cases. The term 'vaginosis' was introduced to indicate that, unlike the specific vaginitides, there is an increased discharge without significant inflammation, as indicated by a relative absence of polymorphonuclear leukocytes. Bacterial vaginosis is not an infection by a single organism, but rather a polymicrobial overgrowth of facultative and anaerobic bacterial flora such as *Mycoplasma hominis*, *Gardnerella vaginalis*, and *Mobiluncus species*.[16] This occurs most frequently when the pH of the vagina is no longer acid, as for example when semen is present or *Lactobacillus* species absent. *G. vaginalis*, a small Gram variable bacillus, is responsible, at least in part, for many occurrences in women of reproductive age,[17] and is important in forming adherent biofilms[18] that affect both genders and is sexually transmitted.[19] The most important diagnostic finding is squamous cells covered with coccobacilli ('clue cells') (Figure 7.19).[20]

The most common cause of vaginitis throughout the reproductive period is *T. vaginalis*, a sexually transmitted flagellate, ovoid protozoon.[21] In fresh, wet, microscopic preparations, the trichomonad shows as a motile organism with several flagella; in dry, fixed films it appears as a small (10–20 μm in diameter), eosinophilic, shield-shaped object, with poorly defined cytoplasmic and nuclear outlines (Figure 7.20). Biopsies are unusual, but show a nonspecific, chronic inflammatory infiltrate in the submucosa. The

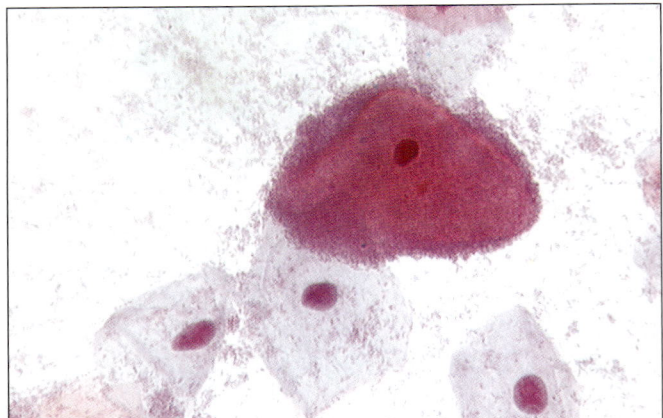

Figure 7.19 Clue cell. Bacteria cover the cells.

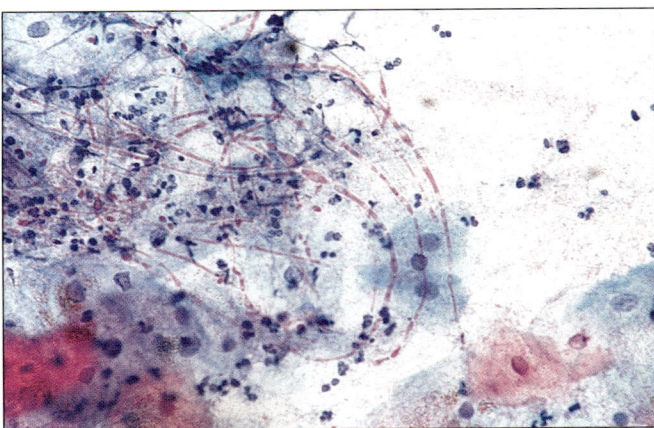

Figure 7.21 *Candida* with pink-staining, spore-bearing hyphae.

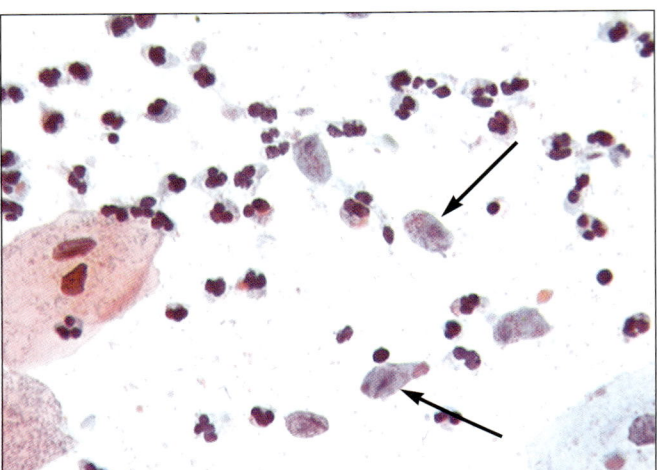

Figure 7.20 *Trichomonas vaginalis*. The organisms appear as small bodies that stain blue and have elongated nuclei (arrows).

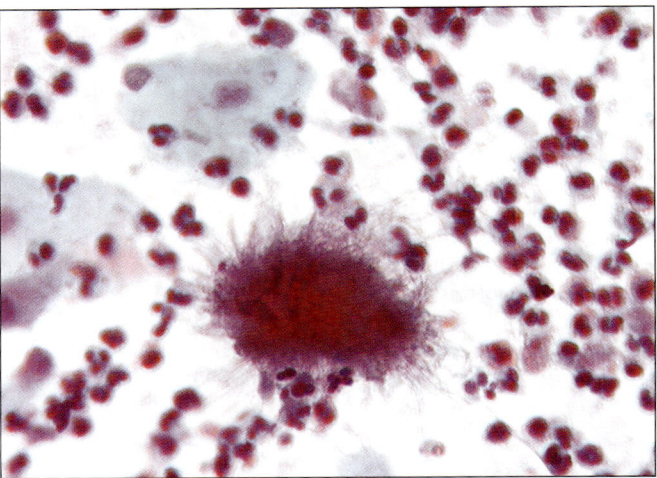

Figure 7.22 *Actinomyces* with characteristic club-like projections.

organisms ingest erythrocytes,[22,23] leukocytes,[23] bacilli,[24] and even vaginal epithelial cells.[25] The average disease is long lasting (3–5 years).[26] *Candida* infection, often as *C. albicans*, is found in a high proportion of women with vaginal discharge. It produces a characteristically cheesy discharge, and its presence can be confirmed by culture, rapid vaginal yeast immunologic assay, and by its recognition in cervicovaginal smears or preparations (Figure 7.21).[27] Factors associated with an increased risk of developing symptomatic *Candida* infection include pregnancy, oral contraceptive use, diabetes mellitus, and antibiotic use. Changes in the vaginal flora likely play a role in the development of candidiasis. In both conditions, trichomoniasis and candidiasis, a biopsy specimen is usually normal, because the organisms normally do not penetrate the mucosa or elicit an inflammatory reaction. Both may resist treatment, particularly if the male partner is not treated at the same time. Coital reinfection in that situation is frequent.

Actinomyces-like organisms are identified in cervicovaginal smears of some women who have noncopper-containing intrauterine contraceptive devices (Figure 7.22). Although sometimes associated with a true inflammatory process, more often the organism is commensal, and its presence, therefore, is of no clinical significance.

Atrophic vaginitis, sometimes called 'senile vaginitis,' occurs usually after menopause. The lack of an estrogenic stimulus results in a thin epithelium composed entirely of parabasal cells. This epithelium is much less resistant to infection than is the thick, well-estrogenized epithelium of a younger woman. The condition may present as postmenopausal bleeding. It responds well to estrogen therapy.

Emphysematous vaginitis is a rare self-limiting disease in which multiple gas-filled cysts are present in the submucosa of the upper vagina and sometimes extending to the ectocervix.[28] It is associated with gas-forming organisms and is typically seen in pregnancy and the puerperium. Histologically, histiocytic giant cells line the gas-filled cysts (Figure 7.23), and the surrounding vaginal wall discloses scattered and a rather inconspicuous inflammatory infiltrate, rendering a picture similar to colitis cystica profunda.

MALAKOPLAKIA

Malakoplakia is an uncommon chronic granulomatous process that most commonly affects the urinary tract, but

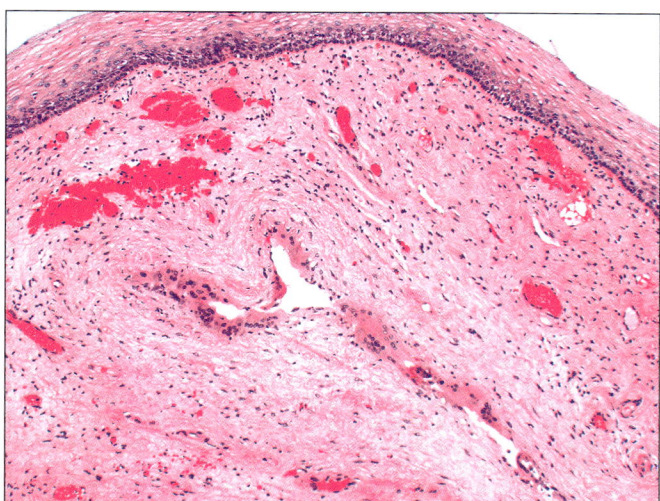

Figure 7.23 Emphysematous vaginitis. Histiocytic giant cells line gas-filled cysts.

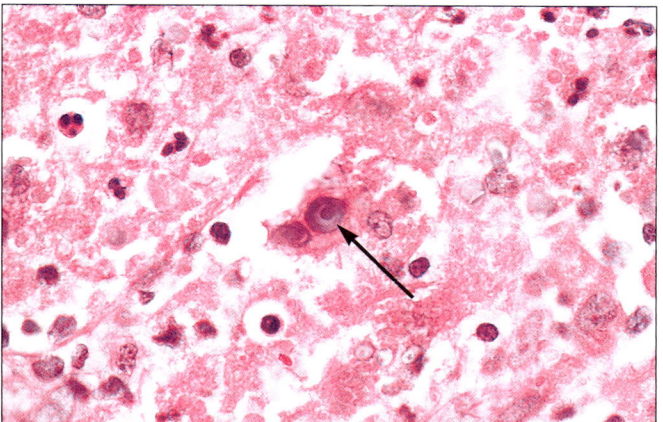

Figure 7.24 Malakoplakia. Michaelis–Gutmann bodies (arrow).

sometimes the vagina.[29] It results from defective macrophage function, manifesting as an inability to destroy ingested bacteria, usually *Escherichia coli*. Within masses of polymorphonuclear leukocytes, lymphocytes, and plasma cells are histiocytes that contain small laminated bodies (Michaelis–Gutmann bodies) (Figure 7.24). These basophilic structures are nuclear sized, sometimes with a bull's eye appearance, and contain stainable iron and calcium. Ultrastructurally, they are electron dense with a variable core of lysosome-like material. The macrophages also exhibit numerous secondary lysosomes filled with partially digested bacteria and neutrophils.

TAMPON-RELATED LESIONS AND TOXIC SHOCK SYNDROME

Vaginal ulcerations in tampon users have been considered a portal of entry for *Staphylococcus aureus* and its toxic products in patients with toxic shock syndrome (TSS). The incidence is about 6 cases per 100,000 menstruating women per year. Fever, a diffuse erythematous rash, and hypotension characterize the syndrome, which results from release of the staphylococcal toxin TSST-1 (toxic shock syndrome toxin-1) into the circulation.[30] The mechanism by which tampon use during menses predisposes to TSS remains somewhat unclear, but it is believed that microulcerations of the vaginal mucosa caused by tampons permit the growth of toxin-producing staphylococci. The lesions healed spontaneously within 2–3 months after discontinuation of tampon usage. Although initially described with tampon use, postoperative cases are being reported increasingly and the syndrome may occur with any staphylococcal infection. Autopsy findings include perivasculitis, predominantly in the skin, lungs, kidneys, vagina, and other mucous membranes. The vaginal mucosa shows edema and ulceration in addition. The severity of the toxic shock syndrome varies from a mild to a rapidly fatal illness, with a mortality rate of about 4%.

NONINFECTIOUS INFLAMMATORY DISEASES

LIGNEOUS VAGINITIS

Ligneous vaginitis is a localized manifestation of a rare, inherited, and potentially life-threatening systemic disease in which affected individuals develop pseudomembranous lesions of mucosal surfaces in the acute phase.[31] The disease results from mutations in the plasminogen leading to a severe type 1 plasminogen deficiency. Clinical manifestations often include ligneous conjunctivitis, ligneous gingivitis, and occasional involvement of the respiratory or gastrointestinal tract. The chronic phase is characterized by asymptomatic yellow-white to red firm masses. Histologically, these represent subepithelial accumulations of amorphic, eosinophilic material that represents fibrin and collagen,[31] which may be accompanied by granulation tissue or chronic inflammatory cells.

VAGINAL CYSTS

Vaginal cysts are uncommon and may be of müllerian (paramesonephric), mesonephric, squamous (traumatic), or urogenital (usually Bartholin gland) origin. Most are asymptomatic. Cysts of the first two varieties are more commonly found in the upper vagina. The last two are usually encountered distally. Except for traumatic cysts, which are usually squamous, most cysts have an embryologic basis. Only when a cyst enlarges to more than a 2–3 cm size, usually due to infection or inspissated secretions, does the patient notice it.

Cysts derived from müllerian epithelium arise from patches of vaginal adenosis and are lined by tuboendometrial- or mucinous-type epithelia, sometimes with metaplastic squamous epithelium. They are seen most frequently in young women who were exposed prenatally to DES (as previously mentioned), but occur rarely in older women. Cysts of mesonephric (Gartner) duct origin are typically found in the lateral walls of the vagina. They are often clinically apparent cysts up to several centimeters in size, and may cause dyspareunia or other symptoms. Frequently, the mesonephric cyst has smooth muscle in its wall. The cells lining the cysts are cuboidal to columnar. The nuclei, which are large, pale, and have bland chromatin, often overlap. The cytoplasm is mucicarmine negative. Eosinophilic and mucicarmine-positive secretions are frequently present in the lumen. Occasionally, atrophic mesonephric ducts are found adjacent to the cysts, providing an additional clue to their origin.

Cysts lined by stratified squamous epithelium are nearly always traumatic in origin. The cysts are usually single and have been reported in all areas of the vagina, although most are caudal. Posterior cysts often result from epithelium trapped during episiotomy. The cause at other sites is less obvious, perhaps from trauma to the vagina during curettage. Urothelial cysts are uncommon and are lined by transitional epithelium or a mixture of stratified cuboidal and columnar epithelium. As these cysts are derived from the urogenital sinus, they are usually situated low in the vagina, close to the urethra.

Rarely, cysts in the upper vagina are inflammatory in nature (see emphysematous vaginitis as discussed earlier). We have seen isolated examples of inflammatory pseudocysts of rectal origin presenting as posterior vaginal wall cysts—a trap more for the clinician than for the pathologist.

CYSTS OF THE INTROITUS

Bartholin duct cysts and mucinous cysts of vulvar origin are often misinterpreted as being of vaginal origin. Bartholin duct cysts, which are common, are recognized by ducts lined by transitional epithelium adjacent to arborized acini lined by mucin-rich cells. The occasional presence of ciliated cells in some Bartholin cysts has been responsible for a misdiagnosis of vaginal adenosis, and hence the erroneous impression that the patient has been exposed prenatally to DES. Mucinous cysts (also sometimes referred to as mucous or dysontogenetic cysts) of the vulvar vestibule likely arise from mucinous glands that are normally present in this site.

TUMOR-LIKE CONDITIONS

FIBROEPITHELIAL POLYPS

Vaginal fibroepithelial polyps are benign growths that likely arise from a stromal layer of hormone-sensitive fibroblastic or myofibroblastic cells.[32–34] Cells with a similar histologic appearance have been described in a band-like subepithelial–stromal zone extending from the endocervix to the vulva of normal females, and may represent the origin of these atypical cells. The polyps commonly develop in the lower vagina of women who are pregnant or on hormone therapy, thus implicating hormonal stimulation as a causative factor. A rare example has developed in a newborn.[35] Grossly, the polyps are single and solid (Figure 7.25), but occasionally villiform with finger-like rubbery projections, and up to 3 cm in size. Their surface is smooth and covered by squamous epithelium. The stroma, which is composed of loose fibroconnective tissue, may contain large atypical stromal cells with delicate, pointed cytoplasmic processes; hyperchromatic, pleomorphic, irregular nuclei; and occasionally prominent nucleoli (Figures 7.26 and 7.27). Mitotic figures are uncommon, but do occur, even with atypical forms. The cells frequently express vimentin, desmin, and receptors for estrogen and progesterone.[32] In the absence of cross-striations, the stromal cells should not be called rhabdomyomatous cells. Ultrastructurally, the stromal cells resemble

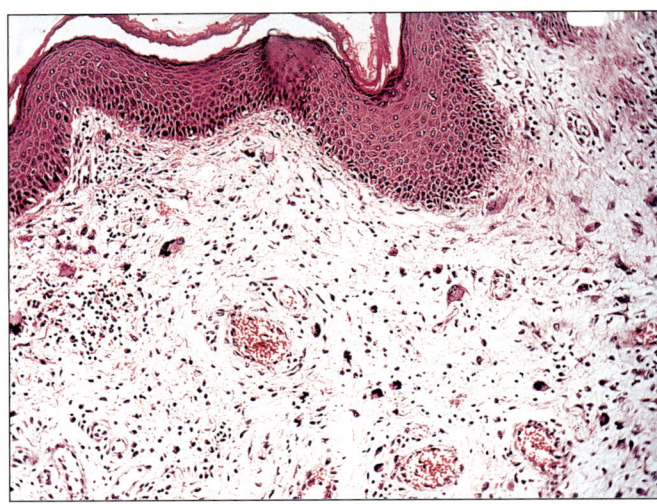

Figure 7.26 Fibroepithelial polyp. Large atypical stromal cells with delicate, pointed cytoplasmic processes are conspicuous.

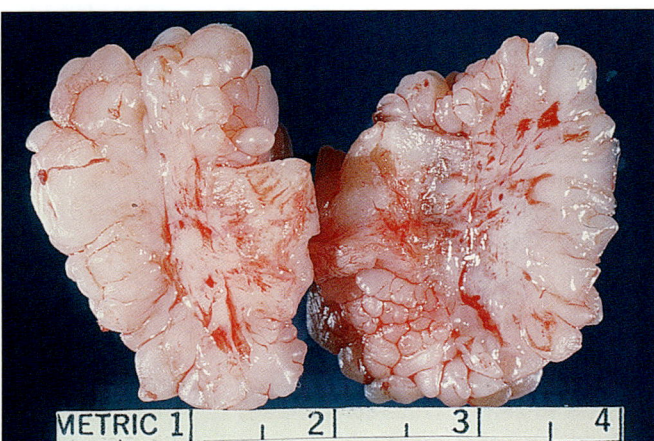

Figure 7.25 Fibroepithelial polyp, solid.

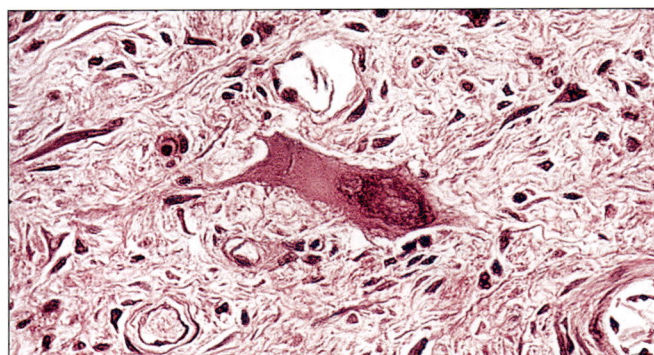

Figure 7.27 Fibroepithelial polyp. Detail of large atypical stromal cells with delicate, pointed cytoplasmic processes.

both fibroblasts and myofibroblasts. Fibroepithelial polyps, which are effectively treated with simple excision, should not be mistaken for a malignant growth, especially embryonal rhabdomyosarcoma, which has a cambium layer, hypercellular stroma, and strap cells, often with cross-striations. Also, embryonal rhabdomyosarcoma usually occurs in children under the age of 4 years whereas most fibroepithelial polyps occur in women over the age of 20.

PROLAPSED FALLOPIAN TUBE

Prolapse of the fallopian tube into the vagina is a rare complication of either vaginal or abdominal hysterectomy.[36] On clinical examination, a red nodule simulating granulation tissue is typically visible at the vaginal apex usually within a few weeks of the operation, but sometimes several months later, and is usually not recognized clinically prior to biopsy. Biopsy shows glandular epithelium, often with a villous pattern suggestive of tubal plicae, with an intense inflammatory cell infiltrate (Figure 7.28). Nuclear crowding and stratification are common, but ciliated or secretory columnar cells may be difficult to identify. The presence of smooth muscle organized as tubal muscularis sometimes aids in the correct diagnosis. Prolapsed fallopian tube may masquerade as a simple vault granulation tissue polyp or as adenocarcinoma, a diagnosis suggested by the architecturally abnormal tubal plicae, reactive stroma, and inflammatory cytologic atypia. Florid reactive stromal proliferations may also masquerade as a vaginal mesenchymal neoplasm.[37] Anecdotally, it is a rare cause of ectopic pregnancy following hysterectomy[38] and of true glandular cells in a posthysterectomy vaginal vault Pap smear.

GRANULATION TISSUE NODULE

Nodules of granulation tissue in the vaginal vault commonly develop following total abdominal hysterectomy. Nearly one-sixth of women will develop nodules greater than 5 mm, one-fifth of which are symptomatic.[39] Grossly, the nodules are red, soft, and sometimes friable. Microscopically, they consist of usually quite immature granulation tissue with extensive numbers of plasma cells. Only about two-thirds of the nodules disappear spontaneously. These lesions are biopsied most often to exclude implanted malignancies, the most common being adenocarcinoma of the endometrium.

POSTOPERATIVE SPINDLE CELL NODULE

Spindle cell nodules resembling sarcomas develop occasionally in the genitourinary tract after surgical procedures.[32,40,41] Clinically, the polypoid nodules, which may be several centimeters in greatest dimension and bleed easily, develop in or about operative sites in the vagina, endocervix, endometrium, prostate, and bladder. Microscopically, they are highly cellular and composed of an unusual proliferation of spindle cells, identified as myofibroblasts. The spindle cells have oval, elongated nuclei with evenly dispersed chromatin and abundant eosinophilic cytoplasm. The vascularity may be pronounced, disclosing a delicate network of small blood vessels, sometimes accompanied by extravasated blood or hemosiderin. Although the mitotic rate is often high, abnormal mitoses and cytologic atypia are absent, features facilitating its differentiation from a spindle cell sarcoma, such as leiomyosarcoma. Negative immunostaining for cytokeratins also distinguishes these lesions from the rare spindle cell squamous cell carcinomas of the cervix or vagina. Local recurrence has not been reported, even after incomplete resection.

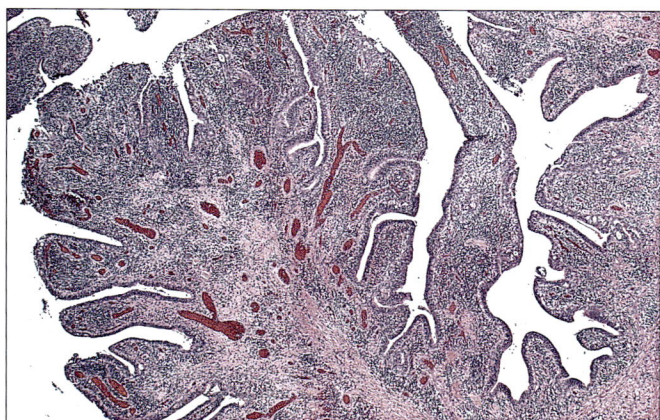

Figure 7.28 Prolapsed fallopian tube into vagina.

MICROGLANDULAR HYPERPLASIA

Microglandular hyperplasia is a benign, usually cervical, lesion composed of microglands lacking intervening stroma and frequently associated with the use of oral contraceptives or pregnancy. Rarely, it may occur in the vagina of young women exposed to DES *in utero* arising in foci of adenosis of the mucinous type. Most of these patients were also pregnant or using oral contraceptives at the time the lesion developed. Grossly, the lesion is soft, granular, tan-yellow, and usually flat. Occasionally, it may be cauliflower-like and multicentric (Figure 7.29). Microscopic examination demonstrates many small, closely packed microglands devoid of intervening stroma (Figure 7.30).

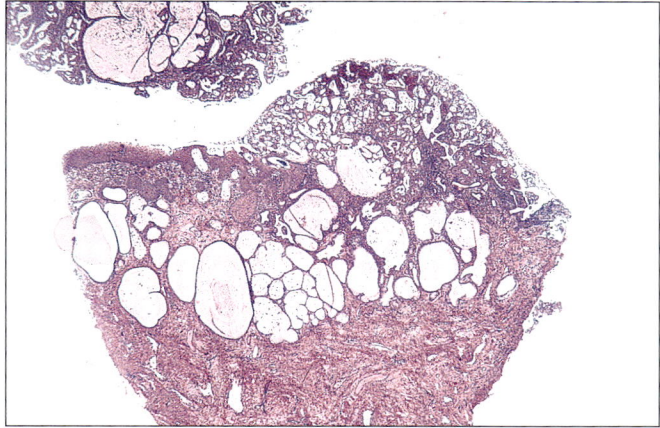

Figure 7.29 Microglandular hyperplasia of vagina. The nodule of microglandular hyperplasia (top) has arisen on a background of mucinous adenosis (larger cysts beneath).

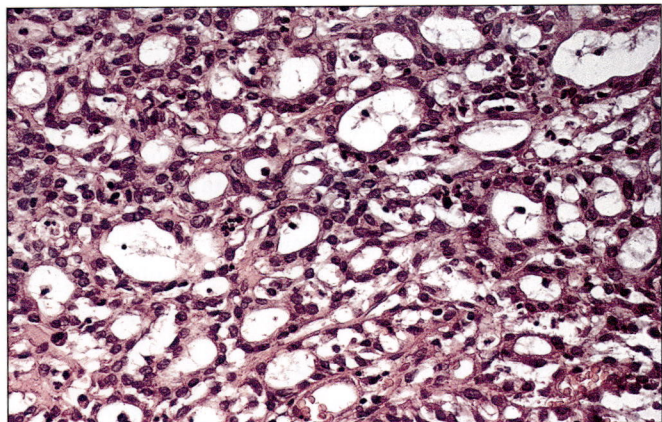

Figure 7.30 Microglandular hyperplasia of vagina. The closely packed glands lack intervening stroma.

The presence of extensive nests of metaplastic squamous cells with pale eosinophilic cytoplasm may make the lesion difficult to distinguish from the solid pattern of clear cell adenocarcinoma. A clue to the diagnosis is the presence of clefts lined by mucinous epithelium that course through the metaplastic squamous epithelium. Microglandular hyperplasia has not been shown to arise from the tuboendometrial type of adenosis. The lesion generally regresses when administration of the oral contraceptive is discontinued.

ENDOMETRIOSIS

Endometriosis is rare in the vaginal wall or squamous mucosa, although less rare in the deep pelvic tissues of the rectovaginal septum (see Chapter 22).

BENIGN TUMORS

Benign epithelial tumors of the vagina are uncommon. It is debatable whether genuine benign squamous papillomas, as distinct from the virus-induced condyloma acuminatum, really exist.

BENIGN MIXED TUMOR

The benign mixed tumor, a rare lesion, consists of biphasic stromal and epithelial components. The neoplasm usually presents as a painless, slowly growing mass of up to 5 cm in diameter, most frequently near the hymen. The origin is uncertain, but the immunoprofile (reactivity of the stromal component with CD10, bcl-2, and estrogen and progesterone receptors) favors a müllerian rather than urothelial origin.[42] The mean age at diagnosis is 30 years. The tumors are well circumscribed but nonencapsulated within the submucosa, and often are misdiagnosed preoperatively as a polyp or cyst. Microscopically, they resemble mixed tumors of the salivary glands (Figure 7.31A). The epithelial component appears as striking nests of highly glycogenated, bland squamous cells (Figure 7.31B). Glands are usually present (Figure 7.31C). The spindle cells, arranged in loosely intersecting fascicles, are immunoreactive with vimentin, smooth

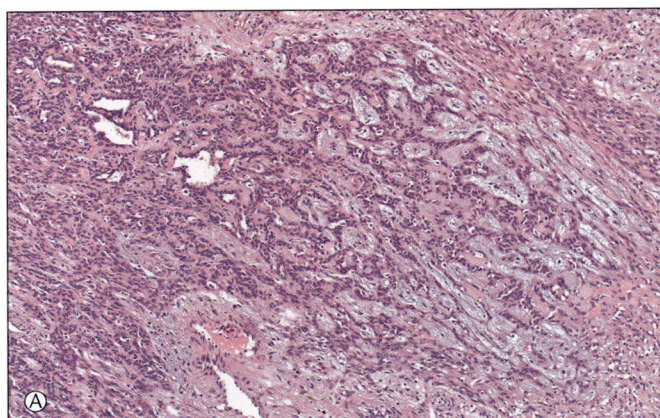
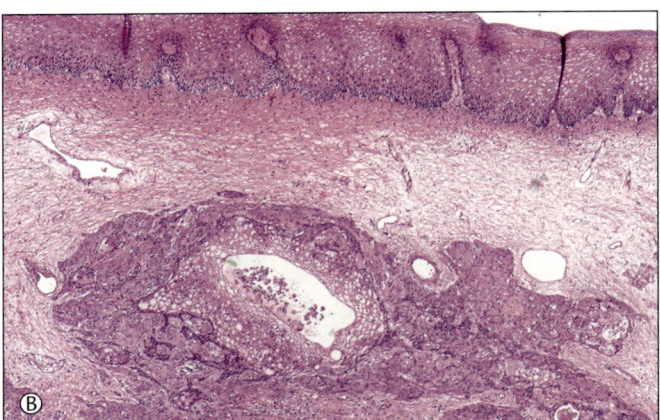
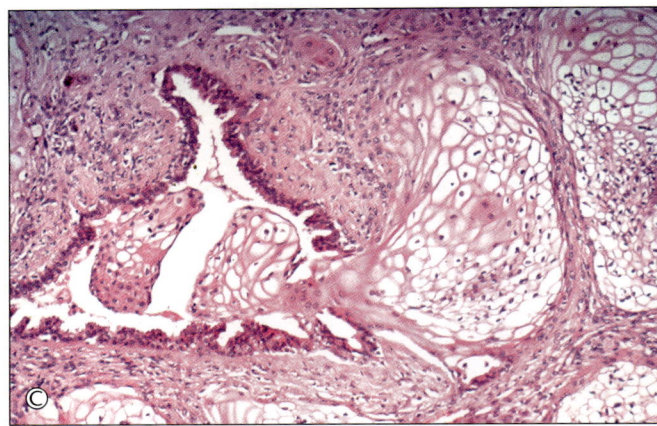

Figure 7.31 Benign mixed tumor. **(A)** Microscopically, the tumor resembles mixed tumors of the salivary glands. **(B)** The epithelial component appears as striking nests of highly glycogenated, bland squamous cells. **(C)** Glands are usually present.

muscle actin, and cytokeratin, and show tonofilaments and desmosomes consistent with epithelial differentiation.[43,44] These tumors are treated by complete excision, but rarely recur.

MÜLLERIAN PAPILLOMA

The müllerian papilloma is a rare tumor composed of a complex arborizing fibrovascular core lined by a mantle of

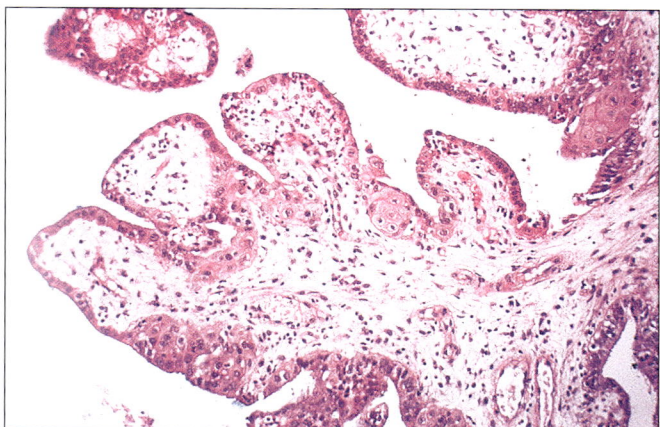

Figure 7.32 Müllerian papilloma of infancy.

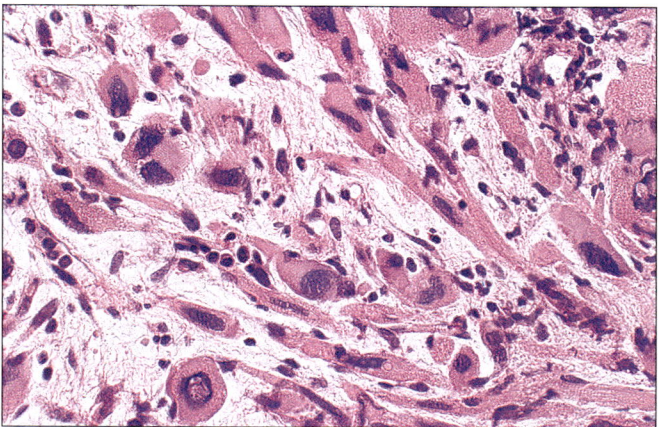

Figure 7.34 Rhabdomyoma.

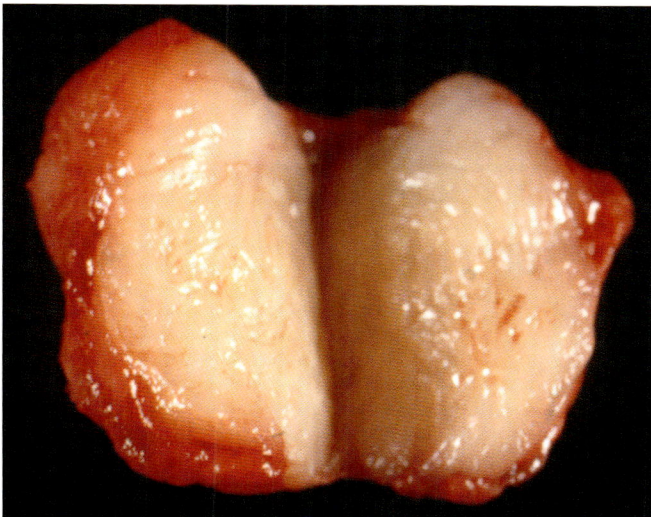

Figure 7.33 Vaginal leiomyoma.

bland glandular epithelium one to two cells thick (Figure 7.32). It occurs in the upper vagina of infants and young children. It is polypoid and should not be confused with embryonal rhabdomyosarcoma in which embryonal rhabdomyoblasts are present in the stroma. Almost all are benign, although rare local recurrences have been reported, and a solitary case after many recurrences progressed to malignancy.[45]

LEIOMYOMA

Of the mesenchymal tumors, benign smooth muscle tumors are the most common and most pedestrian. Leiomyoma, which occurs most frequently in women about 40 years of age but has a wide range, averages 3 cm in size (range <1–15 cm). Small tumors are usually asymptomatic, whereas larger tumors may produce pain, hemorrhage, dystocia, or dyspareunia. Nearly all are well circumscribed (Figure 7.33) and can be locally excised if desired. An occasional tumor, especially if large, may recur. Criteria for malignancy are similar to those for smooth muscle tumors elsewhere in the female genital tract. Tumors with 5 or more mitoses per 10 HPFs, especially if atypia is present, should be considered malignant. Those with 1–4 mitoses per 10 HPFs are best considered potentially malignant. Leiomyomas have been reported to appear during pregnancy, when there has been increased mitotic activity, minimal atypia, and an absence of aggressive behavior. Rare cases of bizarre leiomyoma have also been reported.[46,47]

RHABDOMYOMA

A rare but interesting tumor is the genital rhabdomyoma, a benign neoplasm that displays a high degree of skeletal muscle differentiation and which has a predilection for the vagina. The average age at diagnosis is 42 years (range 25–55 years).[48] The tumor presents as a solitary, polypoid to nodular mass, usually less than 3 cm in diameter, although some reach 11 cm. The overlying squamous mucosa is usually intact since the tumor arises from the wall. The texture is rubbery, and the tumor has a gray, glassy cut surface. Microscopy discloses bland, interlacing, broad strap-like or round striated muscle cells with abundant eosinophilic cytoplasm with distinct cross-striations (Figure 7.34). Although arranged rather haphazardly and showing variation in size and shape, the cells are easily recognizable as benign, differentiated striated muscle of fetal and adult types with an immunoprofile including muscle-specific actin, myoglobin, and desmin, but not smooth muscle actin. Mitoses are absent. The background connective tissue framework is a loose, collagenous to myxoid stroma with fibroblasts and mast cells. Recurrence has not been reported following wide local excision. The differential diagnosis includes embryonal rhabdomyosarcoma, which occurs in the very young, and both carcinosarcoma (malignant mixed müllerian tumor) and metastatic tumors, which occur in older women.

ANGIOMYOFIBROBLASTOMA

Angiomyofibroblastoma of the vagina is a well-circumscribed myofibroblastic neoplasm consisting of ovoid to round myoid tumor cells with scattered multinucleated cells. It is a distinctive benign tumor that has a diverse histologic and immunohistochemical profile. The patients are 23–71 years of age (mean 46 years). The average tumor size is 7 cm.

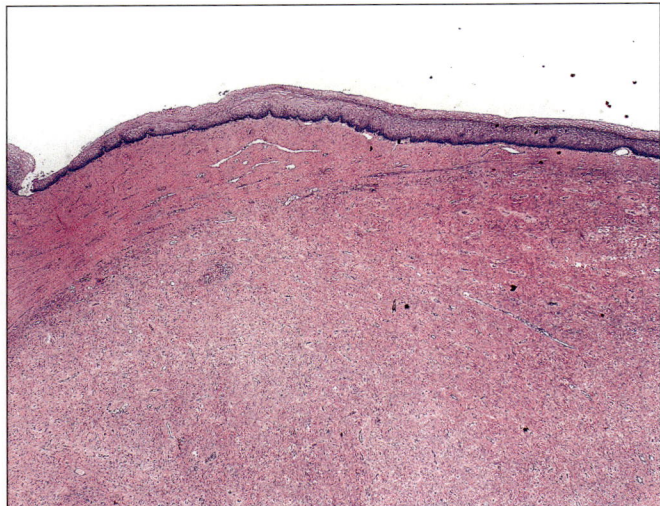

Figure 7.35 Vaginal angiomyofibroblastoma with circumscribed borders.

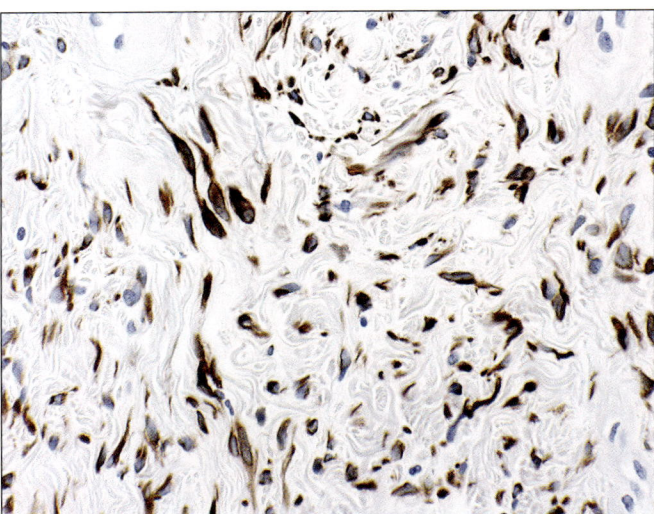

Figure 7.37 Vaginal angiomyofibroblastoma (desmin immunoreaction).

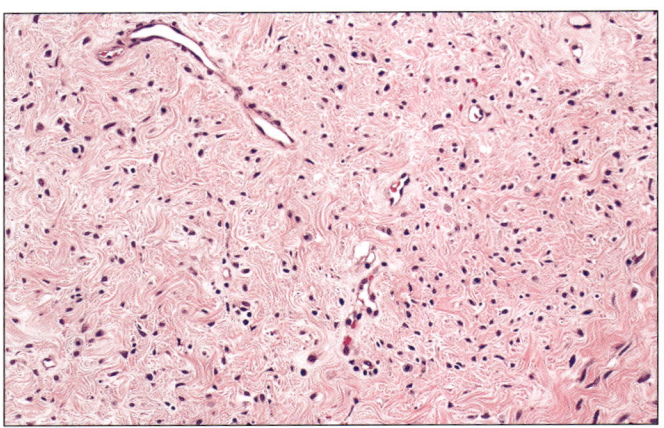

Figure 7.36 Vaginal angiomyofibroblastoma.

Microscopically, the neoplastic cells are spindle-shaped plasmacytoid or epithelioid (Figures 7.35 and 7.36). There is minimal nuclear atypia and no more than a rare mitosis. The tumors contain small to medium sized blood vessels, which are thin walled, and, occasionally, ectatic and branching. Almost all are immunoreactive for vimentin and desmin (Figure 7.37), and some for smooth muscle actin and CD34. These tumors generally have a benign course, although rare recurrences have been reported in the vulva[49] and in the vagina.[50] This tumor forms a continuous morphologic spectrum with the clinically more aggressive angiomyxoma (see Chapter 6).[32,51]

MISCELLANEOUS BENIGN TUMORS

Several benign tumors, such as Brenner tumor,[52] paraganglioma,[53] schwannoma,[54,55] benign mesenchymoma,[56] blue nevi,[57] and mature cystic teratoma dermoid cyst,[58] have been described with gross and microscopic findings similar to those occurring elsewhere.

SQUAMOUS NEOPLASIA

HPV INFECTION

The vaginal mucosa is frequently the site of genital papillomavirus infections, hosting approximately one-fourth of genital condylomata. The lesions may be flat, slightly raised, or verrucous with stromal papillae (asperities). While frequently small and virtually invisible without colposcopic visualization, they usually become more easily identified following application of 3% acetic acid.[59] Biopsy usually discloses cells with a characteristic perinuclear halo (koilocytes). Condylomata acuminata are predominantly HPV 6 or 11 positive,[60] and they are self-limiting. Premalignant changes, which often occur, are reflected by greater degrees of cytologic atypia, mitotic activity, atypical mitotic figures, and lack of squamous maturation, similar to those changes observed in cervical intraepithelial neoplasia (CIN). HPV DNA can be found in about 60% of these lesions, usually type 16. Additionally, HPV types 1, 5, 51, 52, 58, and 66 have been identified in cases of vaginal intraepithelial neoplasia (VaIN).[61]

SQUAMOUS INTRAEPITHELIAL LESION (VaIN)

As discussed in greater detail in Chapter 10, the College of American Pathologists and the American Society for Colposcopy and Cervical Pathology have formally recommended adoption of a unified histopathologic nomenclature for all HPV-associated preinvasive squamous lesions of the lower anogenital tract. The proposed two-tiered nomenclature is to be used for intraepithelial lesions, i.e., low- and high-grade squamous intraepithelial lesions (LSIL and HSIL).[62] SIL replaces VaIN and related terms such as dysplasia and carcinoma *in situ* (CIS) that have been used for many years to describe premalignant lesions that are forerunners of squamous cell carcinoma of the vagina. Lesions considered in the past as VaIN 1 correspond to LSIL, and VaIN 3 lesions correspond to HSIL. VaIN 2 becomes HSIL if the specimen is highly reactive for HPV or if the upper levels of the epithelium show Ki-67 immunoreactivity.

Clinical Features

SIL (VaIN) is far less frequently encountered than the analogous precancerous changes in the cervix and vulva. It gives rise, however, to nearly one-fourth of all vaginal malignancies.[63] The annual incidence of HSIL (VaIN 3) is 0.3/100,000 women, which compares to 38/100,000 for cervical HSIL (CIN 3) and 1/100,000 for high-grade vulvar SIL (VIN 3). The ages of women with vaginal SIL range widely, with a mean of 50 years,[64] which exceeds by 10 years the age of women in whom high-grade cervical SIL is detected.

Vaginal SIL occurs most frequently in association with cervical SIL, either in continuity with it or, more usually, in the vaginal vault after hysterectomy for cervical SIL, when the excision has been insufficiently wide to remove an unsuspected vaginal extension of the cervical SIL. Less frequently, vaginal SIL may be found in the vagina at a site distant from the cervix, which may itself be entirely normal. Multifocal lower genital tract neoplasia occurs and will be dealt with in more detail later. Asynchronous intraepithelial neoplasia may develop in cervix and vagina. Women who have had a hysterectomy for cervical SIL may be found many years later to have a newly developed vaginal SIL (VaIN) at the vaginal vault.[64,65] In one series, 67% of women with vaginal SIL had a prior or concurrent history of cervical SIL.[1-2] The new vaginal disease may represent a field effect, i.e., the squamous epithelium of the entire lower female genital tract is at risk for carcinogenesis. This view is also consistent with the fact that the squamous epithelia of these sites share a common embryonic derivation from the urogenital sinus, and all are susceptible to infection by various HPVs.

Nevertheless, the histogenesis of squamous neoplasia of the vagina, both intraepithelial and invasive, is far from clear. If the squamous epithelia of the cervix, vagina, and vulva form a common field, it might be argued that they should be equally at risk for developing neoplasia when exposed to the same carcinogenic agent. Yet, the actual changes that occur in the vagina (and vulva) may well differ from those in the cervix. Cervical lesions usually develop from the transformation zone. The tissue that is originally columnar undergoes squamous change at the very beginning of its premalignant phase. It is rare for a squamous cell carcinoma of the cervix to arise from the original squamous epithelium. However, no such transformation zone exists in the vagina, so that neoplasia must develop directly from the squamous epithelium. For the field change theory to be accepted, it is necessary to propose that the carcinogens act on the immature metaplastic cells of the cervix and on the original squamous cells of the vagina (and vulva) to produce the same end result of intraepithelial neoplasia.

Several recent investigations have studied the epidemiology of SIL (VaIN). Risk factors in common with cervical cancer include lower socioeconomic status and a history of genital warts. Every patient had demonstrable HPV (more than 1000 viral copies per cell) by blot hybridization, and 80% by immunohistochemistry.[60] The overall risk for developing vaginal CIS as well as squamous cell carcinoma is increased in women with HIV and AIDS.[66] Patients with vaginal SIL often report cancer 5–15 years earlier in other genital organs, most commonly as preinvasive or invasive carcinoma of the uterine cervix.

During the mid-1970s, it was first suggested that DES-exposed offspring might be at risk for increased rates of dysplasia because of the extent of metaplastic tissue present in both the cervix and vagina. Multiple studies of prevalence rates subsequently conducted indicated that the frequency of dysplasia in both the exposed and unexposed populations was approximately the same. In the largest and one of the earliest controlled studies, the DES-unexposed women, in fact, had a higher prevalence rate of dysplasia (4.0%) than the DES-exposed women (1.9%).[67]

Like squamous intraepithelial neoplasia in the cervix and vulva, nearly all LSIL (VaIN 1) are associated with low-risk HPV types,[61] and, as might be expected, over half of the HSILs (VaIN 3) disclose HPV genotype 16. Some vaginal lesions may contain multiple HPV types, but additional testing for viral mRNA shows that only one viral type is transcriptionally active in any individual lesion, indicating that only one is responsible for causing the intraepithelial lesion.[68]

Vaginal SIL affects the upper third of the vagina in over 90% of cases and is multifocal in half of the patients. Although usually asymptomatic, it may be suspected on vaginal smear, colposcopic examination, or biopsy. In one study, approximately 4% of the cases were VaIN 1, 7% VaIN 2, and 43% VaIN 3.[64] Patients with VaIN 1 to VaIN 2 are generally younger than patients with VaIN 3. There is no consensus for optimally treating vaginal SIL. Therapies have included 5-fluorouracil, CO_2 laser, cryotherapy, radiotherapy, partial colpectomy, and observation.[64]

Pathology

SIL in the vagina is not recognizable by gross examination. Its histologic features resemble those of SIL in the cervix (see Chapter 10). One important difference is the absence of gland crypts in the vagina, a feature that is of significance when planning local destructive treatment for vaginal lesions.

Low-grade vaginal SIL (VaIN 1) parallels low-grade cervical SIL (CIN 1) and includes exophytic and flat condyloma. Exophytic condyloma shows characteristic verruca–papillary growth, acanthosis, and superficial koilocytotic atypia; this lesion is associated strongly with HPV types 6 and 11. Flat condyloma shares the superficial distribution of koilocytotic atypia. High-grade vaginal SIL (VaIN 3) shows nuclear abnormalities including enlargement with irregular shape, hyperchromatism, and irregular condensation of chromatin at all epithelial levels. SIL in between, such as those exhibiting maturation at the surface on H&E staining (Figure 7.38), are upgraded to HSIL (VaIN 3) if the epithelium is strongly reactive for HPV or the upper epithelium shows Ki-67 immunoreactivity. SILs nearly always display increased mitotic activity, especially abnormal mitotic figures. Similar to cervical lesions, p16 and Ki-67 are useful in helping to determine that HSIL is present (Figures 7.38 and 7.39).

Differential Diagnosis

The differential diagnosis of SIL (VaIN) includes atrophy, radiation change, and immature squamous metaplasia, all of which may display loss of glycogen and hypercellularity.

The distinction rests mainly on the characteristic nuclear features of SIL (VaIN), which are absent in the other conditions. Radiation changes include nuclear enlargement, smudged chromatin, multinucleation, and vacuolization of cytoplasm, with lack of mitotic activity. Occasionally, there may be significant nuclear atypia associated with inflammatory and reactive processes, but usually this is expressed as regular nuclear enlargement with vesicular chromatin and moderate-sized nucleoli. Such changes are referred to as reactive squamous cell atypia.

Behavior and Treatment

The natural history of SILs (VaIN) is uncertain. In one study, about 5% of SILs (VaIN) progressed to invasive carcinoma, with sequential changes documented by serial biopsies, but this figure probably significantly underestimates the biologic potential of SILs (VaIN) because many lesions were treated.[69] Therapy generally is local excision, although topical 5-fluorouracil, laser vaporization, vaginectomy, and irradiation also have been successfully used. In the referred study of 94 women with SIL (VaIN), 70% achieved remission after a single treatment of any type, but 24% required additional therapy; as indicated above, 5% progressed to invasive squamous carcinoma in spite of therapy and close follow-up.[69]

INVASIVE SQUAMOUS CELL CARCINOMA

An invasive squamous cell carcinoma is an invasive cancer composed entirely of malignant squamous cells.

Clinical Features

Squamous cell carcinoma originating in the vagina is infrequent, accounting for only 1% of all gynecologic malignancies. The age-adjusted incidence is 0.4/100,000 white women in the United States, which is about 1/50th the incidence of cervical squamous cell carcinoma. In fact, the vagina is more commonly involved by secondary spread of tumors from elsewhere than it is by primary cancer. While generally a disease of older women (mean age, 64 years),[70] approximately 10% of women are under 40 years of age and even teenagers are occasionally affected. The International Federation of Gynecology and Obstetrics (FIGO) staging of vaginal cancer is analogous to that of cervical cancer and is based on clinical rather than pathologic examination (Table 7.1). To be considered a primary tumor of the vagina, the neoplasm must be located in the vagina, without clinical or histologic evidence of involvement of the cervix or vulva. The few epidemiologic studies of vaginal carcinoma suggest that the pathogenesis is environmentally related. Interestingly, skin grafts taken from extragenital sites and used to form a neovagina occasionally give rise to histologically

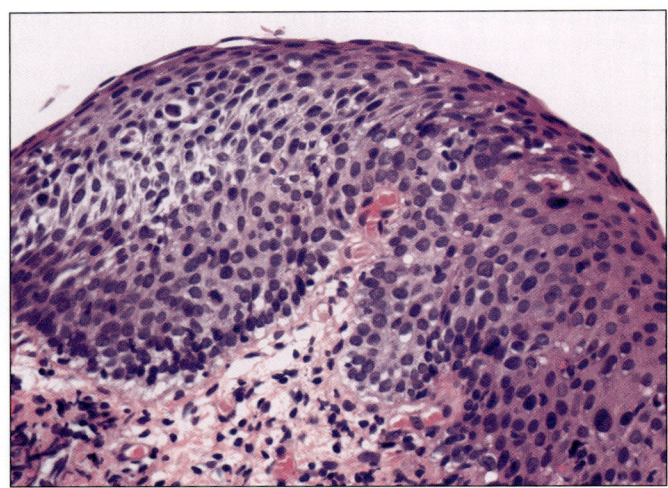

Figure 7.38 HSIL (VaIN 3).

Table 7.1	FIGO Staging of Vaginal Carcinoma (1978)
Stage	**Clinical Status**
0	Intraepithelial
I	Limited to vaginal wall
II	Extends to subvaginal tissue but not to pelvic side wall
III	Extends to pelvic side wall
IV	Extends beyond the true pelvis or involves mucosa of the bladder or rectum (bullous edema does not consign the patient to stage IV)
IVa	Adjacent organs involved
IVb	Distant organs involved

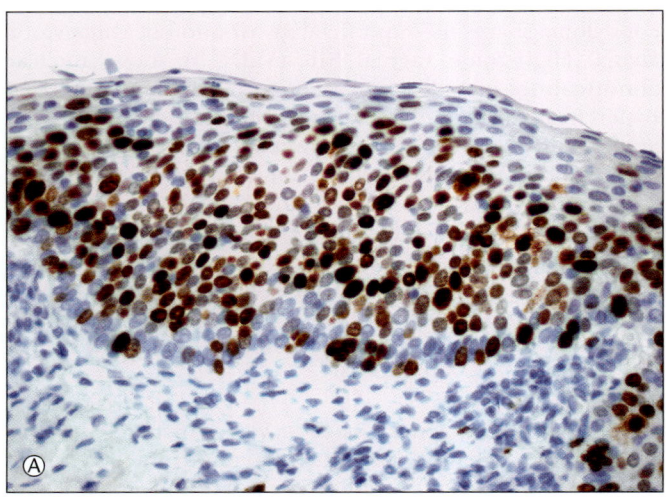
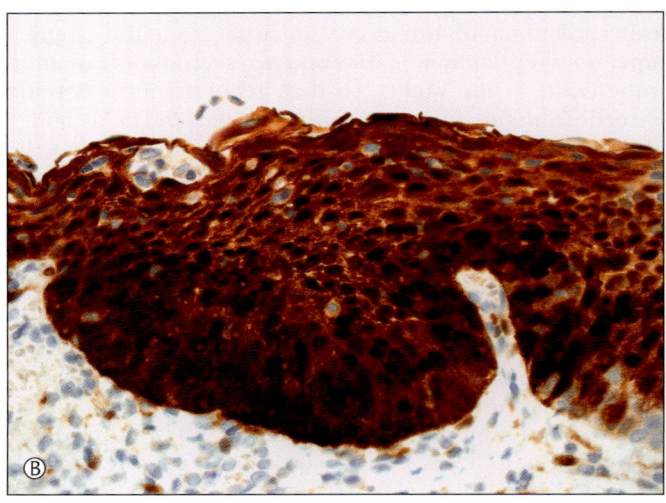

Figure 7.39 HSIL (VaIN 3). **(A)** Ki-67 left **(B)** p16 right.

typical vaginal tumors rather than tumors that usually arise in the original grafted tissue.[71,72] A history of prior hysterectomy is common, quite often for CIN or cervical carcinoma. Between one-fifth and three-fifths of invasive vaginal cancers have demonstrable HPV DNA, usually HPV type 16, confirming the potential role of this virus in vaginal oncogenesis. This is more common in younger than in older patients.[73] However, early age at first intercourse, multiple sexual partners, and a history of smoking were not associated with an elevated risk of neoplasia.[74]

Pathology

As with VaIN, most lesions involve the upper vagina,[75] probably because of a topographical association with CIN. Tumors vary in size from clinically occult to larger than 10 cm. They may be polypoid, fungating, or ulcerated. The histologic appearances of vaginal squamous cell carcinoma are those of squamous cell carcinoma in general, ranging from the keratinizing to the nonkeratinizing poorly differentiated and, in individual cases, are indistinguishable from analogous carcinomas of the vulva or cervix.

Superficially invasive squamous cell carcinoma is not currently a defined entity in the vagina; however, superficially invasive tumors, with less than 3 mm of stromal invasion and no vascular space invasion, appear to have a low risk of lymph node metastasis.

Behavior and Prognosis

The outcome after treatment is poor (5 year survival rates are about 56%).[76] In a review of 300 patients treated over a 40 year interval at one institution, the overall 5 and 10 year survival rates were 60% and 49%, respectively.[77] The most important prognostic indicators included FIGO stage, tumor size, and location in the vagina (with better outcomes for those with lesions in the upper vagina). The relative 5 year survival rate for stage I disease was 73%, 53% for stage II tumors, and only 36% for stages III and IV.[78] Early stage tumors (FIGO I–IIA) tend to recur locally in the vagina, in the immediate paravaginal tissues, or inguinal nodes.[79]

As for metastatic disease, the route of lymphatic spread reflects the cancer's anatomic location. Cancers in the upper third of the vagina tend to spread, like those of the cervix, to the internal pelvic nodes. Those in the lower vagina spread to the inguinal nodes, as do tumors of the vulva. There is too little experience to date to determine the value of sentinel node biopsy.[80]

VERRUCOUS CARCINOMA

The term verrucous carcinoma is applied to a rare vaginal tumor characterized by exophytic growth with a coarsely granular or undulating surface (Figure 7.40). Microscopically, the tumor is composed of uniformly well-differentiated squamous cells with bland cytologic features. The deep margin of the tumor is well circumscribed. In fact, the squamous cells invade in a pushing fashion as broad rounded masses, creating a so-called baggy pants appearance; that is, stromal invasion is pushing rather than destructive (Figure 7.41). If jagged or irregular, the tumor is best regarded as ordinary squamous cell carcinoma. Occasionally, verrucous carcinomas display koilocytosis or surface papillae with central fibrovascular cores, typical of condylomata. Indeed, the distinction of verrucous carcinoma from condyloma or

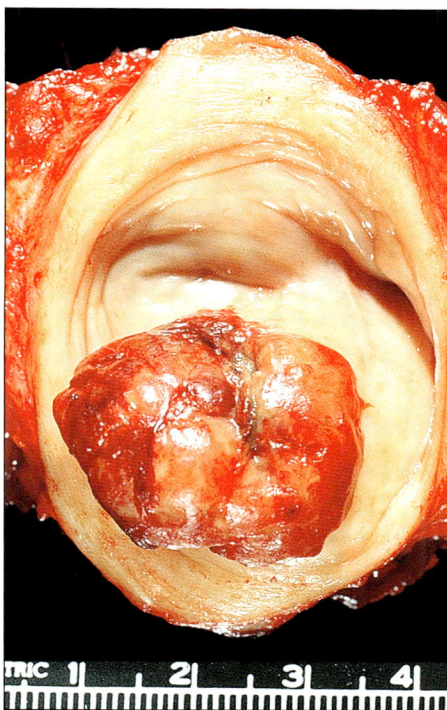

Figure 7.40 Verrucous carcinoma.

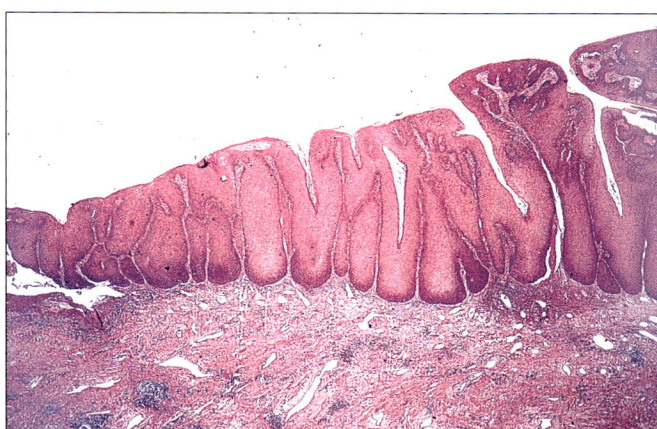

Figure 7.41 Verrucous carcinoma. The deep margin discloses no invasion.

pseudoepitheliomatous hyperplasia may be difficult and even impossible in a superficial biopsy specimen. However, this issue is not important, since the diagnosis is based on the bland cytologic features at the stromal interface.

Verrucous carcinomas display a relatively indolent growth with frequent local recurrence after incomplete excision. Lymph node metastasis occurs rarely. Treatment is usually wide local excision since the neoplasm resists therapeutic radiation. Radiotherapy may in fact transform it to conventional squamous carcinoma. Verrucous carcinoma is also commonly misdiagnosed as giant condyloma, although we are not sure that the two lesions are essentially different. Tumors with a mixed pattern of both verrucous and conventional squamous carcinoma behave with the aggressiveness of typical squamous cancer and should be classified as such.

WARTY CARCINOMA

Warty carcinoma in the vagina is a homolog of the more commonly encountered warty variant of squamous cell carcinoma in the vulva. Microscopy shows marked nuclear abnormalities, koilocytosis and multinucleated cells. The tumor is infiltrative at the stromal interface. Preliminary data from similar tumors in the vulva indicate they may behave in a low-grade malignant fashion. Metastases to regional lymph nodes occur occasionally.

PAPILLARY SQUAMOTRANSITIONAL CELL CARCINOMA

Occasionally, carcinomas that bear a close resemblance to those arising from urothelium may develop in the vagina.[81,82] Grossly, the tumor configuration has been described as polypoid, or exophytic. Microscopically, the tumor shows narrow fibrovascular cores lined by a stratified epithelium that may appear either transitional, squamous, or both. The atypical tumor cells usually contain oval hyperchromatic nuclei, with intranuclear grooves.[83] Mitoses are frequent. Koilocytosis is rare. Stromal invasion is not easily identifiable within the papillae of a superficial biopsy and must be sought at the deeper stromal interface. Unlike transitional cell carcinomas of the urinary bladder, which typically immunoreact with both CK-7 and CK-20, papillary genital tract tumors exclusively express cytokeratin CK-7.[84] The biologic behavior of these carcinomas has been described as either indolent or similar to that of conventional squamous carcinoma.[84]

SMALL CELL CARCINOMA

'Small cell carcinoma' is a term applied ambiguously to two separate lesions, including: (1) nonkeratinizing squamous carcinoma with small cells resembling those of HSIL (VaIN) and (2) carcinomas similar to the small (oat cell) neuroendocrine carcinomas of the cervix and other sites (Figure 7.42). The latter tumors have also been called 'carcinoid tumors,' 'argyrophil cell carcinomas,' 'small cell tumors with neuroepithelial features,' 'oat cell carcinoma,' and 'endocrine cell carcinoma.' These tumors occur in women younger than those with nonkeratinizing squamous carcinoma composed of small cells (36 vs 50 years) and they usually measure several centimeters across. Most neoplasms have spread beyond the vagina at the time of diagnosis.[85] In addition to the light microscopic findings of a small cell neoplasm, the tumor shows reactivity for neuroendocrine markers such as chromogranin, synaptophysin, or neuron-specific enolase (Figure 7.43), and electron microscopy reveals features consistent with neuroendocrine cells such as neurosecretory-type granules, and cytoplasmic processes.[86,87] In recent studies almost all small cell carcinomas have been associated with high-risk HPV types 16 and 18, with type 18 as the most prevalent, detected in 82% of the cases.[141,142]

Distinguishing small cell carcinoma from nonkeratinizing squamous carcinoma with small cells can be difficult. The diagnosis of small cell carcinoma should be reserved for tumors in which squamous or glandular differentiation is absent or minimal. Cytologically, cells of nonkeratinizing squamous carcinoma with small cells resemble those of HSIL and lack the nuclear molding and crush artifact typical

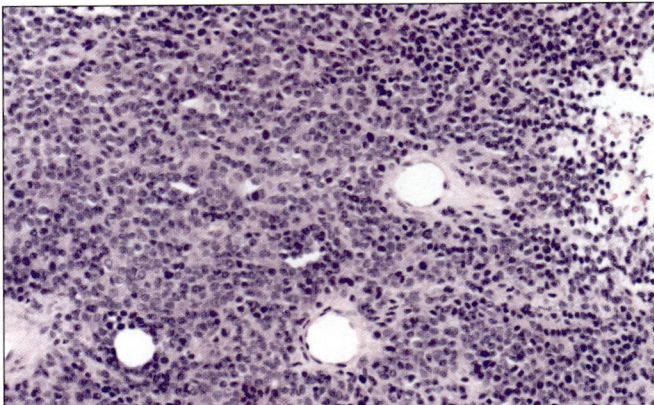

Figure 7.42 Small cell carcinoma. Carcinomas similar to the small (oat cell) neuroendocrine carcinomas of the cervix and other sites may develop in the vagina.

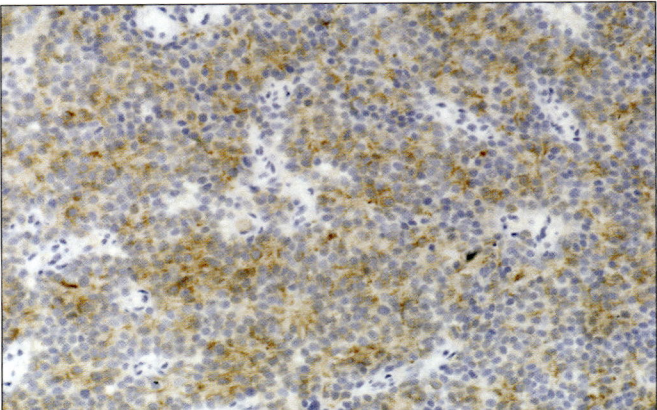

Figure 7.43 Small cell carcinoma. The tumor shows reactivity for neuroendocrine markers such as chromogranin, synaptophysin, or neuron-specific enolase.

of most small cell neuroendocrine carcinomas. Immunohistochemistry for neuroendocrine markers may not be helpful because half of nonkeratinizing squamous carcinomas with small cells immunoreact with neuroendocrine markers and half of small cell carcinomas immunoreact for cytokeratins. Nuclear staining for p63 confirms squamous differentiation in nonkeratinizing small cell carcinomas, while neuroendocrine type small cell carcinomas are negative for this marker. Because of the presence of high-risk HPV in nonkeratinizing small cell carcinomas, they are positive for p16. Small cell carcinoma should be differentiated from lymphoma, which may be difficult to diagnose in a small biopsy with crush artifact, because of different prognostic and therapeutic implications.

CLEAR CELL ADENOCARCINOMA

Clinical Features

More than 750 cases of clear cell adenocarcinoma of the vagina and cervix diagnosed in females born after 1940 have been recorded, with estimates that about 25–50 new cases develop each year.[88] Most are from the United States, but some women with documented exposure to exogenous hormones have been born in Canada, Mexico, Europe, Australia, or Africa. About three-fifths of patients reveal some evidence suggesting exposure *in utero* to DES, hexestrol, or dienestrol. A few women had been exposed to steroidal estrogens or progesterone alone. While the relative risk of a vaginal cancer associated with stilbestrol usage is high,[89,90] many women lack a history of drug exposure, confirming that this tumor may also occur spontaneously.[89,91] For cervical tumors alone, the majority of cases have no history of DES exposure,[92,93] a finding in accord with clear cell adenocarcinoma of the cervix in young women as a well-recognized entity long prior to the DES era. Clear cell adenocarcinoma of the vagina in women under the age of 20 years was also known before the synthesis and use of DES in pregnancy, but less frequently. To date, even with long-term follow-up, no other tumor type has developed in association with DES exposure.

The median age at diagnosis is 19 years, which has remained remarkably uniform regardless of the patient cohort's year of birth. Although a rare patient has been as young as 7 years of age, only after the age of 14 years does the age–incidence curve rise sharply, which strongly suggests a pathogenesis related in part to puberty. It plateaus between ages 17 and 22 years and then declines rapidly,[90] with few women developing this form of cancer in their thirties or forties. Despite the strong association between drug and tumor, clear cell adenocarcinoma develops only rarely in exposed women with a cumulative incidence to date of 0.02% (1/5000),[94] a rarity confirmed by numerous other studies.[95] The greatest numbers of DES-exposed patients with these tumors were born in between 1951 and 1953, the years when the drug was prescribed most frequently for pregnancy support. Epidemiologic studies indicate that the risk of tumor development is higher when the drug was started early in pregnancy or there has been a history of prior miscarriage.[96]

The risk is also increased in women who were taller or more obese than their contemporaries at age 14–15 years,[97] findings of interest since height and body mass are risk factors for endometrial cancer, the most common glandular cancer of the female reproductive tract. Rare reports of tumor development in only one of two monozygotic twins underscore that many factors, including perhaps unidentified environmental ones, operate in carcinogenesis.

The drug only appears to have an effect if administered before week 18 of pregnancy; indeed, most of those affected were exposed in the first trimester.

Pathogenesis

Unlike squamous cell carcinoma, which is linked to HPV, no such viral association has been found with clear cell adenocarcinoma.[98] HPV type 1, an oncogenic type, has been detected in one-fourth of the clear cell cancers, but in none of their metastases. Two-thirds of clear cell carcinomas show overexpression of wild-type p53 protein but no p53 mutations have been found. Similarly, mutations of other genes frequently found in tumors of the female genital tract, such as K-ras and *WT1* have not been identified in clear cell carcinomas. High frequency of microsatellite instability has been found in DES-associated tumors.[99]

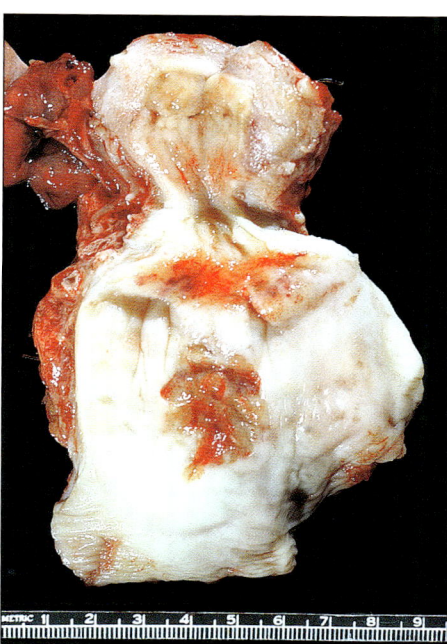

Figure 7.44 Clear cell adenocarcinoma of vagina.

Gross Pathology

The tumor may involve any portion of the vagina and/or cervix (Figure 7.44). Most vaginal tumors arise on the anterior wall, usually in the upper third, corresponding to the most frequent site of adenosis. The lateral and posterior walls and, occasionally, the middle and lower third of the vagina are also involved. On occasion, multicentric tumors have been demonstrated. In many cases, the areas of grossly visible tumor seem discrete, but microscopic examination usually discloses its continuity in the submucosa. Tumors have also been found on the wall opposite the main tumor, presumably as a result of implantation ('kissing lesion').

The tumors have varied in size from microscopic to large. In the years during which the entity was first being recognized, many were of substantial size, reflecting the infrequency of pelvic examinations in asymptomatic and sometimes even symptomatic young women. Most of the larger cancers were polypoid and nodular. Some were flat or ulcerated, having a granular or indurated surface. With increasing awareness that periodic examinations in DES-exposed women should begin early in the teenage period, small tumors were discovered more often. While usually palpable, they may still be invisible on colposcopic examination if confined to the lamina propria and if covered by intact, normal or metaplastic squamous epithelium. Although most cancers are superficial and invade only a few millimeters into the vaginal or cervical wall, some penetrate far more deeply (Figure 7.45) or extend more centrifugally than might be anticipated on gross examination.

Microscopic Pathology

Clear cell adenocarcinomas of both vagina and cervix are identical to müllerian clear cell adenocarcinomas of the ovary and endometrium, the latter two occurring sporadically in older women. Several histologic patterns may be

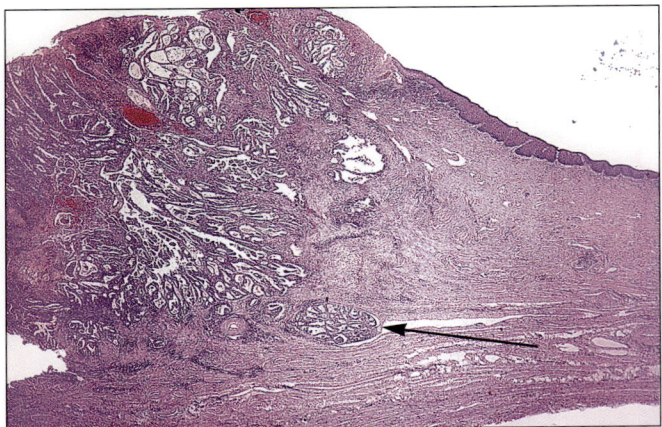

Figure 7.45 Clear cell adenocarcinoma. The large tumor penetrates deeply into the wall and invades a major blood vessel (arrow).

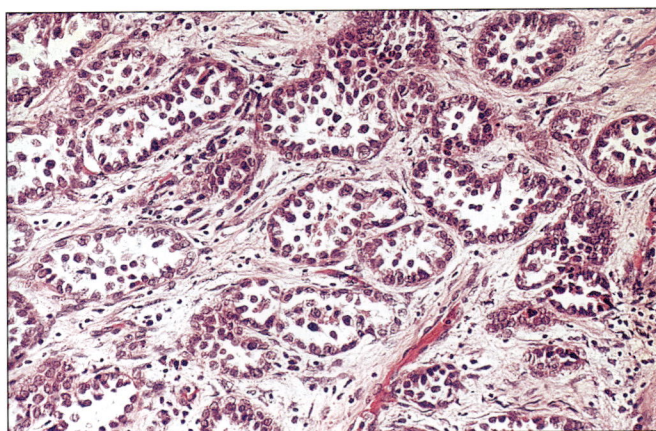

Figure 7.47 Clear cell adenocarcinoma, hobnail cells.

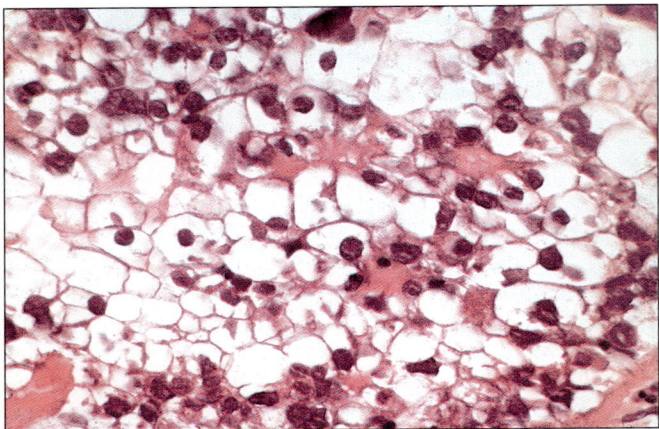

Figure 7.46 Clear cell adenocarcinoma, clear cells.

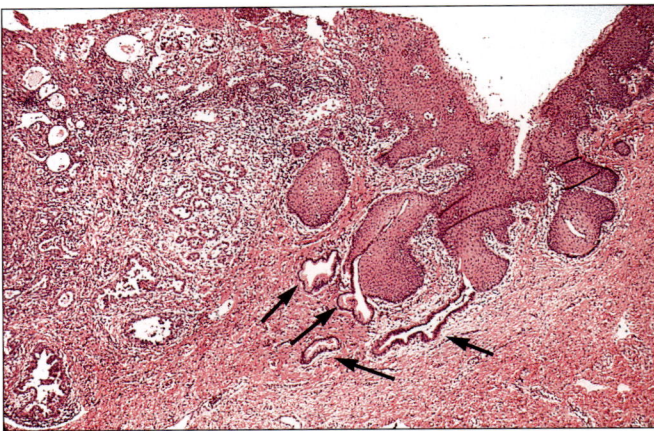

Figure 7.48 Tuboendometrial adenosis. The adenosis (arrows) lies at the edge of the clear cell adenocarcinoma.

observed either alone or in combination. A characteristic pattern, for which the tumor is named, consists of solid sheets of clear cells (Figure 7.46); the clear appearance of the cytoplasm is caused by the dissolution of glycogen when the specimen is processed for microscopic examination. A second pattern, the tubulocystic pattern, exhibits tubules and cysts lined by hobnail cells (Figure 7.47), by flat cells, or by cells that resemble müllerian-type epithelium to varying degrees. The hobnail cell displays a bulbous nucleus that protrudes into the lumen beyond the apparent cytoplasmic limits of the cell. Flat cells often appear innocuous. When only this latter epithelium is present in a small biopsy, it may be difficult to differentiate tumor from adenosis. Less common appearances include a papillary pattern, a tubular pattern resembling endometrial carcinoma, and a pattern composed of cords of cells with eosinophilic cytoplasm. Mitoses are typically infrequent. In any of these patterns, the lumina may contain mucin, but the cytoplasm is mucin free.

Clear cell adenocarcinoma is often detected cytologically, especially in the cervix (80% detection rate in the cervix vs a 3% rate in the vagina).[96] Occasionally, a suspicious or positive smear may be the first indication in an asymptomatic woman. The cancerous cells often resemble large endocervical cells or nonspecific adenocarcinoma cells, but vary greatly and may appear even as undifferentiated carcinoma.

Atypical adenosis, characterized by glands with cellular stratification, nuclear pleomorphism, hyperchromasia, and prominent nucleoli, appears near the periphery of most clear cell carcinomas in which the excised vagina has been serially blocked for microscopic examination.[100] Atypical cells with large, irregular nuclei have also been identified in approximately 0.5% of cervical and vaginal smears from women exposed to DES antenatally. The frequent finding of tuboendometrial-type cells adjacent to the cancers (Figure 7.48), but the rarity of mucinous cells in this location, suggests that the clear cell adenocarcinoma, if it is linked to atypical adenosis, is most likely from the tuboendometrial type.[100] Nevertheless, over time progression from atypical adenosis to adenocarcinoma has not been documented.

Differential Diagnosis

Several conditions are easily confused with clear cell adenocarcinoma. Two are non-neoplastic. Microglandular hyperplasia has been described previously. The Arias-Stella reaction, although usually encountered in the endometrium of pregnant women, is found occasionally in the endocervix and even in vaginal adenosis of the tuboendometrioid type. Characteristically, the Arias-Stella reaction discloses hypersecretory glands where the cells lining the glands have markedly enlarged nuclei and resemble hobnail cells. However, in clear cell adenocarcinoma, the presence of sheets of clear cells or prominent papillae should enable the two lesions to be distinguished. In addition, the hobnail-like nuclei in the Arias-Stella reaction are commonly smudged and appear as degenerative. In contrast to clear cell carcinoma, the Arias-Stella reaction predictably shows low rates of Ki-67 nuclear reactivity and does not overexpress wild-type p53.[101]

Several forms of carcinoma need to be distinguished from clear cell adenocarcinoma. Tumors developing in the distal vagina may resemble transitional cell carcinomas that arise in the urogenital sinus. Metastatic renal cell carcinoma typically displays clear cells and may prove extremely difficult to diagnose without pertinent history.[102,103] Metastatic serous carcinoma of ovarian or other origin may recapitulate the papillary pattern of clear cell carcinoma, and the tumor cells resemble the hobnail cells of the latter.

Natural History and Spread

The tumor spreads locally and metastasizes via both lymphatics and blood vessels. Approximately one-sixth of tumors confined clinically to the lower genital tract (stage I) will have metastasized to the pelvic lymph nodes. The frequency of nodal involvement reaches 50% in clinical stage II tumors. Clear cell adenocarcinoma extends outside the abdominal cavity more frequently than does squamous cell carcinoma of the vagina or cervix. More than one-third of initial recurrences of clear cell carcinomas are in the lung or supraclavicular lymph nodes, in contrast to less than 10% for squamous cell carcinomas.

The survival rate for all patients with clear cell adenocarcinoma is high. It is about 93% at 5 years and 87% at 10 years when the tumor is stage I. If the patient is asymptomatic at diagnosis, survival with appropriate therapy approaches 100%. Other factors associated with a better prognosis are an older age (>19 years) at diagnosis and a tubulocystic pattern.[104] Large size and/or deep invasion into the wall are associated with a poorer prognosis, but small or superficial tumors also may recur or metastasize. While nuclear aneuploidy has no effect on prognosis, nuclear atypia may be associated with a worse prognosis.[96] Pregnancy at the time of diagnosis does not affect outcome adversely.[105] Recurrences develop most often within years after primary therapy, but have been found after nearly two decades. The prognosis for women with clear cell adenocarcinoma who have known exposure to DES *in utero* is significantly better than for those who have no history of DES exposure (5 year survival rates of 84% and 69%, respectively).[143]

ADENOCARCINOMA, NON-CLEAR CELL TYPES

The second most common subtype of vaginal adenocarcinoma is endometrioid adenocarcinoma.[106] Most women present with vaginal bleeding and a tumor in the vaginal apex at a mean age of 60 years. The presence of vaginal endometriosis is a key indication of a primary tumor rather than secondary spread of an endometrial primary. The mucin-secreting adenocarcinoma is a rare tumor that

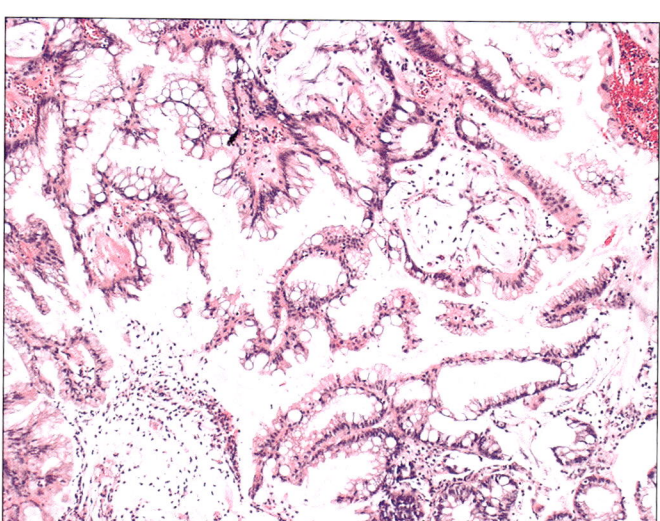

Figure 7.49 Mucinous adenocarcinoma, well differentiated, arising in a vaginal fistulous tract in a patient with Crohn disease.

contains glands resembling intestinal epithelium.[107] Most occur in older women and often involve the lower vagina. A case of low-grade mucinous adenocarcinoma, even to the point of resembling a borderline mucinous tumor, arose in fistulous tracts of women with Crohn disease (Figure 7.49).[108] Also, Paget's disease of vulvar origin can spread to the vagina, occasionally even to the cervix, and can be detected on Pap smears.[109]

OTHER PRIMARY MALIGNANT TUMORS OF THE VAGINA

MALIGNANT MELANOMA

Malignant melanoma is a rare primary tumor in the vagina (incidence 0.03/100,000 per year). Based on a national cancer database,[110] 0.6% of melanomas are genital, of which vulvar and vaginal sites are most common.[111] More than 150 cases have been reported, accounting for less than 5% of the malignant tumors of the vagina. Most appear in women older than 50 years,[112] usually with symptoms such as bleeding or a mass lesion. Some are grossly pigmented and some show convincing junctional activity in or adjacent to the lesion. Microscopically, most tumors disclose sheets of cells that vary from banal in appearance to markedly irregular, but are not readily specific for any common type of primary tumor arising in the vagina. The tumor cells are frequently epithelioid but sometimes spindled or mixed cell (Figure 7.50).[113] Occasionally, the tumor cells infiltrate the submucosa and can be extremely difficult to distinguish from inflammatory cells. S-100 is a useful marker for confirming the diagnosis; Mart-1 can be helpful when S-100 is negative or weakly/focally reactive.[113] An occasional tumor may be amelanotic, but recur as a pigmented melanoma.[114] Because Clark's levels are not appropriate for mucosal melanomas, a system based entirely on tumor thickness has been proposed by Chung et al., as follows: level I, tumor confined to the surface epithelium; level II, invasion of 1 mm or less; level III, invasion of 1–2 mm; and level IV, invasion greater

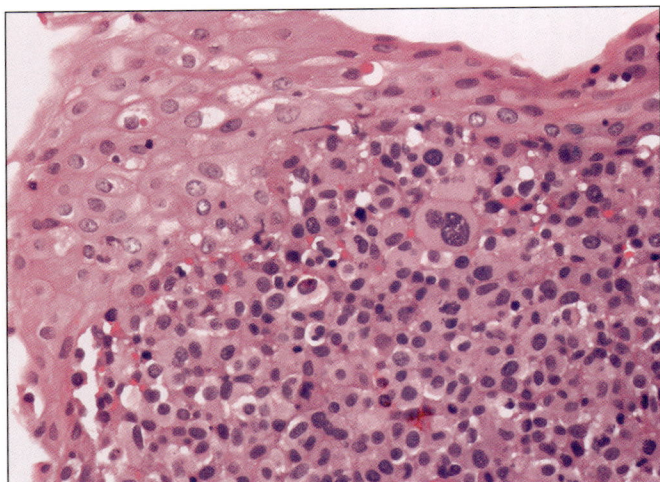

Figure 7.50 Malignant melanoma.

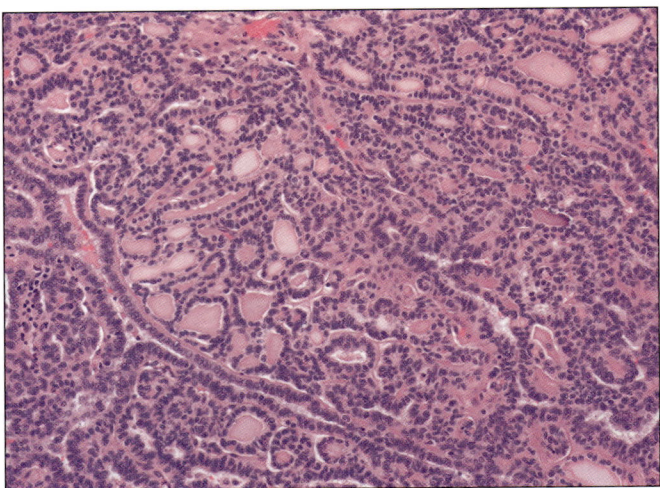

Figure 7.52 Mesonephric carcinoma.

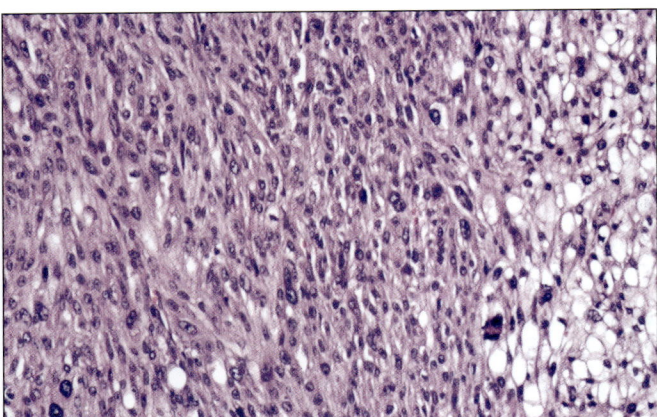

Figure 7.51 Leiomyosarcoma.

than 2 mm.[115] Complete surgical excision[116] and tumors less than 3 cm in greatest dimension[117] have been associated with favorable prognosis. Regional lymph nodes are only infrequently involved. Overall, the median survival is 20 months,[116] with the 5 year survival under 20%.

LEIOMYOSARCOMA

Leiomyosarcoma of the vagina is extremely rare, even though it is the most common form of sarcoma that occurs in this site. As discussed in the previous section Leiomyoma, there is less certainty about the criteria distinguishing benign from malignant lesions than for smooth muscle tumors of the uterus. Tumors greater than 3 cm diameter, with 5 or more mitoses per 10 HPFs or moderate to marked cytologic atypia, or especially when infiltration is present, are best considered as malignant (Figure 7.51).[118]

The tumor occurs over a wide age range (25–86 years) and usually presents with vaginal bleeding. The microscopic features resemble those of uterine leiomyosarcoma. The prognosis generally is poor (35% 5 year survival). The most difficult aspect of therapy is to achieve adequate surgical clearance.

MISCELLANEOUS TUMORS

Most carcinomas reported as arising from mesonephric duct remnants and diagnosed as 'mesonephric carcinoma' actually have been clear cell adenocarcinomas of müllerian type upon review. Most well-documented mesonephric carcinomas have arisen in the cervix. There are exceedingly few documented in the vagina (Figure 7.52).[5]

Other rare malignant primary tumors include transitional cell carcinoma (sometimes also called 'cloacogenic carcinoma'), lymphoepithelioma-like carcinoma,[119] adenoid basal cell carcinoma, basal cell-like carcinoma, basaloid squamous cell carcinoma,[120] angiosarcoma,[121,122] serous adenocarcinoma, aggressive angiomyxoma,[123,124] alveolar soft part sarcoma, carcinosarcoma,[125] malignant peripheral nerve sheath tumor,[126] synovial sarcoma,[127] and other sarcomas.

MALIGNANT VAGINAL TUMORS IN CHILDHOOD

EMBRYONAL RHABDOMYOSARCOMA

Embryonal rhabdomyosarcoma is a tumor composed of embryonal rhabdomyoblasts, thought to arise from the primitive mesenchyme of the lamina propria. Its former name, 'sarcoma botryoides,' reflects the neoplasm's gross appearance as multiple 'grape-like' polyps. While rare in absolute numbers, the tumor is the most common vaginal neoplasm in infants and young children. The mean age at diagnosis is 2 years. Almost all occur in children under the age of 5 years, although occurrences at older ages are known.

The most common symptom is vaginal mass or bleeding. If large, the tumor may distend the lumen of the vagina and protrude through the introitus as a soft, polypoid mass (Figure 7.53).

Pathology

In the vagina, most tumors are of the botryoid (embryonal) subtype. Vaginal rhabdomyosarcomas of the spindle or

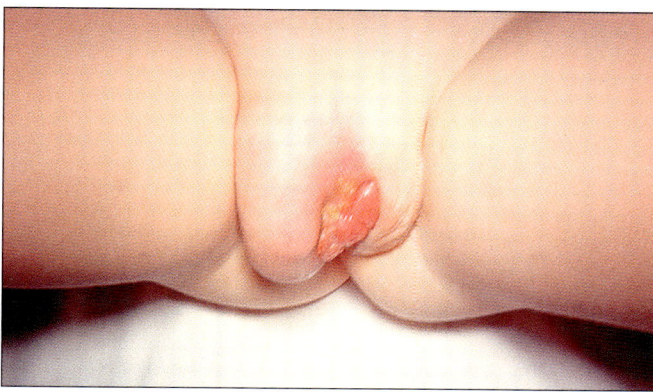

Figure 7.53 Embryonal rhabdomyosarcoma. The polypoid tumor protrudes through the introitus.

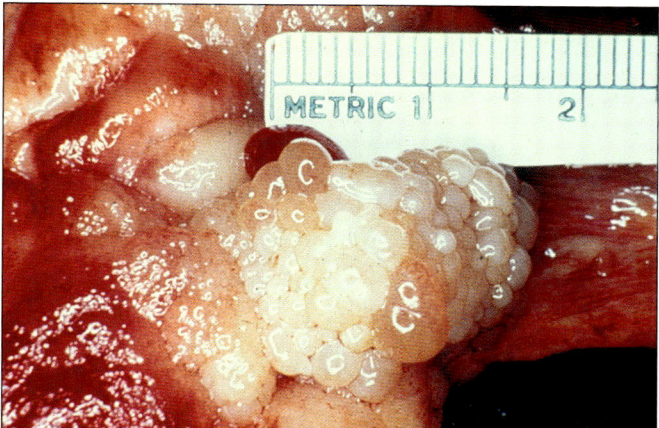

Figure 7.54 Embryonal rhabdomyosarcoma (sarcoma botryoides). The polypoid tumor resembles a bunch of grapes.

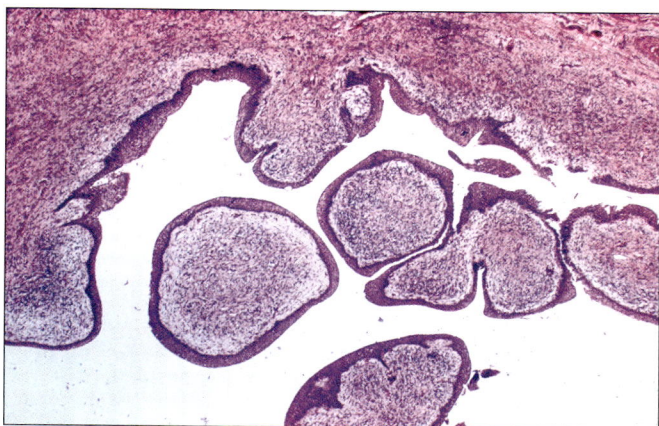

Figure 7.55 Embryonal rhabdomyosarcoma. The cambium layer is a dense zone of rhabdomyoblasts found beneath the surface epithelium. Tumor cells are scattered in a loose myxoid stroma.

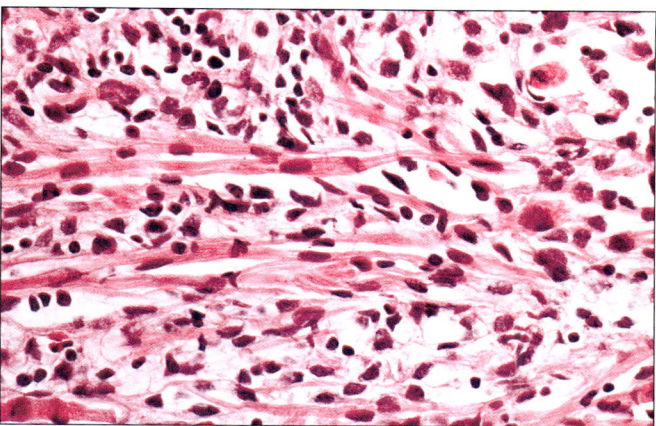

Figure 7.56 Embryonal rhabdomyosarcoma. Rhabdomyoblastic differentiation is prominent as elongate spindle cells with eosinophilic, fibrillary cytoplasm.

alveolar types are extremely rare.[128,129] Grossly, they appear polypoid, soft gray or tan, and edematous resembling a bunch of grapes (Figure 7.54). Microscopic examination shows diffuse thickness of the lamina propria, which appears largely loose, myxoid, and hypocellular, with an overlying intact squamous epithelium. However, the distinctive feature of sarcoma botryoides is the presence of the so-called 'cambium layer,' a condensed layer of neoplastic immature mesenchymal cells just beneath the surface epithelium (Figure 7.55). The botanical term cambium refers to the active growth layer just beneath the bark of trees. The cells in the cambium layer are of round to spindle shape, with oval nuclei, and inconspicuous nucleoli. Rhabdomyoblastic differentiation may be evident as elongated tumor cells with eosinophilic cytoplasm and cross-striations (Figure 7.56). Immunostains for muscle-specific actin, desmin, and myogenin are useful in demonstrating the skeletal muscle nature of the cells. There is immunoreactivity for S-100 protein, which has been reported in about 20% of cases.

Natural History

The tumor grows into the vaginal wall and soft tissue of the pelvis, bladder, or rectum and subsequently metastasizes to lymph nodes, lungs, liver, and bone. Currently, the tumors are staged according to the Intergroup Rhabdomyosarcoma Study (IRS) classification, which is based on combined features of extent of disease, resectability, and microscopic evaluation of margins of excision (Table 7.2).[130] The prognosis has improved greatly since the introduction of multi-agent chemotherapy, especially if the tumor is stage I.[129,131,132] Within this stage, the tumor's growth pattern rather than histologic differentiation appears as the most important prognostic factor. Patients with a polypoid (exophytic) intraluminal tumor, regardless of whether it is the botryoid type with superficially condensed tumor cells or with more evenly distributed cells, survived longer (92% 10 year survival) than if the tumor grew diffusely into the wall (68% 10 year survival). On the other hand, even the focal presence of an alveolar histology confers a worse prognosis.[133] Of surprise, recurrences often display a histologic pattern better than the primary. In one large series, the mitotic count dropped from 8 in the primary to 1.8 per 10 HPFs in the recurrence; the Ki-67 reactivity showed a comparable decrease.[128] To date, there is no convincing evidence that chemotherapy-induced maturation of the tumor cells influences prognosis.

YOLK SAC TUMOR

Even if yolk sac tumors (endodermal sinus tumors) usually arise in the ovary, about 60 cases have been reported in the vagina of infants and children, most under the age of 4 years.[134] The germ cell origin of these tumors is difficult to relate to the infant vagina. Whereas aberrant germ cells may have theoretically 'found' their way to the vagina, this hypothesis does not account for the lack of other malignant germ cell tumors in the vagina.

The tumors present with vaginal bleeding. They are polypoid, soft, and tan to white, and usually fill the vaginal lumen and can be clinically misinterpreted as rhabdomyosarcoma.[135] The most common microscopic pattern is the reticular (honeycomb) pattern. Occasionally some may be focally solid or slightly papillary. Both Schiller–Duval bodies and the polyvesicular pattern are rarely found. The most difficult differential diagnosis is the clear cell adenocarcinoma since the cells of the yolk sac tumor may have clear cytoplasm. Immunostains for α-fetoprotein and α-1-antitrypsin confirm the diagnosis of yolk sac tumor.

The use of adjuvant chemotherapy, usually consisting of vincristine, actinomycin, and cyclophosphamide, has resulted in a 95% disease-free survival.[136] Where the condition was once considered as routinely fatal, long-term survival is now common. New forms of combination chemotherapy and partial but conservative surgery may also permit preservation of fertility.

LYMPHOMA

Vaginal lymphomas, like lymphomas throughout the genital tract, are most commonly secondary to a more generalized spread. About one-fourth[137] to one-half[138] of cases are low stage, and presumably many of these are primary. Lymphomas occur, in general, in women in their forties or older and produce an ill-defined, but very firm thickening of more than one wall and extend toward rectum, bladder, or pelvic walls. At presentation, contiguous structures and/or regional lymph nodes are commonly involved.

Although most are diffuse, large B-cell lymphomas, several have been follicular lymphomas and small lymphocytic lymphomas. In diffuse, large B-cell lymphoma the sheets of neoplastic cells infiltrate deeply in the stroma, producing a dense sclerosis. The lymphoma cells lack tropism for the overlying epithelium and lymphoepithelial lesions are not seen. Rare cases of nasal-type natural killer/T-cell lymphoma, plasmacytoma,[139] and Hodgkin lymphoma have been described. Because the vagina is one of the mucosa-associated lymphoid tissues (MALTs), MALT lymphoma, though rare, must be included in the differential diagnosis of vaginal neoplasms.[140]

The differential diagnosis includes inflammatory conditions, carcinoma, endometrial stromal sarcoma, melanoma, and primitive neuroectodermal tumor.
With the wider availability and routine application of immunohistochemistry to paraffin sections an accurate diagnosis is usually achieved. However, the possibility of lymphoma must be considered first by the pathologist and appropriate immunoreactions performed. Overdiagnosis of lymphoma may occur in cases of so-called 'lymphoma-like lesions,' a term signifying inflammatory lesions mimicking lymphoma.

Table 7.2 IRS Surgical–Pathologic Grouping System

Group	Definition
I	Localized tumor, completely removed with pathologically clear margins and no regional lymph node involvement
II	Localized tumor, grossly removed with (a) microscopically involved margins, (b) involved, grossly resected regional lymph nodes, or (c) both
III	Localized tumor, with gross residual disease after grossly incomplete removal, or biopsy only
IV	Distant metastases present at diagnosis

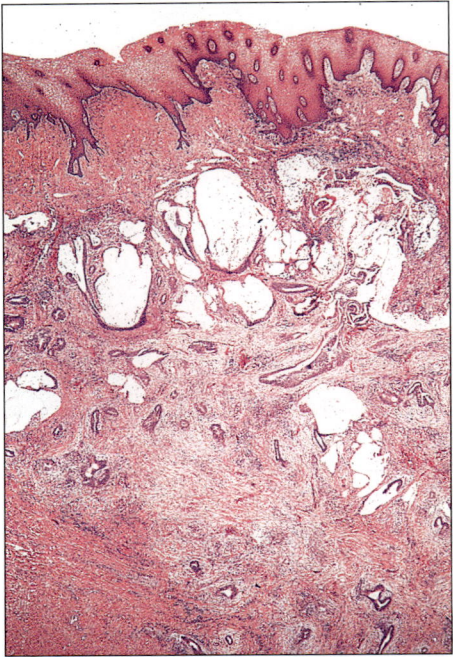

Figure 7.57 Adenocarcinoma of colon, metastatic to vagina.

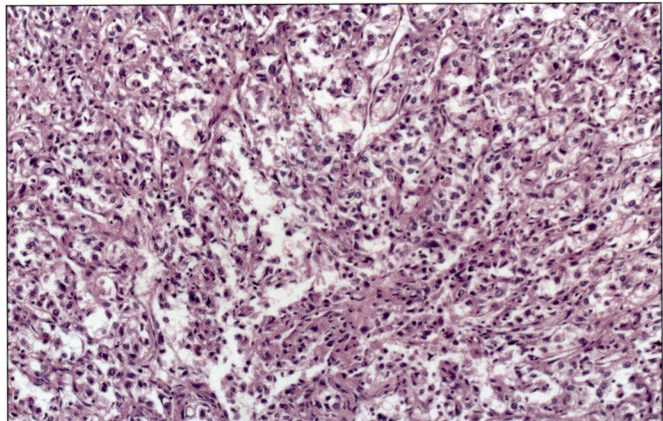

Figure 7.58 Renal cell carcinoma metastatic to vagina.

SECONDARY TUMORS OF THE VAGINA

Secondary tumors of the vagina are four times more common than primary tumors. Most common is direct extension from tumors of adjacent organs, particularly cervix (32%) and endometrium (18%), but metastases from distant organs such as breast, large bowel (Figure 7.57), and left kidney (Figure 7.58) can also be seen. The spread may occur by direct extension, lymphatic spread, or implantation at the time of hysterectomy.

REFERENCES

1. Cunha GR. The dual origin of vaginal epithelium. Am J Anat 1975;143:387–92.
2. Robboy SJ, Taguchi O, Cunha GR. Normal development of the human female reproductive tract and alterations resulting from experimental exposure to diethylstilbestrol. Hum Pathol 1982;13(3):190–8.
3. Patton DL, Thwin SS, Meier A, et al. Epithelial cell layer thickness and immune cell populations in the normal human vagina at different stages of the menstrual cycle. Am J Obstet Gynecol 2000;183(4):967–73.
4. Tai LH, Tavassoli FA. Endometrial polyps with atypical (bizarre) stromal cells. Am J Surg Pathol 2002;26(4):505–9.
5. Bague S, Rodriguez IM, Prat J. Malignant mesonephric tumors of the female genital tract: a clinicopathologic study of 9 cases. Am J Surg Pathol 2004;28(5):601–7.
6. Anderson M, Jordan J, Morse A, Sharp F. Diethylstilbestrol exposure. In: A text and atlas of integrated colposcopy. 2nd ed. London, UK: Chapman and Hall Medical; 1996. p. 240–2.
7. Robboy SJ. A hypothetic mechanism of diethylstilbestrol(DES)-induced anomalies in exposed progeny. Hum Pathol 1983;14(10):831–3.
8. Liang CC, Chang SD, Soong YK. Long-term follow-up of women who underwent surgical correction for imperforate hymen. Arch Gynecol Obstet 2003;269(1):5–8.
9. Wall EM, Stone B, Klein BL. Imperforate hymen: a not-so-hidden diagnosis. Am J Emerg Med 2003;21(3):249–50.
10. Mizia K, Bennett MJ, Dudley J, Morrisey J. Mullerian dysgenesis: a review of recent outcomes at Royal Hospital for Women. Aust N Z J Obstet Gynaecol 2006;46(1):29–31.
11. Guerrier D, Mouchel T, Pasquier L, Pellerin I. The Mayer-Rokitansky-Kuster-Hauser syndrome (congenital absence of uterus and vagina)—phenotypic manifestations and genetic approaches. J Negat Results Biomed 2006;5:1.
12. Li S, Qayyum A, Coakley FV, Hricak H. Association of renal agenesis and mullerian duct anomalies. J Comput Assist Tomogr 2000;24(6):829–34.
13. Pittock ST, Babovic-Vuksanovic D, Lteif A. Mayer-Rokitansky-Kuster-Hauser anomaly and its associated malformations. Am J Med Genet A 2005;135(3):314–6.
14. Gastol P, Baka-Jakubiak M, Skobejko-Wlodarska L, Szymkiewicz C. Complete duplication of the bladder, urethra, vagina, and uterus in girls. Urology 2000;55(4):578–81.
15. Eckert LO. Clinical practice. Acute vulvovaginitis. N Engl J Med 2006;355(12):1244–52.
16. Lamont RF, Sobel JD, Akins RA, et al. The vaginal microbiome: new information about genital tract flora using molecular based techniques. BJOG 2011;118(5):533–49.
17. McGregor JA, French JI. Bacterial vaginosis in pregnancy. Obstet Gynecol Surv 2000;55(5 Suppl 1):S1–19.
18. Swidsinski A, Mendling W, Loening-Baucke V, et al. Adherent biofilms in bacterial vaginosis. Obstet Gynecol 2005;106(5 Pt 1):1013–23.
19. Swidsinski A, Doerffel Y, Loening-Baucke V, et al. Gardnerella biofilm involves females and males and is transmitted sexually. Gynecol Obstet Invest 2010;70(4):256–63.
20. Tokyol C, Aktepe OC, Cevrioglu AS, et al. Bacterial vaginosis: comparison of Pap smear and microbiological test results. Mod Pathol 2004;17(7):857–60.
21. Benchimol M. Trichomonads under microscopy. Microsc Microanal 2004;10(5):528–50.
22. Demirezen S. Phagocytosis of erythrocytes by *Trichomonas vaginalis*: examination of a cervicovaginal smear. Diagn Cytopathol 2001;24(6):435.
23. Demirezen S, Safi Z, Beksac S. The interaction of *Trichomonas vaginalis* with epithelial cells, polymorphonuclear leucocytes and erythrocytes on vaginal smears: light microscopic observation. Cytopathology 2000;11(5):326–32.
24. Demirezen S. Phagocytosis of rod-shaped bacteria and cocci by *Trichomonas vaginalis*: light microscopic observations. Acta Cytol 2001;45(6):1088–9.
25. Chen WL, Chen JF, Zhong XR, et al. Ultrastructural and immunohistochemical studies on *Trichomonas vaginalis* adhering to and phagocytizing genitourinary epithelial cells. Chin Med J (Engl) 2004;117(3):376–81.
26. Bowden FJ, Garnett GP. *Trichomonas vaginalis* epidemiology: parameterising and analysing a model of treatment interventions. Sex Transm Infect 2000;76(4):248–56.
27. Dan M, Leshem Y, Yeshaya A. Performance of a rapid yeast test in detecting *Candida* spp. in the vagina. Diagn Microbiol Infect Dis 2010;67(1):52–5.
28. Sherer DM, Hellmann M, Gorelick C, et al. Transvaginal sonographic findings associated with emphysematous vaginitis at 2 weeks' gestation. J Ultrasound Med 2006;25(4):515–7.
29. Kogulan PK, Smith M, Seidman J, et al. Malakoplakia involving the abdominal wall, urinary bladder, vagina, and vulva: case report and discussion of malakoplakia-associated bacteria. Int J Gynecol Pathol 2001;20(4):403–6.
30. Davis CC, Kremer MJ, Schlievert PM, Squier CA. Penetration of toxic shock syndrome toxin-1 across porcine vaginal mucosa ex vivo: permeability characteristics, toxin distribution, and tissue damage. Am J Obstet Gynecol 2003;189(6):1785–91.
31. Lotan TL, Tefs K, Schuster V, et al. Inherited plasminogen deficiency presenting as ligneous vaginitis: a case report with molecular correlation and review of the literature. Hum Pathol 2007;38:1569–75.
32. McCluggage WG. A review and update of morphologically bland vulvovaginal mesenchymal lesions. Int J Gynecol Pathol 2005;24(1):26–38.
33. Nielsen GP, Young RH. Mesenchymal tumors and tumor-like lesions of the female genital tract: a selective review with emphasis on recently described entities. Int J Gynecol Pathol 2001;20(2):105–27.
34. Nucci MR, Fletcher CD. Vulvovaginal soft tissue tumours: update and review. Histopathology 2000;36(2):97–108.
35. Jallouli M, Trigui L, Gargouri A, Mhiri R. Vaginal polyp in a newborn. Eur J Pediatr 2008;167(5):599–600.
36. de Kroon CD, Bergman I, Westenberg S, et al. Prolapse of the uterine tube after subtotal hysterectomy. BJOG 2003;110(3):333–4.
37. Michal M, Rokyta Z, Mejchar B, et al. Prolapse of the fallopian tube after hysterectomy associated with exuberant angiomyofibroblastic stroma response: a diagnostic pitfall. Virchows Arch 2000;437(4):436–9.
38. Brown WD, Burrows L, Todd CS. Ectopic pregnancy after cesarean hysterectomy. Obstet Gynecol 2002;99(5 Pt 2):933–4.
39. Saropala N, Ingsirorat C. Conservative treatment of vaginal vault granulation tissue following total abdominal hysterectomy. Int J Gynaecol Obstet 1998;62(1):55–8.
40. Guillou L, Gloor E, De Grandi P, Costa J. Post-operative pseudosarcoma of the vagina. A case report. Pathol Res Pract 1989;185(2):245–8; discussion 8–50.
41. Proppe KH, Scully RE, Rosai J. Postoperative spindle cell nodules of genitourinary tract resembling sarcomas. A report of eight cases. Am J Surg Pathol 1984;8(2):101–8.
42. Murdoch F, Sharma R, Al-Nafussi A. Benign mixed tumor of the vagina: case report with expanded immunohistochemical profile. Int J Gynecol Cancer 2003;13(4):543–7.
43. Branton PA, Tavassoli FA. Spindle cell epithelioma, the so-called mixed tumor of the vagina. A clinicopathologic, immunohistochemical, and ultrastructural analysis of 28 cases. Am J Surg Pathol 1993;17(5):509–15.
44. Kang MS, Yoon HK. Mixed tumor of the vagina: a case report. J Korean Med Sci 2002;17(6):845–8.
45. Abu J, Nunns D, Ireland D, Brown L. Malignant progression through borderline changes in recurrent Mullerian papilloma of the vagina. Histopathology 2003;42(5):510–1.

46. Biankin SA, O'Toole VE, Fung C, Russell P. Bizarre leiomyoma of the vagina: report of a case. Int J Gynecol Pathol 2000;19(2):186–7.
47. Vlahos N, Economopoulos K, Skarpidi E, Moraitis D. Bizarre leiomyoma of the posterior vaginal fornix. Int J Gynaecol Obstet 2008;102(3):296–7.
48. Iversen UM. Two cases of benign vaginal rhabdomyoma. Case reports. APMIS 1996;104(7–8):575–8.
49. Nielsen GP, Young RH, Dickersin GR, Rosenberg AE. Angiomyofibroblastoma of the vulva with sarcomatous transformation ("angiomyofibrosarcoma"). Am J Surg Pathol 1997;21(9):1104–8.
50. Saleh MM, Yassin AH, Zaklama MS. Recurrent angiomyofibroblastoma of the vagina: a case report. Eur J Gynaecol Oncol 2007;28(4):324.
51. McCluggage WG, White RG. Angiomyofibroblastoma of the vagina. J Clin Pathol 2000;53(10):803.
52. Gelly-Marty M, Assous D, Padeano MM, Arnould L. [Brenner tumour of the vagina]. Ann Pathol 2007;27(4):310–2.
53. Hassan A, Bennet A, Bhalla S, et al. Paraganglioma of the vagina: report of a case, including immunohistochemical and ultrastructural findings. Int J Gynecol Pathol 2003;22(4):404–6.
54. Dane B, Dane C, Basaran S, et al. Vaginal Schwannoma in a case with uterine myoma. Ann Diagn Pathol 2010;14(2):137–9.
55. Obeidat BR, Amarin ZO, Jallad MF. Vaginal schwannoma: a case report. J Reprod Med 2007;52(4):341–2.
56. Mann S, Russell P, Wills E, et al. Benign vaginal mesenchymoma showing mature skeletal muscle, smooth muscle and fatty differentiation. Int J Surg Pathol 1996;4:49–54.
57. Heim K, Hopfl R, Muller-Holzner E, et al. Multiple blue nevi of the vagina. A case report. J Reprod Med 2000;45(1):42–4.
58. Siu SS, Tam WH, To KF, Yuen PM. Is vaginal dermoid cyst a rare occurrence or a misnomer? A case report and review of the literature. Ultrasound Obstet Gynecol 2003;21(4):404–6.
59. Gagne HM. Colposcopy of the vagina and vulva. Obstet Gynecol Clin North Am 2008;35(4):659–69; x.
60. Sugase M, Matsukura T. Distinct manifestations of human papillomaviruses in the vagina. Int J Cancer 1997;72(3):412–5.
61. Srodon M, Stoler MH, Baber GB, Kurman RJ. The distribution of low and high-risk HPV types in vulvar and vaginal intraepithelial neoplasia (VIN and VaIN). Am J Surg Pathol 2006;30(12):1513–8.
62. Darragh TM, Colgan TJ, Cox JT, et al. The lower anogenital squamous terminology standardization project for HPV-associated lesions: background and consensus recommendations from the College of American Pathologists and the American Society for Colposcopy and Cervical Pathology. J Low Genit Tract Dis, 2012;16:205–42.
63. Creasman WT, Phillips JL, Menck HR. The National Cancer Data Base report on cancer of the vagina. Cancer 1998;83(5):1033–40.
64. Boonlikit S, Noinual N. Vaginal intraepithelial neoplasia: a retrospective analysis of clinical features and colpohistology. J Obstet Gynaecol Res 2010;36(1):94–100.
65. Schockaert S, Poppe W, Arbyn M, et al. Incidence of vaginal intraepithelial neoplasia after hysterectomy for cervical intraepithelial neoplasia: a retrospective study. Am J Obstet Gynecol 2008;199(2):113.e1–5.
66. Frisch M, Biggar RJ, Goedert JJ. Human papillomavirus-associated cancers in patients with human immunodeficiency virus infection and acquired immunodeficiency syndrome. J Natl Cancer Inst 2000;92(18):1500–10.
67. Robboy SJ, Szyfelbein WM, Goellner JR, et al. Dysplasia and cytologic findings in 4,589 young women enrolled in diethylstilbestrol-adenosis (DESAD) project. Am J Obstet Gynecol 1981;140(5):579–86.
68. Stoler MH, Srodon M, Baber GB, Kurman RJ. The frequency and biology of multiple HPV infections in vulvar neoplasia. Mod Pathol 2005;18(Suppl):205A.
69. Sillman FH, Fruchter RG, Chen YS, et al. Vaginal intraepithelial neoplasia: risk factors for persistence, recurrence, and invasion and its management. Am J Obstet Gynecol 1997;176:93–9.
70. Creasman WT. Vaginal cancers. Curr Opin Obstet Gynecol 2005;17(1):71–6.
71. Hiroi H, Yasugi T, Matsumoto K, et al. Mucinous adenocarcinoma arising in a neovagina using the sigmoid colon thirty years after operation: a case report. J Surg Oncol 2001;77(1):61–4.
72. Steiner E, Woernle F, Kuhn W, et al. Carcinoma of the neovagina: case report and review of the literature. Gynecol Oncol 2002;84(1):171–5.
73. Hellman K, Silfversward C, Nilsson B, et al. Primary carcinoma of the vagina: factors influencing the age at diagnosis. The Radiumhemmet series 1956–96. Int J Gynecol Cancer 2004;14(3):491–501.
74. Brinton LA, Nasca PC, Mallin K, et al. Case-control study of in situ and invasive carcinoma of the vagina. Gynecol Oncol 1990;38:49.
75. Otton GR, Nicklin JL, Dickie GJ, et al. Early-stage vaginal carcinoma–an analysis of 70 patients. Int J Gynecol Cancer 2004;14(2):304–10.
76. Lian J, Dundas G, Carlone M, et al. Twenty-year review of radiotherapy for vaginal cancer: an institutional experience. Gynecol Oncol 2008;111(2):298–306.
77. Chyle V, Zagars GK, Wheeler JA, et al. Definitive radiotherapy for carcinoma of the vagina: outcome and prognostic factors. Int J Radiat Oncol Biol Phys 1996; 35:891–905.
78. Creasman WT, Phillips JL, Menck HR. The National Cancer Data Base report on cancer of the vagina. Cancer (Phila) 1998; 83:1033–40.
79. Yeh AM, Marcus Jr RB, Amdur RJ, et al. Patterns of failure in squamous cell carcinoma of the vagina treated with definitive radiotherapy alone: what is the appropriate treatment volume? Int J Cancer 2001;96(Suppl):109–16.
80. van Dam P, Sonnemans H, van Dam PJ, et al. Sentinel node detection in patients with vaginal carcinoma. Gynecol Oncol 2004;92(1):89–92.
81. Gao Z, Bhuiya T, Falkowski O. Papillary squamotransitional cell carcinoma of the vagina: a case report and review of literature. J Obstet Gynaecol 2005;25(1):94–6.
82. Rose P, Stoler M, Abdul-Karim F. Papillary squamotransitional cell carcinoma of the vagina. Int J Gynecol Pathol 1998; 17:372–5.
83. Vesoulis Z, Erhardt CA. Cytologic diagnosis of vaginal papillary squamotransitional cell carcinoma. A case report. Acta Cytol 2001;45(3):465–9.
84. Koenig C, Turnicky R, Kankam C, Tavassoli F. Papillary squamotransitional cell carcinoma of the cervix: a report of 32 cases. Am J Surg Pathol 1997;21:915–21.
85. Hayashi M, Mori Y, Takagi Y, et al. Primary small cell neuroendocrine carcinoma of the vagina. Marked effect of combination chemotherapy: a case report. Oncology 2000;58(4):300–4.
86. Bing Z, Levine L, Lucci JA, et al. Primary small cell neuroendocrine carcinoma of the vagina: a clinicopathologic study. Arch Pathol Lab Med 2004;128(8):857–62.
87. Crowder S, Tuller E. Small cell carcinoma of the female genital tract. Semin Oncol 2007;34(1):57–63.
88. Hanselaar A, Boos E, Shirango H, et al. DES research update 1999: current knowledge, future directions. Publication no. 00-4722 Bethesda, MD: National Institutes of Health; 1999:5.
89. McNall RY, Nowicki PD, Miller B, et al. Adenocarcinoma of the cervix and vagina in pediatric patients. Pediatr Blood Cancer 2004;43(3):289–94.
90. Troisi R, Hatch EE, Titus-Ernstoff L, et al. Cancer risk in women prenatally exposed to diethylstilbestrol. Int J Cancer 2007;121(2):356–60.
91. Frank SJ, Deavers MT, Jhingran A, et al. Primary adenocarcinoma of the vagina not associated with diethylstilbestrol (DES) exposure. Gynecol Oncol 2007;105(2):470–4.
92. Sharp GB, Cole P, Anderson D, Herbst AL. Clear cell adenocarcinoma of the lower genital tract. Correlation of mother's recall of diethylstilbestrol history with obstetrical records. Cancer 1990;66(10):2215–20.
93. Thomas MB, Wright JD, Leiser AL, et al. Clear cell carcinoma of the cervix: a multi-institutional review in the post-DES era. Gynecol Oncol 2008;109(3):335–9.
94. Hatch E, Palmer J, Titus-Ernstoff L, et al. E. DES research update 1999: current knowledge, future directions. Publication no. 00-4722. Bethesda, MD: National Institutes of Health; 1999:7.
95. Trimble EL, Rubinstein LV, Menck HR, et al. Vaginal clear cell adenocarcinoma in the United States. Gynecol Oncol 1996;61(1):113–5.
96. Hanselaar AG, Van Leusen ND, De Wilde PC, Vooijs GP. Clear cell adenocarcinoma of the vagina and cervix. A report of the Central Netherlands Registry with emphasis on early detection and prognosis. Cancer 1991;67(7):1971–8.

97. Sharp GB, Cole P. Identification of risk factors for diethylstilbestrol-associated clear cell adenocarcinoma of the vagina: similarities to endometrial cancer. Am J Epidemiol 1991;134(11):1316–24.
98. Waggoner SE, Anderson SM, Van Eyck S, et al. Human papillomavirus detection and p53 expression in clear-cell adenocarcinoma of the vagina and cervix. Obstet Gynecol 1994;84(3):404–8.
99. Boyd J, Takahashi H, Waggoner SE, et al. Molecular genetic analysis of clear cell adenocarcinomas of the vagina and cervix associated and unassociated with diethylstilbestrol exposure in utero. Cancer 1996;77(3):507–13.
100. Robboy SJ, Young RH, Welch WR, et al. Atypical vaginal adenosis and cervical ectropion. Association with clear cell adenocarcinoma in diethylstilbestrol-exposed offspring. Cancer 1984;54(5):869–75.
101. Vang R, Barner R, Wheeler DT, Strauss BL. Immunohistochemical staining for Ki-67 and p53 helps distinguish endometrial Arias-Stella reaction from high-grade carcinoma, including clear cell carcinoma. Int J Gynecol Pathol 2004;23(3):223–33.
102. Allard JE, McBroom JW, Zahn CM, et al. Vaginal metastasis and thrombocytopenia from renal cell carcinoma. Gynecol Oncol 2004;92(3):970–3.
103. Bozaci EA, Atabekoglu C, Sertcelik A, et al. Metachronous metastases from renal cell carcinoma to uterine cervix and vagina: case report and review of literature. Gynecol Oncol 2005;99(1):232–5.
104. Herbst AL, Anderson S, Hubby MM, et al. Risk factors for the development of diethylstilbestrol-associated clear cell adenocarcinoma: a case-control study. Am J Obstet Gynecol 1986;154(4):814–22.
105. Senekjian EK, Hubby M, Bell DA, et al. Clear cell adenocarcinoma (CCA) of the vagina and cervix in association with pregnancy. Gynecol Oncol 1986;24(2):207–19.
106. Staats PN, Clement PB, Young RH. Primary endometrioid adenocarcinoma of the vagina: a clinicopathologic study of 18 cases. Am J Surg Pathol 2007;31(10):1490–501.
107. Ebrahim S, Daponte A, Smith TH, et al. Primary mucinous adenocarcinoma of the vagina. Gynecol Oncol 2001;80(1):89–92.
108. Moore-Maxwell CA, Robboy SJ. Mucinous adenocarcinoma arising in rectovaginal fistulas associated with Crohn's disease. Gynecol Oncol 2004;93(1):266–8.
109. Gu M, Ghafari S, Lin F. Pap smears of patients with extramammary Paget's disease of the vulva. Diagn Cytopathol 2005;32(6):353–7.
110. Chang AE, Karnell LH, Menck HR. The National Cancer Data Base report on cutaneous and noncutaneous melanoma: a summary of 84,836 cases from the past decade. The American College of Surgeons Commission on Cancer and the American Cancer Society. Cancer 1998;83(8):1564–78.
111. McLaughlin CC, Wu XC, Jemal A, et al. Incidence of noncutaneous melanomas in the U.S. Cancer 2005;103(5):1000–7.
112. DeMatos P, Tyler D, Seigler HF. Mucosal melanoma of the female genitalia: a clinicopathologic study of forty-three cases at Duke University Medical Center. Surgery 1998;124(1):38–48.
113. Gupta D, Malpica A, Deavers MT, Silva EG. Vaginal melanoma: a clinicopathologic and immunohistochemical study of 26 cases. Am J Surg Pathol 2002;26(11):1450–7.
114. Oguri H, Izumiya C, Maeda N, et al. A primary amelanotic melanoma of the vagina, diagnosed by immunohistochemical staining with HMB-45, which recurred as a pigmented melanoma. J Clin Pathol 2004;57(9):986–8.
115. Chung AF, Casey MJ, Flannery JT et al. Malignant melanoma of the vagina: report of 19 cases. Obstet Gynecol 1980;55:720–7.
116. Miner TJ, Delgado R, Zeisler J, et al. Primary vaginal melanoma: a critical analysis of therapy. Ann Surg Oncol 2004;11(1):34–9.
117. Buchanan DJ, Schlaerth J, Kurosaki T. Primary vaginal melanoma: thirteen-year disease-free survival after wide local excision and review of recent literature. Am J Obstet Gynecol 1998;178(6):1177–84.
118. Tavassoli FA, Norris HJ. Smooth muscle tumors of the vagina. Obstet Gynecol 1979;53(6):689–93.
119. McCluggage WG. Lymphoepithelioma-like carcinoma of the vagina. J Clin Pathol 2001;54(12):964–5.
120. Li H, Heller DS, Sama J, et al. Basaloid squamous cell carcinoma of the vagina metastasizing to the lung. A case report. J Reprod Med 2000;45(10):841–3.
121. Morimura Y, Hashimoto T, Soeda S, et al. Angiosarcoma of vagina successfully treated with interleukin-2 therapy and chemotherapy: a case report. J Obstet Gynaecol Res 2001;27(4):231–5.
122. Takeuchi K, Deguchi M, Hamana S, et al. A case of postirradiation vaginal angiosarcoma treated with recombinant interleukin-2 therapy. Int J Gynecol Cancer 2005;15(6):1163–5.
123. Gungor T, Zengeroglu S, Kaleli A, Kuzey GM. Aggressive angiomyxoma of the vulva and vagina. A common problem: misdiagnosis. Eur J Obstet Gynecol Reprod Biol 2004;112(1):114–6.
124. Shahid N, Ahluwalia A, Sahasrabudhe N, Davenport A. Aggressive angiomyxoma of the vagina: a rare differential diagnosis of a lateral vaginal wall cyst. J Obstet Gynaecol 2005;25(6):622–3.
125. Shibata R, Umezawa A, Takehara K, et al. Primary carcinosarcoma of the vagina. Pathol Int 2003;53(2):106–10.
126. Mhaskar R, Mhaskar V, Pritilata R. Malignant peripheral nerve sheath tumour of the vagina. J Obstet Gynaecol 2009;29(4):360.
127. Pelosi G, Luzzatto F, Landoni F, et al. Poorly differentiated synovial sarcoma of the vagina: first reported case with immunohistochemical, molecular and ultrastructural data. Histopathology 2007;50(6):808–10.
128. Leuschner I, Harms D, Mattke A, et al. Rhabdomyosarcoma of the urinary bladder and vagina: a clinicopathologic study with emphasis on recurrent disease: a report from the Kiel Pediatric Tumor Registry and the German CWS Study. Am J Surg Pathol 2001;25(7):856–64.
129. Newton Jr WA. Classification of rhabdomyosarcoma. Curr Top Pathol 1995;89:241–59.
130. Shochat S, Andrassy R, Ransley PG. Progress in the surgical management of vaginal rhabdomycsarcoma: a 25-year review from the Intergroup Rhabdomyosarcoma Study Group. J Pediatr Surg 1999;34:734–5.
131. Andrassy RJ, Wiener ES, Raney RB, et al. Progress in the surgical management of vaginal rhabdomyosarcoma: a 25-year review from the Intergroup Rhabdomyosarcoma Study Group. J Pediatr Surg 1999;34(5):731–4; discussion 4–5.
132. Arndt CA, Donaldson SS, Anderson JR, et al. What constitutes optimal therapy for patients with rhabdomyosarcoma of the female genital tract? Cancer 2001;91(12):2454–68.
133. Qualman S, Coffin C, Newton W, et al. Intergroup rhabdomyosarcoma study: update for pathologists. Pediatr Dev Pathol 1998;1:550–61.
134. Clement PB, Young RH, Scully RE. Extraovarian pelvic yolk sac tumors. Cancer (Phila) 1988;62:620–6.
135. Gangopadhyay M, Raha K, Sinha SK, et al. Endodermal sinus tumor of the vagina in children: a report of two cases. Indian J Pathol Microbiol 2009;52(3):403–4.
136. Handel LN, Scott SM, Giller RH, et al. New perspectives on therapy for vaginal endodermal sinus tumors. J Urol 2002;168(2):687–90.
137. Lagoo AS, Robboy SJ. Lymphoma of the female genital tract: current status. Int J Gynecol Pathol 2006;25(1):1–21.
138. Vang R, Medeiros LJ, Silva EG, et al. Non-Hodgkin's lymphoma involving the vagina: a clinicopathologic analysis of 14 patients. Am J Surg Pathol 2000;24(5):719–25.
139. Torrubia S, Sabate JM, Palmer J, Martinez-Noguera A. Plasmacytoma of the vagina: findings on CT and MR imaging. AJR Am J Roentgenol 2002;178(1):245–7.
140. Yoshinaga K, Akahira J, Niikura H, et al. A case of primary mucosa-associated lymphoid tissue lymphoma of the vagina. Hum Pathol 2004;35(9):1164–6.
141. Horn LC, Lindner K, Szepankiewicz G, et al. p16, p14, p53, and cyclin D1 expression and HPV analysis in small cell carcinomas of the uterine cervix. Int J Gynecol Pathol 2006;25:182–6.
142. Wang HL, Lu DW. Detection of human papillomavirus DNA and expression of p16, Rb, and p53 proteins in small cell carcinomas of the uterine cervix. Am J Surg Pathol 2004;28:901–8.
143. Waggoner SE, Mittendorf R, Biney N, et al. Influence of in utero diethylstilbestrol exposure on the prognosis and biologic behavior of vaginal clear-cell adenocarcinoma. Gynecol Oncol 1994;55:238–44.

8 Cervical Benign and Non-Neoplastic Conditions

Anais Malpica

CHAPTER OUTLINE

Normal Structure	160
Anatomy	160
Native (Original) Squamous Epithelium	160
Native (Original) Cervical Glandular Epithelium	164
Physiologic Changes in the Cervix and the Formation of the Transformation Zone	165
Squamous Metaplasia	166
The Congenital Transformation Zone (CTZ)	169
Histogenesis of the Congenital Transformation Zone	169
Inflammatory Cervicitis and Reactive Changes	170
Infective Cervicitis	170
Epithelial Inflammatory Changes	175
Metaplasias	176
Tubal, Endometrioid, and Tuboendometrioid Metaplasia	176
Intestinal Metaplasia	177
Lesions of the Endocervical Glandular Epithelium	177
Endocervical Tunnel Clusters	177
Deep Nabothian Cysts	179
Lobular Endocervical Glandular Hyperplasia	179
Diffuse Laminar Endocervical Glandular Hyperplasia	180
Lesions Related to Exogenous Stimuli	180
Microglandular Hyperplasia	180
Arias-Stella Reaction	181
Decidual Change	182
Radiation Changes	182
Other Non-Neoplastic Conditions	183
Endometriosis	183
Mesonephric Remnants and Hyperplasia	183
Cervical Polyp	185
Ectopic Tissue	186

NORMAL STRUCTURE

ANATOMY

The cervix is the lower part of the uterus. A fibromuscular junction, usually referred to as the internal cervical os, marks the junction between the muscular corpus and the predominantly fibrous cervix. The cervix projects into the vagina at the vaginal vault and has supravaginal and vaginal portions of approximately equal lengths. The folds of mucosa between vagina and cervix are known as the vaginal fornices. The cervix is roughly cylindrical and is about 3 cm long and 2.5 cm in diameter, although the exact dimensions and shape vary considerably, depending largely on the parity of the woman. The multiparous cervix is larger and more bulbous than the nulliparous and has a transverse and slit-like, rather than circular, external os.

The cervical canal connects the uterine cavity to the vagina and it is flattened from front to back. The external os is a rather imprecise landmark, indicating the point at which the cervical canal opens into the vagina. Tissue that lies outside the external os, on the vaginal portion of the cervix, is referred to as ectocervix or exocervix. That located above the external os, within the canal, is endocervix (Figures 8.1 and 8.2). While strictly incorrect, many histopathologists use these terms to describe the type of tissue found rather than its position. Thus, a biopsy consisting of stroma, glandular surface epithelium, and crypts may be described as endocervical, even though the material may come from a position on the vaginal portion of the cervix, well outside the external os.

NATIVE (ORIGINAL) SQUAMOUS EPITHELIUM

The epithelium covering the cervix is initially of two types, which are laid down during embryologic development. These can be described as the 'native' (or original) squamous and columnar epithelia of the cervix. The interface

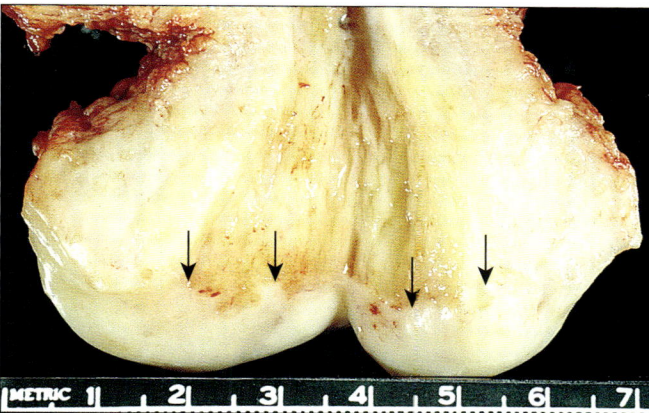

Figure 8.1 Normal cervix. The specimen has been opened to show the rough appearance of the cervical canal in contrast to the smoothness of the ectocervix. The squamocolumnar junction (arrows) is clearly visible.

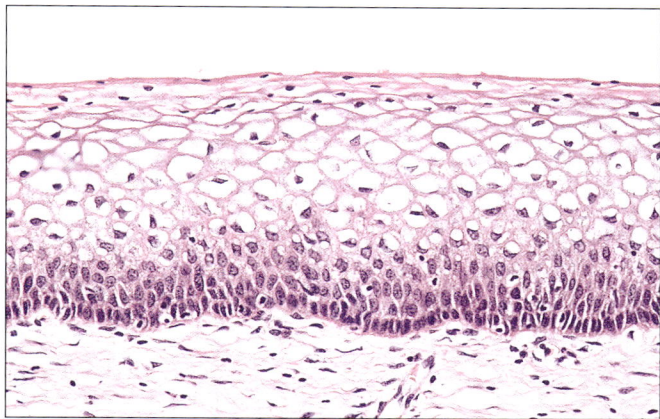

Figure 8.3 Original squamous epithelium in a woman of reproductive age. Maturation of the squamous epithelium is obvious. The basal layer, parabasal zone, intermediate zone, and superficial layer can be clearly distinguished.

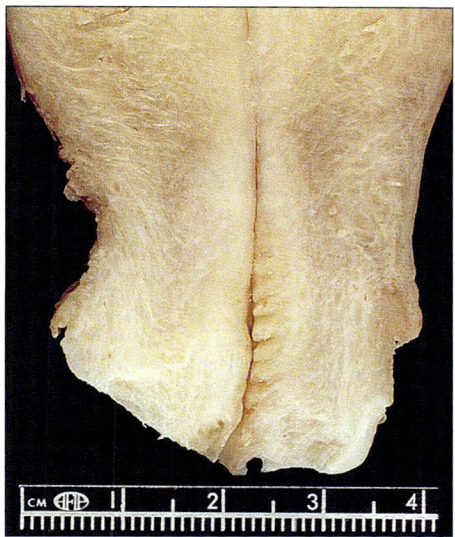

Figure 8.2 Normal cervix. On cross section, the normal cervix has serrated papillary folds that form the plicae of the endocervical canal.

between these two epithelium types is dynamic, and later is the site of the transformation zone.

The squamous epithelium is stratified and nonkeratinizing. It is under the influence of ovarian hormones just as is the vaginal epithelium, although the changes in response to hormonal stimuli are less marked than those encountered in the vagina. The normal appearance in a woman of reproductive age is shown in Figure 8.3.

There is a more or less well-defined layer of basal cells, which have a relatively high nuclear to cytoplasmic ratio, and is usually only one cell thick. The nuclei are slightly oval and oriented vertically, giving a so-called 'picket-fence' appearance; this is an important histologic marker of 'normality' in the squamous epithelium. Lying above this is a layer of parabasal cells, also with large nuclei and sparse, dense cytoplasm. Maturation progresses to form the intermediate zone, in which the cells begin to flatten out. The nuclei of these cells are smaller and darker than those of the parabasal layer, with considerably more cytoplasm. Glycogen, demonstrable in the cytoplasm of the intermediate cells, may take on a characteristic pattern described as 'basket-weave.' The superficial cells have pyknotic nuclei, from which all nuclear detail is lost. The cytoplasm appears, in sections, as a narrow, compressed band of slightly eosinophilic material.

In describing both normal and abnormal squamous epithelium, the terms 'differentiation,' 'maturation,' and 'stratification' are frequently used. These terms are closely interrelated in meaning, but are not quite synonymous.

Terminology

Differentiation. Differentiation, in this context, refers to the process in which the squamous cells become fully functional as a flattened, protective layer. In the skin, which is exposed to the external environment, full differentiation involves keratinization by way of a granular layer, but in the normal cervix, where the surroundings are moist, differentiation does not involve keratinization. The epithelium is said to be 'cornified' and no granular layer is present. In normal epithelium, maturation and differentiation are virtually synonymous, i.e., the cells differentiate as they mature. In abnormal epithelium, in common with other premalignant and malignant states, the term differentiation relates to the degree of morphologic and functional similarity between abnormal and normal cells at all stages of maturation. Therefore, the equivalence of differentiation with maturation diminishes as the epithelium becomes more abnormal.

Maturation. Maturation is closely related to differentiation in meaning, and characterizes the changes seen in cells as they reach the surface of normal squamous epithelium. Thus, a squamous cell that is mature is also well differentiated. An immature squamous cell should also show some degree of differentiation that enables it to be recognized as squamous in type.

Stratification. In squamous epithelium, stratification is a necessary and definitional consequence of maturation and differentiation. It refers to the way in which the epithelium is divided into layers of progressively more mature and flattened cells as the surface is reached.

Cytologic Correlation

Parabasal Squamous Cells. Parabasal cells exhibit a round shape and dense, green/blue cytoplasm. The large nucleus, which approximates 80–90% of the total cell size, is darkly stained with evenly distributed chromatin. Since these cells are immature squamous cells, they are generally seen in smears from postmenopausal women (Figure 8.4) or postpartum.

Intermediate Squamous Cells. As the squamous epithelium responds to hormonal stimuli, the individual cells mature and the intermediate squamous cells reflect this change, both with an increase in the amount of cytoplasm in relation to the nucleus and in terms of total cell size. The cytoplasm becomes more transparent and tends to stain pale blue. Occasionally an area around the nucleus stains yellow, denoting the presence of glycogen. The nucleus is round with pale-staining, finely granular chromatin (Figure 8.5).

Superficial Squamous Cells. With progressing maturation the superficial squamous cells predominate. The cells are large and polyhedral with angled edges. The pink-staining cytoplasm is virtually transparent, and the pyknotic nuclei are small and densely stained with little or no apparent chromatin structure (Figure 8.6). Keratinization does not occur normally in the cervix, although it is associated with several pathologic conditions.

HORMONAL INFLUENCES ON SQUAMOUS EPITHELIUM

After ovulation, when circulating progesterone counteracts the effect of estrogen on the epithelium, the cervical–vaginal smear shows a predominance of intermediate cells and a decreased number of superficial cells. However, this epithelium is often difficult to appreciate in histologic sections. After menopause, when there is a deficiency of ovarian hormones, the squamous epithelium becomes much thinner, and there is no maturation beyond the parabasal level. The thin epithelium is therefore composed entirely of parabasal cells and may appear quite uniform on section (Figure 8.7). The lack of a mature epithelium, coupled with

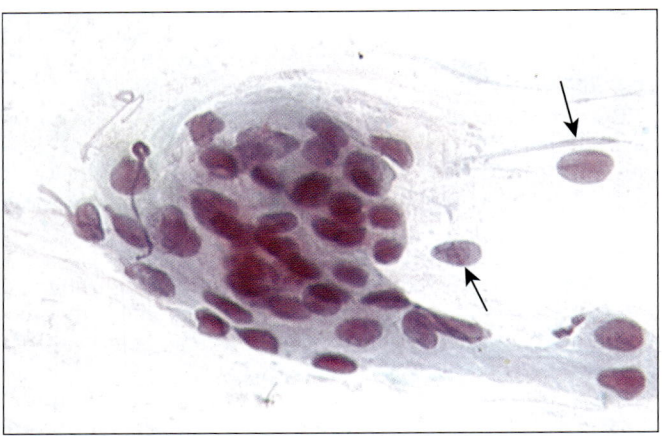

Figure 8.4 Parabasal squamous cells in a cervical smear. Cells with large nuclei with evenly distributed chromatin. Free nuclei (arrows) are present.

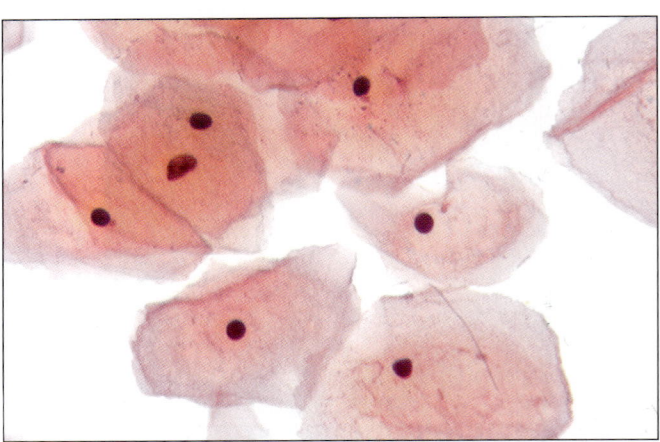

Figure 8.6 Superficial squamous cells in a cervical smear. Large cells with small pyknotic nuclei.

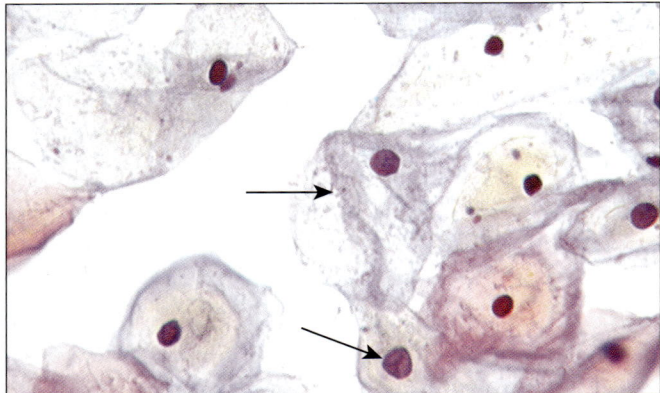

Figure 8.5 Intermediate squamous cells. Cervical smear. Cells show larger nuclei (arrows) than those seen in the superficial cells.

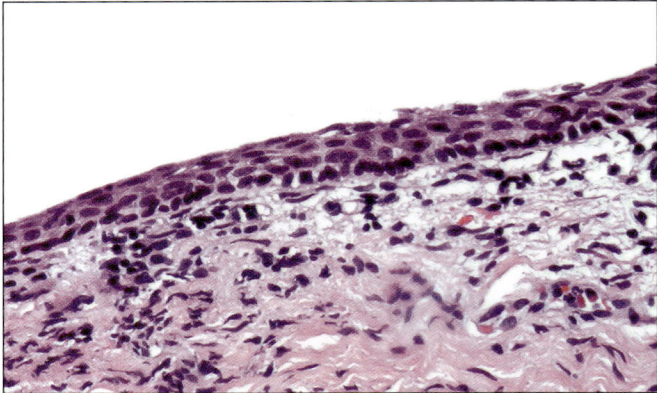

Figure 8.7 Atrophic squamous epithelium. In a postmenopausal woman, the epithelium is thin and the cells do not mature beyond the parabasal stage.

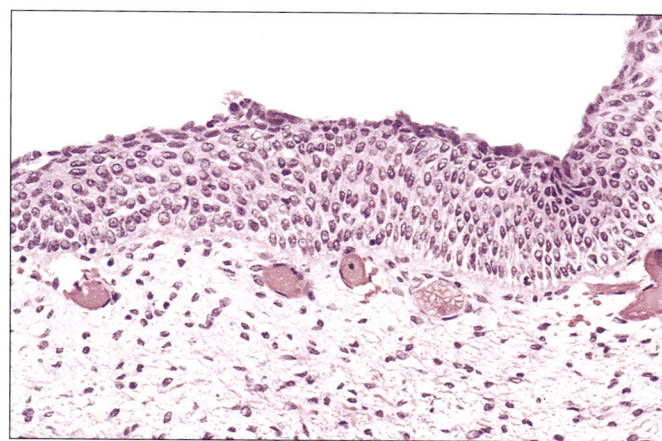

Figure 8.8 Atrophic squamous epithelium in a 6-year-old girl.

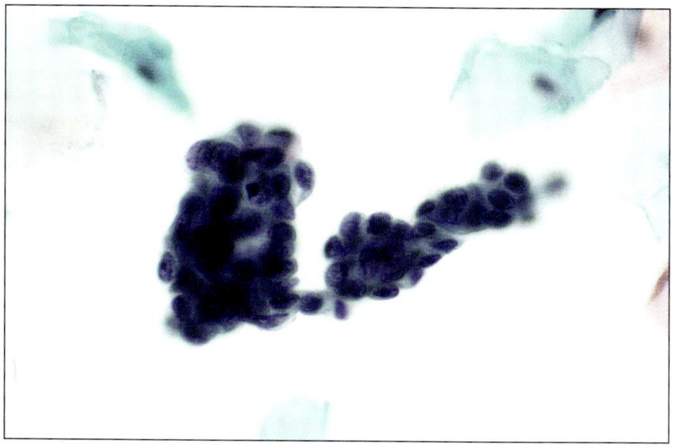

Figure 8.9 Normal endometrial cells in a cervical smear.

the high nuclear to cytoplasmic ratio that the parabasal cells exhibit, can make the distinction from squamous intraepithelial lesion (SIL) difficult (see Chapter 10). However, the regular nuclear contour, the uniform chromatin pattern, and lack of conspicuous mitotic activity point to the correct diagnosis. In difficult cases, the use of immunohistochemical studies will facilitate the correct diagnosis. Atrophic squamous epithelium exhibits little or no proliferative activity, with only focal staining of the basal and parabasal cells with Ki-67 (MIB1). In addition, p16 staining is either negative or minimal.[1] The appearances before puberty are similar (Figure 8.8).

Cytologic Correlation

The proportion of superficial to intermediate squamous cells varies throughout the menstrual cycle. Following menstruation and under the influence of estrogen, the superficial squamous cells predominate. At midcycle the smear may show very few intermediate squamous cells. The background shows few neutrophils and the cells are well separated and clearly displayed. This is the optimum time to take a cervical smear, particularly if the woman is in a cervical screening program.

Following ovulation and under the influence of progesterone, the intermediate cells dominate, forming sheets and clusters of overlapping cells with curled edges. Glycogen can be identified by the yellow staining often seen in the cytoplasm surrounding the nucleus. As this secretory phase continues, the clusters of cells become denser and more ragged looking, and there is an increase in background debris and neutrophils. Not infrequently this renders the smear inadequate for a reliable cytologic evaluation.

Postmenopausal Atrophy. The postmenopausal smear pattern shows a predominance of parabasal and occasional intermediate cell types with no cyclic changes (Figure 8.4). Endocervical cells are frequently not identified. Although a similar pattern is seen postpartum, squamous metaplasia and regenerative changes and endocervical cells are more frequently noted.

Endometrial Cells. Menstrual smears contain increased numbers of leukocytes and varying numbers of red blood cells and endometrial cells. The endometrial cells frequently are found in small darkly stained groups but can be seen in strings or as individual cells, particularly in the late menstrual phase (Figure 8.9). Endometrial cells approximate the size of a neutrophil, with darkly stained coarse chromatin. Nuclei, although normally round, with darkly stained coarse chromatin, often show some irregularity in shape, which may reflect degenerative change. The small amount of cytoplasm usually takes a basophilic stain. Endometrial cells should not normally be seen in a cervical smear after days 10–12 of the menstrual cycle. Not surprisingly, a menstrual smear will frequently be deemed inadequate for reliable assessment, since much cell detail can be obscured.

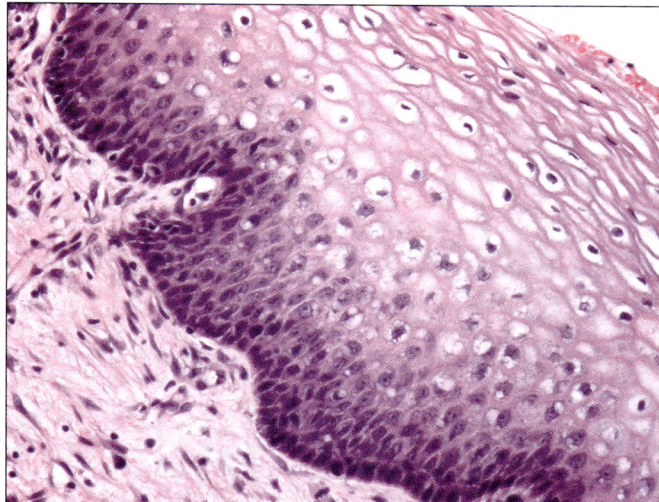

Figure 8.10 Basal cell hyperplasia. The parabasal and basal zones are markedly expanded in an epithelium that is also somewhat thickened. The picket fence appearance of the basal layer is lost.

BASAL CELL HYPERPLASIA

In this condition the basal layer and adjacent part of the parabasal layer form an unusually well-defined stratum that is increased in thickness and is conspicuous because of both nuclear enlargement and cytoplasmic basophilia (Figure 8.10). The oval basal and parabasal nuclei are

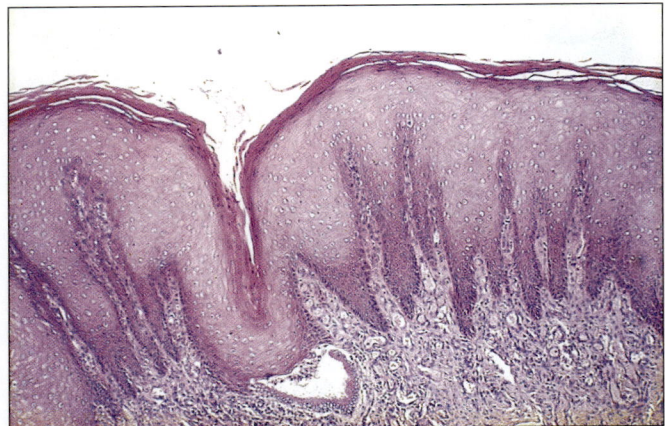

Figure 8.11 Squamous hyperplasia. The epithelium is acanthotic with hyperkeratosis and parakeratosis.

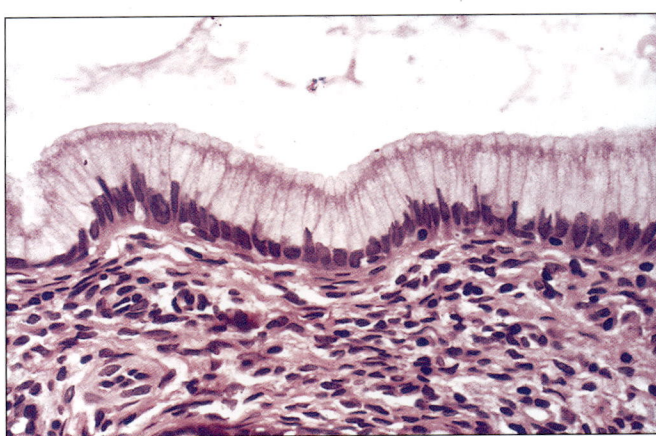

Figure 8.12 Normal endocervical epithelium. The cells are columnar, contain mucin, and the nuclei are basally located.

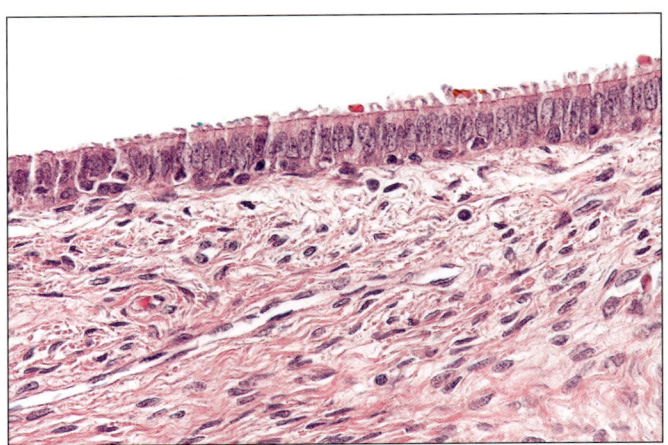

Figure 8.13 Ciliated cells, upper endocervix.

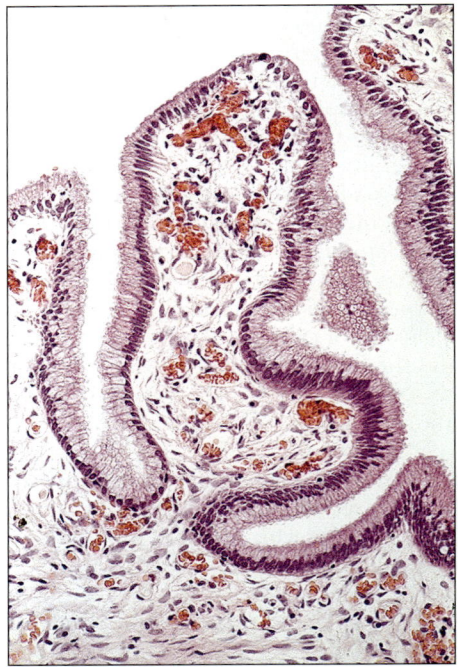

Figure 8.14 Endocervical villi. The papillae exhibit a central fibrous core with blood vessels and a mantle of endocervical mucinous columnar cells.

usually oriented vertically and the picket-fence appearance of a single layer is lost. Nuclear pleomorphism and hyperchromasia are absent. The cells above this stratum are mature and stratified. This condition is usually without import.

SQUAMOUS CELL HYPERPLASIA

The squamous epithelium of the ectocervix becomes thickened when there is uterovaginal prolapse. In these circumstances the epithelium shows acanthosis and there may be an irregularity of the epithelial–stromal junction resembling the rete ridges of the skin. Frequently, there is also hyperkeratosis with/without parakeratosis (Figure 8.11), which may or may not have a granular layer. These changes are the response to mechanical stimulation and take place in the absence of hormonal stimulation. Most prolapses are seen in women after menopause.

Some thickening of the squamous epithelium, often also with keratosis, is frequently seen when the cervix has healed following treatment by laser ablation, laser excision, or large loop diathermy excision. These changes are usually focal and less marked than those seen with prolapse.

NATIVE (ORIGINAL) CERVICAL GLANDULAR EPITHELIUM

Columnar cells line the endocervical canal. The majority of these are tall, thin, mucus-secreting cells with basal nuclei, presenting the familiar picket-fence appearance (Figure 8.12). Ciliated cells are seen in the upper endocervix (Figure 8.13). The epithelium takes the form of villous processes (Figure 8.14) that are seen most dramatically at colposcopy. Although these grape-like villi are characteristic of endocervical tissue colposcopically, they are not always easily seen, particularly in older women. They are, at all ages, more striking when adjacent to the squamocolumnar junction. A further complexity of the endocervical epithelium is the formation of crypts, which are tunnels lined by mucin-secreting epithelium passing into the substance of the cervix, usually to a depth of no more than 3 mm, but on occasion to as much as 1 cm (Figure 8.15). These structures

CHAPTER 8 — CERVICAL BENIGN AND NON-NEOPLASTIC CONDITIONS

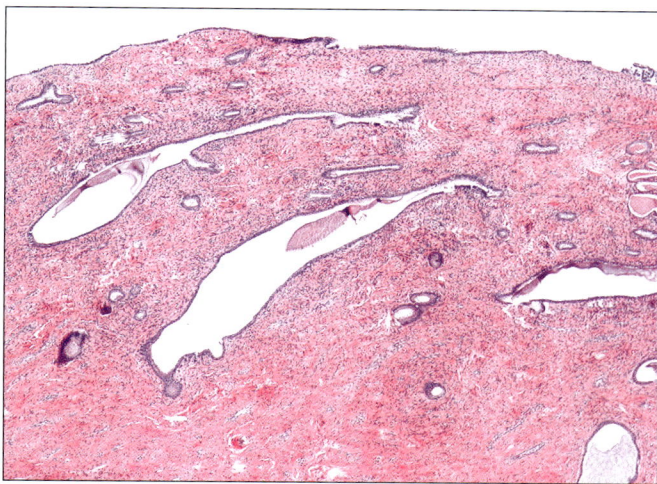

Figure 8.15 Endocervical crypts. Tunnels that are lined by mucinous endocervical columnar epithelium penetrate into the endocervical fibromuscular stroma.

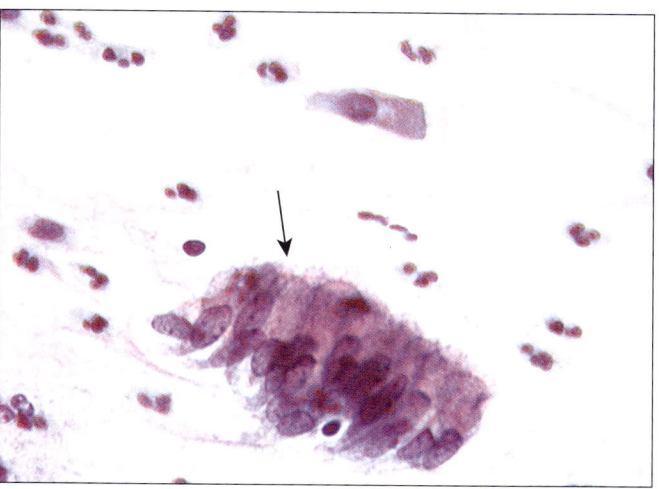

Figure 8.18 Endocervical cells in a cervical smear. Cilia are clearly seen (arrow).

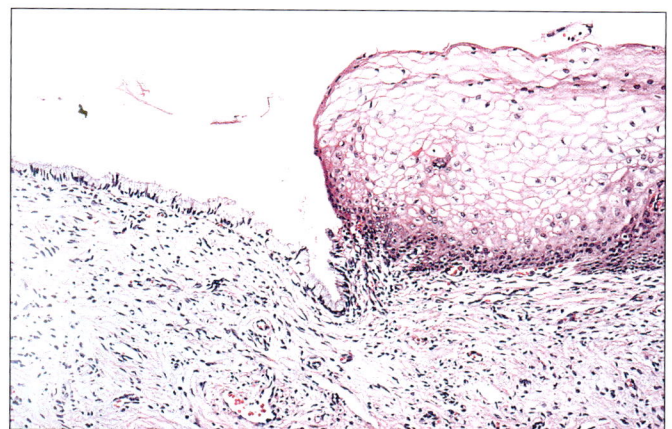

Figure 8.16 Squamocolumnar junction. There is an abrupt transition from squamous to columnar epithelium.

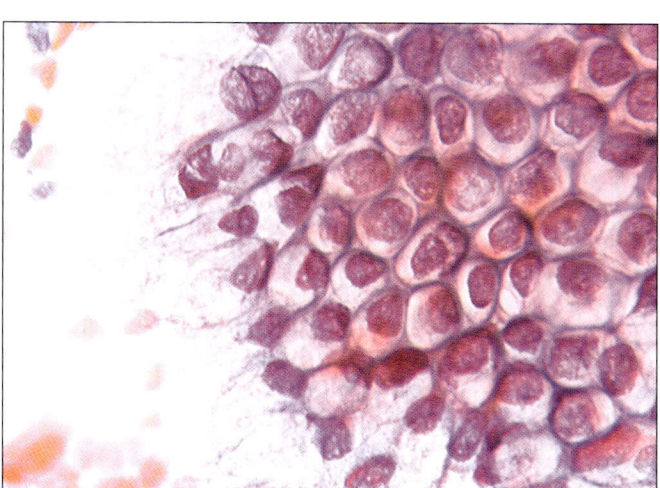

Figure 8.17 Endocervical cells in a cervical smear. Honeycomb arrangement of the cells and mucin in the cytoplasm.

are commonly referred to as 'glands,' but as shown by serial sections they are a system of clefts that may become occluded and thereby form blind-ending tunnels. An awareness that these crypts are present is important when SIL affects the cervix (see Chapter 10). The columnar epithelium of the endocervix meets the squamous epithelium of the ectocervix at the squamocolumnar junction (Figure 8.16). The cytoplasm of the columnar cells stains with mucicarmine and Alcian blue, and is reactive for various mucin antigens, e.g., MUC1, MUC4, and MUC5AC.[2]

Cytologic Correlation

Frequently referred to as 'endocervical cells,' glandular cells of endocervical origin are easily identified in cervical smears. They usually occur in sheets or small groups, although occasionally whole or partial fragments of villi are seen. The nuclei show a finely granular chromatin, sometimes with small nucleoli, and the cells have a cylindrical shape. The pale blue/gray cytoplasm is often vacuolated with poorly defined cell borders (Figure 8.17). Cilia can occasionally be seen with well-defined terminal plates (Figure 8.18). When viewed end on, the round nuclei are centrally placed within the cytoplasm and the close proximity of the cells resembles a honeycomb appearance. Endocervical cells are approximately four to five times larger than endometrial cells, so misinterpretation is uncommon.

PHYSIOLOGIC CHANGES IN THE CERVIX AND THE FORMATION OF THE TRANSFORMATION ZONE

Fundamental to understanding cervical epithelial abnormalities is the formation of the transformation zone. It is in this area of the cervix that SIL and eventually invasive squamous cell carcinoma most commonly develop. The process is represented diagrammatically in Figures 8.19–8.22. Before puberty is reached, the squamocolumnar junction is situated at or near the external cervical os (Figure 8.19). During adolescence the increasing levels of circulating ovarian hormones cause an increase in the bulk both of the body of the uterus and of the cervix, the latter growing proportionally more during this period. A consequence of this increased cervical size is its eversion outward, rather more markedly anteriorly and posteriorly than at the sides. As a result of this change in shape, the endocervical epithelium, together with the underlying crypts and stroma, come to lie on the vaginal portion of the cervix (Figure 8.20). The 'ectopic' endocervical epithelium thus situated on the ectocervix is red and rough. It is red because the columnar epithelium is one cell layer thick and essentially transparent to the rich network of underlying blood vessels. It is rough because of the villous appearance of the endocervical tissue.

The 'transformation zone' is the area where the expected transformation to metaplastic squamous epithelium and abnormal transformation to SIL usually occurs. The process is a rolling outward of the cervical stroma with its crypts and overlying epithelium.

The process of eversion, which gives rise to the transformation zone (ectropion), occurs predominantly during adolescence. Eversion also occurs at other times, notably in the neonatal period and with each pregnancy, after which the squamocolumnar junction regresses to approximately the same position as before that pregnancy. The normal physiologic result of cervical eversion is replacement of the endocervical columnar epithelium by squamous epithelium through the process of squamous metaplasia (Figure 8.21). As menopause approaches, this process reverses, so that the transformation zone tends to pass back into the cervical canal. This process is called 'inversion.' In the postmenopausal woman, the whole transformation zone, whether typical or atypical, may be situated inside the canal and so out of sight both to the naked eye and to colposcopy (Figure 8.22).

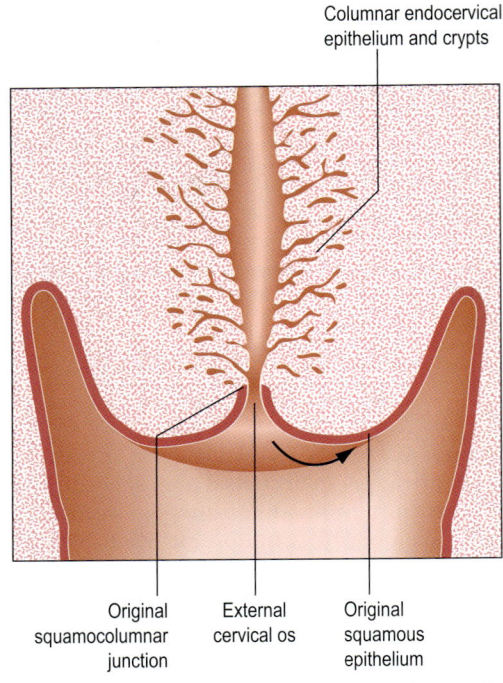

Figure 8.19 Prepubertal cervix. The squamocolumnar junction is situated at the external cervical os. The arrow shows the direction of the movement that takes place as a result of the increase in bulk of the cervix during adolescence.

SQUAMOUS METAPLASIA

This mechanism of squamous metaplasia permits the much tougher and more resistant squamous epithelium to replace

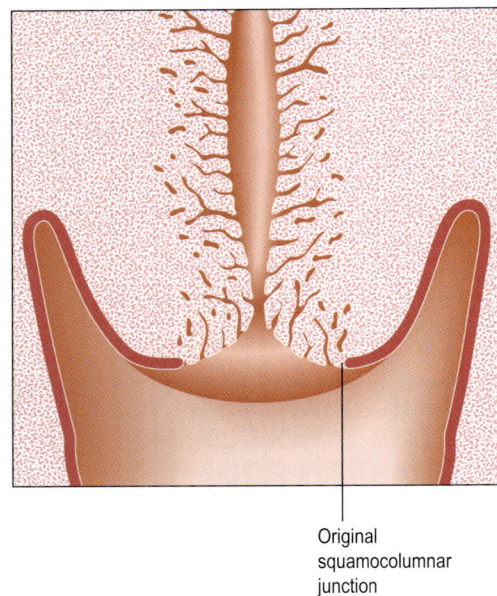

Figure 8.20 The process of eversion. On completion, endocervical columnar tissue lies on the vaginal surface of the cervix and is exposed to the vaginal environment.

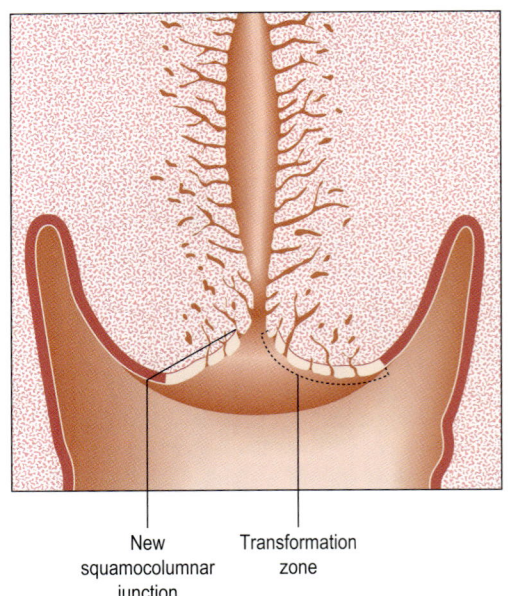

Figure 8.21 Postadolescent cervix. The acidity of the vaginal environment is one of the factors that encourage squamous metaplastic change, replacing the exposed columnar epithelium with squamous epithelium.

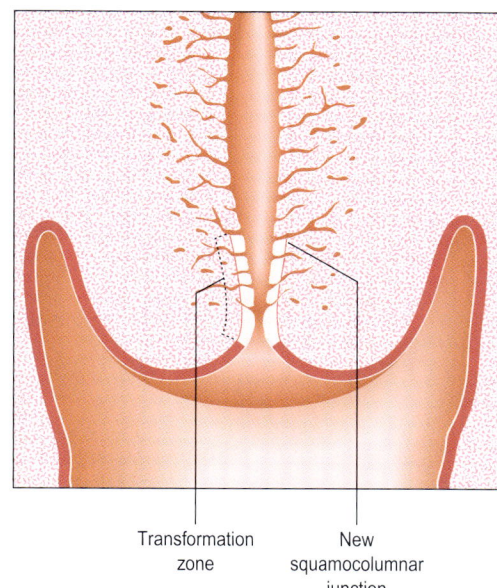

Figure 8.22 Postmenopausal cervix. At this time, cervical inversion occurs. This phenomenon is the reverse of eversion, which was so important in adolescence. The transformation zone is now drawn into the cervical canal, often making it inaccessible to colposcopic examination.

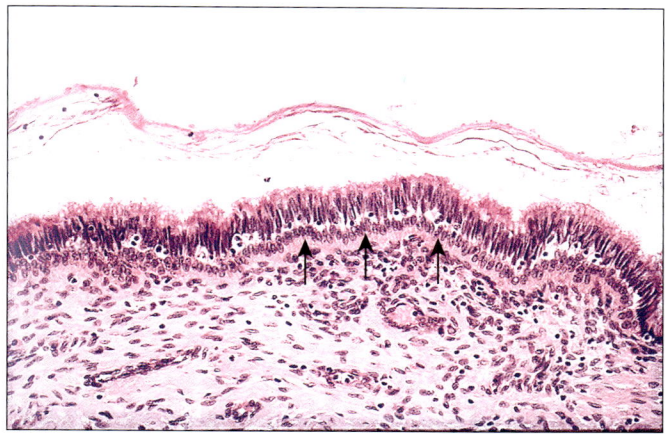

Figure 8.23 Reserve cells. A single row of reserve cells (arrows) is present beneath the columnar epithelium.

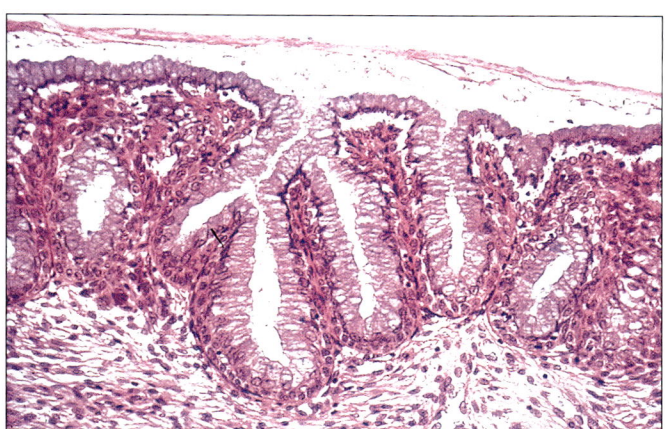

Figure 8.24 Reserve cell proliferation. The reserve cells proliferate to form several layers beneath the still intact columnar epithelium.

the highly specialized, fragile columnar cells of the endocervical epithelium normally present.

The columnar cells do not, of course, transform into squamous cells, as mature epithelial cells of one type cannot change to differentiate and become another cell type. The stimulus to squamous metaplasia in the cervix appears to be the increased acidity of the vaginal environment compared with that of the cervical canal. Figures 8.23–8.33 show stages in the evolution of a metaplastic squamous epithelium. Reserve cells are located beneath the columnar epithelial cells and they give origin to metaplastic squamous cells (Figure 8.23).

The origin of these reserve cells is from a population of cytokeratin 7-positive stem cells located at the transformation zone. It is this population of stem cells that replenishes basal reserve cells, generates the squamous metaplastic cells in the transformation zone, and is the stem cell of cervical SIL and carcinoma.[3] Reserve cells first proliferate as a row of nondescript, small, round cells beneath the columnar epithelium, usually following the contour of the basement membrane (Figure 8.24). Incomplete and immature squamous metaplasia may show columnar cells not totally replaced by squamous cells (Figure 8.25).

As the process continues, the squamous cells make up the whole thickness of the epithelium and start their differentiation to maturity, eventually rendering the metaplastic epithelium indistinguishable from normal, mature, glycogenated squamous epithelium. Metaplastic squamous epithelium may be mistaken for SIL. Figure 8.26 illustrates this dilemma. The epithelium is composed of squamous cells that are immature up to the surface of the epithelium, a feature that is often considered an important diagnostic criterion in the diagnosis of SIL regardless of grade. However, the metaplastic nuclei are regular and round or oval, each with a single, prominent nucleolus, in contrast to SIL where pleomorphism is the rule. The nuclei in metaplastic epithelium lack hyperchromasia and mitotic figures are few, confined to the basal layers, and not abnormal. In addition, normal immature squamous cells are unreactive for p16, which is a surrogate marker for integrated high-risk human papillomavirus (HPV) DNA and almost always seen in high-grade SIL (HSIL).[1,4–6]

In its final state, mature metaplastic squamous epithelium may be histologically indistinguishable from the original squamous epithelium. The only clue to its origin within the transformation zone is the presence of underlying crypts with their mucinous epithelium (Figure 8.27). Squamous metaplasia occurs most notably at the time of adolescence and during pregnancy but may be found in the cervix of women who entered menopause long before.

Although squamous metaplasia is a change that mainly involves the surface epithelium of the cervix, the crypts are also commonly affected (Figure 8.28). Sometimes the crypt

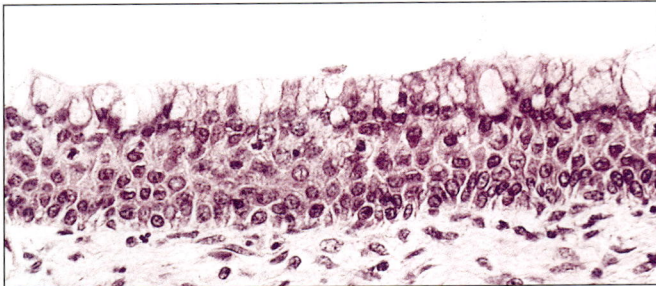

Figure 8.25 Immature squamous metaplasia. As the process progresses, the cells acquire more abundant eosinophilic cytoplasm, stratified into multiple layers, and appear as immature squamous cells lacking intracytoplasmic glycogen. Commonly, a layer of mucinous epithelium lies superficial to the metaplastic cells.

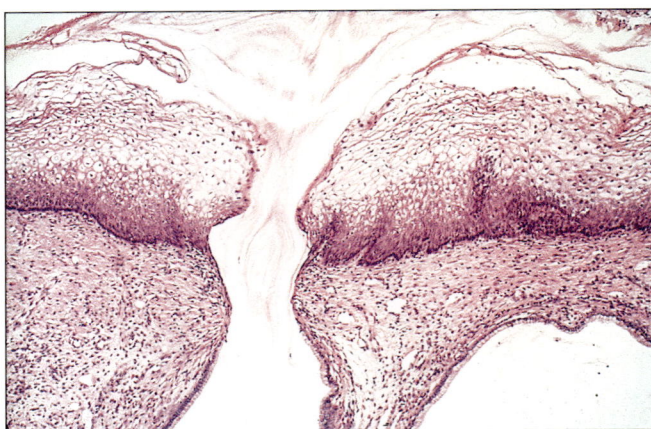

Figure 8.27 Mature squamous metaplasia. The mature metaplastic squamous epithelium here overlies gland crypts, lined by columnar epithelium. Mucin is being discharged from a gland opening.

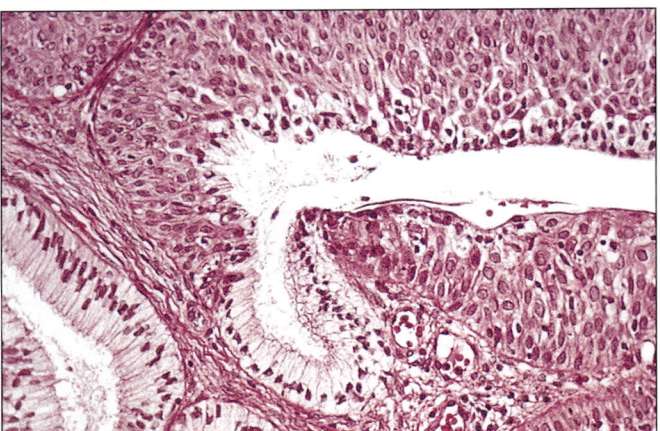

Figure 8.26 Immature squamous metaplasia. The lack of differentiation and maturation can cause confusion with intraepithelial neoplasia.

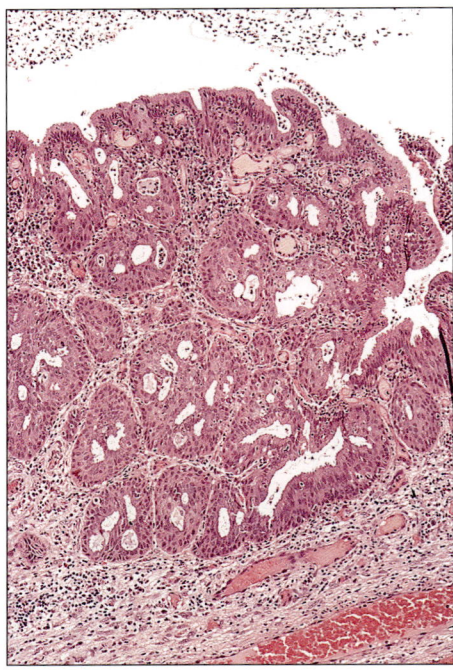

Figure 8.28 Squamous metaplasia in an early stage exhibiting hyperplasia of the reserve cells and immature cells. At this stage, the glandular tissue is only partially replaced. As the metaplastic process continues, the amount of residual glandular tissue will decrease and then disappear.

involvement is sufficiently marked to impart an initial impression of invasive carcinoma. In the cervix, the pathologist should be wary of entertaining a diagnosis of frank malignancy when there is a layer of mucinous columnar epithelium that overlies the questionably cancerous tissue.

Cytologic Correlation

An important aspect associated with recognizing squamous metaplasia cytologically is that metaplastic cells exhibit a wide variety of appearances. Within a single cervical smear, both immature and mature cell types are frequently seen together with the whole spectrum of change (Figures 8.29–8.31). From a cytologic perspective, the terms 'immature' and 'mature' have a slightly different meaning from that used by histopathologists. Cells arising from a histologically mature metaplastic epithelium will be virtually indistinguishable from mature squamous cells. The term mature as used by the cytologist describes cells that show some features of differentiation but still show some characteristics seen in immature metaplastic cells.

In the earliest phase of change, small round cells with a narrow rim of green-staining cytoplasm appear that closely resemble endocervical cells. The nuclei are often hyperchromatic with coarsely clumped chromatin. They are usually seen in small tight groups, a feature that makes recognition easier (Figure 8.29). The cells arising from an area of immature metaplasia are normally round in shape with large, darkly staining nuclei with a coarse chromatin pattern that may contain nucleoli or chromocenters. The cytoplasm is dense with a well-defined cell border and usually stains green (Figure 8.30). Differentiation from HSIL should in most instances be straightforward by attention to the absence of pleomorphism. However, immature metaplasia remains a source of error in diagnosis.

Mature Metaplasia. As the metaplastic epithelium matures, the individual cells assume a squamoid appearance. The cytoplasm becomes more abundant and the cell appears oval or elongated. The cytoplasm may stain either blue or pink but it does not achieve the transparency of a mature squamous cell. Not infrequently the cytoplasm may be pulled out into tails and projections, the remnants of intercellular bridges. The nucleus becomes less dominant with a finer chromatin structure, but it always appears larger in comparison to the nucleus of a squamous cell (Figure 8.31).

THE CONGENITAL TRANSFORMATION ZONE (CTZ)

The congenital transformation zone is a common variant of squamous metaplasia that is found in a position peripheral to the acquired transformation zone. It appears as partially mature squamous epithelium that has an irregular, dentate junction with the stroma.

The CTZ is a variant of squamous metaplasia that exhibits incomplete maturation (Figure 8.32). The deeper layers show the same features as a maturing squamous metaplasia. The nuclei are large but regular, with prominent nucleoli. There is minimal pleomorphism, and mitotic figures, which are infrequent, can usually be found with diligent searching. A layer of hyperkeratosis or parakeratosis is often present, and this layer, when thick, corresponds to the leukoplakia that is a characteristic colposcopic feature of the CTZ. One of the most striking histologic features is the pattern of its lower margin, the epithelial–stromal junction. This is always irregularly dentate, presenting an appearance akin to the rete ridges of the skin. Sometimes the tips of these epithelial incursions into the stroma appear detached from the overlying epithelium, so that they may give the impression of invasive buds. This impression may be heightened when the centers of the processes undergo differentiation, so that a whorl of keratin is seen in the center (Figure 8.33). Attention to the cytologic features will show that the CTZ is not an invasive tumor. It is unusual for there to be any stromal reaction to the CTZ. Another cardinal feature is the absence of cytoplasmic glycogen (i.e., no 'basket-weave' pattern). This causes the epithelium to be iodine negative on examination, further attracting the attention of the colposcopist.

HISTOGENESIS OF THE CONGENITAL TRANSFORMATION ZONE

The colposcopic and histologic appearances of the CTZ are identical to one of the appearances seen in diethylstilbestrol (DES) exposure. It is very likely that the mechanism by

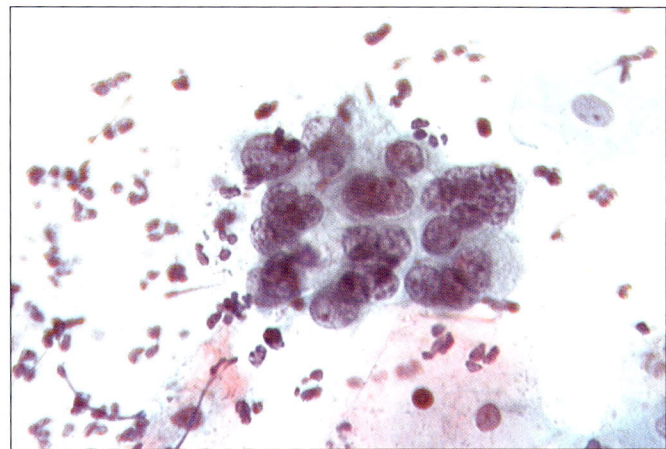

Figure 8.29 Early squamous metaplasia in a cervical smear. The cells, almost indistinguishable from endocervical cells, show clumped chromatin.

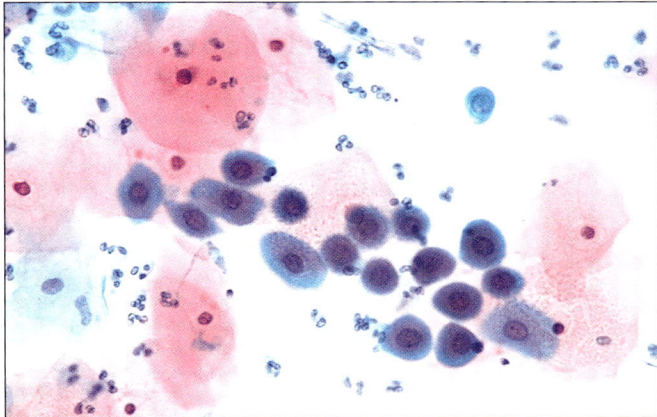

Figure 8.30 Squamous metaplasia in a cervical smear. Darkly stained, small nuclei within basophilic cytoplasm.

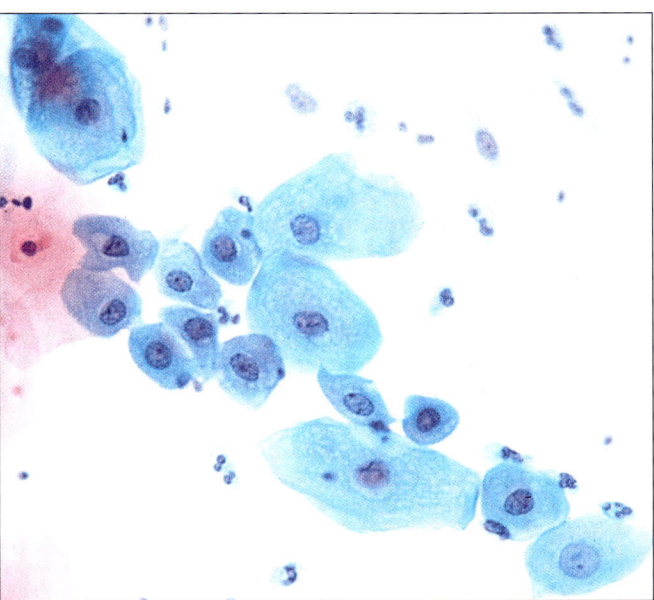

Figure 8.31 Squamous metaplasia in a cervical smear. Some cells show smaller nuclei with an increased amount of cytoplasm and a more squamoid appearance.

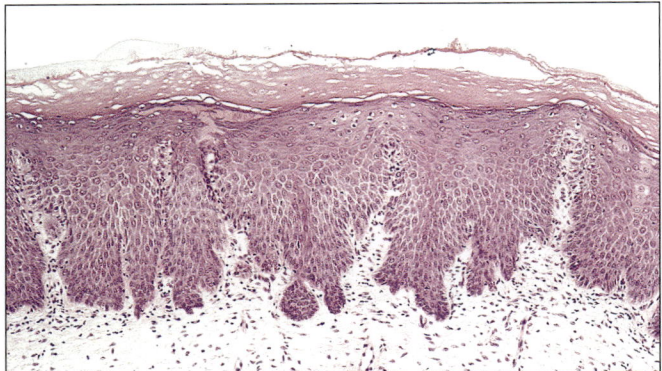

Figure 8.32 Congenital transformation zone. The epithelium has many features of metaplastic squamous epithelium. Highly characteristic is the irregular, dentate outline of the epithelial–stromal junction.

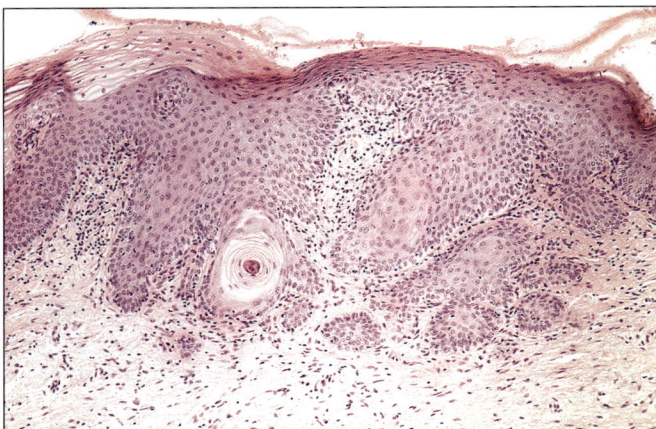

Figure 8.33 Congenital transformation zone. An obvious keratin pearl is present deep within the epithelium.

which the condition develops is the same. As detailed in Chapter 10, during embryogenesis squamous epithelium replaces the glandular epithelium of müllerian type that originally lines the uterovaginal canal. Normally, squamous epithelium advances from below to cover the whole of the vagina and the ectocervix by the time of birth. If arrested for some reason, then some müllerian glandular epithelium remains and is called adenosis in the vagina and ectropion on the ectocervix. This is gradually replaced by squamous epithelium in later intrauterine life and perhaps also for some time after birth.

The product of this late squamous change is seen as the CTZ. The line of demarcation between the CTZ and the original squamous epithelium is the point at which the normal squamous development arrested. As in DES-exposed individuals, this is nearly always a single line. The process hardly ever seems to occur in a patchy fashion, which would leave areas of CTZ in the vagina.

The morphologic appearances of the CTZ through the light microscope are more similar to squamous metaplasia than to SIL, with minimal pleomorphism and few mitotic figures. However, the colposcopic features of the CTZ more closely resemble SIL than a benign condition, often showing an acetowhite color and mosaicism. The behavior of the CTZ, as seen in our own patients who have been followed for many years, has shown no progression toward malignancy, either to SIL or to invasive disease.

Cytologic Correlation

The cytologic features of cells arising from the CTZ are similar in appearance to those arising from squamous metaplasia, although on occasion there may be a predominance of cells showing cytoplasmic keratinization.

INFLAMMATORY CERVICITIS AND REACTIVE CHANGES

The term 'chronic cervicitis' often conveys differing images to the clinician, colposcopist, and pathologist. It describes the clinical appearance of a cervix that is red, inflamed, and irregular on the surface. On colposcopic examination, the 'inflamed' cervix usually shows a wide transformation zone that is red and rough, and the everted glandular epithelium produces excessive mucus. The picture is further enhanced by retention cysts (nabothian cysts), which result when squamous metaplasia obliterates the outlet of cervical crypts. It is almost universal to find some degree of chronic inflammatory cell infiltrate, predominantly plasma cells with some lymphocytes, in the superficial cervical stroma, but it is only when the infiltrate becomes dense that it is justifiable to use the term chronic cervicitis.

INFECTIVE CERVICITIS

The organisms most commonly responsible for active inflammation in the cervix include those that have been discussed in relation to the vagina: *Candida albicans*, *Trichomonas vaginalis*, *Neisseria gonorrhoeae*, *Gardnerella vaginalis*, and herpes simplex virus (HSV). To this list should be added *Chlamydia trachomatis*, HPV, and cytomegalovirus (CMV). Specific forms of chronic cervicitis that may be seen include tuberculous cervicitis and cervical involvement in schistosomiasis, particularly infestation by *Schistosoma haematobium*. The cervix may also be involved in syphilis, granuloma inguinale, and lymphogranuloma venereum.

A cervix that is acutely inflamed is swollen and red, often with a mucopurulent plug exuding from the external os. Histologically, acute cervicitis shows a dense infiltrate of neutrophils in the stroma. They also involve the columnar and the squamous epithelium, as well as the epithelium of the gland crypts. In severe cases, the columnar epithelium may be eroded and partially replaced by granulation tissue. These changes result not only from infection but also from insults such as chemical irritation, copper-containing intrauterine contraceptive devices, inappropriate tampon use, pessaries, and the trauma of parturition or abortion.

True chronic cervicitis shows lymphocytes, histiocytes, and plasma cells in the cervical tissues. If the cells are present only in small or moderate numbers, their presence may represent the normal population of the cervix. If the infiltrate is dense, with lymphoid follicles (Figure 8.34), particularly if there is an admixture of polymorphonuclear

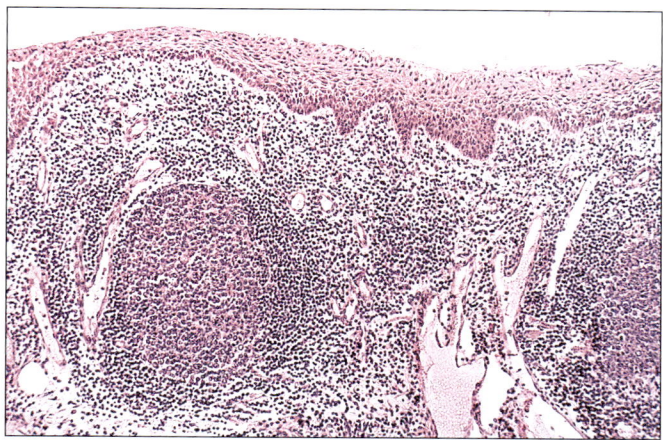

Figure 8.34 Chronic follicular cervicitis. The cervical stroma is densely infiltrated by lymphocytes, with prominent lymphoid follicles.

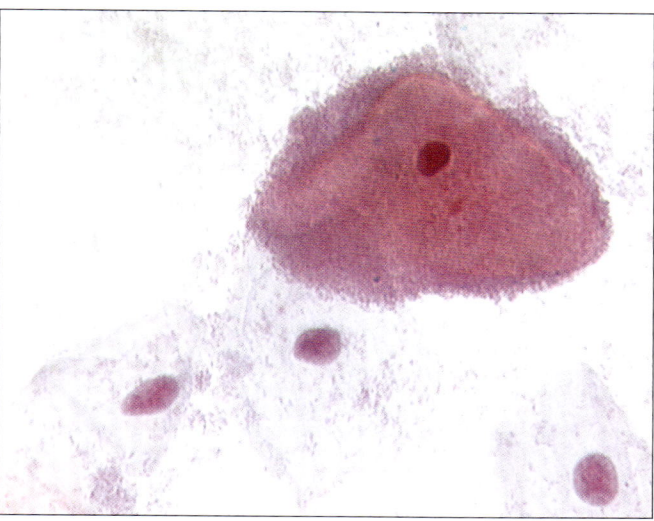

Figure 8.36 Bacterial cervicitis in vaginal smear. Squamous cell covered by bacteria ('clue cell'). A heavy 'coccal' bacterial layer is prominent in the background.

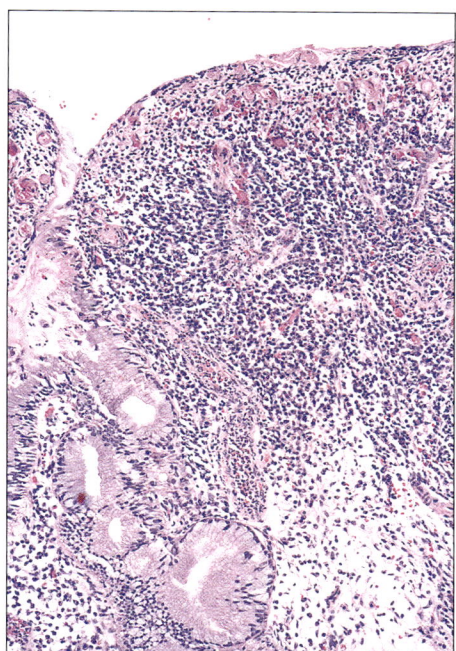

Figure 8.35 Chronic cervicitis. There is a dense infiltrate of lymphocytes and neutrophils with dilated vessels packed with neutrophils.

cells (Figure 8.35), the inflammation is active and is more likely to be pathologic. Many organisms can be isolated from cervices showing chronic cervicitis; indeed, a large number of organisms can be identified in the normal endocervix. Some histologic features may point to specific microorganisms that are responsible for the inflammatory process.[7]

Cytologic Correlation

Cervicitis is a common clinical finding and although often the result of bacterial infection it can be due to trauma, chemical agents, viruses, and radiotherapy. On most occasions it is of little consequence cytologically or clinically.

However, inflammatory changes may mask significant cellular change. The predominance of the inflammation may render dyskaryotic cells more difficult to recognize. The smear is more likely to be inadequate for a reliable assessment in the presence of marked inflammation.

The recognition of bacterial infections in cervical smears is possible and although 'clue cells' (Figure 8.36) have been linked with *G. vaginalis* (bacterial vaginosis) it is not possible to be specific cytologically and microbiologic culture is advisable.

Smears taken from an inflamed cervix may on occasion show numerous bacteria with large numbers of polymorphs. An increase in the number of polymorphs is not in itself an indication of inflammation. Increased numbers of polymorphs can be seen premenstrually and postmenstrually, during pregnancy, with oral contraceptive use, and in the presence of cervical ectropion. Some squamous cells may show mild nuclear enlargement and others may show nuclear pyknosis and karyorrhexis (Figure 8.37). The cells often show eosinophilia or altered staining patterns. Nuclear enlargement of the endocervical glandular cells can occur with occasional small nucleoli and hyperchromasia and rare mitotic figures. The distinction between inflammatory changes and glandular intraepithelial neoplasia can be difficult cytologically.

C. TRACHOMATIS

Infection by *C. trachomatis* initially causes a polymorphonuclear infiltration of both the columnar glandular epithelium and the squamous epithelium, although the inflammation is predominantly endocervical, affecting the crypt field. There may be a focal loss of the surface columnar epithelium. A dense plasma cell infiltrate is found, particularly around the endocervical crypts. Although lymphocytes and histiocytes are always present as well, plasma cells predominate. Germinal center formation is a characteristic feature and this is usually found beneath the surface epithelium and around the gland crypts (Figure 8.38).[7]

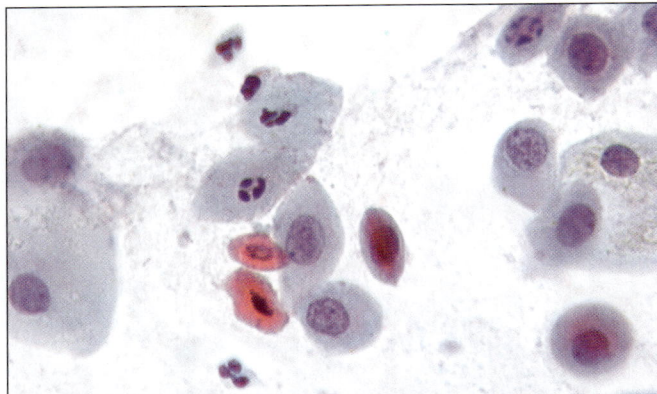

Figure 8.37 Degenerative changes in a cervical smear. Cells show pyknosis and karyorrhexis.

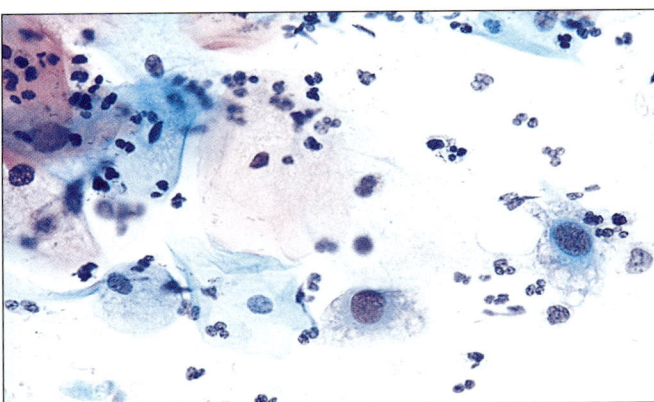

Figure 8.39 Chlamydial infection in a cervical smear. Cells show cytoplasmic vacuolization and a 'moth-eaten' appearance.

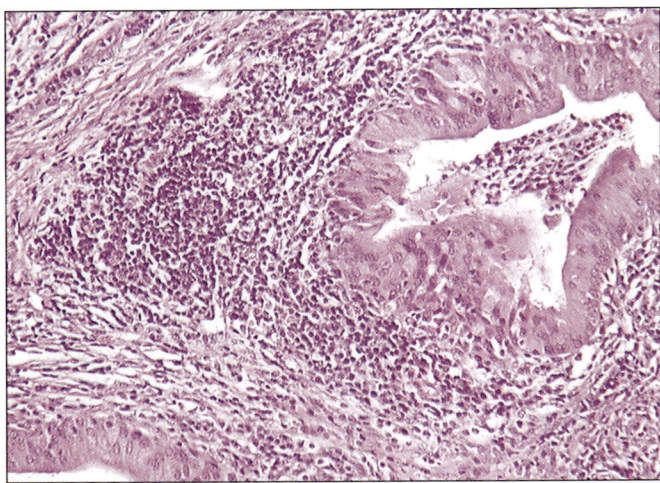

Figure 8.38 Chlamydial cervicitis. A gland crypt surrounded by a dense infiltrate of lymphocytes and plasma cells. The infiltrate also affects the epithelium and is present in the gland lumen.

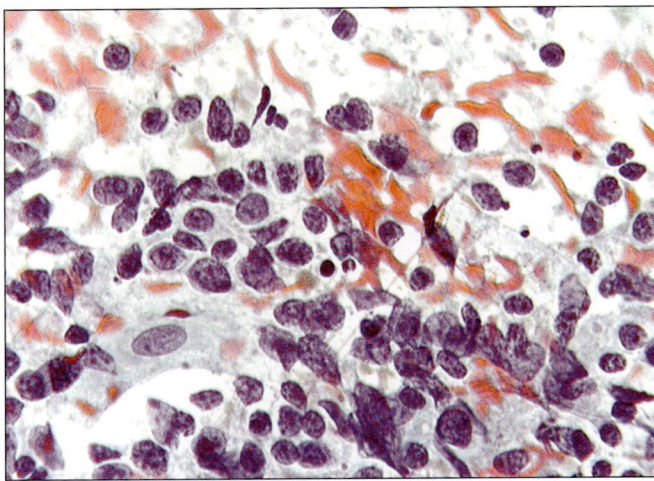

Figure 8.40 Follicular cervicitis in a cervical smear. Immature lymphocytes show variation in size and shape.

Necrosis and destruction of underlying tissue are not features of chlamydial disease.

Cytologic Correlation

The identification of cytoplasmic vacuolization (Figure 8.39) is not a consistent and reliable indicator of the infection. In the presence of *Chlamydia* infection the cervical smear may appear to have a coccal-like background with few polymorphs, and both the squamous and glandular cells show a ragged cytoplasmic border. Because of the association between *Chlamydia* infection and follicular cervicitis, the presence of streaks of lymphocytes, some of which may be immature forms (Figure 8.40), should always raise the suggestion of *Chlamydia* infection, but the diagnosis is best made by culture or molecular diagnostic technology.

TUBERCULOSIS

Cervical tuberculosis is rare in both the United States and the UK. It occurs consequent to infection from upper genital tract disease, which in turn originates from pulmonary tuberculosis. It occurs in about 8% of women with genital tuberculosis.[8,9] The clinical presentation is either as a predominantly hypertrophic lesion that clinically may be mistaken for carcinoma or predominantly ulcerative. Microscopy shows the typical epithelioid cell granulomas of tuberculosis (Figure 8.41), which may be caseating, together with hyperplasia of the epithelial elements; the latter is seen particularly in the hypertrophic variety. Langhans-type giant cells are usually present and the periphery of the tubercle shows a heavy infiltrate of lymphocytes and plasma cells. Acid-fast bacilli can sometimes be demonstrated.

SYPHILIS

Syphilis is a chronic venereal infection caused by *Treponema pallidum*, which gains access directly through the skin and mucosa of the lower genital tract. The primary chancre is usually on the vulva but may be found on the cervix in 10–40% of women with syphilis. The cervix may be firm,

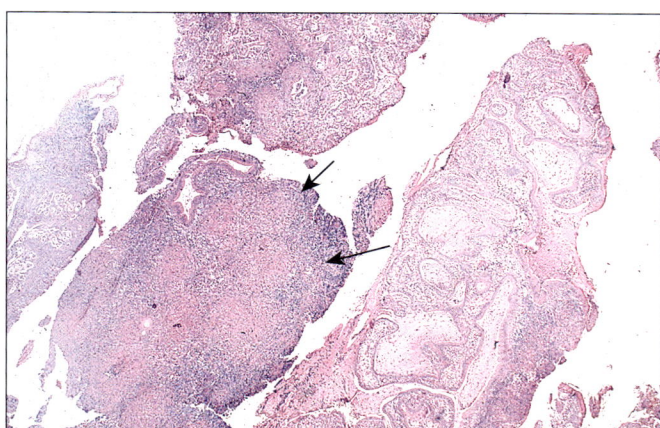

Figure 8.41 Tuberculosis. Curetted material containing fragments of cervical tissue with prominent granulomas containing Langerhans-type giant cells (arrows).

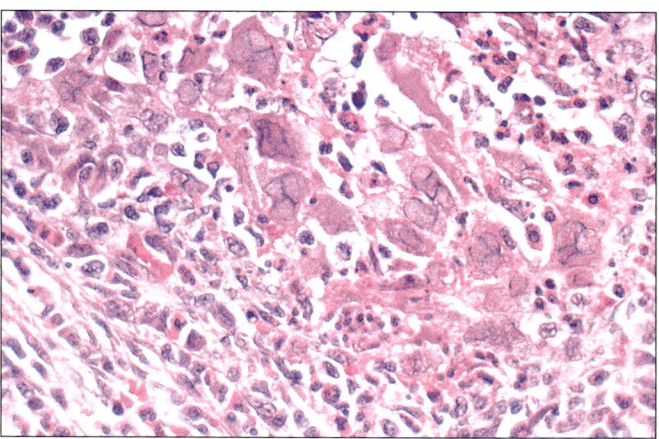

Figure 8.43 Herpes simplex infection. There is lysis of the epithelial tissue. Multinucleated giant cells are present, showing margination of chromatin and a 'ground-glass' appearance of the nuclei.

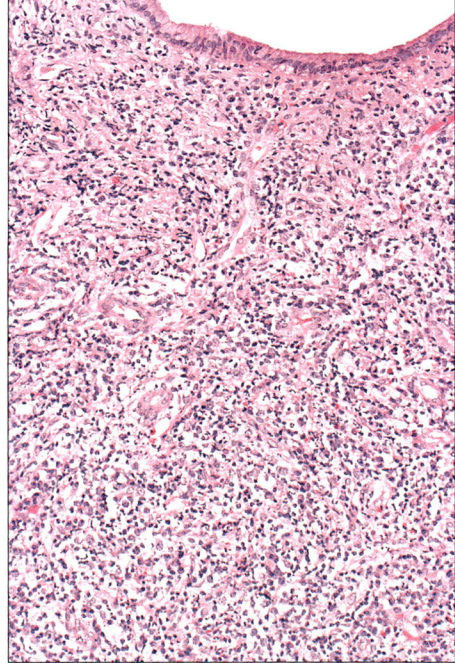

Figure 8.42 Syphilis. A dense plasma cell infiltrate is present, with vasculitis.

nodular, and ulcerating, mimicking cervical carcinoma in some cases. The histologic features are a dense plasma cell infiltration that is most prominent beneath the epithelium (Figure 8.42). Vasculitis, exhibiting plasma cells and lymphocytes together with endothelial cell hyperplasia, is often prominent. Syphilis is one of several venereal infections that a woman may contract today.[10,11] Over one-fifth of women with human immunodeficiency virus (HIV) infection also have syphilis.[12]

HSV

HSV may give rise to an acute infection, which may be severe and necrotizing. The histologic features depend upon the stage of the disease. Even before the small, painful vesicles that are present throughout the lower genital tract appear, the parabasal cells of the squamous epithelium and the columnar endocervical epithelial cells show nuclear enlargement and cytoplasmic swelling accompanied by enlarged nucleoli. Lysis follows after about 36 hours, resulting in vacuoles within the squamous epithelium. Multinucleated giant cells are found around and beneath the vacuoles, but may also be present elsewhere in the epithelium. The multinucleated cells have pleomorphic nuclei with nuclear molding but no overlapping. The nuclear chromatin marginates to give the nuclei a ground-glass appearance (Figure 8.43). Rarely, a single eosinophilic intranuclear rounded inclusion (Cowdry type A inclusion) may be seen. The adjacent epithelium may show basal cell hyperplasia.

Further progression of HSV infection results in acute necrotizing cervicitis where there is extensive necrosis and destruction of stroma, glands, and vessels. These appearances are no longer diagnostic, with a dense stromal infiltrate of mixed acute and chronic inflammatory cells. The inflammation may be distinguished from infection by *C. trachomatis* because it is not localized to the periglandular or subepithelial zone, and extends deep into the underlying tissue, often deeper than the crypt field. Furthermore, plasma cells are not prominent and germinal centers are not encountered.

Cytologic Correlation

HSV is primarily identified by the presence of large multinucleated cells. Multiple nuclei are present that mold one another but do not overlap. The nuclei show variation in size with margination of chromatin and a ground-glass appearance (Figure 8.44). In the late stages of the infection the smear may contain only necrotic debris with few, if any, characteristic multinucleate cells. This necrotizing pattern may resemble that seen in invasive squamous carcinoma.

CYTOMEGALOVIRUS (CMV)

CMV infection of the cervix may be sexually transmitted or it may occur as part of a systemic infection. The

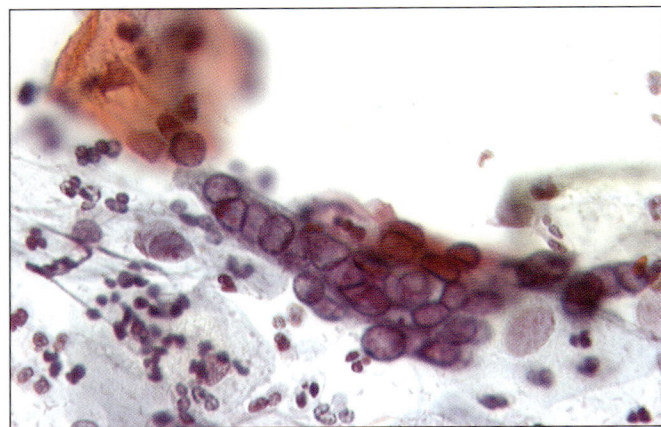

Figure 8.44 HSV in a cervical smear. Molded nuclei with chromatin margination and a 'ground-glass' appearance.

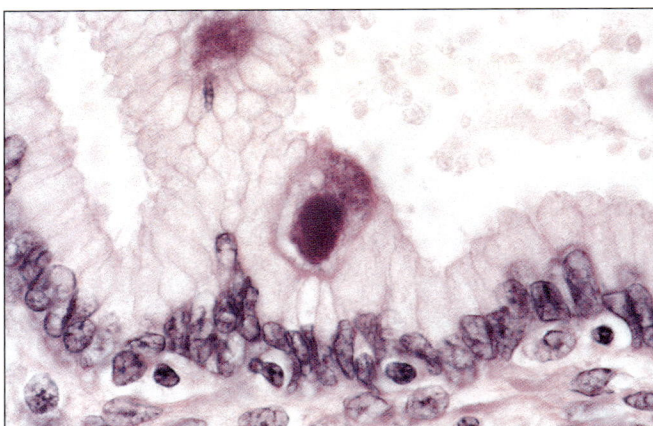

Figure 8.46 CMV infection. A higher magnification of the characteristic CMV intracytoplasmic inclusion.

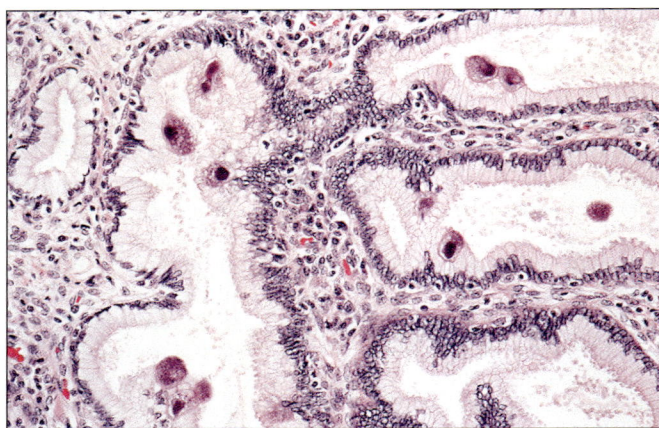

Figure 8.45 CMV infection. Several endocervical cells within the crypt epithelium show large, rounded, basophilic inclusions.

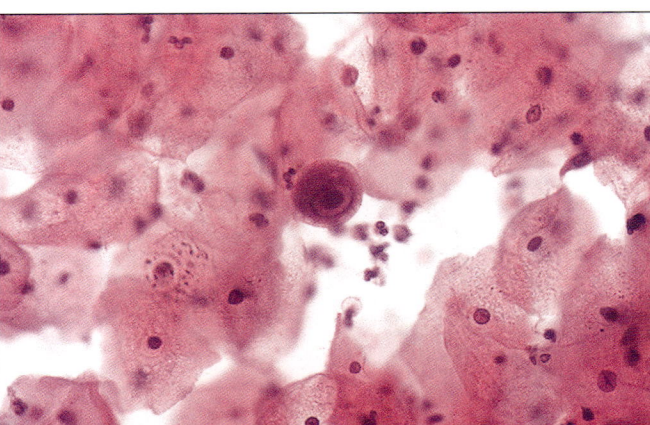

Figure 8.47 CMV infection in a cervical smear. A single cell shows a large central intranuclear inclusion.

characteristic feature is the presence of large, basophilic, intranuclear inclusions, which affect only a minority of epithelial cells in the endocervical crypts (Figures 8.45–8.47) and, occasionally, in endothelial or mesenchymal cells. Associated cytoplasmic inclusions are also found. Associated morphologic features may include fibrin thrombi within small blood vessels, a dense active inflammatory infiltrate, lymphoid follicles, and vacuolated glandular epithelial cells.[13] This appearance is distinctive, and the differential diagnosis from other significant lesions is not difficult. Because the abnormal nuclei are widely separated by normal cells, the distinction from glandular intraepithelial neoplasia is easy.

HUMAN PAPILLOMA VIRUS (HPV)

See Chapters 9 and 10.

SCHISTOSOMIASIS

Although rare in the United States and Western Europe, schistosomiasis is among the most important and widespread of parasitic diseases, and is endemic in tropical and subtropical areas.[14] Schistosomiasis is a cause of infertility when the fallopian tube is involved. The cervical lesions are ulcerative or nodular and may present as papillomatous growths. The ova of the causative organism, *S. haematobium*, become embedded in the tissue and produce a range of tissue reactions (Figure 8.48). The most sensitive diagnostic procedure is a bedside microscopic examination of a wet cervical biopsy crushed between two glass slides, looking for ova.[15] No studies have associated *S. haematobium* infestation with cervical cancer, although infection with the schistosomes seems to favor persistent genital HPV infection, either by traumatizing the genital epithelium and/or by local immunosuppression.[16]

Cytologic Correlation

The ova of this parasite are occasionally found in cervical smears. The thick semitransparent shell can be clearly seen. The spine's location identifies the species: *S. haematobium* has a terminal spike (Figure 8.49) and *S. mansoni* has one that is lateral.

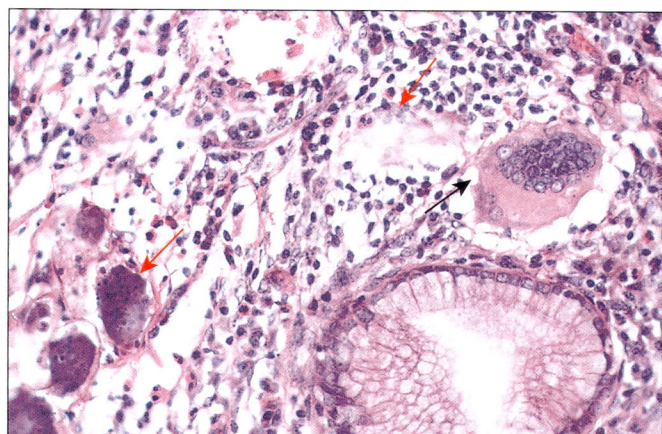

Figure 8.48 Schistosomiasis. The tissue reaction to the ova (red arrows) includes a large, multinucleated, foreign-body giant cell (black arrow).

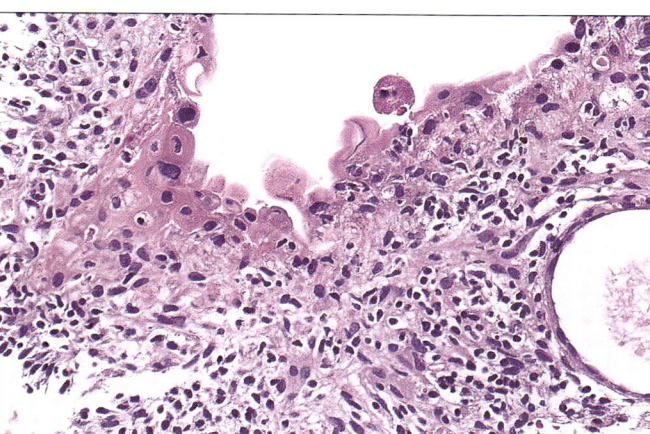

Figure 8.50 Epithelial inflammatory changes. The nuclei are large and hyperchromatic. There is abundant eosinophilic cytoplasm.

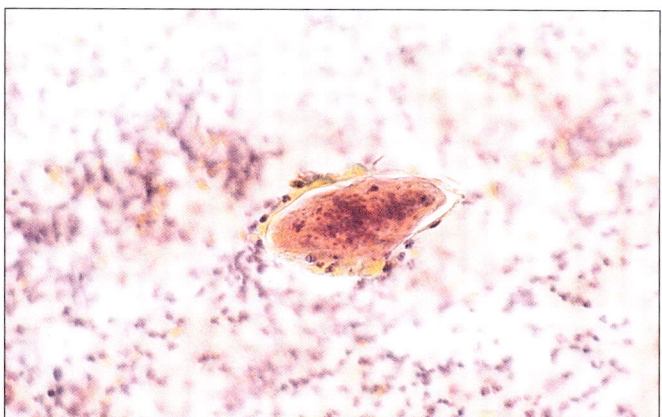

Figure 8.49 Schistosomiasis (*S. haematobium*) in a cervical smear. Ovum with poorly preserved terminal spike.

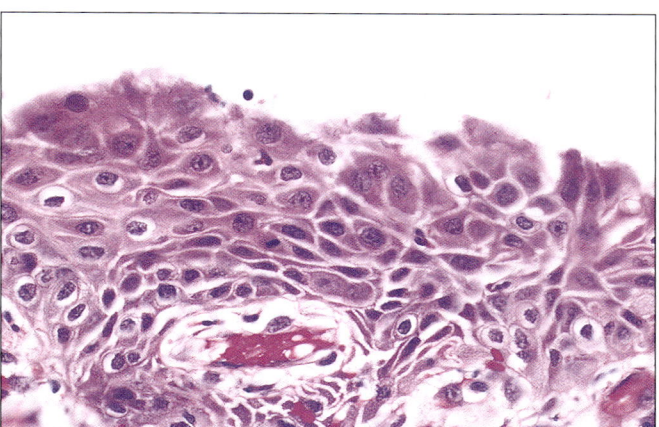

Figure 8.51 Repair. The epithelium has regrown as poorly organized layers of immature squamous cells, lacking maturation at this stage.

EPITHELIAL INFLAMMATORY CHANGES

In the presence of severe inflammatory conditions, the glandular epithelium in the cervix may show some nuclear changes, the most common is slight nuclear enlargement and pleomorphism. Although enlarged and hyperchromatic, the nuclei have an indistinct, degenerating chromatin pattern (Figure 8.50).[17] The cytoplasm is usually abundant and may be eosinophilic. These changes may pose serious problems in the distinction from genuine atypia but are usually mild, without mitotic activity or reduction in cytoplasm.

HEALING/REGENERATING EPITHELIUM

After portions of the cervical epithelium have been eroded from infection or treated for SIL, whether by ablation or excision, re-epithelialization may take place in several ways. In the ideal state, the surface will be recovered by a squamous epithelium that matures over the course of about 3 weeks. This is achieved by cells that migrate in from both edges of the affected area as well as from residual gland crypts. If the environment is acid, differentiation and maturation into squamous epithelium will be encouraged. Often this maturation is impaired, with the result that the healing epithelium morphologically resembles immature squamous epithelium that covers a small or large part of the treated area (Figure 8.51). This reparative atypia may cause the histopathologist exactly the same difficulties in differentiation from SIL as immature squamous metaplasia itself does. Clues to the diagnosis of repair are cells in which the nuclei are uniform and generally have prominent macronucleoli. The stroma is often inflamed.[18]

On the other hand, in an alkaline environment, the new epithelium that will regrow will be columnar (müllerian). This is more likely if the area treated is large as the fluid exudate from the extensively treated surface counteracts the acidity of the vaginal environment. In this case, islands of villous, columnar, endocervical-type epithelium regenerate on the ectocervix or even in the vaginal fornices. This amounts to an iatrogenic adenosis. The biopsy will show inflamed but otherwise normal endocervical-type tissue.

Cytologic Correlation

The cells from a repairing epithelium disclose large hyperchromatic nuclei with prominent chromocenters and nucleoli (Figure 8.52). Mitotic figures are not uncommon and the cytoplasm can appear eosinophilic, although green or blue staining is more likely. Not uncommonly, the cytoplasm appears pulled out in tails, the remnants of intercellular bridges (Figure 8.53). The background usually shows debris and increased numbers of polymorphs and lymphocytes. Plasma cells are rarely seen.

METAPLASIAS

The epithelium that lines the upper female genital tract, i.e., the fallopian tubes, endometrium, and endocervix, derives embryologically from the müllerian (paramesonephric) ducts. Although the epithelium is characteristic for each site, inappropriate müllerian epithelium may be found at any site within the tract. In addition, non-müllerian epithelium (i.e., intestinal) can be seen in the cervix.

TUBAL, ENDOMETRIOID, AND TUBOENDOMETRIOID METAPLASIA

Although initially believed to be a reparative process after a prior cone biopsy, subsequent studies have not provided confirmation.[19] Tubal metaplasia shows tubal-type epithelium composed of ciliated, secretory, and intercalated (peg) cells (Figure 8.54) that replace the normal endocervical epithelium composed of nonciliated secretory and ciliated columnar cells. Its frequency ranges from 21% to 62%.[20] Tubal metaplasia is most commonly seen in premenopausal patients (mean age, 41 years) and is usually an incidental finding, but rarely is found grossly such as the presence of 'spongy mucoid tissue' or an endocervical polyp. It can also be detected on a Pap smear, especially when a cytobrush is used.

Pathology

Tubal (serous) metaplasia occurs mainly in deep glands and in the upper endocervix, but can be seen in the surface epithelium, superficial glands, and lower endocervix.[20] The involved glands are typically small or medium sized but may show variation in size and shape, including branching. The overall cell architecture may show mild atypia. Mitotic figures are rare. The adjacent stroma is often hypercellular, a finding that can be pronounced, but can also be myxoid, loose edematous, or contain focal calcifications.[19] Of interest, a few examples occurring in women exposed prenatally to DES have been extensive, involving all cervical quadrants and reaching a depth of 6.1 mm (pseudoinfiltrative endocervical tubal metaplasia).[21] In these cases, the glands showed a haphazard distribution, variability in shape and size, and were increased in number. Immunohistochemically, tubal metaplasia is unreactive for carcinoembryonic antigen (CEA),[22] and only individual cells are reactive for p16.[23]

Endometrioid metaplasia appears as an epithelium composed of columnar cells, with pseudostratified, oval nuclei (Figure 8.55). Mitotic figures can be seen. Immunohistochemically, the metaplastic endometrioid cells show

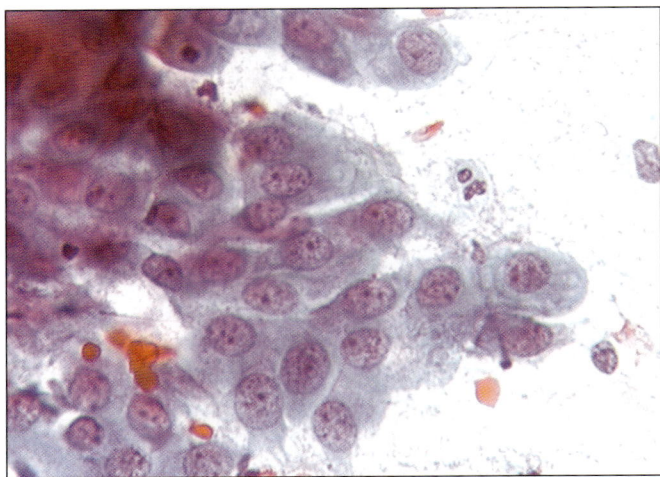

Figure 8.52 Repair in a cervical smear. Cells show prominent nuclei with evenly distributed chromatin with small nucleoli.

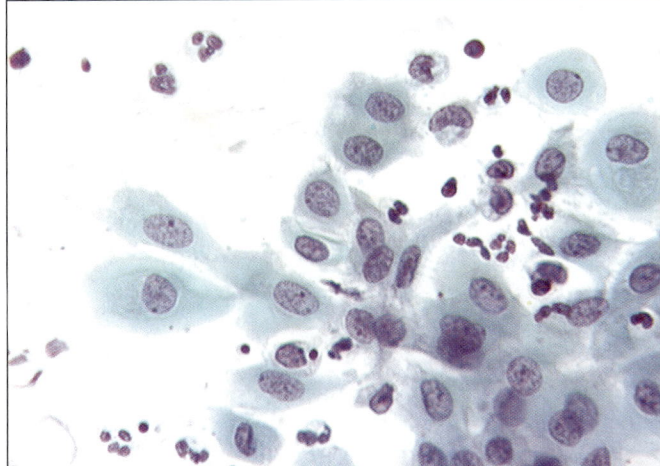

Figure 8.53 Repair in a cervical smear. Elongated cells with 'tails.'

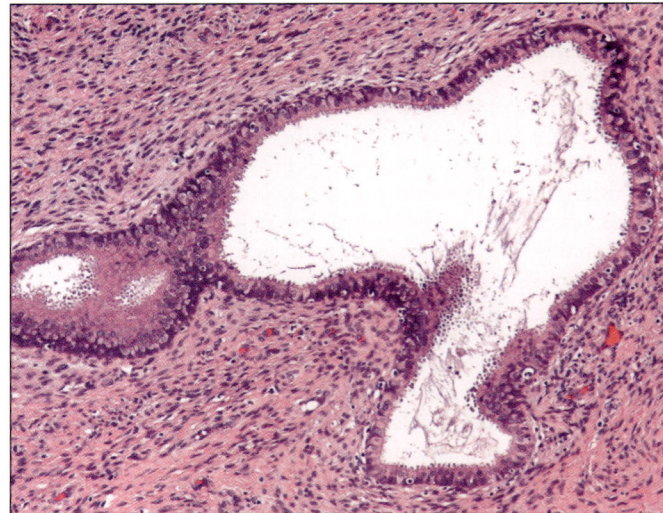

Figure 8.54 Tubal metaplasia.

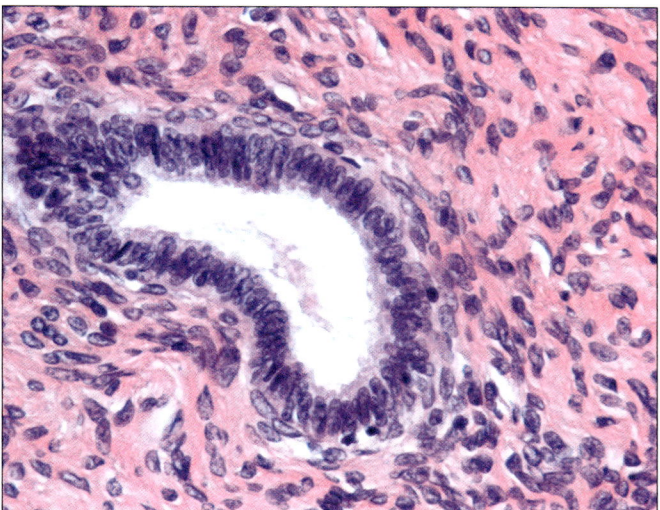

Figure 8.55 Endometrioid metaplasia.

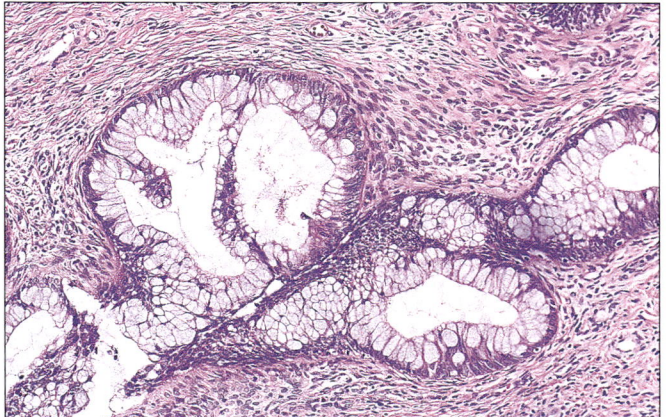

Figure 8.56 Intestinal metaplasia. Goblet cells are prominent.

reactivity for vimentin,[24] but not CEA.[25] In some cases, the metaplastic process mixes tubal and endometrioid cells, which some investigators designate as tuboendometrioid metaplasia. Ki-67 immunostaining shows negligible nuclear proliferation.[13] In addition, bcl-2 is diffusely positive in tuboendometrioid metaplasia and p16 is negative or focally positive.[1]

Differential Diagnosis

The critical differential diagnoses include adenocarcinoma *in situ* (AIS) and invasive adenocarcinoma. The former shows the presence of nuclear abnormalities such as pleomorphism, enlargement, hyperchromasia, conspicuous mitotic activity, and apoptosis. The difficulty arises when AIS develops on a background of tubal metaplasia. This form shows apical cilia in addition to the nuclear abnormalities and mitotic activity mentioned above.[26] Invasive adenocarcinoma can be recognized by the markedly irregular distribution of glands and the presence of frankly malignant cells. The presence of the stromal changes mentioned above may present a confounding factor. While the stroma about invasive adenocarcinomas is typically desmoplastic with an inflammatory infiltrate, this does not always occur. The presence of neoplastic glands in close proximity to thick-walled vessels is highly suggestive of invasive adenocarcinoma.

The cells of minimal deviation adenocarcinoma (adenoma malignum) have a bland cytology and the stroma typically lacks reactive changes. With sufficient sections, foci of marked cytologic atypia and a desmoplastic response are found, at least focally. A better clue to the correct diagnosis is its presence deep in the cervix adjacent to large muscular blood vessels, a location where normal endocervical glands are not found.[27] Finding such diagnostic features is often not possible when examining a limited amount of cervical tissue, i.e., biopsies or loop electrosurgical excision procedure (LEEP) specimens.

INTESTINAL METAPLASIA

Intestinal metaplasia is the rarest form of metaplasia in the uterine cervix, exhibiting goblet and argentaffin cells (Figure 8.56). As this process is most commonly associated with *in situ* or invasive adenocarcinomas, its diagnosis should be made only after careful sampling and microscopic examination to exclude any sign of malignancy (i.e., nuclear atypia, mitotic activity, or the presence of an infiltrative pattern).[17]

LESIONS OF THE ENDOCERVICAL GLANDULAR EPITHELIUM

ENDOCERVICAL TUNNEL CLUSTERS

Tunnel clusters are benign, pseudoneoplastic, glandular proliferations that are relatively common and mostly found in multigravid women over age 30.[28] There are two types, both tending to be multifocal and incidental findings: one (type A) may be small and microscopic only and the second (type B) is usually extensive and can produce marked distortion of the endocervical mucosa and underlying wall due to the presence of cysts that can penetrate up to 1.5 cm into the wall.[29] Type A is maximally 7 mm in greatest dimension and consists of a well-circumscribed, occasionally pseudo-infiltrative, proliferation of oval, round, or angulated glands lined by cells that can be either cuboidal with amphophilic cytoplasm or columnar and mucus secreting (Figure 8.57). The former cells have enlarged nuclei with vesicular chromatin and conspicuous nucleoli (Figure 8.58). Nuclear hyperchromasia, if present, is of the degenerative type. Mitotic figures are absent or rare. The stroma is usually unremarkable although it can be cellular, edematous, or contain inflammatory cells. Occasionally, extravasated mucin can be seen. Localized type A tunnel clusters tend to be associated also with tunnel clusters of the more expansive type (type B), a finding suggesting the latter arises from the former due to obstruction. The expansive tunnel clusters consist of dilated glands forming distinct lobular units that contrast with the usual architectural organization of the endocervical mucosa (Figure 8.59). The cells can be cuboidal or flattened and lack mitotic activity (Figures 8.60 and 8.61). In the cystic variant, the individual clusters can reach up to 18 mm at greatest dimension, and penetrate up to

9 mm into the cervical wall. A rare case associated with nabothian cysts has extended through the cervical wall (1.5 cm). Tunnel clusters are negative for CEA.

Differential Diagnosis

The principal concern is that tunnel cluster is not mistaken for malignancy, either as AIS or as an endocervical adenocarcinoma, especially as the minimal deviation type (adenoma malignum) or microcystic adenocarcinoma. The absence of nuclear pseudostratification and mitotic activity allows the distinction from AIS. The superficial location (inner endocervical wall), lobular configuration, and absence of symptoms, infiltrative pattern, mitoses, and overly malignant cytologic features should help to distinguish tunnel clusters from invasive adenocarcinoma.

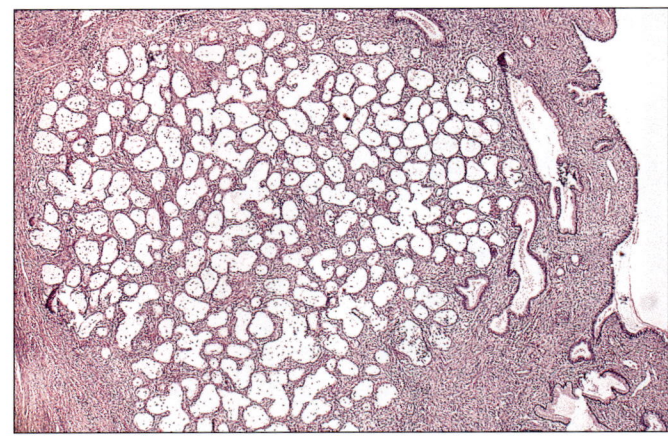

Figure 8.59 Tunnel cluster, type B. Cystic glands in a lobular arrangement.

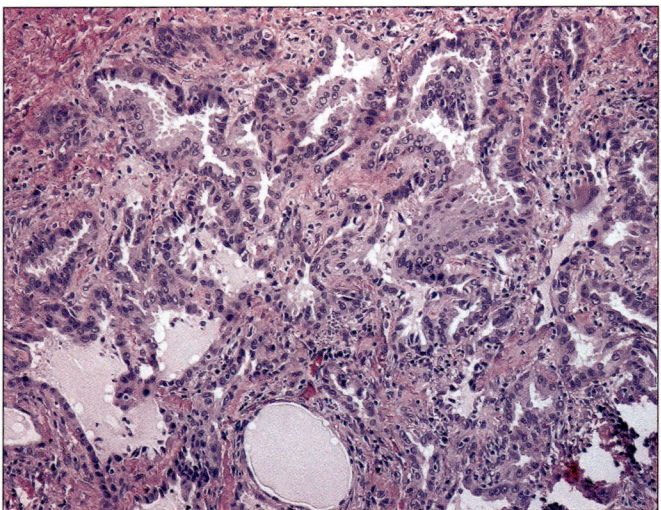

Figure 8.57 Tunnel cluster, type A. Glands have an irregular contour.

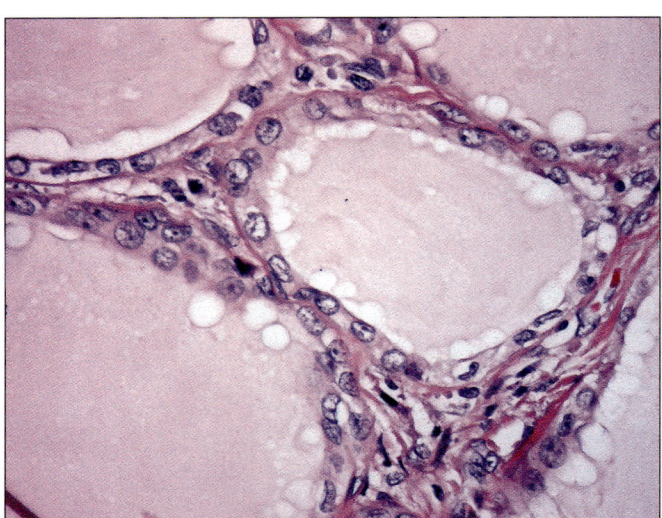

Figure 8.60 Tunnel cluster, type B. Cuboidal epithelium.

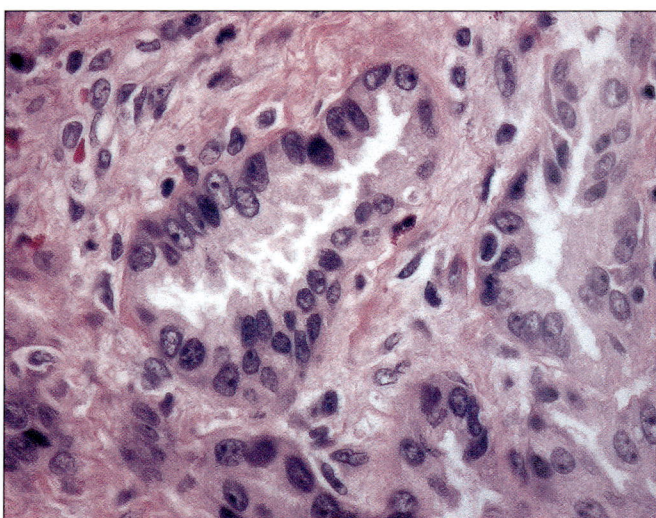

Figure 8.58 Tunnel cluster, type A. Nuclei can be enlarged with vesicular chromatin.

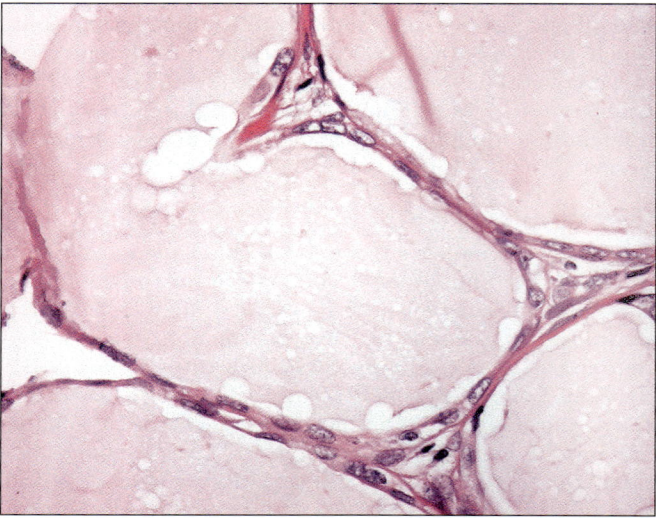

Figure 8.61 Tunnel cluster, type B. Flattened epithelium.

DEEP NABOTHIAN CYSTS

Nabothian cysts, which are a normal finding in multiparous women, are mucus-filled cysts usually 2–10 mm in size located on the surface of the endocervix, corresponding in location to the normal endocervical glands. Occasionally, these cysts are found deep in the wall, almost reaching the outer surface of the uterine cervix or paracervical soft tissue. The cysts form when the duct in the gland neck becomes obstructed, leading to entrapped mucus secretions. Most women are asymptomatic, but some have had long-term chronic cervicitis.

Gross examination discloses the presence of multiple, mucin-filled cysts extending from the mucosa to the deep portion of the wall. Occasionally, the cervix is enlarged.[17] Microscopically, the cysts are either round or with slightly irregular contours (Figure 8.62). They are lined by a single layer of columnar to flattened endocervical cells without atypia or mitotic figures. Nabothian cysts differ from minimal deviation adenocarcinoma (adenoma malignum) by the lack of an obvious mass lesion, markedly irregular glands, desmoplastic response, atypia and mitoses.

LOBULAR ENDOCERVICAL GLANDULAR HYPERPLASIA

This uncommon pseudoneoplastic glandular proliferation, a recently described lesion, has changes suggestive of pyloric gland metaplasia. It occurs in women aged 37–71 years (mean age, 45 years), most of whom are asymptomatic. Some present with a cervical/vaginal discharge or even a cervical mass.[30,31] The cervical smear may show cells interpreted as atypical glandular cells of undetermined significance (AGUS).[32]

Pathology

Grossly, the cervix is commonly unremarkable, but sometimes there is a polypoid mass or multiple cysts within the wall. Microscopically, there is a distinct lobular proliferation of glands ranging in size from small to large and cystic (Figure 8.63). Some lobular aggregates have a centrally located dilated gland surrounded by smaller glands. The glands are mostly round, but can have undulating contours. The lining epithelium is a single layer of columnar, mucin-producing cells with bland, basal nuclei with inconspicuous nucleoli. The nuclei may be slightly enlarged with vesicular chromatin and prominent nucleoli (Figure 8.64). In some cases, mitotic activity is even found (up to 2 mitoses per 10 high power fields). The intervening stroma may be cellular or contain inflammatory cells. The cells of endocervical lobular hyperplasia largely contain neutral mucins (periodic acid–Schiff (PAS) positive), further delineated by reactivity with HIK 1083 and MUC6, both immunomarkers for pyloric gland mucin. These findings have prompted some to designate this lesion as pyloric gland metaplasia.[30,32,33] CEA is reactive.

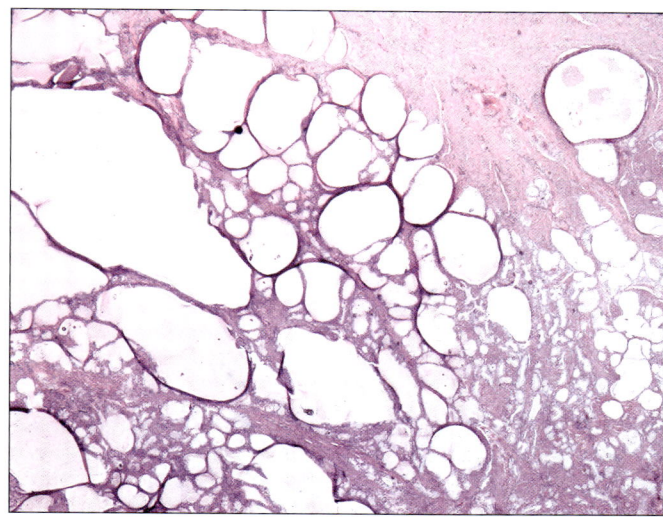

Figure 8.63 Lobular endocervical glandular hyperplasia.

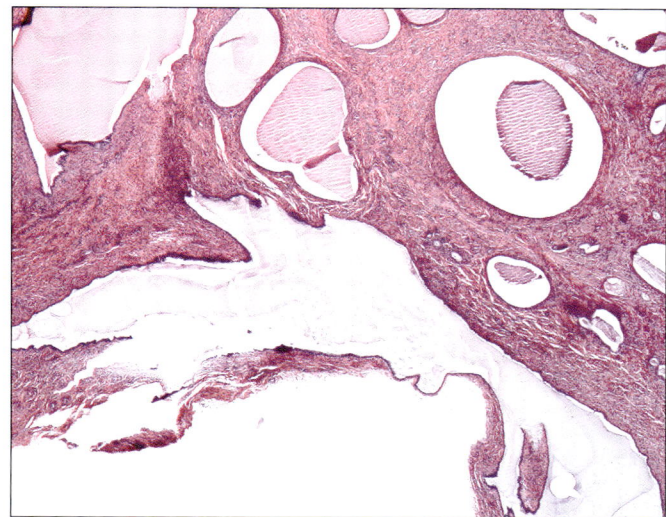

Figure 8.62 Deep nabothian cysts.

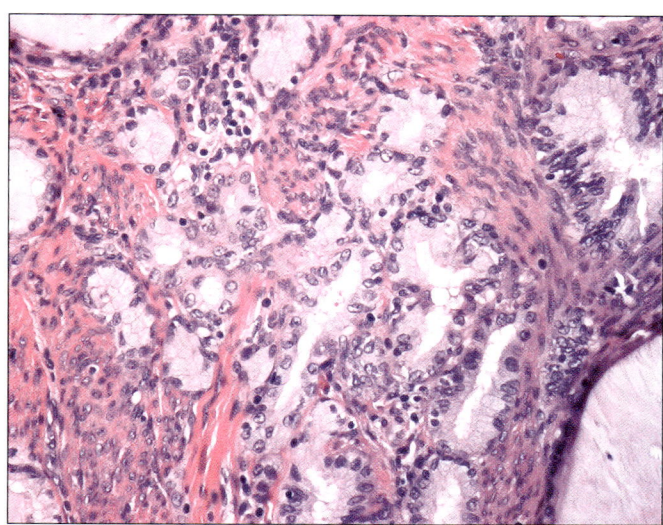

Figure 8.64 Detail of glandular epithelium in lobular endocervical glandular hyperplasia.

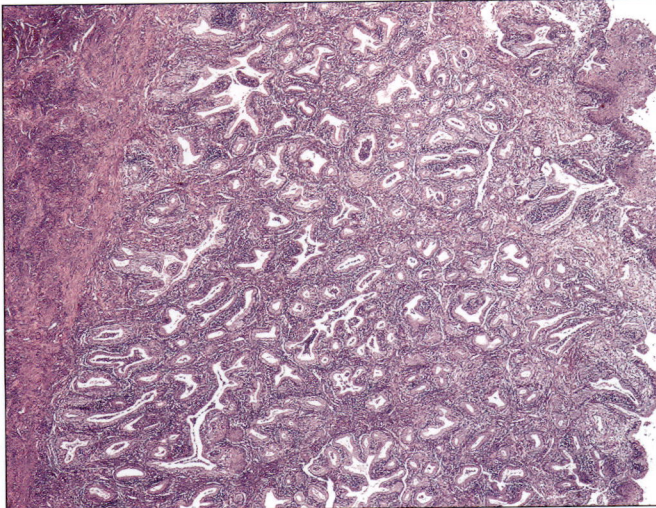

Figure 8.65 Diffuse laminar endocervical glandular hyperplasia.

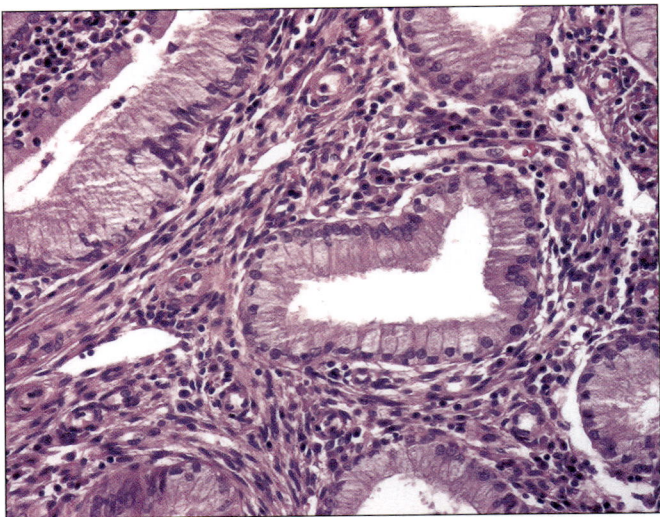

Figure 8.66 Detail of well-differentiated glandular epithelium in diffuse laminar endocervical glandular hyperplasia.

Pathogenesis

Recently, endocervical lobular hyperplasia has been found together with some cases of cervical minimal deviation adenocarcinomas or mucinous adenocarcinomas. As the carcinomas shared the pyloric gland immunophenotype with endocervical lobular hyperplasia, an association between these two entities has been suggested.[32,33]

DIFFUSE LAMINAR ENDOCERVICAL GLANDULAR HYPERPLASIA

This uncommon benign pseudoneoplastic glandular proliferation is seen mostly in premenopausal patients (aged 22–54 years).[34,35] In general, the lesion is an incidental finding, although some produce a watery or mucoid discharge.[34–36] There are no specific macroscopic findings. Microscopically, the lesion, which is clearly demarcated from the subjacent cervical stroma, exhibits a diffuse proliferation of round or abnormally shaped, small or medium sized glands confined to the inner endocervical wall (Figure 8.65). The glands are lined by bland, mucin-containing columnar epithelium (Figure 8.66). In the presence of inflammation, focal reactive changes may show as nuclear enlargement, chromatin clearing, and nucleoli. Mitotic figures are rare. Features helping to distinguish this lesion from minimal deviation adenocarcinoma (adenoma malignum) include its superficial location and well-defined base.

LESIONS RELATED TO EXOGENOUS STIMULI

MICROGLANDULAR HYPERPLASIA

Microglandular hyperplasia refers to a particular form of glandular proliferation encountered mostly in women of reproductive age but occasionally (about 6%) in postmenopausal women. It is commonly associated with exposure to

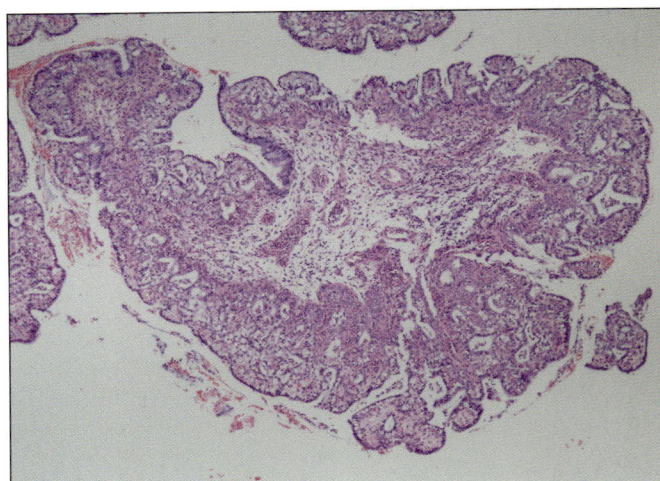

Figure 8.67 Microglandular hyperplasia. A low-power view of microglandular hyperplasia in an endocervical polyp shows proliferation of the glandular elements.

progesterone in the form of oral contraceptive therapy, Depo-Provera, or pregnancy, but in some women no hormonal background can be found. One more recent study has challenged the associations altogether.[37]

Pathology

Most occurrences are found incidentally, but some produce gross abnormalities in the form of ectropions, polyps, or friable raised areas. Microscopically, it can be focal or multifocal. The lesion consists of closely packed glands of variable size and shape, with little intervening stroma (Figure 8.67). Acute inflammatory cells are almost always found within the gland lumens. The epithelium lining the glands is columnar or cuboidal, mucin-producing, and contains supranuclear or subnuclear vacuoles (Figure 8.68). The nuclei are usually uniform, but focal atypia can be encountered. Reserve cell

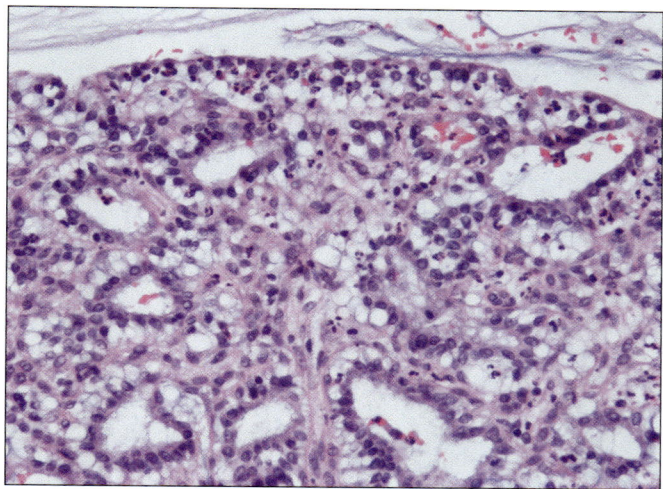

Figure 8.68 Microglandular hyperplasia. Densely crowded small glands appear fused together without intervening stroma. Inflammatory cells are prominent.

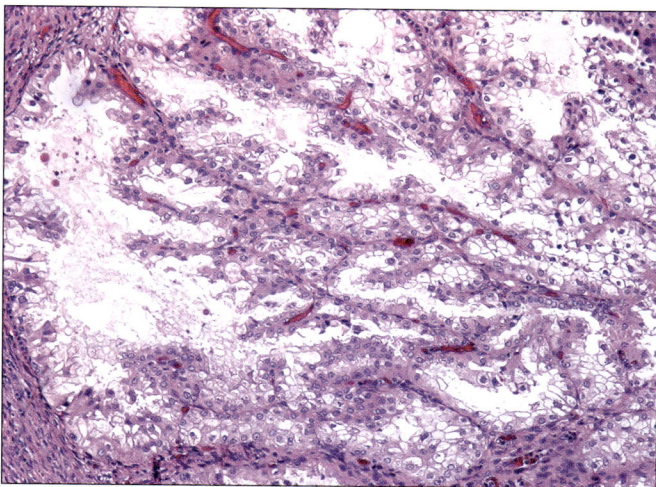

Figure 8.69 Arias-Stella reaction in endocervix. Unusual confluent pattern.

hyperplasia and squamous metaplasia are also seen.[38] Mitotic activity is low.[39,40] Occasionally, microglandular hyperplasia can have focal areas with a solid, pseudoinfiltrative, or reticular pattern, hobnail or signet-ring cells, and stromal hyalinization.[25]

Differential Diagnosis

Clinically important lesions that can be confused with microglandular hyperplasia include clear cell carcinoma and endometrial adenocarcinoma with a microglandular pattern. Clear cell carcinoma is usually associated with a cervical mass, has an infiltrative pattern, and often shows several different patterns within the same tumor, including sheets of clear cells and hobnail cells within tubules. Additionally, it shows greater cytologic atypia than that seen in microglandular hyperplasia. Endometrial adenocarcinoma with a microglandular pattern can represent a true diagnostic challenge that many times cannot be resolved with only a limited tissue sample. Features that favor endometrial adenocarcinoma with a microglandular pattern include transition to other patterns of endometrial adenocarcinoma, and mucinous differentiation in the background endometrium.[40,41] We have not found immunohistochemistry useful in distinguishing these lesions, although some believe vimentin reactivity favors endometrial adenocarcinoma with a microglandular pattern. CEA is unreactive in both entities.[40]

ARIAS-STELLA REACTION

The frequency with which the Arias-Stella reaction occurs in the endocervix of pregnant women ranges between 9% and 37.5%.[42] This reaction may also occur when there is a history of oral contraceptive use, but occasionally no hormonal history can be elicited.[39]

Pathology

Arias-Stella reaction in the cervix can present as involvement of an endocervical polyp or as an incidental finding in cervical tissue obtained for other reasons. It affects superficial and/or deep glands. It is most commonly seen in the upper endocervical canal but can involve glands anywhere in the endocervix.[42] Arias-Stella reaction tends to be focal, but may be extensive, producing a confluent appearance (Figure 8.69). Occasionally, the intraglandular proliferation can be striking, producing a papillary or cribriform pattern.[39] The Arias-Stella reaction exhibits large cells with clear or oxyphilic cytoplasm and large atypical nuclei demonstrating irregularity of the nuclear contour and variability of the chromatin distribution, ranging from even to dense (Figure 8.70). The nuclei typically protrude into the gland lumen, giving the cell a hobnail appearance. A rare mitotic figure can be seen as well as focally decidualized stroma. This lesion is described more fully in Chapter 16.

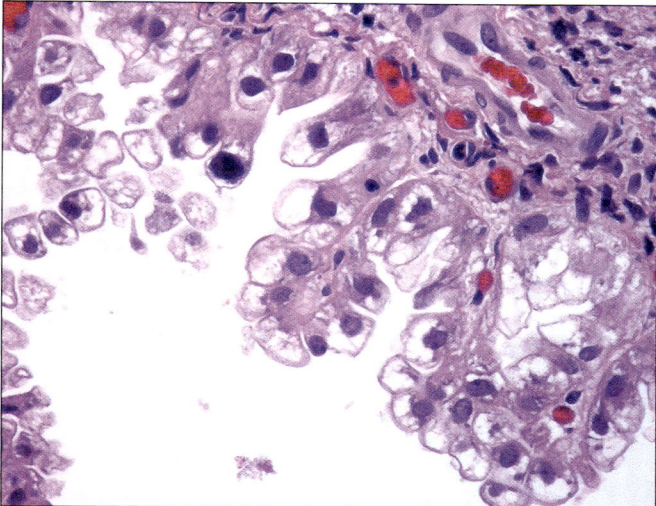

Figure 8.70 Arias-Stella reaction in endocervix. Hobnail clear cells with enlarged, hyperchromatic nuclei.

DECIDUAL CHANGE

Decidual change is a progestin-induced alteration of stromal tissue. Although this hormonal response is usually associated with endometrial stroma, it also affects the superficial stroma of the cervix, the lamina propria of the fallopian tube, the subcortical stroma of the ovary, and the submesothelial stroma of the peritoneum.

Decidual change presents to the naked eye as small, raised, vascular nodules or, less commonly, as sessile polyps. At colposcopy, the appearances can simulate those of invasive carcinoma. The affected area may have a raised, nodular, irregular contour and, in particular, prominent, often rather bizarre, vessels on the surface. Microscopy shows features that are similar to decidual change at more familiar sites (Figures 8.71 and 8.72). The cells of the superficial stroma are enlarged with copious cytoplasm. The nuclei are uniform, small, and central. The change usually affects only a small area of the cervix and may be situated on both the endocervix and ectocervix. The phenomenon of decidual change in the cervix is, of course, of no consequence as it is asymptomatic and regresses soon after the pregnancy finishes.

RADIATION CHANGES

Radiation changes can be acute or long term. Acute changes include erosion; cytoplasmic and nuclear swelling of the squamous and endocervical cells; dilated blood vessels; and stromal changes such as necrosis, edema, and a lymphoplasmacytic infiltrate. In most patients, these acute changes gradually give way to changes associated with the long-term effects of radiation, which can persist for many years. These longer term changes include atrophy of the squamous epithelium (80% of cases); variable degrees of epithelial atypia (two-thirds of cases); and stromal changes encompassing the presence of edema, fibrosis, hyalinization, atypical fibroblasts, multinucleated cells, and focal calcification (Figure 8.73).

The blood vessels may show sclerotic changes, intimal proliferation, and atypical endothelial cells (Figure 8.74).[43] Additionally, the endocervical glands, which decrease in number and have either a tubular or dilated configuration, are lined by enlarged cells with eosinophilic or vacuolated cytoplasm with enlarged nuclei. These endocervical cells are usually cuboidal but can be columnar or flattened. The nuclei enlarge with fine chromatin and visible nucleoli, but

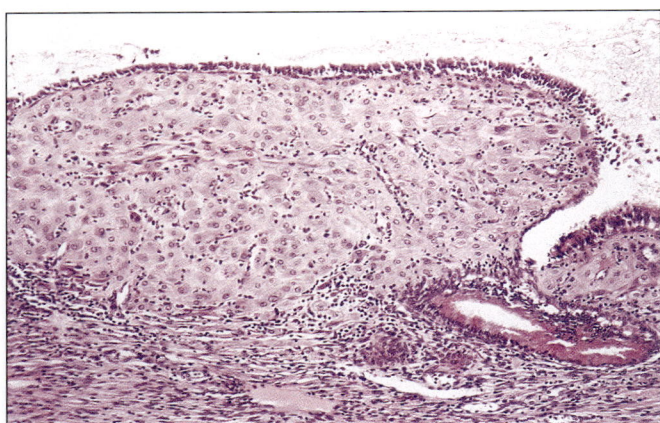

Figure 8.71 Decidual change. A well-defined area of large, pale, decidualized stromal cells is present beneath the surface epithelium.

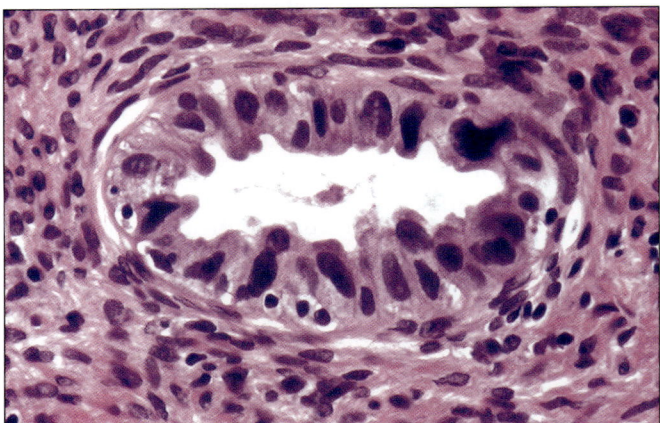

Figure 8.73 Radiation effect with some enlarged nuclei with smudged chromatin.

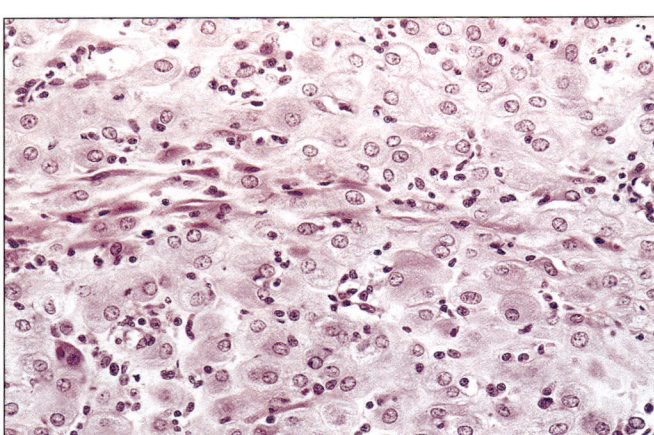

Figure 8.72 Decidual change. At high power, the cells are identical to decidualized endometrial stromal cells.

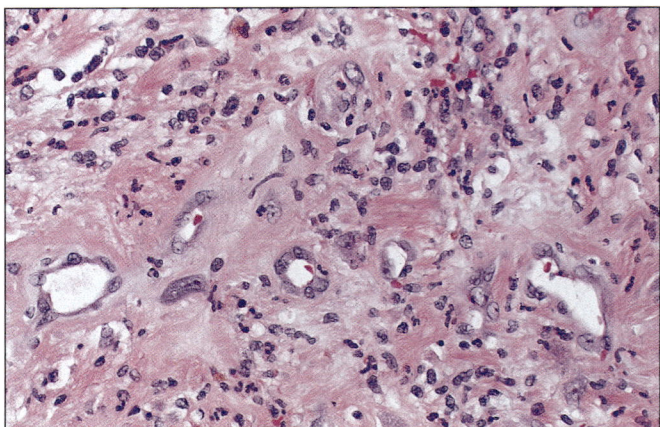

Figure 8.74 Radiation effect. Vessels with plump endothelial cells and reactive fibroblasts in the stroma.

can also be hyperchromatic. The latter are generally scattered through the glands but occasionally are prominent and appear to predominate. These epithelial changes can be focal or extensive. Mitotic figures are absent. In a rare case, multinucleated cells or eosinophilic intranuclear inclusions are present.[44]

Differential Diagnosis

AIS virtually always shows mitoses, a feature absent in radiation change. Clear cell adenocarcinoma may show closely packed invasive glands, mitotic figures, and a combination of architectural patterns (i.e., tubulocystic, papillary, and solid), features also absent in radiation change.

OTHER NON-NEOPLASTIC CONDITIONS

ENDOMETRIOSIS

Endometriosis, described in greater depth in Chapter 22, occurs in the cervix in both deep and superficial forms. The deep form is usually seen in patients with pelvic endometriosis and its recognition does not represent a diagnostic challenge. The superficial form typically consists of endometriotic glands and stroma, but in some instances the glands are sparse or absent (stromal endometriosis). The superficial form can represent a diagnostic dilemma, and forms the basis of the discussion to follow.

Superficial cervical endometriosis is usually seen in premenopausal patients, although the age range is 20–53 years.[45] It is often an incidental finding but may be detected secondary to trauma with subsequent vaginal bleeding from a surgical procedure (curettage, biopsy, loop excision or cone biopsy, and cautery). Grossly, it appears as a mucosal thickening or as nodules, blood-filled blebs, or cysts (up to 2 cm in diameter). The mucosa may appear granular or hemorrhagic.[45] Microscopically, the endometriotic process tends to reside within the inner third of the cervical wall, sometimes producing ulceration. The glands are usually round to oval but occasionally are cystic (Figure 8.75). Hyperplastic or secretory changes and telescoping can be seen. The epithelial cells can show reactive atypia. The mitotic activity tends to be low, although up to three mitoses per gland can be seen. No abnormal mitotic figures are found and apoptotic bodies are rarely seen. The stroma can be focal, which, in addition to the changes listed above, complicates recognition of this lesion.[45] In difficult cases, deeper levels could facilitate the recognition of endometrial stroma. In addition, obtaining the following immunostain results will facilitate the correct diagnosis: (1) Ki-67 (positive in <10% of the cells; (2) bcl-2, vimentin, and estrogen receptor (+); and (3) p16 and CEA (–). CD10 immunostaining is not reliable in this setting since it is not specific for endometrial stroma.[46]

Differential Diagnosis

Superficial cervical endometriosis must be distinguished from AIS. Confounding features rendering the correct diagnosis difficult include mitotic activity within the glandular epithelium (especially in young women), hemorrhage, inflammation, smooth muscle metaplasia, and other reactive changes within the stromal component. The absence of

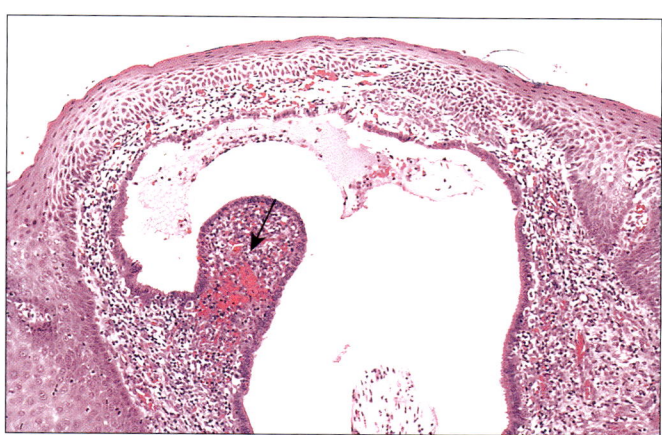

Figure 8.75 Endometriosis. A distended glandular space, lined by endometrial-type epithelium, lies beneath the squamous epithelium of the cervix. Hemorrhagic endometrial stroma (arrows) is also present.

significant cytologic atypia, but the presence of the stromal component, which in some cases will require additional deeper sections, helps to facilitate the correct diagnosis.

Endometriosis can also be misinterpreted as atypical glandular cells of undetermined significance, HSIL, or AIS in cytologic smears.[47]

Rare cases of endometriosis will show exclusively the stromal component. In these instances, the lesion can simulate endometrial stromal sarcoma or Kaposi sarcoma. These latter conditions, however, usually exhibit infiltrative borders and vascular/lymphatic invasion. Kaposi sarcoma also shows spindle cells arranged in short fascicles, slit-like spaces containing red blood cells, and intracellular and extracellular eosinophilic globules. Kaposi sarcoma expresses CD31 and CD34 immunoreactivity.[48–50]

MESONEPHRIC REMNANTS AND HYPERPLASIA

MESONEPHRIC DUCT REMNANTS

Remnants of the embryologic mesonephric duct system are common findings in hysterectomy specimens. They are also occasionally found in cone and even LEEP biopsy specimens. Remnants are found in 22% of adult cervices and in 40% of newborns and children.[51] Not uncommonly, they are detected as an abnormal cervical smear.[52,53]

Mesonephric duct remnants are most commonly found laterally, usually deep in the endocervical wall. Sometimes they are superficial, appearing to open into an endocervical gland.[54] The usual mesonephric duct remnants appear as small groups of glands or tubules, sometimes arranged around a mother duct or a duct branch (Figure 8.76). Some appear as tubules without ducts (Figure 8.77). The lining epithelium is a single layer of cuboidal to columnar cells with scanty clear to slightly eosinophilic cytoplasm. In contrast to müllerian epithelial cells, mesonephric epithelial cells lack both mucinous secretion and cilia. The round, bland nuclei occasionally overlap. Usually there is no mitotic activity. Most of the tubular lumens contain an eosinophilic material, although occasionally it is not found.[51] There is luminal expression of CD10.[1,46] The cytoplasm lacks glycogen (PAS negative), while the luminal contents are PAS positive, diastase resistant.[54]

MESONEPHRIC DUCT HYPERPLASIA

Three different types of hyperplasia arise from the mesonephric remnants: lobular, diffuse, and ductal.[54] The lobular type is the most common type. Its distinction from mesonephric remnants is arbitrary and based on the appearance of the lobules, which are larger, more loosely organized, and more irregularly shaped (Figure 8.78).[53,54] Lobular mesonephric hyperplasia occurs in patients with a mean age of 35 years. Usually, it is an incidental finding, but it can produce nodularity or an indurated cervix. It ranges in size from 4 to 22 mm, retains for the most part a lobular architecture, which can be lost focally, and can extend deep into the cervical wall. The cuboidal or columnar lining epithelium can form small tufts and rare mitotic figures can be found.

The second most common type of mesonephric hyperplasia is the diffuse type. The women are slightly older (mean age, 47 years) and the finding is usually incidental. Extensive disease can result in an irregular cervical shape or hypertrophy and erosion. Most lesions are 13–25 mm in size, extend deeply into the wall, and are not restricted to the lateral walls in the endocervix. Rarely, they expand into the lower uterine segment. Microscopically, there is a diffuse proliferation of mesonephric tubules, with or without ducts (Figure 8.79). A rare mitotic figure is sometimes found, but cytologic atypia is lacking.

The least common form of mesonephric hyperplasia, the ductal type, displays prominent ducts with papillary tufting, but a minimal proliferation of tubules (Figure 8.80).

Differential Diagnosis

Mesonephric hyperplasias must be differentiated from mesonephric adenocarcinoma.[54,55] The latter is usually associated with symptoms and a cervical mass. In addition, the presence of nuclear atypia, conspicuous mitotic

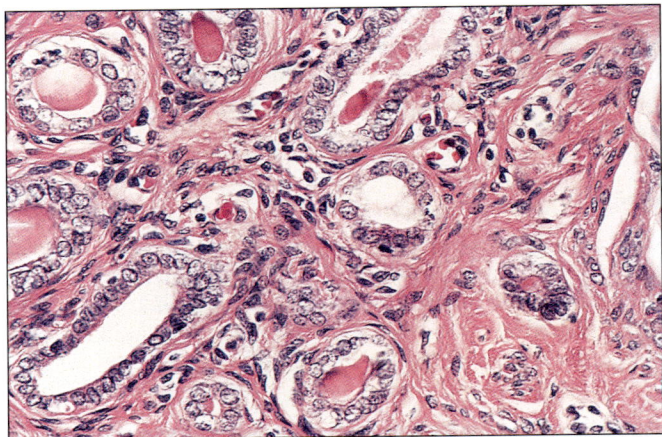

Figure 8.77 Mesonephric remnants. The tubules consist of a single layer of low cuboidal-to-columnar epithelium. The cytoplasm lacks glycogen and is mucin negative. The cells also lack other distinguishing features, such as cilia. The nuclei are bland and large compared to the rest of the cell, and some overlap.

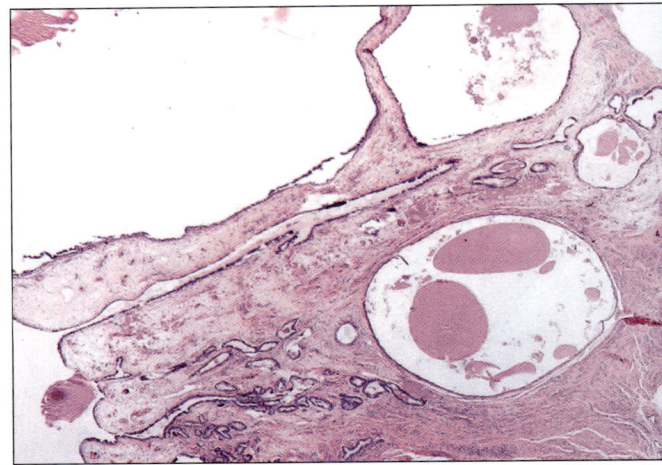

Figure 8.78 Mesonephric hyperplasia, lobular type.

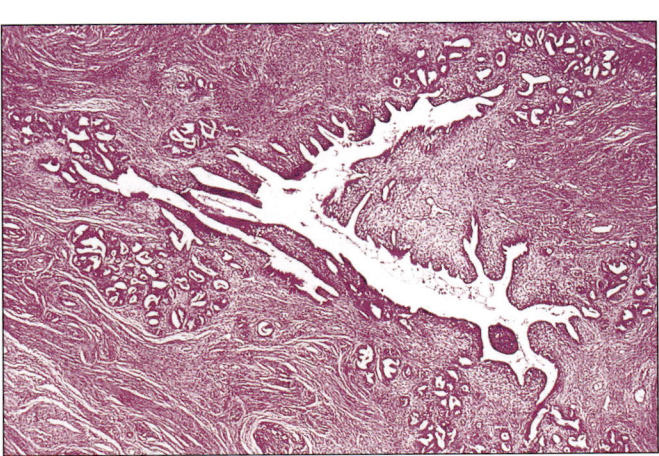

Figure 8.76 Mesonephric remnants. Lobules of smaller tubular glands lie about a main branching duct.

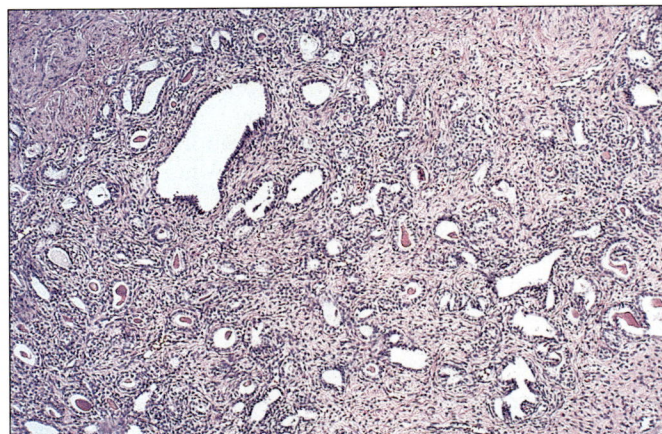

Figure 8.79 Mesonephric duct hyperplasia, diffuse type. The central duct can still be identified but the proliferating tubules have a haphazard arrangement.

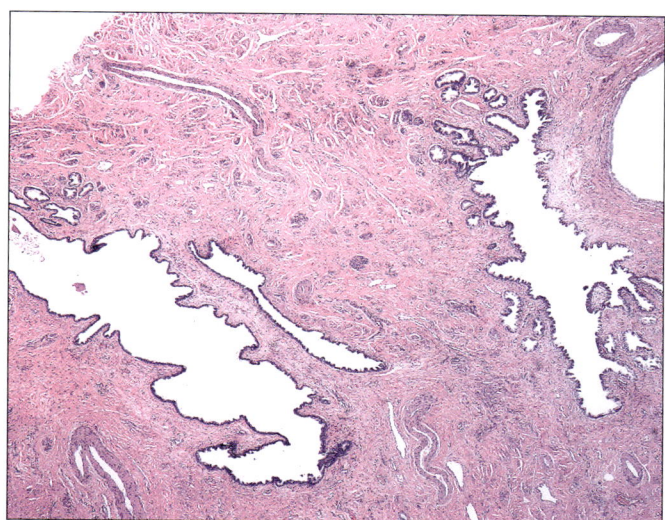

Figure 8.80 Mesonephric hyperplasia, ductal type.

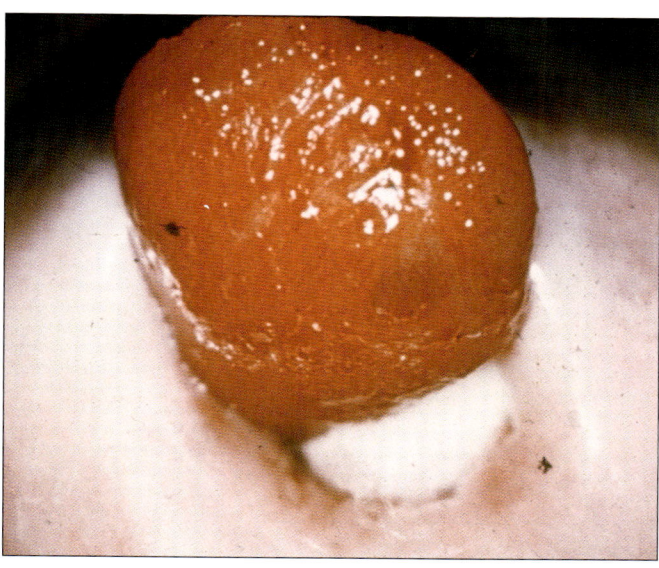

Figure 8.81 Cervical polyp. A large polyp protrudes from the external cervical os. The surface is red and rough, covered by endocervical epithelium. (Courtesy of Dr. Henry J. Norris)

activity, vascular/lymphatic invasion, and other patterns of mesonephric adenocarcinoma, such as solid or ductal, help facilitate the correct diagnosis. Assessment of Ki-67 reactivity is helpful as about 15% of malignant cells are reactive in comparison with 1–2% of hyperplastic mesonephric cells.[56]

CERVICAL POLYP

Cervical polyps, which are common, are localized overgrowths of endocervical tissue (Figures 8.81–8.83). Most do not cause symptoms while others present with spotting or irregular vaginal bleeding. The polyp consists of lamina propria, with surface epithelium and underlying crypts. If the surface epithelium ulcerates, the underlying tissue may take on the character of granulation tissue. This is often seen with symptomatic polyps. The surface epithelium, if present, often shows squamous metaplasia of various degrees of maturity. In addition, inflammatory cells often permeate the superficial stroma with plasma cells predominating. Polyps with squamous metaplasia often contain dilated endocervical crypts. Sometimes a polyp may be composed solely of a few mucus-filled cysts covered by a layer of metaplastic squamous epithelium. Endocervical polyps must be distinguished from polyps arising in the endometrium and from leiomyomatous polyps, both of which may extend into the endocervical canal and protrude through the external os.

Rarely, the surface epithelium of a polyp can have superimposed SIL, usually in association with SIL involving another area of the transformation zone.

'Cervical polyps,' particularly if clinically recurrent, may be a presentation of adenosarcoma or sarcoma. Attention should be given to examination of the stromal as well as to the epithelial component of the polyps. Prolapsed endometrial tissues such as polyps, tumors, or products of

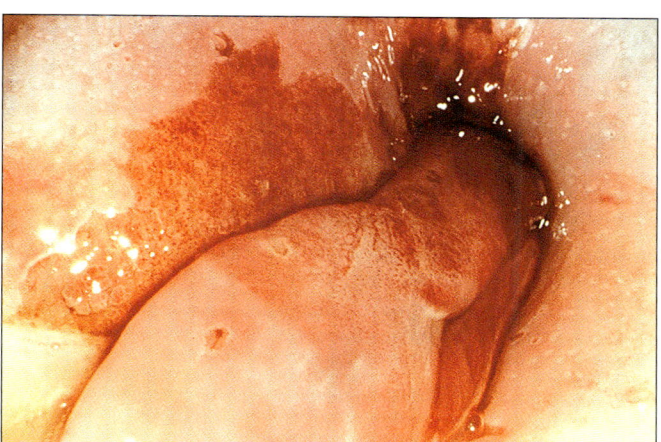

Figure 8.82 Cervical polyp. Bleeding has been caused by mechanical friction of this polyp. The surface is smooth and has undergone squamous metaplasia.

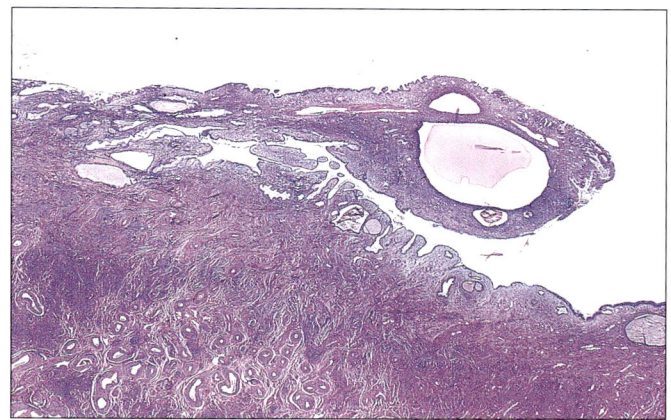

Figure 8.83 Cervical polyp. The stroma contains thick-walled blood vessels. Endocervical crypts, some dilated, are present within the polyp.

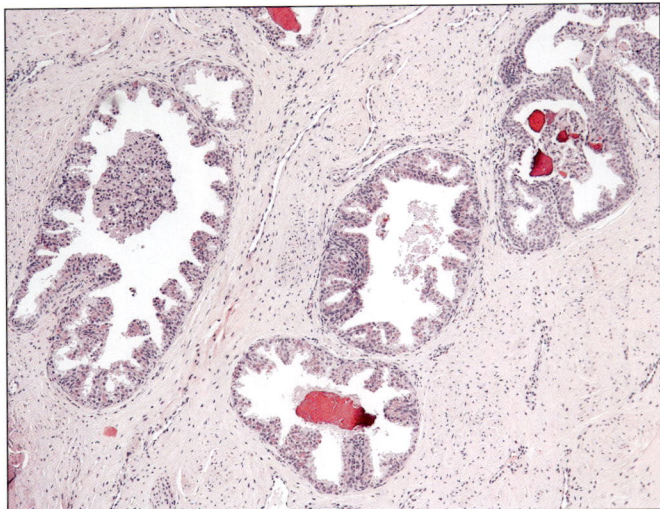

Figure 8.84 Ectopic prostatic tissue.

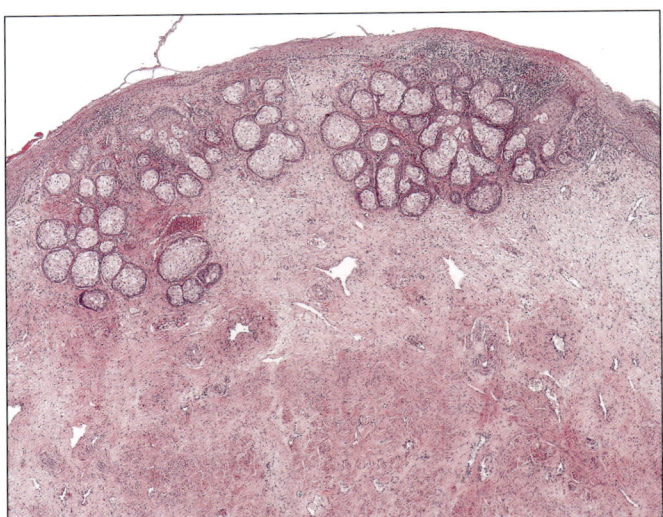

Figure 8.85 Sebaceous hyperplasia in the uterine cervix. (Courtesy of Dr. Denisa Kacerovská.)

conception, may present at the cervical os and be erroneously submitted by the clinician as 'cervical' polyps.

ECTOPIC TISSUE

PROSTATIC TISSUE

On rare occasions, ectopic prostatic tissue can be encountered in the cervix. This is usually an incidental finding in cervical LEEP or cone specimens; although, on a rare occasion, it has been associated with a cervical mass. Patients have a wide age range, early twenties to early sixties. Histologically, the small or middle sized glands do not involve the mucosal surface and are characterized by a double layer of basal and luminal cells, although this distinct arrangement can only be focal (Figure 8.84). The luminal cells are eosinophilic or clear, sometimes with granular cytoplasm, while the basal cells are flattened or cuboidal with little cytoplasm. A cribriform pattern and squamous metaplasia can be seen within the glandular elements. Immunohistochemically, the glands stain with prostatic acid phosphatase and prostatic specific antigen; although the staining can just be focal. CD10 and high molecular cytokeratin 34βE12 are positive in the basal layer. Focal granular cytoplasmic staining for α-methyl acyl-CoA racemase can be seen and p16 is negative.[57]

GLIAL TISSUE

Cases are typically preceded by an instrumental abortion (up to 13 years earlier) and have a polypoid lesion. Microscopically, they show mature glial tissue. Immunohistochemical stains for S-100 and glial fibrillary acidic protein are positive.[58]

SEBACEOUS GLANDS

Sebaceous glands, associated or not with hair follicles, can rarely be seen in the uterine cervix (Figure 8.85). This is usually an incidental finding, although a rare case of cervical sebaceous hyperplasia has been associated with small, yellowish nodules on colposcopic examination.[59]

REFERENCES

1. McCluggage WG. Immunohistochemistry as a diagnostic aid in cervical pathology. Pathology 2007;39:97–111.
2. Baker AC, Eltoum I, Curry RO, et al. Mucinous expression in benign and neoplastic glandular lesions of the uterine cervix. Arch Pathol Lab Med 2006;130:1510–15.
3. Herfs M, Yamamoto Y, Laury A, et al. A discrete population of squamocolumnar junction cells implicated in the pathogenesis of cervical cancer. Proc Natl Acad Sci USA 2012;109:10516–21.
4. Benevolo M, Mottolese M, Marandino F, et al. Immunohistochemical expression of p16(INK4a) is predictive of HR-HPV infection in cervical low-grade lesions. Mod Pathol 2006;19:384–91.
5. Dray M, Russell P, Dalrymple C, et al. P16(INK4a) as a complementary marker of high-grade intraepithelial lesions of the uterine cervix. I: Experience with squamous lesions in 189 consecutive cervical biopsies. Pathology 2005;37:112–24.
6. O'Neill CJ, McCluggage WG. p16 expression in the female genital tract and its value in diagnosis. Adv Anat Pathol 2006;13:8–15.
7. Kiviat NB, Paavonen JA, WolnerHanssen P, et al. Histopathology of endocervical infection caused by Chlamydia trachomatis, herpes simplex virus, Trichomonas vaginalis, and Neisseria gonorrhoeae. Hum Pathol 1990;21:831–7.
8. Chakraborty P, Roy A, Bhattacharya S, et al. Tuberculous cervicitis: a clinicopathological and bacteriological study. J Indian Med Assoc 1995;93:167–8.
9. Lamba H, Byrne M, Goldin R, Jenkins C. Tuberculosis of the cervix: case presentation and a review of the literature. Sex Transm Infect 2002;78:62–3.
10. Aseffa A, Ishak A, Stevens R, et al. Prevalence of HIV, syphilis and genital chlamydial infection among women in North-West Ethiopia. Epidemiol Infect 1998;120:171–7.
11. Dietrich M, Hoosen AA, Moodley J, Moodley S. Urogenital tract infections in pregnancy at King Edward VIII Hospital, Durban, South Africa. Genitourin Med 1992;68:39–41.
12. Clark RA, Brandon W, Dumestre J, Pindaro C. Clinical manifestations of infection with the human immunodeficiency virus in women in Louisiana. Clin Infect Dis 1993;17:165–72.
13. McGalie CE, McBride HA, McCluggage WG. Cytomegalovirus infection of the cervix: morphological observations in five cases of a possibly under-recognised condition. J Clin Pathol 2004;57:691–4.
14. Poggensee G, Feldmeier H. Female genital schistosomiasis: facts and hypotheses. Acta Trop 2001;79:193–210.
15. Poggensee G, Sahebali S, Van Marck E, et al. Diagnosis of genital cervical schistosomiasis: comparison of cytological, histopathological and parasitological examination. Am J Trop Med Hyg 2001;65:233–6.

16. Petry KU, Scholz U, Hollwitz B, et al. Human papillomavirus, coinfection with Schistosoma hematobium, and cervical neoplasia in rural Tanzania. Int J Gynecol Cancer 2003;13:505–9.
17. Young RH, Clement PB. Pseudoneoplastic glandular lesions of the uterine cervix. Semin Diagn Pathol 1991;8:234–49.
18. Yelverton CL, Bentley RC, Olenick S, et al. Epithelial repair of the uterine cervix: assessment of morphologic features and correlations with cytologic diagnosis. Int J Gynecol Pathol 1996;15:338–44.
19. Oliva E, Clement PB, Young RH. Tubal and tubo-endometrioid metaplasia of the uterine cervix: unemphasized features that may cause problems in differential diagnosis. A report of 25 cases. Am J Clin Pathol 1995;103:618–23.
20. Jonasson JG, Wang HH, Antonioli DA, Ducatman BS. Tubal metaplasia of the uterine cervix: a prevalence study in patients with gynecologic pathologic findings. Int J Gynecol Pathol 1992;11:89–95.
21. Vang R, Vinh TN, Burks RT, et al. Pseudoinfiltrative tubal metaplasia of the endocervix: a potential form of in utero diethylstilbestrol exposure-related adenosis simulating minimal deviation adenocarcinoma. Int J Gynecol Pathol 2005;24:391–8.
22. Suh KS, Silverberg SG. Tubal metaplasia of the uterine cervix. Int J Gynecol Pathol 1990;9:122–8.
23. Tringler B, Gup CJ, Singh M, et al. Evaluation of p16INK4a and pRb expression in cervical squamous and glandular neoplasia. Hum Pathol 2004;35:689–96.
24. Kim KR, Park KH, Kim JW, et al. Transitional cell metaplasia and ectopic prostatic tissue in the uterine cervix and vagina in a patient with adrenogenital syndrome: report of a case suggesting a possible role of androgen in the histogenesis. Int J Gynecol Pathol 2004;23:182–7.
25. Young RH, Scully RE. Atypical forms of microglandular hyperplasia of the cervix simulating carcinoma. Am J Surg Pathol 1989;13:50–6.
26. Schlesinger C, Silverberg SG. Endocervical adenocarcinoma in situ of tubal type and its relation to atypical tubal metaplasia. Int J Gynecol Pathol 1999;18:1–4.
27. Wheeler DT, Kurman RJ. The relationship of glands to thick-wall blood vessels as a marker of invasion in endocervical adenocarcinoma. Int J Gynecol Pathol 2005;24:125–30.
28. Jones MA, Young RH. Endocervical type A (noncystic) tunnel clusters with cytologic atypia: a report of 14 cases. Am J Surg Pathol 1996;20:1312–18.
29. Segal GH, Hart WR. Cystic endocervical tunnel clusters. Am J Surg Pathol 1990;14:895–903.
30. Mikami Y, Hata S, Melamed J, et al. Lobular endocervical glandular hyperplasia is a metaplastic process with a pyloric gland phenotype. Histopathology 2001;39:364–72.
31. Nucci MR, Clement PB, Young RH. Lobular endocervical glandular hyperplasia, not otherwise specified—a clinicopathologic analysis of thirteen cases of a distinctive pseudoneoplastic lesion and comparison with fourteen cases of adenoma malignum. Am J Surg Pathol 1999;23:886–91.
32. Kondo T, Hashi A, Murata S, et al. Endocervical adenocarcinomas associated with lobular endocervical glandular hyperplasia: a report of four cases with histochemical and immunohistochemical analyses. Mod Pathol 2005;18:1199–210.
33. Mikami Y, Kiyokawa T, Hata S, et al. Gastrointestinal immunophenotype in adenocarcinomas of the uterine cervix and related glandular lesions: a possible link between lobular endocervical glandular hyperplasia/pyloric gland metaplasia and 'adenoma malignum'. Mod Pathol 2004;17:962–72.
34. Jones MA, Young RH, Scully RE. Diffuse laminar endocervical glandular hyperplasia: a benign lesion often confused with adenoma malignum (minimal deviation adenocarcinoma). Am J Surg Pathol 1991;15:1123–9.
35. Maruyama R, Nagaoka S, Terao K, et al. Diffuse laminar endocervical glandular hyperplasia. Pathol Int 1995;45:283–6.
36. Farlie R, Jylling AMB, Vetner M. Diffuse laminar endocervical glandular hyperplasia—two cases presenting with excessive mucinous cervical discharge. Acta Obstet Gynecol Scand 1998;77:131–3.
37. Greeley C, Schroeder S, Silverberg SG. Microglandular hyperplasia of the cervix: a true 'pill' lesion? Int J Gynecol Pathol 1995;14:50–4.
38. Witkiewicz AK, Hecht JL, Cviko A, et al. Microglandular hyperplasia: a model for the de novo emergence and evolution of endocervical reserve cells. Hum Pathol 2005;36:154–61.
39. Nucci MR, Young RH. Arias-Stella reaction of the endocervix: a report of 18 cases with emphasis on its varied histology and differential diagnosis. Am J Surg Pathol 2004;28:608–12.
40. Qiu WS, Mittal K. Comparison of morphologic and immunohistochemical features of cervical microglandular hyperplasia with low-grade mucinous adenocarcinoma of the endometrium. Int J Gynecol Pathol 2003;22:261–5.
41. Zaloudek C, Hayashi GM, Ryan IP, et al. Microglandular adenocarcinoma of the endometrium: a form of mucinous adenocarcinoma that may be confused with microglandular hyperplasia of the cervix. Int J Gynecol Pathol 1997;16:52–9.
42. Schneider V. Arias-Stella reaction of the endocervix: frequency and location. Acta Cytol 1981;25:224–8.
43. Shield PW. Chronic radiation effects: a correlative study of smears and biopsies from the cervix and vagina. Diagn Cytopathol 1995;13:107–19.
44. Lesack D, Wahab I, Gilks CB. Radiation-induced atypia of endocervical epithelium: a histological, immunohistochemical and cytometric study. Int J Gynecol Pathol 1996;15:242–7.
45. Baker PM, Clement PB, Bell DA, Young RH. Superficial endometriosis of the uterine cervix: a report of 20 cases of a process that may be confused with endocervical glandular dysplasia or adenocarcinoma in situ. Int J Gynecol Pathol 1999;18:198–205.
46. McCluggage WG, Oliva E, Herrington CS, et al. CD10 and calretinin staining of endocervical glandular lesions, endocervical stroma and endometrioid adenocarcinomas of the uterine corpus: CD10 positivity is characteristic of, but not specific for, mesonephric lesions and is not specific for endometrial stroma. Histopathology 2003;43:144–50.
47. Lundeen SJ, Horwitz CA, Larson CJ, Stanley MW. Abnormal cervicovaginal smears due to endometriosis: a continuing problem. Diagn Cytopathol 2002;26:35–40.
48. Cheuk W, Wong KO, Wong CS, et al. Immunostaining for human herpesvirus 8 latent nuclear antigen-1 helps distinguish Kaposi sarcoma from its mimickers. Am J Clin Pathol 2004;121:335–42.
49. Katz IA, De Silva KS, Eckstein RP, Philips J. Stromal endometriosis of the cervix simulating Kaposi's sarcoma. Pathology 1997;29:426–7.
50. Robin YM, Guillou L, Michels JJ, Coindre JM. Human herpesvirus 8 immunostaining: a sensitive and specific method for diagnosing Kaposi sarcoma in paraffin-embedded sections. Am J Clin Pathol 2004;121:330–4.
51. Seidman JD, Tavassoli FA. Mesonephric hyperplasia of the uterine cervix: a clinicopathologic study of 51 cases. Int J Gynecol Pathol 1995;14:293–9.
52. Hejmadi RK, Gearty JC, Waddell C, Ganesan R. Mesonephric hyperplasia can cause abnormal cervical smears: report of three cases with review of literature. Cytopathology 2005;16:240.
53. Welsh T, Fu YS, Chan J, et al. Mesonephric remnants of hyperplasia can cause abnormal pap smears: a study of three cases. Int J Gynecol Pathol 2003;22:121–6.
54. Ferry JA, Scully RE. Mesonephric remnants, hyperplasia, and neoplasia of the uterine cervix: a study of 49 cases. Am J Surg Pathol 1990;14:1100–14.
55. Bague S, Rodriguez IM, Prat J. Malignant mesonephric tumors of the female genital tract—a clinicopathologic study of 9 cases. Am J Surg Pathol 2004;28:601–7.
56. Silver SA, Devouassoux-Shisheboran M, Mezzetti TP, Tavassoli FA. Mesonephric adenocarcinomas of the uterine cervix—a study of 11 cases with immunohistochemical findings. Am J Surg Pathol 2001;25:379–87.
57. McCluggage WG, Ganesan R, Hirschowitz L, et al. Ectopic prostatic tissue in the uterine cervix and vagina. Report of a series with a detailed immunohistochemical analysis Am J Surg Pathol 2006;30:209–15.
58. Siddon A, Hui P. Glial heterotopia of the uterine cervix: DNA genotyping confirmation of its fetal origin. Int J Gynecol Pathol 2010;29:394–7.
59. Kazakov DM, Hejda V, Kacerovska D, Michal M. Hyperplasia of ectopic sebaceous glands in the uterine cervix: Case report. Int J Gynecol Pathol 2010;29:605–8.

9 Biology of Cervical Squamous Neoplasia

Cornelia L. Trimble, Rachel Katzenellenbogen

CHAPTER OUTLINE

Introduction	188	Tissue-Resident Immune Cells	194
HPV Infection	188	HPV Vaccines	194
Low-Grade Squamous Intraepithelial Lesions (CIN1)	191	Primary Prevention: Early Detection and Prophylactic Vaccines	194
High-Grade Squamous Intraepithelial Lesions (CIN 2/3)	191	Secondary Prevention: Immune-Based Therapies	195
Mechanisms of Oncogenesis	192	Vaccine Immunogenicity	195
The HPV E6 and E7 Oncoproteins	192	Future Directions	196
Naturally Occurring Immune Responses to HPV Antigens	193		

INTRODUCTION

In the past half-century, cytologic screening, particularly in high-resource settings, has dramatically decreased the burden of squamous cervical cancers, virtually all of which are caused by tissue-specific, persistent infection with human papillomavirus (HPV). The elucidation of the infectious etiology of this disease led to a Nobel Prize in 2008, and to development of preventative vaccines that became commercially available in 2006. This was a public health milestone; worldwide, chronic infections initiate approximately 20% of human cancers,[1] with HPVs causing more malignancies than any other virus. However, because primary prevention strategies are cumbersome and expensive, cervical cancer is still the third most common cause of cancer death in women.[2] Moreover, the incidence of HPV-associated cancers in other anatomic sites, for which no screening algorithms have been developed, is increasing rapidly.

HPV disease is not restricted to the cervix. A growing body of evidence links persistent HPV infection to squamous cancers of the vagina, vulva, anus, and oropharynx.[3] Almost all vaginal and anal squamous cancers[4] and approximately 20% of squamous cancers of the vulva[5] are caused by HPV. The incidence of preinvasive vulvar disease attributed to HPV has increased by 411% over the past three decades, primarily in women under the age 65.[6] HPVs have been identified in one in four squamous carcinomas of the head and neck; to date, the incidence of HPV-associated oropharyngeal cancers is greater in men than in women.[7] Indeed, in the United States, the incidence of HPV-associated cancers of the oropharynx is approximately equal to that of cervical cancer, and is likely to surpass it soon.[8] Because prophylactic vaccines are not administered to the full target population, cohort-appropriate strategies for preventing and treating HPV disease are needed. A better understanding of the biology of intraepithelial, preinvasive HPV disease will inform strategies for screening, secondary prevention, and treatment.

HPV INFECTION

Like other viruses that cause human cancers, most HPV infections are asymptomatic, eventually cleared, and do not harm the host (Figure 9.1). HPV is an epitheliotropic virus that is essentially endemic. In unvaccinated cohorts, the lifetime risk of acquiring genital HPV at least once is greater than 80%.[9] Over 40 genotypes of HPV can infect the genital tract, 15 of which have been classified as carcinogenic (Table 9.1). These include HPV 16, 18, 31, 33, 35, 39, 45, 51, 52, 56, 58, 59, 66, 68, and 72.[10] Together, HPV 16 and HPV 18 are the most common carcinogenic genotypes worldwide (Figures 9.2 and 9.3).[11]

HPV infects cervical epithelium shortly after sexual debut, and can be detected in up to 50% of young women who have initiated sexual intercourse in the preceding 36 months.[12] Most women clear an incident HPV infection within 1–2 years. Several host cofactors that have been associated with progression of HPV infection to carcinoma are shown in Table 9.2. Older women take longer to clear infections, as do smokers, and women with underlying

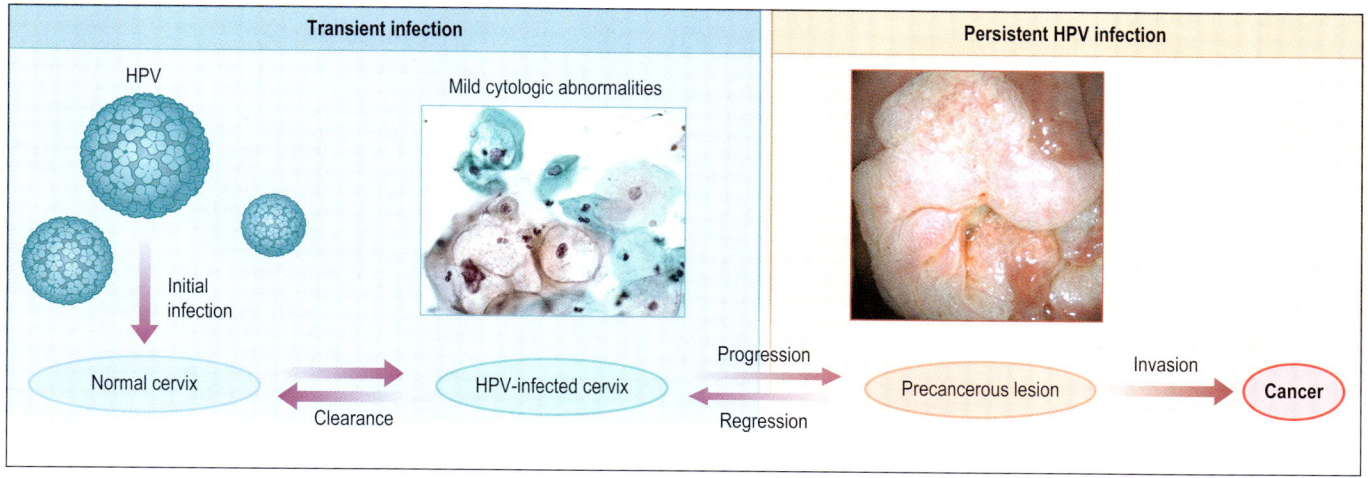

Figure 9.1 Model of HPV-induced cervical pathogenesis, proceeding from HPV infection of the normal cervix to mild cytologic abnormalities, progression to persistent HPV infection and precancerous lesions, and, finally, invasion. Of significance is the ability for precancerous lesions to regress, and the ability of most HPV-infected cervices to clear infection. (Reproduced with permission from Wright and Schiffman.[118])

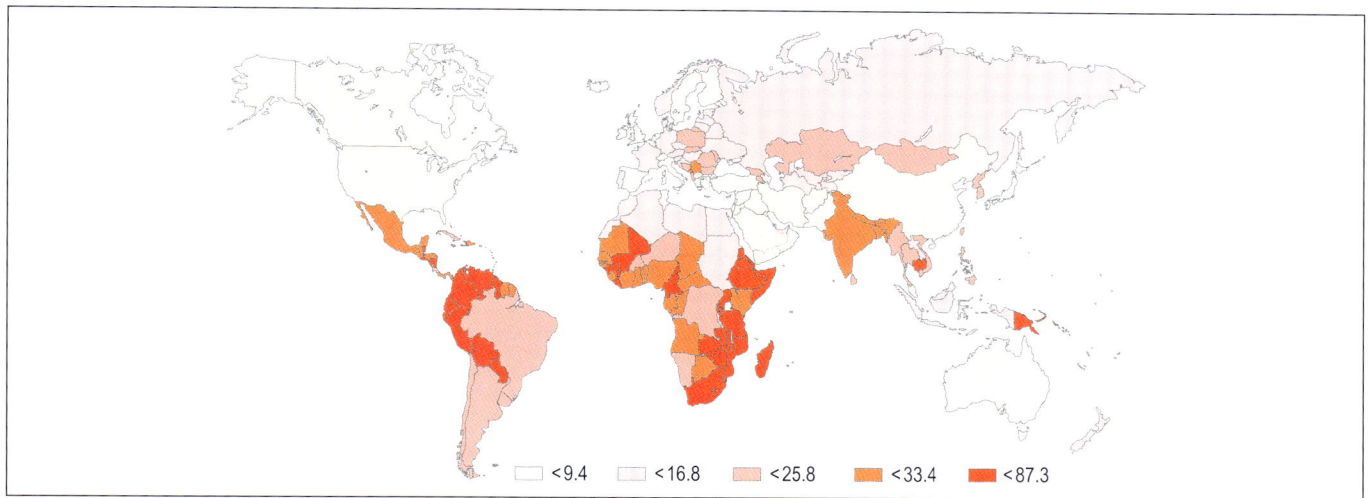

Figure 9.2 Age-standardized incidence rate of cervix uteri per 100,000 women worldwide in the year 2002. The lowest disease burden is largely found among regions with effective screening programs (e.g., North America) and regions where HPV prevalence is low (e.g., China). The greatest disease burden is denoted in red and is found in those countries with high HPV prevalence and without an effective screening program (e.g., East Africa). (Reproduced with permission from Ferlay et al.[119])

Table 9.1 Classification of HPV Types Associated with Genital Lesions

Classification	HPV Type
Oncogenic	16, 18, 31, 33, 35, 39, 45, 51, 52, 56, 58, 59, 68, 73, 82
Putatively oncogenic	26, 53, 66, 70
Non-oncogenic	6, 11, 40, 42, 54, 55, 57, 84

Adapted from Muñoz et al.[13]

HPV infections are limited to the suprabasal compartment of nonsterile barrier epithelia in which the immunologic contributions of the local microbiome are incompletely understood. Viral replication, assembly, and release of virions occur in the context of host cellular maturation and desquamation, without cell lysis, and without systemic viremia. Persistent HPV infections increase susceptibility to malignant transformation by a variety of mechanisms, including enhancing genetic instability and cell proliferation, inducing angiogenesis, interfering with intrinsic and extrinsic apoptotic pathways, downregulating expression of adhesion molecules, abrogating DNA damage responses, and interfering with both innate and adaptive immune responses in the lesion microenvironment. Known virally mediated immune-suppressive mechanisms include interfering with type I interferon responses and Toll-like receptor (TLR) signaling, downregulating cell surface MHC class I expression, enhancing secretion of immunosuppressive immunosuppression.[14] In the cervix, persistent infection is the proximate cause of squamous cancers and their precursors, high-grade squamous intraepithelial lesion (HSIL), or cervical intraepithelial neoplasia (CIN) grade 2 or 3 (CIN 2, CIN 3).

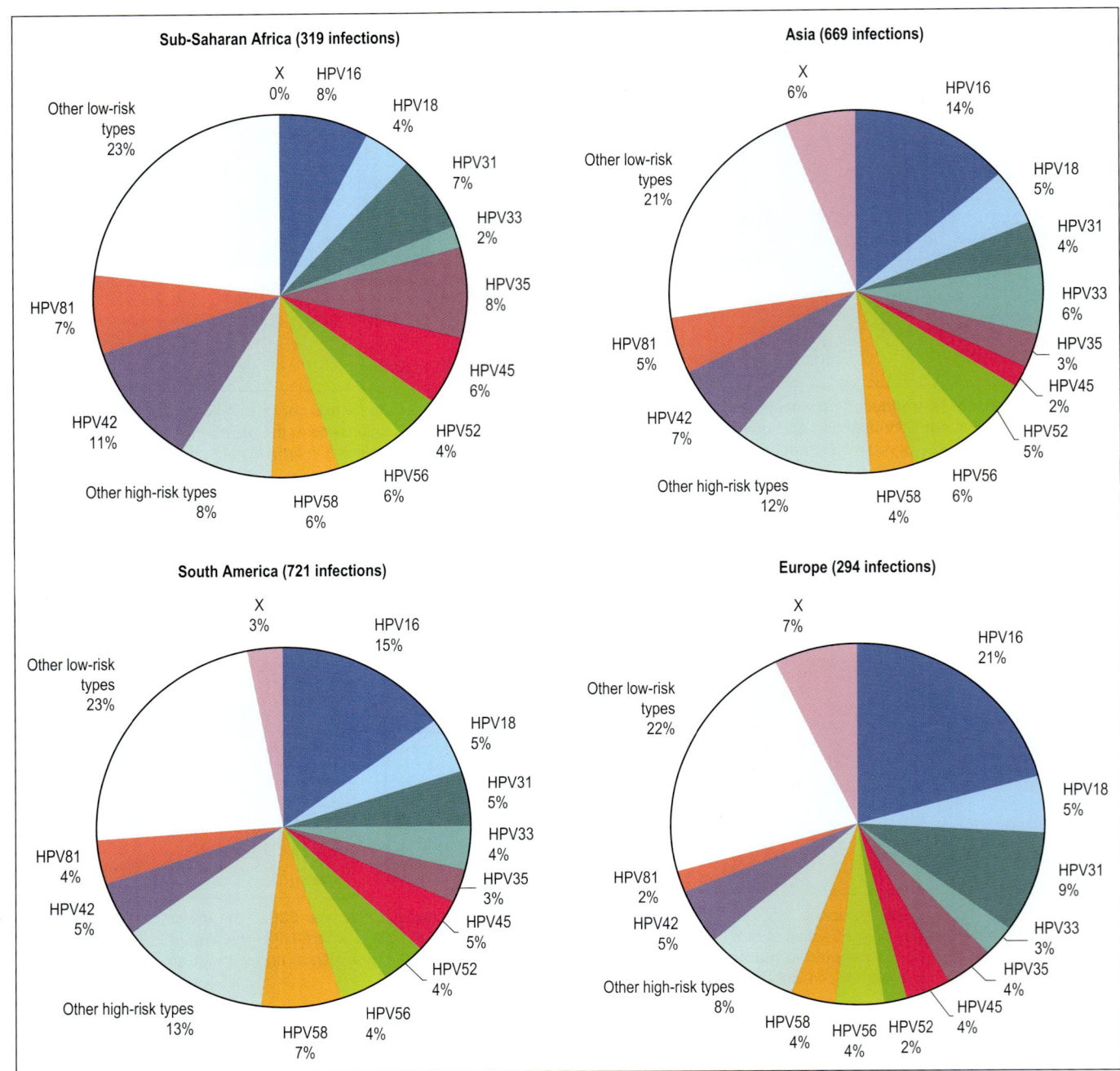

Figure 9.3 Prevalence of HPV types in cytologically normal women worldwide, by geographic region. HPV type-specific burden varies by geography, with HPV 16 prevalence highest (21%) in Europe but HPV 18 prevalence equivalent in all regions. (Reproduced from Clifford et al,[120] with permission from Elsevier)

Table 9.2 Summary of Evaluated HPV Cofactors for Squamous Cell Carcinoma and Adenocarcinoma of the Cervix

HPV Cofactor	Squamous Cell Carcinoma	Adenocarcinoma
Smoking	++ Increased	No association
Parity	++ Increased	No association
Oral contraceptives/hormones	++ Increased	+ Increased
Chlamydia	Increased, but current evidence not significant	No association
Herpes simplex virus 2	Increased, but current evidence not significant	No association
Antioxidants	Decreased, but current evidence not significant	Current evidence not significant
Obesity	No association	+ Increased

cytokines, recruitment of immune cells with suppressive function, and downregulating expression of adhesion molecules in lesional neovascular endothelium.[15–17] Indeed, as we learn more about the immunobiology of persistent infection it becomes less surprising that immune-based therapeutic strategies to date, which have focused solely on eliciting an effector T-cell response to HPV antigens, have failed.

LOW-GRADE SQUAMOUS INTRAEPITHELIAL LESIONS (CIN1)

HPV infects keratinocytes at the basal epithelial layer of the squamocolumnar junction.[18] A productive infection leads to the production of whole infectious virions, and is limited to epithelia that undergo maturation. As HPV does not encode DNA polymerase, host cellular DNA polymerase must be expressed for viral replication. In normal physiologic conditions in stratified squamous epithelium, DNA is copied only in the basal layer. In contrast, in virally infected epithelium, HPV drives DNA replication and cell division in the upper layers of differentiating epithelium, where HPV DNA is packaged into viral capsids, resulting in infectious virions (Figure 9.4).[19] Infectious virions are released not by cell lysis, but in the course of host cell maturation and desquamation, without eliciting an inflammatory response.

HPV infection produces a distinctive cytopathic effect that is recognizable both cytologically and histologically as a sharply demarcated cytoplasmic halo surrounding an enlarged, irregular, hyperchromatic nucleus with uneven chromatin distribution, termed 'koilocytic atypia.'[20] Other findings include multinucleation, parakeratosis, and hyperkeratosis. Histologically, HPV infections can be distinguished by koilocytotic changes in differentiating cells, with increased ratios of nuclear to cytoplasmic area, and mitotically active cells above the basal layer. Clinically, the behavior of cytology interpreted as 'atypical squamous cells of undetermined significance' with a concurrent positive test for oncogenic HPV DNA, cytology interpreted as 'low-grade squamous intraepithelial lesion,' or a tissue biopsy diagnosis of 'low-grade squamous intraepithelial lesion' or 'cervical intraepithelial neoplasia grade I' (CIN 1) is essentially the same; most eventually regress without intervention. Most CIN 1 lesions maintain HPV as an episome, sustain a complete viral replication cycle, and can be thought of as HPV infection.

HIGH-GRADE SQUAMOUS INTRAEPITHELIAL LESIONS (CIN 2/3)

HSILs, or CIN grade 2 or 3 (CIN 2/3), are associated with integration of the viral genome into the host genome, and subsequent constitutive expression of the E6 and E7 viral proteins (Figure 9.5). These proteins are functionally

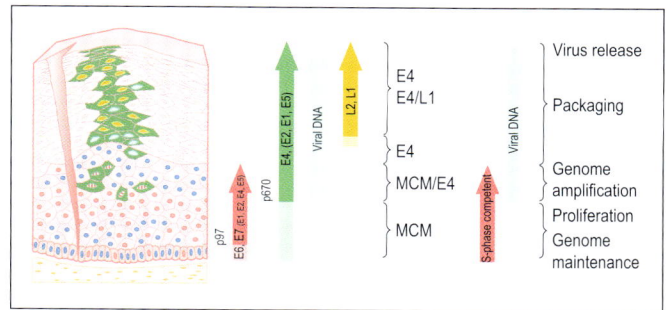

Figure 9.4 HPV gene expression during its life cycle in the genital squamous mucosa, from HPV-infected basal cell and maturation to surface of epithelium. Upon infection, the viral genome is maintained as a low copy number episome. During epithelial differentiation, the p97 promoter directs E6 and E7 expression for S-phase entry (red) and viral replication proteins (E1, E2, E4, E5) increase in abundance (green), facilitating amplification of viral genomes (blue). E4 persists in upper epithelial layers where viral capsid proteins (L1, L2; yellow) are found. (Reproduced with permission from Doorbar.[121])

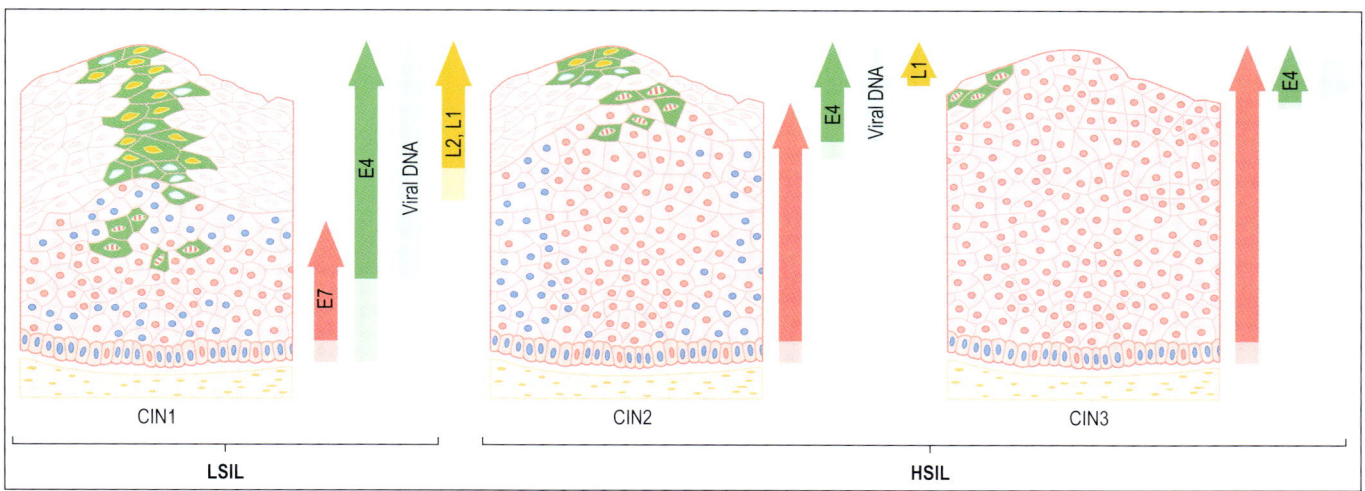

Figure 9.5 HPV early and late gene expression from initial HPV infection through maturation, from CIN 1–3, by evolutionary HPV type. The productive cycle begins close to the basal layer and viral genome amplification begins in the parabasal cell layers. (Reproduced with permission from Doorbar.[121])

required for initiation and persistence of disease.[21,22] Viral integration sites, although randomly distributed within the human genome,[23] occur principally at sites where human DNA is prone to breakage (e.g., fragile sites), and appear to affect only the expression of the HPV genome itself. Specifically, during integration, E1 and/or E2 are frequently disrupted, while the E6 and E7 viral oncogenes are retained, resulting in constitutive expression. Morphologically at the cellular level, HSILs are characterized by a high nuclear to cytoplasmic ratio. Histologically, high-grade lesions display disarray of the basal layer itself, full thickness lack of cell maturation, and are mitotically active.

Although all squamous cervical cancers arise from untreated HSIL, not all HSILs progress to invasive cancer. Approximately 35% of HSILs undergo complete regression in a time frame of 4–6 months.[24,25] Lesions associated with HPV 16 are less likely to regress than lesions associated with other HPV types. Because it is not possible to distinguish HSILs that are likely to regress from those that are not, the standard of care is excision or ablation. Excisional approaches include loop electrocautery excision procedure or cold knife conization. The rate of recurrence is 10%.[26] Iterative excisional procedures are associated with cervical incompetence and subsequent preterm birth.[27,28]

MECHANISMS OF ONCOGENESIS

Mechanisms of oncogenesis can be segregated into those that are directly attributable to viral gene products, which present potential antigenic targets for immune-based prevention or therapy, and those that are indirectly attributable to the effects of viral infection, including immune suppression, type II inflammation, angiogenesis, and genetic instability. These latter pathways present potential druggable targets for secondary prevention strategies targeting tissue microenvironments.

HPV is a small, double-stranded DNA virus with an 8 kb genome comprised of three domains (Figure 9.6): a non-coding upstream regulatory region, an early region containing six genes (E1–E7), and a late region encoding capsid proteins L1 (major capsid) and L2 (minor capsid).[29] The E6 and E7 viral proteins enhance cell proliferation in the face of abrogated DNA damage responses and genetic instability. Additionally, E6 mediates immortalization by activating telomerase. Finally, these oncoproteins compromise both innate and adaptive immune responses in the tissue microenvironment.

Viral persistence is mediated in part by dysregulated innate immunity involving pattern recognition receptor, particularly alterations in expression and function of TLRs in dendritic cells and macrophages. However, as TLRs sense pathogen-associated molecular patterns, including viral genetic material, they are also found in normal cervical epithelial cells.[30,31] While less is known about TLR function in epithelial cells, evidence of dysregulated TLR3 signaling, including dampened expression of genes encoding antimicrobial molecules, chemotactic and pro-inflammatory cytokines, and proteins involved in antigen presentation, has been identified in cervical keratinocytes containing episomal HPV.[32]

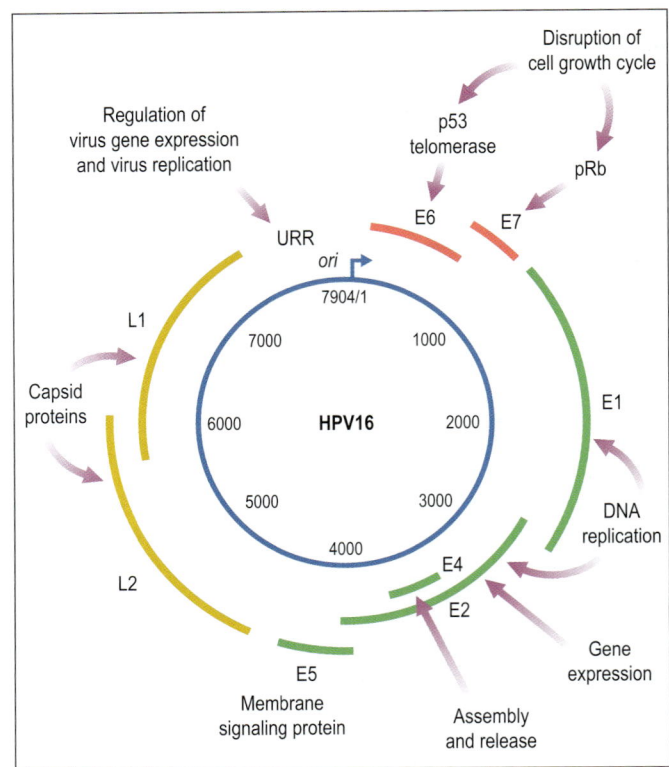

Figure 9.6 HPV genome. (Courtesy Alan Cann, University of Leicester, UK.)

THE HPV E6 AND E7 ONCOPROTEINS

E6 binds to an endogenous E3 ubiquitin ligase, E6 associated protein (E6AP).[33] The E6/E6AP heterodimer binds p53, a tumor suppressor protein that also regulates apoptosis, and targets it for rapid proteasome-mediated degradation.[34] p53 can be stimulated either by genotoxic or cytotoxic damage, or by dysregulated DNA synthesis. These signals would be triggered in an HPV infection, particularly in a persistent infection in which cell cycling continues despite cellular damage.

In infected cells, E6 blocks both the intrinsic and extrinsic apoptosis pathways.[35] The extrinsic apoptosis pathway is triggered by viral infections and activates death receptors on the cell surface. E6 blocks death receptors from interacting with death-inducing signaling complexes, and also degrades signaling proteins, such as FADD and caspase-8.[36,37] The intrinsic apoptosis pathway is activated by DNA damage and oxidative stress. The intrinsic pathway starts in the mitochondria with Bak, and Bak expression in the mitochondrial membrane is blocked by E6.[38] Downstream proteins, such as additional caspases, are degraded by E6, and inhibitors of apoptosis, including NF kappa B, survivin, and c-IAP, are stabilized by E6.[39,40]

E6 also has direct roles in chromosomal instability and DNA damage. Minichromosome maintenance 7 (MCM7) insures there is only a single round of DNA replication in a cell cycle. E6 degrades MCM7, allowing multiple copies of its own DNA to be made.[41] A byproduct of HPV DNA amplification is the risk of excessive cellular chromatin duplication. This aneuploidy normally would be sensed in G2 by p53, triggering cell cycle arrest and apoptosis, but p53 is removed by E6/E6AP. E6 also degrades XRCC1 and O⁶MGMT.[42,43] Both are involved in single-stranded DNA repair, and, without them, stochastic errors that drive cancer development can accrue.

E6 disrupts replicative senescence signals in keratinocytes. With each copy, linear chromosomes lose 100–200 bases of repetitive telomeric DNA. Thus, the age of a cell is inversely proportional to the length of its telomeres. Replicative senescence occurs when somatic cells recognize their intrinsic age.[44] Stem cells express telomerase, a ribonucleoprotein, to extend this DNA, and the catalytic subunit of telomerase, hTERT, is rate determining.[45] By lengthening telomeric DNA, stem cells avoid cellular senescence. Almost all cancers express telomerase to also avoid replicative senescence signals.[46] E6/E6AP enables replicative immortality through hTERT activation. E6/E6AP removes repressors and recruits activators to the normally constitutively repressed promoter of hTERT, and E6 also affects the stability of hTERT mRNA to increase protein production and telomerase activity.[47-52]

E6 degrades proteins involved in cell–cell adhesion and apicobasal polarity. It degrades hScrib, a tight-junction protein, and many postsynaptic density protein 95, *drosophila* disc large tumor suppressor, zonula occludens-1 protein (PDZ) domain-containing proteins.[53-57] Finally E6 binds proteins in the extracellular matrix.[58] These changes are important to allow viral release from cells as they slough off the upper layers of stratified squamous epithelium. They are also important in invasion and metastases.[59,60]

Finally, E6 interferes with innate immune responses. Interferon regulatory factor 3 (IRF-3) is normally activated by a viral infection, but is inhibited by E6.[61] TLR9 is activated by viral DNA motifs and induces cytokine production, but E6 blocks its expression.[62]

The second crucial HPV oncoprotein, E7, destabilizes retinoblastoma protein (pRb) and other pocket proteins by targeting them for proteasome-mediated degradation, resulting in cell cycle progression, as these proteins normally hold cells in G1, not allowing DNA synthesis.[63-65] In E7-driven proliferation, S-phase gene expression ensues, and viral DNA is copied in addition to cellular DNA. E7 drives cell division gene activation and increases the open chromatin structure at gene promoters. E7 also binds histone deacetylases and represses polycomb group complexes, some of which are histone methyltransferases.[66,67]

E7 not only pushes cells to continue to divide, but also helps them to evade growth suppressors. E7 blocks transforming growth factor-beta (TGF-β) and tumor necrosis factor (TNF)-alpha G1.[68,69] TNF-α G1 is a cytokine that induces programmed cell death, and is produced by cytotoxic T-cells to eliminate virally infected cells. Activation of IRFs is also blocked by E7, thereby compromising activation of innate immunity.[70]

E7 also binds to p600, a pRb-associated factor critical for anchorage-dependent growth.[71] E7 increases expression of vascular endothelial growth factor and IL-8, both of which are angiogenic, and enhances transcriptional activity of hypoxia inducible factor 1α (HIF 1α), and disrupts interaction with histone deacetylases.[72-74] Finally E7, like E6, can induce DNA damage at the chromosomal level. E7 increases centrosome amplification early in the viral life cycle.[75,76] This increase in centrosomes can lead to DNA damage, and increases the frequency of DNA integration. As has been demonstrated in cell lines and mouse model systems, E6 and E7 (or equivalently inactivation of p53 and Rb) cooperate to produce full-fledged malignancy.[77]

NATURALLY OCCURRING IMMUNE RESPONSES TO HPV ANTIGENS

In immune-competent hosts, over 90% of genital HPV infections become undetectable without intervention.[78] However, naturally occurring systemic humoral and adaptive responses to HPV antigens, even in cohorts with documented type-specific mucosal infections that have become undetectable, are hard to detect in peripheral blood.[79-81] Type-specific serum antibodies to capsid proteins are detectable in less than half of women in whom cervical HPV infections of known serotype have cleared. Nonetheless, data from cohorts undergoing prophylactic vaccination demonstrate an anamnestic response to a single dose of virus-like particle vaccine in previously infected subjects.[82] Dysplasia is associated with ineffective immune responses to viral nonstructural proteins. Antibody to E7 can be measured in persons with invasive cancer, but not in earlier stage disease.[83]

HSIL (CIN 2/3) is a lesion that should be susceptible to an HPV-specific effector immune response. Expression of viral, non-'self' proteins is functionally required to initiate and maintain the transformed phenotype, thereby providing true tumor-associated antigenic targets.[21,22] Not all cervical HSILs progress to cancer; 25% of established CIN 2/3 lesions caused by HPV 16, the genotype most commonly associated with malignancy, undergo complete regression.[25]

However, women with squamous intraepithelial HPV lesions rarely have systemic T-cell responses to HPV E6 or E7 that can be detected directly *ex vivo*, likely reflecting the tissue compartmentalization of early disease. In contrast to immune responses to other viral infections, the frequency of systemic memory CD8+ T-cells in individuals with a known prior cervical HPV infection, which has subsequently become undetectable, is vanishingly low. For example, using direct *ex vivo* assays, the frequency of systemic virus-specific CD8+ T-cells after primary infection with cytomegalovirus or hepatitis C virus (HCV) can be up to 5%.[84,85] In contrast, in subjects with CIN, the frequency of HPV-specific T-cells is two to three orders of magnitude lower, in the range of 0.1–0.01%.[86] Detection of systemic HPV-specific T-cell responses in subjects with intraepithelial neoplasia requires *ex vivo* sensitization.[87-89] After *in vitro* stimulation with HPV antigens, peptide-specific T-cell frequencies increase in subjects with concurrent disease at the time of blood sampling, compared with subjects with no evidence of disease.[86,90] While amplification can identify qualitative responses to HPV antigens, it is likely to have limited use in accurately distinguishing quantitative differences between individual subjects, either in the course of a natural infection or in subjects with intraepithelial disease. Responses identified only after prolonged *in vitro* restimulation likely represent expansion of previously induced memory immune responses, rather than an ongoing response at the time of sampling.

From a practical standpoint, two conclusions can be drawn concerning T-cell responses in women with squamous intraepithelial lesions: first, natural infection with HPV fails to elicit a potent systemic immune response, and, second, the magnitude of natural HPV-specific T-cell responses measured in the peripheral blood of individual patients does not reliably predict lesion regression. These findings raise the question of whether T-cell responses to these antigens are clinically relevant. Alternatively, responses detected in the blood in the setting of natural infection may not reflect immune responses in the target lesion.

In immune-competent persons with undetectable systemic HPV T-cell responses, dense immune cell infiltrates nonetheless localize at the lesion site, and, in persistent disease, fail to access the lesional epithelium. In contrast, dysplastic lesions that 'permit' CD8+ T-cell access to the epithelial compartment are likely to regress.[17] This observation suggests that, even in the clinical setting of preinvasive, incipient neoplasia, factors in the lesions mitigate the ability of recruited CD8+ T-cells to eliminate disease.

TISSUE-RESIDENT IMMUNE CELLS

Antigen-experienced T-lymphocytes display preferential tropism for the tissue in which they encountered their cognate antigen.[91–94] Constitutive trafficking of antigen-experienced T-lymphocytes in a tissue-specific manner is mediated by distinct sets of chemokines and adhesion molecules. Tissue homing occurs via sequential tethering of leukocyte selectins to vascular endothelium, followed by leukocyte activation by locally expressed chemokines, conformational changes in surface integrins, and subsequent interactions with tissue-localized ligands to mediate firm adhesion and extravasation. This compartmentalization provides a mechanism that is essential for rapid immune recognition of pathogens at the most probable sites of encounter. To date, it has not been possible to study cervical resident T-cell populations in detail, in part because tissues obtained during routine care are small, and because conventional methods of isolating T-cells from tissue biopsies yield only low numbers of cells. Above all, studies on clinical specimens must not compromise the ability to make an accurate diagnosis, or place a study subject at risk from excessive tissue procurement.

The recent development of methods for isolating tissue-resident T-cells from normal and dysplastic primary tissue explants has opened up opportunities to quantitate tissue-specific immunologic parameters. Small tissue cervical mucosal explants cultured short term without cytokine support yield sufficient numbers of tissue T-cells to permit limited characterization of immune cell subset phenotype, and their functional polarization. Like other tissue-resident T-cell populations, cervical T-cells in normal mucosa have an effector memory phenotype (CD45RO+CD62L–CCR7–), and are slightly activated (CD25lo/CD69lo). Virtually all T-cells in both normal and dysplastic cervical mucosa express the α4β7 surface integrin, and the intensity of lesional epithelial CD8+ T-cell infiltrates correlates directly with expression of MAdCAM-1 in lesional epithelial vascular endothelium.[17] Downregulated vascular endothelial expression of adhesion molecules is a common mechanism by which invasive or metastatic human solid tumors evade locally recruited immune effector cells; this finding suggests that endothelial activation is a reasonable therapeutic target in HSILs. Together, this constellation of observations suggests that methods to monitor biologically plausible end points in the target tissue should be validated, as they are likely to provide insights as to the success or failure of immune-based therapies.

HPV VACCINES

PRIMARY PREVENTION: EARLY DETECTION AND PROPHYLACTIC VACCINES

In high-resource settings, the mainstays of cervical cancer prevention include prophylactic vaccination in younger persons, and improved screening, including testing for HPV DNA, in older persons. Because prophylactic vaccination is not universal, age-appropriate screening strategies should be applied. Women over the age of 30 should be screened using a combination of cytology and HPV DNA testing, while young, HPV-naive cohorts will derive more benefit from prophylactic vaccination.

The goal of cervical cancer screening is to identify patients at risk for the development of disease, that is, those with the immediate precursor lesion, HSIL. In high-resource settings, routine screening includes repeated cytologic and HPV screening over the course of a lifetime. Current guidelines issued by the U.S. Preventive Services Task Force recommend age-specific screening strategies; screening should not begin until age 21 regardless of sexual activity. Women aged 21–29 years should be screened every 3 years by cytology alone. In 'older' women aged 30–65 years, co-testing with cytology and HPV testing is recommended at 5 year intervals. More frequent screening is recommended for immunosuppressed patients; women infected with human immunodeficiency virus (HIV); women exposed to diethylstilbestrol *in utero*; and women previously treated for CIN 2, CIN 3, or cancer. Screening may be discontinued in women age 65–70 with three prior consecutively normal Pap smears, and no abnormal Pap smears over a period of 10 years.[95]

Despite the effectiveness of using cytology and HPV DNA testing to detect disease, it is expensive and cumbersome. Many women undergo repetitive Pap smears and colposcopy for evaluation of low-grade dysplastic lesions that are likely to resolve over time. Repetitive clinic visits and testing not only places a psychological burden on the patient, but also places economic strain upon the society providing the screening. In the United States alone, it has been estimated that 6 billion dollars per year are spent on evaluation of low-grade lesions.[96] Recently, the long-term predictive value of HPV testing in a cohort of women followed for up to 18 years has been reported.[97] Women with a baseline prevalent infection, as well as women with incident infections detected over the course of the study were included in this analysis. HPV detection was confirmed using a commercially available diagnostic test that is used routinely in clinical practice. HPV detection stratified risk more accurately than cytology; persons with a baseline negative HPV test were less likely to have a CIN 3 or squamous carcinoma ('CIN 3+') diagnosed than persons who had a normal Pap smear. Conversely, detectable HPV DNA identified women at elevated risk of subsequent CIN 3 or cancer. In the face of a normal Pap smear, detection of either HPV 16 or HPV 18 conferred a higher risk of CIN 3 or cancer than detection of other HPV genotypes. This work is important because it provides data to support risk-based screening, which can be done using tools that are already available as part of routine practice. The implication of using a test that is quantitative and not subjective as a primary screening tool is that it does not need to be performed by a provider with specialized training.

Currently available preventative vaccines, Gardasil (Merck & Co) (HPV 4) and Cervarix (GlaxoSmithKline) (HPV 2), are virtually 100% effective in prevention of high-grade cervical intraepithelial lesions associated with HPV 16 and HPV 18. However, rates of vaccine administration vary widely. For example, in Australia, administration in eligible girls is >80%.[98] In the United States, the Centers for Disease Control reported that, in 2009, less than half (44%) of eligible children had been vaccinated.[99] Rates of vaccine completion, defined as undergoing the full series of three prophylactic vaccinations, is dismal. Among vaccine initiators in the United States, less than one in four complete vaccination.[99] As HPV 4 and HPV 2 elicit type-specific antibody responses to capsid (L1), they have no therapeutic effect whatsoever.

SECONDARY PREVENTION: IMMUNE-BASED THERAPIES

Development of immune therapeutic strategies presents another strategy to decrease the global burden of HPV disease. HPV-infected epithelial cells express viral proteins that should, in theory, provide antigenic targets for therapeutic vaccines. Many therapeutic HPV vaccine constructs, including peptide, protein, recombinant viral vector-based, and DNA vaccines, have elicited antigen-specific effector immune responses that are curative, in preclinical murine models using transplanted E7-expressing epithelial tumor cell lines.[100] To date, clinical success has not been nearly as robust. Several factors are likely to play a role in the pace of translation that has been incremental until relatively recently. Broadly, these include the immunogenicity in humans of vaccines tested, and clinical trial design, including cohort selection, length of study window, and end points assessed.

VACCINE IMMUNOGENICITY

Three broad categories of therapeutic vaccines have been tested to date in subjects with preinvasive HPV disease. These include DNA vaccines, recombinant viral vector-based vaccines, and adjuvanted protein or peptide vaccines. The antigen specificity of DNA vaccines can be engineered precisely, and production can be accomplished relatively simply on a large scale with high purity. Multicomponent vaccines can be engineered to include specific immunogens to amplify immunologic responses. DNA vaccines can be used for repeated administration, as the immunogenicity of plasmid vectors is not influenced by pre-existing neutralizing antibodies.[101] DNA vaccination has been shown to cause minimal if any toxicities or side effects in humans.

In fact, to date, the major drawback of DNA vaccine approaches in clinical translation has been their relatively low potency. The immunogenicity of conventional intramuscular administration is likely to be limited by inefficient uptake of DNA by host cells. Delivery via electroporation, a technology that applies short electrical pulses *in situ*, increases uptake by temporarily permeabilizing cell membranes,[102] which in nonhuman primate models increases immunogenicity of DNA vaccination by 100-fold.[103] Currently, several clinical trials testing electroporation-mediated delivery of DNA vaccines are underway, targeting HIV, HCV, and solid tumor antigens (prostate, carcinoembryonic antigen (CEA), HER2/neu, melanoma), and HPV.[104]

While recombinant viral vector-based vaccines are more immunogenic in humans than DNA vaccines, they cannot be administered sequentially, as immune responses to the vector are likely to outstrip responses to engineered antigenic targets. However, a growing body of preclinical as well as clinical evidence suggests that sequential vaccination consisting of a DNA priming vaccination, followed by a recombinant viral vector-based boost vaccination, is more immunogenic than either strategy used alone.[105] Heterologous prime-boost trials targeting malarial and HIV antigens have demonstrated proof of principle, and studies testing this strategy in HPV disease are underway (National Cancer Institute funded trial NCT00788164).

The third broad category of therapeutic HPV vaccines tested to date includes the use of adjuvanted peptide and proteins. Like DNA vaccines, antigen specificity can be engineered precisely. However, the use of individual peptide targets is restricted by the assumption of immunodominant epitopes. Vaccination with protein or with long peptides has the advantage of allowing antigen processing in the host. Recently, the use of adjuvanted long peptides spanning the length of HPV 16 E6 and E7 has sparked a great deal of interest, as clinical responses were observed in 47% of vaccinated subjects with vulvar intraepithelial neoplasia (VIN).[106]

Similar to other therapeutic cancer vaccines, initially, therapeutic HPV vaccines were tested in cohorts with late-stage disease. More recently, the focus of immune-based therapies for HPV disease has shifted to testing interventions to eliminate preinvasive, intraepithelial disease. Preinvasive HPV lesions provide a potentially informative clinical setting to test proof-of-principle trial designs, for several reasons. Intraepithelial HPV disease is readily accessible, allowing direct monitoring of target lesions as well as topical application of immune response modifiers. HSIL is relatively indolent clinically, and some lesions appear to be susceptible to immune modulation.

Several painstaking studies of immune responses to HPV early antigens, in clinically annotated cohorts, provide important insights for the design and interpretation of clinical trials to test therapeutic HPV vaccines. First, it is clear that weak virus-specific systemic effector responses measured in the peripheral blood in otherwise healthy subjects with preinvasive lesions can be associated with lesion regression.[81,107-109] In vaccinated as well as unvaccinated cohorts, systemic effector immune responses to HPV E6 and E7, even in healthy subjects, have required *ex vivo* expansion for detection.[108,110,111] The fact that women with pre-existing detectable systemic T-cell responses to HPV antigens are more likely to respond clinically to directed manipulations creating a local proinflammatory microenvironment suggests that virus-specific adaptive responses do play a role in lesion clearance.[112]

Mechanisms of immune evasion that have already been identified in invasive or metastatic solid tumors are also likely to play a role in preinvasive HPV disease. The study of effector and homeostatic immune cell infiltrates in HPV-infected epithelia has begun to provide insights that are likely to be useful in directing future clinical investigations. CIN 2/3 lesions are associated with accumulation of Foxp3+ and IDO+ immune-suppressive T-cells, compared with normal cervical tissue.[113,114] Conversely, immune-active CD4 and CD8 T-cell infiltrates in lesional epithelium are identified in regressing lesions.[107,108,112] Lesional stroma is also likely to play a role in immune suppression, particularly in the functional polarization of recruited immune cells, via secretion of immune-suppressive cytokines.[115] Most analyses of clinical tissue samples, however, have been case–control studies, and it is worth stating that preinterventional and postinterventional studies of immunologic parameters in the target tissues should be incorporated into clinical trial design, when possible.

Recent therapeutic trials in healthy cohorts with VIN illustrate the concept of testing combinatorial regimens that include both therapeutic vaccination as well as manipulation of the lesion microenvironment. VIN lesions, although indolent, are also clinically recalcitrant. Currently, the mainstay of treatment for VIN is wide local excision. Recurrence is common, particularly in multifocal disease, requiring additional surgery in approximately 15% of subjects with negative resection margins, 40% of subjects with multifocal disease, and nearly half of subjects with positive margins.[116] Recently, two approaches have demonstrated significant clinical responses that are associated with immune readouts: systemic immunization with long peptides spanning E6 and E7, administered with adjuvant, and local manipulation of the lesion site using topical application of imiquimod, a TLR7 agonist, followed by therapeutic HPV vaccination.

In subjects with HPV 16+ VIN, therapeutic vaccination with long peptides spanning HPV 16 E6 and E7, adjuvanted with montanide, achieved a complete response rate of 45%.[106] This result is remarkable because, unvaccinated, the expected rate of regression in this cohort is well under 5%. In this study, clinical responders had smaller lesions at study entry than nonresponders. Responders also had peripheral blood proliferative responses to vaccine antigens that were broader and of greater magnitude than nonresponders. In contrast, nonresponders had a detectable increase in CD4+CD25+Foxp3+ cells post vaccination in the peripheral blood. However, the magnitude of effector responses in responders overlapped with that identified in nonresponders, which suggests that factors in the lesions themselves may have mitigated the ability of vaccine-induced immune responses to eliminate disease.

Subjects enrolled in a different trial that tested the sequence of lesion manipulation with imiquimod, a topical TLR7 agonist, followed by therapeutic vaccination, achieved a complete response rate of 63%.[112] Similar to previous therapeutic vaccine studies, peripheral blood responses of responders overlapped with those detected in nonresponders. However, responders were nonetheless more likely than nonresponders to have had detectable pre-existing proliferative responses to HPV antigens in the peripheral blood. Similar to subjects in the long peptide trial, responders had postvaccination proliferative responses to vaccine antigens that were broader and of greater magnitude than nonresponders. The fact that, in both of these trials, sophisticated methods using *ex vivo* manipulation were required to detect immune responses suggests that HPV-specific cells identified in the blood were not effector memory cells, which respond immediately, but were more likely to have been central memory cells, which have a longer time frame for response. Quantitative analyses of immune cell subsets in lesional tissue identified increased aggregates of both CD4 and CD8 T-cells in responders, and increased infiltrates of regulatory T-cells in nonresponders.

In both of these studies, clinical responses 'accumulated' over study time frames that extended well beyond the last study vaccination. In both studies, subjects with VIN were monitored for 52 weeks before definitive surgical excision. Although subjects whose lesions underwent regression tended to do so earlier rather than later, these trials suggest that, in subjects whose disease can be monitored safely, allowing immune responses to access lesions may require patience. Second, although both local manipulation to enhance acute inflammation as well as systemic vaccination enhanced the rate of lesion regression, immunologic parameters that could reliably distinguish or predict 'responders' from 'nonresponders' at the outset have yet to be identified. These studies are consistent with animal studies in which clearance of HPV disease requires enabling HPV-specific immune effector cells via tissue-localized acute inflammation.[117] Together these studies emphasize the need to include immunologic parameters in the target tissues as study end points. They also suggest that interventional clinical trials testing systemically administered therapeutic vaccines should be designed to allow a sufficient time frame for responses to accumulate.

FUTURE DIRECTIONS

Much remains to be learned about the effect of the genital mucosal microenvironment on the development of virus-specific effector and suppressor immune responses and their ability to modulate clinical outcomes of HPV infection. Our understanding of the biology of mucosal immune cell trafficking, including the induction and maintenance of tissue-resident T-cells in the genital mucosa, is only beginning. A better understanding of the mechanisms that allow discrimination between potentially harmful pathogens and symbiosis with mucosal commensal flora is likely to inform therapeutic strategies for persistent HPV infections. A prerequisite to realizing these advances is development of improved methods for determination of qualitative and quantitative changes in genital mucosal resident immune cell populations.

REFERENCES

1. Parkin DM, Bray F, Ferlay J, Pisani P. Global cancer statistics, 2002. CA Cancer J Clin 2005;55(2):74–108.

2. Ferlay J, Shin HR, Bray F, et al. Estimates of worldwide burden of cancer in 2008: GLOBOCAN 2008. Int J Cancer 2008;127(12):2893–917.
3. De Vuyst H, Clifford GM, Nascimento MC, et al. Prevalence and type distribution of human papillomavirus in carcinoma and intraepithelial neoplasia of the vulva, vagina and anus: a meta-analysis. Int J Cancer 2009;124(7):1626–36.
4. Parkin DM. The global health burden of infection-associated cancers in the year 2002. Int J Cancer 2006;118(12):3030–44.
5. van de Nieuwenhof HP, van Kempen LC, de Hullu JA, et al. The etiologic role of HPV in vulvar squamous cell carcinoma fine tuned. Cancer Epidemiol Biomarkers Prev 2009;18(7):2061–7.
6. Jones RW, Rowan DM, Stewart AW. Vulvar intraepithelial neoplasia: aspects of the natural history and outcome in 405 women. Obstet Gynecol 2005;106(6):1319–26.
7. Kreimer AR, Clifford GM, Boyle P, Franceschi S. Human papillomavirus types in head and neck squamous cell carcinomas worldwide: a systematic review. Cancer Epidemiol Biomarkers Prev 2005;4(2):467–75.
8. Chaturvedi AK, Engels EA, Pfeiffer RM, et al. Human papillomavirus and rising oropharyngeal cancer incidence in the United States. J Clin Oncol 2011;29(32):4294–301.
9. Baseman JG, Koutsky, LA. The epidemiology of human papillomavirus infections. J Clin Virol 2005;32(Suppl 1):S16–24.
10. Muñoz N, Franco EL, Herrero R, et al. Recommendations for cervical cancer prevention in Latin America and the Caribbean. Vaccine 2008;26(Suppl 11):L96–107.
11. de Sanjose S, Diaz M, Castellsague X, et al. Worldwide prevalence and genotype distribution of cervical human papillomavirus DNA in women with normal cytology: a meta-analysis. Lancet Infect Dis 2007;7(7):453–9.
12. Woodman CB, Collins S, Winter H, et al. Natural history of cervical human papillomavirus infection in young women: a longitudinal cohort study. Lancet 2001;357(9271):1831–6.
13. Muñoz N, Bosch FX, de Sanjose S, et al. Epidemiologic classification of human papillomavirus types associated with cervical cancer. N Engl J Med 2003;348:518–27.
14. Frazer IH, Lowy DR, Schiller JT. Prevention of cancer through immunization: prospects and challenges for the 21st century. Eur J Immunol 2007;37(Suppl 1):S148–55.
15. Visser J, Nijman HW, Hoogenboom BN, et al. Frequencies and role of regulatory T cells in patients with (pre)malignant cervical neoplasia. Clin Exp Immunol 2007;150(2):199–209.
16. Cromme FV, Snijders PJ, van den Brule AJ, et al. MHC class I expression in HPV 16 positive cervical carcinomas is post-transcriptionally controlled and independent from c-myc overexpression. Oncogene 1993;8(11):2969–75.
17. Trimble CL, Clark RA, Thoburn C, et al. Human papillomavirus 16-associated cervical intraepithelial neoplasia in humans excludes CD8 T cells from dysplastic epithelium. J Immunol 2010;185(11):7107–14.
18. Herfs M, Yamamoto Y, Laura A, et al. A discrete population of squamocolumnar junction cells implicated in the pathogenesis of cervical cancer. Proc Natl Acad Sci USA 2012;109(26):10516–21.
19. Doorbar J. Molecular biology of human papillomavirus infection and cervical cancer. Clin Sci (Lond) 2006;110(5):525–41.
20. Koss LG, Durfee, GR. Unusual patterns of squamous epithelium of the uterine cervix: cytologic and pathologic study of koilocytotic atypia. Ann NY Acad Sci 1956;63(1):1245–61.
21. Werness B, Levine A, Howley P. Association of human papillomavirus types 16 and 18 proteins with p53. Science 1990;248:76–9.
22. Hudson JB, Bedell MA, McCance DJ, Laiminis LA. Immortalization and altered differentiation of human keratinocytes in vitro by the E6 and E7 open reading frames of human papillomavirus type 18. J Virol 1990;64(2):519–26.
23. Wang SS, Hildesheim A. Chapter 5: Viral and host factors in human papillomavirus persistence and progression. J Natl Cancer Inst Monogr 2003;(31):35–40.
24. Melnikow J, Nuovo J, Willan AR, et al. Natural history of cervical squamous intraepithelial lesions: a meta-analysis. Obstet Gynecol 1998;92(4 Pt 2):727–35.
25. Trimble CL, Piantadosi S, Gravitt P, et al. Spontaneous regression of high-grade cervical dysplasia: effects of human papillomavirus type and HLA phenotype. Clin Cancer Res 2005;11(13):4717–23.
26. Ramchandani SM, Houck KL, Hernandez E, Gaughan JP. Predicting persistent/recurrent disease in the cervix after excisional biopsy. MedGenMed 2007;9(2):24.
27. Bevis KS, Biggio, JR. Cervical conization and the risk of preterm delivery. Am J Obstet Gynecol 2011;205(1):19–27.
28. Sadler L, Saftlas A, Wang W, et al. Treatment for cervical intraepithelial neoplasia and risk of preterm delivery. JAMA 2004;291(17):2100–6.
29. Laimins LA. The biology of human papillomaviruses: from warts to cancer. Infect Agents Dis 1993;2(2):74–86.
30. Andersen JM, Al-Khairy D, Ingalls RR. Innate immunity at the mucosal surface: role of toll-like receptor 3 and toll-like receptor 9 in cervical epithelial cell responses to microbial pathogens. Biol Reprod 2006;74(5):824–31.
31. DeCarlo CA, Rosa B, Jackson R, et al. Toll-like receptor transcriptome in the HPV-positive cervical cancer microenvironment. Clin Dev Immunol 2012;2012:785825.
32. Karim R, Meyers C, Backendorf C, et al. Human papillomavirus deregulates the response of a cellular network comprising of chemotactic and proinflammatory genes. PLoS One 2011;6(3):e17848.
33. Huibregtse JM, Scheffner M, Howley PM. A cellular protein mediates association of p53 with the E6 oncoprotein of human papillomavirus types 16 or 18. EMBO J 1991;10(13):4129–35.
34. Huibregtse JM, Scheffner M, Howley PM. Cloning and expression of the cDNA for E6-AP, a protein that mediates the interaction of the human papillomavirus E6 oncoprotein with p53. Mol Cell Biol 1993;13(2):775–84.
35. Howie HL, Katzenellenbogen RA, Galloway DA. Papillomavirus E6 proteins. Virology 2009;384(2):324–34.
36. Filippova M, Johnson MM, Bautista M, et al. The large and small isoforms of human papillomavirus type 16 E6 bind to and differentially affect procaspase 8 stability and activity. J Virol 2007;81(8):4116–29.
37. Tungteakkhun SS, Filippova M, Neidigh JW, et al. The interaction between human papillomavirus type 16 and FADD is mediated by a novel E6 binding domain. J Virol 2008;82(19):9600–14.
38. Thomas M, Banks L. Inhibition of Bak-induced apoptosis by HPV-18 E6. Oncogene 1998;17(23):2943–54.
39. James MA, Lee JH, Klingelhutz AJ. Human papillomavirus type 16 E6 activates NF-kappaB, induces cIAP-2 expression, and protects against apoptosis in a PDZ binding motif-dependent manner. J Virol 2006;80(11):5301–7.
40. Borbely AA, Murvai M, Konya J, et al. Effects of human papillomavirus type 16 oncoproteins on survivin gene expression. J Gen Virol 2006;87(Pt 2):287–94.
41. Kuhne C, Bank L. E3-ubiquitin ligase/E6-AP links multicopy maintenance protein 7 to the ubiquitination pathway by a novel motif, the L2G box. J Biol Chem 1998;273(51):34302–9.
42. Iftner T, Elbel M, Schopp B, et al. Interference of papillomavirus E6 protein with single-strand break repair by interaction with XRCC1. EMBO J 2002;21(17):4741–8.
43. Srivenugopal KS, Ali-Osman F. The DNA repair protein, O(6)-methylguanine-DNA methyltransferase is a proteolytic target for the E6 human papillomavirus oncoprotein. Oncogene 2002;21(38):5940–5.
44. Hayflick L. The limited in vitro lifetime of human diploid cell strains. Exp Cell Res 1965;37:614–36.
45. Counter CM, Meyerson M, Eaton EN, et al. Telomerase activity is restored in human cells by ectopic expression of hTERT (hEST2), the catalytic subunit of telomerase. Oncogene 1998;16(9):1217–22.
46. Shay JW, Bacchetti S. A survey of telomerase activity in human cancer. Eur J Cancer 1997;33(5):787–91.
47. Veldman T, Horikawa I, Barrett JC, Schlegel R. Transcriptional activation of the telomerase hTERT gene by human papillomavirus type 16 E6 oncoprotein. J Virol 2001;75(9):4467–72.
48. Katzenellenbogen RA, Vliet-Grett P, Xu M, Galloway D. NFX1-123 increases hTERT expression and telomerase activity posttranscriptionally in human papillomavirus type 16 E6 keratinocytes. J Virol 2009;83(13):6446–56.
49. James MA, Lee JH, Klingelhutz AJ. HPV16-E6 associated hTERT promoter acetylation is E6AP dependent, increased in later passage cells and enhanced by loss of p300. Int J Cancer 2006;119(8):1878–85.
50. Liu X, Yuan H, Fu B, et al. The E6AP ubiquitin ligase is required for transactivation of the hTERT promoter by the human

papillomavirus E6 oncoprotein. J Biol Chem 2005;280(11): 10807–16.
51. McMurray HR, McCance DJ. Human papillomavirus type 16 E6 activates TERT gene transcription through induction of c-Myc and release of USF-mediated repression. J Virol 2003;77(18):9852–61.
52. Oh, ST, Kyo S, Laimins LA. Telomerase activation by human papillomavirus type 16 E6 protein: induction of human telomerase reverse transcriptase expression through Myc and GC-rich Sp1 binding sites. J Virol 2001;75(12):5559–66.
53. Nakagawa S, Huibregtse JM. Human scribble (Vartul) is targeted for ubiquitin-mediated degradation by the high-risk papillomavirus E6 proteins and the E6AP ubiquitin-protein ligase. Mol Cell Biol 2000;20(21):8244–53.
54. Lee SS, Glaunsinger B, Mantovani F, et al. Multi-PDZ domain protein MUPP1 is a cellular target for both adenovirus E4-ORF1 and high-risk papillomavirus type 18 E6 oncoproteins. J Virol 2000;74(20):9680–93.
55. Massimi P, Gammoh N, Thomas M, Banks L. HPV E6 specifically targets different cellular pools of its PDZ domain-containing tumour suppressor substrates for proteasome-mediated degradation. Oncogene 2004;23(49):8033–39.
56. Spanos WC, Hoover A, Harris GF, et al. The PDZ binding motif of human papillomavirus type 16 E6 induces PTPN13 loss, which allows anchorage-independent growth and synergizes with ras for invasive growth. J Virol 2008;82(5):2493–500.
57. Kranjec C, Banks L. A systematic analysis of human papillomavirus (HPV) E6 PDZ substrates identifies MAGI-1 as a major target of HPV type 16 (HPV-16) and HPV-18 whose loss accompanies disruption of tight junctions. J Virol 2011;85(4):1757–64.
58. Du M, Fan X, Hong E, Chen JJ. Interaction of oncogenic papillomavirus E6 proteins with fibulin-1. Biochem Biophys Res Commun 2002;296(4):962–9.
59. Watson RA, Thomas M, Banaks L, et al. Activity of the human papillomavirus E6 PDZ-binding motif correlates with an enhanced morphological transformation of immortalized human keratinocytes. J Cell Sci 2003;116(Pt 24):4925–34.
60. Nguyen ML, Nguyen MM, Lee D, et al. The PDZ ligand domain of the human papillomavirus type 16 E6 protein is required for E6's induction of epithelial hyperplasia in vivo. J Virol 2003;77(12):6957–64.
61. Ronco LV, Karpova AY, Vidal M, Howley PM. Human papillomavirus 16 E6 oncoprotein binds to interferon regulatory factor-3 and inhibits its transcriptional activity. Genes Dev 1998;12(13):2061–72.
62. Hasan UA, Bates E, Takeshita F, et al. TLR9 expression and function is abolished by the cervical cancer-associated human papillomavirus type 16. J Immunol 2007;178(5):3186–97.
63. Dyson N, Howley PM, Munger, K, Harlow E. The human papilloma virus-16 E7 oncoprotein is able to bind to the retinoblastoma gene product. Science 1989;243(4893):934–7.
64. Balsitis S, Dick F, Dyson N, Lambert PF. Critical roles for non-pRb targets of human papillomavirus type 16 E7 in cervical carcinogenesis. Cancer Res 2006;66(19):9393–400.
65. Huh K, Zhou X, Kayakawa H, et al. Human papillomavirus type 16 E7 oncoprotein associates with the cullin 2 ubiquitin ligase complex, which contributes to degradation of the retinoblastoma tumor suppressor. J Virol 2007;81(18):9737–47.
66. Longworth MS, Wilson R, Laimins LA. HPV31 E7 facilitates replication by activating E2F2 transcription through its interaction with HDACs. EMBO J 2005;24(10):1821–30.
67. Burgers WA, Blanchon L, Pradhan S, et al. Viral oncoproteins target the DNA methyltransferases. Oncogene 2007;26(11):1650–5.
68. De Geest K, Bergman CA, Turyk ME, et al. Differential response of cervical intraepithelial and cervical carcinoma cell lines to transforming growth factor-beta 1. Gynecol Oncol 1994;55(3 Pt 1):376–85.
69. Pietenpol JA, Stein RW, Moran E, et al. TGF-beta 1 inhibition of c-myc transcription and growth in keratinocytes is abrogated by viral transforming proteins with pRB binding domains. Cell 1990;61(5):777–85.
70. Park JS, Kim EJ, Kwon HJ, et al. Inactivation of interferon regulatory factor-1 tumor suppressor protein by HPV E7 oncoprotein. Implication for the E7-mediated immune evasion mechanism in cervical carcinogenesis. J Biol Chem 2000;275(10):6764–9.
71. Huh KW, DeMasi J, Ogawa H, et al. Association of the human papillomavirus type 16 E7 oncoprotein with the 600-kDa retinoblastoma protein-associated factor, p600. Proc Natl Acad Sci USA 2005;102(32):11492–7.
72. Nakamura M, Bodily JM, Beglin M, et al. Hypoxia-specific stabilization of HIF-1alpha by human papillomaviruses. Virology 2009;387(2):442–8.
73. Chen W, Li F, Mead L, et al. Human papillomavirus causes an angiogenic switch in keratinocytes which is sufficient to alter endothelial cell behavior. Virology 2007;367(1):168–74.
74. Toussaint-Smith E, Donner DB, Roman A. Expression of human papillomavirus type 16 E6 and E7 oncoproteins in primary foreskin keratinocytes is sufficient to alter the expression of angiogenic factors. Oncogene 2004;23(17):2988–95.
75. Duensing S, Duensing A, Crum CP, et al. Human papillomavirus type 16 E7 oncoprotein-induced abnormal centrosome synthesis is an early event in the evolving malignant phenotype. Cancer Res 2001;61(6):2356–60.
76. Korzeniewski N, Treat B, Duensing S. The HPV-16 E7 oncoprotein induces centriole multiplication through deregulation of Polo-like kinase 4 expression. Mol Cancer 2011;10:61.
77. Hawley-Nelson P, Vousden KH, Hubbert NL, et al. HPV16 E6 and E7 proteins cooperate to immortalize human foreskin keratinocytes. EMBO J 1989;8(12):3905–10.
78. Bosch FX, Burchell AN, Schiffman M, et al. Epidemiology and natural history of human papillomavirus infections and type-specific implications in cervical neoplasia. Vaccine 2008;26(Suppl 10):K1–16.
79. Frazer IH. Interaction of human papillomaviruses with the host immune system: a well evolved relationship. Virology 2009;384(2):410–4.
80. Konya J, Dillner J. Immunity to oncogenic human papillomaviruses. Adv Cancer Res 2001;82:205–38.
81. Carter JJ, Koutsky LA, Hughes JP, et al. Comparison of human papillomavirus types 16, 18, and 6 capsid antibody responses following incident infection. J Infect Dis 2000;181(6):1911–9.
82. Villa LL, Ault KA, Giuliano AR, et al. Immunologic responses following administration of a vaccine targeting human papillomavirus Types 6, 11, 16, and 18. Vaccine 2006;24(27–28):5571–83.
83. Jochmus-Kudielka I, Schneider A, Braun R, et al. Antibodies against the human papillomavirus type 16 early proteins in human sera: correlation of anti-E7 reactivity with cervical cancer. J Natl Cancer Inst 1989;81(22):1698–704.
84. Lechner F, Gruener NH, Urbani S, et al. CD8+ T lymphocyte responses are induced during acute hepatitis C virus infection but are not sustained. Eur J Immunol 2000;30(9):2479–87.
85. Sester M, Sester U, Gartner BC, et al. Dominance of virus-specific CD8 T cells in human primary cytomegalovirus infection. J Am Soc Nephrol 2002;13(10):2577–84.
86. Youde SJ, Dunbar PR, Evans EM, et al. Use of fluorogenic histocompatibility leukocyte antigen-A*0201/HPV 16 E7 peptide complexes to isolate rare human cytotoxic T-lymphocyte- recognizing endogenous human papillomavirus antigens. Cancer Res 2000;60(2):365–71.
87. Kadish AS, Timmins P, Wang Y, et al. Regression of cervical intraepithelial neoplasia and loss of human papillomavirus (HPV) infection is associated with cell-mediated immune responses to an HPV type 16 E7 peptide. Cancer Epidemiol Biomarkers Prev 2002;11(5):483–8.
88. Nimako M, Flander AN, Wilkinson GW, et al. Human papillomavirus-specific cytotoxic T lymphocytes in patients with cervical intraepithelial neoplasia grade III. Cancer Res 1997;57(21):4855–61.
89. van der Burg SH, Ressing ME, Kwappenberg KM, et al. Natural T-helper immunity against human papillomavirus type 16 (HPV16) E7-derived peptide epitopes in patients with HPV16-positive cervical lesions: identification of 3 human leukocyte antigen class II-restricted epitopes. Int J Cancer 2001;91(5):612–8.
90. Bontkes HJ, de Gruijl TD, van den Muysenberg AJ, et al. Human papillomavirus type 16 E6/E7-specific cytotoxic T lymphocytes in women with cervical neoplasia. Int J Cancer 2000;88(1):92–8.
91. Campbell DJ, Butcher EC. Rapid acquisition of tissue-specific homing phenotypes by CD4(+) T cells activated in cutaneous or mucosal lymphoid tissues. J Exp Med 2002;195(1):135–41.
92. Kupper TS, Fuhlbrigge RC. Immune surveillance in the skin: mechanisms and clinical consequences. Nat Rev Immunol 2004;4(3):211–22.
93. Clark RA, Chong B, Mirchandani N. The vast majority of CLA+ T cells are resident in normal skin. J Immunol 2006;76(7):4431–9.

94. Koelle DM, Liu Z, McClurkan CM, et al. Expression of cutaneous lymphocyte-associated antigen by CD8(+) T cells specific for a skin-tropic virus. J Clin Invest 2002;110(4):537–48.
95. Moyer VA. Screening for cervical cancer: U.S. Preventive Services Task Force recommendation statement. Ann Intern Med 2012;156(12):880–91.
96. Follen M, Richards-Kortum R. Emerging technologies and cervical cancer. J Natl Cancer Inst 2000;92(5):363–5.
97. Castle PE, Glass AG, Rush BB, et al. Clinical human papillomavirus detection forecasts cervical cancer risk in women over 18 years of follow-up. J Clin Oncol 2012;30(25):3044–50.
98. Smith MA, Lew JB, Walker RJ, et al. The predicted impact of HPV vaccination on male infections and male HPV-related cancers in Australia. Vaccine 2011;29(48):9112–22.
99. Ioannidis V, Beermann F, Clevers H, Held W. The beta-catenin—TCF-1 pathway ensures CD4(+)CD8(+) thymocyte survival. Nat Immunol 2001;2(8):691–7.
100. Frazer IH. Prevention of cervical cancer through papillomavirus vaccination. Nat Rev Immunol 2004;4(1):46–54.
101. Chattergoon M, Boyer J, Weiner DB. Genetic immunization: a new era in vaccines and immune therapeutics. FASEB J 1997;11(10):753–63.
102. Aihara H, Miyazaki J. Gene transfer into muscle by electroporation in vivo. Nat Biotechnol 1998;16(9):867–70.
103. Luckay A, Sidhu MK, Kjeken R, et al. Effect of plasmid DNA vaccine design and in vivo electroporation on the resulting vaccine-specific immune responses in rhesus macaques. J Virol 2007;81(10):5257–69.
104. van Drunen Littel-van den Hurk S, Hannaman D. Electroporation for DNA immunization: clinical application. Expert Rev Vaccines 2010;9(5):503–17.
105. Hanke T, Goonetilleke N, McMichael AJ, Dorrell L. Clinical experience with plasmid DNA- and modified vaccinia virus Ankara-vectored human immunodeficiency virus type 1 clade A vaccine focusing on T-cell induction. J Gen Virol 2007;88 (Pt 1):1–12.
106. Kenter GG, Welters MJ, Valentijn AR, et al. Vaccination against HPV-16 oncoproteins for vulvar intraepithelial neoplasia. N Engl J Med 2009;361(19):1838–47.
107. Coleman N, Birley HD, Renton AM, et al. Immunological events in regressing genital warts. Am J Clin Pathol 1994;102(6):768–74.
108. Trimble CL, Peng S, Thoburn C, et al. Naturally occurring systemic immune responses to HPV antigens do not predict regression of CIN2/3. Cancer Immunol Immunother 2010;59(5):799–803.
109. Farhat S, Nakagawa M, Moscicki AB. Cell-mediated immune responses to human papillomavirus 16 E6 and E7 antigens as measured by interferon gamma enzyme-linked immunospot in women with cleared or persistent human papillomavirus infection. Int J Gynecol Cancer 2009;19(4):508–12.
110. Nakagawa M, Stites DP, Patel S, et al. Persistence of human papillomavirus type 16 infection is associated with lack of cytotoxic T lymphocyte response to the E6 antigens. J Infect Dis 2000; 182(2):595–8.
111. Frazer IH, Leggatt GR, Mattarollo SR. Prevention and treatment of papillomavirus-related cancers through immunization. Annu Rev Immunol 2011;29:111–38.
112. Daayana S, Elkord E, Winters U, et al. Phase II trial of imiquimod and HPV therapeutic vaccination in patients with vulval intraepithelial neoplasia. Br J Cancer 2010;102(7):1129–36.
113. Kobayashi A, Weinberg V, Darragh T, Smith-McCune K. Evolving immunosuppressive microenvironment during human cervical carcinogenesis. Mucosal Immunol 2008;1(5):412–20.
114. Nakamura T, Shima T, Saeki A, et al. Expression of indoleamine 2, 3-dioxygenase and the recruitment of Foxp3-expressing regulatory T cells in the development and progression of uterine cervical cancer. Cancer Sci 2007;98(6):874–81.
115. El-Sherif AM, Seth R, Tighe PJ, Jenkins D. Quantitative analysis of IL-10 and IFN-gamma mRNA levels in normal cervix and human papillomavirus type 16 associated cervical precancer. J Pathol 2001;195(2):179–85.
116. Lanneau GS, Argenta PA, Lanneau MS, et al. Vulvar cancer in young women: demographic features and outcome evaluation. Am J Obstet Gynecol 2009;200(6):645 e1–5.
117. Frazer IH. Measuring serum antibody to human papillomavirus following infection or vaccination. Gynecol Oncol 2010;118(1 Suppl):S8–11.
118. Wright Jr TC, Schiffman M. Adding a test for human papillomavirus DNA to cervical-cancer screening. N Engl J Med 2003;348(6):489–90.
119. Ferlay JB, Pisani FG, Parkin DM. GLOBOCAN 2000: Cancer incidence, mortality and prevalence worldwide. IARC Cancer Base No.5 2006.
120. Clifford GM, Gallus S, Herrero R, et al. Worldwide distribution of human papillomavirus types in cytologically normal women in the International Agency for Research on Cancer HPV prevalence surveys: a pooled analysis. Lancet 2005;366(9490):991–8.
121. Doorbar J. The papillomavirus life cycle. J Clin Virol 2005;32(Suppl 1):S7–15.

10 Cervical Squamous Intraepithelial Lesions

C. Simon Herrington, Jan P.A. Baak, George L. Mutter

CHAPTER OUTLINE

Introduction	200
Squamous Intraepithelial Lesions (SILs)	202
Nomenclature	202
Features	203
Disease States: Types of SIL	207
LSIL (Condyloma/CIN 1)	208
High-Grade Squamous Intraepithelial Lesions (CIN 2–3)	212
Areas of Diagnostic Difficulty	214
Biomarkers	218
Histologic Features of SIL (CIN) Affecting Management and Prognosis	219
Regression and Progression to Invasive Carcinoma	221
Correlation Between Cytology and Histology	223
Distribution and Site of Origin of SIL	224
Colposcopy	224
Normal Colposcopic Findings	225
Abnormal Colposcopic Findings	226

INTRODUCTION

Human papillomavirus (HPV) infection is now understood to be the underlying cause of squamous carcinogenesis in the cervix.[1-4] Older diagnostic classifications of preinvasive disease based purely on descriptive correlation of histology with clinical behavior included dysplasia/carcinoma *in situ* (CIS; a four-grade system) and cervical intraepithelial neoplasia (CIN; a three-grade system). Each provided a convenient diagnostic spectrum against which patient samples could be matched, and both are still in use to varying degrees.

The clinical goal of segregating individual lesions into dichotomous high- and low-risk categories was furthered by evidence showing that cancer outcomes correlated predominantly with one of two HPV subtype classes. Thus, the two-class Bethesda System of low-grade squamous intraepithelial lesion (LSIL) and high-grade squamous intraepithelial lesion (HSIL) was formally endorsed by the National Cancer Institute (USA) at a workshop held in December 1988.[5] Implementation was recommended for lesions in the cervix and vagina. LSIL was generally equated with condylomata and CIN 1, and HSIL with CIN grades 2 and 3 (CIN 2, CIN 3, or CIN 2–3). This principle of a two-tier system was reaffirmed by consensus of the College of American Pathologists and American Society for Clinical Pathology (ASCP) in 2012, with the additional recommendation that it be extended to all anogenital HPV-related lesions, including those in vulvar and perianal sites.[6]

The initial expectation of the two-tier system was that viral type would be the primary determinant of outcome, and careful correlation of intraepithelial morphology with viral type would yield diagnostic criteria for the new entities of LSIL and HSIL. However, it is now clear that LSIL is the biologic manifestation of productive HPV infection with episomal viral DNA. Therefore, *all* HPVs can generate low-grade morphology as this type of cellular differentiation is required for viral replication to produce viral particles (virions). These infections and their cytohistologic manifestations are almost always transient, resolving on average in less than a year.[7]

HSIL results predominantly from genomic integration of high-risk types of HPV DNA into the host genome of replicating parabasal cells, with consequent deregulation of expression of E6 and E7 viral oncogenes. The parabasal cells become disorganized relative to the underlying basement membrane, with subsequent clonal expansion extending upward toward the epithelial surface (Figure 10.1). Cells containing only integrated viral DNA are virologically noninfectious as no viral particles are produced but the viral genes drive the human (host) cells to proliferate. HSILs may, however, contain both episomal and integrated HPV DNA,[8] which is consistent with the presence of koilocytes in some HSILs.

Of the more than 120 HPV types known to exist,[9] only about 30–40 affect the genital tract. Probably less than 15 are oncogenic; the most common is HPV type 16 and its related viruses 31, 33, 35, and 56 from the α 9 clade (a taxonomic group derived from a common ancestor)[9] and type 18 with its close relations such as type 45 (Table 10.1).[10] They are termed high risk or oncogenic because they are

CHAPTER 10 — CERVICAL SQUAMOUS INTRAEPITHELIAL LESIONS

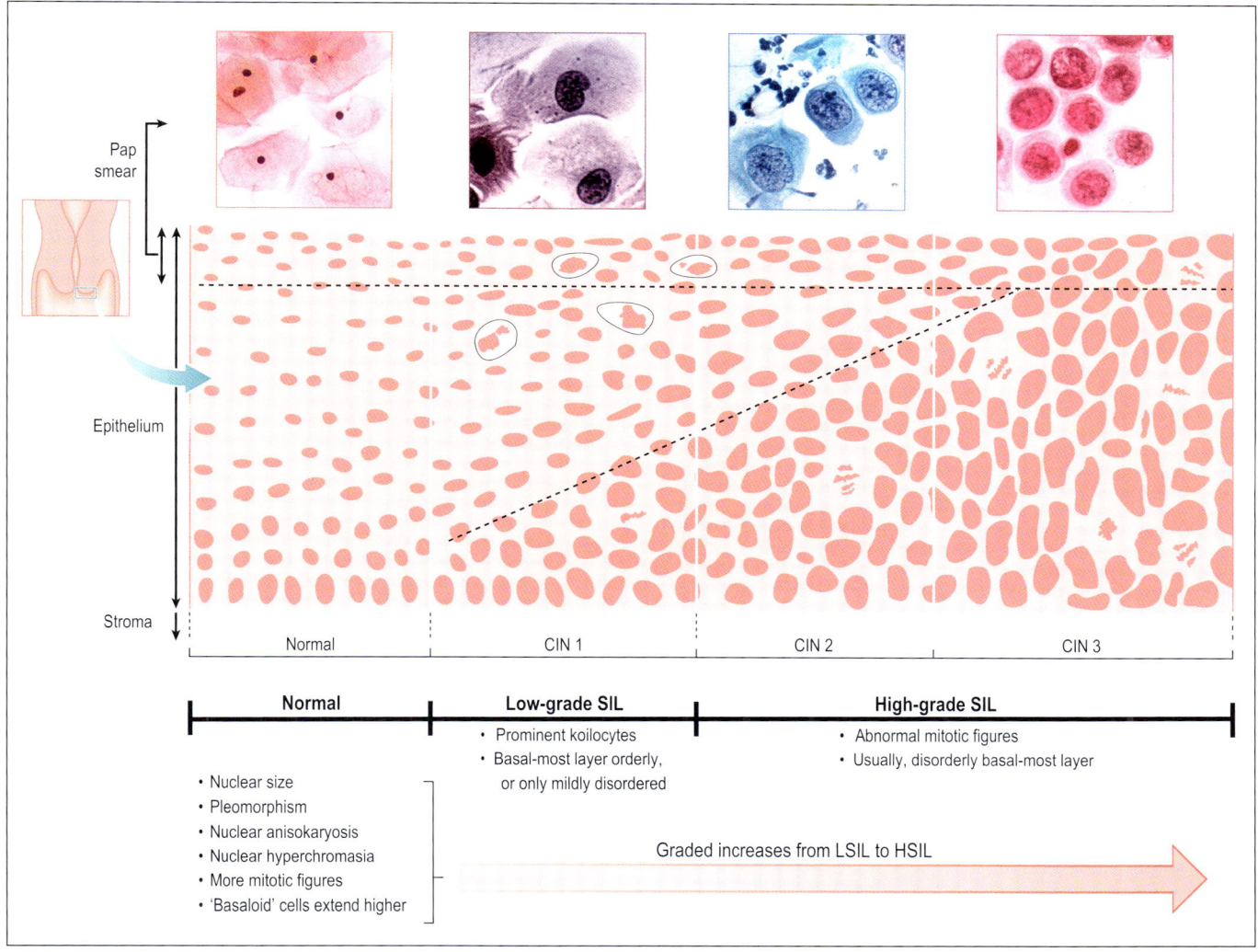

Figure 10.1 Morphologic features and nomenclature of preinvasive cervical disease. The morphologic changes that occur with increasing lesion grade and how the SIL (Bethesda) and CIN systems relate to one another are illustrated. Quantitative features that become increasingly more abnormal with increasing grade are listed, along with those qualitative features that differ across the LSIL–HSIL boundary. The corresponding cytologic smear appearances resulting from exfoliation of the most superficial cells are also illustrated. Note that some pathologists subdivide HSIL into HSIL (CIN 2) and HSIL (CIN 3), which are comparable to CIN 2 and CIN 3 respectively.

Table 10.1 Classification of HPV Types Associated with Genital Lesions[10]

Most Common Types	
6, 11	Condyloma acuminatum, LSIL (condyloma/CIN 1)
16	All grades of SIL, squamous cell carcinoma
18	All grades of SIL, adenocarcinoma, squamous cell carcinoma, small cell carcinoma
Less Common Types	
31, 33, 35, 39, 45, 51, 52, 56	All grades of SIL, squamous cell carcinoma
30, 40, 58, 69	All grades of SIL
42, 43, 44	Condyloma acuminatum, LSIL (condyloma/CIN 1)
53	Normal cervical epithelium, LSIL (condyloma/CIN 1) and sometimes HSIL (CIN 2)
54	Condyloma acuminatum
55	Bowenoid papulosis
59	Vulvar HSIL (usual type vulvar intraepithelial neoplasia)
61, 62, 64, 67	Vaginal HSIL (vaginal intraepithelial neoplasia)
66	Squamous cell carcinoma
70	Vulvar papilloma

Table 10.2 Comparison of HPV Frequency Detected by Laboratory Techniques[11]

	DNA Hybridization (%)	Koilocytosis (%)	Immunocytochemistry for Viral Capsid Protein (%)
LSIL (Condyloma)	100	80	80
LSIL (CIN 1)	100	89	61
HSIL (CIN 2)	86	57	29
HSIL (CIN 3, severe dysplasia)	100	33	17
HSIL (CIN 3, CIS)	100	20	0

the types found in invasive tumors. Progression of high-risk viral infection to HSIL is inefficient and, although high-risk types are the most common cervical HPV infections, most result in only low-grade lesions. The low-risk group constitutes only a minority of cervical infections. The low-risk HPV types are prototypically HPV types 6 and 11 whose biology is one of transient productive infection with only extremely rare examples of progression to carcinoma. The apparent prevalence of HPV infection in cervical lesions of different types and grades depends on the technique used for detection of the virus and the criteria applied for histologic annotation.

Irrespective of HPV type, the viral cytopathic effect (koilocytosis) and the production of viral capsid protein become progressively less frequent with increasing lesion grade (Table 10.2).[11] Indeed, the inability of most high-grade lesions to support productive HPV infection can be viewed in a biologic context as viral failure. Local immune response within the cervical microenvironment is somewhat more common with high-risk HPV infections, and this can be associated with regression of HSILs.[12,13] Conversely, low-grade lesions are, in a sense, 'successful' infections in that they represent productive infections with little or no propensity to kill the host.

Although SILs are capable of changing dynamically over time as a combined function of viral type(s), phase of viral life cycle (especially episomal vs integrated) and host factors, classification of SILs must be accomplished from the morphologic appearance of an individual HPV-infected squamous lesion. Further information about virologic and immunologic dynamics of HPV infection from individual and public health perspectives are available in Chapter 9. Cervical biopsy and cytologic smears each have their own sampling and interpretive errors, occasionally creating discordant results. Both are equally variable and may provide valuable information on disease presence or absence. Even visually directed colposcopic biopsy is imperfect in identifying the area of most severe pathology.[14] Every attempt should be made to reconcile discordances by a combination of interpretive re-review, or further sampling, as clinically appropriate. Evidence-based criteria-driven approaches to diagnosis remain the best way to achieve clinical utility with a minimum of interpretive variation.[15]

In this chapter we will follow a two-class schema of cervical squamous precancers designated as LSIL (condyloma/CIN 1) and HSIL (CIN 2-3), digressing into more specialized distinctions where appropriate.

SQUAMOUS INTRAEPITHELIAL LESIONS (SILs)

NOMENCLATURE

The nomenclature used to describe the precursor conditions of invasive squamous cell carcinoma continues to be a subject of some debate. In the 1950s and into the 1960s, the term 'dysplasia' was equated to a graded lesion something less than CIS, which was diagnosed and managed separately. Both were composed of basal-type cells extending upward in the epithelium, to almost full thickness in the case of severe dysplasia. Flattening of the topmost surface cells, construed as a sign of differentiation, was said to occur in severe dysplasia, but not CIS. These diagnoses led to widely divergent interventions: the former passively followed, and the latter often to hysterectomy. Critical examination of the data subsequently showed that distinction between severe dysplasia and CIS was not only poorly reproducible by pathologists, but, when applied, failed to stratify patients into differing risk groups for invasive carcinoma.[15,16] Lack of clinical significance of the dysplasia/CIS distinction led to the simplified classification of CIN in which three grades of precancerous lesions were acknowledged, but the term 'carcinoma' was reserved for invasive processes. New treatment options for intraepithelial precursor lesions, intended to ablate only the cervical lining, were introduced. These included topically applied liquid nitrogen (cryosurgery), laser ablation, and local excision by electrocautery loop.

Knowledge of the role of HPV infection (see Chapter 9)[1,2,15] and more specifically the roles of individual HPV types, suggested division according to the presence of the low-risk HPV types such as HPV 6 and 11 and the high-risk HPV types, most commonly HPV 16 and 18. Since the late 1980s, the Bethesda classification scheme, introduced for use in reporting cervical cytology smears, has incorporated these concepts into a bimodal classification system of LSIL/HSIL, which differ in their risk for subsequent carcinoma. HPV lesions previously considered condylomata or CIN 1 (mild dysplasia) are grouped into the single category of LSIL. These low-grade lesions have a low growth fraction, koilocytotic atypia (also called 'HPV cytopathic effect'), and are the morphologic manifestation of productive HPV infection. They might perhaps be better called 'low risk for the development of high-grade intraepithelial neoplasia or invasive carcinoma.' All HPV types functionally produce LSIL at some point in their life cycle (or they would not survive).

In contrast, HSILs are the approximate equivalent of CIN 2 and CIN 3 (moderate dysplasia, severe dysplasia, and CIS). HSIL is sometimes subdivided into HSIL-2 and HSIL-3 to reflect this comparison with CIN 2 and CIN 3. The relationship between these various terms is shown in Figure 10.1. A strength of the Bethesda System is that it may be applied to both cytologic and histologic specimens. The cells from an HPV-associated lesion are all included under the umbrella of SIL, as there is no underlying biologic or diagnostic basis to maintain a separate category of non-SIL condyloma.[15] As suggested earlier, the concept of progression is best considered probabilistically, incorporating independent assessment of the results of cytology and biopsy and, when appropriate, HPV testing.[17,18]

The cytopathologist, in contrast to the histopathologist, can only examine cells that have been exfoliated, which tend to be the most superficial cells in the mucosa. Yet, in some ways, the cytologic sample may be more representative of the spectrum of pathology in the cervix because of its ability to sample a much larger surface area compared to the punch biopsy. The fact that smear and biopsy findings from samples obtained during the same patient examination show high degrees of correlation supports the concept that SIL, even when low-grade, affects *all* layers of the epithelium. The sections that follow, therefore, emphasize the quantitative and qualitative changes that occur throughout the epithelium in the various degrees of SIL.

FEATURES

The histopathologic assessment of a cervical biopsy must determine whether SIL is present in a sample of epithelium and, if so, the grade of SIL (Figure 10.2). Both of these decisions may be difficult to make: the former because benign and reactive changes may be mistaken for SIL; the latter because interpretation of features used for grading is complex (Table 10.3).

SIL is divided into grades as a prognostic aid, implying it can be used as a guide in managing the patient. As a result, criteria that are purely morphologic are used to predict the clinical behavior of the abnormal epithelium. The correlation between histologic appearance and behavior is, however, imperfect. This may be in part due to diagnostic imprecision, in addition to modifying host factors not reflected in the classification system itself. An additional complication in the cervix is that the current aim of treatment is to eradicate the disease before it becomes invasive. Thus the clinical outcomes observed are rarely unaltered by therapy, especially for HSILs. True invasion is found only in a minority of SIL cases, even in untreated HSILs, not exceeding 30% after many years.

CHANGES OF HPV INFECTION

In cervical epithelia, all productive HPV infections commonly manifest themselves both cytologically and histologically through a distinctive cytopathic effect. The cell in which this is found has been termed the 'koilocyte' (Figure 10.3). This feature, first recognized more than 50 years ago, was given the term 'koilocytotic atypia' (some use koilocytic) as these cells histologically resembled those in skin warts. Some 20 years later it was recognized that this same cell type occurred in genital warts and was associated with both HPV infection and preinvasive squamous intraepithelial lesions.

The koilocyte is an intermediate cell that has a prominent cytoplasmic space around an atypical nucleus (Table 10.4; Figures 10.3–10.8). Due to an extensively marginated

---

Table 10.3 Histopathologic Features of SIL/CIN

1. Nuclear abnormalities
   a. Nuclear to cytoplasmic ratio (↑)
   b. Hyperchromasia (↑)
   c. Nuclear pleomorphism and anisokaryosis (↑)
   d. Nuclear polarity (↑ irregular)
   e. Wrinkling of nuclear membrane (↑)
2. Mitotic activity
   a. Number of mitotic figures (↑)
   b. Height in epithelium (↑)
   c. Abnormal mitotic figures (↑)
3. Differentiation (maturation, stratification)
   a. Proportion of epithelium showing differentiation (↓)
   b. Proportion of unit area occupied by nuclei (↑)

These features become progressively more prominent with increasing grade.

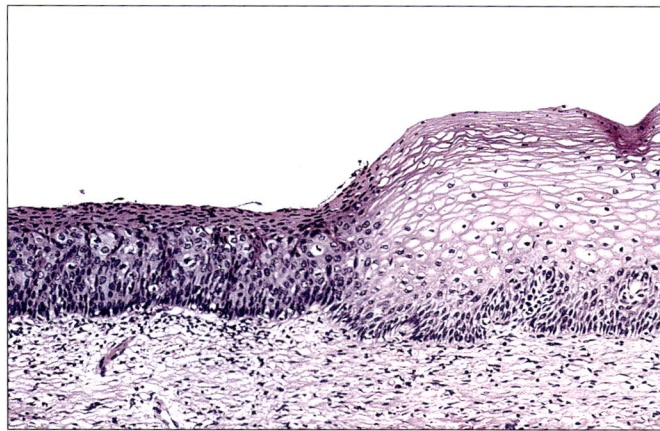

Figure 10.2 Abrupt transition between normal squamous epithelium (right) and an adjacent HSIL (left).

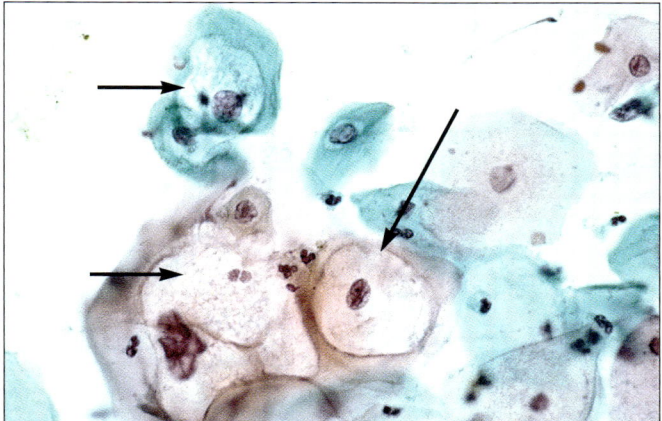

Figure 10.3 Koilocytes (arrows) in a cervical smear.

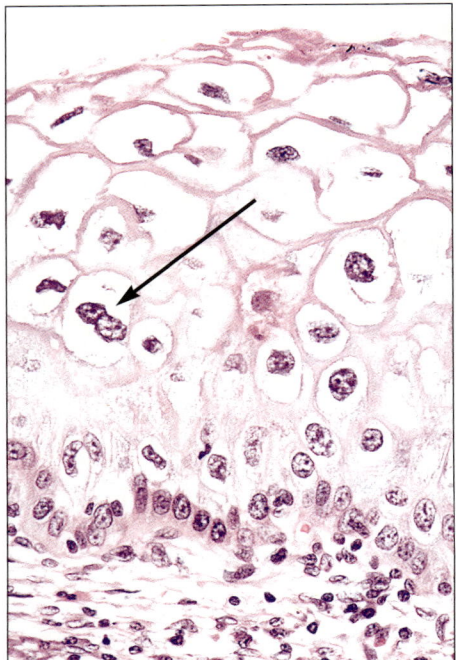

Figure 10.4 HPV-associated koilocytes in an LSIL. The cells in the intermediate layers are ballooned with copious clear cytoplasm. One cell is binucleate (arrow). The lowermost layer of cells against the basement membrane is orderly.

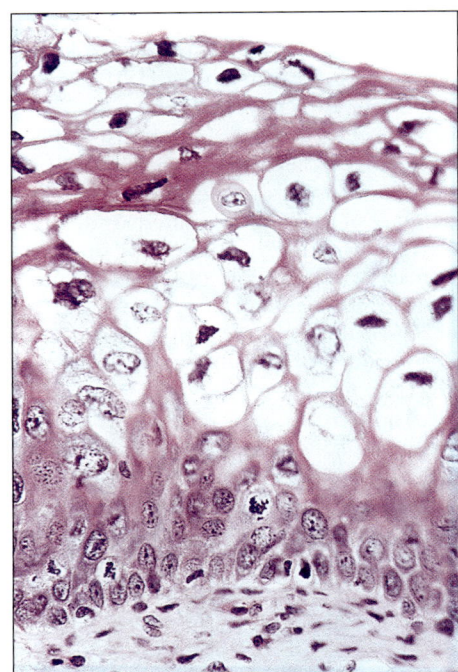

Figure 10.5 LSIL. The basal layer is slightly thickened. Koilocytes are prominent.

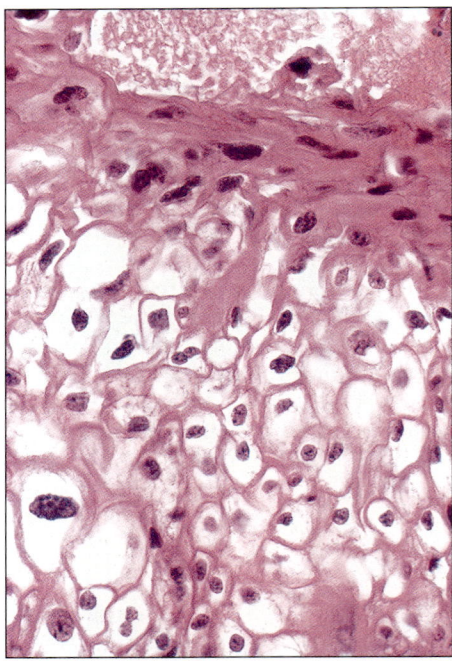

Figure 10.6 LSIL (CIN 1). Several of the koilocytes show nuclear atypia, which persists in the parakeratotic scale. Figures 10.4–10.6 are all low-risk viral lesions.

Table 10.4	Koilocytotic Change: Diagnostic Criteria
Well-defined and exaggerated perinuclear halo	
Cytoplasmic condensation around the halo	
Nuclear area at least 2–3 times that of a normal intermediate cell nucleus	
Increased nuclear to cytoplasmic ratio	
Mild nuclear hyperchromasia (usually)	
Wrinkled nuclear membrane	
Nuclear membrane chromatin condensation	
Degenerative nuclear changes (variable)	

cytoplasm, the halo has a sharp edge. The cytoplasmic change is thought to be due to abundant expression of the HPV E1^E4 fusion protein, which binds with cytoplasmic keratin. Even in the state where the nuclei are not overtly dysplastic by size criteria, they are still, nonetheless, irregular and hyperchromatic and, if near the surface, may show a wrinkled nuclear membrane. The nuclei, which lack nucleoli, are usually two to four times larger in nuclear area than those of the adjacent, nonballooned cells. Koilocytotic atypia, which under the Bethesda classification is considered a low-grade SIL, is the most common definite abnormality in cytologically screened women and is found in up to 4% of all cervical smears.

While the koilocyte is often described to be pathognomonic for HPV infection, perinuclear halos that mimic koilocytotic atypia may be caused by other infectious diseases and at times may be due to artifact. Epstein–Barr virus, when present in the cervix, may be associated with koilocytic change[19] (although this may also be due to coinfection with HPV). Likewise, when the cytoplasmic halo is less than morphologically perfect, i.e., when the borders are smooth or when the nuclei have smooth borders, trichomoniasis may be a consideration. It is therefore important that the presence of a cytoplasmic halo is not overinterpreted as due to

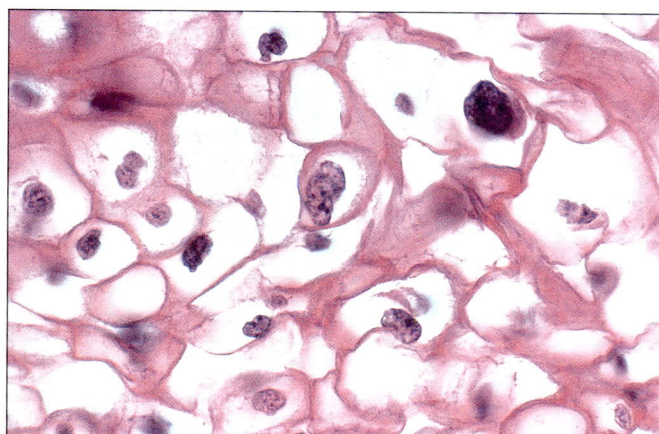

Figure 10.7 The nuclei of koilocytes are wrinkled and enlarged but show neither mitotic activity nor nucleoli.

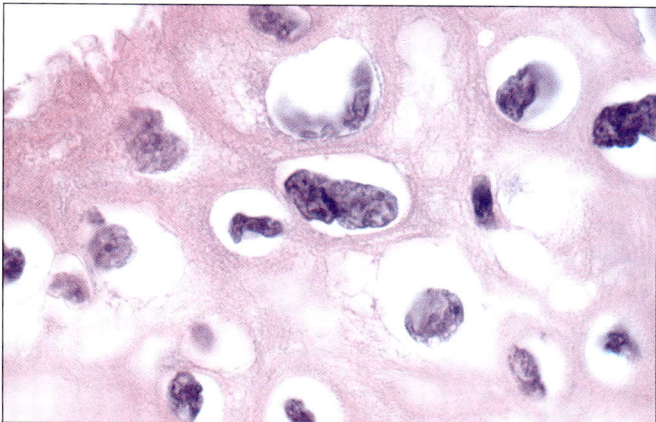

Figure 10.8 High-power magnification of koilocytes. The nuclei are wrinkled and enlarged with coarse chromatin.

HPV infection. Rather, it is the combination of a well-defined halo plus definite nuclear atypia as defined previously that confers specificity to the morphologic findings. Other features associated with HPV infection include binucleation (Figure 10.4) and meganuclei. Both are found in the mid to superficial levels. Some investigators have suggested that the latter feature, or more severely pleomorphic koilocytes, is more associated with high-risk HPV types. However, since over 85% of cervical HPV infections are due to viruses from the high-risk group, this is not a practically useful concept and LSILs of the cervix cannot be reliably genotyped by morphology.

NUCLEAR ABNORMALITIES

The defining hallmarks of SIL are its nuclear abnormalities. These include nuclei that are enlarged, pleomorphic (irregular in size and shape), and often have a wrinkled nuclear membrane. The chromatin is increased in amount (hyperchromasia) and irregularly clumped, often condensing along the inside of the nuclear membrane. Collectively, this constellation of features is described as 'nuclear atypia.' These changes may reflect the polyploid and/or aneuploid DNA content of the cells induced by the action of HPV E6 and E7 on host DNA synthesis and cell cycle checkpoints (see Chapter 9) and are important for the diagnosis of SIL. Neoplastic atypia is distinguished from reactive changes by the heterogeneity of the nuclear changes in SIL, contrasting with the relatively homogeneous changes in reactive atypia. It is of note that nucleoli are rare in preinvasive lesions, especially in smears, but are commonly seen in reactive atypia.

Cytologic atypia must always be interpreted within the local context of level in the epithelium, and by comparison with adjacent cells. It is common for the koilocytes of LSILs, which reflect HPV DNA amplification and viral propagation, to demonstrate bizarre nuclear pleomorphism in an irregular distribution. These are generally confined to the superficial layers, have classic perinuclear halos, and may be polynucleated. Clonal HSILs may contain koilocytes, but their more characteristic feature is an increased nuclear to cytoplasmic ratio which creates a basal-type appearance to cells high in the epithelium. This is in addition to the previously mentioned pleomorphism and chromatin changes, which are also present.

If a particular epithelium is extremely thin, it may be difficult to relate changes in cytology to position within the vertical height of the epithelium, thus confounding evaluation of maturation from base to surface. In this situation, the cytology alone may provide some clues as to grade, or the specimen may be regarded as ungradeable (or the grade undetermined/indeterminate).

MITOTIC ACTIVITY

Mitotic activity is the histologic hallmark of cell proliferation. The conceptual distinction between a normal epithelium and SIL has much to do with the frequency, distribution, and type of mitotic activity. HSIL has a proliferative phenotype. Though LSIL is slightly more proliferative than normal epithelium, it does not display the same viral oncogene-driven proliferation as HSIL: this is related at least in part to the switch to productive HPV infection, which occurs in the suprabasal keratinocytes of low-grade lesions.

In normal epithelium, mitotic figures are rare and are restricted to the parabasal cells. In contrast, SIL shows an increased number of mitoses, and they may be present at any level in the epithelium. The frequency of mitoses in the epithelium increases from normal epithelium to LSIL to HSIL. Moreover, the density of mitotic figures in the superficial third of the epithelium increases with the degree of abnormality. Thus, vertical position in the epithelium at which mitotic figures are found is a useful diagnostic indicator when contemplating the grade of SIL. However, not all SILs show mitoses above the parabasal layer.

Mitotic activity above the basal layer, however, is not always by itself pathognomonic for SIL. A reactive or inflamed but otherwise normal differentiated epithelium may also have increased mitotic activity, but the mitotic figures are concentrated in the basal areas. More problematic are reactive changes in metaplastic squamous areas, such as an inflamed transformation zone, as these may have full thickness mitotic activity and fail to demonstrate the polarization of differentiation. The presence of reactive cytologic features lacking the particular chromatin condensation of SIL may assist in the distinction. Special stains for

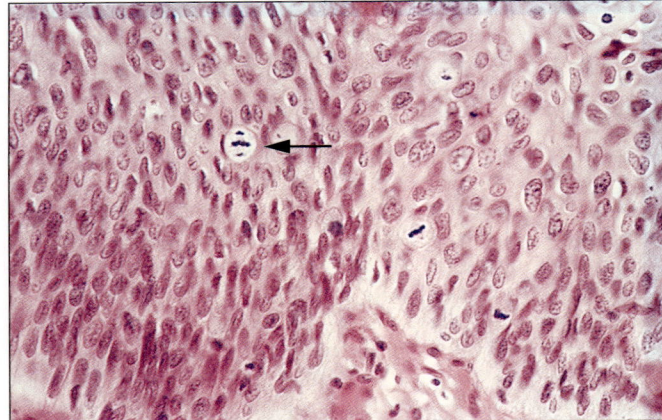

Figure 10.9 Three-group metaphase mitosis (arrow) in HSIL.

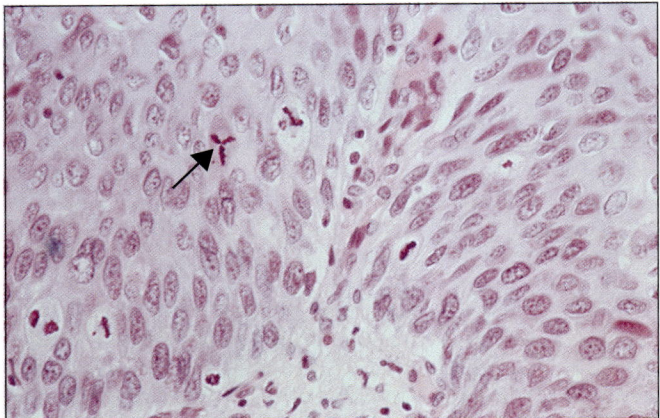

Figure 10.10 Tripolar mitosis (arrow) in HSIL.

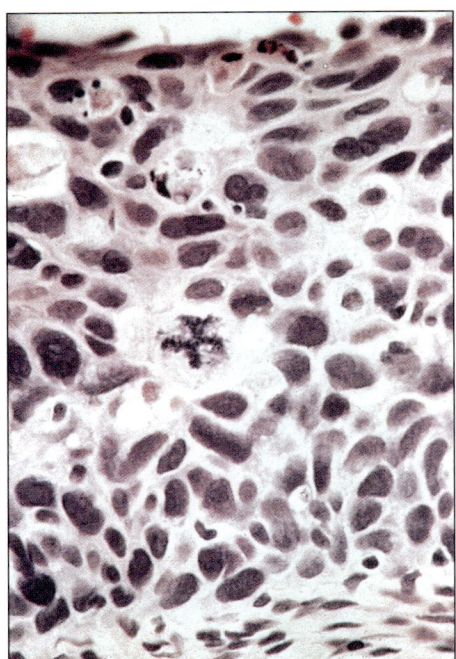

Figure 10.11 Multipolar mitosis in HSIL.

p16, which is positive in epithelia infected with high-risk HPV, may also be helpful in differentiating between reactive metaplasia and SIL.

Abnormal mitotic configurations, which reflect aneuploidy, are common in HSIL, where they account for between 15% and 30% of total mitoses, but rare in LSIL. HSIL associated with HPV type 16 infection has the highest number of mitoses and the most abnormal forms.[20,21] The most common of these abnormal configurations is the lag-type mitosis, which is defined as a metaphase with non-attached chromatin in the area of the mitotic figure. The 'three-group metaphase' (Figure 10.9), which is where the main mass of the chromatin aligns along the equatorial plate and the nonattached condensed chromatin remains laterally at the two polar sites, has been found in 6% of CIN 1–2, 56% of CIN 3, and 93% of high-grade CIN lesions just adjacent to microinvasive carcinoma.[22,23] Two-group metaphases (displaced chromatin at only one polar site) may also be seen. Less common than either of these forms is the multipolar mitotic figure, either as a triaster (tripolar) (Figure 10.10) or as a more bizarre multipolar figure (Figure 10.11). Tripolar mitoses may reflect polyploidy, rather than aneuploidy, and thus may be seen in both HSIL and LSIL.

DIFFERENTIATION, MATURATION, AND STRATIFICATION

'Differentiation' and 'maturation' are terms that, while having slightly different meanings, are often used synonymously and interchangeably in the cervix.

The proportion of epithelial cells showing differentiation is a useful indicator of the grade of SIL, although it must not be taken as the only criterion. For example, while SIL develops by a dysplastic process and may show little if any differentiation, it may be difficult to distinguish from an immature, but nondysplastic metaplastic squamous epithelium that also lacks any substantial degree of cytoplasmic differentiation. In this case, the distinguishing feature is the lack of nuclear atypia in the metaplastic process as well as much less evidence of mitotic activity. Nonetheless, distinction between the two conditions can be difficult and the presence of atypical changes in immature metaplastic squamous epithelium may indicate SIL, as shown by the presence of high-risk HPV types, high Ki-67 proliferation indices, p16 expression, and follow-up studies.[24,25]

As normal cells differentiate and mature and migrate toward the surface, stratification is observed. One means of assessing maturation is to look for a decreasing percentage of nuclear area to overall epithelial area, reflecting a decreasing nuclear to cytoplasmic ratio at increasingly more superficial levels of the epithelium. In smears, which sample superficial cell layers preferentially, this change in ratio is quite dramatic. In normal smears, the nucleus has undergone pyknosis by the time the cell reaches the surface, so that in the smear the nuclear to cytoplasmic ratio is quite low. With increasing grade of SIL, the individual cells have matured progressively less so that the amount of cytoplasm present, as well as its differentiation, is less. Thus, mildly dyskaryotic (a synonym of dysplasia used in cytologic terminology)/LSIL cells present in cervical smears/scrapes have ample cytoplasm with a well-defined polygonal squamous shape, and moderately dyskaryotic/HSIL-2 cells possess less cytoplasm and a less well-defined oval or elliptical squamous shape, whereas in severely dyskaryotic/HSIL-3 cells the rim of cytoplasm that encircles the nucleus is small. These features also occur in histopathologically defined lesions and, in SIL, the proportionally decreasing quantity of cytoplasm contributes far more to the increase in the nuclear to cytoplasmic ratio with increasing lesion grade than does the change in nuclear size. This is consistent with the persistence of nuclear abnormality throughout the epithelial thickness in all grades of SIL.

The presence of surface differentiation, which defined the difference between CIS and severe dysplasia, is poorly reproducible and of no biologic import, as mentioned previously. Thus, with the adoption of the CIN terminology and now with SIL terminology, the former class of squamous CIS is encompassed in CIN 3 and HSIL, respectively.

In smears, the Pap stain accentuates states of maturation. The color of staining, which results in either acidophilic (pink) or basophilic (blue-green) cytoplasm, usually corresponds to normal superficial and intermediate cell types, respectively. Although this helps to distinguish the various grades of SIL, it is not a reliable criterion, being influenced, for example, by stain quality control factors.

DISEASE STATES: TYPES OF SIL

Despite the earlier critical comments about reproducibility, application of discrete diagnostic criteria allows for distinction between benign cervix and SIL, and grading of SILs. SIL is primarily divided into two major classes of LSIL (condyloma/CIN 1) and HSIL (CIN 2–3), using similar terminologies across cytologic and histologic specimens.[6]

We have retained, in this section, separate CIN 2 and 3 descriptions under the umbrella of HSIL for several reasons. First is that specification of an HSIL diagnosis by appending its CIN equivalent, although not essential, remains a common practice. Thus a diagnosis of HSIL (CIN 2), or HSIL (CIN 3), may be rendered in an individual HSIL case. In addition, the CIN system is still used in some healthcare systems, for example the UK cervical screening program. Second, direct translation of legacy CIN 2 and 3 into HSIL remains one of the most widely used implementations of the Bethesda System today. In part this is because many pathologists assume that diagnostic criteria have not really changed since the 1960s when CIN was first defined, but rather the entities have simply been rebundled. This is not strictly true, as the LSIL–HSIL boundary has become the predominant threshold for management, and certainly some diagnostic insights have since been gained by focusing more intently at this junction. For example, disorderly versus orderly arrangement of the deepest layer of epithelial cells may be useful in, respectively, recognizing HSIL compared with LSIL. Also, atypical mitotic figures are more common in HSIL than in LSIL. Neither of these were formal components of CIN grading when first proposed. Third, since the all-important LSIL–HSIL threshold is best understood by comparison of those lesions that flank the boundary, this ends up effectively being a contrast between CIN 1 and 2.

The following discussion should be used as a general guide to the central features of the distinct grades of SIL, since examples of the same SIL grade may have varying appearances. For example, one specimen may show a lack of differentiation and stratification throughout (Figure 10.12), whereas others may show more prominent mitoses, some being abnormal (Figure 10.13), or bizarre nuclei located at superficial levels (Figure 10.14). Many of the

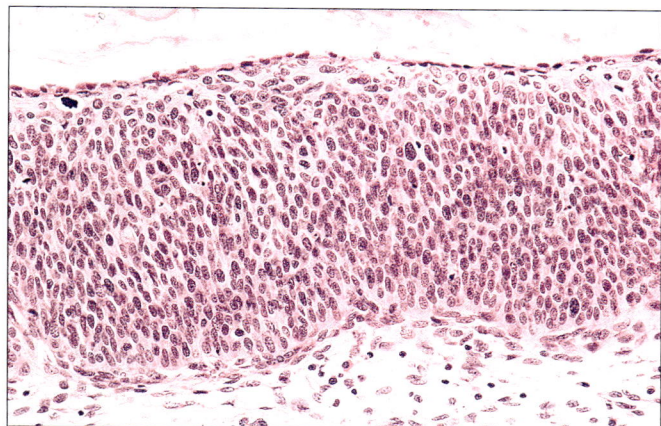

Figure 10.12 HSIL (CIN 3). Maturation is lacking throughout the entire thickness of the epithelium.

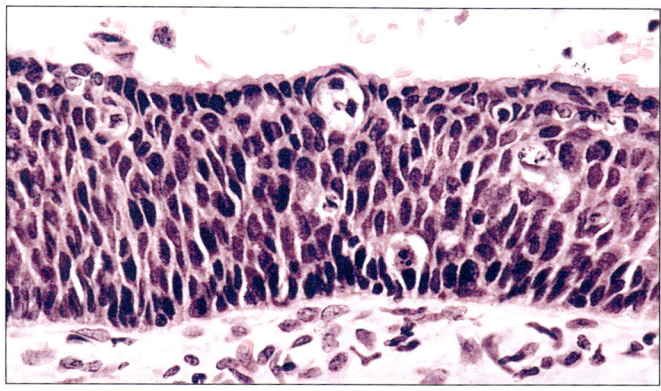

Figure 10.13 HSIL (CIN 3) in which a thin residual layer of mucinous columnar cells is present on the surface.

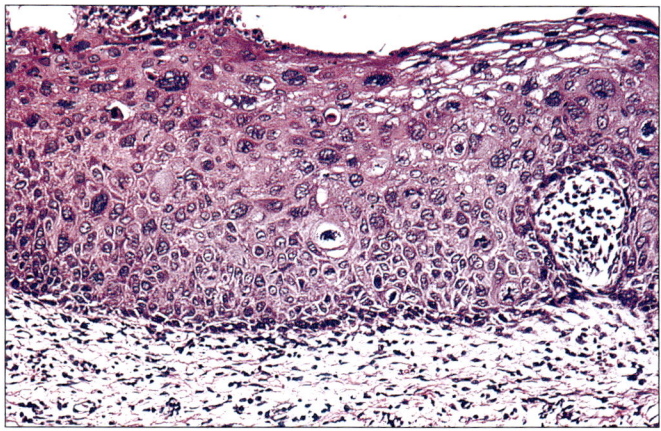

Figure 10.14 HSIL (CIN 3). The superficial nuclei are markedly enlarged and bizarre in shape.

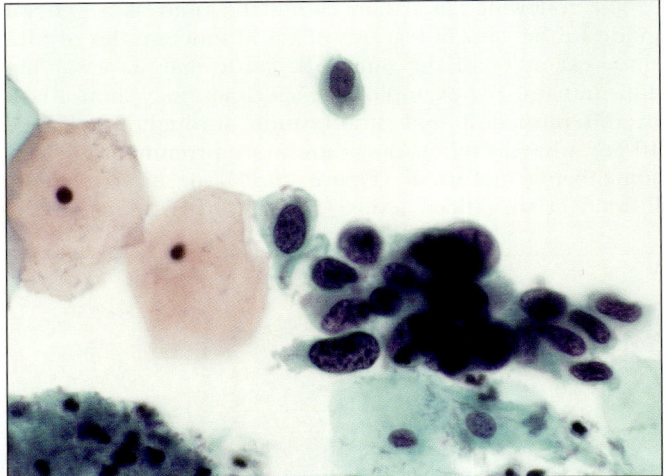

Figure 10.15 HSIL, severe dyskaryosis, on a cervical smear. The atypical cells have a high nuclear to cytoplasmic ratio.

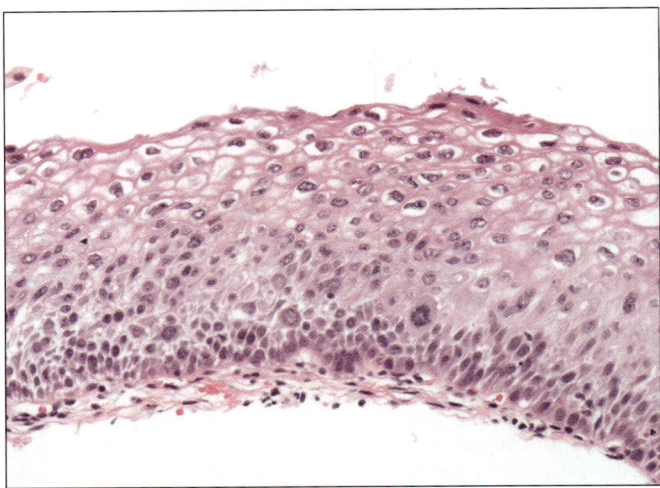

Figure 10.16 LSIL (CIN 1). Cytologic atypia extends throughout the epithelium but there is cytoplasmic maturation and the superficial-most epithelial cells display marked koilocytosis.

histologic features used in the grading of SIL may vary independently of each other, so the emphasis put on each of these criteria may vary from one specimen to another. All of this variation diminishes reproducibility of diagnosis.

Like histology, assignment of an overall grade of SIL to a smear is as subjective as the assessment-based examination of the individual cells. The cervical smear will frequently contain cells showing both grades of SIL, and it is the most severe cell type that determines the grade (Figure 10.15). A smear containing only a few dyskaryotic (dysplastic) cells, all of which show a marked degree of abnormality, almost certainly reflects HSIL. Likewise, a smear containing a majority of dyskaryotic (dysplastic) cells of moderate degree with only occasional severely dyskaryotic (dysplastic) cells, while seemingly suggestive of HSIL (CIN 2), will often disclose HSIL (CIN 3) on biopsy or conization.

LSIL (CONDYLOMA/CIN 1)

LSIL is a term that unifies entities previously referred to as condyloma acuminatum, 'flat condyloma,' and CIN 1. LSIL is the histopathologic presentation of productive episomal HPV propagation, essentially a field effect caused by viral activation in maturing squamous cells. Although a degree of nuclear maturation occurs, abnormal nuclei persist throughout the full thickness of the epithelium (if this were not so, a diagnosis by cytologic smear would not be possible; see earlier sections) (Figures 10.16–10.18). Mitotic figures, if present, are few in number and generally confined to the basal third of the epithelium. Abnormal mitosis forms are uncommon: these usually indicate aneuploidy and thus are more specific for the diagnosis of HSIL. Characteristic LSIL changes are concentrated in the upper part of the epithelium where productive episomal virus propagation in maturing squamous cells forms characteristic koilocytes. These koilocytotic nuclei can be wildly pleomorphic, and are among the largest nuclei seen in any kind of SIL. Upon integration of viral DNA into the genome of host cells, episomal propagation, and their koilocytotic phenotype, are diminished. Thus koilocytes are less common in HSIL (CIN 2 and 3), although they do still occur in these lesions, particularly where surface epithelial maturation is retained.

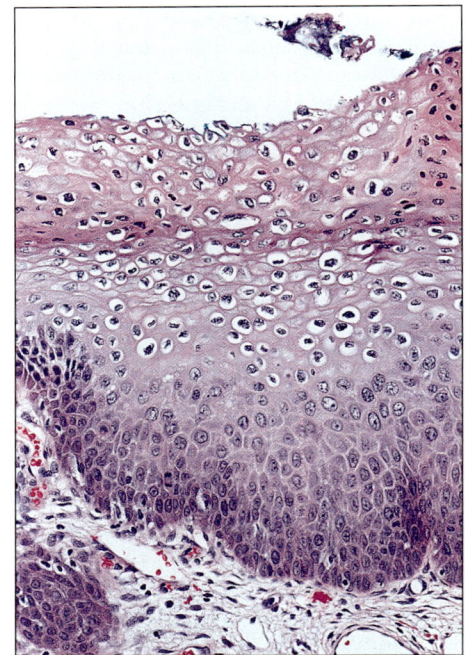

Figure 10.17 LSIL (CIN 1).

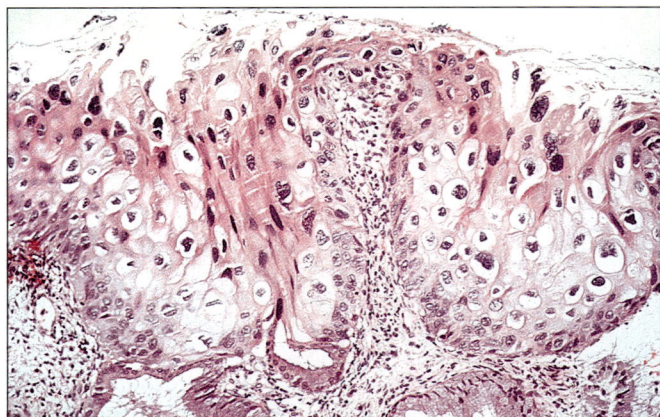

Figure 10.18 LSIL (CIN 1). There is prominent nuclear pleomorphism in koilocytes with extensive cytoplasmic maturation.

LSILs, on occasion, may lie adjacent to high-grade lesions, or occasionally even adjacent to carcinomas. Sometimes this reflects progression of a single viral infection from an episomal to integrated phase across one epithelium, whereas in others it may be due to infection by multiple viral types.

In the past, much attention was paid to distinguishing isolated 'koilocytosis' from 'dysplasia.' These were pressing issues in a premolecular world where histologic–viral correlations were not yet available, and the functional significance of HPV infection was unknown. From a pathologist's perspective, there was no objective gold standard to establish what was actually a koilocyte, or its diagnostic and clinical relationship to what had previously, and separately, been identified as a precancerous process (dysplasia). One solution was to diagnose HPV effects and dysplasia separately, so it was frequent to see a diagnosis of 'koilocytotic change without dysplasia/CIN.' Many of these 'dysplasia-free' koilocytes were overdiagnosed binucleate but otherwise normal-appearing nuclei in a glycogen-rich cell. This has been remedied by more specific criteria for histologic diagnosis of HPV-related koilocytes, which include nuclear size variation, wrinkled contours, and coarse chromatin as defined elsewhere. Other 'dysplasia-free koilocytes' described diagnoses separately applied to the superficial (koilocyte-containing) and basal (dysplasia) zones of one epithelium.

This is no longer strictly necessary, as examination of all features of the epithelium must be considered in rendering a comprehensive diagnosis. Thus, using the diagnostic criteria described later, the distinction of whether an LSIL does or does not have a coexisting dysplasia is no longer clinically or scientifically significant. Rather, distinction of no-SIL from LSIL, and LSIL from HSIL are the key clinical management thresholds.

The basal area of the majority of LSILs lacks any notable architectural changes, more resembling the aligned uniform basal cells of a normal epithelium. When the basal area is affected, and this can be difficult to assess reliably in an inflamed or disoriented specimen, the pleomorphism is minimal, and confined to the deepest aspects. Usually the basal-most cells retain their alignment with the basement membrane in LSILs, a feature that changes with the clonal outgrowth of HSILs. LSILs lack the degree and extent of basal disorganization, which can be seen to creep upward in the epithelium of HSILs.

Several other features are found with low-grade lesions. Nuclei that are binucleate (Figure 10.4), or even sometimes multinucleate, are found in 95% of HPV infections.[26] Occasional cells may show individual cell keratinization (dyskeratosis) (Figures 10.19 and 10.20). In smears, LSIL (mildly dyskaryotic) cells have ample cytoplasm with a well-defined squamous shape (Figure 10.21). Anucleate and nucleate keratinized cells are commonly present in sheets or plaques with poorly defined cell borders.

On a cellular basis, the koilocyte in histologic specimens is usually distinctive although the number of cells with koilocytotic change ranges from few to many (Figure 10.22). Typically, the nucleus is 3–4 times enlarged in area compared to a normal intermediate cell, uniform in size and shape, and has a halo with smooth outer borders. HPV immunostains have shown that typical koilocytes usually react with antibodies to the HPV L1 group-specific capsid protein (Figures 10.23 and 10.24). Since capsid/virion production is a temporally controlled phenomenon linked to both differentiation and lesional age, which likely explains the variability in koilocyte number between lesions, not all cells containing HPV will necessarily stain. Cells less typical

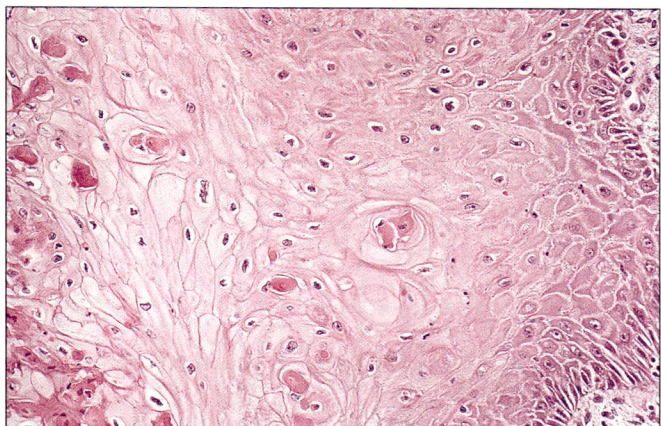

Figure 10.19 Focal individual cell dyskeratosis in LSIL (condyloma).

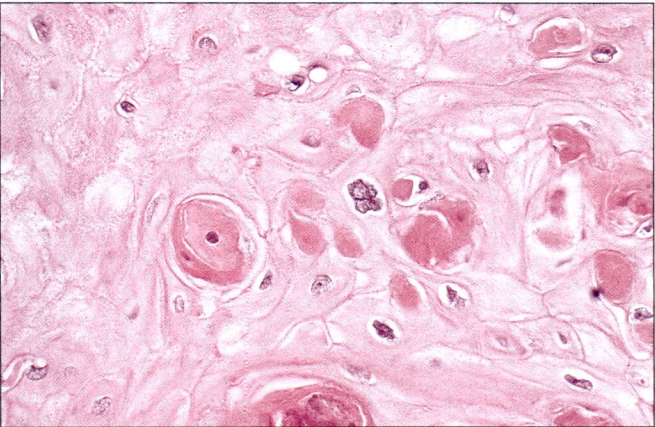

Figure 10.20 Focal individual cell dyskeratosis in LSIL (condyloma), detail.

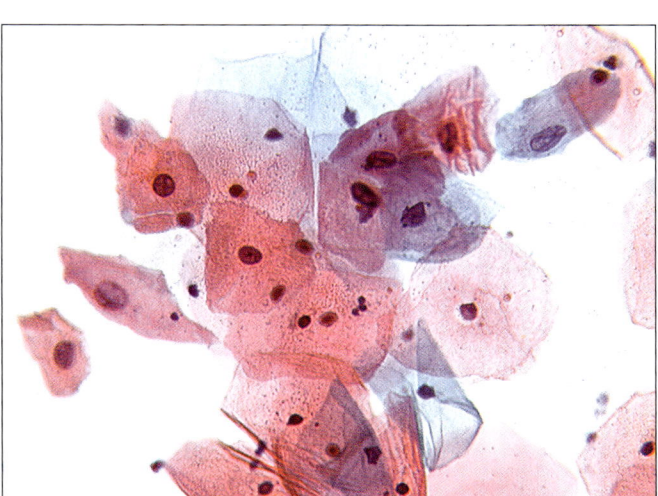

Figure 10.21 LSIL, mild dyskaryosis. Cells show dyskaryotic nuclei with abundant cytoplasm.

for koilocytes are less likely to stain. Because of the potential social stigma often attached to a smear or biopsy specimen that is diagnosed as harboring HPV, prudence dictates that no specimen should be diagnosed as LSIL unless the overall microscopic picture is distinctive.

If left untreated, most LSILs regress but laser vaporization or diathermy also easily eradicates them, although recurrence is common. Condylomata acuminata are a subtype of LSIL, so the patient with a cervical wart must have continued cytologic surveillance. Furthermore, histologic examination of LSIL should, of course, include an assessment of atypia throughout the epithelial thickness, as well as the surrounding epithelium. Sometimes a lesion with prominent superficial koilocytes suggestive of an LSIL contains cells that have sufficient atypia or basal changes to warrant a diagnosis of HSIL.

LSIL (Condyloma Acuminatum)

Condylomata acuminata of the cervix, exophytic papillary lesions caused by HPV (Figure 10.25), are much less common than those with flat architecture. This fact is consistent with the knowledge that the acuminate architecture is somewhat more frequently associated with HPV types 6 and 11 and some other low-risk types, and that these make up only 10–15% of cervical infections. Yet HPV 6/11 account for around 95% of cutaneous genital condylomata. Larger condylomata can be seen with the naked eye, and they may initially be mistaken for carcinoma (Figure 10.26).

The histology of exophytic, or acuminate, LSIL (condyloma) shows papillomatosis, acanthosis, parakeratosis, and hyperkeratosis. At higher magnification, each asperity, i.e., each papillary frond, has a tiny blood vessel at its core. Koilocytotic atypia is usually a prominent feature, with individual cell keratinization (dyskeratosis) and multinucleation. There is often a chronic inflammatory infiltrate in the underlying cervical stroma (Figures 10.27–10.30).

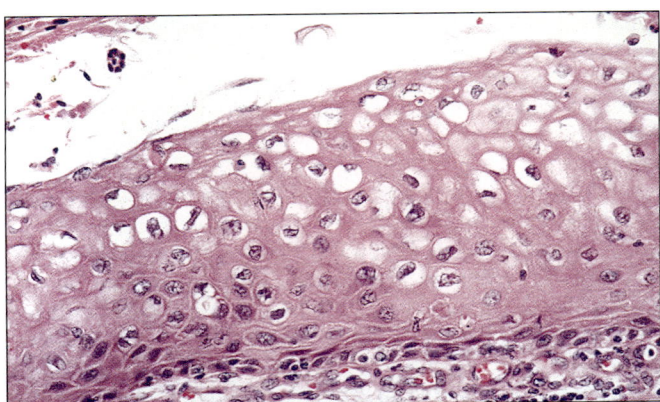

Figure 10.23 LSIL with minimal parabasal hyperplasia.

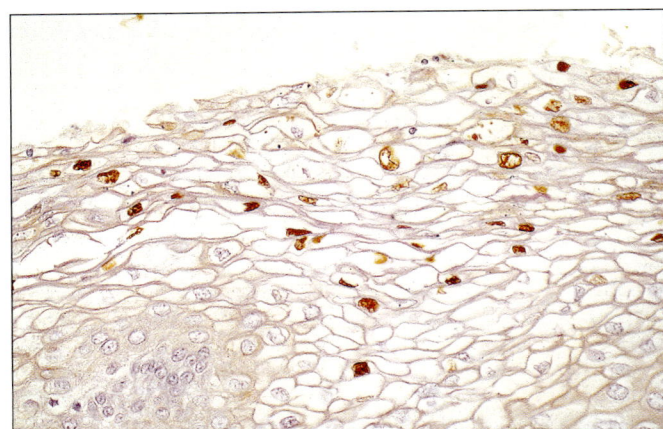

Figure 10.24 LSIL. Immunocytochemical staining shows viral capsid protein in koilocytes.

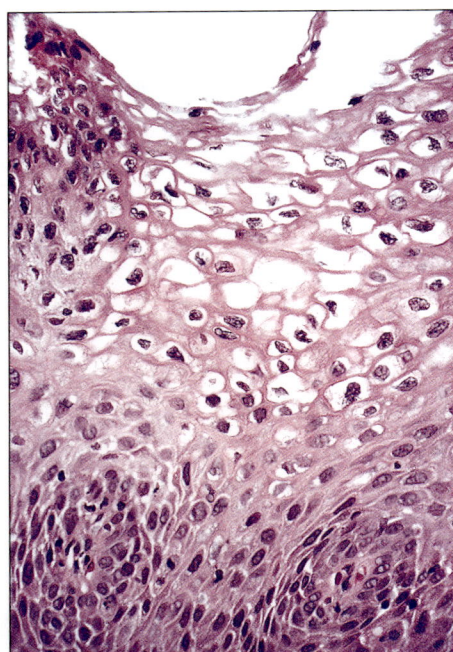

Figure 10.22 Koilocytes in LSIL (CIN 1).

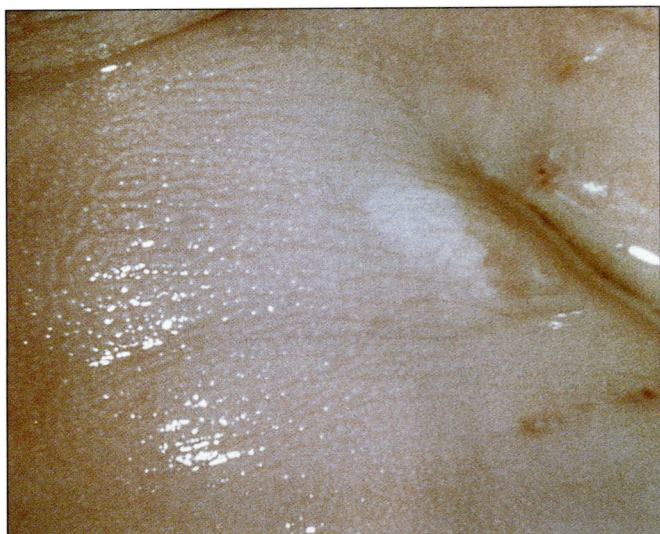

Figure 10.25 LSIL (condyloma acuminatum). The condyloma is exophytic but very small in size. It turned white when 3% acetic acid was applied.

CHAPTER 10 — CERVICAL SQUAMOUS INTRAEPITHELIAL LESIONS   211

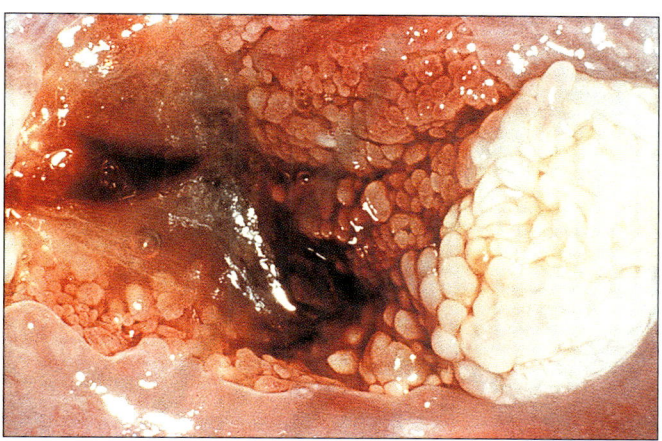

Figure 10.26 LSIL (condyloma acuminatum). This exophytic condyloma acuminatum is large and cauliflower-like.

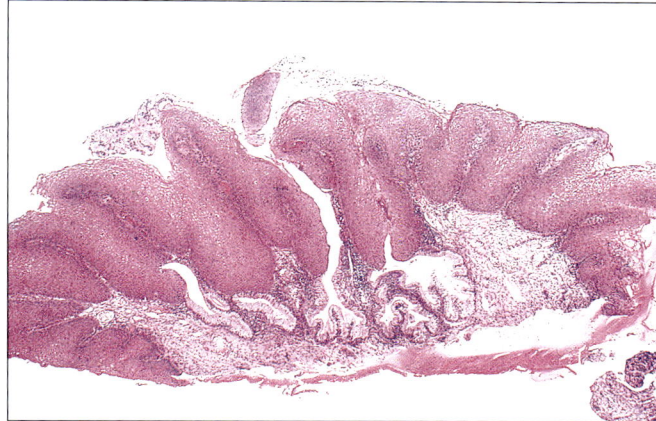

Figure 10.27 LSIL (condyloma acuminatum) that is sessile and broad.

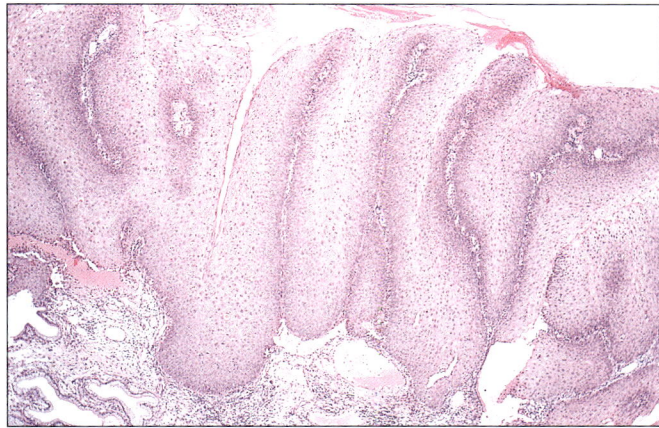

Figure 10.28 LSIL (condyloma acuminatum). Medium magnification of a sessile and broad condyloma.

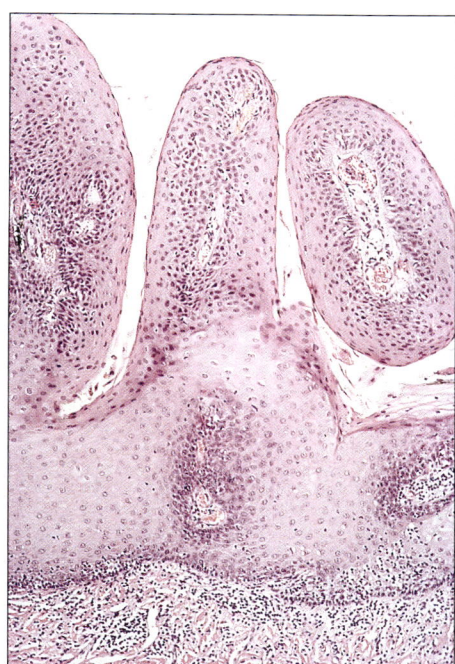

Figure 10.29 LSIL (condyloma) with asperities.

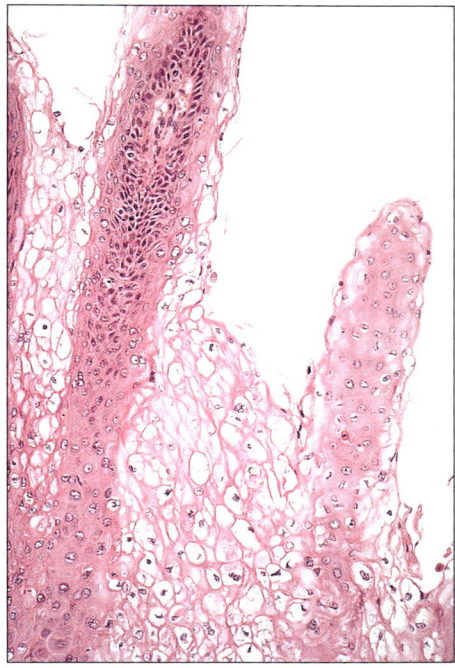

Figure 10.30 LSIL (condyloma) with asperities. High magnification of asperity showing both koilocytes and a fibrovascular core containing a central blood vessel.

LSIL ('Flat Condyloma'/CIN 1)

Flat LSILs that lack the architecture of condyloma acuminatum are recognizable colposcopically, cytologically, and histologically but cannot usually be seen with the naked eye (not to be confused with condylomata lata or flat warts of secondary syphilis, which are external genital lesions) (Figures 10.4–10.6, 10.16–10.18, 10.22–10.24). The colposcopic features are fully described later, but they are not altogether diagnostic. Based on histology, several features in addition to the presence of koilocytes are useful in the detection of HPV infection. On low-power magnification, large areas may be composed of squamous epithelial cells

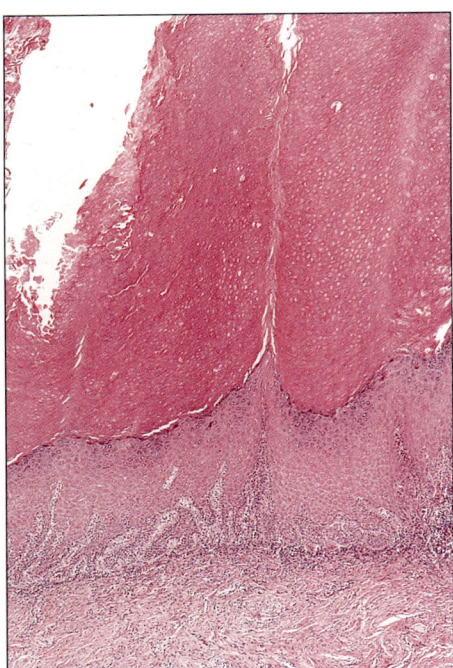

Figure 10.31 LSIL (condyloma) with marked hyperkeratosis. The lesion grossly had the appearance of a cutaneous horn.

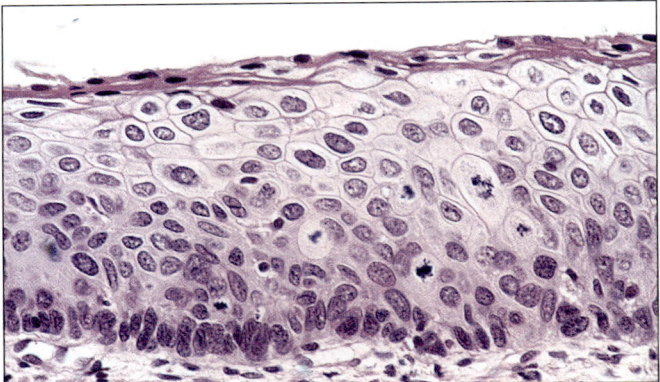

Figure 10.32 HSIL (CIN 2). There are several atypical mitoses in a lesion that exhibits suprabasal cytoplasmic maturation.

lacking glycogen. While suggestive, this feature is nonspecific. The cytoplasm from the basal-most cells to the surface is eosinophilic. Commonly a sharp boundary demarcates the epithelium that is glycogen rich (normal) and glycogen poor (HPV). In addition, the superficial cells in the glycogen-poor zones commonly show acanthosis, parakeratosis, and sometimes even hyperkeratosis. The last, rarely, may be quite striking (Figure 10.31). The term flat condyloma, originally used to describe lesions containing koilocytes but without a condylomatous architecture or CIN 1, is a contradiction and is no longer used, and is now replaced by LSIL. Whether flat lesions with and without CIN 1 can be separated reproducibly, and whether their separation has any clinical meaning, is debatable but some, particularly those using the CIN system, attempt to make this distinction.

HIGH-GRADE SQUAMOUS INTRAEPITHELIAL LESIONS (CIN 2–3)

HSIL is a neoplastic process composed of a clonal outgrowth of cells with genomically integrated HPV. Its characteristic histologic features include jumbled or irregular arrangements of epithelial cells against the basement membrane, and extension of basaloid atypical cells above the lower third of the epithelial thickness with an accompanying reduction in cytoplasmic maturation. These distinguish HSIL from LSIL, which must be diagnosed separately as they often lead to differing patient management. Koilocytotic change may or may not be present within HSIL, and some HSILs coexist with LSIL. The appearance of abnormal mitotic configurations is common, reflecting aneuploidy induced by high-risk viruses, and when present should be considered a basis for upgrading to HSIL.

The category of HSIL encompasses both CIN 2 and 3 as carried forward from the cervical intraepithelial schema. In creating HSIL, the Bethesda System unified high-risk lesions to promote uniform management of these patients, and today these are minimally diagnosed simply as HSIL, or HSIL with a parenthetic reference to the combined CIN 2 and 3 categories (HSIL, CIN 2–3). Nonetheless, there is persistent clinical interest in substratifying HSIL into risk subgroups. This clinical goal has remained somewhat elusive. Not only is there no consensus on precise criteria for this distinction in a given patient, but the magnitude of risk substratification required to justify triaging into differing management options is unclear. Furthermore, there is confusion and disagreement among pathologists regarding whether a reintroduced category of CIN 2 should be defined by diagnostic imprecision in labeling a lesion as LSIL or HSIL (essentially a SIL that is difficult to grade), or whether it is a biologically intermediate entity between LSIL and HSIL. The latter is perhaps a more proactive stance, as true diagnostic improvements might be realized through revised histologic criteria, perhaps integrated with biomarkers or host parameters, to guide management.

HSIL (CIN 2)

In HSIL (CIN 2), the upper two-thirds of the epithelium shows some differentiation and maturation, with, as in LSIL, nuclear atypia persisting to the surface (Figures 10.32–10.38). Nuclear abnormalities are more marked than in LSIL, and more nuclei with greater degrees of abnormality are found high in the epithelium. Examination of the lowermost epithelial layer, abutting the basement membrane, is an important aspect of segregating LSIL from HSIL (CIN 2), with irregular nuclear placement in HSIL (CIN 2) creating a 'jumbled' look. Mitotic figures are present in the basal two-thirds of the epithelium. If attention is focused upon the findings in the upper portion of the epithelium, the changes would be similar qualitatively, but more advanced quantitatively, in comparison to LSIL. More nuclei are pleomorphic in relation to neighboring nuclei, lack polarity to various degrees, have wrinkled nuclear membranes, and show various degrees of hyperchromasia. Overall, the percentage of nuclear area to total epithelial area is roughly 40–60% in the upper half of the epithelium.

CHAPTER 10 — CERVICAL SQUAMOUS INTRAEPITHELIAL LESIONS

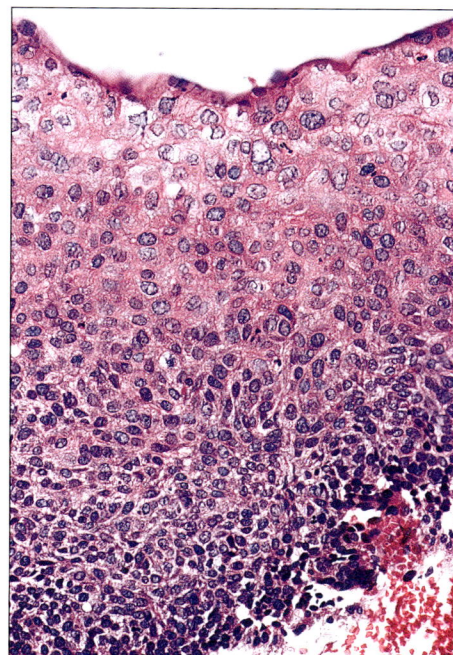

Figure 10.33 HSIL (CIN 2). Cytoplasmic maturation is less than that seen in LSIL, and is largely confined to the upper third of the epithelium. Basal cells are not oriented against the basement membrane.

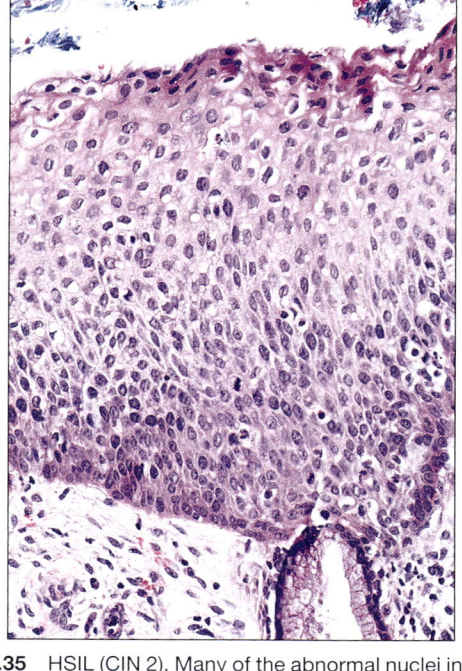

Figure 10.35 HSIL (CIN 2). Many of the abnormal nuclei in the upper epithelium are larger than those seen in the basal epithelium.

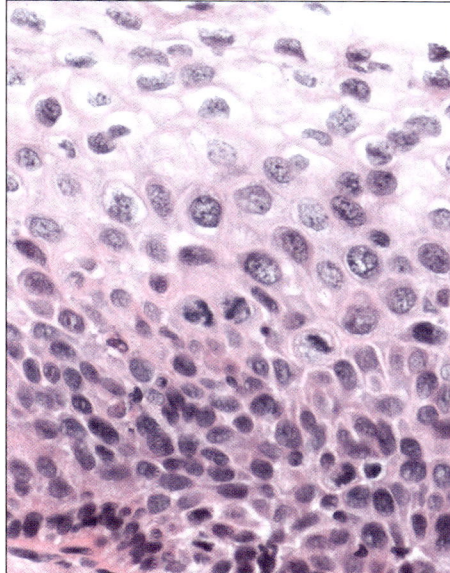

Figure 10.34 HSIL (CIN 2) with abnormal mitotic figures in the middle third of the epithelium.

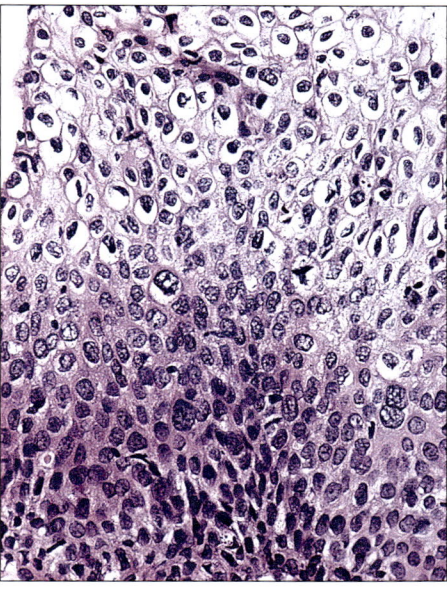

Figure 10.36 HSIL (CIN 2) with koilocytosis. Although cut tangentially, the cells show cytoplasmic maturation and koilocytosis toward the surface.

The diagnosis of CIN 2 is the least reproducible form of CIN. It is viewed by some as an equivocal diagnostic interpretation, by others as a distinctive intermediate biologic state. Across the spectrum of individual examples encountered, it is probably both. By forcing diagnostic reassignment of HSIL (CIN 2) into LSIL and HSIL (CIN 3) categories, approximately one-third are the former and two thirds the latter.[17]

HSIL (CIN 3)

In HSIL (CIN 3), any maturation, if present, is confined to the superficial third of the epithelium. Generally, it is minimal to completely absent. Nuclear abnormalities are marked throughout the whole thickness of the epithelium. Similarly, mitotic figures are found at all levels of the epithelium and may be numerous. The findings in the upper portion of the epithelium include more extensive nuclear

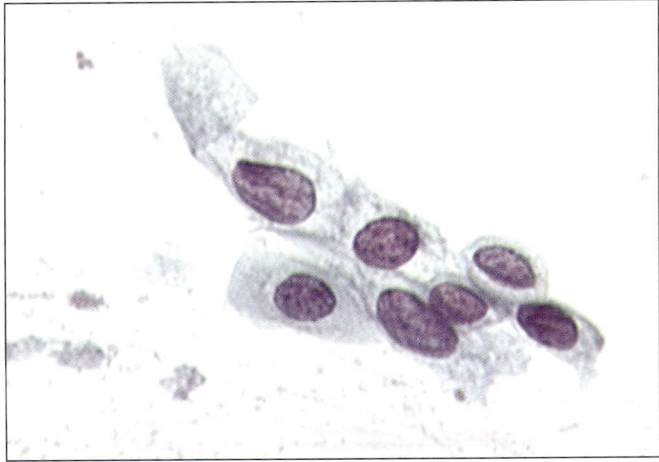

Figure 10.37 HSIL, moderate dyskaryosis. The nuclei are large, occupying more than half the total cell size.

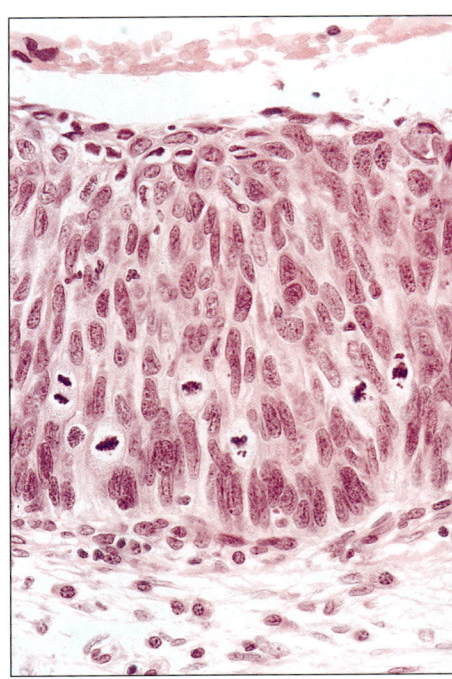

Figure 10.39 HSIL (CIN 3). There is full thickness involvement of the epithelium by undifferentiated epithelial cells.

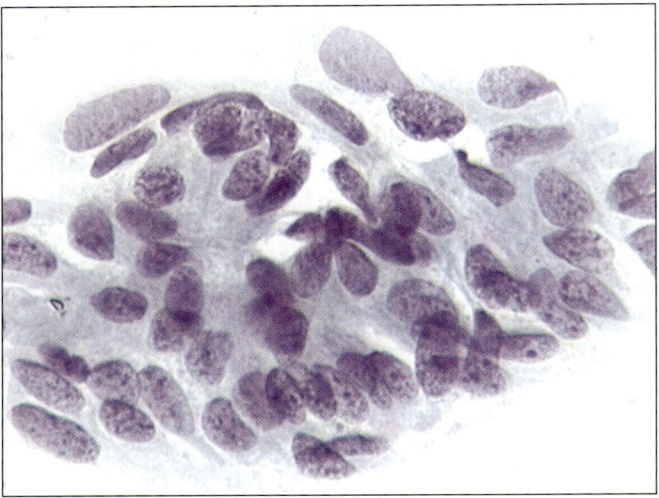

Figure 10.38 HSIL, moderate dyskaryosis. A sheet of cells with atypical nuclei and reduced amounts of cytoplasm showing some differentiation.

changes and the proportion of the lesional area that consists of nuclear material can exceed 60% in the upper half of the epithelium (Figure 10.39). In smears, the rim of cytoplasm is thin, and the nucleus occupies virtually the entire cell (Figure 10.15). As with HSIL (CIN 2), the basal-most layer of cells is disorderly in HSIL (CIN 3).

In some cases of HSIL (CIN 3) the entire epithelium is occupied by monomorphic basal-like cells, and these can easily be mistaken for atrophy, squamous metaplasia, or reactive change. Careful examination of chromatin texture, which is coarse in HSIL, the assessment of mitotic figures, and immunostains for p16 and Ki-67 are useful in this differential diagnosis.

Given the previous discussion, SIL (CIN) terminology will be used from this point onward, except where specific studies using either the dysplasia/CIS or CIN terminologies are cited.

AREAS OF DIAGNOSTIC DIFFICULTY

THE SCANT ENDOCERVICAL CURETTAGE

In the absence of any generally accepted criteria for what constitutes either an adequate or scant specimen, pathologists frequently encounter the problem of what language to use when reporting a curettage specimen where the diagnostic tissue is less than sufficient. This is also true for endometrial samples where only endocervical tissue is present. Many specimens, even with copious amounts of material, consist largely of mucus, which itself is not of diagnostic value. Often the only diagnostic cellular component present consists of little more than a few small strips of mucinous columnar epithelium devoid of any underlying stroma. To diagnose a specimen as 'unsatisfactory' would generally require that the clinician repeat a painful procedure. The recommended approach is to report endocervical curettages (ECCs) descriptively (mucus, mucinous columnar cells, fragments of endocervix, fragments of exocervix) and when necessary with the qualifiers 'scant, rare, miniscule quantities of, etc.' A typical example is 'scant mucus and mucinous columnar epithelium.' When the specimen consists of just a few exfoliated mucinous cells, some use the phraseology 'rare exfoliated mucinous cells, inadequate (or insufficient or suboptimal) for further diagnosis,' which serves as a trigger for the clinician to rethink the issue. A distinction should be made between strips of mucinous columnar cells and rare isolated exfoliated mucinous cells as the former likely reflects the curettage while the latter may represent little more than cells already exfoliated into the mucus. Although the ECC is primarily used to assess the extent of squamous neoplasia, it also helps in evaluating the presence or absence of glandular tumors and their precursors that may involve the endocervix.

LESIONS SUSPICIOUS FOR, BUT SUBDIAGNOSTIC OF, SIL

Conceptually, this is the histologic equivalent of the cytologic diagnosis of atypical squamous cells of undetermined significance (ASCUS/borderline change). Since ASCUS/borderline change is a cytologic equivocation and a risk assessment rather than a biologic entity, there has been no formal translation to a histologic diagnostic entity. Rather, if features are present that raise the possibility of SIL (CIN) but this cannot be diagnosed, the findings should be described. Samples may be subdiagnostic because of adequacy (technical condition or abundance) or interpretive difficulties. Where appropriate, some indication of the basis of diagnostic uncertainty, and recommendation for clinical correlation and follow-up, can be made.

BASAL CELL HYPERPLASIA

Basal cell hyperplasia shows regular replication of basal layers with nuclear enlargement. However, nuclear pleomorphism and hyperchromasia are absent. Differentiation is relatively normal in the upper half of the epithelium. While the significance of basal cell hyperplasia and its long-term implications are unknown, it may reflect the early stages of dysplasia occurring in the 'original' (native rather than metaplastic) squamous epithelium.

In some cases, the distinction between basal cell hyperplasia and HSIL (CIN 2-3) can be difficult to make. Cases exist where the basal and parabasal cells are remarkably abnormal, and yet the upper two-thirds of the epithelium is relatively normal (Figures 10.40 and 10.41). Emphasis on the upper layers leads to a diagnosis of basal cell hyperplasia, whereas emphasis on the basal layers leads to a diagnosis of HSIL (CIN 2-3). Ki-67 (MIB1) and p16 immunohistochemistry can be helpful in making the distinction, with Ki-67 highlighting the increased proliferation and p16 the presence of a high-risk HPV infection in HSIL.

IMMATURE SQUAMOUS METAPLASIA AND ATYPICAL SQUAMOUS METAPLASIA

Squamous metaplasia is a physiologic process characterized by reserve cell hyperplasia, early squamous differentiation, variable polarity, and nuclear enlargement, any component of which may sometimes be quite exaggerated (see Chapter 8). Nuclear pleomorphism and hyperchromasia are absent, thus rendering to the epithelium an appearance of somewhat bland nuclei of uniform size and shape (the nuclei are typically round). During the time when metaplastic squamous cells develop, they may undermine and replace endocervical columnar cells. At times the nuclei can be enlarged and yet be relatively uniform, which elicits differences in diagnoses among pathologists as to whether the lesion represents immature squamous metaplasia or SIL, especially when columnar cells are present on the surface (Figure 10.42). HPV-associated features such as koilocytosis are rarely seen in immature metaplastic squamous epithelium, presumably as a result of the lack of differentiation.

It can be difficult to distinguish immature squamous metaplasia with minimal nuclear changes from SIL (CIN) (Table 10.5). Typically, immature metaplastic squamous cells have abundant cytoplasm and homogeneous round nuclei with fine speckled chromatin and a small nucleolus. The frequency of Ki-67 (MIB1)-reactive nuclei is low and the staining intensity minimal.[27] Cylindrical cells can occur intermingled with, or at the surface of, the immature cells and then are a strong diagnostic criterion, but are not always present. Whenever substantial nuclear pleomorphism is found, SIL (CIN) should be diagnosed even if columnar cells are present on the surface (Figure 10.43). Ki-67 staining is useful in resolving the differential diagnosis, as it is typically unremarkable in immature squamous metaplasia but appears at high density throughout the epithelium in SIL (CIN). Similarly, p16 is typically diffusely expressed in SIL (CIN) but absent or expressed only focally in immature metaplastic squamous epithelium.

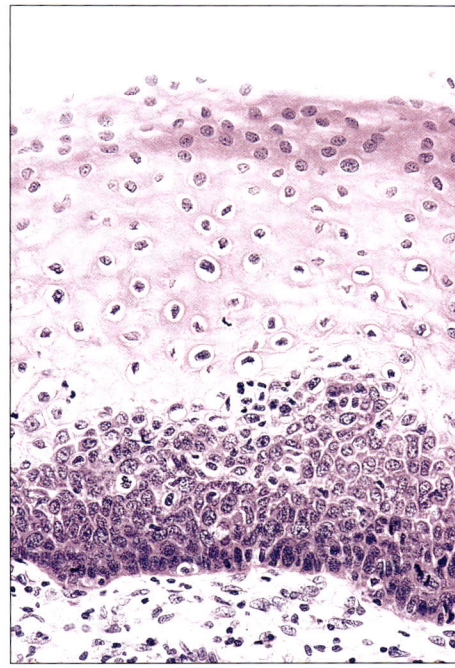

Figure 10.40 'Excessive differentiation.' The basal and parabasal epithelium show features suggesting HSIL (CIN 2-3), but the upper epithelium is normal. The quandary exists whether such a case should be categorized as HSIL (CIN 2-3) or as basal cell hyperplasia.

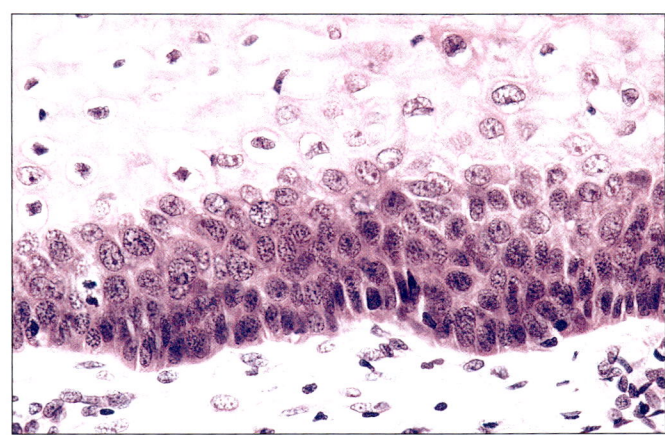

Figure 10.41 High magnification of 'excessive differentiation.'

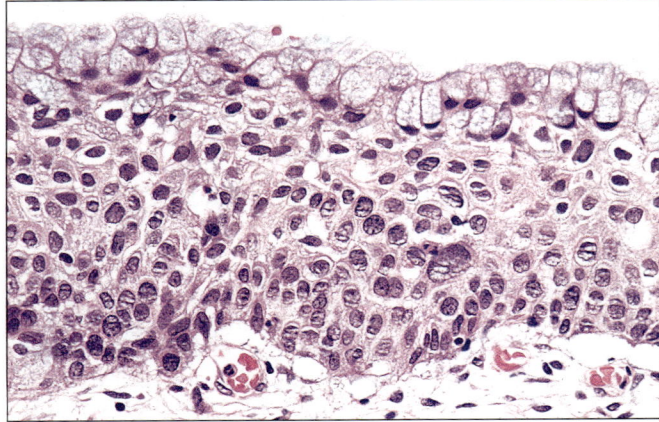

Figure 10.42 Immature squamous metaplasia versus HSIL (CIN 2), with surface columnar epithelium. Ki-67 and p16 immunostaining may help to make this distinction.

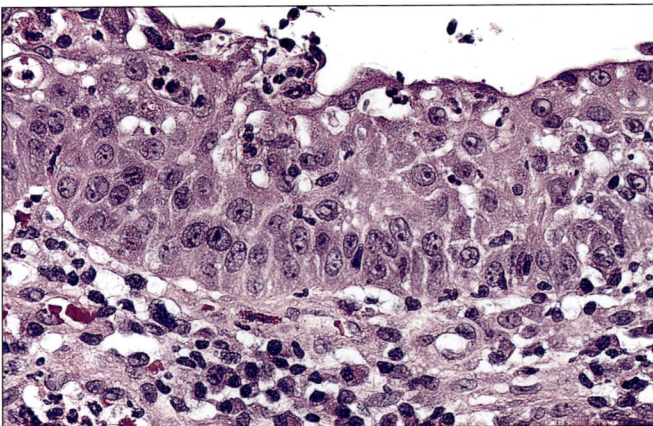

Figure 10.44 Repair. The nuclei lack pleomorphism and contain prominent nucleoli.

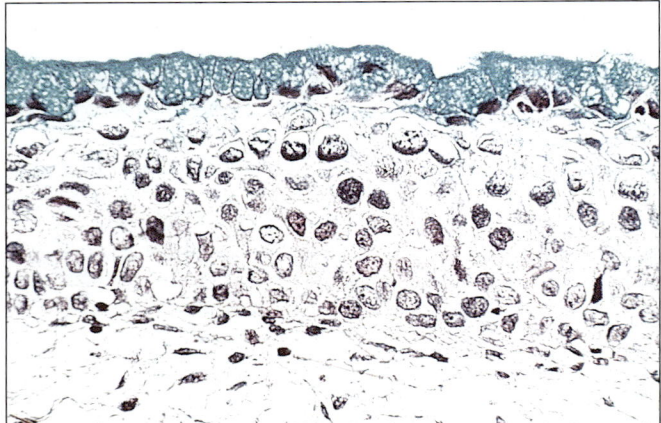

Figure 10.43 HSIL (CIN 2) with pleomorphic nuclei beneath the surface columnar mucinous epithelium. Mucin stain.

Table 10.5 Differential Diagnostic Features of Immature Squamous Metaplasia and SIL (CIN)

Feature	Immature squamous Metaplasia	SIL (CIN)
Nuclei	Round	Variable
Chromatin	Homogeneous	Coarse, clumped
Nucleoli	Single and prominent	Usually inconspicuous. When present, often large and multiple
Cylindrical cells	Useful when present but often absent	Absent
Ki-67 (MIB1)	Scattered positive cells	Often diffusely positive
p16	Negative or focally positive	Diffusely positive

REPAIR (REACTIVE EPITHELIAL CHANGES)

Repair of the squamous epithelium is a condition that commonly mimics the features of SIL (CIN).[28] Unlike SIL (CIN), the stroma in repair is virtually always chronically and often floridly inflamed. The nuclei are uniform, with no or minimal pleomorphism. The chromatin is bland and evenly distributed. Nucleoli of 'bull's eye' or macronucleolar appearance are often easily found (Figure 10.44). The epithelium in SIL (CIN) may be incidentally associated with an intensely inflamed stroma, but can be recognized by nuclei that are pleomorphic and commonly display coarse chromatin and mitoses.

LOW ESTROGEN STATES AND ATROPHY

In low estrogen states (i.e., after menopause), and in high progesterone states (e.g. during pregnancy or as a result of progestogen therapy), the cervical squamous epithelium is usually thin and may be composed entirely of parabasal cells. While mild nuclear hyperchromasia is often seen, the nuclei are uniform in size and shape and a constant amount of cytoplasm surrounds most nuclei. Nuclear pleomorphism is absent. In some postmenopausal women, the cervix may exhibit a spectrum of epithelial alterations, including prominent perinuclear halos, nuclear hyperchromasia, some variation in nuclear size, and multinucleation. In one study, all cases showing these changes were negative for HPV by polymerase chain reaction (PCR) analysis.[29] Several features help to distinguish postmenopausal atrophy from the HPV-associated changes of SIL (CIN). They include less variation in nuclear size and staining intensity, more finely and evenly distributed nuclear chromatin, and greater uniformity of perinuclear halos in the former. Ki-67 (MIB1) expression can also be useful, as positive nuclei are typically limited to the lower layers. However, this must be interpreted with care as very thin epithelium may lack superficial cells and can mimic HSIL (CIN 2-3). However, correlation with HPV testing is important as many studies demonstrate a 'bump' in HPV prevalence in the postmenopausal age group. p16 immunostaining can be helpful as a surrogate marker of high-risk HPV infection in this situation as it is typically diffusely positive in SIL (CIN) but negative in atrophic epithelium. Hence, a combination of Ki-67 and p16 immunostaining may be particularly useful in this context.

THIN EPITHELIUM

In an epithelium that has only a few layers of cells, it is commonly impossible to confidently diagnose the presence of

CHAPTER 10 — CERVICAL SQUAMOUS INTRAEPITHELIAL LESIONS

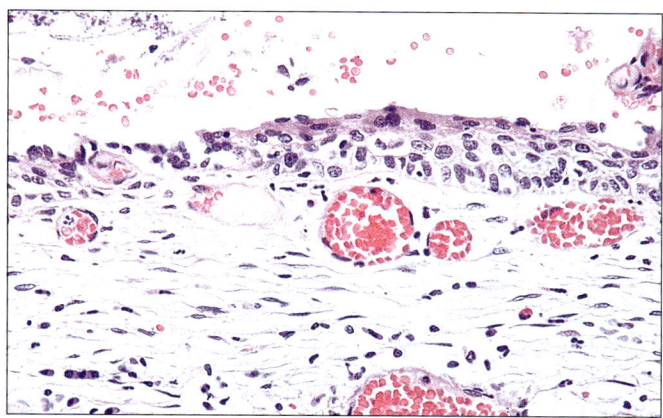

Figure 10.45 Thin epithelium, probably SIL (CIN). The nuclei appear atypical. Immunostaining for Ki-67 and p16 is useful in this situation, as diffuse and widespread expression of these markers, particularly p16, supports a diagnosis of SIL (CIN).

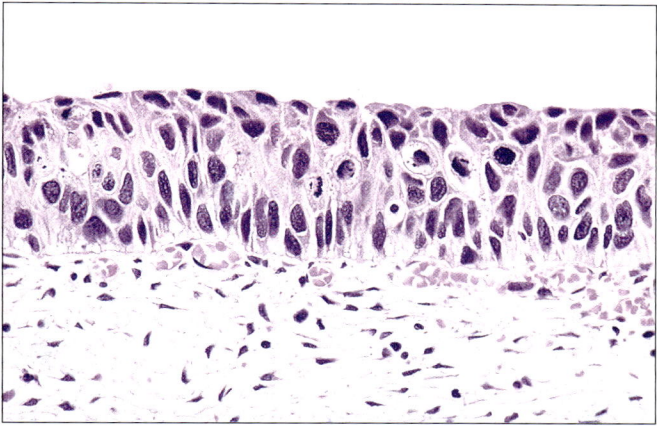

Figure 10.46 Thin epithelium with ungradeable SIL (CIN). The number of cell layers present is sufficient to diagnose SIL (CIN), but further formal definition is precluded. However, the cytologic features including atypical mitoses suggest a high-grade lesion.

SIL (CIN). There is often the concern that the epithelium is not naturally thin, and that some artifactual process is responsible for the removal of multiple superficial layers. In the absence of severe inflammation, SIL (CIN) should usually be diagnosed if there is cytologic atypia (Figure 10.45). Sometimes, the number of cell layers present is sufficient to diagnose SIL (CIN), or even probable HSIL (CIN 2-3), but further definition is precluded (Figure 10.46). It may be helpful to designate these lesions as SIL (CIN) of indeterminate grade (or ungradeable SIL (CIN)), using the cytologic features to indicate whether the lesion is likely to be low or high grade. Correlation with the Pap smear may be useful in this situation, as may immunostaining for Ki-67 and p16, as discussed previously for atrophic epithelium.

INVASIVE SQUAMOUS CELL CARCINOMA

Not uncommonly, one of the most difficult entities to distinguish from HSIL (CIN 2-3) is invasive squamous cell carcinoma. This occurs most commonly if the biopsy is superficial and is devoid of an obvious stromal component. In such examples, the lesion appears as sheets of irregularly folded dysplastic epithelium lying on a thin basement membrane. The most appropriate diagnosis is that of 'at least HSIL (CIN 2-3), cannot exclude invasion. In one study testing for cellular features that distinguish invasive and noninvasive disease, several histologic features found in the cone biopsy specimens were preferentially associated with invasive tumor.[30] These included giant bizarre cells that were irregular, hyperchromatic, and up to five times the size of a basal cell (67% vs 6%), large keratinized cells with distinct cell borders (87% vs 0%), keratin pearls (41% vs 0%), necrosis, often comedo-like (80% vs 8%), and neovascularized tumor cells close to the endothelial lining and lacking intervening connective tissue (57% vs 0%). In 74% of invasive carcinomas, a component of CIN 3 was present, of which 35% showed large keratinized cells or keratin pearls in the *in situ* components. This suggested that the presence of either feature in biopsy specimens showing CIN 3 might signify the presence of invasive lesions elsewhere in the cervical mucosa. In another study, several histologic features were associated with the presence of invasive disease: these included extensive and expansile involvement of endocervical crypts; and the presence of comedo-type necrosis in the center of involved crypts (see later).[31]

It is not unusual for the diagnosis of HSIL (CIN 2-3) to be correct, but for the results of hysterectomy to show the disease process to be more extensive than expected. Occasionally, the surface and the endocervical crypts are involved only by HSIL (CIN 2-3) in a biopsy, as suggested by a history of only HSIL (CIN 2-3) on smears (even when reviewed retrospectively) and the absence of any abnormality clinically. However, the hysterectomy specimen shows that the cervical wall harbors a small carcinoma or on occasion is permeated by a larger carcinoma (see Chapter 11).

ARTIFACT

Fragmentation and thermal artifact in cone, loop electrosurgical excision procedure (LEEP) or loop excision of the transformation zone (LETZ) biopsy specimens are major problems affecting correct diagnosis.[32,33] When specimens are fragmented into multiple small pieces, it is difficult, if not impossible, to evaluate margins. Thermal artifact, which is often caused by low-voltage techniques, results in an epithelium that appears smudged and uninterpretable. Cellular and nuclear details are lost (Figure 10.47). In a LEEP biopsy correctly done, the thermal artifact produces a very thin rim, usually a fraction of a millimeter wide, at the periphery of the specimen. The outermost layer, the carbonization zone, is usually quite thin. The coagulation zone is deeper and is significantly larger and more readily apparent. Unacceptable thermal artifact occurs when the coagulation zone is wide (Figure 10.48), resulting in extensive loss of cellular detail. A randomized controlled trial that evaluated pure cut versus traditional blending settings in large LETZs found no significant differences in thermal artifact. In the deep stroma, however, the blended setting had a thicker thermal artifact band (0.382 mm) than the pure cut setting (0.325 mm).[34]

STRATIFIED MUCIN-PRODUCING INTRAEPITHELIAL LESION

Some intraepithelial lesions show features intermediate between HSIL (CIN) and cervical adenocarcinoma *in situ*

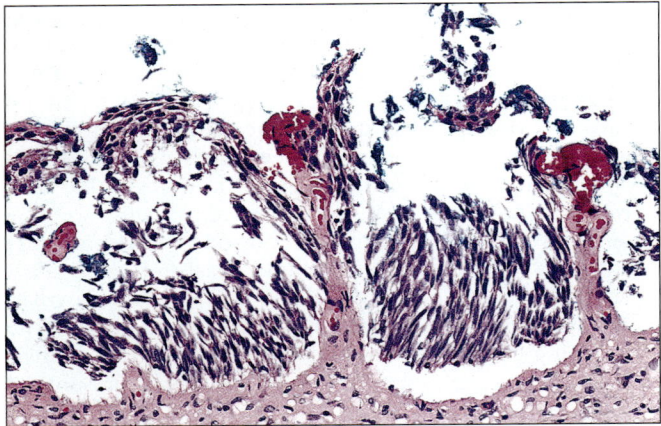

Figure 10.47 Thermal artifact with LEEP biopsy. The epithelium has lost all cellular detail.

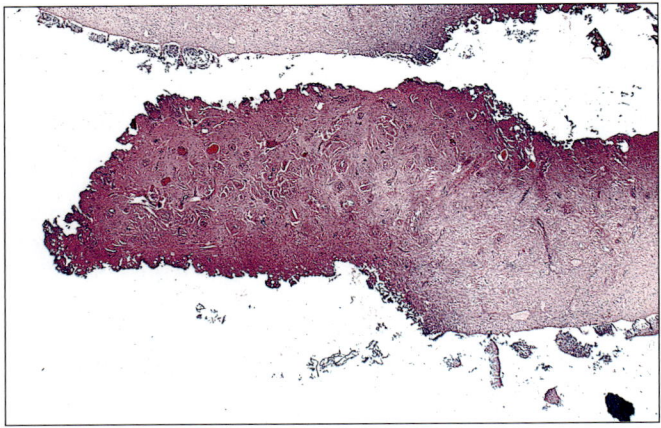

Figure 10.48 Thermal artifact with LEEP biopsy. The stroma shows extensive coagulative changes.

(AIS) (also termed high-grade cervical glandular intraepithelial neoplasia) (see Chapter 12). Where mucin-producing cells are admixed with non-mucin-producing cells in an atypical stratified intraepithelial lesion, the term stratified mucin-producing intraepithelial lesion or SMILE has been proposed.[35] This entity is uncommon[36] and when observed is best diagnosed as a histologic variant of cervical AIS: 'cervical adenocarcinoma *in situ*, stratified mucin-producing intraepithelial type.' In many cases features of 'pure' AIS are also present in the histologic slides.

CONGENITAL TRANSFORMATION ZONE
(See also Chapter 8)

Immature squamous epithelium may be present distal (caudal, vaginal) to the last endocervical gland (discussed later) in an anatomic position, peripheral to the transformation zone, which is normally occupied by native, mature squamous epithelium. Recognition of the appearance of this epithelium, which has been termed the 'congenital transformation zone,' is therefore important. Surface hyperkeratosis or parakeratosis is often present and this can produce a leukoplakic appearance colposcopically. Histologically, the typical features are a relative lack of epithelial maturation of squamous epithelium that has an irregular, dentate, contour. The lack of maturation raises the possibility of SIL (CIN) but cytologic atypia is absent. Specific recognition of this entity is important for colposcopy–histopathology correlation.

MISCELLANEOUS CONDITIONS

One of the more bizarre situations rarely encountered is when the cervix is treated for SIL (CIN), but the results of hysterectomy show the SIL (CIN) process involves more than the cervix. There are rare reported cases where hysterectomy and bilateral salpingo-oophorectomy performed to treat SIL (CIN) disclosed that the disease had extended to the endometrium and fallopian tubes, and there extensively replaced the normal glandular mucosa.[37,38]

BIOMARKERS

p16

The cyclin-dependent kinase 2A inhibitor, $p16^{INK4}$, or simply p16, helps distinguish SIL (CIN) from reactive and atrophic lesions.[39] Since a retinoblastoma protein (pRb)-dependent negative feedback loop regulates p16 expression, continuous inactivation of pRb by high-risk (but not low-risk) HPV E7 results in increased p16 levels. Hence, increased p16 levels may reflect HPV-induced SIL (CIN) with deregulated E7 expression.[40] Marked overexpression of p16 protein, i.e., diffuse and strong immunostaining (Figure 10.49), is present in virtually all cervical squamous cell and adenocarcinomas, and high-grade squamous and glandular preinvasive lesions (HSIL (CIN) and AIS) infected by high-risk HPVs, e.g., types 16, 18, 31, 33, 52, and 58, in contrast to the weak/focal staining in lesions infected with HPV 6/11 or other low-risk HPVs.[41] p16 overexpression is sensitive (84%) and specific (98%) for the detection of high-risk HPV.[42] At low magnification, p16 staining facilitates finding a dysplastic area, especially if the epithelium is heavily infiltrated by leukocytes, as often occurs in SILs (CINs).[39] In addition, overexpressed p16 helps identify individual SIL cells in fluid-based cytologic smears.[43] This biomarker is particularly useful in the distinction between SIL (CIN) and reactive and atrophic epithelia, especially where the epithelium is thin (see earlier).

p16 positivity should not be used directly to grade SIL (CIN), a distinction that must be based upon the diagnostic appearance on H&E as outlined previously. This is because high-risk viruses infect some LSIL epithelia, and these will be p16 positive and should not be overdiagnosed as HSIL. A negative p16 result, however, can be used to rule out an HSIL where the differential diagnosis includes mimics such as atrophy or reactive change. Detailed discussion of the use of p16 is included in reference 6.

Ki-67

The expression of Ki-67 can also be used to support a diagnosis of SIL (CIN) as its expression signifies continued cellular proliferation and, if present beyond the parabasal cells, may indicate SIL (CIN). Used in conjunction with p16 immunostaining, it can help to distinguish between reactive and atrophic states and SIL (CIN).

ProExC

More recently, immunostaining using ProExC, which detects the combination of minichromosome maintenance (MCM)

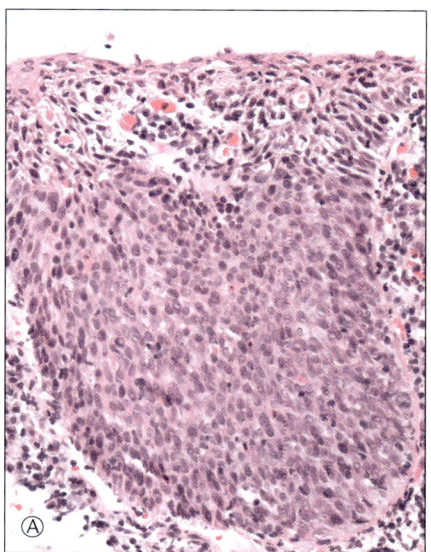 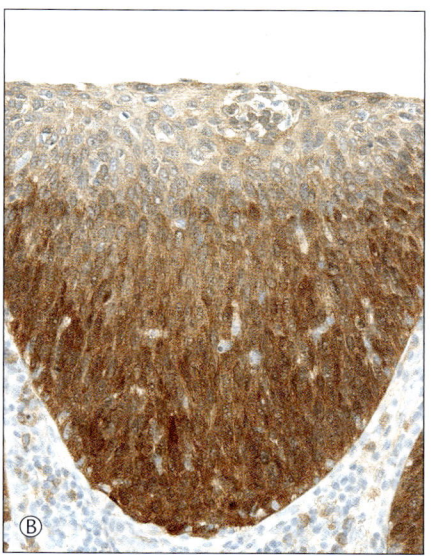 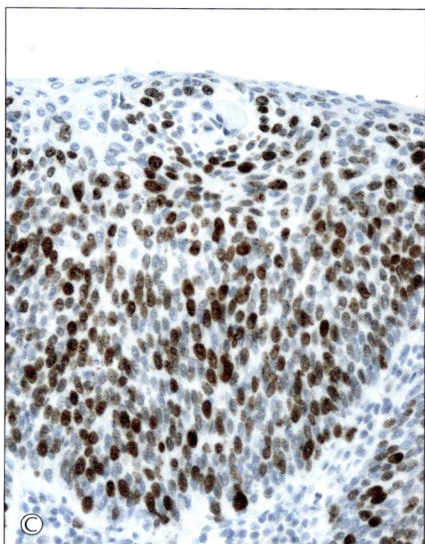

Figure 10.49 There is diffuse, strong p16 and Ki-67 expression in this HSIL (CIN 3). Note that expression becomes less intense and widespread, respectively, in parallel with superficial maturation at the surface of the lesion. **(A)** H&E. **(B)** p16. **(C)** Ki-67.

protein 2 (MCM2) and topoisomerase 2α (TOPO2α), has been suggested as an alternative biomarker for the diagnosis of SIL (CIN). This performs well in some studies[44] and there is some evidence that the combination of ProExC and p16 may be diagnostically useful.[45]

HPV TYPING

There is a large amount of literature addressing the role of HPV testing in cervical screening, particularly the triage of women with low-grade cervical cytologic abnormalities,[46] or during follow-up of patients with SIL (CIN),[47] but the role of HPV typing in the assessment of biopsy material is limited. The detection of HPV DNA by *in situ* hybridization can aid the identification of HPV-associated carcinomas, particularly adenocarcinomas, and in the distinction between cervical and endometrial adenocarcinomas.[48] However, its use in the assessment of SIL (CIN) is limited, particularly in view of the excellent performance of immunohistochemical biomarkers such as p16,[25,49] which are more easily implemented in a routine laboratory context.

HISTOLOGIC FEATURES OF SIL (CIN) AFFECTING MANAGEMENT AND PROGNOSIS

The specification of a biopsy-proven SIL (CIN) as low or high grade greatly influences management, with the former usually eliciting prospective surveillance and the latter ablative therapy. This was reaffirmed in the 2012 consensus recommendations by the College of American Pathologists and the American Society for Colposcopy and Cervical Pathology.[50] There is some controversy, however, regarding whether HSIL (CIN 2) should be managed differently from HSIL (CIN 3), especially in the younger patient. This is fueled by the observation that HSIL (CIN 2) is a less reproducible diagnosis than HSIL (CIN 3), with the implication that some proportion of HSIL (CIN 2) cases are low clinical risk lesions overdiagnosed by the pathologist.

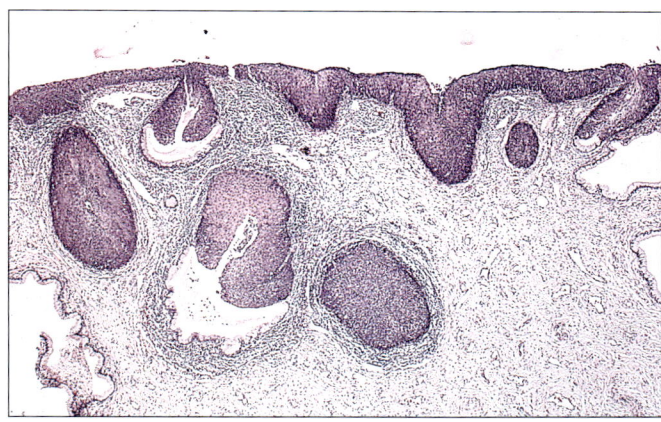

Figure 10.50 HSIL (CIN 3) with endocervical crypt involvement. Several crypts are only partially replaced; the endocervical mucosa remains intact. Where the HSIL (CIN 3) has entirely replaced the crypt, the smooth perimeter indicates that the lesion is *in situ* and has not invaded into the cervical stroma.

INVOLVEMENT OF ENDOCERVICAL GLAND CRYPTS

Consideration of the involvement of endocervical gland crypts in addition to surface epithelium is important for patient management (Figures 10.50–10.52). The number and depth of involved crypts increases with the grade of SIL (CIN). In CIN 3 cone biopsy specimens, nearly 90% had involved crypts.[51] The mean depth of involvement was 1.2 mm, but 5% extended deeper than 3 mm and some reached a depth of over 5.2 mm[52] or even over 6 mm.

Extreme care must be taken not to mistake crypt involvement for invasive carcinoma. When HSIL (CIN 2-3) involves only a portion of the crypt, thus exposing some of the lining composed of mucinous columnar cells, the correct diagnosis is usually obvious. Difficulties arise when SIL (CIN) replaces the crypts in their entirety, especially in a biopsy

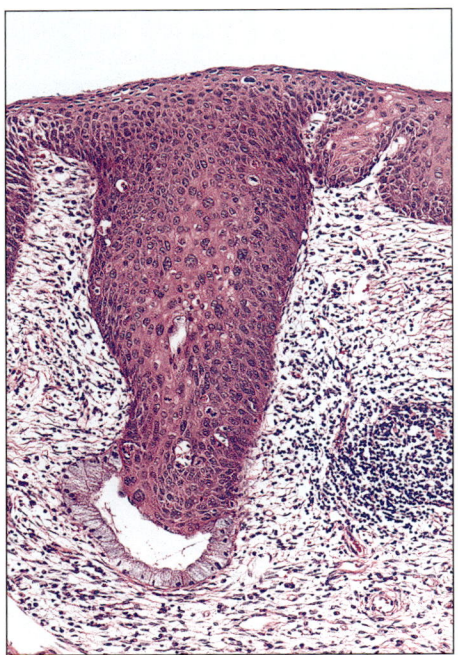

Figure 10.51 HSIL (CIN 3) with endocervical crypt involvement. The perimeter is smooth, indicating that the HSIL (CIN 3) is replacing the gland crypt rather than invading into the underlying stroma.

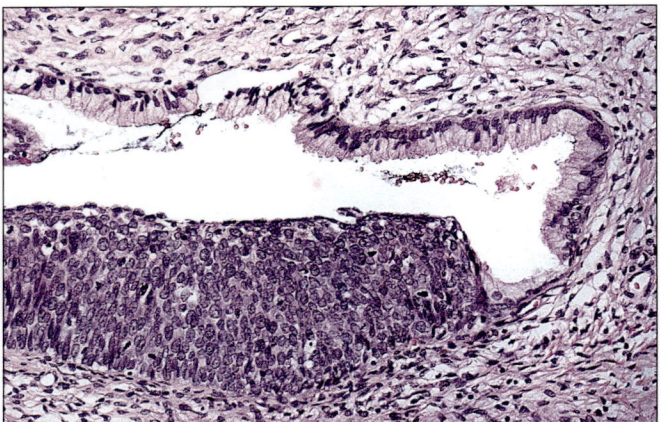

Figure 10.52 HSIL (CIN 3) with endocervical crypt involvement. Note the abrupt transition between the lesion and the adjacent normal endocervical epithelium.

specimen. In this instance the clue that the disease process is not invasive carcinoma, but HSIL (CIN 2-3) that involves a crypt, lies with its shape. Crypts that are involved have perimeters that are round to oblong and smooth, reflecting the fact that the normal crypt lining has been replaced. Sometimes the crypt diameter may be expanded. The stroma around the crypt is often inflamed, and may be edematous, complicating assessment of the epithelial–stromal interface. Tumor that is invasive usually has irregular and sharply angulated borders, and frequently exhibits features of increased squamous differentiation (e.g., increased cytoplasmic eosinophilia, reduced nuclear to cytoplasmic ratio, dyskeratosis) by comparison with the overlying or adjacent SIL (CIN).

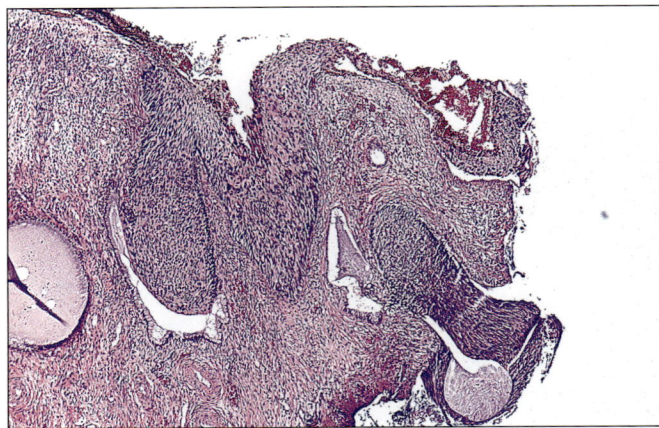

Figure 10.53 HSIL (CIN 3) involving resection margins both on the surface and within endocervical crypts.

RESECTION MARGINS

Not infrequently, LEEP, LETZ, or cone biopsy specimens disclose HSIL (CIN 2-3) that reaches the resection margins either on the surface or in involved endocervical crypts (Figure 10.53), both of which may confer an increased risk of residual disease. Residual CIN has been detected in 8–85% of women with positive margins on cone biopsy and in 0–55% of women with negative margins.[53] In a study of 782 women treated for CIN with large loop excision, 9% of margins were involved but, within 2 years, the treatment failure rate was 30%.[54] With uninvolved margins, 5% of these patients proved still to have residual disease. Endocervical glandular involvement, age exceeding 40 years, and the presence of satellite lesions were all identified as independent risk factors for the appearance of a subsequent lesion. Among a cohort of 390 patients, 22% had recurrent CIN or developed invasive carcinoma after cold knife conization with positive margins. Persistent or recurrent disease was more common in women with both ectocervical and endocervical margin involvement as opposed to singular ectocervical or endocervical positive margins.[55,56]

In another study, if an ECC was positive for CIN, 65% had CIN 2–3 in a cone biopsy.[57] A retrospective study of 152 women who underwent ECC at the time of conization concluded that only the endocervical margin status predicted residual disease (and not ECC).[58]

In one study where hysterectomy was performed soon after the cone biopsy, 61% of patients who had both involved margins and involved crypts had residual CIN: 29% of women with uninvolved margins and crypts also had residual CIN in the hysterectomy specimen.[59] In a second phase of the same investigation, women treated with cone biopsy alone were followed over a long period. Of women with both involved margins and involved crypts, 23% developed a subsequent recurrence, which compared to only 8% of women in whom both the margins and crypts were initially normal. The average time to the first recurrence was 2.2 years. In predicting recurrence, positive margins and involved crypts were each found to be independent prognostic factors with equal predictive value.

It is of note that margin status has been shown to be less sensitive than cytology or high-risk HPV testing in

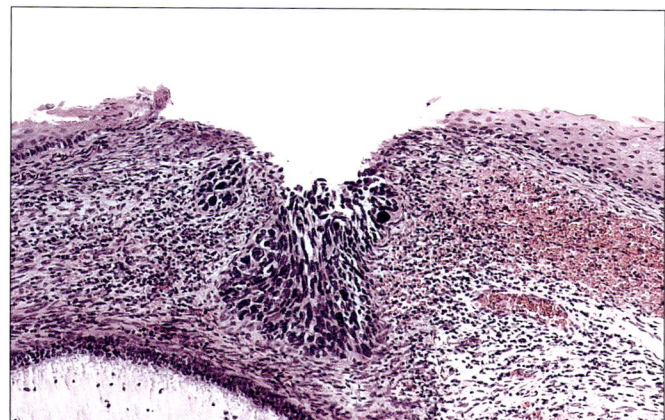

Figure 10.54 A focus of HSL (CIN 3) under 1 mm in total size.

Table 10.6 Occult Invasive Carcinoma as an Unexpected Finding after Biopsy or Conization[52]

Procedure	Total Patients (n)	Patients with More Severe Lesion on Subsequent Surgical Specimen (%)	Invasive Lesions Missed (%)
Punch biopsy	4334	16.7	6.0
Colposcopically directed biopsy	1930	4.0	0.8
Cone biopsy without invasive carcinoma	1734	7	2.1

predicting post-treatment disease.[60,61] In addition, a recent systematic review concluded that high-risk HPV testing had higher sensitivity than, but similar specificity to, cytology for the detection of post-treatment high-grade disease.[47]

With the knowledge that the status of the endocervical margin can have a substantial effect on immediate therapy and later disease progression, a lively debate has ensued over the years about the wisdom of using frozen sections to examine cone biopsy specimens.[62] The consensus has been that complete examination of specimens by frozen section is less thorough than if the specimen is first fixed in formalin and then carefully blocked. It is the common experience that cone specimens cut into 12 or more pieces not infrequently show only a small focus of high-grade disease, which would easily have been missed by frozen section examination. In the example shown, the entire focus of HSIL (CIN 3) was under 1 mm in total size (Figure 10.54). Frozen-section examination of large specimens is also time-consuming and expensive. However, in those institutions where frozen-section evaluation of the endocervical margins is performed routinely, the overall experience has been highly satisfactory.[63] A number of institution also report excellent correlation between the frozen sections and permanent sections in cases of CIN 3[64] and superficial invasive carcinoma.[65] Yet the artifacts and tissue loss at frozen section can compromise the evaluation of early invasion. Furthermore, rarely will the astute gynecologist need to alter the approach based on the finding of superficial invasion. Hence, frozen-section evaluation of conization is generally discouraged.

INVASIVE DISEASE

An obvious concern in the management of SIL (CIN) is to ensure that the therapy is not excessive for the degree of abnormality present. Conversely, it is important not to treat lesions inadequately and miss an occult carcinoma as a result. In a meta-analysis examining the use of various diagnostic techniques, both punch biopsy and cone biopsy with or without colposcopy missed significant numbers of invasive carcinomas (Table 10.6).[52]

In one of the largest case series, 2.7% of 600 patients with CIN 3 had invasive carcinomas detected in a subsequent cone biopsy specimen.[66] Another 1% had microinvasive carcinomas. The major features identified in CIN 3 associated with carcinoma in another study were as follows:[31]

- Extensive involvement of surface epithelium, often with multiquadrant disease
- Deep involvement of endocervical crypts by expansile CIN 3
- Luminal necrosis.

One study has shown that the mean size of CIN 3 lesions exhibiting microinvasion is seven times greater than CIN 3 lesions without invasion and 100-fold greater than CIN 1 lesions.[67] Several studies have shown that care must also be exercised to remove the entire lesion when locally destructive methods are used in the treatment of HSIL (CIN 2-3). In a multicenter retrospective study, the British Society for Colposcopy and Cervical Pathology identified 49 women who subsequently developed invasive carcinoma following therapy with laser vaporization, cold coagulation, diathermy, or cryosurgery.[68] Most of these tumors were ascribed to failure to recognize the early invasive disease at the time the patients were initially assessed. Fortunately, radical reoperation has been performed in such patients with low morbidity and excellent cure rates.[69]

REGRESSION AND PROGRESSION TO INVASIVE CARCINOMA

REGRESSION

Practical data are difficult to find regarding the transit times from SIL (CIN) to invasive carcinoma. In one of the better older studies,[70] the median transit times for progression from mild, moderate, and severe dysplasia to CIS were 5 years (58 months), 3 years (38 months), and 1 year (12 months), respectively. The regression rate for the high-grade abnormality reverting to normal was 6%, a lower number than anticipated, attributed to the fact that biopsies were not taken. It was believed that removing even a small piece of tissue from a field of dysplasia materially altered the disease's natural history. In contrast, others found higher regression rates:[71] 50% of patients followed by cytology and biopsy experienced regression during the next 10

Table 10.7 Natural History of CIN[72,73]

	Regress (%)	Persist (%)	Progress to CIS (%)	Progress to Invasion (%)
HPV without CIN	80	15	5	0
CIN 1	57	32	11	1
CIN 2	43	35	22	5
CIN 3	32	<56	—	>12

years. In the same interval, only 1.4% of all patients with dysplasia showed progression to CIS. In part the rates of progression and regression are related to the initial grade of the CIN, as shown by a meta-analysis of papers published since 1950 (Table 10.7).[72,73]

In a more recent study based on a historical cohort of women whose Pap smear histories were recorded continuously between 1962 and 1980, and during which time CIN was managed conservatively, both CIN 1 and CIN 2 were more likely to regress (usually within 2 years) than to progress. The risk of progression from CIN 1 to CIN 3 or worse was only 1% per year, but the risk of progression from CIN 2 was 16% within 2 years and 25% within 5 years, in agreement with meta-analyses.[72] Most of the excess risk for carcinomas developing from CIN 2 or 3 occurred within the first 2 years after the initial cervical abnormality was identified.[74]

Two decades ago, it was generally assumed that progression through SIL (CIN) grades occurred incrementally, starting as LSIL (CIN 1) and over many years progressing through HSIL (CIN 2) to HSIL (CIN 3) before becoming invasive. However, this is not based on actual observations. The biopsies necessary to confirm the diagnoses on each occasion would destroy the tissue under study and colposcopic observations are insufficiently reliable to diagnostically render such a claim. Moreover, there are very rare reports of cases in which HSIL (CIN 2) and even LSIL (CIN 1) have apparently developed directly into invasive carcinoma, without reaching the stage of HSIL (CIN 3). It is possible that a small, very aggressive, newly formed clone of abnormal cells appearing in the deeper epithelium acquires sufficient molecular abnormality to drive the daughter cells to acquire invasive capacity so that these lesions immediately invade, bypassing HSIL (CIN 3). On the basis of such observations, some have argued for treating all patients who have SIL (CIN), irrespective of its grade, but this would lead to enormous overtreatment and has not been widely adopted. Also, it has never been fully established whether the lower grade SIL (CIN) lesions that appeared to progress rapidly to invasive disease had been adequately sampled.

PROGRESSION

The goal of early treatment is to prevent squamous cell carcinoma by eradicating preinvasive lesions. Cervical screening programs to detect SIL (CIN) by cytology and treat during the preinvasive phase are based on two assumptions: (1) a significant proportion of women with SIL (CIN) would eventually develop invasive carcinoma if not treated and (2) most invasive squamous cell carcinomas are preceded by a demonstrable intraepithelial phase. Despite the fact that cervical screening is the most effective cancer preventive program currently available, total eradication has not been obtained. There are numerous reasons why this hope has not been fully realized, including poor coverage by the screening programs of the population most at risk, poor quality of screening, and the possibility that some invasive carcinomas may not be preceded by a demonstrable preinvasive phase. Even so, a woman who has been screened even once during her lifetime will have a nearly sixfold lower incidence rate of cervical cancer (decreasing from about 34 to 4.2/100,000 women-years).[75]

Several early studies provided insights into the relationship between SIL (CIN) and invasive carcinoma. One highly quoted study showed that 14% of 59 women whose CIS (now HSIL or CIN 3) remained untreated developed invasive carcinoma. It was later admitted that many of the original diagnoses were incorrect and that only 14 of the patients had acceptable CIS. Thus the percentage rose to 57%, i.e., 8 of 14 women developed invasive carcinoma over a period of 10 years. Later still, it was reported that 31 of these women had been followed for at least 12 years and that 22 (71%) of them had developed invasive disease.[76] Other reports from that time were similar.[77] Of 127 women with 'epithelial atypia,' 26% ultimately developed invasive carcinoma. In a fuller account of the same patients, it was admitted that only 67 had a recognizable abnormality still present at the end of the first year of follow-up. Of the 67 who remained in the series, two-thirds eventually developed invasive carcinoma. While the more recent amended rates are rarely quoted, they may well provide a more reliable indication of the malignant potential of SIL (CIN) than their earlier and more widely quoted figures. Most investigations have found that the time for progression from CIN 3 to occult invasive cancer takes between 5 and 25 years, with most series reporting times of over 10 years. Estimates of transit time from CIN to microinvasive/subclinical carcinoma are about 10 years with another 4–5 years elapsing until the tumor causes symptoms.[78]

These estimates are in accord with the average ages when women develop SIL (CIN) (25–40 years), microinvasive carcinoma (43 years), stage 1 squamous cell carcinoma (48 years), and stage 4 squamous cell carcinoma (58 years) (Figure 10.55).

A common issue in evaluating the natural progression of SIL (CIN) is the effect introduced by both biopsy and conization. The former can theoretically affect the diseased tissues that remain in place, while conization certainly can ablate all tissues, removing the entire lesion or even the entire transformation zone. To overcome the difficulty that the method of diagnosis may interfere with the natural history of the disease, 52 women were traced who had positive smears diagnosed at least 2 years previously but had had neither biopsies nor any treatment.[79] Ten of these women (19%) developed invasive carcinoma, including some preclinical invasive carcinomas.

A notable study involved 948 women who had CIS diagnosed by histology, most of whom had cone biopsies.[80,81] Of this group, 131 continued to have abnormal cytology, indicative of residual disease. No further treatment was given to these patients but they were followed closely. After 10 years 18% had developed invasive carcinoma, and after 20 years

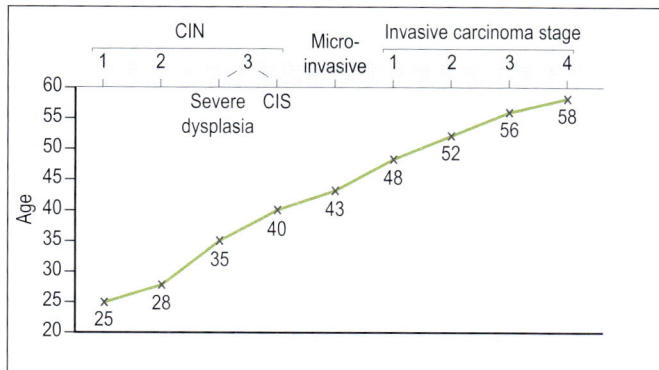

Figure 10.55 Ages of occurrence of squamous cell carcinoma of the cervix and its precursor states. Mean ages are presented for each category.

Table 10.8 Reappearance of Disease after Conization[66]

Results of Follow-Up	Free Margins	Ambiguous Margins	Involved Margins
Women treated by conization for CIS	672	40	6
Abnormal <3 months	3.6%	20%	100%
Abnormal 4 months to 1 year	1.3%	12.5%	—
Abnormal >1.1 year	2.5%	0%	—

the number had risen to 36%. Of those whose cytology was normal after the initial treatment, 1.5% developed invasive carcinoma and 0.8% developed recurrent CIS. One explanation of the latter figures is that the propensity to develop new disease may remain where there is residual or new infection or other promoting factors (relative risk of 3.2). A retrospective study of 33 women revealed that the invasive carcinoma occurred within 5 and 10 years in 67% and 94% of women, respectively, after their CIN was treated.[82]

The figures quoted for the progression from SIL (CIN) to invasive carcinoma thus vary widely, from 0.17% to 71%. Several difficulties exist in characterizing this relationship. First, all reliable methods for diagnosing SIL (CIN) involve the removal of tissue with the associated risk of interfering with the disease's natural progression. Second and more importantly is an ethical consideration. Once it becomes apparent that there is a substantial risk of a woman developing invasive carcinoma from unattended SIL (CIN) it is unthinkable not to provide treatment. Because currently available methods to assess follow-up are destructive (biopsy), progression to cancer cannot be observed and therefore precise rates of progression from SIL (CIN) to invasive carcinoma are now virtually impossible to determine. Another factor to consider when evaluating follow-up studies, making certain conclusions difficult, is that the invasive or higher grade lesions may be unrelated to the original lesion, but caused by reinfection.

In examining the natural history of SIL (CIN) following conization, caution must be exercised in attributing the reappearance of an abnormality to the development of new disease. In one large study, 672 women were treated with conization for CIS and had resection margins free of tumor.[66] Of this group, 4% had abnormal smears detected within 3 months and 5% within 1 year, suggesting that the original tumor had never been fully resected. Another 2.5% developed abnormal smears during the ensuing 2–6 years. In general, the recurrence rate and time of recurrence correlated strongly with the presence or absence of initial disease at the resection margins (Table 10.8).[66]

During the past several decades disquieting new trends have developed. Since the 1960s and the era of the 'sexual revolution,' the average age of SIL (CIN) development has fallen progressively to between 25 and 30 years of age and more recently even further. There is concern that the age when invasive carcinoma will develop is also dropping.

The second issue involves reports of young women developing invasive carcinoma of the cervix after recent prior negative cytology.[26,83] Some of these lesions have been called rapidly progressive cancer, a condition discussed elsewhere (see Chapter 9). There are several explanations for these findings. Some of the smears were probably false negatives that would have been found to contain malignant cells or at least dyskaryotic/dysplastic cells on review. Others may have been genuine false negatives, in which either the cytologic sample was inadequate, the tumor was located high in the endocervical canal, or the tumor did not exfoliate cells and none were present in the smears.[84] However, it is impossible to escape the conclusion that at least some of these women had true progression from normal histology to invasive carcinoma. This has occurred in a short period between the collection of the smear and the diagnosis of the carcinoma, sometimes in less than a year. It seems reasonable to speculate that, although the mean time interval for the progression through SIL (CIN) to invasive carcinoma may be 10–15 years, a few women will fall at the two extremes of the distribution curve of the length of natural history. Some may have such a long natural history that progression to invasion will never occur in the course of their lifetime; these women would be categorized as nonprogressive. On the other hand, there may be those women at the other extreme, in whom the natural history of the disease runs a very rapid course, measured in months rather than years. These may be the patients described in the previous reports. Indeed, very rarely do women under age 20 develop rapidly lethal invasive cancer. This hypothesis presumes that one disease process is occurring and that the difference in the behavior in different women is the result of extreme variations in the length of the natural history of the same disease. Another suggestion for which there are only scant data is that certain HPV types associated with cervical cancer are intrinsically associated with more rapid progression. This may correlate with the finding that HPV type 18 is rarely detected in cases of HSIL (CIN 2-3), but commonly in cervical cancers that have metastasized.[85]

CORRELATION BETWEEN CYTOLOGY AND HISTOLOGY

Since the publication in 1987 by the *Wall Street Journal* about incorrectly read cytology smears, there has been increased awareness of quality and liability issues associated with the Pap smear. Substantial literature has accumulated since that time,[86] one common theme of which has been the question of what constitutes an error or false-negative smear. While most false-negative rates are between 2% and 28%,[87] the issue is often far more subtle. In evaluating these rates, it is important to understand what components are truly being measured. If a patient has cancer but the smear truly contains no abnormal cells, is this a false negative? Equally perplexing is the question of whether to include or exclude consideration of cells considered ASCUS; or those cells showing signs of HPV infection; or even LSIL itself.

A theme implicit in most articles is that histologic findings are always correct and therefore histology is the gold standard. While it is beyond the scope of this chapter to examine this subject in detail, several studies have shown convincingly that the findings in tissue biopsies and cervical smears are complementary.[15] An abnormal finding by either modality should not be dismissed as artifact when not confirmed by the other. In a prospective examination of 3404 paired biopsies and cytologic smears, 481 paired cases (14%) had discordant diagnoses, defined as differing by more than one degree of CIN or as CIN or carcinoma identified by only one modality.[84] Eighteen initial diagnostic differences arose from cytologic screening errors, 16 from interpretive errors by staff pathologists, and one from superficial initial histologic sections. Of these, 33 involved lesions with CIN 1. Only two involved high-grade CIN (0.06%); both smears initially interpreted as atrophy were in fact examples of CIN 3. Perhaps even this could have been prevented by routinely using additional biomarkers, such as Ki-67 and p16, in cases of 'atrophic' smears. The remaining examples of discordance resulted from sampling differences. The cytologic smear contained the diagnostic lesion in 40% of the cases and the surgical biopsy detected the remainder, emphasizing the utility of pairing these sampling techniques in patients at risk for SIL (CIN). Not infrequently, the discordant, but verified, finding of an abnormality on cytopathology alone led to re-examination of the patient and discovery of a preinvasive lesion somewhere in the endocervical canal. Clearly, if cytologic and histologic diagnoses are discordant but valid independently, then the diagnosis of the more advanced disease state should be favored for the purposes of patient safety.

DISTRIBUTION AND SITE OF ORIGIN OF SIL

There is recent evidence that cervical squamous neoplasia arises in most cases from a discrete group of cells in the squamocolumnar junction characterized by a gene expression profile that is conserved in SIL (CIN) and squamous cell carcinoma of the cervix.[88] Uniquely expressed markers include cytokeratin 7, anterior gradient 2, cluster differentiation 63, matrix metalloproteinase 7, and guanine deaminase. HPV-related squamous lesions arising in the vagina and vulva lack this distinctive immunophenotype, suggesting that the cell of origin for most cervical SIL (CIN) is confined to the native cervical squamocolumnar junction. The cervical squamocolumnar junction is not static over time, rather it is moving in a cranial (uterine) direction through a process of endocervical encroachment by advancing squamous metaplasia. Recent demonstration that the immunophenotype is not regenerated during re-epithelization following ablation suggests that it might be permanently destroyed by topical ablation.

The region of endocervix swept by this migrating squamocolumnar junction, called the transformation zone, is an anatomic site that overlaps with, or encroaches upon, virtually all cervical SILs (CINs).[89] Rare carcinomas found outside this zone, on the vaginal aspect of the cervix, more often are keratinizing, suggesting that these tumors have arisen from the basal layer of the original (native) squamous epithelium.

Most studies have shown that SILs (CINs) increase in size with the grade of the disease. CIN 3 lesions have an average linear extent of 6.3 mm and 65% of CIN 3 lesions involve two or more quadrants. Approximately 10–25% of lesions that arise in the transformation zone extend more than 1 cm into the endocervical canal. An occasional case may exceed 4 cm. In one study, nearly all lesions involved the anterior or posterior lips (94%), and fewer the lateral edges (38%),[90] which affects how biopsies are taken.[91] Other more recent studies have shown CIN 2–3 to be randomly distributed,[92] or slightly more common posteriorly than anteriorly, but equally on the right and left sides of the cervix.[93] Based on results from the ASCUS/LSIL Triage Study for Cervical Cancer (ALTS) studies, SIL (CIN) occurred more commonly on the anterior and posterior lips, but the data were confounded by the tendency for these areas to appear acetowhite even when HPV or CIN were not identified.[94] Of course patient age and presenting morphology bias all of these measurements.

COLPOSCOPY

Epithelial abnormalities of the cervix are initially recognized by exfoliative cytology, further evaluated by colposcopy and definitively diagnosed by histology. The indication for referral for colposcopy in nearly all cases is an abnormal cervical smear. This section presents a broad outline of the principles involved and discusses briefly the important part that the colposcopic examination plays in the management of women with preclinical neoplasia of the cervix.

Colposcopy is a technique for examining the cervix using relatively low, stereoscopic magnification and bright illumination. All colposcopes have a movable base, adjustable supporting arm, bright light source, and variable magnification. Many incorporate a camera to allow a visual record of the colposcopic appearances to be kept. The colposcopic examination is usually carried out as an outpatient procedure. The cervix is exposed using a speculum and, after being gently cleaned with saline on a cotton wool ball, is examined with the colposcope. Topography, vascular pattern, color, and surface contour are all observed, both before and after the application of acetic acid. Lugol's iodine is often applied at the end of the colposcopic examination to identify glycogenated (I_2-positive) and nonglycogenated (I_2-negative) epithelium.

Using these features a colposcopist can assess the extent of SIL (CIN) and identify an early invasive carcinoma, at the same time selecting the most appropriate sites for punch biopsy so that a precise histologic diagnosis may be made.

Colposcopy also enables the lesional extent to be determined accurately. An atypical transformation zone may extend off the cervix into the vaginal fornices or even, very occasionally, some way down the vaginal walls.

The uses of colposcopy can be summarized as follows:

- To determine the extent and distribution of the lesion
- To select the sites for directed biopsy
- To confirm the cytologic findings
- To rule out invasive carcinoma.

NORMAL COLPOSCOPIC FINDINGS

The normal colposcopically visible components are the original squamous epithelium, the original columnar epithelium, and squamous metaplasia (the typical transformation zone).

ORIGINAL SQUAMOUS EPITHELIUM

Normal original squamous epithelium presents a uniform, relatively featureless appearance with a smooth surface contour, which does not become white after the application of acetic acid (Figures 10.56 and 10.57). The vessels are usually inconspicuous and are mostly of hairpin type, showing one ascending and one descending branch of very fine caliber, forming a small loop. If the surface epithelium is thin, it is sometimes possible to observe the whole loop by colposcopy. Generally only the tip of the loop is visible, so that these hairpin capillaries are usually seen as regularly and densely arranged small dots.

COLUMNAR EPITHELIUM

Normal columnar epithelium is easily recognized by its characteristic grape-like or villous appearance. Before application of acetic acid, the colposcopist will see that each columnar epithelial villus contains a fine capillary. As the villus is covered by no more than a single layer of columnar cells, the blood in the capillary gives columnar epithelium its typically red appearance. Following application of acetic acid, the villi often appear white and swollen and are more easily recognizable (Figure 10.58).

SQUAMOUS METAPLASIA

The transformation zone in the cervix lies between the native/original squamous epithelium and the current squamocolumnar junction. It is normally covered at least in part by mature squamous metaplasia, but, at some earlier time, was covered by columnar epithelium. The new epithelium results from transformation of columnar to squamous epithelium, through the process of squamous metaplasia.

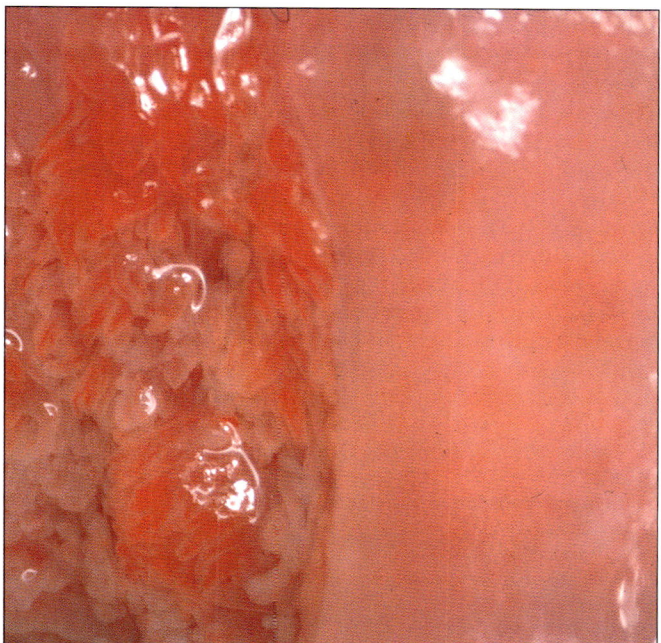

Figure 10.56 Original squamous epithelium. On the right, the original squamous epithelium is smooth, shiny, and featureless. Very fine vessels can just be discerned. The sharp squamocolumnar junction separates the squamous epithelium from the villous endocervix.

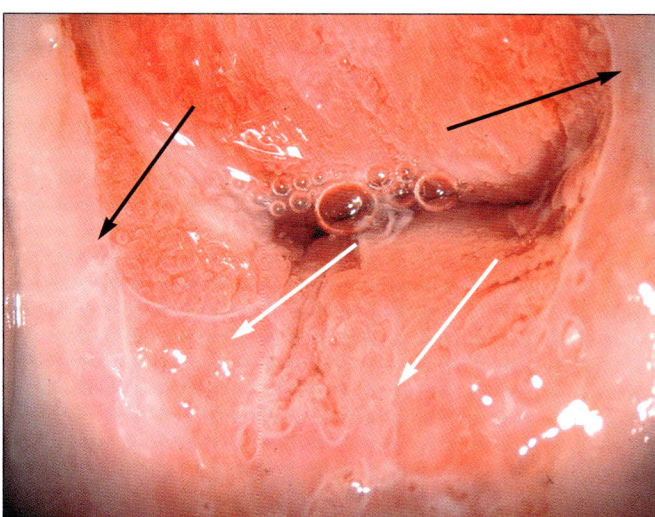

Figure 10.57 Normal cervix. Original squamous epithelium is seen at the two lateral aspects of the cervix (black arrows). Patchy squamous metaplasia is present on the posterior lip (white arrows).

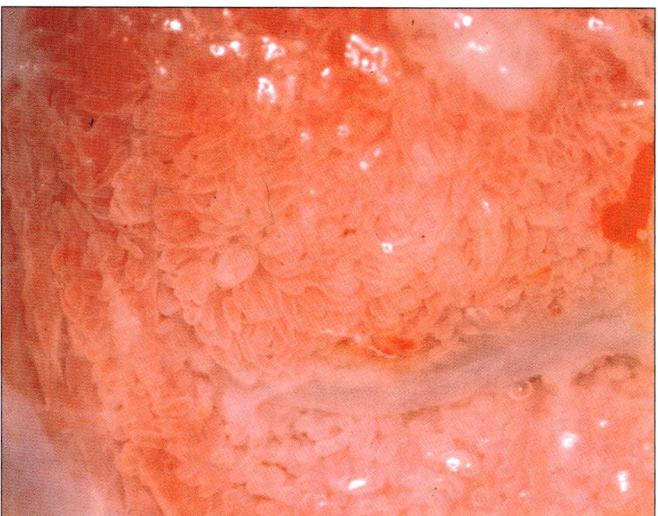

Figure 10.58 Columnar epithelium. After application of acetic acid, the endocervical villi separate, become prominent, and slightly white.

Mature Metaplasia

Fully mature, squamous epithelium of metaplastic origin exhibits gland openings and typical branching vessels (Figure 10.59). The surface contour resembles that of original squamous epithelium so that, in the absence of prominent branching vessels, gland openings, or retention cysts, distinction from original squamous epithelium may be impossible.

Immature Metaplasia

Immature or active metaplasia, which is epithelium that is in the process of being transformed from columnar to squamous, is difficult to fully evaluate colposcopically (Figure 10.60). The epithelium is often acetowhite and is easily confused with abnormal epithelium.

The process of squamous metaplasia occurs in a patchy fashion. Cervical columnar epithelium often appears as a series of ridges and clefts. If this is the case, the epithelium along the surface of the ridges is usually the first to undergo metaplasia.

ABNORMAL COLPOSCOPIC FINDINGS

In SIL (CIN), one or more features of an atypical transformation zone would be expected (Table 10.9). Some of these features may also occur with entities other than SIL (CIN), e.g., immature squamous metaplasia, the normal transformation zone, and HPV infection.

MOSAIC AND PUNCTATION

These are both patterns of the small blood vessels that arise in the stromal plexus beneath the epithelium and pass into the epithelium surrounded by a very sparse stromal core (Figure 10.61). If the vessels branch and anastomose, forming a basket-like pattern around epithelial blocks, a mosaic pattern results (Figures 10.62 and 10.63). On the other hand, if the vessel travels toward the surface and then turns back again without branching, a punctate pattern will be seen (Figures 10.64 and 10.65). The two patterns often

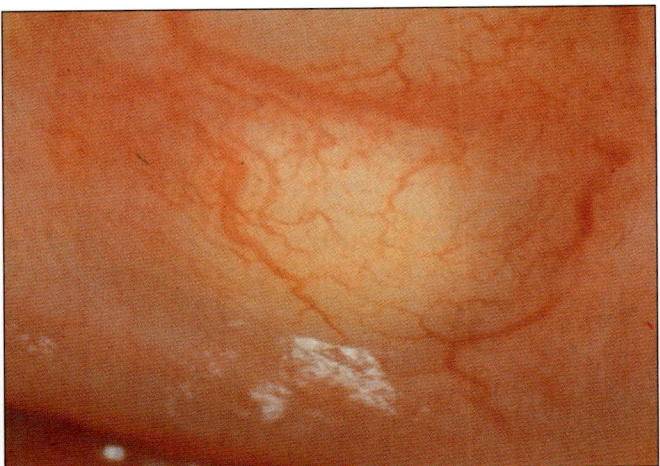

Figure 10.59 Mature squamous metaplasia. The surface is smooth with pale retention cysts beneath it. Branched vessels are prominent.

> **Table 10.9 Abnormal Colposcopic Findings**
>
> **Atypical transformation zone**
> - Mosaic
> - Punctation
> - Acetowhite epithelium
> - Leukoplakia
> - Atypical vessels
>
> **Suspect frank invasive carcinoma**

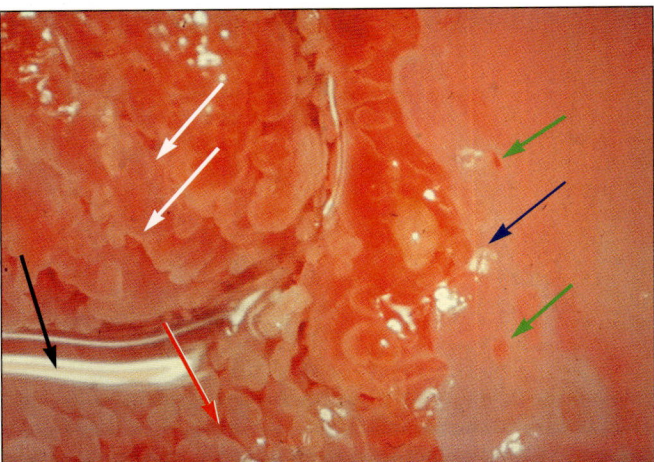

Figure 10.60 Squamous metaplasia. Original squamous epithelium is present on the right and the transverse, slit-like external os (black arrow) is seen on the left. Normal endocervical villi are present on the posterior lip (red arrow). There is an irregular crescent of maturing squamous metaplasia adjacent to the squamocolumnar junction (blue arrow), which is slightly acetowhite and shows gland openings (green arrows). On the anterior lip are diagonal columns of very immature metaplasia (white arrows) where the endocervical villi are fused.

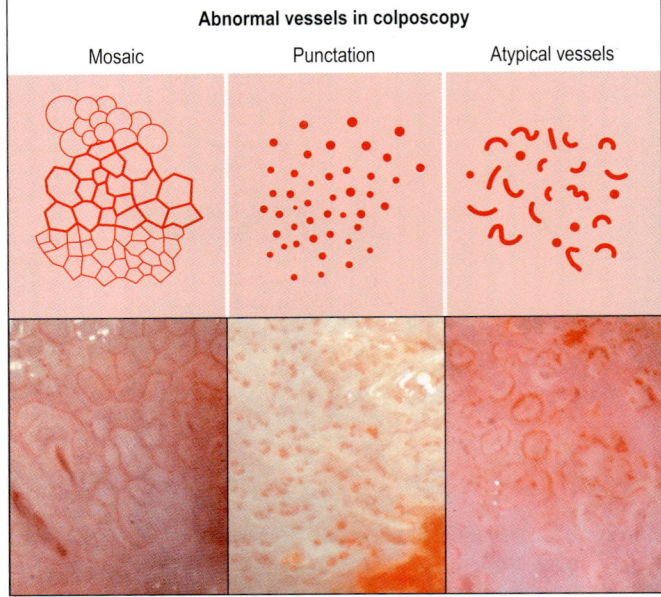

Figure 10.61 Abnormal vascular patterns in colposcopy.

CHAPTER 10 — CERVICAL SQUAMOUS INTRAEPITHELIAL LESIONS 227

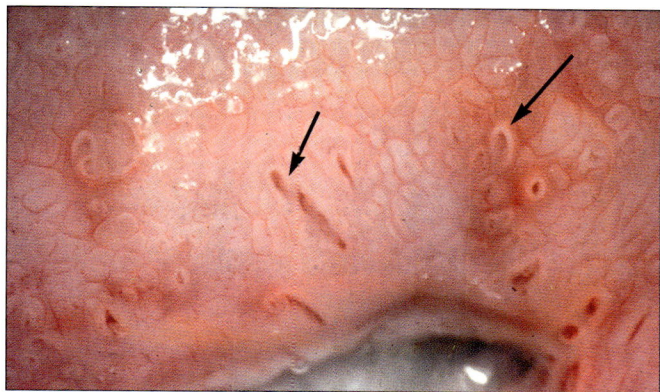

Figure 10.62 Mosaic. The epithelium is acetowhite and there is a prominent abnormal vascular pattern of intercommunicating horizontal vessels just beneath the surface, giving rise to the mosaic appearance. Gland openings (arrows) are obvious. Biopsy showed HSIL (CIN 3).

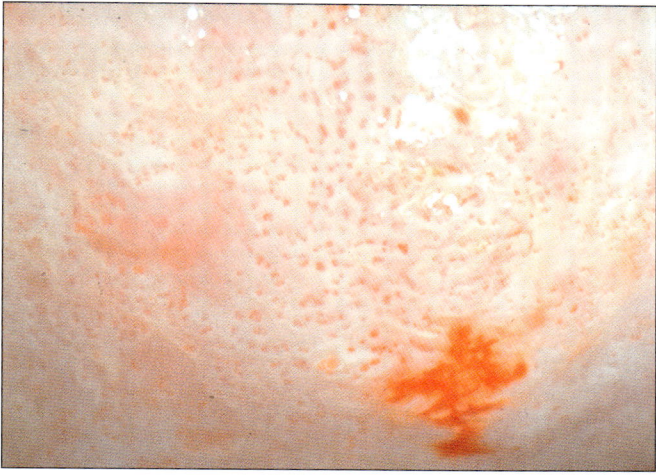

Figure 10.65 Punctation. The epithelium is acetowhite and there is prominent 'stippling' of vessels that do not intercommunicate. Biopsy showed HSIL (CIN 3).

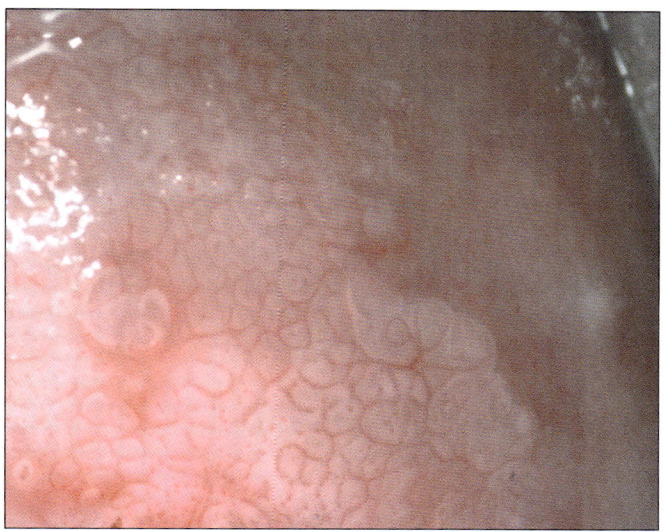

Figure 10.63 Mosaic. Biopsy showed HSIL (CIN 3).

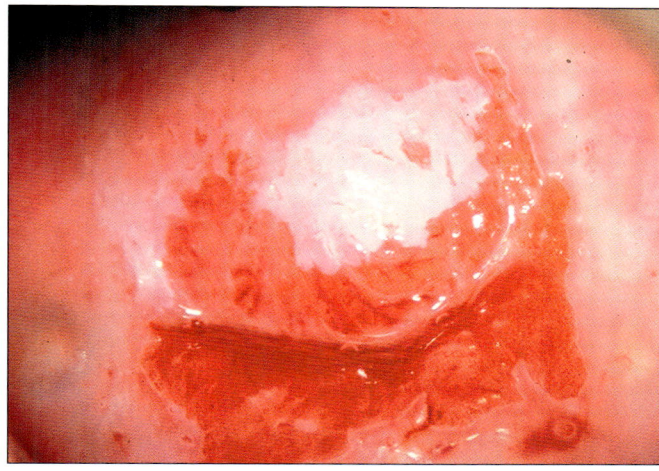

Figure 10.66 Acetowhite epithelium. A small area of abnormal epithelium is sharply defined after the application of acetic acid. Biopsy showed HSIL (CIN 3).

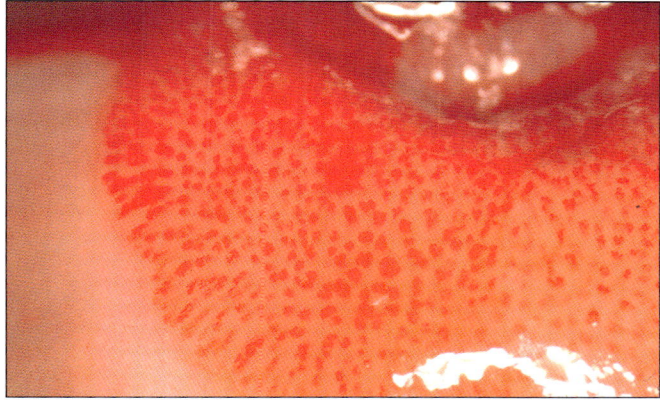

Figure 10.64 Punctation. A sharply defined area of marked punctation is occupying the transformation zone of the posterior lip. Acetic acid has not been applied. Biopsy showed HSIL (CIN 3).

coexist on the same cervix. The degree of histologic abnormality that the epithelium shows may be roughly predicted by the intercapillary distance, the coarseness of the vessels, and the regularity of the pattern. The greater the intercapillary distance, the coarser the vessels and more irregular the pattern, the more severe the histologic grade of SIL (CIN) is likely to be. However, it is wrong to believe that colposcopy itself is capable of making a precise histologic diagnosis of an epithelial abnormality.[14] The final diagnosis must always be histologic.

ACETOWHITE EPITHELIUM

Application of aqueous acetic acid (3–5%) to the cervix causes a color change when SIL (CIN) (or some of the other changes listed earlier) is present. The acetic acid has the effect of making the abnormal epithelium appear white and opaque, whiter than it was before the application of the acetic acid and whiter than the normal epithelium after the application of acetic acid (Figures 10.66 and 10.67). The

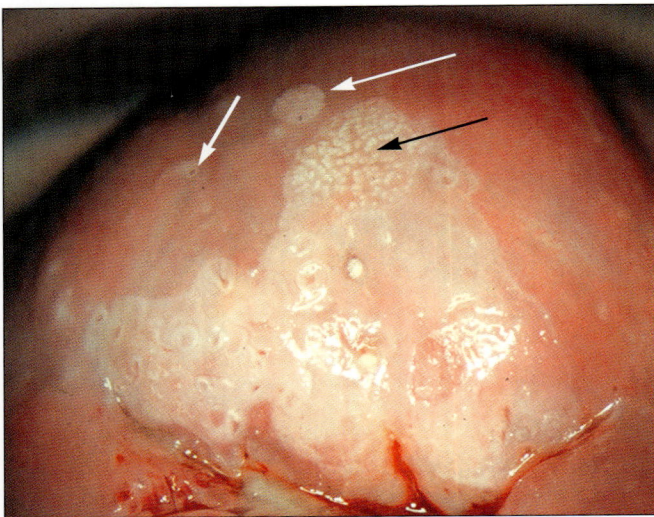

Figure 10.67 Acetowhite epithelium. The abnormal epithelium is apparently confined to the anterior lip. One area shows white, raised 'asperities' (black arrow) and 'satellite' lesions are present (white arrows). Both of these features suggest that HPV infection is present. Biopsy showed HSIL (CIN 3) with koilocytes.

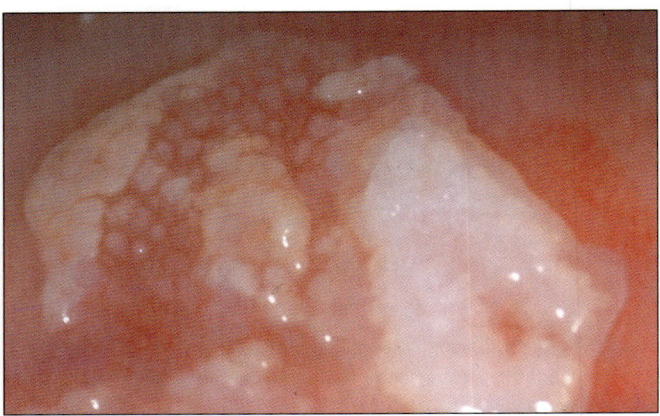

Figure 10.68 Leukoplakia. Raised plaques that are white before the application of acetic acid are present on the anterior lip. Biopsy showed HSIL (CIN 2) with keratosis.

whiteness, usually referred to as 'acetowhite epithelium,' is related to the amount of nuclear material present.

LEUKOPLAKIA

Leukoplakia appears as a well-defined white area, often slightly raised and with a 'waxy,' shiny surface (Figure 10.68). It differs from acetowhite epithelium as it is white before acetic acid application and the acetic acid has no effect on its whiteness.

While the finding of leukoplakia indicates keratinized epithelium, the underlying features that enable the degree of abnormality to be assessed are masked by the keratin. Biopsy is therefore essential as the underlying pathology may range from otherwise normal epithelium with surface keratinization through keratinizing SIL (CIN) to invasive carcinoma.

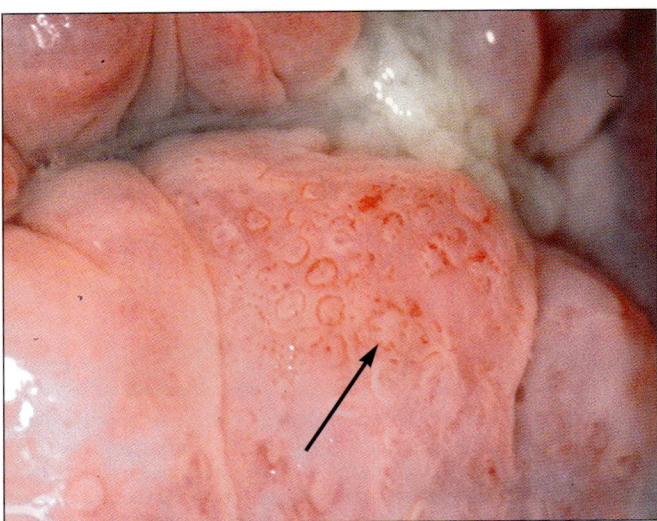

Figure 10.69 Atypical vessels. This extensive atypical transformation zone is markedly acetowhite and shows a vascular pattern on the posterior lip that is basically a mosaic. In places (arrow) the mosaic pattern has broken and there are small, irregular, comma-shaped vessels running parallel to the surface. The surface contour is slightly nodular. These features suggest that the lesion may be more advanced than an SIL (CIN). Biopsy showed microinvasive squamous carcinoma.

ATYPICAL VESSELS

Atypical vessels indicate the possibility of a more advanced abnormality, perhaps early invasive carcinoma. These atypical vessels are basically punctate or mosaic patterns, but turn and run a short way parallel to the surface of the epithelium, forming commas, spirals, and irregular shapes (Figures 10.61 and 10.69).

SUSPECT FRANK INVASIVE CARCINOMA

This term refers to cases where a preclinical invasive carcinoma is present, usually larger than microinvasive carcinoma. The surface contour is irregular and nodular. There is intense acetowhiteness and coarse, bizarre, and irregular vessels (Figure 10.70).

CONGENITAL TRANSFORMATION ZONE

In some patients, immature squamous epithelium is present peripheral to the transformation zone, producing an acetowhite epithelium that is nonglycogenated. These changes are primarily confined to the cervix, but in 4% of women they extend to involve the vagina, usually anteriorly and posteriorly.

This type of transformation zone may develop during intrauterine life, or later but prior to sexual activity, and is not associated with an increased risk of neoplastic change. It is colposcopically significant as it shares some features with SIL (CIN). The epithelium is acetowhite, has a fine mosaic pattern, and is either nonglycogenated or patchily and partially glycogenated. The histologic appearances were discussed previously and are illustrated in Chapter 8.

OTHER COLPOSCOPIC FINDINGS

Acuminate Warts

Colposcopy can identify condylomata acuminata (Figure 10.71), which need to be distinguished from invasive

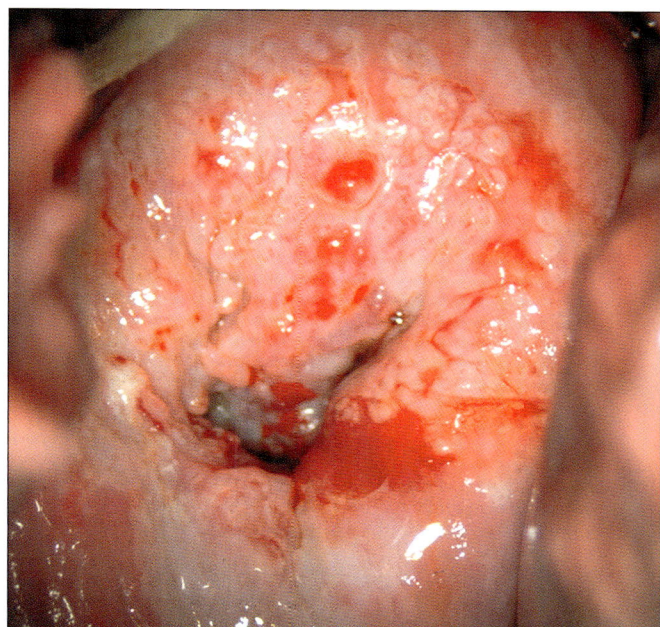

Figure 10.70 Invasive squamous cell carcinoma. The surface is densely acetowhite and nodular, with bizarre vessels and areas of hemorrhage.

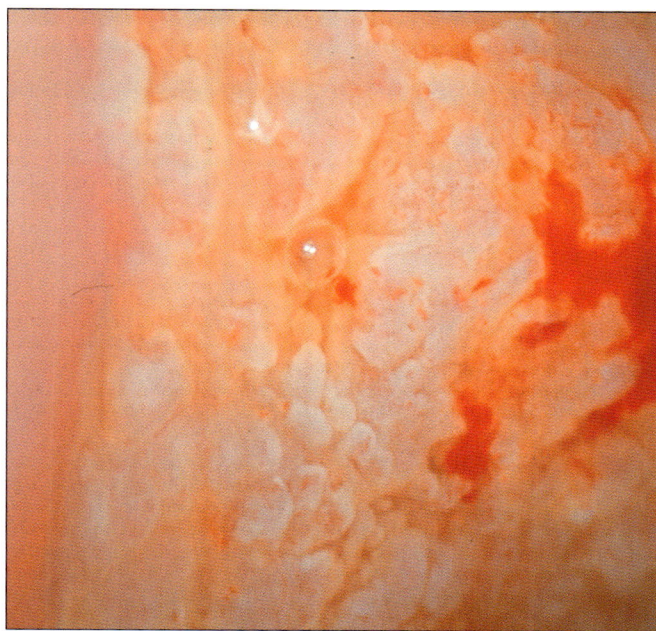

Figure 10.72 Invasive adenocarcinoma. This example shows large, irregular villi that are acetowhite. The tissue is fragile and hemorrhage has occurred.

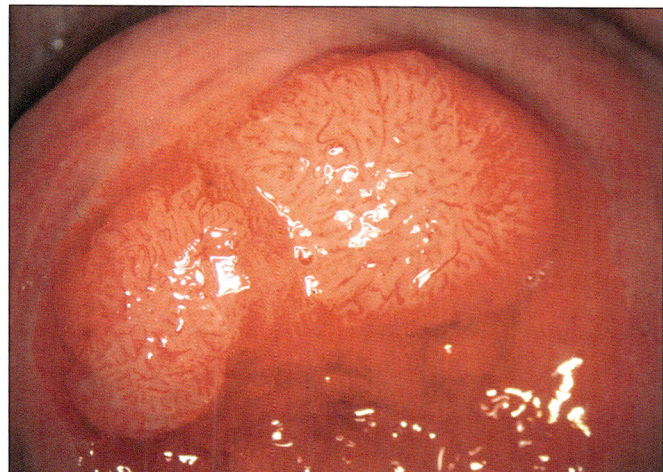

Figure 10.71 LSIL (condyloma acuminatum). Two viral warts are present on the anterior lip. They are composed of delicate, finger-like fronds, each with a central vessel.

carcinoma, because both show nodularity of the surface contour and prominent vasculature. Biopsy of suspected condylomata is mandatory for this reason.

Subclinical HPV Infection

HPV infection may be detected by molecular probes in patients who have unremarkable or nonspecific cervical findings at colposcopy. The cervix may appear entirely normal, without localizing lesions. In other cases acetowhiteness is seen, commonly with a pattern of satellite lesions distinguished from SIL (CIN). In addition, the more marked lesions show changes in surface contour, such as a cerebriform pattern or asperities. It is often the case, however, that colposcopy alone cannot differentiate between SIL (CIN) and non-SIL when all that is seen is an area of otherwise featureless acetowhite epithelium.

Glandular Lesions

AIS (high-grade cervical glandular intraepithelial neoplasia) and invasive adenocarcinoma may show colposcopic abnormalities (Figure 10.72), but distinction from squamous lesions is not usually possible. Moreover, glandular lesions are often not colposcopically visible, necessitating LEEP, LETZ, or cone biopsy to investigate a cervical smear containing abnormal glandular epithelial cells with features suggesting a neoplastic glandular lesion.

Vagina

Vaginal SIL (VaIN) generally shows the same colposcopic features that have been described for cervical SIL (CIN). Acetowhiteness and punctation are often present, but a mosaic pattern is rare. Because of the area involved and the folded nature of the mucosa, full colposcopic examination of the vagina is a lengthy procedure.

REFERENCES

1. Baak JP, Kruse AJ, Robboy SJ, et al. Dynamic behavioural interpretation of cervical intraepithelial neoplasia with molecular biomarkers. J Clin Pathol 2006;59:1017–28.
2. Schiffman M, Castle PE, Jeronimo J, et al. Human papillomavirus and cervical cancer. Lancet 2007;370:890–907.
3. Stoler MH. Human papillomaviruses and cervical neoplasia: a model for carcinogenesis. Int J Gynecol Pathol 2000;19:16–28.
4. Stoler M. The impact of human papillomavirus biology on the clinical practice of cervical pathology. Pathol Case Rev 2005; 10:119–27.

5. The 1988 Bethesda System for reporting cervical/vaginal cytological diagnoses. National Cancer Institute Workshop. JAMA 1989;262: 931–4.
6. Darragh TM, Colgan TJ, Cox JT, et al. The Lower Anogenital Squamous Terminology Standardization Project for HPV-Associated Lesions: background and consensus recommendations from the College of American Pathologists and the American Society for Colposcopy and Cervical Pathology. J Low Genit Tract Dis 2012;16(3):205–42.
7. Ho G, Bierman R, Beardsley L, et al. Natural history of cervicovaginal papillomavirus infection in young women. N Engl J Med 1998;338:423–8.
8. Hudelist G, Manavi M, Pischinger KID, et al. Physical state and expression of HPV DNA in benign and dysplastic cervical tissue: different levels of viral integration are correlated with lesion grade. Gynecol Oncol 2004;92(3):873–80.
9. Bernard H-U, Burk RD, Chen Z, et al. Classification of papillomaviruses (PVs) based on 189 PV types and proposal of taxonomic amendments. Virology 2010;401:70–9.
10. Wright TC, Park TW. Cervical cancer and its precursors—an introduction. In: Langdon SP, Miller WR, Berchuk A, editors. Biology of female cancer. Boca Raton, FL: CRC Press; 1997. p. 221–43.
11. Sato S, Okagaki T, Clark BA, Twiggs LB. Sensitivity of koilocytosis, immunocytochemistry and electron microscopy as compared to DNA hybridization in detecting human papillomavirus in cervical and vaginal condyloma and intraepithelial neoplasia. Int J Gynecol Pathol 1986;5:297–307.
12. Øvestad IT, Gudlaugsson E, Skaland I, et al. Local immune response in the microenvironment of CIN2-3 with and without spontaneous regression. Mod Pathol 2010;23(9):1231–40.
13. Øvestad IT, Gudlaugsson E, Skaland I, et al. The impact of epithelial biomarkers, local immune response and human papillomavirus genotype in the regression of cervical intraepithelial neoplasia grades 2–3. J Clin Pathol 2011;64(4):303–7.
14. Welch WR, Robboy SJ, Kaufman RH, et al. Pathology of colposcopic findings in 2635 diethylstilbestrol-exposed young women. Gynecol Oncol 1985;21:277–86.
15. Stoler MH, Schiffman M. Interobserver reproducibility of cervical cytologic and histologic interpretations: realistic estimates from the ASCUS-LSIL Triage Study. JAMA 2001;285:1500–5.
16. Parker MF, Zahn CM, Vogel KM, et al. Discrepancy in the interpretation of cervical histology by gynecologic pathologists. Obstet Gynecol 2002;100:277–80.
17. Castle PE, Sideri M, Jeronimo J, et al. Risk assessment to guide the prevention of cervical cancer. Am J Obstet Gynecol 2007;197 (356):e1–6.
18. Stoler MH. ASC, TBS, and the power of ALTS. Am J Clin Pathol 2007;127:489–91.
19. Szkaradkiewicz A, Wal M, Kuch A, Pieta P. Human papillomavirus (HPV) and Epstein–Barr virus (EBV) cervical infections in women with normal and abnormal cytology. Pol J Microbiol 2004;53:95–9.
20. Crum CP, Ikenberg H, Richart RM, Gissman L. Human papillomavirus type 16 and early cervical neoplasia. N Engl J Med 1984;310:880–3.
21. Mittal K, Demopoulos RI, Tata M. A comparison of proliferative activity and atypical mitoses in cervical condylomas with various HPV types. Int J Gynecol Pathol 1998;17:24–8.
22. Mourits MJE, Pieters WJLM, Hollema H, Burger MPM. 3-Group metaphase as a morphologic criterion of progressive cervical intraepithelial neoplasia. Am J Obstet Gynecol 1992;167:591–5.
23. Van Leeuwen AM, Pieters WJ, Hollema H, Burger MP. Atypical mitotic figures and the mitotic index in cervical intraepithelial neoplasia. Virchows Arch 1995;427:139–44.
24. Iaconis L, Hyjek E, Ellenson LH, Pirog EC. p16 and Ki-67 immunostaining in atypical immature squamous metaplasia of the uterine cervix: correlation with human papillomavirus detection. Arch Pathol Lab Med 2007;131:1343–9.
25. Kong C, Balzer B, Troxell M, et al. p16INK4A immunohistochemistry is superior to HPV in situ hybridization for the detection of high-risk HPV in atypical squamous metaplasia. Am J Surg Pathol 2007;31:33–43.
26. Prendiville W, Guillebaud J, Bamford P, et al. Carcinoma of the cervix with recent normal Papanicolaou tests. Lancet 1980;ii:835–54.
27. Kruse AJ, Baak JP, Helliesen T, et al. Evaluation of MIB-1-positive cell clusters as a diagnostic marker for cervical intraepithelial neoplasia. Am J Surg Pathol 2002;26:1501–7.
28. Yelverton CL, Bentley RC, Olenick S, et al. Epithelial repair of the uterine cervix: assessment of morphologic features and correlations with cytologic diagnosis. Int J Gynecol Pathol 1996;15: 338–44.
29. Jovanovic AS, Mclachlin CM, Shen LH, et al. Postmenopausal squamous atypia: a spectrum including 'pseudo-koilocytosis.' Mod Pathol 1995;8:408–12.
30. Leung KM, Chan WY, Hui PK. Invasive squamous cell carcinoma and cervical intraepithelial neoplasia III of uterine cervix—morphologic differences other than stromal invasion. Am J Clin Pathol 1994;101:508–13.
31. Al-Nafussi AI, Hughes DE. Histological features of CIN3 and their value in predicting invasive microinvasive squamous carcinoma. J Clin Pathol 1994;47:799–804.
32. dos Santos L, Odunsi K, Lele S. Clinicopathologic outcomes of laser conization for high-grade cervical dysplasia. Eur J Gynaecol Oncol 2004;25:305–7.
33. Ioffe OB, Brooks SE, DeRezende RB, Silverberg SG. Artifact in cervical LLETZ specimens: correlation with follow-up. Int J Gynecol Pathol 1999;18:115–21.
34. Nagar HA, Dobbs SP, McClelland HR, et al. The large loop excision of the transformation zone cut or blend thermal artefact study: a randomized controlled trial. Int J Gynecol Cancer 2004;14: 1108–11.
35. Park J, Sun D, Quade B, et al. Stratified mucin-producing intraepithelial lesions of the cervix: adenosquamous or columnar cell neoplasia? Am J Surg Pathol 2000;24:1414–9.
36. Gupta S, Parsons P, Saha A, Wight C. Follow-up of patients with SMILE (stratified mucin producing intraepithelial lesion) on the cervix—a dilemma. Eur J Obstet Gynecol Reprod Biol 2010;148:207–9.
37. Pins MR, Young RH, Crum CP, et al. Cervical squamous cell carcinoma in situ with intraepithelial extension to the upper genital tract and invasion of tubes and ovaries: report of a case with human papilloma virus analysis. Int J Gynecol Pathol 1997;16:272–8.
38. Sasa H, Imai K, Kudo K, et al. A case of uterine cervical carcinoma in situ with replacement of the entire corpus endometrium. J Low Genit Tract Dis 2007;11:279–80.
39. Klaes R, Benner A, Friedrich T, et al. p16INK4a immunohistochemistry improves interobserver agreement in the diagnosis of cervical intraepithelial neoplasia. Am J Surg Pathol 2002;26:1389–99.
40. Snijders PJ, Steenbergen RD, Heideman DA, Meijer CJ. HPV-mediated cervical carcinogenesis: concepts and clinical implications. J Pathol 2006;208:152–64.
41. Sano T, Oyama T, Kashiwabara K, et al. Expression status of p16 protein is associated with human papillomavirus oncogenic potential in cervical and genital lesions. Am J Pathol 1998;153:1741–8.
42. Benevolo M, Mottolese M, Marandino F, et al. Immunohistochemical expression of p16(INK4a) is predictive of HR-HPV infection in cervical low-grade lesions. Mod Pathol 2006;19:384–91.
43. Klaes R, Friedrich T, Spitkovsky D, et al. Overexpression of p16(INK4A) as a specific marker for dysplastic and neoplastic epithelial cells of the cervix uteri. Int J Cancer 2001;92:276–84.
44. Sanati S, Huettner P, Ylagan LR. Role of ProExC: a novel immunoperoxidase marker in the evaluation of dysplastic squamous and glandular lesions in cervical specimens. Int J Gynecol Pathol 2010;29:79–87.
45. Guo M, Baruch AC, Silva EG, et al. Efficacy of p16 and ProExC immunostaining in the detection of high-grade cervical intraepithelial neoplasia and cervical carcinoma. Am J Clin Pathol 2011;135:212–20.
46. Rebolj M, Bais AG, van Ballegooijen M, et al. Human papillomavirus triage of women with persistent borderline or mildly dyskaryotic smears: comparison of costs and side effects of three alternative strategies. Int J Cancer 2007;121:1529–35.
47. Kocken M, Uijterwaal MH, de Vries ALM, et al. High-risk human papillomavirus testing versus cytology in predicting post-treatment disease in women treated for high-grade cervical disease: A systematic review and meta-analysis. Gynecol Oncol 2012;125:500–7.
48. Kong CS, Beck AH, Longacre TA. A panel of 3 markers including p16, ProExC, or HPV ISH is optimal for distinguishing between primary endometrial and endocervical adenocarcinomas. Am J Surg Pathol 2010;34:915–26.
49. Galgano MT, Castle PE, Atkins KA, et al. Using biomarkers as objective standards in the diagnosis of cervical biopsies. Am J Surg Pathol 2010;34:1077–87.

50. Saslow D, Solomon D, Lawson HW, et al. American Cancer Society, American Society for Colposcopy and Cervical Pathology, and American Society for Clinical Pathology screening guidelines for the prevention and early detection of cervical cancer. Am J Clin Pathol 2012;137(4):516–42.
51. Anderson MC, Hartley RB. Cervical crypt involvement by intraepithelial neoplasia. Obstet Gynecol 1980;55:546–50.
52. Sze EHM, Rosenzweig BA, Birenbaum DL, et al. Excisional conization of the cervix uteri. J Gynecol Surg 1989;5:235–68.
53. Jakus S, Edmonds P, Dunton C, King SA. Margin status and excision of cervical intraepithelial neoplasia: a review. Obstet Gynecol Surv 2000;55:520–7.
54. Paraskevaidis E, Lolis ED, Koliopoulos G, et al. Cervical intraepithelial neoplasia outcomes after large loop excision with clear margins. Obstet Gynecol 2000;95:828–31.
55. Narducci F, Occelli B, Boman F, et al. Positive margins after conization and risk of persistent lesion. Gynecol Oncol 2000;76:311–14.
56. Reich O, Lahousen M, Pickel H, et al. Cervical intraepithelial neoplasia III: long-term follow-up after cold-knife conization with involved margins. Obstet Gynecol 2002;99:193–6.
57. Massad LS, Chronopoulos FT, Cejtin HE. Correlating cone biopsy histology with operative indications. Gynecol Oncol 1997;65:286–90.
58. Ramchandani SM, Houck KL, Hernandez E, Gaughan JP. Predicting persistent/recurrent disease in the cervix after excisional biopsy. MedGenMed 2007;9:24.
59. Demopoulos RI, Horowitz LF, Vamvakas EC. Endocervical gland involvement by cervical intraepithelial neoplasia grade III: predictive values for residual and/or recurrent disease. Cancer 1991;68:1932–6.
60. Alonso I, Torné A, Puig-Tintoré LM, et al. Pre- and post-conization high-risk HPV testing predicts residual/recurrent disease in patients treated for CIN 2–3. Gynecol Oncol 2006;103(2):631–6.
61. Zielinski GD, Bais AG, Helmerhorst TJ, et al. HPV testing and monitoring of women after treatment of CIN 3: review of the literature and meta-analysis. Obstet Gynecol Surv 2004;59:543–53.
62. Baker P, Oliva E. A practical approach to intraoperative consultation in gynecologic pathology. Int J Gynecol Pathol 2008;27:353–65.
63. Behtash N, Karimi Zarchi M, Hamedi B, et al. The value of frozen sectioning for the evaluation of resection margins in cases of conization. Arch Gynecol Obstet 2007;276:529–32.
64. Gu M, Lin F. Efficacy of cone biopsy of the uterine cervix during frozen section for the evaluation of cervical intraepithelial neoplasia grade 3. Am J Clin Pathol 2004;122:383–8.
65. Giuntoli RL 2nd, Winburn KA, Silverman MB, et al. Frozen section evaluation of cervical cold knife cone specimens is accurate in the diagnosis of microinvasive squamous cell carcinoma. Gynecol Oncol 2003;91:280–4.
66. Larsson G. Conization for cervical dysplasia and carcinoma in situ: long term follow-up of 1013 women. Ann Chir Gynaecol 1981;70:79–85.
67. Tidbury P, Singer A, Jenkins D. CIN-3—the role of lesion size in invasion. Br J Obstet Gynaecol 1992;99:583–6.
68. Anderson MC. Invasive carcinoma of the cervix following local destructive treatment for cervical intraepithelial neoplasia. Br J Obstet Gynaecol 1993;100:657–63.
69. Ayhan A, Otegen U, Guven S, Kucukali T. Radical reoperation for invasive cervical cancer found in simple hysterectomy. J Surg Oncol 2006;94:28–34.
70. Richart RM, Barron BA. A follow-up study of patients with cervical dysplasia. Am J Obstet Gynecol 1969;105:386–93.
71. Johnson LD, Nickerson RJ, Easterday CL, et al. Epidemiological evidence for the spectrum of change from dysplasia through carcinoma in situ to invasive cancer. Cancer 1968;22:901–14.
72. Ostor AG. Natural history of cervical intraepithelial neoplasia—a critical review. Int J Gynecol Pathol 1993;12:186–92.
73. Syrjanen KJ. Condyloma acuminatum and other HPV-related squamous cell tumors of the genitoanal area. In: Gross G, Vonkrogh G, editors. Human papillomavirus infections in dermatovenereology. Boca Raton, FL: CRC Press; 1997. p. 151–80.
74. Holowaty P, Miller AB, Rohan T, To T. Natural history of dysplasia of the uterine cervix. J Natl Cancer Inst 1999;91:252–8.
75. Fidler HK, Boyes DA, Worth AJ. Cervical cancer detection in British Columbia. J Obstet Gynaecol Br Commonwealth 1968;75:392–404.
76. Kottmeier HL. Evolution et traitement des epitheliomas. Rev Fr Gynecol Obstet 1961;56:821–6.
77. Petersen O. Spontaneous course of cervical precancerous conditions. Am J Obstet Gynecol 1956;72:1063–71.
78. Herrero R, Muñoz N. Human papillomavirus and cancer. Cancer Surv 1999;33:75–98.
79. Kinlen LJ, Spriggs AI. Women with positive cervical smears but without surgical intervention. Lancet 1978;ii:463–5.
80. McIndoe WA, McLean MA, Jones RW, Mullins PR. The invasive potential of carcinoma in situ of the cervix. Obstet Gynecol 1984;64:451–4.
81. Paul C. The New Zealand cervical cancer study: could it happen again? Br Med J 1988;297:533–9.
82. Gornall RJ, Boyd IE, Manolitsas T, Herbert A. Interval cervical cancer following treatment for cervical intraepithelial neoplasia. Int J Gynecol Cancer 2000;10:198–202.
83. Berkeley AS, LiVolsi VA, Schwartz PE. Advanced squamous cell carcinoma of the cervix with recent normal Papanicolaou tests. Lancet 1980;ii:375–6.
84. Ibrahim SN, Krigman HR, Coogan AC, et al. Prospective correlation of cervicovaginal cytologic and histologic specimens. Am J Clin Pathol 1996;106:319–24.
85. Kurman RJ, Schiffman MH, Lancaster WD, et al. Analysis of individual human papillomavirus types in cervical neoplasia: a possible role for type 18 in rapid progression. Am J Obstet Gynecol 1988;159:293–6.
86. Kline TS. The Papanicolaou smear—a brief historical perspective and where we are today. Arch Pathol Lab Med 1997;121:205–9.
87. Naryshkin S. The false-negative fraction for Papanicolaou smears: how often are 'abnormal' smears not detected by a 'standard' screening cytologist? Arch Pathol Lab Med 1997;121:270–2.
88. Herfs M, Yamamoto Y, Laury A, et al. A discrete population of squamocolumnar junction cells implicated in the pathogenesis of cervical cancer. Proc Natl Acad Sci USA 2012;109:10516–21.
89. Burghardt E, Ostor AG. Site and origin of squamous cervical cancer: a histomorphologic study. Obstet Gynecol 1983;62:117–27.
90. Heatley M. Distribution of cervical intraepithelial neoplasia: are hysterectomy specimens sampled appropriately? J Clin Pathol 1995;48:323–4.
91. Allard JE, Rodriguez M, Rocca M, Parker MF. Biopsy site selection during colposcopy and distribution of cervical intraepithelial neoplasia. J Low Genit Tract Dis 2005;9:36–9.
92. Lurie S, Eliaz M, Boaz M, et al. Distribution of cervical intraepithelial neoplasia across the cervix is random. Am J Obstet Gynecol 2007;196(125):e1–3.
93. Pretorius RG, Zhang X, Belinson JL, et al. Distribution of cervical intraepithelial neoplasia 2, 3 and cancer on the uterine cervix. J Low Genit Tract Dis 2006;10:45–50.
94. Guido RS, Jeronimo J, Schiffman M, Solomon D. The distribution of neoplasia arising on the cervix: results from the ALTS trial. Am J Obstet Gynecol 2005;193:1331–7.

11 Cervical Squamous Cell Carcinoma

Thomas C. Wright, Jr.

CHAPTER OUTLINE

Epidemiology and Staging	232	Effects of Radiotherapy on Cervical Carcinoma	245
Types of Cervical Malignancies	233	Micrometastasis	246
Superficially Invasive Squamous Cell Carcinoma	233	'Mucin-Secreting' Carcinoma	246
Depth of Invasion	234	**Histologic Variants**	**246**
Morphologic Features	235	Verrucous Squamous Cell Carcinoma	246
Squamous Cell Carcinoma	238	Warty Squamous Cell Carcinoma	247
Microscopic Features Used in Classification	239	Papillary Squamous Cell Carcinoma	247
Clinicopathologic Correlation	242	Lymphoepithelioma-Like Squamous Cell Carcinoma	247
Prognostic Features	243	Papillary Squamotransitional Cell Carcinoma	248
Special Considerations	245		
Cervical Stump Carcinoma	245		

EPIDEMIOLOGY AND STAGING

Epidemiology

Cancer of the cervix is the second most common cancer in women worldwide after cancer of the breast. Each year, approximately 529,828 new cases are diagnosed worldwide.[1] In the United States in 2012, cervical cancer was a distant third most common neoplasm of the female genital tract (12,170 cases, or about 14% of all genital cancers), after endometrium (47,130 cases) and ovary (22,280 cases).[2] Breast cancer, by comparison, is 22 times more common (229,060 cases in the United States in 2012). Cervical cancer caused about 4220 deaths in 2012 in the United States (2.0 deaths/100,000 women). It is responsible for 1.6% of all deaths from neoplasia and 14% of all deaths from genital tract cancer. This compares with 39,510 deaths annually from breast cancer, 15,500 from ovarian cancer, and 8010 from cancer of the uterine corpus.[2]

The lifetime risk of a woman developing cervical cancer is 3% worldwide and 1.1% in the United States. The incidence rates for cervical cancer show a wide geographic variation, which is partially explained by differences in healthcare systems, intensity of screening programs, and exposure to major risk factors. A nearly eightfold difference exists between the lowest age-adjusted incidence rate (4.5/100,000 in western Asia) and the highest rate (34.5/100,000 women in eastern Africa).[1] The age-adjusted incidence rate in the United States is 10.3/100,000 for African/American women, 11.4/100,000 for Hispanic women, but only 6.7/100,000 for non-Hispanic White women.[3] During the past 50 years, both incidence and mortality rates for cervical cancer have declined precipitously in most developed countries. In the United States, the incidence has declined nearly 75% (from 34/100,000 in 1947) while the mortality rate has declined by more than 60%. The single most important factor in this decline is the success of screening with cervical cytology. Studies from both the Nordic countries and British Columbia demonstrate a significant reduction in cervical cancer incidence after only two cervical cytology tests.[4] Repeated studies have shown the single most common factor associated with the development of cervical cancer is the history of not having undergone recent cytologic screening.[5,6] The marked variations in cervical cancer rates in different regions of the globe relate to environmental, socioeconomic, and cultural factors, but, most importantly, to access to screening programs.

Staging

The most widely adopted staging system for cervical cancers worldwide is that of the International Federation of Gynecologists and Obstetricians (FIGO) (Table 11.1), which was last updated in 2009.[7] This is a four-stage system that is in large part clinically determined, as opposed to pathologically determined. Stage I tumors are tumors that are confined to the uterus and are subdivided into two subcategories: those that are not macroscopically visible and invade 5 mm or less into the stroma and tumors that are macroscopically visible and/or invade more than 5 mm into the stroma. Stage II tumors invade beyond the uterus, but not to the pelvic sidewall or the lower third of the vagina. Stage III tumors extend to the pelvic sidewall and/or involve the lower third of the vagina and/or cause hydronephrosis or a nonfunctioning kidney. Stage IV tumors extend beyond the true pelvis or involve the mucosa of the bladder or rectum.

TYPES OF CERVICAL MALIGNANCIES

The World Health Organization (WHO) currently recognizes three general histologic subtypes of cervical cancer: squamous cell carcinoma, adenocarcinoma, and 'other epithelial carcinomas.'[8] While squamous cell carcinoma accounted for upward of 90% of primary neoplasms several decades ago, the overall frequency has now dropped to about 60–70%.[9,10] The various histologic variants of adenocarcinoma constitute much of the remainder of cervical cancers. The remaining primary malignancies of the cervix include sarcomas, lymphomas, and melanomas. Endometrial tumors frequently spread to the cervix, but it is unusual to find other tumors metastasizing to the cervix.

SUPERFICIALLY INVASIVE SQUAMOUS CELL CARCINOMA

Superficially invasive squamous cell carcinoma (SISCCA), or 'microinvasive carcinoma,' a concept introduced over 50 years ago, refers to cancer of the cervix that demonstrates a minimal degree of stromal invasion, and as such has a prognosis much better than that of more invasive cervical carcinomas. In 2012, lower anogenital squamous terminology (LAST) for human papillomavirus (HPV)-associated lesions (LAST consensus recommendations by the College of American Pathologists and American Society of Clinical Pathologists; CAP/ASCP) unified microinvasive lesions under the moniker 'superficially invasive squamous cell carcinoma,' further designated by site-specific definitions. Thus, SISCCA of the cervix is defined as invasion ≤3 mm from the basement membrane point of origin, and horizontal spread ≤7mm.[92] The critical point with regards to SISCCA is that these tumors, although locally invasive, present a negligible risk for having extended beyond the cervical conization specimen being examined, or of having metastasized to regional lymph nodes. As a result, patients with

Table 11.1 2009 Modification of FIGO Staging of Carcinoma of the Cervix[7]

Stage I	Cervical carcinoma confined to uterus (extension to the corpus should be disregarded)
IA	Invasive carcinoma that can be diagnosed only by microscopy with deepest invasion ≤5 mm and largest diameter ≤7.0 mm
IA1	Measured stromal invasion ≤3.0 mm in depth and diameter of ≤7.0 mm
IA2	Measured stromal invasion >3.0 mm but not greater than 5 mm with a diameter of ≤7.0 mm
IB	Clinically visible lesion confined to the cervix uteri or preclinical cancers greater than stage IA.*
IB1	Clinically visible lesion ≤4 cm in greatest dimension
IB2	Clinically visible lesion >4 cm in greatest dimension
Stage II	Cervical carcinoma invades beyond the uterus but not to the pelvic wall or to lower third of the vagina
IIA	Without parametrial invasion
IIA1	Clinically visible lesion ≤4 cm in greatest dimension
IIA2	Clinically visible lesion >4 cm in greatest dimension
IIB	With obvious parametrial invasion
Stage III	Tumor extends to the pelvic wall and/or involves lower third of the vagina and/or causes hydronephrosis or nonfunctioning kidney
IIIA	Tumor involves lower third of the vagina; no extension to pelvic wall
IIIB	Extension to pelvic wall and/or causes hydronephrosis or nonfunctioning kidney
Stage IV	The carcinoma has extended beyond the true pelvis or has involved (biopsy proven) the mucosa of the bladder or rectum. A bullous edema, as such, does not permit a case to be allotted to stage IV
IVA	Spread of the growth to adjacent organs
IVB	Spread to distant organs

*All macroscopically visible lesions, even with superficial invasion, are allocated to stage IB. Invasion is limited to a measured stromal invasion with a maximal depth of 5 mm and horizontal extension of not >7 mm. Depth of invasion should not be >5 mm taken from the base of the epithelium of the original tissue, superficial or glandular. The depth of invasion should always be reported in millimeters, even in those cases with 'early (minimal) stromal invasion' (<1 mm). The involvement of vascular/lymphatic spaces should not change the stage allotment.

cervical SISCCA can be treated in a less radical manner without jeopardizing their chance for curative resection than women with more deeply invasive carcinomas. This is important because SISCCA accounts for about 20% of all cervical cancers and the majority of cases occur in women aged 35–46 years.[11,12] SISCCA is now most often diagnosed in women presenting with abnormal smears interpreted as high-grade squamous intraepithelial lesion (HSIL).

DEPTH OF INVASION

Among the many literature reports on SISCCA, whether presenting the findings of an individual series of patients or meta-analyses of all published articles, there is a general agreement that depth of invasion is a key prognostic indicator. Tumors that invade <1 mm into the underlying stroma are virtually never associated with lymph node metastases, although exemptions have been occasionally reported.[13] Moreover, if we take 50–100 sections from a conization specimen performed for HSIL we are much more likely to find small epithelial buds extending <1 mm into the stroma than if we take only 10–15 sections. However, excellent clinical outcomes are achieved in both settings.[7] Thus there is uniform agreement that tumors with very superficial stromal invasion (<1 mm) can be safely treated with conservative measures. There is more controversy with respect to the management of tumors with 1–5 mm of invasion. Although most studies have shown that the risk of lymph node metastases and the development of recurrent disease after conservative treatment are relatively low for carcinomas that invade ≤5 mm the risk is clearly not zero. For example, one study examining lesions invading <3 mm found that the recurrence rate was 6% during the 10 year follow-up period.[14] Clinicopathologic analyses of carcinomas that invade ≤5 mm have shown a distinct difference between tumors invading ≤3 mm and those with 3–5 mm of invasion (Table 11.2).[15–25] Tumors that invade to a depth of 3–5 mm are associated with lymph node metastases in about 8% of cases whereas those that invade ≤3 mm have only a 1–2% risk of lymph node metastases. The threshold of 3 mm invasion has now been formally adopted by the LAST group to define the maximum depth of invasion in SISCCA of the cervix.

TUMOR VOLUME AND LATERAL EXTENT OF SPREAD

Although, as discussed above, it is generally accepted that depth of the invasion correlates with prognosis, other studies have documented that the tumor volume might be an even better prognostic measure. In order to accurately determine tumor volume, an excisional specimen needs to be serially step sectioned. When this is done and the distance between the sections is known, tumor volume can be calculated. This approach was first advocated by Burghardt and Holtzer,[26] who reported no pelvic lymph node metastases in patients with <420 mm^3 of cancer unless lymphovascular space involvement was identified. However, performing serial step sections to assess tumor volume is not practical for most laboratories. Thus FIGO has recommended that the greatest lateral extent of the tumor be measured as a surrogate for tumor volume. The usefulness of lateral tumor extension as a prognosticator was shown in an analysis of 402 women with squamous cell carcinomas by Takeshima et al.[27] In this study, the incidence of nodal metastases was only 1.2% among patients with ≤3 mm of invasion but increased to almost 7% among women with 3–5 mm of invasion. However, in both groups, almost all recurrences occurred in women with >7 mm of horizontal spread. Based on these and other data showing the importance of lateral tumor extension, the FIGO staging system now requires stage IA tumors to be ≤7 mm in greatest diameter. This was reaffirmed by the LAST group, which defines SISCCA of the cervix as having no more than 7 mm in maximal extent.[28]

LYMPHOVASCULAR INVASION

The role of lymphovascular invasion (LVI) as a prognostic indicator is more controversial than that of the depth of invasion and lateral extent of tumor. Although it would seem reasonable to assume that a tumor with LVI is more likely to have lymph node metastases than one without, the data are conflicting. In part, this stems from the relatively poor reproducibility of a pathologic diagnosis of LVI, especially when not extensive. It is well documented that the stroma in which foci of invasion lie can retract during preparation of the tissue sections for microscopic examination. A clear space can easily be mistaken for LVI. Another problem with the reporting of LVI is the fact that the finding is contingent on the number of sections that are examined. In one study serial step sections were examined from 30 cervices diagnosed with cervical carcinoma having only 2–5 mm of invasion. Thirty percent of the women had 'capillary-like space' involvement based on the first cut of tissue from the blocks, but this increased to 57% when the serial step sections were examined. All of the women in this study had been treated with radical hysterectomy with lymph node dissection. No lymph node metastases were found, regardless of the presence or absence of LVI. This study concluded that the presence of tumor in lymphatic spaces was of no value by itself in predicting which patients are likely to have lymph node metastases.[29] However, other studies have reported that the presence of LVI is an important prognostic indicator.[30,31] For example, a recent literature review of carcinomas with <3 mm of invasion reported recurrent cancer in 3.1% (3 of 96) of conservatively managed

Table 11.2 Impact of Depth of Invasion on Nodal Status, LVI, and Recurrence[15–25]

Adverse Indicator	Number of Cases	Depth of Invasion	
		<3 mm	3.1–5 mm
Presence of LVI	1494	10.6%	19.7%
Pelvic node metastases	1308	1.5%	7.6%
Recurrent cancer after therapy	1256	0.4%	4.6%

Modified from sources.

patients with LVI versus only 0.6% (3 of 486) of those without LVI.[32] Overall, LVI has been reported in 0–10% of carcinomas invading <1 mm and 3–30% of those invading 1–3 mm.

MORPHOLOGIC FEATURES

STROMAL INVASION

A diagnosis of SISCCA is made based on finding buds or tongues of malignant cells penetrating the basement membrane and extending into the stroma. The earliest stage at which invasion can be recognized is when a well-defined, tiny bud of invasive cells emanates from the base of HSIL on the surface of the cervix or in endocervical glands (Figure 11.1). The bud projects into the stroma, clearly having disrupted the adjacent smooth basement membrane. In one large series a single bud accounted for one-third of all the microinvasive cancers.[33] However, in other cases, multiple small buds and sometimes individual tumor cells extend into the stroma.

A number of different histologic patterns of SISCCA have been described. In very early foci of invasion the tumor cells are often separated by <1 mm from the nearest involved surface or glandular basement membrane. Cases with <1 mm tumor invasion were previously referred to as 'early stromal invasion,' which was the original definition of the FIGO substage IA1 in the 1985 FIGO classification. Another common pattern of growth is when microinvasive cancers appear as tiny nests of cells extending into the stroma that are totally separated from the overlying surface (Figures 11.2 and 11.3). This pattern of invasion has been referred to as a 'spray bud' pattern. The spray bud pattern of growth is usually <1–2 mm deep. As the foci of invasion become larger, the growths become broader and longer and eventually, as the tumor becomes more advanced, a 'confluent' pattern develops (Figure 11.4). In these larger lesions the invasive foci often form intertwining cords, much like thick

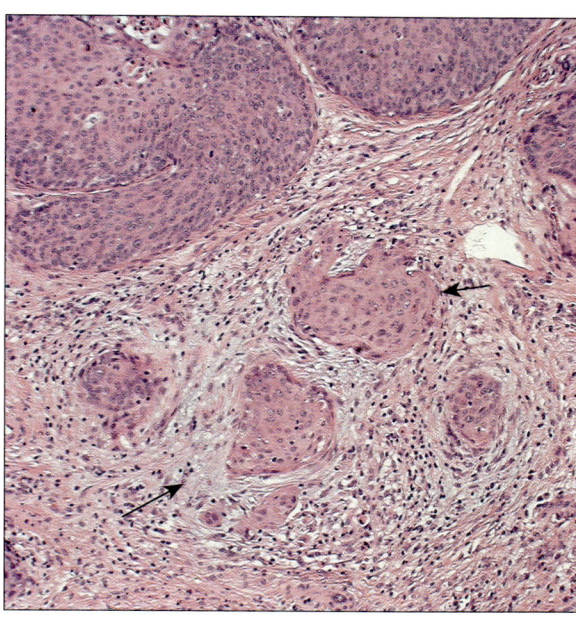

Figure 11.2 Microinvasive carcinoma. A focus of stromal invasion (arrows) that is separated by <1 mm from the overlying HSIL. In this instance multiple small tumor nests are totally separated from the surface epithelium.

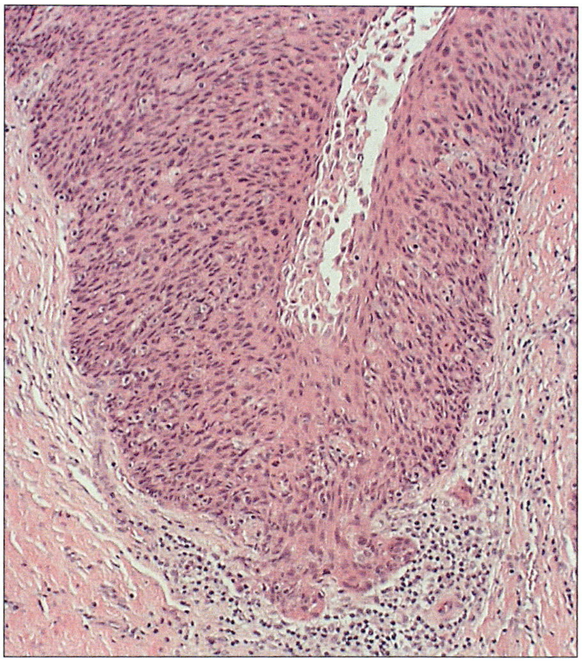

Figure 11.1 Microinvasive carcinoma. A tiny focus of stromal invasion that is barely perceptible arises from an extensive HSIL that fills an endocervical gland.

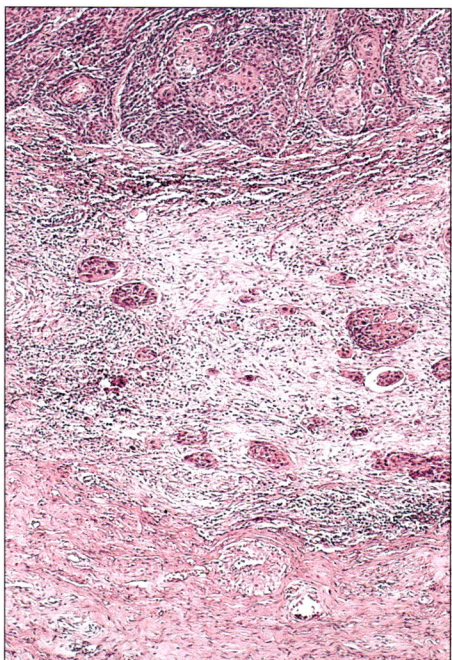

Figure 11.3 Microinvasive carcinoma, spray bud pattern. At high magnification, numerous clusters composed of small numbers of tumor cells are present in a desmoplastic stroma with a mild inflammatory infiltrate. Stromal retraction secondary to processing artifact creates the false impression of lymphovascular space invasion.

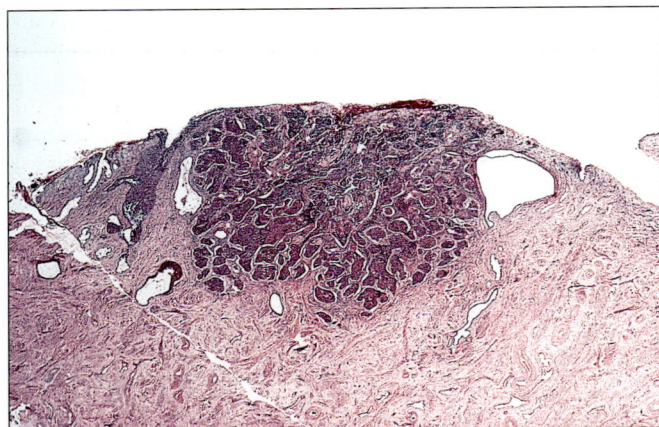

Figure 11.4 Microinvasive carcinoma, confluent pattern. The depth of invasion is slightly greater than 3 mm so this tumor is staged as FIGO stage IA2.

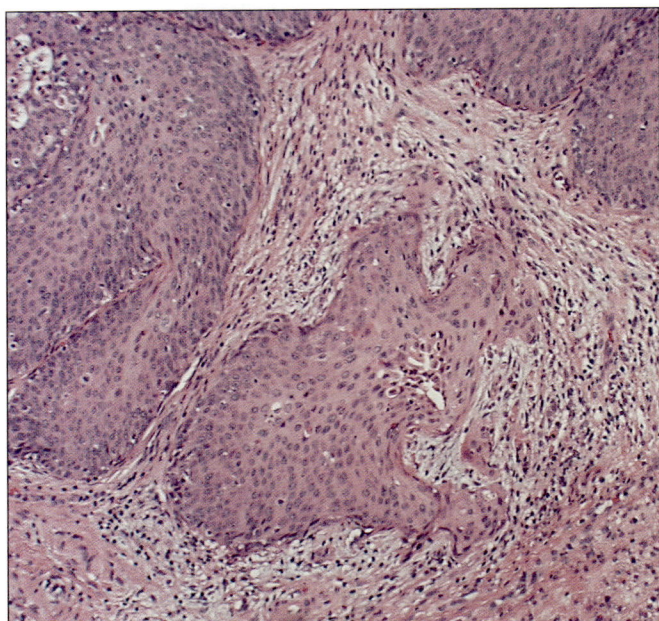

Figure 11.5 Microinvasive carcinoma. The invasive foci have an irregular or 'scalloped' margin that clearly distinguishes it from the sharp margin of the adjacent HSIL.

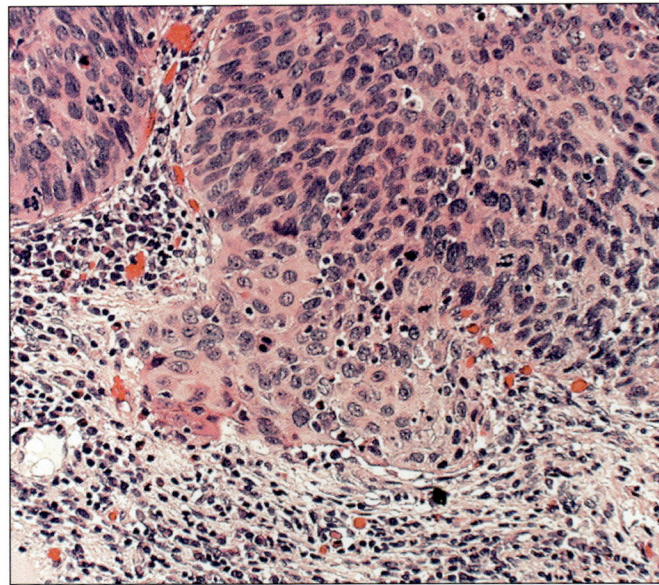

Figure 11.6 Microinvasive carcinoma. Cells in the invasive foci have developed abundant eosinophilic cytoplasm compared to the adjacent HSIL. Individual dyskeratotic cells are present in the invasive foci.

Table 11.3 Histopathologic Features of SISCCA

Qualitative Features:

Irregular, ragged, or even scalloped epithelial margin
Increased cellular maturation compared with adjacent HSIL
Nuclei of invasive cells show clearing of chromatin and prominent nucleoli
Stromal reaction to tumor with desmoplasia and prominent lymphocytic infiltrate

Quantitative Features[28]

Depth of invasion ≤3 mm from basement membrane of point of origin
Horizontal spread ≤7 mm maximal extent

tangled roots of a tree. It is important to stress that reproducible definitions of different patterns of invasion such as spray bud and confluent have proven difficult to develop and, not surprisingly, most studies have shown that the pattern of invasion does not influence clinical outcome independently of depth of invasion.[30]

It is frequently difficult to determine whether a given focus represents SISCCA or instead is HSIL that extends into endocervical glands. There are four qualitative histopathologic features that can help with the diagnosis of SISCCA, in addition to measured limits of extent (Table 11.3).[28] The first is presence of an epithelial margin that can be described as irregular, ragged, or even scalloped in appearance (Figure 11.5). This irregular margin develops because the adjacent smooth basement membrane has been disrupted. The second histopathologic feature is increased cellular maturation compared to the adjacent HSIL. The cells in the invasive foci often have abundant eosinophilic cytoplasm and are paradoxically keratinized (Figure 11.6). The third feature is that the nuclei of the invasive cells frequently show clearing of the chromatin and develop prominent nucleoli (Figure 11.7). The fourth feature is a stromal reaction to the SISCCA. Invasive foci are often surrounded by a prominent lymphoplasmacytic infiltrate and the stroma frequently has a desmoplastic response (Figure 11.3).

MEASURING DEPTH OF INVASION AND LATERAL EXTENT OF SPREAD

Of all the variables evaluated during the assessment of SISCCA, depth of invasion is the one that is universally considered the easiest to measure and the most objective. The interobserver variability in assessing depth of invasion is also considered to be the lowest among the various features considered to have prognostic value. In order to

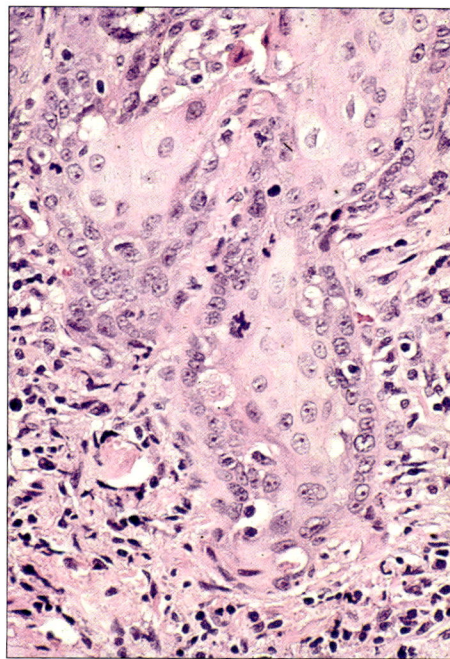

Figure 11.7 Microinvasive carcinoma. The nuclei of cells in the invasive foci show clearing of their chromatin and have developed prominent nucleoli.

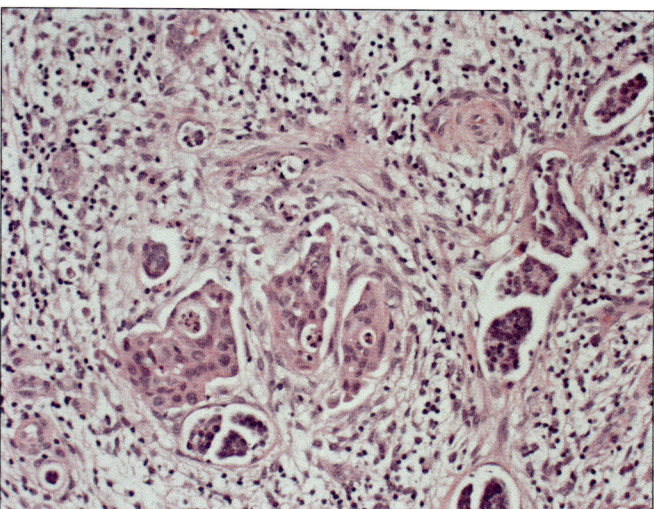

Figure 11.8 LVI in microinvasive carcinoma. Multiple foci of LVI are present at the leading edge of this tumor. Sparse endothelial cells line many of the channels.

accurately determine the maximum depth of invasion, loop electrosurgical excision procedure (LEEP) and conization specimens should be sectioned along the long axis of the cervical canal in a clockwise fashion while trying to avoid tangential sections, which invariably result in inaccurate measurement of the depth of invasion. The current FIGO/LAST staging method recommends that measurement of depth of invasion be made from the base of the epithelium where invasion occurs to the deepest point of carcinoma in a vertical line. In most SISCCAs, invasion either occurs from the base of the surface squamous epithelium or originates from both the surface epithelium and endocervical glands simultaneously. In such cases, measurement should be made from the base of the surface epithelium involved by HSIL. In some cases invasion is limited to the periphery of a few endocervical glands without surface involvement. In these cases, measurement is made from the base of the glands to the deepest point. The deepest measurement should be reported when multiple foci of SISCCA are present.

The lateral extent of SISCCA is usually measured directly from the microscopic slides using a micrometer or ruler as well as by determining the number of contiguous tissue sections that have microinvasive carcinoma. Since most tissue blocks submitted for histologic processing are 2–3 mm in thickness, if three separate, contiguous tissue blocks show SISCCA it is highly probable that the diameter of the tumor is more than 7 mm and the lesion no longer fits the criteria for superficial invasion, or a FIGO stage IA tumor.

ASSESSING PRESENCE OF LVI

Even though the 2009 FIGO staging system does not take into account the presence or absence of LVI, most gynecologic oncologists want to know this information so that treatment can be individualized. Therefore the pathologist should always provide this information in the pathology report. Lymphatic space involvement was defined back in the 1960s as endothelial-lined (capillary-like) spaces containing tumor cells that are contiguous with the stroma. Until the recent introduction of the antibody D2-40 that specifically identifies lymphatic vessels, it was impractical to tell the difference between lymphatic and blood vessels under microscopy. Therefore the term lymphovascular space involvement, or invasion, came into widespread use when discussing cervical small vessel invasion by tumor, be it capillary or lymphatic. Identification of LVI, especially when only several foci are present, can be quite challenging. There is general agreement that LVI should be diagnosed whenever tumor is seen within endothelial-lined spaces at the leading edge of the tumor or beyond (Figure 11.8). Although it is preferable to identify tumor cells attached to the endothelium, this is not always possible. It is well documented that the stroma in which foci of invasion lie can retract during preparation of the tissue sections for microscopic examination. A clear space can easily be mistaken for LVI. Various immunohistochemical markers such as CD34, a marker for endothelium, and D2-40, a marker of lymphatic epithelium, can assist in identifying LVI in some instances. However, it should be remembered that there are a variety of markers available and the results obtained with them can be discordant. Moreover, it is unclear whether LVI, as determined by immunohistochemical markers, correlates with clinical outcomes.[34] Therefore, the standard for assessing the presence or absence of LVI in the cervix remains H&E staining alone.

ASSESSING SURGICAL MARGINS

Although the 2009 FIGO staging system does not take into account the status of the surgical margins of a conization or LEEP specimen, assessment of the surgical margins of excision is one of the most important contributions of the pathologist to management of women with SISCCA. This is because women with either HSIL or SISCCA on the surgical margin are much more likely to have a residual invasive cervical cancer than are women with clear margins. Inking of LEEP specimens is optional since a thermal artifact is universally present in the resection margin. However, a cold-knife cone requires application of ink at the margins, preferably one color at the endocervical and another on peripheral or deep margins.[35]

Diagnosis

SISCCA is a diagnosis based almost wholly on microscopic examination and it usually is an incidental finding in either a cold-knife conization or LEEP specimen obtained for the treatment of HSIL. Most experts believe that a diagnosis of SISCCA should only be made on a LEEP or conization specimen for which the margins of excision are free of both HSIL and SISCCA. This is because the depth of invasion seen on a cervical biopsy specimen or a LEEP/conization specimen with a positive margin may not represent the maximal depth of invasion. SISCCA is a condition that is easily misdiagnosed. Almost 50% of cases diagnosed as SISCCA during routine clinical care are either cases of carcinoma in situ that have been overcalled or cases of invasive carcinoma that have been missed. For example, in a series of 265 cases of SISCCA submitted to a reference pathology panel as part of a Gynecologic Oncology Group (GOG) study, 132 (approximately 50%) were reclassified as something other than SISCCA.[15] Similarly, in a UK study of 286 cases of SISCCA that underwent pathologic review, 41% were incorrectly diagnosed.[36]

One of the more common pathologic pitfalls in the diagnosis of SISCCA, made on conization or LEEP specimens after a prior colposcopy with punch biopsy, is the misclassification of nests of HSIL that have become embedded into the stroma at the site of previous punch biopsy as SISCCA. Distinguishing SISCCA from artifacts secondary to previous biopsy is made more difficult by the fact that the site of a recent biopsy frequently has a prominent lymphoplasmacytic infiltrate. Another common pitfall is to misclassify either immature squamous metaplasia or HSIL with extensive gland involvement as SISCCA. Features that help distinguish foci SISCCA in these instances are a prominent desmoplastic response, increased maturation of the invasive foci, and the presence of an irregular or scalloped margin.

The utility of immunohistochemistry in the diagnosis of SISCCA has been evaluated for a double-staining method combining collagen IV or laminin antibodies to identify the basement membrane and pan cytokeratin antibodies to identify invasive squamous cells.[37] Although in some equivocal cases this approach appears to be useful, since it identified clear-cut invasion in 4 of 10 cases originally reported as 'suspicious for invasion,' it does not always clarify whether or not invasion is actually present.

Cytologic Findings

The cytology of microinvasive carcinoma is controversial. Most cytologists believe that the distinction between HSIL and the earliest stages of invasion cannot be made on cell appearances alone, and for this reason SISCCA is not included as a specific entity in the Bethesda System.[38]

Clinical Management

For the last two decades conservative management of women desirous of childbearing who have SISCCA has been undergoing dramatic changes. In the 1970s most women with SISCCA underwent radical hysterectomy unless they were very young, had ≤3 mm of stromal invasion, and had no LVI. Today, clinicians are much more receptive to a less aggressive approach to SISCCA, especially in women desirous of maintaining their fertility. This argues that the role of the pathologist in assessing specimens with SISCCA is to provide the clinician with all of the information that they require in order to individualize a patient's therapy. This includes depth of invasion, lateral extent of tumor, presence or absence of LVI, and the status of the surgical margins.

The treatment for stage IA1 lesions is typically a LEEP, cold-knife conization, or a simple hysterectomy. With these approaches the cure rate approaches 100%.[39,40] The presence or absence of LVI as well as the exact depth of invasion will impact the treatment approach for stage IA1 tumors. Tumors with <1 mm of invasion almost never have pelvic lymph node metastasis whereas tumors with 1–3 mm invasion or with LVI have a low, but measurable, rate of nodal involvement. If fertility is not a consideration and a woman has adverse prognostic features such as LVI or involved margins, simple hysterectomy is the standard form of definitive treatment. The management of stage IA2 tumors is more controversial. In the United States, women with stage IA2 tumors and LVI are usually not considered candidates for conservative management and they are typically treated with a modified radical hysterectomy and pelvic lymphadenectomy. There is a growing trend, however, to tailor the management for patients desirous of maintaining fertility who present with stage IA2 tumors without LVI and with negative conization margins.[41]

SQUAMOUS CELL CARCINOMA

Squamous Cell Carcinoma is a malignant neoplasm composed of squamous cells. While generally derived from stratified squamous epithelium, it may occur in sites, such as the endocervix, where columnar epithelium is normally present. WHO recognizes nine histologic variants of squamous cell carcinoma (Table 11.4).[35]

Gross Features

To the unaided eye, early stage invasive squamous cell carcinoma is not easy to diagnose. The tumor may present as a rough, raised, red granular area that bleeds on manipulation. However, it is usually difficult to macroscopically distinguish an early invasive carcinoma from ectropion, which is where endocervical-type epithelium lines the ectocervix. The gross features of a more advanced tumor depend upon its site of origin, the pattern of growth, and the rate of necrosis. Most squamous cell carcinomas, by the time they become clinically apparent, involve the external os and are visible on speculum examination (Figure 11.9). However, there are some patients who show no grossly observable tumor, but clearly have tumor diffusely present in the wall of the cervix (Figures 11.10 and 11.11). A few squamous cell carcinomas remain entirely within the canal so that they are not visible until they expand the endocervix to produce a 'barrel-shaped' cervix (defined as a diameter greater than 4 cm). Thus, the growth pattern of a squamous cell carcinoma may be either predominantly exophytic, in which case it grows out from the surface, often as a polypoid excrescence (Figure 11.12), or mainly endophytic so that it infiltrates into the surrounding structures, without much surface growth. Infiltrative lesions that extensively permeate the stroma often result in hard lesions with minimal surface change. If necrosis is marked, ulceration occurs. Ulcerative examples usually involve the ectocervix and sometimes the upper vaginal vault.

MICROSCOPIC FEATURES USED IN CLASSIFICATION

Although no histologic classification system currently in use for invasive squamous cell carcinoma provides reliable prognostic correlations, a number of classification systems are in use that emphasize the type and degree of differentiation of the predominant cell. WHO terminology divides pure squamous cell lesions into the following:[35]

1. *Keratinizing carcinomas*, which account for one-sixth of cases, by definition require the presence of keratin pearl formation (Figure 11.13). Keratin pearls are circular whorls of squamous epithelium with central nests of

Table 11.4 Histologic Variants of Squamous Cell Carcinoma Recognized by WHO[35]

Keratinizing
Nonkeratinizing
Basaloid
Verrucous
Warty
Papillary
Lymphoepithelioma like
Squamotransitional

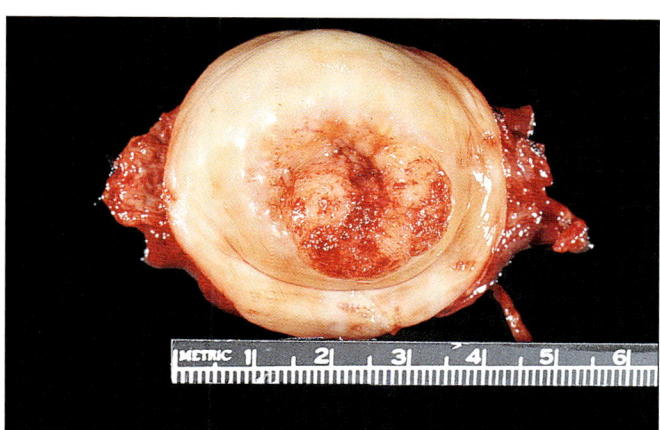

Figure 11.9 Squamous cell carcinoma. Tumor protrudes through the external os and involves the exocervix.

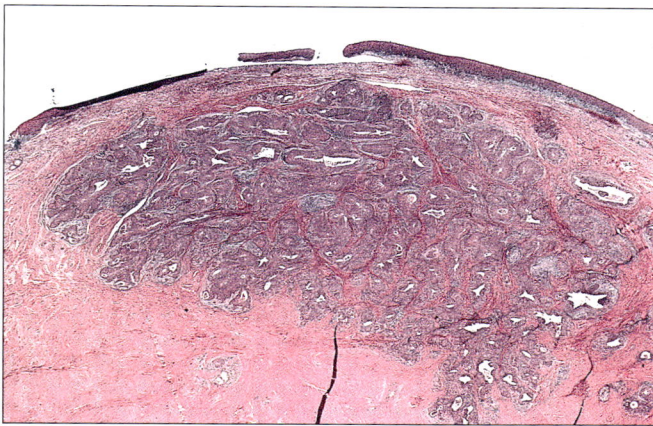

Figure 11.11 Macroscopically invisible 'occult' squamous cell carcinoma. The tumor diffusely involves the wall. The overlying epithelium is relatively normal. The tumor in this instance was not obvious to the clinician, who noted at the time of examination only that the cervix might be slightly more firm than normal.

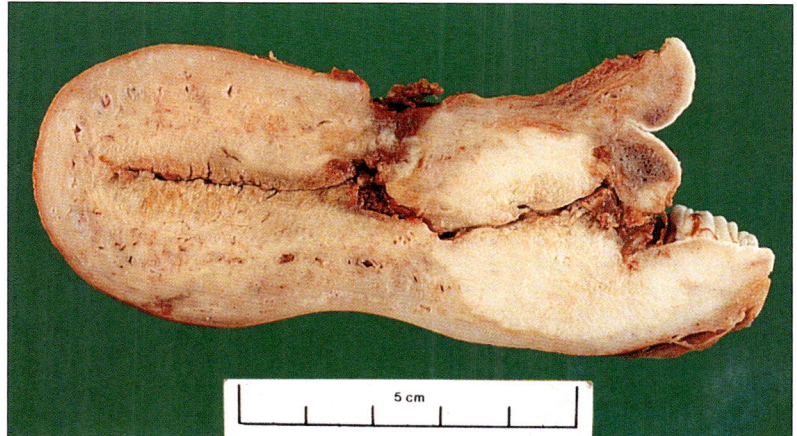

Figure 11.10 Squamous cell carcinoma. The uterus, cut in cross section, discloses an extensive tumor infiltrating throughout the wall of the endocervix (white).

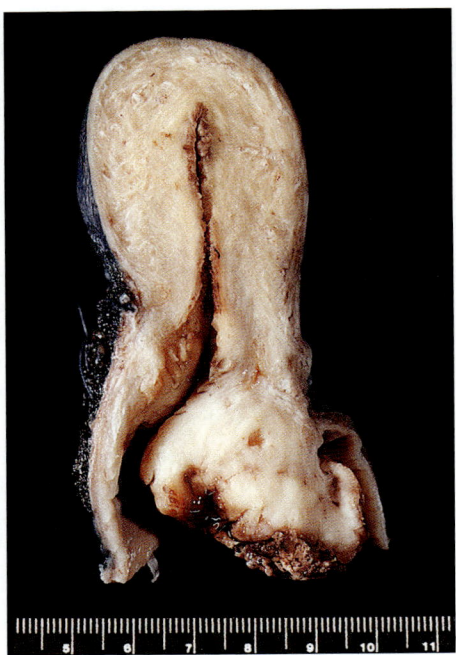

Figure 11.12 Squamous cell carcinoma. The tumor replaces the entire posterior wall of the cervix.

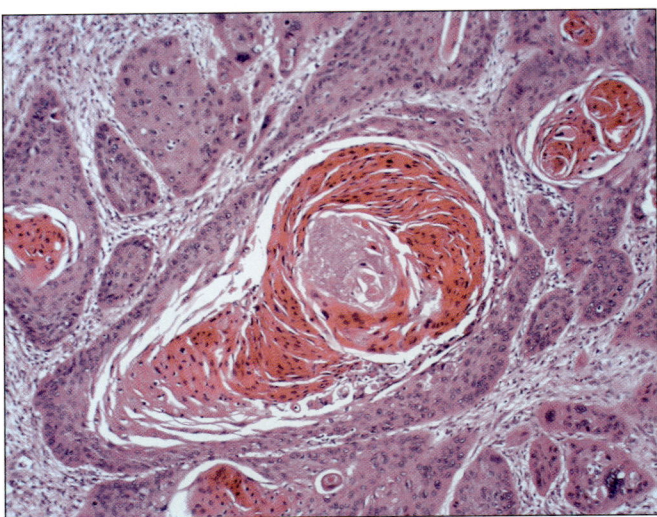

Figure 11.14 Squamous cell carcinoma, keratinizing type. Higher magnification showing keratin pearls. This tumor has many bizarre multinucleated cells.

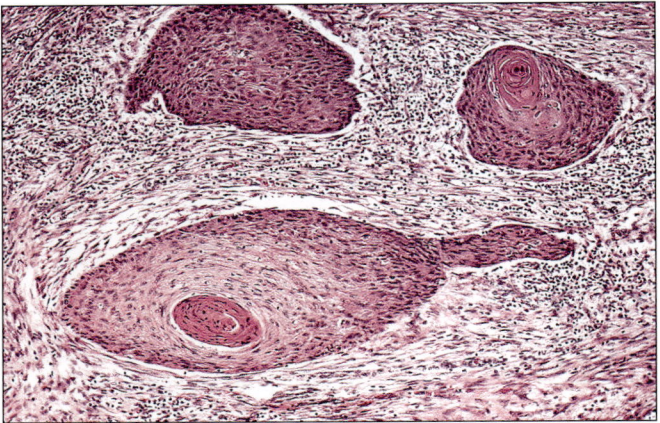

Figure 11.13 Squamous cell carcinoma, keratinizing type. Keratin pearls are present. The irregular angulations that protrude from the tumor nests into the stroma are indicative of invasion.

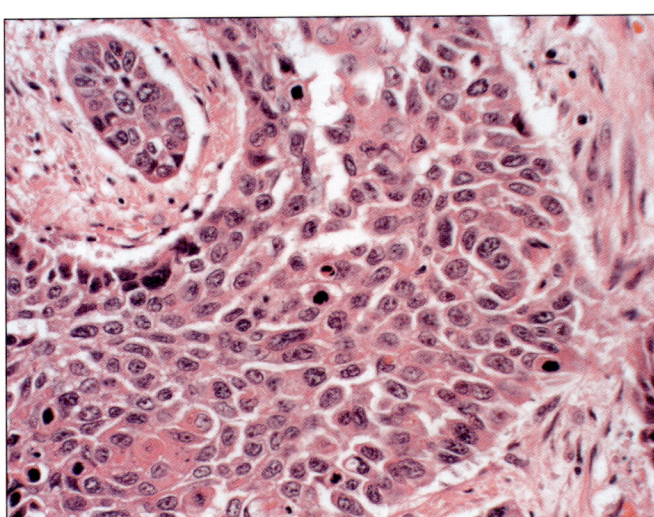

Figure 11.15 Squamous cell carcinoma, nonkeratinizing type. The nuclei are highly pleomorphic and many mitoses are present, suggesting the tumor is poorly differentiated. Although classified as a nonkeratinizing type, individual cells are keratinized.

acellular keratin. Usually, the tumor cells appear mature and are organized in nests or cords. Individual squamous cells are large and usually show abundant eosinophilic cytoplasm. The cells are tightly adherent and may show prominent intercellular bridges. The nuclei may be enlarged or pyknotic (Figure 11.14). Mitotic activity is relatively sparse compared with the other tumor types. While individual cell keratinization (dyskeratosis) may occur, squamous pearls, or broad expanses of keratinization, are required to establish the diagnosis of the keratinizing subtype.

2. *Nonkeratinizing carcinomas*, which account for two-thirds of cases, contain cells that are generally recognizable as squamous from their polygonal shape. There may be individual cell keratinization, but keratin pearls are not seen. Cellular and nuclear pleomorphism is typically more prominent than in the well-differentiated keratinizing tumors, and mitotic figures may be quite numerous (Figure 11.15). Cell borders may be distinct, sometimes with intercellular bridges. An occasional tumor may focally show differentiation as if it were mimicking the normal squamous lining of the exocervix. The more poorly differentiated cells involve deeper stromal areas of tumor while the more superficial portions show cytoplasmic differentiation with accumulation of extensive intracytoplasmic glycogen (not to be confused with clear cell adenocarcinoma, where the tumor is uniform throughout) (Figure 11.16).

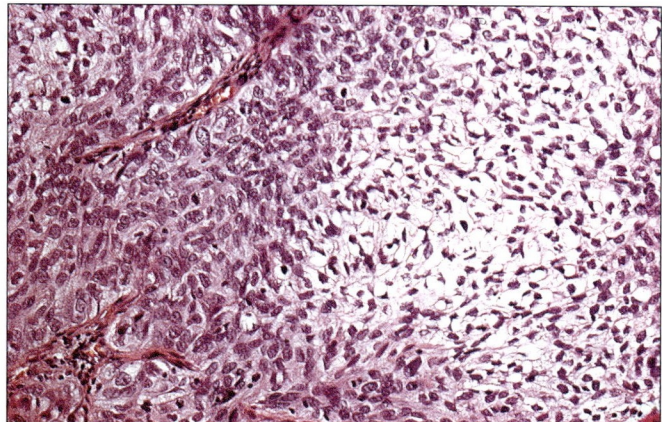

Figure 11.16 Glycogen-rich squamous cell carcinoma, nonkeratinizing type. Much of the tumor shows cellular differentiation with glycogen accumulation, reminiscent of the maturation that occurs in the normal squamous epithelium of the cervix.

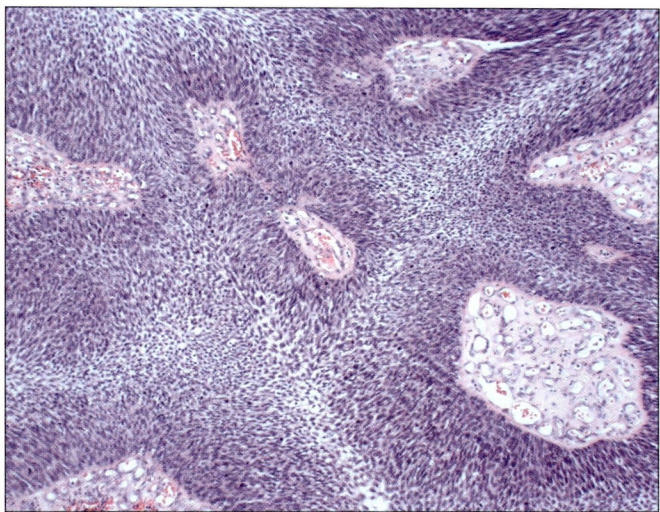

Figure 11.17 Basaloid squamous cell carcinoma. The cells contain minimal cytoplasm and resemble the cells of a HSIL.

3. *Basaloid squamous cell carcinomas* account for approximately one-sixth of cases. They consist of small, oval-shaped basaloid cells with scant cytoplasm (resembling the cells commonly seen in HSILs) that grow in masses and nests (Figure 11.17).[42] The nuclei are usually fairly uniform, hyperchromatic, small, and display abundant mitotic activity. Necrosis is frequently observed. While foci of squamous differentiation and keratinization may sometimes be present, keratin pearls are rarely present. These tumors resemble the vaginal and vulvar tumors designated as basaloid carcinoma, and, by definition, lack the characteristic argyrophilic, immunohistochemical, and ultrastructural features of endocrine carcinomas, also often called 'small cell carcinoma.'[43] Except for their size and growth pattern, there is little to characterize these latter tumors as squamous cell. This variant of squamous cell carcinoma is under-recognized and is an aggressive tumor. Basaloid squamous cell carcinomas together with adenoid cystic carcinoma form one end of the spectrum of basaloid tumors of the cervix. The other end of the spectrum consists of adenoid basal carcinomas, which are low-grade carcinomas. Therefore to prevent confusion, it is recommended that the basaloid squamous cell carcinomas always be referred to by their complete name and the term 'basaloid carcinoma' be avoided.[43]

MICROSCOPIC GRADING

The most widely utilized grading system for squamous cell carcinoma is a modification of the Broder system, which was originally introduced in 1920.[35] This grading system takes into account the degree of keratinization, cellular atypia, and mitotic activity.

1. *Well-differentiated (Grade 1)* tumors have individual cell keratinization (dyskeratosis) that is characterized by intense cytoplasmic eosinophilia. Mitotic figures are often present, but are primarily at the edge of tumor nests. Well-differentiated tumors typically have keratin pearls, which are deposits of acellular keratin found within tumor nests.
2. *Moderately differentiated (Grade 2)* tumor cells are more pleomorphic than in Grade 1 tumors with less cytoplasm and larger irregular nuclei. The cell borders are often indistinct. Although keratin pearls are uncommon, individual tumor cells, especially those in the center of tumor nests, are often keratinized. Mitotic activity is greater than in Grade 1 tumors.
3. *Poorly differentiated (Grade 3)* tumor cells are primitive appearing with hyperchromatic oval nuclei and scant indistinct cytoplasm that resemble the cells of HSILs. Mitoses are common and there often is extensive necrosis. Evidence of keratinization is difficult to identify. Occasionally, Grade 3 tumors consist of large pleomorphic cells with bizarre nuclei and abnormal mitotic figures. Grade 3 tumors can also present as spindle-shaped cells resembling a sarcoma.

In general, the grade of squamous cell carcinoma has little impact on overall patient survival. A GOG study carefully evaluated the clinical impact of tumor grade determined by a number of different grading systems, including the modified Broder's system described above in a group of surgically treated stage IB cervical cancers.[44] Although there was good reproducibility of tumor grade between different pathologists, none of the grading systems had a significant impact on prognosis. Moreover, when analyzed individually, neither extent of keratinization, nuclear grade, pattern of infiltration nor mitotic activity influenced prognosis.[44]

ADDITIONAL MICROSCOPIC FEATURES

Tumors classified as squamous cell carcinoma of the cervix often show extensive variation in patterns of growth, cell types, and degrees of cellular differentiation. Most carcinomas infiltrate as networks of anastomosing bands with intervening stroma that on section appear as irregular islands, some rounded and some angular and spiked. Often, particularly in the early tumors, a HSIL may be found on the surface and at the edge of the invasive tumor. Occasionally it may be difficult to distinguish between invasive nests of tumor in the stroma and HSIL in the gland crypts. Useful clues of invasive cancer are an irregular outer perimeter, the

242 PATHOLOGY OF THE FEMALE REPRODUCTIVE TRACT

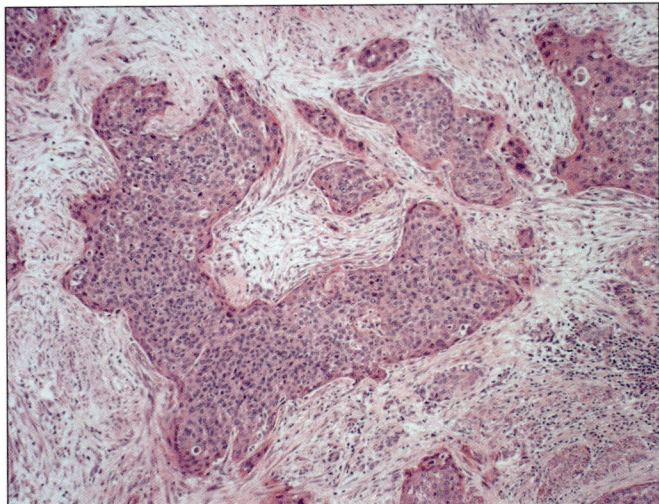

Figure 11.18 Squamous cell carcinoma, invasive. The angulated tumor buds are diagnostic of invasion.

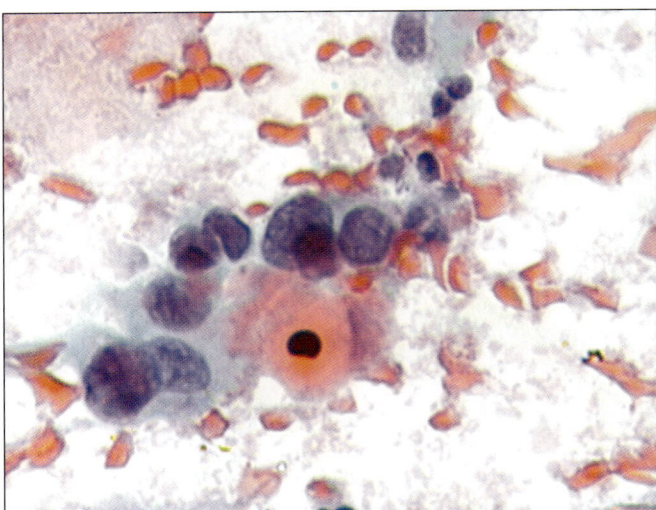

Figure 11.20 Squamous cell carcinoma, nonkeratinizing type. The tumor cells have large, pale pleomorphic nuclei.

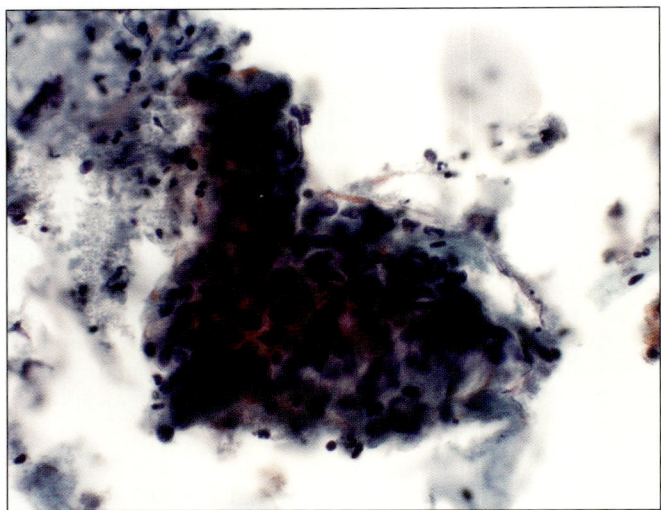

Figure 11.19 Squamous cell carcinoma, invasive. The tumor cells form a sheet of cells and are difficult to visualize. There is necrotic and inflammatory debris present (tumor diathesis) together with pink-staining keratin.

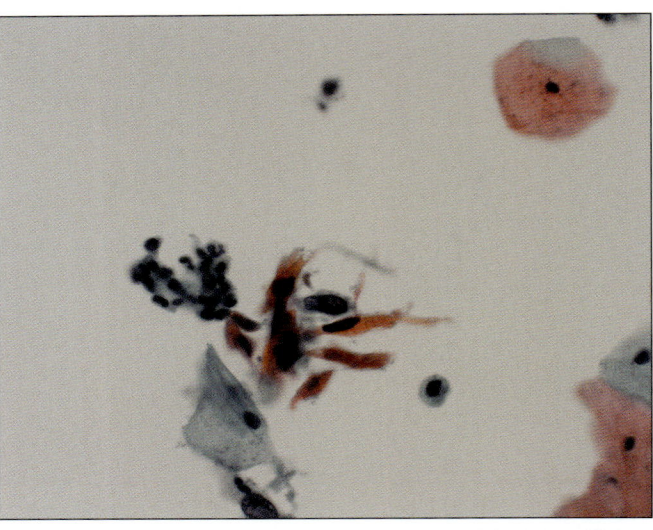

Figure 11.21 Squamous cell carcinoma, keratinizing type. Bizarre keratinized cells with enlarged hyperchromatic nuclei.

presence of a desmoplastic stromal response, or sharp angulations of the tumor suggesting invasive growth through stromal planes (Figure 11.18).

Cytology

The cytologic features associated with invasive squamous cell carcinoma are well described, although invasive carcinoma is under-recognized cytologically.[38] One reason for this is the preconceived impression that many have bizarre keratinizing cells. However, the actual cytologic pattern associated with most cases is that of poorly preserved cells in a background of cell necrosis and inflammatory changes (Figure 11.19). Often the background is as important as the cytology of the cells. Small, highly keratinized cells or cells showing a wide variation in size and shape are important to recognize. Some cells may show hyperchromasia, but others appear pale and insignificant (Figure 11.20). Careful evaluation of all these features is essential.

Keratinizing carcinoma may show bizarre, elongated, and 'tadpole' forms, often associated with excessive keratinization (Figure 11.21). Well-differentiated carcinoma cells may be confused with regenerative tissue cells or squamous metaplasia. When few cells are present, screening becomes more challenging and subtle cytologic detail more important.

CLINICOPATHOLOGIC CORRELATION

Cervical cancer has several modes of presentation, each of which reflects the extent of tumor spread. Depending upon the level of routine medical care received, the majority of patients present initially with an abnormal cervical cytology. The age in a woman's life when cervical cancer presents has become lower in recent decades. Currently, the mean age of women with stage I tumors is 47 years, whereas it is 57 years for women with stage III and IV tumors.[45] 30% of stage I tumors occur in women under 40 years of age; 4.6% occur in women 30 years of age or younger.

About 60% of patients with early stage disease present with intermittent painless vaginal bleeding, which is usually postmenopausal, but is sometimes postcoital. With more advanced disease, bleeding may become continuous and accompanied by a malodorous discharge. As the endopelvic fascia envelops the cervix in an anterior–posterior fashion and therefore serves as a natural barrier, cervical cancer preferentially grows within the parametria and involves the ureters before it infiltrates the bladder or rectum.[46] Ureteral obstruction and death from renal failure mark the natural course of untreated cervical cancer. Pain, present in <10% of cases, frequently refers to the flank or leg, indicating that tumor may have invaded the pelvic wall or lumbosacral nerve roots. Edematous lower extremities signify involved lymphatics. During the late stages in the evolution of the cancer, dysuria, hematuria, rectal bleeding, or constipation may herald bladder or rectal involvement.

Clinical Behavior

Squamous cell carcinomas spread primarily by local extension and lymphatic invasion. Local extension includes adjacent vaginal mucosa, parametrial soft tissue and pelvic wall, corpus uteri, bladder, and rectum. Spread into the peritoneum is uncommon, and, when grossly absent, the peritoneal cytologic wash is almost always negative (98.3%).[47] Lymphatic spread primarily involves parametrial, paracervical, obturator, hypogastric, external iliac, and sacral lymph nodes and, secondarily, common iliac, inguinal, and para-aortic nodes. A close correlation exists among stage, frequency, and location of lymph node metastasis. Thus, tumor is found in pelvic lymph nodes in 15%, 30%, and 40% of patients with stage I, II, and III/IV disease, respectively. About one-third of patients with para-aortic node involvement have metastases to the scalene nodes. Most recurrences are local and occur within 3 years of the initial diagnosis (Figure 11.22).

PROGNOSTIC FEATURES

Numerous prognostic factors have been studied in patients with cervical carcinoma. Stage, which relates to the anatomic extent of the disease and is largely a function of tumor size, is generally considered to be the single most important determinant of outcome (Table 11.5).[45] The 5 year survival of stage I patients ranges from 97.5% for those with stage IA1, tumors to 75.7% for those with stage IB2.[45] For women with stage III disease, overall 5 year survival is about 40%.

HISTOPATHOLOGIC PROGNOSTIC FEATURES

Histologic type and tumor grade have been shown to have little impact on prognosis. In women with early stage tumors (stages IB and IIA) that have been surgically treated, tumor size, depth of invasion, parametrial involvement, and nodal invasion and LVI have all been shown to significantly impact survival.[44,48,49] Depth of invasion, a feature easily obtained in a surgically removed specimen, is proportional to the volume of tumor present. In stage I tumors, depth of invasion is a reasonably reliable indicator of survival (Table 11.6).

The finding of LVI has long been recognized as an adverse prognostic sign (Figure 11.23).[50] However, the critical question is whether this feature is independent, or simply secondary to overall tumor size. Some other factor, such as the quantity of positive LVI, might be a more important predictor.[51] While it has been reported that the survival of patients with and without LVI is not significantly different, a correlation exists between the presence of tumor in lymphatic

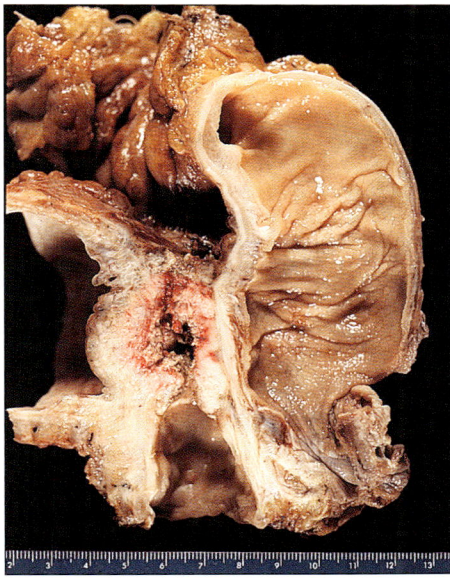

Figure 11.22 Squamous cell carcinoma, recurrent. Hysterectomy has been previously performed. The local recurrence at the site of the removed cervix indents the rectum posteriorly and bladder wall anteriorly.

Table 11.5 FIGO Stage and 5 Year Survival[45]

FIGO Stage	5 Year Survival (%)
IA1	97.9
IA2	94.6
IB	87.5
IIA	74.8
IIB	67.4
III	43.7
IV	16.3

Table 11.6 Depth of Invasion in Stage I Tumors

Depth of Invasion (mm)	Vascular Invasion (%)	Positive Lymph Nodes (%)	5 Year Survival (%)
<3	3	3	99
4–5	11	5	96
6–10	21	6	91
11–15	65	31	72
>19	69	47	63

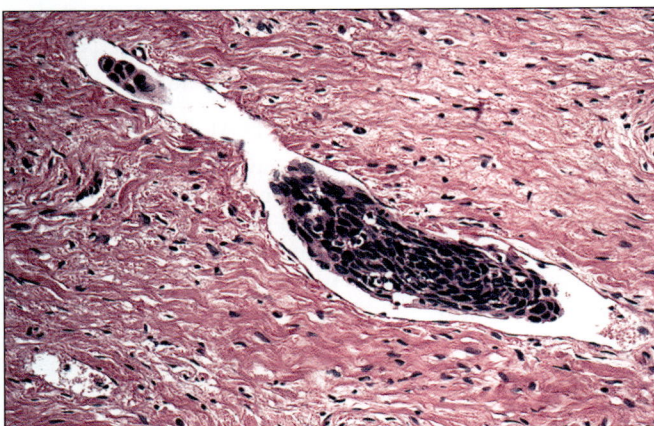

Figure 11.23 Lymphovascular channel with tumor. Endothelial cells line the vessel.

channels and lymph node metastases, even when corrected for size of clinical tumor.[52]

It is generally agreed that the presence and number of lymph node metastases, the number of nodal groups involved, and the size of the metastases themselves are of prognostic significance.[53] While these features may reflect the size of the primary cervical tumor, some report that the presence of nodal metastases is in itself an independent prognostic factor.[54] Survival rates decrease with increasing numbers of involved nodes. One series of low-stage tumors reported a 90% survival rate with no involved nodes, 70% with one to three involved nodes, and 38% with over four involved nodes.[55] For patients with positive nodes, survival was better if the cervical tumor was small rather than large (82% vs 48%). Lymph node metastases smaller than 2 mm were associated with much higher survival rates than if the metastases exceeded 2 cm (85% vs 38%, respectively).[55]

TUMOR SIZE

In large part tumor size determines tumor stage, at least for stage I and II tumors, and, as expected, tumor size correlates with prognosis. In most studies, size has been defined using the diameter of the tumor, which is based on two-dimensional measurements.[56] When used as a continuous variable, it is a good predictor of survival.[57] In some studies, size has also been measured in terms of volume and this has been found to be a key prognostic index.[55,58] Tumors with a volume <2 cm^3 had 5 year survival rates of about 90% in contrast to those with volumes >30 cm^3 (~65% survival). Volumes of 2 and 30 cm^3 roughly equate to tumor diameters of 1.6 and 3.8 cm, respectively. With the availability of magnetic resonance imaging (MRI) techniques, precise volumetric measurement has now become routine in recent years, regardless of whether the patient is treated with radical surgery or radiotherapy.

PERITUMORAL LYMPHATIC VESSEL DENSITY

Peritumoral lymphatic density as evaluated using immunohistochemistry with D2-40 antibodies (selective marker for lymphatic endothelium) or antibodies against lymphatic vessel hyaluronan receptor 1 appears to be a prognostic marker in early stage cervical cancer. High peritumoral lymphatic vessel density is associated with increased lymph node metastases and poor survival.[59,60] Similarly, increased amounts of the vascular endothelial growth factor (VEGF), which promotes angiogenesis, have been associated with higher stage and an increase in lymph node metastases, as well as a shorter survival in some but not other studies.[61–63] A recent GOG study reported that elevated microvessel density as measured using CD31 immunohistochemical staining, but not VEGF levels, was an independent prognostic factor in high-risk, early stage cervical cancers.[63]

BIOMARKERS

Recent studies have evaluated a number of biochemical markers as prognostic factors including specific high-risk HPV genotype. Even though any of the 14 high-risk HPV genotypes can cause squamous cell carcinomas of the cervix, just two, HPV 16 and 18, are found in two-thirds of cases.[64] Several studies have evaluated the impact of specific HPV genotype on survival in cervical cancer and, in general, HPV 18 is associated with a worse prognosis than the other genotypes. For example, a recent study of 1067 patients with stage IA–IIA disease identified HPV 18 in 16.5% of the cases. In patients with stage II disease, deep stromal invasion, parametrial extension, and HPV 18 were all significant predictors for death.[65] Similarly, a study of 296 stage IB or greater cervical cancers found that HPV 18 was associated with an approximately threefold increase in death for women with stage IB cancers.[66] In another study, the 5 year disease-free survival rate was reported as 58% for patients with HPV 16-positive tumors but only 38% for patients with HPV 18-positive tumors. Patients with HPV 18-associated tumors had a relative risk of death 2.4 times greater than that for patients with HPV 16, and 4.4 times greater than that for patients with tumors associated with a viral type different from HPV 16/18.[67]

Other investigations have examined oncogene and tumor suppressor gene expression, cell cycle protein expression, cell adhesion molecules, loss of heterogeneity, and microsatellite instability.[59,68–71] Some of these studies have attempted to discern the changes important in pathogenesis from those that may reflect progression of the cancer. Some of the most interesting potential biomarkers include cyclooxygenase 2 (COX-2) expression, epidermal growth factor receptor (EGFR) expression, and expression of the transmembrane protein, leucine-rich repeats, and immunoglobin-like domains 1 (LRIG1), which has been shown to restrict growth factor signaling by degradation of EGFR. EGFR is expressed in approximately three-fourths of cervical cancers and correlates with a poor prognosis.[72] High COX-2 expression has been associated with poor survival in several studies, as has synchronous co-expression of COX-2 and EGFR, which is reported in only one-third of cancers.[69] However, there currently is insufficient data to warrant the use of specific biomarkers in assessing the prognosis or response to treatment of individual patients.

DIFFERENTIAL DIAGNOSIS

The differential diagnosis for invasive squamous cell carcinoma includes squamous metaplasia, condyloma acuminatum, HSIL with extensive involvement of endocervical glands, gestational decidual reaction of the cervical stroma, trophoblastic lesions such as epithelioid trophoblastic tumor, and granulomatous diseases such as lymphogranuloma venereum with associated reparative reactions. Now that p16 immunostaining is widely available for the identification of HPV-associated squamous intraepithelial lesion (SIL) and invasive cancers, it is much easier to differentiate between squamous metaplasia involving endocervical glands, which stains negatively with p16, and squamous cell carcinoma, which stains diffusely positive with p16. Similarly, condyloma acuminatum, which is usually associated with low-risk HPV genotypes (HPV 6 or 11), typically stains negatively for p16, as do gestational decidual reactions and granulomatous diseases. Histologic features that allow HSIL extending into endocervical glands from invasive squamous cell carcinoma are discussed in the section on SISCCA.

A number of other tumors can be difficult to distinguish from squamous cell carcinoma. When squamous cell carcinomas are of the basaloid histologic type, they can be confused with a small cell neuroendocrine tumor, primitive neuroendocrine tumors, melanomas, and lymphomas. Most small cell neuroendocrine cancers have a distinctive growth pattern. Small nests and typically individual cells diffusely infiltrate the stroma. Sometimes they differentiate toward rosettes, trabeculae, and ribbons. The cytoplasm is scant. The round to spindle-shaped nuclei lack prominent nucleoli and are intensely hyperchromatic. The smudged chromatin obscures nuclear and nucleolar details. A characteristic crush artifact is frequently present. Immunostains exhibit reactivity for chromogranin, synaptophysin, neuron-specific enolase, and S-100 protein. In contrast, squamous cell carcinomas composed of small cells have oval-shaped nuclei and granular chromatin arranged in cohesive nests; squamous differentiation is found occasionally in the center of some nests. Primitive neuroendocrine tumors stain negatively for p63 and have membranous staining for CD99 and nuclear staining for FLI-1.

The cells of squamous cell carcinoma may diffusely contain extensive intracytoplasmic glycogen (Figure 11.16). Unlike clear cell adenocarcinomas where the change is uniform throughout, the glycogenated elements in squamous cell carcinoma are confined only to superficial portions of the epithelium. Clear cell adenocarcinoma, in addition to solid areas, usually has a papillary portion or tubulocystic areas with hobnail cells.

Epithelioid trophoblastic tumor frequently involves the endocervix and lower uterine segment.[73] This tumor displays a nodular proliferation of a monomorphic population of intermediate-sized epithelioid trophoblasts with eosinophilic or clear cytoplasm, forming nests and cords. The center of tumor nests often displays an area of hyalinization or eosinophilic debris, resembling keratinous material in a squamous cell carcinoma. Occasionally, epithelioid trophoblast tumor shows focal replacement of the surface and/or glandular epithelium with stratified neoplastic cells, simulating HSIL. A high index of suspicion, a clinical presentation in a young woman having a relatively low, but definitely elevated level of serum human chorionic gonadotropin (hCG; <2500 mIU/ml), and/or an intrauterine mass identified by ultrasound help to make a correct diagnosis. Histologically, the absence of a definite HSIL, the presence of decidualized stromal cells in the neighborhood, reactivity for a-inhibin, human placental lactogen (hPL), and cytokeratin 18 (CK18) help to confirm the diagnosis of epithelioid trophoblast tumor.

When utilizing immunohistochemical staining to distinguish between squamous cell carcinomas and other tumors it must be remembered that, although strong diffuse p16 positivity is a marker for high-risk HPV-associated neoplasia, positive immunostaining for p16 can be seen in many non-HPV-related neoplasms. Immunostaining for p63 (marker for squamous differentiation) can also be quite helpful in difficult cases. One study of 250 invasive cervical tumors found strong diffuse staining for p63 in 97% of the squamous cell carcinomas.[74] Neuroendocrine carcinomas, melanomas, and lymphomas all stained negatively for p63. Similarly, *in situ* hybridization for high-risk HPV can be a useful marker when trying to confirm that a given lesion is cervical in origin. Again it should be cautioned that, because many cervical cancers have a low number of HPV copies, a negative high-risk HPV *in situ* hybridization does not rule out that a given lesion is HPV associated.

SPECIAL CONSIDERATIONS

CERVICAL STUMP CARCINOMA

Recently supracervical or subtotal hysterectomies have come back into favor, and in the future there will be a considerable number women with a cervix post hysterectomy. The cancers that occur in the residual cervix have been referred to as 'cervical stump carcinomas.' Currently, cervical stump carcinomas account only for about 2% of all cervical cancers and occur on average about 17 years post subtotal hysterectomy.[75] The proportion of squamous cell carcinoma to adenocarcinoma, and other clinical pathologic features, resemble those of cervical carcinoma in general. However, carcinomas of the cervical stump show a worse stage profile than do cancer cases with an intact uterus.[75]

EFFECTS OF RADIOTHERAPY ON CERVICAL CARCINOMA

Biopsies are often taken during and after a course of radiotherapy to assess the response of the tumor to the treatment. The initial gross change is a decrease in tumor size. The rapidity of this change is quite variable, although most tumors will have regressed within 3 months of the cessation of treatment. During this period of regression, the tumor is initially hyperemic, then becomes necrotic. The necrotic slough separates and contraction of the underlying tissue ensues because of fibrosis.

Microscopically, the effect on cell division that radiation induces is reflected in reduced numbers of mitotic figures. Those that remain often appear even more abnormal than before radiation. At the same time, the same cells tend to exhibit better differentiation, with more abundant cytoplasm that may appear keratinized. Degenerative changes are superimposed, with hyperchromatic nuclei that are sometimes pyknotic and sometimes enlarged and bizarre in shape (Figure 11.24). Vacuolization is seen both in the cytoplasm and in the nuclei. The stroma shows a variable inflammatory infiltrate composed of both acute and chronic inflammatory cells, with fibrosis. Endothelial proliferation may be prominent and is often seen to progress to complete obliteration of the lumen of many arterioles. Areas of

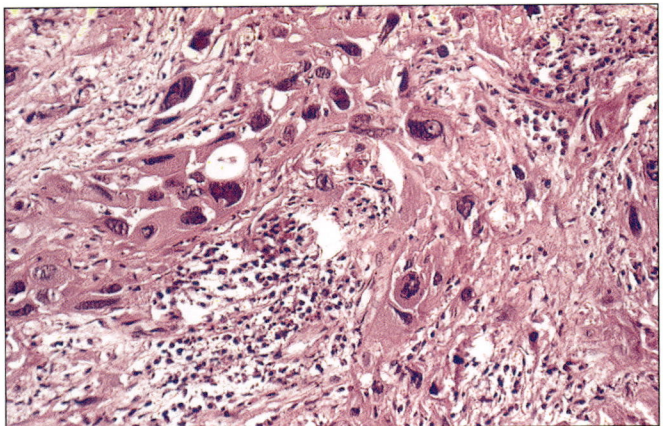

Figure 11.24 Squamous cell carcinoma with radiation change. The nuclei are enlarged, pleomorphic, and have smudged chromatin.

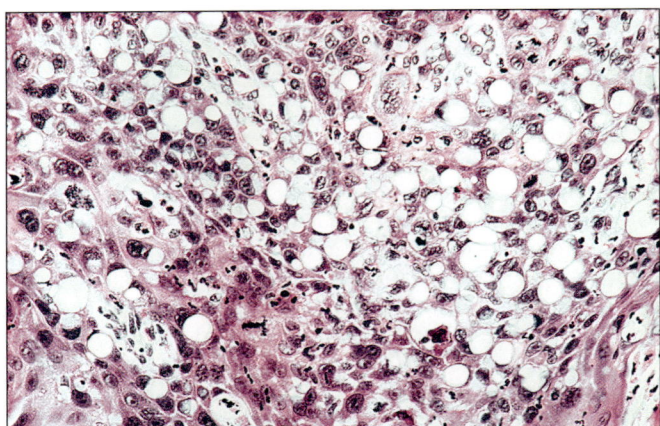

Figure 11.25 Squamous cell carcinoma with intracellular mucin. Most tumors display less mucin.

necrosis are almost universal; sometimes the biopsies consist entirely of necrotic material. Assessment should, of course, be made on the least degenerated areas.

MICROMETASTASIS

Immunohistochemical analysis is currently used for the detection of breast cancer micrometastasis in sentinel lymph nodes, and this procedure is being actively investigated as a staging procedure for cervical cancer.[76] However, the incidence and, more importantly, the clinical significance of micrometastases detected by immunohistochemical methods in cervical cancer are still being defined.[77] The term micrometastasis is used to describe small foci of metastases (0.2–2.0 mm), found only microscopically. The process of sentinel node biopsy combined with multiple sections and immunohistochemical staining with cytokeratins is sometimes referred to as 'ultrastaging.' In one recent large study of 645 patients with early stage cervical cancer, macrometastasis (>2 mm), micrometastasis (0.2–2.0 mm), and isolated tumor cells (<0.2 mm) were detected in 14.7%, 10.1%, and 4.5% of patients, respectively.[77] The presence of isolated tumor cells did not appear to have an impact on either recurrence-free survival or overall survival. However, the presence of micrometastases conveyed a similar risk as did the presence of macrometastasis. In two other studies, immunohistochemical analyses identified 8–15% of patients with lymph node micrometastasis not initially identified by H&E analysis.[78,79] These data were conflicting as to whether the patients with micrometastases did or did not have a statistically significant probability of having other high-risk factors, including LVI.

'MUCIN-SECRETING' CARCINOMA

Approximately 25–35% of carcinomas lacking definitive glandular structures have intracellular mucin demonstrable with the use of mucin stains. Some have named this as 'mucin-secreting squamous cell carcinoma,' or sometimes 'mucoepidermoid carcinoma' (Figure 11.25). It has been suggested that these tumors are slightly more aggressive than the typical squamous cell carcinoma, but this has not been borne out uniformly.[80,81] In the absence of any substantial information indicating that these tumors have a significantly different clinical pathologic behavior from the typical squamous carcinoma, these lesions are not classified as a distinct entity. For this reason, we see no value in the routine staining for mucin in invasive squamous cell carcinomas to identify these tumors.

HISTOLOGIC VARIANTS

VERRUCOUS SQUAMOUS CELL CARCINOMA

Verrucous squamous cell carcinoma is a rare variant of well-differentiated squamous cell carcinoma that can be confused with the more common papillary squamous cell carcinoma. It occurs preferentially in older women, and is found anywhere throughout the lower genital tract or perivulvar regions.[82] Only a small number of cases of verrucous carcinoma of the cervix have been described in the literature. These tumors were previously referred to as giant condyloma acuminatum of Buschke and Lowenstein. Unlike other cervical carcinomas, these tumors can be associated with either low-risk or high-risk types of HPV.[83] Clinically they are usually large, bulky, and exophytic but sometimes are warty, fungating, or even ulcerated. Their deceptively benign cytologic features distinguish them from more common forms of invasive squamous cell carcinoma. Verrucous squamous cell carcinoma typically grows slowly in size, encroaching on adjoining structures. On sectioning, the sessile tumor commonly invades into the stroma at its base, but the deep margin characteristically is broad and sharply circumscribed. As the tumor invades along a wide front in a 'pushing' fashion, it keeps a well-defined deep margin.

The high degree of differentiation of verrucous carcinoma is striking on both low- and high-power microscopic examination. Other than for its immense bulk and the fact that it can recur, the cells are so well differentiated that they often appear benign, or at most only slightly atypical (Figure 11.26). Not infrequently, it is misdiagnosed initially as a condyloma, hence the name 'verrucous.' The atypia is also

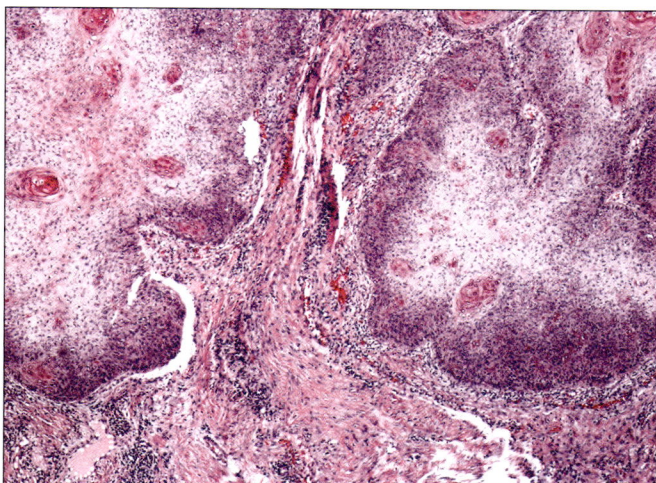

Figure 11.26 Verrucous carcinoma.

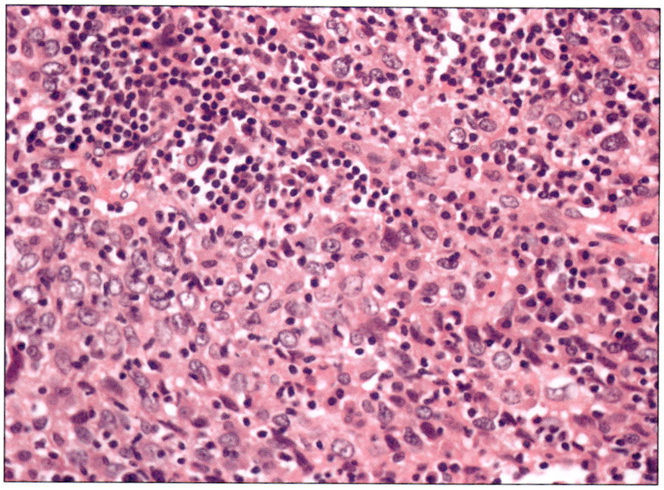

minimal in the basal layers adjacent to the basement membrane. The tumor base shows pushing nests of tumor extending into the stroma and typically surrounded by a dense stromal inflammatory infiltrate. Laminated keratin whorls are sometimes present within the epithelium. Mitotic activity is low, and if present it is usually confined to the basal cells. An accurate diagnosis can only be made if the biopsy is sufficiently large to include the base of the lesion as well as the more superficial, well-differentiated, keratotic areas. The correct diagnosis is impossible if only the surface layers are examined. While the tumor rarely metastasizes, obviating the need for lymphadenectomy, local recurrences are common and occasionally the tumor can be deeply invasive and extend into the adjacent pelvic tissues. Rarely it pursues a relentless course manifested by uncontrolled local recurrence.

WARTY SQUAMOUS CELL CARCINOMA

Warty carcinoma is a well-differentiated variant of squamous cell carcinoma that has marked condylomatous features.[42] These tumors are distinguished from verrucous carcinomas by the fact that the tumor cells in the lower portion of the epithelium resemble typical squamous cell carcinomas. They are typically associated with high-risk HPV genotypes. Koilocytes, which are rarely found on cervical cytology when women have typical squamous cell carcinomas, are often seen in women with warty carcinoma.[84]

PAPILLARY SQUAMOUS CELL CARCINOMA

These are another rare variant of squamous cell carcinoma that resemble a transitional cell carcinoma of the bladder.[85] The tumor consists of papillae with fibrovascular cores covered by several layers of atypical epithelial cells that in many instances resemble HSIL, but in other instances the cells are oval with their long axis perpendicular to the surface and resemble transitional cells.[86] The importance of these lesions is that, like verrucous carcinomas, the invasive nature of the lesion is frequently not recognized with superficial biopsies. Papillary squamous cell carcinomas can be distinguished from warty squamous cell carcinomas by their lack of koilocytosis and minimal keratinization.

Figure 11.27 Lymphoepithelioma.

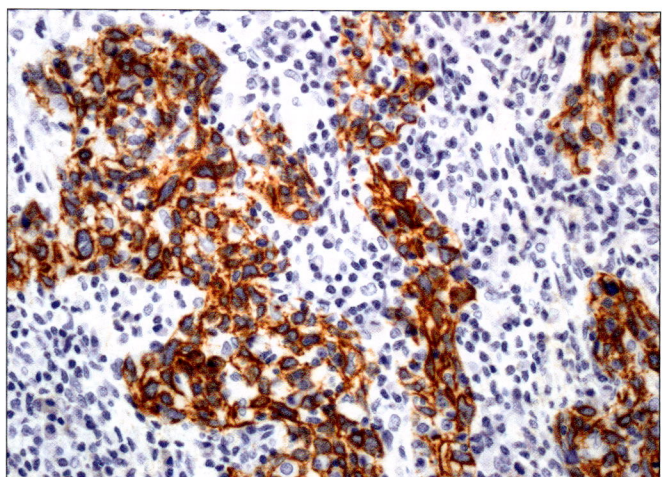

Figure 11.28 Lymphoepithelioma. The squamous component reacts with cytokeratin.

LYMPHOEPITHELIOMA-LIKE SQUAMOUS CELL CARCINOMA

Lymphoepithelial carcinoma has a histologic appearance similar to that of nasopharyngeal lymphoepithelioma-like squamous cell carcinomas. They exhibit malignant squamous cells enveloped in an intense stromal chronic inflammatory infiltrate (Figure 11.27). The cells have moderate cytoplasm, and often vesicular nuclei with prominent nucleoli.[87] The epithelial nature of the tumor is obvious when the cells are aggregated into nests or examined for cytokeratin filaments (Figure 11.28), but, when scattered in small clusters or even individual cells, differentiation from lymphoma can be difficult. This tumor is rare in Caucasian women, but has been described more commonly in Japanese women. The Epstein–Barr virus, which is common in this tumor when in the nasopharynx, has not been identified in most cases from the cervix and most cervical tumors are associated with HPV.[82,88] The frequency of nodal metastasis is low and the prognosis is generally favorable.[89]

PAPILLARY SQUAMOTRANSITIONAL CELL CARCINOMA

This is another rare form of cervical cancer that is reported to be essentially indistinguishable from similar tumors occurring in the urinary bladder.[90] The tumors have a tendency to present at advanced stage and tend to be recurrent and have metastases. The finding of HPV 16 in many tumors, the finding that they may show allelic loss at chromosome 3p, and the fact they are uroplakin III negative suggest that these tumors are cervical, as opposed to urinary bladder, in origin.[91] Grossly, the tumor size may range from 0.7 to 6 cm, and the clinical stages may range from intraepithelial to IIIB. Microscopically, the prominent features are a papillary architecture with fibrovascular cores lined by a multilayered, atypical epithelium that is predominantly squamous, mixed squamous, and transitional, or predominantly transitional, and resembles a HSIL of the cervix.[92] Nearly all tumors are immunoreactive for CK7 and about 10% are reactive for CK20.[90] These potentially aggressive malignant tumors need to be distinguished from the far more common and benign papillary lesions of the cervix. An additional consideration in the differential diagnosis of such neoplasms includes villoglandular carcinomas of the cervix. However, unlike papillary squamotransitional cell carcinomas, villoglandular lesions, as the name implies, are stratified columnar adenocarcinomas without any squamous features.

REFERENCES

1. Burden of cervical cancer globally. WHO/ICO Information Center on HPV and Cervical Cancer 2011.
2. American Cancer Society. Cancer facts & figures. http://www.cancer.org/acs/groups/content/@epidemiologysurveilance/documents/document/acspc-031941.pdf, 2012 [accessed 24.07.12].
3. SEER. Cancer statistics. Bethesda, MD: National Cancer Institute. http://seer.cancer.gov/ [accessed 01.03.11].
4. Miller AB, Knight J, Narod S. The natural history of cancer of the cervix and the implications for screening policy. In: Miller AB, Chamberlain J, Day NE, et al, editors. Cancer screening. Cambridge, UK: Cambridge University Press; 1991. p. 141–52.
5. Leyden WA, Manos MM, Geiger AM, et al. Cervical cancer in women with comprehensive health care access: attributable factors in the screening process. J Natl Cancer Inst 2005;97:675–83.
6. Andrae B, Kemetli L, Sparen P, et al. Screening-preventable cervical cancer risks: evidence from a nationwide audit in Sweden. J Natl Cancer Inst 2008;100:622–9.
7. Pecorelli S. Revised FIGO staging for carcinoma of the vulva, cervix, and endometrium. Int J Gynaecol Obstet 2009;105:103–4.
8. Tavassoli FA, Devilee P, editors. Pathology and genetics of tumours of the breast and female genital organs. Lyons, France: IARC Press; 2003.
9. Smith HO, Tiffany MF, Qualls CR, Key CR. The rising incidence of adenocarcinoma relative to squamous cell carcinoma of the uterine cervix in the United States—a 24-year population-based study. Gynecol Oncol 2000;78:97–105.
10. Vizcaino AP, Moreno V, Bosch FX, et al. International trends in incidence of cervical cancer: II. Squamous-cell carcinoma. Int J Cancer 2000;86:429–35.
11. Cairns M, Cruickshank M. A review of women with microinvasive cervical cancer in the Grampian region. J Low Genit Tract Dis 2007;11:290–3.
12. Mobius G. Cytological early detection of cervical carcinoma: possibilities and limitations. Analysis of failures. J Cancer Res Clin Oncol 1993;119:513–21.
13. Kohlberger P, Edwards L, Hacker NF. Microinvasive squamous cell carcinoma of the cervix: immunohistochemically detected prognostic factors in a case with poor clinical outcome. Gynecol Oncol 2003;90:443–5.
14. Raspagliesi F, Ditto A, Quattrone P, et al. Prognostic factors in microinvasive cervical squamous cell cancer: long-term results. Int J Gynecol Cancer 2005;15:88–93.
15. Sedlis A, Sall S, Tsukada Y, et al. Microinvasive carcinoma of the uterine cervix: a clinical-pathologic study. Am J Obstet Gynecol 1979;133:64–74.
16. Bohm JW, Krupp PJ, Lee FY, Batson HW. Lymph node metastasis in microinvasive epidermoid cancer of the cervix. Obstet Gynecol 1976;48:65–7.
17. Copeland LJ, Silva EG, Gershenson DM, et al. Superficially invasive squamous cell carcinoma of the cervix. Gynecol Oncol 1992;45:307–12.
18. Attanoos R, Nahar K, Bigrigg A, et al. Primary adenocarcinoma of the cervix. A clinicalpathologic study of prognostic variables in 55 cases. Int J Gynecol Cancer 1995;5:179–86.
19. Ehrmann RL, Dwyer IM, Yavner D, Hancock WW. An immunoperoxidase study of laminin and type IV collagen distribution in carcinoma of the cervix and vulva. Obstet Gynecol 1988;72:257–62.
20. Hasumi K, Sakamoto A, Sugano H. Microinvasive carcinoma of the uterine cervix. Cancer 1980;45:928–31.
21. Maiman M, Fruchter RG, DiMaio TM, Boyce JG. Superficially invasive squamous cell carcinoma of the cervix. Obstet Gynecol 1988;72:399–403.
22. Morgan PR, Anderson MC, Buckley CH, et al. The Royal College of Obstetricians and Gynaecologists micro-invasive carcinoma of the cervix study: preliminary results. Br J Obstet Gynaecol 1993;100:664–8.
23. Simon NL, Gore H, Shingleton HM, et al. Study of superficially invasive carcinoma of the cervix. Obstet Gynecol 1986;68:19–24.
24. van Nagell JR, Greenwell N, Powell DF, et al. Microinvasive carcinoma of the cervix. Am J Obstet Gynecol 1983;145:981–91.
25. Sevin BU, Nadji M, Averette HE, et al. Microinvasive carcinoma of the cervix. Cancer 1992;70:2121–8.
26. Burghardt E, Holzer E. Diagnosis and treatment of microinvasive carcinoma of the cervix uteri. Obstet Gynecol 1977;49:641–53.
27. Takeshima N, Yanoh K, Tabata T, et al. Assessment of the revised International Federation of Gynecology and obstetrics staging for early invasive squamous cervical cancer. Gynecol Oncol 1999;74:165–9.
28. Darragh TM, Colgan TJ, Cox JT, et al. The Lower Anogenital Squamous Terminology Standardization Project for HPV-Associated Lesions: background and consensus recommendations from the College of American Pathologists and the American Society for Colposcopy and Cervical Pathology. Arch Pathol Lab Med 2012;136:1266–97.
29. Roche WD, Norris HJ. Microinvasive carcinoma of the cervix. The significance of lymphatic invasion ans confluent patterns of stromal growth. Cancer 1975;36:180–6.
30. Benedet JL, Anderson GH. Stage IA carcinoma of the cervix revisited. Obstet Gynecol 1996;87:1052–9.
31. Marana HR, de Andrade JM, Matthes AC, et al. Microinvasive carcinoma of the cervix. Analysis of prognostic factors. Eur J Gynaecol Oncol 2001;22:64–6.
32. Witkiewicz AK, Wright TC, Ferenczy A, et al. Carcinoma and other tumors of the cervix. In: Kurman RJ, Hedrick Ellenson L, Ronnett BM, editors. Blaustein's pathology of the female genital tract. 6th ed. New York: Springer; 2011. p. 254–95.
33. Ostor AG, Rome RM. Micro-invasive squamous cell carcinoma of the cervix: A clinico-pathologic study of 200 cases with long-term follow-up. Int J Gynecol Cancer 1994;4:257–64.

34. Bean SM, Kurtycz DF, Colgan TJ. Recent developments in defining microinvasive and early invasive carcinoma of the uterine cervix. J Low Genit Tract Dis 2011;15:146–57.
35. Wells M, Ostor AG, Franceschi S, et al. Epithelial tumors of the uterine cervix. In: Tavassoli FA, Devilee P, editors. Tumors of the breast and female genital organs. Lyons, France: IARC Press; 2003. p. 221–32.
36. Morgan PR, Anderson MC, Buckley CH, et al. The Royal College of Obstetricians and Gyneecologists micro-invasive carcinoma of the cervix study: preliminary results. Br J Obstet Gynaecol 1993;100:664–8.
37. Rush D, Hyjek E, Baergen RN, et al. Detection of microinvasion in vulvar and cervical intraepithelial neoplasia using double immunostaining for cytokeratin and basement membrane components. Arch Pathol Lab Med 2005;129:747–53.
38. Solomon D, Davey D, Kurman R, et al. The 2001 Bethesda System: terminology for reporting results of cervical cytology. JAMA 2002;287:2114–19.
39. Kolstad P. Follow-up study of 232 patients with stage IA1 and 411 patients with stage IA2 squamous cell carcinoma of the cervix (microinvasive carcinoma). Gynecol Oncol 1989;33:265–72.
40. Morris M, Mitchell MF, Silva EG, et al. Cervical conization as definitive therapy for early invasive squamous carcinoma of the cervix. Gynecol Oncol 1993;51:193–6.
41. Gadducci A, Sartori E, Maggino T, et al. The clinical outcome of patients with stage Ia1 and Ia2 squamous cell carcinoma of the uterine cervix: a Cooperation Task Force (CTF) study. Eur J Gynaecol Oncol 2003;24:513–16.
42. Kurman RJ, Toki T, Schiffman MH. Basaloid and warty carcinomas of the vulva. Distinctive types of squamous cell carcinoma frequently associated with human papillomaviruses. Am J Surg Pathol 1993;17:133–45.
43. Grayson W, Cooper K. A reappraisal of "basaloid carcinoma" of the cervix, and the differential diagnosis of basaloid cervical neoplasms. Adv Anat Pathol 2002;9:290–300.
44. Zaino RJ, Ward S, Delgado G, et al. Histopathologic predictors of the behavior of surgically treated stage IB squamous cell carcinoma of the cervix. Cancer 1992;69:1750–8.
45. Quinn MA, Benedet JL, Odicino F, et al. Carcinoma of the cervix uteri. FIGO 26th Annual Report on the Results of Treatment in Gynecological Cancer. Int J Gynaecol Obstet 2006;95(Suppl 1):S43–103.
46. Nguyen HN, Averette HE. Biology of cervical carcinoma. Semin Surg Oncol 1999;16:212–16.
47. Takeshima N, Katase K, Hirai Y, et al. Prognostic value of peritoneal cytology in patients with carcinoma of the uterine cervix. Gynecol Oncol 1997;64:136–40.
48. Delgado G, Bundy B, Zaino R, et al. Prospective surgical-pathological study of disease-free interval in patients with stage IB squamous cell carcinoma of the cervix: a Gynecolgic Oncology Group study. Gynecol Oncol 1990;38:352–7.
49. Kristensen GB, Abeler VM, Risberg B, et al. Tumor size, depth of invasion, and grading of the invasive tumor front are the main prognostic factors in early squamous cell cervical cancer. Gynecol Oncol 1999;74:245–51.
50. Delgado G. Lymphovascular space involvement in cervical cancer: an independent risk factor. Gynecol Oncol 1998;68:219.
51. Roman LD, Felix JC, Muderspach LI, et al. Influence of quantity of lymph-vascular space invasion on the risk of nodal metastases in women with early-stage squamous cancer of the cervix. Gynecol Oncol 1998;68:220–5.
52. Zhang Y, Yan M, He J, et al. Significant effects of lymph and blood vascular invasion on the prognosis of early-stage cervical squamous cell carcinoma. J Obstet Gynaecol Res 2010;36:1015–22.
53. Okazawa M, Mabuchi S, Isohashi F, et al. The prognostic significance of multiple pelvic node metastases in cervical cancer patients treated with radical hysterectomy plus adjuvant chemoradiotherapy. Int J Gynecol Cancer 2012;22:490–7.
54. Fyles AW, Pintilie M, Kirkbride P, et al. Prognostic factors in patients with cervix cancer treated by radiation therapy: results of a multiple regression analysis. Radiother Oncol 1995;35:107–17.
55. Pickel H, Haas J, Lahousen M. Prognostic factors in cervical cancer. Eur J Obstet Gynecol Reprod Biol 1997;71:209–13.
56. Lambin P, Kramar A, Haie-Meder C, et al. Tumour size in cancer of the cervix. Acta Oncol 1998;37:729–34.
57. Finan MA, DeCesare S, Fiorica JV, et al. Radical hysterectomy for stage IB1 vs IB2 carcinoma of the cervix: does the new staging system predict morbidity and survival? Gynecol Oncol 1996;62:139–47.
58. Kinney WK, Hodge DO, Egorshin EV, et al. Identification of a low-risk subset of patients with stage IB invasive squamous cancer of the cervix possibly suited to less radical surgical treatment. Gynecol Oncol 1995;57:3–6.
59. Zhang SQ, Yu H, Zhang LL. Clinical implications of increased lymph vessel density in the lymphatic metastasis of early-stage invasive cervical carcinoma: a clinical immunohistochemical method study. BMC Cancer 2009;9:64.
60. Gombos Z, Xu X, Chu CS, et al. Peritumoral lymphatic vessel density and vascular endothelial growth factor C expression in early-stage squamous cell carcinoma of the uterine cervix. Clin Cancer Res 2005;11:8364–71.
61. Loncaster JA, Cooper RA, Logue JP, et al. Vascular endothelial growth factor (VEGF) expression is a prognostic factor for radiotherapy outcome in advanced carcinoma of the cervix. Br J Cancer 2000;83:620–5.
62. Cheng WF, Chen CA, Lee CN, et al. Vascular endothelial growth factor and prognosis of cervical carcinoma. Obstet Gynecol 2000;96:721–6.
63. Randall LM, Monk BJ, Darcy KM, et al. Markers of angiogenesis in high-risk, early-stage cervical cancer: a Gynecologic Oncology Group study. Gynecol Oncol 2009;112:583–9.
64. de Sanjose S, Quint WG, Alemany L, et al. Human papillomavirus genotype attribution in invasive cervical cancer: a retrospective cross-sectional worldwide study. Lancet Oncol 2010;11:1048–56.
65. Lai CH, Chang CJ, Huang HJ, et al. Role of human papillomavirus genotype in prognosis of early-stage cervical cancer undergoing primary surgery. J Clin Oncol 2007;25:3628–34.
66. Schwartz SM, Daling JR, Shera KA, et al. Human papillomavirus and prognosis of invasive cervical cancer: a population-based study. J Clin Oncol 2001;19:1906–15.
67. Lombard I, Vincent-Salomon A, Validire P, et al. Human papillomavirus genotype as a major determinant of the course of cervical cancer. J Clin Oncol 1998;16:2613–19.
68. Baykal C, Ayhan A, Al A, Yuce K. Overexpression of the c-Met/HGF receptor and its prognostic significance in uterine cervix carcinomas. Gynecol Oncol 2003;88:123–9.
69. Kim GE, Kim YB, Cho NH, et al. Synchronous coexpression of epidermal growth factor receptor and cyclooxygenase-2 in carcinomas of the uterine cervix: a potential predictor of poor survival. Clin Cancer Res 2004;10:1366–74.
70. Goff BA, Sallin J, Garcia R, et al. Evaluation of p27 in preinvasive and invasive malignancies of the cervix. Gynecol Oncol 2003;88:40–4.
71. Skomedal H, Kristensen GB, Lie AK, Holm R. Aberrant expression of the cell cycle associated proteins TP53, MDM2, p21, p27, cdk4, cyclin D1, RB, and EGFR in cervical carcinomas. Gynecol Oncol 1999;73:223–8.
72. Kersemaekers AM, Fleuren GJ, Kenter GG, et al. Oncogene alterations in carcinomas of the uterine cervix: overexpression of the epidermal growth factor receptor is associated with poor prognosis. Clin Cancer Res 1999;5:577–86.
73. Fadare O, Parkash V, Carcangiu ML, Hui P. Epithelioid trophoblastic tumor: clinicopathological features with an emphasis on uterine cervical involvement. Mod Pathol 2006;19:75–82.
74. Wang TY, Chen BF, Yang YC, et al. Histologic and immunophenotypic classification of cervical carcinomas by expression of the p53 homologue p63: a study of 250 cases. Hum Pathol 2001;32:479–86.
75. Hellstrom AC, Hellman K, Pettersson BF, Andersson S. Carcinoma of the cervical stump: fifty years of experience. Oncol Rep 2011;25:1651–4.
76. Darlin L, Persson J, Bossmar T, et al. The sentinel node concept in early cervical cancer performs well in tumors smaller than 2 cm. Gynecol Oncol 2010;117:266–9.
77. Cibula D, Abu-Rustum NR, Dusek L, et al. Prognostic significance of low volume sentinel lymph node disease in early-stage cervical cancer. Gynecol Oncol 2012;124:496–501.
78. Juretzka MM, Jensen KC, Longacre TA, et al. Detection of pelvic lymph node micrometastasis in stage IA2-IB2 cervical cancer by immunohistochemical analysis. Gynecol Oncol 2004;93:107–11.

79. Lentz SE, Muderspach LI, Felix JC, et al. Identification of micrometastases in histologically negative lymph nodes of early-stage cervical cancer patients. Obstet Gynecol 2004;103:1204–10.
80. Samlal RA, Ten Kate FJ, Hart AA, Lammes FB. Do mucin-secreting squamous cell carcinomas of the uterine cervix metastasize more frequently to pelvic lymph nodes? A case-control study? Int J Gynecol Pathol 1998;17:201–4.
81. Husniye Dilek F, Kucukali T. Mucin production in carcinomas of the uterine cervix. Eur J Obstet Gynecol Reprod Biol 1998;79:149–51.
82. Wong WS, Ng CS, Lee CK. Verrucous carcinoma of the cervix. Arch Gynecol Obstet 1990;247:47–51.
83. Frega A, Lukic A, Nobili F, et al. Verrucous carcinoma of the cervix: detection of carcinogenetic human papillomavirus types and their role during follow-up. Anticancer Res 2007;27:4491–4.
84. Ng WK, Cheung LK, Li AS. Warty (condylomatous) carcinoma of the cervix. A review of 3 cases with emphasis on thin-layer cytology and molecular analysis for HPV. Acta Cytol 2003;47:159–66.
85. Brinck U, Jakob C, Bau O, Fuzesi L. Papillary squamous cell carcinoma of the uterine cervix: report of three cases and a review of its classification. Int J Gynecol Pathol 2000;19:231–5.
86. Odida M. Papillary squamous cell carcinoma of the cervix in Uganda: a report of 20 cases. Afr Health Sci 2005;5:291–4.
87. Reich O, Pickel H, Purstner P. Exfoliative cytology of a lymphoepithelioma-like carcinoma in a cervical smear. A case report. Acta Cytol 1999;43:285–8.
88. Martorell MA, Julian JM, Calabuig C, et al. Lymphoepithelioma-like carcinoma of the uterine cervix. Arch Pathol Lab Med 2002;126:1501–5.
89. Kaul R, Gupta N, Sharma J, Gupta S. Lymphoepithelioma-like carcinoma of the uterine cervix. J Cancer Res Ther 2009;5:300–1.
90. Koenig C, Turnicky RP, Kankam CF, Tavassoli FA. Papillary squamotransitional cell carcinoma of the cervix: a report of 32 cases. Am J Surg Pathol 1997;21:915–21.
91. Maitra A, Wistuba II, Gibbons D, et al. Allelic losses at chromosome 3p are seen in human papilloma virus 16 associated transitional cell carcinoma of the cervix. Gynecol Oncol 1999;74:361–8.
92. Kokka F, Verma M, Singh N, et al. Papillary squamotransitional cell carcinoma of the uterine cervix: report of three cases and review of the literature. Pathology 2006;38:584–6.

Cervical Glandular Neoplasia

Emanuela D'Angelo, Jaime Prat

CHAPTER OUTLINE

Preinvasive Glandular Lesions	251	Villoglandular Adenocarcinoma	265
Adenocarcinoma *In Situ*	251	Endometrioid Adenocarcinoma	267
Adenocarcinoma	257	Minimal Deviation Adenocarcinoma, Endometrioid Type	267
Microinvasive (Early Invasive) Adenocarcinoma	257	Clear Cell Adenocarcinoma	267
Invasive Adenocarcinoma	259	Serous Adenocarcinoma	268
Adenocarcinoma, Usual-type	259	Mesonephric Adenocarcinoma	269
Mucinous Adenocarcinoma, Intestinal-type	262	Adenosquamous Carcinoma	270
Mucinous Adenocarcinoma, Signet-Ring Cell-type	262	Glassy Cell Carcinoma	271
Mucinous Adenocarcinoma Gastric-type (Minimal Deviation Adenocarcinoma)	263		

PREINVASIVE GLANDULAR LESIONS

Terminology

In keeping with the terminology used for squamous cervical intraepithelial neoplasia (CIN), earlier investigators recognized three grades of cervical glandular intraepithelial neoplasia (CGIN),[1] but this has proven unrealistic. Three grades (glandular atypia, glandular dysplasia, and atypical hyperplasia), with only subtle differences among them, are not reproducible, and far less so than for corresponding squamous lesions. Even squamous intraepithelial lesions, in the Bethesda System, for example, are grouped into two categories for this reason.[2] A more practical approach is to divide the spectrum of glandular changes into two grades. These are variously referred to as low-grade CGIN and high-grade CGIN, or endocervical glandular dysplasia and adenocarcinoma *in situ* (AIS).[3]

The 2003 World Health Organization (WHO) classification included, among the precursors of invasive cervical adenocarcinoma, glandular dysplasia and AIS; however, their morphologic distinction remains unclear.[4] Endocervical glandular dysplasia (atypical hyperplasia) refers to 'glandular lesions characterized by significant nuclear abnormalities that are more striking than those in glandular atypia but fall short of the criteria for adenocarcinoma *in situ*.'[4] In other words, glandular dysplasia closely resembles AIS but differs in that the nuclei are not cytologically malignant and mitoses are less numerous. However, because of its rarity, the lack of diagnostic reproducibility, and the uncommon coexistence with AIS, the clinical and biologic significance of glandular dysplasia has not been established.[5] Among the biomarkers used to clarify the relationship between glandular dysplasia and AIS are p16^{INK4A}, Ki-67/MIB1, and human papillomavirus (HPV) DNA determination, but results have been controversial.[6–8] Besides, the relationship of HPV infection to glandular precursors differs from that of HPV and squamous precursor lesions. Whereas productive HPV infection is represented morphologically by low-grade squamous intraepithelial lesion (LSIL; mild dysplasia), a comparable lesion does not occur in glandular epithelium. Thus, it appears that productive HPV infection is closely associated with squamous but not glandular epithelium. Rather than using the term glandular dysplasia, it has been recommended to evaluate the atypical glandular lesions that fall short of AIS with p16^{INK4A} and Ki-67/MIB1.[6,7] Lesions negative for p16^{INK4A} and showing a low Ki-67/MIB1 proliferation index should be diagnosed as reparative changes; on the other hand, lesions expressing a strong and diffuse p16^{INK4A} immunoreaction and a high Ki-67/MIB1 labeling index should be classified as AIS.

ADENOCARCINOMA *IN SITU*

Definition

AIS is characterized by replacement of glandular epithelium by cytologically malignant epithelial cells with preservation of the glandular architecture. Involvement of more than one gland is required for the diagnosis.[9,10]

Etiology

The evidence in favor of AIS being a precursor lesion for invasive adenocarcinoma includes the following: (1) patients with AIS are about 10–15 years younger than those with invasive adenocarcinoma, (2) AIS is commonly found in the vicinity of invasive adenocarcinoma, (3) similar HPV types are identified in both AIS and invasive adenocarcinoma,[11] and (4) occasional cases of AIS have been documented to progress to adenocarcinoma.[12]

General Features

AIS represents 10–20% of cervical adenocarcinomas.[13] Compared to high-grade squamous intraepithelial lesions (HSILs), AIS is much less common, with reported ratios varying from 1:26 to 1:237.[14,15] In the Surveillance, Epidemiology and End Results (SEER) registry, of 121,793 (82%) cervical lesions classified as in situ, 120,317 (99%) were squamous cell carcinoma in situ (CIS) and only 1476 (1%) were AIS.[14] In contrast to squamous cervical lesions, the incidence of invasive glandular lesions is higher than that of noninvasive glandular lesions.[16] The median age at diagnosis in a recent large series was 35 years compared with 41 years for women with invasive adenocarcinoma.[17] Most AIS are asymptomatic and found in patients with abnormal cervical smears. AIS does not produce a grossly visible lesion, nor does it have a characteristic lesion like SIL by colposcopy. It involves both the surface and glands of the transformation zone in 65% of cases and is predominantly unifocal.[13,18] It can extend for a distance of up to 3 cm into the endocervical canal.[18] SIL or invasive squamous cell carcinoma coexists with AIS in 24–75% of cases and the exfoliated atypical cells lead to clinical investigation helping to identify AIS.[19] Most AIS are associated with HPV DNA and HPV 16 and 18 are the most commonly encountered types.[20]

Pathology

Microscopically, AIS spreads along the surface of the endocervix and does not extend below normal glands. There is neither stromal invasion nor desmoplasia. Part or all of the epithelium lining the glands shows nuclear stratification with elongated, cigar-shaped, hyperchromatic nuclei and increased mitotic activity. Based on cytoplasmic features, four subtypes of AIS have been described: (1) endocervical or mucinous type, (2) intestinal type, (3) endometrioid type, and (4) adenosquamous type. In addition, rare examples of clear cell[21] and tubal type have been described. Although these histologic types do not have biologic significance, their distinction helps the pathologist to recognize AIS.

The most common form of AIS is the endocervical type,[22] in which the cells resemble those of the endocervix, and glands show nuclear pseudostratification, nuclear atypia, small to moderate amounts of juxtaluminal cytoplasm containing mucin, scattered juxtaluminal mitoses (normal and/or abnormal), and apoptotic bodies (Figures 12.1–12.5).[22,23] Typically, there is a sharp demarcation of AIS from closely uninvolved glands and from the uninvolved epithelium of the same gland (Figure 12.6). The glands of AIS can show numerous outpouchings and complex papillary infoldings and may exhibit a cribriform pattern. Intestinal-type AIS, a form of intestinal metaplasia, is characterized by the presence of goblet cells (Figure 12.7). Occasionally,

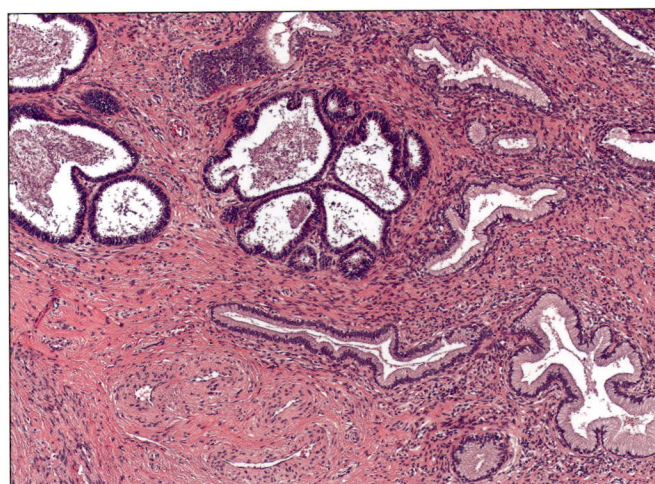

Figure 12.1 AIS compared with normal glands. The glands involved by AIS show little mucin in comparison to normal endocervical glands.

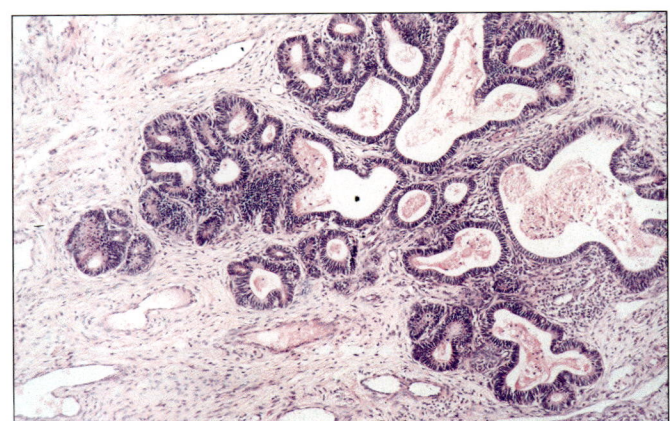

Figure 12.2 AIS. Clusters of glands involved by AIS

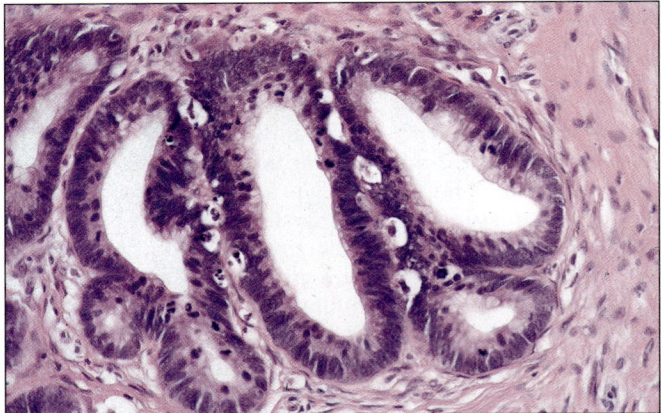

Figure 12.3 AIS endocervical type with numerous mitoses and apoptosis.

neuroendocrine cells, which are argentaffin positive, and even Paneth cells may also be present.[22] Nuclear atypia is not as evident because the mucin globules compress the nuclei, reducing the degree of nuclear enlargement and pseudostratification. Endometrioid AIS is characterized by glands resembling proliferative or hyperplastic endometrium

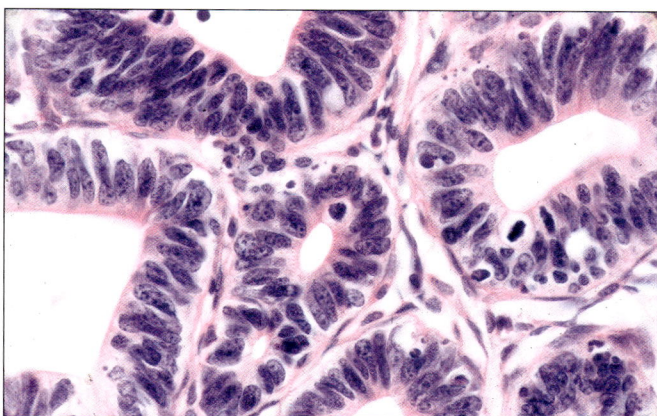

Figure 12.4 AIS. Stratification with elongated, cigar-shaped, hyperchromatic nuclei.

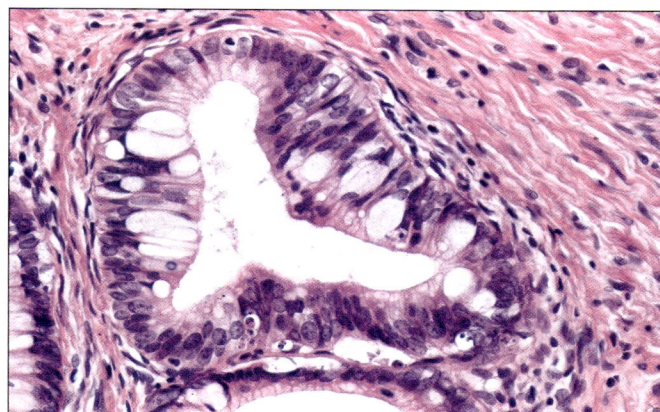

Figure 12.7 AIS, intestinal type with numerous goblet cells.

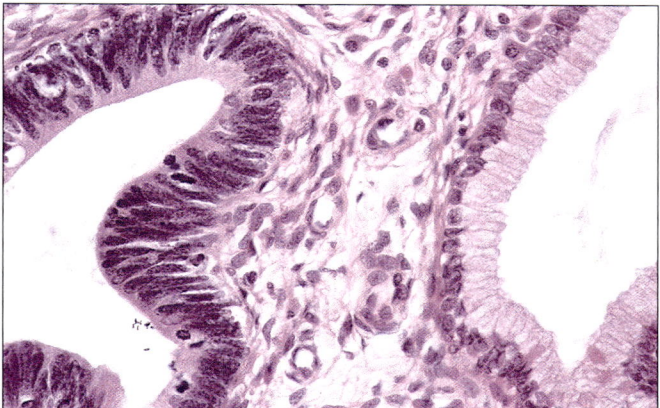

Figure 12.5 AIS compared with normal endocervical gland.

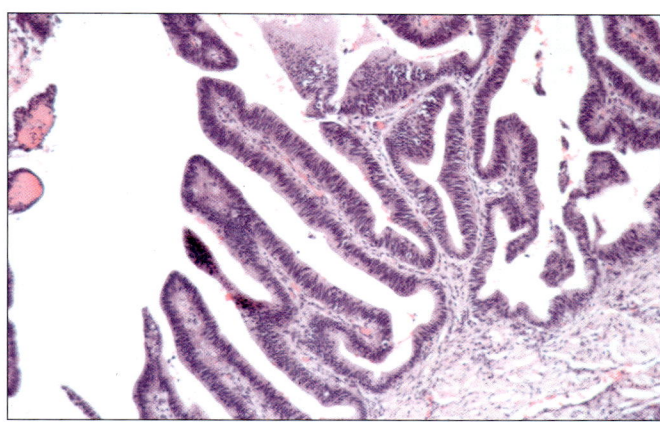

Figure 12.8 Villoglandular AIS.

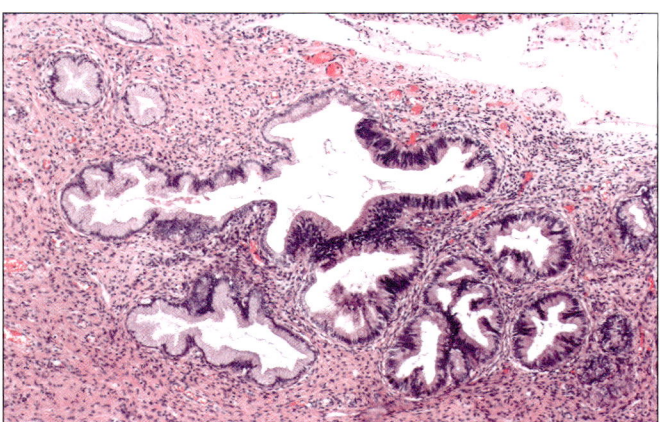

Figure 12.6 AIS. Sharp demarcation from closely uninvolved glands and from the uninvolved epithelium of the same gland.

and exhibits marked nuclear pseudostratification and absent cytoplasmic mucin or mucin staining confined to the luminal border.[22] In many ways, this distinction between endocervical and endometrioid AIS is artificial as the endometrioid features represent endocervical-type cells that have lost their intracytoplasmic mucin. Endometrioid AIS is most distinctive when it exhibits villoglandular architecture (Figure 12.8). The adenosquamous type is characterized by glands containing cells exhibiting both glandular and squamous features. It is important to distinguish adenosquamous CIS from AIS, which coexists but is separate from an adjacent HSIL. The tubal type of AIS is diagnostically challenging because of its similarity to tubal metaplasia, but the cells have pseudostratification, nuclear enlargement, coarse chromatin, apoptotic bodies, and mitotic figures.

Immunohistochemistry

Most cases of AIS show diffuse nuclear and/or cytoplasmic immunoreactivity for p16^{INK4A} (Figure 12.9) whereas normal endocervix demonstrates no reactivity.[24] Overexpression of p16^{INK4A} is induced when high-risk HPV DNA integrates into the cell genome. Another useful marker is Ki-67/MIB1. The majority of AIS cells exhibit nuclear reactivity for Ki-67 and the proliferation index is usually over 30% (Figure 12.10).[25] In contrast, p53 is expressed only focally in 20% of cases.[26] In fact, a strong p53 reaction should alert the possibility of serous carcinoma, either extending from the endometrium or as a primary endocervical tumor. Since AIS typically shows significant degrees of apoptosis, the anti-apoptotic marker bcl-2 is usually negative or only focally positive.[25,26] Possibly, Ki-67/MIB1, p16^{INK4A}, and bcl-2 may serve as

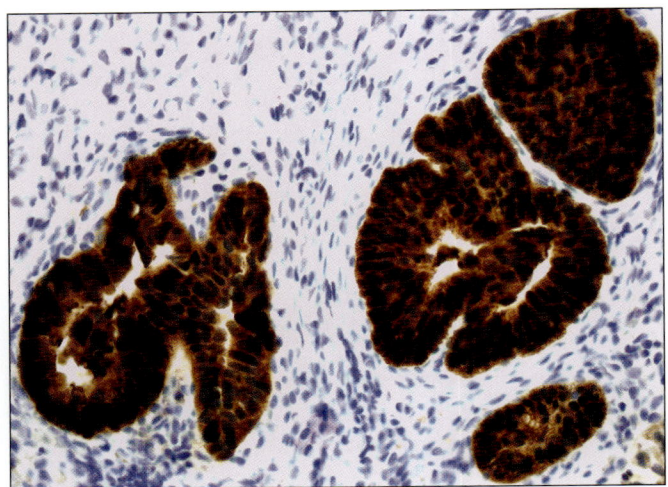

Figure 12.9 AIS. Overexpression of p16^{INK4A}.

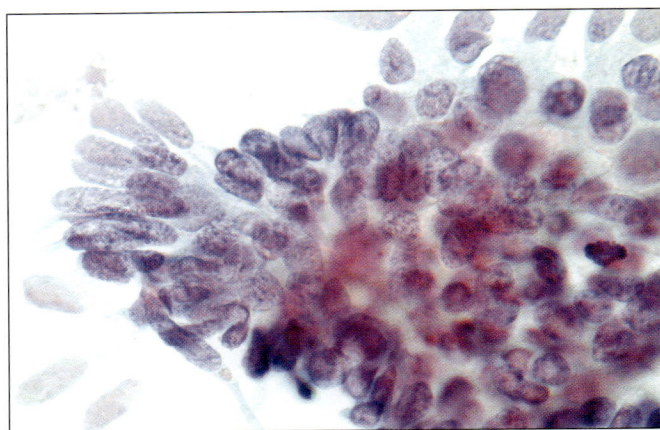

Figure 12.11 AIS, endocervical type (Pap smear). A crowded sheet with ragged edges. Hyperchromatic elongated nuclei show palisading and feathering at the edges of the sheet.

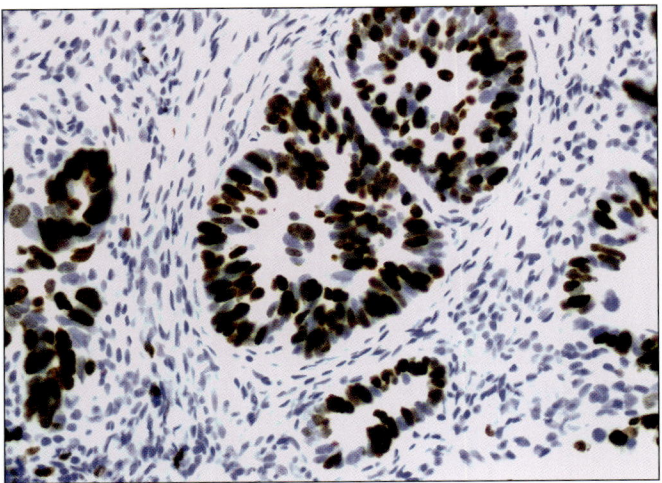

Figure 12.10 AIS. Nuclear reactivity for Ki-67.

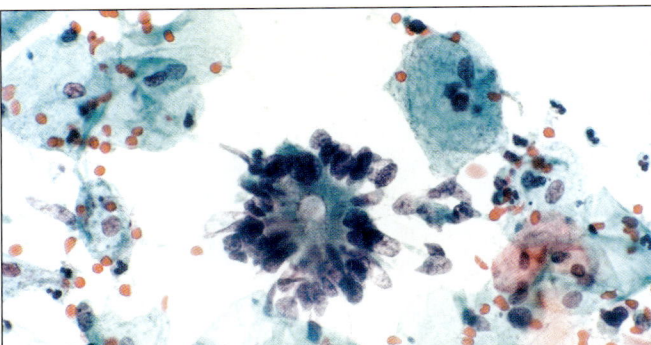

Figure 12.12 AIS, endocervical type (Pap smear). A rosette displays a central lumen and a ragged periphery.

a diagnostic panel.[25] Carcinoembryonic antigen (CEA) immunoreactivity occurs in 63–78% of AIS cases,[27,28] whereas the endocervical epithelium is either negative or shows only luminal reaction. Vimentin immunostaining is negative. As indicated earlier, accurate application of these markers may clarify whether an atypical glandular lesion is a reparative condition or a precursor to endocervical glandular malignancy. Moreover, while these ancillary tests are useful, the mainstay of diagnosis should be careful morphologic examination.[25]

Cytologic Findings

Cytologic ability to detect cervical glandular lesions is limited by both sampling and interpretation. The historical view that the Pap smear has low sensitivity for AIS is changing.[29] While relevant studies are few, emerging evidence indicates that the sensitivity of the cervical smear for detecting AIS is in the range of 40–69%.[29–32] This compares favorably with sensitivity for CIN 3, which has been reported as ranging between 43% and 75%.[31] In the 2001 Bethesda System 'AIS' became a separate category.[2] Cases showing some features suggestive but not diagnostic of AIS are 'atypical endocervical cells, favor neoplastic.' The lowest reporting category for abnormal endocervical cells is 'atypical endocervical cells, NOS' (not otherwise specified). Typical architectural features include crowded sheets of columnar cells with palisading and feathering of nuclei at group edges, pseudostratification, small strip-off sheets, and gland openings within the sheets (Figure 12.11). In addition, rosettes are also a characteristic feature (Figure 12.12). The nuclei are typically enlarged and oval shaped with coarse granular chromatin. Mitoses and apoptosis are helpful features if seen. With the use of liquid-based cytology (LBC), the cytologic appearances are different. Glandular groups with this methodology are more three-dimensional than with the usual cervical smear and show attenuation of several typical architectural features of AIS. Nuclear features are better preserved in samples collected in fluid medium.[33,34] An advantage of this new methodology is the opportunity to perform immunohistochemical stains, such as p16^{INK4A} on the original cytology samples.[24,35]

Differential Diagnosis

Several benign glandular lesions simulate AIS. The most common is tubal metaplasia, which displays in varying proportions a mixture of ciliated, secretory, and resting

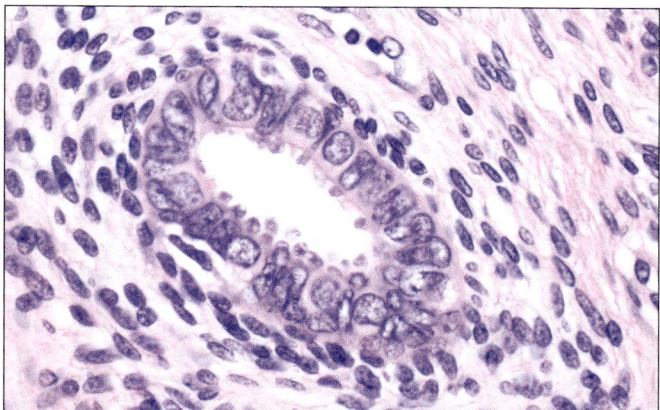

Figure 12.13 Tuboendometrioid metaplasia.

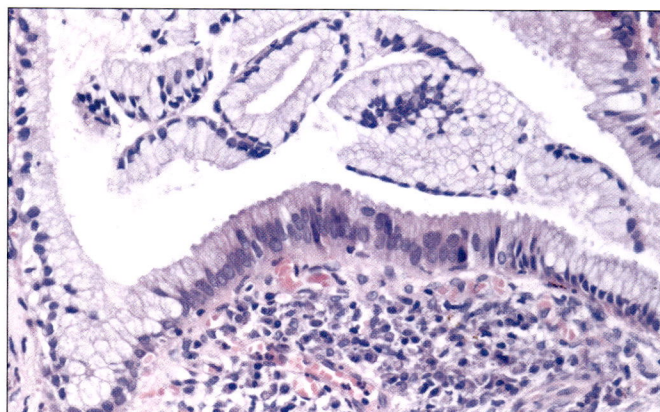

Figure 12.15 Endocervical gland showing inflammatory changes.

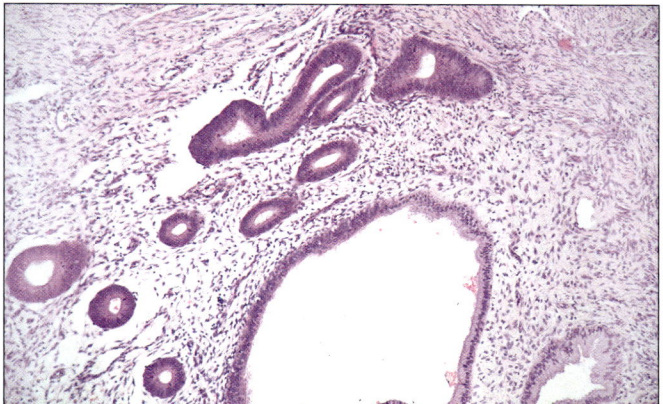

Figure 12.14 Superficial cervical endometriosis.

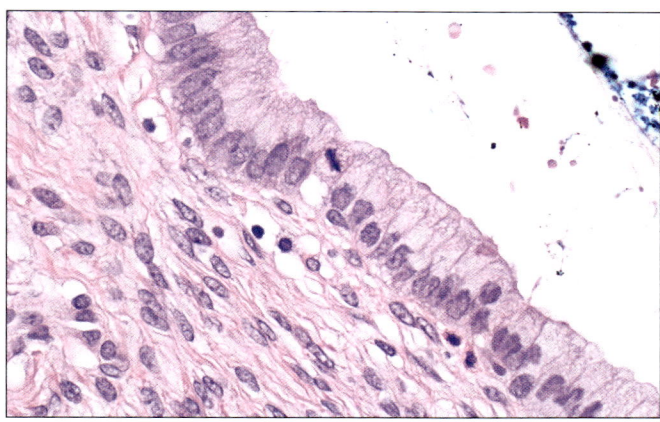

Figure 12.16 Normal endocervical gland showing a mitotic figure.

(intercalary or peg) cells, even within a single case (Figure 12.13). Glands exhibiting tubal metaplasia lack nuclear atypia and mitoses are seen only occasionally. Apoptotic bodies are inconspicuous. The glands may be associated with endometrioid-type stroma. Endometrioid metaplasia also shows bland nuclei that lack significant mitotic activity. CD10-positive endometrioid stroma may also be present. Immunohistochemically, tuboendometrioid metaplasia shows a low Ki-67/MIB1 immunoreactivity and strong widespread reaction for bcl-2.[25,26] It also exhibits p16^{INK4A} in 62% of cases, but, unlike AIS, the reactivity is only focal.[25] Tuboendometrioid metaplasia may show reactivity for CEA in 39% of cases, but, unlike AIS, expresses vimentin.[27] The presence of cilia usually implies a benign process, but, of note, ciliated AIS also occurs.[36]

Superficial cervical endometriosis (Figure 12.14) may be confused with AIS histologically, particularly in patients followed with cytologic smears after cone biopsy.[37] The endometriotic foci are usually confined to the inner third of the cervical wall. The endometrioid glands are typically evenly spaced, show bland cytologic features, and are surrounded, at least focally, by endometrial-type stroma, which may show focal hemosiderin deposition. Inflammation and hemorrhage may obscure the stromal cells. Mitotic figures are seen in 37% of cases.[37]

Endocervical glands may show a variety of architectural and cytologic changes in response to inflammation. This may lead to a suspicion of AIS. In inflammatory/reparative changes, the nuclei become enlarged and show chromatin clearing and prominent nucleoli. Nuclear pleomorphism may occur, but the chromatin is often smudged (Figure 12.15). Pseudostratification and mitotic activity are minimal. Apoptotic bodies are generally absent. p16^{INK4A} and Ki-67/MIB1 immunoreactions are usually negative. Endocervical glands in some patients may also show mild morphologic changes during the menstrual cycle. Occasionally, a normal-appearing mitosis can be found in normal endocervical glands and should not raise concern (Figure 12.16).

Radiation therapy results in widely spaced endocervical glands that are often dilated and lined by cells showing nuclear enlargement and pleomorphism, but the cytoplasm is finely vacuolated or granular (Figure 12.17). There is often loss of nuclear polarity and the nuclei show dispersed chromatin and one or two prominent eosinophilic nucleoli. Focal cytoplasmic CEA reactivity occurs and does not distinguish it from AIS.[38]

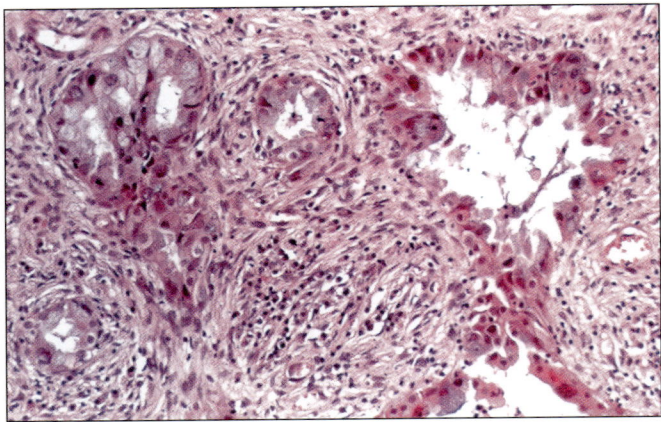

Figure 12.17 Radiation changes. The endocervical glands show hyperchromatic nuclei.

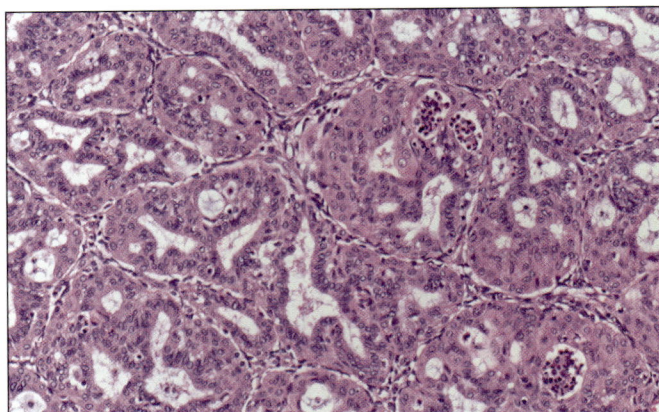

Figure 12.19 Microglandular hyperplasia. The small glands lack significant nuclear atypia, pseudostratification, and mitotic figures.

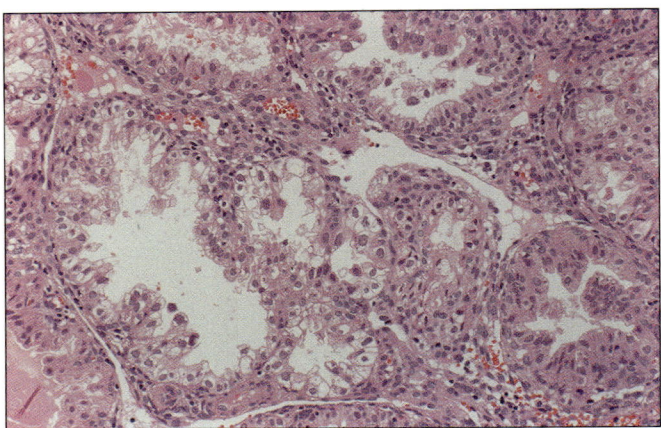

Figure 12.18 Arias-Stella reaction. Hyperchromatic 'hobnail' nuclei protruding into the gland lumina.

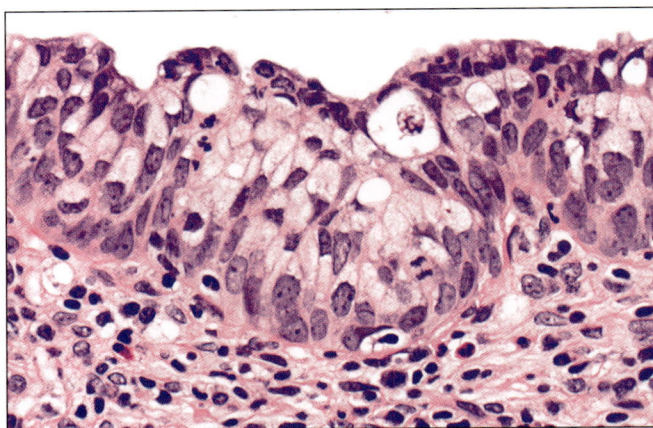

Figure 12.20 SMILE in a case also with AIS and CIN 3 elsewhere in the cervix.

The Arias-Stella reaction involves the endocervical glands in 10% of gravid uteri (Figure 12.18). Superficial glands are more commonly involved than deep glands. The involved glands typically have a single layer of enlarged hyperchromatic pleomorphic nuclei that protrude into the lumen producing a 'hobnail' appearance. The glandular cells may also show intranuclear cytoplasmic inclusions as well as optically clear nuclei. Mitoses are exceedingly rare or absent.[39]

In contrast to AIS, microglandular hyperplasia lacks significant nuclear atypia (Figure 12.19), lacks pseudostratification, has rare mitotic figures, and p16^{INK4A} immunoreaction is negative. AIS, however, may occasionally involve areas of microglandular hyperplasia and, in such cases, the presence of residual microglandular hyperplasia uninvolved by AIS is the key to establishing the diagnosis. Similarly, AIS may also extend into other benign endocervical glandular lesions, such as tunnel clusters.

A stratified mucin-producing intraepithelial lesion (SMILE) exhibits stratified epithelium resembling CIN in which there is conspicuous mucin production (Figure 12.20). Mucin is present throughout the epithelium, varying from indistinct cytoplasmic clearing to discrete vacuoles. The lesion shows a rounded or lobulated contour at the epithelial–stromal interface and a high Ki-67/MIB1 index. SMILE is an unusual cervical intraepithelial lesion best regarded as a variant of cervical columnar cell neoplasia based on phenotype. SMILE is frequently associated with CIN, AIS, or invasive carcinoma.[40]

Biologic Behavior and Treatment

AIS is treated either by conization or by hysterectomy. Because of the multicentric distribution of AIS, recurrence occurs more often after conization than after hysterectomy, particularly if the lesion involves the margins of the cone.[41] Even though in young women who are desirous of preservation of fertility cone biopsy may be selected, currently the definitive therapy for AIS remains hysterectomy.[42] In a meta-analysis, 27% of patients treated with conization where the margins were free of abnormality had residual AIS in the subsequent hysterectomy specimen.[43] This figure reached 59% if the margins on cone biopsy were positive.[44–48] Some authors believe that the disease-free endocervical margin in a cone biopsy must be at least 10 mm to consider the lesion completely excised.[45] If a lesser procedure is performed, cold knife or laser cone biopsy is more effective than loop electrosurgical excision, especially for the endocervical margin.[49,50] Furthermore, patients with AIS and positive margins on cone biopsy are at moderate risk of harboring an occult invasive endocervical adenocarcinoma that has already developed. The optimal management of the atypical glandular lesions that fall short of AIS is even more controversial, with treatment options including cytologic follow-up or management along the lines of AIS.

ADENOCARCINOMA

In developed countries, adenocarcinoma currently accounts for 15–20% of all carcinomas of the uterine cervix.[51,52] Prior to 1970, it represented only 5% of cervical carcinomas. The relative frequency has increased due to a decrease in that of invasive squamous cell carcinoma, which is much more readily identified in its preinvasive stages by cytologic examination than adenocarcinoma. Nevertheless, there is evidence of an absolute increase in the incidence of adenocarcinoma in both the United States and Northern Europe, particularly in women under the age of 35 years.[51–53]

Almost 60% of cervical adenocarcinomas are associated with SIL or invasive squamous cell carcinoma.[54,55] Also, several reports have suggested that HPV 16, 31, and, particularly, 18 may have a significant role in the causation of cervical adenocarcinomas. These HPV types have been identified in adenocarcinomas and adenosquamous carcinomas with a frequency of 80% or more.[56–58] The HPV status, however, is not predictive of disease outcome. An association with prior use of oral contraceptive, particularly those with a strong progestogen component, has been described but it has not been totally proved. It is noteworthy that the introduction of oral contraceptive in the 1960s was followed a few years later by the recognition of microglandular hyperplasia, a proliferative cervical lesion that develops in women using oral contraceptive.[59] Although the similar temporal association suggested the possibility of a causal relationship between oral contraceptive and cervical adenocarcinoma, the association was diminished when adjusted for HPV.[17] On the other hand, use of hormone replacement therapy, especially unopposed estrogens, in older women may be associated with an increased risk of cervical adenocarcinoma.[60] Yet other reports indicate that cervical adenocarcinomas share some epidemiologic associations with endometrial carcinoma, including a slight tendency toward patient obesity, hypertension, and nulligravidity.[61]

Intrauterine exposure to diethylstilbestrol (DES) (administered in the 1950s and 1960s to pregnant women in the United States and Western Europe) resulted in a subset of young patients developing clear cell adenocarcinomas of the cervix and upper vagina several years later. The occurrence of these tumors has decreased following the withdrawal of DES from the market about 30 years ago.

Patients with adenocarcinoma of the cervix, particularly those with minimal-deviation mucinous adenocarcinoma, tend to develop mucinous tumors of the ovary and some of them have the Peutz–Jeghers syndrome.[62]

Adenocarcinoma of the cervix is almost always a tumor of adult life; it is rare in the first decade and uncommon in the second decade.[51] The average age ranges from 47 to 53 years.[52] The patients present with abnormal uterine bleeding in 80–90% of cases. Occasional patients complain of vaginal discharge or pain. The tumor is asymptomatic in up to 20% of cases and is usually discovered in such cases because of an abnormal Pap smear. The diagnostic ability of cytopathology for detecting cervical adenocarcinoma varies according to the expertise of the pathologist and the sampling techniques used. Most patients with adenocarcinoma of the cervix have cytologic abnormalities. At the time of diagnosis, 67.8% of tumors are FIGO stage I, 23.8% stage II, 7.4% stage III, and 1% stage IV. The older the age group, the higher the proportion of cases with a more advanced FIGO stage.[63]

MICROINVASIVE (EARLY INVASIVE) ADENOCARCINOMA

Definition

Microinvasive adenocarcinoma refers to the earliest form of invasive adenocarcinoma and is classified generally in a manner similar to microinvasive squamous cell carcinoma.

Pathology

In contrast to microinvasive squamous cell carcinoma, the glandular counterpart has received little attention in the literature. The ideal definition of microinvasive adenocarcinoma should guarantee the safety of conservative therapy; it should describe an invasive adenocarcinoma small enough not to be associated with metastasis. The main diagnostic problems are, first, to distinguish microinvasive adenocarcinoma from AIS and, second, how to measure the depth of invasion.[64]

The criteria for microinvasion include: (1) obvious stromal invasion by epithelial finger-like processes arising from glands involved by AIS or detached cellular clusters with abundant pink cytoplasm lying free in the stroma; (2) obliteration of the normal endocervical crypts; (3) complex intraglandular cribriform or papillary growth patterns; (4) stromal edema, inflammation, and desmoplasia; and (5) extension below the deep margin of normal endocervical glands[64] (Figures 12.21 and 12.22). If the distance between

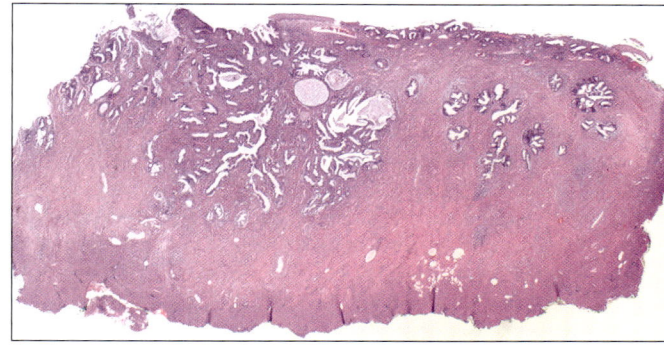

Figure 12.21 Microinvasive adenocarcinoma. The irregular growth pattern and irregular outlines of the glands are indicative of early invasive carcinoma.

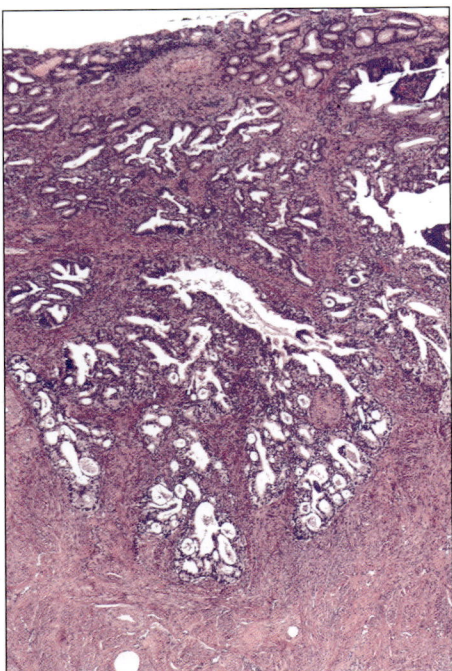

Figure 12.22 Microinvasive adenocarcinoma. Numerous irregular glands with cribriform pattern.

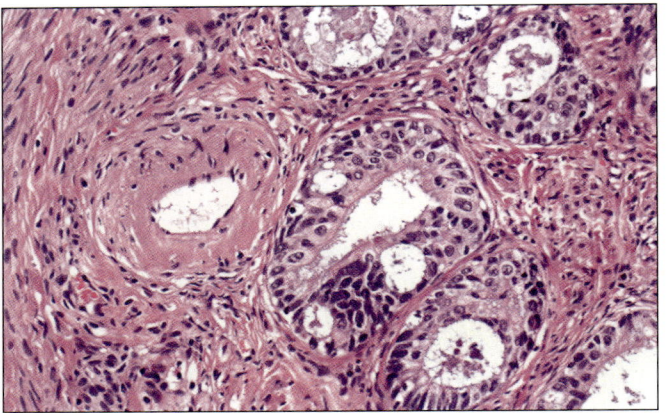

Figure 12.23 Microinvasive adenocarcinoma. A tumor gland appears adjacent to a thick-walled blood vessel.

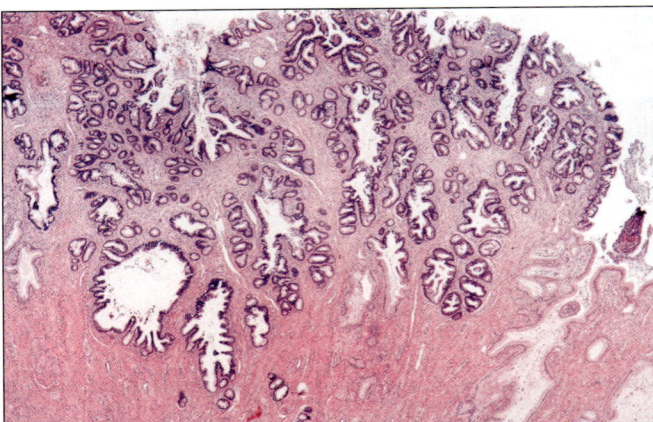

Figure 12.24 Microinvasive adenocarcinoma. In some cases it may be difficult to distinguish AIS from invasive adenocarcinoma. The deeply invasive glands suggest this tumor is invasive.

neoplastic glands and thick-walled blood vessels is less than the thickness of the vessel wall, invasion should be suspected[65] (Figure 12.23). Not all of these features are present in every case and invasion is indicated by the gland pattern and haphazard distribution on low-power examination. The depth of invasion is usually measured from the surface epithelium (tumor thickness) rather than from the point of origin. This is due to the difficulty to determine where AIS ends and stromal invasion begins[64] (Figure 12.24). Indeed, the identification of early invasion in cervical glandular lesions may not always be possible, and in approximately 10–15% of patients the pathologist may be uncertain.

The FIGO system (2009) for staging carcinoma of the cervix makes no distinction between squamous and glandular lesions. Stage IA1 defines invasion to less than 3 mm in depth and less than 7 mm in width; stage IA2 defines invasion between 3 and 5 mm in depth and less than 7 mm in width. Vascular space invasion does not alter the stage.

Cytologic Correlation

Microinvasive adenocarcinoma can sometimes be predicted cytologically. Features include those of AIS, which are always present. Syncytia of glandular cells, small cells in supercrowded sheets, papillary groupings, and dissociated cells are suggestive of the diagnosis. Nuclear features include pleomorphism with irregular chromatin and nucleoli. Tumor diathesis may also be present. Collectively, these criteria help predict microinvasion in over two-fifths of cases.[66,67] In practical terms, microinvasion can be accurately defined only histologically. The major role of cytology in this circumstance is identifying the existence of high-grade neoplasia of endocervical columnar cell origin.

Biologic Behavior and Treatment

It appears that microinvasive adenocarcinoma behaves in the same way as its squamous counterpart. What is uncertain is the maximum size at which less than radical treatment is safe. When microinvasive adenocarcinoma does not invade beyond 5 mm, the margins are free, and the conization specimen has been totally embedded, conservative treatment is acceptable.[64] A review of the literature revealed that only five (2%) of 219 patients with microinvasive adenocarcinoma invading less than 5 mm were found to have metastasis after pelvic lymph node dissection.[64] Of these patients, 3.4% developed recurrences and 1.4% died. No patient treated by radical hysterectomy had parametrial involvement.[63] The relationship of capillary–lymphatic space involvement, lymph node metastasis, and recurrence remains uncertain. Conization is considered acceptable treatment only if the specimen has been adequately sampled and the margins free. Fifty percent of patients with positive margins had residual disease in the subsequent hysterectomy specimen.[64]

In a SEER database review of 301 cases of microinvasive adenocarcinoma of which 131 were FIGO stage IA1 and 170 were stage IA2, only one of 140 women who had lymphadenectomy had a single positive lymph node. This patient had stage IA2 disease. Moreover, of four women with tumor-related deaths, three were stage IA2. Overall, the prognosis for microinvasive adenocarcinoma is excellent and, in 96 cases, simple hysterectomy alone proved adequate.[68] In a more recent study evaluating depth of invasion, none of 48 patients with tumor under 5 mm invasion had involved parametria or nodes; whereas eight of the 36 with invasion greater than 5 mm had nodal metastases. None of the former developed a recurrence whereas one-sixth of the latter had recurrent disease.[69] These data argue that, for patients with tumor less than 5 mm invasion and negative margins, pelvic lymphadenectomy may be omitted.[69] Similarly, in a study of 32 patients with FIGO stage IA1 and IA2 adenocarcinomas of the cervix where invasion was strictly defined, the method of measurement was standardized and villoglandular, serous, and clear cell carcinomas were excluded, no recurrences have been reported to date.[70] Clearly, some young women with early invasive adenocarcinomas might best be served by treating the tumor in the same way as microinvasive squamous cell carcinoma.

INVASIVE ADENOCARCINOMA

Although less common than squamous cell carcinomas, adenocarcinomas generally cause greater diagnostic difficulty because of their relative rarity, their varied patterns, and the potential for confusing them with several non-neoplastic lesions. Some variants are associated with a distinctive biologic behavior. A classification of these tumors is presented in Table 12.1.

The 2014 WHO classification divides these tumors into usual-type adenocarcinoma, mucinous adenocarcinomas (including intestinal-type, signet-ring cell type, gastric-type or minimal deviation adenocarcinoma, and NOS), villoglandular adenocarcinoma, endometrioid adenocarcinoma, clear cell adenocarcinoma, serous adenocarcinoma, and mesonephric adenocarcinoma.[4] A number of uncommon variants will also be covered in this chapter.

ADENOCARCINOMA, USUAL-TYPE

Whereas cervical adenocarcinoma is often referred to as mucinous adenocarcinoma, it is not always overtly mucinous. In fact, it is commonly mucin poor due to less than a high degree of differentiation and instead is composed of cells with eosinophilic cytoplasm. Therefore, the designation 'endocervical adenocarcinoma of usual type' is also used.

Definition

An adenocarcinoma in which the tumor cells resemble those lining the endocervical glands and contain varying amounts of cytoplasmic mucin. This is the most common type of adenocarcinoma accounting for almost 80% of all cervical adenocarcinomas.

Pathology

Grossly, half of cervical adenocarcinomas are exophytic, usually as a polypoid or papillary mass. Some may be nodular, with diffuse enlargement (Figure 12.25) or ulceration, and some tumors present as a barrel-shaped cervix. About one-sixth are small and not visible, usually because of their location within the endocervical canal. Even in the absence of visible signs or symptoms, the tumor may infiltrate deeply into the wall (Figure 12.26). Generally, the gross appearance is not helpful in predicting the histologic appearance.

As indicated earlier, most tumors are moderately differentiated and show little intracytoplasmic mucin; thus, the tumor glands resemble those of endometrioid carcinoma or exhibit a mixed endocervical and endometrioid appearance. This has led to confusion, with these tumors regarded as endometrioid adenocarcinomas. Gland size may vary from small to cystic, and the glands may be widely spaced

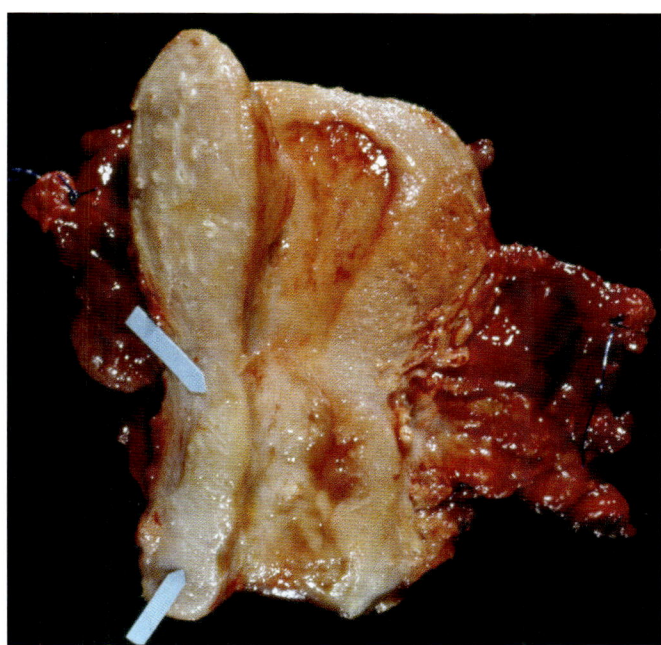

Figure 12.25 Adenocarcinoma. Diffuse enlargement of the cervical wall.

Table 12.1 Modified WHO Histologic Classification of Adenocarcinomas of the Uterine Cervix

AIS	8140/2
Early invasive adenocarcinoma	8140/3
Adenocarcinoma, usual-type	8140/3
Mucinous adenocarcinoma	8480/3
Intestinal-type	8482/3
Signet-ring cell type	8144/3
Gastric-type (minimal deviation adenocarcinoma)	8490/3
NOS	8480/3
Villoglandular	8262/3
Endometrioid adenocarcinoma	8380/3
Clear cell adenocarcinoma	8310/3
Serous adenocarcinoma	8441/3
Mesonephric adenocarcinoma	9110/3
Adenosquamous carcinoma	8560/3
Glassy cell variant	8015/3

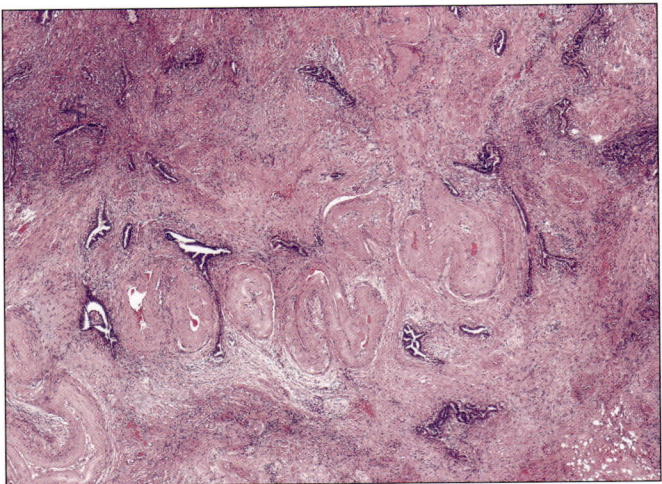

Figure 12.26 Adenocarcinoma. Perivascular infiltration deep into the cervical wall.

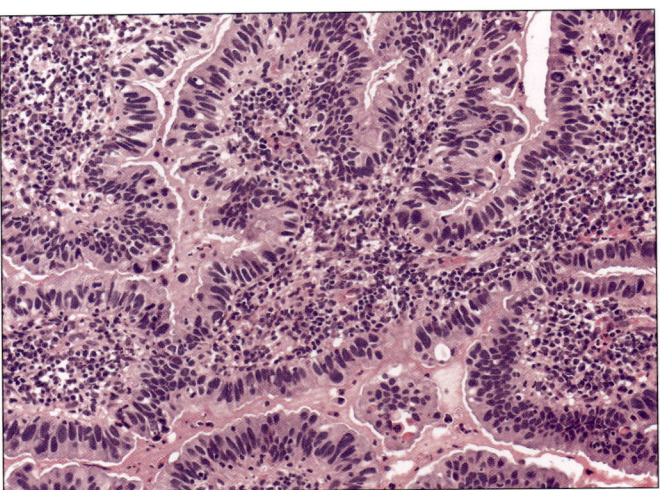

Figure 12.28 Adenocarcinoma, usual-type. The papillae are lined by stratified epithelial cells showing numerous mitoses and apoptotic bodies. The stroma contains abundant chronic inflammatory cells.

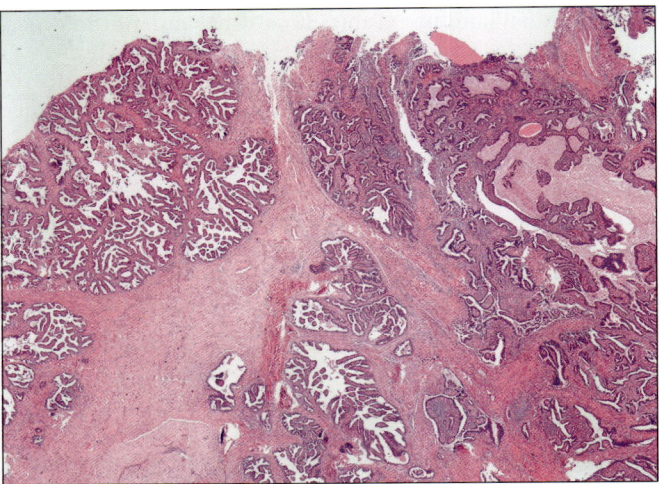

Figure 12.27 Adenocarcinoma, usual-type. The glands are arranged in a complex pattern. Stroma is abundant.

Table 12.2	Distinction of Endocervical Adenocarcinomas from Endometrioid Adenocarcinomas of the Corpus	
	Endocervical Adenocarcinoma	Endometrioid Adenocarcinoma of the Corpus
Intracellular mucin	+++	+/−
Fibrous stroma	Abundant	Scanty
Villoglandular architecture	+	+++
HPV DNA	+	−
P16^{INK4A}	+++	− or +/−
Estrogen receptor	− or +/−	+++
Vimentin	−	++

or closely packed, often with a cribriform pattern. Papillae may be present, but are rarely conspicuous (Figure 12.27). Mitoses are readily found and apoptotic bodies are commonly seen (Figure 12.28). The tumors are usually associated with a desmoplastic or a prominent fibromatous stroma. Some tumors show prominent numbers of acute inflammatory cells within both the stroma and the gland lumens.

Well-differentiated endocervical adenocarcinomas show complex glandular arrangement resembling the tunnel configuration of the normal endocervical mucosa. The tumor cells have basal nuclei and abundant pale cytoplasm, which stains positively with mucicarmine stains. There is significant nuclear atypia and mitotic figures. Large amounts of mucin may be found in the stroma, forming mucin lakes or pools in the so-called colloid carcinoma.

Grading of the tumors follows the general FIGO system for glandular tumors as described elsewhere for endometrium and ovary. Grade 1 tumors (well-differentiated tumors) grow in glandular formations with less than 5% of areas being solid. Grade 3 tumors (poorly differentiated tumors) are more than 50% composed of solid tumor nests; the cells may show pseudorosette formation or palisading of nuclei.

The distinction of endocervical adenocarcinomas from endometrial adenocarcinomas may be difficult particularly when a fractional curettage has not been performed or when tumor is present in both samples of the curettage. The presence of abundant intracellular mucin favors an endocervical origin, but most endometrial adenocarcinomas show focal mucinous differentiation and some of them are largely mucinous. The stroma of the tumor may be helpful; in cervical tumors it is typically fibrous whereas endometrial carcinomas usually contain very little stroma. Hysteroscopy is often helpful in identifying the site of origin of the tumor (Table 12.2).

Coexistent CIN occurs in up to 40% of cases[54], and AIS is also common. Synchronous mucinous tumors may be found elsewhere in the female genital tract.[71,72]

Immunohistochemistry

Approximately 90% of endocervical adenocarcinomas are HPV related and show diffuse and moderate/strong immunoreaction for p16^{INK4A} (Figure 12.29A). Apparently, high-risk E6 and E7 HPV transforming proteins interact with cell cycle regulatory proteins (p53, Rb) and cause p16^{INK4A} overexpression. In contrast, endometrioid carcinomas are etiologically unrelated to HPV and exhibit usually patchy p16^{INK4A} immunoreaction of variable intensity.[73] Typical endocervical adenocarcinomas are often, but not always, cytoplasmic CEA positive and are negative for vimentin (Figure 12.29B). Estrogen (ER) and progesterone (PR) receptors are also generally negative (Figure 12.29C); however, focal weak reactivity for ER may be present. In contrast, primary endometrial adenocarcinomas of endometrioid type are strongly immunoreactive for both vimentin and ER and PR and are negative for CEA. However, endometrial tumors showing mucinous differentiation may be strongly positive for CEA.

Thus, it appears that tumors that show strong positive immunoreaction for vimentin and ER, and weak or negative immunostaining for p16^{INK4A}, are almost invariably of endometrial origin.[73,74]

In situ Hybridization

In situ hybridization for high-risk HPV types is the most specific test available for distinguishing endocervical from endometrial adenocarcinoma. At least 90% of cervical adenocarcinomas contain high-risk HPV types,[58,75] whereas endometrial carcinomas are negative.

Cytologic Correlation

Invasive endocervical adenocarcinoma shares many features with AIS. Features helpful in correctly predicting histologic invasion include: heavy blood staining, abundant abnormal glandular epithelium, supercrowding of sheets, small three-dimensional groups, papillary clusters, tumor diathesis, single malignant cells with nuclear pleomorphism and macronucleoli, and mitotic figures (Figure 12.30).[76,77] LBC may be more sensitive than conventional cytology in detection of cervical adenocarcinoma.[33,34] The reduction in screening false negatives has been attributed to enhanced cytologic detail and the elimination of obscuring elements such as blood.[33,34]

Differential Diagnosis

The histologic differential diagnosis of cervical adenocarcinoma includes benign glandular lesions (see Chapter 8) including tunnel clusters (types A and B), microglandular hyperplasia, lobular endocervical glandular hyperplasia, diffuse laminar endocervical glandular hyperplasia, and deep nabothian cysts, as well as secondary adenocarcinoma metastatic to the cervix. In general, when faced with a problematic endocervical glandular lesion, features that favor a benign lesion include: (1) superficial location and lack of deep infiltration, (2) lobulation, (3) well-defined margins, (4) bland nuclear features, (5) inconspicuous mitotic and apoptotic activity, and (6) absence of a stromal reaction. However, benign glandular lesions may coexist with adenocarcinoma and, ultimately, assessment of the overall cytologic and architectural features facilitates the correct diagnosis.[78]

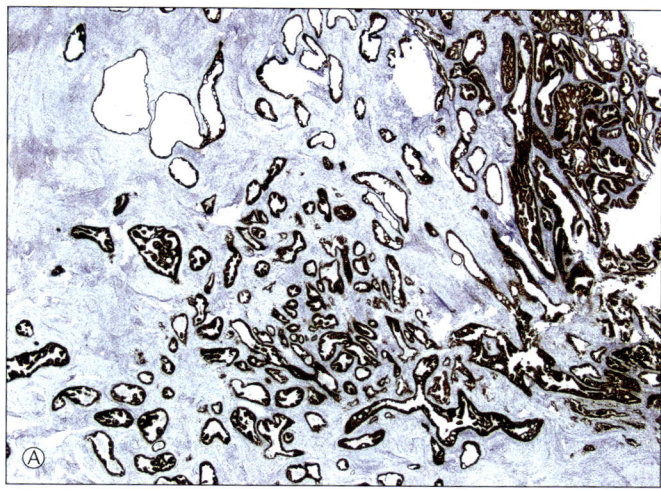

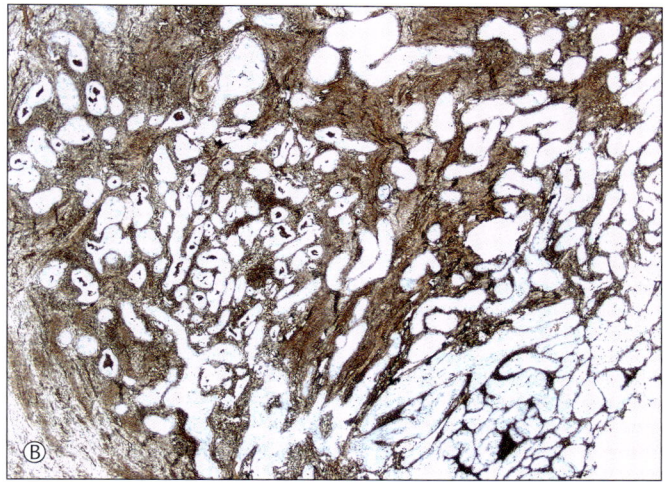

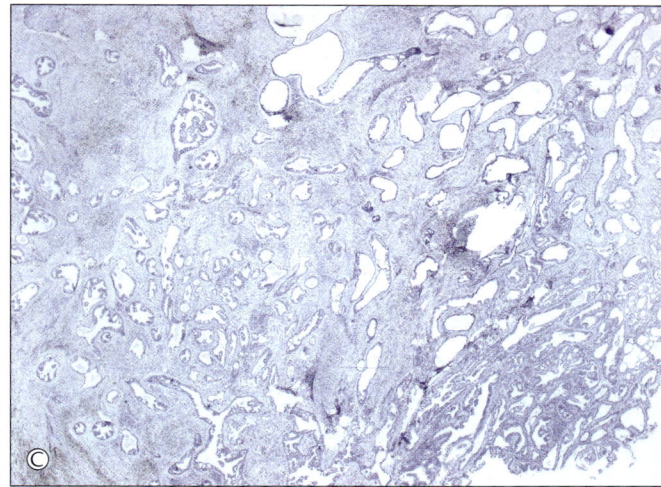

Figure 12.29 Adenocarcinoma. **(A)** Diffuse and strong immunoreaction for p16. **(B)** Negative vimentin. **(C)** Negative estrogen receptors.

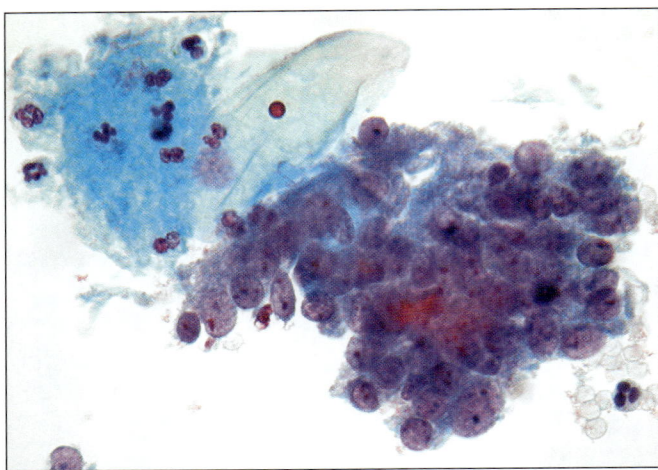

Figure 12.30 Adenocarcinoma (ThinPrep) showing a group of malignant glandular cells with lysed blood in the background.

An Arias-Stella reaction involving endocervical glands is found in 10–50% of pregnant uteri. These glands show markedly pleomorphic cells with large abnormal nuclei; prominent nucleoli; and pale, vacuolated cytoplasm.[79] Knowledge of the patient's pregnant status is very important to prevent a false-positive diagnosis of adenocarcinoma. Occasionally glandular changes similar to the Arias-Stella reaction occur in nonpregnant women, usually in patients taking exogenous hormones. Whereas the characteristic nuclear atypicality may suggest malignancy, lack of mitoses and partial gland involvement help to establish the correct diagnosis. Both atypical oxyphilic metaplasia and radiation-induced atypia show enlarged, hyperchromatic nuclei exhibiting smudged chromatin, cytoplasmic vacuolation, and preservation of the nuclear to cytoplasmic ratio.[38,80]

Tunnel clusters mimic cervical adenocarcinoma with a microcystic pattern.[81] High-power examination, however, reveals the presence of cytologic atypia and the malignant nature of the lesion. Other benign lesions that may simulate invasive adenocarcinoma of the cervix are microglandular hyperplasia and hyperplastic mesonephric remnants. Microglandular hyperplasia tends to occur in young women and is frequently polypoid. In contrast to cervical adenocarcinoma, microglandular hyperplasia is composed of small and uniform glands lined by a single layer of bland epithelium with few mitoses. Mesonephric remnants show lobular arrangement in the vicinity of mesonephric ducts, and are deep in the cervical stroma. The epithelium lining the tubules is usually cuboidal, lacks mucin, and shows minimal cytologic atypia.[82]

Endometrial carcinoma may extend to the endocervix, but, when it does, it has usually invaded the myometrium and has become sufficiently bulky to enlarge the uterus. Microscopically, endocervical adenocarcinoma can be distinguished from endometrial adenocarcinoma extending to the cervix by the presence of squamous metaplasia and foamy histiocytes in the latter. Immunohistochemical stains may be helpful in difficult cases (see earlier) (Table 12.2). Metastatic adenocarcinoma of the cervix usually occurs in patients with known widely spread tumors and typically shows lack of surface involvement and widespread lymphovascular invasion. Metastatic carcinomas involving the cervix arise most commonly from gastrointestinal tract, ovary, and breast and are characterized by a clean background. In contrast, bowel and bladder carcinomas, which directly invade the female genital tract, often have a necroinflammatory diathesis due to fistula formation. In assessing whether a carcinoma is of primary endocervical origin or is metastatic in the cervix, the finding of a transition between *in situ* and invasive carcinoma provides the strongest evidence for a primary cervical origin and is found in approximately 50% of cases.

Biologic Behavior and Treatment

Although older studies suggested that the prognosis of adenocarcinomas of the cervix was worse than that of squamous cervical cancer, more recent studies adjusting for depth, stage, and therapy have not found a significant difference.[83,84] Collectively, the prognosis for adenocarcinoma is essentially that of squamous carcinoma or slightly worse, and, in general, both squamous carcinomas and adenocarcinomas are treated similarly.[85–87] Differences in survival rates for squamous cell carcinoma and adenocarcinoma in stage I and II disease may be due to the relative ineffectiveness of radiotherapy as a primary treatment in cases of adenocarcinoma.[88] The features that influence prognosis are similar to those for squamous cell carcinoma, mainly histologic grade, tumor size, depth of invasion, lymphatic–capillary space involvement, stage, age, and lymph node status.[63,88] In addition, the ratio of mitotic index to apoptotic index is also of prognostic significance.[89] Young age at presentation has been associated with a good prognosis in several series.[90] Infection with HPV 18 has been associated with poor survival.[91] The 5 year survival for adenocarcinoma according to stage is stage IA1, 100%; stage IA2, 93%; stage IB, 83%; stage II, 37–62.9%; stage III, 13–31%; and stage IV, 0–6%.[86,88] Longest survival is seen in patients with early stage disease, younger patients, and those treated with primary surgery.[88]

MUCINOUS ADENOCARCINOMA, INTESTINAL-TYPE

These tumors resemble adenocarcinoma of the large intestine. Intestinal-type change may be found diffusely or only focally within a mucinous carcinoma. The tumor cells tend to be pseudostratified, and contain only small amounts of intracytoplasmic mucin. They can either form glands with papillae or infiltrate throughout the stroma in a pattern similar to that of colonic adenocarcinoma (Figures 12.31 and 12.32). There are goblet cells and less frequently endocrine and Paneth cells. It is presumed that these tumors arise from intestinal-type AIS. The main differential diagnosis is with metastatic intestinal adenocarcinoma. Primary endocervical adenocarcinoma of intestinal type is generally reactive with keratin 7 and nonreactive with keratin 20 and Cdx-2.

MUCINOUS ADENOCARCINOMA, SIGNET-RING CELL-TYPE

Primary signet-ring cell adenocarcinomas occurring either in a pure form or, more frequently, as part of a poorly differentiated endocervical or intestinal carcinoma are

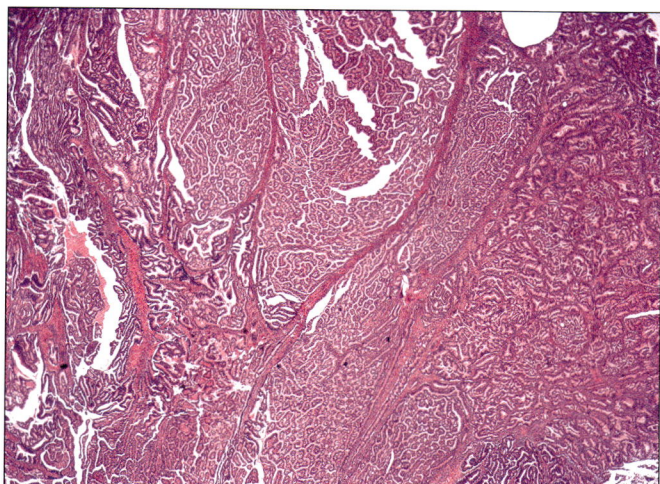

Figure 12.31 Mucinous adenocarcinoma, intestinal-type. Confluent papillary pattern similar to that of colonic adenocarcinoma.

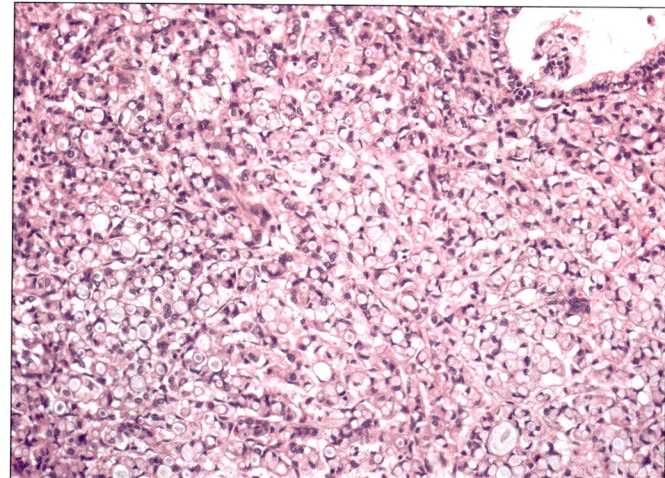

Figure 12.33 Mucinous adenocarcinoma, signet-ring cell type. The tumor cells exhibit eccentric nuclei and cytoplasmic vacuoles filled with mucin.

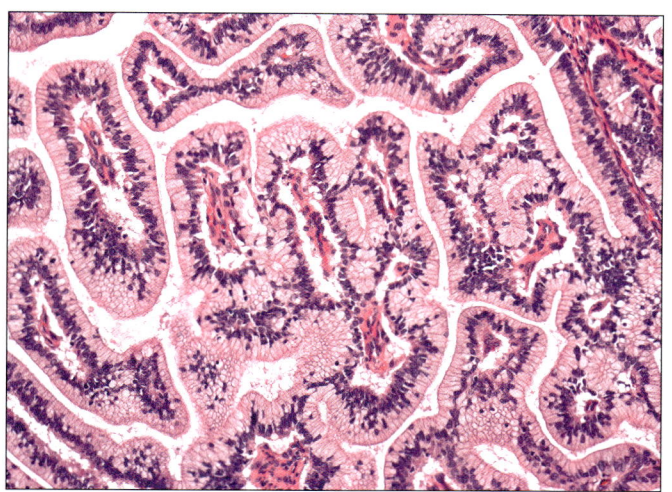

Figure 12.32 Mucinous adenocarcinoma, intestinal-type. The papillae are lined by numerous goblet cells with basally located nuclei.

uncommon.[101] Typically, cells with eccentric nuclei and pale, mucin-filled cytoplasm growing singly, in clusters, nests, or in columns are present (Figure 12.33). The differential diagnosis includes metastatic adenocarcinoma from the gastrointestinal tract.[92]

MUCINOUS ADENOCARCINOMA GASTRIC-TYPE (MINIMAL DEVIATION ADENOCARCINOMA)

Definition

This unusually well-differentiated mucinous adenocarcinoma was initially designated as *adenoma malignum* to emphasize its bland histologic appearance in spite of its highly malignant behavior.[93,94] Today, the term 'minimal deviation adenocarcinoma' is often used synonymously with 'adenoma malignum.' The concept of minimal deviation adenocarcinoma has been expanded to include endometrioid and clear cell variants.[95]

Recent studies have shown that minimal deviation adenocarcinoma frequently exhibits a gastric immunophenotype, as demonstrated by immunoreactivity for HIK1083 and/or anti-MUC6 antibodies which recognize pyloric gland mucin.[96–98]

Clinical Features

It is a rare tumor accounting for only 1–3% of adenocarcinomas of the cervix.[93,99] The age range of patients is 25–72 years (mean age, 42 years).[99] Synchronous or metachronous ovarian mucinous tumors with histologic features resembling cystadenoma, borderline tumor, and well-differentiated adenocarcinoma may also occur and have been interpreted as representing independent primary ovarian tumors or metastases.[94] A minority of cases are associated with the Peutz–Jeghers syndrome.[94,100] Other ovarian neoplasms associated with minimal deviation adenocarcinoma of the cervix in patients with the Peutz–Jeghers syndrome are sex cord tumors with annular tubules.[101] In these patients, benign mucinous epithelium may be seen in the endometrium and fallopian tubes and should not be interpreted as metastasis. Therefore, close follow-up of patients with Peutz–Jeghers syndrome is recommended, including periodic endocervical cytologic examination and curettage. The most common presenting sign, as with most cervical carcinomas, is abnormal vaginal bleeding. A mucoid, watery, or purulent vaginal discharge may be present.

Pathology

Grossly, adenoma malignum resembles and is indistinguishable from other types of endocervical adenocarcinoma. It may be polypoid or ulcerative and the cervical wall is typically firm or indurated. In early lesions, the cervix may even look normal. The mucosa is usually hemorrhagic, friable, or mucoid. On section, the cervix usually shows thickening by yellow or tan-white tumor tissue and mucin-filled cysts are occasionally prominent (Figure 12.34).[93,94]

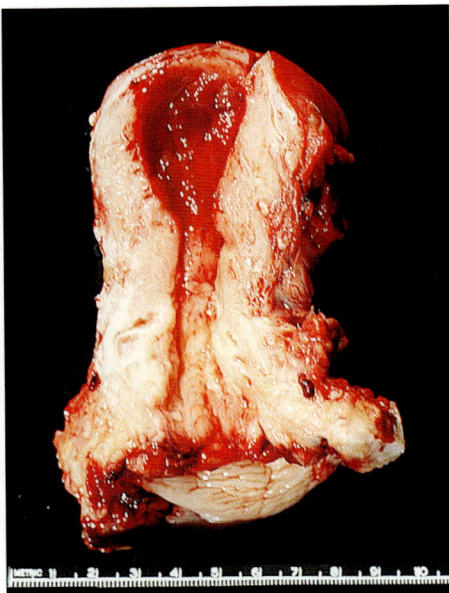

Figure 12.34 Minimal deviation adenocarcinoma ('adenoma malignum'). The tumor diffusely infiltrates the entire thickness of the cervical wall.

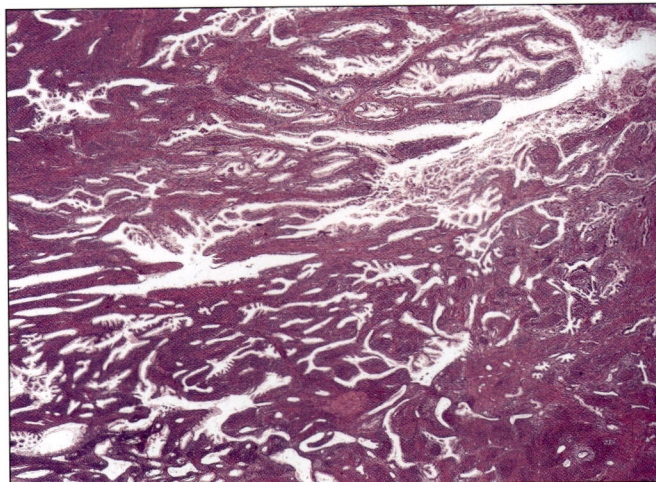

Figure 12.35 Gastric-type or minimal deviation adenocarcinoma ('adenoma malignum'). There are numerous branching glands of varying size and shape.

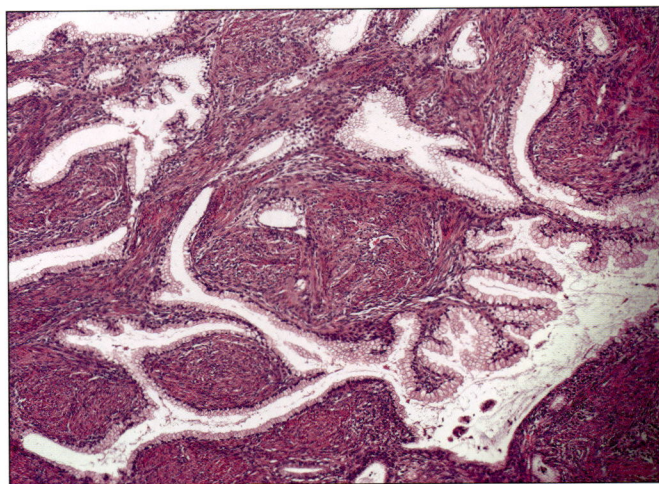

Figure 12.36 Gastric-type or minimal deviation adenocarcinoma ('adenoma malignum'). Well-differentiated and excessively convoluted endocervical-type glands.

The tumor shows glands lined by a single layer of columnar cells with clear and/or pale eosinophilic and voluminous cytoplasm, with distinct cell borders and basal uniform nuclei with inconspicuous nucleoli. Features that help in arriving at the correct diagnosis include: (1) variability in gland shape and size, often exhibiting large branching glands (Figures 12.35 and 12.36); (2) desmoplastic or edematous stroma; and (3) mitotic figures. Nevertheless, large areas of invasive tumor may be devoid of any stromal reaction. In such areas, the presence of glands adjacent to thick-walled blood vessels is a helpful finding in determining that stromal invasion is present (Figure 12.37). Furthermore, areas of clearly malignant glands, vascular invasion, or perineural invasion (Figure 12.38), which help to confirm the diagnosis, are present in approximately half of the cases. In most cases the tumor deeply invades the cervical wall and spreading to the parametrium is seen in approximately 40% of patients. The most reliable criterion to assess the malignant nature of minimal deviation adenocarcinoma is the haphazard arrangement of glands that extend beyond the level of normal endocervical glands (over 8 mm). Thus, a histologic diagnosis of minimal deviation adenocarcinoma may be impossible in small superficial biopsies; it instead requires cone biopsy or hysterectomy specimen.[93,94]

Cytologic diagnosis of adenoma malignum is challenging. Smears display many large branching sheets of enlarged glandular cells with retention of the honeycomb pattern and peripheral palisading. Nuclei can be enlarged but are uniform, with smooth nuclear membranes, occasional irregularities in shape, and fine chromatin. Small nucleoli may be present.[102,103] Cytoplasm is abundant and vacuolated or lacy.[102] The presence of more usual type adenocarcinoma cells with increased nuclear atypia and pleomorphism may provide a useful clue.[99,102]

Immunohistochemistry

Immunohistochemical staining for estrogen and progesterone receptors is uniformly negative in minimal deviation adenocarcinoma, and this finding helps to distinguish these tumors from variants of normal endocervical glands.[94,104] Stains for p16^{INK4A} are negative or only focally positive since minimal deviation adenocarcinoma is not associated with high-risk HPV infection and the Ki-67/MIB1 proliferation index is often low.[75] HIK1083 and MUC6, two markers for pyloric gland phenotype, are frequently positive with 75% and 65% rates, respectively. Up to 95% of cases are positive for at least one of these two markers.[96–98] MUC6 can also be positive in intestinal-type adenocarcinoma.

Somatic Genetics

Somatic mutations of the *STK11* gene, the gene responsible for Peutz–Jeghers syndrome, are characteristic of minimal deviation adenocarcinoma.[105] They were found in 55% of

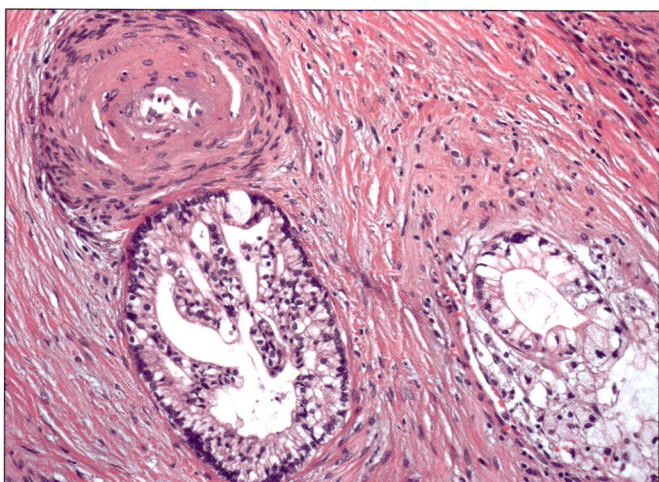

Figure 12.37 Gastric-type or minimal deviation adenocarcinoma ('adenoma malignum'). Tumor gland adjacent to thick-walled blood vessel.

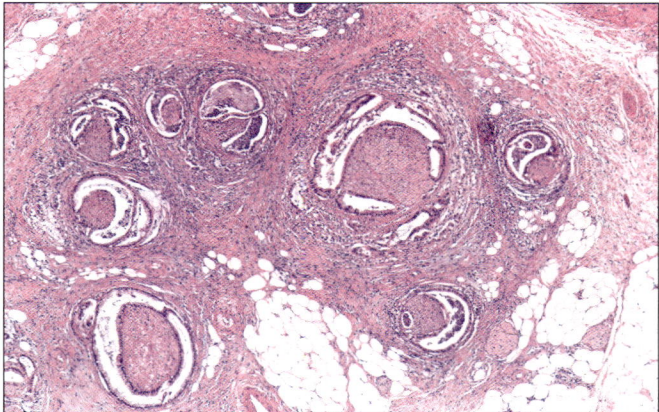

Figure 12.38 Gastric-type or minimal deviation adenocarcinoma ('adenoma malignum'). Extensive perineural invasion.

patients with minimal deviation adenocarcinoma and in only 5% of other types of mucinous adenocarcinoma of the cervix. In the sporadic form of adenoma malignum, a putative tumor suppressor gene is located at D19S216 on chromosomal band 19p13.3 and plays an important role in adenoma malignum tumor genesis.[105]

DNA measurements of the glands of adenoma malignum disclose patterns similar to those of normal endocervical glands. Reports of HPV identification strongly suggest that HPV is involved in only rare cases.[57,75,106]

Differential Diagnosis

Benign lesions which must be distinguished from adenoma malignum include tunnel clusters, deep nabothian cysts, diffuse laminar endocervical glandular hyperplasia, microglandular hyperplasia, and mesonephric hyperplasia.

Tunnel clusters are benign, lobulated proliferations of small, nondilated, closely packed glands found virtually always as an incidental finding. While most glands are arranged around a central primary or secondary endocervical cleft and as a group are well circumscribed, occasionally the borders may be irregular and have a pseudoinvasive appearance. Rarely, some areas may show cytologic atypia.[107]

Diffuse laminar endocervical glandular hyperplasia is also an incidental finding in hysterectomy or cone biopsy specimens.[108] Moderate-sized, evenly spaced, extremely well-differentiated endocervical glands are present within the inner one-third of the cervical wall and are sharply demarcated from the underlying cervical stroma. A marked inflammatory response is often present. Occasionally, entirely normal endocervical glands can be found deep in the wall as an incidental finding. Usually the glands are few in number, but rarely may be florid.

Endocervicosis, a condition that usually involves the urinary bladder, but may also involve the deep cervix, is of unknown pathogenesis. In the few cases described, the lesion grossly consisted of firm rubbery masses 1–2.5 cm in size, and was located in the outer half of the anterior cervical wall and separate from the normal endocervical glands lining the endocervix. Microscopically, the mucinous glands are of variable size and shape, and exhibit endocervical-type glands with bland cytologic features. Desmoplasia is absent.[109]

Histochemistry using a combined Alcian blue (pH 2.5)/periodic acid–Schiff (PAS) stain may be useful. Normal endocervical glands with their high content of acid and neutral mucins stain a purple to violet color, whereas the glands of cervical adenoma malignum (and conventional adenocarcinomas) stain red because of the almost exclusive presence of neutral mucin.[110]

In a recent study, both adenoma malignum and well-differentiated adenocarcinoma of usual type could be distinguished from endocervical glandular hyperplasia by identifying surrounding α-smooth muscle actin-positive stromal cells and by the absence or decreased number of ER-positive stromal cells in the malignant tumors.[111]

Biologic Behavior and Treatment

Despite its histologically bland appearance, adenoma malignum invades deeply and commonly metastasizes to lymph nodes. In a literature review of tumors that were clinically staged before treatment, 50% of patients with stage I tumors and 80% of patients with stage II tumors died of recurrent tumor despite radical treatment in most cases.[94] Hematogenous dissemination of tumor is exceptional and tumor recurrence is most commonly in the abdominopelvic region.[94]

VILLOGLANDULAR ADENOCARCINOMA

Definition and Clinical History

Villoglandular adenocarcinoma is an uncommon variant of cervical adenocarcinoma that shows well-differentiated villoglandular fronds resembling villoglandular adenoma of the colon.[112] It occurs mostly in young women (average age, 35–45 years) and is associated with excellent prognosis.[112,113] A link with oral contraceptive use has been suggested.[113]

Pathology

The tumor is grossly distinctive and usually appears as a broad-based, papillary, and friable cervical polyp (Figure 12.39). Microscopically, it shows by a surface

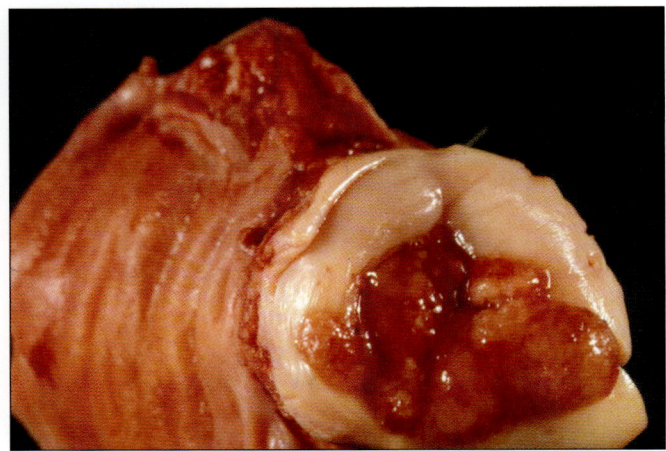

Figure 12.39 Villoglandular adenocarcinoma. The tumor appears as a broad-based, papillary, and friable cervical polyp.

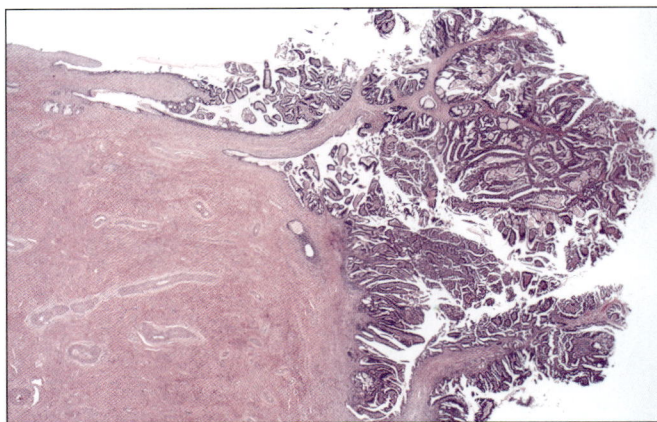

Figure 12.40 Villoglandular adenocarcinoma. Surface papillary component without obvious stromal invasion.

papillary component of variable thickness (Figure 12.40). The papillae are long and slender, occasionally short and broad, and covered by endocervical, endometrioid, or intestinal epithelia with at most mild to moderate cytologic atypia (Figures 12.41–12.43). The amount of stroma in the villi may be substantial or minimal, and often contains many acute and chronic inflammatory cells. The epithelium may be pseudostratified, but lacks tufting and solid areas. The invasive portion of the tumor, if present, is composed of elongated branching glands separated by a fibrous stroma like that seen in the stroma of the papillae but sometimes it may be myxoid or desmoplastic. Most tumors are either entirely exophytic or show only superficial invasion, confined to the inner third of the cervical wall. The tumor cells usually exhibit mild to moderate nuclear atypicality and contain scattered mitotic figures. Lymphatic or vascular invasion is rarely observed. Associated SIL or AIS is common. Lymph node metastases are rare.[113–115]

A tumor should not be placed in this group if any adverse prognostic feature, e.g., presence of coexisting serous carcinoma or small cell carcinoma is present.[114,115] As a cautionary note, we have seen cases where the superficial tumor, seen on biopsy, was villoglandular, but where the deeper tumor found in the subsequent hysterectomy specimen was a typical invasive adenocarcinoma. The differential diagnosis of villoglandular adenocarcinoma also includes benign lesions such as papillary endocervicitis, müllerian papilloma, and müllerian adenofibroma.[115] All three of these lesions lack the degree of nuclear atypia that is present in villoglandular adenocarcinomas. Also, in contrast to villoglandular adenocarcinoma, müllerian adenofibroma and müllerian papilloma typically show a more prominent stromal component. Villoglandular adenocarcinoma should also be distinguished from serous carcinoma of the cervix. Serous carcinomas exhibit more irregular papillae, which are lined by cells with nuclear anaplasia and numerous mitoses. Cellular tufts are also frequent.

Villoglandular adenocarcinoma has distinct cytologic appearances.[116,117] Smears contain many large cohesive sheets, with crowded nuclei and loss of the normal honeycomb structure. Most characteristic are true papillary structures with stromal cores covered by palisaded columnar cells

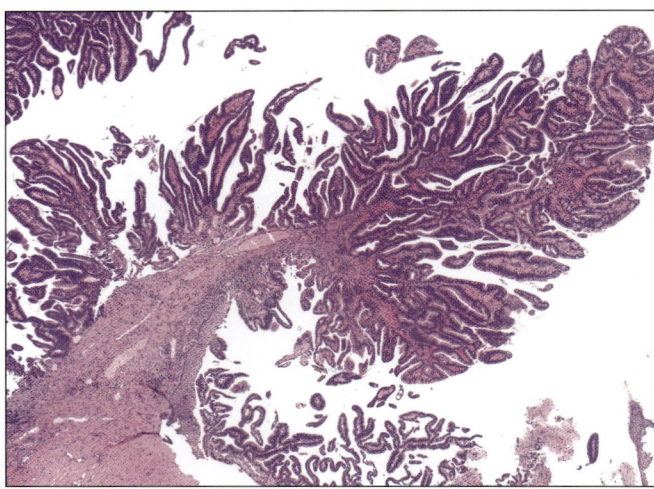

Figure 12.41 Villoglandular adenocarcinoma. The tumor resembles a villous adenoma of the colon.

with intact cytoplasm. Nuclei are small, moderately hyperchromatic, and round to oval with minimal pleomorphism and small or absent nucleoli. The nuclear features are not clearly malignant and, if close attention is not paid to the architectural features, the diagnosis may be missed.

Somatic Genetics and Immunohistochemistry

Villoglandular adenocarcinomas are associated with HPV (type 16 more commonly than type 18)[58,75,118] but do not carry *K-ras-2* and *p53* gene point mutations.[118] Immunohistochemically, they overexpress Ki-67/MIB1, and lack reactivity for *p53* and estrogen and progesterone receptors.[119]

Biologic Behavior and Treatment

The young age of the patients and the excellent prognosis of these tumors suggest that they may be managed by a cone biopsy and careful follow-up, if the tumor is superficial and well differentiated, without vascular space invasion or involvement of resection margins.[112,113] In the two largest series reported, all patients, including those treated by cone biopsy, were alive and well with no evidence of recurrent

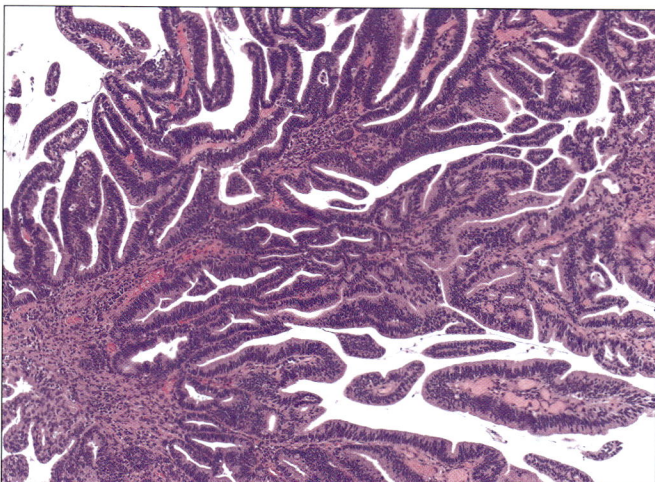

Figure 12.42 Villoglandular adenocarcinoma. The papillae are covered by epithelia showing endocervical, endometrioid, or intestinal features.

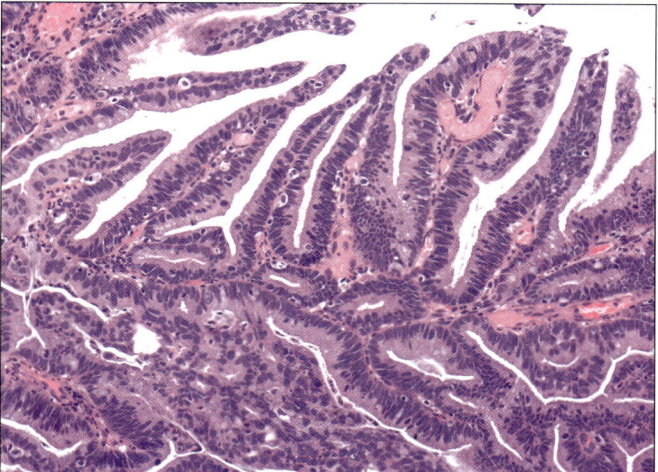

Figure 12.43 Villoglandular adenocarcinoma. The epithelium shows moderate cytologic atypia.

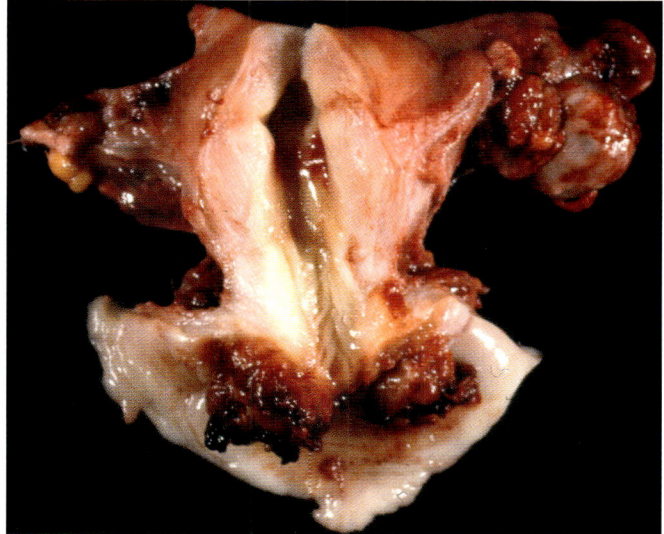

Figure 12.44 Clear cell adenocarcinoma involving the exocervix.

disease after 7–77 months.[112,113] Nevertheless, two cases of 'villous adenoma' of the uterine cervix associated with underlying invasive adenocarcinoma have been reported.[120] The presence of an underlying invasive carcinoma in these cases indicates that the finding of a villoglandular lesion of the cervix, even if it is lined by only slightly atypical cells, should warrant investigation to exclude an underlying adenocarcinoma.

ENDOMETRIOID ADENOCARCINOMA

Endometrioid adenocarcinomas of the cervix resemble primary adenocarcinomas of the uterine corpus. The reported frequency of cervical endometrioid adenocarcinoma ranges from 7% to 50% and such discrepancy is related to whether mucin-poor tumors are included within the classification of mucinous endocervical-type adenocarcinoma or as the specific 'endometrioid' variant. As indicated previously, endocervical-type adenocarcinomas that contain relatively little intracytoplasmic mucin may resemble endometrioid adenocarcinomas of endocervical origin. In such cases, however, endocervical extension from an adenocarcinoma of the corpus has to be ruled out. Tumors of the uterine corpus have frequently invaded the myometrium by the time they extend to the cervix and therefore cause uterine enlargement. Immunohistochemically, adenocarcinomas that show strong positive immunoreaction for vimentin and ER, and weak or negative immunostaining for $p16^{INK4A}$, are most likely of endometrial origin.

MINIMAL DEVIATION ADENOCARCINOMA, ENDOMETRIOID TYPE

The term minimal deviation adenocarcinoma of the endometrioid type refers to the occasional endometrioid adenocarcinoma of the cervix that has a deceptively benign histologic appearance. This definition expands upon the original description of adenoma malignum that is confined to the mucinous tumor and resembles normal endocervical epithelium. In these cases the architecture and distribution of the glands and the presence of at least low-grade nuclear atypia help achieve the correct diagnosis. Cilia and/or apical snouts are commonly seen in these tumors.[95]

CLEAR CELL ADENOCARCINOMA

Definition

Clear cell adenocarcinoma is composed mainly of clear or hobnail cells arranged in solid, tubulocystic, or papillary patterns or a combination. This tumor is histologically similar to clear cell adenocarcinoma of the ovary, endometrium, and vagina, where they are more common.[121–123] Clear cell adenocarcinoma accounts for only 2–4% of cervical adenocarcinomas. Although well known because of its association in young women with a history of *in utero* exposure to DES, currently its peak frequency is in the postmenopausal group.[121–123]

Pathology

Grossly, the tumors may involve the exocervix or the endocervix (Figure 12.44). Microscopically, the tumor cells have abundant clear cytoplasm due to the accumulation of

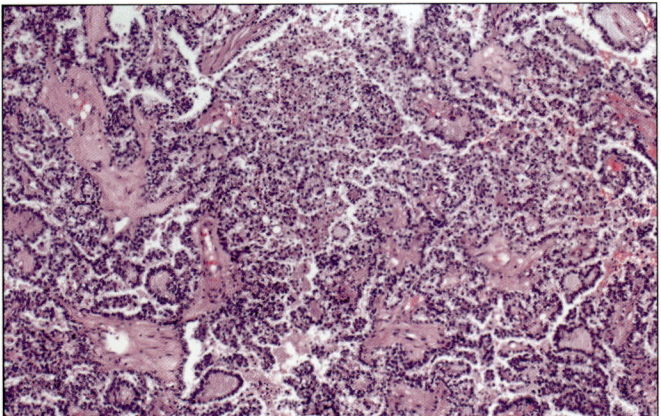

Figure 12.45 Clear cell adenocarcinoma. The tumor cells show clear cytoplasm and prominent 'hobnail' nuclei.

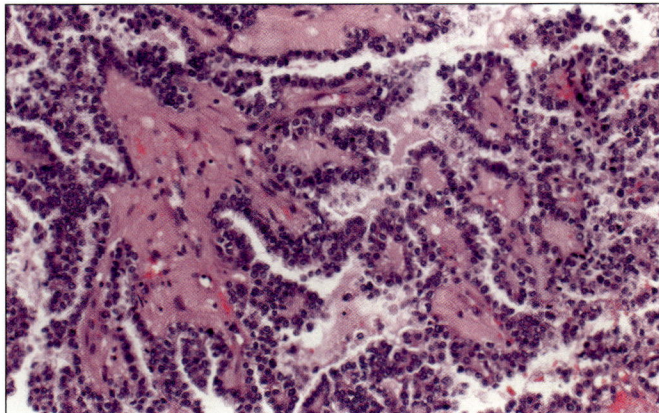

Figure 12.46 Clear cell adenocarcinoma. The papillae have hyalinized cores.

glycogen or granular eosinophilic cytoplasm, with prominent nuclei that project into the lumen of the cysts and tubules beyond the apparent limits of the cytoplasm (Figure 12.45). The papillae often have hyalinized cores (Figure 12.46). Tumor nuclear grade is usually 2 or 3 and mitoses are infrequent. Intraluminal but not intracytoplasmic mucin may be present. On Pap smear, clear cell adenocarcinoma may display large nuclei with prominent single nucleoli and variable hyperchromasia.[124]

Genetic instability as manifested by somatic mutation of microsatellite repeats was investigated in these tumors, with evidence of microsatellite instability in all DES-associated tumors examined, and in 50% of those tumors not associated with DES exposure.[125]

Differential Diagnosis

The differential diagnosis of clear cell carcinoma includes other types of cervical adenocarcinoma as well as benign cervical lesions such as the Arias-Stella reaction, microglandular hyperplasia, and hyperplasia of mesonephric remnants. Microglandular hyperplasia develops in women of reproductive age, lacks severe nuclear atypia, and usually contains mucin. In the Arias-Stella reaction the nuclei tend to be dark and homogeneous and there is no mitotic activity.

Similarly, mesonephric hyperplasia does not reveal clear or hobnail cells.

In young children, the rare yolk sac tumor of the cervix contains clear cells and may be confused with clear cell adenocarcinoma. The presence of a reticular pattern with Schiller–Duval bodies, the positivity of α-fetoprotein, and the primitive appearance of the tumor cells facilitate the diagnosis. Finally, the rare primary alveolar soft part sarcoma of the cervix should not be confused with a clear cell carcinoma. The distinctive architecture of the former tumor and its characteristic PAS-positive intracytoplasmic crystals help in the differential diagnosis.

Biologic Behavior and Treatment

More than 85% of clear cell carcinomas are stage I or II when diagnosed.[126] Treatment is either radical hysterectomy and vaginectomy or radiation. Metastasis occurs in about 18% of patients with stage I disease, but in nearly 50% of stage II tumors. The 10 year survival rate is 57%.[127] Survival of patients with stage I disease is about 90%. Metastasis to distant sites (lung or supraclavicular nodes) occurs more frequently (36%) than with squamous cell carcinoma (10%). Features associated with a better prognosis include small size of the tumor, shallow depth of invasion, and older age (19+ years) of the patient.[126]

SEROUS ADENOCARCINOMA

Definition

Carcinomas histologically identical to serous carcinomas of the endometrium or ovary seldom occur in the cervix. The diagnosis of primary serous carcinoma of the cervix should be made only after tumor spread from the ovary, fallopian tube, or endometrium has been excluded. Serous carcinoma accounts for 3% of cervical adenocarcinomas (in either pure form or mixed with another type of adenocarcinoma) and has a bimodal age distribution, with one peak occurring before the age of 40 years and the second after the age of 65.[128] Serous carcinoma usually presents with abnormal vaginal bleeding, an abnormal cervical smear, or a watery vaginal discharge.

Pathology

Grossly it resembles other types of cervical adenocarcinoma and microscopically shows a complex pattern of papillae with cellular budding, grade 3 nuclei, and sometimes psammoma bodies. An *in situ* component may be present. Nearly half of cases exhibit a second admixed pattern, most commonly low-grade villoglandular adenocarcinoma but endocervical, clear cell, and endometrioid adenocarcinoma may be admixed.[128] Serous adenocarcinoma of the cervix is frequently CEA positive in contrast to this tumor when arising in other sites.

Cytologically, serous carcinoma shows pseudopapillary clusters and balls of atypical cells as well as single cells displaying extreme cytologic atypia with enlarged irregular nuclei and large nucleoli.[129]

Biologic Behavior and Treatment

Forty percent of patients die with widespread metastases within 5 years of diagnosis.[15] Patients with stage I tumors have a similar outcome to those with usual-type cervical adenocarcinoma, while those with advanced stage disease have a poor prognosis.[128] While most metastases are to pelvic and para-aortic lymph nodes, other sites involved are lung, peritoneum (with production of ascites), liver, and skin. Features associated with a poor prognosis include age <65 years, stage II and higher tumors, tumor size >2 cm, depth of tumor invasion >10 mm, lymph node metastases, and elevated serum CA125.

MESONEPHRIC ADENOCARCINOMA

Definition

Mesonephric adenocarcinoma is one of the rarest subtypes of cervical adenocarcinoma. The tumor originates from mesonephric remnants and there are fewer than 40 well-documented cases in the literature.[130–133] In the past, mesonephric carcinomas were confused with clear cell adenocarcinomas of the cervix.

Pathology

Microscopic examination usually reveals a tubuloglandular pattern (Figures 12.47–12.49). The tubules and glands are small and round and typically contain bright pink or red hyaline material, which is negative on mucin staining (Figure 12.50). Rarely, the tumor forms solid sheets, slit-like spaces, and papillary structures resembling serous carcinoma. In some cases a spindle cell component is present. These tumors are frequently immunoreactive for CD10 (Figure 12.51) as well as for vimentin, calretinin, low molecular weight keratins, and epithelial membrane antigen. Mesonephric carcinomas usually invade the cervical wall and mesonephric hyperplasia is often present at the periphery of the tumor.[130–133]

Biologic Behavior and Treatment

In two reported series, the prognosis of mesonephric carcinomas was better than that of müllerian carcinomas at the same stage.[131,133] Nine cases of malignant mixed mesonephric tumors have also been reported.[130,131] They are aggressive tumors that may present in advanced stage, similar to malignant mixed müllerian tumors.[130] Surgery alone is the treatment of choice.

Differential Diagnosis

The most difficult differential diagnosis of mesonephric carcinoma is with mesonephric hyperplasia. Hyperplastic tubules may extend deeply into the cervical wall and even into the uterine corpus.[130] However, in cases of carcinoma,

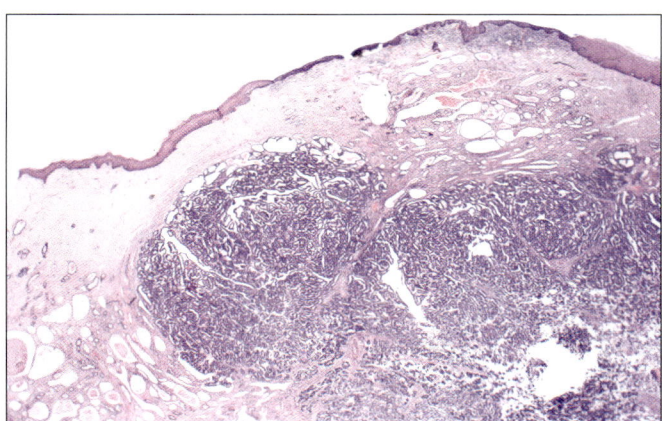

Figure 12.47 Mesonephric adenocarcinoma surrounded by mesonephric hyperplasia.

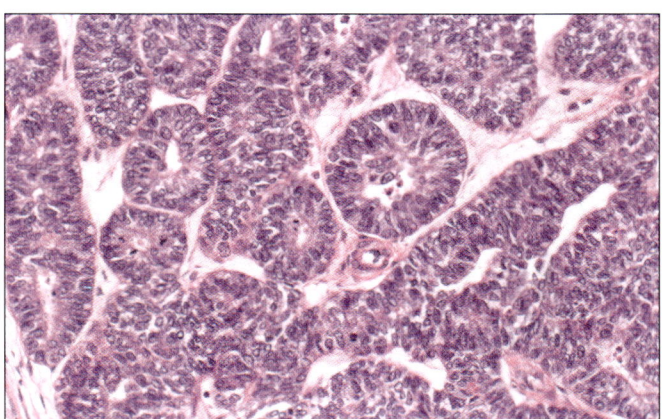

Figure 12.49 Mesonephric adenocarcinoma. Stratified hyperchromatic nuclei with numerous mitoses. The tumor cells lack cytoplasmic mucin.

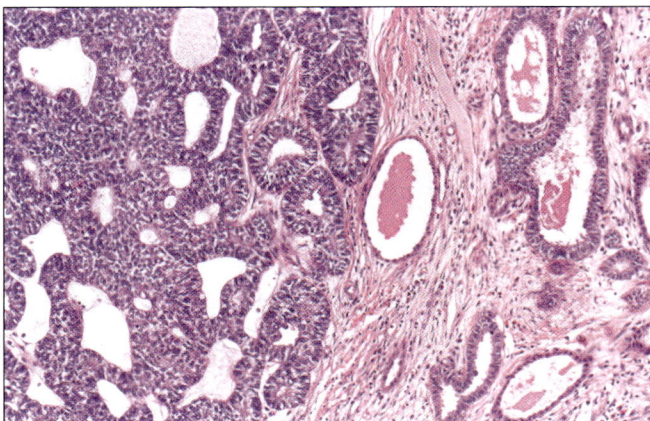

Figure 12.48 Mesonephric adenocarcinoma (left side) adjacent to mesonephric hyperplasia (right side).

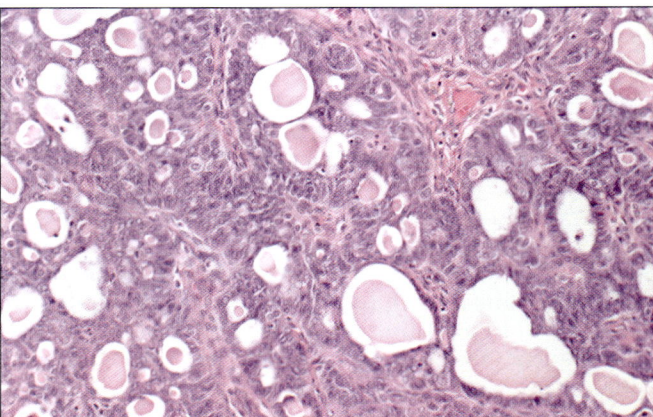

Figure 12.50 Mesonephric adenocarcinoma. The tumor glands typically contain bright pink or red secretion.

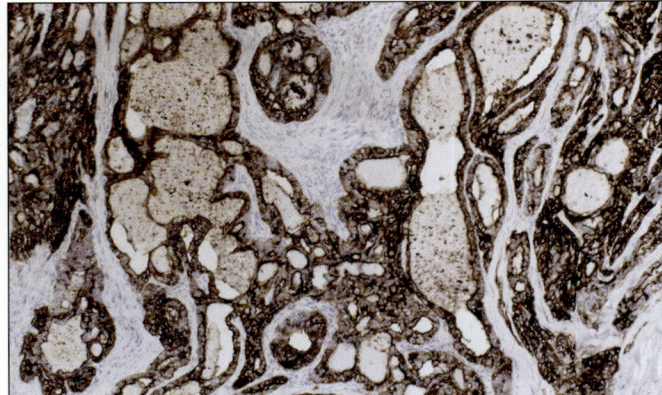

Figure 12.51 Mesonephric adenocarcinoma. CD10 immunoreaction.

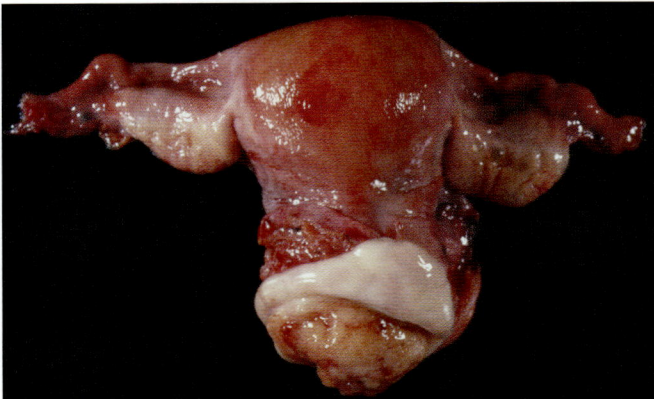

Figure 12.52 Adenosquamous carcinoma. Barrel-shaped tumor with exocervical growth.

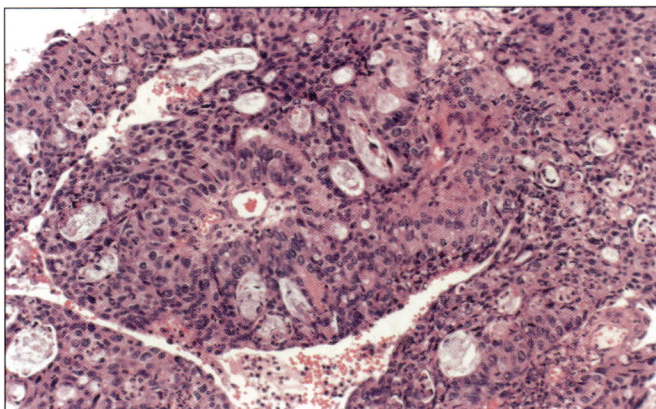

Figure 12.53 Adenosquamous carcinoma. The tumor is composed of various amounts of glands and squamous epithelium which are intimately admixed.

a back-to-back pattern of tubular glands is present, along with significant cytologic atypia and mitotic activity. Mesonephric carcinoma must be distinguished from other adenocarcinomas of the cervix such as minimal deviation adenocarcinoma, endometrioid carcinoma, and clear cell carcinoma.[130–133]

ADENOSQUAMOUS CARCINOMA

Definition

Adenosquamous carcinoma shows both glandular and squamous cell differentiation, with each component clearly visible on H&E-stained slides without special histochemical stains.[4] The occurrence of scattered mucin-producing cells in an otherwise typical-appearing squamous cell carcinoma has been referred to as mucoepidermoid carcinoma, an unnecessary term. There is no convincing evidence that such tumors behave differently.

Clinical Features

Adenosquamous carcinoma accounts for approximately 4% of all cervical cancer.[139] They occur in both old and young women, often in association with pregnancy. The risk factors are more like those of squamous cell carcinoma of the cervix than those of adenocarcinoma, e.g., multiple sexual partners. HPV types 16 and 18 are frequently identified.[134]

Pathology

The tumor may be polypoid, ulcerated, or nodular, and grossly indistinguishable from cervical adenocarcinoma and squamous cell carcinoma (Figure 12.52). On microscopic examination, adenosquamous carcinomas are composed of various amounts of glands and squamous epithelium, which are intimately admixed (Figures 12.53 and 12.54). The glandular component is usually of endocervical type, but may include mucinous signet-ring type. Tumors with an endometrioid appearance and bland (non-malignant)-appearing squamous differentiation should be classified as endometrioid adenocarcinomas of the cervix with squamous differentiation. In practice, most tumors are poorly differentiated and the presence of either component, but especially the glandular component, may not be readily apparent with a superficial glance.

Differential Diagnosis

In some tumors the squamous component may show prominent cytoplasmic glycogen accumulation. A gradient from basal cells that are glycogen poor to more superficial cells that are progressively more glycogen rich helps distinguish it from clear cell carcinoma where the glycogen content is uniform throughout. Adenosquamous carcinoma is usually easy to distinguish from adenoid basal carcinoma as the latter cells are uniform, with generally bland nuclear features, exhibit peripheral palisading, and have scant cytoplasm.

Biologic Behavior and Treatment

The belief that adenosquamous carcinoma has a poorer prognosis than squamous cell carcinoma or adenocarcinoma has been repeatedly challenged.[135–137] In one large series, patients with adenocarcinoma, squamous cell carcinoma, and adenosquamous carcinoma had no significant difference in 5 year survival in any clinical stage except American Joint Committee on Cancer stage II, where squamous cell carcinoma had a better survival. Of interest, patients with adenosquamous carcinoma and positive lymph nodes had the highest 5 year survival rate, whereas women with adenocarcinoma and positive nodes had a sharply reduced survival rate.[135–137] Recent data suggest that patients

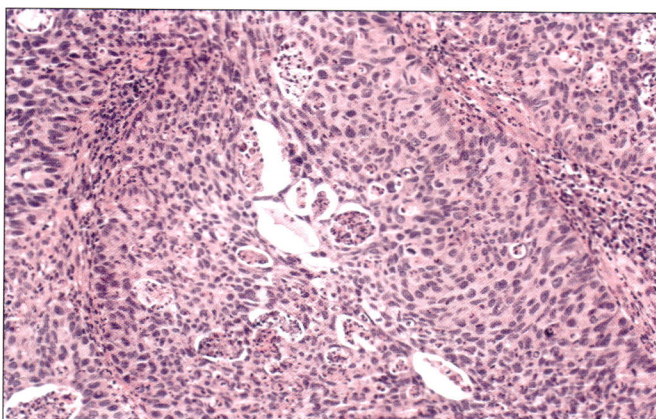

Figure 12.54 Adenosquamous carcinoma. Predominantly squamous cell component.

with adenosquamous carcinoma have a better prognosis than endocervical adenocarcinoma in patients who are stage I, and sometimes stage II.[135] Regardless, adenosquamous histology, like most cancers, predicts a poor outcome for patients with advanced-stage disease.[135]

GLASSY CELL CARCINOMA

Definition
Glassy cell carcinoma, the undifferentiated form of adenosquamous carcinoma of the cervix, exhibits cells with abundant, granular, lightly eosinophilic cytoplasm imparting a so-called ground-glass appearance.[138]

General Features
These tumors, which account for only 1–2% of all cervical carcinomas, occur in younger patients (mean age, 31–41 years) than those with ordinary squamous cell or adenocarcinoma of the cervix and are commonly associated with HPV 18 and occasionally with HPV 16.[138,139]

Pathology
Tumors are usually bulky, exophytic masses, ranging from 3 to 7 cm in size (Figure 12.55). Microscopically, they are characterized by invasive nests and sheets of large cells with abundant eosinophilic or amphophilic, ground-glass cytoplasm, prominent cell borders, large nuclei with prominent nucleoli, and a high mitotic rate (Figure 12.56). A striking inflammatory infiltrate composed predominantly of eosinophils and plasma cells is present. Rare foci of squamous or glandular differentiation and intracellular mucin may be seen.

Biologic Behavior and Treatment
Although the earliest studies of glassy cell carcinomas considered these tumors to be aggressive with a uniformly poor survival rate, subsequent studies have demonstrated that survival is related to stage of the disease at diagnosis.[139] The treatment for glassy cell carcinoma is the same as that for invasive squamous cell carcinoma and adenocarcinoma of the same stage. More recently patients treated with neoadjuvant chemotherapy have been reported to have longer survival.[140]

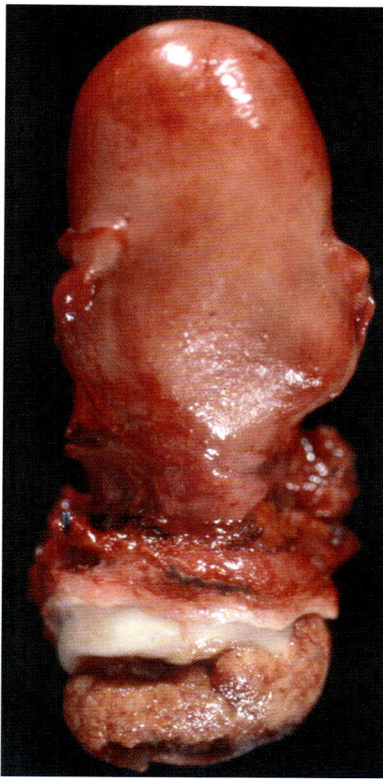

Figure 12.55 Glassy cell carcinoma. Exophytic tumor. The corpus contains a leiomyoma.

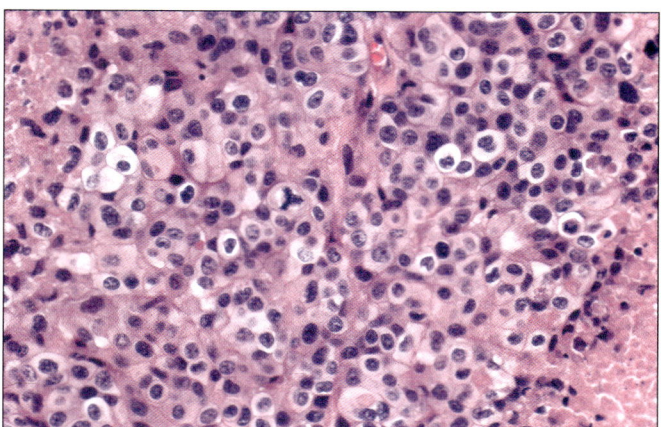

Figure 12.56 Glassy cell carcinoma. The tumor cells show abundant eosinophilic or amphophilic, ground-glass cytoplasm, with prominent cell borders, large nuclei with prominent nucleoli, and a high mitotic rate. Necrosis is seen at the lower right corner.

Differential Diagnosis
The main differential diagnosis is with large cell nonkeratinizing squamous cell carcinoma. The latter tumor lacks a ground-glass appearance of the cell cytoplasms, does not exhibit the prominent nucleoli, and shows more than a minor degree of squamous differentiation. In a recent study, large cell nonkeratinizing squamous cell carcinomas were found to have a prognosis similar to that of glassy cell carcinoma.

REFERENCES

1. Gloor E, Hurlimann J. Cervical intraepithelial glandular neoplasia (adenocarcinoma in situ and glandular dysplasia). A correlative study of 23 cases with histologic grading, histochemical analysis of mucins, and immunohistochemical determination of the affinity for four lectins. Cancer 1986;58:1272–80.
2. Solomon D, Davey D, Kurman R, et al. The 2001 Bethesda System: terminology for reporting results of cervical cytology. JAMA 2002;287:2114–9.
3. Jaworski RC. Endocervical glandular dysplasia, adenocarcinoma in situ, and early invasive (microinvasive) adenocarcinoma of the uterine cervix. Semin Diagn Pathol 1990;7:190–204.
4. Wells M, Ostor AG, Crum CP, et al. Epithelial tumours of the uterine cervix. In: Tavassoli FA, Devilee P, editors. World Health Organization Classification of Tumours. Pathology and genetics. Tumors of the breast and female genital organs. Lyon, France: IARC Press; 2003. p. 260–79.
5. Lee KR. Symposium part 4: should pathologists diagnose endocervical preneoplastic lesions 'less than' adenocarcinoma in situ? Counterpoint. Int J Gynecol Pathol 2003;22:22–4.
6. Lee KR, Sun D, Crum CP. Endocervical intraepithelial glandular atypia (dysplasia): a histopathologic, human papillomavirus, and MIB-1 analysis of 25 cases. Hum Pathol 2000;31:656–64.
7. Murphy N, Heffron CC, King B, et al. p16INK4A positivity in benign, premalignant and malignant cervical glandular lesions: a potential diagnostic problem. Virchows Arch 2004;445:610–5.
8. Riethdorf L, Riethdorf S, Lee KR, et al. Human papillomaviruses, expression of p16, and early endocervical glandular neoplasia. Hum Pathol 2002;33:899–904.
9. Friedell G, McKay D. Adenocarcinoma in situ of the endocervix. Cancer 1953;6:887–97.
10. Christopherson W, Nelson N, Gray L. Noninvasive precursor lesions of adenocarcinoma and mixed adenosquamous carcinoma of the cervix uteri. Cancer 1979;44:975–83.
11. Farnsworth A, Laverty C, Stoler MH. Human papillomavirus messenger RNA expression in adenocarcinoma in situ of the uterine cervix. Int J Gynecol Pathol 1989;8:321–30.
12. Boddington MM, Spriggs AI, Cowdell RH. Adenocarcinoma of the uterine cervix: cytological evidence of a long preclinical evolution. Br J Obstet Gynaecol 1976;83:900–3.
13. Ostor AG, Pagano R, Davoren RA, et al. Adenocarcinoma in situ of the cervix. Int J Gynecol Pathol 1984;3:179–90.
14. Anonymous (2001) SEER Program—National Cancer Institute, USA. http://www-seer.ims.nci.nih.gov/ScientificSystems/. 2003, 2009 [accessed 20.03.03, 20.03.09].
15. Wang SS, Sherman ME, Hildesheim A, et al. Cervical adenocarcinoma and squamous cell carcinoma incidence trends among white women and black women in the United States for 1976–2000. Cancer 2004;100:1035–44.
16. Plaxe SC, Saltzstein SL. Estimation of the duration of the preclinical phase of cervical adenocarcinoma suggests that there is ample opportunity for screening. Gynecol Oncol 1999;75:55–61.
17. Wang SS, Sherman ME, Silverberg SG, et al. Pathological characteristics of cervical adenocarcinoma in a multi-center US-based study. Gynecol Oncol 2006;103:541–6.
18. Bertrand M, Lickrish GM, Colgan TJ. The anatomic distribution of cervical adenocarcinoma in situ: implications for treatment. Am J Obstet Gynecol 1987;157:21–5.
19. Denehy TR, Gregori CA, Breen JL. Endocervical curettage, cone margins, and residual adenocarcinoma in situ of the cervix. Obstet Gynecol 1997;90:1–6.
20. Duggan MA, Benoit JL, McGregor SE, et al. Adenocarcinoma in situ of the endocervix: human papillomavirus determination by dot blot hybridization and polymerase chain reaction amplification. Int J Gynecol Pathol 1994;13:143–9.
21. Hasumi K, Ehrmann RL. Clear cell carcinoma of the uterine endocervix with an in situ component. Cancer 1978;42:2435–8.
22. Jaworski RC, Pacey NF, Greenberg ML, Osborn RA. The histologic diagnosis of adenocarcinoma in situ and related lesions of the cervix uteri. Adenocarcinoma in situ. Cancer 1988;61:1171–81.
23. Biscotti CV, Hart WR. Apoptotic bodies: a consistent morphologic feature of endocervical adenocarcinoma in situ. Am J Surg Pathol 1998;22:434–9.
24. Negri G, Egarter-Vigl E, Kasal A, et al. p16INK4a is a useful marker for the diagnosis of adenocarcinoma of the cervix uteri and its precursors: an immunohistochemical study with immunocytochemical correlations. Am J Surg Pathol 2003;27:187–93.
25. Cameron RI, Maxwell P, Jenkins D, McCluggage WG. Immunohistochemical staining with MIB1, bcl2 and p16 assists in the distinction of cervical glandular intraepithelial neoplasia from tubo-endometrial metaplasia, endometriosis and microglandular hyperplasia. Histopathology 2002;41:313–21.
26. McCluggage G, McBride H, Maxwell P, Bharucha H. Immunohistochemical detection of p53 and bcl-2 proteins in neoplastic and non-neoplastic endocervical glandular lesions. Int J Gynecol Pathol 1997;16:22–7.
27. Marques T, Andrade LA, Vassallo J. Endocervical tubal metaplasia and adenocarcinoma in situ: role of immunohistochemistry for carcinoembryonic antigen and vimentin in differential diagnosis. Histopathology 1996;28:549–50.
28. Nanbu Y, Fujii S, Konishi I, et al. Immunohistochemical localizations of CA 125, carcinoembryonic antigen, and CA 19-9 in normal and neoplastic glandular cells of the uterine cervix. Cancer 1988;62:2580–8.
29. Mitchell H, Hocking J, Saville M. Cervical cytology screening history of women diagnosed with adenocarcinoma in situ of the cervix: a case-control study. Acta Cytol 2004;48:595–600.
30. Lee KR, Minter LJ, Granter SR. Papanicolaou smear sensitivity for adenocarcinoma in situ of the cervix. A study of 34 cases. Am J Clin Pathol 1997;107:30–5.
31. Schoolland M, Segal A, Allpress S, et al. Adenocarcinoma in situ of the cervix. Cancer 2002;96:330–7.
32. Shin CH, Schorge JO, Lee KR, Sheets EE. Cytologic and biopsy findings leading to conization in adenocarcinoma in situ of the cervix. Obstet Gynecol 2002;100:271–6.
33. Belsley NA, Tambouret RH, Misdraji J, et al. Cytologic features of endocervical glandular lesions: comparison of SurePath, ThinPrep, and conventional smear specimen preparations. Diagn Cytopathol 2008;36(4):232–7.
34. Hecht JL, Sheets EE, Lee KR. Atypical glandular cells of undetermined significance in conventional cervical/vaginal smears and thin-layer preparations. Cancer 2002;96:1–4.
35. Murphy N, Ring M, Killalea AG, et al. p16INK4A as a marker for cervical dyskaryosis: CIN and cGIN in cervical biopsies and ThinPrep smears. J Clin Pathol 2003;56:56–63.
36. Schlesinger C, Silverberg SG. Endocervical adenocarcinoma in situ of tubal type and its relation to atypical tubal metaplasia. Int J Gynecol Pathol 1999;18:1–4.
37. Baker PM, Clement PB, Bell DA, Young RH. Superficial endometriosis of the uterine cervix: a report of 20 cases of a process that may be confused with endocervical glandular dysplasia or adenocarcinoma in situ. Int J Gynecol Pathol 1999;18:198–205.
38. Lesack D, Wahab I, Gilks CB. Radiation-induced atypia of endocervical epithelium: a histological, immunohistochemical and cytometric study. Int J Gynecol Pathol 1996;15:242–7.
39. Nucci MR, Young RH. Arias-Stella reaction of the endocervix: a report of 18 cases with emphasis on its varied histology and differential diagnosis. Am J Surg Pathol 2004;28:608–12.
40. Park JJ, Sun D, Quade BJ, et al. Stratified mucin-producing intraepithelial lesions of the cervix: adenosquamous or columnar cell neoplasia? Am J Surg Pathol 2000;24:1414–9.
41. Hopkins MP, Roberts JA, Schmidt RW. Cervical adenocarcinoma in situ. Obstet Gynecol 1988;71:842–4.
42. Hopkins MP. Adenocarcinoma in situ of the cervix—the margins must be clear. Gynecol Oncol 2000;79:4–5.
43. Salani R, Puri I, Bristow RE. Adenocarcinoma in situ of the uterine cervix: a metaanalysis of 1278 patients evaluating the predictive value of conization margin status. Am J Obstet Gynecol 2009;200:182e1–5.
44. Azodi M, Chambers SK, Rutherford TJ, et al. Adenocarcinoma in situ of the cervix: management and outcome. Gynecol Oncol 1999;73:348–53.
45. Goldstein NS, Mani A. The status and distance of cone biopsy margins as a predictor of excision adequacy for endocervical adenocarcinoma in situ. Am J Clin Pathol 1998;109:727–32.
46. Ostor AG, Duncan A, Quinn M, Rome R. Adenocarcinoma in situ of the uterine cervix: an experience with 100 cases. Gynecol Oncol 2000;79:207–10.

47. Shin CH, Schorge JO, Lee KR, Sheets EE. Conservative management of adenocarcinoma in situ of the cervix. Gynecol Oncol 2000;79:6–10.
48. Zaino RJ. Symposium part I: adenocarcinoma in situ, glandular dysplasia, and early invasive adenocarcinoma of the uterine cervix. Int J Gynecol Pathol 2002;21:314–26.
49. Kennedy AW, Biscotti CV. Further study of the management of cervical adenocarcinoma in situ. Gynecol Oncol 2002;86:361–4.
50. Widrich T, Kennedy AW, Myers TM, et al. Adenocarcinoma in situ of the uterine cervix: management and outcome. Gynecol Oncol 1996;61:304–8.
51. Bulk S, Visser O, Rozendaal L, et al. Cervical cancer in the Netherlands 1989–1998: decrease of squamous cell carcinoma in older women, increase of adenocarcinoma in younger women. Int J Cancer 2005;113:1005–9.
52. Smith HO, Tiffany MF, Qualls CR, Key CR. The rising incidence of adenocarcinoma relative to squamous cell carcinoma of the uterine cervix in the United States—a 24-year population-based study. Gynecol Oncol 2000;78:97–105.
53. Saraiya M, Ahmed F, Krishnan S, et al. Cervical cancer incidence in a prevaccine era in the United States, 1998–2002. Obstet Gynecol 2007;109:360–70.
54. Parazzini F, La Vecchia C. Epidemiology of adenocarcinoma of the cervix. Gynecol Oncol 1990;39:40–6.
55. Maier RC, Norris HJ. Coexistence of cervical intraepithelial neoplasia with primary adenocarcinoma of the endocervix. Obstet Gynecol 1980;56:361–4.
56. Andersson S, Rylander E, Larsson B, et al. The role of human papillomavirus in cervical adenocarcinoma carcinogenesis. Eur J Cancer 2001;37:246–50.
57. Castellsague X, Diaz M, de Sanjosé S, et al. Worldwide human papillomavirus etiology of cervical adenocarcinoma and its cofactors: implications for screening and prevention. J Natl Cancer Inst 2006;98:303–15.
58. Pirog EC, Kleter B, Olgac S, et al. Prevalence of human papillomavirus DNA in different histological subtypes of cervical adenocarcinoma. Am J Pathol 2000;157:1055–62.
59. Taylor H, Irey N, Norris HJ. Atypical endocervical hyperplasia in women taking oral contraceptives. JAMA 1967;202:185–90.
60. Lacey Jr JV, Brinton LA, Barnes WA, et al. Use of hormone replacement therapy and adenocarcinomas and squamous cell carcinomas of the uterine cervix. Gynecol Oncol 2000;77:149–54.
61. Kjaer SK, Brinton LA. Adenocarcinomas of the uterine cervix: the epidemiology of an increasing problem. Epidemiol Rev 1993;15:486–98.
62. Connolly DC, Katabuchi H, Cliby WA, Cho KR. Somatic mutations in the STK11/LKB1 gene are uncommon in rare gynecological tumor types associated with Peutz-Jegher's syndrome. Am J Pathol 2000;156:339–45.
63. Chen RJ, Chang DY, Yen ML, et al. Prognostic factors of primary adenocarcinoma of the uterine cervix. Gynecol Oncol 1998;69:157–64.
64. Östör AG. Early invasive adenocarcinoma of the uterine cervix. Int J Gynecol Pathol 2000;19:29–38.
65. Wheeler DT, Kurman RJ. The relationship of glands to thickwall blood vessels as a marker of invasion in endocervical adenocarcinoma. Int J Gynecol Pathol 2005;24:125–30.
66. Ayer B, Pacey F, Greenberg M. The cytologic diagnosis of adenocarcinoma in situ of the cervix uteri and related lesions. II. Microinvasive adenocarcinoma. Acta Cytol 1988;32:318–24.
67. Mulvany N, Ostor A. Microinvasive adenocarcinoma of the cervix: a cytohistopathologic study of 40 cases. Diagn Cytopathol 1997;16:430–6.
68. Webb JC, Key CR, Qualls CR, Smith HO. Population-based study of microinvasive adenocarcinoma of the uterine cervix. Obstet Gynecol 2001;97(5 Pt 1):701–6.
69. Balega J, Michael H, Hurteau J, et al. The risk of nodal metastasis in early adenocarcinoma of the uterine cervix. Int J Gynecol Cancer 2004;14:104–9.
70. Ceballos KM, Shaw D, Daya D. Microinvasive cervical adenocarcinoma (FIGO stage 1A tumors): results of surgical staging and outcome analysis. Am J Surg Pathol 2006;30:370–4.
71. Kaminski PF, Norris HJ. Coexistence of ovarian neoplasms and endocervical adenocarcinoma. Obstet Gynecol 1984;64:553–6.
72. Young RH, Scully RE. Mucinous ovarian tumors associated with mucinous adenocarcinomas of the cervix. A clinicopathological analysis of 16 cases. Int J Gynecol Pathol 1998;7:99–111.
73. Yemelyanova A, Vang R, Seidman JD, et al. Endocervical adenocarcinomas with prominent endometrial or endomyometrial involvement simulating primary endometrial carcinomas: utility of HPV DNA detection and immunohistochemical expression of p16 and hormone receptors to confirm the cervical origin of the corpus tumor. Am J Surg Pathol 2009;33:914–24.
74. Kamoi S, AlJuboury AI, Akin MR, Silverberg SG. Immunohistochemical staining in the distinction between primary endometrial and endocervical adenocarcinomas: another viewpoint. Int J Gynecol Pathol 2002;21:217–23.
75. An HJ, Kim KR, Kim IS, et al. Prevalence of human papillomavirus DNA in various histological subtypes of cervical adenocarcinoma: a population-based study. Mod Pathol 2005;18:528–34.
76. Boon ME, Ouwerkerk-Noordam E, van Leeuwen AW, et al. How to improve cytologic screening for endocervical adenocarcinoma? Eur J Gynaecol Oncol 2002;23:481–5.
77. DiTomasso JP, Ramzy I, Mody DR. Glandular lesions of the cervix. Validity of cytologic criteria used to differentiate reactive changes, glandular intraepithelial lesions and adenocarcinoma. Acta Cytol 1996;40:1127–35.
78. Young RH, Clement PB. Endocervical adenocarcinoma and its variants: their morphology and differential diagnosis. Histopathology 2002;41:185–207.
79. Benoit JL, Kini SR. 'Arias-Stella reaction'-like changes in endocervical glandular epithelium in cervical smears during pregnancy and postpartum states—a potential diagnostic pitfall. Diagn Cytopathol 1996;14:349–55.
80. Jones MA, Young RH. Atypical oxyphilic metaplasia of the endocervical epithelium: a report of six cases. Int J Gynecol Pathol 1997;16:99–102.
81. Tambouret R, Bell DA, Young RH. Microcystic endocervical adenocarcinomas: a report of eight cases. Am J Surg Pathol 2000;24:369–74.
82. Ferry JA, Scully RE. Mesonephric remnants, hyperplasia, and neoplasia in the uterine cervix. A study of 49 cases. Am J Surg Pathol 1990;14:1100–11.
83. Vesterinen E, Forss M, Nieminen U. Increase of cervical adenocarcinoma: a report of 520 cases of cervical carcinoma including 112 tumors with glandular elements. Gynecol Oncol 1989;3349–53.
84. Look KY, Brunetto VL, Clarke-Pearson DL, et al. An analysis of cell type in patients with surgically staged stage IB carcinoma of the cervix: a Gynecologic Oncology Group study. Gynecol Oncol 1996;63:304–11.
85. Ayhan A, Al RA, Baykal C, et al. A comparison of prognoses of FIGO stage IB adenocarcinoma and squamous cell carcinoma. Int J Gynecol Cancer 2004;14:279–85.
86. Pecorelli S. Annual report on the results of treatment in gynecological cancer. Int J Gynecol Obstet 2003;25(Suppl 1):1–211.
87. Recoules-Arche A, Rouzier R, Rey A, et al. [Does adenocarcinoma of uterine cervix have a worse prognosis than squamous carcinoma?] Gynecol Obstet Fertil 2004;32:116–21.
88. Baalbergen A, Ewing-Graham PC, Hop WC, et al. Prognostic factors in adenocarcinoma of the uterine cervix. Gynecol Oncol 2004;92:262–7.
89. Leung TW, Xue WC, Cheung AN, et al. Proliferation to apoptosis ratio as a prognostic marker in adenocarcinoma of uterine cervix. Gynecol Oncol 2004;92:866–72.
90. Attanoos R, Nahar K, Bigrigg A, et al. Primary adenocarcinoma of the cervix. A clinicopathological study of prognostic variables in 55 cases. Int J Gynecol Cancer 1995;5:179–86.
91. Nakagawa S, Yoshikawa H, Onda T, et al. Type of human papillomavirus is related to clinical features of cervical carcinoma. Cancer 1996;78:1935–41.
92. Haswani P, Arseneau J, Ferenczy A. Primary signet ring cell carcinoma of the uterine cervix: a clinicopathologic study of two cases with review of the literature. Int J Gynecol Cancer 1998;8:374–9.
93. Kaminski P, Norris H. Minimal deviation carcinoma (adenoma malignum) of the cervix. Int J Gynecol Pathol 1983;2:141–52.
94. Gilks C, Young R, Aguirre P, et al. Adenoma malignum (minimal deviation adenocarcinoma) of the uterine cervix. A clinicopathological and immunohistochemical analysis of 26 cases. Am J Surg Pathol 1989;13:717–29.
95. Young RH, Scully RE. Minimal-deviation endometrioid adenocarcinoma of the uterine cervix. A report of five cases of a distinctive neoplasm that may be misinterpreted as benign. Am J Surg Pathol 1993;17:660–5.

96. Mikami Y, Kiyokawa T, Hata S, et al. Gastrointestinal immunophenotype in adenocarcinomas of the uterine cervix and related glandular lesions: a possible link between lobular endocervical glandular hyperplasia/pyloric gland metaplasia and 'adenoma malignum'. Mod Pathol 2004;17:962–72.

97. Kojima A, Mikami Y, Sudo T, et al. Gastric morphology and immunophenotype predict poor outcome in mucinous adenocarcinoma of the uterine cervix. Am J Surg Pathol 2007;31:664–72.

98. Kusanagi Y, Kojima A, Mikami Y, et al. Absence of high-risk human papillomavirus (HPV) detection in endocervical adenocarcinoma with gastric morphology and phenotype. Am J Pathol 2010;177:2169–75.

99. Hirai Y, Takeshima N, Haga A, et al. A clinicocytopathologic study of adenoma malignum of the uterine cervix. Gynecol Oncol 1998;70:219–23.

100. McGarrity TJ, Kulin HE, Zaino RJ. Peutz–Jeghers syndrome. Am J Gastroenterol 2000;95:596–604.

101. Young RH, Welch WR, Dickersin GR, Scully RE. Ovarian sex cord tumor with annular tubules: review of 74 cases including 27 with Peutz–Jeghers syndrome and four with adenoma malignum of the cervix. Cancer 1982;50:1384–402.

102. Granter SR, Lee KR. Cytologic findings in minimal deviation adenocarcinoma (adenoma malignum) of the cervix. A report of seven cases. Am J Clin Pathol 1996;105:327–33.

103. Ishii K, Katsuyama T, Ota H, et al. Cytologic and cytochemical features of adenoma malignum of the uterine cervix. Cancer 1999;87:245–53.

104. Toki T, Shiozawa T, Hosaka N, et al. Minimal deviation adenocarcinoma of the uterine cervix has abnormal expression of sex steroid receptors, CA125, and gastric mucin. Int J Gynecol Pathol 1997;16:111–16.

105. Lee JY, Dong SM, Kim HS, et al. A distinct region of chromosome 19p13.3 associated with the sporadic form of adenoma malignum of the uterine cervix. Cancer Res 1998;58:1140–3.

106. Fukushima M, Shimano S, Yamakawa Y, et al. The detection of human papillomavirus (HPV) in a case of minimal deviation adenocarcinoma of the uterine cervix (adenoma malignum) using in situ hybridization. Jpn J Clin Oncol 1990;20:407–12.

107. Jones MA, Young RH. Endocervical type A (noncystic) tunnel clusters with cytologic atypia. A report of 14 cases. Am J Surg Pathol 1996;20:1312–8.

108. Jones MA, Young RH, Scully RE. Diffuse laminar endocervical glandular hyperplasia. A benign lesion often confused with adenoma malignum (minimal deviation adenocarcinoma). Am J Surg Pathol 1991;15:1123–9.

109. Young RH, Clement PB. Endocervicosis involving the uterine cervix: a report of four cases of a benign process that may be confused with deeply invasive endocervical adenocarcinoma. Int J Gynecol Pathol 2000;19:322–8.

110. Hayashi I, Tsuda H, Shimoda T. Reappraisal of orthodox histochemistry for the diagnosis of minimal deviation adenocarcinoma of the cervix. Am J Surg Pathol 2000;24:559–62.

111. Mikami Y, Kiyokawa T, Moriya T, Sasano H. Immunophenotypic alteration of the stromal component in minimal deviation adenocarcinoma ('adenoma malignum') and endocervical glandular hyperplasia: a study using oestrogen receptor and alpha-smooth muscle actin double immunostaining. Histopathology 2005;46:130–6.

112. Young RH, Scully RE. Villoglandular papillary adenocarcinoma of the uterine cervix. A clinicopathologic analysis of 13 cases. Cancer 1989;63:1773–9.

113. Jones MW, Silverberg SG, Kurman RJ. Well-differentiated villoglandular adenocarcinoma of the uterine cervix: a clinicopathological study of 24 cases. Int J Gynecol Pathol 1993;12:1–7.

114. Kaku T, Kamura T, Shigematsu T, et al. Adenocarcinoma of the uterine cervix with predominantly villogladular papillary growth pattern. Gynecol Oncol 1997;64:147–52.

115. Young RH, Clement PB. Endocervical adenocarcinoma and its variants: their morphology and differential diagnosis. Histopathology 2002;41:185–207.

116. Ballo MS, Silverberg SG, Sidawy MK. Cytologic features of well-differentiated villoglandular adenocarcinoma of the cervix. Acta Cytol 1996;40:536–40.

117. Chang WC, Matisic JP, Zhou C, et al. Cytologic features of villoglandular adenocarcinoma of the uterine cervix: comparison with typical endocervical adenocarcinoma with a villoglandular component and papillary serous carcinoma. Cancer 1999;87:5–11.

118. Jones MW, Kounelis S, Papadaki H, et al. Well-differentiated villoglandular adenocarcinoma of the uterine cervix: oncogene/tumor suppressor gene alterations and human papillomavirus genotyping. Int J Gynecol Pathol 2000;19:110–7.

119. Polat A, Dusmez D, Pata O, et al. Villoglandular papillary adenocarcinoma of the uterine cervix with immunohistochemical characteristics. J Exp Clin Cancer Res 2002;21(3):425–7.

120. Michael H, Sutton G, Huil MT, Roth LM. Villous adenoma of the uterine cervix associated with invasive adenocarcinoma: a histologic, ultrastructural, and immunohistochemical study. Int J Gynecol Pathol 1986;5:163–9.

121. Robboy SJ, Young RH, Welch WR, et al. Atypical vaginal adenosis and cervical ectropion. Association with clear cell adenocarcinoma in diethylstilbestrol-exposed offspring. Cancer 1984;54:869–75.

122. Matias-Guiu X, Lerma E, Prat J. Clear cell tumors of the female genital tract. Semin Diagn Pathol 1997;14:233–9.

123. Hanselaar A, van Loosbroek M, Schuurbiers O, et al. Clear cell adenocarcinoma of the vagina and cervix. An update of the central Netherlands registry showing twin age incidence peaks. Cancer 1997;79:2229–36.

124. Geisinger KR, Stanley MW, Raab SS, et al. Invasive glandular malignancies of the gynecologic tract. In: Geisinger KR, Stanley MW, Raab SS, et al., editors. Modern cytopathology. Philadelphia: Churchill Livingstone; 2004. p. 167–96.

125. Boyd J, Takahashi H, Waggoner SE, et al. Molecular genetic analysis of clear cell adenocarcinomas of the vagina and cervix associated and unassociated with diethylstilbestrol exposure in utero. Cancer 1996;77:507–13.

126. Reich O, Tamussino K, Lahousen M, et al. Clear cell carcinoma of the uterine cervix: pathology and prognosis in surgically treated stage IB-IIB disease in women not exposed in utero to diethylstilbestrol. Gynecol Oncol 2000;76:331–5.

127. Kaminski PF, Maier RC. Clear cell adenocarcinoma of the cervix unrelated to diethylstilbestrol exposure. Obstet Gynecol 1983;62:720–7.

128. Zhou C, Gilks CB, Hayes M, Clement PB. Papillary serous carcinoma of the uterine cervix: a clinicopathologic study of 17 cases. Am J Surg Pathol 1998;22:113–20.

129. Zhou C, Matisic JP, Clement PB, Hayes MM. Cytologic features of papillary serous adenocarcinoma of the uterine cervix. Cancer 1997;81:98–104.

130. Ferry JA, Scully RE. Mesonephric remnants, hyperplasia, and neoplasia in the uterine cervix. A study of 49 cases. Am J Surg Pathol 1990;14:1100–11.

131. Clement PB, Young RH, Keh P, et al. Malignant mesonephric neoplasms of the uterine cervix: a report of eight cases, including four with a malignant spindle cell component. Am J Surg Pathol 1995;19:1158–71.

132. Silver SA, Devouassoux-Shisheboran M, Mezzeti TP, et al. Mesonephric adenocarcinomas of the uterine cervix: a study of 11 cases with immunohistochemical findings. Am J Surg Pathol 2001;25:379–87.

133. Bagué S, Rodríguez IM, Prat J. Malignant mesonephric tumors of the female genital tract. A clinicopathologic study of 9 cases. Am J Surg Pathol 2004;28:601–7.

134. Ueda Y, Miyatake T, Yoshino K. Clonality and HPV infection analysis of concurrent glandular and squamous lesions and adenosquamous carcinomas of the uterine cervix. Am J Clin Pathol 2008;130:389–400.

135. Farley JH, Hickey KW, Carlson JW, et al. Adenosquamous histology predicts a poor outcome for patients with advanced-stage, but not early-stage, cervical carcinoma. Cancer 2003;97:2196–202.

136. Lea JS, Coleman RL, Garner EO, et al. Adenosquamous histology predicts poor outcome in low-risk stage IB1 cervical adenocarcinoma. Gynecol Oncol 2003;91:558–62.

137. Helm CW, Kinney WK, Keeney G, et al. A matched study of surgically treated stage IB adenosquamous carcinoma and adenocarcinoma of the uterine cervix. Int J Gynecol Cancer 1993;3:245–9.

138. Littman P, Ciement PB, Henriksen B, et al. Glassy cell carcinoma of the cervix. Cancer 1976;37:2238–46.

139. Tamini HK, Ek M, Hesla J, et al. Glassy cell carcinoma of the cervix redefined. Obstet Gynecol 1988;71:837–41.

140. Nagai T, Okubo T, Sakaguchi R, et al. Glassy cell carcinoma of the uterine cervix responsive to neoadjuvant intraarterial chemotherapy. Int J Clin Oncol 2008;13:541–4.

Miscellaneous Cervical Neoplasms

13

Anais Malpica

CHAPTER OUTLINE

Epithelial Tumors	275	Rhabdomyosarcoma	283
Adenoid Basal Carcinoma (Adenoid Basal Epithelioma)	275	Smooth Muscle Tumors (Leiomyoma and Leiomyosarcoma)	283
Adenoid Cystic Carcinoma	277	Malignant Peripheral Nerve Sheath Tumor	283
Neuroendocrine Tumors	277	Primitive Neuroectodermal Tumor/ Ewing Sarcoma	284
Typical (Classic) Carcinoid Tumor	277	Alveolar Soft Part Sarcoma	284
Atypical Carcinoid Tumor	277	Blue Nevus	284
Small Cell Neuroendocrine Carcinoma	278	Malignant Melanoma	284
Large Cell Neuroendocrine Carcinoma	280	Lymphoma and Leukemia	285
Biphasic Tumors	281	Metastatic Tumors to the Cervix	286
Adenofibroma	281	Other Types of Cervical Neoplasms	287
Adenomyoma	281		
Adenosarcoma	281		
Carcinosarcoma (Malignant Mixed Müllerian Tumor)	282		

EPITHELIAL TUMORS

ADENOID BASAL CARCINOMA (ADENOID BASAL EPITHELIOMA)

Definition

Adenoid basal carcinoma (adenoid basal epithelioma) is composed of bland, uniform, basaloid cells arranged in nests with a variable amount of glandular and squamous differentiation.[1] Based on their favorable outcome, there is a proposal to designate this tumor as 'epithelioma,' rather than carcinoma.[1,2]

General Features

Adenoid basal carcinoma (epithelioma) accounts for less than 1% of cervical cancers and usually develops in post-menopausal women with a median age of 66.5 years and a wide age range, from 19 to 91 years.[2,3] Most patients are asymptomatic and the tumor is frequently an incidental finding in a surgical specimen obtained after the diagnosis of high-grade squamous intraepithelial lesion on a Pap smear. In rare cases, patients can complain of vaginal bleeding, hematuria, or dysuria.[1,2] The tumor appears to arise from reserve cells and is usually associated with human papillomavirus (HPV) 16.[2]

Pathology

Grossly, the tumor is usually invisible; however, induration, erosion, ulceration, and abnormalities of the cervical mucosa have been described in rare cases.[2] Adenoid basal carcinoma (epithelioma) is composed of multiple, small, round to oval nests of bland, uniform, basaloid cells with peripheral palisading (Figures 13.1 and 13.2). The tumor nests are haphazardly distributed in the cervical stroma without eliciting a desmoplastic response although focal edema and mild chronic inflammation may be seen.[1] The tumor typically does not reach the surface of the endocervical canal; however, occasionally it appears in continuity with an overlying dysplastic squamous epithelium.[4] Clearing of the cytoplasm due to the accumulation of glycogen may be seen.[5] There is a variable degree of glandular and squamous differentiation (Figure 13.3). The former is characterized by the presence of columnar or cuboidal cells with bland nuclei surrounding a distinct lumen while the latter shows bland squamous cells in the center of the nests with preservation of a peripheral rim of basaloid cells. Occasionally, a

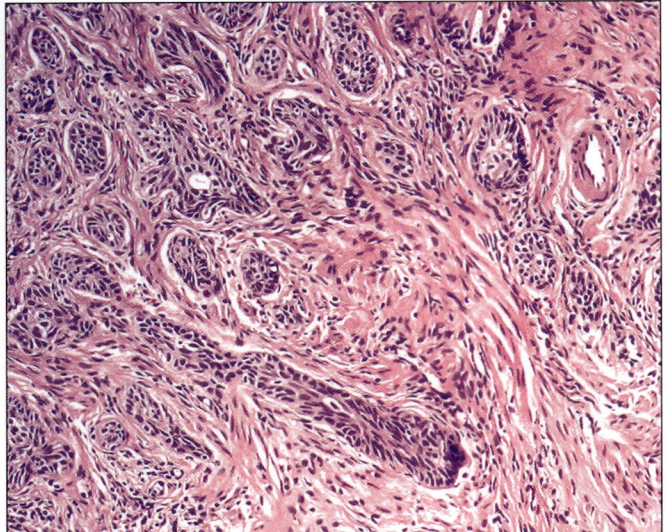

Figure 13.1 Adenoid basal carcinoma (epithelioma) composed of round, oval, or slightly distorted nests.

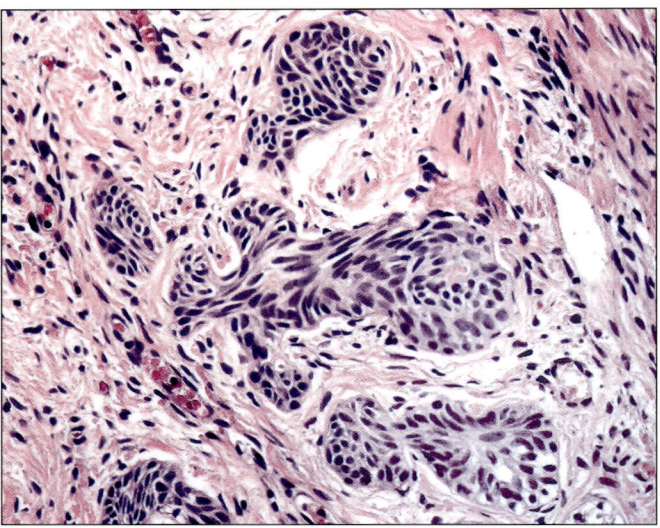

Figure 13.2 Adenoid basal carcinoma (epithelioma) with bland cytology and peripheral palisading.

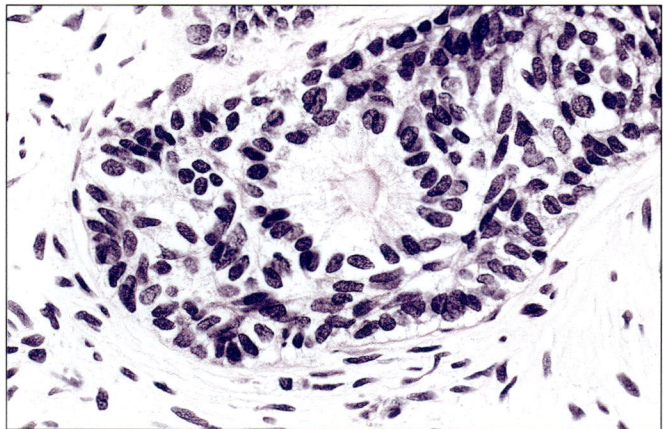

Figure 13.3 Adenoid basal carcinoma (epithelioma) with focal glandular formation.

cribriform pattern can be noted. The mitotic index is usually low, although it may vary from 0 to 9 mitoses per 10 high power fields (HPFs). There is no necrosis or lymphovascular or perineural invasion.[1,4] Although the tumor is typically associated with a high-grade squamous intraepithelial lesion, rarely, it can be associated with a superficially or frankly invasive squamous carcinoma, adenoid cystic carcinoma, adenosquamous carcinoma, clear cell carcinoma, neuroendocrine carcinoma, or carcinosarcoma.[3–6]

Immunohistochemistry

Adenoid basal carcinoma (epithelioma) is usually immunoreactive for keratin AE1/AE3, CK902 (against cytokeratin 8 and 18), epithelial membrane antigen (EMA), carcinoembryonic antigen (CEA), CAM 5.2, p16, p53, and p63. S-100 can be positive in a few cases.[2] A limited number of cases of adenoid basal carcinoma (epithelioma) has been tested for CD117 (c-kit) and found to be negative.[7]

Differential Diagnosis

Adenoid basal hyperplasia is a superficial lesion with epithelial nests smaller than those seen in adenoid basal carcinoma (epithelioma). The nests reside within 0.5 mm of the basement membrane of the overlying or adjacent epithelium and are connected to it.

Adenoid cystic carcinoma tends to produce symptoms and a grossly visible mass. Microscopically, it contains tumor nests that are larger than those seen in adenoid basal carcinoma (epithelioma) and characteristically show a cribriform pattern containing either amorphous, hyaline, eosinophilic basement membrane-like material, or basophilic mucinous or eosinophilic secretion. Necrosis and stromal changes are often seen as well as lymphovascular invasion.

Squamous carcinoma can represent a diagnostic difficulty since adenoid basal carcinoma (epithelioma) can have florid squamous metaplasia with marked expansion of the tumor nests, thus mimicking an invasive squamous carcinoma. In addition, focal dysplastic changes can be noted in the areas of squamous metaplasia. Recognition of a residual rim of bland basaloid cells, which can be highlighted with the use of CAM 5.2 immunoreaction, will facilitate the proper identification of adenoid basal carcinoma (epithelioma) with extensive squamous metaplasia.[3]

Basaloid squamous carcinoma, a rare type of cervical tumor, usually produces a symptomatic tumor mass.[8] Microscopically, this tumor is composed of moderately pleomorphic, basaloid cells arranged in nests and cords. There is also peripheral palisading. Mitotic activity and necrosis are conspicuous. Larger cells with eosinophilic cytoplasm as well as a cribriform pattern can be seen. Hyalinization or myxoid change of the stroma is also common.[9]

Clinical Behavior and Management

Morphologically pure adenoid basal carcinomas (epitheliomas) behave in a benign fashion without metastases to lymph nodes or other sites, local recurrences, or death.[2,3] Microscopic examination of the entire tumor is necessary to exclude the presence of an associated neoplasm that could have an adverse impact on the prognosis. Cases of morphologically pure adenoid basal carcinoma (epithelioma) are treated with a loop electrosurgical excision procedure or cold knife cone with negative margins. In cases where the neoplasm extends to the margins, a comment should be included in the report about the possible association with another tumor type that could affect the prognosis.

ADENOID CYSTIC CARCINOMA

Definition
Cervical adenoid cystic carcinoma is a neoplasm with histologic features mimicking those of similar tumors of the salivary glands and upper respiratory tract.

General Features
This tumor is rare and mostly seen in postmenopausal women (mean age, 72 years),[4] but it is occasionally detected in younger women in the third or fourth decades of life.[10,11] Uterine bleeding is the most common presentation with a rare case diagnosed incidentally.[4] This neoplasm appears to originate from reserve cells and is usually associated with HPV 16.[5,12]

Pathology Features
The tumor has a variable appearance from small polypoid lesions to large exophytic, friable masses or deeply invasive endophytic tumors.[4] Microscopically, it is composed of mildly pleomorphic basaloid cells arranged in nests, sheets, cords, and trabeculae. Clear cell changes may be present.[5] A distinct cribriform pattern containing either an amorphous hyaline eosinophilic basement membrane-like material or basophilic mucinous or eosinophilic secretion is usually seen (Figure 13.4). Mitotic activity is variable, ranging from scanty to very high.[4,5] Necrosis is often present and extensive. Stromal changes are typically prominent, ranging from hyalinization to myxoid or fibroblastic change. The solid variant lacks the typical cribriform pattern, but the tumor is recognized by the presence of abundant periodic acid–Schiff (PAS)-positive basement membrane material around the tumor cells that grow in solid nests, cords, and trabeculae.[13] Small foci of squamous differentiation may be seen. Adenoid cystic carcinoma can be associated with adenoid basal carcinoma (epithelioma), *in situ* or invasive squamous cell carcinoma, adenosquamous carcinoma, or adenocarcinoma.[5,11] Adenoid cystic carcinoma tends to involve lymphovascular spaces and develops lymph node metastasis early.[11]

Immunohistochemistry
Tumor cells are reactive for wide spectrum cytokeratin (CK), CAM 5.2, and EMA. S-100 protein reactivity occurs in some cases[5] while others are unreactive or just focally and weakly reactive.[4,13] A rare case of cervical adenoid cystic carcinoma has been tested for CD117 (c-kit) and was found to be strongly reactive in approximately 5% of the cells. This finding does not compare with the common expression of CD117 (c-kit) in adenoid cystic carcinoma of the salivary glands, which is seen in 80–100% of cases.[7]

Clinical Behavior and Management
Adenoid cystic carcinoma is an aggressive tumor. In one series, nearly half of the patients died of local recurrence or metastatic disease within 8 months to 8 years of diagnosis.[4] Treatment options include radiotherapy, surgery, surgery and adjuvant radiotherapy, or chemotherapy.[11]

NEUROENDOCRINE TUMORS

Neuroendocrine tumors of the uterine cervix are rare.[14] According to the nomenclature system proposed in 1997 by the College of American Pathologists and the National Cancer Institute, they are classified as typical (classic) carcinoid tumors, atypical carcinoid tumors, small cell neuroendocrine carcinomas, and large cell neuroendocrine carcinomas.[15] These tumors may originate from cells containing neuroendocrine granules, seen in 20% of normal cervices, or from reserve cells.[16–18]

Additionally, an association with HPV 18 or 16 has been described in atypical carcinoids, small cell neuroendocrine carcinoma, and large cell neuroendocrine carcinoma.[17,18,20–22]

TYPICAL (CLASSIC) CARCINOID TUMOR
The least common of the neuroendocrine tumors[14,17] is composed of uniform cells forming nests, trabeculae, cords, or glands. The chromatin is finely granular. Mitoses are rare (at the most 3 mitoses per 10 HPFs) and there is no necrosis (Figure 13.5).[23] Immunohistochemical studies show that the tumor cells are positive for neuroendocrine markers such as neuron-specific enolase, CD56, chromogranin, or synaptophysin.

The experience with this tumor, when arising in the cervix, is limited to delineating its behavior and optimal treatment.

ATYPICAL CARCINOID TUMOR
The second least common of the neuroendocrine tumors[14,17] is distinguished from the typical (classic) carcinoid on the basis of a mitotic index above 3 mitoses per 10 HPFs (but fewer than 10 mitoses per 10 HPFs) and/or necrosis, usually comedo-type (Figures 13.6 and 13.7).[23]

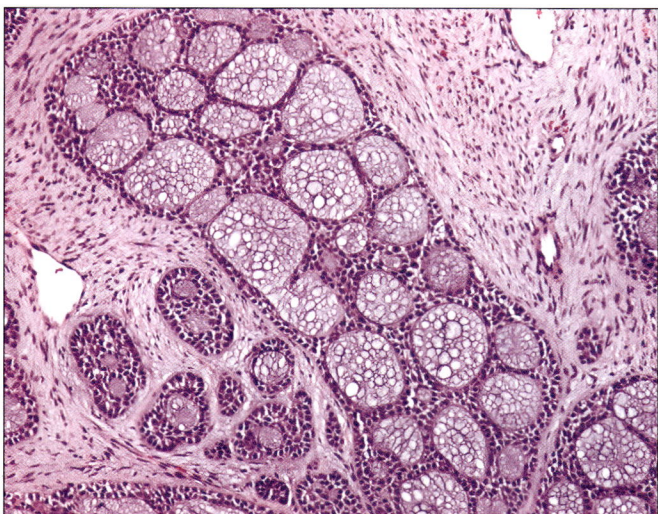

Figure 13.4 Adenoid cystic carcinoma.

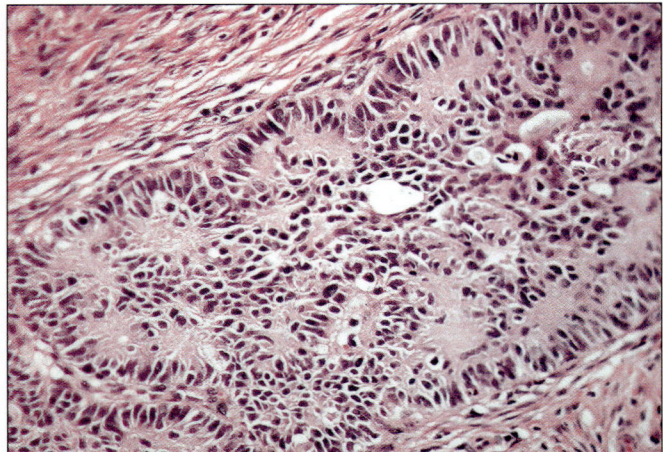

Figure 13.5 Typical (classic) carcinoid tumor.

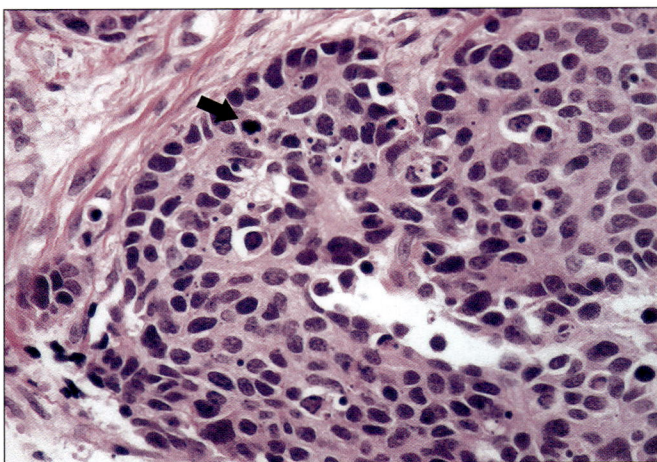

Figure 13.7 Atypical carcinoid tumor with mitotic figure (arrow).

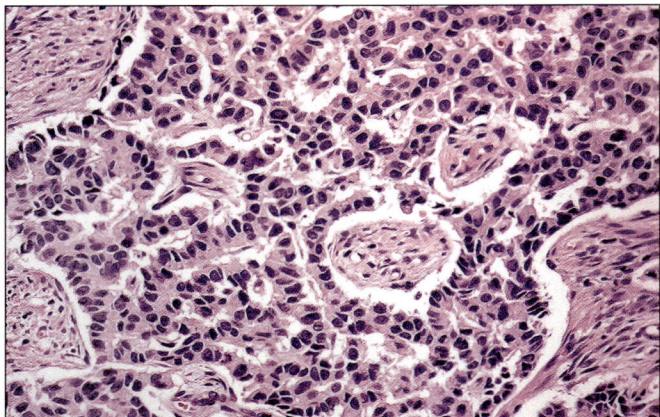

Figure 13.6 Atypical carcinoid tumor with trabecular pattern.

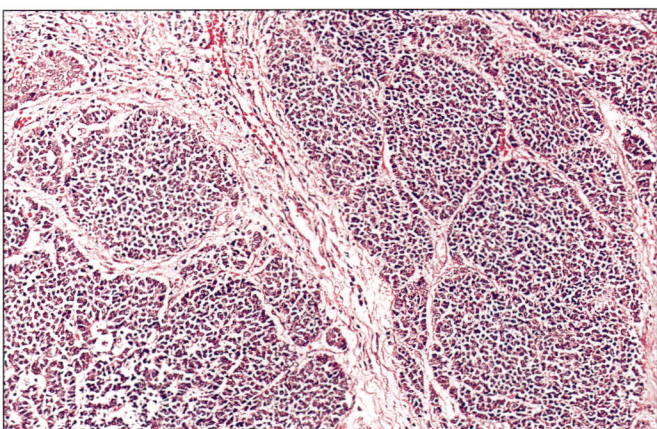

Figure 13.8 Neuroendocrine carcinoma, small cell type. Nests and trabeculae of tumor cells.

Immunohistochemical studies show that the tumor cells are positive for the neuroendocrine markers listed above. Similarly to the typical carcinoid tumor, the experience with atypical carcinoid tumor of the cervix is limited. Therefore, its behavior and optimal treatment are undetermined.

SMALL CELL NEUROENDOCRINE CARCINOMA

Definition

This tumor is composed of uniform small cells with a high nuclear to cytoplasmic ratio, similar to small cell carcinoma of the lung.

General Features

This tumor accounts for less than 5% of the cervical carcinomas;[24] however, it represents the most frequent neuroendocrine neoplasm of the uterine cervix.[14] Patients' ages range from 20 to 87 years (mean, 45 years).[19,24,25] Vaginal bleeding is the most common symptom followed by pain.[25,26] A rare case has been detected in an abnormal Pap smear.[27] Occasionally, patients have developed paraneoplastic syndromes, including Cushing's syndrome, hypoglycemia, inappropriate antidiuretic hormone production, carcinoid syndrome, and Eaton–Lambert syndrome.[19,27–29] Most tumors are International Federation of Gynecology and Obstetrics (FIGO) stage I or II.[19,24,25]

Pathology

Tumors range in size from 1 to 10 cm.[24] A rare case has presented in a normal-appearing cervix.[27] Microscopically, small cell carcinoma is composed of oval or spindled cells with scanty cytoplasm, dark nuclei, and no apparent nucleoli. The cells are arranged in nests, trabeculae, and cords (Figures 13.8 and 13.9). Focal gland formation can be noted. There are numerous mitoses and apoptotic bodies. Molding of the nuclei, crush artifact, and necrosis are common. Occasionally, deposition of hematoxylin-stained material around vessels walls (Azzopardi phenomenon) is seen. Lymphovascular invasion is commonly seen. Associated large cell neuroendocrine carcinoma, *in situ* or invasive squamous cell carcinoma, or adenocarcinoma may be found.[26,27]

Immunohistochemical Studies

In most cases, the tumor cells express at least one neuroendocrine marker, such as synaptophysin, chromogranin, NSE, or CD56[24,30,31] (Figure 13.10A and B). The tumor cells are diffusely positive for p16.[32] Up to 87% of the cases are reactive for TTF-1. In addition, the tumor cells may react for keratin 20, neurofilament, and CD99.[32] There are conflicting reports on the expression of c-kit in these tumors. Whereas in one study up to 43% of the tumors expressed c-kit,[33] only one tumor of another series expressed c-kit diffusely.[34]

Differential Diagnosis

Poorly differentiated squamous cell carcinomas can be composed of small cells with scanty cytoplasm resembling a small cell neuroendocrine carcinoma. However, squamous carcinoma typically lacks the abundant apoptotic bodies, nuclear molding, and crush artifact that are commonly seen in small cell neuroendocrine carcinoma. The use of neuroendocrine markers such as synaptophysin, chromogranin, and CD56 will facilitate the correct diagnosis as small cell carcinoma should be positive for at least one of these markers. It should be noted that markers traditionally used to prove squamous differentiation (i.e., p63 and CK 5/6) can be positive in neuroendocrine carcinomas.[32,35]

Lymphoma and melanoma require standard immunohistochemical studies to distinguish them from small cell neuroendocrine carcinoma.

Primitive neuroectodermal tumor can share histologic and immunohistochemical features with small cell neuroendocrine carcinoma. Molecular studies for HPV together with CD99, keratin, and neuroendocrine marker immunoreactions are required to ascertain the correct diagnosis as cervical neuroendocrine carcinomas are HPV associated whereas primitive neuroectodermal tumors are not.[32]

Clinical Behavior and Management

Small cell carcinoma is an aggressive neoplasm that tends to develop widespread metastases (i.e., bone, liver, lung, lymph nodes, and soft tissue) and has an overall 5 year survival rate of only 29%. Patients with early stage disease are treated with radical hysterectomy. In addition, adjuvant cisplatinum and etoposide-based chemotherapy and radiotherapy are used for distant and local control of the disease. Patients with advanced stage disease are treated with radiotherapy and chemotherapy.[24]

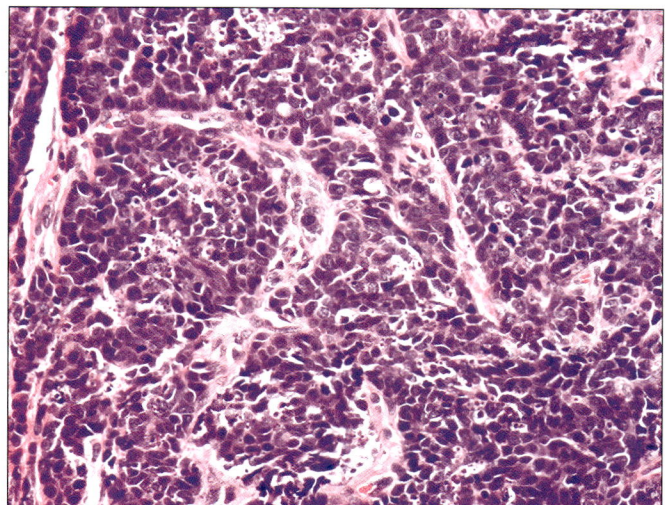

Figure 13.9 Neuroendocrine carcinoma, small cell type.

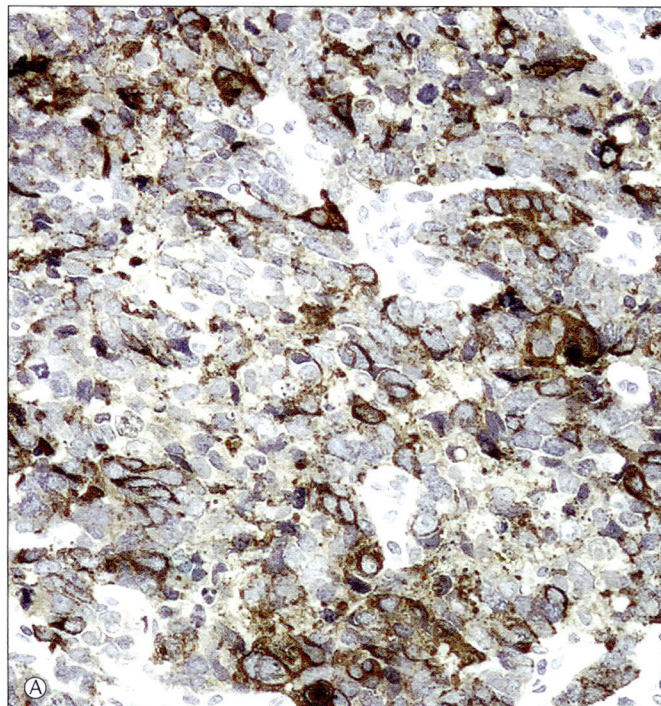
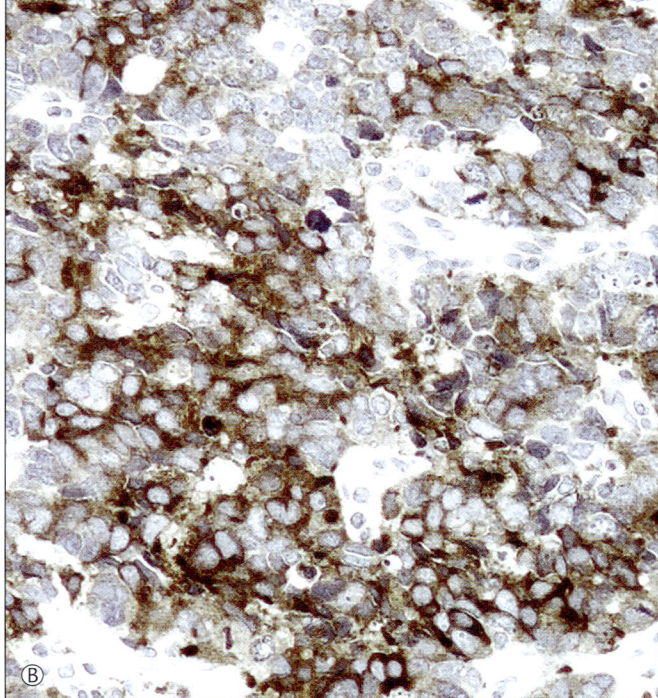

Figure 13.10 Neuroendocrine carcinoma, small cell type, reactive for chromogranin (**A**) and synaptophysin (**B**).

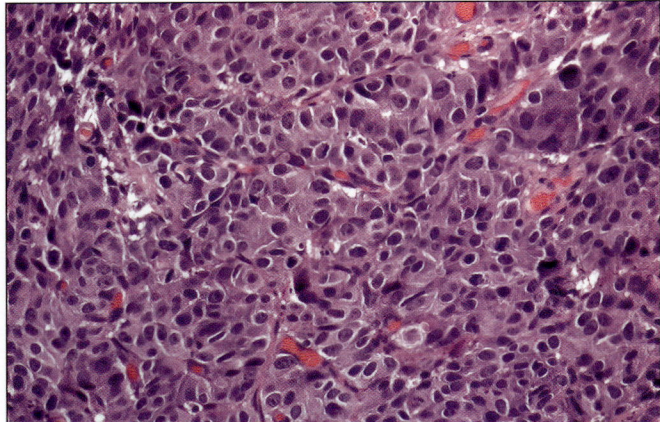

Figure 13.11 Neuroendocrine carcinoma, large cell type.

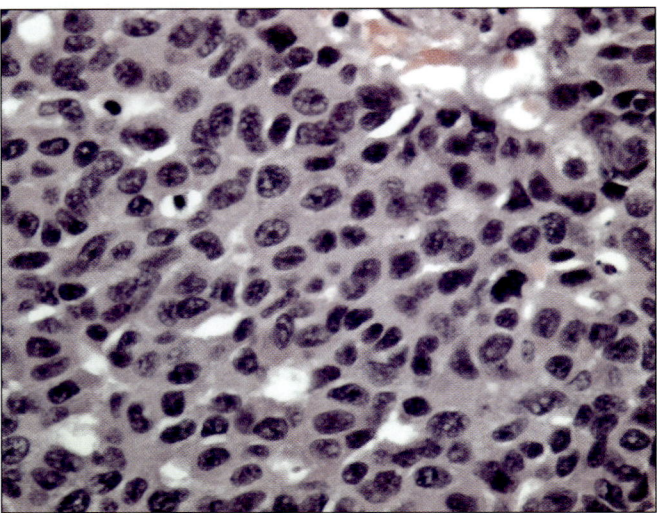

Figure 13.12 Neuroendocrine carcinoma, large cell type. Focal glandular differentiation.

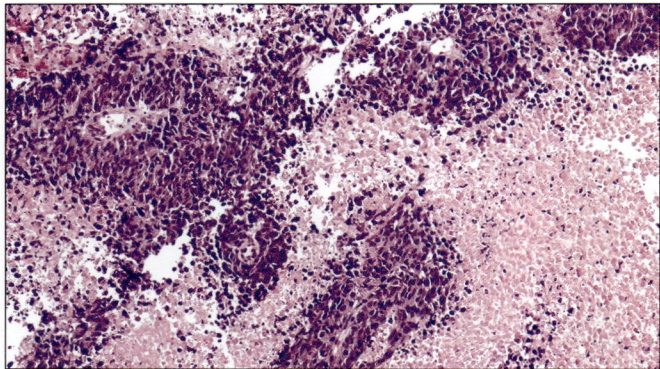

Figure 13.13 Neuroendocrine carcinoma, large cell type, showing geographic necrosis.

LARGE CELL NEUROENDOCRINE CARCINOMA

Definition

This high-grade tumor is composed of cells with a moderate or abundant cytoplasm, visible nucleoli, and neuroendocrine differentiation.

General Features

Large cell neuroendocrine carcinoma is the second most common type of neuroendocrine tumor of the uterine cervix and accounts for 0.6% of the invasive cervical carcinomas.[14,17,36] The mean age of patients is 37 years (age range, 21–75 years).[36] The most common symptom is vaginal bleeding, but some tumors are detected as a result of an abnormal Pap smear. The tumors are usually FIGO stage I or II.[16,36,37]

Pathology

The tumor is usually polypoid or exophytic, although it may be ill defined and not even grossly visible. The tumor can be up to 6 cm in greatest dimension and shows a variable cut surface, ranging from tan-brown to yellow-gray or white, with areas of hemorrhage or necrosis.[16,37] Microscopically, the tumor cells have a moderate or abundant amount of cytoplasm, moderately or markedly atypical nuclei with vesicular or finely granular chromatin, and visible nucleoli (Figure 13.11). They are arranged in nests, trabeculae, or solid sheets. Glandular formation can be seen (Figure 13.12). The mitotic index is high (more than 10 mitoses per 10 HPFs). Geographic necrosis and lymphovascular invasion are typically present (Figure 13.13). The tumor can be associated with adenocarcinoma *in situ*, invasive adenocarcinoma (mucinous or endometrioid type), and small cell carcinoma.[16,17,37,38]

Immunohistochemistry

All tumors express at least one neuroendocrine marker, such as synaptophysin, chromogranin, or CD56. All cases are reactive for p16. The tumor cells can also express TTF-1, p63, keratin 20, neurofilament, and CD99.[16,32]

Differential Diagnosis

Small cell neuroendocrine carcinoma has cells with scanty cytoplasm, hyperchromatic nuclei, and no nucleoli.

Adenocarcinoma may be erroneously diagnosed due to the presence of focal glandular differentiation in large cell neuroendocrine carcinoma, or the association with either an adenocarcinoma *in situ* or invasive adenocarcinoma. Attention to the architectural patterns (i.e., insular or trabecular) and the presence of geographic necrosis as well as the use of neuroendocrine markers will allow the proper diagnosis. It is important to bear in mind that focal expression of neuroendocrine markers can be seen in an otherwise typical adenocarcinoma or adenosquamous carcinoma of the uterine cervix.[16]

Poorly differentiated squamous cell carcinoma shows at least focal evidence of keratin production or intercellular bridges.

Melanoma requires standard immunohistochemical studies to be distinguished from large cell neuroendocrine carcinoma.

Clinical Behavior and Management

The outcome for patients with large cell neuroendocrine carcinoma is poor. Survival across all stages is dismal with 67% of patients dying of disease. Intra-abdominal/intra-pelvic and distant metastasis, including liver, kidney, adrenal gland, lymph nodes, lung, bone, and brain, are usually seen.[16,36,37] Treatment includes surgery with adjuvant radiotherapy and chemotherapy.[36]

BIPHASIC TUMORS

ADENOFIBROMA

This rare neoplasm is composed of benign glands embedded in a fibromatous stroma. The glands are lined by columnar or cuboidal epithelium with endocervical or endometrioid differentiation. The stroma shows no atypia or condensation around the glands, and the mitotic index is very low (<2 mitoses per 10 HPFs;[39] Figure 13.14). The tumor does not invade into the cervical stroma.[40] A confident diagnosis of adenofibroma requires the examination of the entire lesion to rule out the more common adenosarcoma; therefore, the diagnosis of adenofibroma cannot be made on curetted material or biopsy.[41]

ADENOMYOMA

This uncommon biphasic tumor is composed of benign glands admixed with a variable amount of smooth muscle and fibrous tissue. Patients range in age from 21 to 55 years (mean, 40 years) and, although usually asymptomatic, can present with vaginal bleeding or discharge. The tumors are well circumscribed, frequently polypoid, and range in size from 2.5 to 8.0 cm. Most are found in the upper cervical canal with a rare case arising in its lower end. The tumor glands are usually lined by endocervical epithelium. However, a few glands can be lined by endometrioid or tubal epithelium. The glands range from regular, small, round to oval to irregular and dilated with papillary infoldings. A vague lobular pattern is usually present. Atypia is not found in the epithelial or the stromal component. Less than 1 mitosis per 10 HPFs is seen in the epithelial component whereas the stromal component lacks mitotic activity. Cytoplasmic CEA immunoreaction can be focally detected in the glandular epithelium.[42] The differential diagnosis includes: (1) minimal deviation adenocarcinoma, endocervical type (adenoma malignum), an ill-defined tumor that grossly expands the cervical wall and contains numerous glands, haphazardly distributed in the cervical stroma with at least focal desmoplasia, cytologic atypia, and lymphovascular invasion; (2) adenosarcoma, which shows minimal or no smooth muscle differentiation, intracystic or surface papillary stromal projections, and at least focal periglandular stromal condensation, stromal atypia, and 2 or more mitoses per 10 HPFs; or (3) endocervicosis, which lacks the smooth muscle stroma, lobular organization, and gross circumscription seen in adenomyoma.

ADENOSARCOMA

Definition

This tumor has a benign, although occasionally atypical, epithelial component and a malignant mesenchymal component.

General Features

Adenosarcomas of the uterine cervix are less common than their counterparts in the uterine corpus.[43,44] The patients are aged 11–67 years (mean, 36 years) and usually present with abnormal bleeding and the finding of a 'cervical polyp.'[43,44]

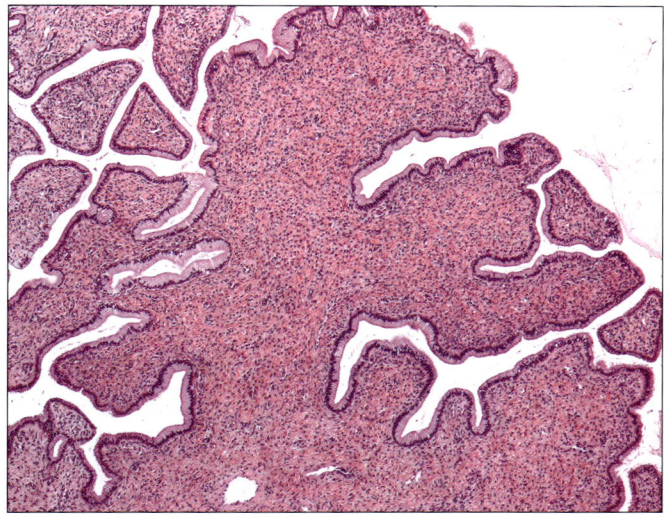

Figure 13.14 Adenofibroma.

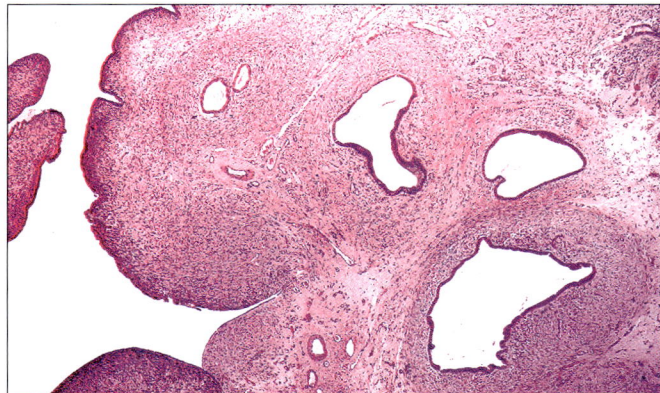

Figure 13.15 Adenosarcoma with prominent periglandular cuffing.

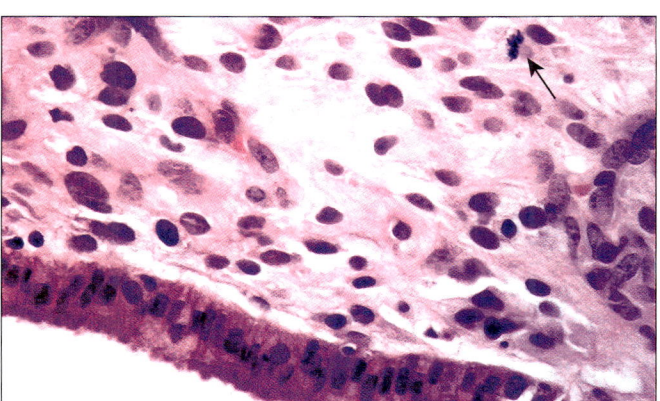

Figure 13.16 Adenosarcoma with stromal atypia and a rare mitotic figure (arrow).

Pathology

Cervical adenosarcomas range in size from 1.5 to 20 cm and usually have a polypoid configuration. Most are solitary but may be multiple.[43,44] Characteristically, they show relatively bland, occasionally atypical, glands intermixed with a low-grade homologous sarcoma. A leaf-like pattern due to growth of the stromal component into dilated glands and/or the tumor surface is characteristic. Most cases show a distinctive band of hypercellular stroma surrounding the glandular epithelium (periglandular cuffing). It has been stated that the diagnosis of adenosarcoma requires one or more of the following findings: marked nuclear atypia of the stromal cells; 2 or more stromal mitoses per 10 HPFs; and stromal hypercellularity, usually forming periglandular cuffs.[39] However, most cases display at least two of these features (Figures 13.15 and 13.16). Usually, the epithelial component is endocervical type with focal squamous metaplasia, although endometrioid or tubal-type epithelia may be seen. In nearly all cases, there is focal epithelial atypia. The glandular epithelial cells show irregularly shaped abundant eosinophilic cytoplasm and enlarged nuclei. By definition, however, these features are insufficient to diagnose adenocarcinoma. Occasionally, the sarcomatous component shows heterologous elements in the form of skeletal muscle, cartilage, lipoblasts, or bone.[43,44] A minority of cases show 'sarcomatous overgrowth,' defined as the presence of sarcoma occupying at least 25% of the tumor volume and frequently high grade.[39] From a prognostic viewpoint, finding sarcomatous overgrowth is important since it indicates potential aggressive behavior.[45] In fact, in our experience, foci of high-grade sarcoma even representing <25% of the tumor may also indicate an aggressive behavior.

Immunohistochemistry

Adenosarcomas with sarcomatous overgrowth often show strong immunoreaction for Ki-67 and p53 and loss of CD10 and progesterone receptor immunoexpression. Immunoreactivity for these markers is similar in classic adenosarcomas and adenofibromas.[41]

Differential Diagnosis

Adenofibromas are composed of benign epithelial and stromal components, and, particularly, lack hypercellularity, nuclear atypia, or mitotic activity in the stroma. As discussed in Chapter 20, many pathologists doubt adenofibromas even exist or can be diagnosed with certainty, since adenosarcomas may appear histologically so well differentiated, and yet may behave aggressively. We recommend a low threshold in the diagnosis of adenosarcomas when pathologic doubt exists or there is a clinical history of 'recurrent polyps.'

Endocervical polyps usually lack the leaf-like pattern and the microscopic features of adenosarcoma. Malignant mixed müllerian tumors (carcinosarcomas) have a malignant epithelial component, usually high grade, and a clearly malignant sarcomatous component, frequently with heterologous elements.

Embryonal rhabdomyosarcomas have a characteristic hypercellular layer of immature tumor cells beneath the covering epithelium (so-called cambium layer), not dissimilar to adenosarcomas, but this fades quickly into looser mesenchyme containing small, dark, mitotically active cells with focally demonstrable cross-striations, and lack the distinct leaf-like pattern so commonly seen in adenosarcomas. Reactivity with myxoid markers (myogenin and myo-D1) confirms the diagnosis.

Clinical Management and Prognosis

Cervical adenosarcomas are usually treated by hysterectomy. If less than hysterectomy is done in a young patient willing to preserve fertility, close and reliable follow-up is mandatory. Local resection of a polypoid adenosarcoma followed by recurrence in the corpus several years postoperatively has been fatal.[41] Adjuvant radiotherapy may be considered in cases with invasion into the cervical wall. Cases with sarcomatous overgrowth should be treated like other high-grade sarcomas of the uterus.[39]

The presence of deep cervical wall invasion and sarcomatous overgrowth are adverse prognostic factors; however, recurrences can be seen in cases lacking these features.

CARCINOSARCOMA (MALIGNANT MIXED MÜLLERIAN TUMOR)

Carcinosarcoma consists of admixed but distinct malignant epithelial and stromal elements (Figures 13.17 and 13.18).

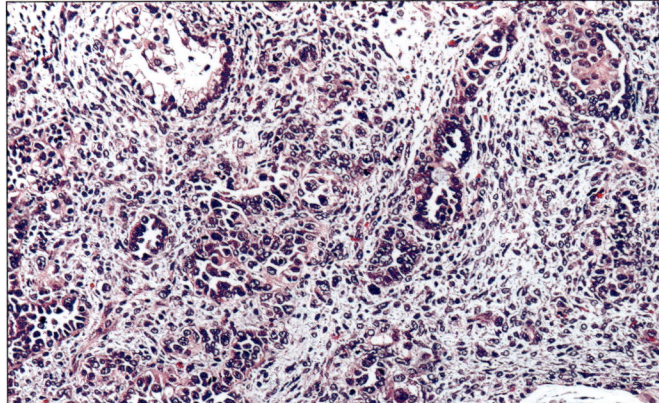

Figure 13.17 Carcinosarcoma (malignant mixed müllerian tumor).

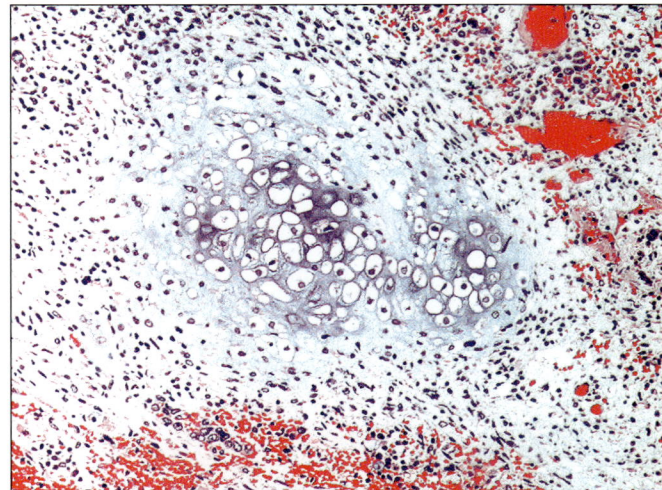

Figure 13.18 Carcinosarcoma with cartilaginous differentiation.

It is rarely found in the cervix.[46] Most patients are elderly (mean age, 60 years), but the tumor may develop in children and the very old.[46–48] HPV 16 has been identified in a few cases.[46] The most common symptoms at presentation are vaginal bleeding or spotting, with an occasional asymptomatic case being detected by a cervical smear. Grossly, the tumor is generally polypoid and ranges in size from 1 to 10 cm. Microscopically, the epithelial component may be an endometrioid adenocarcinoma, squamous cell carcinoma, basaloid squamous carcinoma, adenoid cystic carcinoma, or adenoid basal carcinoma, while the mesenchymal component may be homologous (fibrosarcoma, endometrial stromal sarcoma, high-grade spindle cell sarcoma) or heterologous (rhabdomyosarcoma, chondrosarcoma). The differential diagnosis includes adenosarcoma, as discussed above, and sarcomatoid carcinoma. Most cases present with FIGO stage I disease.[46–48] Although the experience with cervical carcinosarcomas is limited, prognosis seems to be better than that of similar tumors of the corpus.[46,47]

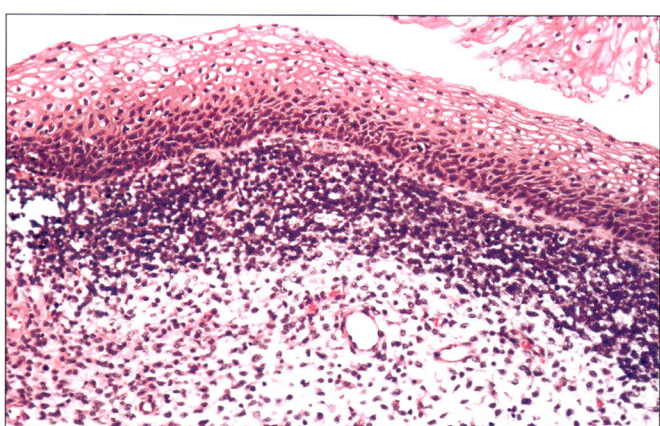

Figure 13.19 Embryonal rhabdomyosarcoma with prominent cambium layer.

RHABDOMYOSARCOMA

Embryonal rhabdomyosarcoma with classic botryoid features is the most common sarcoma of the uterine cervix.[49] It mostly affects young women aged 12–26 years (average, 18 years).[50] However, it is occasionally seen in older patients, up to 58 years of age.[51] The most common symptom is vaginal bleeding. In some cases, a mass protrudes through the introitus or the tumor is detected during a routine gynecologic examination. Grossly, the tumors are polypoid and measure 2–10 cm in size.[50] Microscopically, they show a 'cambium layer,' i.e., a subepithelial condensation of embryonal rhabdomyoblasts (Figure 13.19). The tumor cells vary in appearance, ranging from small cells to cells with definitive rhabdomyoblastic differentiation.[50] The cells are usually reactive for desmin (Figure 13.20), myo-D1, and myogenin. However, nuclear staining for myo-D1 and myogenin may be absent or sparse in some embryonal rhabdomyosarcomas.[52] The prognosis of cervical sarcoma botryoides is more favorable than that of other types of rhabdomyosarcoma. Surgery, including fertility-sparing procedures in selected cases, combined with chemotherapy is the treatment of choice.[53]

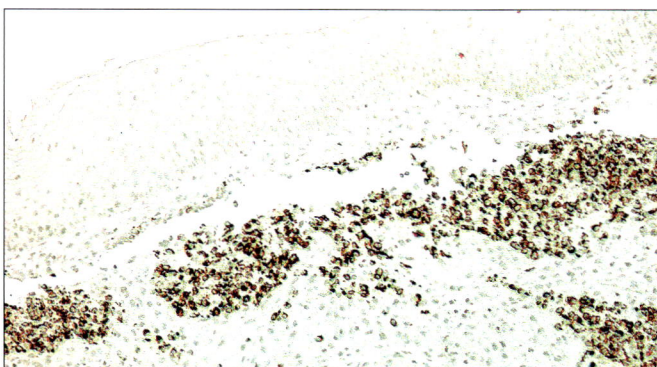

Figure 13.20 Embryonal rhabdomyosarcoma, cambium layer reactive for desmin.

SMOOTH MUSCLE TUMORS (LEIOMYOMA AND LEIOMYOSARCOMA)

Leiomyomas are uncommon in the uterine cervix.[54] They are usually an incidental finding and may occur in all the variants that have been described in the uterine corpus. Cervical leiomyosarcomas are also uncommon. They occur in perimenopausal or postmenopausal women, with a rare case seen in a pediatric patient. These tumors are usually large.[49] They can be spindle cell (conventional) type, epithelioid, or myxoid. The diagnostic criteria to distinguish these malignant tumors from their benign counterparts are those used for smooth muscle tumors of the corpus; thus, the diagnosis of conventional (spindle cell) leiomyosarcoma is based on the presence of two of the three following features: (1) diffuse severe nuclear atypia, (2) coagulative tumor cell necrosis, and (3) a mitotic index of ≥10 mitoses per 10 HPFs.[55] In contrast, the diagnostic criteria for epithelioid leiomyosarcomas are not well established. These tumors usually show a combination of nuclear atypia (either grade 2 or 3) and a mitotic index of at least 4 mitoses per 10 HPFs.[56] Myxoid leiomyosarcomas are frequently large tumors with infiltrative margins, mild to moderate nuclear atypia, and very few mitoses. Tumor necrosis may or may not be present.[57,58] Since the experience with cervical leiomyosarcoma is limited, no specific therapy has been recommended.

MALIGNANT PERIPHERAL NERVE SHEATH TUMOR

This tumor, also known as 'malignant schwannoma,' 'neurogenic sarcoma,' or 'neurofibrosarcoma,' is composed of cells of the peripheral nerve sheath. Eight cases have been reported in the cervix. Patients ranged in age from 25 to 73 years (mean, 50 years) and had no history of neurofibromatosis. The tumors were polypoid, measured 3–4 cm, and were composed of atypical and mitotically active spindle cells arranged in a herringbone, nodular, or storiform patterns. Epithelioid as well as pigmented areas have been described. This tumor has a variable expression of S-100 and is negative for desmin, myoglobin, and actin. Three of the four cases with available follow-up of 1–2 years were free of disease, while one patient developed abdominal metastases less than 2 years after diagnosis.[49]

PRIMITIVE NEUROECTODERMAL TUMOR/ EWING SARCOMA

This is a primitive round cell tumor showing varying degrees of neuroectodermal differentiation. Ten cases arising in the uterine cervix have been reported. Patients ranged in age from 21 to 51 years. Vaginal bleeding was the most common symptom. The tumor ranged from 5 to 7 cm. Most patients with localized disease at presentation were free of disease after an average follow-up of 19 months. Treatment included surgery with neoadjuvant or adjuvant chemotherapy.[49]

ALVEOLAR SOFT PART SARCOMA

This is a tumor of uncertain origin composed of uniform, large cells with eosinophilic granular cytoplasm arranged in alveolar and/or solid nests (Figure 13.21). The patients range in age from 8 to 39 years (mean, 29.9 years). Vaginal bleeding is the most common symptom, although some cases can be incidental findings. Grossly, the tumor is well circumscribed and ranges from 0.2 to 4 cm in size. Mitotic activity is usually low. A rare case has metastasized to a pelvic lymph node. Most patients have been treated with hysterectomy, with a few patients treated with radiotherapy or chemotherapy. Although experience with alveolar soft part sarcomas of the cervix is limited, they seem to have a better prognosis than their soft tissue counterparts. So far, no pulmonary or brain metastases or death has been reported.[49]

BLUE NEVUS

Cervical blue nevus of the common type is seen mostly in patients in their fifth or sixth decades of life as an incidental finding. Grossly, it consists of single or multiple, 0.1–0.4 mm, blue to gray macules located in the endocervix. Microscopically, it shows slender, wavy, and dendritic melanin-containing cells arranged in irregular clusters in the superficial cervical stroma (Figure 13.22). These cells are S-100 positive. A rare case of cellular blue nevus has been reported in the cervix.[59]

MALIGNANT MELANOMA

Malignant melanomas arising in the cervix are exceptionally rare.[60] While the age range is wide (19–78 years), most women are postmenopausal.[61] The most common symptom is vaginal bleeding. Occasional tumors are detected during routine clinical examination by cervical smear or the discovery of a distant metastasis.[61,62]

Pathology

The tumors are usually polypoid and red, brown, gray, black, or blue. Frequently, they are ulcerated. About 25% of cases are amelanotic. The neoplastic cells are usually epithelioid or spindle (Figure 13.23). Intranuclear inclusions and multinucleated tumor giant cells are common. Occasional variants include desmoplastic melanoma[63] and a clear cell type with polygonal cells that contain glycogen and mimic

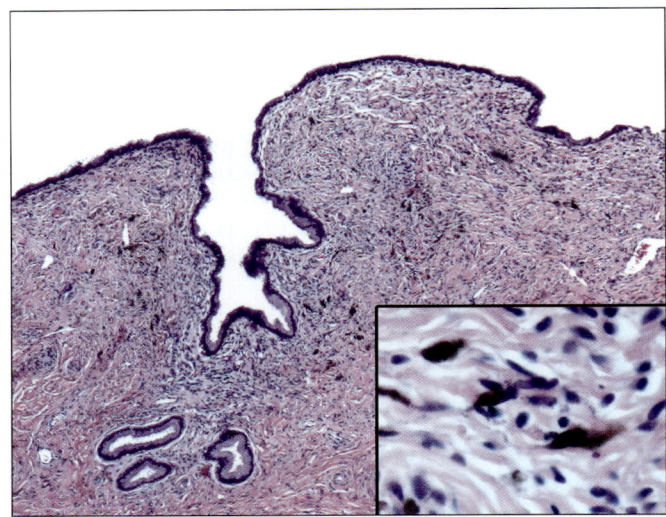

Figure 13.22 Blue nevus.

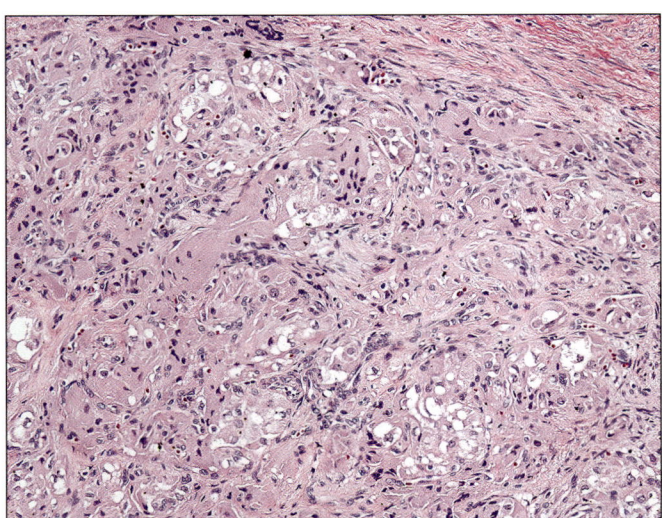

Figure 13.21 Alveolar soft part sarcoma.

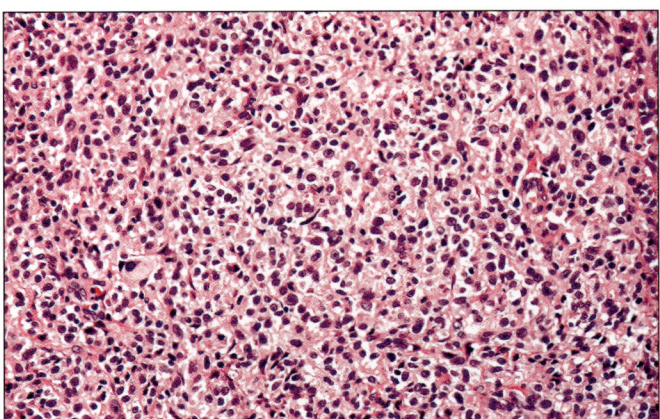

Figure 13.23 Malignant melanoma, epithelioid cells.

CHAPTER 13 — MISCELLANEOUS CERVICAL NEOPLASMS

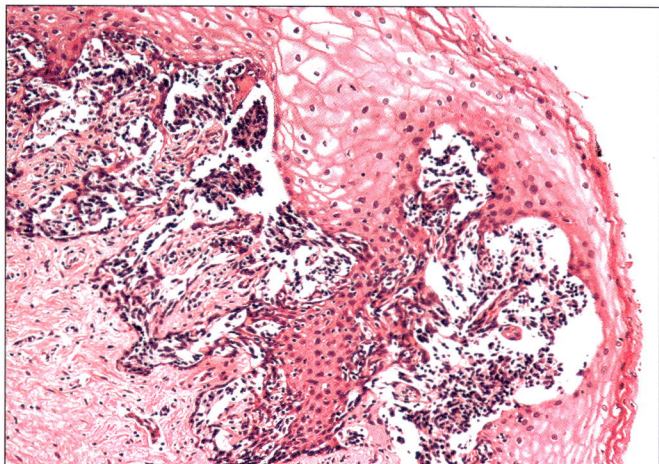

Figure 13.24 Malignant melanoma, junctional component.

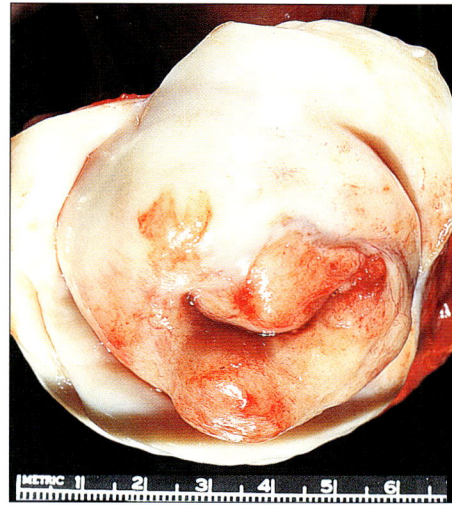

Figure 13.25 Lymphoma. A rubbery, fleshy mass diffusely enlarges the cervix.

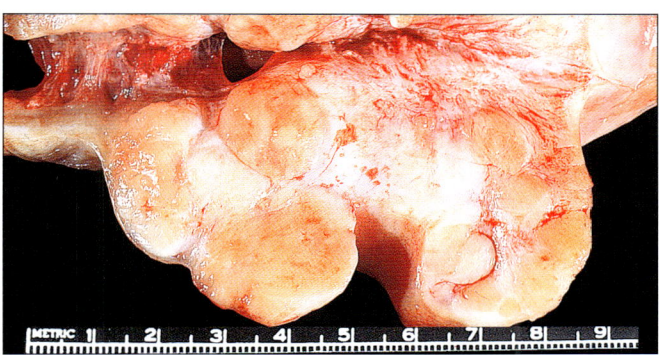

Figure 13.26 Lymphoma. The tumor, cut in cross section, is fleshy and rubbery without necrosis.

those of clear cell carcinoma.[64] Criteria that favor a primary cervical origin include the presence of a junctional component (Figure 13.24), melanosis in the squamous or glandular epithelium, and absence of a primary or regressed melanoma elsewhere, especially in the skin, uveal tract, and other mucosal sites.[61]

Immunohistochemistry

The tumor cells are always reactive for either S-100 protein or HMB45, or both.[61,63,65]

Clinical Behavior and Management

Most cases of cervical melanoma present with FIGO stage I or II tumors. Malignant melanomas are aggressive tumors. The 5 year survival rates for patients with stage I, II, and III/IV tumors are 25%, 14%, and 0%, respectively. The mean overall survival rate for all cervical melanomas is 2.4 years.[61] There is no standard treatment for melanoma of the cervix. However, treatment with radical hysterectomy, pelvic lymphadenectomy, and partial vaginectomy with or without adjuvant radiation therapy has been recommended.[66]

LYMPHOMA AND LEUKEMIA

Definition

Malignant lymphoproliferative or hematopoietic tumors that arise in the cervix or involve the cervix secondarily.

General Features

Most cases of lymphoma or leukemia involving the uterine cervix represent a manifestation of widespread disease. Occasionally, however, lymphomas arise in the cervix and most are diffuse large B-cell lymphoma. The second most common type is follicular lymphoma.[67–69] Much more rare are cases of mantle cell lymphoma, Burkitt lymphoma, natural killer (NK)/T-cell lymphoma of the nasal type, peripheral T-cell lymphoma, and Hodgkin lymphoma.[68–72] Although occurring over a wide age range (20–80 years), cervical lymphomas are predominantly seen in premenopausal women (median age, 41 years). Bleeding is the most common symptom, although occasionally atypical lymphoid cells on a routine cervical smear have led to detection.[70]

Pathology: Macroscopic Features

The cervix is typically diffusely enlarged and barrel shaped[70] (Figure 13.25), and often appears as a polyp or a tumor mass. Only rarely is the mucosa abnormal due to tumor ulceration. The tumor cut surface is usually fleshy, rubbery, or firm, and homogeneous or white to tan (Figure 13.26). Focal necrosis or hemorrhage may be seen. Granulocytic sarcomas may give a green color when freshly cut, thus the term 'chloroma.'

Pathology: Microscopic Features

Most cases extend deep into the wall. In diffuse large B-cell lymphomas, neoplastic cells separate or surround endocervical glands without destroying the endocervical or squamous epithelium. Characteristically, a collagenous stroma separates the tumor from the ectocervical epithelium. The neoplastic cells are moderate to large, mostly rounded, with slightly pleomorphic nuclei, containing vesicular chromatin, small nucleoli, and numerous mitoses (Figures 13.27

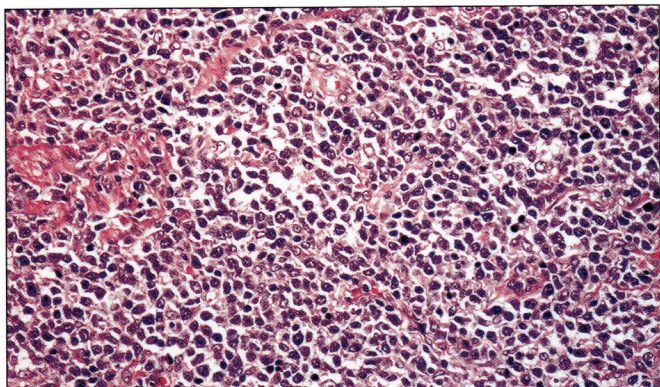

Figure 13.27 Diffuse large B-cell lymphoma.

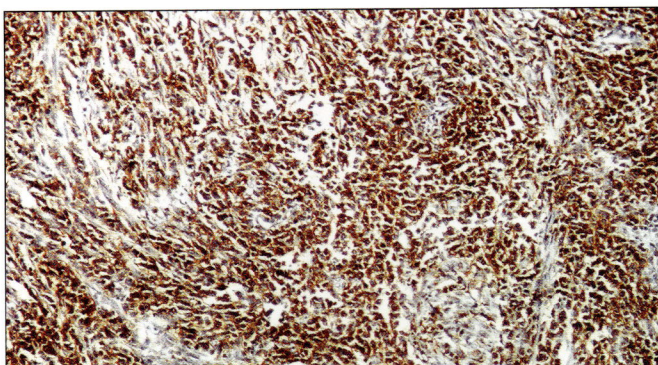

Figure 13.29 Diffuse large B-cell lymphoma, reactive for CD20.

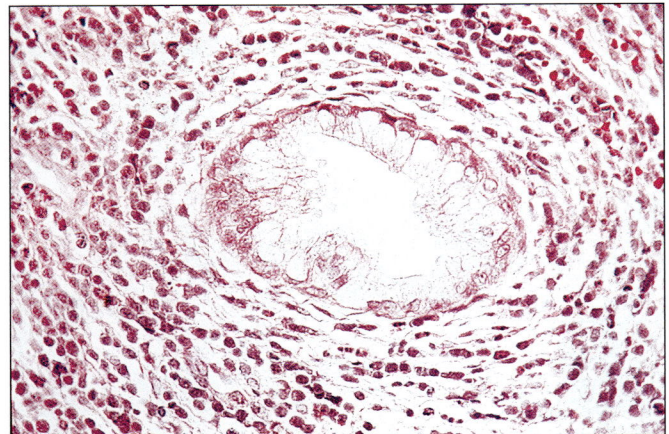

Figure 13.28 Lymphoma. The tumor infiltrates about, but does not replace or destroy, the endocervical glands.

and 13.28). Follicular lymphomas tend to infiltrate along the blood vessel walls at the periphery of the tumor.[70]

Pathology: Immunohistochemical Features

- A screening panel consisting of CD3, CD20, CD45, and keratin is useful to ascertain whether the tumor is a B-cell lymphoma (CD20+) (Figure 13.29), T-cell lymphoma (CD3+), granulocytic sarcoma (only CD45+), or carcinoma (keratin).
- In lymphomas composed of small cells, a panel consisting of CD5, CD10, cyclin D1, CD23, bcl-2, and bcl-6 helps to distinguish follicular lymphoma (CD10+, bcl-6+, bcl-2+) from follicular hyperplasia (bcl-2−), or chronic lymphocytic leukemia/small lymphocytic lymphoma (CD5+, CD23−, cyclin D1+).
- For B-cell proliferations with large or intermediate cells or blasts, reactivity for CD10, CD79a, cyclin D1, bcl-6, Ki-67, T-cell lymphoblastic lymphoma (TdT), Epstein–Barr virus-latent membrane protein (EBV–LMP), and EBNA2 suggests precursor B-acute lymphoblastic lymphoma (CD79a+, CD10±, TdT±), diffuse large B-cell lymphoma (CD10±, bcl-6±, Ki-67 reactivity in >90% of nuclei), blastic variant of mantle cell lymphoma (cyclin D1+), and Burkitt lymphoma (CD10+, TdT−, Ki-67 reactivity in >99% of nuclei).
- CD15 and CD30 are necessary to confirm the diagnosis of classic Hodgkin lymphoma and CD57 for the lymphocyte-predominant variant.
- The uncommon NK/T-cell neoplasms are better defined with antibodies to CD30 and ALK1 (anaplastic large cell lymphoma), CD1a and TdT, and TIA-1 and EBV antigens (cytotoxic T-cells and nasal-type NK cell tumors).
- To diagnose granulocytic sarcoma, testing with myeloperoxidase, CD4, CD68, and CD117 is required.[70]

Differential Diagnosis

Patients with a lymphoma-like lesion tend to be in the fourth decade of life, and experience bleeding and pelvic pain. Although a cervical mass is usually absent, erosion, erythema, bleeding at touch, nodularity, or a friable exophytic growth may be seen. Some patients have had the Epstein–Barr virus.[73] Commonly, the infiltrate is superficial, rarely extending deeper than the endocervical glands. The infiltrate may be diffuse or nodular and contains a mixture of mature lymphocytes, polyclonal plasma cells, and polymorphonuclear cells with numerous mitoses. Immunohistochemically, B-cells predominate and the plasma cells exhibit polyclonality. Rare cases have monoclonal B-cells by polymerase chain reaction. A cervical cone may be necessary to rule out the presence of deep invasion.[70]

Poorly differentiated carcinomas and neuroendocrine carcinomas are distinguished from lymphomas and leukemias by reactivity for keratin and neuroendocrine markers such as CD56, synaptophysin, and chromogranin.

Primitive neuroectodermal tumors (PNETs) may cause diagnostic difficulties and attention to features such as the presence of fibrillary material and rosettes, as well as the use of immunomarkers such as synaptophysin, facilitate the diagnosis. CD99 is not specific for PNETs as it may often be detected in lymphoblastic lymphomas.[70]

METASTATIC TUMORS TO THE CERVIX

Secondary involvement of the uterine cervix is commonly seen as a result of contiguous spread from carcinoma arising in the endometrium.[74] Metastases to the uterine cervix are infrequent.[75,76] In decreasing order of frequency, the primary sites of the metastatic tumors are ovaries, large bowel,

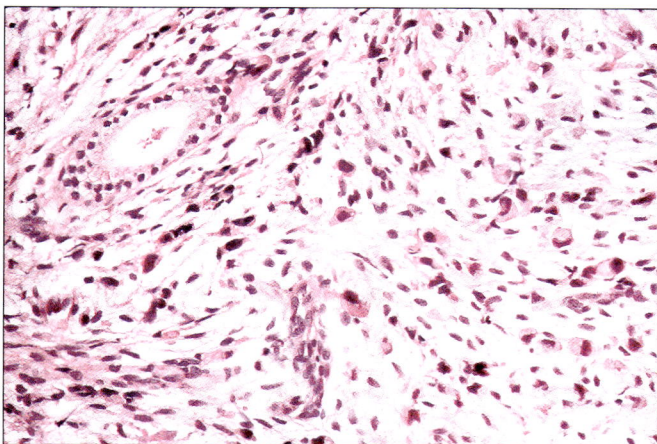

Figure 13.30 Metastatic gastric carcinoma with signet-ring cell features.

stomach, breast, and kidneys. Occasionally, tumors arising in the lungs, pancreaticobiliary tract, and fallopian tubes, as well as appendiceal carcinoids, mesotheliomas, or melanomas may metastasize to the cervix.[74,75] Metastases to the cervix are usually detected after the primary tumor has been diagnosed; however, they may be the initial presentation of the tumor. In certain cases, the disease is discovered after an abnormal Pap smear.[74] Pathologic features that raise the possibility of metastatic tumor include extensive signet ring cells (Figure 13.30), a permeative growth pattern without destruction of the endocervical glands, multinodular growth, Indian file pattern, absence of an *in situ* component, predominant involvement of the outer cervical wall, numerous psammoma bodies, prominent lymphovascular involvement, extensive dirty necrosis, and a low mitotic activity in an invasive adenocarcinoma involving the cervix.[74,77] Noticeably, some metastatic tumors may extend to the surface of the endocervical mucosa mimicking an *in situ* component. The use of immunohistochemistry, *in situ* hybridization for high-risk HPV, and clinical correlation will allow a correct diagnosis.

OTHER TYPES OF CERVICAL NEOPLASMS

Cases of neurilemmoma (schwannoma), neurofibromatosis, lipoma, liposarcoma, perivascular epithelioid cell tumor, angiosarcomas, undifferentiated sarcoma, and endometrial stromal sarcoma have been described in the uterine cervix.[49,78–82]

REFERENCES

1. Brainard JA, Hart WR. Adenoid basal epitheliomas of the uterine cervix: a reevaluation of distinctive cervical basaloid lesions currently classified as adenoid basal carcinoma and adenoid basal hyperplasia. Am J Surg Pathol 1998;22:965–75.
2. Russell MJ, Fadare O. Adenoid basal lesions of the uterine cervix: evolving terminology and clinicopathological concepts. Diagn Pathol 2006;1:18.
3. Hart WR. Symposium part II: special types of adenocarcinoma of the uterine cervix. Int J Gynecol Pathol 2002;21:327–46.
4. Ferry JA, Scully RE. 'Adenoid cystic' carcinoma and adenoid basal carcinoma of the uterine cervix. A study of 28 cases. Am J Surg Pathol 1988;12:134–44.
5. Grayson W, Taylor LF, Cooper K. Adenoid cystic and adenoid basal carcinoma of the uterine cervix: comparative morphologic, mucin, and immunohistochemical profile of two rare neoplasms of putative 'reserve cell' origin. Am J Surg Pathol 1999;23:448–58.
6. Parwani AV, Smith Sehdev AE, Kurman RJ, et al. Cervical adenoid basal tumors comprised of adenoid basal epithelioma associated with various types of invasive carcinoma: clinicopathologic features, human papillomavirus DNA detection, and P16 expression. Hum Pathol 2005;36:82–90.
7. Chen TD, Chuang HC, Lee LY. Adenoid basal carcinoma of the uterine cervix: clinicopathologic features of 12 cases with reference to CD117 expression. Int J Gynecol Pathol 2012;31:25–32.
8. Kwon YS, Kim YM, Choi GW, et al. Pure basaloid squamous cell carcinoma of the uterine cervix: a case report. J Korean Med Sci 2009;24:542–5.
9. Banks ER, Frierson Jr HF, Mills SE, et al. Basaloid squamous cell carcinoma of the head and neck. A clinicopathologic and immunohistochemical study of 40 cases. Am J Surg Pathol 1992;16:939–46.
10. King LA, Talledo OE, Gallup DG, et al. Adenoid cystic carcinoma of the cervix in women under age 40. Gynecol Oncol 1989;32:26–30.
11. Koyfman SA, Abidi A, Ravichandran P, et al. Adenoid cystic carcinoma of the cervix. Gynecol Oncol 2005;99:477–80.
12. Grayson W, Taylor L, Cooper K. Detection of integrated high risk human papillomavirus in adenoid cystic carcinoma of the uterine cervix. J Clin Pathol 1996;49:805–9.
13. Albores-Saavedra J, Manivel C, Mora A, et al. The solid variant of adenoid cystic carcinoma of the cervix. Int J Gynecol Pathol 1992;11:2–10.
14. McCusker ME, Cote TR, Clegg LX, et al. Endocrine tumors of the uterine cervix: incidence, demographics, and survival with comparison to squamous cell carcinoma. Gynecol Oncol 2003;88:333–9.
15. Albores-Saavedra J, Gersell D, Gilks CB, et al. Terminology of endocrine tumors of the uterine cervix: results of a workshop sponsored by the College of American Pathologists and the National Cancer Institute. Arch Pathol Lab Med 1997;121:34–9.
16. Gilks CB, Young RH, Gersell DJ, et al. Large cell neuroendocrine [corrected] carcinoma of the uterine cervix: a clinicopathologic study of 12 cases. Am J Surg Pathol 1997;21:905–14.
17. Mannion C, Park WS, Man YG, et al. Endocrine tumors of the cervix: morphologic assessment, expression of human papillomavirus, and evaluation for loss of heterozygosity on 1p,3p, 11q, and 17p. Cancer 1998;83:1391–400.
18. Stoler MH, Mills SE, Gersell DJ, et al. Small-cell neuroendocrine carcinoma of the cervix. A human papillomavirus type 18-associated cancer. Am J Surg Pathol 1991;15:28–32.
19. Abeler VM, Holm R, Nesland JM, et al. Small cell carcinoma of the cervix. A clinicopathologic study of 26 patients. Cancer 1994;73:672–7.
20. Ambros RA, Park JS, Shah KV, et al. Evaluation of histologic, morphometric, and immunohistochemical criteria in the differential diagnosis of small cell carcinomas of the cervix with particular reference to human papillomavirus types 16 and 18. Mod Pathol 1991;4:586–93.
21. Grayson W, Rhemtula HA, Taylor LF, et al. Detection of human papillomavirus in large cell neuroendocrine carcinoma of the uterine cervix: a study of 12 cases. J Clin Pathol 2002;55:108–14.
22. Wistuba II, Thomas B, Behrens C, et al. Molecular abnormalities associated with endocrine tumors of the uterine cervix. Gynecol Oncol 1999;72:3–9.
23. Moran CA, Suster S, Coppola D, et al. Neuroendocrine carcinomas of the lung: a critical analysis. Am J Clin Pathol 2009;131:206–21.
24. Viswanathan AN, Deavers MT, Jhingran A, et al. Small cell neuroendocrine carcinoma of the cervix: outcome and patterns of recurrence. Gynecol Oncol 2004;93:27–33.
25. Cohen JG, Kapp DS, Shin JY, et al. Small cell carcinoma of the cervix: treatment and survival outcomes of 188 patients. Am J Obstet Gynecol 2010;203(4):347e341–6.
26. Conner MG, Richter H, Moran CA, et al. Small cell carcinoma of the cervix: a clinicopathologic and immunohistochemical study of 23 cases. Ann Diagn Pathol 2002;6:345–8.

27. Gersell DJ, Mazoujian G, Mutch DG, et al. Small-cell undifferentiated carcinoma of the cervix. A clinicopathologic, ultrastructural, and immunocytochemical study of 15 cases. Am J Surg Pathol 1988;12:684–98.
28. Ishibashi-Ueda H, Imakita M, Yutani C, et al. Small cell carcinoma of the uterine cervix with syndrome of inappropriate antidiuretic hormone secretion. Mod Pathol 1996;9:397–400.
29. Seckl MJ, Mulholland PJ, Bishop AE, et al. Hypoglycemia due to an insulin-secreting small-cell carcinoma of the cervix. N Engl J Med 1999;341:733–6.
30. Straughn Jr JM, Richter HE, Conner MG, et al. Predictors of outcome in small cell carcinoma of the cervix. A case series. Gynecol Oncol 2001;83:216–20.
31. Zivanovic O, Leitao Jr MM, Park KJ, et al. Small cell neuroendocrine carcinoma of the cervix: Analysis of outcome, recurrence pattern and the impact of platinum-based combination chemotherapy. Gynecol Oncol 2009;112:590–3.
32. McCluggage WG, Kennedy K, Busam KJ. An immunohistochemical study of cervical neuroendocrine carcinomas: Neoplasms that are commonly TTF1 positive and which may express CK20 and P63. Am J Surg Pathol 2010;34:525–32.
33. Ohwada M, Wada T, Saga Y, et al. C-kit overexpression in neuroendocrine small cell carcinoma of the uterine cervix. Eur J Gynaecol Oncol 2006;27:53–5.
34. Wang HL, Lu DW. Overexpression of c-kit protein is an infrequent event in small cell carcinomas of the uterine cervix. Mod Pathol 2004;17:732–8.
35. Serrano MF, El-Mofty SK, Gnepp DR, et al. Utility of high molecular weight cytokeratins, but not p63, in the differential diagnosis of neuroendocrine and basaloid carcinomas of the head and neck. Hum Pathol 2008;39:591–8.
36. Embry JR, Kelly MG, Post MD, et al. Large cell neuroendocrine carcinoma of the cervix: prognostic factors and survival advantage with platinum chemotherapy. Gynecol Oncol 2011;120:444–8.
37. Sato Y, Shimamoto T, Amada S, et al. Large cell neuroendocrine carcinoma of the uterine cervix: a clinicopathological study of six cases. Int J Gynecol Pathol 2003;22:226–30.
38. Yun K, Cho NP, Glassford GN. Large cell neuroendocrine carcinoma of the uterine cervix: a report of a case with coexisting cervical intraepithelial neoplasia and human papillomavirus 16. Pathology 1999;31:158–61.
39. Clement PB, Scully RE. Mullerian adenosarcoma of the uterus: a clinicopathologic analysis of 100 cases with a review of the literature. Hum Pathol 1990;21:363–81.
40. Zaloudek CJ, Norris HJ. Adenofibroma and adenosarcoma of the uterus: a clinicopathologic study of 35 cases. Cancer 1981;48:354–66.
41. Gallardo A, Prat J. Mullerian adenosarcoma: a clinicopathologic and immunohistochemical study of 55 cases challenging the existence of adenofibroma. Am J Surg Pathol 2009;33:278–88.
42. Gilks CB, Young RH, Clement PB, et al. Adenomyomas of the uterine cervix of endocervical type: a report of ten cases of a benign cervical tumor that may be confused with adenoma malignum [corrected]. Mod Pathol 1996;9:220–4.
43. Jones MW, Lefkowitz M. Adenosarcoma of the uterine cervix: a clinicopathological study of 12 cases. Int J Gynecol Pathol 1995;14:223–9.
44. Kerner H, Lichtig C. Mullerian adenosarcoma presenting as cervical polyps: a report of seven cases and review of the literature. Obstet Gynecol 1993;81:655–9.
45. Clement PB. Mullerian adenosarcomas of the uterus with sarcomatous overgrowth. A clinicopathological analysis of 10 cases. Am J Surg Pathol 1989;13:28–38.
46. Grayson W, Taylor LF, Cooper K. Carcinosarcoma of the uterine cervix: a report of eight cases with immunohistochemical analysis and evaluation of human papillomavirus status. Am J Surg Pathol 2001;25:338–47.
47. Clement PB, Zubovits JT, Young RH, et al. Malignant mullerian mixed tumors of the uterine cervix: a report of nine cases of a neoplasm with morphology often different from its counterpart in the corpus. Int J Gynecol Pathol 1998;17:211–22.
48. Sharma NK, Sorosky JI, Bender D, et al. Malignant mixed mullerian tumor (MMMT) of the cervix. Gynecol Oncol 2005;97:442–5.
49. Fadare O. Uncommon sarcomas of the uterine cervix: a review of selected entities. Diagn Pathol 2006;1:30.
50. Daya DA, Scully RE. Sarcoma botryoides of the uterine cervix in young women: a clinicopathological study of 13 cases. Gynecol Oncol 1988;29:290–304.
51. Ferguson SE, Gerald W, Barakat RR, et al. Clinicopathologic features of rhabdomyosarcoma of gynecologic origin in adults. Am J Surg Pathol 2007;31:382–9.
52. Riedlinger WF, Kozakewich HP, Vargas SO. Myogenic markers in the evaluation of embryonal botryoid rhabdomyosarcoma of the female genital tract. Pediatr Dev Pathol 2005;8:427–34.
53. Karaman E, Akbayir O, Kocaturk Y, et al. Successful treatment of a very rare case: locally treated cervical rhabdomyosarcoma. Arch Gynecol Obstet 2011;284:1019–22.
54. Tiltman AJ. Leiomyomas of the uterine cervix: a study of frequency. Int J Gynecol Pathol 1998;17:231–4.
55. Bell SW, Kempson RL, Hendrickson MR. Problematic uterine smooth muscle neoplasms. A clinicopathologic study of 213 cases. Am J Surg Pathol 1994;18:535–58.
56. Prayson RA, Goldblum JR, Hart WR. Epithelioid smooth-muscle tumors of the uterus: a clinicopathologic study of 18 patients. Am J Surg Pathol 1997;21:383–91.
57. Atkins K, Bell S, Kempson R Hendrickson MR. Myxoid smooth muscle neoplasm of the uterus. Mod Pathol 2001;14:772.
58. Kindelberger D, Hollowell M, Otis C, et al. Myxoid leiomyosarcoma: a clinicopathologic study of ten cases. Mod Pathol 2002;20:203A.
59. Craddock KJ, Bandarchi B, Khalifa MA. Blue nevi of the Mullerian tract: case series and review of the literature. J Low Genit Tract Dis 2007;11:284–9.
60. DeMatos P, Tyler D, Seigler HF. Mucosal melanoma of the female genitalia: a clinicopathologic study of forty-three cases at Duke University Medical Center. Surgery 1998;124:38–48.
61. Clark KC, Butz WR, Hapke MR. Primary malignant melanoma of the uterine cervix: case report with world literature review. Int J Gynecol Pathol 1999;18:265–73.
62. Cantuaria G, Angioli R, Nahmias J, et al. Primary malignant melanoma of the uterine cervix: case report and review of the literature. Gynecol Oncol 1999;75:170–4.
63. Ishikura H, Kojo T, Ichimura H, et al. Desmoplastic malignant melanoma of the uterine cervix: a rare primary malignancy in the uterus mimicking a sarcoma. Histopathology 1998;33:93–4.
64. Furuya M, Shimizu M, Nishihara H, et al. Clear cell variant of malignant melanoma of the uterine cervix: a case report and review of the literature. Gynecol Oncol 2001;80:409–12.
65. Kristiansen SB, Anderson R, Cohen DM. Primary malignant melanoma of the cervix and review of the literature. Gynecol Oncol 1992;47:398–403.
66. Sugiyama VE, Chan JK, Kapp DS. Management of melanomas of the female genital tract. Curr Opin Oncol 2008;20:565–9.
67. Au WY, Chan BC, Chung LP, et al. Primary B-cell lymphoma and lymphoma-like lesions of the uterine cervix. Am J Hematol 2003;73:176–9.
68. Kosari F, Daneshbod Y, Parwaresch R, et al. Lymphomas of the female genital tract: a study of 186 cases and review of the literature. Am J Surg Pathol 2005;29:1512–20.
69. Vang R, Medeiros JL, Ha CS, Deavers M. Non-Hodgkin's lymphoma involving the uterus: a clinicopathologic analysis of 26 cases. Mod Pathol 2000;13:19–28.
70. Lagoo AS, Robboy SJ. Lymphoma of the female genital tract: current status. Int J Gynecol Pathol 2006;25:1–21.
71. Mhawech P, Medeiros LJ, Bueso-Ramos C, et al. Natural killer-cell lymphoma involving the gynecologic tract. Arch Pathol Lab Med 2000;124:1510–3.
72. Pomares Arias E, Payeras Mas M, Conchillo Armendariz MA, et al. Linfoma difuso de células T de cervix uterino: una localización inusual de un tumor poco frecuente. An Med Interna 2000;17:432–3.
73. Hachisuga T, Ookuma Y, Fukuda K, et al. Detection of Epstein-Barr virus DNA from a lymphoma-like lesion of the uterine cervix. Gynecol Oncol 1992;46:69–73.
74. Clement PB. Miscellaneous primary tumors and metastatic tumors of the uterine cervix. Semin Diagn Pathol 1990;7:228–48.
75. Lemoine NR, Hall PA. Epithelial tumors metastatic to the uterine cervix. A study of 33 cases and review of the literature. Cancer 1986;57:2002–5.

76. Mazur MT, Hsueh S, Gersell DJ. Metastases to the female genital tract. Analysis of 325 cases. Cancer 1984;53:1978–84.
77. Malpica A, Deavers MT. Ovarian low-grade serous carcinoma involving the cervix mimicking a cervical primary. Int J Gynecol Pathol 2011;30:613–9.
78. Boardman CH, Webb MJ, Jefferies JA. Low-grade endometrial stromal sarcoma of the ectocervix after therapy for breast cancer. Gynecol Oncol 2000;79:120–3.
79. Fadare O, Parkash V, Yilmaz Y, et al. Perivascular epithelioid cell tumor (PEComa) of the uterine cervix associated with intraabdominal 'PEComatosis': a clinicopathological study with comparative genomic hybridization analysis. World J Surg Oncol 2004;2:35.
80. Folpe AL, Mentzel T, Lehr HA, et al. Perivascular epithelioid cell neoplasms of soft tissue and gynecologic origin: a clinicopathologic study of 26 cases and review of the literature. Am J Surg Pathol 2005;29:1558–75.
81. LeMaire WJ, Kreiss C, Commodore A, et al. Neurilemmoma: an unusual benign tumor of the cervix. Alaska Med 2002;44:63–5.
82. Morrel B, Mulder AF, Chadha S, et al. Angiosarcoma of the uterus following radiotherapy for squamous cell carcinoma of the cervix. Eur J Obstet Gynecol Reprod Biol 1993;49:193–7.

14 The Normal Endometrium

Rex C. Bentley, George L. Mutter, Stanley J. Robboy

CHAPTER OUTLINE

Components of the Normal Endometrium	290	Late Secretory Phase, Days 22–28: Predecidual Change	301
Surface Epithelium	292	Endometrium after Menopause	303
Glandular Cells	292	Methods of Endometrial Sampling	304
Stromal Cells	293	Dilatation and Curettage	304
Endometrial Lymphocytes	294	Vabra Aspirator	304
Blood Vessels	295	Pipelle Biopsy	305
Endometrium During the 28 Day Idealized Normal Menstrual Cycle	295	Cytologic Evaluation of the Endometrium	305
Menstrual Endometrium (Days 1–3 of 28)	297	Hysteroscopy	305
Proliferative Phase (Days 4–15 of 28)	298	Endometrial Resection and Ablation	305
Interval Endometrium (Day 16 of 28)	299	Problems in Interpretation of Endometrial Specimens	307
Secretory Endometrium (Days 17–28 of 28)	299	Adequacy	307
Early Secretory Phase, Days 16–18: Changing Vacuolar Patterns	299	Dissociation Artifact	307
		Telescoping Artifact	308
Mid-secretory Phase, Days 19–21: Increasing Stromal Edema	300	Fixation Artifact	308
		Legitimate Tissue Contaminants	308

COMPONENTS OF THE NORMAL ENDOMETRIUM

The mucosal lining of the uterus consists of glands, stroma, and blood vessels. The function of the endometrium is to form a receptive site for pregnancy. This is initially accomplished through a nutrient effect of the glands and their secretions on the blastocyst in the 24 hours or so before implantation takes place (on or about day 7 post ovulation). Once nidation has occurred, the relationship between the conceptus and its mother is primarily between extraembryonic trophoblast and the decidualized endometrial stroma. Glandular changes are the most easily observed and common pathologic conditions in the uterus.

The endometrium merges with the mucosa of the fallopian tube at its upper extreme and with the endocervical epithelium at its lower end. The junction with the fallopian tube epithelium is usually abrupt, although the exact position may vary considerably. Uncommonly, endometrium may line the tube some centimeters lateral to the cornu, a condition referred to as 'endometrialization' (to be distinguished from endometriosis, Chapter 22). At the junction of the endometrium with the endocervical epithelium, however, there is a gradual transition from one type of mucosa to the other, sometimes over a distance of as much as 1 cm. This is the lower uterine segment, which contains glands with features between those of the endometrium proper and the endocervix (Figure 14.1). Not uncommonly, endometrial glands will be found deep to the endocervical lining. Glands of the lower uterine segment show practically none of the morphologic effects that hormonal stimulation elicits in the fundus. Care must be taken to recognize this tissue for what it is, so that the inactivity in these pieces is not taken to mean that the endometrium as a whole is not being stimulated or is not responding. Glands in this area are prone to be partly lined by epithelium containing a mixture of undistinguished columnar cells admixed with ciliated cells. The stroma of the lower uterine segment differs from that of the endometrium proper in being rather more fibrous and displaying cells that are generally more spindled. The glands are typically flattened and slit-like and the epithelial cells lack mucus.

The endometrium from the uterine body and fundus is generally fairly uniform from one area to another. There is, however, variation within the endometrial thickness

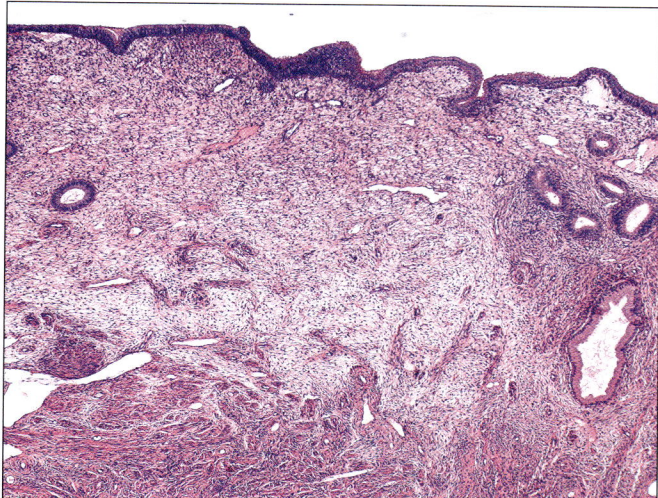

Figure 14.1 Lower uterine segment mucosa, or 'isthmic endometrium.' In a hysterectomy specimen, the isthmic endometrium is seen as a zone of poorly developed glands in fibrous stroma, which lack the cyclical hormonally induced changes of endometrium within the uterine corpus.

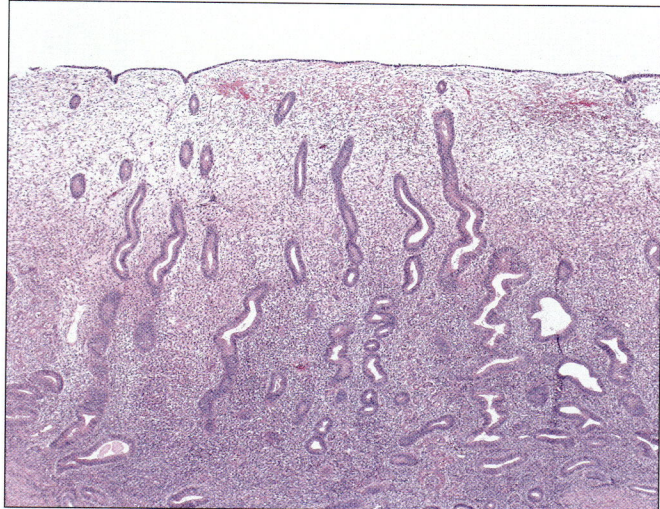

Figure 14.2 Normal proliferative endometrium, low power.

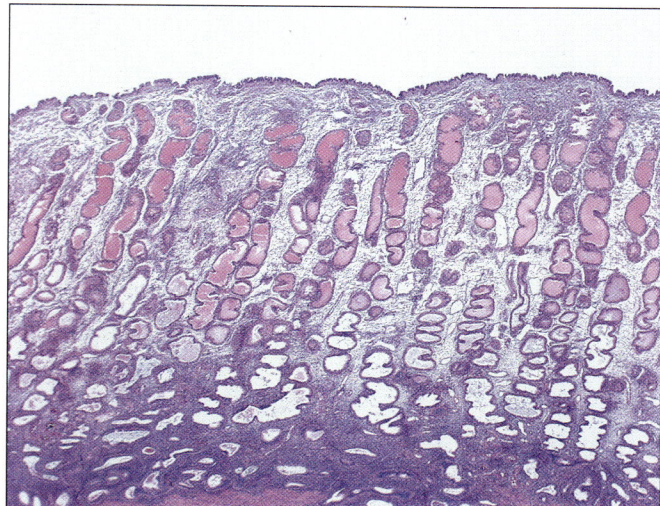

Figure 14.3 Mid-secretory phase endometrium (day 22).

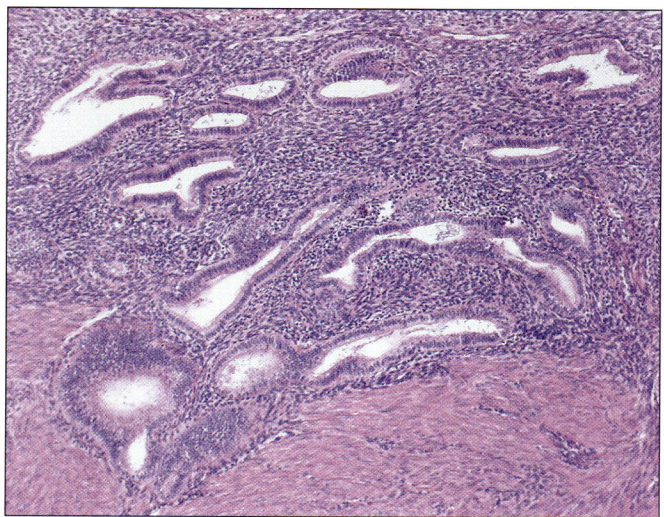

Figure 14.4 Basal zone. Normal secretory endometrium.

depending on the vertical position of the tissue in relation to the surface epithelium and the endometrial–myometrial junction (Figure 14.2). These layers become more pronounced as the menstrual cycle progresses (Figure 14.3). The basal layer (stratum basalis) is adjacent to the myometrium, and consists of tubular glands, occasionally branching, lined by simple to pseudostratified epithelium in a more basophilic, compact stroma (Figure 14.4). The glandular epithelium shows no evidence of secretory activity whatever the phase of the cycle, and there is no or minimal mitotic activity in either glands or stroma. As the overall volume of glands is small compared with that in the functional layer, the stroma is relatively more prominent. The stroma also appears more cellular as it is composed of largely spindled nuclei with only scant, inapparent cytoplasm.

The remaining endometrium is the functional zone (stratum functionalis), which is further subdivided into the superficial compact layer (stratum compactum) and the deeper spongy layer (stratum spongiosum). This distinction only becomes striking in the late secretory (postovulatory or luteal) phase (Figure 14.5). At that time the spongy layer consists of glands showing maximal secretory activity but a relatively unresponsive stroma that does not develop a good predecidual response apart from the immediate vicinity of the spiral arterioles. Stroma in the more superficial compact layer, on the other hand, responds remarkably to hormonal stimulation with a prominent predecidual reaction and numerous granulated lymphocytes (see later). Glands in this zone are stretched thin by the expanding stroma, and demonstrate less secretory activity. It is apparent therefore that the morphology of the endometrial stromal and glandular cells is a function not only of the systemic hormonal environment, but also of the position in the corpus or lower uterine segment, and vertical location within the endometrial layers. As material from all of these layers routinely appears in curettings, the pathologist must be aware of

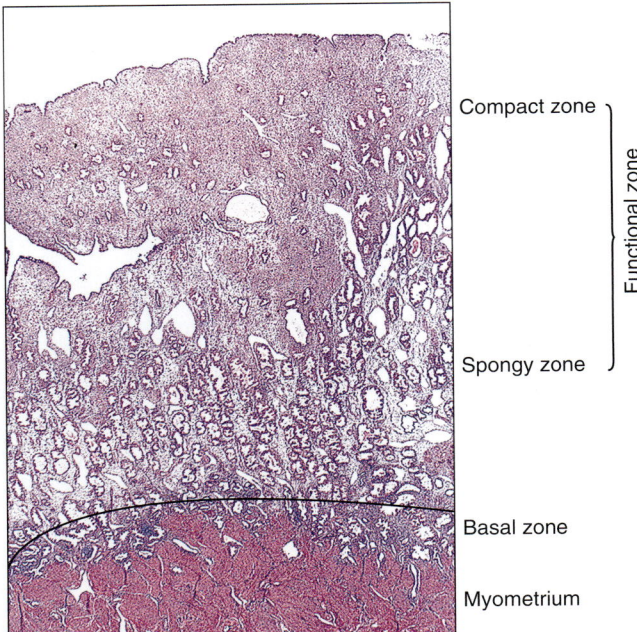

Figure 14.5 Late secretory phase endometrium (day 27). The stratification is demonstrated.

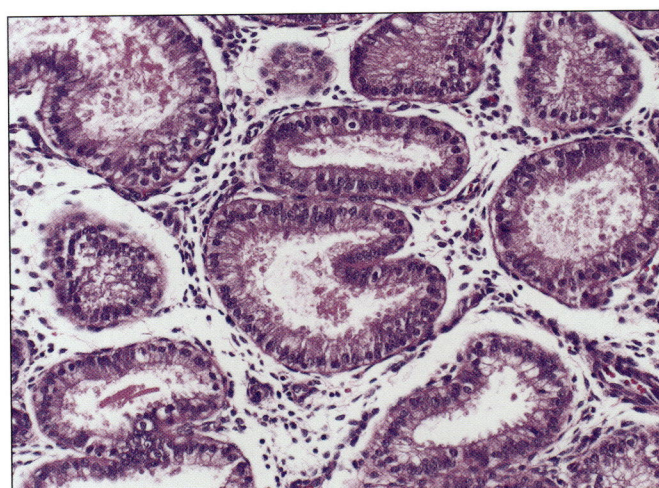

Figure 14.7 Secretory epithelial changes in secretory phase endometrium.

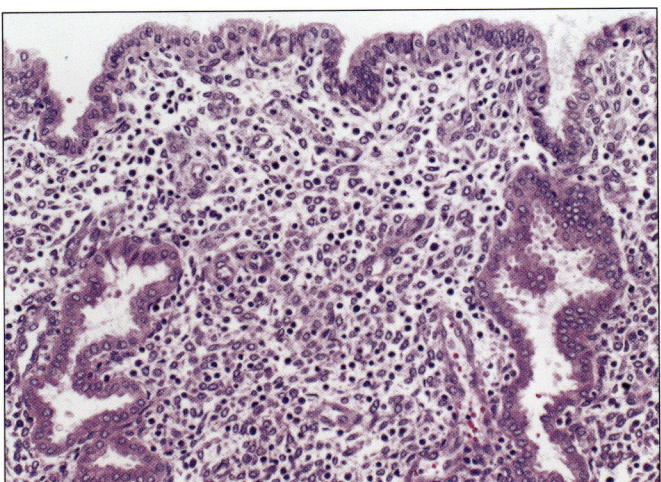

Figure 14.6 Surface epithelium, late secretory endometrium. Note contrast of surface at top to glands below.

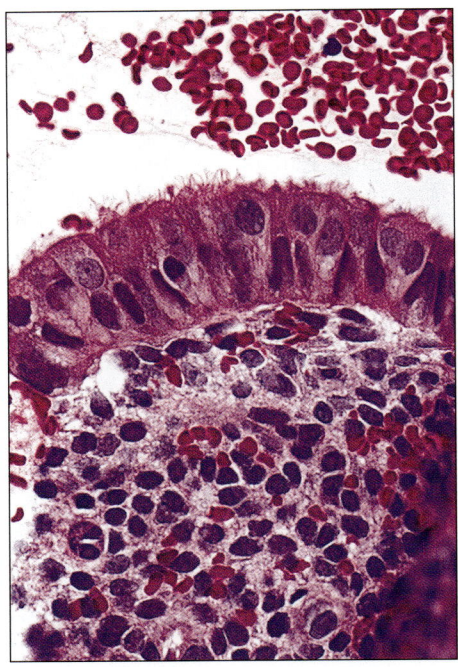

Figure 14.8 Ciliated epithelium.

characteristic appearances at all sites throughout the menstrual cycle.

SURFACE EPITHELIUM

The surface epithelium of the endometrium is continuous with the glandular epithelium and is generally similar. However, the constituent cells show less marked cyclical variation than the cells in the glands (Figure 14.6), responding relatively weakly to circulating sex steroids, and are frequently ciliated. Although subnuclear vacuolation and mitotic activity are seen, these features do not always accurately reflect the time of the cycle. There is usually no problem in identifying surface epithelium in curettings, but the few small epithelial strips that may constitute an entire biopsy sample in an atrophic endometrium can be difficult if not impossible to characterize with any degree of certainty.

GLANDULAR CELLS

There are three types of endometrial glandular cells: the secretory cell (Figure 14.7), the ciliated cell (Figure 14.8), and the clear cell (Figure 14.9).

- The secretory cells are by far the most abundant and their morphology varies with the time of the menstrual cycle. The various appearances will be covered when the phases of the cycle are described.

CHAPTER 14 — THE NORMAL ENDOMETRIUM 293

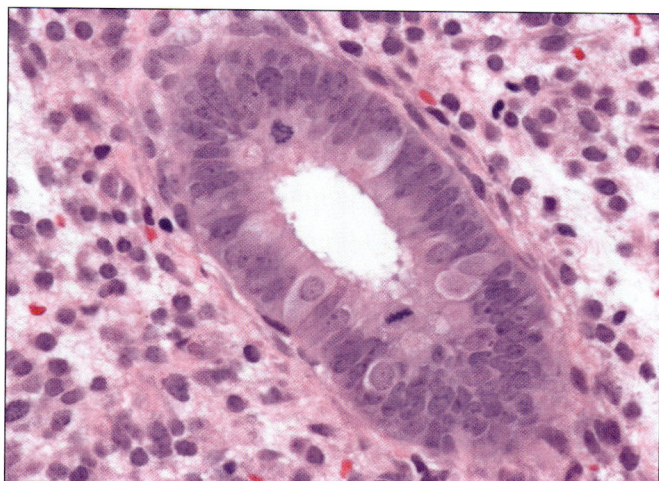

Figure 14.9 Clear cells in glandular epithelium.

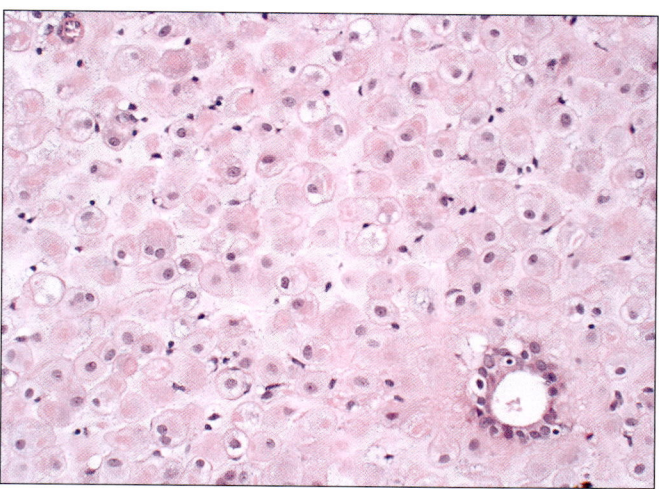

Figure 14.12 Markedly decidualized endometrium after exogenous progestin therapy.

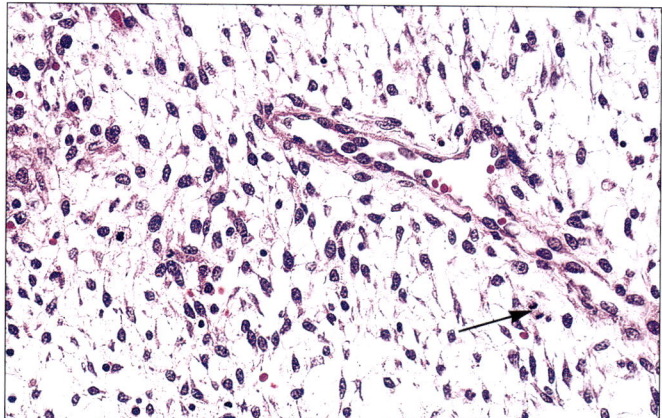

Figure 14.10 Endometrial stroma. Proliferative phase. Stromal mitotic activity (arrow) is seen. Part of a spiral arteriole is present.

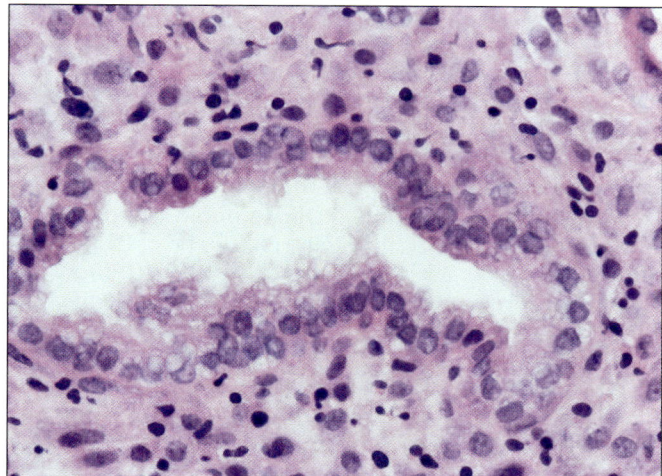

Figure 14.11 Endometrial stroma. Late secretory phase (day 27), compact layer. The stromal cells surrounding the gland show predecidual change and have abundant cytoplasm. Granulated lymphocytes are present.

- The ciliated cells are more frequent near the cornua and toward the endocervix as well as being quite common in the surface epithelium. Although a normal constituent of the endometrium, the ciliated cells are particularly under the influence of estrogens and become more prominent in conditions of estrogen excess (e.g., anovulatory cycles).[1] As ciliated cells are so common, they must be considered as normal and not as 'ciliated metaplasia' as described elsewhere in the literature. Furthermore, in specimens, where only strips of cells are produced, the presence of cilia is useful to suspect that an estrogenic milieu is present whether from endogenous or exogenous sources and that the specimen is not atrophic.
- The clear cells are much less common and are thought to be precursors of the ciliated cells. They are most frequently seen in the proliferative phase.

STROMAL CELLS

The morphology of the endometrial stromal cells varies dramatically throughout the menstrual cycle. During the proliferative phase, the stromal cells are small and mostly compact, with oval, hyperchromatic nuclei and inapparent cytoplasm. In the mid-proliferative phase, at the preovulatory peak of serum estrogen levels, stromal cells are separated by increased intercellular edema. At the end of the proliferative phase the nuclei become slightly larger and their chromatin a little less dense (Figure 14.10). The stroma again becomes edematous in the middle of the secretory phase, reaching a peak at about the 22nd day of a normalized 28 day cycle (again due to an estrogen peak), after which the cells of the compact zone progressively undergo predecidual change, developing into polygonal cells with vesicular nuclei and abundant, pale cytoplasm with well-defined cell borders (Figure 14.11) The terms 'predecidua' and 'pseudodecidua' are often used to describe this change in the morphology of the stromal cells as a response to endogenous and exogenous progesterone, respectively. The term 'decidua' is properly reserved for the change seen in pregnancy, but in practice many pathologists

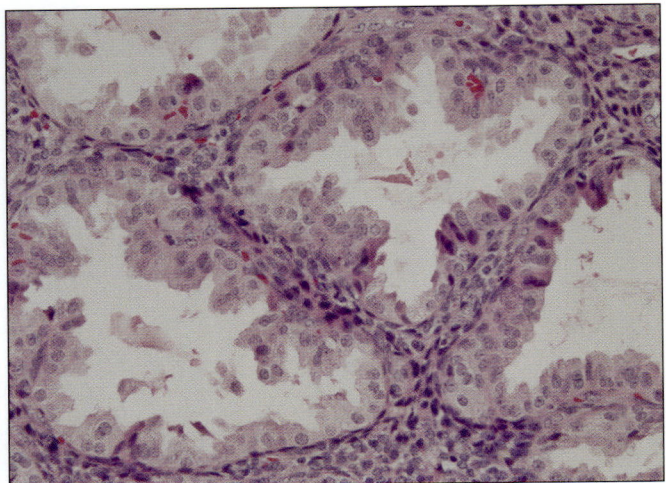

Figure 14.13 Endometrial stroma. Late secretory phase (day 27), spongy layer. The glands are active but the stromal cells are small with no decidual change.

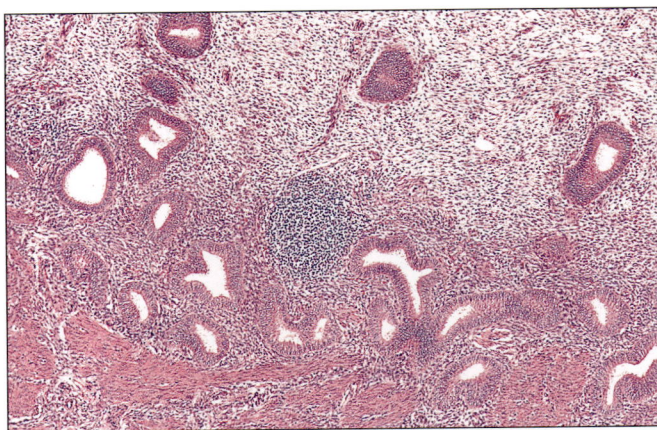

Figure 14.15 Normal endometrium. Lymphoid aggregate.

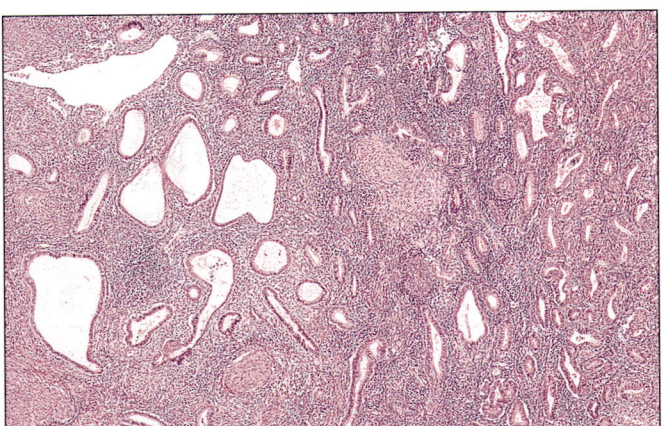

Figure 14.14 Smooth muscle in endometrial stroma.

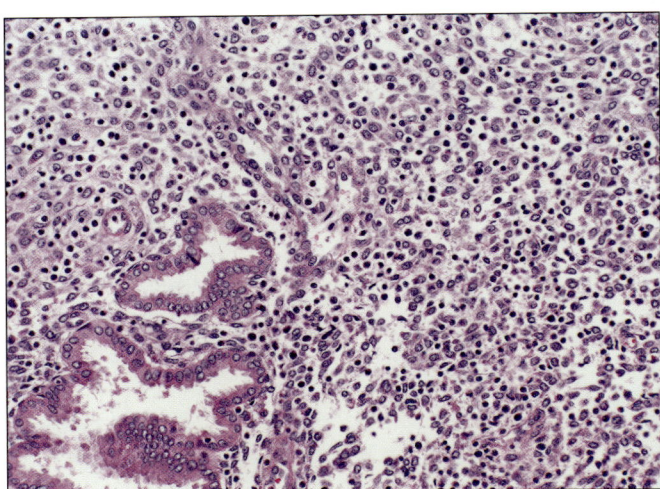

Figure 14.16 Endometrial lymphocytes in late secretory endometrium.

use the terms interchangeably. While it is true that the morphologic changes in the cells are qualitatively the same whether it has been brought about by physiologic levels of progesterone or by synthetic progestins (as in oral contraceptives), there usually is a quantitative difference in both the amount of cytoplasm present in any given cell and the proportion of stromal cells with the change. In general, decidual change is more extensive and uniform in pregnancy and in patients receiving exogenous progestins (Figure 14.12), whereas in premenstrual endometrium a significant proportion of the cells are only minimally or partially affected (compare with Figure 14.11). Decidual change is first apparent adjacent to the spiral arterioles but toward the end of the secretory phase and in pregnancy the change becomes diffuse. The stromal cells that are situated deeper in the endometrium, lying between the active glands of the spongy layer, show little, if any, decidual change and remain fairly nondescript (Figure 14.13). Occasionally, small bundles of smooth muscle may be found in the endometrial stroma (Figure 14.14). The decidual cells of the endometrial stroma, together with an exponential increase in granulated lymphocytes and natural killer (NK) cells, and the synthesis of a variety of cytokines and extracellular matrix proteins including laminin and fibronectin play a central role in the process of nidation (see Chapter 32).

ENDOMETRIAL LYMPHOCYTES

Several subpopulations of T-lymphocytes reside in the normal endometrium, and small lymphoid aggregates are normal, particularly in the basal zone (Figure 14.15). CD4+ and CD8+ T-cells are randomly scattered throughout the functional layer and, in the absence of an inflammatory process, show only a modest variation in density throughout the menstrual cycle, increasing toward menstruation.[2] In any form of endometritis, they aggregate near and around glands and can be seen within the gland lumens along with CD68+ or CD163+ macrophages. Macrophages are normally found in all areas of the functional and basal zones.

In contrast, small, rounded cells with hyperchromatic nuclei that are usually kidney-shaped or segmented increase in number in the endometrial stroma in the second half of the cycle (Figures 14.16 and 14.17). These cells are known

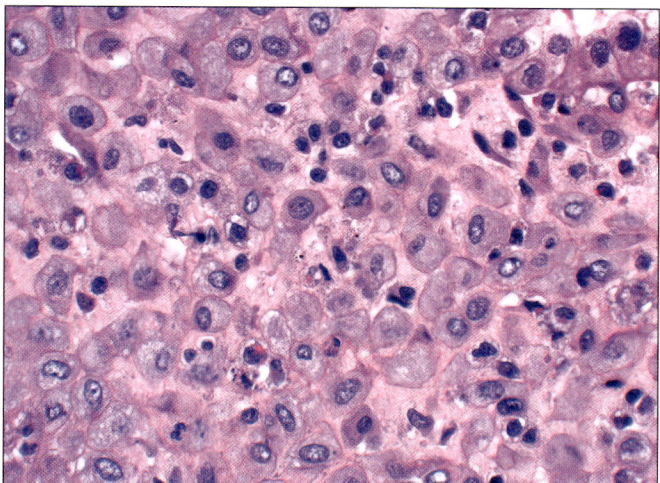

Figure 14.17 Large granular lymphocytes in predecidua of normal late secretory endometrium. The cells have hyperchromatic, kidney-shaped nuclei and eosinophilic granules in the cytoplasm.

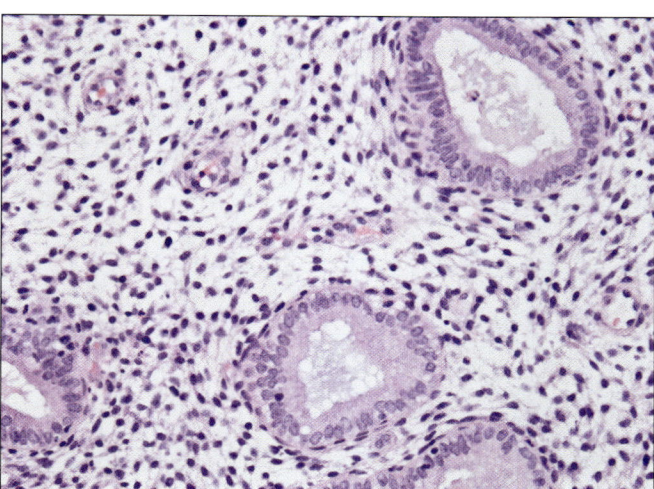

Figure 14.18 Spiral arterioles in the early secretory phase.

as endometrial granulocytes, endometrial granular cells, or K-cells. The cytoplasm contains eosinophilic granules of variable size, so that the cells are also often mistaken for infiltrating polymorphonuclear leukocytes, particularly in the presence of early or imminent menstrual fragmentation (neutrophils are not seen in a normal endometrium until menstruation is well established and their presence at other times of the cycle indicates inflammation). These cells are large granulated lymphocytes that, on flow cytometric analysis, exhibit the unusual T-cell phenotype CD56+, CD3−, CD16−, and also have an NK function. Endometrial NK cells increase in number dramatically in the late secretory phase of the menstrual cycle, sometimes reaching a population density exceeding 25% of all stromal cells. If conception and implantation occur, they continue to increase in number and make up about 70% of the stromal lymphocytes in the first trimester of pregnancy. Endometrial and decidual NK cells are distinct from other classes of NK cells, having both a major immune regulatory function and a critical role in remodeling of the endometrium after implantation.[2,3] Our expanding understanding of the important role of decidual NK cells is leading to the possibility of infertility therapies aimed at disorders in their function.[4]

In comparison to T-lymphocytes, B-lymphocytes are normally sparse in the endometrium. Whether rare plasma cells can be seen in normal endometrium remains a controversial topic, as observations differ according to the population studied and detection method employed. One of the few studies to rigorously select normal women used a sensitive methyl-green pyronine stain to identify small numbers of plasma cells in about one-third of normal endometria.[5]

BLOOD VESSELS

The arterial supply of the endometrium is from the radial arteries that arise from the arcuate arteries in the myometrium. The radial arteries branch near the endometrial–myometrial interface, forming the basal arteries. As these ascend through the functionalis to the endometrial surface, they become the spiral arterioles (Figure 14.18). The spiral arterioles respond to the varying levels of ovarian hormones and become prominent in the second half of the secretory phase, under the influence of progesterone. Coiling becomes most pronounced when the stromal edema is re-absorbed prior to menstruation. In the proliferative phase, the arterioles show little coiling and are confined to the deeper levels of the functionalis. There is an irregular network of venous channels with the veins frequently intersecting, forming venous lakes. Lymphatic vessels are present in normal endometrium, but disappear in decidualized endometrium during pregnancy.[6]

ENDOMETRIUM DURING THE 28 DAY IDEALIZED NORMAL MENSTRUAL CYCLE

The endometrium undergoes a complex and orchestrated series of changes during menstrual cycle progression that when properly interpreted can provide useful information about the patient's hormonal state.[7–11] The main features throughout the cycle are summarized and illustrated in Figure 14.19. The endometrial cycle is renewed with menses, and then customarily divided into two sequential phases, the proliferative (preovulatory or follicular) and the secretory (postovulatory or luteal) phases. This division of the cycle is related, of course, to the hormones stimulating it, with estrogen predominating in the proliferative phase and progesterone in the secretory phase. The endometrial cycle is often standardized in pathology reports as an idealized 28 day cycle beginning on the first day of clinical menses, followed by a proliferative phase with ovulation on day 14. Physiologic differences in total cycle length between women are generally caused by variation in the duration of menses and the proliferative phase, as the postovulatory temporal sequence is a remarkably consistent 14 days. In dating the endometrium it is important to remember that there is a delay of 2–3 days between ovulation and appearance of

Endometrial phase	Menstrual	Proliferative	'Interval'	Secretory Early		Mid	Late	
Day, of 28 day cycle (ovulation on D14)	1–3	4–15	~16	17	18	19–21	22–24	25–28
Key feature	Stromal crumbling	Mitoses	Subnuclear vacuoles, staggered, with mitoses	Subnuclear vacuoles, regular, with mitoses	Sub- and supra-nuclear vacuoles. No mitoses	Stromal edema	Focal predecidua around spiral arteries	Predecidua involves surface
Microscopic features of functional zone — Stroma	Stromal aggregates. 'Blue balls' hemorrhage	Loose stroma. Mitoses	Loose stroma. Mitoses	Loose stroma, scanty mitoses	Loose stroma, scanty mitoses	Stromal edema increases from D19–21	Perivascular 'naked nuclei' (D22) form predecidual cuffs (D23) that bridge vessels (D24)	Focal (D25) then extensive (D26) surface predecidua extends downwards (D26–28). Prominent granulated lymphocytes
Microscopic features of functional zone — Glands	Collapsed epithelium and displaced secretory glands	Straight to tightly coiled tubules. Mitoses	Some staggered subnuclear vacuoles. Many mitoses	'Piano key' subnuclear vacuoles. Some mitoses	Some staggered subnuclear vacuoles. No mitoses	Dilated glands with irregular outlines. Luminal secretion	'Saw tooth' glands	Prominent 'saw tooth' glands
Appearances	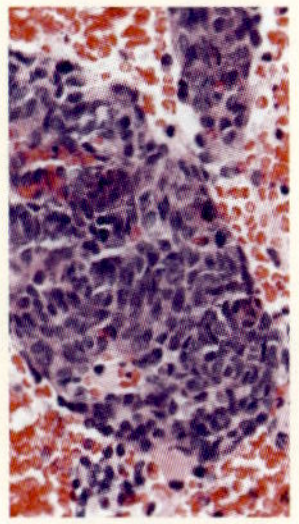	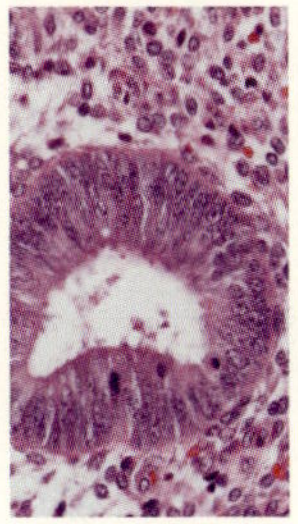	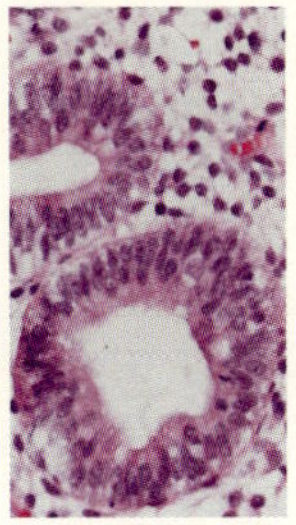	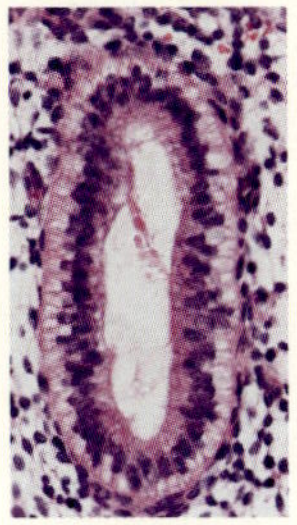	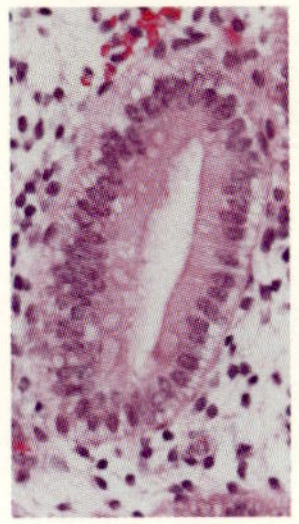	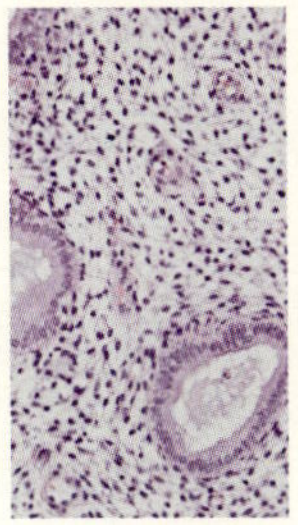	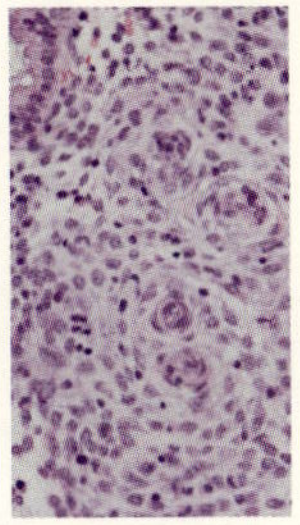	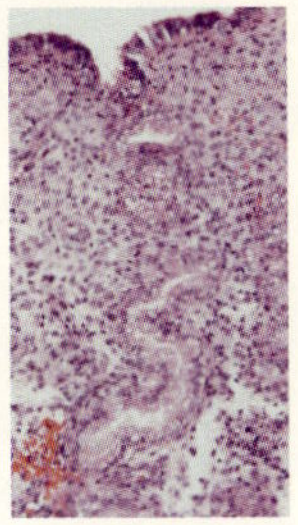

Figure 14.19 Main histologic features of the menstrual cycle. Histologic classification stages, according to 28 day idealized cycle in which day 1 is the first day of clinical menses and ovulation occurs on day 14.

diagnostic postovulatory histologic changes. This is caused by progressively rising progesterone levels and time necessary for the endometrium to respond. Thus, although clinical ovulation is assumed to occur on day 14, there is a brief 'interval phase' corresponding to days 15–16, before definitive progestational effects are evident.

In the following description we summarize histopathologic endometrial features seen on particular days according to an idealized 28 day cycle (e.g., secretory endometrium, 24 days), starting with the first day of menses. The more physiologic approach of directly referencing the date of ovulation (e.g., postovulatory day 10) is an alternative.

MENSTRUAL ENDOMETRIUM (DAYS 1–3 OF 28)

If conception and implantation have not occurred by day 24 (postovulatory day 10), the corpus luteum involutes, leading to a marked fall in progesterone output. The late secretory phase then leads inevitably to the menstrual phase, which defines cycle day 1. This is recognized histologically by very fine crumbling or fragmentation of the stroma and glandular collapse (Figure 14.20), with abundant blood and neutrophils in the background. Two very characteristic changes, especially when seen in combination, are compact balls of stromal cells which, with hematoxylin, have an unusually deep blue color (Figure 14.21), and which are covered by a layer of epithelial cells that appear eosinophilic and reactive. A third change, often seen, is the presence of plump epithelial glandular cells that are frequently multilayered, the so-called 'papillary syncytial metaplasia' (Figure 14.22).

The appearances of menstrual endometrium can confuse inexperienced pathologists because the stromal crumbling results in irregular, collapsing glands often coming together to give a 'back-to-back' pattern that may be misinterpreted as hyperplasia or even malignancy. Attention to the rest of the material on the slide will show the remains of secretory glands and, perhaps, some areas where the stroma remains intact and shows predecidual change (Figures 14.21 and 14.23). In addition, the highly cellular stromal balls are occasionally misinterpreted as small cell carcinoma of either endometrium or cervix due to the very high nuclear to cytoplasmic ratios and prominent nuclear molding and apoptosis.

Histologic examination of curettings taken during menstruation is usually uninformative, as architecture is obscured by fragmentation and the true morphology of the epithelium is replaced by the degenerative changes that take place very rapidly once menstruation commences. From the configuration of the larger intact fragments, and the appearances of the glandular cells, especially by the presence of secretory change, it is often possible to indicate whether the cycle just finishing has been ovulatory. Mitotic figures are not seen at the time of menstruation, but some residual stromal aggregates remaining after cessation of clinical

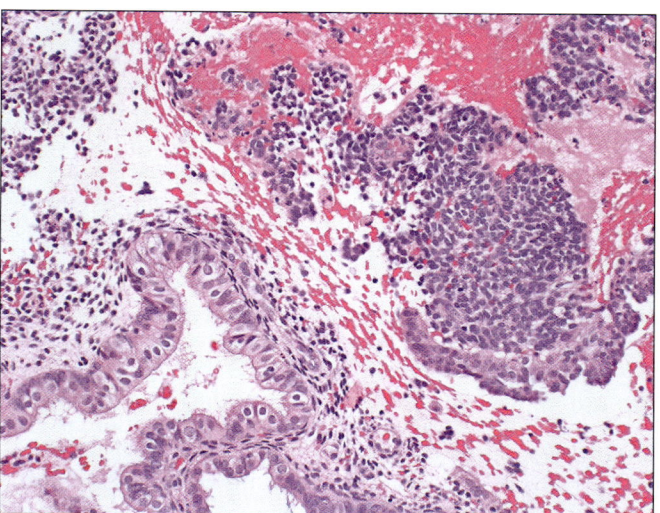

Figure 14.21 Menstrual endometrium, secretory glands, and detached stromal aggregate ('blue ball').

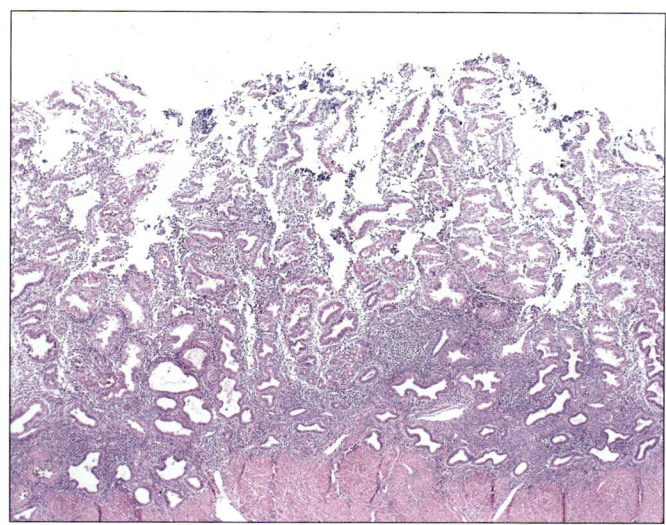

Figure 14.20 Menstrual endometrium, fragmentation of the endometrium.

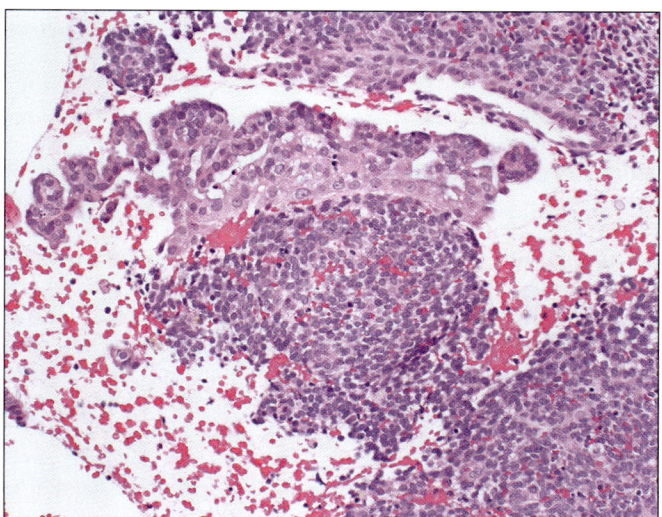

Figure 14.22 Menstrual endometrium, stromal ball, and collapsed overlying redundant epithelium, 'papillary syncytial metaplasia.'

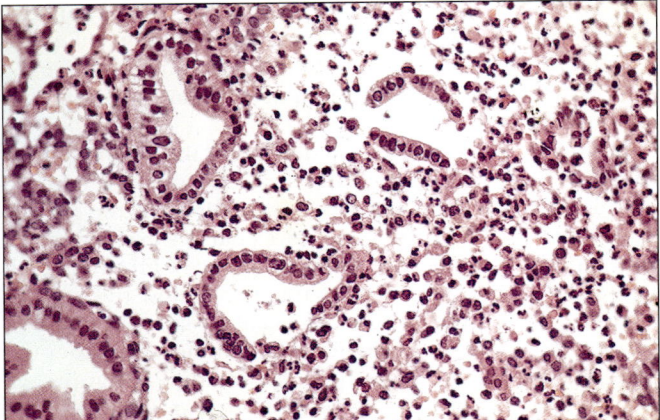

Figure 14.23 Menstrual phase endometrium. Inflammation is present in the background and the endometrial glands are extensively fragmented, but disaggregated stromal cells are not formed into balls, and gland epithelium has not collapsed.

bleeding may coexist with occasional mitoses during transition to the proliferative phase. In general, if the curettage is undertaken to diagnose a suspected underlying hormonal abnormality or cause of infertility, it is best performed when intact tissue can be obtained, outside of menses. On the other hand, if a woman has abnormal bleeding, then curettage can be done while bleeding is occurring.

Menstruation follows a chain of events that begins with involution of the corpus luteum. Falling levels of estradiol and progesterone have direct effects upon vascular, stromal, and glandular elements, which then develop a secondary cascade of dynamic interactions. Stromal breakdown, the pathognomonic histologic feature of menstruation, is initiated by the progesterone drop, which forces stromal cells into apoptosis.[12,13] At the same time, intracapillary and intravenular hydrostatic pressure declines, with reabsorption of stromal edema fluid and a rapid decrease in the endometrial thickness. Spiral arterioles, which are structured as irregular spirals, collapse and kink, resulting in ischemia of the overlying endometrial tissue. Thrombus formation is not part of the normal process. About 20 hours after menstruation starts, intense prostaglandin-induced vasoconstriction controls the blood loss.[12,14]

It follows from this outline that true menstruation cannot occur in the absence of ovulation. The complete process depends on falling levels of both estrogen and progesterone. From a morphologic point of view, fragments of endometrial epithelium showing secretory changes are diagnostic of ovulation, and these samples may be designated 'menstrual endometrium, ovulatory type.' By late menses, even in postovulatory patients, these glands with diagnostic secretory changes may already be completely passed and it may no longer be possible to confirm ovulation. These can be diagnosed as 'late menstrual endometrium,' with a note or qualifier that ovulation cannot be confirmed in the late phase of shedding. One clue of a preceding anovulatory cycle is the presence of fibrin thrombi, not normally seen in a true menstrual phase endometrium, but in itself it is not diagnostic.

The remaining basal layer and a variable, narrow band of the spongy zone is then ready to begin proliferating again

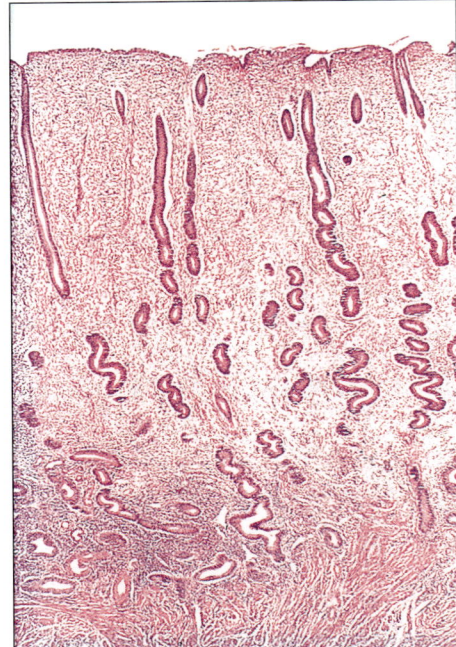

Figure 14.24 Proliferative endometrium. Low power.

at the start of the next cycle. In fact, it is usually possible to appreciate an overlap between the menstrual breakdown and beginning proliferation; curettings taken after menstruation is well established will often contain crumbling tissue, intact basal endometrium, and early proliferating endometrium. A further feature of the endometrium at menstruation is the presence of a neutrophil polymorph infiltrate, which is seen as a response to necrotic tissue and does not indicate acute infection.

PROLIFERATIVE PHASE (DAYS 4–15 OF 28)

This part of the cycle generally lasts for 11–12 days, but may vary considerably between patients with cycles of differing lengths. Proliferative activity commences before menstrual bleeding from the previous cycle has finished, when the endometrium is thin with sparse, small, straight glands and a loose stroma of spindled cells. At 8–10 days, the endometrial thickness increases, mainly as a result of stromal edema induced by estrogen (Figure 14.24), which reaches a peak at about the 10th day. Continued growth of the glands overtakes that of the stroma, so that they become slightly tortuous. This process becomes more exaggerated close to the time of ovulation (Figure 14.25). Glandular epithelium takes on a 'pseudostratified' appearance, with nuclei staggered at various heights in the cell, although most are in the basal half. The epithelial cells have smooth, sharp luminal borders and basophilic or amphophilic cytoplasm (Figure 14.26). Mitoses are frequent in both glands and stroma, and are a direct result of stimulation by estrogen. Accurate dating of the proliferative endometrium as early, mid, or late proliferative is rarely possible using morphologic criteria or, indeed, necessary, as in most cases a diagnosis of 'proliferative endometrium' is sufficient.

CHAPTER 14 — THE NORMAL ENDOMETRIUM

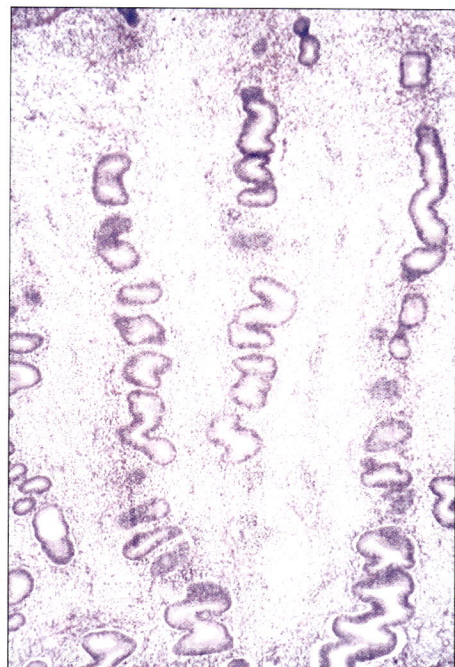

Figure 14.25 Proliferative endometrium with tortuous coiled glands just prior to ovulation.

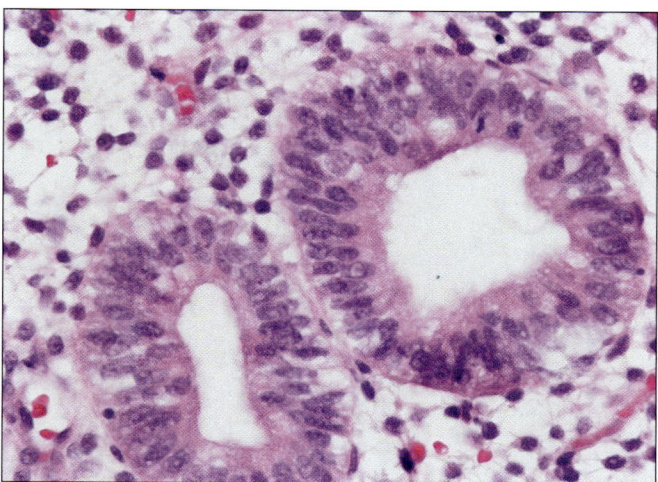

Figure 14.27 'Interval phase' endometrium, day 16. Scattered poorly developed subnuclear vacuoles in glands that still have some proliferative activity.

in states of chronic estrogen stimulation such as anovulation. Histologic confirmation of ovulation requires extensive formation of regular and uniform vacuoles at day 17, or subsequent patterns as described next.

SECRETORY ENDOMETRIUM (DAYS 17–28 OF 28)

After ovulation, which occurs on day 14, the development and involution of the corpus luteum is controlled in a very precise way. The response of the endometrium to changing levels of both estrogen and progesterone follows a predictable pattern so that the appearances seen in the secretory phase of the cycle allow accurate dating. Initial endometrial changes are nonspecific (interval phase, see earlier), but starting at day 17 they become pathognomonic of ovulation, which can be communicated to the clinician as 'secretory endometrium, x days' where 'x' is the corresponding day in a 28 day cycle. The secretory phase is often divided into early, mid, and late phases, but these phases are variably (and arbitrarily) defined by different authorities.

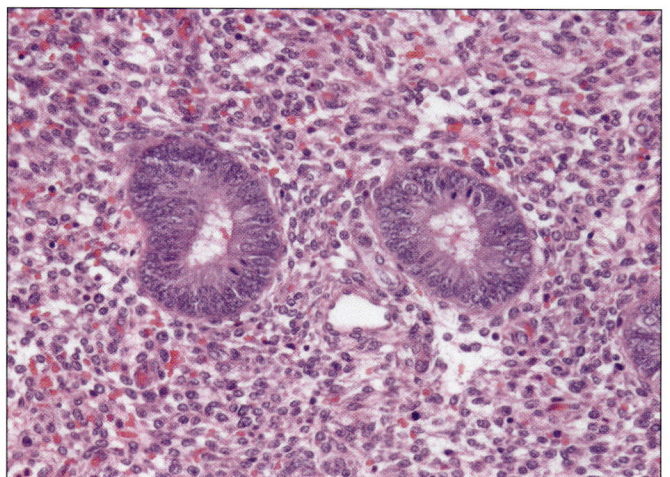

Figure 14.26 Proliferative phase endometrium. Mitotic figures are present in the glandular epithelium and in the stroma. A spiral arteriole is present.

EARLY SECRETORY PHASE, DAYS 16–18: CHANGING VACUOLAR PATTERNS

The appearance of subnuclear vacuolation in interval phase endometrium at day 16 heralds the onset of the early secretory phase. By the third day after ovulation (day 17), the changes are sufficiently developed to be diagnostic of ovulation. Prominent uniformly sized basal vacuoles push the nuclei into alignment (loss of nuclear pseudostratification) in the middle of the cell (Figure 14.28). The combination of clear basal vacuoles and aligned dark nuclei resemble a row of 'piano keys.' The glands become more tortuous during this part of the cycle and the glands become more crowded, with an approximately 1:1 gland–stroma ratio. By day 18, the subnuclear vacuoles are less regular and similar secretory vacuoles are additionally present in the cytoplasm on the luminal side of the nucleus (Figure 14.29). Both 16

INTERVAL ENDOMETRIUM (DAY 16 OF 28)

A short period centered on day 16, caused by rising serum progesterone levels and an incomplete endometrial response, is termed the 'interval phase,' or, simply, '16 day endometrium.' Epithelial mitoses combined with scattered glands containing poorly formed staggered basal secretory vacuoles are seen in this phase (Figure 14.27). It seems odd that secretory vacuoles first appear in a basal position, when it has eventually to be discharged into the lumen. These are not diagnostic of ovulation, as a similar change can be seen scattered in occasional glands at any time of the cycle, and

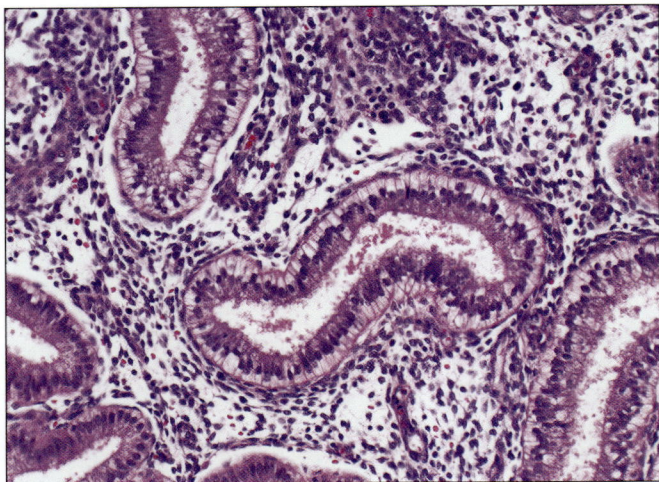

Figure 14.28 Secretory endometrium, day 17. The glands are becoming tortuous and subnuclear vacuolation is prominent.

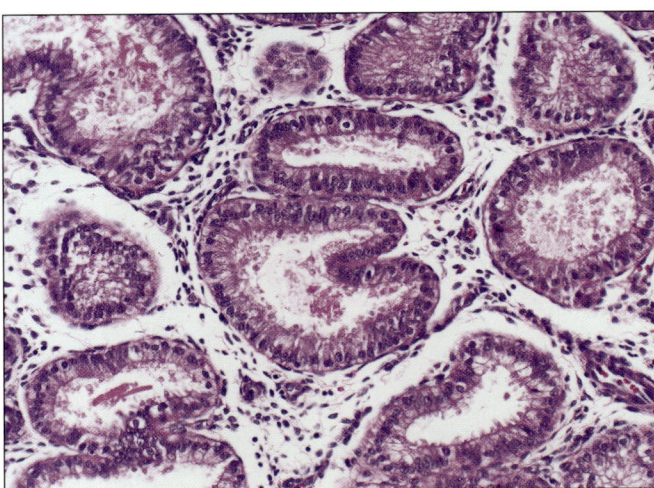

Figure 14.30 Secretory endometrium, days 18–19. The secretory vacuoles are now mostly on the luminal side or almost disappeared, and apical secretion is more prominent. The nucleus has returned to a basal location and mitoses are rare or absent.

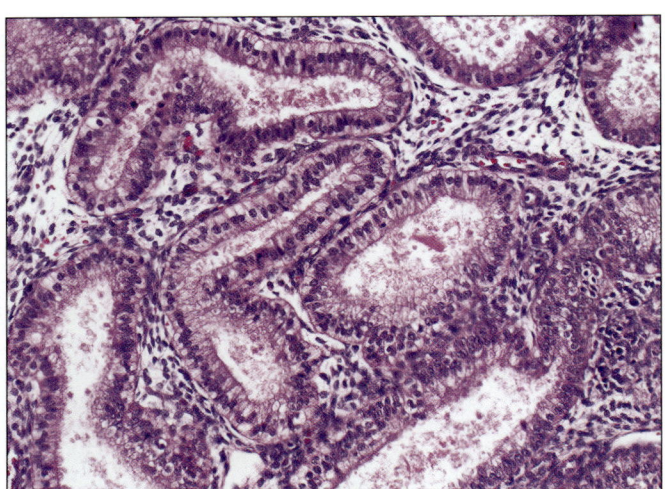

Figure 14.29 Secretory endometrium, day 18. The subnuclear vacuolation is less prominent and less regular. Secretory vacuoles are also seen on the luminal side of the nucleus.

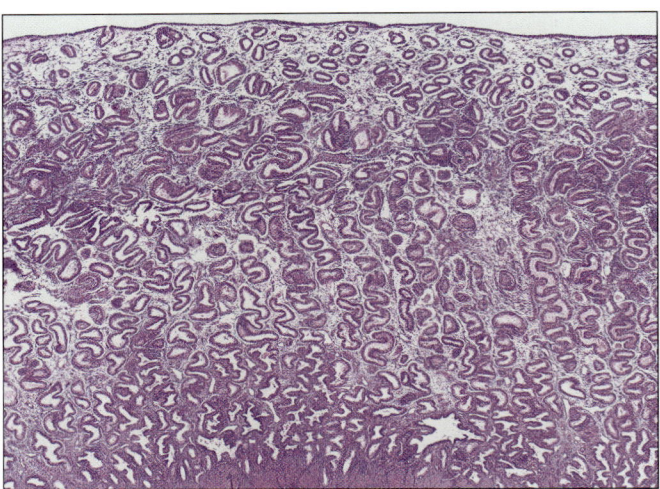

Figure 14.31 Secretory endometrium, day 19, low power. Glands appear 'crowded.'

day endometrium and 18 day endometrium have pseudostratified nuclei and variably sized basal vacuoles, but can readily be distinguished by the paucity of mitoses and presence of supranuclear glycogen at day 18.

MID-SECRETORY PHASE, DAYS 19–21: INCREASING STROMAL EDEMA

The mid-secretory phase lasts from cycle day 19 to cycle day 21, following disappearance of cytoplasmic vacuoles, but before development of stromal predecidual change. The histologic changes within this time reflect changes in the degree of stromal edema and the amount of intraluminal secretory material. By day 19, the glycogen vacuoles are largely absent and the nuclei have returned to the base of the glandular cells. There is evidence of apical decapitation secretion, and mitoses are rare (Figure 14.30). The glands in this time have a coiled tubular morphology that can be easily confused with proliferative endometrium. Stromal edema has not yet separated glands, which appear with an increased gland to stroma ratio (Figure 14.31). Stromal changes, in response to ovulation and rising serum progesterone levels, begin with edema in the functional zone on day 19. Edema is greatest at days 20–21, coinciding with the second estrogen peak in the menstrual cycle and with a peak in eosinophilic luminal secretions (Figures 14.32–14.35). Dating within the 20–22 day window is particularly difficult, both because the histologic appearance of edema may be modified by artifact and because of the paucity of confirmatory discrete glandular benchmarks. From a practical standpoint, it is often difficult to determine whether a given biopsy is at the 'peak' of stromal edema or luminal secretion, and providing a date range is often appropriate for mid-secretory endometrium. At the same time, and partly as a result of these changes,

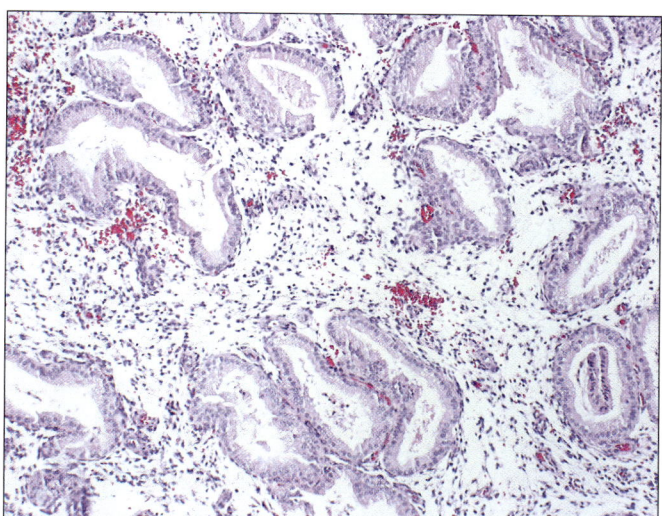

Figure 14.32 Secretory endometrium, day 21. Stromal edema.

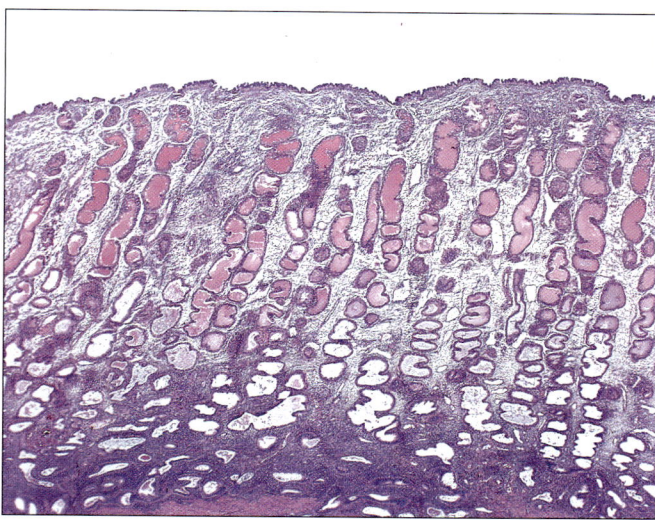

Figure 14.34 Secretory endometrium, days 20–22. Peak of intraluminal secretions.

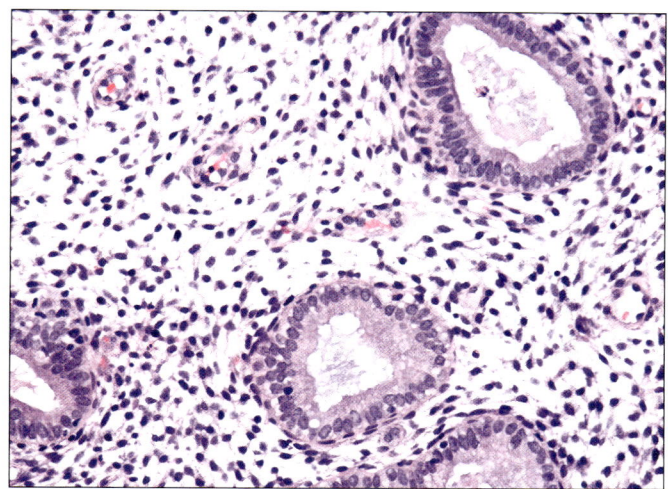

Figure 14.33 Secretory endometrium, day 21. Stromal edema.

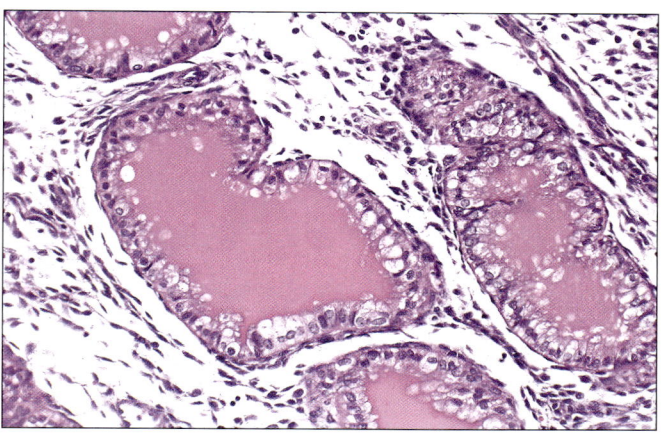

Figure 14.35 Secretory endometrium, days 20–22. Peak of intraluminal secretions. Detail.

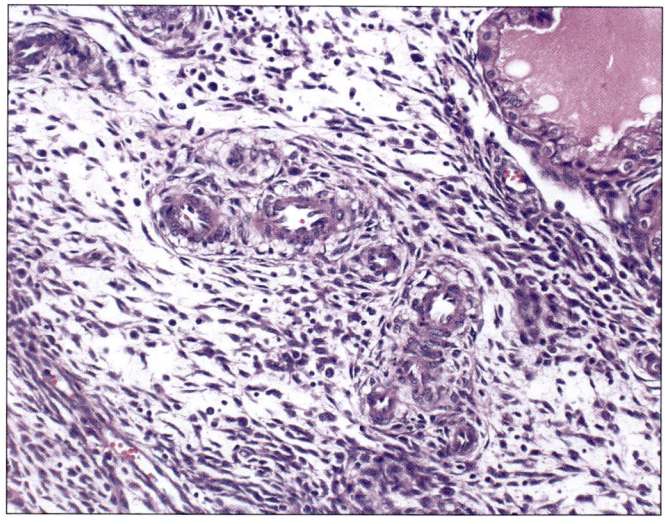

Figure 14.36 Secretory endometrium, day 22. Earliest predecidual cuffing of stromal cells around a spiral arteriole. Stromal cells have poorly defined cytoplasmic boundaries, appearing as 'naked nuclei.'

the endometrial layers become more apparent. The basal layer is now clearly distinguished from the functional endometrium (Figure 14.34).

LATE SECRETORY PHASE, DAYS 22–28: PREDECIDUAL CHANGE

During the late secretory phase (days 22–28) dating is based primarily on the development of stromal predecidual changes. This begins at 22 days when the edema starts to regress, especially in a perivascular distribution that leaves a stromal cell concentration of 'naked' nuclei without discrete cytoplasmic boundaries (Figure 14.36). At day 23, the stromal cells commence decidualization in the immediate vicinity of the spiral arterioles. When decidualization occurs beneath the surface epithelium it is primarily perivascular. Somewhat paradoxically, mitoses are frequently seen in the stromal cells, peaking at day 23. The previously 'naked' spiral arterioles are now cuffed by predecidua (decidualized

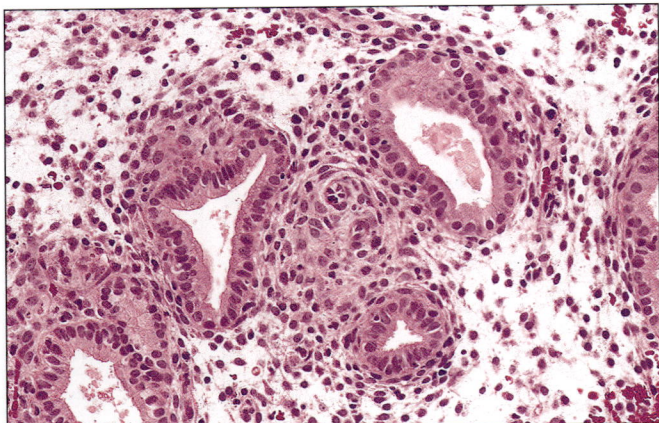

Figure 14.37 Secretory endometrium, day 23. Predecidual cuff around spiral arteriole.

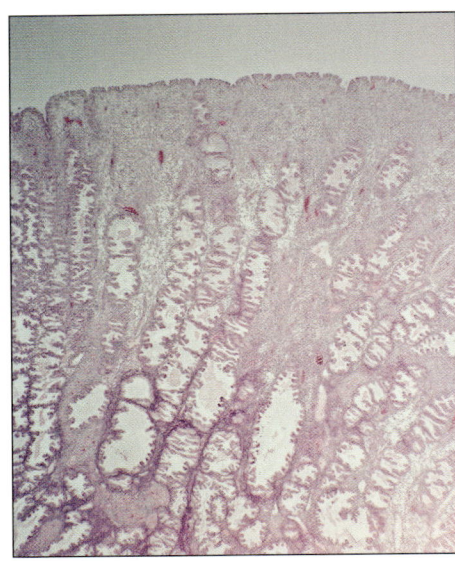

Figure 14.39 Secretory endometrium, day 26. Predecidua is present underneath the uterine lining, in a band-like pattern. Deeper involvement is nonuniform, being concentrated between vascular groups.

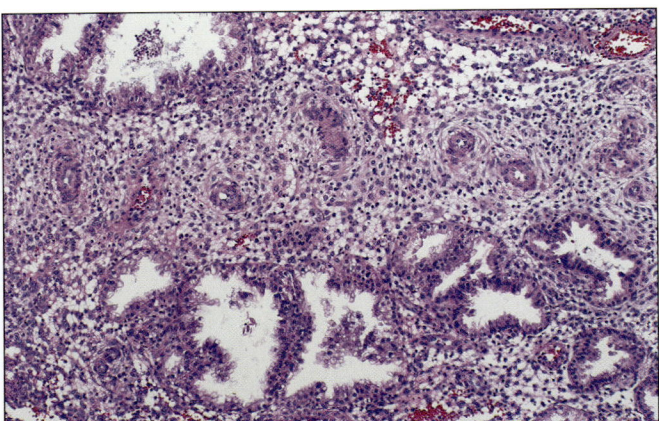

Figure 14.38 Secretory endometrium, day 24. Predecidua bridges vascular groups.

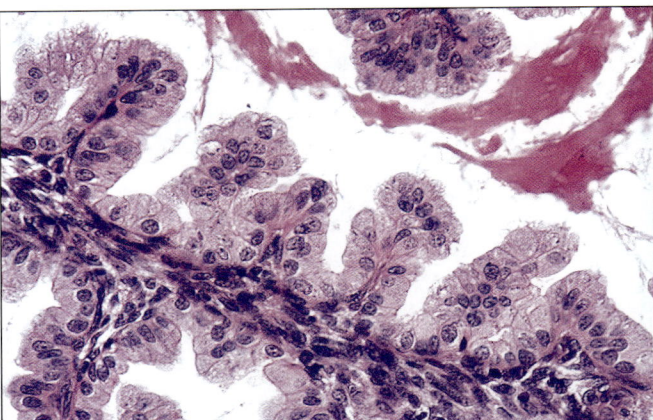

Figure 14.40 Secretory endometrium, days 27–28. Saw-tooth pattern.

stromal cells), but still suspended in the otherwise loose, edematous stroma (Figure 14.37). At 24 days predecidua extends to bridge vascular elements (Figure 14.38). The stromal edema is progressively reabsorbed as predecidua begins to focally form a layer under the surface epithelium at day 25 and extends continuously under the surface by day 26 (Figure 14.39).

Several changes occur in the character of the glands beginning on day 23 and become progressively more developed over the following days. In cross section, the outlines of the glands become larger in diameter and markedly irregular, in striking contrast to the round or oval pattern seen in the proliferative phase. The lining epithelium also changes character and begins to develop slight papillary infoldings. This progresses together with the dilated outline to give the so-called 'saw-tooth pattern' (Figures 14.38 and 14.40). There is no longer the pseudostratified appearance of the nuclei that typifies the late proliferative phase, and mitoses cease to be apparent. At day 26, the stroma just under the endometrial lining epithelium shows a band of continuous predecidual change (Figure 14.39). This diffusely projects more deeply to include all of the stratum compactum by day 27, when numerous granulated lymphocytes are evident (Figures 14.16, 14.17, and 14.41). The

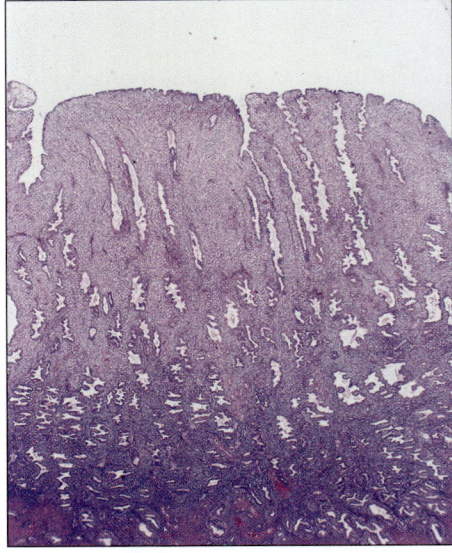

Figure 14.41 Secretory endometrium, day 27. Extensive, confluent predecidual change.

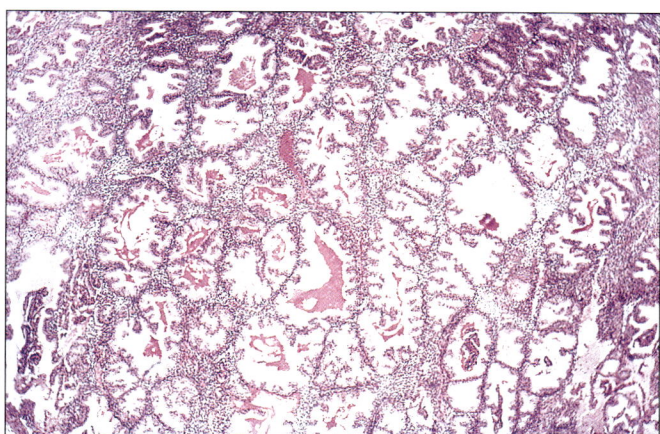

Figure 14.42 Secretory endometrium, days 27–28. Spongy or deep zone.

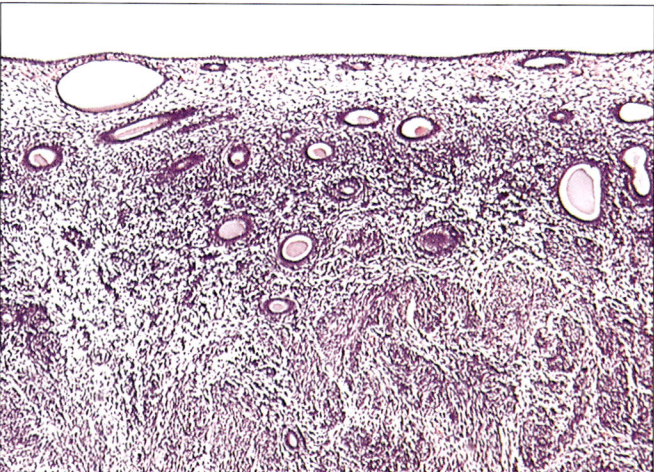

Figure 14.44 Atrophic postmenopausal endometrium.

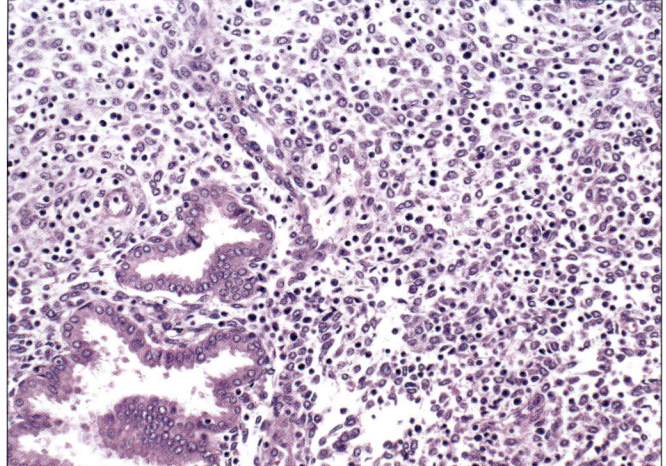

Figure 14.43 Secretory endometrium, day 28. Numerous stromal granulocytes and very early condensation of stromal cells into cords that will soon form aggregates.

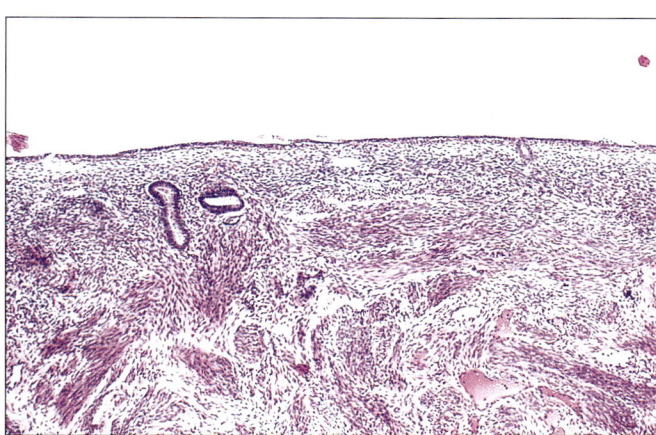

Figure 14.45 Atrophic postmenopausal endometrium, with only rare remaining glands.

stroma in the deeper spongy zone does not undergo predecidual change, and remains undifferentiated. The glands also show differences according to their position relative to the surface. In the central, spongy part of the endometrium the glands have a characteristic saw-tooth appearance (Figure 14.42). The epithelial cells are now full of secretion and are of a moderately tall, columnar type (Figure 14.40). The glands of the stratum compactum, on the other hand, appear to be fewer in number (an illusion, as each gland in the spongy layer must have an opening onto the surface) and are lined by flat to cuboidal cells with some luminal membrane breakdown (the beginning of 'secretory exhaustion') (Figure 14.43).

With the onset of stromal breakdown, the cycle returns to day 1.

ENDOMETRIUM AFTER MENOPAUSE

Once the ovaries cease their cyclical production of estrogen and progesterone, the endometrium is no longer subject to its normal stimulation and undergoes atrophy. The endometrium after the menopause is usually thin and inactive, although varying somewhat in thickness (Figures 14.44 and 14.45), and becoming quite atrophic in the elderly. The glands are typically small and sparse and are often not evenly distributed throughout the tissue. They exhibit an epithelium composed of cuboidal or flattened cells. The stroma becomes fibrous and the stromal cells lose virtually all their cytoplasm with the result that the stroma of the postmenopausal endometrium may appear remarkably cellular (Figure 14.46). Commonly, the endometrium is so thin and meager in amount that biopsy specimens yield only strips of atrophic surface endometrial epithelium (Figure 14.47).

Some common variants of the pattern just described should be mentioned, in particular the so-called 'cystic atrophy' pattern. The endometrium in this state has glands that are distended, often only slightly (Figure 14.48), but sometimes strikingly so (Figure 14.49). The epithelium lining the distended glands is flattened and inactive and the lumens contain material that is partly nonspecific secretion

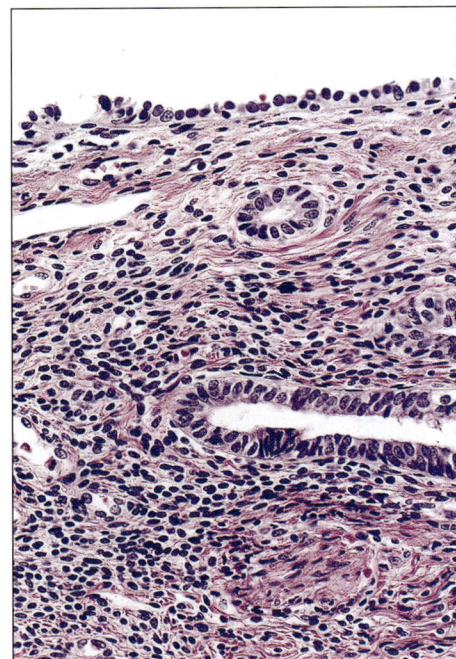

Figure 14.46 Atrophic postmenopausal endometrium. Low cuboidal epithelial and fibrous stroma.

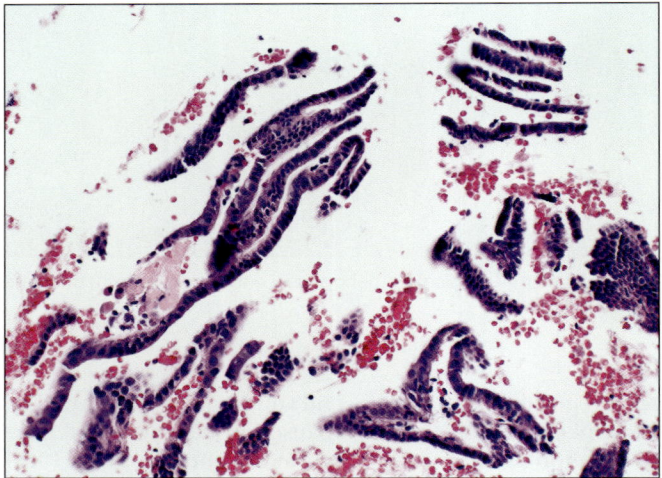

Figure 14.47 Atrophic postmenopausal endometrium, curettings. Strips of atrophic surface epithelium.

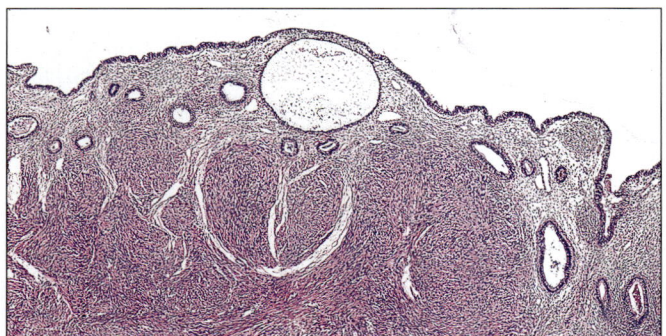

Figure 14.48 Atrophic postmenopausal endometrium, with some cystic dilatation.

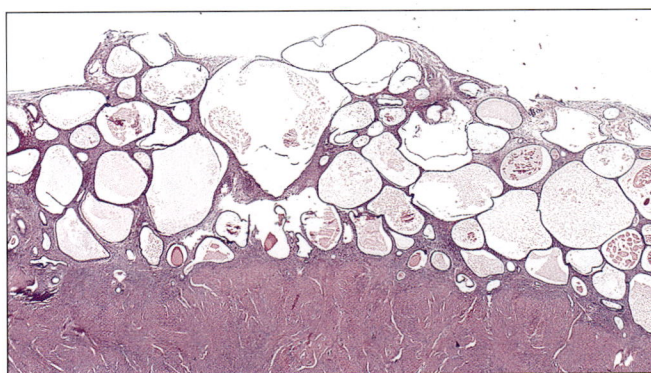

Figure 14.49 Cystic atrophy in a postmenopausal endometrium.

and partly transudate. This change may occasionally be so marked and widespread as to be apparent to the naked eye on opening the uterus (so-called 'Swiss cheese endometrium'). This condition may arise in two ways: (1) as a result of non-atypical hyperplasia present at the time of the menopause regressing as its hormonal support diminishes, with the architectural cystic pattern remaining without the accompanying cellular activity, and (2) as a simple obstruction of the endometrial gland ostia by the stromal fibrosis that occurs after the menopause. It must be remembered that the epithelium of the endometrium not only secretes in response to progesterone but also produces a nonspecific seromucinous secretion at other times: before puberty, after the menopause, and in the first half of the menstrual cycle. Obstruction of the glands will therefore always produce an accumulation of this secretion in the lumens, resulting in distension. It is, of course, paramount to distinguish cystic atrophy from postmenopausal hyperplasia; the atrophic appearance of the epithelium and the lack of mitotic figures in glands and stroma of the former condition distinguish the two. The presence of a proliferative endometrium in a woman past the age of 60 years is abnormal.

METHODS OF ENDOMETRIAL SAMPLING

DILATATION AND CURETTAGE

For decades, the diagnostic curettage has been one of the most common operations performed on women. The procedure is not without its limitations. Hemorrhage, infection, and uterine perforation may occur and, because cervical dilatation is painful, the risks associated with the necessary general anesthetic are also present. Furthermore, although a carefully performed curettage should involve sampling most of the endometrium, this ideal is rarely achieved. Consequently, as many as 5% of hyperplasias or carcinomas remain undetected in curettage immediately preceding hysterectomy.[15,16] Most specimens, however, are adequate for a reliable histologic assessment.

VABRA ASPIRATOR

This is a suction curette device composed of a 3–4 mm diameter steel cannula that has an opening on one side of its bent tip. The endometrial tissue is obtained by suction with an attached syringe. The amount of material this procedure captures varies from specimens that are as abundant as a curettage, usually in women of reproductive age, to blood and minute fragments, often in a postmenopausal woman, which may not be adequate for histologic assessment.

PIPELLE BIOPSY

This is probably the most widely used outpatient method used today in the United States and Europe to sample the endometrial cavity. The device is a flexible plastic tube, 3.1 mm in outer diameter, with a solid tip and a side port. A vacuum is created by the withdrawal of a piston from the cannula and, as the device is gently rotated and moved from side to side as it is withdrawn from the uterus, endometrial tissue is sucked into the 2.6 mm internal diameter cannula by the slight negative pressure. This procedure is quick and while causing significantly less pain than the Novak curette or Vabra aspirator, it is nonetheless uncomfortable, especially if the cervix must be dilated. Although it produces less tissue, the diagnostic accuracy of the Pipelle biopsy is similar to that of the Vabra aspirator.[17] It is no less reliable than other techniques for identifying endometrial carcinoma,[18,19] although some studies have suggested a poor pick-up rate for early, low-volume tumors.[20]

CYTOLOGIC EVALUATION OF THE ENDOMETRIUM

Cervical smears, while generally inadequate and unreliable for the recognition of endometrial adenocarcinoma, let alone subtly assessing endometrial status, may on occasion disclose the presence of malignant endometrial cells.[21,22] The presence of normal endometrial cells up to days 10–12 of the menstrual cycle is within normal limits and cytologists rarely report them. It is good cytologic practice to report morphologically normal endometrial cells seen beyond days 10–12 or in postmenopausal women. Identifying endometrial intraepithelial neoplasia (EIN) and differentiating it from proliferative and secretory endometrial cells are unrealistic possibilities using conventional cervical smears. It should also be noted that endometrial epithelium in cervical smears can easily be misinterpreted as endocervical adenocarcinoma *in situ*.[23]

DIRECT ENDOMETRIAL CYTOLOGIC SAMPLING

Direct endometrial cytology presents special sampling and interpretive challenges, along with risks attendant to transcervical placement of a surgical device. Although it has not become a practice standard in the United States, there is significant literature supporting its use in Japan and Europe.[24,25] The Tao brush, a low-morbidity device optimized for endometrial cytology, is capable of collecting aggregates of epithelial and stromal cells, a sort of 'microbiopsy.' It can be an effective technique for the discovery and diagnosis of malignant states[24,26] (Figure 14.50).

HYSTEROSCOPY

In recent years, hysteroscopy has become a valuable additional method for assessing the uterine cavity. Hysteroscopy,

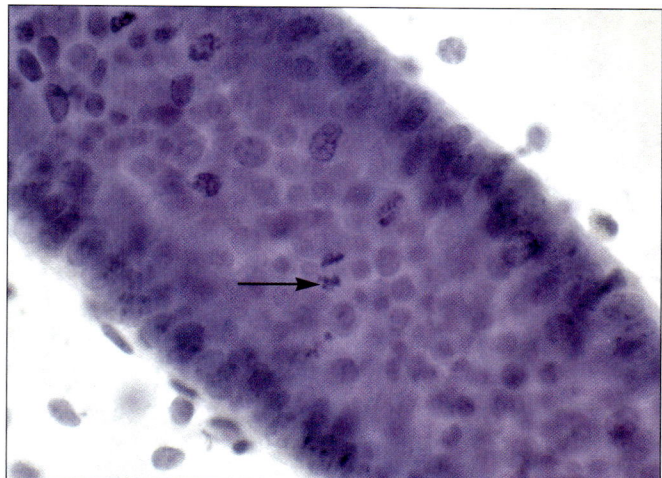

Figure 14.50 Endometrial 'microbiopsy' by direct cytologic sampling with the smear with mitosis (arrow) in proliferative endometrium. Tao Brush technique. Normal proliferative gland with mitoses.

accompanied where necessary by biopsy, curettage, or Pipelle aspiration, is rapidly replacing the curettage in the investigation of menstrual disorders, with significant cost benefits.[27,28] The hysteroscope is a rigid or flexible optical instrument of sufficiently narrow diameter that it can be passed into the uterine cavity through the endocervical canal. During hysteroscopic examination, the instrument is introduced through the cervix, with either electrolyte (saline) or nonconductive solutions (commonly sugars or carbohydrates) used as distension media depending on the clinical need. Exposure to some of these solutions, especially when hypertonic or hypotonic, can create significant histologic artifact if the tissue is not rapidly fixed.

ENDOMETRIAL RESECTION AND ABLATION

The advent of hysteroscopy as a reliable method of accessing the uterine cavity has led the way to conservative methods of treating abnormal uterine bleeding. If certain qualifying criteria are met, including biopsy-proven absence of hyperplasia or malignancy, the patient may be treated by endometrial resection or ablation rather than hysterectomy.[29–32]

Although most centers treating patients by endometrial ablation employ hysteroscopy, this is not an absolute prerequisite. The technique aims to destroy the entire endometrium, including the basal layer, thereby preventing regrowth by inducing a therapeutic Asherman's syndrome, where synechiae form and the anterior and posterior walls become adherent. Many different modalities have been used, including hot or cold fluids, electrocautery rollers, and microwaves. All are effective if properly applied.

Endometrial resection uses the cutting loop of a resecting hysteroscope to excise the endometrial lining. The depth of cut with a resection loop is 3–4 mm. Because the endometrial thickness varies from 3 to 12 mm during the menstrual cycle, the endometrium may first be suppressed with either danazol or gonadotropin-releasing hormone analogs, This hormonal manipulation must be taken into account by the histopathologist interpreting the resected material.

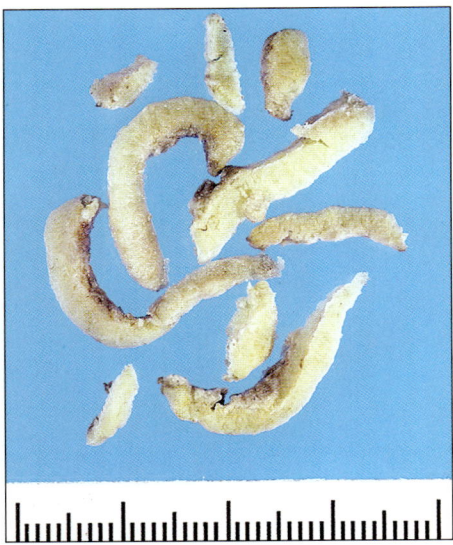

Figure 14.51 Endometrial resection specimen, removed using a hot loop at hysteroscopy.

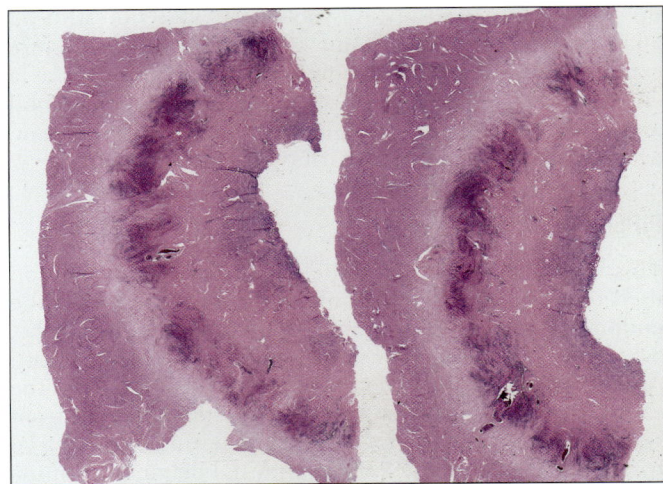

Figure 14.52 Uterus, whole-mount sections 1 month after thermal ablation. Inner half of myometrium is completely necrotic.

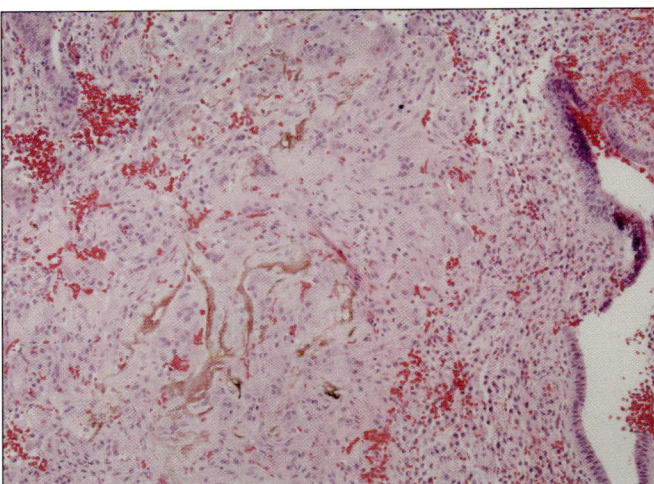

Figure 14.53 Myometrium, several months after ablation. Denatured proteins have caused granulomatous inflammation, and surface epithelium is regrowing.

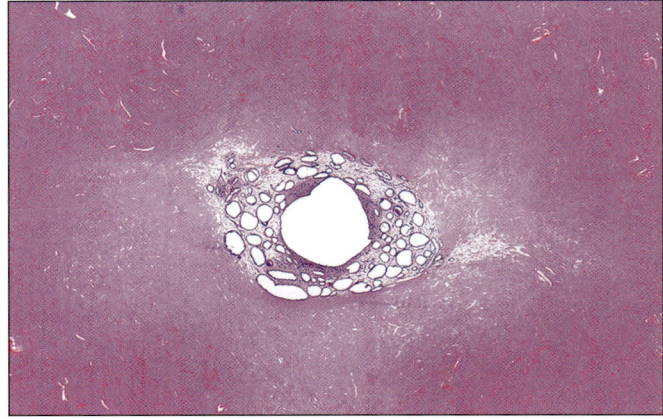

Figure 14.54 Failed endometrial ablation. A narrow uterine cavity is present with somewhat disorganized residual endometrium present in the myometrium. Deep to this is a zone of fibrosis in the central myometrium.

Endometrial resection produces a specimen that looks rather like bulky endometrial curettings but, as it consists largely of myometrium, the tissue is firmer than curettings in the fixed state (Figure 14.51). Microscopic examination confirms that the tissue is composed predominantly of myometrium, most pieces being covered by thin, inactive endometrium if the patient has been hormonally prepared (e.g., with danazol). Endocervical tissue is often present. Diathermy artifact frequently hinders histologic interpretation, particularly at the edges of the fragments. It is important to look for hyperplasia and carcinoma, although these should both have been excluded before the procedure was undertaken.[29] The presence of adenomyosis correlates with a poor outcome following endometrial ablation[33] due to the superficial adenomyotic islands regenerating into pockets of functioning endometrium. Whether this diagnosis can be made with any confidence in the resected material is debatable, because of random orientation of the pieces of tissue and the normal irregularity of the endometrial–myometrial junction. Despite these mitigating factors, a histologic suspicion of adenomyosis in the endomyometrial strips should be communicated to the surgeon in the ultimate interests of managing patient expectations.

Several reports describe large series of patients who have undergone endometrial ablation or resection.[30] Over 80% of patients have been satisfied with the procedure.[34] In unsatisfactory cases, a repeat procedure can sometimes be performed without resorting to hysterectomy. Women in whom the procedure fails to cure the symptoms may then be treated by hysterectomy. If performed within weeks of ablation, often there is a foreign-body giant cell reaction and carbonaceous debris affecting the lining of the cavity (Figures 14.52–14.53). This debris is cleared over the course of ensuing months, when gross examination of the uterus usually shows a narrow cavity often with patches of endometrium visible. Microscopy may show residual endometrium, often poorly organized, and a zone of fibrosis in the underlying myometrium (Figure 14.54). In some patients, a functionally normal endometrial cavity eventually regenerates, and numerous successful pregnancies have been reported after ablation.[35]

PROBLEMS IN INTERPRETATION OF ENDOMETRIAL SPECIMENS

The endometrium is a composite tissue. Glands, stroma, blood vessels, and lymphocytes all contribute to the physiologic and nonphysiologic changes that together enable a histologic diagnosis to be made. If any of these components is lacking or if the relations among them are disrupted, the validity of a histologic diagnosis is compromised. To definitively identify the phase of the menstrual cycle requires intact endometrial functionalis capable of being oriented. Problems therefore arise in interpreting the endometrial tissue if the specimen is scanty, fragmented, or distorted during its collection.

ADEQUACY

A scanty specimen may be a problem with any method of collection. If the endometrium is abundant, as it is during the late proliferative and secretory phase of a normal cycle as well as in many cases where there is hyperplasia or carcinoma, an adequate, diagnostic sample is likely to be obtained, irrespective of the method of sampling.

If little endometrial tissue is present in the uterus, as in postmenopausal atrophy, a very scanty specimen usually results irrespective of the method of collection. The scanty specimen may consist of mucus and blood with tiny broken strips of surface and glandular epithelium, sometimes with a little stroma attached, but often with no stroma at all (Figures 14.47 and 14.55), and frequently cervical tissue removed *en passant*.

In these circumstances, it is tempting simply to dismiss the specimen as inadequate and unsuitable for diagnosis. A diagnosis of endometrial epithelium or tissue, however scant, confirms that the device reached the uterine cavity.

The epithelium may be classified as inactive if it is cuboidal or columnar without evidence of mitotic figures or secretory vacuoles, or proliferative if even only one mitotic figure is seen. If secretory vacuoles are present, either subnuclear or supranuclear, the epithelium may be designated as secretory in type. For specimens taken in the course of monitoring women on hormone replacement therapy, for example, comments such as these can be helpful. It is important to avoid the statement that the specimen is 'inadequate for histologic assessment,' since the expected result in an atrophic endometrium is a scant specimen. The statement of inadequacy may force the gynecologist in this instance to unnecessarily repeat the procedure. In postmenopausal women, 'inadequate' should be reserved for those specimens where there is literally no endometrial tissue at all, and a statement that no endometrial tissue was seen should be included. We find it useful in these cases simply to report the tissue components that are present and note that the material is scant, allowing the individual gynecologist to decide what other diagnostic work-up, if any, is indicated.

DISSOCIATION ARTIFACT

If the stroma between endometrial glands is disrupted or lost, then the relations of the glands to each other become disturbed. This usually means that the glands lie closer together than normal (Figure 14.56) but sometimes they are widely separated by mucus or clear space. This false crowding may be sufficiently marked to give a back-to-back appearance and an erroneous impression of hyperplasia or even carcinoma. A commonly encountered situation in which this phenomenon occurs is in menstrual endometrium, when due allowance can usually be made because the phase of the cycle is obvious (Figure 14.57). Dissociation artifact is more of a problem when traumatic sampling damages the stroma at other times in the cycle. The changes are usually focal, so that at least some of the endometrium appears normal but groups of glands are crowded, without intervening stroma. Careful examination will show that the stroma

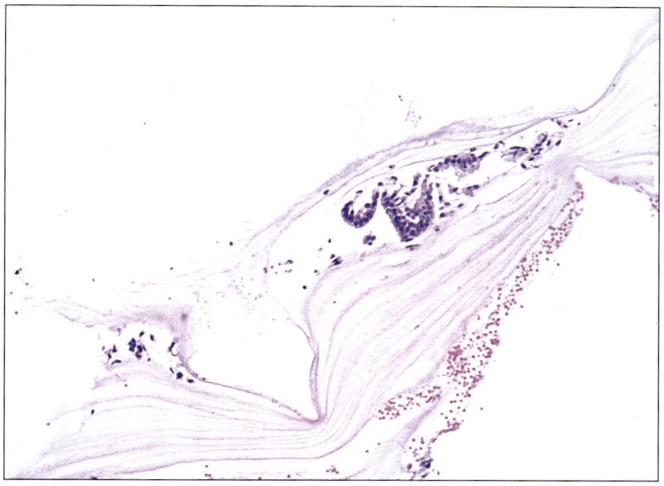

Figure 14.55 Pipelle aspiration specimen. A single strip of epithelium is present amongst the cervical mucus.

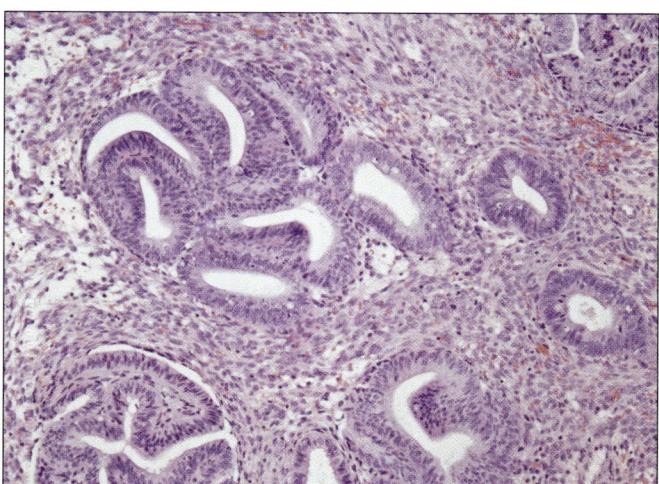

Figure 14.56 Endometrial curettings. The glands are artifactually crowded because of traumatic fragmentation of the stroma. These appearances must not be mistaken for hyperplasia or EIN.

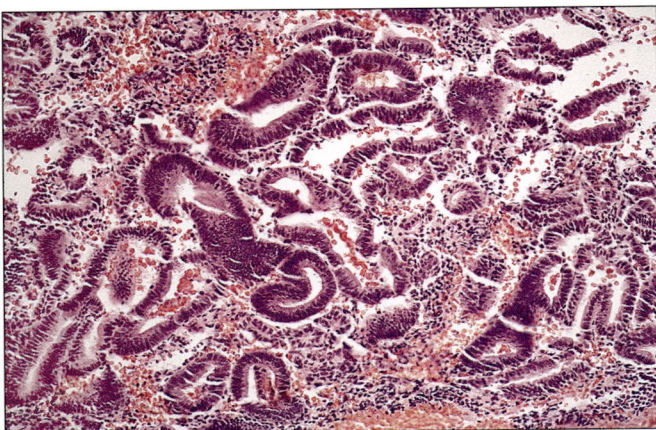

Figure 14.57 Endometrial curettings. The glands are artifactually crowded because of menstrual breakdown of the stroma.

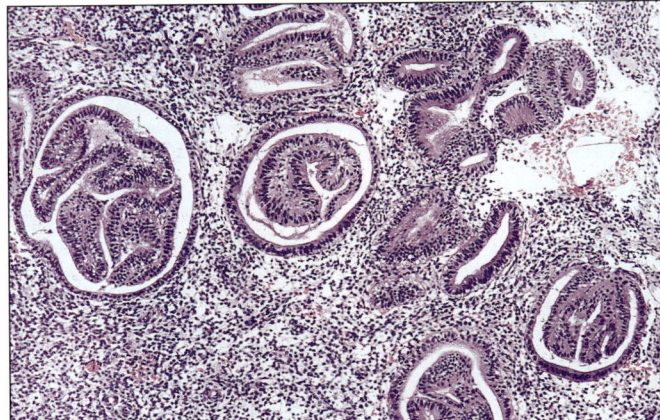

Figure 14.59 Endometrial curettings. Telescoping artifact. This apparently complicated pattern is most probably the result of glandular epithelium intussuscepting as the curettage is performed. The presence of a complete epithelial circle surrounding the unit allows hyperplasia to be excluded.

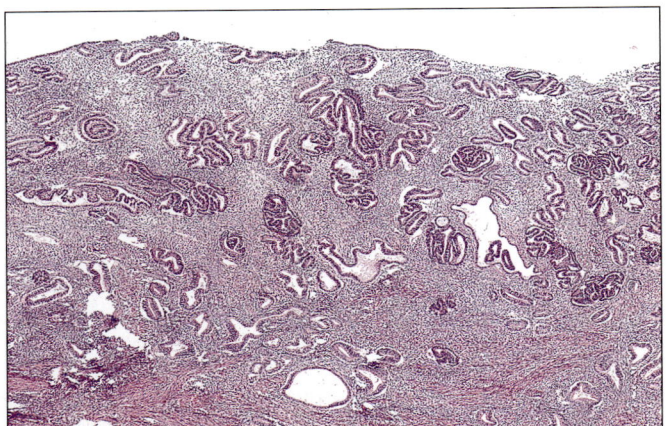

Figure 14.58 Endometrial curettings. Telescoping artifact. Low power.

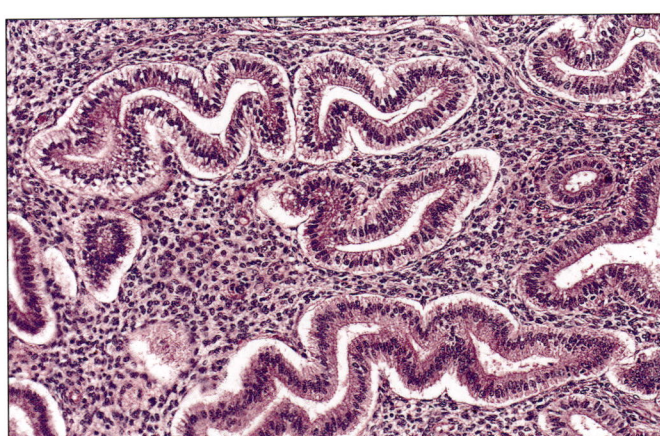

Figure 14.60 Endometrium. Fixation artifact.

between and around these glands has been disrupted, so that the abnormal architectural pattern can be disregarded. Additionally, there is rarely if ever any significant complexity to the crowded glandular structures (multiple lumens, irregular outlines, etc.) that are common in neoplasia and their precursors. Sometimes, however, even careful examination may fail to resolve the dilemma.

TELESCOPING ARTIFACT

This is another effect of trauma on the endometrium brought about at the time of sampling, whereby the glands undergo intussusception, producing a gland-within-gland appearance. The result is what appears, at first sight, to be a complex glandular pattern at low magnification (Figure 14.58). An erroneous diagnosis of hyperplasia or even carcinoma may be made. Closer examination shows that each of these apparently complex glandular structures is completely surrounded by a circle of epithelium representing the original gland outline (Figure 14.59).

FIXATION ARTIFACT

If fixation of the endometrial specimen is poor or delayed, the stroma may retract from the glands, leaving an artifactual clear space around the glands. At low magnification, this may give a false impression of subnuclear vacuolation and so compromise accurate dating of the sample (Figure 14.60). Careful examination under the high power allows this artifact to be recognized. Endometrium autolyzes rapidly and timely exposure to fixative is important in hysterectomy specimens to avoid a major 'laboratory' error from which no recovery is possible. Many pathology services recommend the surgeon open the uterus before placing it in adequate fixative.

LEGITIMATE TISSUE CONTAMINANTS

Nonendometrial components are frequently and legitimately found in curettings. Endocervical tissue is common; it is nearly always easy to identify and should not cause any problems. Cervical microglandular hyperplasia, however, is not always easily recognizable and care must be taken not to mistake it for endometrial pathology because of its superficial resemblance to hyperplasia or carcinoma. Endocervical stroma containing plasma cells can, if not correctly identified, mislead the pathologist to diagnose endometritis, particularly if the clinical notes indicate 'removal of intrauterine contraceptive device' or some such. Stratified squamous epithelium from the ectocervix or vagina is also seen quite often. Occasionally, but of great import, the diagnosis of cervical squamous intraepithelial lesion is first made as a result of cervical contamination of endometrial curettings.

Fragments of smooth muscle may represent normal myometrium or a submucous leiomyoma, a distinction that it is not always possible to make from the pattern of the muscle bundles. The presence of adipose tissue in endometrial curettings means that the uterus has likely been perforated, although a rare uterine tumor such as lipoleiomyoma can contain fat. This information should immediately be communicated to the clinician (although, in our experiences, clinicians often already know that perforation has happened or report that the patient is not having any detectable adverse effects). Fetal tissues (bone, cartilage, neural tissue) may be found unexpectedly, without clinical reference to a recent miscarriage.

REFERENCES

1. Nicolae A, Preda O, Nogales FF. Endometrial metaplasias and reactive changes: a spectrum of altered differentiation. J Clin Pathol 2011;64:97–106.
2. Tilburgs T, Claas FH, Scherjon SA. Elsevier Trophoblast Research Award Lecture: unique properties of decidual T cells and their role in immune regulation during human pregnancy. Placenta 2010;31(Suppl):S82–6.
3. Manaster I, Mandelboim O. The unique properties of uterine NK cells. Am J Reprod Immunol 2010;63:434–44.
4. Toth B, Wurfel W, Germeyer A, et al. Disorders of implantation—are there diagnostic and therapeutic options? J Reprod Immunol 2011;90:117–23.
5. Achilles SL, Amortegui AJ, Wiesenfeld HC. Endometrial plasma cells: do they indicate subclinical pelvic inflammatory disease? Sex Transm Dis 2005;32:185–8.
6. Volchek M, Girling JE, Lash GE, et al. Lymphatics in the human endometrium disappear during decidualization. Hum Reprod 2010;25:2455–64.
7. Heller DS. The normal endometrium. New York: Igaku-Shoin Medical; 1994.
8. Mazur MT, Kurman RJ. Normal endometrium and infertility evaluation. New York: Springer-Verlag; 1995.
9. Zaino RJ. The logical patterns of the normal endometrial cycle. Interpretation of endometrial biopsies and curettings. Philadelphia: Lippincott-Raven; 1996. p. 53–99.
10. Dallenbach-Hellweg G, Schmidt D, Dallenbach F. Atlas of endometrial histopathology. 3rd ed. Berlin, Germany: Springer-Verlag; 2010.
11. Nucci M, Oliva E. Gynecologic pathology: a volume in foundations in diagnostic pathology series. Philadelphia: Churchill Livingstone; 2009.
12. Lockwood CJ. Mechanisms of normal and abnormal endometrial bleeding. Menopause 2011;18:408–11.
13. Henriet P, Gaide Chevronnay HP, Marbaix E. The endocrine and paracrine control of menstruation. Mol Cell Endocrinol; 2012; 385(2):197–207.
14. Jabbour HN, Sales KJ. Prostaglandin receptor signalling and function in human endometrial pathology. Trends Endocrinol Metab 2004;15:398–404.
15. Vorgias G, Lekka J, Katsoulis M, et al. Diagnostic accuracy of prehysterectomy curettage in determining tumor type and grade in patients with endometrial cancer. MedScape General Med 2003;5:7.
16. Bradley LD. Diagnosis of abnormal uterine bleeding with biopsy or hysteroscopy. Menopause 2011;18:425–33.
17. Manganiello PD, Burrows LJ, Dain BJ, Gonzalez J. Vabra aspirator and pipelle endometrial suction curette—a comparison. J Reprod Med 1998;43:889–92.
18. Guido RS, Kanbourshakir A, Rulin MC, Christopherson WA. Pipelle endometrial sampling: sensitivity in the detection of endometrial cancer. J Reprod Med 1995;40:553–5.
19. Ong S, Duffy T, Lenehan P, Murphy J. Endometrial pipelle biopsy compared to conventional dilatation and curettage. Irish J Med Sci 1997;166:47–9.
20. Tanriverdi HA, Barut A, Gun BD, Kaya E. Is pipelle biopsy really adequate for diagnosing endometrial disease? Med Sci Monit 2004;10:CR271–4.
21. DuBeshter B. Endometrial cancer: predictive value of cervical cytology. Gynecol Oncol 1999;72:271–2.
22. Mitchell H, Giles G, Medley G. Accuracy and survival benefit of cytological prediction of endometrial carcinoma on routine cervical smears. Int J Gynecol Pathol 1993;12:34–40.
23. Risse EK, Ouwerkerk-Noordam E, Boon ME. Endometrial cells in liquid-based cervical cytology: a diagnostic pitfall solved by preparing cytohistology from the residual thin layer sample. Acta Cytol 2011;55:327–33.
24. Mossa B, Ebano V, Marziani R. Reliability of oupatient endometrial brush cytology vs biopsy in postmenopausal symptomatic women. Eur J Gynaecol Oncol 2010;31:621–6.
25. Norimatsu Y, Kouda H, Kobayashi TK, et al. Utility of liquid-based cytology in endometrial pathology: diagnosis of endometrial carcinoma. Cytopathology 2009;20:395–402.
26. Maksem JA, Meiers I, Robboy SJ. A primer of endometrial cytology with histological correlation. Diagn Cytopathol 2007;35:817–44.
27. Goldstein SR. Modern evaluation of the endometrium. Obstet Gynecol 2010;116:168–76.
28. Marsh F, Duffy S. The technique and overview of flexible hysteroscopy. Obstet Gynecol Clin North Am 2004;31:655–68, xi.
29. Lewis BV. Guidelines for endometrial ablation. Br J Obstet Gynaecol 1994;101:470–3.
30. Lethaby A, Hickey M, Garry R, Penninx J. Endometrial resection/ablation techniques for heavy menstrual bleeding. Cochrane Database Syst Rev 2009:CD001501.
31. Zarek S, Sharp HT. Global endometrial ablation devices. Clin Obstet Gynecol 2008;51:167–75.
32. Practice Committee of American Society for Reproductive Medicine. Indications and options for endometrial ablation. Fertil Steril 2008;90:S236–40.
33. McCausland V, McCausland A. The response of adenomyosis to endometrial ablation/resection. Hum Reprod Update 1998;4:350–9.
34. Munro MG. Endometrial ablation for heavy menstrual bleeding. Curr Opin Obstet Gynecol 2005;17:381–94.
35. Yin CS. Pregnancy after hysteroscopic endometrial ablation without endometrial preparation: a report of five cases and a literature review. Taiwan J Obstet Gynecol 2010;49:311–9.

15 Exogenous Hormones and their Effects on the Endometrium

Rex C. Bentley

CHAPTER OUTLINE

Introduction	310
Estrogens	310
Progestins	312
Oral Contraceptives	313
Combined OCs	314
Pure Progestin OCs ('Mini-pill')	315
Long-term, Progestin-only OCs	315
Hormone Replacement Therapy	315
Unopposed Estrogen HRT	316
Cyclic Estrogen–progesterone HRT	316
Combined Estrogen–progesterone HRT	317
Other Hormonal Agents	318
Tamoxifen	318
Other Selective Estrogen Receptor Modulators	319
Aromatase Inhibitors	319
Phytoestrogens and other Dietary Agents	319
Clomiphene/Ovulation Induction Therapy	320
Progesterone Receptor Modulators	320
GnRH Agonists and Antagonists	321
Gonadotropins	321
Corticosteroids	321
Danazol	321
Treatment of Endometrial Lesions with Progestins	321
Progestin Therapy of Persistent Estrogen States (Hyperplasia)	322
Progestin Therapy of Neoplastic Lesions: EIN and Carcinoma	322

INTRODUCTION

Exogenous hormonal agents represent one of the most commonly prescribed medications in women. Hormonal therapies are used for a wide range of indications, including birth control, postmenopausal hormone replacement, dysfunctional uterine bleeding, endometriosis, infertility, and the treatment of malignant and premalignant lesions of the endometrium and breast. These drugs can be administered by many methods, including oral, parenteral, transdermal, transvaginal, and subcutaneous, vaginal, or intrauterine implants. Consequently, a significant proportion of endometrial specimens that the surgical pathologist evaluates show the effects of these exogenous hormonal agents. At first glance, the spectrum of changes seen with hormone therapy appears excessively broad, and it is certainly true that nearly any endometrial appearance can be attributed to therapy with hormones. With a basic understanding of the effects of estrogens and progestins on the normal endometrium, however, substantial order emerges from this confusing pathologic array. Essentially, it is possible to predict the common appearances of hormone therapy based on the known effects of the endogenous steroid hormones on normal endometrium.

ESTROGENS

The basic effect of estrogens on the endometrium is to induce proliferation of the endometrial glands and stroma, including vascular endothelium. The degree of proliferation can vary in proportion to the estrogenic stimulus. Very low levels of estrogen or a very weak estrogen will lead to an inactive or atrophic endometrium. Higher levels lead to proliferation, which when excessive can produce a hyperplastic endometrium (Figure 15.1). The degree of proliferative activity can usually be assessed by the mitotic activity in both the glandular epithelium and the stroma. Women who are many years postmenopausal demonstrate profound endometrial atrophy, secondary to lack of estrogen, but even atrophic endometrium remains estrogen responsive to quite advanced age (Figure 15.2). A number of estrogenic drugs on the market are listed in Table 15.1.[1]

Persistent exposure to a significant estrogenic stimulus, such as occurs in anovulation, leads to a pattern of continued, unrelieved proliferation. The endometrium cannot support such continued growth. Whether the estrogen source is endogenous or exogenous, the histologic consequence is the same: a combination of proliferative endometrium with episodic coexisting stromal breakdown,

CHAPTER 15 — EXOGENOUS HORMONES AND THEIR EFFECTS ON THE ENDOMETRIUM

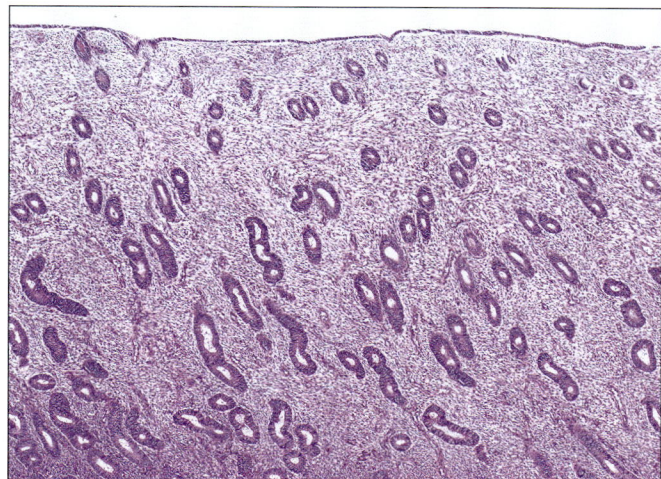

Figure 15.1 Normal proliferative endometrium (normal estrogen effect).

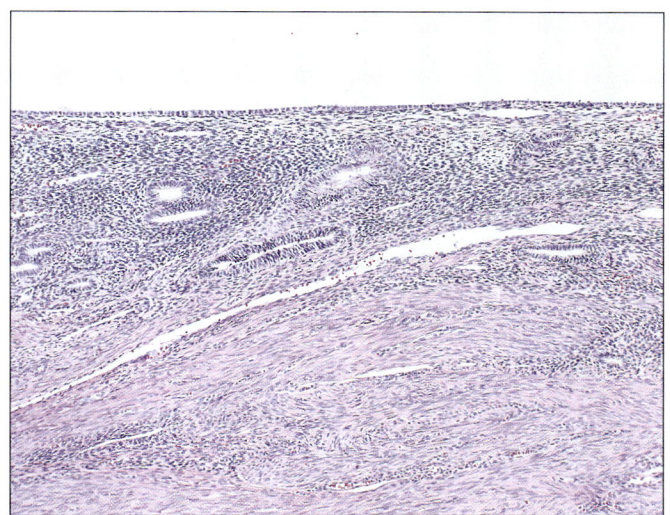

Figure 15.2 Atrophic endometrium. The few glands present have minimal cytoplasm and small nuclei. The endometrial stroma is dense.

Table 15.1 Representative Estrogenic Agents Available in the United States

Generic Name	U.S. Brand Name
Estradiol	Estrace
Estradiol valerate	Delestrogen, Gynogen, Valergen
Estradiol (transdermal)	Estraderm, Climara, Fempatch
Diethylstilbestrol	
Conjugated equine estrogens	Premarin
Synthetic conjugated estrogens	Cenestin, Enjuvia
Mestranol	
Ethinyl estradiol	Estinyl
Estropipate	Ogen, Ortho-Est

Adapted from Schimmer and Parker (2012).[1]

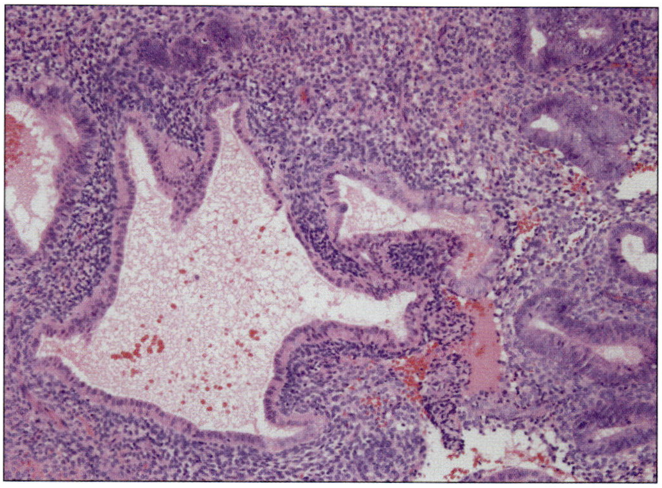

Figure 15.3 'Persistent' proliferative endometrium with unopposed estrogen effect and secondary breakdown. Present is proliferative endometrium with scattered cysts and stromal breakdown forming stromal balls and collapsed eosinophilic epithelium. Often associated with fibrin thrombi, this pattern differs from a physiologic late menstrual–early proliferative endometrium in nonuniform distribution of breakdown throughout a thickened, dense, nonspindly stroma.

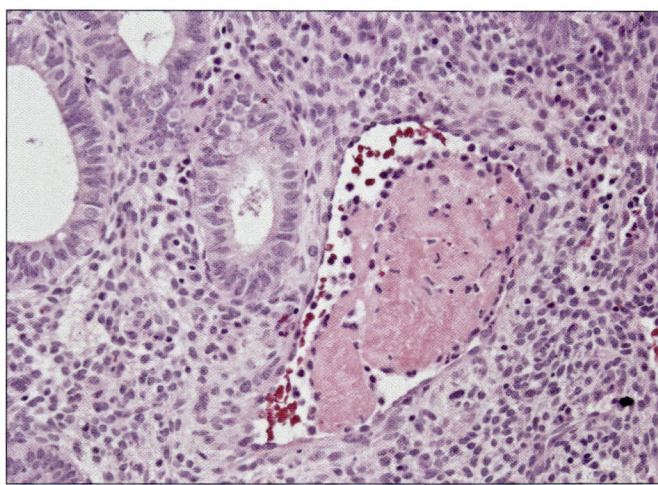

Figure 15.4 Fibrin thrombi in endometrium with anovulatory bleeding.

or shedding, which accounts for the clinical presentation of irregular bleeding (Figure 15.3). This pattern is also called 'anovulatory bleeding' or 'anovulatory shedding.' Because the endometrial vessels become abnormally large, bleeding can also be quite severe. Some pathologists mistakenly refer to the shedding endometrium as 'menstrual,' but it is important to distinguish this appearance from the appearance of menstrual endometrium occurring at the end of a normal cycle. In normal endometrium, the endometrial glands transform soon after ovulation to a secretory pattern and by the time menstrual bleeding begins will still show some residual changes, most commonly secretory exhaustion (see Chapter 14). This change is absent in anovulatory-type bleeding or where the drug administered is progestin poor. Another common difference is the presence of large fibrin thrombi in the vessels of anovulatory shedding endometrium (Figure 15.4). They are absent from menstrual endometrium because of the marked fibrinolytic activity typical of normal menstruation.

With prolonged estrogen exposure, the proliferating glands tend to lose their uniformity of size, shape, and distribution, leading to so-called disordered proliferative endometrium. Cystic dilatation of glands and 'tubal' metaplasia are commonly present. With continued, longer term, unopposed estrogen exposure, a high proportion of patients will ultimately develop non-atypical endometrial hyperplasia. A small number will also go on to develop endometrial intraepithelial neoplasia (EIN) (also called 'atypical hyperplasia') or even adenocarcinoma (see Chapters 17 and 18).

PROGESTINS

The effect of progestins on the endometrium depends on 'priming' by estrogen, which induces progesterone receptors in the endometrial cells. One important feature of progestins is that they act to downregulate estrogen and progesterone receptors; in other words, they reduce the sensitivity of the endometrium to both of these hormones. Prolonged exposure to progestins can thus lead to a histologic picture that is paradoxically similar to the atrophy seen in a postmenopausal or hormone-suppressed patient. Some commonly used progestins are shown in Table 15.2.[1]

In the short term, however, progestins induce secretory differentiation in endometrial glands and decidual-type change in the stroma, i.e., the classic changes of a normal secretory endometrium. The glands develop large glycogen vacuoles that are then secreted into the increasingly complex gland lumina (Figures 15.5 and 15.6). At the same time, the stromal cells enlarge strikingly, acquire an abundant cytoplasm, and appear relatively cohesive (Figure 15.7). Even when pathology is present, the stroma may demonstrate pseudodecidual changes, but progesterone responsiveness is often diminished in disease states such as endometritis, and in polyps.

With continued exposure or repeated cycles, the receptor downregulation causes the glands to lose their sensitivity to estrogens and progestins, leading to progressively less

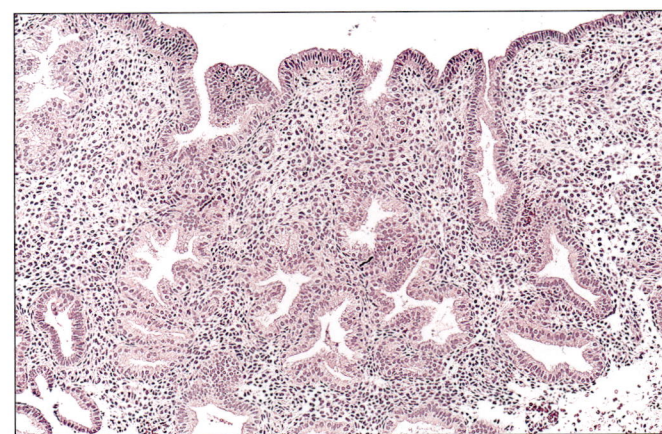

Figure 15.5 Secretory endometrium, demonstrating exogenous progesterone effect. The appearance is indistinguishable from a normal cycle. The woman, who was older, had received progesterone for 20 days.

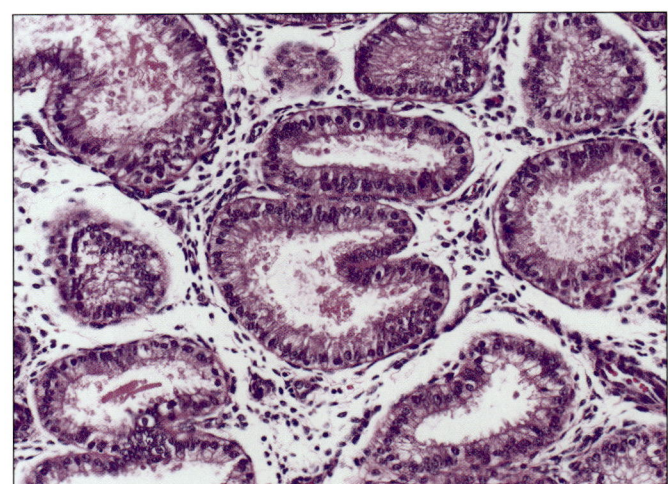

Figure 15.6 Vacuolated secretory glandular changes in response to short-term progestin therapy.

Table 15.2 Representative Progestational Agents Available in the United States

Generic Name	Brand Name
Progesterone	Prometrium, Crinone
Hydroxyprogesterone	Hylutin, Makena
Medroxyprogesterone	Provera, Prodrox, Cycrin, Amen, Curretab
Megestrol acetate	Megace
Norgestrel	Neogest
Drospirenone	
Levonorgestrel	Norplant, Plan B
Norethindrone	Aygestin
Norethynodrel	
Desogestrel	Cerazette
Norgestimate	

Adapted from Schimmer and Parker (2012).[1]

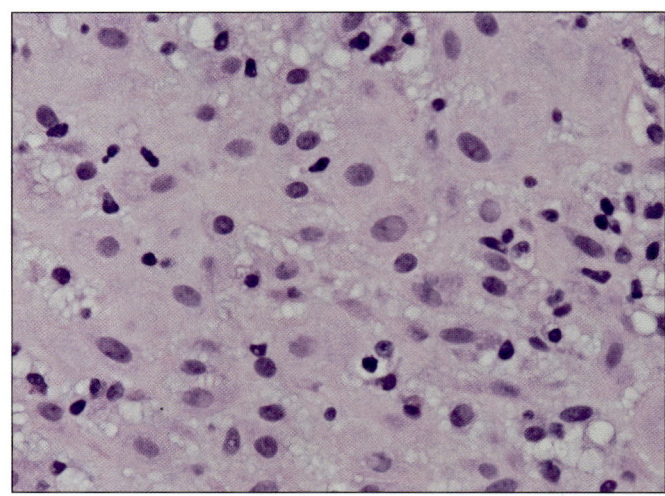

Figure 15.7 Stromal pseudodecidualization, response to progesterone therapy.

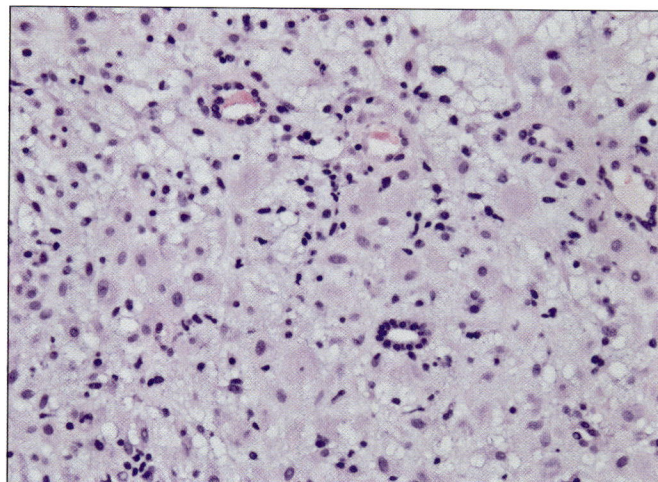

Figure 15.8 Atrophic gland in decidualized stroma in a woman receiving progesterone.

Table 15.3 Composition of Representative OCs Available in the United States

Generic Class/Name	Brand Name
Combination Monophasic	
Ethinyl estradiol/desogestrel	Desogen, Ortho-Cept
Ethinyl estradiol/drospirenone	Yasmin, Yaz
Ethinyl estradiol/ethynodiol	Demulen, Zovia
Ethinyl estradiol/norethindrone	Loestrin, Femcon, Junel, Brevicon, Norinyl, Ortho-Novum, Ovcon
Ethinyl estradiol/levonorgestrel	Alesse, Levlite, Lybrel, Nordette
Ethinyl estradiol/norgestrel	Lo/Ovral, Ovral, Cryselle
Ethinyl estradiol/norgestimate	Ortho-Cyclen
Mestranol/norethindrone	Norinyl, Ortho-Novum, Genora, Nelova
Biphasic	
Ethinyl estradiol/norethindrone	Ortho-Novum, Jenest, Necon
Ethinyl estradiol/desogestrel	Mircette, Kariva
Triphasic	
Ethinyl estradiol/norethindrone	Ortho-Novum, Tri-Norinyl, Estrostep, Aranelle
Ethinyl estradiol/norgestimate	Ortho Tri-Cyclen, Ortho Tri-Cyclen Lo
Ethinyl estradiol/levonorgestrel	Tri-Levlen, Triphasil, Trivora
Ethinyl estradiol/desogestrel	Cyclessa
Combination Extended Cycle	
Ethinyl estradiol/drospirenone	Yaz
Ethinyl estradiol/levonorgestrel	Lybrel, Seasonale, Seasonique
Ethinyl estradiol/norethindrone	Loestrin
Progestin-Only (Mini-Pill)	
Norethindrone	Micronor, Nor-QD
Norgestrel	Ovrette

Adapted from Schimmer and Parker (2012).[1]

secretory change ('secretory exhaustion'), such that they ultimately appear atrophic. At this stage, which only occurs after prolonged exposure or multiple cycles, the appearance is that of decidualized stroma with widely dispersed atrophic glands, often referred to as a 'pill' endometrium (Figure 15.8). More slowly, the decidualized stroma also begins to be suppressed by the receptor downregulation, and over months to years will become attenuated and atrophic, ultimately losing most of its decidual features. At this point, the appearance resembles endometrial atrophy due to menopause or hormone suppression.

Exposure to high-dose progestins (often given for dysfunctional uterine bleeding and usually with a good initial response) can, paradoxically, cause secondary necrosis of the superficial endometrium, often in the form of wedge-shaped infarcts, and renewed bleeding. The hysteroscopic appearances are often alarming. Both the continued bleeding and the hysteroscopic findings lead the clinician to perform a dilatation and curettage to exclude hyperplasia or malignancy and yielding abundant, macroscopically suspicious tissue fragments. Occasionally, patients will spontaneously pass large intact sheets of decidualized endometrium ('decidual casts').

ORAL CONTRACEPTIVES

Oral contraceptives (OCs) are one of the most widely used medications in the developed world. They are used as treatment for several common medical problems in addition to contraception, including dysfunctional uterine bleeding and endometriosis. A variety of formulations and administration schedules have been developed (Table 15.3).[1] Sequential OCs contain only estrogen during the first half of the cycle, with progestin added during the second half. Because of the increased risk of endometrial cancer with some sequential formulations,[2] the most commonly used types today are combined estrogen–progestin and progestin-only formulations administered over 21 consecutive days of the cycle, followed by 7 days of placebo tablets yielding a withdrawal week. Combined pills can be monophasic, in which there is a fixed dose of estrogen and a progestin in combination for the 21 days of each cycle, or they can be biphasic or triphasic, depending on whether the progestin dose is altered once or twice during the cycle. In contrast to some sequential OCs and estrogen-only hormone replacement regimens, which increase the risk of endometrial carcinoma, combined OCs are protective, with the degree of protection increasing with the length of therapy. Patients with 10 years of OC use have about a 75% reduction in endometrial carcinoma.[3,4] OC use is also associated with a 30–50% decrease in the risk of ovarian carcinoma; this lowered risk persists for at least 20 years after cessation of their use and is also seen in *BRCA1* and *BRCA2* mutation carriers.[5] Recently, a variety of extended cycle (91 day) and even continuous cycle (365 day) OCs have been introduced that appear to have similar effectiveness to traditional OCs.[6] The histologic effects of these newer formulations have not been well studied.

COMBINED OCs

The histologic appearance of the endometrium in a patient on combined OCs is extremely variable, but is dominated by the progestin effects. It depends on various factors, some poorly understood, including the type of pill, the duration of therapy, precise dose of the individual pill, levels of compliance with the regimen, and endogenous hormone synthesis and metabolism.[7–9] Certain generalizations are possible, however. Within the first several cycles of a combined OC, there is a mixture of proliferative and secretory features seen in the endometrium ('asynchronous' or 'discordant' endometrium). The glands tend to remain relatively straight and narrow, resembling proliferative endometrial glands but with cuboidal rather than columnar epithelium, and with very minimal mitotic activity. Subnuclear vacuoles may be seen, especially during the first 2 weeks of the cycle. Decidual change can be seen early but is usually more evident after several cycles have been completed (Figures 15.9 and 15.10). Despite the stromal changes, spiral arterioles do not develop normally.[10] With prolonged therapy over many cycles the glands develop secretory exhaustion and become increasingly small, inactive, and ultimately atrophic. As this occurs, the stromal decidual changes become increasingly well developed, until the endometrium is uniformly decidualized, with only rare, atrophic-appearing glands (Figures 15.11 and 15.12). This is the classic appearance of the so-called 'pill' endometrium. Prominent ectatic thin-walled veins are also seen, which often contain thromboses in patients having breakthrough bleeding (Figure 15.13). The classic pill endometrium is not seen in all patients, and there is a spectrum from well-developed stromal changes to complete atrophy, with only a very thin endometrium showing little or no identifiable decidual change. The atrophic changes are seen more frequently with some of the lower dose regimens.[8]

Formulations that include short estrogen-only periods have been used in an attempt to lower the overall dose of

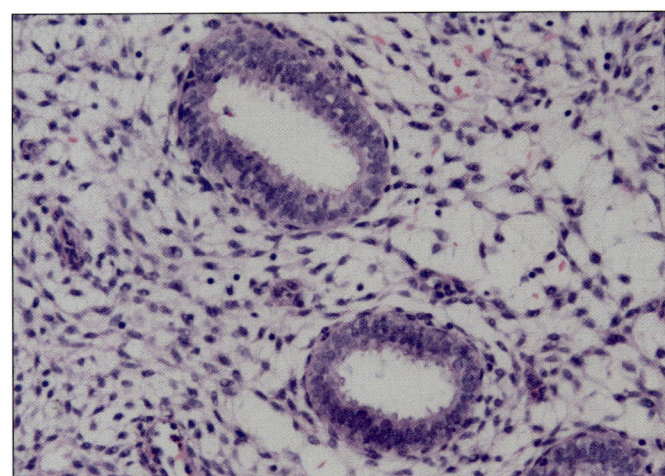

Figure 15.10 Combined OC, secretory exhaustion. The glands are small and show only rudimentary evidence of secretory activity in the form of apical snouts.

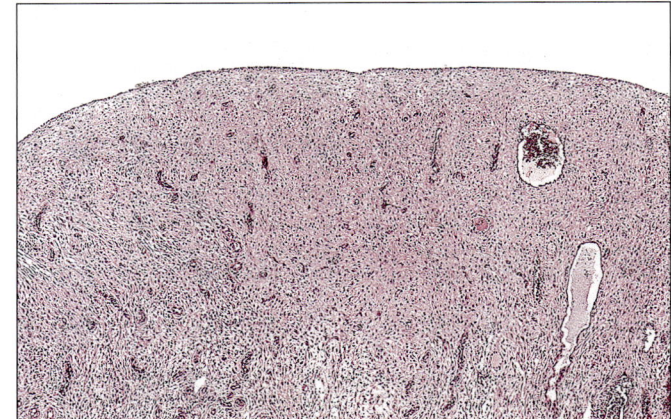

Figure 15.11 Combined OC (Loestrin), with classic pill endometrium. The stroma is massively decidualized and contains widely scattered, atrophic glands.

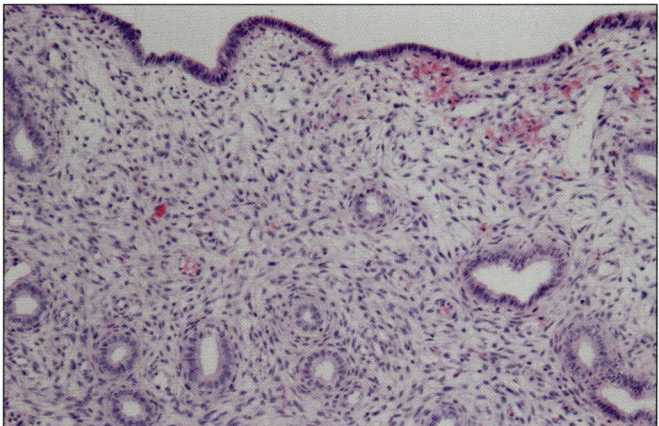

Figure 15.9 Gland atrophy with combined OC. The stromal decidual response is minimal.

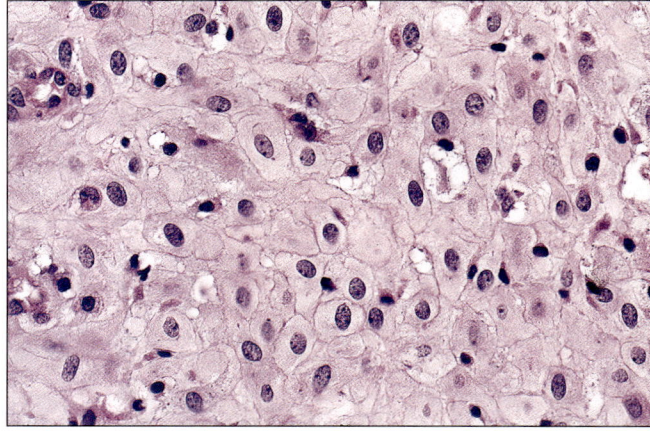

Figure 15.12 Combined OC (Loestrin) with well-developed decidual change (high magnification).

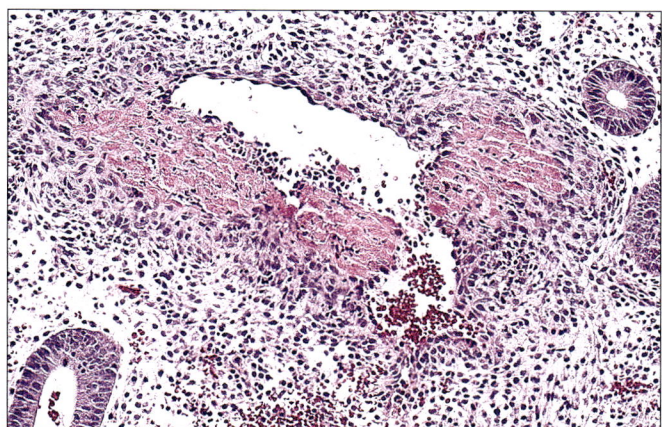

Figure 15.13 Thrombi in prominent ectatic thin-walled veins (combined OC).

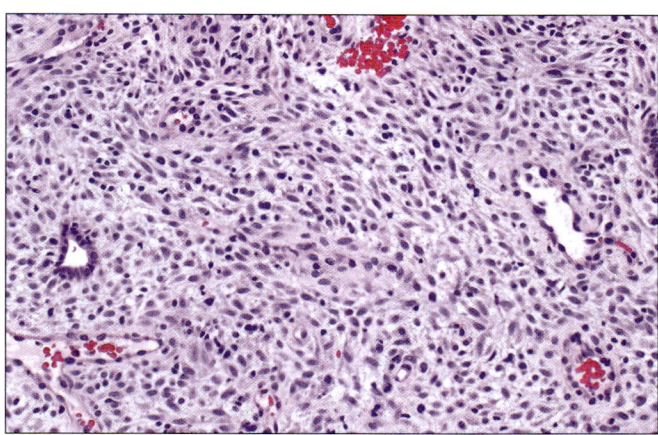

Figure 15.14 Decidualized endometrium with long-term Depo-Provera use.

hormones. Mircette, for example, has 21 days of combination treatment followed by a 2 day, hormone-free interval and 5 days of unopposed estrogen. Technically, this is a sequential OC, but to date it has not had the safety issues associated with the older, higher dose sequential therapies. This formulation has a distinctly different histologic pattern than the combined OCs. Biopsies taken during the estrogen-only portion of the cycle show proliferative endometrium while biopsies taken during the combined portion of the cycle show secretory endometrium.[11]

PURE PROGESTIN OCs ('MINI-PILL')

In contrast to the combined OCs, the pure progestin OC (the mini-pill, 300 μg norethisterone) is taken daily without interruption during the cycle. The mechanism of contraception differs from combined OCs in that ovulation is not consistently suppressed. Instead, contraception is due to the production of relatively thick cervical mucus that is impermeable to sperm, and to the atrophic endometrium that will not support implantation. The endometrial changes seen with the mini-pill are not distinctly different from those seen with combined OCs, but marked atrophy is more common and biopsy frequently yields only scanty material. In addition, proliferative endometrium is not infrequently seen, and this correlates with abnormal bleeding.[12]

LONG-TERM, PROGESTIN-ONLY OCs

Several systems have been developed for long-term, progestin-only contraception. Medroxyprogesterone acetate microcrystals in an aqueous solution (Depo-Provera) are used as an intramuscular injection. The slow dissolution of the crystals maintains effective progestin levels for several months, allowing for an injection schedule of every 3 months. Levels of progestin are typically higher than with the mini-pill. Early after injection, some women develop exaggerated hypersecretory changes that resemble gestational endometrium, including the presence of Arias-Stella reaction. By 3–6 months these changes have resolved and stromal decidual changes develop, resembling those seen with combined OCs as described earlier. Long-term treatment can result in atrophy or pure decidua-like change (Figure 15.14), just as with combined OCs.[8,13]

The Norplant system consists of several Silastic tubes containing levonorgestrel. The tubes are slightly permeable to steroids, and the progestin is slowly released for a period of 3–5 years. As in other progestin-only regimens, ovulation occurs in about one-third of cycles, and contraception is by production of thick cervical mucus and an endometrium inimical to implantation. There are relatively few studies on the histologic findings with Norplant,[14,15] but the findings seem to be similar to other progestin-only regimens, with atrophy being the most common finding. Proliferative endometrium can also be seen, and correlates with irregular bleeding patterns.[16]

Devices that supply progestins directly to the endometrium are also used. The most common of these uses a slow-release formulation of levonorgestrel in combination with an intrauterine device (Mirena). Although physically located within the endometrium, absorption is systemic and they can be used for treatment of extrauterine disease such as endometriosis as well as abnormal uterine bleeding.[17–19] Histologically, the endometrium shows extensive decidualization.[20]

HORMONE REPLACEMENT THERAPY

Three general types of hormone replacement therapy (HRT) have been used clinically: unopposed estrogen, cyclic estrogen and progestin, and combined estrogen and progestin formulations. Because of the markedly increased risk of endometrial cancer with unopposed estrogen, only the last two are in common use today. While the exact agents used and their dosage can vary, within each of these groups the histologic findings tend to be similar, and thus they will be discussed as categories.

The number of patients receiving long-term (>5 years) HRT dropped precipitously after large studies showed an increase in cardiovascular risk rather than the predicted protective effects.[21] In the United States, the number of prescriptions for HRT in the national Medicaid program fell by 57% between 2002 and 2004.[22] Nonetheless, HRT continues to be commonly used as short-term therapy for symptoms related to menopause.

UNOPPOSED ESTROGEN HRT

Historically, estrogen alone was given as hormone replacement for postmenopausal women, and the beneficial effects of this therapy in preventing osteoporosis and cardiovascular disease have been well documented. Then a series of case–control studies subsequently demonstrated a markedly increased risk of endometrial adenocarcinoma in women using long-term estrogens unopposed by progestins. Patients receiving unopposed estrogens for 5 years or more have an approximately sixfold increase in endometrial carcinoma. With the addition of progestins, the risk of endometrial carcinoma fell to near control levels.[23–25] The risk of endometrial carcinoma is dose related, but low-dose estrogens (0.3 mg conjugated estrogens or equivalent) continue to be associated with a risk of carcinoma if not combined with a progestin.[26] Even estrogens applied as vaginal creams have sufficient systemic absorption to increase the risk.[27] Although current practice is treatment with combined therapy, occasional patients are still treated with estrogen alone. It should be noted that, although addition of a progestin reduces the risk of endometrial cancer from HRT, combined HRT is associated with a significant increase in the risk of breast cancer.[28]

The endometrium from a woman being treated with unopposed estrogens will most commonly appear proliferative, and may in fact be indistinguishable from a normal proliferative endometrium in a premenopausal patient. If the estrogen dose is low, there may also be a lesser degree of proliferation that is described as weakly proliferative.[29] If the patient is bleeding, the endometrium will often have proliferative glands with associated stromal breakdown deep below the uterine surface lining (Figure 15.3), a feature that specifically suggests unopposed estrogen exposure. Unfortunately, conventional microscopy cannot distinguish these changes due to exogenous estrogens from the effects of endogenous estrogen, as in anovulatory bleeding, or from the effects of other agents that may act as estrogenic agents in the endometrium. These include tamoxifen, various drugs and pharmaceutical agents such as digitalis or phenothiazines, and herbal preparations such as ginseng.

Long-term estrogen exposure can lead to a full spectrum of appearances, ranging from disordered proliferative changes to non-atypical endometrial hyperplasia, EIN, or even adenocarcinoma.[7] Disordered proliferative endometrium shows a basic pattern of proliferative endometrium, with the addition of irregularly dilated and focally branched glands. This condition is most commonly seen in untreated women during the perimenopause and is not felt to be premalignant (see Chapter 17). Tubal metaplasia is common. The hallmark of non-atypical endometrial hyperplasia is the development of endometrial compartment-wide irregular gland shape and distribution, which in many areas has glandular crowding to more than a 1:1 gland to stroma ratio. EIN may emerge from non-atypical endometrial hyperplasia as a localized lesion with discrete cytology.[30] Adenocarcinomas are of the endometrioid type, exhibit severe glandular crowding, usually with a cribriform or papillary architecture, and at least mild nuclear atypia (see Chapter 18). Tumors developing from unopposed estrogen exposure, whether endogenous or exogenous, are usually low grade with high long-term survival rates. Patients who develop adenocarcinomas usually have a minimum of 2–3 years of unopposed estrogen use. The risk increases over time, with the highest risk in patients who have taken estrogens for 10 or more years.[9]

CYCLIC ESTROGEN–PROGESTERONE HRT

Because unopposed estrogens elevate the risk of endometrial adenocarcinoma, HRT today nearly always includes a progestin (if the patient has a uterus). The most commonly used agents are conjugated equine estrogen (Premarin) in combination with medroxyprogesterone acetate (Provera). Cyclic or sequential HRT uses daily estrogen for the first 21–25 days of the month with daily progestin added for the last 10–13 days. Consistent reduction of mitotic rates in glandular epithelium is found after generally only 9 or more days of progesterone administration in each cycle.[31,32] This regimen mimics to some degree the normal progression of these hormones during a menstrual cycle and typically results in a withdrawal bleed at the end of each cycle. Longer cycle lengths (i.e., 12 instead of 4 weeks) have shown a decrease in the protective effect of the progestin and are not generally recommended.[33]

The pathologic findings in the endometrium are somewhat but not entirely predictable based on our understanding of normal endometrial cycles. Not surprisingly, biopsies taken from the estrogen-only portion of the cycle typically have a proliferative appearance, and may be histologically identical to a normal proliferative endometrium (Figures 15.15–15.17). Biopsies taken after the initiation of the progestin are more variable. Most show some degree of secretory change, beginning about 3 days after the beginning of the progestin therapy, but the changes lack the well-ordered daily progression seen in normal secretory endometrium and cannot be 'dated' in the same fashion (see Chapter 14).[34–36] Frequently, the glandular component develops no further than an early secretory appearance, with variably developed glycogen vacuoles persisting even late into the artificial cycle. The stroma shows a variable response to the progestin, and may develop a spotty decidual response by day 10 after progestin initiation. This is often described in pathology reports as gland–stromal asynchrony, and can be

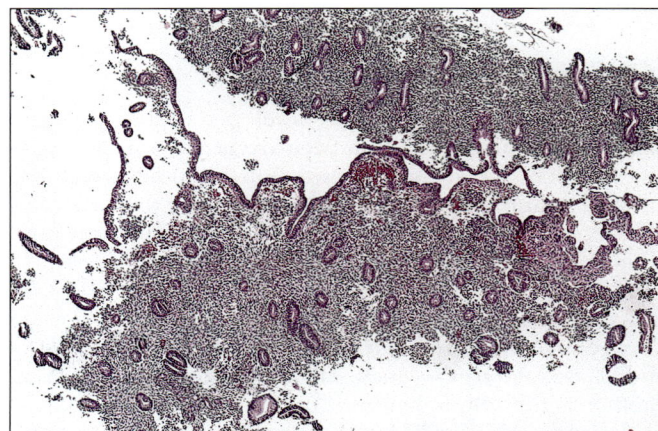

Figure 15.15 Cyclic HRT, weakly proliferative pattern.

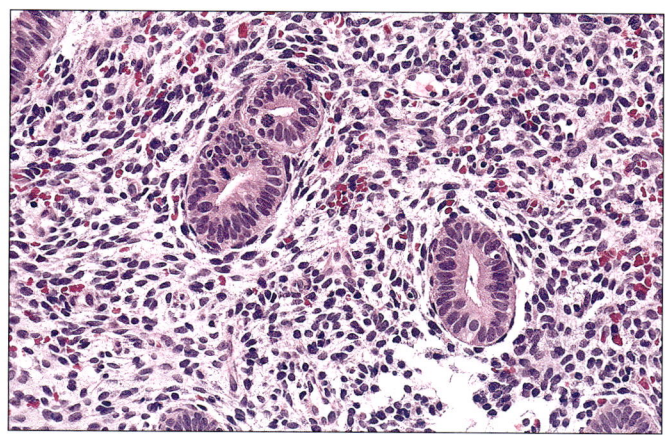

Figure 15.16 Cyclic HRT, weakly proliferative pattern (high magnification).

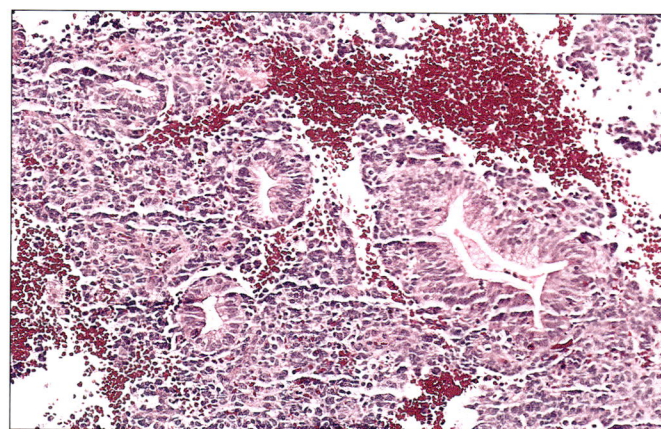

Figure 15.18 Normal menstrual endometrium with focal secretory changes in a woman receiving HRT.

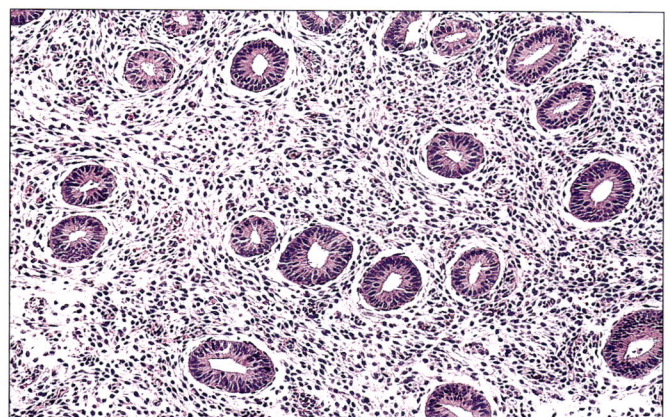

Figure 15.17 Proliferative endometrium with cyclic HRT.

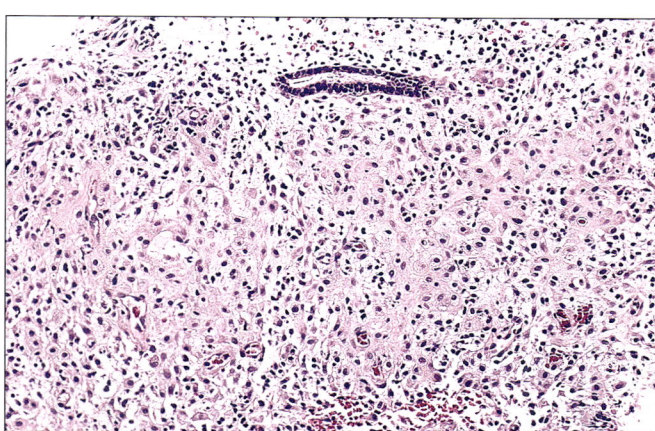

Figure 15.19 Combined HRT (Prempro), extensive stromal decidual change. The stroma shows a well-developed decidual change, with inactive glands. This pattern can mimic "pill" endometrium.

due to various other factors, including intrauterine devices (IUDs), OCs, underlying mass lesions such as leiomyomas or polyps, chronic endometritis, and other types of hormone such as mifepristone, clomiphene, and gonadotropins. Although this sequence of incomplete cycling is the most common picture with cyclic HRT, other patterns are not infrequent. Some patients will have normal menstrual changes (Figure 15.18) impossible to distinguish from women who have never taken HRT. Up to one-fifth of patients will have an inactive endometrium. This group of patients generally does not experience monthly withdrawal bleeds.

Our understanding of precisely why the endometrium responds so variably to cyclic HRT is poor, but presumably reflects multiple host factors (age, years post menopause, level of endogenous hormones) and medication-specific factors (precise drug, dose, and duration).

COMBINED ESTROGEN–PROGESTERONE HRT

Continuous combined estrogen–progestin HRT protects against the carcinogenic effects of unopposed estrogen. These regimens generally have a relatively predictable and uniform effect on the endometrium. As described previously, the continuous long-term use of progesterone leads to downregulation of both estrogen and progesterone receptors, diminishing the responsiveness of the endometrium. This leads to the most common appearance, namely an atrophic or inactive endometrium.[8,37] There may be weak, poorly developed decidual change in the stromal cells, and the glandular component may show a few glycogen vacuoles suggesting progestin effect in the glands, but these findings are variable. Least common, there is a well-developed stromal decidual change, similar to that seen with OCs (Figure 15.19). Metaplastic changes such as tubal metaplasia, eosinophilic metaplasia, squamous metaplasia, and papillary syncytial metaplasia are more common with combined continuous HRT.[7]

A clearly proliferative pattern in the endometrium would suggest an inadequate dose of the progestational agent, especially if there is ongoing breakdown (i.e., an anovulatory-like pattern) (Figures 15.20 and 15.21).

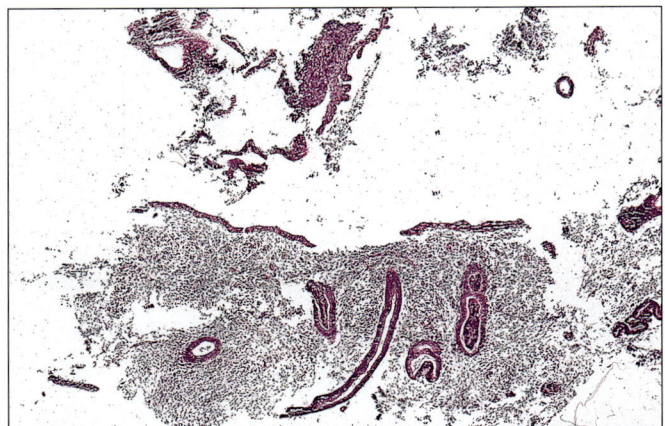

Figure 15.20 Combined HRT (Prempro), proliferative with breakdown. This unusual pattern is identical to that seen with anovulation in the premenopausal patient. It indicates continuous estrogen stimulation to the endometrium with an insufficient opposing level of progestin.

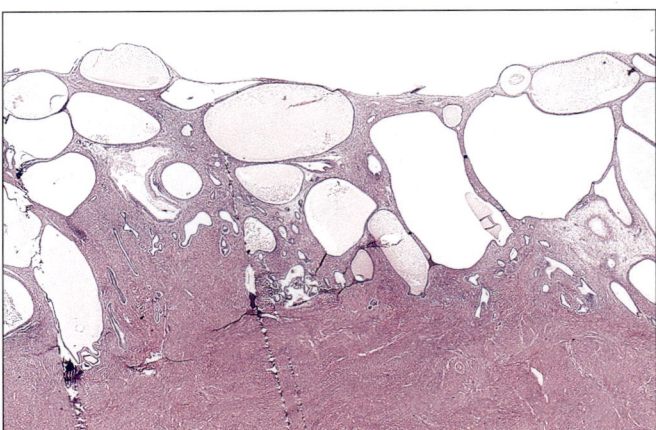

Figure 15.22 Tamoxifen, cystic atrophy. Large cystic glands are present in the endometrium. (Courtesy of Dr. H. Krigman, University of Minnesota.)

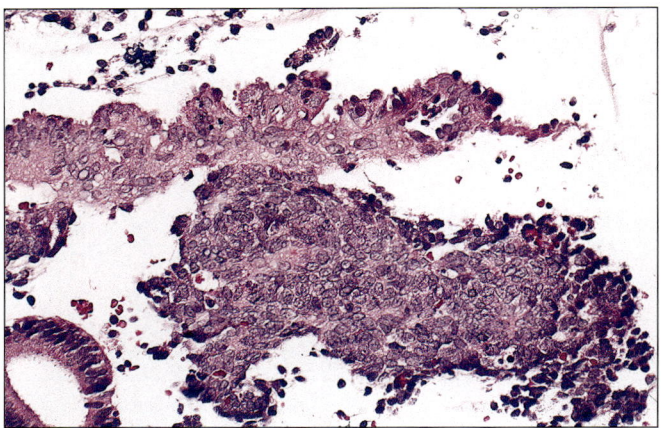

Figure 15.21 Detail of stromal breakdown with combined HRT (Prempro).

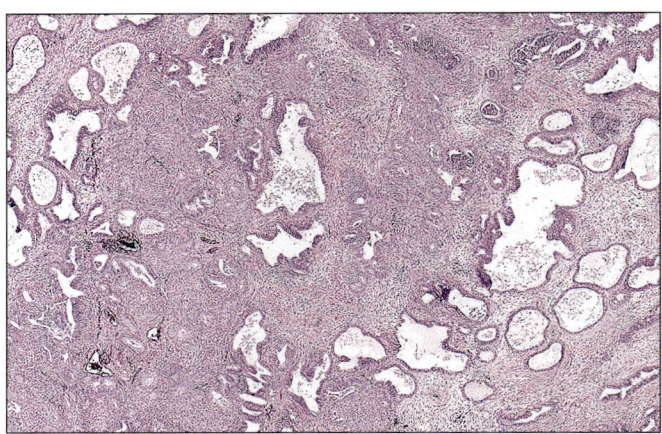

Figure 15.23 Tamoxifen, polyp. This polyp also showed extensive squamous metaplasia, a not uncommon finding.

OTHER HORMONAL AGENTS

TAMOXIFEN

Tamoxifen has been widely used in the treatment and now the prevention of breast cancer, where it functions as an antiestrogen.[38] Toremifene is a closely related agent that is available in several countries; it will be considered together with tamoxifen as they have very similar actions.[39] In the endometrium, tamoxifen is a strong competitive inhibitor of circulating estrogens, but also a weak estrogen agonist. In the presence of high estrogen levels, as found in premenopausal women, it competes for receptors, thereby reducing overall estrogen stimulation. In the presence of very low ambient estrogen levels, i.e., in the postmenopausal patient, the agonist activity of tamoxifen can result in mild activation of the endometrial estrogen receptor.[40] While most postmenopausal women will continue to have atrophic or (regular or cystic) inactive endometrium (Figure 15.22), a few will develop the pathologic changes associated with chronic unopposed estrogen stimulation.[41] As might be expected, women receiving tamoxifen who are symptomatic have far greater frequencies of endometrial pathologies than women who are asymptomatic (93% vs 25%).[42–44]

Multiple reports have described unusual-appearing endometrial polyps in tamoxifen-treated patients, with cystically dilated glands sometimes containing luminal secretions, a variety of metaplasias, massive fibrosis and, more rarely, decidualized stroma (Figures 15.23 and 15.24).[44,45] Some of these changes may be dose related.[46] Many of the polyps are 20 mm or more in size, which is larger than seen with any other form of HRT. No studies have yet to indicate why this drug alone has such a peculiar effect on the endometrial stroma. Malignancies are occasionally found in polyps associated with tamoxifen therapy and at rates much higher than in healthy nonusers (3% vs 0.5%).[46]

Endometrial carcinomas arise at approximately the same rate as with unopposed estrogen and at far greater rates than women not receiving HRT. The risk is related to the duration of therapy, and is increased approximately

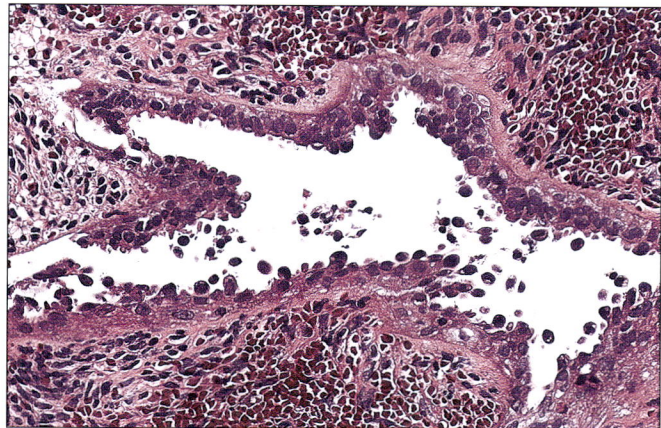

Figure 15.24 Tamoxifen, serous-like epithelial atypia in polyp. (Courtesy of Dr. H. Krigman, University of Minnesota.)

fourfold in patients exposed to tamoxifen for more than 5 years.[47] Some initial anecdotal reports and small series suggested that tamoxifen-induced carcinomas might be more frequently high grade,[48] but larger subsequent series including results from the NSABP B-14 study have shown a similar proportion of high-grade tumors to those arising sporadically.[49,50] Most cancers are low-grade, low-stage endometrioid adenocarcinomas. Uterine sarcomas also occur rarely in association with tamoxifen therapy,[51] but most of these examples are carcinosarcomas that the current body of opinion places into the category of 'metaplastic carcinomas' (see Chapter 18).

OTHER SELECTIVE ESTROGEN RECEPTOR MODULATORS

There are at least two types of estrogen receptors that are differentially active between reproductive and somatic target organs. This has led to the development of selective estrogen receptor modulators (SERMs), designed for relatively tissue-specific effects.[39] Clinically beneficial compounds would minimize the stimulatory effect in endometrial tissue while retaining the beneficial effects in bone and the cardiovascular system. The first of these to come into wide use was tamoxifen, but in recent years a number of additional SERMs have become available.

Raloxifene, an antiestrogen designed initially for breast cancer treatment, has selective beneficial effects on bone and cardiovascular systems, while lacking any evident estrogenic activity within the endometrium itself. Endometrial biopsies from postmenopausal women taking raloxifene show atrophy or inactive endometrium,[52] and treated patients show no increase in endometrial thickness as measured by ultrasound.[53] Long-term follow-up studies now confirm that patients receiving raloxifene have neither increased endometrial hyperplasia nor carcinoma when compared with control groups,[54–56] although there has been an increase in endometrial polyps.

A number of other SERMS are entering clinical use or have shown promise in clinical trials, including lasofoxifene, arzoxifene, bazedoxifene, ospemifene and fulvestrant. None of these have had detailed, long-term evaluations of their endometrial effects, but at least one (lasofoxifene) has been shown to be associated with increased endometrial thickness and polyps.[55] It appears that each of these agents has a unique combination of activities and their effects on the endometrium will need to be documented individually rather than as a single class of drugs.

AROMATASE INHIBITORS

Aromatase inhibitors are a class of endocrine agents that block the peripheral conversion of steroids into estradiol by inhibiting the aromatase enzyme. Letrozole, anastrozole, and exemestane are the three mostly thoroughly studied members of this drug class. These drugs are used primarily to treat estrogen receptor-positive breast cancers in postmenopausal women (in this situation they are highly effective)[57,58] and, more recently, endometriosis[59] and ovulation induction for *in vitro* fertilization.[60,61] Because they reduce circulating estrogen levels to near zero, the primary effect on the endometrium is atrophy, and the rate of endometrial carcinoma is lower than in tamoxifen-treated patients.[52] As measured by transvaginal ultrasound, aromatase inhibitors do not increase endometrial thickness. Some preliminary evidence suggests that aromatase inhibitors could even help treat pre-existing endometrial hyperplasias.[63] Although aromatase inhibitors effectively shut down endometrial proliferation, endometrial polyps continue to develop, an observation that contradicts current dogma that endometrial polyps are estrogen induced.

PHYTOESTROGENS AND OTHER DIETARY AGENTS

Dietary and herbal remedies are widely used worldwide for relief of menopausal symptoms. Commonly used herbs include black cohosh (*Cimicifuga racemosa*), chaste tree berry (*Vitex agnus-castus*), dong quai (*Angelica sinensis*), ginseng (*Panax ginseng* and other *Panax* species), evening primrose oil (*Oenothera biennis*), motherwort (*Leonurus cardiaca*), red clover (*Trifolium pratense*), and licorice (*Glycyrrhiza glabra*). In many cases the active ingredients of these herbal preparations have not been clearly identified.[64]

Phytoestrogens, new forms of SERM still being evaluated, are plant estrogens that occur naturally as constituents of many plants, most notably beans and a variety of grains and seeds. Soybeans and flaxseed are commonly cited in the lay literature as sources of phytoestrogens,[65,66] which have a weak estrogen-like effect in the body. One tantalizing observation is that Asian women, who are known to have a much lower incidence of endometrial carcinoma than Western women, consume much higher amounts of phytoestrogen-rich foods, such as soy and tofu. Human studies suggest that a diet high in phytoestrogens may protect against endometrial adenocarcinoma and provide benefits in bone density.[67] Nationwide population-based studies, while not specifically evaluating phytoestrogens, suggest that a diet with a low fruit and vegetable intake is associated with higher rates of endometrial cancer.[68]

The most common types of phytoestrogen in plants and foods are the isoflavones. The richest sources in nature are the leaves of the subterranean red clover with levels of up to 5 g/100 g dry weight, and soybeans with levels up to 300 mg/100 g dry weight. The most commonly studied

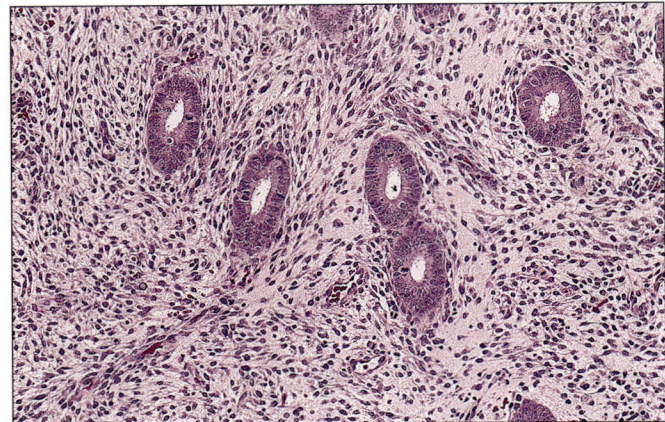

Figure 15.25 Phytoestrogen, with well-developed proliferative endometrium.

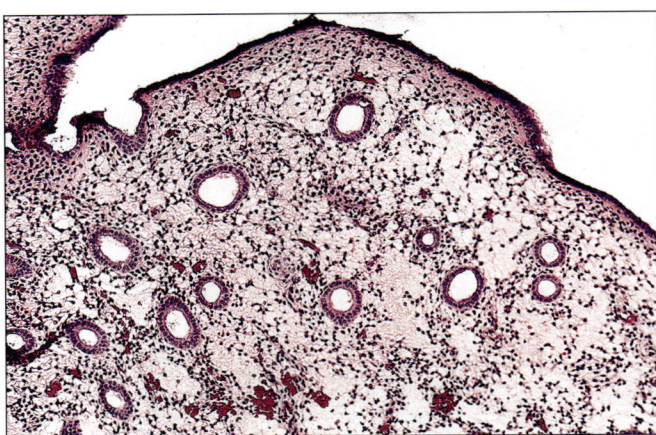

Figure 15.26 Markedly edematous stroma (clomiphene). (Courtesy of Dr. Karen Ireland, Liberty Lake, WA.)

phytoestrogens within this group are genistein and daidzein.

The initial data available on the effects on the endometrium itself suggest that phytoestrogens likely function as weak estrogen agonists. Long-term exposure to high doses may increase the risk of endometrial hyperplasia in postmenopausal women, but most evidence suggests that short-term exposure to lower doses has no discernible histologic effect on endometrium.[69,70] In premenopausal women, the endometrium appears to cycle normally (Figure 15.25).

Wild yam preparations contain diosgenin, which can be converted to progesterone in a laboratory but not in the human body. Whether dietary supplementation with wild yams has any histologic effects on the endometrium is unknown.[66]

CLOMIPHENE/OVULATION INDUCTION THERAPY

Clomiphene citrate (Clomid) is an agent with strong affinity for the estrogen receptor. It binds essentially irreversibly to the receptor, reducing turnover. Its clinical usefulness stems from its effects on the hypothalamus, which interprets this activity as a low level of estrogen, causing increased gonadotropin-releasing hormone (GnRH) stimulation of the pituitary, and hence increased follicle-stimulating hormone (FSH) production. This increases ovarian estrogen production, which then feeds back to the pituitary and causes a luteinizing hormone (LH) surge, followed by ovulation.[8] This drug, used to induce ovulation, is usually given on cycle days 5–10, with ovulation occurring 5–10 days after its administration. The increased stimulation of the dominant follicle results in higher serum estrogen and progesterone levels during the resulting secretory phase.

The effects of clomiphene on the endometrium are relatively subtle.[71,72] Some, but not all, studies suggest that, in a clomiphene-induced secretory phase, the glandular development is delayed relative to the time of ovulation (Figure 15.26). Although delayed, the early secretory changes are unusually well developed, with large, uniform subnuclear glycogen vacuoles that persist longer than in a normal cycle. Later in the cycle, decidual changes in the stroma are less prominent, and a coiled glandular architecture persists. These findings probably represent the antiestrogenic effects of clomiphene in combination with the high circulating levels of estrogen and progesterone.[73]

In more recent years, ovulation induction has involved more complex regimens, generally involving administration of GnRH agonists and antagonists, FSH, human chorionic gonadotropin, and aromatase inhibitors. There are few treatment-specific studies on endometrial morphology, and it is difficult to extrapolate results between regimens. At least some studies suggest a relative delay in secretory phase maturation, similar to that seen with clomiphene. Other studies show in-phase or even advanced date endometrium.[74,75] The alterations in endometrial function may be responsible for the reduced rate of successful implantation seen in some patients.

PROGESTERONE RECEPTOR MODULATORS

This class of agents modulates the activity of the progesterone receptor. Although developed originally as progesterone receptor antagonists, their actions *in vivo* appear to be more complex, varying by agent and modified by the hormonal environment of the individual patient. The most widely known agent in the United States is mifepristone, which is primarily used as an agent of very early abortion ('morning after pill'), but these agents are also effective in the treatment of a variety of common conditions such as endometriosis and leiomyomata.[76] Other drugs in this category include asoprisnil, and Proellex (CDB-4124). Several studies have shown unique histologic changes in the endometrium in patients receiving progesterone receptor modulators (PRMs), and a National Institutes of Health-sponsored workshop has suggested the term 'progesterone receptor modular associated endometrial changes' (PAEC) as a name for this constellation of findings.[77–79] Common findings include the development of multiple cysts, and glandular epithelium with nonphysiologic combinations of estrogen and progesterone effects: mitoses with apoptosis, or secretory vacuoles with proliferative activity (Figures 15.27 and 15.28). Stromal predecidual change is rare, and they differ from unopposed estrogens in lacking fibrin thrombi. PAEC changes are not seen in every treated patient,

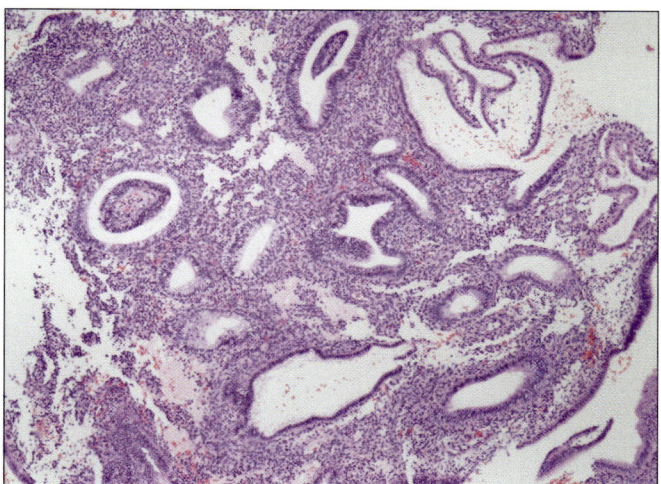

Figure 15.27 Effects of progesterone blockade on the premenopausal endometrium. PAEC caused by CDB-4124 includes epithelial–stromal dyssynchrony, evident as scattered cysts. (Courtesy Repros Therapeutics, Woodlands, TX)

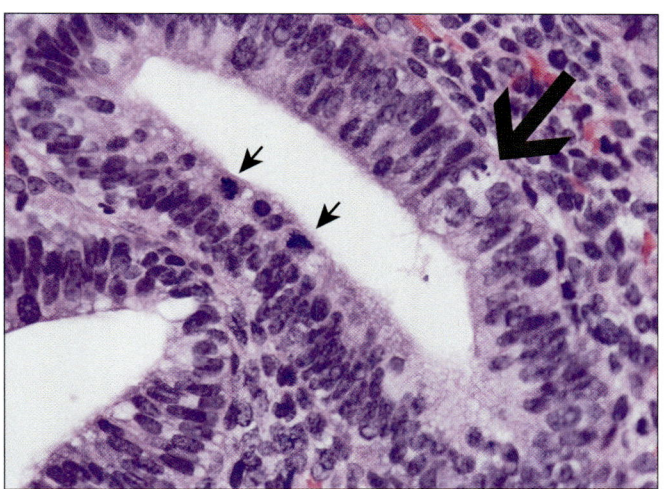

Figure 15.28 Closer view of CDB-4124-treated endometrium shows nonphysiologic combinations of mitoses (small arrows), apoptotic change (large arrow), and secretory vacuoles within glands. (Courtesy Repros Therapeutics, Woodlands, TX)

some of whom have proliferative or atrophic endometria that lack any distinctive features that would suggest exposure to a PRM. Long-term clinical outcomes are generally unknown or poorly understood, as the majority are newly introduced agents. However, as PRMs become more widely used, it will be important for pathologists to be aware of these changes so they are not confused with polyps or unopposed estrogen effects.

GnRH AGONISTS AND ANTAGONISTS

Pulsatile release of GnRH from the hypothalamus is the normal stimulus to the pituitary to secrete FSH and LH. Paradoxically, chronic nonpulsatile treatment has the opposite effect and results in the inhibition of FSH and LH secretion (after an initial surge), apparently via downregulation of the GnRH receptors in the pituitary. Several GnRH agonists make use of this pathway to suppress pituitary gonadotropin secretion, including leuprolide acetate, buserelin acetate, triptorelin, nafarelin, and goserelin acetate. More recently, direct GnRH antagonists have been developed (cetrorelix, ganirelix) that have similar suppressive effects but without the initial surge in FSH and LH secretion. Administering these agents blocks ovarian follicle development and induces a marked reduction in estrogen and progesterone levels, comparable to a postmenopausal state. Indeed, long-term treatment with these agents is limited due to the side effects of marked hypoestrogenemia, including profound bone density loss.

Currently, GnRH agonists and antagonists are used to reduce the size of uterine leiomyomas and endometrial stromal sarcomas.[80] They are also used in the diagnosis and treatment of endometriosis, and in the suppression of ovulation during oocyte harvest for *in vitro* fertilization. Histologically, it is not surprising that the endometrium from patients treated chronically with GnRH shows profound atrophy.[81]

GONADOTROPINS

Gonadotropins are used primarily to treat infertility. Human menopausal gonadotropins, LH and FSH, are extracted from the urine of postmenopausal women. Human chorionic gonadotropin is closely related to LH, and can be used to simulate the mid-cycle LH surge in ovulation induction. The effects of these agents on the endometrium are not clear. Various conflicting findings report delayed, normal, or advanced histologic maturation relative to the clinical dates, as well as hypersecretory changes similar to Arias-Stella reactions.[8,9,82]

CORTICOSTEROIDS

High doses of corticosteroids can have a progestational effect on the endometrium. Presumably, this is due to a weak affinity for the progesterone receptor. The histologic appearance is similar to other progestational agents. Chronic lower dose therapy will eventually result in endometrial atrophy.

DANAZOL

Danazol is a weak androgen that is structurally related to testosterone and is used to treat endometriosis and endometrial hyperplasia. The endometrial changes resemble those seen with progestational agents. As with progestins, long-term therapy usually leads to atrophy[83,84] or a reduction in the severity of hyperplasia.[85]

TREATMENT OF ENDOMETRIAL LESIONS WITH PROGESTINS

Hormonal therapy, primarily high-dose progestin therapy, has long been used to treat lesions diagnosed as endometrial hyperplasia, EIN, and even well-differentiated adenocarcinomas in women who are poor surgical candidates or who wish to preserve fertility. Relatively high doses of progestins are used, typically 20–40 mg/day oral medroxyprogesterone acetate (Provera), 80 mg/day megestrol acetate (Megace), or intramuscular depo-medroxyprogesterone acetate (Depo-Provera). Levonorgestrel-releasing IUDs are also effective. Repeat biopsy is usually obtained (typically at around 3 months) to evaluate response to therapy. The histologic response to this therapy requires progesterone receptors within lesional tissue, a condition met in almost all non-atypical endometrial hyperplasias and EIN, and well-differentiated adenocarcinomas.[7]

Endometrium treated with high-dose progestins shows typical secretory changes in the first weeks of therapy. By 3 months, the endometrium in patients who respond completely shows diffuse and profound decidualization, with widely scattered atrophic-appearing glands similar to the decidua seen in pregnancy. A variety of metaplastic epithelial changes are commonly seen with progestin therapy, including squamous, mucinous, secretory, or eosinophilic.[86]

PROGESTIN THERAPY OF PERSISTENT ESTROGEN STATES (HYPERPLASIA)

Non-atypical endometrial hyperplasia, or benign endometrial hyperplasias, can be viewed as a primary endocrine abnormality of unopposed estrogens. In this circumstance even a functionally 'normal' endometrium responds by hyperplastic growth, and, eventually, development of symptoms of irregular menses and bleeding. Clinical management incorporates several elements, including establishing an underlying endocrine mechanism (anovulation, polycystic ovary syndrome, for example), assessment of intrinsic endometrial risk for neoplasia (to be ruled out on pathologic sampling), and symptomatic relief. Although symptomatic relief is often achieved through short- or medium-term progestin therapy and synchronized shedding of affected tissues, the condition may recur if the causal estrogen excess persists.

Short-term therapy with oral progestins leads to the formation of secretory vacuoles within the maintained architectural structure of the pre-existing lesion (Figure 15.29). Stromal decidualization and secretory exhaustion follows, but initially with the cysts and irregular glands of the underlying lesion (Figure 15.30). Eventually, and especially if a withdrawal shedding is allowed to occur, the hyperplastic architecture is lost (Figure 15.31). Incomplete responses are common, and may be caused by patient noncompliance, inadequate dose or duration, or lack of endometrial responsiveness. Adequacy of treatment can be assessed by repeat endometrial sampling, in conjunction with clinical symptoms.

If the underlying production of persistent estrogens is not remedied, the endometrium will revert to an anovulatory, or hyperplastic, appearance upon cessation of progestin therapy. Direct intrauterine delivery of progestins by placement of a hormonally impregnated IUD can provide long-term (years) endometrial treatment with the additional advantage of reducing the level of systemic exposure (Figure 15.32).

PROGESTIN THERAPY OF NEOPLASTIC LESIONS: EIN AND CARCINOMA

The histologic response of neoplastic (EIN and endometrioid type adenocarcinoma) endometrial tissues to progestin therapy is discussed in Chapters 17 and 18, respectively.

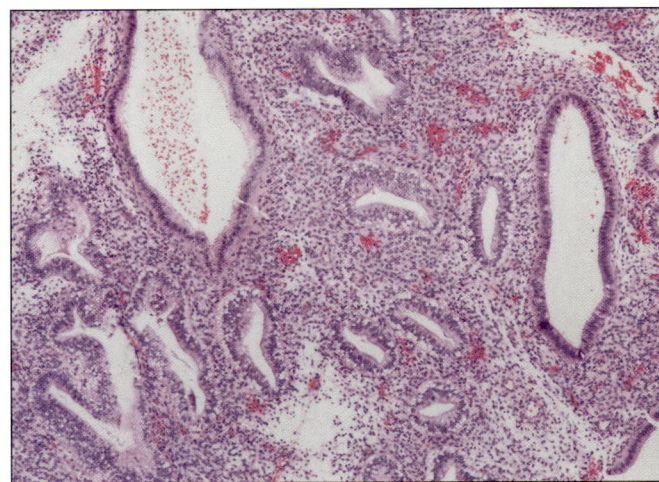

Figure 15.29 Short-term (days) oral progestin treatment of an anovulatory (unopposed estrogen type) endometrium retains the architecture of cysts and disordered glands, but with development of secretory vacuoles. Mitotic activity is not yet suppressed.

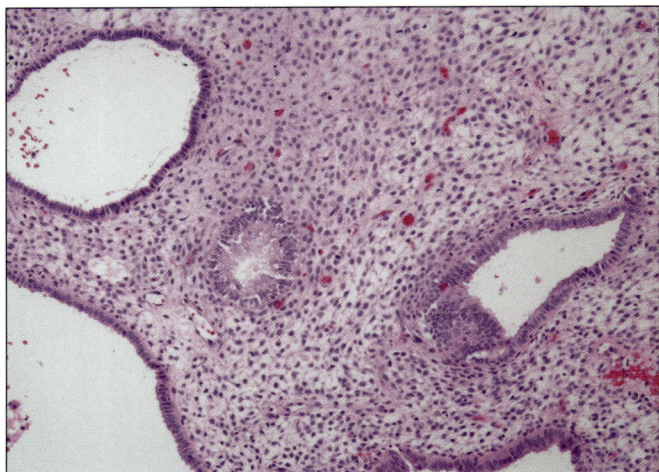

Figure 15.30 Anovulatory (unopposed estrogen type) endometrium treated for 1 week with oral progestins still retains the architecture of cysts and disordered glands, but now the secretory vacuoles are gone and the stroma is developing decidual change.

Generally, the therapeutic goal is to stabilize or ablate lesional tissues, and when successful the histologic appearance is dominated by hormonally altered background endometrium, which may revert to normal after cessation of therapy. Presently there are no clinically useful parameters to predict which lesions will, or will not, respond to therapy. A decision to treat medically is thus made on a clinical basis once a specific qualifying diagnosis is rendered.

Progestin-altered glands of persistent premalignant EIN lesions and adenocarcinoma may become widely separated by an expanded decidualized stroma, and acquire a bland nuclear cytology. This can make persistent disease difficult to recognize in biopsies taken while the patient is still receiving hormonal therapy. Close follow-up is always warranted even when there has been an apparently complete histologic response.[87]

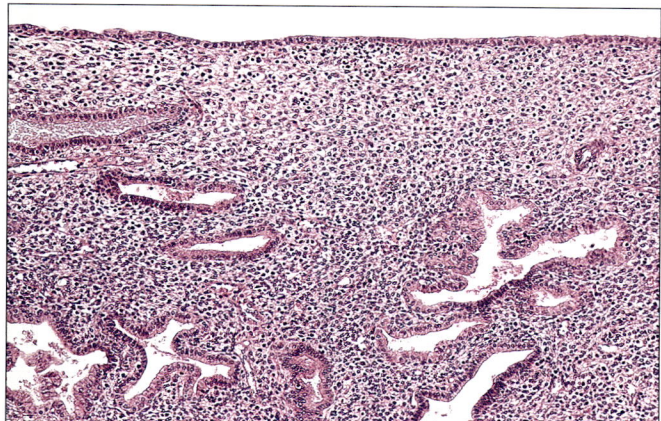

Figure 15.31 Changes in an endometrium treated with progesterone for simple hyperplasia. This woman had initially used high-dose Premarin over a long period, with shedding or involution of the hyperplastic glands. After a short period of receiving Depo-Provera, some of the endometrial glands show secretory changes. The stroma has become decidualized.

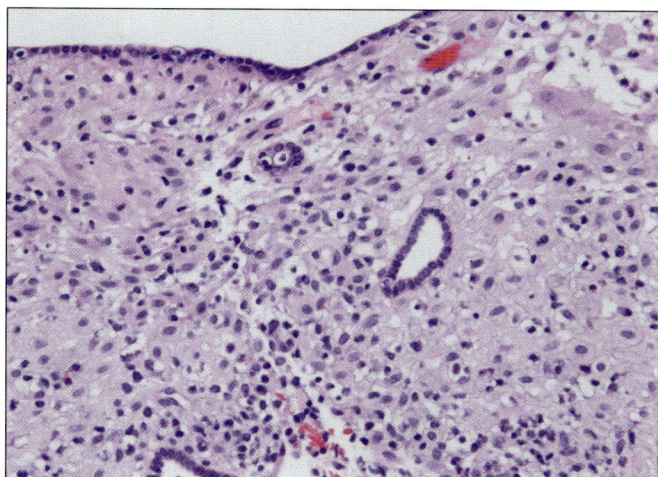

Figure 15.32 Stroma decidual changes, similar to pill endometrium, in a patient treated with a levonorgestrel IUD (Mirena). Long-term treatment has, in some areas, resulted in atrophic glands in a decidualized stroma.

REFERENCES

1. Schimmer BP, Parker KL. Contraception and Pharmacotherapy of Obstetrical and Gynecological Disorders. In: Brunton L, Chabner B, Knollmann B, editors. Goodman and Gilman's the pharmacological basis of therapeutics. 12th ed. New York: McGraw-Hill; 2011.
2. Weiss NS, Sayvetz TA. Incidence of endometrial cancer in relation to the use of oral contraceptives. N Engl J Med 1980;302:551–4.
3. Hannaford PC, Selvaraj S, Elliott AM, et al. Cancer risk among users of oral contraceptives: cohort data from the Royal College of General Practitioner's oral contraception study. BMJ 2007;335:651.
4. Bernstein L. The risk of breast, endometrial and ovarian cancer in users of hormonal preparations. Basic Clin Pharmacol Toxicol 2006;98:288–96.
5. Iodice S, Barile M, Rotmensz N, et al. Oral contraceptive use and breast or ovarian cancer risk in BRCA1/2 carriers: a meta-analysis. Eur J Cancer 2010;46:2275–84.
6. Rodolakis A, Thomakos N, Akrivos N, et al. Clinicopathologic insight of simultaneously detected primary endometrial and ovarian carcinomas. Arch Gynecol Obstet 2012;285(3):817–21.
7. Deligdisch L. Hormonal pathology of the endometrium. Mod Pathol 2000;13:285–94.
8. Ireland K, Zaino RJ. Iatrogenic patterns: what hath the physician wrought? In: Zaino RJ, editor. Interpretation of endometrial biopsies and curettings. New York: Lippincott-Raven; 1996. p. 143–73.
9. Mazur MT, Kurman RJ. Effects of hormones. Diagnosis of endometrial biopsies and curettings: a practical approach. New York: Springer-Verlag; 1995. p. 109–30.
10. Wynants P, Ide P. Endometrial morphology during a normophasic and a triphasic regimen: a comparison. Contraception 1986;33:149–57.
11. Archer DF. Endometrial histology during use of a low-dose estrogen-desogestrel oral contraceptive with a reduced hormone-free interval. Contraception 1999;60:151–4.
12. Kim-Bjorklund T, Landgren BM, Johannisson E. Morphometric studies of the endometrium, the fallopian tube and the corpus luteum during contraception with the 300 micrograms norethisterone (NET) minipill. Contraception 1991;43:459–74.
13. Rivera R, Yacobson I, Grimes D. The mechanism of action of hormonal contraceptives and intrauterine contraceptive devices. Am J Obstet Gynecol 1999;181:1263–9.
14. Hickey M, Simbar M, Young L, et al. A longitudinal study of changes in endometrial microvascular density in Norplant implant users. Contraception 1999;59:123–9.
15. Oliveira-Ribeiro M, Petta CA, De Angelo Andrade LA, et al. Correlation between endometrial histology, microvascular density and calibre, matrix metalloproteinase-3 and bleeding pattern in women using a levonorgestrel-releasing intrauterine system. Hum Reprod 2004;19:1778–84.
16. Rhoton-Vlasak A, Chegini N, Hardt N, Williams RS. Histological characteristics and altered expression of interleukins (IL) IL-13 and IL-15 in endometria of levonorgestrel users with different uterine bleeding patterns. Fertil Steril 2005;83:659–65.
17. Abou-Setta AM, Al-Inany HG, Farquhar CM. Levonorgestrel-releasing intrauterine device (LNG-IUD) for symptomatic endometriosis following surgery. Cochrane Database Syst Rev 2006:CD005072.
18. Busfield RA, Farquhar CM, Sowter MC, et al. A randomised trial comparing the levonorgestrel intrauterine system and thermal balloon ablation for heavy menstrual bleeding. BJOG 2006;113:257–63.
19. Roberts TE, Tsourapas A, Middleton LJ, et al. Hysterectomy, endometrial ablation, and levonorgestrel releasing intrauterine system (Mirena) for treatment of heavy menstrual bleeding: cost effectiveness analysis. BMJ 2011;342:d2202.
20. Jones RL, Critchley HO. Morphological and functional changes in human endometrium following intrauterine levonorgestrel delivery. Hum Reprod 2000;15 Suppl 3:162–72.
21. Anderson GL, Limacher M, Assaf AR, et al. Effects of conjugated equine estrogen in postmenopausal women with hysterectomy: the Women's Health Initiative randomized controlled trial. JAMA 2004;291:1701–12.
22. Udell JA, Fischer MA, Brookhart MA, et al. Effect of the Women's Health Initiative on osteoporosis therapy and expenditure in Medicaid. J Bone Miner Res 2006;21:765–71.
23. Effects of hormone replacement therapy on endometrial histology in postmenopausal women. The Postmenopausal Estrogen/Progestin Interventions (PEPI) Trial. The Writing Group for the PEPI Trial. JAMA 1996;275:370–5.
24. Weiderpass E, Adami HO, Baron JA, et al. Risk of endometrial cancer following estrogen replacement with and without progestins. J Natl Cancer Inst 1999;91:1131–7.
25. Beral V, Bull D, Reeves G. Endometrial cancer and hormone-replacement therapy in the Million Women Study. Lancet 2005;365:1543–51.
26. Cushing KL, Weiss NS, Voigt LF, et al. Risk of endometrial cancer in relation to use of low-dose, unopposed estrogens. Obstet Gynecol 1998;91:35–9.
27. Labrie F, Cusan L, Gomez JL, et al. Effect of one-week treatment with vaginal estrogen preparations on serum estrogen levels in postmenopausal women. Menopause 2009;16:30–6.

28. Calcagno A, Grassi T, Mariuzzi L, et al. Expression patterns of Aurora A and B kinases, Ki-67 and the estrogen and progesterone receptors determined using an endometriosis tissue microarray model. Hum Reprod 2011;26(10):2731–41.
29. Ettinger B. Rationale for use of lower estrogen doses for postmenopausal hormone therapy. Maturitas 2007;57:81–4.
30. Mutter GL, Zaino RJ, Baak JP, et al. Benign endometrial hyperplasia sequence and endometrial intraepithelial neoplasia. Int J Gynecol Pathol 2007;26:103–14.
31. Moyer DL, Felix JC. The effects of progesterone and progestins on endometrial proliferation. Contraception 1998;57:399–403.
32. Moyer DL, de Lignieres B, Driguez P, Pez JP. Prevention of endometrial hyperplasia by progesterone during long-term estradiol replacement: influence of bleeding pattern and secretory changes. Fertil Steril 1993;59:992–7.
33. Cerin A, Heldaas K, Moeller B. Adverse endometrial effects of long-cycle estrogen and progestogen replacement therapy. N Engl J Med 1996;334:668–9.
34. Carranza-Lira S, Martinez-Chequer JC, Santa Rita MT, et al. Endometrial changes according to hormone replacement therapy schedule. Menopause 1998;5:86–9.
35. Habiba MA, Bell SC, Al-Azzawi F. Endometrial responses to hormone replacement therapy: histological features compared with those of late luteal phase endometrium. Hum Reprod 1998;13:1674–82.
36. Vandermooren MJ, Hanselaar AGJM, Borm GF, Rolland R. Changes in the withdrawal bleeding pattern and endometrial histology during 17 beta-estradiol—dydrogesterone therapy in postmenopausal women: a 2 year prospective study. Maturitas 1994;20:175–80.
37. Piegsa K, Calder A, Davis JA, et al. Endometrial status in postmenopausal women on long-term continuous combined hormone replacement therapy (Kliofem). A comparative study of endometrial biopsy, outpatient hysteroscopy and transvaginal ultrasound. Eur J Obstet Gynecol Reprod Biol 1997;72:175–80.
38. Jordan VC, Brodie AM. Development and evolution of therapies targeted to the estrogen receptor for the treatment and prevention of breast cancer. Steroids 2007;72:7–25.
39. Ye J, Hameed O, Findeis-Hosey J, et al. Diagnostic utility of PAX8, TTF-1 and napsin A for discriminating metastatic carcinoma from primary adenocarcinoma of the lung. Biotech Histochem 2012;87(1):30–4.
40. Cohen I, Beyth Y, Altaras MM, et al. Estrogen and progesterone receptor expression in postmenopausal tamoxifen-exposed endometrial pathologies. Gynecol Oncol 1997;67:8–15.
41. Suh-Burgmann EJ, Goodman A. Surveillance for endometrial cancer in women receiving tamoxifen. Ann Intern Med 1999;131:127–35.
42. Seoud M, Shamseddine A, Khalil A, et al. Tamoxifen and endometrial pathologies: a prospective study. Gynecol Oncol 1999;75:15–9.
43. Deligdisch L, Kalir T, Cohen CJ, et al. Endometrial histopathology in 700 patients treated with tamoxifen for breast cancer. Gynecol Oncol 2000;78:181–6.
44. Kennedy MM, Baigrie CF, Manek S. Tamoxifen and the endometrium: review of 102 cases and comparison with HRT-related and non-HRT-related endometrial pathology. Int J Gynecol Pathol 1999;18:130–7.
45. Schlesinger C, Kamoi S, Ascher SM, et al. Endometrial polyps: a comparison study of patients receiving tamoxifen with two control groups. Int J Gynecol Pathol 1998;17:302–11.
46. Cohen I, Perel E, Tepper R, et al. Dose-dependent effect of tamoxifen therapy on endometrial pathologies in postmenopausal breast cancer patients. Breast Cancer Res Treat 1999;53:255–62.
47. Bernstein L, Deapen D, Cerhan JR, et al. Tamoxifen therapy for breast cancer and endometrial cancer risk. J Natl Cancer Inst 1999;91:1654–62.
48. Bland AE, Calingaert B, Secord AA, et al. Relationship between tamoxifen use and high risk endometrial cancer histologic types. Gynecol Oncol 2009;112:150–4.
49. Silva EG, Tornos CS, Follenmitchell M. Malignant neoplasms of the uterine corpus in patients treated for breast carcinoma—the effects of tamoxifen. Int J Gynecol Pathol 1994;13:248–58.
50. Treilleux T, Mignotte H, Clement-Chassagne C, et al. Tamoxifen and malignant epithelial-nonepithelial tumours of the endometrium: report of six cases and review of the literature. Eur J Surg Oncol 1999;25:477–82.
51. Arenas M, Rovirosa A, Hernandez V, et al. Uterine sarcomas in breast cancer patients treated with tamoxifen. Int J Gynecol Cancer 2006;16:861–5.
52. Boss SM, Huster WJ, Neild JA, et al. Effects of raloxifene hydrochloride on the endometrium of postmenopausal women. Am J Obstet Gynecol 1997;177:1458–64.
53. Davies GC, Huster WJ, Shen W, et al. Endometrial response to raloxifene compared with placebo, cyclical hormone replacement therapy, and unopposed estrogen in postmenopausal women. Menopause 1999;6:188–95.
54. DeMichele A, Troxel AB, Berlin JA, et al. Impact of raloxifene or tamoxifen use on endometrial cancer risk: a population-based case-control study. J Clin Oncol 2008;26:4151–9.
55. Pinkerton JV, Goldstein SR. Endometrial safety: a key hurdle for selective estrogen receptor modulators in development. Menopause 2010;17:642–53.
56. Grady D, Herrington D, Bittner V, et al. Cardiovascular disease outcomes during 6.8 years of hormone therapy: Heart and Estrogen/progestin Replacement Study follow-up (HERS II). JAMA 2002;288:49–57.
57. Lonning PE. Adjuvant endocrine treatment of early breast cancer. Hematol Oncol Clin North Am 2007;21:223–38.
58. Smith IE, Dowsett M. Aromatase inhibitors in breast cancer. N Engl J Med 2003;348:2431–42.
59. Ferrero S, Venturini PL, Ragni N, et al. Pharmacological treatment of endometriosis: experience with aromatase inhibitors. Drugs 2009;69:943–52.
60. Wagman I, Levin I, Kapustiansky R, et al. Clomiphene citrate vs. letrozole for cryopreserved-thawed embryo transfer: a randomized, controlled trial. J Reprod Med 2010;55:134–8.
61. Pritts EA. Letrozole for ovulation induction and controlled ovarian hyperstimulation. Curr Opin Obstet Gynecol 2010;22:289–94.
62. Eisen A, Trudeau M, Shelley W, et al. Aromatase inhibitors in adjuvant therapy for hormone receptor positive breast cancer: a systematic review. Cancer Treat Rev 2008;34:157–74.
63. Li HZ, Chen XN, Qiao J. Letrozole as primary therapy for endometrial hyperplasia in young women. Int J Gynaecol Obstet 2008;100:10–2.
64. Borrelli F, Ernst E. Alternative and complementary therapies for the menopause. Maturitas 2010;66:333–43.
65. Nicolae A, Goyenaga P, McCluggage WG, et al. Endometrial intestinal metaplasia: a report of two cases, including one associated with cervical intestinal and pyloric metaplasia. Int J Gynecol Pathol 2011;30:492–6.
66. Suh S, Kim KW. Diabetes and cancer: is diabetes causally related to cancer? Diabetes Metab J 2011;35:193–8.
67. Tanaka T, Bai T, Utsunomiya H, et al. STAT3 enhances intracellular Fas-mediated apoptotic signals in HHUA human endometrial epithelial cells. Mol Med Report 2011;4:307–12.
68. Wrenn DC, Saigal K, Lucci JA 3rd, et al. A Phase I Study using low-dose fractionated whole abdominal radiotherapy as a chemopotentiator to full-dose cisplatin for optimally debulked stage III/IV carcinoma of the endometrium. Gynecol Oncol 2011;122:59–62.
69. Tempfer CB, Froese G, Heinze G, et al. Side effects of phytoestrogens: a meta-analysis of randomized trials. Am J Med 2009;122:939–46.e9.
70. Bandera EV, Williams MG, Sima C, et al. Phytoestrogen consumption and endometrial cancer risk: a population-based case-control study in New Jersey. Cancer Causes Control 2009;20:1117–27.
71. Sereepapong W, Suwajanakorn S, Triratanachat S, et al. Effects of clomiphene citrate on the endometrium of regularly cycling women. Fertil Steril 2000;73:287–91.
72. Marotti JD, Glatz K, Parkash V, Hecht JL. International Internet-based assessment of observer variability for diagnostically challenging endometrial biopsies. Arch Pathol Lab Med 2011;135:464–70.
73. Benda JA. Clomiphene's effect on endometrium in infertility. Int J Gynecol Pathol 1992;11:273–82.
74. Tropea A, Miceli F, Minici F, et al. Endometrial evaluation in superovulation programs: relationship with successful outcome. Ann N Y Acad Sci 2004;1034:211–8.
75. Simon C, Oberye J, Bellver J, et al. Similar endometrial development in oocyte donors treated with either high- or standard-dose

GnRH antagonist compared to treatment with a GnRH agonist or in natural cycles. Hum Reprod 2005;20:3318–27.
76. Spitz IM. Clinical utility of progesterone receptor modulators and their effect on the endometrium. Curr Opin Obstet Gynecol 2009;21:318–24.
77. Ioffe OB, Zaino RJ, Mutter GL. Endometrial changes from short-term therapy with CDB-4124, a selective progesterone receptor modulator. Mod Pathol 2009;22:450–9.
78. Mutter GL, Bergeron C, Deligdisch L, et al. The spectrum of endometrial pathology induced by progesterone receptor modulators. Mod Pathol 2008;21:591–8.
79. Fiscella J, Bonfiglio T, Winters P, et al. Distinguishing features of endometrial pathology after exposure to the progesterone receptor modulator mifepristone. Hum Pathol 2011;42:947–53.
80. Lethaby A, Vollenhoven B, Sowter M. Pre-operative GnRH analogue therapy before hysterectomy or myomectomy for uterine fibroids. Cochrane Database Syst Rev 2001:CD000547.
81. Sowter MC, Lethaby A, Singla AA. Pre-operative endometrial thinning agents before endometrial destruction for heavy menstrual bleeding. Cochrane Database Syst Rev 2002:CD001124.
82. Heller DS. Hormonal effects on the endometrium—dysfunctional uterine bleeding, iatrogenic hormonal effects, and luteal phase defects. New York: Igaku-Shoin Medical Publishing; 1994.
83. Matias-Guiu X, Oliva E. Pathology of the endometrium. Introduction. Semin Diagn Pathol 2010;27:197–8.
84. Cheng W, Wang YJ, Zhang X, Gao XM. [The effect on angiogenesis of endometrium after transcervical resection of polyp]. Sichuan Da Xue Xue Bao Yi Xue Ban 2010;41:854–7.
85. Gomez-Lopez N, Vadillo-Perez L, Nessim S, et al. Choriodecidua and amnion exhibit selective leukocyte chemotaxis during term human labor. Am J Obstet Gynecol 2011;204:364.e9–16.
86. Miranda MC, Mazur MT. Endometrial squamous metaplasia: an unusual response to progestin therapy of hyperplasia. Arch Pathol Lab Med 1995;119:458–60.
87. Wheeler DT, Bristow RE, Kurman RJ. Histologic alterations in endometrial hyperplasia and well-differentiated carcinoma treated with progestins. Am J Surg Pathol 2007;31:988–98.

16 Endometritis, Metaplasias, Polyps, and Miscellaneous Changes

George L. Mutter, Joseph W. Carlson

CHAPTER OUTLINE

Inflammatory and Infectious Processes	326	Metaplasias to Nonspecific Cell Types	340
Endometritis	326	Mesenchymal Metaplasias	342
Nonspecific Endometritis	327	Endometrial Polyps	342
Specific Forms of Endometritis	328	Atypical Polypoid Adenomyoma	345
Other Forms of Endometritis	330	Miscellaneous Conditions	345
Endometrial Metaplasias	331	Asherman's Syndrome	345
Epithelial Metaplasias	332	Radiation Effect	346
Tubal Metaplasia	332	The Effects of the IUD on the Endometrium	346
Squamous Metaplasia	333	Endometrial Ablation	347
Mucinous Metaplasia	336		
Secretory Metaplasia	339		

INFLAMMATORY AND INFECTIOUS PROCESSES

Infections of the gynecologic tract are relatively common, and cause an enormous health impact. It is estimated that there are 19 million cases of sexually transmitted diseases (STDs) in the United States, with a total healthcare cost of roughly $16.4 billion.[1] These infections can be both symptomatic and asymptomatic, and it is believed that up to 24,000 cases of infertility in the United States are related to STDs. Symptomatic infections are most commonly diagnosed based on the clinical examination and basic laboratory studies, and, as such, a tissue biopsy is generally not needed. Approximately 20% of cases of STD can result in pelvic inflammatory disease (PID), which is inflammation of the uterus, fallopian tubes, or ovaries. An unknown fraction of STDs lead to asymptomatic infections, or to signs that are not recognized to be related to infection, such as dysfunctional uterine bleeding. Chronic endometritis has been shown to interfere with local expression of estrogen and progesterone receptors in the endometrium, which may also contribute to infertility.[2] It is especially in the evaluation of women with bleeding that a diagnosis of infection is critical. STDs can be readily treated, and proper treatment can prevent later complications. In a minority of cases the pattern of inflammation in the endometrium is indicative of a specific organism (Table 16.1). In the majority of cases the pattern of inflammation is nonspecific.

Endometrial inflammation is recognized, as in other organs, primarily by the presence of inflammatory cells. However, as the endometrium may normally contain inflammatory cells, the diagnosis of endometritis is often not straightforward. Lymphocytes, even when focally collected around blood vessels, are not necessarily indicative of endometritis. As plasma cells are seldom found in a normal endometrium, their presence is indicative of chronic endometritis. Neutrophil polymorphonuclear leukocytes may also be found in the normal cycle, especially in appreciable numbers once menstruation is well established. Granulated lymphocytes, or CD56+ uterine natural killer cells, present in the stroma during the second half of the cycle, and especially in predecidua, are easily mistaken for neutrophils.[3,4] Macrophages are always present in the normal endometrium, but in their usual appearance resemble endometrial stromal cells, rendering separation difficult.

ENDOMETRITIS

Patients with endometritis often present with the clinical features of PID. They will have a history of fever and lower abdominal pain, with leukocytosis and bilateral adnexal or cervical motion tenderness on bimanual pelvic

Table 16.1 Classification of Endometritis

Specific microorganism
    Neisseria
    Tuberculosis
    Chlamydia
    Mycoplasma
    Cytomegalovirus (CMV)
    Herpes simplex virus (HSV)
No specific microorganism
    Associated with intrauterine contraceptive device
    Granulomatous (excluding tuberculosis)
    Histiocytic
    Postpartum
    Postabortal
    Pyometra
    Not otherwise specified (chronic nonspecific)

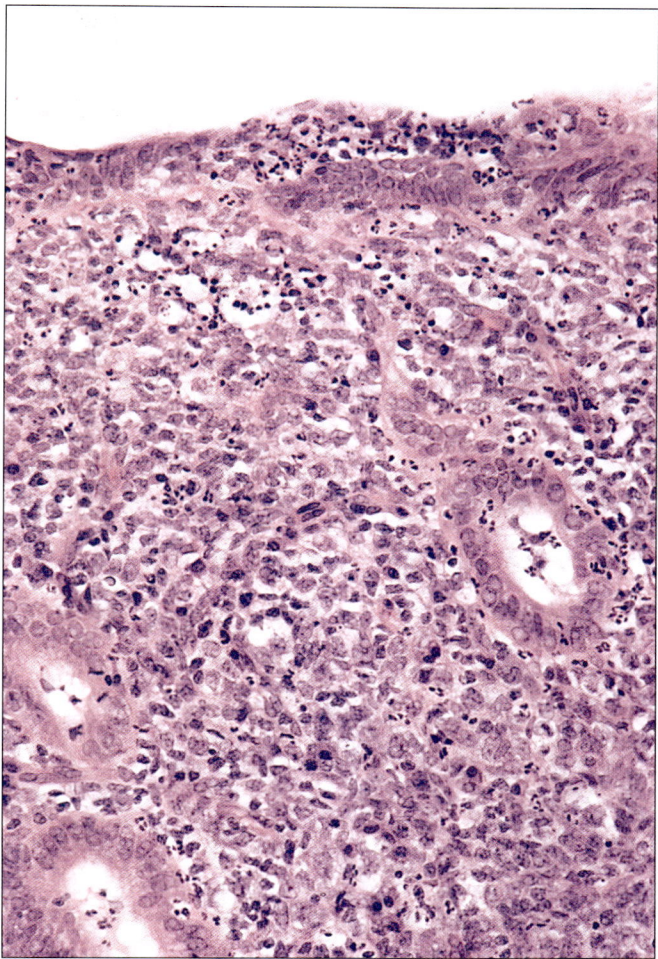

Figure 16.1 Acute endometritis. Polymorphs are present in the surface epithelium and throughout the stroma.

examination. If the infecting organism is less virulent or if the disease is early in its natural history, the symptoms, such as menstrual abnormalities, pelvic pain, or infertility, may not initially indicate the clinical diagnosis of endometritis. Although most cases of acute salpingitis are accompanied by endometritis, it is not known how often endometritis occurs in isolation, without involving the fallopian tubes. The diagnosis of endometritis is therefore often a histologic one that, particularly in the case of nonspecific endometritis, is not associated with a specific clinical presentation or cause.

NONSPECIFIC ENDOMETRITIS

Microscopic Features

The histologic diagnosis of acute endometritis is made when significant numbers of neutrophils are present in the endometrial stroma at a time other than menstruation (Figure 16.1). Isolated or rare neutrophils are insufficient for a diagnosis of acute endometritis. The usual pattern is that of patchy distribution, with or without microabscesses. As with all forms of endometritis, it is not only the presence of a particular inflammatory cell that is important, but also the reaction pattern of the endometrium. A common appearance in the patient of reproductive age is glandular dyssynchrony in response to circulating sex hormones. In the case of acute endometritis it should be accompanied by other features of inflammation and repair, including edema, hemorrhage, venule ectasia, microabscesses, or pus-filled glands. In the case of menstrual endometrium other features of menstruation are typically seen, including secretory vacuoles in the glandular epithelium and predecidual change of the stroma with diffuse stromal breakdown. It may not always be possible to distinguish between acute endometritis and menstrual endometrium.

The acute inflammation seen in acute endometritis is often confined to the upper layers of the functionalis, leading to shedding of the inflamed tissue during menstruation. Assuming that the organism that precipitated the endometritis is no longer present, a new functionalis can develop from a healthy basalis layer. If the infection is not treated then the inflammation will proceed to chronic endometritis.

If plasma cells are present, often seen together with aggregates of lymphocytes and/or germinal centers, then a diagnosis of chronic endometritis is made (Figure 16.2). A not uncommon problem occurs when only a rare plasma cell is identified or it is a minor component of the infiltrate. If on a low-power magnification the endometrium looks 'dirty' with numerous lymphocytes (Figure 16.3), a careful search under higher magnification often shows scattered plasma cells that justify a diagnosis of chronic endometritis. Areas worthy of particular attention include glands engorged with inflammatory cells. As plasma cells may be a normal component within the stroma of the endocervix and lower uterine segment, care must be taken to ensure that only the functionalis is assessed.

Glands may be involved in the inflammatory process in two ways. There may be an infiltrate of inflammatory cells, predominantly neutrophils, affecting the epithelium of the glands and the lumina may contain pus. In addition, as the process becomes more advanced, the glandular response to hormonal stimulation becomes impaired, the glands appearing inactive, with neither proliferation nor secretion. Once

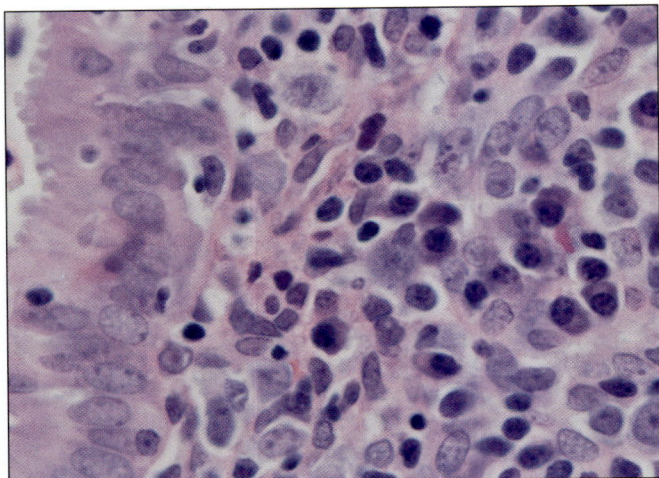

Figure 16.2 Chronic endometritis. Plasma cells are prominent in the stroma.

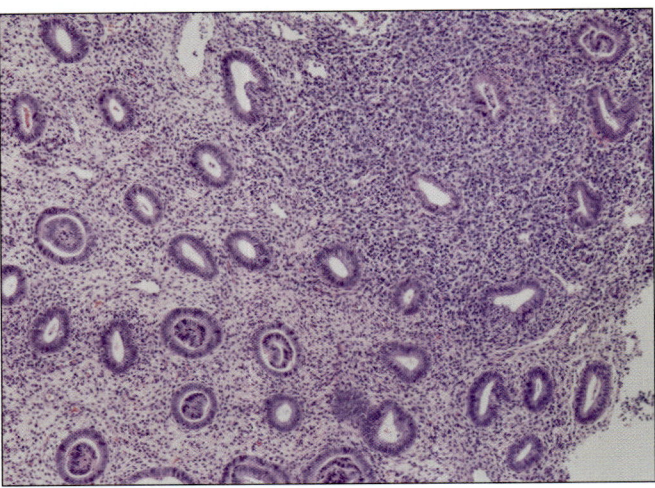

Figure 16.3 Chronic endometritis. At low magnification, the presence of a patchy infiltrate of inflammatory cells makes the stroma appear dirty.

Table 16.2 Histologic Features of Endometritis
Neutrophil infiltrate in microabscesses or gland lumens
Plasma cell infiltrate
Lymphocyte infiltrate (focal collections with germinal centers)
Edema
Vascular ectasia
Necrosis and fragmentation of stroma
Suppression of glandular hormonal response

an endometrium shows signs of endometritis, precise dating is not possible. It is probably not even reliable to categorize the endometrium as either proliferative or secretory. Dating is unnecessary in a patient who has significant endometritis. The histologic features of endometritis are summarized in Table 16.2.

Routine Biomarkers of Clinical Relevance

Several studies have investigated the use of biomarkers (both histochemical and immunohistochemical methods) to aid in the identification of plasma cells. Because rare plasma cells can be identified in the background of women without the other diagnostic features of chronic endometritis described earlier, the routine use of these methods is not currently recommended. Instead, a careful histologic examination by routine H&E stain using the previous criteria is recommended.

Differential Diagnosis

The most difficult aspect in the diagnosis of endometritis is simply recognizing it and, when necessary, initiating a search for plasma cells and other histologic features consistent with the diagnosis. The differential diagnosis includes normal menstrual endometrium, where (nonplasma cell) inflammatory cells are widespread, and plasma-cell-bearing fragments of cervix or lower uterine segment, which are mistaken for endometrial tissue.

SPECIFIC FORMS OF ENDOMETRITIS

CHLAMYDIA TRACHOMATIS AND *NEISSERIA GONORRHOEAE*

Many upper genital tract infections result from the sexually transmitted organisms *Chlamydia trachomatis* and *Neisseria gonorrhoeae*.[5,6] Infection by *C. trachomatis* exhibits supranuclear, intracytoplasmic vacuoles containing inclusions, but these are not readily apparent by microscopic examination. Immunohistologic or molecular methods are usually required for confirmation of chlamydial infection. Polymerase chain reaction identifies *C. trachomatis* in one-fourth of plasma cell endometritis specimens, and these can also be cultured.[7,8] Endometritis due to either *Chlamydia* or *Neisseria* has large numbers of plasma cells in the endometrial stroma, neutrophils in the endometrial surface epithelium, and lymphoid aggregates with transformed lymphocytes,[9] thus providing clues to the diagnosis. Intraluminal neutrophils and subepithelial hemorrhages are also usually present, but these findings are less specific. Histopathology alone can suggest, but not reliably distinguish between, these organisms. Prominent lymphoid follicles with transformed lymphocytes points more to chlamydial infection while extensive stromal fragmentation favors gonococcal infection.[5]

MYCOPLASMA

Infection with the mycoplasma *Ureaplasma urealyticum* produces subtle but distinctive changes that may be easily missed. *Mycoplasma* is the second most common etiologic agent after common bacteria.[10] The changes are focal, composed of lymphocytic clusters with histiocytes and occasional neutrophils. Plasma cells are not prominent. These focal collections often lie beneath the surface epithelium, around glands, and surrounding spiral arterioles. In many of these patients, *U. urealyticum* also has been cultured from the uterine cervix, suggesting an ascending infection. *Mycoplasma genitalium* is a common pathogen associated with acute endometritis.[11]

CYTOMEGALOVIRUS

Cytomegalovirus (CMV) infection of the endometrium has been reported rarely and may be associated with pregnancy

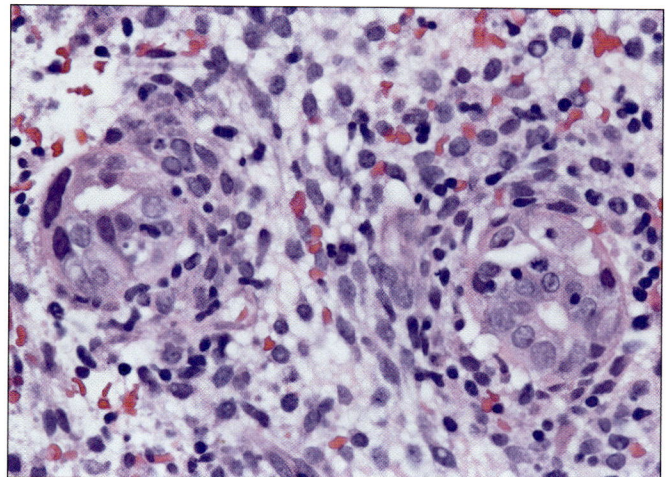

Figure 16.4 Cytomegalovirus infection. Cells with grossly enlarged nuclei are present in small glands.

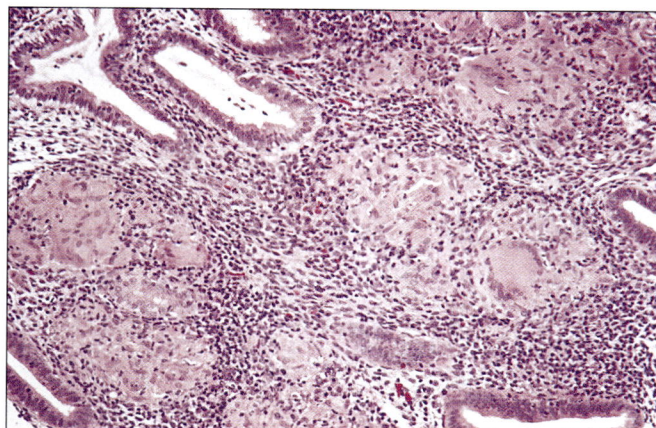

Figure 16.5 Tuberculous endometritis. Noncaseating granulomas are distributed throughout the stroma.

and immunosuppression as well as being found in women with no known underlying disorder. The affected epithelial and sometimes endothelial cells are grossly enlarged and each contains a usually single large, basophilic intranuclear inclusion that is surrounded by a narrow clear space separating it from the nuclear membrane (Figure 16.4).

HERPES SIMPLEX VIRUS

Like CMV infection, herpes simplex virus (HSV) infection of the endometrium is rare. It may occur as an ascending process associated with cervical infection or result from disseminated virus in immunosuppressed patients. It may cause postpartum endometritis in cases where infants have died from disseminated HSV infection.[5] Infection of the endometrium produces changes similar to those associated with HSV elsewhere, namely extensive acute inflammation with necrosis. Cowdry type A inclusions and, occasionally, multinucleated giant cells with ground-glass nuclei may be identified in glandular epithelium or in the stroma.

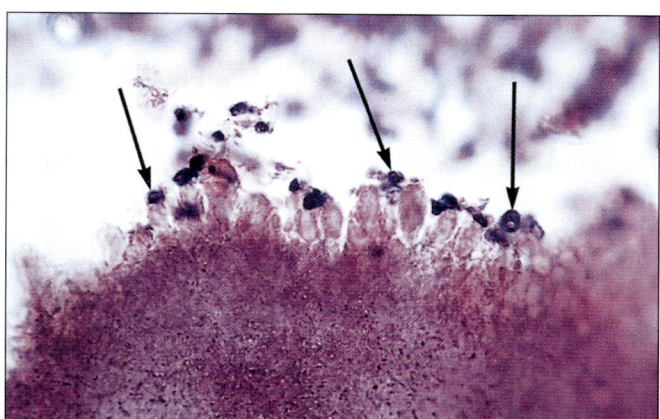

Figure 16.6 Intrauterine device. *Actinomyces*. Sulfur granule with clubs (arrows).

TUBERCULOUS ENDOMETRITIS

Although tuberculosis has become infrequent in the United States, it remains an endemic disease in some parts of the world[12] and more may be seen in the future as a result of the emergence of drug-resistant strains of *Mycobacterium tuberculosis* and the immunosuppression of AIDS. Tuberculosis of the female genital tract is virtually always secondary to disease of the lungs or gastrointestinal tract, which often occurred many years previously. About three-fourths of women with tuberculosis of the genital tract have endometrial involvement. The fallopian tubes are almost always involved and the endometrium is affected secondarily by passage of the bacteria down the tube into the uterine cavity.

The disease may present without gynecologic symptoms or it may be associated with infertility, irregular bleeding, or amenorrhea. The principal histologic feature is the epithelioid cell granuloma. These may be sparse, so that a thorough search of the material is required if tuberculosis is suspected clinically. The granulomas are usually small and central caseation is unusual, especially in women who have normal, or near normal, menstrual cycles. Caseation is found only when there is amenorrhea or after menopause, for it is only when the endometrium no longer periodically sheds that there is sufficient time for the granuloma to develop *de novo* and then caseate. The disease process affects all layers of the endometrium.

The granuloma of tuberculous endometritis contains a central collection of epithelioid cells with both Langhans and foreign body-type giant cells (Figure 16.5). There is usually a peripheral collar of lymphocytes. Because caseation is absent, the granulomas more closely resemble those of sarcoidosis, a feature reinforced because they are well circumscribed. Uterine sarcoidosis rarely presents without proven sarcoidosis elsewhere in the body.

Culture of the endometrial tissue best confirms the diagnosis. In a classic study that has not been repeated, acid-fast bacilli were demonstrated in less than 2% of 1134 women with culture-proven organisms.[13] More recently molecular methods have been developed that allow the specific detection, and strain classification, of *M. tuberculosis* in formalin-fixed paraffin-embedded materials at a level of sensitivity exceeding that of special stains.[14–16]

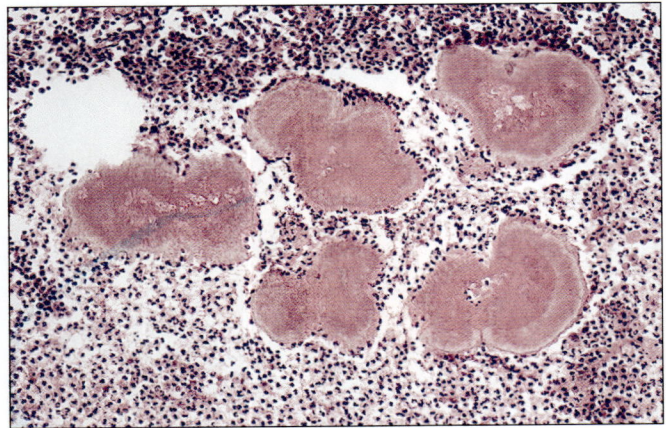

Figure 16.7 Intrauterine device. *Actinomyces*. Sulfur granules surrounded by pus.

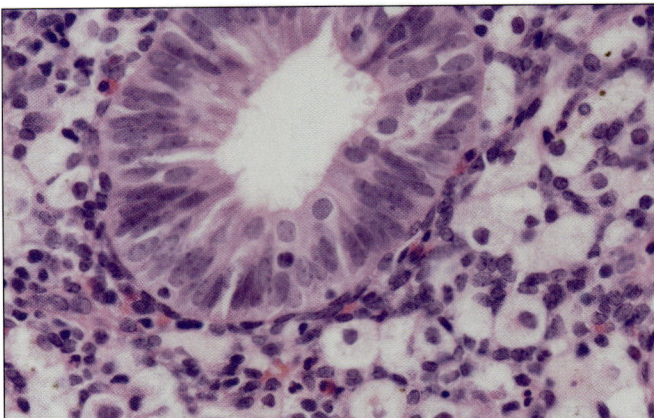

Figure 16.8 Histiocytic endometritis.

ACTINOMYCES ISRAEILII

Infection by *Actinomyces israeilii* has long been associated with intrauterine contraceptive device (IUD) usage.[17] This organism is a slow-growing, filamentous, Gram-positive anaerobe that is not normally found in the lower genital tract (Figure 16.6). When found in cervical smears or curettings, half the women lack symptoms. Microscopic examination of the curettings shows densely matted filaments of the Gram-positive organisms (Figure 16.7). Gomori methenamine silver stain is positive in *Actinomyces*, which is a useful means of identifying noninfectious pseudoactinomycotic radiate granules (negatively staining) that are even more common than actual organisms in women with an IUD.[18,19] There is usually some degree of associated endometritis, with a dense infiltrate of neutrophils. The infection may progress to pelvic actinomycosis. The risk of infection by *A. israeli* relates less to the type of IUD in use than the length of time it has been in place in the uterine cavity; 85% of cases occur when the IUD has been worn for 3 or more years.

OTHER FORMS OF ENDOMETRITIS

GRANULOMATOUS ENDOMETRITIS

The finding of granulomas in an endometrial biopsy can be caused by a variety of diseases. In a recent review granulomas were identified in 0.15% of endometrial biopsies.[20] Focal granulomas, that is the finding of a single granulomatous focus, were significantly associated with a prior history of cesarean section or dilatation and curettage, and none of the women had any signs of a systemic disorder or infection upon follow-up. In terms of infection, granulomas can be caused by tuberculosis (as described previously), atypical mycobacteria, endemic mycosis, actinomycosis, and parasites.[20,21] Noninfectious causes can include a reaction to foreign material, Crohn disease, sarcoidosis, or lymphoma. Granulomas can also be seen postsurgically. Sarcoidosis is associated with well-formed, clearly demarcated epithelioid cell granulomas lacking central necrosis. It occurs usually, but not always, in women with known systemic disease. However, as necrosis is unusual in tuberculous endometritis, endometrial sarcoid should only be diagnosed if the disease is present elsewhere in the body. An effort should be made to identify a treatable, infective cause if it is present. Fungi may be identified using periodic acid–Schiff (PAS) or Grocott stains, but it is questionable whether a time-consuming search for acid-fast bacilli is worth undertaking because of the very low chance of identifying the organism, even in culture-proven cases.[13] The identification of pigment or birefringence under polarized light points to a foreign body reaction. A clinical history may also be useful in coming to a conclusion.

HISTIOCYTIC ENDOMETRITIS

On rare occasions, the endometrium discloses a massive infiltrate of histiocytes that contain abundant lipid, together with multinucleated giant cells, hemosiderin, cholesterol clefts, plasma cells, lymphocytes, and occasional neutrophils (Figure 16.8). This may occur in association with pyometra, due to postmenopausal cervical stenosis, or in association with an endometrial glandular neoplasm. The terms 'pseudoxanthoma' and 'xanthogranuloma' have also been used but the term 'histiocytic endometritis' is preferred. The condition bears no relation to the focal clusters of foamy macrophages sometimes found in the stroma of endometrial carcinomas. Appearances similar to histiocytic endometritis may be seen in the fallopian tube. Malakoplakia is a rare variant of histiocytic endometritis. The appearances are generally similar to those already described but in addition Michaelis–Gutmann bodies are present. These are small, round, laminated calcospherules that may be found both in the cytoplasm of the histiocytes and also extracellularly.

POSTPARTUM AND POSTABORTAL ENDOMETRITIS

Endometritis occurs in 2–5% of women following vaginal delivery, 20–55% of women following cesarean section, and 1–8% of women having termination of pregnancy in a hospital setting.[22] The risk of endometritis is even higher in women with retained products of conception. Plasma cell infiltrates, which are not a normal postpartum response, are characteristic of postpartum chronic endometritis

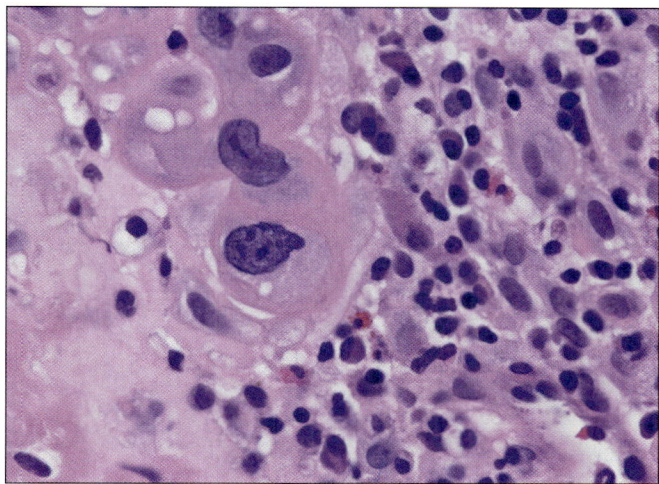

Figure 16.9 Postabortal chronic endometritis. Plasma cells are adjacent to a recent nodular implantation site.

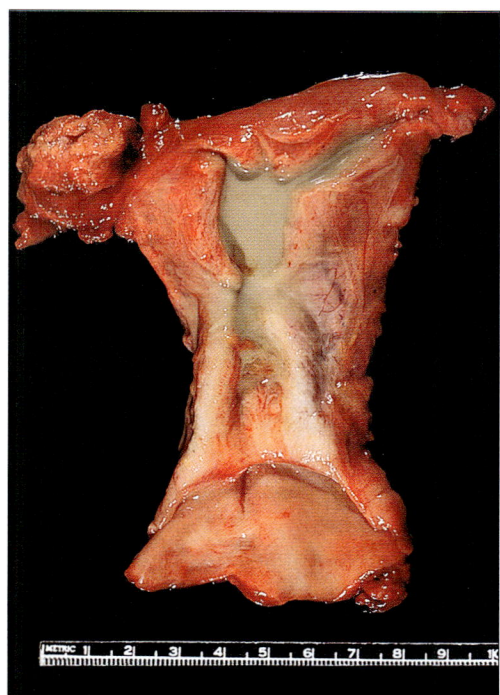

Figure 16.10 Pyometrium.

(Figure 16.9). Microbiologic examination shows that the infection is caused by two or more microorganisms, the most frequently cultured being *U. urealyticum* and *Gardnerella vaginalis*. The latter is most commonly associated with bacterial vaginosis and clinical evidence of bacterial vaginosis is associated with a sixfold increase in the risk of post-cesarean endometritis.[23] Furthermore, recent studies have shown that bacterial vaginosis is associated with a higher risk of endometritis[9] and upper genital tract infection in the nonpregnant state.[24]

Following elective and spontaneous abortion, the infective organisms are more likely to be the usual pathogens, *Escherichia coli*, *Staphylococcus aureus*, *N. gonorrhoeae*, and *Streptococcus viridans*.

The histopathologic features of the endometrium in these forms of endometritis are usually those of an acute infection, with prominence of neutrophils and tissue necrosis. Organisms are often identified by Gram stain.

PYOMETRA

Inflammation of the endometrium is most dramatic when pyometra, pus filling the uterine cavity, develops (Figure 16.10). This is often due to a blocked cervical canal in conditions such as cervical carcinoma or, more frequently, postmenopausal stenosis. Introduction of foreign material through fistulous tracts is another common cause. As the term implies, the cavity of the distended uterus is filled with pus and the endometrium usually shows the features of severe acute and chronic inflammation (Figure 16.11). Squamous metaplasia may develop in the surface epithelium and glands, and at its most extreme is known as ichthyosis uteri.[25] Squamous cell carcinoma, rarely, may also occur.

ENDOMETRIAL METAPLASIAS

Endometrial metaplasia is a change in cellular differentiation to a type that is not present in the normal endometrium. Terms such as metaplasia, differentiation, and 'change' are

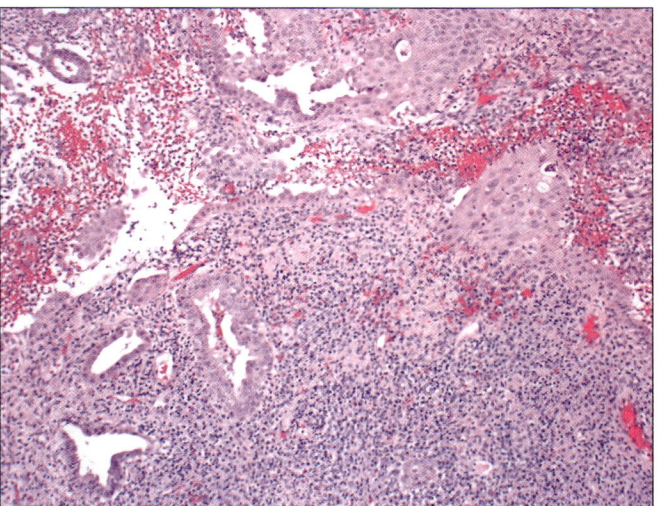

Figure 16.11 Acute inflammatory infiltrate and severe epithelial reactive change in pyometrium.

used, often interchangeably, to reflect the wide variety of cell types that can be seen in the endometrium. These can include alterations in cytoplasm, nuclei, and even architecture. Metaplasia most commonly involves the epithelial compartment but can also involve the stromal compartment. Because altered differentiation may be seen in benign, premalignant, or malignant endometria, a simple diagnosis of endometrial metaplasia is rarely sufficient to fully convey the lesion's clinical significance. Endometrial metaplasias are best considered a spectrum of altered differentiation states in which the pathologist should attempt to determine the underlying mechanism, and use terminology that clearly communicates clinical significance to the referring physician.

EPITHELIAL METAPLASIAS

The epithelium of the upper female genital tract, whether endocervical, endometrial, or tubal, is all of paramesonephric (müllerian) origin, but each area shows its own characteristic cell type: mucus secreting in the cervix, ciliated in the fallopian tube, and columnar with secretory potential in the endometrium. The most common forms of endometrial metaplasia are those in which endometrial glands assume a morphology resembling that seen elsewhere along the müllerian duct, such as serous, mucinous, or squamous. Müllerian-derived structures thus maintain an element of plasticity in which any of a number of pathogenetic mechanisms may incite differentiation inappropriate for the particular anatomic location. The resultant metaplasia is accompanied by the appearance of differentiated structures and protein expression patterns usually associated with a specific nonendometrial cell type, such as intracellular mucin in mucinous metaplasia, cilia in tubal metaplasia, or keratin in squamous metaplasia. In practice, use of the term 'metaplasia' is not constrained to a change in differentiation, having been extended as a descriptive label for some nonspecific degenerative changes.

Etiology

The term metaplasia applies to a broad range of cytologic appearances caused by degenerative, hormonal, or neoplastic processes (Table 16.3). The overall low-magnification topography of metaplastic changes within the endometrial compartment, combined with the local histologic context, are extremely useful in ascertaining a likely cause.[26,27] Degenerative changes can be localized to areas of inflammation, stromal breakdown, or recent surface repair.

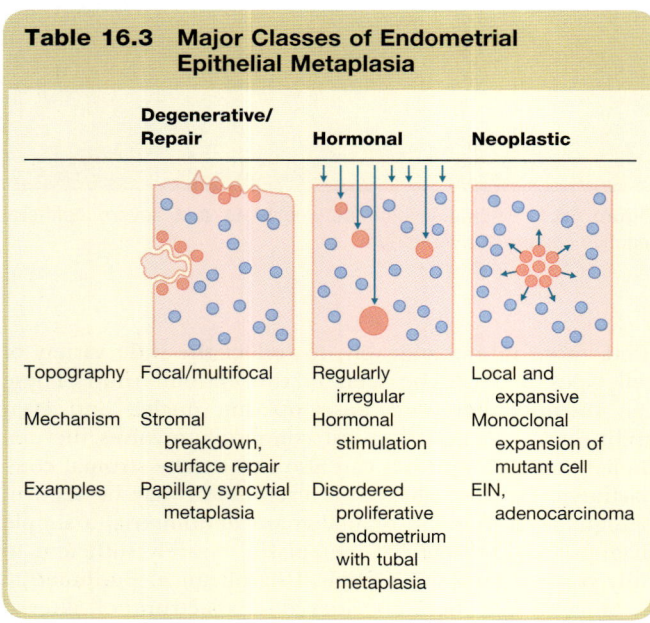

Table 16.3 Major Classes of Endometrial Epithelial Metaplasia

	Degenerative/Repair	Hormonal	Neoplastic
Topography	Focal/multifocal	Regularly irregular	Local and expansive
Mechanism	Stromal breakdown, surface repair	Hormonal stimulation	Monoclonal expansion of mutant cell
Examples	Papillary syncytial metaplasia	Disordered proliferative endometrium with tubal metaplasia	EIN, adenocarcinoma

Hormonally induced changes tend to be diffusely and randomly scattered throughout the upper endometrial compartment (functionalis), whereas premalignant and malignant processes are monoclonal expansions that begin as localizing lesions offset by the normal background. The genetic underpinnings of müllerian metaplasia are just now emerging. Genetic mediators of müllerian differentiation include members of the homeobox gene superfamily, HOX, where coordinate expression of HOX genes determines differentiation state.[28] Altered HOX gene expression, through hormonal[29,30] or epigenetic mechanisms,[31,32] is capable of re-determining differentiation state. For example, HOXA11 expression can be induced by progestins and in müllerian epithelium is associated with acquisition of mucinous differentiation.[33]

Many instances of degenerative metaplasia will show an underlying cause, such as physical irritation due to an intrauterine mass lesion (submucous fibroid, polyp), inflammatory conditions (endometritis), or breakdown of endometrial stroma. Most are not true metaplasias demonstrating features of specialized altered differentiation, but rather histologic mimics where use of the term descriptively augments a more specific diagnosis of endometritis or breakdown. An example is 'papillary syncytial metaplasia,' which exhibits papillary fronds of epithelium that have lost nuclear polarity and can be seen in association with breakdown of supporting stroma, irritation of the uterine lining epithelium, or as part of a reparative process.

Hormonally induced metaplasias are common and not always abnormal, particularly in the case of estrogen-induced tubal change. Estrogens may induce tubal metaplasia of endometrial glands in a random interspersed pattern throughout the entire endometrial compartment at a density depending on dose and duration of exposure. Estrogen-induced tubal metaplasia is most frequently seen in women around the time of menopause and just afterward, and is associated with abnormal uterine bleeding.

A particular pitfall in dealing with endometrial neoplasms with altered (metaplastic) differentiation is the incorrect assumption that metaplasia and neoplasia are mutually exclusive processes. Squamous, mucinous, tubal, or secretory differentiation may be acquired features intrinsic to a premalignant (endometrial intraepithelial neoplasia; EIN) or malignant (adenocarcinoma) neoplastic clone.[34-37] In these instances, altered differentiation is best noted descriptively appended to a primary diagnosis of EIN or adenocarcinoma (Table 16.4). Individual examples of EIN or adenocarcinoma can demonstrate quite unstable differentiation states in which admixed cytologies line individual glands or populate different regions of the neoplastic field.[34,38,39] In the case of metaplastic premalignant lesions, all EIN criteria must be met (Chapter 17),[40] with the observed change in cellular differentiation sometimes contributing to the altered cytology requirement. Overtly malignant processes, especially mucinous and secretory adenocarcinomas, may have unusually bland nuclei as part of their altered differentiation state.

TUBAL METAPLASIAS

Tubal differentiation is the most commonly encountered form of endometrial metaplasia, accounting for 60% of

CHAPTER 16 — ENDOMETRITIS, METAPLASIAS, POLYPS, AND MISCELLANEOUS CHANGES

Table 16.4 Diagnostic Terminology of Benign, Premalignant, and Malignant Endometrial Epithelial Metaplasias

Differentiation	Benign	Premalignant	Malignant
Tubal	• Normal proliferative endometrium with tubal metaplasia • Disordered proliferative endometrium with tubal metaplasia • Non-atypical endometrial hyperplasia with tubal metaplasia	• EIN with tubal differentiation	• Endometrial adenocarcinoma, endometrioid type, with tubal differentiation
Squamous	• Chronic endometritis with squamous differentiation (ichthyosis uteri) • Isolated squamous morules (requires follow-up)	• EIN with morular squamous differentiation	• Endometrial adenocarcinoma, endometrioid type, with squamous (morular/non-morular) differentiation
Mucinous	• Mucinous degenerative changes • Polyp, mixed endometrial and endocervical type • Benign mucinous differentiation	• EIN with mucinous differentiation	• Endometrial adenocarcinoma, endometrioid type, with mucinous differentiation
Secretory	• Secretory endometrium, mixed type • Hypersecretory endometrium (includes Arias-Stella)	• EIN with secretory differentiation	• Endometrial adenocarcinoma, endometrioid type, with secretory differentiation

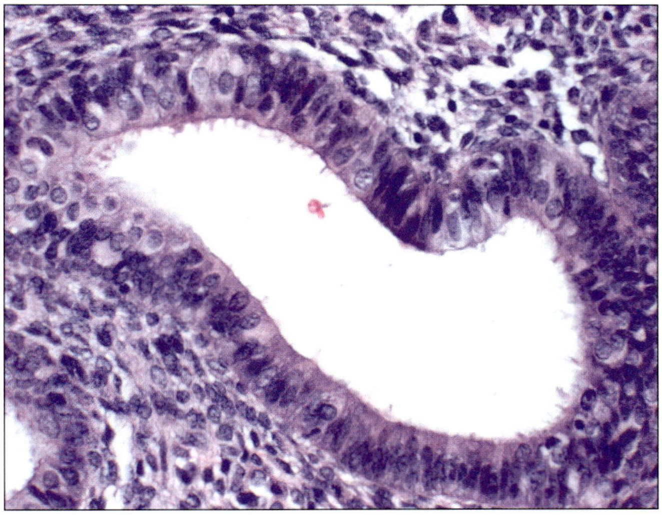

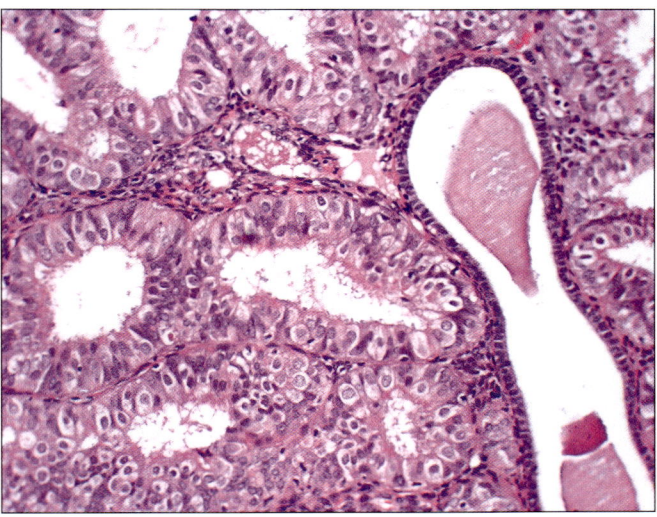

Figure 16.12 Tubal (ciliated cell) metaplasia.

Figure 16.13 EIN with ciliated tubal differentiation. The long vertical gland on the right is an overrun normal gland.

examples of metaplasia in the endometrium. Cilia are the most distinctive manifestation, but changes evident even at low magnification are increased cytoplasmic volume and eosinophilic staining. Interspersed between cuboidal ciliated cells are occasional round secretory cells in a pattern resembling that of the normal fallopian tube. The density of cilia varies greatly, and even a cilia-poor epithelium that demonstrates characteristic cytoplasmic properties of admixed round and columnar cells may be considered serous like ('seroid') or tubal in character (Figure 16.12). Some cilia-depleted tubal metaplasias display such prominent micropapillary or eosinophilic features that they may be considered mixed-type metaplasias.

Tubal differentiation may be induced by estrogen exposure or be a manifestation of a neoplastic clone. It is frequent in the normal proliferative endometrium, especially the uterine lining, suggesting that this can be a normal physiologic finding indicative of an underlying estrogenic milieu. An endometrial field altered by unopposed estrogens demonstrates tubal metaplasia in irregularly scattered occasional glands rather than in tight clusters. It also occurs in half of endometrial adenocarcinomas and 20% of precancerous EIN lesions demonstrating localized clonal architecture (Figure 16.13).[37,41] When tubal glands are present within an EIN lesion, cilia formation is usually variable (Figure 16.14), admixed with micropapillary or endometrioid cytologies (Figure 16.15) in flanking glands. Some EIN lesions with tubal differentiation occur within an inactive or even atrophic background, implying that estrogens, while common, are not essential for tubal differentiation within neoplastic clones.

SQUAMOUS METAPLASIA

Squamous metaplasia may be seen as a stratified epithelium lining the uterine cavity, or as expansile round morules

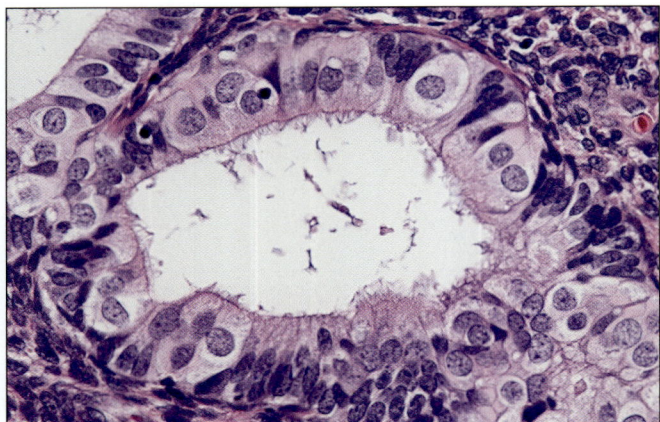

Figure 16.14 Detail of cilia in EIN with ciliated tubal differentiation.

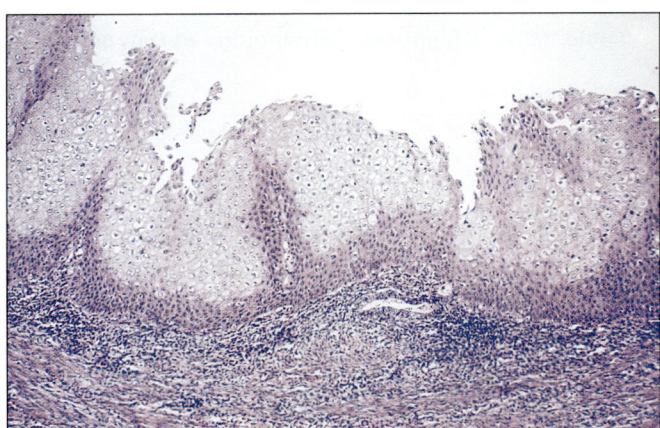

Figure 16.16 Ichthyosis uteri, in which the surface of the endometrium is replaced by stratified squamous epithelium.

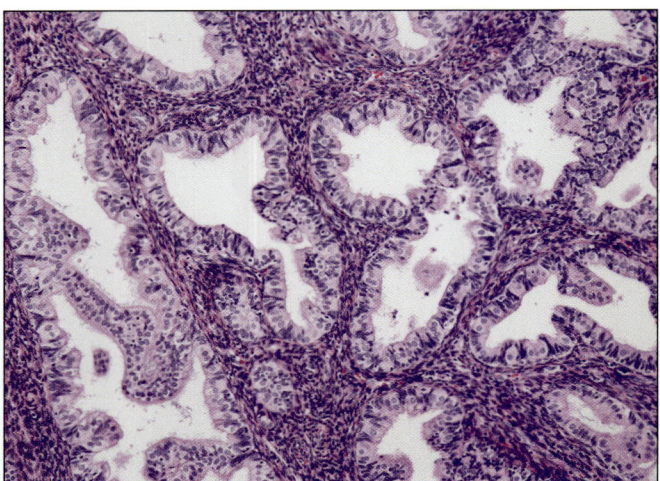

Figure 16.15 EIN with tubal–micropapillary differentiation.

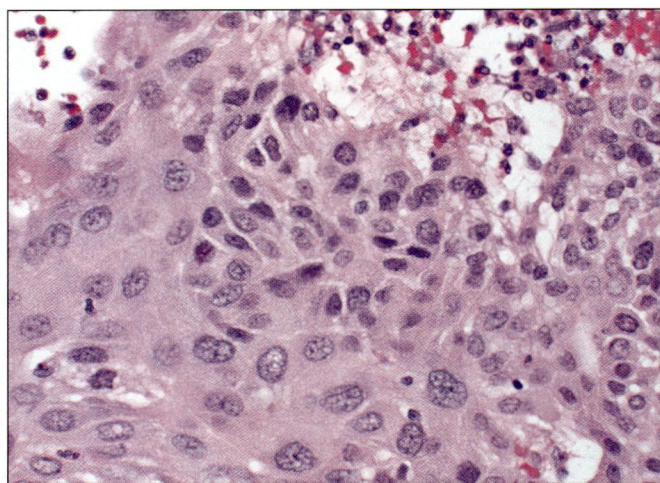

Figure 16.17 Well-differentiated squamous cells in chronic endometritis.

within individual glands. When there is an isolated finding, the former typically results from chronic irritation or infection. Squamous morules have a rather unique appearance and have not been described outside of the uterus. These round balls of somewhat immature epithelium are quite distinct, though, and are usually easily identified when present. Squamous morules are an interesting form of metaplasia, because they are quite frequently associated with neoplasia but are not malignant.

Squamous differentiation within endometrial glands occurs in 18% of premalignant EIN[34] lesions and approximately 25% of adenocarcinomas.[37,40] Not uncommonly, one or several foci of isolated squamous morules is found in a small biopsy specimen, but proves to be located at the periphery of an EIN lesion. This has prompted the clinical recommendation that follow-up sampling be performed when such unexplained morules are found.

ICHTHYOSIS UTERI

Ichthyosis uteri defines a stratified squamous uterine lining epithelium (Figure 16.16) that extends downward to individual glands and demonstrates intercellular bridges and even keratin pearls.[25,42] Chronic endometritis of several years' duration is almost always the antecedent condition (Figure 16.17). Much more common in the pre-antibiotic era, ichthyosis uteri is now rare and most commonly encountered in women with anatomic abnormalities favoring recurrent infection, such as fistulous tracts into the uterine cavity. We have encountered cases in which primary squamous cell carcinoma of the endometrium has been associated with ichthyosis uteri of the adjacent, non-malignant endometrium, although there is no evidence that ichthyosis itself is premalignant.

EIN WITH SQUAMOUS MORULES

Even though morules may be an intimate component of a premalignant EIN lesion, it is the glandular element that has biologic potential to progress to carcinoma (Figure 16.18).[43] Conserved molecular markers such as β-catenin mutation in both the squamous and glandular elements of EIN as well as the adenocarcinoma suggests all are derived from a common clone.[44] Loss of estrogen and progesterone receptors and reduced mitotic activity occurs specifically in

CHAPTER 16 — ENDOMETRITIS, METAPLASIAS, POLYPS, AND MISCELLANEOUS CHANGES   335

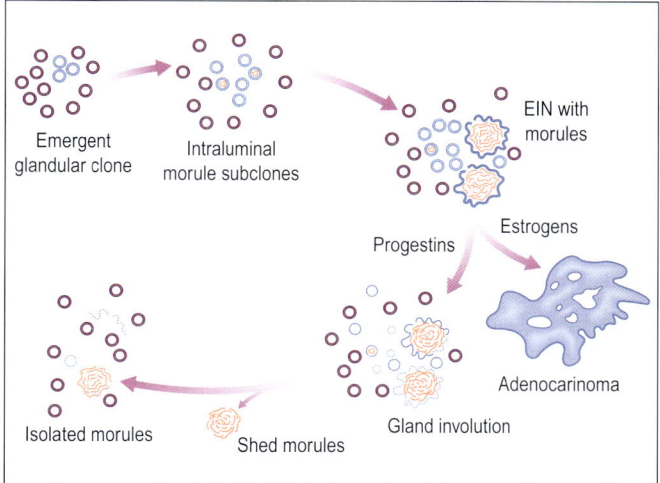

Figure 16.18 Natural history of endometrial squamous morules.

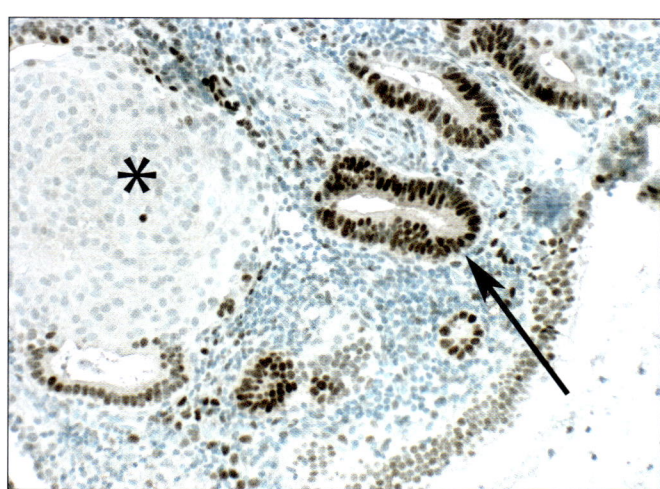

Figure 16.20 Squamous morules in EIN lose estrogen responsiveness. Immunohistochemistry showing estrogen receptors in glands (arrow) but not in squamous morules (asterisk).

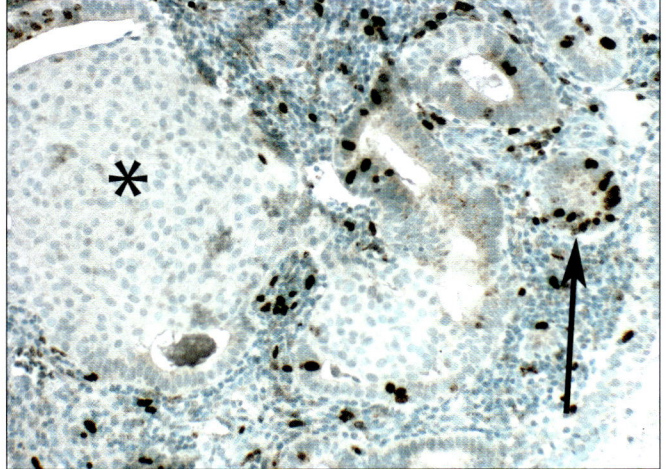

Figure 16.19 Squamous morules in EIN are mitotically quiescent. Mitotic activity shown by Ki-67 (MIB1) immunohistochemistry is high in glands (arrow) but not in squamous morules (asterisk).

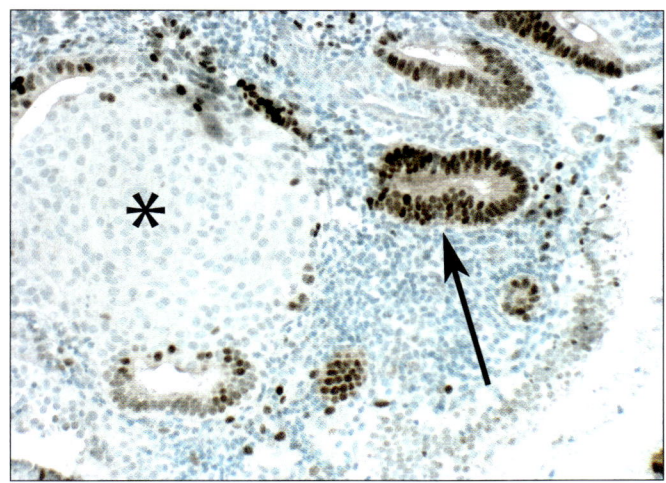

Figure 16.21 Squamous morules in EIN lose progesterone responsiveness. Immunohistochemistry showing progesterone receptors in glands (arrow) but not in squamous morules (asterisk).

the squamous but not glandular elements[44,45] (Figures 16.19–16.21), suggesting that squamous differentiation confers a terminal differentiation state with behavior and biologic potential quite different than that of the accompanying glands. Progestin-treated EIN lesions may demonstrate response within the glandular component, with relative sparing of the progesterone receptor-deficient morules (Figures 16.22 and 16.23).

A diagnosis of EIN is made exclusively by careful evaluation of the glandular cytology and architecture, which must meet all criteria specified in Chapter 17, including size greater than 1 mm, cytologic change, and area of glands exceeding that of stroma. Intermingled morules, which are hormonally unresponsive and lack mitotic activity, should not be incorporated into the size and area estimates. This can be accomplished either by focusing upon a morule-depleted area of the glandular lesion or by mentally subtracting the interposed squamous areas.

Squamous morules within the gland tracts of EIN lesions are not always easily recognizable as well-differentiated squamous cells. The morules form central, rounded epithelial aggregates that are usually continuous at the periphery with the endometrial glandular epithelium (Figure 16.24). The morules may appear to enlarge into sheets with multiple glands arranged radially around the periphery (Figure 16.25). These should not be confused with cribriform adenocarcinoma. Key features are peripheral glands displaced by an expansile solid central component, and transition from glandular to squamous cytology within individual lumens. Central comedo necrosis of squamous morules is common (Figure 16.26) in the context of EIN, but of no clinical or diagnostic significance.

ISOLATED SQUAMOUS MORULES

Not uncommonly, the presence of isolated squamous morules is the only clue that something more serious may be present

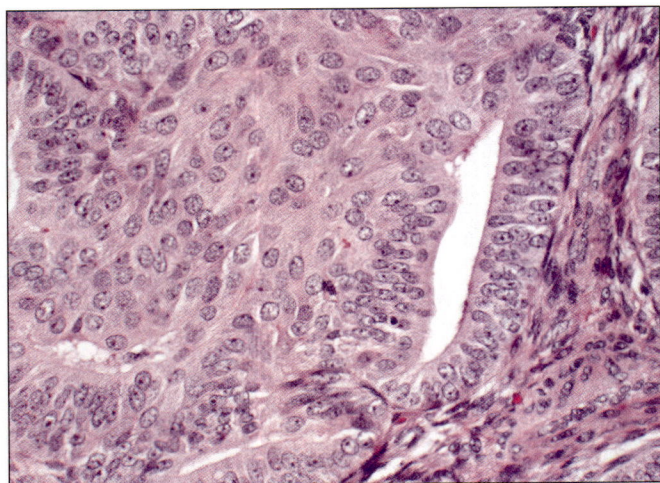

Figure 16.22 EIN with squamous morules, before progestin therapy.

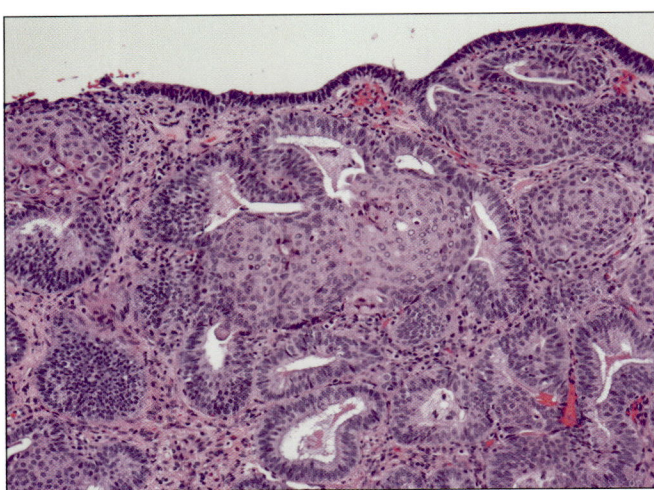

Figure 16.24 Squamous morules in EIN.

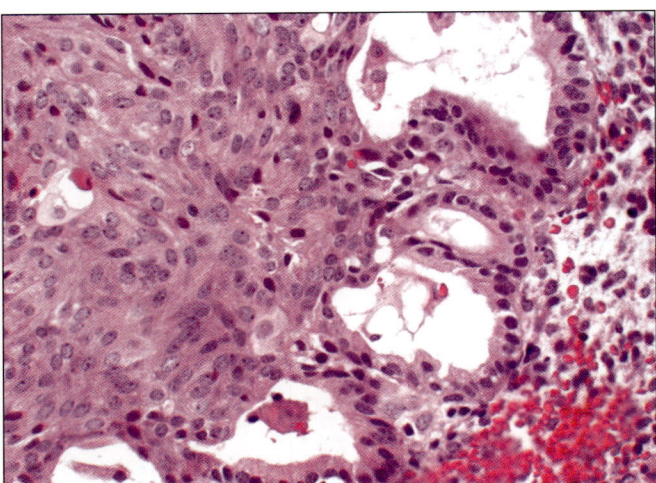

Figure 16.23 Re-biopsy of Figure 16.22 case after 4 months of therapy with progestins. The squamous components are unchanged, but cells of the glandular epithelium demonstrate reduction of epithelial thickness and nuclear size.

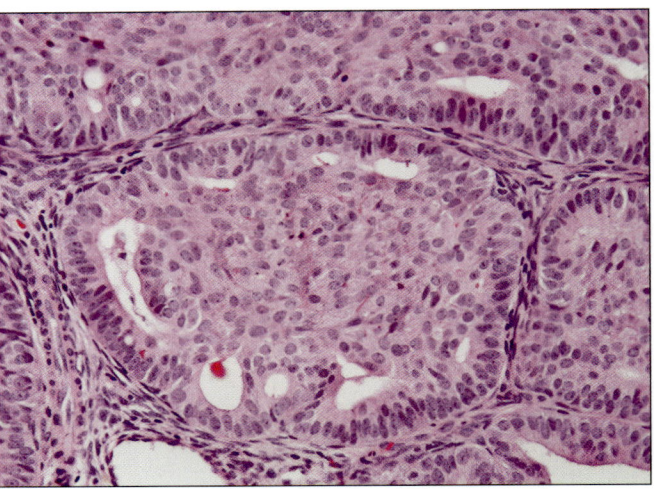

Figure 16.25 Squamous morules with marginal glands, EIN mimicking cribriform adenocarcinoma.

elsewhere in the endometrium (Figures 16.27 and 16.28). The endometrium may be proliferative or secretory; the glands small and uniform with little nuclear atypia and a low mitotic count. Possible mechanisms for presentation of isolated squamous morules in an otherwise unremarkable endometrial biopsy include morule persistence following involution of a previous glandular lesion (Figure 16.18), or morule shedding from a coexisting glandular lesion missed due to sampling error. Isolated morules should always be clearly described, with diagnosis of the underlying glandular pattern and careful clinical correlation or follow-up.

MUCINOUS METAPLASIA

Mucinous metaplasia is a relatively common form of metaplasia that can vary in appearance from extracellular mucin to extensive intracellular mucin droplets. Mucinous metaplasia is almost uniformly of endocervical type. It can be seen in benign and degenerative conditions, and as a result

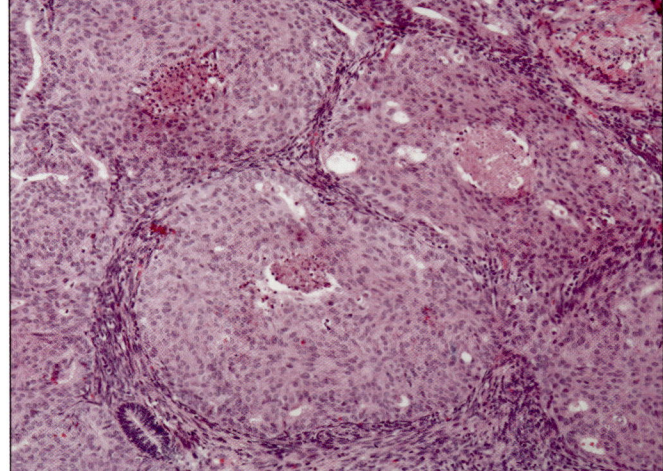

Figure 16.26 Central necrosis in a squamous morule.

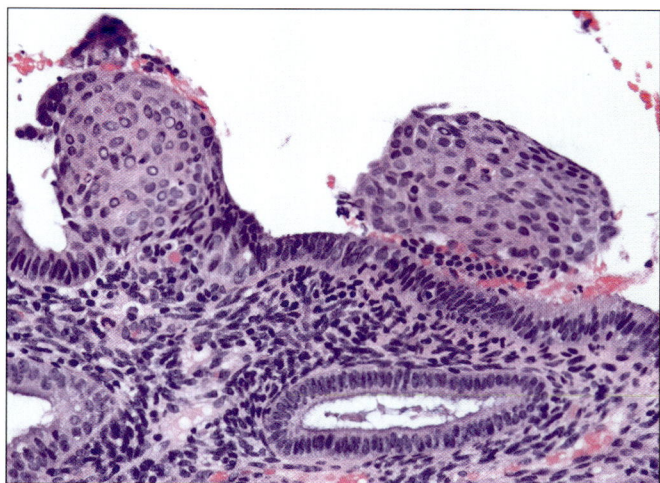

Figure 16.27 Squamous morules shedding from the luminal surface.

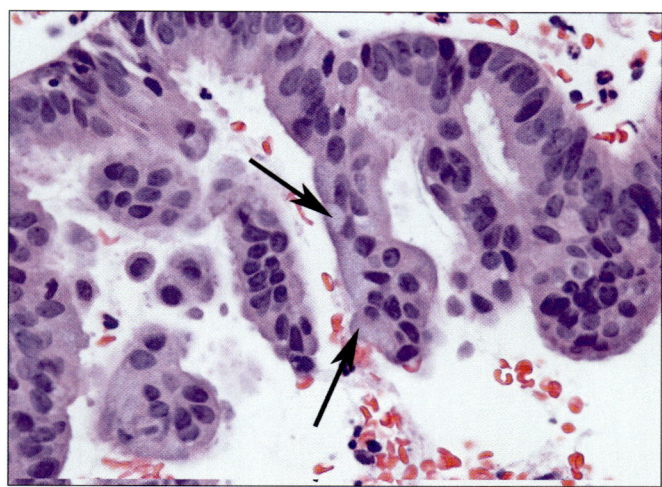

Figure 16.29 Degenerative mucinous change. Cytoplasmic droplets (arrows).

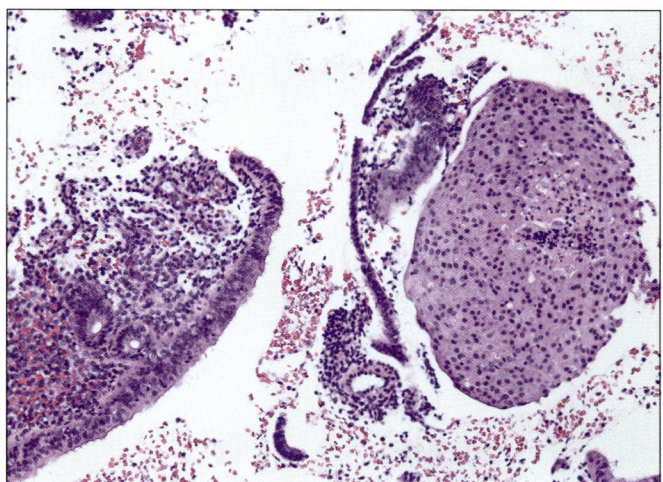

Figure 16.28 Isolated squamous morule.

of hormone therapy. Additionally, mucinous differentiation can be frequently seen in intraepithelial neoplasia and adenocarcinoma. Evaluation of mucinous epithelium is made more difficult by the fact that mucinous epithelium, whether part of a benign or malignant process, almost never shows any cytologic atypia. In general, it is the cases with prominent or regimented intracellular mucinous vacuoles that are most problematic. These are separated by architecture into different clinical outcome, and thus diagnostic, categories.[46,47]

Resemblance of some endometrial mucinous metaplasias to normal endocervical epithelium and bland cytology of many endometrial mucinous neoplasms creates diagnostic challenges for the pathologist. This is particularly so when scanty amounts of mucinous epithelium, especially those with prominent aligned cytoplasmic vacuoles, are too fragmented to evaluate the underlying architecture. General familiarity with the varied appearances of normal endocervical epithelium is most helpful in these circumstances, and fractional dilatation and curettage may assist in discriminating between an endometrial and endocervical site of origin.

Not uncommonly, a layer of basal reserve cells exhibiting cytoplasmic eosinophilia identifies the tissue as normal endocervix with squamous metaplasia. Tissue from the lower uterine segment or fragments of mixed endometrial–endocervical polyps are banal examples of mucinous epithelium presenting in association with endometrial stroma within an endometrial sample. Aside from these obviously benign contexts, the presence of well-differentiated mucinous epithelium within endometrial tissue fragments is a significant abnormality that requires explanation.

BENIGN MUCINOUS CHANGES

Mucin droplets may be seen in association with degenerative changes or syncytial repair associated with stromal breakdown. In these cases, there are disorganized cellular aggregates of cuboidal to columnar eosinophilic cells with mucinous vacuoles or entrapped extracellular mucin droplets (Figure 16.29). A minor degree of architectural complexity as evidenced by multilayering of the cells and irregular slit-like spaces can be seen in association with reparative changes and should be distinguished from the more worrisome architectural features associated with mucinous metaplasia as outlined later.

Benign tubular glands or flat uterine lining surface sometimes show mucinous epithelium with a simple architecture. These may be single layers of columnar epithelium with either focal cytoplasmic mucin droplets or less commonly rows of tall, columnar cells that are identical to those seen in the endocervix with basally located nuclei and abundant vacuolated, mucin-rich cytoplasm. Goblet cells may also occasionally be seen. The presence of endometrial-type stroma between the glands enables differentiation from endocervical contaminants. Most examples are fragments of partly sampled or unrecognized mixed endometrial–endocervical polyps or lower uterine segment, but others involve glands within the native endometrium. Lack of glandular crowding and absence of complex exophytic architecture are key elements in discrimination from a neoplastic process.

'Complex hyperplastic papillary proliferations of the endometrium' are a special type of papillary mucinous

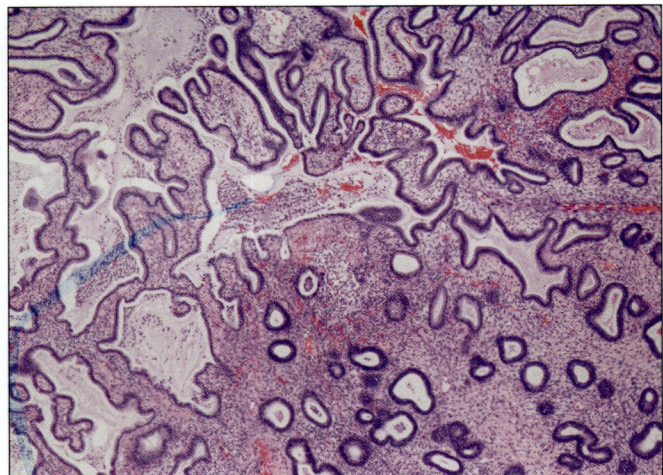

Figure 16.30 Complex hyperplastic papillary proliferation of the endometrium. Blunt fibrous cores with folded epithelium merging with tubular glands.

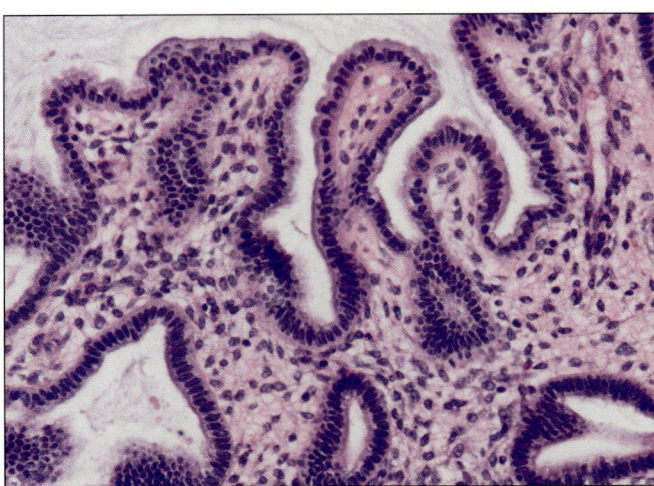

Figure 16.31 Complex hyperplastic papillary proliferation of the endometrium. Bland single layer of mucinous to endometrioid epithelium.

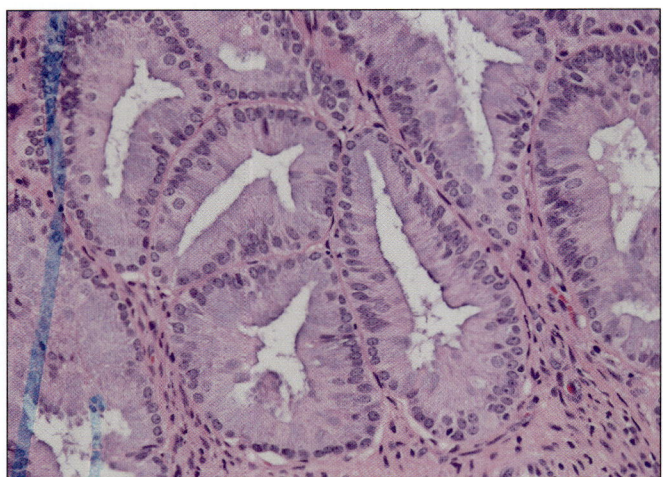

Figure 16.32 EIN with mucinous differentiation.

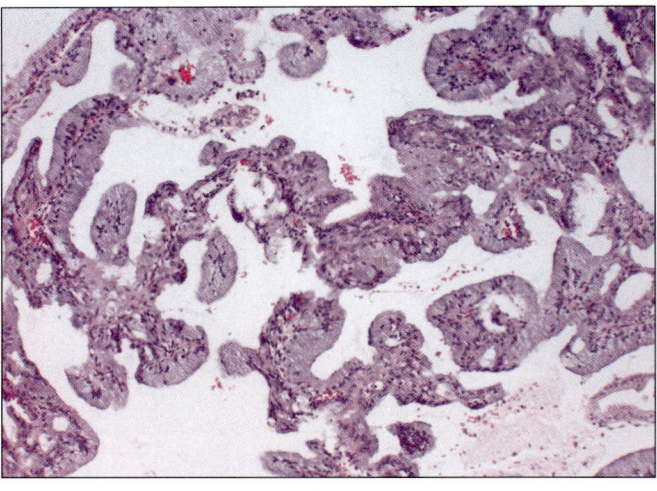

Figure 16.33 Well-differentiated endometrial adenocarcinoma, endometrioid type, with mucinous differentiation. Filiform pattern.

lesion composed of blunt stromal cores covered by a single layer of bland flat endometrioid to mucinous epithelium. Papillary components may anastomose at their base with underlying tubal glands (Figures 16.30 and 16.31). Most are within endometrial polyps. These have been shown in a limited series to have a benign course.[48]

EIN AND ADENOCARCINOMA WITH MUCINOUS DIFFERENTIATION

EIN may demonstrate mucinous metaplasia within the crowded glands that define the lesion (Figure 16.32). The extent of mucinous differentiation varies between adjacent, and even within individual, EIN glands. Intermediate extents of vacuole formation are common, phasing in and out between areas of mucinous and endometrioid differentiation. When gland-lining epithelium is simple, and architecture restricted to tubular or slightly branching forms, these are unlikely to be confused with carcinoma. Papillary redundant folds within mucinous EIN lesions are typically intraglandular, allowing them to be distinguished from the more complex folded sheets or meandering gland lumens of carcinoma.

Very well differentiated endometrial adenocarcinomas with mucinous differentiation are most readily distinguished from EIN by the presence of a conspicuous exophytic surface papillary (Figure 16.33) or microglandular cribriform architectural component.[49] Cytology may be bland, and alternating endometrioid and mucinous differentiation within individual surfaces (Figure 16.34) is a clue to its nonendocervical origin. The papillary fronds of well-differentiated adenocarcinoma are supported by a complicated delicate branching stromal support network, and may appear in a biopsy or curettage as detached 'free-floating' filiform fragments, often admixed with a microglandular component. These microglandular mucinous proliferations show small glands with rigid, 'punched out' lumens superficially resembling microglandular hyperplasia of the endocervix

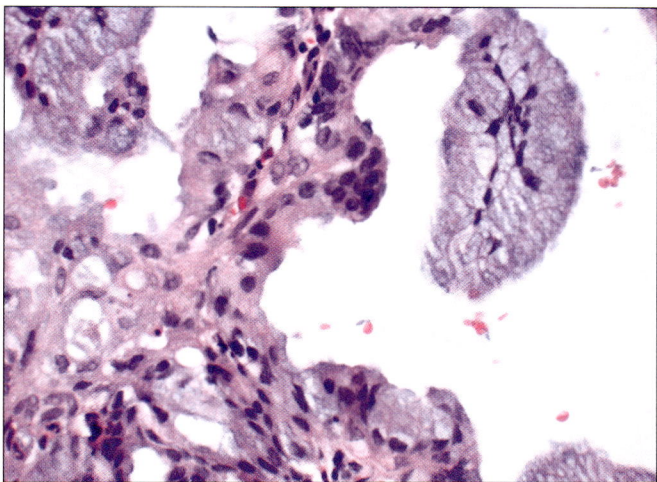

Figure 16.34 Detail of mucinous epithelium in filiform mucinous adenocarcinoma, showing alternating mucinous and non-mucinous differentiation.

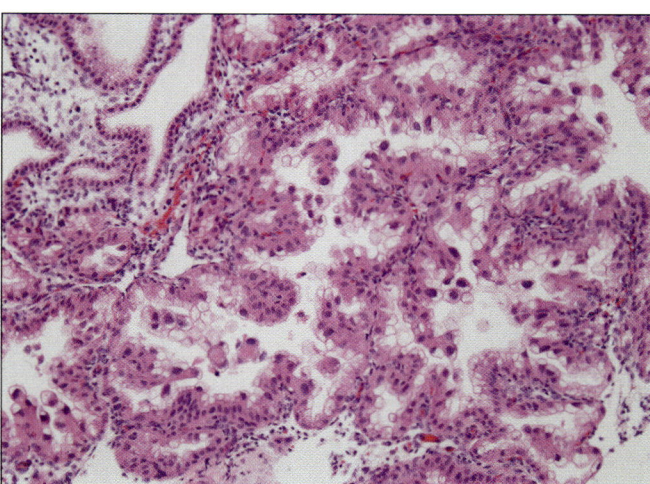

Figure 16.36 Arias-Stella phenomenon.

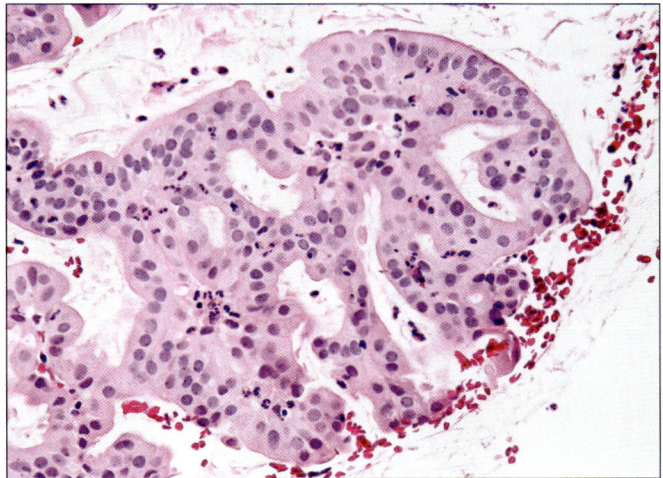

Figure 16.35 Well-differentiated endometrial adenocarcinoma, endometrioid type, with mucinous differentiation. Microglandular pattern.

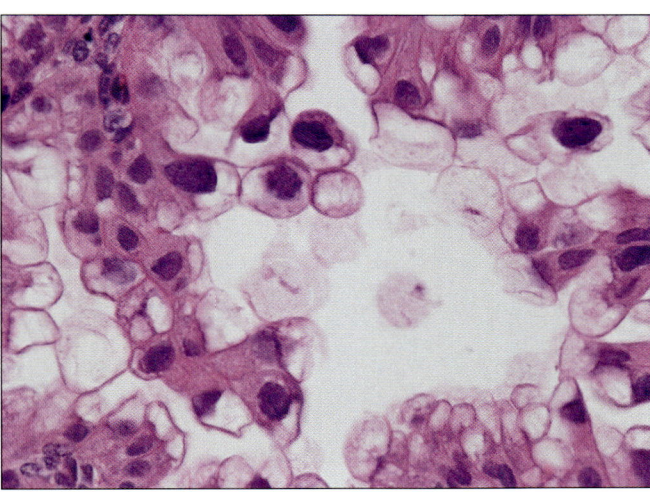

Figure 16.37 Papillary hobnail cells in Arias-Stella phenomenon.

(Figure 16.35). Very small or highly fragmented pieces of tissue with this appearance may or may not represent a well-differentiated mucinous adenocarcinoma of the endometrium, the diagnosis of which depends on the amount of tissue, its preservation, and fragmentation. In scanty specimens, we diagnose a 'complex mucinous epithelial proliferation' and advise a follow-up endometrial sampling.

SECRETORY METAPLASIA

Secretory change, a normal response of endometrial glands to circulating progesterone, is accompanied also by a characteristic change in the stromal cells to a cell resembling decidua. These changes, strictly speaking, are physiologic and not metaplastic. Normal secretory phase glands can focally have little intervening stroma and can show a variety of artifacts that can lead to an erroneous diagnosis of neoplasia. Hypersecretory change, also referred to as Arias-Stella phenomenon, is a result of high levels of progesterone accompanying pregnancy (Figure 16.36). Because the secretory glands can have irregular hyperchromatic nuclei they can be mistaken for neoplastic epithelium (Figure 16.37). This mistake is most easily made in sites other than the endometrium; for example, in the cervix or fallopian tube. However, the change is entirely benign.

Neoplastic glands of EIN and adenocarcinoma may be capable of mounting a secretory response to progestins, and this may appear as subnuclear vacuoles in patients who have recently ovulated or received hormonal therapy (Figures 16.38 and 16.39). Not all secretory changes, however, are caused by progestational stimulation.[69] A subset of neoplastic lesions develop prominent cytoplasmic secretory vacuoles as an integral feature of their neoplastic growth, independent of ambient progestational exposure (Figure 16.40). In those instances the stroma is free of pseudodecidual changes, and secretory change is confined to

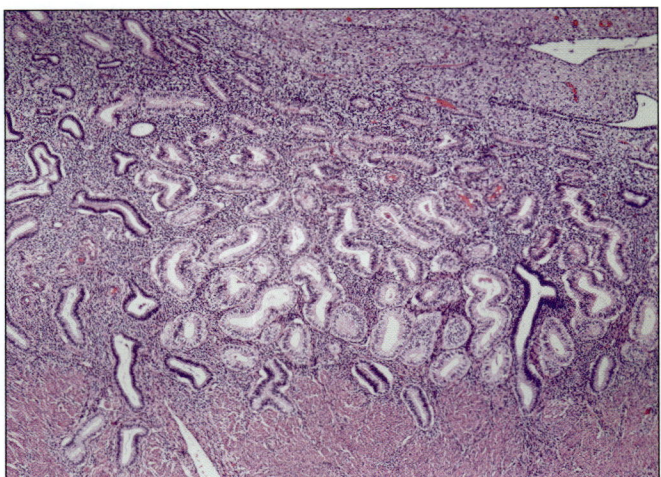

Figure 16.38 Residual EIN with secretory differentiation, in basalis following progestin therapy.

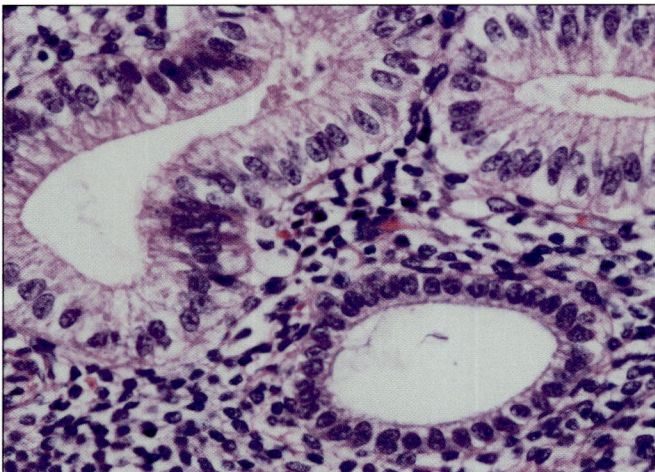

Figure 16.39 Residual EIN glands with secretory changes (top) following withdrawal of progestin therapy.

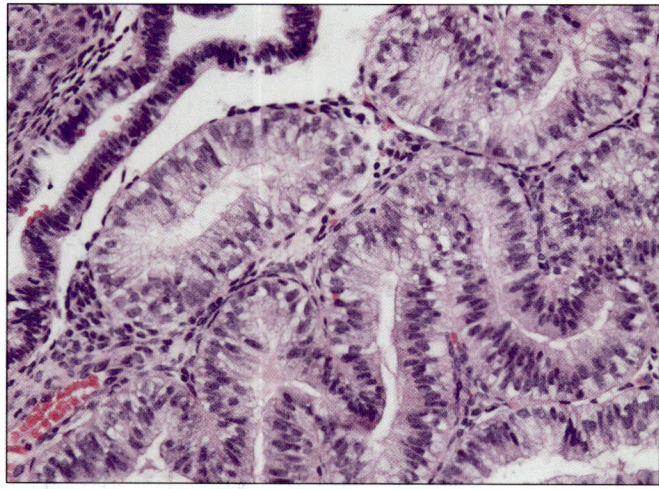

Figure 16.40 EIN glands with secretory differentiation, occurring without progestin exposure. Comparison background gland in upper left.

architecturally and cytologically abnormal glands. These can be diagnosed as EIN or adenocarcinoma, with secretory differentiation.

METAPLASIAS TO NONSPECIFIC CELL TYPES

Some changes in endometrial epithelial appearance do not resemble any particular differentiated müllerian cell type, and thus cannot be properly considered metaplasias. Nonetheless, the term metaplasia is sometimes loosely applied to these processes to indicate their unusual appearance, but they are usually best diagnosed using more specific terminology.

EOSINOPHILIC METAPLASIA

An eosinophilic change can be associated with a variety of endometrial alterations such as ciliated cell metaplasia, squamous metaplasia, papillary metaplasia, and adenocarcinoma, and, as such, it is fair to question its status as a true metaplasia. Many eosinophilic metaplasias contain features overlapping with other altered differentiation states, such as mucin expression (85% of cases),[50] or micropapillary architecture. The metaplasia can take several forms. When focal and associated with a simple lining epithelium, the change is always benign. This change is most commonly encountered within endometrial polyps, but occurs within the endometrial glands of the functionalis, usually in an inflammatory setting.

More commonly, the term 'eosinophilic metaplasia' refers to a change that is also known as oxyphil or oncocytic metaplasia. The cells showing eosinophilic metaplasia, which may be either on the surface or in the glands, are of a tall columnar type with abundant eosinophilic cytoplasm that ranges from homogeneous to granular and a bulging surface membrane similar to the oncocytes seen in other organs such as the salivary glands, pancreas, thyroid, and kidney. The nuclei are centrally placed, large, and round to oval with a delicate chromatin pattern. The eosinophilia corresponds to myriads of mitochondria as shown by electron microscopy.[48] Like most other metaplasias, this change can be associated with a spectrum of endometrial changes ranging from benign to malignant.

As with other types of metaplasia, eosinophilic change is worrisome when associated with architectural complexity. In particular, intraglandular papillary proliferations exhibiting eosinophilic change can be associated with EIN.

MICROPAPILLARY METAPLASIA

Papillary metaplasia is a descriptive term without any specific cellular basis. It involves glandular tissue thrown into papilla and is principally used to reflect degenerative processes that may involve endometrial glands and epithelial surfaces,[47] in addition to a tufted pattern of intraglandular differentiation in EIN (Figure 16.41) and adenocarcinoma. It lacks the pleomorphic nuclear cytology and coarse chromatin seen in serous adenocarcinomas, which also show papillary tufting. It is of practical diagnostic significance because endometria with this histologic feature may present an unusually broad differential diagnosis, including degenerative, reactive, and neoplastic processes.

EIN lesions may show micropapillary differentiation where a crowded focus of glands is distinguished by small

CHAPTER 16 — ENDOMETRITIS, METAPLASIAS, POLYPS, AND MISCELLANEOUS CHANGES

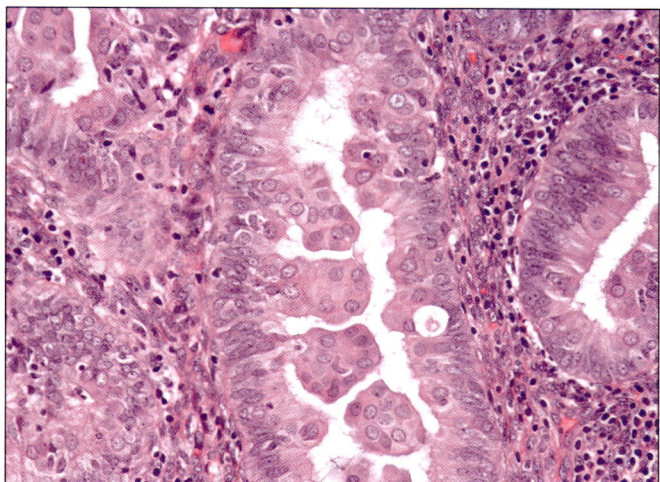

Figure 16.41 EIN with eosinophilic micropapillary differentiation.

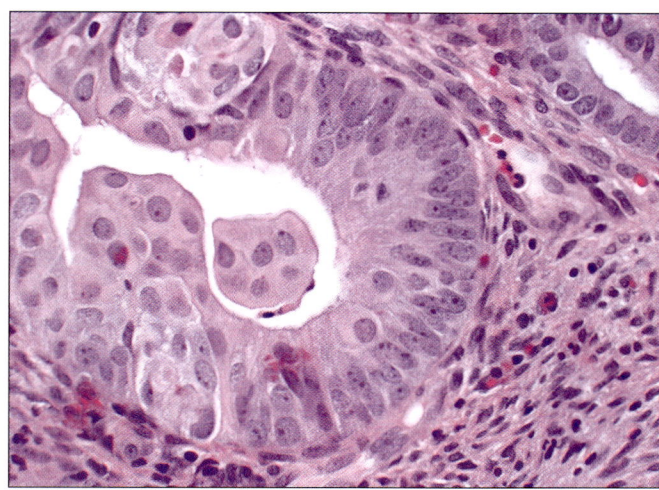

Figure 16.43 EIN with alternating endometrioid and micropapillary differentiation in a single gland.

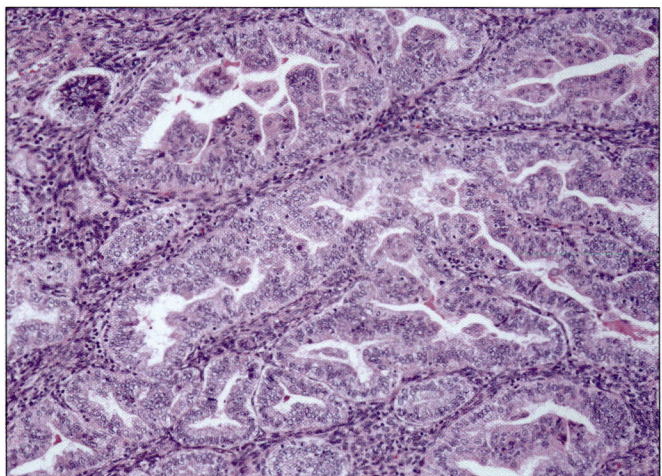

Figure 16.42 EIN with micropapillary differentiation. Complex intraglandular redundant folds.

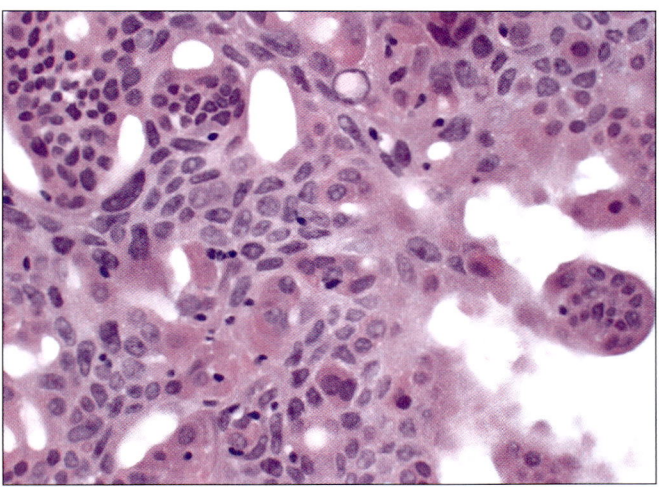

Figure 16.44 Papillary syncytial metaplasia, a mimic of squamous differentiation.

intraluminal tufts protruding from a flat simple epithelium. These can be confused with adenocarcinoma when tufting defines a complicated luminal architecture mimicking a maze-like or cribriform architecture (Figure 16.42). Tangential sectioning artifacts of the papillary areas create numerous clefts communicating to the central lumen, and redundant 'saw-tooth' folds contained within the boundaries of an encasing basement membrane. Nuclear cytology is round and bland or monomorphic, unlike the highly atypical exfoliative nuclei characteristic of the papillary branching typifying an adenocarcinoma as serous. Micropapillary areas are often admixed with, or blend into, other EIN glands with tubal or endometrioid differentiation (Figure 16.43).

PAPILLARY SYNCYTIAL METAPLASIA

This epithelial change is a misnomer because the papillary areas are not a true syncytium, nor do they resemble any specific normal epithelium. Rather, papillary syncytial metaplasia is a degenerative process in which collapsed sheets of epithelium with abundant pink cytoplasm resemble squamous cells, but lack true squamous differentiation (Figure 16.44). This has also been called 'surface syncytial change' and 'eosinophilic syncytial metaplasia.' It is found in nearly one-fifth of curettage specimens and appears as aggregates of eosinophilic, cuboidal to spindly epithelial cells.[50] The underlying stroma is nondescript to tight balls, indicative of menstruation or anovulatory bleeding (Figure 16.45). Supportive fibrovascular cores are not seen.

MICROPAPILLARY 'HOBNAIL' METAPLASIA

This form of metaplasia is rare, and likely represents a variety of etiologies including degenerative changes associated with underlying necrosis, artifacts, pseudo-Arias-Stella-like changes and changes associated with endometrial polyps. On morphologic grounds, hobnail cell metaplasia exhibits glandular cells with rounded nuclear protrusions into the gland lumina. These can be artificially created by

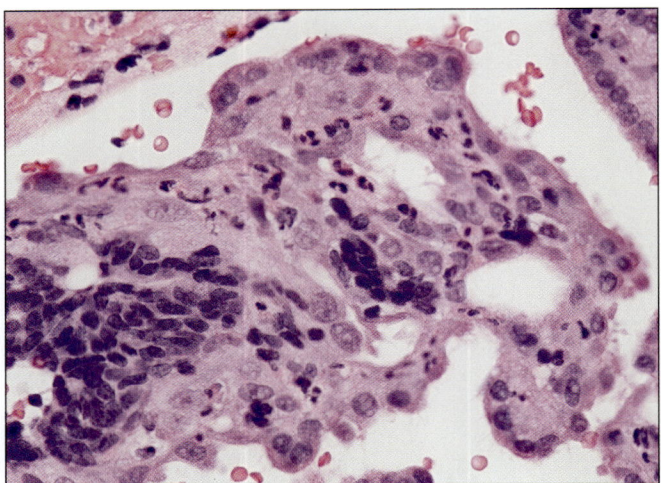

Figure 16.45 Papillary syncytial metaplasia overlying stromal breakdown, and entrapping stromal aggregates.

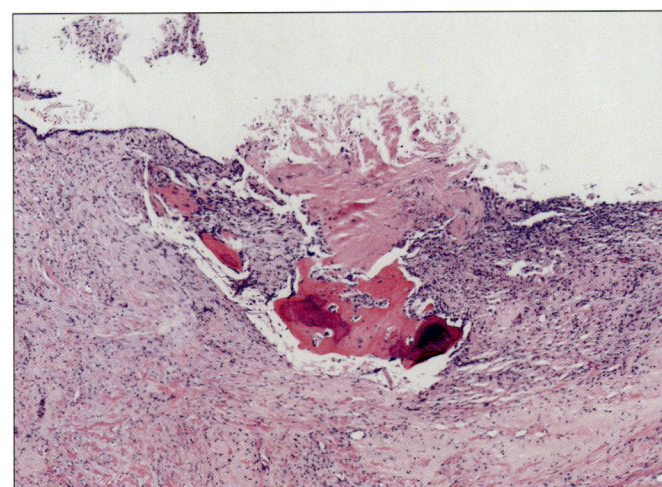

Figure 16.47 Osseous metaplasia following endometrial ablation.

ENDOMETRIAL EXTRAMEDULLARY HEMOPOIESIS

Extramedullary hemopoiesis is a rare finding associated with hematologic disease, and thus not strictly a metaplastic condition. The finding of endometrial extramedullary hemopoiesis may herald the presence of an underlying hematologic abnormality.[55]

ENDOMETRIAL POLYPS

Endometrial polyps are biphasic growths of endometrial glands and stroma with blood vessels, sometimes also containing smooth muscle, which protrude into the uterine cavity.

Etiology and Natural History

Polyps arise as monoclonal overgrowths of genetically altered endometrial stromal cells with secondary induction of polyclonal benign glands through as yet undefined stromal–epithelial interactive mechanisms.[56] Chromosomal analysis of polyp stroma shows in the majority of cases clonal translocations, involving 6p21–p22, 12q13–15, or 7q22 regions.[57] One breakpoint gene, the *HMGIC* gene at 12q15, is also rearranged in uterine leiomyomas, lipomas, pleomorphic adenomas, and pulmonary chondroid hamartomas.[58]

Endometrial polyps variably respond to circulating estrogens and progesterone. Most commonly the polyp is nonfunctional, lacking those normal cyclical changes seen in the adjacent normal endometrium. The glands are frequently entirely inactive, showing neither proliferative nor secretory activity. Some or many of the glands may be dilated, slightly branching, or irregularly distributed. Functioning polyps are less common than those already described and are composed of glands that show secretory activity during the secretory phase. When present, the secretory changes in the polyp either lag behind or are less well developed and dyssynchronous relative to the normal endometrium. An irregular gland pattern is common and should not give cause for concern or be separately

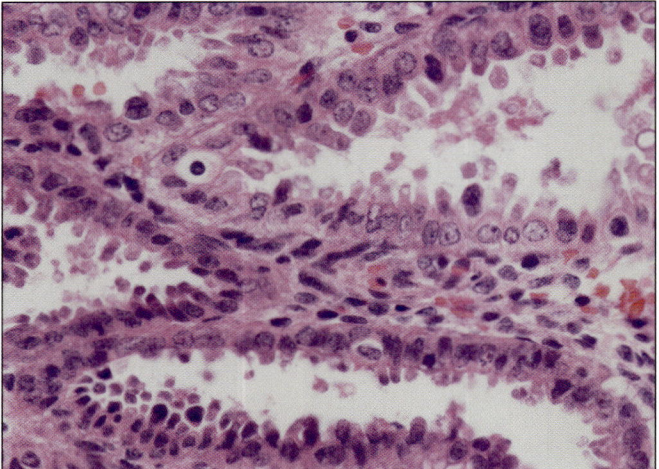

Figure 16.46 Exfoliation artifact caused by hypertonic fluid instillation at hysteroscopy.

exfoliation in response to nonphysiologic fluid instillation during hysteroscopy or placement of a specimen in hypotonic medium (Figure 16.46). When the cytoplasm is abundant and clear, the differential diagnosis is with clear cell carcinoma. Lack of mitotic activity and atypia, and the fact that the change is focal, assists in recognizing it as a benign process.

MESENCHYMAL METAPLASIAS

OSSEOUS METAPLASIA

Osseous tissue in the endometrial stroma is a rarely encountered condition that is often associated with a previous history of abortion or instrumentation (Figure 16.47). Some may be residual fetal bone incorporated into the endometrium. Others are doubtless genuine metaplasia, albeit sometimes induced by the retention of fetal bones.[51,52] Most cases occur in women aged between 20 and 40 years and are associated with infertility.[53] It occurs also in post-menopausal women.[54]

CHAPTER 16 — ENDOMETRITIS, METAPLASIAS, POLYPS, AND MISCELLANEOUS CHANGES

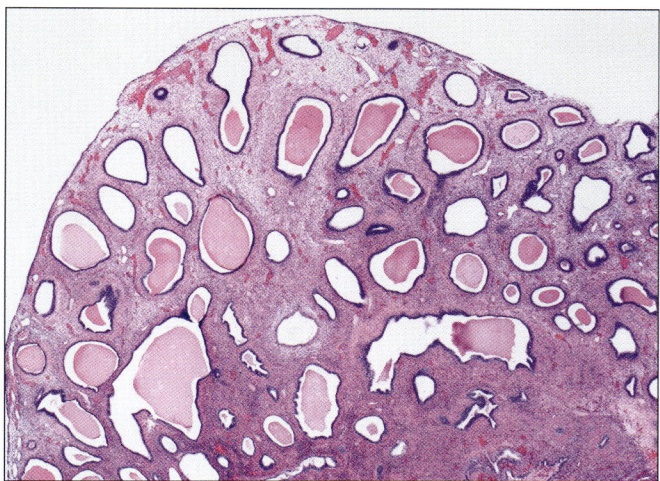

Figure 16.48 Endometrial polyp with fibrous stroma and irregular cystic glands.

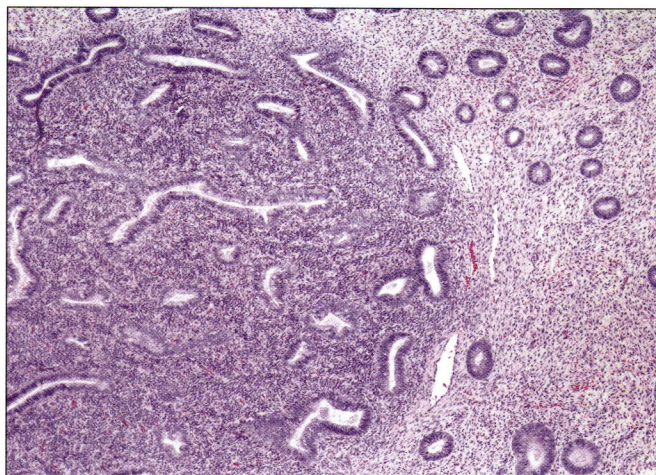

Figure 16.49 Nodular stromal expansion in an early endometrial polyp.

diagnosed as an endometrial hyperplasia, especially when it is uniformly distributed throughout the entire polyp (Figure 16.48).

There have been numerous reports of endometrial polyps occurring in women treated with tamoxifen for breast cancer. It is clear that women on tamoxifen have a higher incidence of endometrial polyps than the rest of the population and that their polyps are likely to be much larger, more fibrotic, more likely to show mucinous metaplasia, and more likely to contain hyperplasia or carcinoma than women not on tamoxifen treatment.[59,60]

Clinical Features

Endometrial polyps may be found at any age, but are most frequent around and shortly after menopause. They are present in about 13–17% of women.[61] Polyps may cause abnormal bleeding, a finding that may be explained when hemorrhage or necrosis is demonstrated on pathologic examination. Use of a rigid curette to completely shear away the polyp may be both diagnostic and therapeutic at the same time, although diagnostic material is often rendered by flexible sampling devices (Pipelle). Because they are typically removed in fragments and difficult to orient, surgical margins are difficult to assess within most polyp specimens. If EIN or adenocarcinoma is found in what is thought to be a polyp at curettage, the patient should generally be managed in exactly the same way as would have been done had the changes been in a nonpolypoid area.

Gross Features

Early in their development, clonal stromal proliferations destined to become bulky endometrial polyps may not be grossly evident. These can be seen microscopically as a localized stromal component with interposed distorted glands within the endometrial functionalis (Figure 16.49). More commonly, at the time of diagnosis endometrial polyps range in size from a slightly rounded protuberance to a large, broad-based or pedunculated, oval structure filling the uterine cavity. They may also expand the cervical canal and present at the external cervical os. Pedunculated polyps

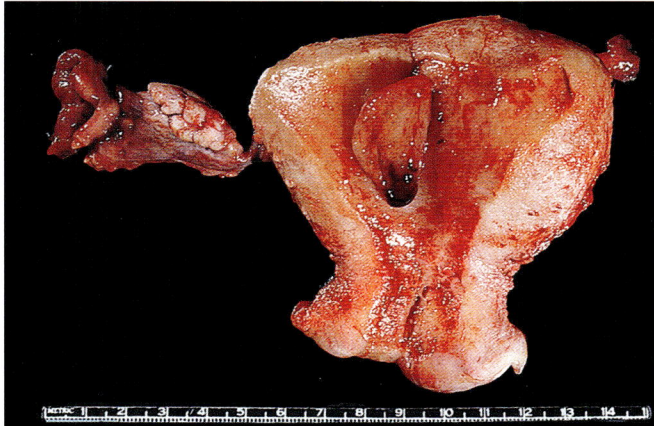

Figure 16.50 Endometrial polyp. The polyp arises on a narrow pedicle at one cornu and has a hemorrhagic tip.

are the easiest to recognize and often attract the most attention (Figure 16.50). Many polyps are sessile and have a broad base of attachment to the internal surface of the uterus. Some sessile polyps are only slightly raised and are easy to miss on gross examination. About 20% of polyps are multiple. The surface may be smooth and shiny and there is often hemorrhage, particularly at the tip. Necrosis is sometimes present, although this is uncommon in benign polyps. The cut surface may be uniform or it may show cysts, hemorrhage, and necrosis.

Microscopic Features

The diagnosis of a polyp in a curetting depends upon the finding of at least two of three particular histologic features, in addition to exclusion of mimics. These include: (1) irregularly shaped and positioned glands, (2) stroma altered by fibrosis or excessive collagen, and (3) thick-walled blood vessels (Figures 16.51 and 16.52). In addition, as polyps elongate, the glands often get stretched such that parallel glands with intervening fibrous stroma becomes a useful

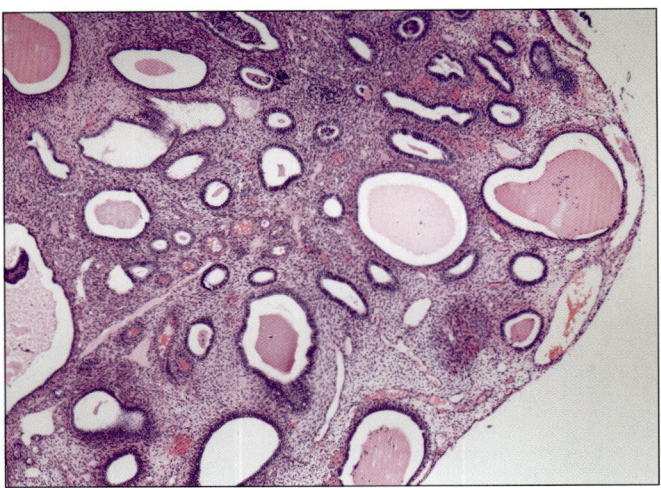

Figure 16.51 Endometrial polyp. Irregular bland glands with cysts and fibrous stroma.

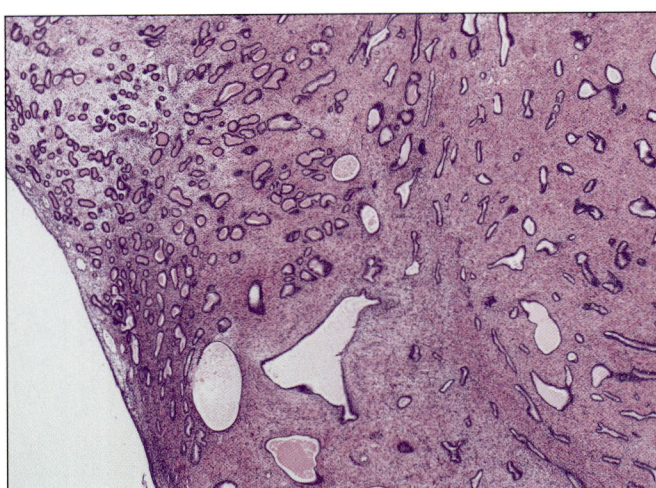

Figure 16.53 Endometrial polyp. Irregular gland density within the polyp and at the interface with adjacent endometrium. Some compressed glands are parallel to the surface.

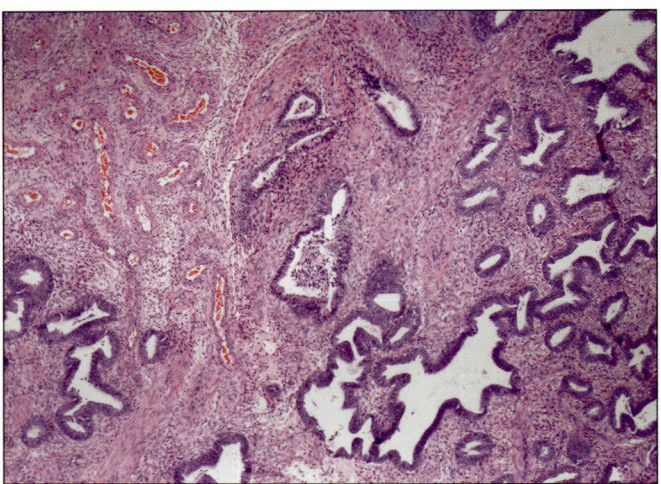

Figure 16.52 Endometrial polyp. Fibrous stroma, with prominent vessels.

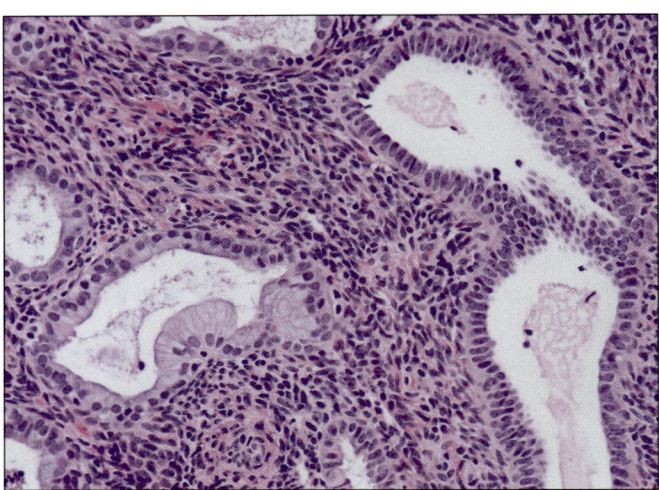

Figure 16.54 Mucinous differentiation in mixed endometrial–endocervical type endometrial polyp.

clue to the diagnosis (Figure 16.53).[62] There are two polyp mimics that should be excluded before the diagnosis of an endometrial polyp can be made. The first is fragments of basalis, which can be ruled out if at least one of the polyp fragments shows surface epithelium. The second is lower uterine segment, which typically has a lower gland density, a more collagenous stroma, mucinous and tubal differentiation, and a lack of endometrial stroma. It is important to note that the identification of polypoid endometrial mucosa with surface epithelium on three sides is not sufficient for the diagnosis of an endometrial polyp if the previously mentioned features are lacking. Many fragments of normal epithelium can be artifactually cut in such a way as to have a 'polypoid' appearance.

Admixtures of mucinous and endometrial-type glands can be seen within endometrial polyps (Figure 16.54). The mucinous component demonstrates cytoplasmic mucin resembling that of the normal endocervix. When mucinous glands are prominent, occasional interspersed endometrial glands, commingled endometrial stroma, and lack of overlying squamous metaplasia are useful in distinguishing them from cervical polyps.

In postmenopausal women, the polyps are usually composed of dilated cysts (Figure 16.55) lined by atrophic epithelium (Figure 16.56). They are sometimes called 'senile' polyps. These are clearly a remnant of the time when the endometrium was active, and the pattern described represents a regressed state following a period of growth, perhaps many years previously.

EIN, when seen in polyps, may be recognized as a discrete geographic focus of crowded glands with a cohesive cytology that differs from the background polyp (Figure 16.57). Polyps with EIN need to be distinguished from a carcinoma arising in a pre-existing polyp and a polypoid carcinoma, which depends on finding a benign fibrous stalk or benign glandular elements in the polypoid mass.

CHAPTER 16 — ENDOMETRITIS, METAPLASIAS, POLYPS, AND MISCELLANEOUS CHANGES   345

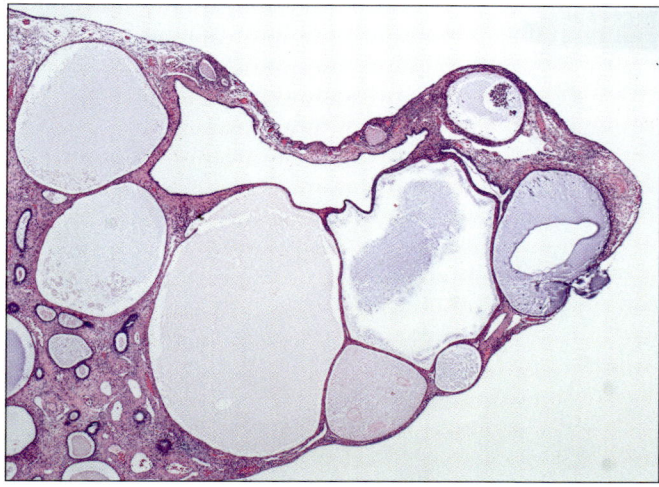

Figure 16.55 Endometrial polyp, senile type. The glands are cystic with flaccid walls.

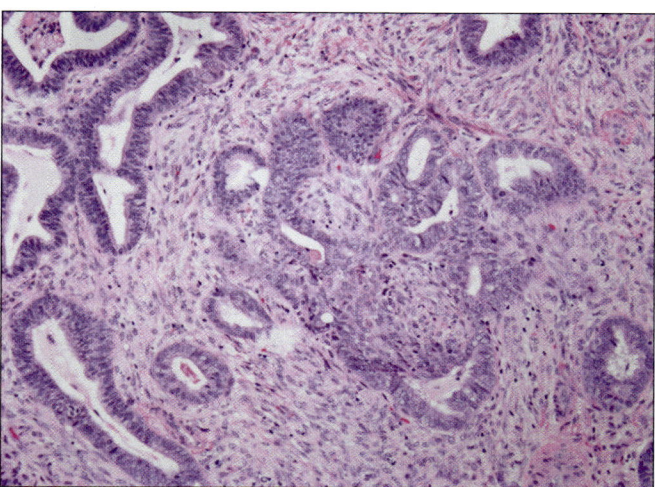

Figure 16.58 Atypical polypoid adenomyoma. Muscle with admixed glands having squamous morules.

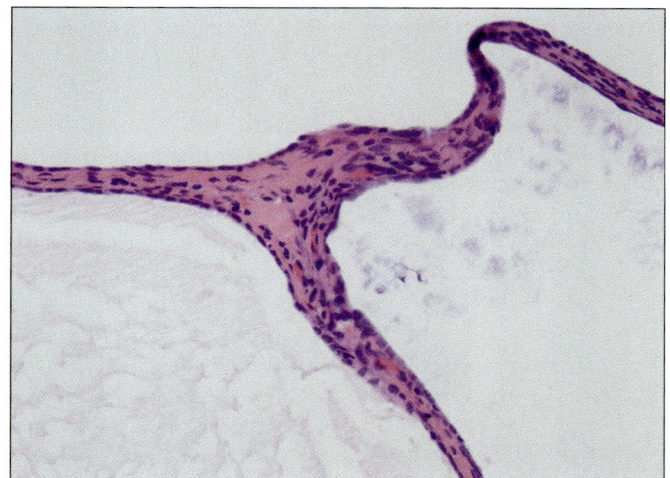

Figure 16.56 Endometrial polyp, senile type. Cystic glands are lined by flattened epithelium.

ATYPICAL POLYPOID ADENOMYOMA

Atypical polypoid adenomyomas are admixtures of smooth muscle and atypical endometrial glands which form an exophytic, usually broad-based, projection into the uterine cavity.[63] These tumors occur primarily in reproductive age women, and are only rarely diagnosed in patients after menopause. When encountered within a fragmented endometrial sample, the disordered arrangement of atypical glands among a dense muscular stroma can easily be confused as myoinvasive adenocarcinoma. The presence of characteristic and extensive morular squamous metaplasia (present in >90% of examples; Figure 16.58), lack of cribriform or solid architecture, and absence of stromal desmoplasia are helpful in excluding adenocarcinoma. Approximately half persist or recur locally after conservative treatment by curettage.[63]

Atypical polypoid adenomyomas have been associated with endometrioid adenocarcinoma and its precursor lesions (EIN or atypical endometrial hyperplasia), either of which may be present within the main polypoid mass or elsewhere in the endometrium.[64,65] It is therefore important to look carefully for coexisting carcinoma, and examine the native endometrium for EIN. If either are present, they should be separately diagnosed.

MISCELLANEOUS CONDITIONS

ASHERMAN'S SYNDROME

Asherman's syndrome, defined as synechiae within the endometrial cavity, often causes menstrual disorders and infertility (62% and 43% of patients, respectively).[66] The most common causes are curettage after a missed abortion or during the puerperium. Genital tuberculosis, in countries where this disease is still common, is a principal causative factor. Hysterosalpingography and hysteroscopy are the usual methods of definitive diagnosis.

There are no gross features as the specimens usually consist of fragments of fibrous tissue with varying amounts

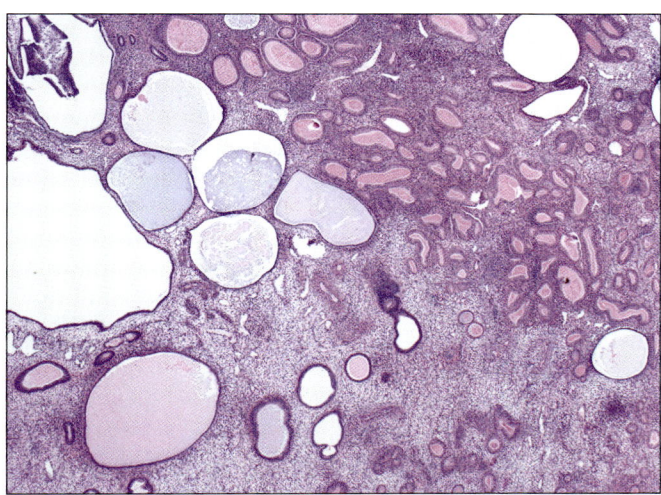

Figure 16.57 EIN in endometrial polyp. Increased gland density and cytologic change are seen within the EIN focus (upper right).

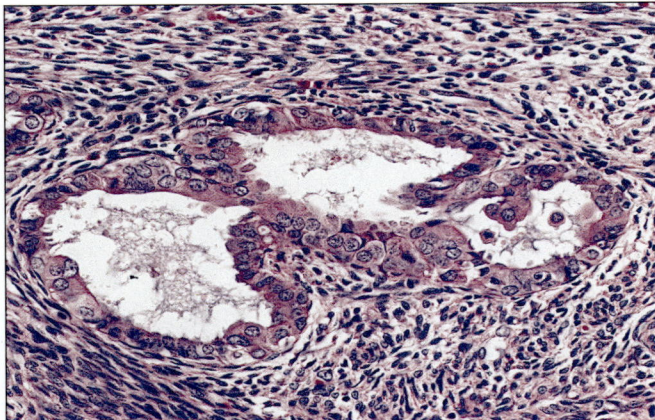

Figure 16.59 Radiation changes.

of entrapped residual endometrial glands. The rare hysterectomy specimen discloses massive fibrosis of the residual 'endometrium.'

Treatment usually consists of lysing the adhesions followed by immediate insertion of an IUD, together with a course of estrogens. The usual measure of successful treatment is the ability to achieve a term delivery.[67,68] Placenta accreta is not an uncommon complication during the subsequent pregnancy, usually because the endometrium is absent and the placental villi have implanted directly into the myometrium.

RADIATION EFFECT

Radiation delivered for therapy of cervical or other pelvic malignancies may alter the histology of what initially was normal endometrium. Grossly, no changes are seen, unless the absence of lush endometrium 2–3 mm thick is considered abnormal. The endometrium is usually paper thin, and more akin to an atrophic endometrium. The chief microscopical features are glands in which the nuclei are irregular in size and shape, but in which the chromatin is usually smudged (Figure 16.59). Mitoses are absent. The glands are either normal or slightly irregular in shape, but lack any evidence of any usual features of carcinoma with which it is commonly mistaken. Normal glands affected by radiotherapy lack signs of invasion or a cribriform arrangement of the cells. The glands are also usually spaced as normal glands.

THE EFFECTS OF THE IUD ON THE ENDOMETRIUM

Often, the IUD (Figure 16.60) appears to have no demonstrable effect on the endometrium, although subtle, local changes are almost invariable. Focally compressed endometrium may be seen at the site of contact, which may vary between a slight indentation of the surface to deep implantation almost through the endometrium or even into the myometrium (Figure 16.61). Rarely, an IUD may penetrate the uterine wall and even lie in the peritoneal cavity. Commonly, near the point where the IUD is in contact with the endometrium, a fibroblastic overgrowth will develop to isolate the IUD as if it were a foreign body. The surface

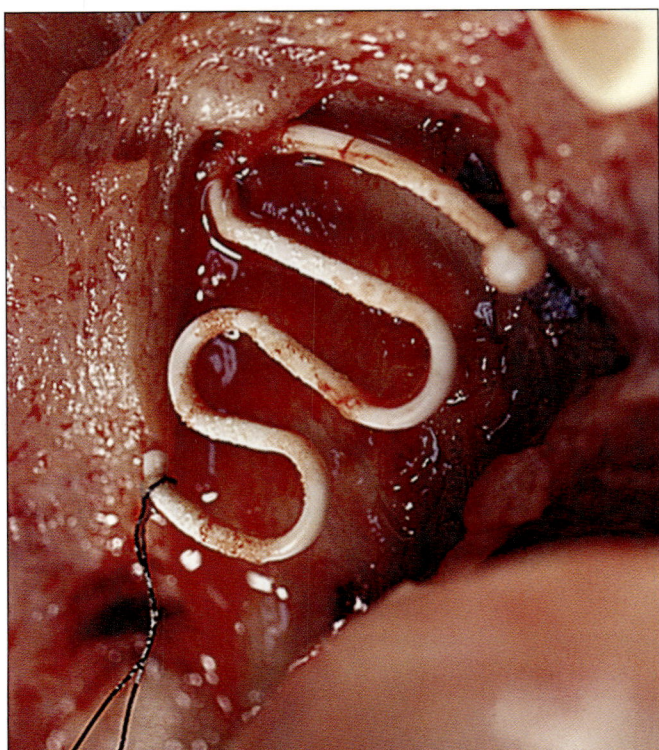

Figure 16.60 IUD. A Lippes loop in position in an opened uterus. Adhesions are attached to the loop.

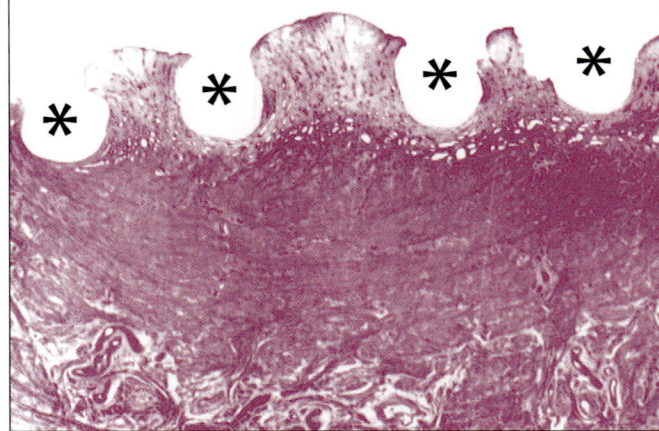

Figure 16.61 IUD. Imprint of a Lippes loop in the endometrium. The endometrium is normal between the depressions (asterisks) caused by the IUD itself.

epithelium at the point of contact with the IUD may also show atypical features, with loss of cellular polarity and nuclear enlargement and pleomorphism. Squamous metaplasia of the surface epithelium has been seen on occasion. The stroma may exhibit focal edema and dilated blood vessels. Small foci of an exaggerated decidual-like response to progesterone may also be evident.

Inflammation is the most important complication of an IUD in the endometrium, particularly with the noncopper-containing types. It is common to observe a sparse, focal

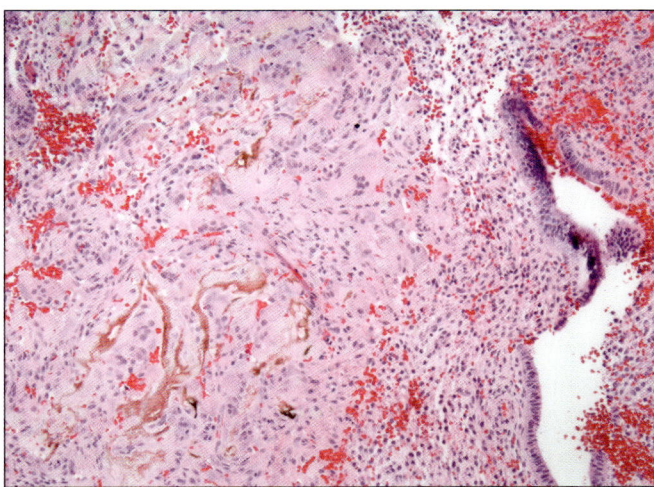

Figure 16.62 Re-epithelialized surface with underlying coagulative debris and giant cells 2 years after endometrial ablation.

scattering of neutrophils in the superficial stroma close to the contact point with the device, as well as neutrophils and nuclear debris in gland lumina. These minor local inflammatory changes are thought more often to result from irritation rather than infection, as the uterine cavity becomes sterile again within 48 hours after the device has been inserted. Even so, some organisms are probably introduced with it. More widespread and severe inflammatory changes, however, result from infection. In these circumstances, the full picture of acute or chronic endometritis may be seen with a stromal infiltrate of neutrophils, plasma cells and lymphocytes, pus in the gland lumina, and suppression of the glandular hormonal cyclical response.

ENDOMETRIAL ABLATION

Procedures for endometrial ablation have grown in popularity as a method to treat benign symptomatic disease. Diffuse coagulative necrosis lacking any granulomatous component dominates the histologic picture for the first few weeks. It closely resembles the artifact commonly seen on the periphery of surgical specimens obtained by cauterizing sampling devices, but is more extensive and uniform. As collagen replaces the necrotic tissue, the appearance varies from well-formed noncaseating granulomas, which are difficult to distinguish from those of infective origin, to surrounding foreign-body giant cells and debris (Figure 16.62). Not all endometrial epithelium is destroyed during ablation, and residual glands that regrow may be inaccessible to future biopsy attempts because of obscuring adhesions. For this reason endometrial ablation is not advised for treatment of premalignant disease, where complete sampling during follow-up surveillance biopsies is desired.

REFERENCES

1. Centers for Disease Control and Prevention. Sexually transmitted disease surveillance 2009. http://www.cdc.gov/std/stats09/default.htm. 2009 [accessed 2012].
2. Mishra K, Wadhwa N, Guleria K, Agarwal S. ER, PR and Ki-67 expression status in granulomatous and chronic non-specific endometritis. J Obstet Gynaecol Res 2008;34:371–8.
3. Disep B, Innes BA, Cochrane HR, et al. Immunohistochemical characterization of endometrial leucocytes in endometritis. Histopathology 2004;45:625–32.
4. Searle RF, Jones RK, Bulmer JN. Phenotypic analysis and proliferative responses of human endometrial granulated lymphocytes during the menstrual cycle. Biol Reprod 1999;60:871–8.
5. Kiviat NB, Wolner-Hanssen P, Eschenbach DA, et al. Endometrial histopathology in patients with culture-proved upper genital tract infection and laparoscopically diagnosed acute salpingitis. Am J Surg Pathol 1990;14:167–75.
6. Peeling RW, Brunham RC. Chlamydiae as pathogens: new species and new issues. Emerg Infect Dis 1996;2:307–19.
7. Mount S, Mead P, Cooper K. Chlamydia trachomatis in the endometrium: can surgical pathologists identify plasma cells? Adv Anat Pathol 2001;8:327–9.
8. Paukku M, Puolakkainen M, Paavonen T, Paavonen J. Plasma cell endometritis is associated with Chlamydia trachomatis infection. Am J Clin Pathol 1999;112:211–15.
9. Korn AP, Bolan G, Padian N, et al. Plasma cell endometritis in women with symptomatic bacterial vaginosis. Obstet Gynecol 1995;85:387–90.
10. Cicinelli E, De ZD, Nicoletti R, et al. Chronic endometritis: correlation among hysteroscopic, histologic, and bacteriologic findings in a prospective trial with 2190 consecutive office hysteroscopies. Fertil Steril 2008;89:677–84.
11. Haggerty CL. Evidence for a role of Mycoplasma genitalium in pelvic inflammatory disease. Curr Opin Infect Dis 2008;21:65–9.
12. Kumar P, Shah NP, Singhal A, et al. Association of tuberculous endometritis with infertility and other gynecological complaints of women in India. J Clin Microbiol 2008;46:4068–70.
13. Nogales-Ortiz F, Tarancon I, Nogales Jr FF. The pathology of female genital tuberculosis. A 31-year study of 1436 cases. Obstet Gynecol 1979;53:422–8.
14. Patzina RA, de Andrade Jr HF, de Brito T, et al. Molecular and standard approaches to the diagnosis of mycobacterial granulomatous lymphadenitis in paraffin-embedded tissue. Lab Invest 2002;82:1095–7.
15. Selva E, Hofman V, Berto F, et al. The value of polymerase chain reaction detection of Mycobacterium tuberculosis in granulomas isolated by laser capture microdissection. Pathology 2004;36:77–81.
16. Salian NV, Rish JA, Eisenach KD, et al. Polymerase chain reaction to detect Mycobacterium tuberculosis in histologic specimens. Am J Respir Crit Care Med 1998;158:1150–5.
17. Valicenti Jr JF, Pappas AA, Graber CD, et al. Detection and prevalence of IUD-associated Actinomyces colonization and related morbidity. A prospective study of 69,925 cervical smears. JAMA 1982;247:1149–52.
18. Boyle DP, McCluggage WG. Combined actinomycotic and pseudoactinomycotic radiate granules in the female genital tract: description of a series of cases. J Clin Pathol 2009;62:1123–6.
19. Pritt B, Mount SL, Cooper K, Blaszyk H. Pseudoactinomycotic radiate granules of the gynaecological tract: review of a diagnostic pitfall. J Clin Pathol 2006;59:17–20.
20. Almoujahed MO, Briski LE, Prysak M, et al. Uterine granulomas: clinical and pathological features. Am J Clin Pathol 2002;117:771–5.
21. Knuth KR, Fraiz J, Fisch JA, Draper TW. Pinworm infestation of the genital tract. Am Fam Physician 1988;38:127–30.
22. Zaino RJ. Endometritis. In: Silverberg S, editor. Interpretation of endometrial biopsies and curettings. Philadelphia: Lippincott-Raven; 1996. p. 241–61.
23. Watts DH, Krohn MA, Hillier SL, Eschenbach DA. Bacterial vaginosis as a risk factor for post-cesarean endometritis. Obstet Gynecol 1990;75:52–8.
24. Peipert JF, Montagno AB, Cooper AS, Sung CJ. Bacterial vaginosis as a risk factor for upper genital tract infection. Am J Obstet Gynecol 1997;77:1184–7.
25. Bewtra C, Xie QM, Hunter WJ, Jurgensen W. Ichthyosis uteri: a case report and review of the literature. Arch Pathol Lab Med 2005;129:e124–5.
26. Mutter GL, Ince TA. Molecular pathogenesis of endometrial cancer. In: Fuller A, Seiden MV, Young R, editors. Uterine cancer:

American Cancer Society atlas of clinical oncology. Hamilton, ON Canada: B.C. Decker; 2004. p. 10–21.
27. Mutter GL. Endometrial carcinogenesis: an integrated molecular, histologic, and functional model of a dualistic disease. In: Giordano A, Bovicelli A, Kurman R, editors. Molecular pathology of gynecologic cancer. Totowa, NJ, USA: Humana; 2006.
28. Deutchman ME, Hartman KJ. Postpartum pyometra: a case report. J Fam Pract 1993;36:449–52.
29. Naora H. Developmental patterning in the wrong context: the paradox of epithelial ovarian cancers. Cell Cycle 2005;4:1033–5.
30. Samuel S, Naora H. Homeobox gene expression in cancer: insights from developmental regulation and deregulation. Eur J Cancer 2005;41:2428–37.
31. Block K, Kardana A, Igarashi P, Taylor HS. In utero diethylstilbestrol (DES) exposure alters Hox gene expression in the developing mullerian system. FASEB J 2000;14:1101–8.
32. Taylor HS, Arici A, Olive D, Igarashi P. HOXA10 is expressed in response to sex steroids at the time of implantation in the human endometrium. J Clin Invest 1998;101:1379–84.
33. Yoshida H, Broaddus R, Cheng W, et al. Deregulation of the HOXA10 homeobox gene in endometrial carcinoma: role in epithelial-mesenchymal transition. Cancer Res 2006;66:889–97.
34. Jovanovic AS, Boynton KA, Mutter GL. Uteri of women with endometrial carcinoma contain a histopathologic spectrum of monoclonal putative precancers, some with microsatellite instability. Cancer Res 1996;56:1917–21.
35. Cheng W, Liu J, Yoshida H, et al. Lineage infidelity of epithelial ovarian cancers is controlled by HOX genes that specify regional identity in the reproductive tract. Nat Med 2005;11:531–7.
36. Taylor HS, Igarashi P, Olive DL, Arici A. Sex steroids mediate HOXA11 expression in the human peri-implantation endometrium. J Clin Endocrinol Metab 1999;84:1129–35.
37. Carlson JW, Mutter GL. Endometrial intraepithelial neoplasia is associated with polyps and frequently has metaplastic change. Histopathology 2008;53:325–32.
38. Mutter GL. Histopathology of genetically defined endometrial precancers. Int J Gynecol Pathol 2000;19:301–9.
39. Mutter GL. Diagnosis of premalignant endometrial disease. J Clin Pathol 2002;55:326–31.
40. Silverberg SG, Mutter GL, Kurman RJ, et al. Tumors of the uterine corpus: epithelial tumors and related lesions. In: Tavassoli FA, Stratton MR, editors. WHO classification of tumors: pathology and genetics of tumors of the breast and female genital organs. Lyon, France: IARC Press; 2003. p. 221–32.
41. Kaku T, Silverberg SG, Tsukamoto N, et al. Association of endometrial epithelial metaplasias with endometrial carcinoma and hyperplasia in Japanese and American women. Am J Pathol 1993;12:297–300.
42. Crum CP, Richart RM, Fenoglio CM. Adenoacanthosis of endometrium: a clinicopathologic study in premenopausal women. Am J Surg Pathol 1981;5:15–20.
43. Lin MC, Lomo L, Baak JPA, et al. Squamous morules are functionally inert elements of premalignant endometrial neoplasia. Mod Pathol 2009;22:167–74.
44. Saegusa M, Okayasu I. Frequent nuclear beta-catenin accumulation and associated mutations in endometrioid-type endometrial and ovarian carcinomas with squamous differentiation. J Pathol 2001;194:59–67.
45. Brachtel EF, Sanchez-Estevez C, Moreno-Bueno G, et al. Distinct molecular alterations in complex endometrial hyperplasia (CEH) with and without immature squamous metaplasia (squamous morules). Am J Surg Pathol 2005;29:1322–9.
46. Vang R, Tavassoli FA. Proliferative mucinous lesions of the endometrium: analysis of existing criteria for diagnosing carcinoma in biopsies and curettings. Int J Surg Pathol 2003;11:261–70.
47. Nucci M, Crum CP, Prasad C, Mutter GL. Mucinous endometrial epithelial proliferations: a morphologic spectrum of changes with diverse clinical significance. Mod Pathol 2000;12:1137–42.
48. Lehman MB, Hart WR. Simple and complex hyperplastic papillary proliferations of the endometrium—a clinicopathologic study of nine cases of apparently localized papillary lesions with fibrovascular stromal cores and epithelial metaplasia. Am J Surg Pathol 2001;25:1347–54.
49. Bergeron C, Ferenczy A. Oncocytic metaplasia in endometrial hyperplasia and carcinoma. Int J Gynecol Pathol 1988;7:93–5.
50. Zaman SS, Mazur MT. Endometrial papillary syncytial change. A nonspecific alteration associated with active breakdown. Am J Clin Pathol 1993;99:741–5.
51. Basu M, Mammen C, Owen E. Bony fragments in the uterus: an association with secondary subfertility. Ultrasound Obstet Gynecol 2003;22:402–6.
52. Bolaji I, Saridogan E, Hasan N, et al. Prolonged retention of fetal bones with osseous metaplasia of the endometrium. Int J Gynaecol Obstet 1995;50:65–6.
53. Bahceci M, Demirel LC. Osseous metaplasia of the endometrium: a rare cause of infertility and its hysteroscopic management. Hum Reprod 1996;11:2537–9.
54. Shimizu M, Nakayama M. Endometrial ossification in a postmenopausal woman. J Clin Pathol 1997;50:171–2.
55. Creagh TM, Bain BJ, Evans DJ, et al. Endometrial extramedullary haemopoiesis. J Pathol 1995;176:99–104.
56. Fletcher J, Pinkus J, Lage J, et al. Clonal 6p21 rearrangement is restricted to the mesenchymal component of an endometrial polyp. Genes Chromosomes Cancer 1992;5:260–3.
57. Dal Cin P, Vanni R, Marras S, et al. Four cytogenetic subgroups can be identified in endometrial polyps. Cancer Res 1995;55:1565–8.
58. Bol S, Wanschura S, Thode B, et al. An endometrial polyp with a rearrangement of HMGI-C underlying a complex cytogenetic rearrangement involving chromosomes 2 and 12. Cancer Genet Cytogenet 1996;90:88–90.
59. Cohen I. Endometrial pathologies associated with postmenopausal tamoxifen treatment. Gynecol Oncol 2004;94:256–66.
60. Deligdisch L, Kalir T, Cohen CJ, et al. Endometrial histopathology in 700 patients treated with tamoxifen for breast cancer. Gynecol Oncol 2000;78:181–6.
61. Kim KR, Peng R, Ro JY, Robboy SJ. A diagnostically useful histopathologic feature of endometrial polyp: the long axis of endometrial glands arranged parallel to surface epithelium. Am J Surg Pathol 2004;28:1057–62.
62. Reslova T, Tosner J, Resl M, et al. Endometrial polyps. A clinical study of 245 cases. Arch Gynecol Obstet 1999;262:133–9.
63. Longacre TA, Chung MH, Rouse RV, Hendrickson MR. Atypical polypoid adenomyofibromas (atypical polypoid adenomyomas) of the uterus. A clinicopathologic study of 55 cases. Am J Surg Pathol 1996;20:1–20.
64. Ota S, Catasus L, Matias-Guiu X, et al. Molecular pathology of atypical polypoid adenomyoma of the uterus. Hum Pathol 2003;34:784–8.
65. Clement PB, Young RH. Endometrioid carcinoma of the uterine corpus: a review of its pathology with emphasis on recent advances and problematic aspects. Adv Anat Pathol 2002;9:145–84.
66. Fernandez H, Al-Najjar F, Chauveaud-Lambling A, et al. Fertility after treatment of Asherman's syndrome stage 3 and 4. J Minim Invasive Gynecol 2006;13:398–402.
67. Roy KH, Mattox JH. Advances in endometrial ablation. Obstet Gynecol Surv 2002;57:789–802.
68. Mencaglia L, Tonellotto D. Endometrial ablation: a review. In: Blanc B, Marty R, DeMontgolfier R, editors. Office and operative hysteroscopy. Paris, France: Springer-Verlag; 2002. p. 197–202.
69. Parra-Herran CE, Monte NM, Mutter GL. Endometrial intraepithelial neoplasia with secretory differentiation: Diagnostic features and underlying mechanisms. Mod Pathol 2013;26:868–73.

Endometrial Hyperplasia without Atypia and EIN

George L. Mutter

CHAPTER OUTLINE

Introduction and Terminology	349	EIN, Atypical Hyperplasia	357
Two Diseases	350	Cancer Outcomes in Women with EIN	358
The Spectrum of Non-Atypical Endometrial Hyperplasias	350	Molecular Etiology and Natural History	358
Disordered Proliferative Endometrium: a Prelude to Non-Atypical Hyperplasia	352	Specific EIN Diagnostic Criteria	360
		Common EIN Diagnostic Problems	364
Non-Atypical Hyperplasia	353	Non-Endometrioid EIN	366
Non-Atypical Hyperplasia with Superimposed Progestin Effect	355	Hormonally Treated EIN	366
		Special Studies for EIN Diagnosis	367
Withdrawal Shedding Following Non-Atypical Hyperplasia	355	Biomarkers: *PAX2* and *PTEN*	367
		Quantitative Histomorphometry	367
Normal Endometrium	356	Management of EIN	368
Endometrial Polyps	356	Hysterectomy	368
Postmenopausal Cystic Atrophy	356	Hormonal Therapy	368
Exclusion of EIN	357		

INTRODUCTION AND TERMINOLOGY

The meaningful resolution of endometrial hyperplasias, a mixed group of diseases, has challenged pathologists for decades. Long envisioned as a continuous spectrum of morphologic changes of increasing severity, in reality they encompass only two discrete disease states, which can and should be diagnosed independently of carcinoma (Table 17.1). This consensus has now been endorsed by the Clinical Practice Committee of the Society of Gynecologic Oncologists[1] and the World Health Organization (WHO).[2] Endometrial hyperplasia without atypia is a functionally normal endometrium which has developed changes in response to an abnormal hormonal environment, usually unopposed estrogens. EIN, endometrial (or, endometrioid) intraepithelial neoplasia, also known as atypical hyperplasia, is a monoclonal proliferation of mutated glands that increases the likelihood of carcinoma through malignant transformation of its component cells. We have used the terms non-atypical hyperplasia and EIN throughout this chapter, corresponding to the respective WHO 2014[2] categories of hyperplasia without atypia, and Endometrioid Intraepithelial Neoplasia. The supportive evidence base for EIN has already been published extensively,[3,4] and has been clinically implemented since 2001 as part of a two-class system.[5]

All examples of endometrial hyperplasia are abnormal in having too many glands, with distinction between non-atypical endometrial hyperplasia and EIN based upon the character and architectural context of those cytologic changes that are present. The intrinsic plasticity of the endometrium, and its dynamic response over time to a large number of internal and external factors, contributes a great deal of variation to the appearances of individual lesions between patients. It has been the examination of many examples of functionally classified disease that has provided a new evidence base for their diagnosis.[6] As several of the most informative diagnostic criteria available today were unknown at the time of the formulation of the 1993 four-class WHO system (simple non-atypical, simple atypical, complex non-atypical, complex atypical),[7] the current 2014 version is a replacement for, rather than condensation of, the prior system.

Table 17.1 Diagnostic Entities and Terminology (WHO, 2014)

Nomenclature*	Topography	Functional Category	Cancer Risk	Treatment
Hyperplasia without Atypia	Diffuse	Prolonged estrogen effect	2–4×[18–21]	Hormonal therapy, symptomatic
EIN (atypical hyperplasia)	Focal progressing to diffuse	Precancerous	45×[14]	Hormonal or surgical
Endometrioid adenocarcinoma	Focal progressing to diffuse	Malignant	—	Surgical stage-based

*In WHO 2014 terminology, EIN and atypical hyperplasia are alternative, synonymous, terms.

TWO DISEASES

Endometrial hyperplasia is a nonspecific histopathologic term indicating an abundance of glands and increase in tissue bulk (Figure 17.1). Historically, it came to encompass a bewildering array of lesions that were further subdivided by morphology and suspected to include precancers as one of its subsets. New possibilities emerged in the last two decades, as molecular tools were applied to the problem of precancers. It became possible to query growth patterns (polyclonal, monoclonal), develop markers to highlight lesions against the backdrop of their tissue of origin, and track cell lineages between premalignant and malignant phases. As a result of these changes, a National Institutes of Health workshop convened in 2004 to define features of epithelial precancers that are shared across multiple tissues.[8] These included: (1) the lesion is different from normal tissues,[9] (2) the lesion is different from cancer,[10,11] (3) the lesion can be diagnosed,[12] (4) there is lineage continuity between cells of the precancer and cancer,[6,11] and (5) patients with the lesion have increased rates of cancer.[13,14] All of these evidence-based criteria had already been met by EIN, as indicated by citations inserted into the preceding numbered list. Field effects, such as the general response of a tissue to hormonal, irradiation, or infectious factors, do not meet the definition of a precancerous lesion, as these are intrinsically normal tissues reacting to external influences (failed criterion 1) and it is not possible to identify specific cells that will become cancer (failed criterion 4).

The neoplastic character of EIN, originally documented by nonrandom X chromosome inactivation,[15] has since been shown to bear clonal abnormalities of PTEN,[10] PAX2,[16] KRAS2,[17] and altered microsatellites.[6,11] In the case of those markers which can be studied in situ by immunohistochemistry, PTEN and PAX2, staining of informative lesions has been useful in defining lesion distribution.[16] Most importantly, the localized clonal character of premalignant lesions affords an opportunity to compare lesional with background cytology in a robust internally controlled assessment of cytologic alteration. Such a standard holds across shifting hormonal states, and between patients, in whom the lesions themselves may have a variety of absolute cytologies. Additionally, large-scale 'topographic' features are informative in distinguishing localized precancers from the diffuse field effects of hormonal change. Morphometry of biologically defined precancers (monoclonal, in a continuous lineage to cancer) has contributed precise definition of gland

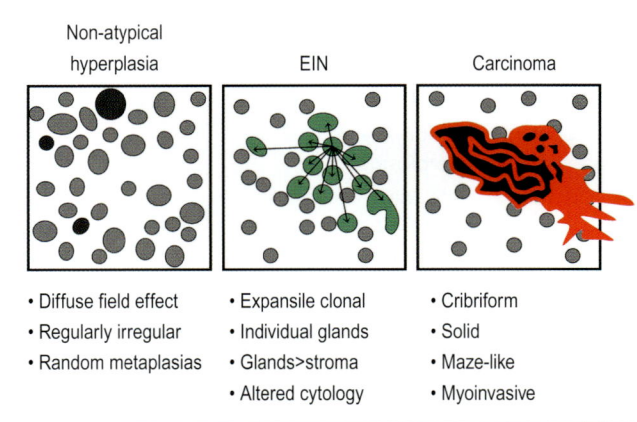

Figure 17.1 General features that distinguish EIN from non-atypical hyperplasia and carcinoma. (For carcinoma, see also Figure 18.12.)

crowding in precancers. These simple insights provide a new evidence base for revision of precancer diagnostic criteria as presented below.

Prolonged estrogen exposure unmitigated by opposing progestins and the appearance of an abnormal endometrial histology have long been associated with an increased risk for endometrioid (type I) endometrial adenocarcinoma. The risk, which is two- to four-fold increased,[18–20] has been calculated from large epidemiologic studies of cancer outcomes in women of known hormonal exposure. The histologic appearance of the endometrium modified by unopposed estrogens is initially dependent on dose and duration of exposure, but uniform throughout the field. These can be heavily modified when the estrogens decline or are subsequently countered by progestins. The resultant spectrum of histologies, which we have described as a dynamic sequence of change over time, is discussed below as non-atypical endometrial hyperplasia.

THE SPECTRUM OF NON-ATYPICAL ENDOMETRIAL HYPERPLASIAS

Non-atypical endometrial hyperplasia is a spectrum of hormonally induced pan-endometrial changes, characterized by increased gland density and variation in gland size and shape. Glands may branch slightly. Cytologic change, when it occurs, is most often metaplastic and distributed in a scattered, non-geographic or random fashion. Areas of stromal breakdown and epithelial collapse may be present. This appearance changes dynamically as a function of interval and amount of unopposed estrogens,[21] may persist in altered form after the exposure ends, and can be modified by superimposed secondary hormonal effects such as by progestins.[22]

Non-atypical hyperplasia of the endometrium has many synonyms including simple or complex non-atypical hyperplasia,[23] endometrial hyperplasia,[4] and benign endometrial hyperplasia.[22] It is related to disordered proliferative and anovulatory endometrium, which are lesser changes seen with shorter estrogen exposures (see Chapter 15).

Clinical Features

Non-atypical hyperplasia is encountered most frequently around the time of perimenopause when the normal cycle of sequentially regulated estrogen and progesterone is perturbed. Changes may carry forward into menopause or develop *de novo* in the hormonally stimulated postmenopausal patient. In a woman of childbearing age, there is characteristically prolonged or excessive bleeding at irregular intervals. As the endometrial bulk increases through proliferation, the bleeding may become more frequent and almost continuous. The causes of excessive bleeding are multiple. Dilated and delicate superficial blood vessels undergo thrombosis, which contributes to intermittent bleeding. Because the condition depends upon estrogen stimulation for its development, the fluctuation of estrogenic support results in irregular episodes of extensive apoptotic endometrial stromal cell death and breakdown of the tissue.

Persistent estrogen production may be associated with ovarian abnormalities such as granulosa cell tumors, thecomas, polycystic ovary disease, or exogenous administration of estrogens. Most patients eventually become symptomatic and present with abnormal vaginal bleeding. An unknown proportion has no symptoms and the abnormality only becomes apparent when baseline biopsies are taken for hormone replacement therapy.

The two- to four-fold increased risk of endometrioid endometrial cancer in patients with non-atypical hyperplasia is referable to the extent of estrogen exposure.[18-21] Clinical treatment is focused on symptomatic relief, and identification and control of estrogens. This can be a difficult task, especially when the underlying condition is a chronic state, such as obesity or polycystic ovarian syndrome.

Etiology

In the first half of a normal cycle, unopposed estrogen brings about proliferation, with mitotic activity of both glands and stroma. Ovulation occurs at day 14, followed by secretion of progesterone, the effect of which is to stimulate secretory activity in the endometrium and, at the same time, to inhibit proliferation through downregulation of estrogen receptors. If ovulation does not occur until much later than day 14 or does not happen at all, the estrogen remains unopposed and proliferation continues. This prolonged proliferation as a result of anovulation first gives rise to disordered proliferative endometrium after a period of about 3 weeks. The serum levels of estrogens are not necessarily raised, although in some circumstances they may be.

Longer intervals of estrogen stimulation cause an even greater exaggeration of the proliferative phase, with an increasingly irregular distribution of individually variable endometrial glands, which are known as non-atypical hyperplasia. Looked at in this way, disordered proliferative endometrium and non-atypical hyperplasia may be regarded as a physiologic response of a normal endometrium to prolonged and unopposed estrogen stimulation. Microinfarcts and estrogen withdrawal are responsible for symptomatic bleeding.[24,25] Both mechanisms may be effective at different times in patients with non-atypical hyperplasia. Patchy stromal breakdown secondary to estrogen-induced microthrombi can produce intermittent spotting.

The pharmacologic administration of estrogen, or estrogenic compounds, can cause a persistent proliferative state in the postmenopausal patient.[26] As with anovulation, the root cause is the systemic hormonal imbalance, and the endometrial response a frequent source of symptomatic bleeding.

Although the causal event in non-atypical hyperplasia is unopposed estrogen, the histologic appearance at diagnosis may be heavily modified by subsequent loss of estrogen or introduction of superimposed effects of other hormones. Rapid withdrawal of estrogen stimulation causes apoptosis of the endometrial glands and stroma of the hypertrophied functionalis, and resultant heavy shedding. Occasionally, decline in estrogen levels is sufficiently gradual that generalized apoptosis and shedding fail to take place leaving behind an architecturally altered endometrium composed of inactive glands.

Superimposition of progesterone upon a non-atypical hyperplasia occurs in women with delayed or intermittent ovulation, or therapeutic administration of progestins following an extended follicular phase. Downregulation of estrogen receptors by progestins leads to a dominant progestational effect, regardless of the presence or absence of continued estrogen production. In this environment menstrual shedding is delayed, as progestins have the capacity to directly support the endometrium. Progesterone-related stromal and secretory glandular changes develop within the setting of irregular glands previously formed under the influence of estrogens.

Gross Features

Initial changes, seen after only 3 weeks of unopposed estrogens (1 week beyond expected ovulation date), are subtle. The endometrium may be moderately but uniformly thickened with a smooth surface lining. Scattered microcysts, although often present, are not apparent on gross examination. With further estrogen exposure, the uterus may enlarge and the endometrium often is irregularly thickened, pale to tan, and sometimes sessile polypoid (Figure 17.2). Endometrial curettage in a woman who has non-atypical hyperplasia is likely to generate abundant curettings that require two or more cassettes for adequate processing. Foci of hemorrhage may be present in the areas of breakdown. Ultrasound may help identify the thickened endometrium.[27]

Microscopic Features

The histologic changes of non-atypical hyperplasia are conceptually and morphologically well represented as a disease spectrum related to unopposed estrogens.

Table 17.2 Histologic Features of Non-Atypical Hyperplasia (Not All Are Present in Every Case)

Feature	Comment	Disordered Proliferative	Non-Atypical Hyperplasia[1] Active Phase	Non-Atypical Hyperplasia[1] Inactive Phase	Non-Atypical Hyperplasia[1] Superimposed Progestin	Shedding Following Non-Atypical Hyperplasia[2]
Mitotic activity	Similar to normal proliferation	+	+			
Scattered cysts	Within functionalis, random placement	+	+	+	+	
Tubal metaplasia	Randomly involves scattered tubular or cystic glands, ± cilia	+	+	+	+	
Variable gland density	'Regularly irregular' Secondary to gland proliferation and remodeling		+	+	+	
Bulky specimen	Reflects prolonged proliferative activity		+	+	+	
Fibrin thrombi	Often separate or displaced		+	+	+	+
Microinfarcts with epithelial change	Randomly placed, multifocal, with intervening intact		+	+	+	
Low or absent mitoses	Reflects decline in estrogen			+	+	+
Secretory change	Variable extent depending on exposure				+	+
Stromal pre-decidualization	May be patchy or lacking, depending on progestin exposure				+	+
Global breakdown	Architectural clues obscured, cytology degenerative					+

[1] Diagnosis is 'non-atypical hyperplasia.' Subphases need not be specified.
[2] Indistinguishable from menstrual endometrium, with or without confirmation of ovulation. If present, fibrin thrombi can be described as a feature consistent with a hormonally abnormal antecedent cycle.

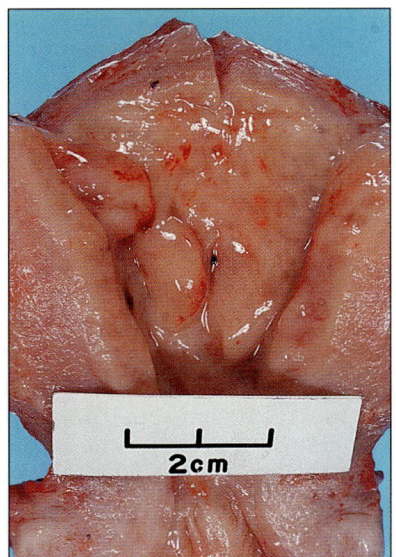

Figure 17.2 Non-atypical hyperplasia. The endometrium is diffusely thickened with a nodular surface but no overt polyp formation. Microscopy showed non-atypical hyperplasia with multiple cysts.

The morphologic features are characteristically diffuse and widespread, as would be expected for a tissue responding uniformly to an underlying systemic hormonal cause. Individual examples differ by time line and amount of estrogen exposure, and may be further modified by degenerative changes or other sex hormones such as progestins (Table 17.2). The range of possible histologic changes is thus broad, with few specimens demonstrating them all. Aside from providing some measure of the patient's hormonal state at the time of biopsy, discrimination among the various histologic subtypes of non-atypical hyperplasia discussed below is of little immediate clinical importance. Much more critical is that non-atypical hyperplasia is not confused with EIN (Figure 17.1). These are not mutually exclusive in the individual patient, however, as non-atypical hyperplasia is a common comorbidity in women with EIN. The sections below provide a functional framework to describe the histologic varieties of commonly encountered non-atypical endometrial hyperplasia.

DISORDERED PROLIFERATIVE ENDOMETRIUM: A PRELUDE TO NON-ATYPICAL HYPERPLASIA

Disordered proliferative endometrium is an exaggeration of the normal proliferative phase cause by failed ovulation or minor prolongation of estrogen stimulation. The pathognomonic feature is cystic changes of individual glands distributed randomly throughout the entire hormonally responsive region of the endometrium (superficial functionalis) (Figure 17.3). The overall ratio of glands to stroma is not significantly increased from that of a normal proliferative phase, and mitotically active glands are proliferative with a simple but often pseudostratified epithelium (Figure 17.4). The stroma is usually dense, cellular, and abundant, thus

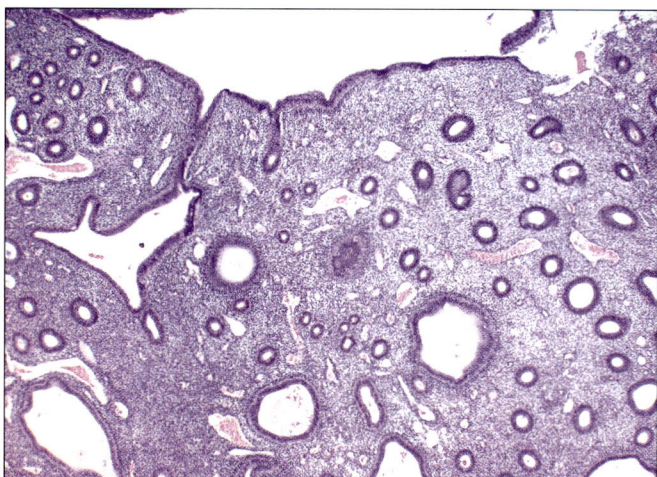

Figure 17.3 Disordered proliferative endometrium demonstrating glands at low density with scattered cyst formation. Placement of glands is quite regular, and branching is slight, indicating a minimal extent of remodeling.

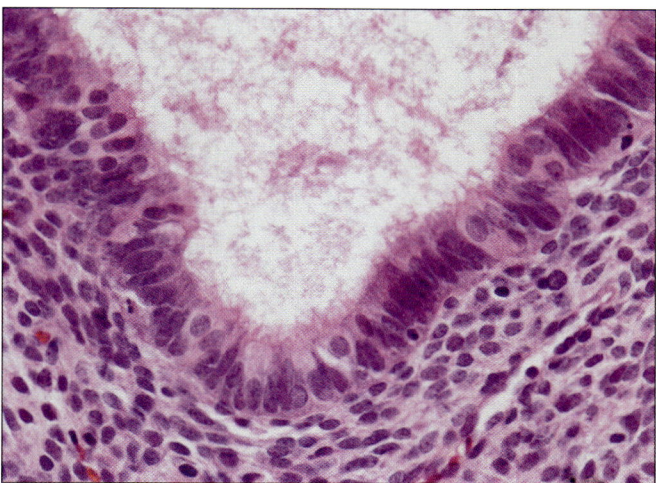

Figure 17.5 Tubal differentiation with cilia formation, interposed round epithelial cells, and eosinophilic cytoplasm is a common estrogen effect in disordered proliferative endometrium and non-atypical hyperplasia.

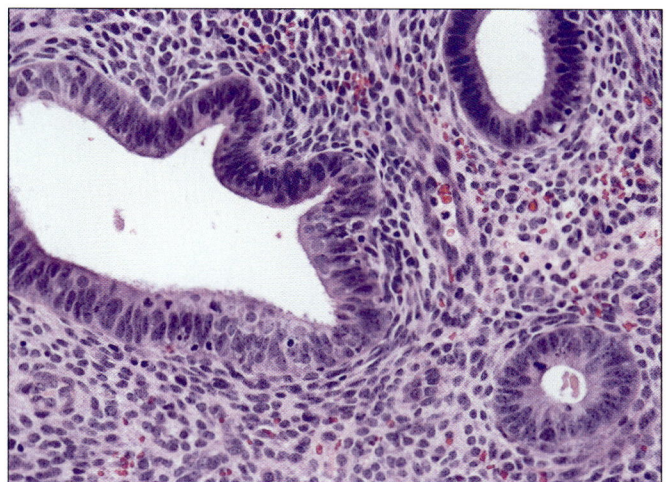

Figure 17.4 Cytology of disordered proliferative glands resembles that of normal proliferative endometrium, surrounded by a dense stroma.

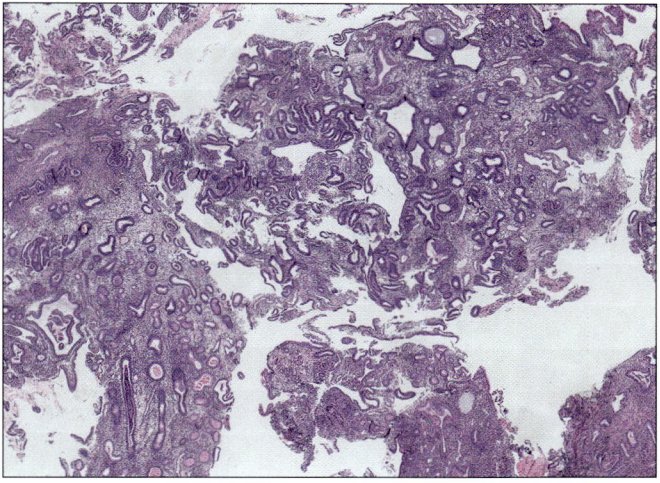

Figure 17.6 Macroscopic view of non-atypical hyperplasia showing randomly distributed cysts and variable gland spacing across multiple fragments. This presents a 'regularly irregular' pattern, in which there is a broad symmetry among fragments at very low magnification, which disappears at smaller scales where each field looks different.

separating the glands. Gland density is low. Some background tubular glands are slightly irregular and minimal budding and branching is commonly seen.

Ciliated cell change (tubal metaplasia) of endometrial glandular cells is common, reflecting estrogen's pivotal role in the process (Figure 17.5). Characteristically, glands affected by tubal differentiation are randomly interspersed among proliferative glands, and they may demonstrate tubular, branching, or cystic architecture.

NON-ATYPICAL HYPERPLASIA

Non-atypical hyperplasia develops from disordered proliferative endometrium under the continued influence of unopposed estrogens. The entire endometrial compartment contains variable gland densities caused by remodeling of stroma and glands to the extent that in some areas the gland to stroma ratio exceeds 1. It is the change in gland density that offsets non-atypical hyperplasia from disordered proliferative endometrium. Individual glands may be tubular, cystic, or branching, and these forms are commingled throughout. On a large scale the endometrium appears uniformly affected; however, at medium magnification local admixtures of individually variable glands present quite differing appearances between separate microscopic fields. This combination of low-magnification uniformity, made up of variable medium magnification fields, can be described as 'regularly irregular' (Figure 17.6).

The cytology of non-atypical hyperplasia does not change between architecturally crowded and uncrowded areas. This reflects the systemic hormonal etiology of the process, which similarly exposes the entire endometrium, and allows

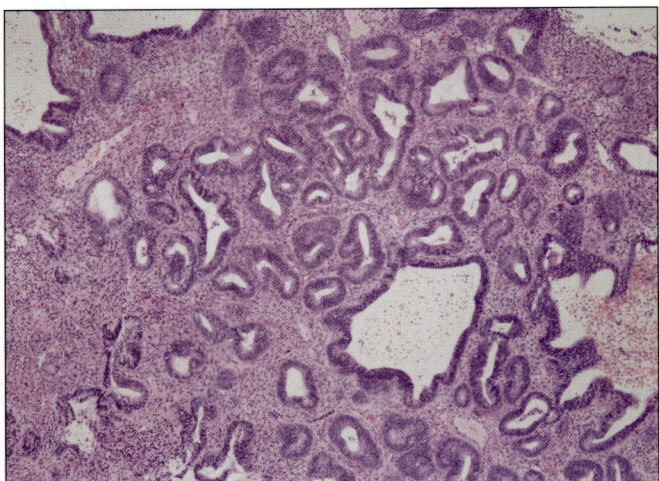

Figure 17.7 Non-atypical hyperplasia with randomly interspersed cystic and tubular glands. The entire endometrial compartment is involved, but local remodeling of glands with stroma creates regional heterogeneity of gland density. Glands are tubular, cystic, and branching.

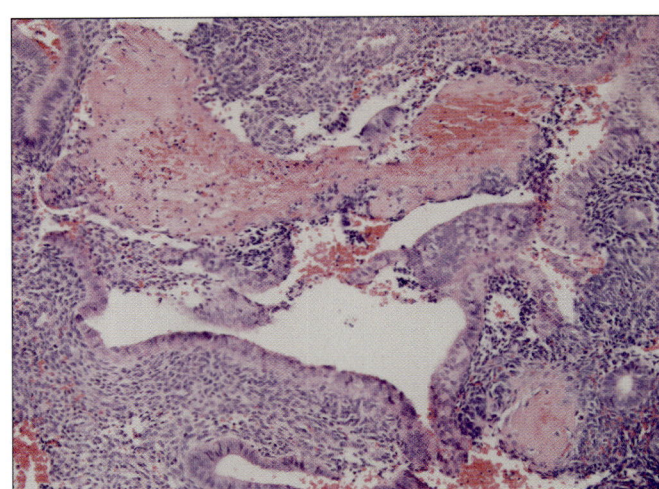

Figure 17.9 Fibrin thrombi can be seen in superficial blood vessels of non-atypical hyperplasia, causing local breakdown.

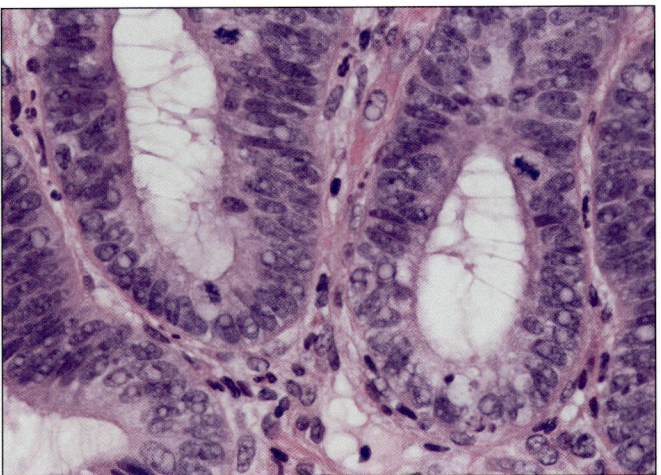

Figure 17.8 Non-atypical endometrial hyperplasia, detail. Proliferative glands indicate an active phase of estrogen stimulation.

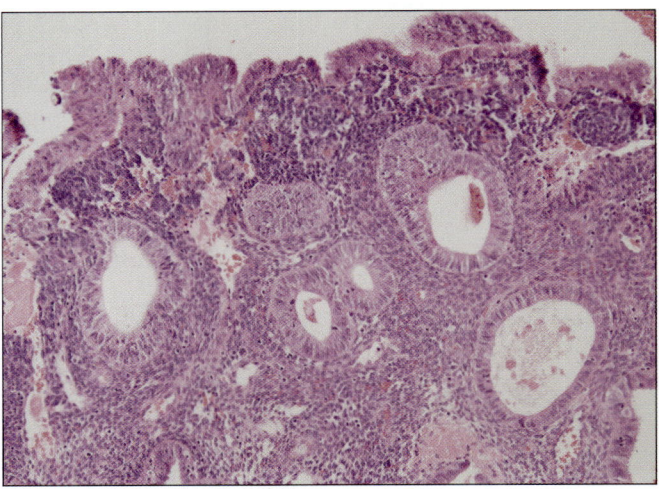

Figure 17.10 Stromal breakdown in non-atypical hyperplasia alters the cytology of the adjacent epithelium, and may lead to gland displacement.

its distinction from EIN. Absolute cytologic presentation may change over time with the evolving hormonal state of the patient, and superimposition of local factors such as breakdown and repair. During the established phase of active estrogen exposure glands are proliferative and interposed tubal metaplasia is common (Figures 17.7 and 17.8).

Sometime after initiation of cystic gland dilatation the endothelial lining of ectatic superficial endometrial vessels may be damaged and occlusive luminal fibrin thrombi form (Figure 17.9). Unopposed estrogen states are the most common setting in which fibrin thrombi are seen in the intact endometrial functionalis.[24] Fibrin thrombi are rarely seen in architecturally normal late secretory endometrium, and there is no evidence that vascular thrombosis is a primary mechanism of cyclical synchronized menstrual shedding. Thrombi are often intimately associated with discrete areas of surrounding stromal breakdown, which has been interpreted as either a cause or effect of the vascular lesion. Whatever the sequence and mechanism of events, the two are linked in non-atypical hyperplasias, and are responsible for patchy non-synchronous endometrial breakdown and resultant symptoms of spotting and intermenstrual bleeding. Collapse of intervening broken down stroma may lead to close apposition of endometrial glands, degenerative epithelial changes (Figure 17.10), and dislodgement of vascular thrombi from their tissue context. It is the close association of these epithelial changes with stromal breakdown that permits their distinction from EIN.

Estrogen production from persistent follicles or by peripheral conversion following the menopause is inconstant. When the estrogen level declines slowly, massive breakdown does not occur and the glands lose mitotic activity and enter an inactive phase. These endometria retain the

CHAPTER 17 — ENDOMETRIAL HYPERPLASIA WITHOUT ATYPIA AND EIN

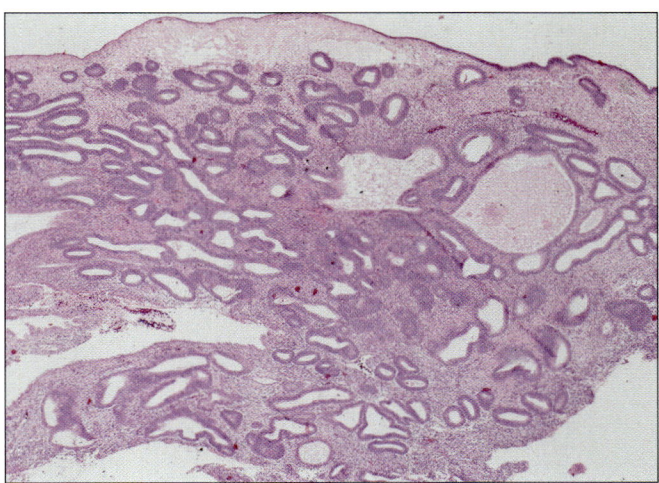

Figure 17.11 Non-atypical hyperplasia, inactive phase. Irregular and cystic glands are present at high density.

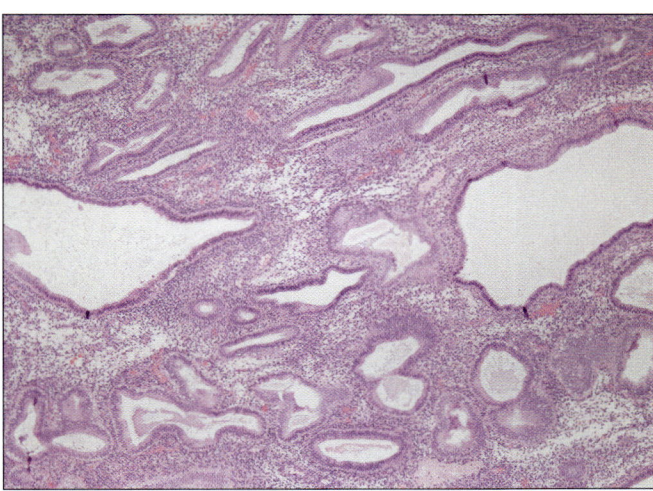

Figure 17.13 Delayed ovulation following protracted estrogen stimulation superimposes secretory change upon pre-existing cystic architecture.

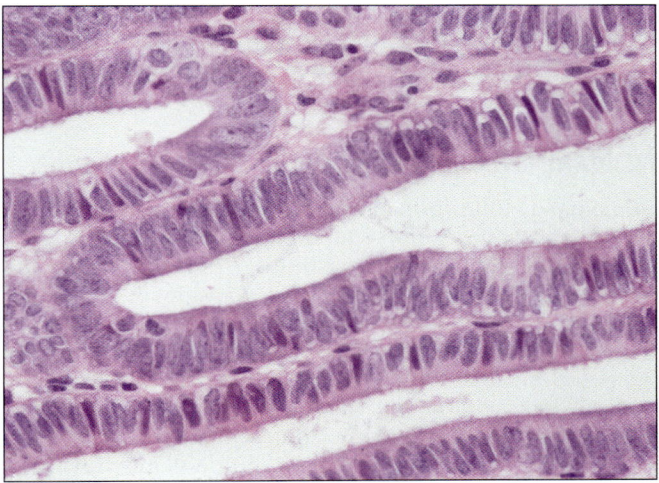

Figure 17.12 Non-atypical hyperplasia, detail of inactive phase. Amitotic epithelium, indicating that high estrogen levels are no longer present.

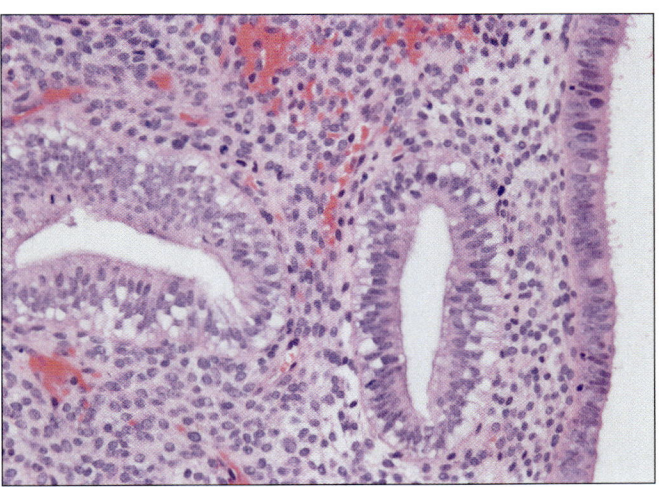

Figure 17.14 Detail of delayed ovulation in non-atypical endometrial hyperplasia showing vacuoles, which indicate progesterone effect. The progesterone is of short duration, as mitoses are not yet suppressed.

architectural features of a bulky endometrium with altered gland architecture, but the glands lack mitotic activity (Figures 17.11 and 17.12) and may become karyorrhectic. With prolonged low estrogen levels, endometrial bulk declines toward an atrophic pattern, sometimes with cysts.

NON-ATYPICAL HYPERPLASIA WITH SUPERIMPOSED PROGESTIN EFFECT

Superimposition of endogenous or exogenous progestins upon non-atypical hyperplasia shuts down mitotic activity, and may initiate secretory change. The most common endogenous progesterone source is delayed ovulation in a perimenopausal woman, where the corpus luteum is typically unable to elaborate normal quantities and duration of progesterone (Figures 17.13 and 17.14). The process is widespread throughout the endometrial compartment, although the secretory response of glands may be patchy or irregular when progestin levels are subphysiologic. More profound progestin effects, including secretory exhaustion and extensive stromal pseudodecidualization, can be seen with exogenous hormonal therapy (Figure 17.15).

WITHDRAWAL SHEDDING FOLLOWING NON-ATYPICAL HYPERPLASIA

Cessation of estrogenic stimulation, such as occurs systemically upon shutdown or exhaustion of the persistently active ovarian follicle, leads to rapid endometrial-wide stromal breakdown and heavy menses. This occurs through a direct apoptotic effect upon endometrial stromal and epithelial cells, rather than thrombosis-initiated infarction responsible for breakdown during the estrogen-rich period. Architectural features of cysts and irregular gland distribution are

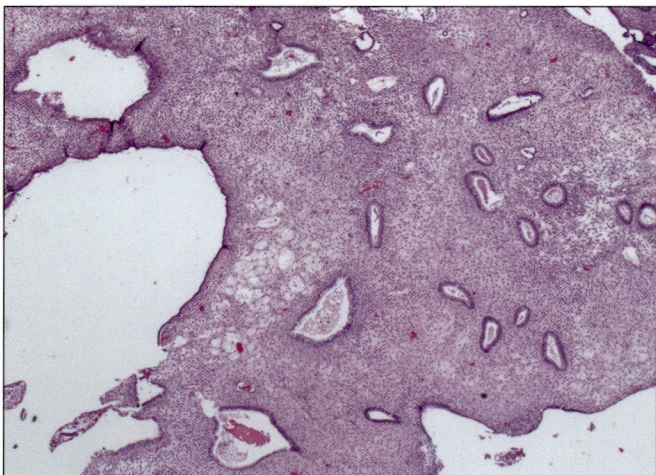

Figure 17.15 Endometrial hyperplasia following 1 week of progestin treatment. This 49-year-old woman had not ovulated in 6 months and had intermittent bleeding and a thickened endometrium on ultrasound. Stromal pseudodecidualization is superimposed on preexisting cystic architecture.

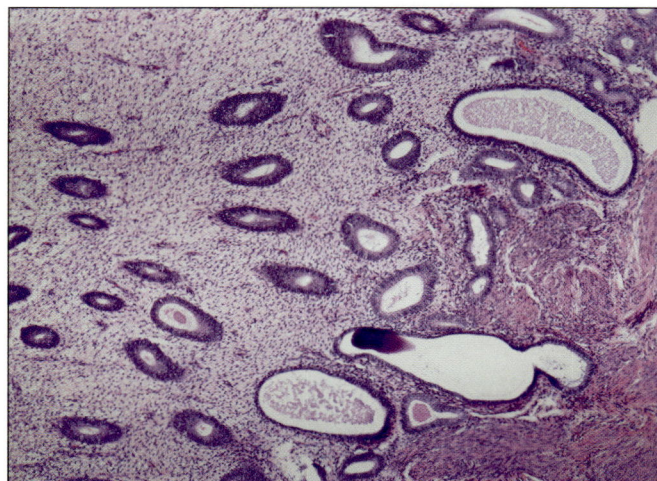

Figure 17.17 The glands of normal basal endometrium may be cystic but they are localized to the endomyometrial junction.

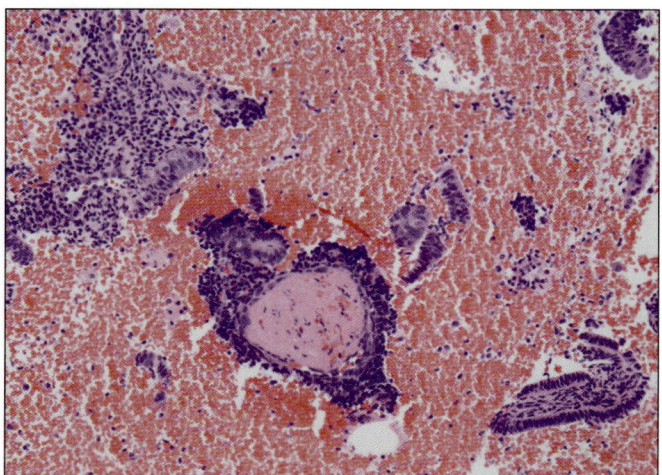

Figure 17.16 Withdrawal shedding of non-atypical hyperplasia is caused by rapid decline of supportive sex hormones. Fibrin thrombi scattered among nondescript stromal aggregates may be the only identifiable residua, as more specific diagnostic features are obscured or 'erased' by massive breakdown.

increasingly obscured by stromal collapse, eventually yielding a nondescript collection of degenerative individual glands. For these reasons, it can be difficult to confirm in the late stages of shedding whether the preceding cycle was normal or abnormal, or whether a non-atypical hyperplasia was present or not. Fibrin thrombi may remain, but their presence in itself is nonspecific and insufficient for a diagnosis of non-atypical endometrial hyperplasia (Figure 17.16).

Differential Diagnosis

It is necessary to distinguish non-atypical hyperplasia from a variety of conditions, both physiologic and pathologic. These include EIN (atypical hyperplasia), changes induced by artifacts during the gathering of the specimen, misinterpretation of a variety of normal appearances, and other pathologic states.

NORMAL ENDOMETRIUM

Immediately following menses and at the beginning of the proliferative phase, the endometrial functionalis is thin, with endometrial basalis constituting the majority of the tissue seen. Irregularly spaced and occasionally branching glands of the basalis must be distinguished from non-atypical hyperplasia. The glands of basal endometrium are dark and irregular and may be cystic but they are localized to the endomyometrial junction (Figure 17.17). The basal stroma is dense and cellular. Endometrium sampled between cessation of menses and onset of proliferation is much scantier than that of non-atypical hyperplasias, and there is usually evidence of recent repair along the luminal surface.

ENDOMETRIAL POLYPS

Endometrial polyps (see Chapter 16), especially when fragmented, are commonly misdiagnosed. Within individual polyp fragments, the irregularly distributed and occasionally branching glands with occasional cysts bear some resemblance to non-atypical hyperplasia. Thick-walled blood vessels and fibrous stroma commonly seen in polyps are lacking in non-atypical hyperplasia. Further clues are provided by careful examination of all available fragments. Because polyps are localizing lesions, specimens obtained by undirected biopsy or curettage typically contain commingled native endometrium with a completely different polyp pattern. This is not the case with non-atypical hyperplasia where the entire functionalis is affected.

POSTMENOPAUSAL CYSTIC ATROPHY

A commonly encountered pattern that may be mistaken for non-atypical hyperplasia is seen during the perimenopausal and postmenopausal periods and is composed of prominent cystically dilated glands in scant, often septated, fibrous stroma. In the past this was one of two patterns often called 'Swiss cheese endometrium.' The terms 'cystic atrophy' or 'cystic atrophic endometrium' accurately describe these appearances and show cuboidal or flattened and inactive cells lining the distended glands. In contrast the epithelium of non-atypical hyperplasia is thicker and may be pseudostratified. Furthermore, the glands in cystic atrophy lack budding and infoldings.

EXCLUSION OF EIN

Distinction of non-atypical hyperplasia from EIN is critical because the former will result in symptomatic hormonal management, and the latter aggressive attempts at lesion ablation by surgery or high-dose progestin therapy. Non-atypical hyperplasia is a diffuse condition in which the cytology of crowded glands resembles that of uncrowded areas. Locally random admixtures of tubal or reactive (adjacent to stromal breakdown) glands are common in non-atypical hyperplasia. In contrast, EIN lesions demonstrate coordinated changes in cytology within crowded areas of glands that offset them from the background.

Treatment

The underlying cause of unopposed estrogens in a patient with non-atypical hyperplasia will commonly determine appropriate clinical management. Endogenous sources in the young and perimenopausal patient include failed or delayed ovulation. Anovulatory women of reproductive age should be evaluated by a reproductive endocrinologist to determine whether there is a primary endocrine abnormality, or if anovulation is secondary to other treatable factors such as stress or low body weight. Resultant infertility can be treated by hormonal induction of ovulation, or through a variety of assisted reproductive techniques. Most women experience occasional anovulatory or delayed ovulatory menstrual cycles during perimenopause with onset of erratic ovarian responsiveness to gonadotropins. The symptom of irregular bleeding in these patients can to a certain extent be treated by progestins, which when withdrawn cause shedding of the overstimulated endometrium. A non-atypical hyperplasia in the postmenopausal woman without a history of exogenous (pharmacologic) estrogen use requires explanation. Elaboration of estrogenic compounds by hormonally active ovarian tumors should be considered especially in this group, but may also occur in the younger patient.

Clinical evaluation of the risk for cancer will determine the appropriate follow-up and need for endometrial re-biopsy following a diagnosis of non-atypical hyperplasia. Women with intractable chronic anovulation, such as that caused by polycystic ovarian syndrome or associated with obesity, may have years of unopposed estrogen. If exposure lasts for more than a decade, cancer risk soars 10-fold.[18]

EIN, ATYPICAL HYPERPLASIA

EIN is a monoclonal premalignant glandular lesion whose component cells are prone to malignant transformation to endometrioid (type 1) endometrial adenocarcinoma. EIN is composed of crowded aggregates of cytologically altered tubular, cystic, or slightly branching glands. Within the geographic confines of the lesion, the area of glands exceeds that of stroma, and there is a change in cytology relative to the background. EIN may emerge within a pre-existing endometrial polyp, contain metaplastic differentiation as part of its altered cytology, or extend diffusely throughout the endometrium at presentation. If significant solid, cribriform, maze-like, or villoglandular architecture is present, or if myoinvasion is seen, a diagnosis of carcinoma should be considered (see Chapter 18).

Other terms that have been applied to EIN include atypical endometrial hyperplasia, simple atypical hyperplasia, complex atypical hyperplasia, adenomatous hyperplasia, anaplasia, and glandular hyperplasia with atypical epithelial proliferation.[28] None of these previously described entities explicitly includes all of the diagnostic elements used today for EIN diagnosis, although the new term 'atypical hyperplasia,' unqualified by simple or complex architecture, has been designated as equivalent to EIN by the WHO.[2]

Clinical Features

EIN is uncommon, and is present as a new diagnosis in only 1.2% of all endometrial samples.[5] Because there are no systematic endometrial screening programs, and the Pap smear is ineffective for screening, EIN is almost always detected in an endometrial biopsy performed in response to patient symptoms or incidental to work-up of an unrelated disorder or when monitoring women receiving hormone replacement therapy.[5] Postmenopausal bleeding or irregular menses in the perimenopausal period are most common signs. Especially in perimenopausal women, a coexisting condition such as non-atypical hyperplasia or adenocarcinoma may lead to the bleeding. The postmenopausal patient with a non-cycling atrophic endometrium may experience symptomatic bleeding directly from an EIN lesion.

The average age of women presenting with EIN is 53 years, which is about 9 years earlier than the average age of 62 for endometrioid endometrial adenocarcinoma in the same patient population.[5] The interval for progression from EIN to adenocarcinoma can be more directly estimated in individual patients who undergo protracted surveillance following an EIN diagnosis. Once patients with concurrent adenocarcinoma are excluded (defined as cancer found within the first year of follow-up), the average interval to diagnosis of adenocarcinoma is 4 years.[14] Demographic analysis of patients with EIN shows the following characteristics (percentage affected, of a sample of 142): 66% obese (BMI ≥25), 48% postmenopausal, 5% polycystic ovarian syndrome, 5% tamoxifen use, and 3% presenting with infertility.[5]

Hormonal risk factors for EIN include estrogens as promoters and progestins as protectors. In the Postmenopausal Estrogen/Progestin Interventions (PEPI) Trial, 12% of women receiving unopposed estrogens developed atypical hyperplasia over the 3 year surveillance period compared to 0% of placebo controls.[21] Estrogen risks are obviated by addition of progestins such as medroxyprogesterone acetate, which protects against endometrial lesions,[21,29] and when administered in a combined low-dose oral contraceptive formulation may reduce endometrial cancer risk below that of the population background.[30,31]

CANCER OUTCOMES IN WOMEN WITH EIN

All patients with EIN are at high risk for endometrial cancer, as there are no histologic subdivisions or 'grades' of EIN that further stratify risk. Women newly diagnosed with EIN are usually treated by hysterectomy within a few months (83% in one United States study),[5] and these show carcinoma within the hysterectomy specimen in one-third of cases.[5,13] These should be considered concurrent instances of carcinoma, as the cancer was most likely already present in the patient at the time of EIN diagnosis but missed by sampling error. Longer term follow-up data, acquired by surveillance resampling of 477 women with EIN not having a hysterectomy in the first year, shows a 45-fold increased risk of cancer in the women with EIN compared to those with non-atypical hyperplasia[14] (Figure 17.18). Absence of EIN in an initial representative biopsy, including those showing non-atypical hyperplasia, has a very high (99%) negative predictive value for concurrent or future adenocarcinoma (Figure 17.18, blue line).[14] EIN lesions that do not progress to cancer may involute, or stably persist for protracted periods of time.[5]

There are characteristics of certain patients that may influence the course of disease once EIN is diagnosed. A case-control analysis of women newly diagnosed with EIN showed that obese women with EIN (BMI ≥25) are at three-fold increased risk for cancer compared to the non-obese patient with EIN.[5] This is consistent with the model that the hyperestrogenic state in obese patients is a risk factor for both EIN and carcinoma, facilitating progression from one to the other. Progestins have long been known to have an antitumorigenic effect in the endometrium, reducing endometrial cancer occurrences by half when taken by the young patient as oral contraceptives.[31,32] One study examined outcomes of EIN in women with a secretory endometrium in the background, indicating presence of circulating progesterone. They tend to be younger (averaging 45 years) than the typical patient with EIN (53 years), and maintain menstrual cycles as an intermittent source of progesterone. For this group, involution of EIN during follow-up was more frequent (81%, 17/21) than historical averages of all women with EIN (25%, 36/142).[33] These results suggest a potential role for endogenous progesterone, as well as therapeutic progestins, in modulating EIN outcomes.

MOLECULAR ETIOLOGY AND NATURAL HISTORY

MUTATION AND CLONAL GROWTH IN EIN

EIN lesions begin as localized monoclonal outgrowths of mutated endometrial cells with a changed cytology and architecture that enables their recognition when compared to the background source polyclonal field.[6,15] Monoclonal growth is a generalizable feature of premalignant epithelial lesions, which is also present in precancers originating at other sites.[8]

Each EIN lesion is the end result of multiple mutations that occur in varying combinations and order of invocation between patients. Within individual patients, however, particular changes seen in EIN are carried forward to the resultant cancer, thereby establishing lineage continuity between these phases of disease.[6,11] Comparison of the extent and range of genomic damage between premalignant and malignant phases shows a greater cumulative mutational load in cancers, a feature that must contribute to their differing morphology and behavior. For example, while 55% of EIN lesions have demonstrable inactivating events (mutation and/or deletion)[34] of the *PTEN* tumor suppressor gene, the proportion rises to 83% in cancers that follow.[10] Similarly, for those lesions with microsatellite instability, the burden of altered microsatellite alleles increases between EIN and carcinoma.[6,11]

All genes known to be altered in EIN have been shown to be similarly abnormal in endometrioid (type 1) endometrial cancers. This is to be expected in a continuous progression lineage where many events occur 'early,' or prior to malignant transformation. These include inactivation of the *PTEN* tumor suppressor gene (44–63%[10,35]), inactivation of the morphogenesis gene *PAX2* (71%[16]), mutation of k-RAS (16%[17]), and acquisition of a microsatellite instability phenotype (20–25%[6,11,36]). Late genetic events seen in endometrioid carcinomas, such as p53 mutation, are not present in EIN precursor lesions. These genetic changes are acquired somatically within the endometrial tissues during regeneration. Rare exceptions are heritable cancer syndromes where germline transmission of defective genes predisposes to neoplasia. Patients with hereditary nonpolyposis colon cancer (HNPCC) syndrome, also known as Lynch syndrome, have defective DNA mismatch repair genes that confer a 22–43% lifetime endometrial cancer risk.[37] HNPCC-associated endometrial cancers are usually of the endometrioid type, and may include a premalignant phase of EIN.[38]

The minimum number of accumulated mutations required to create EIN is unknown, but certainly one is inadequate, and at least 3–5 is likely. This is based on the observation of a high rate of single mutations in normal appearing glands (estimated at >50% of women, 'latent precancers,' below), and knowledge that only a small proportion of these will ever progress to endometrial cancer (lifetime risk is only 2.5%).[39] Thus, individually, neither

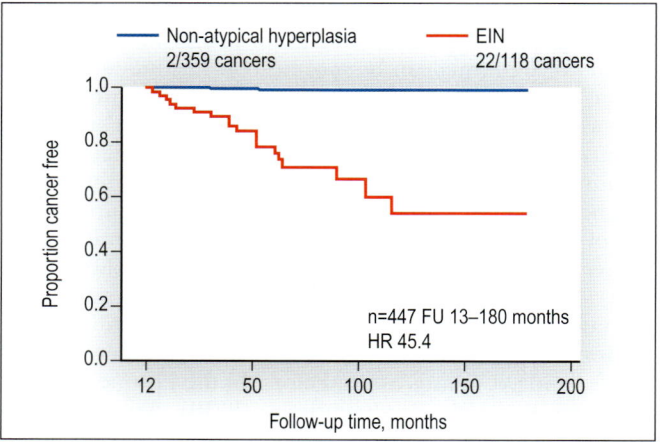

Figure 17.18 Proportion of patients with EIN and non-atypical hyperplasia on biopsy who remain cancer free during clinical follow-up (FU). Those with concurrent cancers (within 12 months of entry) are excluded. There is a 45-fold elevated prospective cancer risk in women with EIN (red) compared to women with non-atypical hyperplasia endometria (blue). EIN diagnoses in this study were made objectively by morphometry, and these have been shown to be highly concordant with those made subjectively using criteria from Table 17.3.[12,13]

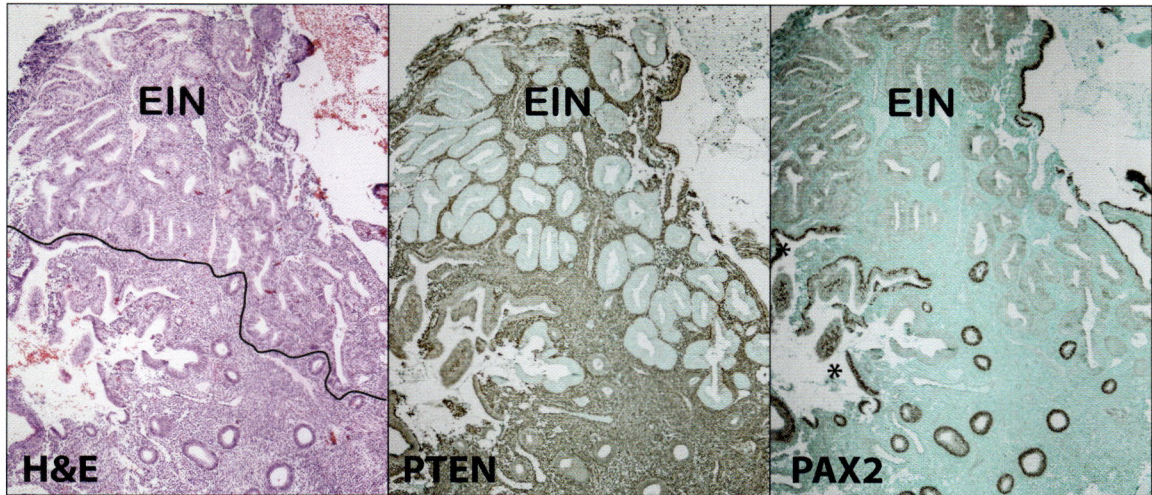

Figure 17.19 Classic features of EIN are highlighted by *PTEN* (middle) and *PAX2* (right), which are both clonally lost in lesional glands. The lesion is an expansile aggregate of densely packed tubular glands lacking cribriform, solid, or maze-like architecture, which commingles with, and overruns, normal proliferative glands at its perimeter. EIN glands have an altered cytology. Immunostains show a brown reaction product and green counterstain.

PTEN nor *PAX2* inactivation is sufficient to cause EIN. Inactivation of both in the same cells is, however, a common and specific feature of neoplastic endometrial glands rarely encountered in normal tissues but seen in 31% of EIN and 55% of endometrioid cancers (Figure 17.19).[16]

LATENT PRECANCERS—A PRECLINICAL PHASE WITHIN NORMAL TISSUES

Independent mutations of many genes occur randomly and independently during physiologic endometrial proliferation, within small numbers of glands that are morphologically virtually indistinguishable from their genetic wild-type counterparts nearby.[35] These have been designated 'latent precancers' and they have been detected using *PTEN* and *PAX2* as markers in 49% and 36%, respectively, of normal women.[16] The burden of mutated glands in affected patients is quite small, only 1.3% and 0.46% for *PTEN* and *PAX2*, respectively, of the hundreds of glands present in the typical biopsy. Independence of these different genetic events is shown by their infrequent co-occurrence in the same individual gland—estimated at 0.01% (15 glands of 149,744 examined in 199 patients). Thus, although the individual genetic events themselves may occur dozens of times each month, they are distributed within such a vast tissue field that only rarely do they happen to take place within the same cell.

Once mutated, affected 'normal' glands are susceptible to hormonal selection, as they maintain high levels of nuclear estrogen and progesterone receptors.[35] Native *PTEN* expression is greatest in an estrogenic environment, when its antimitotic effects are most needed.[40] *PTEN* inactivation under these circumstances confers a selective proliferative advantage. In contrast, upon progesterone exposure native *PTEN* protein is shut down with the result that latent precancers with mutant *PTEN* genes no longer have an advantage and disappear in competition with wild-type glands.[41,42] Ablation of latent precancers from 'normal' tissues by progestational therapy is one possible mechanism for reduced endometrial cancer risk in the women who have a histologically unremarkable endometrium. Longitudinal studies of the fate of latent endometrial precancers under differing hormonal and clinical circumstances are required before their clinical implications can be fully understood.

Gross Features

Most EIN lesions are grossly inapparent. They expand by interactively remodeling the stroma relative to the neoplastic glands unaccompanied by gross distortion or compression of the flanking normal tissues. One circumstance in which EIN may be seen grossly is when a thin atrophic background endometrium lacks the bulk necessary to contain the expanding EIN lesion. Thus some EIN lesions in postmenopausal patients are visible as local thickenings. The background endometrium in which an EIN arises is often itself abnormal, and this can dominate the appearance on gross examination. Non-atypical hyperplasia is a common background, which can have a thickened and multicystic appearance. EIN may also present within otherwise grossly unremarkable sessile or pedunculated endometrial polyps.

The pathologist should sample grossly visible lesions, while keeping in mind that EIN is a disease that is most often detected by random sampling of undistinguished regions of the endometrium. Thoroughness of sampling is therefore a key element in successful detection of EIN lesions, especially those that are physically small and localized at the time of diagnosis.

Microscopic Features of EIN

Focal origin of EIN lesions explains why most are represented in only some of the many tissue fragments that constitute a typical endometrial biopsy or curettage specimen. The first step in diagnosis is thus low-magnification scanning of all tissue fragments in search of outlier architectural patterns that visually punctuate a more uniform background (Figures 17.1 and 17.20). These are usually regions of increased gland density. Closer examination will show a change in cytology of the crowded focus relative to the background endometrium, in addition to all other features listed in Table 17.3 and discussed in detail in the following sections.

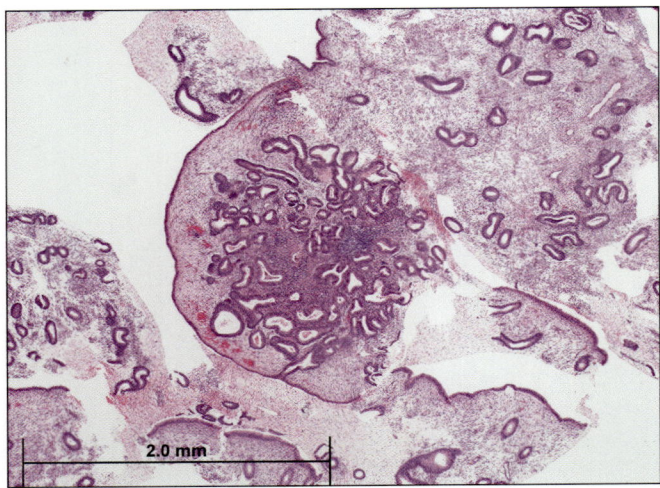

Figure 17.20 This discrete EIN lesion is readily visible under low magnification as a 1.5 mm diameter region of crowded glands against a regular background of proliferative endometrium. Only one tissue fragment was involved. The patient was diagnosed with endometrioid endometrial adenocarcinoma 2 years later.

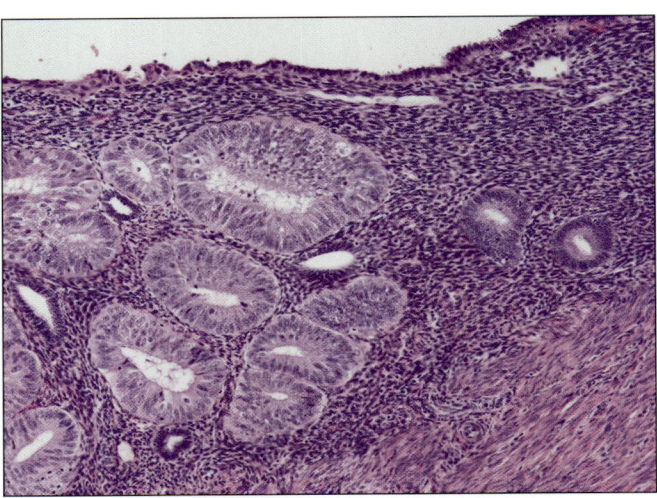

Figure 17.21 Growth of EIN lesions occurs through percolation of affected peripheral glands between and among overrun normal glands. Extension is lateral rather than exophytic, preserving a smooth uterine cavity surface lining which obscures recognition of EIN at gross examination.

Table 17.3 Diagnostic Features of EIN (All Must be Met)

EIN Criterion	Comments
Architecture	• Area of glands exceeds that of stroma (glands/stroma > 1) • Lesion composed of individual glands which may branch slightly and vary in shape
Cytology	• Nuclear and/or cytoplasmic features of epithelial cells differ between architecturally crowded glands and normal background glands • May include change in nuclear polarity, nuclear pleomorphism, or altered cytoplasmic differentiation state • If no normal glands present, highly abnormal cytology
Size	• Maximum linear dimension exceeds 1 mm
Exclude mimics	• Benign conditions with overlapping criteria: disordered proliferative, non-atypical hyperplasia, basalis, secretory, polyps, repair, etc.
Exclude cancer	• Carcinoma if maze-like glands, solid areas, or significant cribriforming (see Figure 18.12)

Large-scale topography has been greatly underestimated as a useful feature in endometrial precancer diagnosis. It is the geographic aggregation of similarly altered endometrial glands, a reflection of clonal growth, which offsets EIN from non-atypical hyperplasia. Secondly, the cytologic changes of EIN can most reliably be recognized when comparing lesions with adjacent or interposed background endometrial glands. This requires awareness, on a large scale, of which fragments and regions should be compared.

EIN lesions are composed of aggregates of individual tubular or slightly branching glands, in which the surface area of glands is greater than that of the stroma which contains them (Figure 17.19). The 'crowded' appearance of these clusters is what makes localizing EIN lesions so readily visible under low magnification. Expanses of obviously benign cysts, commonly encountered in the atrophic endometrium of the postmenopausal patient or within the non-atypical hyperplasia from which an EIN has arisen, should be avoided in this assessment.

EIN lesions interact with endometrial stroma, having an expansile rather than compressing interface with adjacent tissues. A peripheral spray of EIN glands projects between and among overrun normal glands (Figure 17.20). When present as wholly visible discrete lesions, there may be an 'epicenter' of maximally concentrated glands that becomes less densely distributed towards the periphery. Non-invasive remodeling between glands and stroma, rather than invasion, changes gland density (Figure 17.21).[43,44] The stroma intervening between glands of EIN will have an appearance dependent on the regional and hormonal context, ranging from the lush stroma of the functionalis to more fibrous non-cycling stroma within the basalis or a polyp. Attempts to interpret endometrial stroma as 'desmoplastic' or altered in response to 'invasion' are of no diagnostic benefit because of the irreproducible[45] nature of that determination.

SPECIFIC EIN DIAGNOSTIC CRITERIA

EIN diagnostic criteria (Table 7.3) include the presence of conserved features and exclusion of benign mimics and carcinoma. It is the latter that requires experience to recognize, as familiarity with a broad range of entities that share some features with EIN is a prerequisite to avoid misdiagnosis. It is the combined application of multiple diagnostic features that confers robustness to an EIN diagnosis. All five EIN criteria listed must be met in a single fragment, in each case, to maintain a high level of diagnostic specificity and clinical predictive value. These criteria were developed and validated[5,12–14] in biopsy and curetting specimens, and are thus applicable to fragmented specimens.

The precise criteria as listed in Table 17.3 yield highly reproducible EIN classification between experts (interobserver kappas 0.54–0.63[12]). A large EIN diagnostic reproducibility study was recently carried out between two subspecialty experts and 20 practicing community pathologists of varying experience and training.[46] The two experts were highly concordant across the 62 circulated cases, with interobserver kappas of 0.74. Additionally, 79% of all community diagnoses were in agreement with the reference expert diagnostic consensus, and the weighted interobserver kappas between the 20 community pathologists averaged 0.72 (range 0.45–0.84). The most discordant cases all had identifiable 'problems' (e.g., poor technical preparation, presence of non-endometrioid differentiation, borderline size) to which the participants responded in a manner reflecting their own diagnostic style. Pathologist diagnostic style was characterized by different levels of aggressiveness in diagnosis of cancer and EIN, and varying response to suboptimal specimens. Interobserver variation in EIN diagnosis is thus not entirely random, but rather a complex combination of the qualities of the material and individual bias of the pathologist.

Several of the criteria listed were empirically defined by correlation of computerized morphometric assessments of lesion cancer outcomes[47–49] and clonal growth.[6] This includes the gland crowding threshold of 50%, and minimum size of 1 mm. Others, such as cytology interpretation against a relative internal standard, became possible only with demonstration of the clonal character of EIN within a background field. Similarly, a minimum size requirement was not indicated in older models where transformation of the field, rather than localized emergence, was assumed to be the manner of genesis.

Architecture

The area of glands exceeds that of stroma. The endometrial compartment can be thought of as glands (combined epithelium and internal lumina) distributed within supportive stroma, and the extent of crowding expressed as the percentage occupied by glands. EIN lesions have >50% glands, which can intuitively be translated to 'gland area exceeds stromal area.' When evaluating the extent of gland crowding awareness of an intact stromal compartment will prevent misinterpretation of sheared or disrupted specimens.

The 50% threshold can be learned and applied through use of reference graphics (Figure 17.22), or viewing of calibrated training sets online (at www.endometrium.org). Alternatively, a rapid and easy form of morphometry can be performed using inexpensive ocular grids with 50–100 regularly placed points indicated by intersecting lines (number of points over glands/number of points over glands and stroma).

Cytology

The cytology of EIN changes relative to the background endometrium from which it has arisen. A comparison of background with EIN cytology makes it possible to recognize a changed cytology at the contrasting interface despite a variable appearance of EIN cytology between patients (Figure 17.23). The term 'cytologic demarcation' is a good description of this feature, where cytology as well as

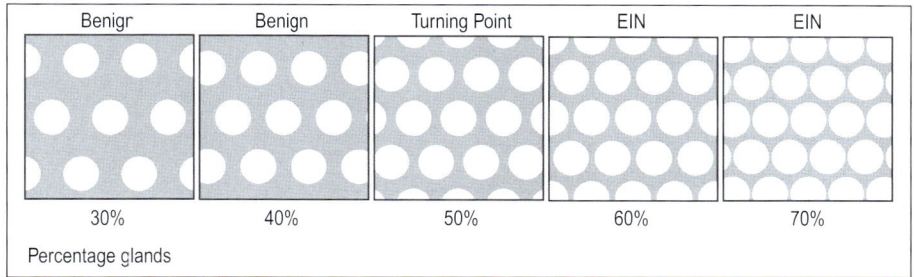

Figure 17.22 Appearance of glands (white) packed at different densities within endometrial stroma (gray).

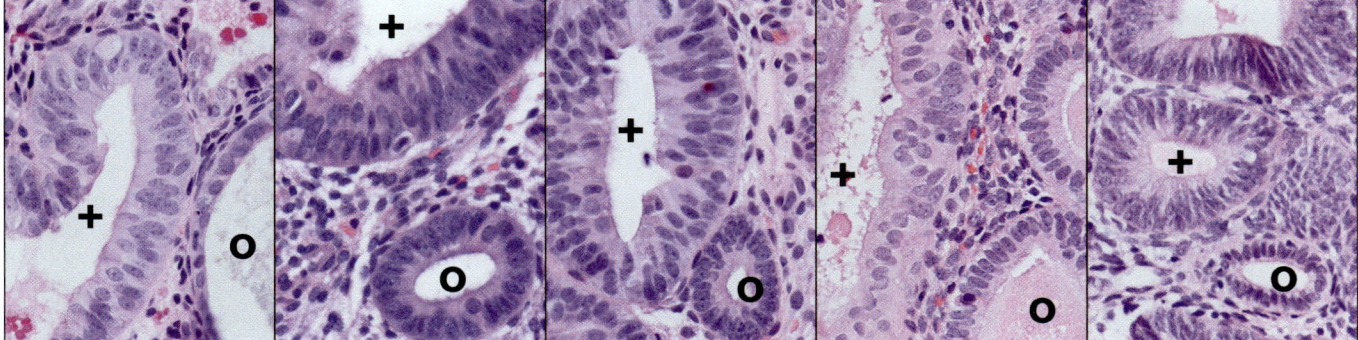

Figure 17.23 Spectrum of EIN cytology (+) compared to internal background non-lesional glands (o) in five different patients (400× magnification). Criteria of EIN, including architectural features, were present in each case (not shown), and all developed endometrioid endometrial adenocarcinoma during follow-up.

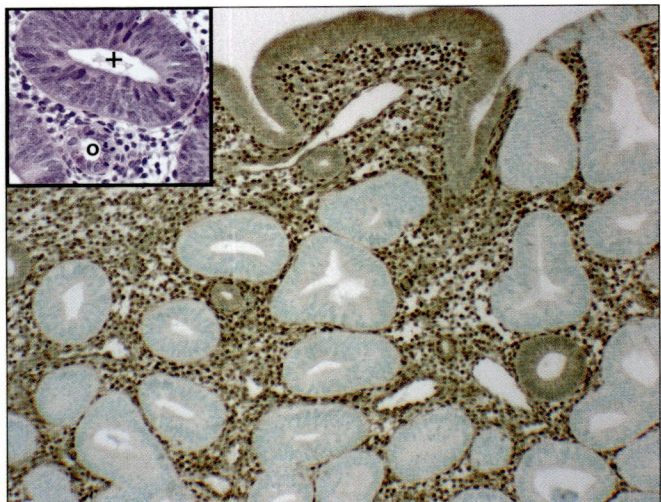

Figure 17.24 Overrun background glands within an EIN lesion. PTEN immunohistochemistry highlights stroma and normal glands in brown. Neoplastic glands of EIN have a different cytology (+) than overrun background glands (o).

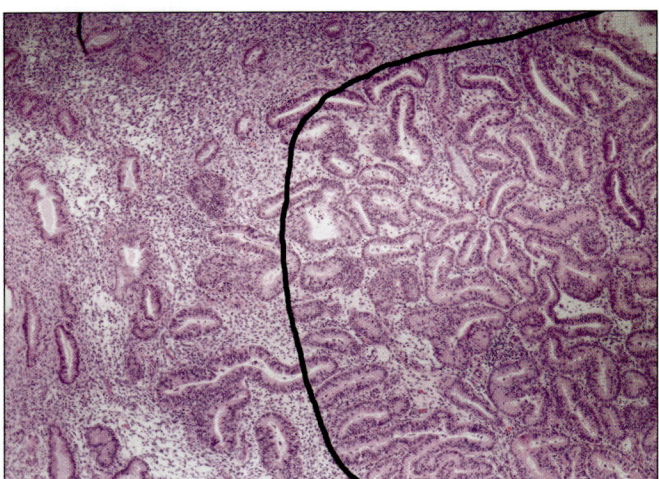

Figure 17.25 The perimeter of an EIN lesion used to measure maximum linear extent should be drawn at the margin of a suitably dense arrangement of cytologically altered glands, a position that is often internal to the outermost distribution of individual neoplastic glands, which become rarified on the periphery. The epicenter of this EIN lesion is to the right.

architecture demarcates the perimeter of the lesion. For lesions that are no longer localized, or do not have readily identifiable perimeters, individually overrun normal glands may be available for comparison (Figure 17.24). This is discussed further in the section that follows.

Cytologic change can include nuclear and/or cytoplasmic components. EIN lesions may have round non-stratified, or elongated pseudostratified, nuclei. Round non-polarized nuclear morphology with prominent nucleoli, although often present, is not required for EIN diagnosis. The cytoplasm may retain endometrioid differentiation or acquire non-endometrioid differentiation of tubal, mucinous, secretory, or eosinophilic epithelium.[56] The latter are discussed in detail in Chapter 16 on endometrial 'metaplasias,' a subset of which are premalignant EIN lesions.

EIN, like endometrioid adenocarcinoma, generally lacks the markedly pleomorphic hobnailed nuclei seen in serous or clear cell adenocarcinoma of the endometrium. In the presence of such cytology, a non-endometrioid neoplasm or surface spread from an adjacent high-grade carcinoma should be considered. The p53 immunohistochemistry, usually positively staining in serous endometrial adenocarcinomas, may help in recognizing this process.

Size

The lesion must be at least 1 mm in dimension. The perimeter of an EIN lesion used for measurement should be drawn at the margin of a suitably dense arrangement of cytologically altered glands, a position often located internal to the outermost distribution of individual neoplastic glands, which can become rarified on the periphery (Figure 17.25). The 1 mm size needs to be present in only one linear measurement. Elongated or irregularly shaped lesions may have other axes of lesser extent. Separate foci cannot be added to achieve this minimum size—it must be met in a single focus.

Cancer outcome prediction is dependent on the ability to reliably measure the extent of gland crowding, a difficult task unless a critical mass of representative glands are included in the assessment. There are many processes, such as estrogen-induced tubal metaplasia, and local reactive changes, where tiny clusters of three to four glands may demonstrate an altered cytology unrelated to premalignant change. The minimum size considerably reduces the likelihood of overreacting to these processes. Lesions smaller than 1 mm, or excessively fragmented specimens with few or no individual fragments 1 mm in dimension, represent a class of endometria subdiagnostic for EIN that are discussed below.

EXCLUSION OF BENIGN MIMICS

Glands artifactually pushed together or telescoped into a crowded discrete focus may have angular contours due to extrinsic compression, and will lack the cytologic change of EIN (Figure 17.26). Normal tissues with irregularly placed glands such as lower uterine segment or uterine basalis can usually be identified by their more fibrous stromal context and quiescent epithelium. The gland density of late secretory endometrium may be very high in the deep functionalis where the predecidual change is minimal (Figure 17.27). When the endometrium breaks down, either in the normal menstrual phase of the cycle or as a result of estrogen withdrawal, the glands collapse and the stroma crumbles. This frequently results in irregular glands lacking much stromal separation and there is a real danger of misinterpretation as EIN. When an EIN-like area is focal, it is important that the surrounding stroma is intact and the cytology of the localizing lesion differs distinctly from the background.

EIN lesions may arise within an otherwise benign endometrial polyp, as discussed later. Polyps usually exhibit altered stroma, thick vessels, and random irregular glands (Figure 17.28). EIN lesions within polyps usually stand out as a

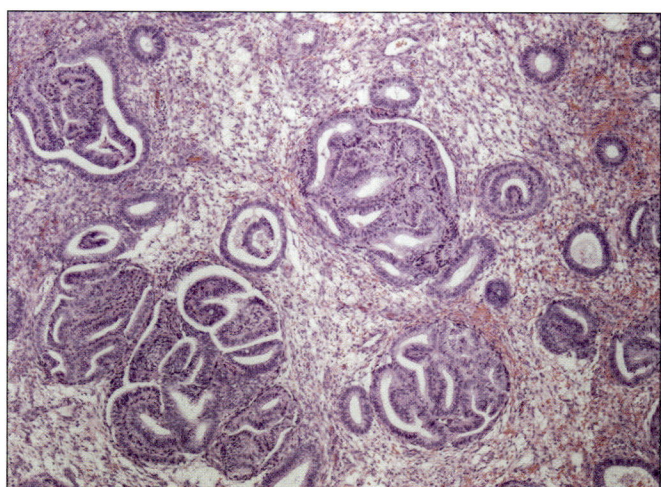

Figure 17.26 Glands artifactually pushed together or telescoped into a crowded discrete focus will have sharp angled corners and lack the cytologic change of EIN.

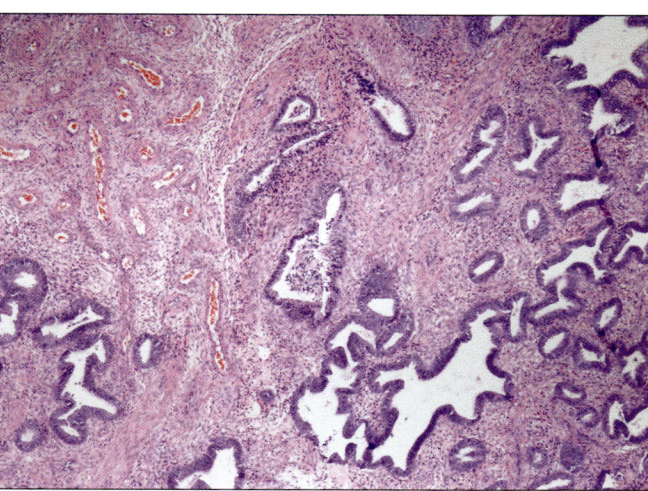

Figure 17.28 Polyps may have regions of high gland density, but the cytology of these areas is usually similar to that seen elsewhere in the polyp. Polyps can be recognized by their altered stroma, thick vessels, and random irregular glands

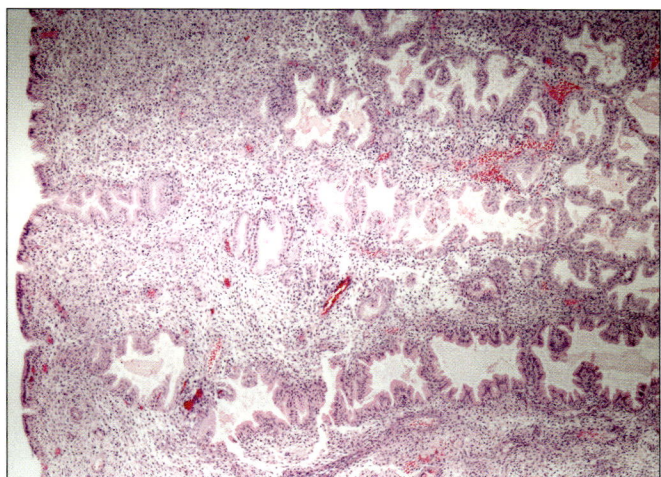

Figure 17.27 Density of secretory endometrial glands in this 27 day normal endometrium is very high in the deep functionalis (right) where there is less predecidual change than toward the luminal surface (left). Gradual transition and recognition of the sawtooth configuration of lumens assists in discrimination from EIN.

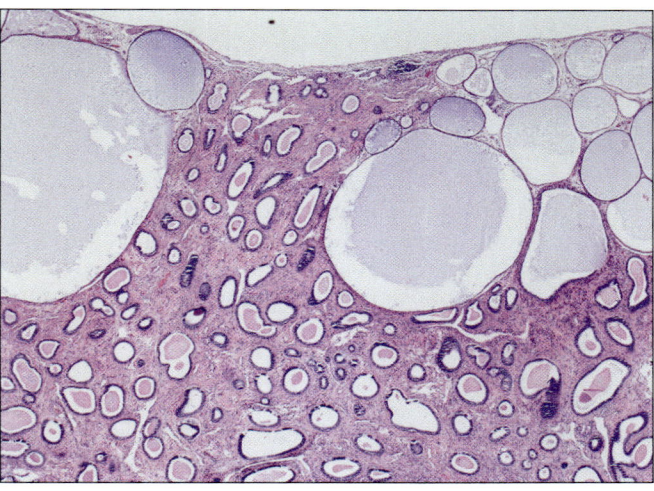

Figure 17.29 Collections of bland endometrial cysts may be seen in atrophic endometria or senile polyps, and these will have a very low stromal density and lining epithelium with a more attenuated cytology than uninvolved areas.

discrete focus in comparison with the remaining polyp. These are discussed in the following section.

Non-atypical hyperplasia should not be confused with EIN, although EIN lesions often arise in that context. Non-atypical hyperplasia changes involve the entire endometrial compartment, and have an irregular random pattern of architectural and cytologic alterations unlike the localizing and expansile features of EIN (Figure 17.1).

Collections of bland endometrial cysts may be seen in atrophic endometria or senile polyps, and these will have a very low stromal density and lining epithelium with a more attenuated cytology than uninvolved areas (Figure 17.29). They have a sufficiently distinctive appearance unlikely to be confused with EIN, but which may otherwise meet the formal architectural and size criteria for EIN.

EXCLUSION OF CARCINOMA

Distinction between EIN and adenocarcinoma is of clinical importance. Not uncommonly, foci of adenocarcinoma will appear to have developed from the EIN, in which case both entities should be included in the final diagnosis.

EIN lesions are composed of clusters of individually recognizable glands with a simple lining epithelium, whereas adenocarcinomas may have one or more specific patterns not seen in EIN, such as solid, cribriform, or complex interlacing maze-like growth (Figure 17.1). These architectural changes of endometrial cancer are discussed further in Chapter 18, and illustrated in Figure 18.12. EIN lesions with non-endometrioid differentiation, especially those with squamous morular or micropapillary change, may have epithelial stratification in the absence of malignant

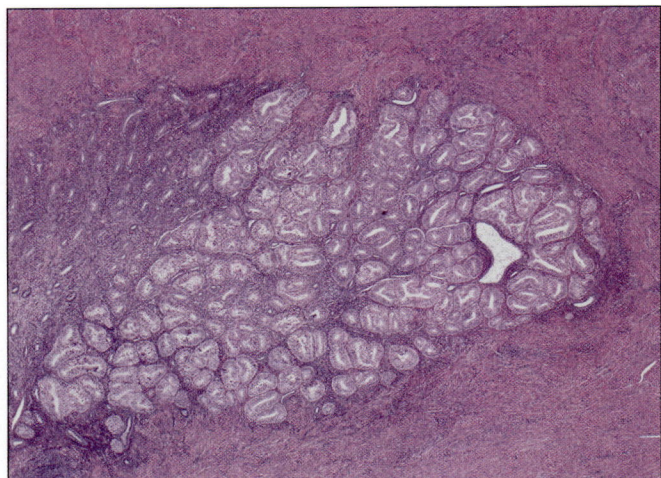

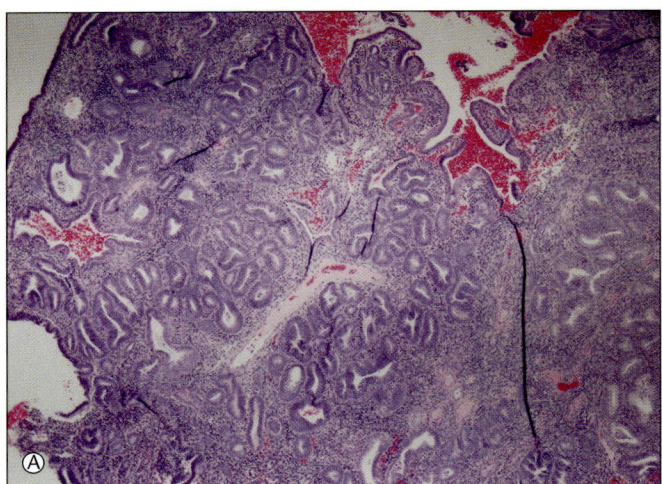

Figure 17.30 EIN extending into an area of adenomyosis. Within the myometrium, the area is surrounded by endometrial stroma and normal glands remain.

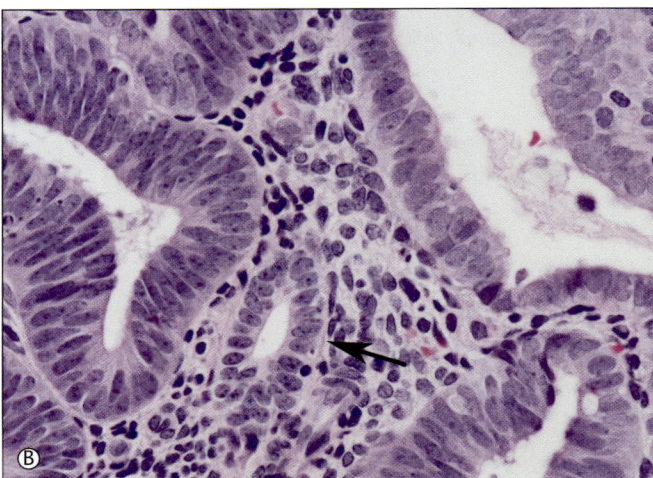

Figure 17.31 **(A and B)** EIN lesion occupying the entire endometrial compartment, which is difficult to diagnose because it lacks boundaries with areas of normal endometrium. It can be recognized as an EIN by the high gland density **(A)** and evidence of cytologic change when compared to interspersed 'overrun' normal glands (**B**, arrow). This 47-year-old patient was diagnosed at hysterectomy 8 months later with well-differentiated adenocarcinoma.

behavior. Precise criteria for defining the precancer–cancer threshold in metaplastic EINs are dependent on the differentiation state. This is discussed in the next section and in Chapter 16.

EIN lesions with tightly packed glands may be difficult to distinguish from adenocarcinoma. Lesions composed of confluent glands separated by thread-like strands of intervening connective tissue, with abutting glands having a septate appearance resembling fitted elements of a mosaic, are candidates for a diagnosis of adenocarcinoma. Caution must be exercised, however, to avoid overinterpretation of artifactually compressed or displaced EIN glands as adenocarcinoma.

In those instances where myometrium is included, the presence of myoinvasion is diagnostic of carcinoma. The absence of myometrial invasion does not, however, preclude a diagnosis of carcinoma as up to 30% of carcinomas may be confined to the endometrium, and myoinvasion usually is not represented in a superficial biopsy. EIN may occasionally affect endometrial glandular elements in foci of adenomyosis within the myometrium, so that EIN glands are present deep in the myometrium (Figure 17.30). Stromal response to invasion, desmoplasia, is a useful diagnostic feature, if present, in cases of myoinvasion but of no benefit in distinction between EIN and carcinoma within the endometrial compartment itself. Commonly, even extensive myoinvasion shows no desmoplastic reaction.

COMMON EIN DIAGNOSTIC PROBLEMS

Some specimens elude diagnosis. The condition of the specimen may be suboptimal, confounding factors present, or it may have a presentation new to the diagnostician. Most important in these cases is to clearly convey to the clinician the non-diagnostic nature of the case, while specifically identifying the particular problem. Strategies for dealing with specific diagnostic difficulties are presented in the following sections.

NON-LOCALIZING (WIDESPREAD) EIN

One-fifth of EIN lesions are diffuse and non-localizing by the time of initial presentation. This is not an indication of malignancy as, even when widespread, EIN may remain confined to the endometrial compartment for prolonged periods or even undergo complete involution in response to progestin therapy. Complicating the diagnosis is that these fragments lack clear geographic interfaces of lesion and background for interpreting the cytologic change. As such, they can easily be confused with the global field effects of non-atypical hyperplasia. It is usually possible to recognize the EIN either by (1) interspersed 'overrun' normal glands can be used as an internal reference to confirm significant cytologic change within the EIN lesion (Figures 17.24 and 17.31) or by (2) an obviously complicated architecture and greatly abnormal cytology that excludes a benign process, and rather must be distinguished from carcinoma.

EIN WITHIN AN ENDOMETRIAL POLYP

For the one-fifth of EIN cases that occur within an endometrial polyp, the usual diagnostic criteria apply with one caveat—the reference point for recognition of cytologic change must be the uninvolved areas of polyp, rather than comparison to non-polypoid endometrial surface. Almost all EIN lesions within polyps are recognized under low magnification as a defined focus. The presence of EIN within a polyp does not change the risk of concurrent cancer compared to EIN in the native endometrium, even when seemingly localized to one fragment (Figure 17.32). See Chapter 16 for further discussion and examples of EIN within polyps.

A dense, fibrous stroma within the polyp may influence the pattern by which the neoplastic glands grow outward. Sometimes EIN glands are channeled by dense collagen fibers into a loose spray that may be difficult to distinguish from invasive carcinoma. The presence of cribriform or maze-like lumens favors a diagnosis of adenocarcinoma.

LOCALIZING LESIONS SUBDIAGNOSTIC FOR EIN

Lesions suspicious for, but not diagnostic of, EIN are rare, occurring at about one-third the frequency of readily diagnosable EINs. These can present as large fragments of endometrial tissue with discrete dense clusters of cytologically altered endometrial glands that fail to meet size (1 mm) and/or gland density (>50% glands) requirements (Figure 17.33). Some represent an early phase of EIN development in which the disease burden has not yet achieved a sufficient level to appear in fully diagnostic form, whereas others are tangentially sectioned regions of peripheral aspects of a lesion. Deeper sections (levels) of the tissue block should be considered, but infrequently resolve these possibilities.

A clinical outcome study of 143 such lesions with short-term follow-up showed most (77%) had an unremarkable benign outcome, whereas 19% showed EIN and 4% carcinoma.[50] Based on this, our current practice is to make a descriptive diagnosis of 'microscopic focus of crowded, cytologically altered endometrial glands—see note,' then in the note state that it is subdiagnostic of EIN but resampling in 3–6 months is advised.

EXCESSIVELY FRAGMENTED TISSUE

Definitive diagnosis of highly fragmented tissue is always difficult. The problem is greatest when multiple small tissue fragments contain neoplastic glands from edge to edge. In some cases the aggregate tissue is sufficiently abundant so as not to be confused with a benign process, but insufficient to discriminate between EIN and well-differentiated adenocarcinoma. The latter may be suspected if very high grade nuclei or cribriform or solid neoplastic epithelium are present.

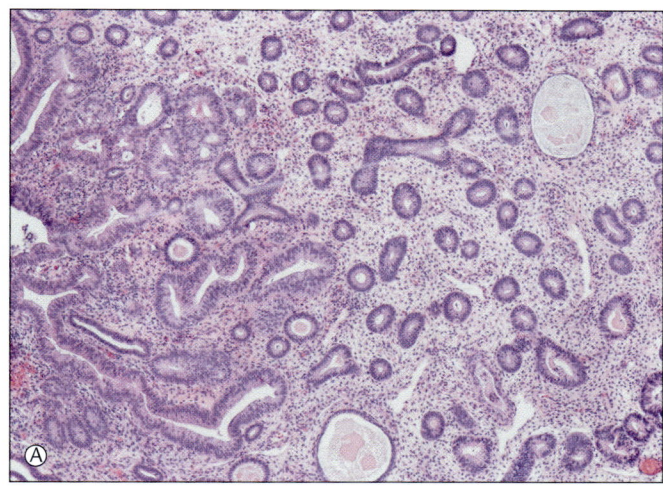

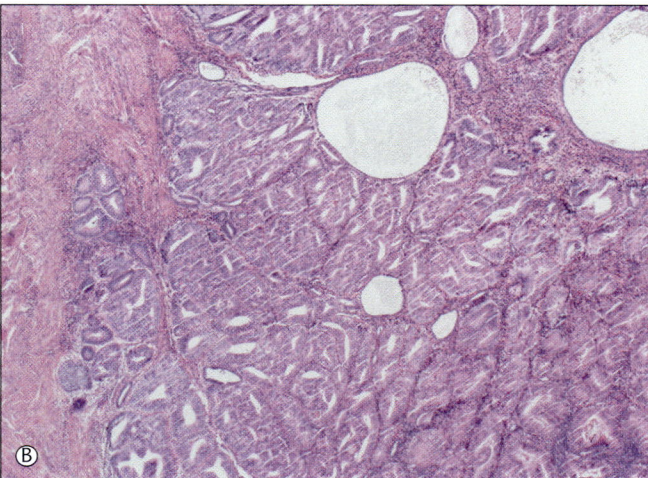

Figure 17.32 Localizing EIN (left), arising within an endometrial polyp **(A)**. The interface is expanding to the right and could be outlined continuously within the fragment. Endometrioid carcinoma was diagnosed at hysterectomy 60 days later **(B)**.

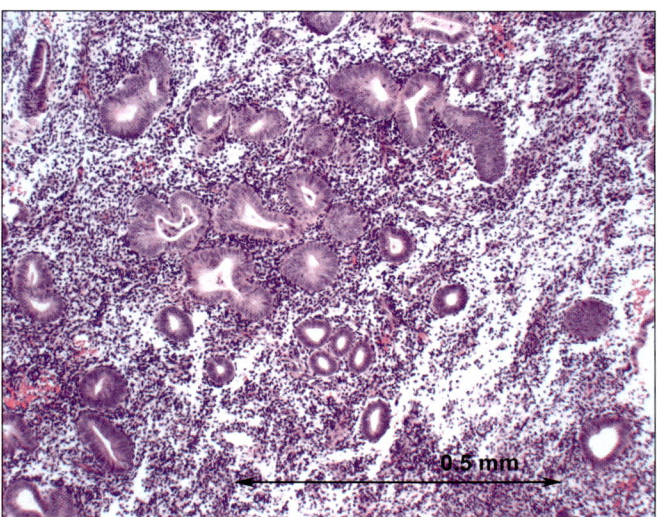

Figure 17.33 Small, non-compact cluster of cytologically altered glands subdiagnostic of EIN. This should not be diagnosed as EIN because the affected glands in the center of the field are too loosely arranged, fail to meet the criterion of gland area exceeding stromal area, and are too small in linear dimension. These can be diagnosed descriptively.

NON-ENDOMETRIOID EIN

Not all EIN lesions maintain endometrioid differentiation, with some displaying complete, or more often partial, mucinous, squamous morular, tubal, eosinophilic, or micropapillary differentiation (Figure 17.34).[56] A rule of thumb is that the usual EIN diagnostic criteria apply, and that the altered differentiation state is only one of the many ways in which lesion cytology can be offset from the background. The change in cytology may involve the cytoplasm primarily, with a variable degree of nuclear change. To some extent, the specific type of altered differentiation dictates additional elements that must be incorporated into the diagnosis. For example, the morular component of EIN with squamous morules should be ignored in calculating the ratio of glands to stroma. Morules are functionally inert, and it is the abundance of glandular elements relative to stroma that determines cancer risk. Morules surrounded by glands present a cribriform-like appearance that should not be confused with adenocarcinoma. Metaplastic EIN lesions are discussed and illustrated in detail, for each differentiation state, in Chapter 16.

HORMONALLY TREATED EIN

There are no formal modified criteria for the diagnosis of premalignant endometrial lesions while under the active influence of progestins. Administration of high-dose progestins such as Megace is an increasingly common clinical intervention that greatly alters the appearance of the EIN itself, often making it non-diagnostic. The extent of stromal pseudodecidual change is often the only clue to the presence of this confounding factor. Glands are pushed apart by stromal pseudodecidualization, and nuclei become smaller and less mitotically active (Figure 17.35). Combined, these changes dramatically alter the appearance of a post-therapy EIN lesion. 'Improvement' in cytology or lessening of gland crowding cannot be viewed as evidence of

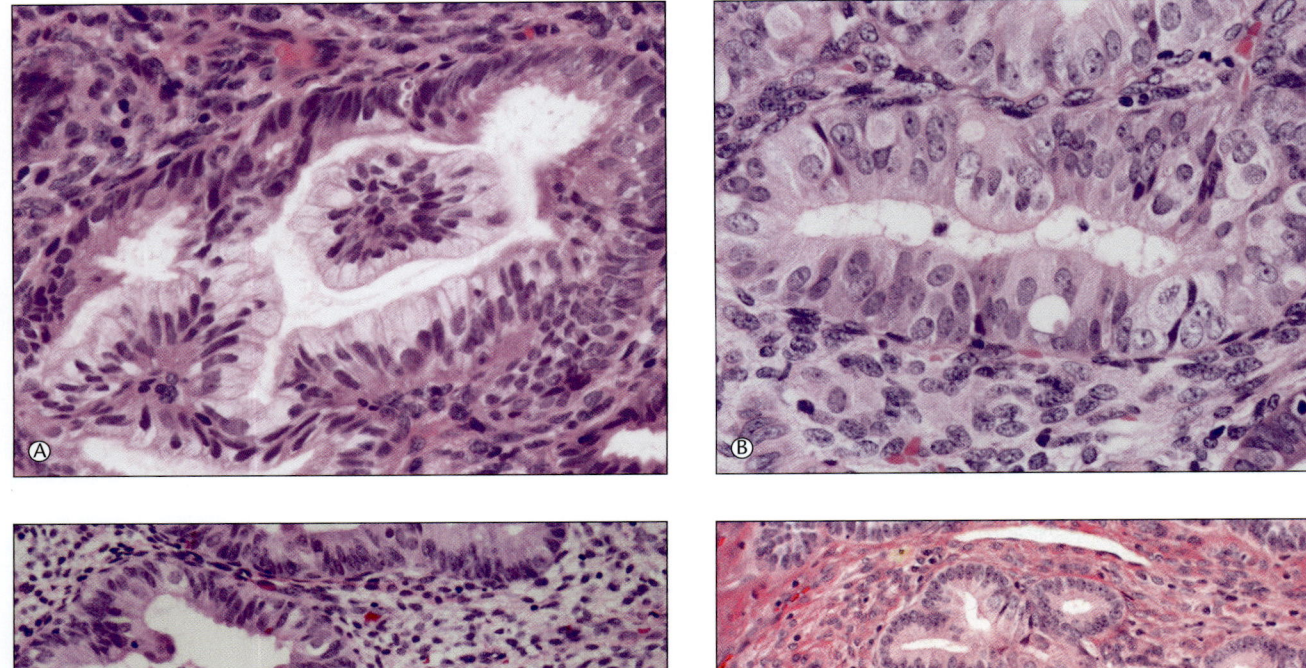

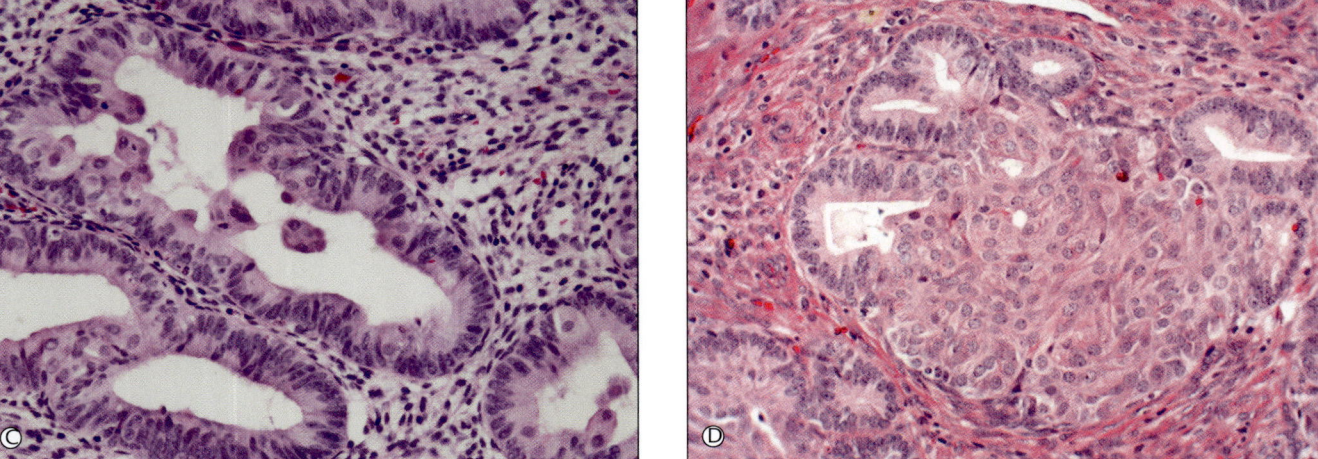

Figure 17.34 Cytology of non-endometrioid EIN lesions may include complete, or more often partial, mucinous **(A)**, tubal **(B)**, micropapillary **(C)**, or squamous morular **(D)** differentiation. Altered differentiation, primarily a cytoplasmic feature, is the nature of the cytologic change that characterizes these EIN lesions. Non-endometrioid lesions present specific interpretive difficulties. Squamous morules surrounded by glands have a cribriform-like appearance that should not be confused with adenocarcinoma.

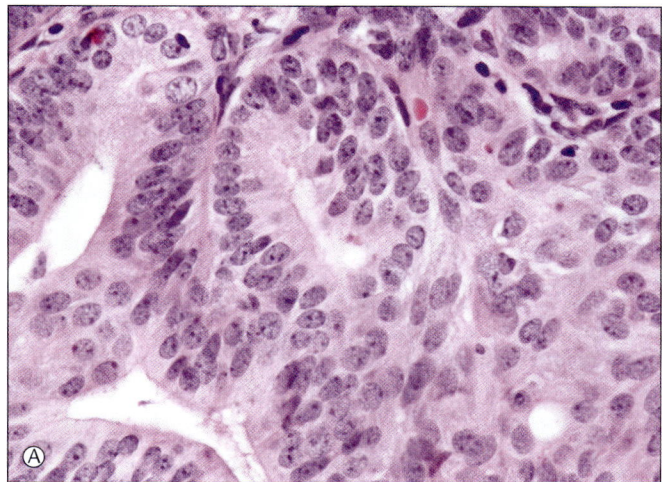

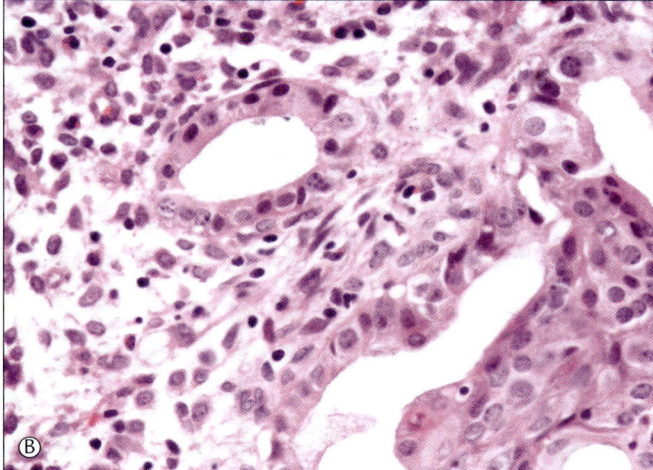

Figure 17.35 EIN cytology altered by 3 months of high-dose progestin (Megace) therapy. Pre-therapy glands **(A)** have plump nuclei and a moderately thick epithelium. After therapy **(B)**, persistent EIN glands are pushed apart by stromal pseudodecidualization, and nuclei become smaller and less mitotically active. Magnification of both images is identical.

and glandular changes of progestin therapy' can be made. The best way to resolve any diagnostic uncertainty introduced by hormonal therapy is to re-biopsy 2–4 weeks following a withdrawal bleed. The hormonal effects will no longer be present, thereby permitting accurate assessment of the presence or absence of residual EIN.

SPECIAL STUDIES FOR EIN DIAGNOSIS

Specialized biomarkers and formal morphometric image analysis have played a crucial role in defining the entity of EIN, and remain useful teaching elements. These have been presented here as part of the evidence base that redefined precancerous lesions. In the end, insights from these tools have changed the way pathologists routinely look at, and interpret, endometrial tissues. None of the specialized evaluations are essential in routine diagnosis, which is done in our and most practices simply by a pathologist equipped with a standard microscope applying the criteria in Table 17.3 to H&E-stained slides.

There are no serum biomarkers of EIN that have value as an early detection system, and cytology-based approaches lack sensitivity. Most important, for an ancillary study to be of practical benefit it must offer information which augments or exceeds at reasonable cost that already available by routine microscopy. This is a tough standard which in the author's opinion has not been met for most special studies in common practice settings. We offer some comments on those of greatest investigational value, and interest.

BIOMARKERS: *PAX2* AND *PTEN*

PAX2 and *PTEN* are clonally inactivated in 71% and 44% of EIN lesions, respectively, and co-inactivation of both occurs in 31% (see Figure 17.19).[16] Either stain permits visual delineation of informative EIN lesions but neither is sensitive or specific enough for routine clinical diagnostic decision making in the individual patient. A problem is that these genes are independently inactivated sporadically in otherwise normal tissues (see the previous section Latent precancers—a preclinical phase within normal tissues), long before clinical disease develops. The second difficulty is that 70% of EIN lesions will express one or both of these markers, so individually they are insensitive. Dual knockout of *PTEN* and *PAX2* is much more specific (but less sensitive) for neoplastic disease, but does not allow discrimination between EIN and carcinoma. Our laboratory experience is that *PAX2* is a much more technically robust marker than *PTEN*, and easier to interpret. If applied to paraffin sections attention must be paid to the reagents chosen, as not all antibodies work in this format. We use (1) polyclonal rabbit anti-*PAX2* directed against a GST-Pax-2 fusion protein derived from the C-terminal domain (amino acids 188–385) of the murine Pax-2 protein and (2) murine anti-human *PTEN* clone 6H2.1.[16]

QUANTITATIVE HISTOMORPHOMETRY

The D-score as measured by an interactive computerized morphometric workstation from H&E-stained slides provides a stable reference tool for objective EIN diagnosis, and

clearance of an EIN lesion when the follow-up biopsy is taken in the presence of active progestational agent. Furthermore, re-biopsy of a hormonally treated EIN while still on progestins may be a premature endpoint to assess lesion involution, as the patient has not yet had the benefit of withdrawal shedding.

There are a few diagnostic strategies that are useful for managing these patients. First, if either adenocarcinoma or (criteria-meeting) EIN is present, it should be diagnosed with a mention of the noted progestational effects. Second, if there are any architecturally localizing cytologically distinctive glandular lesions, they should be described and a comment made that, although subdiagnostic, EIN cannot be excluded while the patient is under active progestin therapy. Third, if the entire endometrium is decidualized with a very low density of secretorily exhausted uniformly appearing glands, a diagnosis of 'endometrium with stromal in some environments is used as part of the routine EIN diagnosis workflow.[49,51] Variables of volume percentage stroma, gland outer surface density, and standard deviation of shortest nuclear axis are algorithmically combined to generate the D-score,[52] a threshold function diagnostic of EIN at values less than 1. Morphometry must be performed on an area selected by a pathologist, who must also exclude any of several confounding conditions likely to give erroneous results (normal secretory endometrium, endometrial polyps). The high clinical outcome predictive value, reproducibility, and commercial availability of analytical systems (QProdit system, Leica, Cambridge, UK) combine to make it of practical value for some groups.

MANAGEMENT OF EIN

EIN is a premalignant lesion whose high likelihood of progression to cancer requires intervention.[1] The first consideration for the managing physician is ruling out a coexisting occult carcinoma. Thirty-nine percent of EIN lesions coexist with well-differentiated adenocarcinoma that may not be evident on the initial biopsy.[14] Tissue-sampling devices, which access the endometrium via the uterine lumen, cannot obtain access to blind luminal pockets, and have a tendency to under-represent tissues deep to the surface lining. Myoinvasive cancers are easily missed if the bulk of tumor is below the endometrial–myometrial interface. Women with abnormally configured luminal cavities or extensive intrauterine adhesions can be difficult to sample adequately. There is no sure way to do this short of hysterectomy, but additional diagnostic procedures such as re-biopsy, imaging studies, or hysteroscopy, all can provide more information.

HYSTERECTOMY

Management of women with a diagnosis of EIN centers on two objectives: (1) exclusion of a coexisting carcinoma, the management of which would supersede that of the EIN itself, and (2) ablation of EIN as a cancer preventative strategy. Hysterectomy fulfills both goals. Topical endometrial ablation by thermal or cautery-mediated devices applied directly to the endometrial lining is not recommended as a treatment option because it may leave residual islands of lesional tissue behind and create intrauterine adhesions, which hinders post-treatment surveillance by re-biopsy.

HORMONAL THERAPY

Although current practice favors hysterectomy for EIN in women past childbearing age, there is an active interest and evolving experience with uterus-sparing alternatives for younger women and those who present unfavorable surgical risks.[1,53] Progestin-based hormonal therapies capable of ablating EIN lesions offer the best alternative to surgery, but the optimal regimens, preferred delivery vehicle (oral, injected, impregnated intrauterine device), expected clinical response, and attendant risks remain to be defined.[1] Progestational therapy is based upon data showing that essentially all EIN lesions contain detectable progesterone receptors,[35] and progestins can produce apoptosis of neoplastic endometrial glandular cells.[54,55] Wholesale shedding of the endometrium after drug withdrawal is another mechanism of removal. The largely anecdotal clinical experience is difficult to aggregate because of significant differences between studies in diagnostic criteria applied, patient mix, agent and administration regimen, and outcome measures. Interested readers are referred to existing reviews on the subject.[1] It is evident that some patients do respond to progestin therapy, but it is not possible to identify responding individuals in advance, nor is the response efficacy known. In our own practice, 21% of newly diagnosed EINs are treated with progestins, sometimes as an interim measure before surgery. This intervention is most common in younger nulliparous patients desiring to maintain fertility, and associated with decreased risk for EIN persistence (OR 0.11), or progression to carcinoma (OR 0.24).[5]

REFERENCES

1. Trimble CL, Method M, Leitao M, et al. Management of endometrial precancers. Obstet Gynecol 2012;120:1160–75.
2. Zaino RJ, et al. Tumours of the uterine corpus: epithelial tumours and precursor lesions. In: Kurman RJ, Carcangiu ML, Herrington S, Young RH, editors. WHO classification of tumours of the female reproductive organs. Lyon, France: IARC Press; 2014.
3. Jarboe EA, Mutter GL. Endometrial intraepithelial neoplasia. Semin Diagn Pathol 2010;27:215–25.
4. Mutter GL. The Endometrial Collaborative Group. Endometrial intraepithelial neoplasia (EIN): Will it bring order to chaos? Gynecol Oncol 2000;76:287–90.
5. Semere LG, Ko E, Johnson NR, et al. Endometrial intraepithelial neoplasia clinical correlates and outcomes: A practice-based experience. Obstet Gynecol 2011;118(1):21–8.
6. Mutter GL, Baak JPA, Crum CP, et al. Endometrial precancer diagnosis by histopathology, clonal analysis, and computerized morphometry. J Pathol 2000;190:462–9.
7. Scully RE, Bonfiglio TA, Kurman RJ, et al. Uterine corpus. Histological typing of female genital tract tumors. New York: Springer-Verlag; 1994. p. 13–31.
8. Berman JJ, bores-Saavedra J, Bostwick D, et al. Precancer: A conceptual working definition. Results of a Consensus Conference. Cancer Detect Prev 2006;30:387–94.
9. Jovanovic AS, Boynton KA, Mutter GL. Uteri of women with endometrial carcinoma contain a histopathologic spectrum of monoclonal putative precancers, some with microsatellite instability. Cancer Res 1996;56:1917–21.
10. Mutter GL, Lin MC, Fitzgerald JT, et al. Altered PTEN expression as a diagnostic marker for the earliest endometrial precancers. J Natl Cancer Inst 2000;92:924–30.
11. Mutter GL, Boynton KA, Faquin WC, et al. Allelotype mapping of unstable microsatellites establishes direct lineage continuity between endometrial precancers and cancer. Cancer Res 1996;56:4483–6.
12. Hecht JL, Ince TA, Baak JP, et al. Prediction of endometrial carcinoma by subjective endometrial intraepithelial neoplasia diagnosis. Mod Pathol 2005;18:324–30.
13. Mutter GL, Kauderer J, Baak JPA, Alberts DA. Biopsy histomorphometry predicts uterine myoinvasion by endometrial carcinoma: A Gynecologic Oncology Group Study. Hum Pathol 2008;39:866–74.
14. Baak JP, Mutter GL, Robboy S, et al. The molecular genetics and morphometry-based endometrial intraepithelial neoplasia classification system predicts disease progression in endometrial hyperplasia more accurately than the 1994 World Health Organization classification system. Cancer 2005;103(11):2304–12.
15. Mutter GL, Chaponot M, Fletcher J. A PCR assay for non-random X chromosome inactivation identifies monoclonal endometrial cancers and precancers. Am J Pathol 1995;146:501–8.

16. Monte NM, Webster KA, Neuberg D, et al. Joint loss of PAX2 and PTEN expression in endometrial precancers and cancer. Cancer Res 2010;70:6225–32.
17. Mutter GL, Wada H, Faquin W, Enomoto T. K-ras mutations appear in the premalignant phase of both microsatellite stable and unstable endometrial carcinogenesis. Mol Pathol 1999;52:257–62.
18. Parazzini F, La Vecchia C, Bocciolone L, Franceschi S. The epidemiology of endometrial cancer. Gynecol Oncol 1991;41:1–16.
19. Shapiro S, Kelly JP, Rosenberg L, et al. Risk of localized and widespread endometrial cancer in relation to recent and discontinued use of conjugated estrogens. N Engl J Med 1985;313:969–72.
20. Zeleniuch-Jacquotte A, Akhmedkhanov A, Kato I, et al. Postmenopausal endogenous oestrogens and risk of endometrial cancer: results of a prospective study. Br J Cancer 2001;84:975–81.
21. Writing Group for the PEPI Trial. Effects of hormone replacement therapy on endometrial histology in postmenopausal women. The Postmenopausal Estrogen/Progestin Interventions (PEPI) Trial. JAMA 1996;275:370–5.
22. Mutter GL, Zaino RJ, Baak JPA, et al. The benign endometrial hyperplasia sequence and endometrial intraepithelial neoplasia. Int J Gynecol Pathol 2007;26:103–14.
23. Silverberg SG, Mutter GL, Kurman RJ, et al. Tumors of the uterine corpus: epithelial tumors and related lesions. In: Tavassoli FA, Stratton MR, editors. WHO classification of tumors: pathology and genetics of tumors of the breast and female genital organs. Lyon, France: IARC Press; 2003. p. 221–32.
24. Ferenczy A. Pathophysiology of endometrial bleeding. Maturitas 2003;45:1–14.
25. Song J, Rutherford T, Naftolin F, et al. Hormonal regulation of apoptosis and the Fas and Fas ligand system in human endometrial cells. Mol Hum Reprod 2002;8:447–55.
26. Boerrigter PJ, van de Weijer PH, Baak JP, et al. Endometrial response in estrogen replacement therapy quarterly combined with a progestogen. Maturitas 1996;24:63–71.
27. Shipley III CF, Simmons CL, Nelson GH. Comparison of transvaginal sonography with endometrial biopsy in asymptomatic postmenopausal women. J Ultrasound Med 1994;13:99–104.
28. Zaino RJ. Endometrial hyperplasia: is it time for a quantum leap to a new classification? Int J Gynecol Pathol 2000;19:314–21.
29. Woodruff JD, Pickar JH. Incidence of endometrial hyperplasia in postmenopausal women taking conjugated estrogens (Premarin) with medroxyprogesterone acetate or conjugated estrogens alone. Am J Obstet Gynecol 1994;170:1213–23.
30. Stanford JL, Brinton LA, Berman ML, et al. Oral contraceptives and endometrial cancer: do other risk factors modify the association. Int J Cancer 1993;54:243–8.
31. Weiderpass E, Adami HO, Baron JA, et al. Use of oral contraceptives and endometrial cancer risk (Sweden). Cancer Causes Control 1999;10:277–84.
32. Grimes DA, Economy KE. Primary prevention of gynecologic cancers. Am J Obstet Gynecol 1995;172:227–35.
33. Parra-Herran CE, Monte NM, Mutter GL. Endometrial intraepithelial neoplasia with secretory differentiation: diagnostic features and underlying mechanisms. Mod Pathol 2013;26:868–73.
34. Esteller M, Catasus L, Matias-Guiu X, et al. hMLH1 promoter hypermethylation is an early event in human endometrial tumorigenesis. Am J Pathol 1999;155:1767–72.
35. Mutter GL, Ince TA, Baak JPA, et al. Molecular identification of latent precancers in histologically normal endometrium. Cancer Res 2001;61:4311–14.
36. Faquin WC, Fitzgerald JT, Lin MC, et al. Sporadic microsatellite instability is specific to neoplastic and preoplastic endometrial tissues. Am J Clin Pathol 2000;113:576–82.
37. Millar AL, Pal T, Madlensky L, et al. Mismatch repair gene defects contribute to the genetic basis of double primary cancers of the colorectum and endometrium. Hum Mol Genet 1999;8:823–9.
38. Sutter C, Ienbach-Hellweg G, Schmidt D, et al. Molecular analysis of endometrial hyperplasia in HNPCC-suspicious patients may predict progression to endometrial carcinoma. Am J Pathol 2004;23:18–25.
39. Ries LAG, Melbert D, Krapcho M, et al. SEER cancer statistics review, 1975–2005. Bethesda, MD: National Cancer Institute. <http://seer cancer gov/csr/1975_2005/2008>; 2005.
40. Mutter GL, Lin MC, Fitzgerald JT, et al. Changes in endometrial PTEN expression throughout the human menstrual cycle. J Clin Endocrinol Metab 2000;85:2334–8.
41. Zheng W, Baker HE, Mutter GL. Involution of PTEN-null endometrial glands with progestin therapy. Gynecol Oncol 2004;92:1008–13.
42. Lin MC, Burkholder KA, Viswanathan AN, et al. Involution of latent endometrial precancers by hormonal and non hormonal mechanisms. Cancer 2009;115:2111–18.
43. Hopfer H, Rinehart Jr CA, Vollmer G, Kaufman DG. In vitro interactions of endometrial stromal and epithelial cells in Matrigel: reorganization of the extracellular matrix. Pathobiology 1994;62:104–8.
44. Osteen KG, Rodgers WH, Gaire M, et al. Stromal-epithelial interaction mediates steroidal regulation of metalloproteinase expression in human endometrium. Proc Natl Acad Sci USA 1994;91:10129–33.
45. Bergeron C, Nogales F, Masseroli M, et al. A multicentric European study testing the reproducibility of the WHO Classification of endometrial hyperplasia with a proposal of a simplified working classification for biopsy and curettage specimens. Am J Surg Pathol 1999;23:1102–8.
46. Usubutun A, Mutter GL, Saglam A, et al. Reproducibility of endometrial intraepithelial neoplasia diagnosis is good, but influenced by the diagnostic style of pathologists. Mod Pathol 2012;25:877–84.
47. Baak JPA, Nauta J, Wisse-Brekelmans E, Bezemer P. Architectural and nuclear morphometrical features together are more important prognosticators in endometrial hyperplasias than nuclear morphometrical features alone. J Pathol 1988;154:335–41.
48. Dunton C, Baak J, Palazzo J, et al. Use of computerized morphometric analyses of endometrial hyperplasias in the prediction of coexistent cancer. Am J Obstet Gynecol 1996;174:1518–21.
49. Baak JP, Orbo A, van Diest PJ, et al. Prospective multicenter evaluation of the morphometric D-score for prediction of the outcome of endometrial hyperplasias. Am J Surg Pathol 2001;25:930–5.
50. Huang EC, Mutter GL, Crum CP, Nucci MR. Clinical outcome in diagnostically ambiguous foci of 'gland crowding' in the endometrium. Mod Pathol 2010;23:1486–91.
51. Orbo A, Baak JP, Kleivan I, et al. Computerised morphometrical analysis in endometrial hyperplasia for the prediction of cancer development. A long-term retrospective study from northern Norway. J Clin Pathol 2000;53:697–703.
52. Baak JP, Mutter GL. EIN and WHO94. J Clin Pathol 2005;58:1–6.
53. Minig L, Franchi D, Boveri S, et al. Progestin intrauterine device and GnRH analogue for uterus-sparing treatment of endometrial precancers and well-differentiated early endometrial carcinoma in young women. Ann Oncol 2011;22:643–9.
54. Dahmoun M, Boman K, Cajander S, et al. Apoptosis, proliferation, and sex hormone receptors in superficial parts of human endometrium at the end of the secretory phase. J Clin Endocrinol Metab 1999;84:1737–43.
55. Mertens HJ, Heineman MJ, Evers JL. The expression of apoptosis-related proteins Bcl-2 and Ki67 in endometrium of ovulatory menstrual cycles. Gynecol Obstet Invest 2002;53:224–30.
56. Carlson JW, Mutter GL. Endometrial intraepithelial neoplasia is associated with polyps and frequently has metaplastic change. Histopathology 2008;53:325–32.

18 Endometrial Adenocarcinoma

George L. Mutter, Jaime Prat

CHAPTER OUTLINE

Introduction	370	Serous Carcinoma	387
An Oversimplified View of Endometrial Adenocarcinoma: Types 1 and 2	370	Serous Endometrial Intraepithelial Carcinoma (EIC)	389
Molecular Pathology of Type 1 and 2 Cancers	372	Clear Cell Adenocarcinoma	391
		Mixed Types of Carcinoma	393
Classification of Endometrial Adenocarcinoma	372	Carcinosarcoma	393
Risk Factors in Endometrial Carcinoma	373	Other Types of Endometrial Carcinoma	394
Estrogens and Estrogen-Associated Conditions	373	Undifferentiated Carcinoma	394
Obesity	373	Squamous Cell Carcinoma	394
Diabetes	373	Synchronous Endometrial and Ovarian Carcinoma	395
Polycystic Ovary Syndrome	373	Tumors Metastatic to the Endometrium	395
Ovarian Sex Cord–Stromal Tumors	373	Prognostic Factors in Endometrial Carcinoma	396
Other Risk Factors	373	Histologic Type	396
Heritable Risk	373	Histologic Grade	396
Tamoxifen	374	Stage and Depth of Myometrial Invasion	396
Reproductive Factors	374	Lymphovascular Invasion	397
Cigarette Smoking	374	Age	397
Endometrioid Adenocarcinoma and Its Variants	374	Steroid Hormone Receptors	397
Precursor Lesions: Endometrial Intraepithelial Neoplasia/Atypical Hyperplasia	381	The Spread of Endometrial Carcinoma	398
Variants of Endometrioid Carcinoma	382		

INTRODUCTION

Endometrial adenocarcinomas are a heterogeneous group of tumors derived from endometrial glandular epithelial cells. Most maintain a resemblance to endometrial glands ('endometrioid') but even in these cases mucinous or squamous differentiation occurs frequently. A much less common group of endometrial carcinomas shows non-endometrioid histology and includes clear cell and serous carcinomas. This chapter provides an overview of current diagnostic criteria as well as relevant molecular genetic findings.

Adenocarcinoma of the endometrium is the most common gynecologic cancer in the United States, having a lifetime occurrence risk of 2.5%[1] with 44,000 new cases and 7950 deaths annually.[2] The median age at presentation is 63 years, of which 90% of cases are found in women past menopause and only 1% are under age 40 years. The absolute prevalence of endometrial cancer is affected by the background hysterectomy rate,[3] which varies greatly between populations, and is 40% by age 60 in the United States.[4]

AN OVERSIMPLIFIED VIEW OF ENDOMETRIAL ADENOCARCINOMA: TYPES 1 AND 2

A two-type view of endometrial adenocarcinoma combines epidemiologic, clinical, histologic, and molecular genetic data, and provides a useful pathogenetic model supported by multiple lines of evidence (Figure 18.1). The two types are: endometrioid carcinomas and their variants (type 1) and the non-endometrioid (type 2) carcinomas.

For many years endometrial cancers were subdivided according to histologic grade into well, moderately, and poorly differentiated groups. This was the case until serous carcinoma, the most aggressive type of endometrial cancer, was recognized in 1982,[5] and soon found to be unassociated with unopposed estrogens, the risk factor tightly linked to other endometrial carcinomas. Based on this finding, a proposal was made to separate endometrial adenocarcinomas into two distinct groups designated as types 1 and 2 (Table 18.1).[6] It was a division into either indolent estrogen-induced or aggressive estrogen-independent tumors, respectively. Type 1 was further designated as 'endometrioid' and type 2 'non-endometrioid' to reflect their divergent histologies, thereby suggesting that the noted functional differences might be extrapolated to their histologic classification.[7]

Molecular genetic analyses of well-differentiated endometrioid and serous carcinomas support this dualistic model of endometrial tumorigenesis (Figure 18.2).[8] Studies using cDNA microarrays confirm that these two tumor types have distinctively different gene expression profiles.[9] Increasing genetic damage can be seen in precursor lesions within the endometrioid pathway, beginning with *PTEN* or *PAX2* inactivation in normal-appearing glands (latent precancers), followed by positive hormonal selection and clonal outgrowth as endometrial intraepithelial neoplasia (EIN; also known as atypical hyperplasia or AH), and then cancer (Figure 18.3).[10] Comparable gradations are less evident in the serous carcinoma pathway, where a noninvasive form of disease, serous endometrial intraepithelial carcinoma

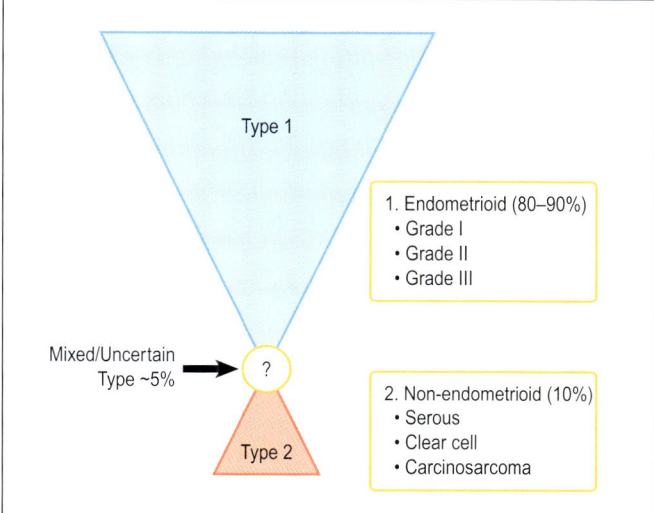

Figure 18.1 Types of endometrial carcinoma, and their clinically significant subdivisions. Endometrioid (type 1) tumors include many histologic variants, but it is tumor grade that is most important in risk prognostication. Non-endometrioid tumors (type 2) are ungraded, but histotypes should be diagnosed separately as each has a distinctive natural history.

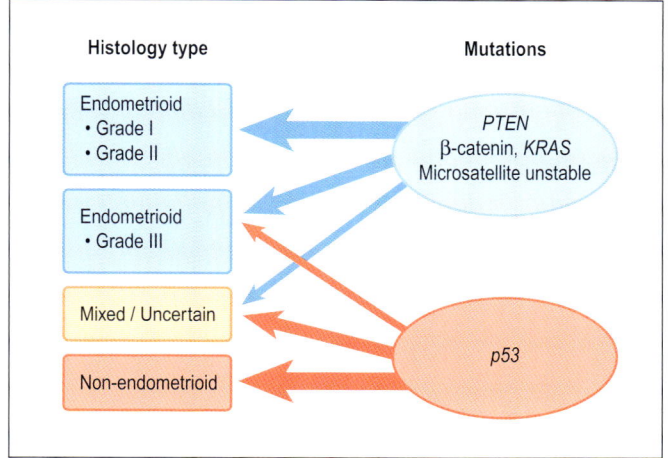

Figure 18.2 Type 1 and 2 endometrial carcinoma differ in the frequency of specific mutations, but there is substantial crossover especially in the grade III endometrioid and mixed categories. p53 inactivation is present in about 90% of serous carcinomas, and much less in clear cell carcinomas and carcinosarcomas.

Table 18.1 Differences between Endometrioid and Non-Endometrioid Endometrial Carcinomas

Feature	Endometrioid (Type 1)	Non-Endometrioid (Type 2)	Refs
Histologic pattern(s)	Endometrioid, mucinous, adenosquamous, secretory	Serous	51,167
Grade	1–3	Not applicable	
Behavior	Indolent	Aggressive	
Average age	59	66	8,168
Risk factors	Endocrine (unopposed estrogen)	Unknown	
Precursor lesion	EIN	Serous EIC	169
p53 mutation	5–10%	>90%	164,168,170
PTEN inactivation	55%	11%	164
KRAS mutation	13–26	0–10%	171,172
PIK3CA mutations	24–39%	12%	
PIK3CA amplification	–	Frequent	
CTNNB1 (β-Catenin mutation)	25–38%	Rare	170
MLH-1 inactivation	17%	5%	68
ARID1A mutation	29–39%	18–26%	
Loss of estrogen and progesterone receptors	27–30%	76–81%	

Note: Clear cell carcinoma and carcinosarcoma are non-endometrioid tumors by exclusion, but are non-equivalent to serous carcinomas.

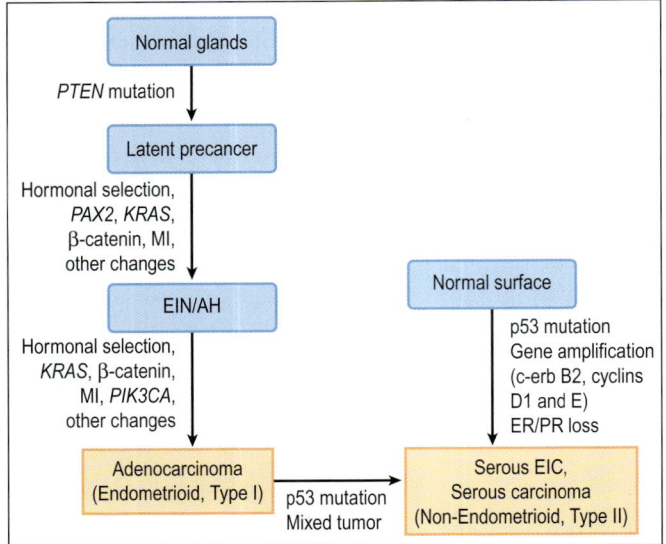

Figure 18.3 Molecular changes during endometrial carcinogenesis, by histologic type.

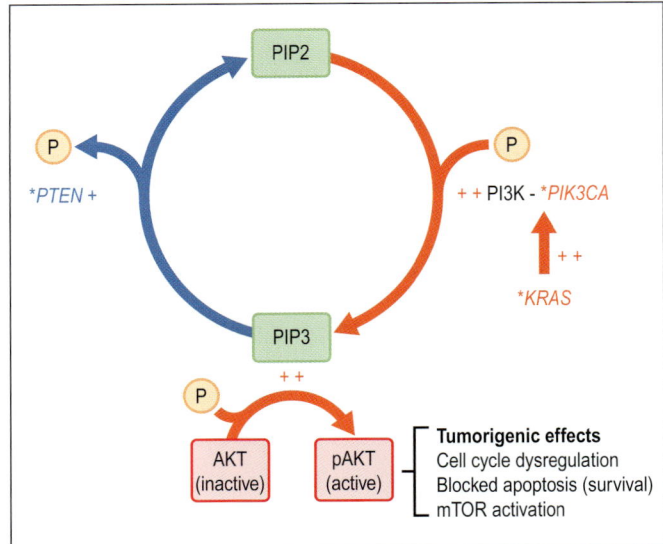

Figure 18.4 Activation of the AKT pathway in endometrioid (type 1) tumorigenesis. Activation of AKT by PIP-mediated phosphorylation is augmented by primary mutations (*), which activate the *KRAS* and/or *PIK3CA* genes, or inactivate *PTEN*. The combination of increased PIP3 production (red) with diminished PIP3 dephosphorylation (blue) has the net effect of increasing PIP3. pAKT has numerous downstream effects including activation of the mTOR pathway, changes in cell cycle regulation, blockade of apoptosis, and prolonged cell survival.

(serous EIC), is genetically identical to its invasive counterpart and also capable of metastasizing.

Although the dualistic model is applicable to a high proportion of endometrial carcinomas, not all tumors fit in. In fact, a gray zone exists between the two broad types, with a significant number of tumors showing overlapping clinical, morphologic, and molecular features (Figures 18.1 and 18.2). Moreover, there is an ongoing debate about whether a histologic subset of endometrioid carcinomas (those that are poorly differentiated or have high nuclear grade) should be assigned to the type 2 group. Furthermore, it is now accepted that a non-endometrioid component may emerge from a pre-existing endometrioid carcinoma. The probable mechanism for this is development of genetic heterogeneity within elements of a type 1 tumor, and progressive expansion of a particularly aggressive tumor subclone with genetic and behavioral features resembling those of type 2 tumors[9] (Figure 18.2).

Some unique tumor histotypes, such as clear cell carcinomas and carcinosarcomas, demonstrate clinical and molecular features that do not fit into either of the prototype endometrioid and non-endometrioid categories.[133] These other histologic types may achieve even greater significance if and when specific therapeutic agents are developed to their peculiar molecular genetic alterations.

There is one aspect of the type 1/2 divide that has been extended to clinical care. Histologic grade of endometrioid (type 1) carcinomas has independent value in determining prognosis and should be included in the diagnosis, whereas all of the type 2 tumors (serous, clear cell, carcinosarcoma) are sufficiently aggressive that subclassification by grade is unnecessary.

MOLECULAR PATHOLOGY OF TYPE 1 AND 2 CANCERS

Estrogen-related type 1 tumors frequently demonstrate one or more of the following: microsatellite instability, inactivated *PTEN* tumor suppressor gene, *KRAS* mutations, and activation of the β-catenin gene (*CTNNB1*).[11] In contrast, the estrogen-independent type 2 tumors show loss of heterozygosity at different loci, altered p53, and abnormalities in genes regulating mitotic checkpoints.[9] However, p53 mutations are found in approximately 10% of endometrioid carcinomas, most frequently in grade 3 and occasionally in grade 2 tumors. Overall, p53 mutations occur in 50% of grade 3 tumors, but not in grade 1 tumors or EIN/AH. This finding suggests that p53 is involved in the progression, but not the initiation, of endometrioid carcinoma.

Our understanding of synergies between multiple independent genetic events that produce endometrioid (type 1) carcinoma centers upon the PI3K pathway, and its ability when perturbed to activate AKT (Figures 18.2–18.4). It is estimated that more than 80% of endometrioid carcinomas have an abnormality in the PI3K pathway,[12] which act to increase levels of PIP3, an activator of AKT. Thus *PTEN* inactivation (60% of cases), or constitutive activation of *KRAS* (10–30%) or *PIK3CA* (30%) act in concert to accumulate PIP3, which in turn activates AKT by phosphorylation.[13] Once activated, pAKT initiates a cascade of tumorigenic events that includes stimulation of the mTOR pathway, deregulation of cell cycle control, blocking of apoptosis, and prolonged cell survival.[13] This model presents new downstream targets for suppression by pharmacologic inhibitors, such as the mTOR pathway.

CLASSIFICATION OF ENDOMETRIAL ADENOCARCINOMA

Recognition of histologic subtypes is an important factor in planning treatment and predicting clinical outcome. A histologic classification of endometrial carcinomas is given in Table 18.2, and this chapter is organized according to these diagnostic categories.

Table 18.2 Histopathologic Classification of Endometrial Carcinoma

Endometrioid adenocarcinoma
    Variants
        Endometrioid adenocarcinoma with squamous differentiation
        Mucinous adenocarcinoma
        Secretory adenocarcinoma
        Ciliated cell adenocarcinoma
        Villoglandular adenocarcinoma
        Endometrioid carcinoma with sertoliform differentiation
Serous carcinoma
Clear cell adenocarcinoma
Carcinosarcoma (MMMT)
Undifferentiated carcinoma
Neuroendocrine carcinoma
Small cell carcinoma
Squamous cell carcinoma
Miscellaneous types

RISK FACTORS IN ENDOMETRIAL CARCINOMA

ESTROGENS AND ESTROGEN-ASSOCIATED CONDITIONS

The overriding stimulus behind the development of EIN/AH and the endometrioid type of endometrial carcinoma is the effect of estrogens, both endogenous and exogenous. These are not mirrored in non-endometrioid tumors, with the exception of carcinosarcomas. Beginning in 1969, a notable rise in the number of endometrial cancers occurred, which coincided with a fourfold increase in the use of estrogens for the alleviation of perimenopausal and postmenopausal symptoms in women. The relative risk of developing endometrial carcinoma in women taking unopposed estrogens is elevated 3- to 6-fold,[14] rising to 9.5-fold if unopposed estrogen has been used for 10 years or longer.[15] The increased risk persists for several years after the estrogen is discontinued.[16] The risk is roughly similar whether the estrogens are taken continuously or cyclically. The additional administration of progestins for several days of each month reduces the risk of carcinoma to baseline population levels. Although progestins are usually prescribed for either 7 or 10 days per month in women taking estrogen-replacement therapy, the protection from endometrial cancer is much greater if progestins are used for at least 10 days or given continuously as combined estrogen-progestin therapy.

OBESITY

The overall relative risk for an obese woman to develop endometrial cancer increases proportionally with increasing body mass index, up to sixfold for the morbidly obese (BMI > 40).[17-19] This risk can be reduced to near baseline levels with bariatric surgery and successful weight reduction.[20] Endometrial cancer is only one of the many comorbidities seen in the obese patient. The association in women past menopause is commonly explained in terms of increased aromatization of androgens to estrogens (estrone and estradiol) in adipose tissue, this being the major source of estrogens in women of this age group. A woman who completes surgical therapy for stage 1 endometrial cancer is more likely to die of cardiovascular disease than any other cause including her cancer.[21]

DIABETES

The magnitude of endometrial cancer risk in patients with type 2 diabetes has been difficult to measure because of a high frequency of coexisting risk factors such as obesity and polycystic ovarian disease. However, improved quantitative markers have confirmed a positive association of diabetes with endometrial cancer. Insulin resistance, as measured by the (inversely proportional) serum surrogate marker adiponectin, correlates highly with endometrial cancer risk even when corrected for obesity.[22,23]

POLYCYSTIC OVARY SYNDROME

Polycystic ovary syndrome (PCOS) is a constellation of endocrine disorders expressing at least two of the following features: anovulation or infrequent ovulation, androgen excess, and polycystic ovaries.[24] Ovarian cysts typically are theca–lutein follicles with prominent luteinization of the theca interna and an inconspicuous granulosa cell layer. Primary endocrine defects in PCOS are peripheral insulin resistance and excess ovarian production of androgens.[25] The population of affected women is enriched for risk factors such as obesity, with endometrial findings indicating a hyperestrogenic state.[26] Endometrial carcinoma occurs at 2.7-fold increased risk in women with PCOS,[27] but, as the women are all young, this number comprises a significant proportion of endometrial carcinomas in women under age 45 years.

OVARIAN SEX CORD–STROMAL TUMORS

Granulosa cell tumor is a relatively uncommon tumor that mainly affects women shortly after menopause. Most tumors produce increased estrogens and about half the women affected present with postmenopausal bleeding, one-third having proliferative endometrium. Endometrial carcinomas occur in 9–13% of women with granulosa cell tumors.[28]

OTHER RISK FACTORS

HERITABLE RISK

Women with hereditary non-polyposis colorectal carcinoma syndrome (HNPCC), Lynch syndrome, a condition affecting about 1% of the population, have a 70% lifetime risk of endometrial adenocarcinoma.[29] They tend to develop disease 15 years earlier than sporadic occurrences and the prognosis is favorable.[30] Their tumors show many of the histopathologic and genetic features of endometrioid endometrial adenocarcinomas,[31] including transit through a premalignant EIN/AH phase,[32] and genetic alterations in mismatch repair genes (mainly *MSH-2*, *MSH-6*, and *MLH-1*)[33,34] and *PTEN*.[35] Immunohistochemistry for DNA mismatch repair proteins is often abnormal in endometrial cancers of Lynch syndrome patients, and has been suggested as a screening test for this heritable condition. Immunohistochemistry is nonspecific, however, because it is a somatically acquired non-heritable feature in 18% of all sporadic endometrial carcinomas. One cost–benefit study has recommended restricting immunotesting of primary endometrial tumors to those patients having additional clinical risk factors, such as one first-degree relative with a Lynch-associated carcinoma.[36]

Germline BRCA mutation, which increases breast and ovarian cancer occurrences, does not significantly alter endometrial cancer risk.[37] There may be a small indirect effect on endometrial cancer incidence in those patients managed by prophylactic tamoxifen administration.[38]

TAMOXIFEN

The antiestrogen tamoxifen is widely used as an adjuvant therapy for women with breast cancer. Tamoxifen is a nonsteroidal compound that competes with estrogen for estrogen receptors (ERs). In women of childbearing age it antagonizes endogenous estrogens and induces endometrial inactivity or atrophy, but in postmenopausal women, who are normally hypoestrogenic, it may have a weak estrogenic effect. Tamoxifen administration is associated with an overall slightly increased risk (2–3 times) of endometrial adenocarcinoma.[39] Carcinoma occurrences are mainly of early stage and low grade, but a small subset of aggressive high-grade endometrioid carcinomas, clear cell carcinomas, or carcinosarcomas are disproportionately increased.[40,41] Placement of a levonorgestrel-impregnated intrauterine device in tamoxifen-treated patients has not yet demonstrated statistically significant protection from tamoxifen-related endometrial cancers.[42]

In addition to the increased risk of endometrial carcinoma, women treated with tamoxifen are particularly prone to developing endometrial polyps, especially ones of gigantic size (see Chapter 15).

REPRODUCTIVE FACTORS

Most studies have shown an association between early age at menarche, late age at natural menopause, and total length of ovulation span,[43] although these findings are not universal. The use of oral contraceptives reduces the risk of endometrial cancer, in some studies by half.

Nulliparity is a strong independent risk factor for endometrial carcinoma.[43] Women with endometrial carcinoma are less likely to have had children than normal controls and, if they are parous, they will have had fewer children. Infertility, particularly that associated with anovulation and progesterone insufficiency, is also associated with the risk of developing endometrial carcinoma.[45] Nulliparity is significant only when the endometrial carcinoma develops before menopause and not after.[46] This suggests that the hormonal disturbances that prevent conception also encourage malignant change in the endometrium. The protective effect of pregnancy applies only to full-term pregnancy.[47]

CIGARETTE SMOKING

Cigarette smoking reduces the risk of endometrial carcinoma. The effect is limited primarily to women whose disease is detected after menopause and, among these women, current smokers show the greatest reduction in risk, and former smokers are less affected.[48] The mechanism whereby cigarette smoking reduces risk is not clear. One study has shown that serum estrogen levels were unaffected but that androstenedione levels were slightly higher in smokers.[49] Paradoxically, women with advanced stage endometrial carcinoma (stages II–IV) were more likely to be smokers than women with early stage disease (stages 0–I).[50]

ENDOMETRIOID ADENOCARCINOMA AND ITS VARIANTS

Endometrioid carcinoma is the most common type of endometrial cancer accounting for approximately 60% of cases. The term 'endometrioid' derives from the tumor's predominant glandular pattern, which resembles proliferative-phase endometrium. Nevertheless, its histologic variants may have a minor, or even predominant, mucinous, secretory, squamous, ciliated, or sex cord-like pattern.

Clinical Features

Most tumors develop slowly in the setting of hyperestrogenism against a background of non-atypical endometrial hyperplasia, although some arise in atrophic endometrium.[51] Endometrioid carcinoma is predominantly a disease of the sixth and seventh decades and 75% of cases occur after the menopause. Only 5% occur in women less than 40 years old. They are low-grade, non-myoinvasive, associated with a good prognosis and often develop after a long history of anovulatory cycles or estrogen therapy. Endometrial carcinoma rarely occurs in pregnancy.[52]

Women with endometrioid carcinoma most often present with abnormal vaginal bleeding, which means in the majority of cases postmenopausal bleeding. The fact that they bleed, however, simply means that the tumor is often large or advanced. Smaller carcinomas may be asymptomatic. Surprisingly frequently, asymptomatic tumor is documented in women who have an endometrial biopsy before instituting hormone replacement therapy, or had the tumor discovered initially at autopsy.[53] Patients with advanced disease may complain of pelvic pain, which reflects tumor spread.

The diagnosis is made by endometrial biopsy or curettage, but imaging techniques and hysteroscopy are being used more and can play an important role. Outpatient endometrial sampling techniques (Pipelle biopsy) have an excellent diagnostic rate for endometrial carcinoma, similar to that for curettage.[54]

Gross Features

Endometrioid carcinoma can present variously to the naked eye when the uterus is opened. The uterus may be slightly or grossly enlarged but it may be of normal size or even

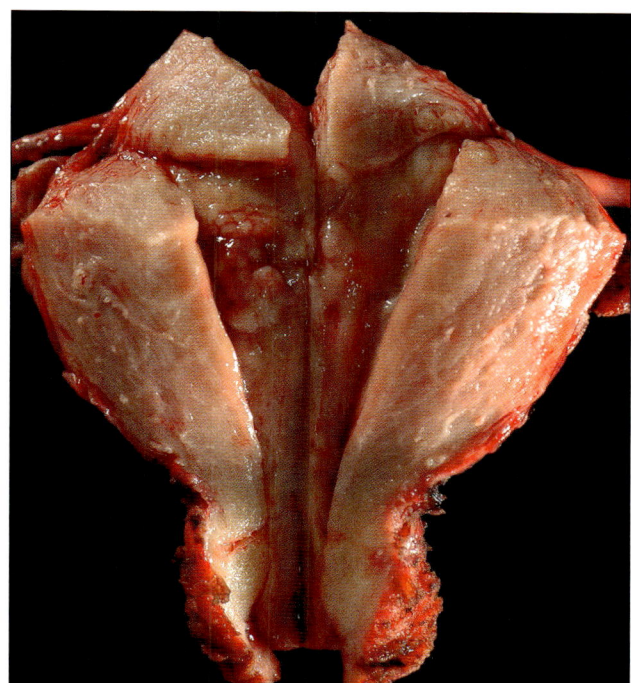

Figure 18.5 Endometrial adenocarcinoma. The tumor involves only part of the endometrium and appears as apparently separate foci.

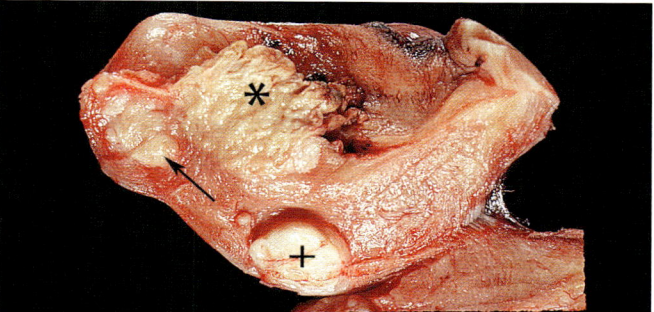

Figure 18.6 Endometrial adenocarcinoma. A section through the wall of a uterus shows carcinoma protruding into the lumen (*) and invading deeply into the myometrium (black arrow). A leiomyoma is also present (+).

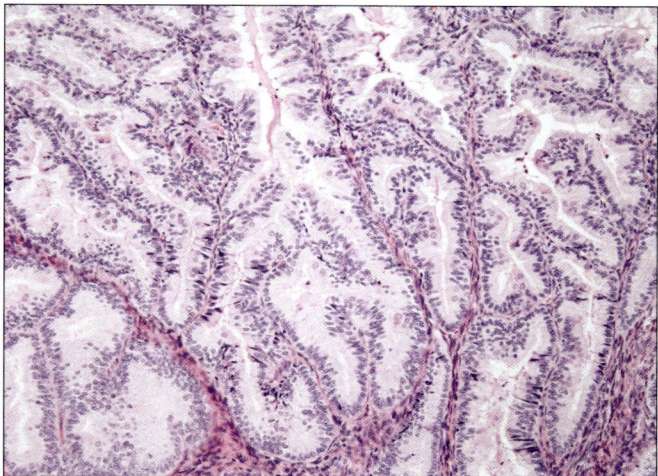

Figure 18.7 Endometrial adenocarcinoma, endometrioid type, grade 1 (well differentiated). The branching glands with maze-like lumens indicate an architecture of folded sheets of neoplastic epithelium, rather than dense packing of tubular structures.

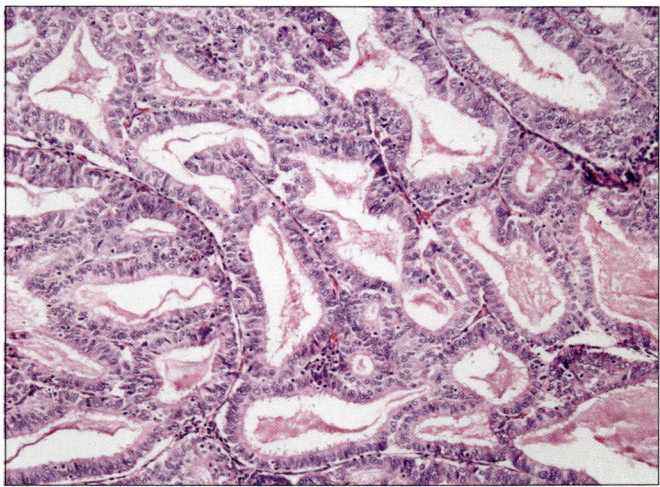

Figure 18.8 Endometrial adenocarcinoma, endometrioid type. Well-differentiated (grade 1) tumor with confluent glands.

small and atrophic, particularly in a postmenopausal woman. Most tumors arise in the corpus but some originate in the lower uterine segment. The tumor may present as a single mass or there may be multiple separate masses (Figure 18.5) or a diffuse thickening of the endometrium. Carcinomas are situated more frequently on the posterior than the anterior wall. The most common appearance is of an exophytic, rough, perhaps papillary area of the endometrium with a shaggy surface and ulceration (Figure 18.6). Sometimes the tumor is polypoid, with a fairly narrow base. When this is the case, its surface may be smooth and hemorrhagic and the uterine cavity distended, with concomitant thinning of the uterine wall. When the tumor is polypoid, the remaining endometrium usually appears thin. Myometrial invasion may be obvious to the naked eye (Figure 18.6), with either pushing or infiltrating borders, but frequently it is difficult to appreciate the degree of myometrial invasion grossly. There seems to be no correlation between the degree of exophytic growth of the tumor within the uterine cavity and the presence of myometrial invasion.[55] However, a tumor diameter of more than 2 cm generally is associated with poorer prognosis and a higher frequency of distant failure.[57]

Microscopic Features

The glandular pattern and cellular features generally resemble the proliferative endometrium. Carcinoma is recognized within the endometrial compartment by the presence of at least one of the following: meandering interconnected lumens formed by folded sheets of neoplastic epithelium (Figure 18.7), irregular angulated and tapering glandular contours (Figure 18.8), a cribriform pattern of the glands

(Figures 18.9 and 18.10), or a solid area of glandular epithelium (Figures 18.10 and 18.11). Several features may be present together. These points are summarized in Figure 18.12.

Stratification of epithelial cells is almost always seen. Occasionally, cribriform fragments have a microglandular appearance easily confused with a cervical lesion (Figure 18.13). The individual epithelial cells are larger than would be expected in the proliferative phase. Compared with the normal endometrium, the carcinoma cells have a distinctly altered cytology that varies between cases and even within areas of a single tumor, but may include rounded nuclei, clumped chromatin, and prominent nucleoli. Individual tumors frequently show patchy changes in differentiation to mucinous, squamous, tubal, or other cytologies, and in these cases cytoplasmic as well as nuclear features stand out from the normal background. Some endometrioid adenocarcinomas secrete abundant mucin ('mucin-rich' variant), and these may or may not have identifiable intracytoplasmic mucin. Mitotic figures are usually present but may be scanty in well-differentiated tumors.

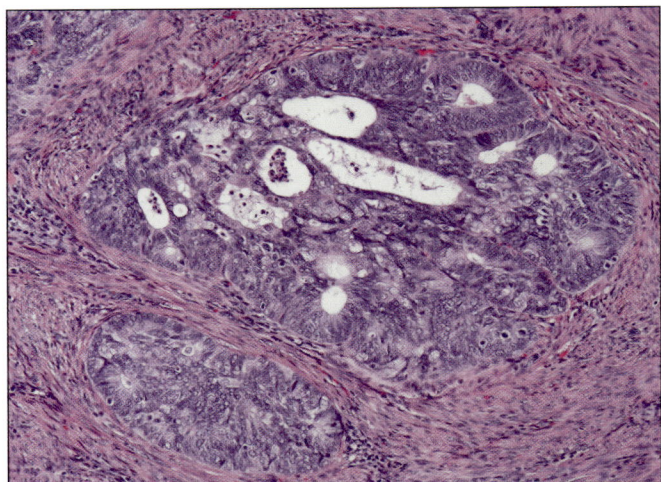

Figure 18.10 Endometrial adenocarcinoma, endometrioid type. Moderately differentiated (grade 2) tumor, with solid and cribriform areas.

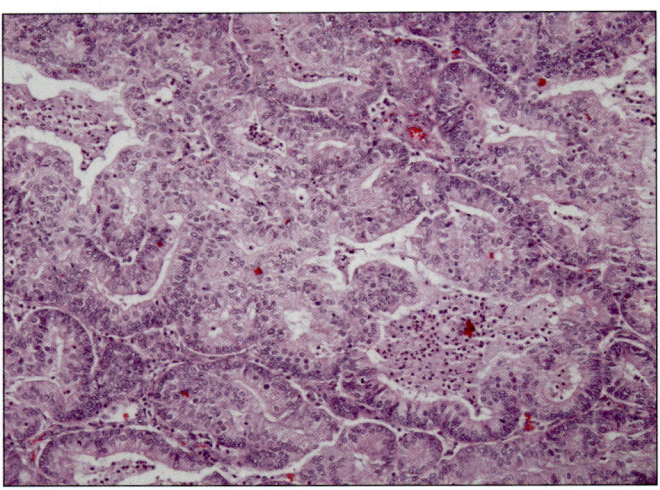

Figure 18.9 Endometrial adenocarcinoma, endometrioid type. Moderately differentiated (grade 2) tumor, with solid and cribriform areas.

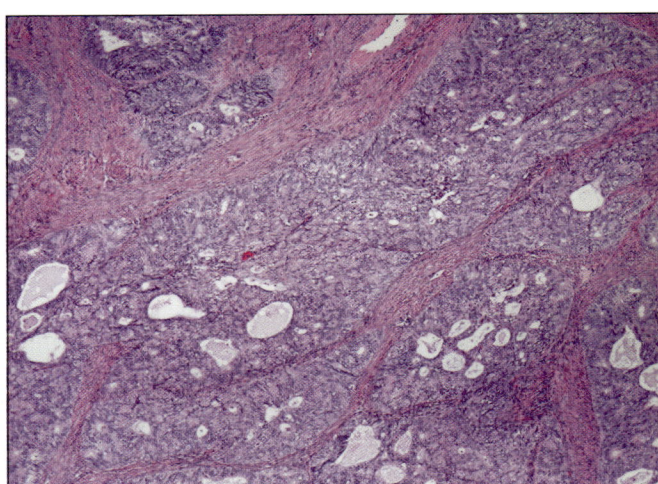

Figure 18.11 Endometrial adenocarcinoma, endometrioid type. Poorly differentiated (grade 3) tumor.

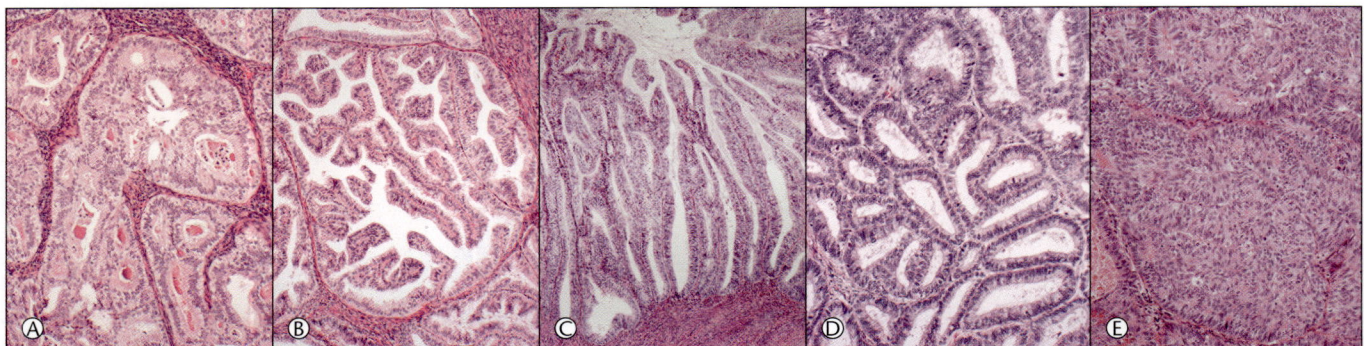

Figure 18.12 **(A–E)** Intraendometrial adenocarcinoma. Glandular architectural patterns that may be seen in non-myoinvasive areas. **(A)** Cribriform glands; **(B)** Maze-like or meandering lumens; **(C)** Villoglandular; **(D)** Confluent polygonal molded glands; **(E)** Solid growth.

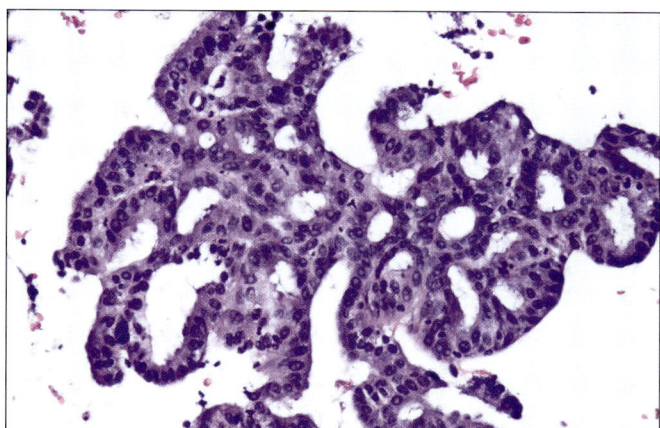

Figure 18.13 Endometrial adenocarcinoma, endometrioid type, with microglandular cribriform architecture. These delicate lesions tend to be exophytic, and may appear highly fragmented in biopsy specimens.

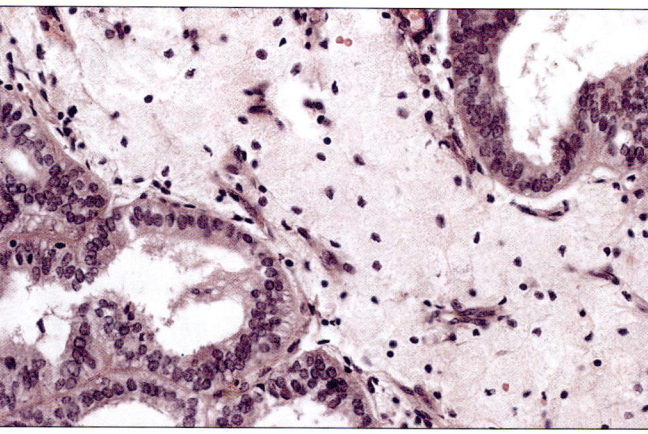

Figure 18.14 Endometrial adenocarcinoma. Foam cells in the stroma.

Endometrioid adenocarcinomas, like their precursor EIN lesions, spread within the endometrial compartment by extension of newly formed, well-differentiated neoplastic glands into the adjacent stroma (centripetal growth). In turn, the adjacent endometrial stroma responds by remodeling, rarely showing a desmoplastic change. For this reason, qualitatively assessing the character of the endometrial stroma within the endometrial compartment itself is noncontributory in distinguishing noninvasive from invasive carcinoma.

Foamy histiocytes are commonly seen in the endometrial stroma of patients with a carcinoma. Nearly one-fifth of cases contain stromal cells laden with lipid (Figure 18.14), but there is no correlation between the presence of these cells and the grade of the tumor or the survival of the patient.[56] This change is simply a reactive response to tumor cells. The presence of such histiocytic cells in endometrial biopsies showing EIN should always lead to further diagnostic work-up for coexistent carcinoma.

Histologic Grading

The most commonly used histologic grading system is that of the International Federation of Gynecology and Obstetrics (FIGO) and is recommended by the World Health Organization (WHO; Table 18.3).[57] This three-tiered grading system is applied to endometrioid adenocarcinomas which are classified, as well differentiated (grade 1), moderately differentiated (grade 2), or poorly differentiated (grade 3). The grading procedure is based on the amount of solid non-squamous areas within a tumor. Squamous components are excluded. Grade 1 tumors (Figure 18.15) show 5% or less solid growth and often there is no solid tumor at all. Grade 2 tumors (Figure 18.16) show solid growth in 6–50% of the tumor. More than 50% solid growth is considered grade 3 (Figure 18.17). Most endometrioid adenocarcinomas are grade 1 or 2.

Although the FIGO grading system of endometrioid carcinoma relies first and foremost on the architectural pattern of the glands, the histologic grade should be raised by one level beyond that determined by architecture alone in those

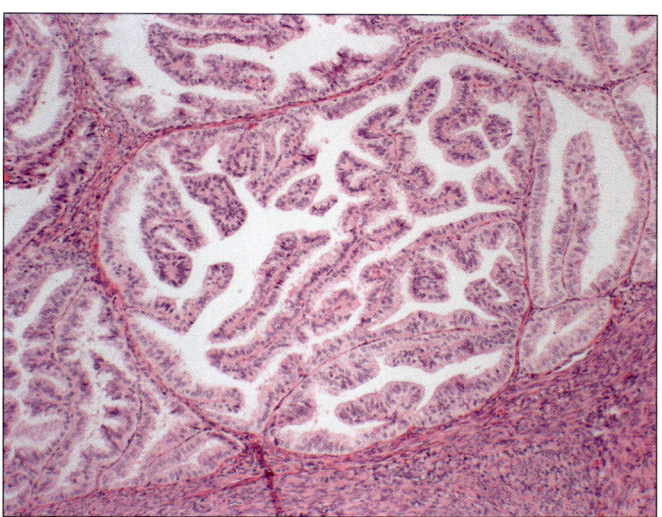

Figure 18.15 Endometrial adenocarcinoma, endometrioid type, grade 1 (well differentiated). Grade 1 tumors have less than 5% solid growth.

Table 18.3 Grading of Endometrioid Endometrial Carcinoma (Note: Serous, Clear Cell, and Carcinosarcoma Tumors Are Not Graded)

Grade 1	5% or less of non-squamous solid growth
Grade 2	6–50% of non-squamous solid growth
Grade 3	More than 50% of non-squamous solid growth

Notable nuclear atypia inappropriately severe for the architectural grade of the tumor raises the grade by one (to a maximum of grade 3).
In tumors with squamous differentiation, grading is based on the glandular component.

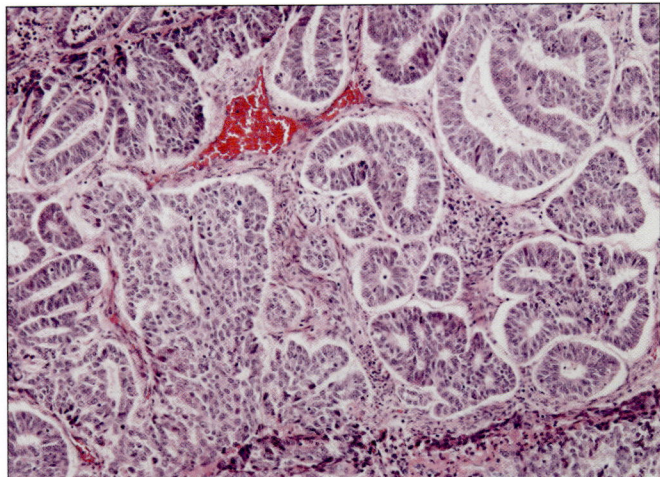

Figure 18.16 Endometrial adenocarcinoma, endometrioid type, grade 2 (moderately differentiated). Grade 2 tumors have between 5% and 50% solid areas.

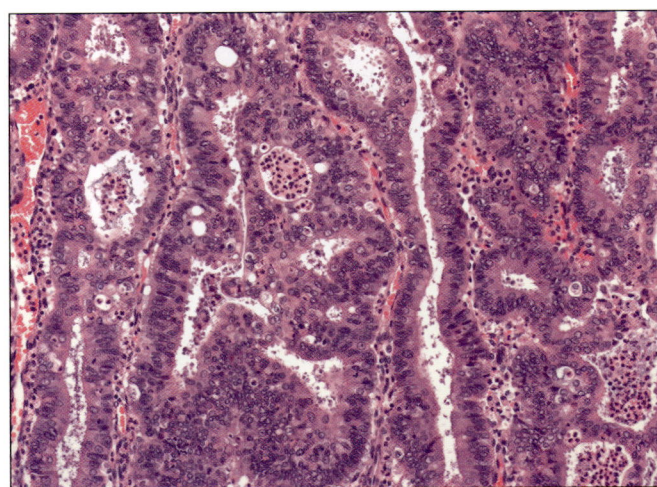

Figure 18.18 High-grade nuclear atypia in this tumor with no solid growth (grade 1 architecture) is the basis to increase the reported grade by one unit, to grade 2 (moderately differentiated).

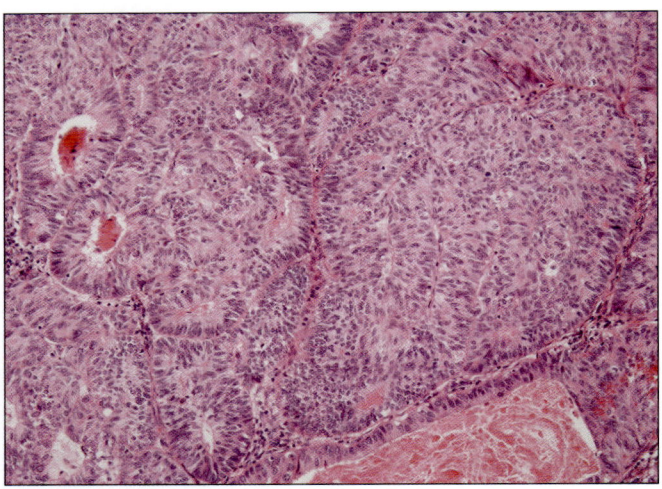

Figure 18.17 Endometrial adenocarcinoma, endometrioid type, grade 3 (poorly differentiated). Grade 3 tumors have more than 50% (non-squamous) solid growth.

Table 18.4 Nuclear Grading of Endometrial Carcinoma

Low Grade	High Grade (Severe Atypia)
Little variation in shape	Marked variation in shape
Little variation in size	Marked variation in size (some markedly enlarged)
Hypochromasia	Marked hyperchromasia (may be focal)
No variation in staining intensity	Marked variation in staining intensity
Evenly distributed chromatin	Coarsely clumped chromatin
Nucleoli not prominent	Prominent nucleoli
Sparse mitoses	Frequent mitoses with abnormal forms

cases exhibiting severe nuclear atypia (Table 18.4[58] and Figure 18.18). Usually the architectural and nuclear grades correspond, but, when at variance, the nuclear grade is often the more reliable indicator of prognosis.[57] When the final grade is elevated due to severe nuclear atypia, a note should appear in the report so that the clinician is alerted that the patient falls into this special category.

Myoinvasion

Myoinvasion is diagnosed when the malignant glands have transgressed the endomyometrial junction and extend into the underlying myometrium. The normal junction, however, is not a straight line, but a rather vague and irregular border. Thus, in many cases, tumors confined to the endometrium cannot be distinguished microscopically from tumors invading the superficial myometrium. In fact, myoinvasion is overdiagnosed in routine practice in as much as 25% of cases; in contrast, failure to diagnose true myoinvasion is extremely rare.[59] This is supported by recent FIGO data, which indicate almost identical 5 year survival rates for women with noninvasive tumors and those with tumors invading less than half of the myometrial thickness.[59] In contrast, the distinction of inner half invasion from outer half invasion is usually straightforward, and the probability of recurrence is markedly increased for women with deeply invasive tumors. Thus, in the 2009 FIGO staging classification of endometrial carcinoma, tumors with no myometrial invasion and tumors with less than 50% invasion are combined under stage IA.[60]

Occasionally, endometrial carcinoma appears confined to foci of adenomyosis. Adenomyosis is really a 'diverticulum' of endometrium deep into the myometrium, and carcinoma can extend into these foci without invading the myometrium.[59] Tumor involvement of adenomyotic foci occurs in about 25% of cases and is not associated with an adverse prognosis.[61,62] When tumor cells extend outward into the myometrium, depth of invasion is measured not from the point of transgression in adenomyosis, but from the superficial endomyometrial junction.

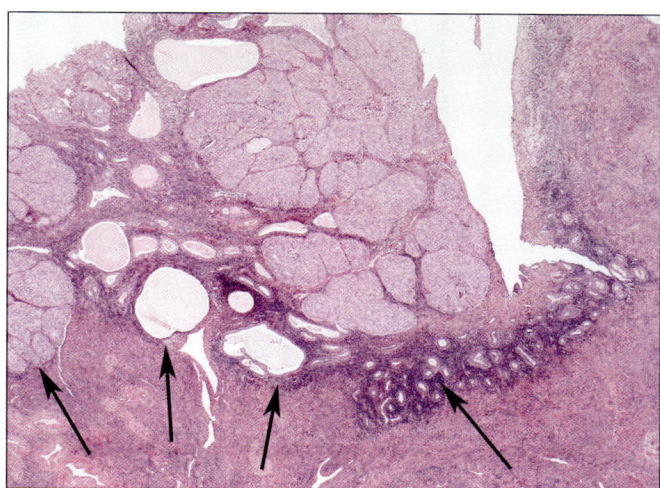

Figure 18.19 This tumor is entirely intraendometrial, but the irregular junction between the endometrium and myometrium imparts a false impression of myoinvasion. Endometrial stroma (arrows) surrounds the tumor.

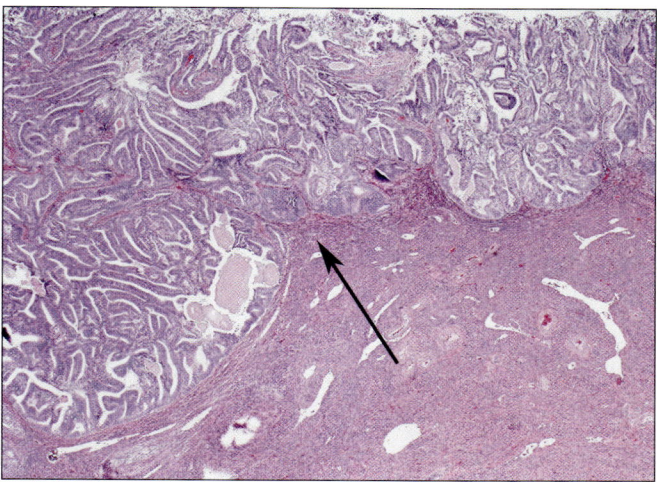

Figure 18.20 Broad front myoinvasion, showing a 'shoulder' (arrow) between myoinvasive (left) and surface (right) involvement.

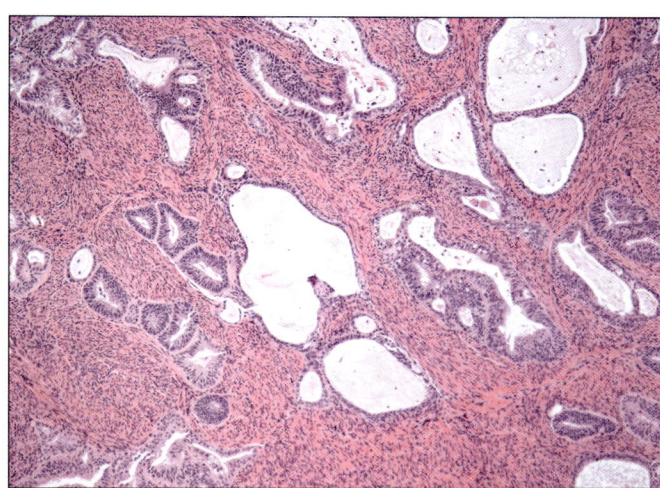

Figure 18.21 Irregular infiltrating glands with no stromal response. (Courtesy of Dr. Marisa R. Nucci.)

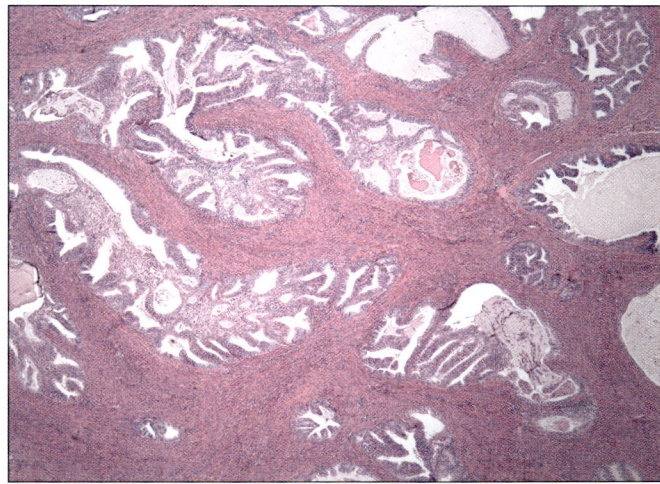

Figure 18.22 Myoinvasion by blunt tumor structures in an 'adenomyosis-like' pattern. (Courtesy of Dr. Marisa R. Nucci.)

The decision to perform pelvic and para-aortic lymph node dissection is largely based on depth of myometrial invasion (also on cell type and histologic grade). Intraoperatively, the pathologist may be requested to assess these features by frozen section.

Maximum depth of myoinvasion is measured in millimeters from the endomyometrial junction, and expressed as the percentage of the total myometrial thickness. Problems arise, however, when the boundary is distorted by the tumor itself or other lesions such as leiomyomas. Residual areas of normal endometrium (Figure 18.19) or overrun normal glands are informative landmarks, when available. Bulky exophytic tumors can be difficult to orient in a single histologic section and, in such cases, assessment of the endomyometrial boundary at the site of deepest invasion requires a combination of gross and histologic evaluation.

Myoinvasion is assessed by evaluation of the topographical distribution of glands and the appearance of adjacent stroma.[63] Invasion across a broad front (21% of cases) may be difficult to distinguish from an irregular endomyometrial interface unless it can be compared to the adjacent uninvolved endomyometrium. This is sometimes evident by a 'shoulder' formed at the juncture of a zone of myoinvasion with an area of surface involvement (Figure 18.20, arrow). Most common (67%) are irregular groups of glands with or without a stromal response (Figure 18.21). 'Adenomyosis-like' invasion (7% of cases) (Figure 18.22) can be distinguished from non-myoinvasive tumor extending into foci of adenomyosis (Figures 18.23 and 18.24) by its lack of accompanying endometrial stroma. Unfortunately, CD10 immunoreaction occurs focally in the cells surrounding tumor clusters in the myometrium of women without adenomyosis, and this limits utility. A distinctive pattern of microcystic, elongated or slit-like, and fragmented (MELF) invasive glands is often accompanied by individual invading cells and a loose stromal response with marked inflammation (Figures 18.25 and 18.26). The MELF pattern of invasion has some features of epithelial–mesenchymal transition,

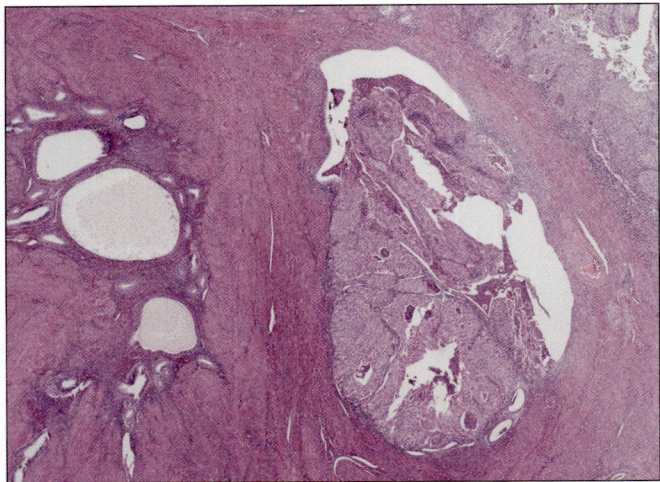

Figure 18.23 Tumor extension into adenomyosis, non-myoinvasive. Two areas of adenomyosis are seen, one with only benign glands (left), and one with extension of adenocarcinoma from the surface (right).

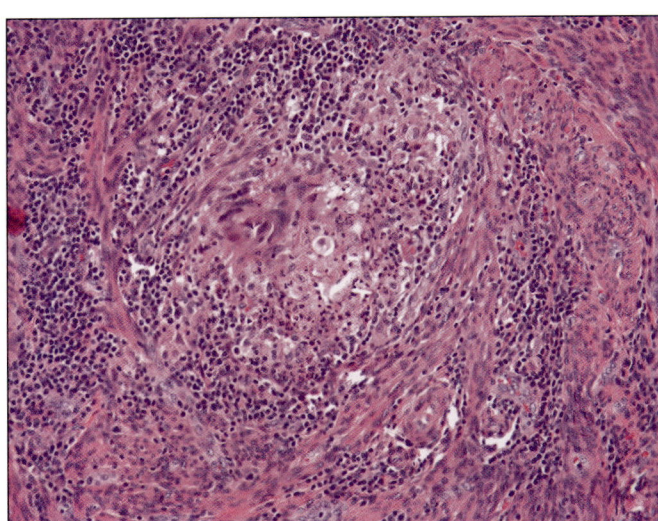

Figure 18.26 Individual invasive cells in MELF-type invasion are eosinophilic or squamous like, and somewhat obscured by the combined stromal and inflammatory response. (Courtesy of Dr. Marisa R. Nucci.)

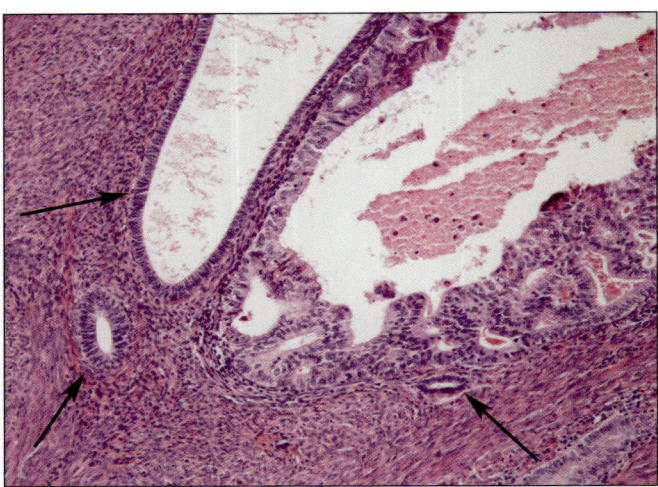

Figure 18.24 Tumor extension into adenomyosis, non-myoinvasive. Detail showing focus of carcinoma and benign glands. A thin layer of intervening stroma is seen.

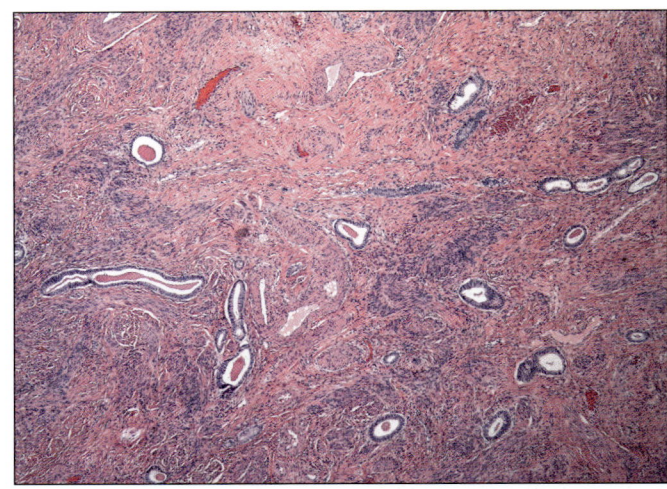

Figure 18.27 'Adenoma malignum' pattern of myoinvasion. (Courtesy of Dr. Marisa R. Nucci.)

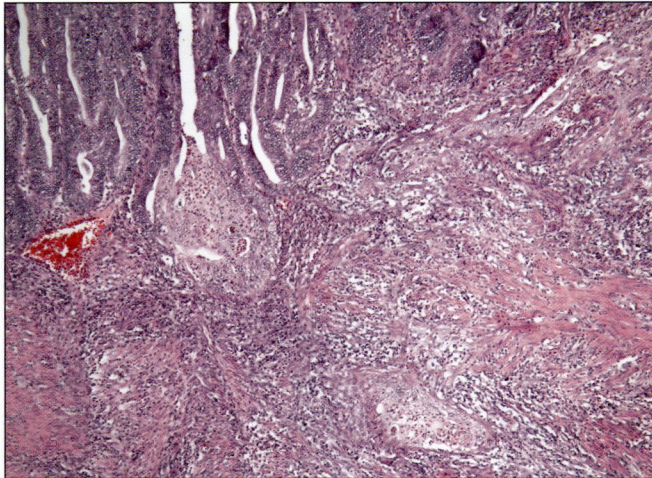

Figure 18.25 Myoinvasion by microcystic elongated (slit-like) glands (MELF). (Courtesy of Dr. Marisa R. Nucci.)

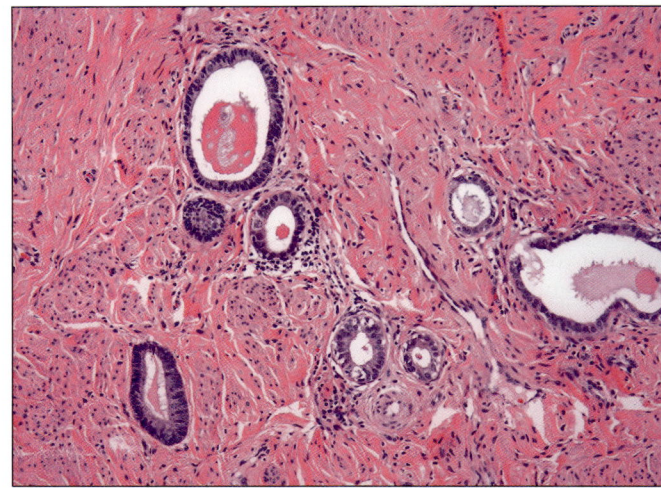

Figure 18.28 There is little stromal response to these well-differentiated adenoma malignum-type invasive glands. (Courtesy of Dr. Marisa R. Nucci.)

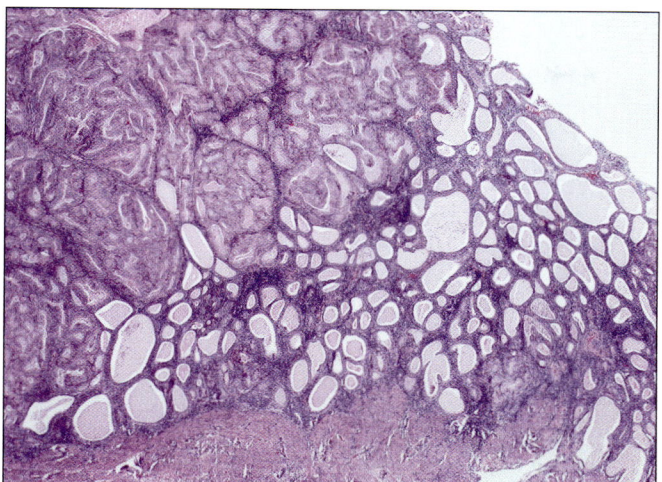

Figure 18.29 Endometrial adenocarcinoma, intraendometrial (left). The endometrium on the right is a premalignant EIN composed of packed round glands.

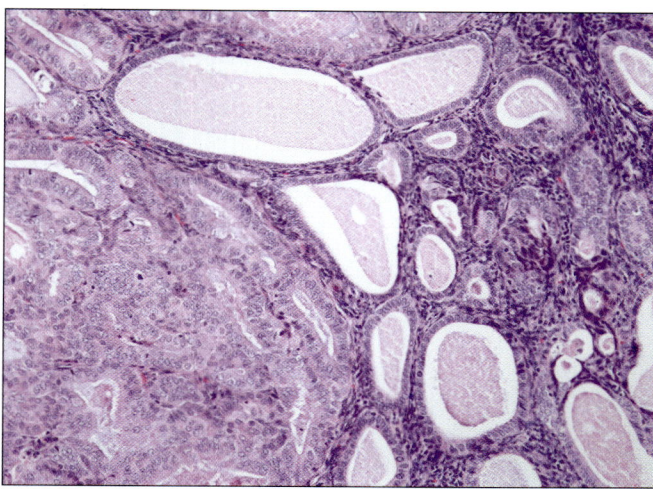

Figure 18.30 Endometrial adenocarcinoma, intraendometrial. Individual tubular glands of EIN are present on the right and adenocarcinoma, with cribriform glands, on the left.

including a greatly reduced proliferative activity and acquisition of a cytokeratin (CK)7-positive immunophenotype.[64] Least common of all (1%) are widely spaced individual glands lacking any stromal response, akin to adenoma malignum of the endocervix (Figures 18.27 and 18.28).

Accessibility of sampling devices to deeper tissues limits the ability to diagnose myoinvasive disease by biopsy or curettage, even when present.

PRECURSOR LESIONS: ENDOMETRIAL INTRAEPITHELIAL NEOPLASIA/ ATYPICAL HYPERPLASIA

Endometrial intraepithelial neoplasia (also known as atypical hyperplasia or AH) is an immediate precursor to endometrioid endometrial adenocarcinoma, which is discussed at length in Chapter 17. It is a clonal expansion of mutated glands, which can be seen as cytologically altered crowded areas of endometrial glands lacking the architectural (solid, cribriform, maze-like, myoinvasive) characteristics of adenocarcinoma (Figure 18.12). Often residual EIN is present within the endometrium at the time of presentation with carcinoma (Figures 18.29 and 18.30).

Cytologic Correlation

There are no established guidelines for routine endometrial cytologic screening, but exfoliated neoplastic endometrial cells are sometimes encountered in cervical Pap smears. Up to two-thirds of women with endometrial adenocarcinoma have malignant cells in their cervical cytology specimen and high-grade as well as high-stage tumors seem to be detected more frequently.[65] In cervical smears, malignant endometrial cells characteristically appear as small clusters with darkly stained nuclei (Figure 18.31) or perhaps as single discrete cells that are easily overlooked. On rare occasions following the recognition of malignant glandular cells in a cervical Pap smear, the endocervical curettage and endometrial biopsy may be negative. The possibility of an ovarian lesion should be considered and excluded.

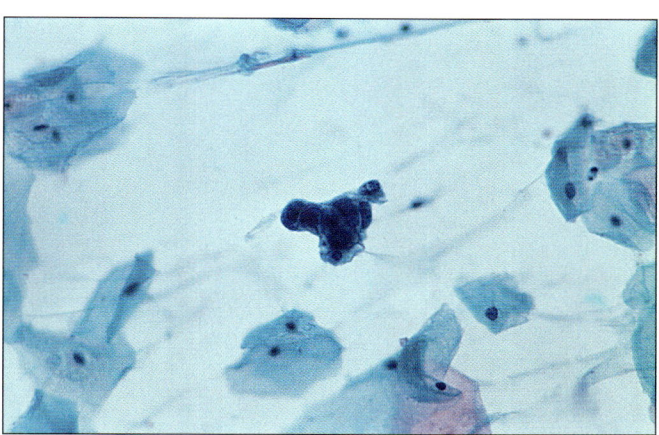

Figure 18.31 Endometrial adenocarcinoma, cytology. Malignant glandular cells in a cervical smear.

Transcervical cytology sampling devices such as the Tao brush have been designed to directly access the endometrium.[66] With this device malignant cells in an endometrial brushing are freshly removed and rapidly fixed so the features are well preserved. Appearance is widely variable, from large single cells to small clusters as well as sheets (Figure 18.32). Although superior to a cervical Pap smear specimen, transcervical instrumentation with a brush introduces many of the potential morbidities of the Pipelle biopsy while yielding less tissue.

Shed tumor DNA incidentally collected by liquid cervical Pap smear may be sequenced to demonstrate mutations known to be present in a coincident endometrial carcinoma.[67] Because the DNA may be shed from anywhere above it is not possible to localize a lesion, nor is the sensitivity and specificity of such a screen known when large

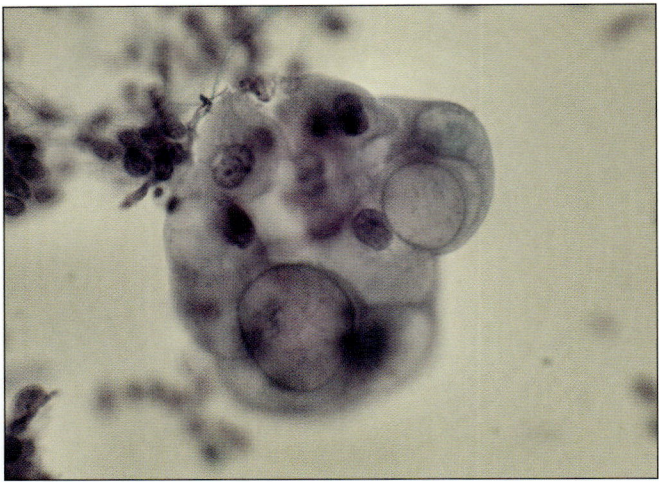

Figure 18.32 Transcervical brush cytology of endometrioid endometrial adenocarcinoma. Carcinoma showing bubble-like mucin-filled cytoplasm. (Courtesy of John Maksem.)

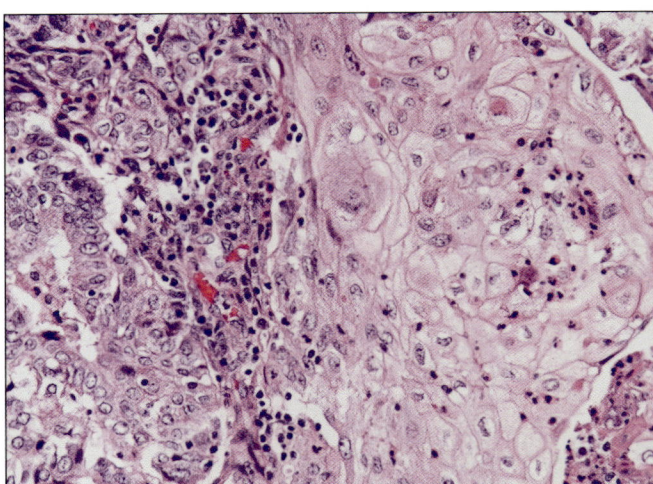

Figure 18.34 Endometrial adenocarcinoma, endometrioid type, with squamous change.

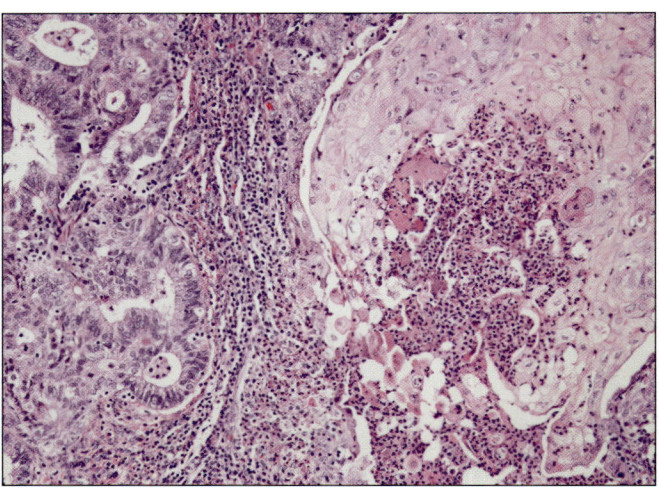

Figure 18.33 Endometrial adenocarcinoma, endometrioid type, with squamous change.

numbers of mutations are screened in the asymptomatic patient.

VARIANTS OF ENDOMETRIOID CARCINOMA

Several histologic variants of endometrioid adenocarcinoma are recognized.

Endometrioid carcinoma with squamous differentiation (one-fourth of endometrial adenocarcinomas) display focal squamous differentiation (Figures 18.33 and 18.34). Formerly, the distinction was made between tumors where the squamous component was well or poorly differentiated. The former tumors were called 'adenoacanthomas' and the latter 'adenosquamous carcinomas.' Several studies have confirmed that prognosis relates largely to the grade of the glandular component. In fact, the glandular component is much easier to grade in a reproducible fashion, and superior in predicting lymph node metastasis and 5 year survival.

Therefore, it is recommended that endometrioid carcinomas with squamous epithelium are classified as endometrioid carcinoma with squamous differentiation and graded, on the basis of the glandular component, as well, moderately, or poorly differentiated (grade 1, 2, or 3, respectively). Besides, the clinical features of adenocarcinoma containing squamous epithelium and those of endometrioid adenocarcinoma are essentially the same.

While the squamous component is often reported as 'benign' or even as 'squamous metaplasia,' it is in reality both neoplastic and metaplastic, as shown by conservation of β-catenin mutations in both squamous and glandular elements. The squamous elements generally have low mitotic activity and lack ERs and thus may be described as being 'terminally differentiated' and 'hormonally incompetent.'

Well-differentiated tumors (grade 1) are composed of glands and squamous nests but usually the glandular component predominates. Squamous epithelium can appear in strips or sheets (Figure 18.34), and when present as oval nests within gland lumens it is referred to as morules. Intercellular bridges and keratin deposits may be seen. The nuclei of the squamous cells are uniform, and lack prominent nucleoli (Figure 18.35). Mitotic figures are rare. In poorly differentiated tumors, the squamous cells show grade 2 or 3 nuclear atypia and are not confined to the lumens of glands. Occasionally, the squamous cells have a spindle morphology, simulating a sarcoma, and may invade the myometrium or vascular spaces. Keratin pearls are often found. Care must be taken in distinguishing between squamous differentiation and solid foci of adenocarcinoma. The undifferentiated epithelial component should be considered glandular unless intercellular bridges are seen or the cells show ample eosinophilic cytoplasm with well-defined borders (Table 18.5).[68]

Foreign-body-type granulomas may form in the peritoneum in response to the keratin component of endometrioid carcinomas with squamous differentiation. These lesions do not seem to affect the prognosis adversely in the absence of viable-appearing tumor cells. The granulomas

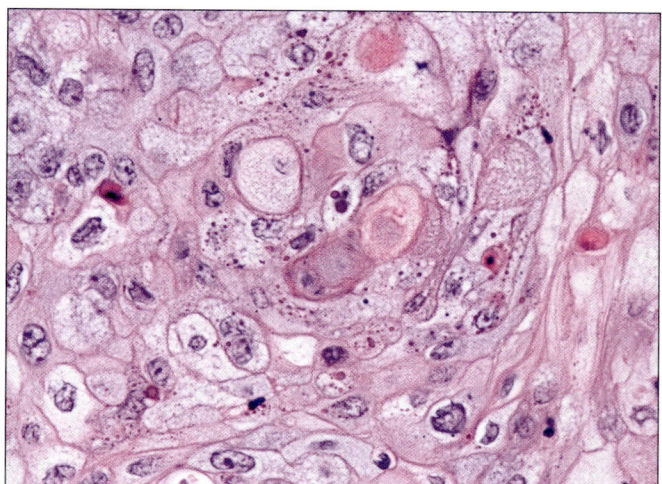

Figure 18.35 Endometrial adenocarcinoma, endometrioid type, with squamous change. High-power view of squamous component.

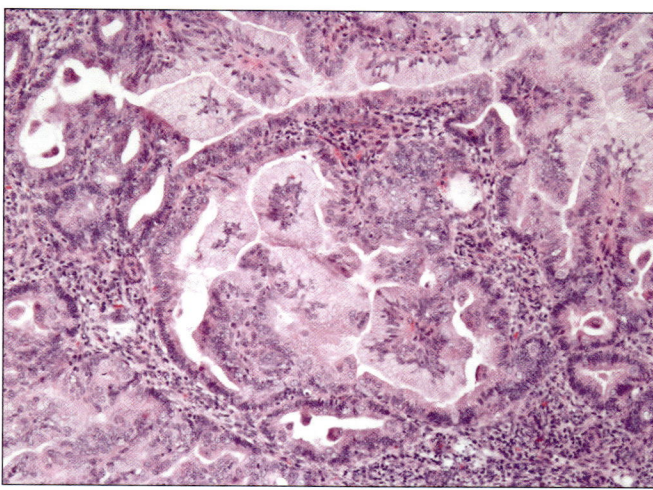

Figure 18.36 Endometrial adenocarcinoma, endometrioid type, with mucinous differentiation. An area of mucinous carcinoma is present in the center.

probably result from transtubal spread of exfoliated necrotic tumor cells.

Mucinous carcinoma in pure form is an uncommon variant of endometrial carcinoma with cells containing prominent intracytoplasmic mucin, resembling the mucinous carcinoma of the endocervix. Mucinous carcinoma constitutes 1–9% of all endometrial carcinomas.[69,70] Patients range in age from 47 to 89 years and their clinical features are similar to those of patients with endometrioid carcinoma. Most patients present with stage I disease.

More commonly mucinous endometrial adenocarcinomas arise in conjunction with an endometrioid component and develop in endometrial polyps in approximately one-fourth of cases. A higher frequency of mucinous adenocarcinomas has been reported in patients receiving tamoxifen and synthetic progestogens[71] suggesting that there might be a different histogenetic mechanism for this tumor, namely progestogens encouraging mucinous metaplasia.[72] The tumors lack distinctive macroscopic features.

Microscopically, the tumors show a glandular architectural pattern or a villoglandular configuration (Figure 18.36). The epithelial cells lining the glands and papillae are tall with basal nuclei, prominent intracytoplasmic mucin, and minimal stratification (Figure 18.37). Nuclear atypia is mild to moderate, and mitotic activity is not prominent. Mucicarmine, periodic acid–Schiff (PAS) and Alcian blue staining can highlight the mucin, but this is rarely necessary for diagnosis. Sometimes, mucinous differentiation is associated with squamous differentiation. Most mucinous carcinomas are well differentiated (grade 1) but grade 2 and grade 3 tumors are occasionally described.[69] More likely than not, poorly differentiated tumors lose their ability to produce mucin. Lymph node metastases may be extremely well differentiated.

Sometimes, complex filiform papillary fragments of mucinous endometrial adenocarcinoma are encountered in biopsy specimens (Figure 18.38). An extremely bland cytology, rare mitoses, and tendency to break apart into small fragments make these tumors extremely difficult to

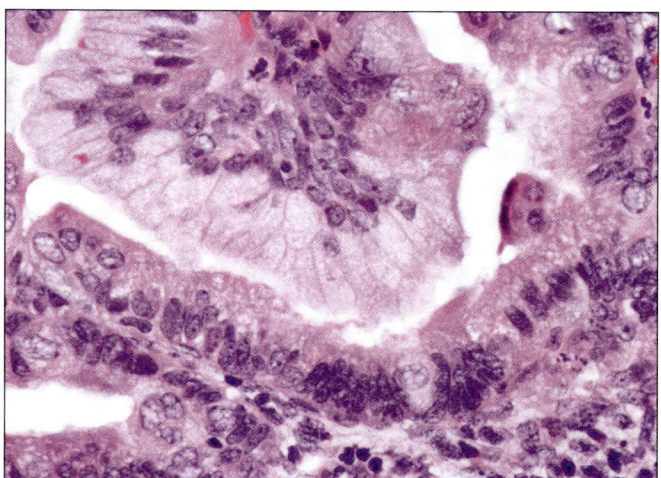

Figure 18.37 Endometrial adenocarcinoma, endometrioid type, with mucinous differentiation. Detail of columnar cells with cytoplasmic mucin.

Table 18.5 Criteria for Identifying Squamous Differentiation in Endometrioid Adenocarcinoma

Squamous differentiation is suggested by the presence of any of the following:
- Keratin or keratin pearls demonstrated without special stains
- Intercellular bridges
- At least three of the following:
  - Sheet-like growth without gland formation or palisading;
  - Distinct cell margins;
  - Deeply eosinophilic or 'glassy' cytoplasm;
  - A decreased nuclear to cytoplasmic ratio compared with the rest of the tumor

recognize, as they resemble endocervical epithelium. The abundance of mucinous epithelium, delicate supportive stroma, and alternating mucinous and non-mucinous differentiation often coexisting with a microglandular cribriform component (Figure 18.39)[73] are characteristic of carcinoma.[74] At hysterectomy, a non-exophytic tumor component may be found, and this may or may not retain the extensive mucinous differentiation of the surface papillary tumor (Figure 18.40). Minor quantities of mucinous elements in an otherwise typical endometrioid adenocarcinoma do not warrant a diagnosis of mucinous adenocarcinoma. Tumors showing typical endometrioid carcinoma with less than 50% of a mucinous component are best designated as endometrioid carcinomas with mucinous differentiation.

The behavior of mucinous carcinomas is similar to that of endometrioid carcinomas. Mucinous carcinomas, however, tend to be low grade and minimally invasive and therefore are associated with an excellent prognosis.

Secretory carcinoma is an uncommon variant of endometrioid adenocarcinoma composed of well-differentiated glands resembling those of early or midsecretory endometrium (Figure 18.41).[75] It accounts for only 1–2% of endometrial carcinomas. The most common changes are subnuclear and/or supranuclear vacuolation in unstratified columnar cells usually exhibiting grade 1 nuclei. The secretory appearance may be focal or diffuse, and not infrequently is admixed with endometrioid carcinoma.

There are two types of secretory carcinoma: those in which the secretory change is induced by circulating progestins, and those in which secretory differentiation is an intrinsic feature of the neoplasm independent of the background hormonal state. The presence or absence of

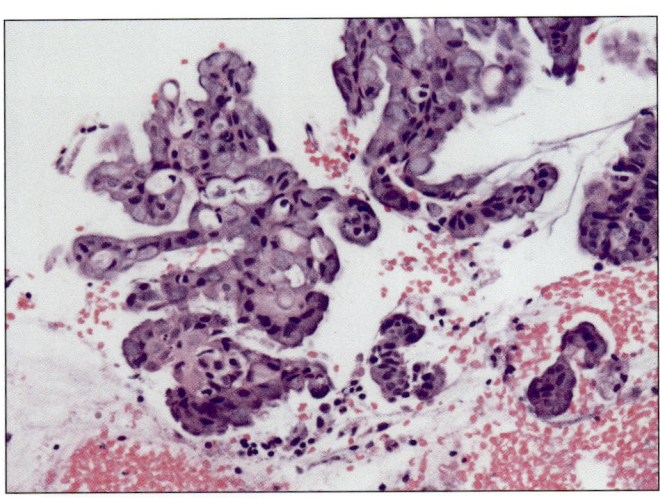

Figure 18.38 Endometrial adenocarcinoma, endometrioid type, with mucinous differentiation. Exophytic fronds of branching mucinous epithelium contain micro cribriform structures.

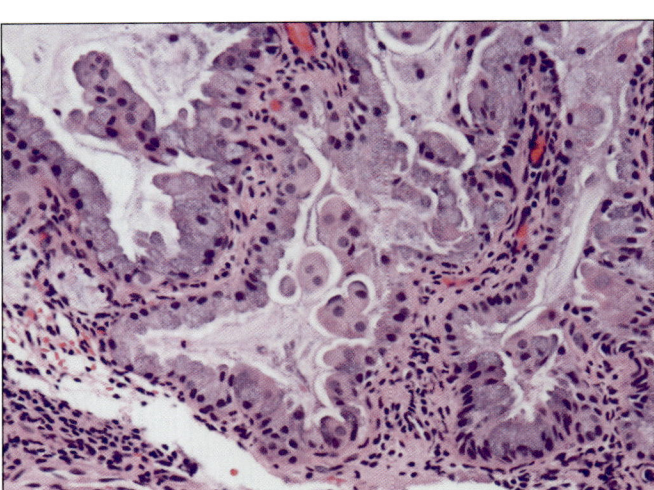

Figure 18.40 Endometrial adenocarcinoma, endometrioid type, with mucinous differentiation. Non-exophytic component of the same tumor as in Figure 18.39 showing a greater degree of endometrioid differentiation and scattered intracytoplasmic mucin.

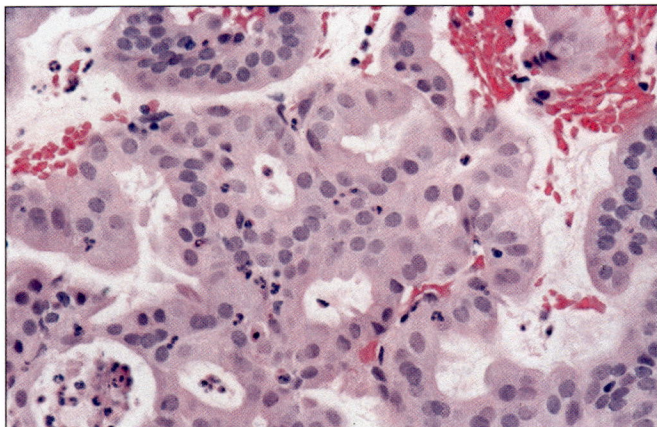

Figure 18.39 Microglandular cribriform architecture in an endometrial adenocarcinoma, endometrioid type, with mucinous differentiation.

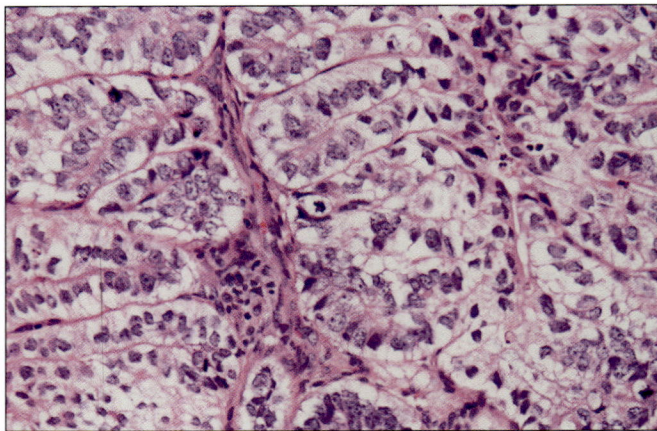

Figure 18.41 Endometrial adenocarcinoma, endometrioid type, with secretory differentiation. This tumor resembles a day 17 secretory endometrium with characteristic and prominent subnuclear vacuoles.

progestin-induced stromal change, and the menopausal status of the patient, distinguishes both types.[76]

Secretory carcinoma must be distinguished from clear cell carcinoma in view of the excellent prognosis of the former and the adverse prognosis of the latter. At times a secretory carcinoma can become solid and mimic clear cell carcinoma. However, contrary to clear cell carcinoma, secretory carcinoma shows a glandular architecture like endometrioid carcinoma, is rarely papillary or cystic, and usually is not solid. The columnar cells of secretory carcinoma are similar to those in endometrioid carcinoma, except that they have supranuclear or subnuclear vacuoles. Clear cell carcinoma, however, usually exhibits tubulocystic and/or papillary architecture. The cells have severe nuclear atypia (grade 3), with rounded nuclei often exhibiting hobnail morphology, smudgy chromatin, and prominent nucleoli. Strong nuclear HNF-1β immunoreaction and negative estrogen/progesterone receptors (ER/PR) favor the diagnosis of clear cell carcinoma. Clear squamous cells tend to be polygonal and usually merge with more typical squamous cells with abundant eosinophilic cytoplasm.

Secretory adenocarcinomas are associated with a good prognosis.[68] Treatment is the same as that for endometrioid carcinoma of the same stage and grade.

Ciliated carcinoma is rare.[77] Ciliated cells are uncommon in adenocarcinomas of the endometrium but occasionally individual ciliated cells can be found with diligent searching. More rarely, extensive ciliated differentiation is present throughout (Figure 18.42). Only if at least 75% of the tumor cells are ciliated should the tumor be termed a 'ciliated cell carcinoma.'[78] Some well-differentiated ciliated tumors may be difficult to distinguish from premalignant EIN/AH lesions. Thus the diagnosis of ciliated cell carcinoma should be made with caution. In some cases only the presence of myometrial or lymphatic invasion establishes the diagnosis. Ciliated carcinoma has an association with exogenous estrogen treatment. The tumors are well differentiated and have a good prognosis.[78]

Villoglandular carcinomas are characterized by long, slender, villous papillae with thin fibrovascular cores usually admixed with typical glandular endometrioid carcinoma (Figure 18.43).[79] The cytologic features are the same as those of typical endometrioid carcinoma (Figure 18.44). Myometrial invasion usually is superficial. Clinical outcomes are based on grade, and are comparable to those seen for other types of endometrioid adenocarcinomas.

Endometrioid adenocarcinomas with sertoliform differentiation[80] are tumors with areas composed of glands resembling sex cord–stromal tumors. The glands are in the form of closely packed tubules or trabeculae with basally oriented nuclei and clear to fibrillary cytoplasm (Figure 18.45). The non-sertoliform areas of the tumors consist of typical endometrioid adenocarcinoma.

Differential Diagnosis

Well-differentiated endometrioid adenocarcinoma may be difficult to distinguish from EIN/AH. This problem has

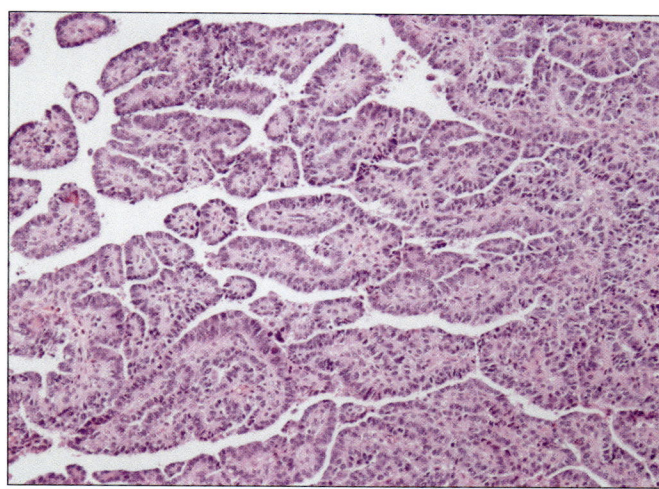

Figure 18.43 Villoglandular architecture in an endometrioid carcinoma, which can be distinguished from its serous counterpart by its simple to pseudostratified rather than exfoliating epithelium.

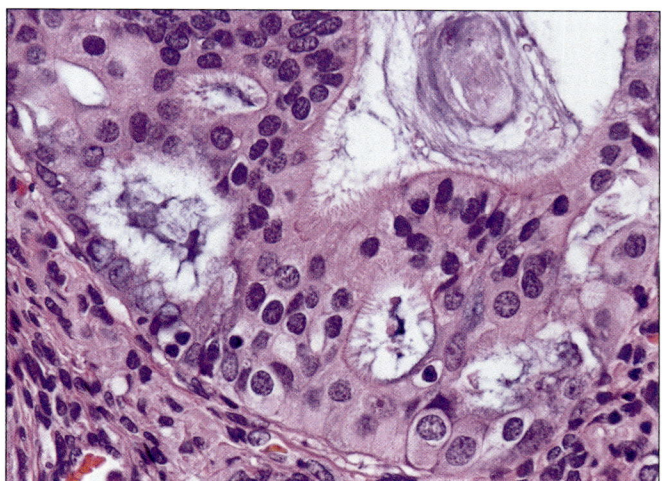

Figure 18.42 Endometrial adenocarcinoma, ciliated type. High-magnification view of cilia.

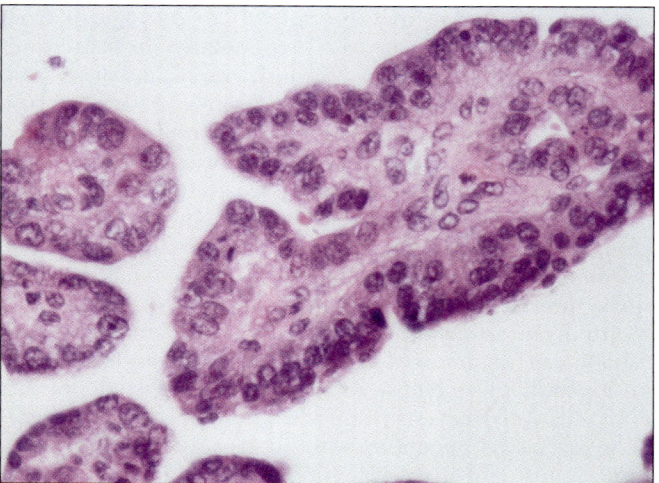

Figure 18.44 Detail of villoglandular endometrioid carcinoma with moderate degree of cytologic atypia. Same case as Figure 18.43.

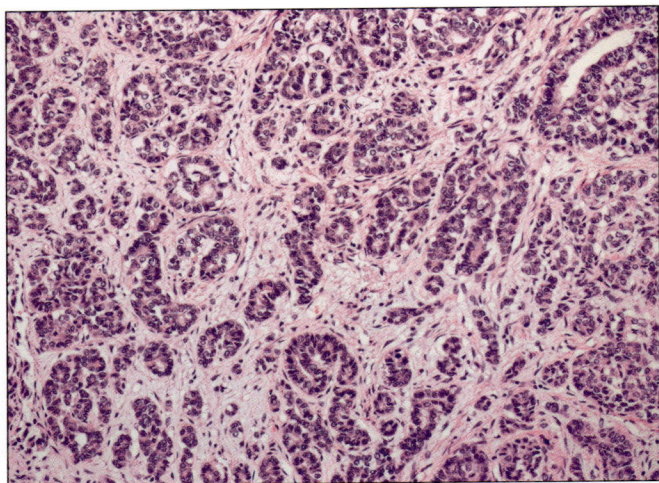

Figure 18.45 Endometrial adenocarcinoma, endometrioid type, sertoliform pattern.

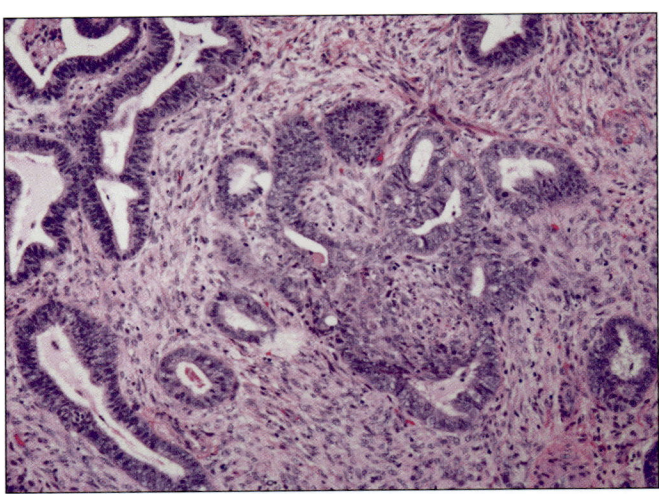

Figure 18.46 Atypical polypoid adenomyoma. Neoplastic glands with squamous morules are offset by a densely muscular stroma.

been discussed in detail in Chapter 17. EIN consists of individual lumen-bearing glands grouped together, whereas a cribriform pattern, solid growth, meandering interconnected lumens, or villoglandular architecture (Figure 18.12) generally are diagnostic of adenocarcinoma.

Myoinvasion clearly favors a diagnosis of carcinoma, but as biopsy and curettage devices rarely sample the myometrial wall it is a criterion only available in hysterectomy specimens and therefore only of use in establishing the final diagnosis. Several groups have systematically examined endometrial biopsy material in women with and without myoinvasive adenocarcinoma to discover features associated with myoinvasion. Variation in nuclear size (anisokaryosis, measured as standard deviation of nuclear diameter) emerged as the single variable most associated with deep myoinvasion. This finding confirms the earlier observation that the presence of extreme nuclear pleomorphism worsens clinical outcome relative to that expected by architectural features alone.[58]

Well-differentiated endometrioid adenocarcinoma with myometrial invasion may be difficult to distinguish from *atypical polypoid adenomyoma*, particularly in curettings (Figure 18.46). This is an obviously important distinction since most atypical polypoid adenomyomas are treated conservatively. Postmenopausal age of the patient and marked nuclear atypia favor a myoinvasive adenocarcinoma, because atypical polypoid adenomyoma usually shows no more than mild to moderate nuclear atypia. In contrast to the elongated fibers of the normal myometrium, the stromal component of atypical polypoid adenomyoma grows in short interlacing fascicles. Furthermore, in curettings or biopsy from an atypical polypoid adenomyoma, there are usually also fragments of normal background endometrium; in contrast, on a biopsy of an endometrioid adenocarcinoma, it would be most unusual to obtain only fragments of myoinvasive neoplasm without free tumor fragments. Immunohistochemistry is helpful in distinguishing between atypical polypoid adenomyoma and a myoinvasive endometrioid adenocarcinoma; whereas the stromal component of atypical polypoid adenomyoma is CD10 negative, the myoinvasive glands of endometrioid adenocarcinoma are typically surrounded by CD10 immunoreactive stromal cells.[81]

Although atypical polypoid adenomyoma has an excellent prognosis, there is a risk of recurrence (around 45%) if curettage or polypectomy is undertaken. There is also a small, but definite, risk of transition to endometrioid adenocarcinoma, which has been estimated at 8.8% in one meta-analysis.[82]

Metaplastic changes as described in Chapter 16 may be seen in benign, premalignant (EIN/AH), or carcinoma states.[83] Hormonally induced metaplasias, such as tubal metaplasia resulting from estrogen stimulation, have a distinctive topography in which metaplastic glands are diffusely interspersed among non-metaplastic glands. This differs from the expanding geographic foci of premalignant and malignant neoplastic processes in which the metaplastic component itself may be cohesive and geographic. Even if metaplastic changes are frequently associated with cancer, the benign cytologic features, architectural pattern, and lack of invasion help to make the correct diagnosis of hormonally induced metaplasias.

Poorly differentiated carcinomas composed of extensive solid tumor may show spindled cells and give a 'pseudo-sarcomatous' appearance. Just the presence of recognizable glands does not mean the tumor is biphasic and, in such cases, a diagnosis of *carcinosarcoma* would be unjustified. Conversely, it is also apparent that the mesenchymal and epithelial elements of carcinosarcomas may both show reactivity with cytokeratins and vimentin.[84] Thus, cytokeratin reactivity in the stromal element does not necessarily mean that a carcinomatous component is present in a sarcoma and, in some cases, a distinction is impossible to make.

The interpretation of *menstrual endometrium* or endometrium with glandular and stromal breakdown in curettings may be difficult, especially in distinguishing it from adenocarcinoma. The absence of stroma between the glandular elements may give the impression of confluent glands or in some cases even of solid epithelial growth. The piled up epithelium may lose nuclear polarity and acquire prominent nucleoli. However, the coarse chromatin and nuclear pleomorphism of malignancy are lacking and a genuine cribriform pattern and invasion are never present. Mitoses are also lacking. Furthermore, the glands of menstrual endometrium regularly exhibit some residual secretory change and a careful search will identify typical areas of stromal fragmentation as opposed to areas of coagulative necrosis (see Chapter 14).

The distinction between endometrial adenocarcinoma and *endocervical adenocarcinoma* may be difficult, if not impossible, to make in curettings. Fractional curettage assists in delimiting the site of involvement, but surface extension along the lower uterine segment may occur. Even though most endometrial carcinomas are of endometrioid type and most endocervical carcinomas are of mucinous type, endometrioid carcinomas may arise in the cervix and mucinous adenocarcinomas not uncommonly arise in the endometrium. The stroma of the tumor may also help; in cervical adenocarcinomas it is typically fibrous whereas endometrial carcinomas usually contain very little stroma. An immunostain panel of three markers can be used in the differential diagnosis. ER and vimentin are more likely to be expressed in endometrial than cervical adenocarcinomas, whereas cervical adenocarcinomas more frequently show strong immunoreactivity for p16.[84,85] In endometrial adenocarcinomas p16 immunostaining is weak or patchy.[86] Reactivity for integrated human papillomavirus (HPV) in DNA isolated from tumor tissue strongly supports a cervical origin, as it is present in 80–90% of cervical, and essentially no endometrial, adenocarcinomas.[87] Tissue processing and HPV polymerase chain reaction testing for this purpose are not generally available, however.

The term 'papillary carcinoma' is imprecise and should not be used for endometrial tumors. Villoglandular endometrioid adenocarcinoma, serous carcinoma, clear cell adenocarcinoma, and mucinous adenocarcinoma may all have a papillary architecture. Villoglandular endometrioid adenocarcinoma shows the columnar and darkly staining cells characteristic of endometrioid carcinoma. Nuclear grade is usually low. The cells of serous carcinoma tend to be small and cuboidal rather than columnar, and nuclear atypia is marked. Indeed, an immediately obvious discrepancy between high-grade nuclear changes in an apparently well-differentiated adenocarcinoma (irrespective of growth pattern) should alert the pathologist to the possibility of a serous carcinoma (see below). Clear cell adenocarcinomas rarely show papillary areas exclusively. Usually tubulocystic areas with a 'hobnail' pattern or solid areas of clear cells are frequently present. The morphology of the epithelial cells in mucinous adenocarcinoma, with regular, basal nuclei and abundant, mucinous cytoplasm allows the distinction to be made easily.

Behavior and Treatment

Endometrioid adenocarcinoma and its variants present early as postmenopausal bleeding, which is both obvious and alarming. Eighty percent of patients present with clinical stage 1 disease, although some patients are found to have more advanced disease at surgery. Five year survival rates are currently 96% for stage 1 disease, 67% for stage 2, and 23%

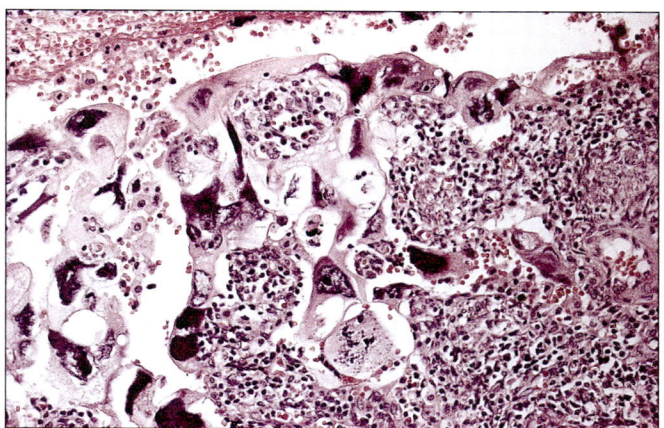

Figure 18.47 Endometrial adenocarcinoma. Appearance following radiation.

for stage 3.[1] The behavior of the endometrioid histologic variants is the same, grade for grade, as that of typical endometrioid adenocarcinoma.[88]

The standard treatment is surgical, consisting of hysterectomy with bilateral salpingo-oophorectomy, with or without adjuvant radiotherapy. Practices vary regionally regarding pelvic and para-aortic lymph node dissection. It is doubtful whether lymphadenectomy has any added benefit in the patient whose primary lesion is well differentiated and superficially invasive.[89,90] Lymph node dissections are commonly carried out, however, if frozen section of the hysterectomy specimen demonstrates deep myometrial invasion, cervical involvement, or a non-endometrioid histology. Local delivery of high-dose progestins by hormone-impregnated intrauterine devices may be effective in controlling well-differentiated local disease with a low rate of systemic complications.[91] Systemic treatment with progestins may be beneficial but, as the tumors that respond are those with ER and PRs that are of early stage and low grade with a favorable outcome anyway, practical use of these agents is limited.[92] Chemotherapy and adjuvant radiotherapy are used for advanced and recurrent disease.[93,94]

Appearances Following Radiation

Curetted specimens may be received following radiation therapy for endometrial carcinoma. Currently, however, this is an infrequent event since radiotherapy is predominantly given postoperatively. The tumor's histologic response to radiation varies and sometimes no changes can be detected. Changes may be seen in both neoplastic and non-neoplastic epithelial cells. Most prominent among these are nuclear enlargement, pleomorphism, and hyperchromasia, often resulting in markedly bizarre forms (Figure 18.47). As these alterations are seen in both benign and malignant cells, identifying residual carcinoma can be difficult.

SEROUS CARCINOMA

Serous carcinoma is an aggressive form of endometrial cancer exhibiting a predominantly papillary architecture composed of exfoliative bulbous hobnail-like cells with

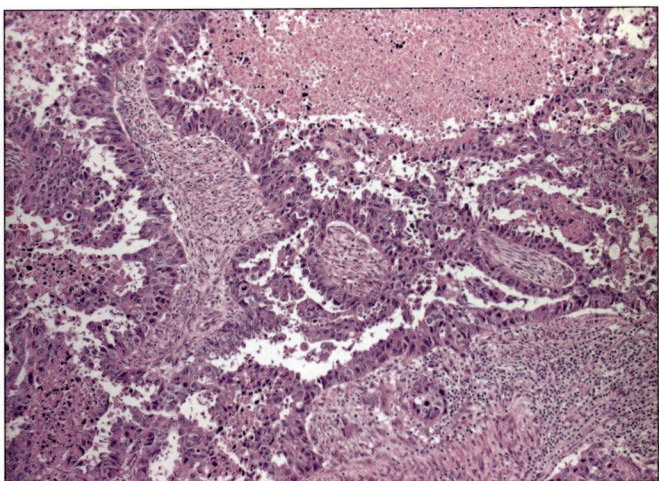

Figure 18.48 Endometrial carcinoma, serous type.

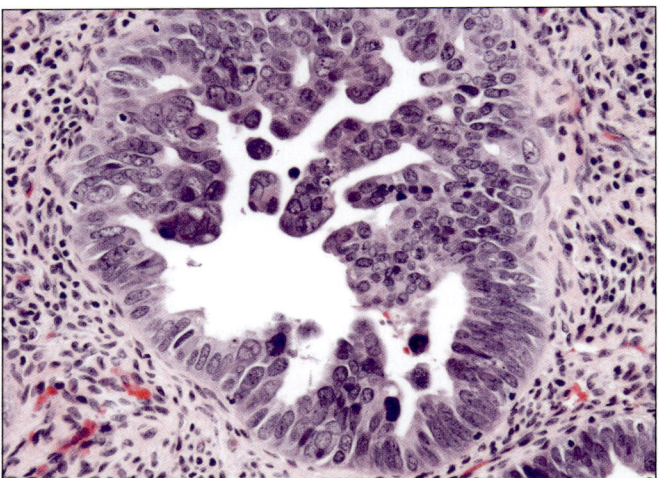

Figure 18.49 Endometrial carcinoma, serous type. High-grade nuclei with exfoliation in a 'hobnail' pattern.

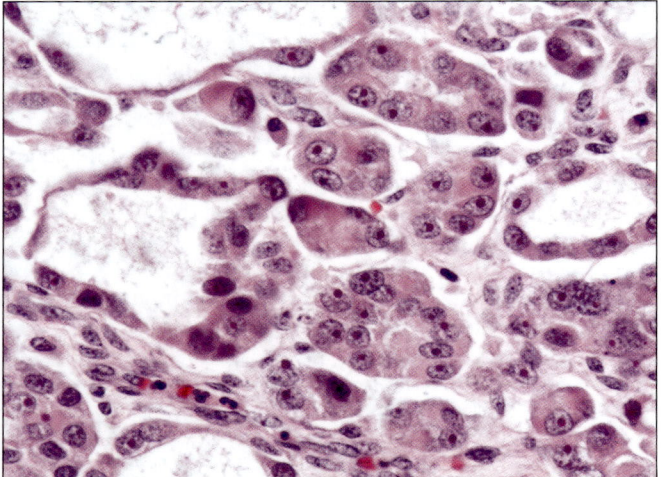

Figure 18.50 Endometrial carcinoma, serous type. Abundant exfoliated cells lie between papillae.

marked nuclear atypia.[5,95] It is the uniformly severe nuclear atypia that distinguishes serous carcinoma from other less aggressive papillary endometrial carcinomas. Therefore, the term 'serous carcinoma' is preferred to 'papillary' serous carcinoma.

Clinical Features

The tumor accounts for 1–10% of all endometrial cancers. It is lower in population-based studies but higher in reports from gynecologic oncology centers.[95] The patients are generally about 4–10 years older than women with endometrioid carcinomas, rarely have received exogenous estrogen therapy, and lack previous or concurrent EIN or AH.[96] Most women are parous (90%). Few are obese (10%) or have diabetes.[97] Typically they have normal serum estrogen levels.[98]

Gross Features

Serous carcinomas generally have the same gross features as endometrioid carcinomas, i.e., exophytic and papillary; however, many tumors appear bulky and necrotic.[8] The uterus is more frequently atrophic as compared with endometrioid carcinomas. Not infrequently the tumor is confined to an endometrial polyp.

Microscopic Features

Histologically, serous carcinomas closely resemble the more common ovarian high-grade serous carcinomas (see Chapter 25). They typically have complex, branching papillae with broad, thick fibrovascular cores, but occasionally thin to delicate cores (Figure 18.48). The papillae are covered by a stratified epithelium with a prominent and very characteristic tufting or budding pattern (Figure 18.49), with many groups of detached cells lying free between the papillae (Figure 18.50). This pattern notwithstanding, serous carcinoma may also show a glandular or solid pattern. Unlike endometrioid adenocarcinoma, the glandular structures are irregularly shaped and often lined by polygonal rather than columnar cells.[95] The tumor cells are often hobnail and contain abundant granular eosinophilic or clear cytoplasm. The nuclei are usually high grade, with marked pleomorphism and large macronucleoli along with occasional bizarre and hyperchromatic giant nuclei. Mitotic figures are numerous and abnormal mitoses are easily identified. Psammoma bodies are found in about 25% of cases (Figure 18.51).[99] A high percentage of cases exhibit striking lymphovascular invasion (Figure 18.52) and deep myometrial invasion.[5] The invasive component can show contiguous downgrowth of papillary processes, or solid masses or glands. Serous endometrial carcinomas also have a higher incidence of cervical and lower uterine segment involvement.[100] The uninvolved endometrium adjacent to serous carcinoma is atrophic in 76% of the cases and hyperplastic in only 5%.[115]

Serous carcinoma of the endometrium may occur in a pure form or associated with other types of endometrial carcinoma, such as endometrioid or clear cell adenocarcinoma.[8,101]

Mixed tumors where at least 25% of the tumor has features of serous differentiation behave as serous cancers and should be treated as such.[95] There is less data and thus some controversy regarding how to manage patients with lesser quantities of admixed serous cancer. In these cases, a clear

CHAPTER 18 — ENDOMETRIAL ADENOCARCINOMA

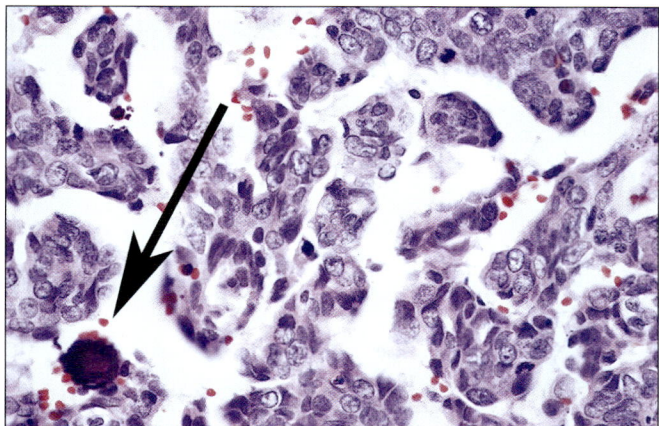

Figure 18.51 Endometrial carcinoma, serous type. A psammoma body (arrow) is present.

indication of the amount of serous component present should be mentioned in the report. Unlike its ovarian counterpart, serous carcinoma of the endometrium is not graded but considered high grade by definition.[102]

Immunohistochemistry

The molecular changes of p53 mutation in 80–90% of serous carcinomas is reflected in p53 immunohistochemistry, which typically shows a diffuse and intense nuclear staining pattern involving almost all tumor cells (Figure 18.53).[8,103] Less frequently, p53 frameshift mutations lead to a truncated protein that is not detected by the antibodies, creating a 'null phenotype' that can be recognized compared to the low level of intermittent staining seen in adjacent normal tissues that serve as an internal positive control for the stain.[103] Ki-67 immunohistochemistry shows a high labeling index (about 40%) in serous carcinoma and ERs and PRs are absent or only weakly expressed in most tumors.[104] The *PTEN* gene is intact, and expressed in normal levels in most serous carcinomas.[105] Strong and diffuse p16 immunoreaction occurs in serous carcinomas without implying HPV infection. Like endometrioid adenocarcinoma, serous carcinoma usually expresses epithelial membrane antigen (EMA), CK7, CA125, Ber EP4, B72.3, and vimentin. WT1 expression occurs infrequently (20% of cases).[106,107]

SEROUS ENDOMETRIAL INTRAEPITHELIAL CARCINOMA (EIC)

In over 90% of cases of serous carcinoma, the surface epithelium adjacent to the carcinoma is replaced by one or several layers of markedly atypical cells lying in the vicinity of atrophic endometrial glands (Figure 18.54). This lesion, which has been designated serous EIC, can extend into the underlying glands without apparent stromal invasion. However, the cells of EIC resemble the cells of the adjacent invasive serous tumor and, like them, show strong nuclear immunoreactivity for p53 (Figure 18.55), high Ki-67 index,

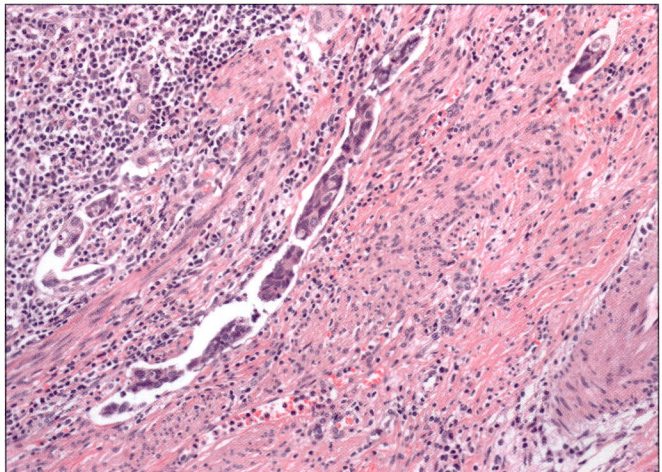

Figure 18.52 Endometrial carcinoma, serous type. Tumor in a myometrial lymphatic.

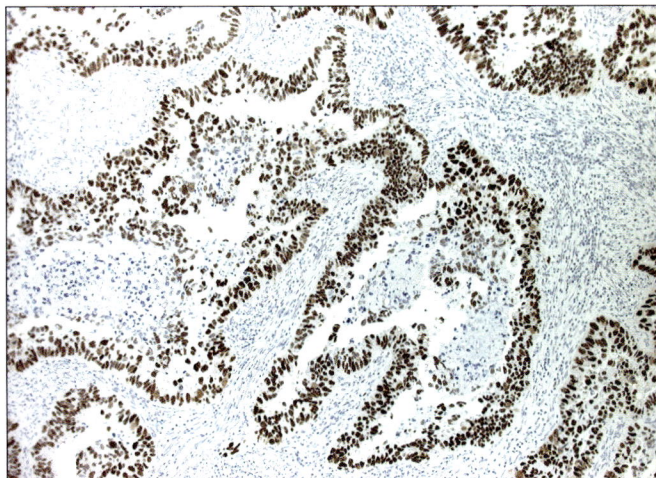

Figure 18.53 Endometrial carcinoma, serous type. Intense nuclear p53 staining of almost all tumor cells indicates clonal p53 mutation.

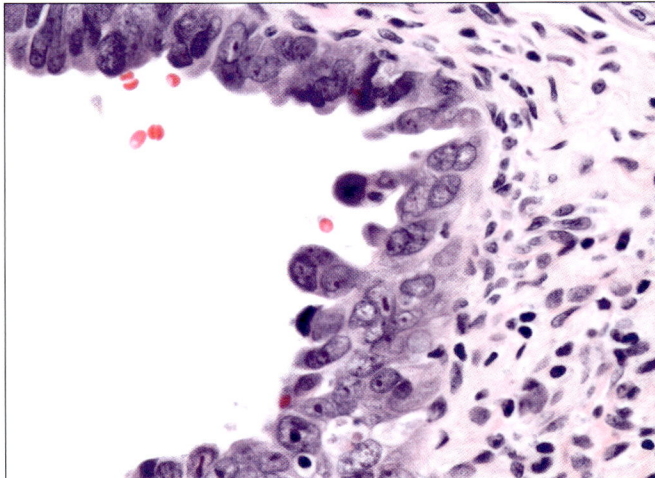

Figure 18.54 Serous EIC. An *in situ*, or surface spreading pattern of serous adenocarcinoma.

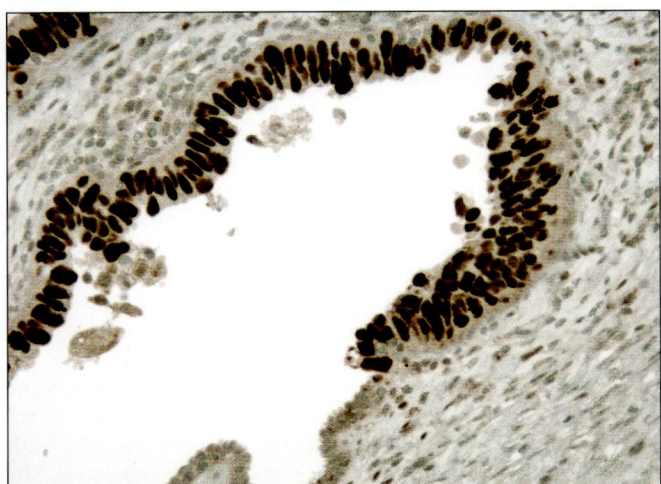

Figure 18.55 Serous EIC. Lesional cells are highlighted on the surface and within overtaken glands by p53 immunohistochemistry.

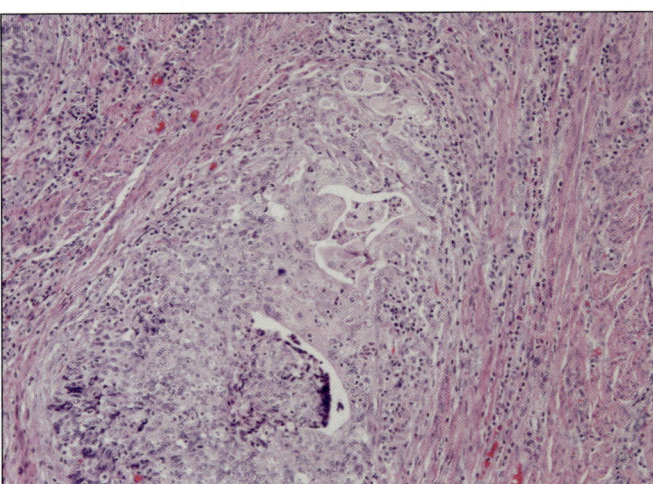

Figure 18.56 Area of invasive poorly differentiated endometrioid carcinoma with separating clefts that resemble serous adenocarcinoma.

and loss of ERs and PRs.[8] Serous EIC may also be observed in association with clear cell adenocarcinoma.[104] Cases of isolated serous EIC without evidence of invasive serous carcinoma are rare, and often confined to endometrial polyps.[108] Extensive serous EIC may cover most of the surface and the glands of the endometrium and, thus, hardly be distinguished from minimally invasive serous carcinoma.

Even in the absence of local uterine myoinvasion, serous EIC has been associated with metastasis in the ovary, peritoneum, or omentum, probably resulting from implantation of exfoliated tumor cells, which pass through the fallopian tube.[109] Thus, serous EIC cannot be considered a precursor lesion but rather an intraepithelial stage of carcinoma capable of spreading to distant sites.

Differential Diagnosis

Serous carcinomas with predominant glandular pattern lacking papillary features can be misinterpreted as high-grade endometrioid carcinoma. However, grade 3 endometrioid carcinoma is almost always solid, not glandular. On the other hand, discohesive solid areas of poorly differentiated endometrioid tumor may develop cleft-like separations that mimic the architecture of serous carcinoma. In these cases, however, the nuclear features help in distinguishing both tumors. The glands and cleft-like fractures in serous carcinoma are lined by cells with high-grade nuclei, often hobnail shaped, whereas the glands in endometrioid carcinoma are lined by columnar cells with grade 1 or 2 nuclei (Figure 18.56). Serous carcinomas almost always (90–95%) have an abnormal p53 immunoreaction, so if this is normal it is unlikely to be serous. Positive p53 staining is not, however, specific for serous cancers, as 40% of poorly differentiated endometrioid carcinomas are p53 abnormal.[110]

Serous carcinoma must be distinguished from its endometrioid counterpart with villoglandular architecture.[79] Architecturally, villoglandular adenocarcinoma exhibits long, convoluted glands usually covered by flat columnar epithelium with pseudostratified nuclei (Figure 18.44), whereas serous carcinoma shows plump papillary excrescences with tufting (Figure 18.49). Nuclear atypia is only mild to moderate in villoglandular endometrioid carcinoma compared to the marked nuclear atypia in serous carcinoma.

Aside from mixed carcinomas, overlap of cellular features exists between serous and clear cell carcinomas.[95] In particular, hobnail-shaped cells, which are characteristic of clear cell carcinoma, may also occur in serous carcinoma but they are usually larger. In contrast to clear cell carcinomas, serous carcinomas lack a tubulocystic or a solid pattern as well as stromal hyalinization and lack a considerable amount of cells with clear cytoplasm. Compared to clear cell carcinomas, serous carcinomas may also show substantial nuclear polymorphism and frequent mitoses. p53 mutation is infrequent (<10%[111]) in clear cell carcinomas compared to (>90%) serous carcinomas.[112]

An artifact that can be confused with serous carcinoma is caused by intracavitary infusion of hypertonic mannitol or electrolyte solutions during uterine hysteroscopy. These nonphysiologic electrolyte solutions can cause exposed epithelia to exfoliate in a hobnail-like manner (Figure 18.57). Hyperchromatic nuclei appear bland and condensed, rather than enlarged with coarse chromatin. Widespread distribution throughout the specimen, along with minimal to absent pleomorphism, is a clue to its benign character.

Behavior and Treatment

The most striking feature of endometrial serous carcinoma is its aggressive behavior leading to a poor overall prognosis. The 5 and 10 year actuarial survival rates for all stages are 36% and 18%, respectively.[113] The 5 year survival for pathologic stage I carcinoma is 40%.[114]

This poor outcome particularly relates to frequent extrauterine disease at the time of diagnosis; 72% of patients whose disease preoperatively appears confined to the uterus already have extrauterine disease found at operation.[97] Even minimal myometrial invasion is frequently associated with widespread disease.[115] Early clinical studies have shown poor outcome for stage I cases, but this may be due in part to incomplete staging procedure.[116] Cancer death may even

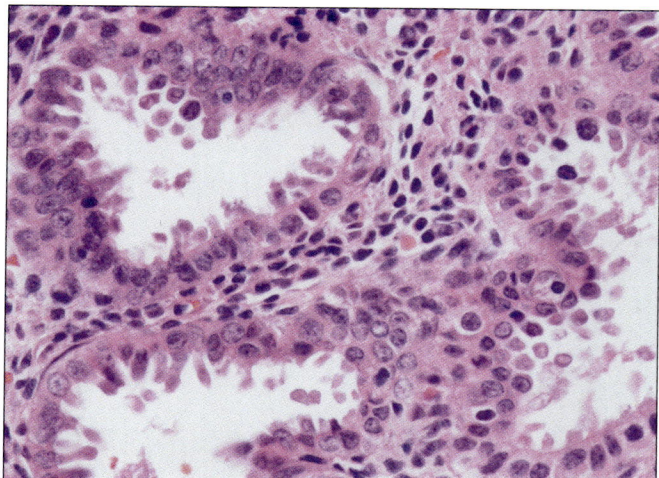

Figure 18.57 Exfoliation artifact induced by exposure to non-isotonic fluids shows nuclear condensation of shed cells that are loosely cohesive.

occur in stage IA disease.[117] Unlike endometrioid carcinomas, grade and depth of myometrial invasion of serous carcinomas are not significant predictors for peritoneal spread of disease. Several studies have demonstrated that serous carcinomas that have not invaded the myometrium can be associated with extrauterine disease or recur after the initial treatment.[104] Most likely, this reflects spread via tubal reflux and subsequent peritoneal carcinomatosis,[118] which is unusual for other forms of endometrial cancer. There is no evidence that endometrial serous carcinoma is a component of a multifocal disease process arising independently in the endometrium, and pelvic and abdominal serosa. On the other hand, spread of serous carcinoma between these sites, including tube and endometrium, has been documented.[119] Not surprisingly, a disproportionately large fraction of patients with relapsed endometrial carcinomas have serous carcinoma. Whereas serous carcinomas constitute less than 10% of endometrial carcinomas, they account for about 50% of treatment failures.[5]

Lymphovascular space invasion, often seen within the myometrium, cervix, parametrium, fallopian tubes, and ovaries, is associated with a high frequency of extrauterine disease. Metastasis to the para-aortic lymph nodes is found in 13% of serous carcinomas confined to the endometrium.[104] Similarly, 6 of 10 serous carcinomas discovered in endometrial polyps with little or no myometrial invasions recurred, and four patients died of disease.[101]

First-line treatment for women with endometrial serous carcinoma is surgery including total abdominal hysterectomy with bilateral salpingo-oophorectomy along with omentectomy and careful surgical staging, including peritoneal cytology and pelvic and para-aortic lymph node sampling. Because this tumor is aggressive, some form of adjunctive therapy is desirable for all tumors except those that qualify as minimal uterine serous carcinoma. In a series of 21 cases with pure serous EIC or minimal serous carcinoma (less than 1 cm of intraendometrial carcinoma) all 14 patients whose tumors lacked myometrial or vascular invasion and who had no evidence of extrauterine disease survived without adjuvant treatment.[118] Patients with early stage disease have a survival advantage, underlining the need for precise staging procedures.[120]

CLEAR CELL ADENOCARCINOMA

Endometrial clear cell carcinoma is similar to those occurring more frequently in the vagina, cervix, and ovary. Its occurrence in the endometrium is evidence of its müllerian derivation.

Clinical Features

Clear cell adenocarcinomas account for 1–6% of endometrial carcinomas and occur at an older age (mean age 65–69 years) than endometrioid adenocarcinoma.[121] The women generally are less often obese, less often have diabetes mellitus, and less frequently have taken hormone replacement therapy.[122] Like all other forms of endometrial cancer, bleeding is the most common initial clinical manifestation.

Gross Features

There are no gross features that distinguish clear cell adenocarcinoma from other varieties of endometrial carcinoma but like serous carcinoma it develops more frequently on a background of an atrophic endometrium.

Microscopic Features

As in other locations along the female genital tract, endometrial clear cell carcinoma may show papillary (Figures 18.58 and 18.59), solid, and tubulocystic (Figure 18.60) patterns. Most clear cell adenocarcinomas have a mixture of at least two of these patterns. The epithelial cells lining the cysts in the tubulocystic areas have discharged their glycogen and have scanty cytoplasm; thus, they show enlarged and pleomorphic nuclei that appear to protrude into the lumens, the hobnail cells (Figure 18.61). Cystic spaces are often lined by flattened cells. However, the most striking feature of the tumor is the clear cytoplasm in many cells (although not necessarily the majority). Nothing in the cytoplasm stains with hematoxylin and eosin (H&E) for the glycogen is leached out during fixation and processing. Mucin, if present, is found only in the lumens of the glands and not in the cell cytoplasm. The stroma may be dense and hyalinized, particularly in tubulocystic areas. The hyalinized stroma is a disorganized type of basement membrane material secreted by tumor cells, which replaces a 'mucoid' material that may persist in some areas (Figure 18.60).[123] Nuclear atypia is often marked and the tumors show a high nuclear grade. Nucleoli are prominent and the frequency of mitotic figures variable. PAS-positive, diastase-resistant intracellular and extracellular hyaline bodies are found in approximately two-thirds of clear cell carcinomas. Clear cell carcinomas are not graded, as all are considered high grade by definition.[102]

Immunohistochemistry

Like endometrioid and serous carcinomas, most clear cell carcinomas express pan-cytokeratins, EMA, CK7, BerEP4, B72.3, CA125, and vimentin, while they are negative for CK20 and WT1. Clear cell carcinomas are typically ER/PR negative and show p53, p16, and Ki-67 expression,

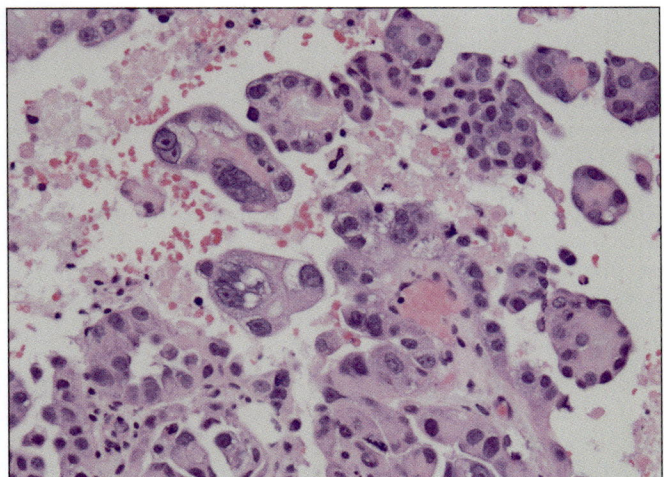

Figure 18.58 Endometrial adenocarcinoma, clear cell type. Papillary pattern with partly hyalinized cores.

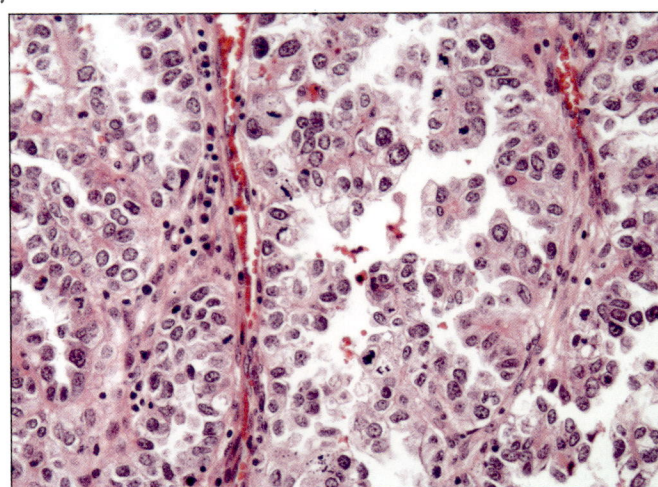

Figure 18.61 Endometrial adenocarcinoma, clear cell type. A papillary area with 'hobnailing.'

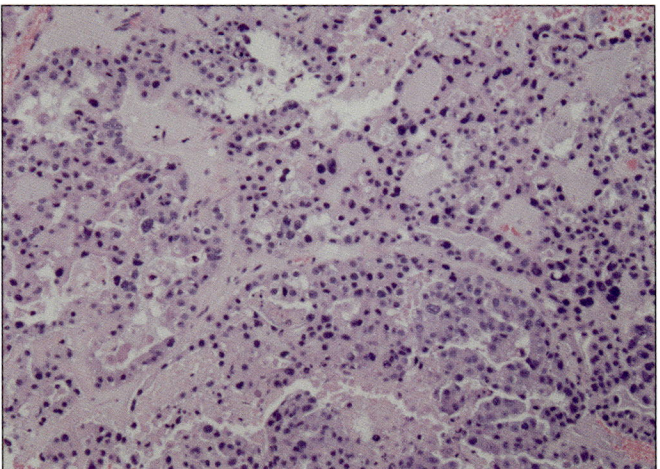

Figure 18.59 Endometrial adenocarcinoma, clear cell type. Glandular pattern.

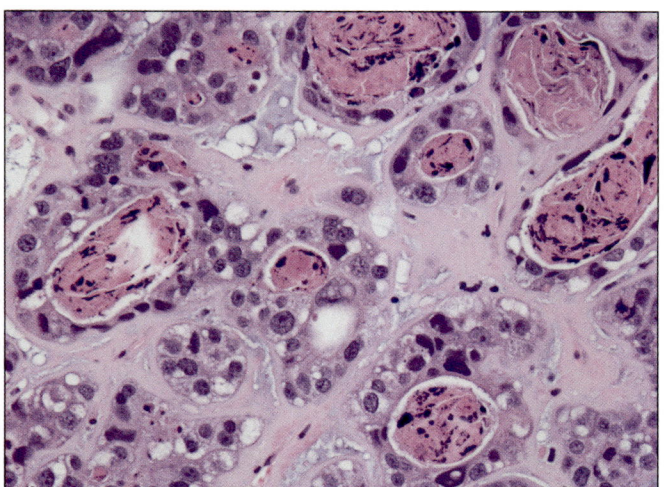

Figure 18.60 Endometrial adenocarcinoma, clear cell type, tubulocystic pattern. Note the hyalinized stroma with 'mucoid' spaces interspersed.

which are intermediate between endometrioid and serous carcinomas.

Rare cases associated with the HNPCC syndrome lack expression of *MSH-2* and *MSH-6*.

Differential Diagnosis

Clear cell adenocarcinoma has to be distinguished particularly from secretory and serous endometrial carcinoma as well as from yolk sac tumor. The differential diagnosis of the secretory carcinoma has been previously discussed. Although clear cell and serous carcinomas share high-grade nuclei and hobnail cells, in contrast to clear cell carcinoma, serous carcinoma is rarely solid and does not show a tubulocystic pattern. It also lacks more than a few cells with clear cytoplasm. However, in cases of mixed serous and clear cell carcinomas there may be overlapping histologic features. Due to their similar clinical behaviors, the distinction between serous and clear cell carcinomas is far less important than the separation of secretory from clear cell carcinomas.

Yolk sac tumors, particularly with clear cytology, are rare in the uterus and exceedingly rare in the endometrium.[124] In contrast to clear cell carcinoma, which typically occurs in postmenopause, the patients are young, in the third or fourth decade. As Schiller–Duval bodies are seen in only a 20% minority of yolk sac tumors, immunoreaction for α-fetoprotein (AFP) or glypican-3 as well elevated serum AFP are helpful diagnostic tools.

Clear cell adenocarcinomas may at times be exceedingly difficult to distinguish from Arias-Stella change in the endometrium (Figure 18.62), but the distinction is critical as therapy differs significantly. While both show bulbous nuclear enlargement, pleomorphism, and hyperchromasia, there is less pleomorphism within flat areas of epithelium in Arias-Stella. Nuclear chromatin is often smudged in Arias-Stella change, whereas the chromatin material in at least some areas in clear cell adenocarcinoma should be crisp. Other signs are often useful. Arias-Stella change is often associated with decidua and in women who are usually young, whereas clear cell adenocarcinoma may show solid areas composed of clear cells and the patients are invariably past menopause.

Behavior and Treatment

Clear cell carcinomas are high-grade, invasive tumors that tend to present at an advanced stage. Like serous carcinomas, clear cell carcinomas are more often associated with deep myometrial invasion, lymphovascular space invasion, and pelvic lymph node metastasis than ordinary endometrioid carcinomas. Thus, the prognosis for women with endometrial clear cell adenocarcinoma is poorer than for endometrioid carcinoma, with 5 and 10 year disease-free survival rates reported as 43–68% and 39% respectively.[115,125] Two-thirds of patients suffer relapses outside the pelvis. Pathologic stage and age are the two most important prognostic factors.[125] Stage I tumors, particularly if confined to an endometrial polyp, are associated with better prognosis.[115] Although treatment is primarily surgical, because of the poor prognosis and high nuclear grade of the tumors, adjuvant therapy is often administered.

MIXED TYPES OF CARCINOMA

An endometrial carcinoma may show a mixture of two or more histologic types within a single endometrial lesion. The term 'mixed carcinoma' is reserved for coexistence of patterns, which individually differ in their natural history or outcome: either endometrioid carcinoma and serous carcinoma, or different subtypes of non-endometrioid histology (e.g., clear cell and serous). Admixtures of histologic variants of endometrioid adenocarcinoma, such as endometrioid carcinoma with squamous differentiation, mucinous carcinoma, or endometrioid carcinoma with variation in solid growth, are not considered mixed carcinomas. If malignant mesenchymal elements are present, a unifying diagnosis of carcinosarcoma should be entertained.

Although arbitrarily chosen, 10% of a minor component is an amount that can readily be recognized and thus a practical and commonly applied guideline for designation as a 'mixed carcinoma.' If a diagnosis of mixed carcinoma is made, the components present should always be specified along with their approximate volume percentage. Mixed endometrioid and serous carcinomas containing at least 25% of a serous component behave as pure serous carcinomas.[95] However, it is unclear how the presence of 10–25% of tumor elements of an unfavorable histologic type affects prognosis.

Because multiple components may not be evenly distributed, accurate diagnosis of mixed carcinomas is prone to sampling error in a biopsy, and potential revision upon availability of the hysterectomy specimen.

CARCINOSARCOMA

Uterine carcinosarcomas are epithelial malignancies with a malignant mesenchymal component that may include homologous or heterologous sarcomatous elements (Figures 18.63 and 18.64). Long known as malignant mixed müllerian tumors (MMMT) or sometimes as malignant mixed mesodermal tumors, they were renamed carcinosarcomas by the WHO in 2003 to reflect current understanding that they are primarily epithelial tumors that have developed a mesenchymal component mimicking epithelial to mesenchymal transition.[126–128] Evidence suggests that carcinosarcomas share some molecular and epidemiologic risk factors with endometrioid-type endometrial carcinoma, including PTEN mutation,[129] microsatellite instability,[130] obesity, use of exogenous hormones, and nulliparity.[131] Carcinosarcomas, however, may demonstrate an expression profile independent of other forms of endometrial cancer,[132] and have a worse prognosis than other high-grade endometrial carcinomas.[133] Many studies have attempted to document a prognostic effect of the extent or type of heterologous elements, but there is no consistent conclusion.[134] One

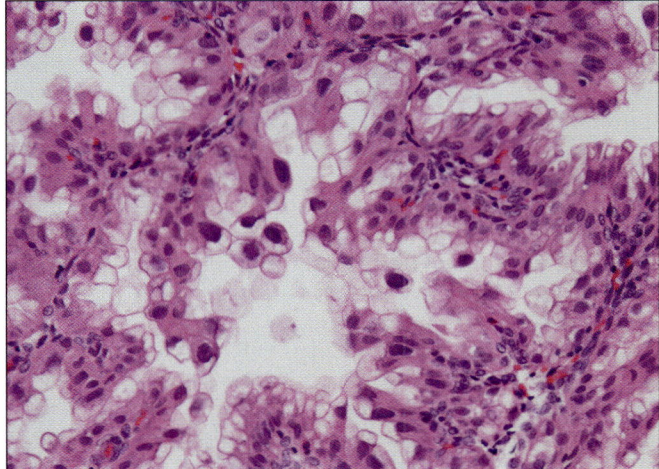

Figure 18.62 Focus of Arias-Stella phenomenon where the cells have pleomorphic, enlarged, and hyperchromatic nuclei that protrude into the glandular lumen, resulting in a 'hobnail' appearance. Non-hobnail cells are less pleomorphic. At times, this change is difficult to distinguish from clear cell adenocarcinoma. Mitoses are extremely rare if not absent.

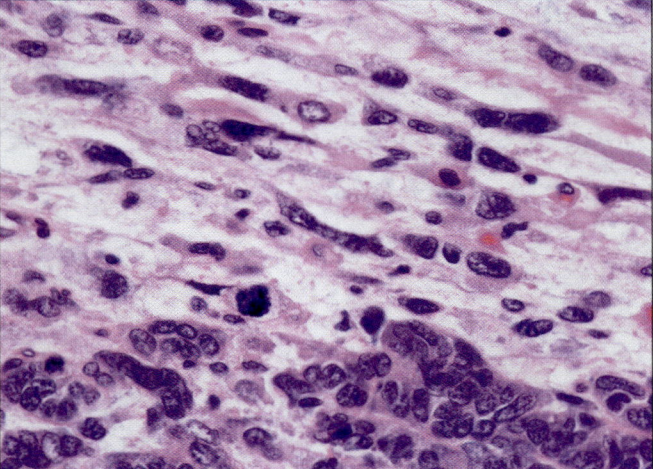

Figure 18.63 Endometrial carcinosarcoma. Nests of high-grade epithelial carcinoma (bottom) are admixed with malignant cells that have undergone sarcomatous transformation (top).

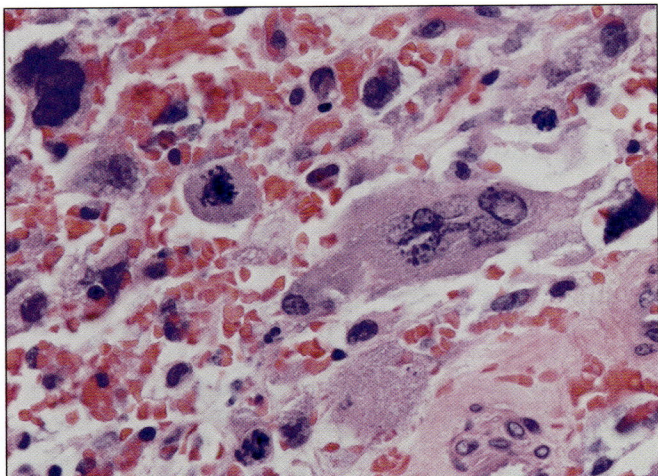

Figure 18.64 Endometrial carcinosarcoma. Sarcomatous elements within endometrial carcinosarcoma demonstrating rhabdoid differentiation.

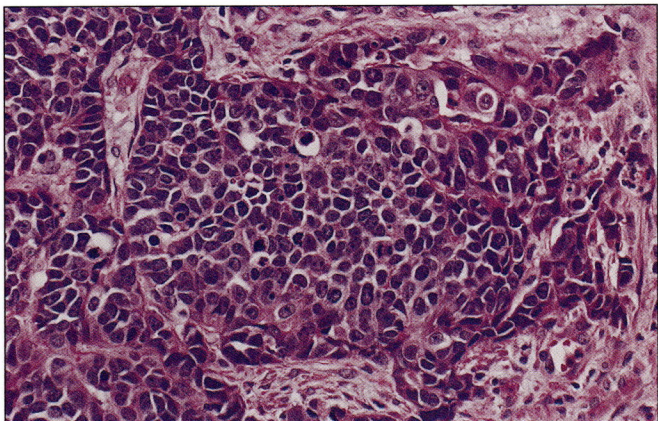

Figure 18.65 Small cell carcinoma.

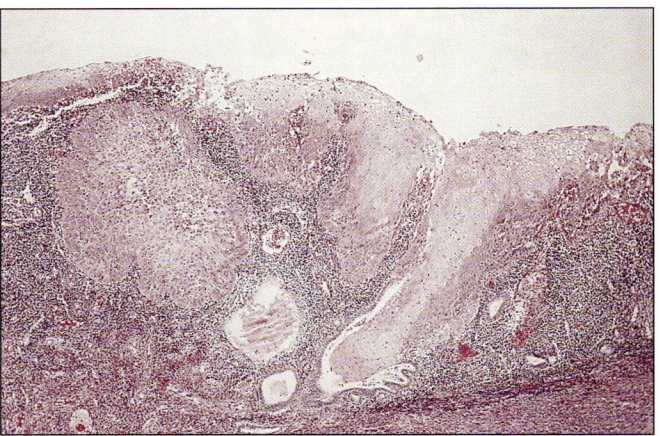

Figure 18.66 Squamous cell carcinoma, arising in a field of squamous metaplasia ('ichthyosis uteri').

recent study suggested that the effect is stage dependent, with the presence of heterologous elements as an adverse indicator in stage 1 disease.[135] Carcinosarcoma is sufficiently distinctive that it might be considered a separate entity of its own rather than a subset within the type 2 class.

OTHER TYPES OF ENDOMETRIAL CARCINOMA

UNDIFFERENTIATED CARCINOMA

This term, while semantically incorrect, is applied, by common usage, to those neoplasms that are demonstrably epithelial in nature but not otherwise differentiated. Less than 2% of endometrial tumors are classified as undifferentiated carcinomas.[88,136] Some of these are of large cell type and may show some attempt at gland formation. These are therefore probably the most anaplastic examples of the tumors described above. The most common tumor considered in the differential diagnosis is grade 3 endometrioid adenocarcinoma with only focal glandular differentiation.

Undifferentiated endometrial carcinomas may contain foci of moderately or well-differentiated endometrioid adenocarcinoma. These tumors have been named 'de-differentiated endometrial carcinoma.'[137] In these neoplasms, the glandular or differentiated components are superficial, whereas the undifferentiated areas are deeper in the endomyometrium and clearly separated the differentiated tumor.

Neuroendocrine carcinomas are classified separately, even though no difference in survival has been shown between large cell and small cell types.[136] In addition to a characteristic neuroendocrine histology, positive staining for a neuroendocrine marker (chromogranin, CD56, synaptophysin) should be seen in 10% or more of the tumor.

Small cell carcinomas (Figure 18.65), both with[138] and without[139] positive neuroendocrine markers, have been reported, some associated with paraneoplastic syndromes.[140] The prognosis is poor.

SQUAMOUS CELL CARCINOMA

Pure squamous cell carcinoma of the endometrium is rare (Figure 18.66). Earlier reports included a high proportion of women who had endometritis and pyometra but this has been less apparent for the last four decades.[141] Many cases are associated with benign squamous metaplasia of the endometrium (ichthyosis uteri; Figure 18.67), a condition encountered only in older women, often in association with intrauterine infection. The diagnosis should be made only if there is no evidence of coexistent adenocarcinoma and if careful examination of the cervix excludes a primary tumor in that organ. Where squamous cell carcinoma is present synchronously in both the uterine body and cervix, the assumption has been that the tumor originated in the cervix and spread upward. More recent views suggest that sometimes the opposite may be true.[142]

The prognosis of squamous cell carcinoma of the endometrium is exceedingly poor,[68] with 26% of reported cases surviving only a median of 9 months after diagnosis.[141] Treatment is primarily by surgery. Adjuvant radiotherapy does not improve survival. The addition of cisplatin-based chemotherapy to postoperative radiotherapy may prolong survival in some patients.[143]

Signet-ring cell carcinoma,[144] *transitional cell carcinoma*,[145] *glassy cell carcinoma*,[146] *mucinous adenocarcinoma of intestinal type*,[73,147] and *lymphoepithelioma-like carcinoma*[148] have also been reported.

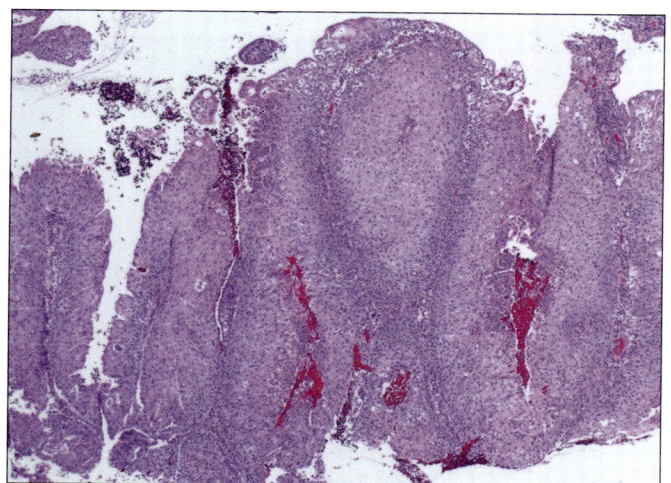

Figure 18.67 Ichthyosis uteri, extensive squamous metaplasia. Most of the endometrium, with the exception of a few basal glandular elements, is replaced by stratified squamous epithelium.

Another rare variant is *endometrial adenocarcinoma with trophoblastic differentiation*.[149] These tumors are poorly differentiated endometrial adenocarcinomas containing syncytiotrophoblast-like giant cells that are reactive for the β-subunit of human chorionic gonadotropin (hCG), some patients also having raised levels of serum β-hCG.[149] The behavior of these tumors is aggressive.

SYNCHRONOUS ENDOMETRIAL AND OVARIAN CARCINOMA

A perplexing problem encountered all too often by the practicing pathologist is to determine whether a tumor involving the endometrium and one or both ovaries has arisen in one organ and metastasized to the other(s) or whether the tumors are independent synchronous primaries.[150] This distinction can be very difficult when the histologies are similar but not exact, or if the tumor in the second organ occurs at a subsequent time. This distinction, however, is of great clinical importance, due to the significantly better prognosis of patients with synchronous primary tumors.[151]

Several histologic features help distinguish primary from metastatic tumors in the endometrium and ovaries.[152] The presence of a precancerous lesion is strong evidence of *in situ* genesis. If the cancer is endometrioid, this would include EIN/AH. Serous carcinomas do not have such a definitive counterpart for this purpose, because the presumed precursor lesion (serous EIC) is closely mimicked by secondary surface spread outward from a main tumor mass. Potentially precancerous processes in the ovary, such as endometriosis or a pre-existing benign or borderline tumor of similar histologic type, suggest *de novo* development of the cancer in the ovary. Disparate histologic types (but not grade) of synchronous endometrial and ovarian tumors are also good evidence of independent primaries. On the other hand, similar histology cannot be taken as evidence of metastasis from one organ to the other. About 15–25% of ovarian tumors with endometrioid histology are associated with a histologically similar lesion in the endometrium. These lesions are usually regarded as well-differentiated independent neoplasms due to their high survival rates.

Multinodular implants on the surface of both ovaries favors metastatic disease rather than an ovarian primary. Synchronous tumors that are regarded as metastases are usually of high histologic grade, e.g., poorly differentiated endometrioid carcinomas, carcinosarcomas, and non-endometrioid carcinomas (serous and clear cell). Metastases from the ovary to the endometrium also occur, and most of these are surface spread of serous cancer via the fallopian tube. In these cases the uterus shows small tumor nodules perched on the superficial endometrium as might be expected of an implant. Such lesions are rare.

While many molecular genetic tests are useful, most lack the specificity needed to distinguish primary tumors from metastases. Conservation of highly specific molecular genetic changes, such as unique point mutations, in tumors occurring at different sites supports metastasis of a single primary tumor.[153] There are, however, two fundamental barriers in applying this in practice: (1) the most commonly performed tests (immunohistochemistry) examine nonspecific protein endpoints without characterizing more specific underlying genetic changes and (2) independent primary tumors may share genetic alterations that are common for a particular histotype. An excellent example is p53 immunohistochemistry of synchronous ovarian and endometrial serous carcinomas. Irrespective of origin, most of these will abnormally accumulate p53 protein in their nuclei. DNA sequencing to characterize underlying mutations as shared or different is required to resolve them as metastatic (unicentric) versus independent (multicentric) carcinomas. Such specialized, and expensive, sequence confirmation of mutations that serve as clonal 'markers' is not routine practice in most pathology departments today. Furthermore, there is the additional complication that metastases may acquire additional changes resulting from tumor progression, thereby diverging from the primary tumor. It must be emphasized, however, that the results of the molecular genetic analyses should always be interpreted in the light of the clinicopathologic findings.

TUMORS METASTATIC TO THE ENDOMETRIUM

The most common tumors that metastasize to the endometrium are those that arise in the pelvis, with cervical and ovarian carcinoma the most frequent. Uterine metastases from extrapelvic sites are distinctly uncommon and only a minority of these affect the endometrium, with most confined to the myometrium. Carcinomas of the breast (particularly lobular carcinoma), colon, stomach, and pancreas are the most frequent tumors to metastasize to the uterus but less common metastases have been reported from kidney, bladder, gallbladder, thyroid, and cutaneous malignant melanoma.

The metastatic tumor in the endometrium frequently has a characteristic appearance that enables the primary tumor to be identified. For instance, lobular carcinoma from the breast often presents a characteristic 'single-cell' pattern. Metastatic signet-ring cell carcinomas of the stomach or

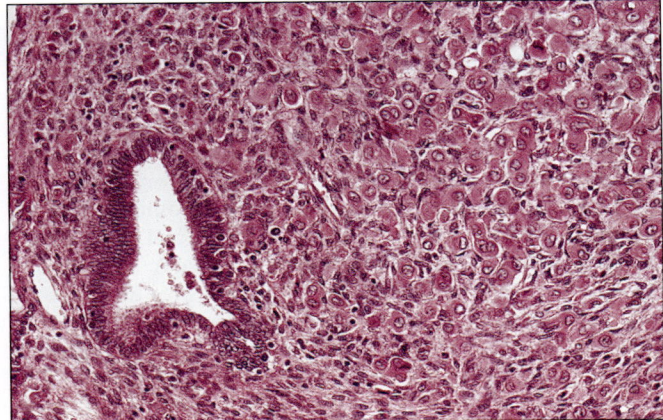

Figure 18.68 Metastatic carcinoma. Tumor cells diffusely permeate the stroma.

colon are equally characteristic. More often, however, the metastatic tumor cells have no diagnostic features and are diffusely distributed through the stroma (Figure 18.68).

PROGNOSTIC FACTORS IN ENDOMETRIAL CARCINOMA

The prognosis in a patient with endometrial carcinoma depends on multiple factors, including histologic type and grade, depth of myometrial invasion, vascular channel involvement, age at diagnosis, and, of course, the tumor stage. Other factors, such as steroid hormone receptor status and genetic and molecular changes, are currently being examined in detail.

HISTOLOGIC TYPE

It is clear from the above descriptions that some histologic types are associated with a better prognosis than others. Endometrioid adenocarcinoma, including its variants of villoglandular adenocarcinoma, secretory carcinoma, mucinous adenocarcinoma, ciliated cell carcinoma, and endometrioid adenocarcinoma with squamous differentiation, are associated with a relatively good prognosis. On the other hand, all non-endometrioid carcinomas, including serous carcinoma, clear cell adenocarcinoma, and undifferentiated carcinoma, have unfavorable outcomes. Pure squamous cell carcinoma of the endometrium also bears a poor prognosis.

HISTOLOGIC GRADE

Histologic grading is clinically prognostic and thus required for all varieties of endometrioid endometrial carcinomas as has been covered in the previous section on endometrioid carcinoma. In contrast, virtually all non-endometrioid endometrial adenocarcinomas including serous, clear cell, and carcinosarcoma subtypes are high-grade tumors associated with aggressive behavior. For this reason, non-endometrioid endometrial carcinomas are not graded.

Table 18.6 Surgical Staging of Carcinoma of the Corpus Uteri (FIGO 2009)[60]

Stage	
Stage I	Tumor confined to the corpus uteri
IA	No or less than half myometrial invasion
IB	More than half myometrial invasion
Stage II	Tumor invades cervical stroma, but does not extend beyond the uterus
Stage III	Local and/or regional spread of the tumor
IIIA	Tumor invades the serosa of the corpus uteri and/or adnexa[a]
IIIB	Vaginal and/or parametrial involvement[a]
IIIC	Metastases to pelvic and/or para-aortic lymph nodes[a]
IIIC1	• Positive pelvic nodes
IIIC2	• Positive para-aortic lymph nodes with or without positive pelvic lymph nodes
Stage IV	Tumor invades bladder and/or bowel mucosa, and/or distant metastases
IVA	Tumor invasion of bladder and/or bowel mucosa
IVB	Distant metastases, including intra-abdominal metastases and/or inguinal lymph nodes

[a]Positive cytology should be reported separately in stage II tumors, without changing the stage.

STAGE AND DEPTH OF MYOMETRIAL INVASION

A critical determinant in the outcome of a woman with endometrial carcinoma is the stage of the tumor at the time of diagnosis.[154] This is true for all tumor types. The staging system most widely used is that of FIGO as revised in 2009,[57] and since adopted by the International Union Against Cancer (UICC).[155]

Several significant changes were made in the 2009 revision (Table 18.6) including:

- *Stage I disease confined to the corpus.* Three tiers of myoinvasion were collapsed to two (1A, 1B), across a 50% myoinvasion threshold.
- *Stage II disease extension to cervix uteri.* Cervical involvement is considered present only when tumor invades into the cervical stroma. Noninvasive intraglandular/surface extension along the cervical canal is not a scored feature.
- *Stage III local and/or regional spread.* Positive peritoneal cytologies are no longer part of the staging system, but should be reported separately. Uterine serosal involvement is stage IIIA. Vaginal and/or parametrial extension is stage IIIB. Lymph node involvement (stage IIIC) is stratified by positive pelvic nodes (IIIC1) and positive para-aortic nodes with or without positive pelvic nodes (stage IIIC2).

Precise histologic assessment of myometrial depth of invasion and cervical stromal involvement is crucial for the staging of early disease in FIGO 2009.

Stage IA tumors are those confined to the uterine corpus with up to 50% depth of myoinvasion. This has improved intraoperative assessments, by increasing accuracy (87%) of assessment across a 50% myoinvasion threshold, compared to that (77%) for any invasive disease.[156] Patients with more than 50% myometrial thickness invasion, those with stage 1B disease, are at increased risk for extrauterine metastases, including pelvic and para-aortic lymph node metastases.

These patients often require more aggressive surgical staging,[157] which may include pelvic and para-aortic lymphadenectomy as well as postoperative adjuvant therapy.

Myoinvasion is measured within the uterine corpus, to the maximum depth from the endometrial–myometrial junction, and reported as a percentage of total myometrial thickness. This is described in detail earlier in the section on endometrioid carcinomas.

Cervical involvement upstages the patient to stage II only when it invades the endocervical stroma. This can be difficult to determine both because of the lack of precise anatomical landmarks delimiting the uterine corpus from the cervix and because of interpretative difficulties in deciding whether the tumor has invaded the stroma or extended to involve endocervical glands only. When present, a desmoplastic stromal response is diagnostic, but this is not always the case in invasive tumors.

Physical displacement of fragmented tumor, either during the surgical procedure or within the pathology laboratory during processing, should not be misinterpreted as tumor spread and a reason to upstage the patient. Detached fragments are commonly squeezed into the fallopian tube lumen or adhere to uterine serosa. Evidence of invasion, encasement of the tumor in reactive exudates, or modeling against the adjacent tissue is all evidence of tumor spread rather than displacement. The introduction of robotic laparoscopic hysterectomy has created new artifacts.[158,159] During these procedures a rigid manipulator is inserted through the cervical os and a high-pressure balloon inflated against the endometrial surface to stabilize the device. The resultant forces can cause deep myometrial fractures perpendicular to the endometrial surface (Figure 18.69), through which extruded tumor fragments enter the myometrium and vessels (Figure 18.70), or fallopian tube.

LYMPHOVASCULAR INVASION

Vascular and lymphatic channel invasion are seen in approximately one-fifth of endometrial carcinomas and the finding correlates significantly with depth of myometrial invasion and histologic grade.[117,160] Patients with lymph node metastasis have a significantly higher incidence of vascular invasion than those without. The presence of vascular invasion has been shown to be an independent indicator for increased risk of recurrence[160] and diminished survival in patients with clinical stage I endometrial adenocarcinoma.[136] Women with stage I endometrial adenocarcinoma who have vascular invasion are candidates for adjuvant therapy.[56]

These statistics belie the considerable difficulty in making a determination of vascular involvement in the individual patient. In addition to the tumor displacement and 'floater' artifacts described previously, myoinvasive tumor retracted from its adjacent stroma can appear to be within a vascular space. Great care must be exercised in determining what true vascular invasion is. We prefer to see several unequivocal foci before diagnosing lymphatic invasion as being present.

AGE

The patient's age at the time of diagnosis is often a critical factor in determining the prognosis of a patient with endometrial carcinoma.[136] Generally, endometrial carcinoma in younger women, particularly before menopause, is associated with a 5 year survival approaching 100%. One study found a 5 year survival of 96% for women aged 40–49 years compared with only 53% for women of 70–79 years.[166] Increasing age is associated with a higher grade and stage of endometrioid tumors, and likelihood of a non-endometrioid type tumor, but this only accounts for part of the difference in survival. An additional factor may be that a relative lack of immunocompetence may be more prevalent in older patients.

STEROID HORMONE RECEPTORS

Essentially all endometrioid carcinomas are reactive for ERs, whereas PR levels depend on the histologic grade of the tumor; well-differentiated carcinomas generally have higher

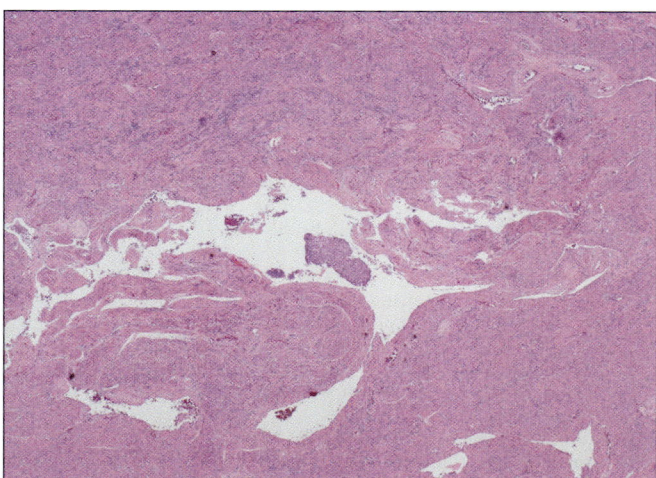

Figure 18.69 Operative myometrial fracture by a robotic manipulator with avulsion of tumor fragments into the artifactual cleft. This well-differentiated carcinoma had no true myoinvasion and was confined to the endometrium.

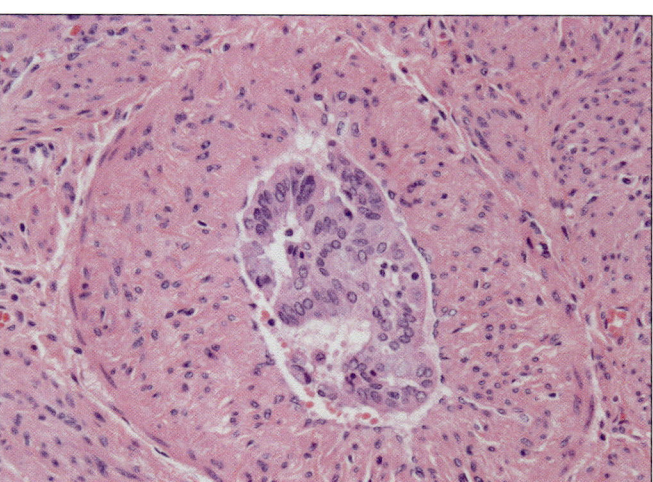

Figure 18.70 Artifactual intravascular extrusion of tumor shards from the myometrial fractures in the same case as in Figure 18.69. The epithelium is torn but not degenerated, and there is no thrombus or adhesion to the endothelial lining.

PR concentrations than poorly differentiated tumors.[110,164] There is some evidence that immunohistochemical determination of PRs may identify an independent predictor of clinical course in patients with endometrioid carcinoma, and receptor studies may prove to be of some value to help determine which patients might or might not be suitable for hormonal therapy.[162] A multitude of recently described ER and PR subtypes has increased the complexity of possible hormonal responses beyond a simple one-hormone, one-receptor model. Relevance of receptor subtypes to disease course and management is not yet completely understood, and is a subject of ongoing investigation.

THE SPREAD OF ENDOMETRIAL CARCINOMA

The most common route of spread, especially for endometrioid tumors, is by direct extension, although sometimes lymphatic spread, especially with high-grade endometrioid and serous tumors, is observed. Endometrial carcinoma spreads initially by invading the myometrium and cervix. Advanced tumors may penetrate fully the myometrium and spread to the adnexa. They may further infiltrate adherent small bowel. Infiltration of the broad ligament, as in cervical carcinoma, also happens occasionally. Lymphatic spread is to the external iliac and internal iliac (hypogastric) lymph nodes and thence to the common iliac and para-aortic groups. If the tumor extends to involve the cervix, the lymphatic spread will be to the internal iliac and obturator lymph nodes as well.

An alternate route of tumor dissemination is by exfoliated carcinoma cells passing retrograde through the fallopian tube and gaining access to the peritoneal cavity. Intra-abdominal spread of serous carcinomas may occur without any myoinvasion at the primary endometrial site.[165] The ovary is involved in 10–15% of advanced cases of endometrial carcinoma. When the ovary contains an appreciable amount of tumor of endometrial pattern, the possibility of a coexistent but separate primary ovarian tumor of endometrioid type must be borne in mind.

Disease distribution at the time of death by disease is similar for endometrioid and non-endometrioid tumor types, with 32% and 40%, respectively, having non-pelvic abdominal disease (liver in 35% of affected cases) and 56% and 51%, respectively, having disease outside the abdomen.[165]

REFERENCES

1. Ries, L, Eisner AG, Kosary MP, et al. SEER cancer statistics review, 1975–2002. Bethesda, MD: National Cancer Institute; 1975.
2. Jemal A, Siegel R, Xu J, Ward E. Cancer statistics, 2010. CA Cancer J Clin 2010;60:277–300.
3. Sherman ME, Carreon JD, Lacey Jr JV, Devesa SS. Impact of hysterectomy on endometrial carcinoma rates in the United States. J Natl Cancer Inst 2005;97:1700–2.
4. Merrill RM. Hysterectomy surveillance in the United States, 1997 through 2005. Med Sci Monit 2008;14:CR24–31.
5. Hendrickson M, Martinez A, Ross J, et al. Uterine papillary serous carcinoma, a highly malignant form of endometrial adenocarcinoma. Am J Surg Pathol 1982;6:93–108.
6. Bokhman J. Two pathogenetic types of endometrial carcinoma. Gynecol Oncol 1983;15:10–17.
7. Lax SF, Kurman RJ. A dualistic model for endometrial carcinogenesis based on immunohistochemical and molecular genetic analyses. Verh Dtsch Ges Pathol 1997;81:228–32.
8. Sherman ME, Bur ME, Kurman RJ. p53 in endometrial cancer and its putative precursors: Evidence for diverse pathways of tumorigenesis. Hum Pathol 1995;26:1268–74.
9. Moreno-Bueno G, Sanchez-Estevez C, Cassia R, et al. Differential gene expression profile in endometrioid and nonendometrioid endometrial carcinoma: STK15 is frequently overexpressed and amplified in nonendometrioid carcinomas. Cancer Res 2003;63:5697–702.
10. Monte NM, Webster KA, Neuberg D, et al. Joint loss of PAX2 and PTEN expression in endometrial precancers and cancer. Cancer Res 2010;70:6225–32.
11. Matias-Guiu X, Prat J. Molecular pathology of endometrial carcinoma. Histopathology 2013;62:111–23.
12. Cheung LW, Hennessy BT, Li J, et al. High frequency of PIK3R1 and PIK3R2 mutations in endometrial cancer elucidates a novel mechanism for regulation of PTEN protein stability. Cancer Discov 2011;1:170–85.
13. Matias-Guiu X, Prat J. Molecular pathology of endometrial cancer. In: Cheng L, Eble JN, editors. Molecular surgical pathology. New York: Springer; 2013.
14. Brinton LA, Hoover RN. Estrogen replacement therapy and endometrial cancer risk: unresolved issues. The Endometrial Cancer Collaborative Group. Obstet Gynecol 1993;81:265–71.
15. Grady D, Gebretsadik T, Kerlikowske K, et al. Hormone replacement therapy and endometrial cancer risk: a meta-analysis. Obstet Gynecol 1995;85:304–13.
16. Pike MC, Peters RK, Cozen W, et al. Estrogen-progestin replacement therapy and endometrial cancer. J Natl Cancer Inst 1997;89:1110–16.
17. Calle EE, Rodriguez C, Walker-Thurmond K, Thun MJ. Overweight, obesity, and mortality from cancer in a prospectively studied cohort of U.S. adults. N Engl J Med 2003;348:1625–38.
18. Reeves GK, Pirie K, Beral V, et al. Cancer incidence and mortality in relation to body mass index in the Million Women Study: cohort study. BMJ 2007;335:1134.
19. Lindemann K, Vatten LJ, Ellstrom-Engh M, Eskild A. Body mass, diabetes and smoking, and endometrial cancer risk: a follow-up study. Br J Cancer 2008;98:1582–5.
20. Adams TD, Stroup AM, Gress RE, et al. Cancer incidence and mortality after gastric bypass surgery. Obesity (Silver Spring) 2009;17:796–802.
21. Ward KK, Shah NR, Saenz CC, et al. Cardiovascular disease is the leading cause of death among endometrial cancer patients. Gynecol Oncol 2012;126:176–9.
22. Schmandt RE, Iglesias DA, Co NN, Lu KH. Understanding obesity and endometrial cancer risk: opportunities for prevention. Am J Obstet Gynecol 2011;205:518–25.
23. Cust AE, Kaaks R, Friedenreich C, et al. Plasma adiponectin levels and endometrial cancer risk in pre- and postmenopausal women. J Clin Endocrinol Metab 2007;92:255–63.
24. Rotterdam ESHRE/ASRM-Sponsored PCOS Consensus Workshop Group. Revised 2003 consensus on diagnostic criteria and long-term health risks related to polycystic ovary syndrome (PCOS). Hum Reprod 2004;19:41–7.
25. Ehrmann DA. Polycystic ovary syndrome. N Engl J Med 2005;352:1223–36.
26. Park JC, Lim SY, Jang TK, et al. Endometrial histology and predictable clinical factors for endometrial disease in women with polycystic ovary syndrome. Clin Exp Reprod Med 2011;38:42–6.
27. Chittenden BG, Fullerton G, Maheshwari A, Bhattacharya S. Polycystic ovary syndrome and the risk of gynaecological cancer: a systematic review. Reprod Biomed Online 2009;19:398–405.
28. Malmstrom H, Hogberg T, Risberg B, Simonsen E. Granulosa cell tumors of the ovary: prognostic factors and outcome. Gynecol Oncol 1994;52:50–5.
29. Watson P, Vasen HFA, Mecklin JP, et al. The risk of endometrial cancer in hereditary nonpolyposis colorectal cancer. Am J Med 1994;96:516–20.
30. Bandera CA, Boyd J. The molecular genetics of endometrial carcinoma. Prog Clin Biol Res 1997;396:185–203.
31. Renkonen-Sinisalo L, Butzow R, Leminen A, et al. Surveillance for endometrial cancer in hereditary nonpolyposis colorectal cancer syndrome. Int J Cancer 2007;120:831–4.

32. Sutter C, Dullenbach-Hellweg G, Schmidt D, et al. Molecular analysis of endometrial hyperplasia in HNPCC-suspicious patients may predict progression to endometrial carcinoma. Am J Pathol 2004;23:18–25.
33. Hutter P, Couturier A, Membrez V, et al. Excess of hMLH1 germ-line mutations in Swiss families with hereditary non-polyposis colorectal cancer. Int J Cancer 1998;78:680–4.
34. Peel DJ, Ziogas A, Fox EA, et al. Characterization of hereditary nonpolyposis colorectal cancer families from a population-based series of cases. J Natl Cancer Inst 2000;92:1517–22.
35. Zhou XP, Kuismanen S, Nystrom-Lahti M, et al. Distinct PTEN mutational spectra in hereditary non-polyposis colon cancer syndrome-related endometrial carcinomas compared to sporadic microsatellite unstable tumors. Hum Mol Genet 2002;11:445–50.
36. Kwon JS, Scott JL, Gilks CB, et al. Testing women with endometrial cancer to detect Lynch syndrome. J Clin Oncol 2011;29:2247–52.
37. Levine DA, Lin O, Barakat RR, et al. Risk of endometrial carcinoma associated with BRCA mutation. Gynecol Oncol 2001;80:395–8.
38. Beiner ME, Finch A, Rosen B, et al. The risk of endometrial cancer in women with BRCA1 and BRCA2 mutations. A prospective study. Gynecol Oncol 2007;104:7–10.
39. Cohen I. Endometrial pathologies associated with postmenopausal tamoxifen treatment. Gynecol Oncol 2004;94:256–66.
40. Bland AE, Calingaert B, Secord AA, et al. Relationship between tamoxifen use and high risk endometrial cancer histologic types. Gynecol Oncol 2009;112:150–4.
41. Hoogendoorn WE, Hollema H, van Boven HH, et al. Prognosis of uterine corpus cancer after tamoxifen treatment for breast cancer. Breast Cancer Res Treat 2008;112:99–108.
42. Chin J, Konje JC, Hickey M. Levonorgestrel intrauterine system for endometrial protection in women with breast cancer on adjuvant tamoxifen. Cochrane Database Syst Rev 2009;CD007245.
43. McPherson CP, Sellers TA, Potter JD, et al. Reproductive factors and risk of endometrial cancer. The Iowa Women's Health Study. Am J Epidemiol 1996;143:1195–202.
44. Schlesselman JJ. Risk of endometrial cancer in relation to use of combined oral contraceptives. A practitioner's guide to meta-analysis. Hum Reprod 1997;12:1851–63.
45. Escobedo LG, Lee NC, Peterson HB, Wingo PA. Infertility-associated endometrial cancer risk may be limited to specific subgroups of infertile women. Obstet Gynecol 1991;77:124–8.
46. La Vecchia C, Franceschi S, Decarli A, et al. Risk factors for endometrial cancer at different ages. J Natl Cancer Inst 1984;73:667–71.
47. Brinton LA, Berman ML, Mortel R, et al. Reproductive, menstrual, and medical risk factors for endometrial cancer: Results from a case-control study. Am J Obstet Gynecol 1992;167:1317–25.
48. Al-Zoughool M, Dossus L, Kaaks R, et al. Risk of endometrial cancer in relationship to cigarette smoking: results from the EPIC study. Int J Cancer 2007;121:2741–7.
49. Austin H, Drews C, Partridge EE. A case-control study of endometrial cancer in relation to cigarette smoking, serum estrogen levels, and alcohol use. Am J Obstet Gynecol 1993;169:1086–91.
50. Daniell HW. More advanced-stage tumors among smokers with endometrial cancer. Am J Clin Pathol 1993;100:439–43.
51. Mutter GL, Baak JPA, Crum CP, et al. Endometrial precancer diagnosis by histopathology, clonal analysis, and computerized morphometry. J Pathol 2000;90:462–9.
52. Schneller JA, Nicastri AD. Intrauterine pregnancy coincident with endometrial carcinoma: a case study and review of the literature. Gynecol Oncol 1994;54:87–90.
53. Horwitz RI, Feinstein AR, Horwitz SM, Robboy SJ. Necropsy diagnosis of endometrial cancer and detection-bias in case/control studies. Lancet 1981;2:66–8.
54. Dijkhuizen FP, Mol BW, Brolmann HA, Heintz AP. The accuracy of endometrial sampling in the diagnosis of patients with endometrial carcinoma and hyperplasia: a meta-analysis. Cancer 2000;89:1765–72.
55. Mariani A, Webb MJ, Keeney GL, et al. Surgical stage I endometrial cancer: predictors of distant failure and death. Gynecol Oncol 2002;87:274–80.
56. Connelly PJ, Alberhasky RC, Christopherson WM. Carcinoma of the endometrium. III. Analysis of 865 cases of adenocarcinoma and adenoacanthoma. Obstet Gynecol 1982;59:569–75.
57. Creasman W. Revised FIGO staging for carcinoma of the endometrium. Int J Gynaecol Obstet 2009;105:109.
58. Zaino RJ, Kurman RJ, Diana KL, Morrow CP. The utility of the revised International Federation of Gynecology and Obstetrics histologic grading of endometrial adenocarcinoma using a defined nuclear grading system: a Gynecologic Oncology Group study. Cancer 1995;75:81–6.
59. Silverberg SG. Problems in the differential diagnosis of endometrial hyperplasia and carcinoma. Mod Pathol 2000;13:309–27.
60. Mutch DG. The new FIGO staging system for cancers of the vulva, cervix, endometrium and sarcomas. Gynecol Oncol 2009;15:325–8.
61. Creasman WT, Odicino F, Maisonneuve P, et al. Carcinoma of the corpus uteri. Int J Gyneol Obstet 2003;83:79–118.
62. Hall JB, Young RH, Nelson Jr JH. The prognostic significance of adenomyosis in endometrial carcinoma. Gynecol Oncol 1984;17:32–40.
63. Quick CM, May T, Horowitz NS, Nucci MR. Low-grade, low-stage endometrioid endometrial adenocarcinoma: a clinicopathologic analysis of 324 cases focusing on frequency and pattern of myoinvasion. Int J Gynecol Pathol 2012;31:337–43.
64. Stewart CJ, Little L. Immunophenotypic features of MELF pattern invasion in endometrial adenocarcinoma: evidence for epithelial-mesenchymal transition. Histopathology 2009;55:91–101.
65. Schorge JO, Hossein SM, Hynan L, Ashfaq R. ThinPrep detection of cervical and endometrial adenocarcinoma: a retrospective cohort study. Cancer 2002;96:338–43.
66. Maksem JA. Performance characteristics of the Indiana University Medical Center endometrial sampler (Tao Brush) in an outpatient office setting, first year's outcomes: recognizing histological patterns in cytology preparations of endometrial brushings. Diagn Cytopathol 2000;22:186–95.
67. Kinde I, Bettegowda C, Wang Y, et al. Evaluation of DNA from the Papanicolaou test to detect ovarian and endometrial cancers. Sci Transl Med 2013;5:167ra4.
68. Silverberg S, Kurman R. Endometrial carcinoma. Tumors of the uterine corpus and gestational trophoblastic disease. Washington, DC: Armed Forces Institute of Pathology; 1991. p. 47–89.
69. Melhem MF, Tobon H. Mucinous adenocarcinoma of the endometrium: a clinico-pathological review of 18 cases. Am J Pathol 1987;6:347–55.
70. Ross JC, Eifel PJ, Cox RS, et al. Primary mucinous adenocarcinoma of the endometrium. A clinicopathologic and histochemical study. Am J Surg Pathol 1983;7:715–29.
71. Dallenbach-Hellweg G, Hahn U. Mucinous and clear cell adenocarcinomas of the endometrium in patients receiving antiestrogens (tamoxifen) and gestagens. Int J Gynecol Pathol 1995;14:7–15.
72. Cheng W, Liu J, Yoshida H, et al. Lineage infidelity of epithelial ovarian cancers is controlled by HOX genes that specify regional identity in the reproductive tract. Nat Med 2005;11:531–7.
73. Zaloudek C, Hayashi GM, Ryan IP, et al. Microglandular adenocarcinoma of the endometrium: a form of mucinous adenocarcinoma that may be confused with microglandular hyperplasia of the cervix. Am J Pathol 1997;16:52–9.
74. Nucci M, Crum CP, Prasad C, Mutter GL. Mucinous endometrial epithelial proliferations: a morphologic spectrum of changes with diverse clinical significance. Mod Path 2000;12:1137–42.
75. Clement PB, Young RH. Endometrioid carcinoma of the uterine corpus: a review of its pathology with emphasis on recent advances and problematic aspects. Adv Anat Pathol 2002;9:145–84.
76. Parra-Herran CE, Monte NM, Mutter GL. Endometrial intraepithelial neoplasia with secretory differentiation: diagnostic features and underlying mechanisms. Mod Pathol 2013.
77. Lax SF, Pizer ES, Ronnett BM, Kurman RJ. Comparison of estrogen and progesterone receptor, Ki-67, and p53 immunoreactivity in uterine endometrioid carcinoma and endometrioid carcinoma with squamous, mucinous, secretory, and ciliated cell differentiation. Hum Pathol 1998;29:924–31.
78. Hendrickson MR, Kempson RL. Ciliated carcinoma–a variant of endometrial adenocarcinoma: a report of 10 cases. Int J Gynecol Pathol 1983;2:1–12.
79. Zaino RJ, Kurman RJ, Brunetto VL, et al. Villoglandular adenocarcinoma of the endometrium: a clinicopathologic study of 61 cases: a gynecologic oncology group study. Am J Surg Pathol 1998;22:1379–85.

80. Eichhorn JH, Young RH, Clement PB. Sertoliform endometrial adenocarcinoma: a study of four cases. Am J Pathol 1996;15:119–26.
81. Ohishi Y, Kaku T, Kobayashi H, et al. CD10 immunostaining distinguishes atypical polypoid adenomyofibroma (atypical polypoid adenomyoma) from endometrial carcinoma invading the myometrium. Hum Pathol 2008;39:1446–53.
82. Heatley MK. Atypical polypoid adenomyoma: a systematic review of the English literature. Histopathology 2006;48:609–610.
83. Carlson JW, Mutter GL. Endometrial intraepithelial neoplasia is associated with polyps and frequently has metaplastic change. Histopathology 2008;53:325–32.
84. McCluggage WG. Recent advances in immunohistochemistry in gynaecological pathology. Histopathology 2002;40:309–26.
85. Alkushi A, Irving J, Hsu F, et al. Immunoprofile of cervical and endometrial adenocarcinomas using a tissue microarray. Virchows Arch 2003;442:271–7.
86. Ansari-Lari MA, Staebler A, Zaino RJ, et al. Distinction of endocervical and endometrial adenocarcinomas—immunohistochemical p16 expression correlated with human papillomavirus (HPV) DNA detection. Am J Surg Pathol 2004;28:160–7.
87. Moreira MA, Longato-Filho A, Taromaru E, et al. Investigation of human papillomavirus by hybrid capture II in cervical carcinomas including 113 adenocarcinomas and related lesions. Int J Gynecol Cancer 2006;16:586–90.
88. Sherman ME, Silverberg SG. Advances in endometrial pathology. Clin Lab Med 1995;15:517–43.
89. Dowdy SC, Borah BJ, Bakkum-Gamez JN, et al. Prospective assessment of survival, morbidity, and cost associated with lymphadenectomy in low-risk endometrial cancer. Gynecol Oncol 2012;127:5–10.
90. Kitchener H, Swart AM, Qian Q, et al. Efficacy of systematic pelvic lymphadenectomy in endometrial cancer (MRC ASTEC trial): a randomised study. Lancet 2009;373:125–36.
91. Montz FJ, Bristow RE, Bovicelli A, et al. Intrauterine progesterone treatment of early endometrial cancer. Am J Obstet Gynecol 2002;186:651–7.
92. Randall TC, Kurman RJ. Progestin treatment of atypical hyperplasia and well-differentiated carcinoma of the endometrium in women under age 40. Obstet Gynecol Surv 1997;90:434–40.
93. Shaeffer DT, Randall ME. Adjuvant radiotherapy in endometrial carcinoma. Oncologist 2005;10:623–31.
94. Vaidya AP, Littell R, Krasner C, Duska LR. Treatment of uterine papillary serous carcinoma with platinum-based chemotherapy and paclitaxel. Int J Gynecol Cancer 2006;16(Suppl 1):267–72.
95. Sherman ME, Bitterman P, Rosenshein NB, et al. Uterine serous carcinoma. A morphologically diverse neoplasm with unifying clinicopathologic features. Am J Surg Pathol 1992;16:600–10.
96. Hendrickson MR, Longacre TA, Kempson RL. Uterine papillary serous carcinoma revisited. Gynecol Oncol 1994;54:261–3.
97. Goff BA, Kato D, Schmidt RA, et al. Uterine papillary serous carcinoma: patterns of metastatic spread. Gynecol Oncol 1994;54:264–8.
98. Sherman ME, Sturgeon S, Brinton LA, et al. Risk factors and hormone levels in patients with serous and endometrioid uterine carcinomas. Mod Pathol 1997;10:963–8.
99. Demopoulos RI, Genega E, Vamvakas E, et al. Papillary carcinoma of the endometrium: morphometric predictors of survival. Am J Pathol 1996;15:110–18.
100. Longacre TA, Chung MH, Jensen DN, Hendrickson MR. Proposed criteria for the diagnosis of well-differentiated endometrial carcinoma. A diagnostic test for myoinvasion. Am J Surg Pathol 1995;19:371–406.
101. Silva EG, Jenkins R. Serous carcinoma in endometrial polyps. Mod Pathol 1990;3:120–8.
102. Tavassoli FA, Stratton MR. Tumors of the breast and female genital organs. Lyons, France: IARC Press; 2003.
103. Lax SF, Kendall B, Tashiro H, et al. The frequency of p53, K-ras mutations, and microsatellite instability differs in uterine endometrioid and serous carcinoma: evidence of distinct molecular genetic pathways. Cancer 2000;88:814–24.
104. Lax SF, Pizer ES, Ronnett BM, Kurman RJ. Clear cell carcinoma of the endometrium is characterized by a distinctive profile of p53, Ki-67, estrogen, and progesterone receptor expression. Hum Pathol 1998;29:551–8.
105. Darvishian F, Hummer AJ, Thaler HT, et al. Serous endometrial cancers that mimic endometrioid adenocarcinomas: a clinicopathologic and immunohistochemical study of a group of problematic cases. Am J Surg Pathol 2004;28:1568–78.
106. Acs G, Pasha T, Zhang PJ. WT1 is differentially expressed in serous, endometrioid, clear cell, and mucinous carcinomas of the peritoneum, fallopian tube, ovary, and endometrium. Int J Gynecol Pathol 2004;23:110–18.
107. Goldstein NS, Uzieblo A. WT1 immunoreactivity in uterine papillary serous carcinomas is different from ovarian serous carcinomas. Am J Clin Pathol 2002;117:541–5.
108. Zheng W, Khurana R, Farahmand S, et al. p53 immunostaining as a significant adjunct diagnostic method for uterine surface carcinoma: precursor of uterine papillary serous carcinoma. Am J Surg Pathol 1998;22:1463–73.
109. Baergen RN, Warren CD, Isacson C, Ellenson LH. Early uterine serous carcinoma: clonal origin of extrauterine disease. Am J Pathol 2001;20:214–19.
110. Lax SF. Molecular genetic pathways in various types of endometrial carcinoma: from a phenotypical to a molecular-based classification. Virchows Arch 2004;444:213–23.
111. Okuda T, Otsuka J, Sekizawa A, et al. p53 mutations and overexpression affect prognosis of ovarian endometrioid cancer but not clear cell cancer. Gynecol Oncol 2003;88:318–25.
112. An HJ, Logani S, Isacson C, Ellenson LH. Molecular characterization of uterine clear cell carcinoma. Mod Pathol 2004;17:530–7.
113. Abeler VM, Kjorstad KE. Serous papillary carcinoma of the endometrium: a histopathological study of 22 cases. Gynecol Oncol 1990;39:266–71.
114. Carcangiu ML, Chambers JT. Uterine papillary serous carcinoma: a study on 108 cases with emphasis on the prognostic significance of associated endometrioid carcinoma, absence of invasion, and concomitant ovarian carcinoma. Gynecol Oncol 1992;47:298–305.
115. Carcangiu ML, Chambers JT. Early pathologic stage clear cell carcinoma and uterine papillary serous carcinoma of the endometrium: comparison of clinicopathologic features and survival. Int J Gynecol Pathol 1995;14:30–8.
116. Gitsch G, Friedlander ML, Wain GV, Hacker NF. Uterine papillary serous carcinoma: a clinical study. Cancer 1995;75:2239–43.
117. Carcangiu ML, Tan LK, Chambers JT. Stage IA uterine serous carcinoma: a study of 13 cases. Am J Surg Pathol 1997;21:1507–14.
118. Snyder MJ, Bentley R, Robboy SJ. Transtubal spread of serous adenocarcinoma of the endometrium: an underrecognized mechanism of metastasis. Int J Gynecol Pathol 2006;25:155–60.
119. Jarboe EA, Miron A, Carlson JW, et al. Coexisting intraepithelial serous carcinomas of the endometrium and fallopian tube: frequency and potential significance. Int J Gynecol Pathol 2009;28:308–15.
120. Kato DT, Ferry JA, Goodman A, et al. Uterine papillary serous carcinoma (UPSC): a clinicopathologic study of 30 cases. Gynecol Oncol 1995;59:384–9.
121. Abeler VM, Kjorstad KE. Clear cell carcinoma of the endometrium: a histopathological and clinical study of 97 cases. Gynecol Oncol 1991;40:207–17.
122. Kanbour-Shakir A, Tobon H. Primary clear cell carcinoma of the endometrium: a clinicopathologic study of 20 cases. Int J Gynecol Pathol 1991;10:67–78.
123. Kato N, Takeda J, Fukase M, Motoyama T. Hyalinized stroma in clear cell carcinoma of the ovary: how is it formed? Hum Pathol 2012;43:2041–6.
124. Spatz A, Bouron D, Pautier P, et al. Primary yolk sac tumor of the endometrium: a case report and review of the literature. Gynecol Oncol 1998;70:285–8.
125. Abeler VM, Vergote IB, Kjorstad KE, Trope CG. Clear cell carcinoma of the endometrium. Prognosis and metastatic pattern. Cancer 1996;78:1740–7.
126. Fujii H, Yoshida M, Gong ZX, et al. Frequent genetic heterogeneity in the clonal evolution of gynecological carcinosarcoma and its influence on phenotypic diversity. Cancer Res 2000;60:114–20.
127. Silverberg SG, Mutter GL, Kurman RJ, et al. Tumors of the uterine corpus: epithelial tumors and related lesions. In: Tavassoli FA, Stratton MR, editors. WHO classification of tumors: pathology and genetics of tumors of the breast and female genital organs. Lyons, France: IARC Press; 2003. p. 221–32.
128. Castilla MA, Moreno-Bueno G, Romero-Perez L, et al. Micro-RNA signature of the epithelial-mesenchymal transition in endometrial carcinosarcoma. J Pathol 2011;223:72–80.
129. Amant F, de la Rey M, Dorfling CM, et al. PTEN mutations in uterine sarcomas. Gynecol Oncol 2002;85:165–9.

130. Taylor NP, Zighelboim I, Huettner PC, et al. DNA mismatch repair and TP53 defects are early events in uterine carcinosarcoma tumorigenesis. Mod Pathol 2006;19:1333–8.
131. Inthasorn P, Carter J, Valmadre S, et al. Analysis of clinicopathologic factors in malignant mixed Mullerian tumors of the uterine corpus. Int J Gynecol Cancer 2002;12:348–53.
132. Maxwell GL, Chandramouli GV, Dainty L, et al. Microarray analysis of endometrial carcinomas and mixed mullerian tumors reveals distinct gene expression profiles associated with different histologic types of uterine cancer. Clin Cancer Res 2005;11:4056–66.
133. Vaidya AP, Horowitz NS, Oliva E, et al. Uterine malignant mixed mullerian tumors should not be included in studies of endometrial carcinoma. Gynecol Oncol 2006;103:684–7.
134. Lopez-Garcia MA, Palacios J. Pathologic and molecular features of uterine carcinosarcomas. Semin Diagn Pathol 2010;27:274–86.
135. Ferguson SE, Tornos C, Hummer A, et al. Prognostic features of surgical stage I uterine carcinosarcoma. Am J Surg Pathol 2007;31:1653–61.
136. Abeler VM, Kjorstad KE. Endometrial adenocarcinoma in Norway. A study of a total population. Cancer 1991;67:3093–103.
137. Silva EG, Deavers MT, Bodurka DC, Malpica A. Association of low-grade endometrioid carcinoma of the uterus and ovary with undifferentiated carcinoma: a new type of dedifferentiated carcinoma? Int J Gynecol Pathol 2006;25:52–8.
138. van Hoeven KH, Hudock JA, Woodruff JM, Suhrland MJ. Small cell neuroendocrine carcinoma of the endometrium. Am J Pathol 1995;14:21–9.
139. Huntsman DG, Clement PB, Gilks CB, Scully RE. Small-cell carcinoma of the endometrium. A clinicopathological study of sixteen cases. Am J Surg Pathol 1994;18:364–75.
140. Campo E, Brunier MN, Merino MJ. Small cell carcinoma of the endometrium with associated ocular paraneoplastic syndrome. Cancer 1992;69:2283–8.
141. Kennedy AS, Demars LR, Flannagan LM, Varia MA. Primary squamous cell carcinoma of the endometrium: a first report of adjuvant chemoradiation. Gynecol Oncol 1995;59:117–23.
142. Dalrymple JC, Russell P. Squamous endometrial neoplasia-are Fluhmann's postulates still relevant? Int J Gynecol Cancer 1995;5:421–5.
143. Sorosky JI, Kaminski PF, Kreider J, et al. Endometrial squamous cell carcinoma following whole pelvic radiation therapy: response to carboplatin. Gynecol Oncol 1995;57:426–9.
144. Mooney EE, Robboy SJ, Hammond CB, et al. Signet-ring cell carcinoma of the endometrium: a primary tumor masquerading as a metastasis. Am J Pathol 1997;16:169–72.
145. Fukunaga M, Ushigome S. Transitional cell carcinoma of the endometrium. Histopathology 1998;32:284–6.
146. Hachisuga T, Sugimori H, Kaku T, et al. Glassy cell carcinoma of the endometrium. Gynecol Oncol 1990;36:134–8.
147. McCluggage WG, Roberts N, Bharucha H. Enteric differentiation in endometrial adenocarcinomas: a mucin histochemical study. Int J Gynecol Pathol 1995;14:250–4.
148. Vargas MP, Merino MJ. Lymphoepitheliomalike carcinoma: an unusual variant of endometrial cancer. A report of two cases. Am J Pathol 1998;17:272–6.
149. Bradley CS, Benjamin I, Wheeler JE, Rubin SC. Endometrial adenocarcinoma with trophoblastic differentiation. Gynecol Oncol 1998;69:74–7.
150. Zaino R, Whitney C, Brady MF, et al. Simultaneously detected endometrial and ovarian carcinomas—a prospective clinicopathologic study of 74 cases: a gynecologic oncology group study. Gynecol Oncol 2001;83:355–62.
151. Liu Y, Li J, Jin H, et al. Clinicopathological characteristics of patients with synchronous primary endometrial and ovarian cancers: a review of 43 cases. Oncol Lett 2013;5:267–70.
152. Robboy SJ, Datto MB. Synchronous endometrial and ovarian tumors: metastatic disease or independent primaries? Hum Pathol 2005;36:597–9.
153. Irving JA, Catasus L, Gallardo A, et al. Synchronous endometrioid carcinomas of the uterine corpus and ovary: alterations in the beta-catenin (CTNNB1) pathway are associated with independent primary tumors and favorable prognosis. Hum Pathol 2005;36:605–19.
154. Kato T, Watari H, Endo D, et al. New revised FIGO 2008 staging system for endometrial cancer produces better discrimination in survival compared with the 1988 staging system. J Surg Oncol 2012;106:938–41.
155. Ugaki H, Kimura T, Miyatake T, et al. Intraoperative frozen section assessment of myometrial invasion and histology of endometrial cancer using the revised FIGO staging system. Int J Gynecol Cancer 2011;21:1180–4.
156. Ali A, Black D, Soslow RA. Difficulties in assessing the depth of myometrial invasion in endometrial carcinoma. Am J Pathol 2007;26:115–23.
157. Inoue Y, Obata K, Abe K, et al. The prognostic significance of vascular invasion by endometrial carcinoma. Cancer 1996;78:1447–51.
158. Krizova A, Clarke BA, Bernardini MQ, et al. Histologic artifacts in abdominal, vaginal, laparoscopic, and robotic hysterectomy specimens: a blinded, retrospective review. Am J Surg Pathol 2011;35:115–26.
159. Delair D, Soslow RA, Gardner GJ, et al. Tumoral displacement into fallopian tubes in patients undergoing robotically assisted hysterectomy for newly diagnosed endometrial cancer. Int J Gynecol Pathol 2013;32:188–92.
160. Gal D, Recio FO, Zamurovic D, Tancer ML. Lymphvascular space involvement—a prognostic indicator in endometrial adenocarcinoma. Gynecol Oncol 1991;42:142–5.
161. Satyaswaroop PG, Mortel R. Sex steroid receptors in endometrial carcinoma. Gynecol Oncol 1993;50:278–80.
162. Fukuda K, Mori M, Uchiyama M, et al. Prognostic significance of progesterone receptor immunohistochemistry in endometrial carcinoma. Gynecol Oncol 1998;69:220–5.
163. Kerner H, Sabo E, Friedman M, et al. An immunohistochemical study of estrogen and progesterone receptors in adenocarcinoma of the endometrium and in the adjacent mucosa. Int J Gynecol Cancer 1995;5:275–81.
164. Matias-Guiu X, Catasus L, Bussaglia E, et al. Molecular pathology of endometrial hyperplasia and carcinoma. Hum Pathol 2001;32:569–77.
165. Barlin JN, Wysham WZ, Ferda AM, et al. Location of disease in patients who die from endometrial cancer: a study of 414 patients from a single institution. Int J Gynecol Cancer 2012;22:1527–31.
166. Connelly PJ, Alberhasky RC, Christopherson WM. Carcinoma of the endometrium. III. Analysis of 865 cases of adenocarcinoma and adenoacanthoma. Obstet Gynecol 1982;59:569–575.
167. Ambros RA, Sherman ME, Zahn CM, et al. Endometrial intraepithelial carcinoma: a distinctive lesion specifically associated with tumors displaying serous differentiation. Hum Pathol 1995;26:1260–7.
168. Berchuck A, Boyd J. Molecular basis of endometrial cancer. Cancer 1995;76(Suppl):2034–40.
169. Mutter GL. PTEN, a protean tumor suppressor. Am J Pathol 2001;158:1895–8.
170. Kounelis S, Kapranos N, Kouri E, et al. Immunohistochemical profile of endometrial adenocarcinoma: a study of 61 cases and review of the literature. Mod Pathol 2000;13:379–88.
171. Faquin WC, Fitzgerald JT, Lin MC, et al. Sporadic microsatellite instability is specific to neoplastic and preoplastic endometrial tissues. Am J Clin Pathol 2000;113:576–82.
172. Esteller M, Levine R, Baylin SB, et al. MLH1 promoter hypermethylation is associated with the microsatellite instability phenotype in sporadic endometrial carcinomas. Oncogene 1998;17:2413–17.

19 Uterine Smooth Muscle Tumors

Emanuela D'Angelo, Bradley J. Quade, Jaime Prat

CHAPTER OUTLINE

Introduction	402	Unusual Growth Patterns of Leiomyomas	411
Leiomyoma	402	Diffuse Leiomyomatosis and Myometrial Hypertrophy	411
Variants of Leiomyoma	405	Intravenous Leiomyomatosis	411
Mitotically Active Leiomyoma	405	Benign Metastasizing Leiomyoma	412
Cellular Leiomyoma	405	Disseminated Peritoneal Leiomyomatosis	413
Hemorrhagic Cellular Leiomyoma and Hormone-Induced Changes	406	Leiomyosarcoma	414
Degenerated Leiomyoma	406	Histologic Diagnosis of Leiomyosarcoma	416
Leiomyoma Treated by Interventional Radiology	407	Diagnostic Criteria	417
		Molecular Genetics	418
Leiomyoma with Bizarre Nuclei (So-Called 'Atypical' Leiomyoma)	408	Prognosis and Treatment	419
Epithelioid Leiomyoma	409	Atypical Smooth Muscle Tumors (So-Called Smooth Muscle Tumors of Uncertain Malignant Potential)	420
Myxoid Leiomyoma	410		
Leiomyomas with Heterologous Elements	411		

INTRODUCTION

Smooth muscle tumors of the uterus are very common and the vast majority are benign leiomyomas. In contrast, leiomyosarcomas are rare and constitute only 1.3% of uterine malignancies (Figure 19.1). Nevertheless, leiomyosarcoma is the most frequent malignant mesenchymal tumor of the uterus, accounting for almost 60% of uterine sarcomas.

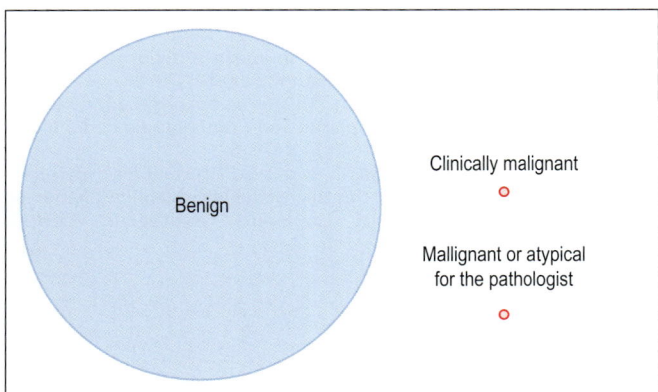

Figure 19.1 Estimated comparative frequency of benign, atypical, and malignant smooth muscle tumors of the uterus.

Whereas almost all leiomyosarcomas are high-grade tumors and their diagnosis is straightforward, a small fraction of uterine smooth muscle tumors show atypical histologic features that are insufficient for the diagnosis of malignancy or have an unpredictable clinical behavior. The term *smooth muscle tumors of uncertain malignant potential* (STUMP) has been used to describe these neoplasms; however, we prefer to call them *atypical smooth muscle tumors* in view of their favorable behavior in most cases. The latter term simply describes the morphologic findings avoiding the words 'uncertain' and 'malignant,' which undoubtedly create unnecessary concern for the patient. A classification of smooth muscle tumors of the uterus is given in Table 19.1.

LEIOMYOMA

Leiomyoma is a benign smooth muscle tumor that most commonly occurs in the uterus, but may also be found in the cervix, uterine ligaments, and, rarely, the ovary or fallopian tube.

Incidence

Leiomyomas are clinically evident in 20–30% of women over 30 years of age,[1,2] rising to more than 40% in those over 40 years old.[3] In a series of 1000 uteri that were serially

> **Table 19.1 Classification of Smooth Muscle Tumors**
>
> Leiomyoma
>   Variants of leiomyoma
>   Mitotically active leiomyoma
>   Cellular leiomyoma
>   Hemorrhagic leiomyoma and hormone-induced changes
>   Leiomyoma with bizarre nuclei (atypical leiomyoma)
>   Epithelioid leiomyoma
>   Myxoid leiomyoma
>   Leiomyomas with heterologous elements
>   Unusual growth patterns
>   Diffuse (intrauterine) leiomyomatosis
>   Intravenous leiomyomatosis
>   Benign metastasizing leiomyoma
>   Disseminated peritoneal leiomyomatosis
> Atypical leiomyoma (smooth muscle tumors of uncertain malignant potential is a term to be discouraged)
> Leiomyosarcoma
>   Variants of leiomyosarcoma
>   Epithelioid leiomyosarcoma
>   Myxoid leiomyosarcoma

examined, over 56% contained leiomyomas.[4] In other studies, 69–77% of women who underwent hysterectomy for non-cancerous conditions were found to have leiomyomas.[5,6] The clinical presentation depends on their size and location.[1] Most are asymptomatic while others present abnormal uterine bleeding, pain, and/or abdominal enlargement.

Leiomyomas are more common in black than in Caucasian women.[6,7] Recently, a higher prevalence for genetic polymorphisms in the estrogen receptor (ER)-α and catechol-O-methyltransferase (an enzyme involved in estrogen metabolism) was observed in black women with leiomyomas, but it is unknown whether these polymorphisms account for the higher tumor incidence in these patients.[8,9] In fact, a number of nuclear receptors are differentially expressed by leiomyomas in black women compared to other ethnic groups.[10]

Like the contribution of race, familial patterns of inheritance also suggest that genetic risk factors are important in the pathogenesis of leiomyomas.[11,12]

Etiology

The precise etiology of leiomyomas is unknown, but the hormonal milieu is pivotal.[13] Recent evidence confirms that estrogens and progesterone receptors (ERs and PRs) are important in their pathogenesis.[14] Studies comparing gene expression in leiomyomas with that in normal myometrium show that leiomyomas maintain a high level of sensitivity to estrogen during the estrogen-dominated proliferative phase of the menstrual cycle.[15] Furthermore, cultured cells from leiomyomas have a significantly higher response to estrogen than do matched cultures of myometrial cells from the same patient, particularly if the tissue is taken for culture in the proliferative phase.[16] Semiquantitative immunohistochemistry for ERs and PRs correlates with tumor growth rate.[17] Accelerated growth, sufficient to require hysterectomy, also occurs in women taking tamoxifen for breast cancer treatment.[18,19]

Further information on the origin of leiomyomas has come from studying their clonality. Originally, glucose-6-phosphate dehydrogenase isoforms were used as a marker for X chromosome inactivation,[20,21] but this has been supplanted by newer molecular biologic techniques that exploit methylation differences between polymorphic loci on the active and inactive X chromosomes.[22–24] These methods confirm that each leiomyoma derives from a single transformation event.[25] Interestingly, these studies also suggest that each tumor is a distinct clone, reinforcing the notion that smooth muscle tumorigenesis is an exceedingly common event.

The genetic mechanisms by which initiation and growth of leiomyomas occur so frequently are not fully understood. Cytogenetic analysis of these benign smooth muscle tumors, however, has revealed important clues.[12] Nearly one-half of leiomyomas have chromosomal rearrangements large enough to be seen in G-banded karyotypes. These chromosomal rearrangements are generally simple, which is in sharp contrast to the aberrations seen in leiomyosarcoma. To date, recurrent aberrations have allowed the definition of seven cytogenetic subgroups: t(12;14)(q14–15;q23–24), del(7)(q22q32), rearrangements of 6p21 and 10q22, trisomy 12, and deletions of 3q and 1p.[12,26] Of these, the translocation between chromosomes 12 and 14 and the rearrangements involving chromosome 6 are perhaps the best understood. Both rearrangements involve genes for two closely related non-histone chromatin proteins: *HMGA1* at 6p21 and *HMGA2* at 12q15.[27–29] Rearrangements involving *HMGA1* and *HMGA2* are also associated with lipomas, endometrial polyps, vulvar aggressive angiomyxoma, and several other benign mesenchymal neoplasms.[30,31] Evidence suggests that inappropriate expression of AT-hook DNA binding domains from *HMGA2* are relevant in uterine leiomyoma.[32,33] Interestingly, rearranged 10q22 disrupts a gene for another class of chromatin protein, namely the histone acetyltransferase *MYST4*, which raises the possibility that chromatin regulation more broadly is important in the pathogenesis of uterine leiomyoma.[34] Beyond such mechanistic insights, cytogenetic studies may also have some practical significance. Tumors with chromosomal rearrangements are on average larger and often within the uterine wall.[35] In addition, some aberrations are associated with specific variants of uterine leiomyomas.

An autosomal dominant syndrome, Reed syndrome[36] (Mendelian Inheritance in Man #150800 and #605839), exhibits a predisposition toward cutaneous and uterine leiomyomas as well as renal cell carcinoma. This syndrome has inactivated fumarate hydratase,[37,38] an enzyme of the Krebs cycle. Germline fumarate hydratase mutations behave like those in classical tumor-suppressor genes. Some non-syndromic (i.e., typical 'garden variety') leiomyomas also have a subset, particularly those from symptomatic younger women, which may have deleted fumarate hydratase.[11,39,40]

Transcriptional profiling has been used to study uterine smooth muscle tumors.[33,41,42] While lists of dysregulated genes produced by various groups overlap to some degree, and while much more study is needed to understand fully the significance of these transcriptional profiles, it seems that the transcriptional profiles for uterine leiomyomas are much closer to myometrium than to leiomyosarcoma and atypical leiomyomas, and that malignant transformation appears to coincide in downregulation of gene expression more frequently than upregulation.[43] Three potential mechanisms proposed to account for differential gene regulation in the smooth muscle transcriptome include: (1) differential expression of non-histone chromatin proteins such as *HMGA2* and *MYST4*; (2) altered expression of tuberin and the glucocorticoid receptor;[10] and (3) abnormal regulation of micro-RNAs, which in turn might regulate *HMGA2*.[44]

Gross Features

Leiomyomas occur anywhere within the myometrium and are multiple in about two-thirds of cases. They also occur occasionally in the cervix (see Chapter 13). The most frequent location is within the myometrial wall where, if numerous or large, they can also grossly distort the uterus (Figure 19.2). Those situated close to the endometrium or the serosa are referred to as submucosal and subserosal, respectively. Submucosal leiomyomas are frequently ulcerated and may lead to intermenstrual bleeding (Figure 19.3). A subserosal, pedunculated leiomyoma may, on rare occasions, lose its connection with the uterus and become attached to another pelvic structure, such as the omentum, bowel, or peritoneum ('parasitic' leiomyoma), which must not be mistaken for a metastasis from a malignant smooth muscle tumor. Leiomyomas are round, firm, and rubbery and they rise above the surrounding myometrium from which they are easily shelled out. The cut surface is typically white to tan, with a whorled, spiral pattern. A striking feature is the very sharp demarcation between it and the surrounding normal myometrium. Several degenerative changes may occur in leiomyomas. Hemorrhage and necrosis are frequent in leiomyomas, particularly if they are large or occur in women who are pregnant or receiving progestogen. Whereas the hemorrhagic areas appear dark, necrotic zones are yellow. Cystic change and calcification also occur.

Microscopic Features

A leiomyoma consists of intersecting bundles of smooth muscle cells. The margins are well circumscribed (Figure 19.4). The smooth muscle cells are markedly elongated and have eosinophilic cytoplasm and tapered, cigar-shaped nuclei. In a typical leiomyoma, the nuclei are uniform and mitotic figures absent or sparse (Figure 19.5).

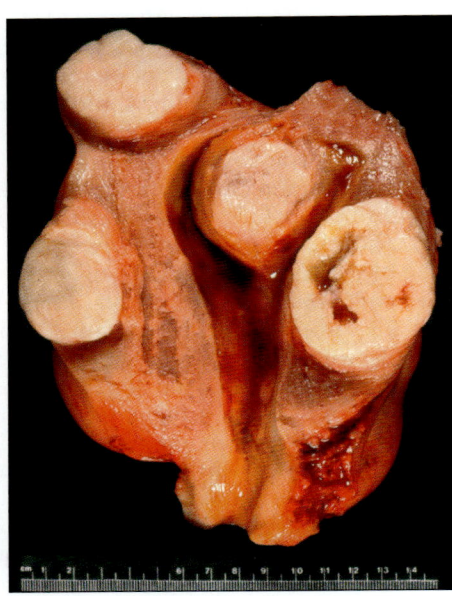

Figure 19.2 Multiple leiomyomas. On cut section, the tumors have a whorled white-tan surface that bulges above the normal myometrium. Three leiomyomas are intramural and one submucosal.

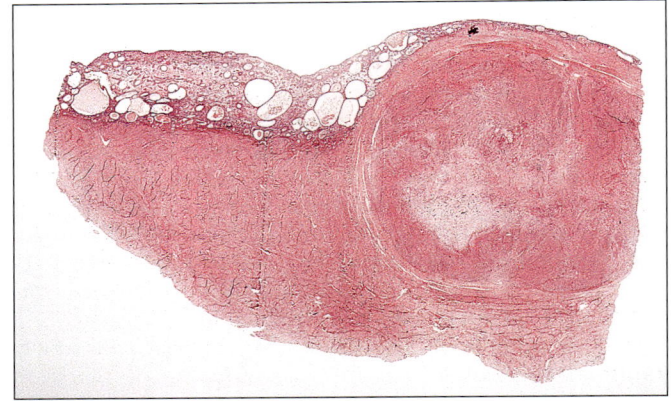

Figure 19.4 Submucosal leiomyoma. At this low magnification the sharp line of demarcation between the leiomyoma and the surrounding myometrium is clearly shown. The overlying endometrium is compressed and atrophic.

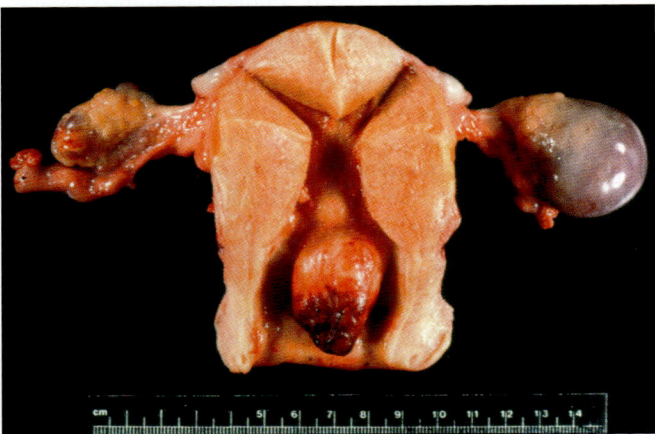

Figure 19.3 Polypoid leiomyoma. A prolapsed submucosal leiomyoma protrudes into the endocervical canal. The vaginal surface of the leiomyoma is hemorrhagic and the cause of bleeding.

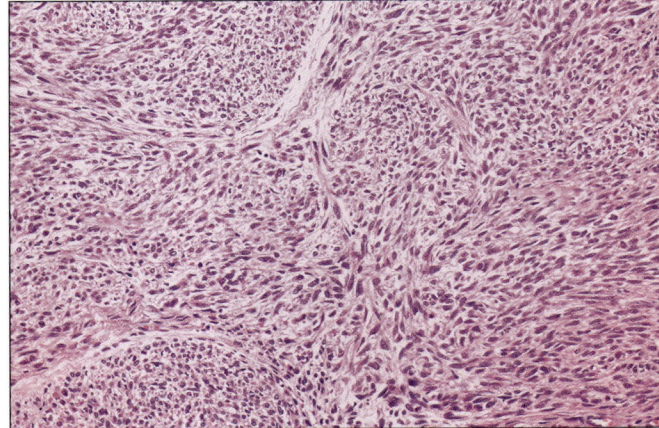

Figure 19.5 Leiomyoma. Intersecting bundles of elongated smooth muscle cells exhibiting eosinophilic cytoplasm and cigar-shaped nuclei. The nuclei are uniform and mitotic figures absent.

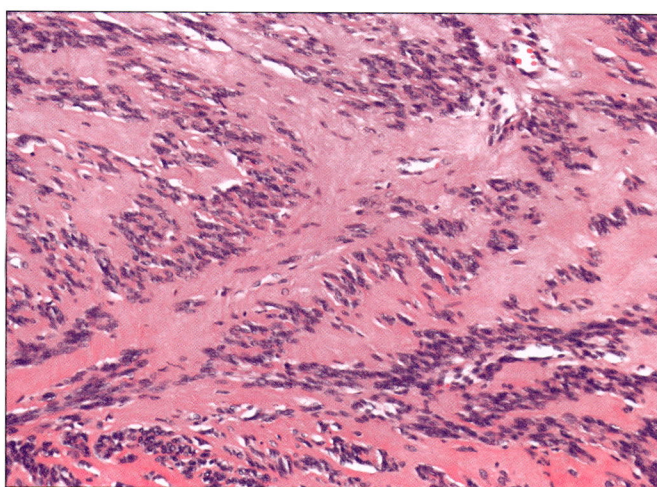

Figure 19.6 Leiomyoma. Nuclear palisading (plexiform tumorlet).

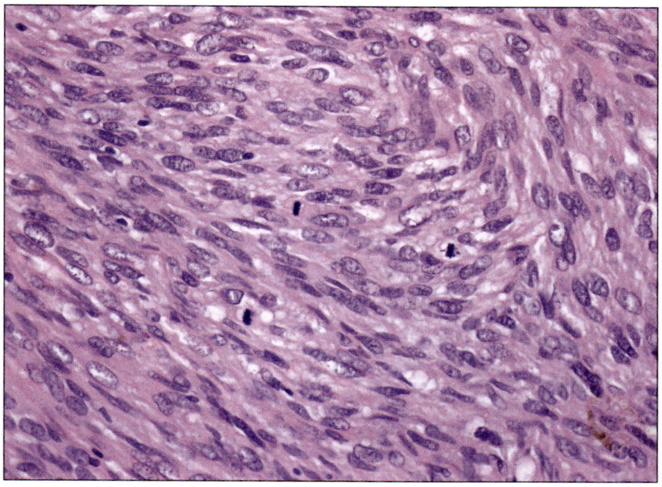

Figure 19.7 Mitotically active leiomyoma. Normal mitotic figures are seen in this otherwise ordinary leiomyoma. Nuclear atypia is lacking.

Abundant reticulin is present. The smooth muscle cells of a leiomyoma are usually more closely packed than those of the surrounding myometrium, so that the tumor usually appears more cellular and the small blood vessels appear compressed and less randomly distributed. Such increased cellularity is often particularly striking in women past menopause. The nuclei in a leiomyoma are generally arranged in a fascicular fashion, but occasionally there is palisading resulting in a pattern similar to that seen in a neurilemmoma (schwannoma) (Figure 19.6).

Marked attenuation of overlying endometrium may be seen in some mucosal leiomyomas (Figure 19.4). By extension, the presence of aglandular functionalis in curettings is a hint that dysfunctional uterine bleeding might be due to a nearby leiomyoma.

Hyaline change is common in leiomyomas, particularly in postmenopausal women, and edema or marked hydropic change is found in half of them. The areas of hemorrhage are usually well circumscribed. Hypercellularity, hemorrhage, edema, and myxoid change occur in leiomyomas in women who are pregnant or taking progestogens. Progestational agents are associated with increased mitotic activity but mitoses appear normal.

VARIANTS OF LEIOMYOMA

MITOTICALLY ACTIVE LEIOMYOMA

In premenopausal women, otherwise typical leiomyomas may occasionally show 5 or more mitotic figures per 10 HPF. These tumors have a benign clinical course (even when treated by myomectomy).[45–47] They are typically small (<10 cm) and have a benign gross appearance. Approximately 60% of mitotically active leiomyomas are submucosal. Microscopically, they have 5–14 mitotic figures per 10 HPF when counted in the most active area. This increased proliferative rate is frequently, but not always, diffusely distributed (Figure 19.7). In submucosal leiomyomas, ulceration, inflammation, or necrosis may be accompanied by a focal increase of proliferation and mitotic activity. Increased

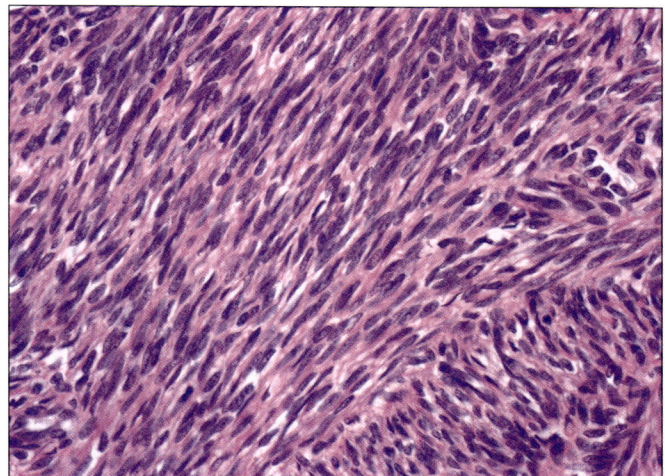

Figure 19.8 Cellular leiomyoma. The nuclear features are the same as those of a typical leiomyoma but the nuclei are more closely packed.

proliferation has also been associated with higher progestin levels, such those seen during the secretory phase.[48] Malignant tumors exhibiting severe nuclear atypia, abnormal mitoses, or geographic necrosis should not be diagnosed as mitotically active leiomyomas.

CELLULAR LEIOMYOMA

A cellular leiomyoma is a benign smooth muscle tumor that has a cellularity greater than the surrounding myometrium and the majority of leiomyomas.[49,50] Grossly, cellular leiomyoma may resemble typical leiomyoma but often has a fleshier and softer sectioned surface and the color tends to be tan or creamy yellow rather than pinkish white. Microscopically, cellular leiomyomas almost always have <5 mitotic figures per 10 HPF and are cytologically bland. A fascicular pattern is present in some areas. The tumor is markedly cellular, and the cells are small and round to spindle shaped (Figure 19.8). The blood vessels are typically large with thick muscular walls and cleft-like spaces are often seen, possibly representing compressed vessels or edema.[50] Unlike the usual leiomyoma, cellular leiomyomas often show focal extensions into and appear to merge with the adjacent myometrium.

Differential Diagnosis

Cellular leiomyomas may resemble endometrial stromal tumors.[50] Helpful features in the differential diagnosis include: (1) coexistence of the highly cellular areas with a fascicular growth pattern typical of smooth muscle tumors; (2) reticulin stains with fibers that tend to parallel the cell bundles in leiomyomas but surround individual tumor cells in endometrial stromal tumors; (3) vessels of large caliber with thick muscular walls, in contrast to the prominent network of small blood vessels typical of endometrial stromal tumors; (4) presence of cleft-like spaces and the absence of foamy histiocytes, which are often present in endometrial stromal tumors; and (5) strong and multifocal or diffuse immunoreactivity for smooth muscle markers such as desmin and h-caldesmon.

In the absence of vascular invasion, the distinction is between two benign lesions, i.e., cellular leiomyoma and endometrial stromal nodule. However, when there is intravascular tumor, the differential is clinically relevant, i.e., intravenous leiomyomatosis versus endometrial stromal sarcoma. In young women wishing to retain their fertility or in older women with high surgical risk, hysteroscopy, imaging studies, or repeat sampling should be considered before hysterectomy.

The cellular leiomyoma must also be distinguished from leiomyosarcoma. The cellular leiomyoma lacks geographic tumor cell necrosis, nuclear atypia, and mitotic activity, all characteristic of leiomyosarcoma.

Cytogenetic Features

The cellular variant may be associated with two chromosomal aberrations: deletion of 1p and rearranged 10q22.[34,51] Whether all cellular leiomyomas have these or related chromosomal aberrations is unknown.

HEMORRHAGIC CELLULAR LEIOMYOMA AND HORMONE-INDUCED CHANGES

Hemorrhagic cellular leiomyoma, or 'apoplectic leiomyoma,' occurs in pregnancy and during treatment with oral contraceptive or gonadotrophin-releasing hormone agonists (GnRHa). Grossly, hemorrhage and cystic change are frequently seen (Figure 19.9).[52,53] Microscopically, the leiomyoma is densely cellular and contains stellate zones of recent hemorrhage. Mitotic activity may be increased (up to 8 mitotic figures per 10 HPF), but there is no atypia and necrosis generally is not present. Vascular changes may be prominent. Leiomyomas treated with GnRHa, to reduce their size prior to their removal, may exhibit the features of apoplectic leiomyomas and vascular changes (i.e., myxoid change, fibrinoid change, mural thickening, luminal narrowing, and thrombosis). Leiomyomas removed several weeks after withdrawal of GnRHa treatment may have increased mitotic activity.[54]

The most striking feature that may be present is geographic (coagulative) necrosis exhibiting nuclear

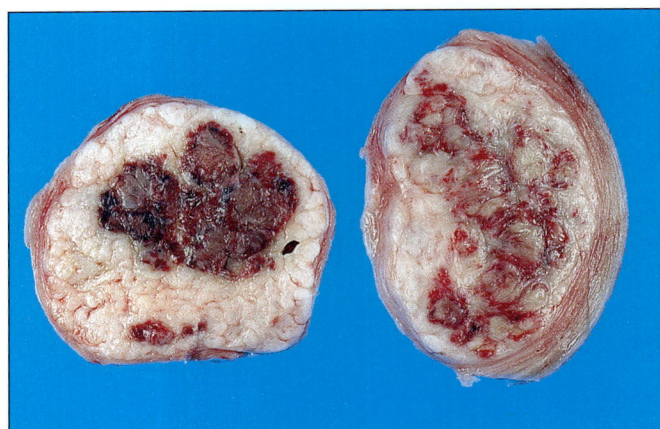

Figure 19.9 After treatment with GnRH agonists, the leiomyoma shows focal areas of hemorrhagic necrosis.

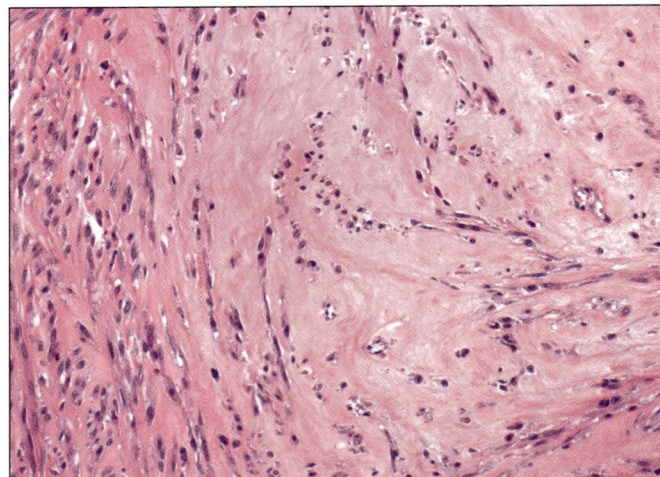

Figure 19.10 Leiomyoma with hyaline change. The tumor shows a uniform, eosinophilic, ground-glass appearance.

pyknosis, karyorrhexis, karyolysis, and markedly increased cytoplasmic eosinophilia.[55] This may affect a small group of cells or extensive areas within the leiomyoma and be surrounded by a rim of inflammatory cells. Apoptosis may be prominent.[56] Changes in cellularity are not significant and both decreased[57] and increased[55] cellularity have been reported. A massive lymphocytic infiltration[58] and thickening of blood vessel walls with narrowing of the lumen may also be seen.[57] A study of cell proliferation indices (Ki-67 and proliferating cell nuclear antigen) suggests that the reduction in size of leiomyomas treated by GnRHa is due to a reduction in the number of cycling cells, presumably secondary to reduced levels of ERs and PRs.[59]

DEGENERATED LEIOMYOMA

A variety of degenerative changes can occur in leiomyomas. By far the most common form of degeneration is *hyaline change* whereby expanded septa have lost their fibrillary structure, assuming a uniform, pale eosinophilic, ground-glass appearance (Figure 19.10). This change may be localized or it may affect extensive areas of the tumor, occasionally even the whole of it. This form of degeneration may be accompanied by surviving muscle cells oriented into lacework patterns. The blood vessels within an area of hyaline necrosis undergo the same change and can be seen as pale outlines, a point of distinction from the geographic tumor cell necrosis seen in leiomyosarcoma where the vessels are often spared.[60] Degenerated areas may liquefy, resulting in *hydropic* or *cystic degeneration*. When extreme, such a degenerated leiomyoma may take on a peculiar multinodular appearance.[61] *Mucoid* and *myxoid degeneration* are also common. In myxoid change, the scattered nuclei are embedded in an amorphous, slightly amphophilic matrix whereas in mucoid degeneration the matrix appears to be mucinous in nature. The mucoid and myxoid forms of degeneration lack practical importance and the two terms are often used interchangeably.

Red degeneration (*necrobiosis*), on the other hand, occurs characteristically but not exclusively in pregnancy and often causes pain and fever. Necrobiosis results in the cut surface taking on a more homogeneous look with loss of the whorled appearance. At the same time, the color becomes a deeper pink or red (due to staining by fresh blood pigment) and the consistency softer (Figure 19.11). Over time, the periphery of a leiomyoma that has undergone red degeneration may become white and calcified. Unlike hyaline change, the microscopic appearance in red degeneration shows the ghosts of the muscle cells and their nuclei. Uncommonly, a leiomyoma may undergo necrosis, resulting in a soft, structureless, pale gray mass. This change is seen most often in submucous leiomyomas that protrude into the endometrial cavity.

Calcific degeneration is seen more frequently in women after the menopause.

Fatty degeneration is rare. In most circumstances fat in a myometrial mass is part of a lipoleiomyoma. In these tumors, the fat is within recognizable adipocytes; in contrast, fatty degeneration discloses the lipid in the smooth muscle cells themselves or in histiocytes.

In general, benign forms of necrosis tend to be unifocal, centrally located, rounded in shape, and relatively uniform in color and consistency of the gross cut surface. The microscopic border exhibits a gradual transition from viable to fully necrotic tumor. Inflammation, granulation, and early hyaline change may be found in these transitional areas. Atypical ghost cells should not be present. Vascular sparing within larger areas of degeneration is unusual. Not infrequently, thrombosis may be seen in the tumor. The overall impression rendered is that of an ongoing or chronic process with a corresponding host reaction. These features are important to recognize and distinguish degenerated leiomyomas from the geographic pattern of necrosis found in leiomyosarcomas.

LEIOMYOMA TREATED BY INTERVENTIONAL RADIOLOGY

Besides conservative medical treatment with GnRH analogs and selective ER modulators (e.g., raloxifene) and less invasive surgical procedures such as laparoscopic or hysteroscopic myomectomy, recent advances in interventional radiology have been made for the management of uterine leiomyomas. In some cases, these techniques are unsuccessful and hysterectomy ensues. As these minimally invasive technologies become more widespread, pathologists often encounter surgical specimens from these cases and need to distinguish treatment effects from other types of degeneration as well as from the tumor cell necrosis frequently found in leiomyosarcomas.

Selective arterial embolization is one such conservative method for treating uterine leiomyomas.[62] The complication most interesting to pathologists is the delay in diagnosis of leiomyosarcoma.[63-65] In about 80–90% of women who underwent embolization, the symptoms improved sufficiently for surgical treatment to be avoided.[62] Gross examination of hysterectomy specimens may sometimes reveal distended small arteries occluded by small aggregates of translucent spheres that might conjure up the notion of a bizarre parasitic infection to the unaware examiner. Such occluded vessels may be found throughout the specimen, and not necessarily in proximity to leiomyomas. Microscopically, a foreign-body giant cell reaction surrounds the amorphous spheroids after the initial period following instillation.[66] The leiomyomas themselves may show various patterns of necrosis, including hyaline, coagulative, and suppurative types, or they may show no apparent change at all.[66]

Another emerging technology for the noninvasive treatment of leiomyoma is ablation by magnetic resonance (MR)-guided focused ultrasound (FUS or MRgFUS).[67] Patients are placed in a specialized MR scanner that has been modified to include a large panel of ultrasound transducers. The ultrasound emissions interfere in a small focus and result in very rapid tissue heating and thermal necrosis, which may grossly mimic the geographic tumor necrosis seen in leiomyosarcoma. One clue that distinguishes this treatment effect from malignant-type geographic tumor necrosis is the firmness of the tissue section. Sudden thermal ablation results in massive protein denaturation, resulting in a hard, unyielding cut surface, whereas necrosis in leiomyosarcomas produces additional softening in tissue. Microscopic inspection of the FUS treatment effect is also notable for the sharp transition from viable to nonviable tissue, at least in the short term following treatment. In contrast to leiomyosarcoma, the necrosis following FUS comprises a remarkably bland eosinophilia typical of thermal denaturation.

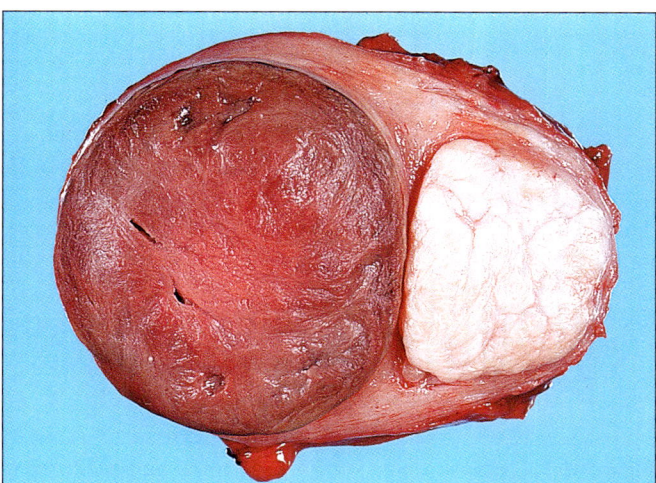

Figure 19.11 Red degeneration (necrobiosis). The cut surface of the leiomyoma on the left is red and more homogeneous, with loss of the whorled appearance.

LEIOMYOMA WITH BIZARRE NUCLEI (SO-CALLED 'ATYPICAL' LEIOMYOMA)

Even if nuclear atypia is necessary for the diagnosis of malignancy in uterine smooth muscle tumors, as an isolated finding, it is insufficient for that purpose. Furthermore, leiomyomas may occasionally show giant cells with pleomorphic nuclei and little or no mitotic activity.[68] The terms 'symplastic leiomyoma,' 'bizarre leiomyoma,' and 'pleomorphic leiomyoma' are older synonyms for leiomyomas exhibiting this striking change in the absence of tumor cell necrosis and abnormal mitotic figures. Most occur during reproductive age (mean age 40.7 years). In a series of 24 cases in which most patients were treated by hysterectomy and a minority by myomectomy, no deaths or recurrences were recorded after a prolonged follow-up, underscoring the benign nature of this histologic variant of leiomyoma.[69,70] In other words, this peculiar type of nuclear atypia differs from that encountered in leiomyosarcomas; it is not 'premalignant' as implied by the term 'atypia' in most precancerous lesions, and should be categorized separately.

Grossly, bizarre tumors may resemble conventional leiomyomas or show yellow or tan areas, hemorrhage, softening, cavitation or myxoid change (Figure 19.12).[69] In contrast with the large size of most leiomyosarcomas, bizarre leiomyomas are usually small (<5.5 cm).

Microscopically, nuclear atypia is easily appreciated at lower magnification (i.e., with 4 or 10× objectives) in most cases. The pleomorphic cells with abundant eosinophilic cytoplasm and atypical nuclei with prominent pseudoinclusions (invaginations of brightly eosinophilic cytoplasm) may appear unifocal, multifocal, or diffusely distributed (Figure 19.13). Many of these cells are multinucleated or have multilobed nuclei, but large hyperchromatic mononuclear cells are also common. Some of the nuclear features are degenerative, including smudged chromatin, vacuolation, karyorrhexis, and pyknosis; however, most tumors also contain cells with ominous nuclear features such as coarsely clumped or granular chromatin with areas of clearing and enlarged nucleoli;[69] yet, in alternate bands of tumor uninvolved by the pleomorphic cells, the spindled smooth muscle cells are uniform and show bland nuclei, as seen in ordinary leiomyomas[69] (Figure 19.13A). This 'zebra-like' pattern helps in the distinction between bizarre leiomyoma and leiomyosarcoma. Mitotic activity in bizarre leiomyomas is usually low. In the series mentioned earlier,[69] the mean mitosis count was only 1.6 mitotic figures per 10 HPF by the highest count method and 0.8 mitotic figures per 10 HPF by the average count method.[69] However, one tumor had up to 7 mitotic figures per 10 HPF.[47,69,70] Most bizarre leiomyomas have 0–4 mitotic figures per 10 HPF. The mitotic figures are only rarely atypical (e.g., multipolarity or extreme polyploidy). Furthermore, these tumors may show degeneration, edema, and hyaline change, with the bizarre cells typically present at the edge of the degenerating areas and around blood vessels (Figure 19.14).

Leiomyomas with bizarre nuclei are distinguished from leiomyosarcomas by an absence of tumor cell necrosis and mitotic counts of <10 mitotic figures per 10 HPFs. A mitotic index higher than 10 mitotic figures per 10 HPF in

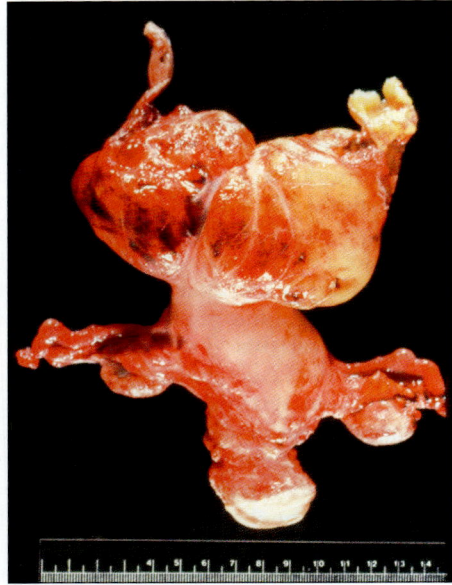

Figure 19.12 Bizarre leiomyoma. The subserosal tumor shows yellow areas and extensive hemorrhage.

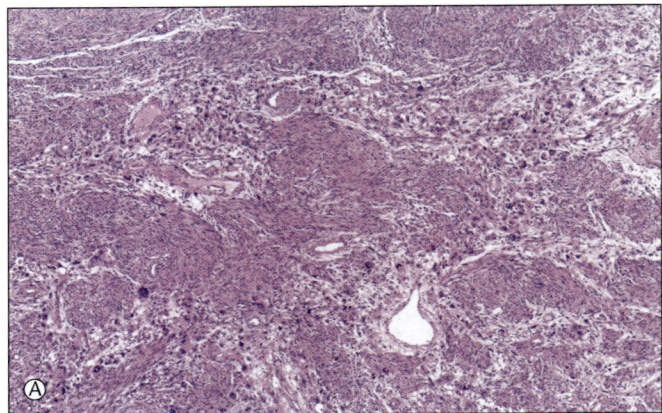

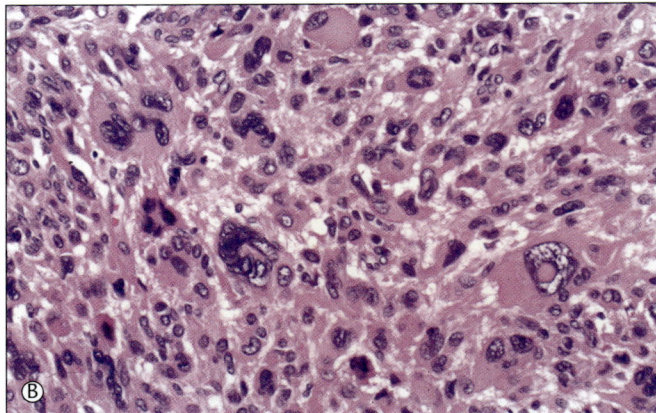

Figure 19.13 Bizarre leiomyoma. **(A)** 'Zebra-like' pattern. Zones of bizarre smooth muscle cells alternate with bands of uninvolved ordinary leiomyoma. **(B)** Cluster of bizarre smooth muscle cells with hyperchromatic and hyperlobated nuclei containing prominent eosinophilic cytoplasmic pseudoinclusions. No mitotic figures are present.

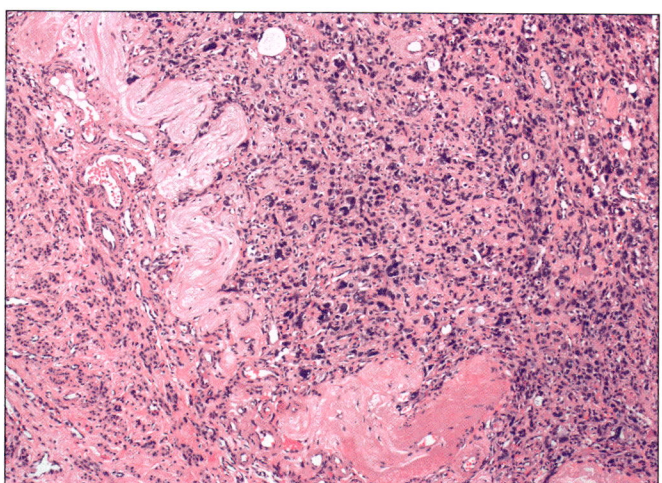

Figure 19.14 Bizarre leiomyoma. The pleomorphic cells are seen in the vicinity of blood vessels.

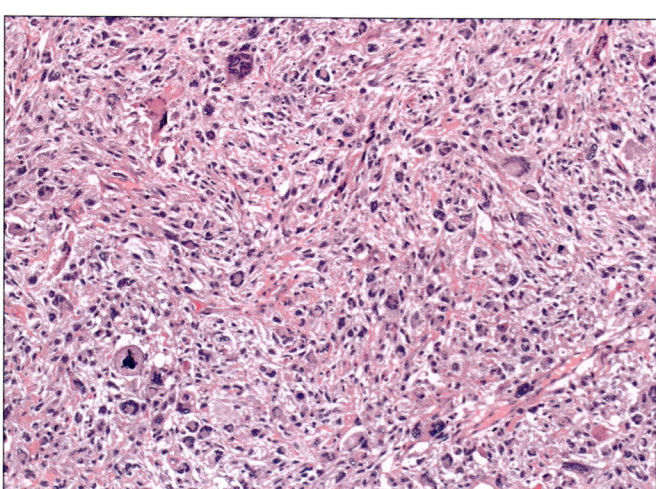

Figure 19.15 Leiomyosarcoma. Focally, this pleomorphic leiomyosarcoma may resemble a bizarre leiomyoma, but the presence of abnormal mitoses is indicative of malignancy.

an atypical uterine smooth muscle tumor is diagnostic of malignancy. However, otherwise clear-cut leiomyosarcomas may contain areas indistinguishable from bizarre leiomyomas. In such cases, the finding of atypical mitotic figures and tumor cell necrosis helps in establishing the correct diagnosis (Figure 19.15).

Unfortunately, in the 2003 World Health Organization (WHO) classification of mesenchymal neoplasms of the uterus, 'leiomyoma with bizarre nuclei' was renamed as 'atypical leiomyoma.' Furthermore, uterine smooth muscle tumors with borderline atypia and mitotic activity were designated as STUMP.[71] This change of terminology has created controversy and is not universally accepted. Whereas the bizarre nuclear changes of leiomyomas are qualitative and readily identified microscopically, the term 'atypical' leiomyoma best describes a smooth muscle tumor exhibiting nuclear atypicality and mitotic activity quantitatively insufficient for the diagnosis of leiomyosarcoma, i.e., STUMP. In fact, we think the term 'atypical smooth muscle tumor' is preferable to STUMP because it avoids the word 'malignant,' does not imply uncertainty, and does not cause unnecessary concern to patients.

Immunohistochemical and Cytogenetic Features

Most bizarre leiomyomas are immunoreactive for p16 (86.5%) and approximately 60% immunoreact for p53. Nearly half of these tumors show over 10% of cells positive for Ki-67. Thus, because of significant overlapping staining patterns between leiomyosarcoma and bizarre leiomyoma, immunoreactions for p16, p53, and Ki-67 have a limited role in distinguishing these two tumors.[72]

Nearly half of bizarre leiomyomas show loss of heterozygosity for loci on the short arm of chromosome 1, suggesting that they might harbor a tumor suppressor gene for atypical smooth muscle tumors on 1p.[51] Interestingly, the expression profiles of bizarre leiomyomas with 1p more closely resemble that of leiomyosarcomas than the profiles of myometrium and leiomyomas of the usual histologic type.[51]

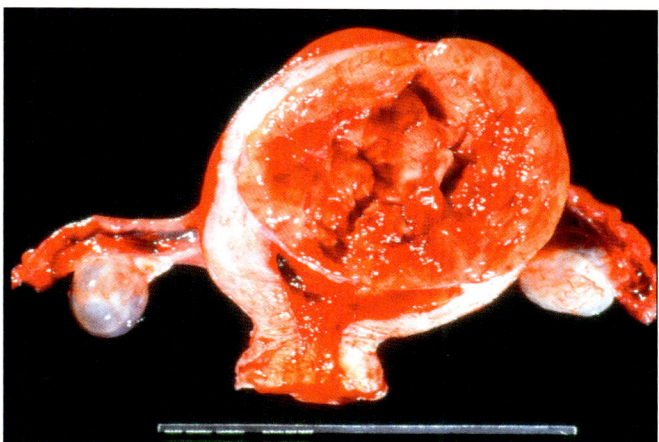

Figure 19.16 Epithelioid leiomyoma. Compared to the ordinary leiomyoma, the tumor appears fleshy and shows yellow and hemorrhagic areas.

EPITHELIOID LEIOMYOMA

Epithelioid leiomyomas are composed of rounded or polygonal cells rather than the usual spindle-shaped cells of ordinary leiomyomas. They are also known as leiomyoblastomas, clear cell leiomyomas, or plexiform leiomyomas.[73–75]

Grossly, these tumors may resemble typical leiomyomas or appear fleshy due to their high cellularity. They may be softer and more yellow than the ordinary non-epithelioid type leiomyoma (Figure 19.16). The average diameter is 6–7 cm. The tumor cells are usually arranged in nests or cords, and show abundant cytoplasm, rounded nuclei with finely stippled chromatin, and a single nucleolus (Figure 19.17). *Leiomyoblastomas* contain rounded cells with ample eosinophilic cytoplasm (Figure 19.18). The cells in *clear cell leiomyomas* are polygonal and have abundant clear cytoplasm, which may contain glycogen (Figure 19.19).

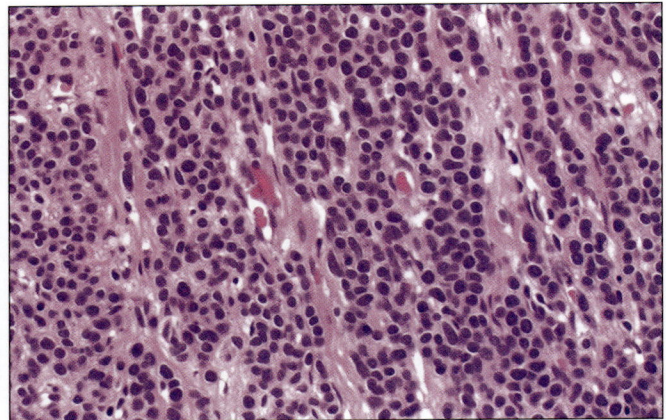

Figure 19.17 Epithelioid leiomyoma. The tumor cells are arranged in nests or cords and show abundant cytoplasm, rounded nuclei with finely stippled chromatin, and a single nucleolus.

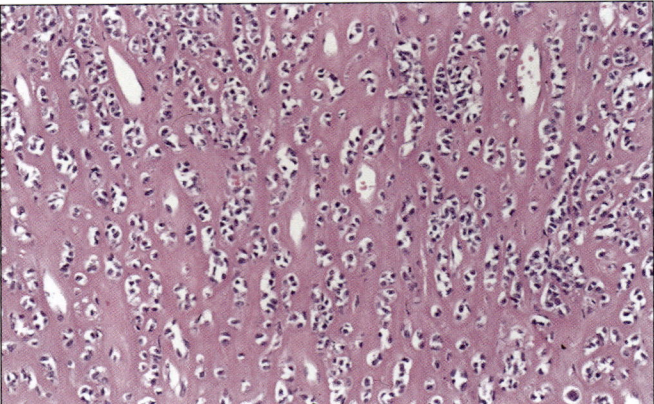

Figure 19.19 Epithelioid leiomyoma, clear cell type. Polygonal cells with abundant clear cytoplasm in a hyalinized stromal background.

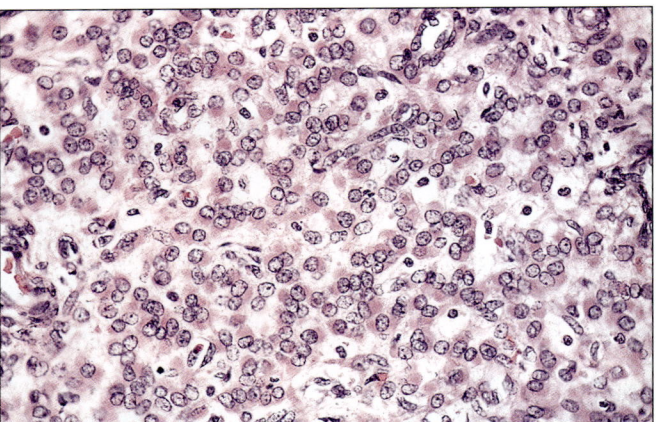

Figure 19.18 Epithelioid leiomyoma, leiomyoblastoma type. The tumor is composed of uniform, round cells with eosinophilic cytoplasm.

Sometimes the nucleus is eccentric, resulting in a signet-ring appearance. *Plexiform leiomyomas* show cords or nests of rounded cells with scanty to moderate amounts of cytoplasm. These tumors may appear as multiple, microscopic foci, which have been referred to as 'plexiform tumorlets.' The histologic phenotype of plexiform tumors may be more a result of abundant elaboration of extracellular matrix material than of epithelioid differentiation. A transition to more typical spindled smooth muscle cells is frequently seen within an epithelioid leiomyoma and mixtures of the various patterns are common.

The smooth muscle nature of these variants of epithelioid leiomyoma has been confirmed by immunohistochemistry and electron microscopy.[73] Ultrastructural studies have revealed features of smooth muscle differentiation such as parallel cytoplasmic filaments, dense bodies, and basal lamina.

Because of the rarity of epithelioid smooth muscle tumors, criteria predictive of their malignant behavior are less well established than those for spindle-cell smooth muscle tumors.[72] In an old study of 26 cases, small size, expansile margin, presence of clear cytoplasm, extensive hyalinization, and lack of tumor cell necrosis were parameters associated with a favorable prognosis; in contrast, larger tumors (>6 cm) that exhibited >5 mitotic figures per 10 HPF were designated as epithelioid leiomyosarcomas based on their metastatic potential.[75] Intermediate tumors with moderate to severe atypia, without necrosis, and <5 mitotic figures per 10 HPF should be classified as atypical or borderline leiomyomas (so-called STUMPs) and patients should be followed.[76] In summary, extensive epithelioid differentiation of a uterine smooth muscle tumor is a disturbing finding because the absence of nuclear atypia and tumor cell necrosis does not warrant a favorable behavior when the tumor contains 5 mitotic figures per 10 HPF.[77] However, the risk of recurrence is probably low. Epithelioid leiomyomas should be distinguished from carcinomas, especially those composed of eosinophilic or clear cells, PEComas, placental site trophoblastic tumors (PSTTs) or epithelioid trophoblastic tumors (ETTs), and low-grade endometrial stromal sarcomas. Desmin immunoreactivity; absence of the characteristic features of PEComa, PSTT, and ETT; and lack of vascular space invasion typically found in low-grade endometrial stromal sarcoma facilitate the correct diagnosis.

MYXOID LEIOMYOMA

Myxoid leiomyoma is a benign smooth muscle tumor with extensive myxoid change that may occur during pregnancy.[78,79] Grossly, it resembles an extrauterine myxoma. Microscopically, it shows well-defined borders and contains abundant, acellular, pale-staining material rich in acid mucins that stain with Alcian blue or colloidal iron. The tumor cells may be elongated or stellate in shape and are widely separated by the extracellular material. Cytologic features are bland and mitotic figures are rare. In curettage specimens, distinction between myxoid leiomyoma and myxoid leiomyosarcoma may be difficult. Non-myxoid portions of the leiomyoma may be erroneously interpreted as evidence of myometrial invasion. In an unpublished study,[78] a mitotic index of <2 mitotic figures per 10 HPF in the absence of tumor cell necrosis or severe cytologic atypia favored the diagnosis of myxoid leiomyoma. However, large myxoid smooth muscle tumors and those with an infiltrating margin, exhibiting moderate to severe nuclear atypia, with or without necrosis and any mitotic index, should be regarded as myxoid leiomyosarcomas.

LEIOMYOMAS WITH HETEROLOGOUS ELEMENTS

The most common heterologous element in a well-circumscribed leiomyoma-like uterine mass consists of endometrial glands and stroma.[80] This is termed an *adenomyoma*, but it is not clear whether the lesion represents focal adenomyosis with reactive smooth muscle proliferation or a truly neoplastic leiomyoma with benign heterologous elements.

Grossly, adenomyomas may be less well circumscribed than typical leiomyomas and punctate hemorrhagic foci may be recognized.[80] When this mass protrudes into the uterine cavity it is best referred to as an adenomyomatous polyp, to avoid confusion with the atypical polypoid adenomyoma (see Chapter 20). Otherwise typical leiomyomas may rarely contain other more exotic mature heterologous elements. Of these, the most common is the *lipoleiomyoma* (Figures 19.20 and 19.21).[81] In this tumor, the lipid is present within adipocytes, which distinguishes it from the very rare fatty degenerate leiomyoma where the lipid resides within the degenerating smooth muscle cells themselves or in histiocytes. The tumor should also be distinguished from the even rarer lipoma and liposarcoma of the uterus, although the latter may not occur as a primary tumor in the uterus.[82] If a vascular component is also present, it is designated as an angiolipoleiomyoma. As noted elsewhere, dysregulated *HMGA2* may be found in cutaneous lipoma and uterine leiomyoma and lipoleiomyoma.[83]

Examples of *osseous*, *chondroid*,[84] and *skeletal muscle*[85] *metaplasia* have also been reported. A *sex cord-like pattern* has been described in a single case of disseminated peritoneal leiomyomatosis.[86] Sex cord-like differentiation also occurs in uterine leiomyomas; however, when extensive, a variant of endometrial stromal tumor should be considered, i.e., the so-called 'uterine tumor resembling ovarian sex cord tumor' (UTROSCT).[87]

UNUSUAL GROWTH PATTERNS OF LEIOMYOMAS

Leiomyomas may have a number of special and unusual growth patterns: diffuse leiomyomatosis, intravenous leiomyomatosis, benign metastasizing leiomyoma, and disseminated peritoneal leiomyomatosis. Although of considerable biologic interest, their rarity precludes a lengthy discussion.

DIFFUSE LEIOMYOMATOSIS AND MYOMETRIAL HYPERTROPHY

Diffuse leiomyomatosis is a rare condition characterized by symmetrical uterine enlargement due to innumerable small smooth muscle nodules.[88,89] The uterus is enlarged, weighing up to 1 kg.[90] The nodules range from microscopic to 3 cm in diameter. They are composed of uniform, cytologically bland, mitotically inactive, spindled smooth muscle cells and are less circumscribed than typical leiomyomas. Differential diagnosis includes rare cases of uterine involvement by lymphangioleiomyomatosis, usually in patients with tuberous sclerosis (autosomal dominant disorder; facial angiofibromas, retinal hamartomas, and renal angiomyolipomas).[91] In such cases, the myometrium is grossly normal but contains numerous microscopic ill-defined nodules of smooth muscle surrounding lymphatics and protruding into their lumens. Typically, there is involvement of lung and lymph nodes. The smooth muscle cells of lymphangiomyomatosis are immunoreactive for HMB-45.[91] In diffuse leiomyomatosis, leiomyomas of the usual type may also be present. Recently, a case of diffuse uterine leiomyomatosis, complicated by uterine rupture and 'benign' lytic bone metastasis during pregnancy, has been reported.[92] In myometrial hypertrophy, the myometrium is thickened and the uterus is also symmetrically enlarged. However, no specific gross or microscopic abnormality is found; the only abnormality is the uterine size. The upper normal weight of the uterus is 130 g for nulliparous women and between 210 and 250 g for parous women.

INTRAVENOUS LEIOMYOMATOSIS

Intravenous leiomyomatosis is a rare condition in which masses of benign-appearing smooth muscle are found within venous channels. If the invasion is of microscopic proportion only and confined to the limits of a leiomyoma,

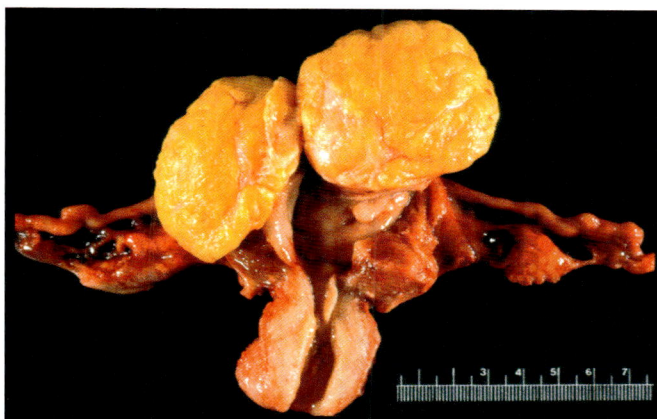

Figure 19.20 Lipoleiomyoma. Depending on the fat content, these leiomyomas are seen grossly as yellow, well-circumscribed, intramural masses.

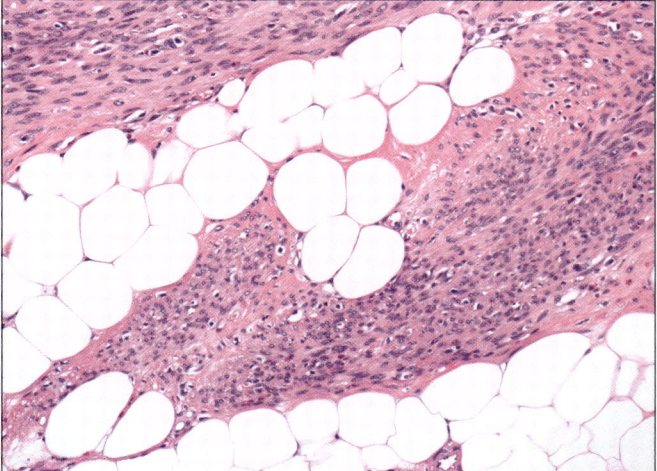

Figure 19.21 Lipoleiomyoma. Few adipocytes appear scattered throughout the smooth muscle.

then the term 'leiomyoma with vascular invasion' is used and the lesion is of no consequence. In contrast, the intravascular growth in intravenous leiomyomatosis extends outside the uterus into the pelvic veins in 80% of cases and along the inferior vena cava in 10%. Rarely, it may even reach the right side of the heart.[93–97] The median age of patients is 45 years. Patients present with the same symptoms as women with ordinary leiomyomas, i.e., abnormal bleeding and pelvic pain. Most patients have a pelvic mass.

Dysregulated *HMGA2* and simple chromosomal aberrations similar to those found in typical uterine leiomyoma have been noted in intravenous leiomyomatosis, but the molecular mechanism responsible for this angioinvasive phenotype remains unclear.[98,99]

Intravenous leiomyomatosis is usually apparent on gross examination. The uterus is enlarged and, when cut across, the intravenous elements may pop up as 'worm-like' coils of firm, rubbery tissue. Uterine leiomyomas may or may not be present. When present, continuity may sometimes be demonstrated between the leiomyomas and the intravascular component. Some cases lack an extravascular component and the smooth muscle merges with the vessel wall, perhaps indicating a vascular origin.[100,101] Arteries are not involved. The intravascular smooth muscle tissue usually resembles that of an ordinary leiomyoma, although it often shows numerous thick-walled blood vessels, fibrosis, and hyalinization (Figure 19.22). Mitotic figures are usually rare but cellular intravenous leiomyomatosis may contain up to 4 mitotic figures per 10 HPF. Several histologic patterns of leiomyoma have been described in intravenous leiomyomatosis including cellular, epithelioid, bizarre, myxoid, and lipoleiomyoma.[102,103] The clinical behavior of these cases is the same as that of ordinary intravenous leiomyomatosis.

Intravenous leiomyomatosis is distinguished from endometrial stromal sarcoma by the thick-walled blood vessels of its intravascular component and the presence of desmin-positive smooth muscle cells. Rarely, leiomyosarcoma may exhibit a florid intravenous component that simulates intravenous leiomyomatosis,[104] However, intravenous leiomyomatosis differs from leiomyosarcoma by the lack of mitotic activity, atypia, and tumor cell necrosis. Treatment is by total hysterectomy and bilateral salpingo-oophorectomy, along with removal of as much of the extrauterine tumor as possible. Intravascular tumor remaining after hysterectomy may need further surgical treatment. Intravenous leiomyomatosis is an estrogen-dependent tumor and progression is more likely in surgically treated patients in whom the ovaries have been preserved. This has prompted treatment by GnRH analogs or tamoxifen for controlling unresectable tumors.[94,105] Prognosis is largely determined by the degree of hemodynamic compromise. The only deaths reported have been associated with intracardiac involvement.[106]

BENIGN METASTASIZING LEIOMYOMA

This is a very rare phenomenon in which histologically benign smooth muscle tumors are present at distant sites, particularly the lungs (Figure 19.23) or the lymph nodes (Figure 19.24), and thought to be 'metastasis' from benign uterine leiomyomas.[107–110]

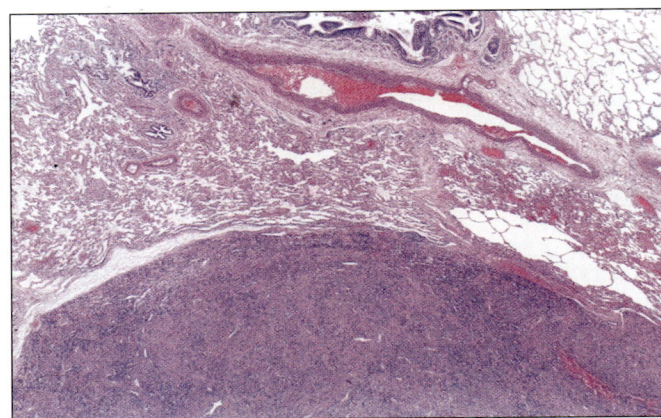

Figure 19.23 Benign metastasizing leiomyoma. A well-circumscribed leiomyoma is present in the lung.

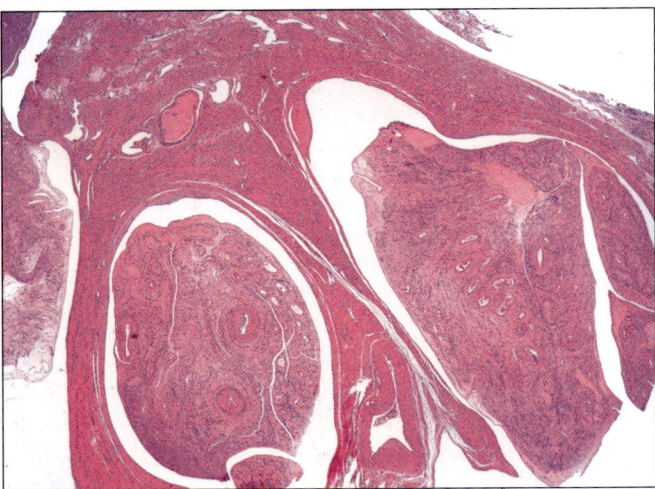

Figure 19.22 Intravenous leiomyomatosis. The intravascular smooth muscle tissue typically shows numerous thick-walled blood vessels.

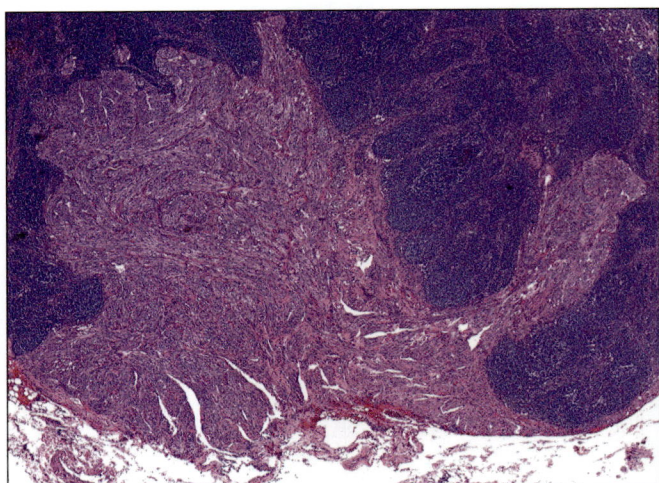

Figure 19.24 Benign metastasizing leiomyoma. Cytologically bland smooth muscle tissue is present in a pelvic lymph node.

However, critical analysis of the reported cases shows that few can be accepted as genuine examples of 'benign' metastasis. The allegedly primary tumor, typically removed years before the metastases are detected, often has been inadequately studied. Mitotic counts on the uterine tumors are not recorded in many reports and, where multiple uterine leiomyomas have been present, not all have been histologically sampled, factors that raise doubts over their benign nature. A high proportion of women with benign metastasizing leiomyomas, however, had a prior dilatation and curettage, myomectomy, or hysterectomy, raising the possibility that surgery had predisposed them to the subsequent spread. Pulmonary metastasis both before and after resection of intravenous leiomyomatosis has been reported;[94,111] this observation raises the possibility that benign metastasizing leiomyoma originates from unrecognized intravenous leiomyomatosis. It is also possible that some cases, in which concomitant leiomyomas of the uterus and smooth muscle tumors in the lungs have been found, represent independent primary tumors.

The pulmonary tumor is grossly evident and usually solitary. It differs from the multifocal, microscopic smooth muscle proliferations of lymphangioleiomyomatosis that occurs in the lungs of women with tuberous sclerosis.[111–113] Cytogenetic analysis of five cases of benign metastasizing leiomyoma revealed deletion of 19q and 22q in all five cases; a subset of cases also showed deletions of 1p or 13q as well as 6p arrangement.[114]

Favoring the secondary nature of benign metastasizing leiomyoma are the facts that primary smooth muscle tumors of the lung are exceedingly rare, ERs are found in the pulmonary tumors, and response to hormonal treatment has been documented.[115] Treatment is by the removal of as much of the 'metastatic' tumor as is feasible, but hormonal treatment using progestins, luteinizing hormone-releasing hormone analogs, and raloxifene[116] has also been tried. Progression is slow.

DISSEMINATED PERITONEAL LEIOMYOMATOSIS

This rare condition is characterized by the presence of multiple small, white or tan nodules of benign-appearing smooth muscle on the peritoneal surfaces in women of reproductive age (see Chapter 31). The widespread nodules, which involve mainly the uterine serosa, fallopian tubes, ovaries, and omentum (Figure 19.25A), simulate metastatic leiomyosarcoma.[117,118] Most cases are associated with hormonal stimulation, as many patients are pregnant, puerperal, or taking oral contraceptives at the time of diagnosis. The most common presentation is as an incidental finding at the time of cesarean section.

The peritoneal nodules are distributed randomly, and most of them are less than 1 cm in diameter. They are firm, well-circumscribed, and have a tan, often whorled, cut surface, similar to that of uterine leiomyomas. In contrast, the peritoneal metastases of leiomyosarcoma tend to be fewer, larger, and invasive into adjacent tissues. Microscopically, the nodules of disseminated peritoneal leiomyomatosis consist of collagen, fibroblasts, myofibroblasts, smooth muscle cells (Figure 19.25B), and, in pregnancy or the postpartum period, decidual cells. Foci of endometrial glands and stroma may occasionally be found and such an

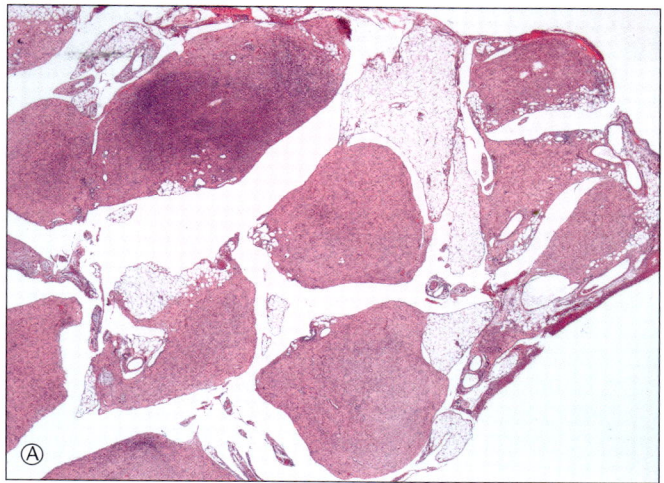

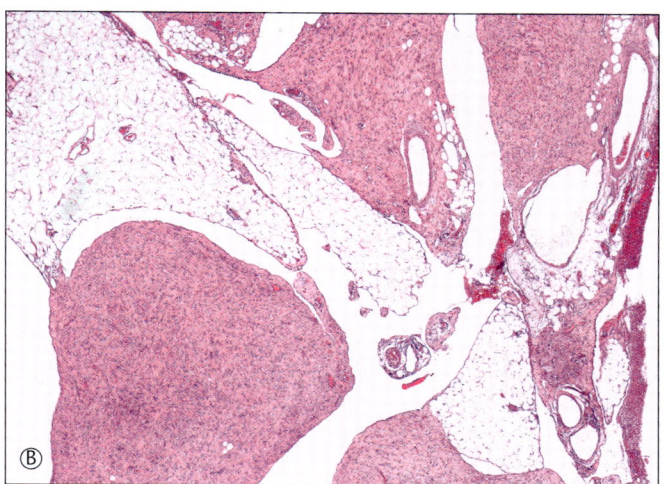

Figure 19.25 Peritoneal leiomyomatosis. **(A)** Multiple small nodules of smooth muscle are scattered throughout the omentum. **(B)** At higher magnification, the whorled nature of the smooth muscle bundles can be appreciated.

adenomyomatous appearance poses an interesting question as to their origin.

Specifically, disseminated peritoneal leiomyomatosis was thought to represent fibrosis and smooth muscle metaplasia of ectopic nodules of decidua found in the omentum and peritoneum during pregnancy. Similar peritoneal lesions have been produced experimentally in animals by administration of estrogen alone or in combination with progestins, raising the possibility of a multicentric origin involving metaplasia of subperitoneal mesenchymal stem cells to smooth muscle, fibroblasts, myofibroblasts, and decidual cells. A study undertaking clonality analysis based on patterns of X chromosome inactivation, however, has shown that the same parental X chromosome was non-randomly inactivated in all of the peritoneal smooth muscle tumors in each of the four patients analyzed.[118] This finding would not be expected if the condition were metaplastic, but rather is consistent with either metastasis from a single primary tumor or selection for an X-linked allele in clonal multicentric lesions.

Nearly all reported cases of disseminated peritoneal leiomyomatosis have run a benign course. However, six cases of leiomyosarcoma are known to have developed in diffuse peritoneal leiomyomatosis.[119] One patient developed bony metastatic lesions and died within 2 years.[120]

LEIOMYOSARCOMA

After excluding carcinosarcoma (malignant mixed müllerian tumor), leiomyosarcoma represents the most common type of uterine sarcoma (more than 50%), accounting for 1–2% of uterine malignancies.[121] The incidence of leiomyosarcoma is 0.3–0.4/100,000 women per year.[122] Approximately 1 of every 800 smooth muscle tumors of the uterus is a leiomyosarcoma.[122,123] The tumor is more common in black than in white women, but the difference is less than that estimated for leiomyoma.[124] The incidence in women who are on tamoxifen therapy for breast cancer is increased compared with those who are not.[124]

Clinical Features

Most leiomyosarcomas occur in women over 50 years of age who usually present with abnormal vaginal bleeding (56%), palpable pelvic mass (54%), and pelvic pain (22%). Signs and symptoms resemble those of the far more common leiomyoma and preoperative distinction between the two tumors may be difficult. Nevertheless, malignancy should be suspected when tumor growth is detected in menopausal women who are not on hormone replacement therapy.[125] Occasionally, the presenting manifestations are related to tumor rupture (hemoperitoneum), extrauterine extension (one-third to one-half of cases), or metastases. Only very rarely does a leiomyosarcoma originate from a leiomyoma. Unlike carcinosarcoma, leiomyosarcoma is almost never associated with a history of pelvic radiation therapy.

Gross Features

Leiomyosarcomas are either single masses or, when associated with leiomyomas, the largest mass. They are typically voluminous tumors with a mean diameter of 10 cm. Only 25% of cases are <5 cm in size. About two-thirds of leiomyosarcomas are intramural, one-fifth are submucosal, and one-tenth subserosal; 5% arise in the cervix. The cut surface is typically soft, bulging, fleshy, necrotic, and hemorrhagic (Figure 19.26) and lacks the prominent whorled appearance of leiomyomas. Leiomyosarcomas tend to be less circumscribed than leiomyomas and a sharp line of demarcation separating the tumor from the normal myometrium is not seen. The irregular margin denotes invasion and is not always so apparent in early tumors. When a myometrial tumor shows an unusual gross appearance, thorough sampling is recommended (at least one section per centimeter in diameter) including the interface with the adjacent myometrium. However, there is overlap in appearance between leiomyosarcoma and ischemic degeneration of leiomyomas and most smooth muscle neoplasms that have a peculiar gross appearance are found to be benign.

Microscopic Features

Most uterine leiomyosarcomas are high grade and obviously malignant tumors. Compared with leiomyomas, they are usually more cellular (Figure 19.27), show moderate to severe nuclear atypia (Figure 19.28), and contain frequent mitotic figures (Figure 19.29). The mitotic rate is usually of 10 or more mitotic figures per 10 HPF, and over 90% of cases have >15 mitotic figures per 10 HPF. The degree of smooth muscle differentiation varies both between tumors and within an individual leiomyosarcoma. Well-differentiated leiomyosarcomas consist of elongated smooth muscle cells with regular nuclei that may differ little from those of leiomyoma. At the other end of the spectrum, a poorly differentiated leiomyosarcoma shows rounded and

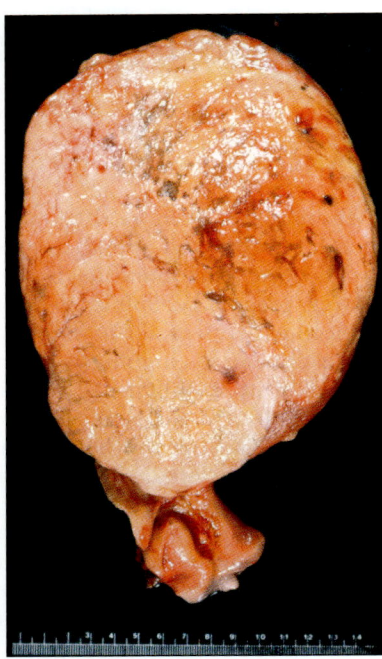

Figure 19.26 Leiomyosarcoma. The cut surface appears fleshy and heterogeneous with extensive necrosis and hemorrhage.

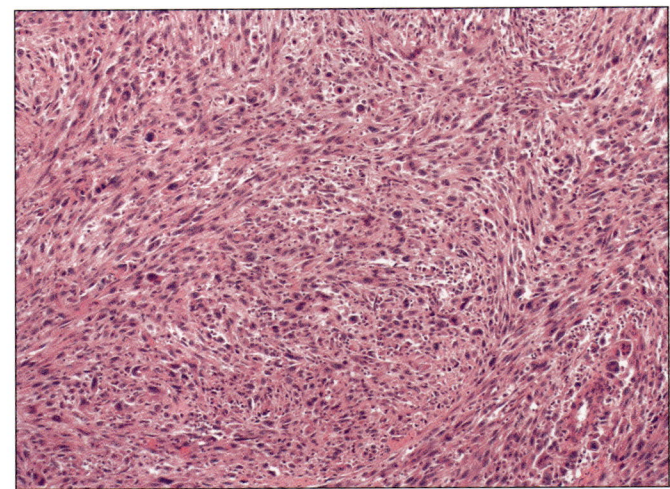

Figure 19.27 Leiomyosarcoma. Hypercellular bundles of pleomorphic smooth muscle cells with numerous mitotic figures.

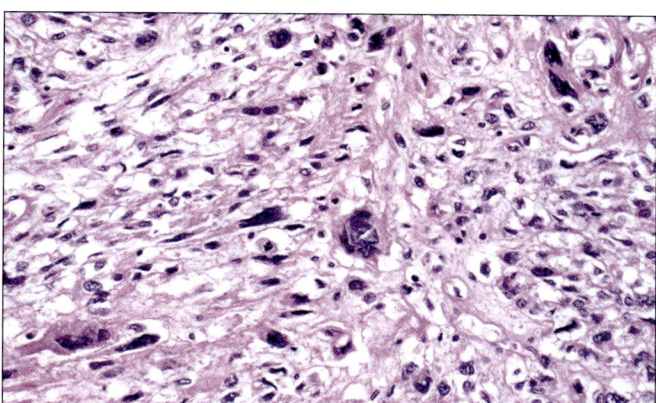

Figure 19.28 Leiomyosarcoma. Severe nuclear atypia.

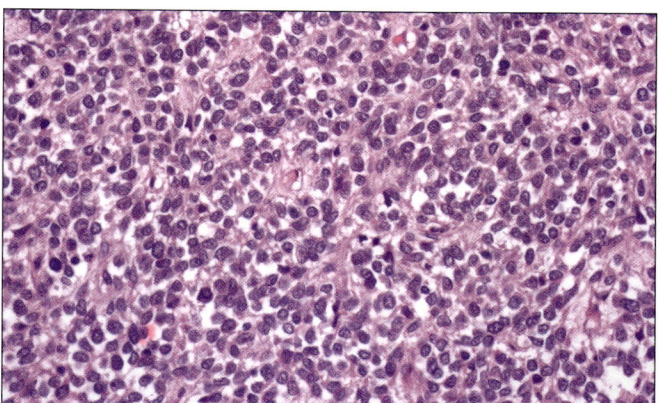

Figure 19.31 Epithelioid leiomyosarcoma. The tumor cells are polygonal with pale cytoplasm and atypical nuclei. Mitoses are not numerous.

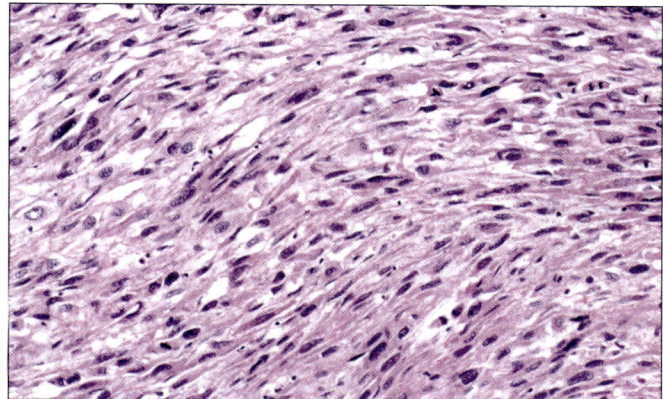

Figure 19.29 Leiomyosarcoma. High mitotic activity.

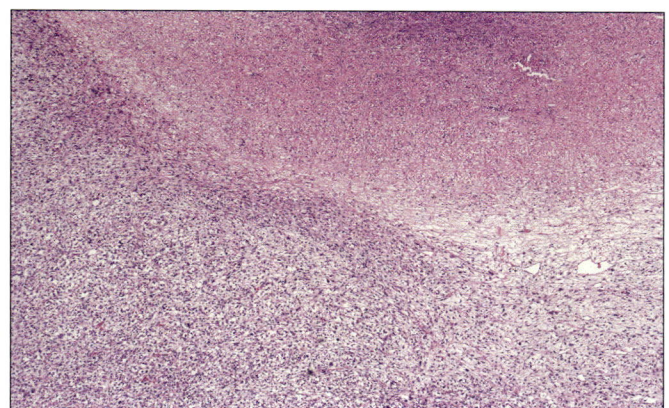

Figure 19.30 Tumor cell necrosis. There is a sharp line of demarcation between the area of necrosis and the viable tumor.

pleomorphic cells that have virtually no resemblance to normal smooth muscle cells. Nuclear as well as cellular pleomorphism, nuclear hyperchromasia, and giant cells are indicative of increasing anaplasia. Multinucleated tumor cells are found in 50% of leiomyosarcomas and osteoclast-like cells are occasionally seen. Areas of tumor cell necrosis (Figure 19.30) and hemorrhage, which are already seen macroscopically, are common. Frequently, leiomyosarcomas have invaded the adjacent myometrial tissue at the time of diagnosis, even to the extent of breaking through the serosal surface of the uterus and involving other pelvic organs. Vascular invasion is found in 10–20% of cases.

Tumor cell necrosis is a characteristic feature of leiomyosarcoma, but its presence is not necessary for establishing the diagnosis. Nevertheless, tumor cell necrosis, nuclear atypia, and high mitotic rate are thought to be the stronger histologic criteria and the presence of two of three is considered sufficient for the diagnosis.[60]

Epithelioid and myxoid leiomyosarcomas are two rare histologic variants that lack the severe nuclear atypia and high mitotic activity of the usual spindle-shaped leiomyosarcomas.

Epithelioid leiomyosarcomas are composed predominantly or entirely of round or polygonal cells exhibiting eosinophilic or clear cytoplasm (Figure 19.31).[74,76] Tumor cells grow diffusely in nests, cords, or forming a plexiform pattern. Although nuclear pleomorphism is usually mild, some tumors show moderate to marked nuclear atypia. The mitotic rate is generally <3 mitotic figures per 10 HPF. Most tumors infiltrate the adjacent myometrium but vascular invasion is rare. Tumor cell necrosis may be absent. Three of 26 epithelioid smooth muscle tumors in one series recurred or metastasized.[75] The malignant tumors exhibited one or more of the following features: eosinophilic cells, infiltrating margins, necrosis, diameter greater than 6 cm, and absence of hyaline stroma.[75] In a larger but still unpublished series of 80 cases, features indicative of malignancy were the presence of necrosis, vascular invasion, significant nuclear pleomorphism, and a mitotic count of >3 mitotic figures per 10 HPF.[126] If none of these four features was present, the tumor behaved in a malignant fashion in under 10% of cases; however, if one, two, or three features were identified, malignant behavior was observed in 42%, 56%, and 88% of patients, respectively. Nearly 1 in 10 epithelioid tumors that showed no necrosis, no vascular invasion, no significant nuclear pleomorphism, and mitotic counts of less than 3 per 10 HPF still behaved in a malignant fashion.

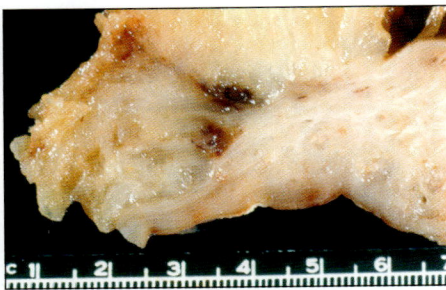

Figure 19.32 Myxoid leiomyosarcoma. The tumor is large, gelatinous, and apparently well circumscribed.

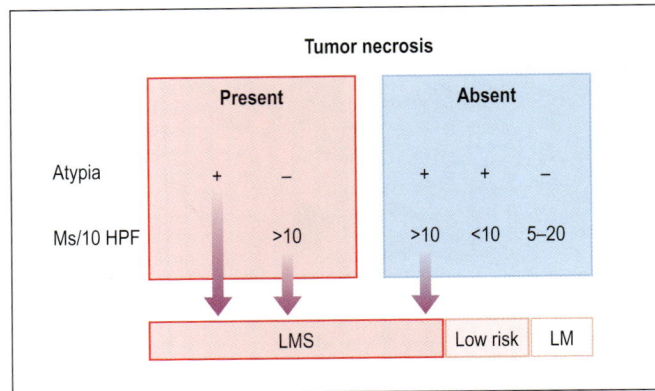

Figure 19.34 Practical approach for the diagnosis of leiomyosarcoma.[60] LM, leiomyoma; LMS, leiomyosarcoma; Ms, mitosis.

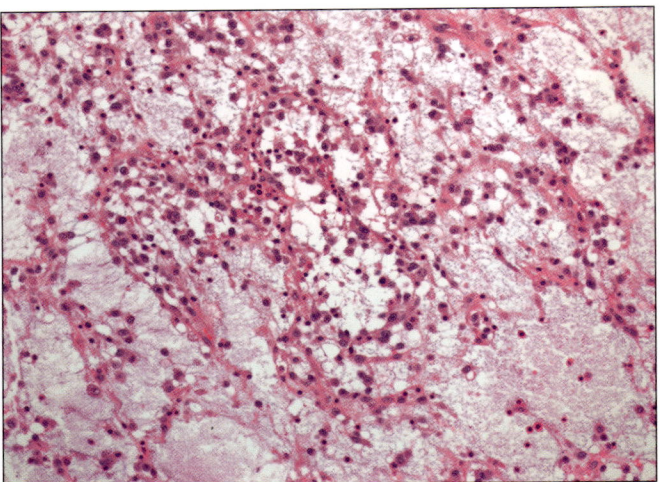

Figure 19.33 Myxoid leiomyosarcoma. The cells are widely separated by myxoid material and have bland nuclear features.

Myxoid leiomyosarcomas are rare smooth muscle tumors with abundant myxoid stroma. On gross examination, the tumors are usually large, gelatinous, and apparently well circumscribed (Figure 19.32). Microscopically, they differ from conventional leiomyosarcomas and have a hypocellular and myxoid appearance (Figure 19.33).[127] Despite low mitotic rates and bland nuclear features, myxoid leiomyosarcomas are almost always clinically malignant. Of the first six tumors reported,[127] all had mitotic indices from 0 to 2 per 10 HPF but, in subsequent cases, about one-fourth contained 5 or more mitoses per 10 HPF.[128] A single example had as many as 30 abnormal mitotic figures per 10 HPF.[129] The typically low mitotic count in these tumors is largely due to the separation of cells by the abundant myxoid stroma, so that there are few nuclei in each HPF. Along with the myxoid appearance, other microscopic features that suggest the diagnosis of leiomyosarcoma include infiltrative margins and vascular-space invasion. The basophilic or eosinophilic myxoid matrix reacts strongly with Alcian blue and colloidal iron. Smooth muscle markers are detected immunohistochemically in <25% of tumor cells.[72,130] Myxoid tumors of the uterus must be regarded with suspicion, and any myxoid smooth muscle tumor with nuclear atypia, regardless of the mitotic activity or the presence or absence of necrosis, should be diagnosed as leiomyosarcoma. Myxoid leiomyosarcoma should be distinguished from the far more common hydropic changes seen in degenerating leiomyomas. The former tumor is histologically reminiscent of myxoid malignant fibrous histiocytoma of soft tissues.

HISTOLOGIC DIAGNOSIS OF LEIOMYOSARCOMA

As indicated previously, the histologic features that play a role in the diagnosis of leiomyosarcoma and its distinction from leiomyoma include mitotic activity, nuclear atypia, tumor cell necrosis, degree of cellularity, degree of differentiation, presence of tumor giant cells, atypical mitotic figures, vascular invasion, and invasion of the surrounding myometrium. The last two are unquestionably diagnostic of malignancy (with the exception of intravenous leiomyomatosis; see earlier). If a smooth muscle tumor is well circumscribed, composed of cells that are uniform in size and shape, has no intravascular component, cytologic atypia and necrosis are lacking, and the mitotic index is less than 5 mitotic figures per 10 HPF, then the tumor is a leiomyoma. On the other hand, if the tumor has infiltrative margins, intravascular growth, marked cytologic atypia and geographic tumor cell necrosis, a mitotic index greater than 10 mitotic figures per 10 HPF, and abnormal mitotic figures, then it is an obvious leiomyosarcoma. It is when a smooth muscle neoplasm has features somewhere between these extremes that difficulty and controversy exist.

Initially, mitotic count, and specifically 10 mitotic figures per 10 HPF, was the recommended threshold for the diagnosis of leiomyosarcoma[131] and, consequently, diagnosis was based almost exclusively on mitotic count regardless of the degree of atypia.[3] However, it has become clear over the last three decades that mitotic activity is only one of several parameters to be evaluated when assessing the potential malignancy of smooth muscle tumors. From all histologic features, mitotic activity, degree of nuclear atypia, and the presence or absence of tumor cell necrosis emerged as the most important predictors of malignant behavior. By employing these three variables in the assessment of smooth muscle tumors, the diagnostic strategy moves away from complete dependence on mitotic count. This is shown graphically in Figure 19.34.

DIAGNOSTIC CRITERIA

Mitotic Activity

Mitotic counting (without rigor or standardization) is not reliable or reproducible, and could not be used as a precise basis for diagnosis, prognosis, or treatment. There are many variables in mitotic counting: (1) the number of sections taken from the tumor, (2) the thickness of the sections, (3) mitotic figures unrecognized or mistaken for pyknotic or otherwise degenerating nuclei, (4) different number and size of HP used, and (5) the rapidity of fixation.

Only definite mitotic figures should be counted, while questionable figures should be ignored. Recent exposure to progestins can increase mitotic activity of smooth muscle tumors and this information should be sought from clinicians or the medical record in difficult cases. Likewise, ischemic change or proximity to an inflamed or ulcerated mucosa can induce a reactive increase in mitotic count. Atypical mitotic figures are often found in leiomyosarcomas (Figure 19.35). Examples of atypical mitotic figures include spindle poles in excess of two (i.e., tripolar and tetrapolar metaphases), chromosomes lagging far behind the separating groups in later phases of division (as they may be damaged by cycles of chromosomal fusion and subsequent breakage), and extreme polyploidy (which admittedly is a subjective appraisal as accurate enumeration requires other cytogenetic or molecular techniques). Each of these forms of atypia reflects cytogenetic aberrations that characterize malignant smooth muscle tumors and a mechanism to generate genomic instability.

Atypia

Paramount is nuclear pleomorphism, with a variable increase in nuclear size, irregularities of nuclear membrane, chromatin clumping, and prominent nucleoli also taken into account. An increase in the number of nuclei, when none of these features is present, does not constitute atypia. Crowded normal nuclei are seen in a cellular leiomyoma. Significant atypia (moderate or severe) can be identified readily under the low power of the microscope. Mild atypia is subtler, requires evaluation under a higher power, and does not carry the same diagnostic import, as do greater degrees of atypia. One difficulty in applying this approach occurs when the nuclear atypia is very uniform from tumor cell to tumor cell. The monomorphic quality of such tumors suggests that there is less intratumoral genetic heterogeneity than typical for leiomyosarcoma. This difficulty in recognizing nuclear atypia can be overcome when one compares the tumor nuclei to nuclei in the adjacent myometrium. This comparison reveals the increases in nuclear size, chromasia, and chromatin distribution in rare cases of low-grade or well-differentiated leiomyosarcomas.

Necrosis

Tumor cell necrosis is highly characteristic of leiomyosarcomas. It is characterized by an abrupt transition from the viable cells to the necrotic cells without an interposed zone of granulation tissue or fibrous tissue (Figure 19.36). Preserved nuclei with marked pleomorphism and hyperchromasia can still be seen within the necrotic areas and often there is a perivascular growth of viable tumor cells. Tumor cell necrosis should be distinguished from infarct-type

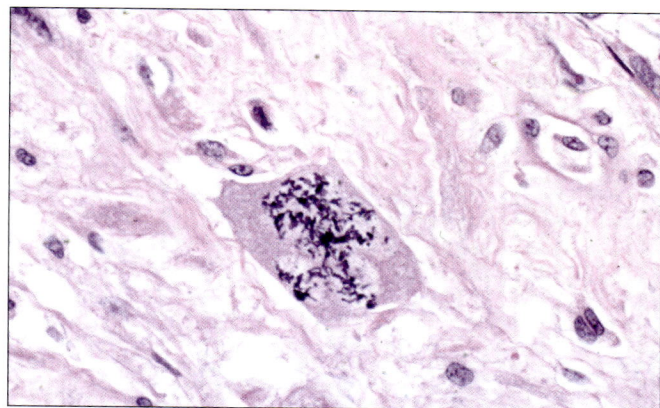

Figure 19.35 Leiomyosarcoma. Atypical mitotic figure.

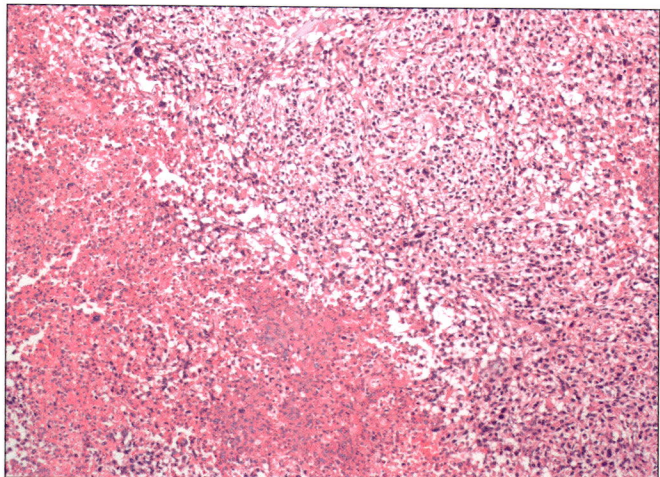

Figure 19.36 Tumor cell necrosis. Ghost-like outlines of necrotic atypical cells can still be seen abruptly separated from preserved tumor cells.

necrosis (which may be seen in benign or malignant smooth muscle tumors) and is characterized by a transition zone composed of granulation or fibrous (hyalinized) tissue (Figure 19.37) depending upon the age of the infarct. The necrotic tissue has a mummified and homogeneous appearance, areas of hemorrhage are common, and no perivascular growth of tumor cells is seen. In some cases, distinguishing between tumor cell necrosis and infarct-type necrosis may be difficult. The 'geographic' tumor cell necrosis is often multifocal and distributed throughout the tumor. In contrast, benign necrosis typically consists of a single, often centrally located region with a simple, rounded border.

Coagulative necrosis is a feature of leiomyomas treated with GnRH analogs. The distinction between this type of necrosis and the necrosis found in leiomyosarcomas may be difficult. Treatment with GnRH analogs does not result in nuclear atypia elsewhere in the tumor and thick-walled blood vessels may be prominent.[56,58] Focused ultrasound effect, used in the ablation of 'fibroids,' may mimic the pattern of necrosis found in leiomyosarcoma. Gross tissue hardening, as well as histologic blandness and hypereosinophilia associated with thermal denaturation, should provide the clues needed to correlate with the clinical history and arrive at the correct diagnosis.

However, the histologic features typical of ischemic or hormonally induced degeneration and subsequent host tissue reaction found in leiomyomas may also occasionally be seen in leiomyosarcoma. Consequently, the presence of such benign degenerative changes cannot be used to exclude malignancy.

Other Factors that Favor Malignancy

Along with high mitotic activity, significant nuclear atypia, and tumor cell necrosis, the finding of a tumor larger than 3 cm in diameter and, to a lesser extent, patient age over 50 years are factors associated with metastasis and mortality. Tumors under 3 cm almost never metastasize.[77]

Immunohistochemistry

Although immunohistochemistry is not necessary for the diagnosis of leiomyosarcoma, it may occasionally help to distinguish leiomyosarcoma from other uterine malignancies such as high-grade endometrial sarcoma or sarcomatoid carcinoma.[72,132–140] Leiomyosarcomas usually express smooth muscle markers such as desmin, h-caldesmon, smooth muscle actin, and histone deacetylase 8 (HDCA8). However, immunoreaction for one or more of these markers can be lost or may be weak in poorly differentiated leiomyosarcomas or in the epithelioid and myxoid variants. Also, leiomyosarcomas are often immunoreactive for CD10 and epithelial markers including keratin and epithelial membrane antigen (the latter is more frequently positive in the epithelioid variant). Conventional leiomyosarcomas express ERs, PRs, and androgen receptors in 30–40% of cases. Whereas a variable proportion of uterine leiomyosarcomas has been reported as being immunoreactive for c-KIT, no c-KIT mutations have been identified.[141] Recent studies have shown statistically significant higher levels of Ki-67 in uterine leiomyosarcomas (Figure 19.38) compared with benign smooth muscle tumors.[72,135–138] Mutation and overexpression of p53 have been described in a significant minority of uterine leiomyosarcomas (25–47%) (Figure 19.39) but not in leiomyomas.[72,137,138] Intermediate rates have been found in bizarre and atypical (STUMP) leiomyomas. Overexpression of p16 has been described in uterine leiomyosarcomas (Figure 19.40) and may prove to be a useful adjunct immunomarker for distinguishing between benign and malignant uterine smooth muscle tumors.[136–138] Strong and diffuse p16 immunoreaction, especially when accompanied by strong staining for p53, favors the diagnosis of leiomyosarcoma.

MOLECULAR GENETICS

Although the vast majority of uterine leiomyosarcomas are sporadic, patients with germline mutations in fumarate hydratase are believed to be at increased risk for developing uterine leiomyosarcomas as well as uterine leiomyomas.[142,143] The oncogenic mechanisms underlying the development of uterine leiomyosarcomas remain elusive. Uterine leiomyosarcoma is a genetically unstable tumor that has complex

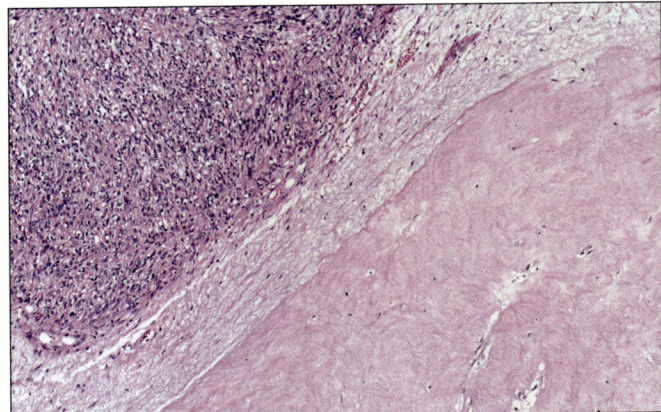

Figure 19.37 Ischemic necrosis. An area of ischemic necrosis is separated from viable spindle-shaped tumor cells by a zone of hyalinized collagen.

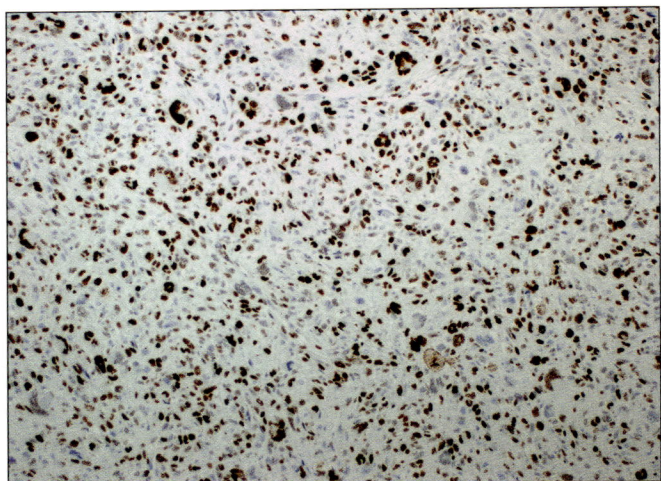

Figure 19.38 Leiomyosarcoma. Positive nuclear immunoreaction for Ki-67.

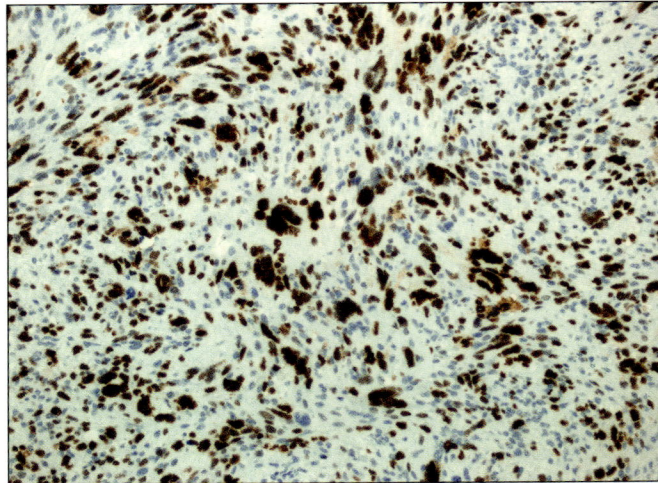

Figure 19.39 Leiomyosarcoma. Positive nuclear immunoreaction for p53.

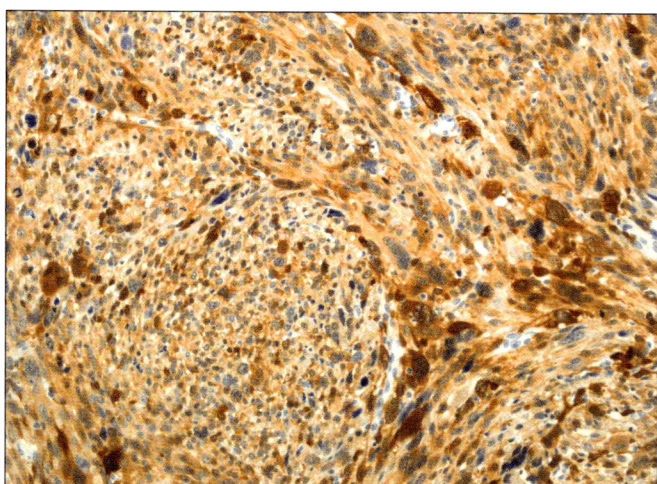

Figure 19.40 Leiomyosarcoma. Positive nuclear and/or cytoplasmic immunoreaction for p16.

structural chromosomal abnormalities and highly disturbed gene regulation, which likely reflects the end state of accumulation of multiple genetic defects. Extrapolating from experiences in soft-tissue leiomyosarcomas, it is unlikely that recurrent disease-driven genetic aberrations (i.e., gene mutation or translocation events) will be found. In comparison with other more common uterine cancers, uterine leiomyosarcomas bear some resemblance to type 2 endometrial carcinomas and high-grade serous carcinomas of ovary/fallopian tube origin, based on their genetic instability, frequent p53 abnormalities, aggressive behavior, and resistance to chemotherapy. Therefore, therapies that exploit the underlying genetic instability of uterine leiomyosarcomas may prove to be an effective therapeutic strategy.

Overexpression of the *c-myc* proto-oncogene occurs in about 50% of both leiomyomas and leiomyosarcomas, and does not correlate with survival.[144] *K-ras* is overexpressed in a small minority of leiomyomas but not at all in leiomyosarcomas.[145] The *MDM2* gene, in contrast, is overexpressed in some leiomyosarcomas but not in leiomyomas.[145] The lack of gamma-smooth muscle isoactin gene, in a pilot study, correlated 100% with a histologic diagnosis of leiomyosarcoma.[146] Abnormalities of the retinoblastoma–cyclin D pathway have been found in about 90% of leiomyosarcomas,[147] which is not surprising considering that the retinoblastoma gene is deleted in about three-fourths of leiomyosarcomas.[148] These different patterns of molecular alterations in leiomyomas and leiomyosarcomas may lead to the conclusion that they are different entities.[145]

Recently, p16, also known as INK4 or cyclin-dependent kinase inhibitor 2A (CDKN2A), has been implicated in the genesis of leiomyosarcoma.[134,149] The p16 protein binds the CDK4–cyclin D complex and acts as a negative cell cycle regulator. Consequently, p16 deletion results in a loss of tumor suppression phenotype.

Proliferation Markers

Proliferating cell nuclear antigen (PCNA) is a protein involved with copying DNA and therefore in cell division. It can be demonstrated immunohistochemically using the antibody PC10. The Ki-67 antigen identifies proliferating normal and neoplastic cells in histologic sections, using the MIB1 antibody. This is a more reliable indication of cell division and proliferation than the mitotic index. Recently, statistically significant higher levels of PCNA and Ki-67 have been shown in uterine leiomyosarcomas compared with leiomyomas.[150,151] In one study, the percentage of MIB1-positive tumor cells helped predict prognosis and extent of tumor spread.[150]

Flow Cytometry, Cytogenetics, and Molecular Genetics

Analysis of leiomyosarcomas by flow cytometry has produced mixed results. Studies show that between about 55% and 70% of the tumors are aneuploid.[151] While most studies report that neither ploidy nor S-phase fraction offers additional value to clinical and histologic factors already described,[152,153] one concluded that DNA ploidy helped identify cases that might have an adverse prognosis.[151]

Cytogenetic analyses show that leiomyosarcomas have both complex numerical and structural chromosomal aberrations.[154,155] The large variability in aberrations found among the metaphases from the same leiomyosarcoma also suggests, in contrast to benign leiomyoma, that genomic instability is a hallmark of malignancy in uterine smooth muscle tumors.[154] Loss of heterozygosity analysis and comparative genomic hybridization, two different means to assess allelic imbalance, also detect complex genomic aberrations. In particular, frequent losses of 10q and 13q as well as occasional gain of 17p and losses of 2p and 16q have been observed.[148,156] At least some leiomyosarcomas have X inactivation that differs from their accompanying leiomyomas, suggesting that the benign and malignant tumors arose from independent transformations and that the genesis of leiomyosarcoma occurs *de novo*. Whether malignant transformation of certain leiomyomas (e.g., bizarre leiomyoma) occurs remains to be proven fully.

PROGNOSIS AND TREATMENT
(see Appendix A, p. 847)

Leiomyosarcomas diagnosed according to the 2003 WHO criteria are associated with poor prognosis even when confined to the uterus[139,157] and even if diagnosed at an early stage; recurrence rate ranges from 53% to 71%.[158] First recurrences occur in the lungs in 40% of patients and in the pelvis in only 13%. Overall survival rate ranges from 15% to 25% with a median survival of only 10 months in one study. In the Norwegian series,[157] patients with leiomyosarcomas limited to the uterus had poor prognosis with a 5 year overall survival of 51% at stage I and 25% at stage II (by the 1988 FIGO staging classification). All patients with tumor spread outside the pelvis died within 5 years.

There has been no consistency among various studies regarding correlation between survival and patient age, clinical stage, tumor size, type of border (pushing vs infiltrative), presence or absence of necrosis, mitotic rate, degree of nuclear pleomorphism, and vascular invasion.[132,139,159–164] One study, however, found tumor size to be a major prognostic parameter:[159] five of eight patients with tumors <5 cm in diameter survived, whereas all patients with tumors >5 cm in diameter died of tumor. In this study of 208 uterine leiomyosarcomas, the only other parameters predictive of prognosis were tumor grade and stage.[159] Histologic grade, however, has not been consistently identified as a significant prognostic parameter. In the report from Norway,[157] including 245 leiomyosarcomas confined to the uterus, tumor size and mitotic index were significant prognostic factors and allowed for separation of patients into three risk groups with marked differences in prognosis. Ancillary parameters including p53, p16, Ki-67, and Bcl-2 have been used in leiomyosarcomas trying to predict outcome.[139,140] However, it is not clear whether they act independently of stage, which still is the most significant prognostic factor for uterine sarcomas.

Treatment of leiomyosarcomas includes total abdominal hysterectomy and debulking of tumor if present outside the uterus. Removal of the ovaries and lymph node dissection remain controversial as metastases to these organs occur in a small percentage of cases and are frequently associated with intra-abdominal disease.[159] Ovarian preservation may be considered in premenopausal patients with early-stage leiomyosarcomas.[159] Lymph node metastases have been identified in 6.6% and 11% of two series of patients with leiomyosarcoma who underwent lymphadenectomy.[159,165] In the first series, the 5 year disease-specific survival rate was 26% in patients who had positive lymph nodes compared with 64.2% in patients who had negative lymph nodes ($p < 0.001$).[165] The influence of adjuvant therapy on survival is uncertain. Radiotherapy may be useful in controlling local recurrences and chemotherapy with doxorubicin or docetaxel/gemcitabine is now used for advanced or recurrent disease, with response rates ranging from 27% to 36%.[166,167] Some patients may respond to hormonal treatment.[168]

ATYPICAL SMOOTH MUSCLE TUMORS (SO-CALLED SMOOTH MUSCLE TUMORS OF UNCERTAIN MALIGNANT POTENTIAL)

Uterine smooth muscle tumors that cannot be histologically diagnosed as unequivocally benign or malignant should be designated atypical smooth muscle tumors (Figures 19.34 and 19.41).[60,170] This group is largely defined by the presence of nuclear atypia and <10 mitotic figures per 10 HPF in the absence of tumor cell necrosis.[169] The accepted degree of nuclear atypia varies from mild[46] to moderate or

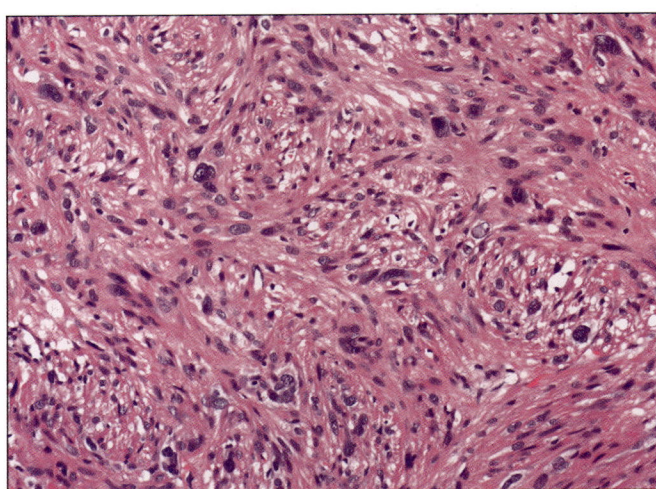

Figure 19.41 Atypical smooth muscle tumor (STUMP). There is obvious moderate nuclear atypia that is not of the 'bizarre' type. In this tumor, mitoses were sparse and tumor cell necrosis absent.

Table 19.2 A Comparison of Features Seen in Groups of Smooth Muscle Tumors[170]

Parameter	Leiomyoma	Atypical Smooth Muscle Tumor[a]		Leiomyosarcoma
		Probably Benign	Probably Malignant	
Age (average)	30s	30s	50s	50s
Invasiveness	None	Rare	Many	All
Tumor margins	Distinct	Distinct	Variable	Indistinct
Vascular invasion	None	None	33%	33%
Size (average)	<5 cm	6 cm	5–15 cm	>10 cm
Incised surface	Bulging	Bulging	Variable	Soft, irregular
Necrosis	None	33%	All	All
Nuclear atypia	None	Mild	Marked	Marked
Mitoses—atypia absent[b]	<5	5–14	5–14	≥10
Mitoses—atypia present	<5	5–10	5–10	≥10
Abnormal mitoses	None	Rare	Occasional	Frequent
Adjunct from the Literature, Not to Supplant Histologic Features				
p16[133,136]	10%	20%	>20%	>50%
Ki-67[72,136]	Low (<5%)	Intermediate (5–10%)	Intermediate (5–10%)	High (≥15%)

[a]Includes lesions variously described as atypical leiomyomas, smooth muscle tumors of uncertain malignant potential, and smooth muscle tumors of low malignant potential.
[b]Mitotic activity is expressed as the number of readily identifiable mitotic figures per 10 HPF in the most proliferative areas. The evaluation of mitotic activity differs when nuclear atypia is present or absent.

severe,[60] depending upon the mitotic index (5–9 or <10 mitotic figures per 10 HPF, respectively). Furthermore, atypical smooth muscle tumors were subdivided into three groups:[60]

1. Atypical smooth muscle tumor with *low risk of recurrence*, which shows diffuse moderate to severe nuclear atypia, <10 mitotic figures per 10 HPF, and no tumor cell necrosis. Only one of 46 such tumors was clinically malignant.[60]
2. Atypical smooth muscle tumor *with limited experience*, characterized by focal moderate to severe nuclear atypia, <20 mitotic figures per 10 HPF, and no tumor cell necrosis. All five cases in this group were clinically benign. Three of the five tumors had <5 mitotic figures per 10 HPF and would be considered leiomyomas with bizarre nuclei by most investigators. The other two tumors had 10–19 mitotic figures per 10 HPF.[60]
3. Smooth muscle tumors *of low malignant potential*, which had tumor cell necrosis, <10 mitotic figures per 10 HPF, and none to mild nuclear atypia. One of four tumors in this group was clinically malignant, again underscoring the importance of tumor cell necrosis.

The unpredictable behavior of some of these tumors has led some to introduce the concept of the STUMP, a term to be discouraged for the reasons given earlier. Nevertheless, most tumors classified as STUMP have been associated with favorable prognosis and, in these cases, only follow-up of the patients is recommended.[171] In two recent studies of 41 and 16 cases of STUMP, only 3 (7%) and 2 (12%) patients developed recurrences, respectively. Recurrence occurred, several years after hysterectomy, in the form of STUMP in three cases and as leiomyosarcoma in the other two.[171,172] All five patients were alive and disease free after prolonged follow-up. As indicated previously, when account is taken of mitotic count, myometrial invasion, nuclear atypia, tumor cell necrosis, size of tumor, and age of patient, tumors can be allocated to benign or malignant categories with greater certainty and the term 'of uncertain malignancy' can be avoided in most cases (Table 19.2).[170]

REFERENCES

1. Stewart EA. Uterine fibroids. Lancet 2001;357:293–8.
2. Payson M, Leppert P, Segars J, et al. Epidemiology of myomas. Obstet Gynecol Clin North Am 2006;33:1–11.
3. Hendrickson MR, Kempson RL. Smooth muscle neoplasms. In: Surgical Pathology of the Uterine Corpus. Philadelphia: Saunders; 1980. p. 472.
4. Tiltman AJ. Adenomatoid tumours of the uterus. Histopathology 1980;4:437–43.
5. Cramer SF, Patel A. The frequency of uterine leiomyomas. Am J Clin Pathol 1990;94:435–8.
6. Kjerulff KH, Langenberg P, Seidman JD, et al. Uterine leiomyomas. Racial differences in severity, symptoms and age at diagnosis. J Reprod Med 1996;41:483–90.
7. Baird DD, Dunson DB, Hill MC, et al. High cumulative incidence of uterine leiomyoma in black and white women: ultrasound evidence. Am J Obstet Gynecol 2003;188:100–7.
8. Al-Hendy A, Salama SA. Catechol-O-methyltransferase polymorphism is associated with increased uterine leiomyoma risk in different ethnic groups. J Soc Gynecol Invest 2006;13:136–44.
9. Al-Hendy A, Salama SA. Ethnic distribution of estrogen receptor-alpha polymorphism is associated with a higher prevalence of uterine leiomyomas in black Americans. Fertil Steril 2006;86:686–93.
10. Wei JJ, Chiriboga L, Arslan AA, et al. Ethnic differences in expression of the dysregulated proteins in uterine leiomyomata. Hum Reprod 2006;21:57–67.
11. Gross KL, Panhuysen CI, Kleinman MS, et al. Involvement of fumarate hydratase in nonsyndromic uterine leiomyomas: genetic linkage analysis and FISH studies. Genes Chromosomes Cancer 2004;41:183–90.
12. Ligon AH, Morton CC. Leiomyomata: heritability and cytogenetic studies. Hum Reprod Update 2001;7:8–14.
13. Marsh EE, Bulun SE. Steroid hormones and leiomyomas. Obstet Gynecol Clin North Am 2006;33:59–67.
14. Sozen I, Arici A. Cellular biology of myomas: interaction of sex steroids with cytokines and growth factors. Obstet Gynecol Clin North Am 2006;33:41–58.
15. Andersen J, Barbieri RL. Abnormal gene expression in uterine leiomyomas. J Soc Gynecol Invest 1995;2:663–72.
16. Andersen J, DyReyes VM, Barbieri RL, et al. Leiomyoma primary cultures have elevated transcriptional response to estrogen compared with autologous myometrial cultures. J Soc Gynecol Invest 1995;2:542–51.
17. Ichimura T, Kawamura N, Ito F, et al. Correlation between the growth of uterine leiomyomata and estrogen and progesterone receptor content in needle biopsy specimens. Fertil Steril 1998;70:967–71.
18. Attilakos G, Fox R. Regression of tamoxifen-stimulated massive uterine fibroid after conversion to anastrozole. J Obstet Gynaecol 2005;25:609–10.
19. Le Bouedec G, De Latour M, Dauplat J. Tamoxifen and uterine fibroids. Eur J Cancer 1998;34:S19–21.
20. Linder D, Gartler SM. Glucose-6-phosphate dehydrogenase mosaicism: utilization as a cell marker in the study of leiomyomas. Science 1965;150:67–9.
21. Townsend DE, Sparkes RS, Baluda MC, McClelland G. Unicellular histogenesis of uterine leiomyomas as determined by electrophoresis by glucose-6-phosphate dehydrogenase. Am J Obstet Gynecol 1970;107:1168–73.
22. Hashimoto K, Azuma C, Kamiura S, et al. Clonal determination of uterine leiomyomas by analyzing differential inactivation of the X-chromosome-linked phosphoglycerokinase gene. Gynecol Obstet Invest 1995;40:204–8.
23. Mashal RD, Fejzo ML, Friedman AJ, et al. Analysis of androgen receptor DNA reveals the independent clonal origins of uterine leiomyomata and the secondary nature of cytogenetic aberrations in the development of leiomyomata. Genes Chromosomes Cancer 1994;11:1–6.
24. Zhang P, Zhang C, Hao J, et al. Use of X-chromosome inactivation pattern to determine the clonal origins of uterine leiomyoma and leiomyosarcoma. Hum Pathol 2006;37:1350–6.
25. Lobel MK, Somasundaram P, Morton CC, et al. The genetic heterogeneity of uterine leiomyomata. Obstet Gynecol Clin North Am 2006;33:13–39.
26. Stewart EA, Morton CC. The genetics of uterine leiomyomata: what clinicians need to know. Obstet Gynecol 2006;107:917–21.
27. Gattas GJ, Quade BJ, Nowak RA, Morton CC. HMGIC expression in human adult and fetal tissues and in uterine leiomyomata. Genes Chromosomes Cancer 1999;25:316–22.
28. Sornberger KS, Weremowicz S, Williams AJ, et al. Expression of HMGIY in three uterine leiomyomata with complex rearrangements of chromosome 6. Cancer Genet Cytogenet 1999;114:9–16.
29. Williams AJ, Powell WL, Collins T, Morton CC. HMGI(Y) expression in human uterine leiomyomata. Involvement of another high-mobility group architectural factor in a benign neoplasm. Am J Pathol 1997;150:911–18.
30. Kazmierczak B, Dal Cin P, Wanschura S, et al. HMGIY is the target of 6p21.3 rearrangements in various benign mesenchymal tumors. Genes Chromosomes Cancer 1998;23:279–85.
31. Tallini G, Dal Cin P. HMGI(Y) and HMGI-C dysregulation: a common occurrence in human tumors. Adv Anat Pathol 1999;6:237–46.
32. Quade BJ, Weremowicz S, Neskey DM, et al. Fusion transcripts involving HMGA2 are not a common molecular mechanism in uterine leiomyomata with rearrangements in 12q15. Cancer Res 2003;63:1351–8.

33. Zaidi MR, Okada Y, Chada KK. Misexpression of full-length HMGA2 induces benign mesenchymal tumors in mice. Cancer Res 2006;66:7453–9.
34. Moore SD, Herrick SR, Ince TA, et al. Uterine leiomyomata with t(10;17) disrupt the histone acetyltransferase MORF. Cancer Res 2004;64:5570–7.
35. Rein MS, Powell WL, Walters FC, et al. Cytogenetic abnormalities in uterine myomas are associated with myoma size. Mol Hum Reprod 1998;4:83–6.
36. Reed WB, Walker R, Horowitz R. Cutaneous leiomyomata with uterine leiomyomata. Acta Derm Venereol 1973;53:409–16.
37. Tomlinson IP, Alam NA, Rowan AJ, et al. Germline mutations in FH predispose to dominantly inherited uterine fibroids, skin leiomyomata and papillary renal cell cancer. Nat Genet 2002;30:406–10.
38. Wei MH, Toure O, Glenn GM, et al. Novel mutations in FH and expansion of the spectrum of phenotypes expressed in families with hereditary leiomyomatosis and renal cell cancer. J Med Genet 2006;43:18–27.
39. Kiuru M, Lehtonen R, Arola J, et al. Few FH mutations in sporadic counterparts of tumor types observed in hereditary leiomyomatosis and renal cell cancer families. Cancer Res 2002;62:4554–7.
40. Lehtonen R, Kiuru M, Vanharanta S, et al. Biallelic inactivation of fumarate hydratase (FH) occurs in nonsyndromic uterine leiomyomas but is rare in other tumors. Am J Pathol 2004;164:17–22.
41. Roth TM, Klett C, Cowan BD. Expression profile of several genes in human myometrium and uterine leiomyoma. Fertil Steril 2007;87:635–41.
42. Skubitz KM, Skubitz AP. Differential gene expression in uterine leiomyoma. J Lab Clin Med 2003;141:297–308.
43. Quade BJ, Wang TY, Sornberger K, et al. Molecular pathogenesis of uterine smooth muscle tumors from transcriptional profiling. Genes Chromosomes Cancer 2004;40:97–108.
44. Wang T, Zhang X, Obijuru L, et al. A micro-RNA signature associated with race, tumor size, and target gene activity in human uterine leiomyomas. Genes Chromosomes Cancer 2007;46:336–47.
45. Dgani R, Piura B, Ben Baruch G, et al. Clinical-pathological study of uterine leiomyomas with high mitotic activity. Acta Obstet Gynecol Scand 1998;77:74–7.
46. O'Connor DM, Norris HJ. Mitotically active leiomyomas of the uterus. Hum Pathol 1990;21:223–7.
47. Prayson RA, Hart WR. Mitotically active leiomyomas of the uterus. Am J Clin Pathol 1992;97:14–20.
48. Wu X, Blanck A, Olovsson M, et al. Apoptosis, cellular proliferation and expression of p53 in human uterine leiomyomas and myometrium during the menstrual cycle and after menopause. Acta Obstet Gynecol Scand 2000;79:397–404.
49. Oliva E, Clement PB, Young RY. Mesenchymal tumors of the uterus: selected topics emphasizing diagnostic pitfalls. Curr Diagn 2002;8:268–82.
50. Oliva E, Young RH, Clement PB, et al. Cellular benign mesenchymal tumors of the uterus. A comparative morphologic and immunohistochemical analysis of 33 highly cellular leiomyomas and six endometrial stromal nodules, two frequently confused tumors. Am J Surg Pathol 1995;19:757–68.
51. Christacos NC, Quade BJ, Dal CP, Morton CC. Uterine leiomyomata with deletions of 1p represent a distinct cytogenetic subgroup associated with unusual histologic features. Genes Chromosomes Cancer 2006;45:304–12.
52. Myles JL, Hart WR. Apoplectic leiomyomas of the uterus. A clinicopathologic study of five distinctive hemorrhagic leiomyomas associated with oral contraceptive usage. Am J Surg Pathol 1985;9:798–805.
53. Norris HJ, Hilliard GD, Irey NS. Hemorrhagic cellular leiomyomas ('apoplectic leiomyoma') of the uterus associated with pregnancy and oral contraceptives. Int J Gynecol Pathol 1988;7:212–24.
54. Shaw RW. Gonadotropin hormone-releasing hormone analogue treatment of fibroids. Baillières Clin Obstet Gynaecol 1998;12:245–68.
55. Colgan TJ, Pendergast S, LeBlanc M. The histopathology of uterine leiomyomas following treatment with gonadotropin-releasing hormone analogues. Hum Pathol 1993;24:1073–7.
56. Higashijima T, Kataoka A, Nishida T, Yakushiji M. Gonadotropin-releasing hormone agonist therapy induces apoptosis in uterine leiomyoma. Eur J Obstet Gynecol Reprod Biol 1996;68:169–73.
57. Demopoulos RI, Jones KY, Mittal KR, Vamvakas EC. Histology of leiomyomata in patients treated with leuprolide acetate. Int J Gynecol Pathol 1997;16:131–7.
58. Bardsley V, Cooper P, Peat DS. Massive lymphocytic infiltration of uterine leiomyomas associated with GnRH agonist treatment. Histopathology 1998;33:80–2.
59. Vu K, Greenspan DL, Wu TC, et al. Cellular proliferation, estrogen receptor, progesterone receptor, and bcl-2 expression in GnRH agonist-treated uterine leiomyomas. Hum Pathol 1998;29:359–63.
60. Bell SW, Kempson RL, Hendrickson MR. Problematic uterine smooth muscle neoplasms. A clinicopathologic study of 213 cases. Am J Surg Pathol 1994;18:535–58.
61. Clement PB, Young RH, Scully RE. Diffuse, perinodular, and other patterns of hydropic degeneration within and adjacent to uterine leiomyomas. Problems in differential diagnosis. Am J Surg Pathol 1992;16:26–32.
62. Ravina JH, Aymard A, CiraruVigneron N, et al. Selective arterial embolization for hemorrhagic uterine leiomyomas. Presse Med 1998;27:299–303.
63. Goldberg J, Burd I, Price FV, Worthington-Kirsch R. Leiomyosarcoma in a premenopausal patient after uterine artery embolization. Am J Obstet Gynecol 2004;191:1733–5.
64. Joyce A, Hessami S, Heller D. Leiomyosarcoma after uterine artery embolization. A case report. J Reprod Med 2001;46:278–80.
65. Papadia A, Salom EM, Fulcheri E, Ragni N. Uterine sarcoma occurring in a premenopausal patient after uterine artery embolization: a case report and review of the literature. Gynecol Oncol 2007;104:260–3.
66. Colgan TJ, Pron G, Mocarski EJ, et al. Pathologic features of uteri and leiomyomas following uterine artery embolization for leiomyomas. Am J Surg Pathol 2003;27:167–77.
67. Stewart EA, Rabinovici J, Tempany CM, et al. Clinical outcomes of focused ultrasound surgery for the treatment of uterine fibroids. Fertil Steril 2006;85:22–9.
68. Scully RE, Bonfiglio TA, Kurman RJ, et al. Histological typing of female genital tract tumours. World Health Organization International Histological Classification of Tumours. 2nd ed. Berlin: Springer-Verlag; 1994.
69. Downes KA, Hart WR. Bizarre leiomyomas of the uterus: a comprehensive pathologic study of 24 cases with long-term follow-up. Am J Surg Pathol 1997;21:1261–70.
70. Downes KA, Hart WR. Uterine bizarre ('symplastic') leiomyomas: morphology and behavior. Lab Invest 1997;76:99A.
71. Hendrickson MR, Tavassoli FA, Kempson RL, et al. Mesenchymal tumours and related lesions. In: Tavassoli FA, Devilee P, editors. Pathology and Genetics of Tumours of the Breast and Female Genital Organs. Lyon, France: IARC Press; 2003. p. 233–44.
72. Chen L, Yang B. Immunohistochemical analysis of p16, p53, and Ki-67 expression in uterine smooth muscle tumors. Int J Gynecol Pathol 2008;27:326–32.
73. Hyde KE, Geisinger KR, Marshall RB, Jones TL. The clear-cell variant of uterine epithelioid leiomyoma. An immunohistologic and ultrastructural study. Arch Pathol Lab Med 1989;113:551–3.
74. Prayson RA, Goldblum JR, Hart WR. Epithelioid smooth-muscle tumors of the uterus: a clinicopathologic study of 18 patients. Am J Surg Pathol 1997;21:383–91.
75. Kurman RJ, Norris HJ. Mesenchymal tumors of the uterus. VI. Epithelioid smooth muscle tumors including leiomyoblastoma and clear-cell leiomyoma. A clinical and pathological analysis of 26 cases. Cancer 1976;37:1853–65.
76. Atkins K, Bell S, Kempson R, Hendrickson M. Epithelioid smooth muscle of the uterus. Mod Pathol 2001;14:132A.
77. Jones MW, Norris HJ. Clinicopathologic study of 28 uterine leiomyosarcomas with metastasis. Int J Gynecol Pathol 1995;14:243–9.
78. Atkins K, Bell S, Kempson M, Hendrickson M. Myxoid smooth muscle tumors of the uterus. Mod Pathol 2001;14:132A.
79. Mazur MT, Kraus FT. Histogenesis of morphologic variations in tumors of the uterine wall. Am J Surg Pathol 1980;4:59–74.

80. Tahlan A, Nanda A, Mohan H. Uterine adenomyoma: a clinicopathologic review of 26 cases and a review of the literature. Int J Gynecol Pathol 2006;25:361–5.
81. Wang X, Kumar D, Seidman JD. Uterine lipoleiomyomas: a clinicopathologic study of 50 cases. Int J Gynecol Pathol 2006;25: 239–42.
82. Hendrickson MR, Kempson RL. Pure mesenchymal neoplasms of the uterine corpus. In: Fox H, Wells M, editors. Haines and Taylor Obstetrical and Gynaecological Pathology. 4th ed. New York: Churchill Livingstone; 1995. p. 519–86.
83. Pedeutour F, Quade BJ, Sornberger K, et al. Dysregulation of HMGIC in a uterine lipoleiomyoma with a complex rearrangement including chromosomes 7, 12, and 14. Genes Chromosomes Cancer 2000;27:209–15.
84. Volpe R, Canzonieri V, Gloghini A, Carbone A. 'Lipoleiomyoma with metaplastic cartilage' (benign mesenchymoma) of the uterine cervix. Pathol Res Pract 1992;188:799–801.
85. Martin-Reay DG, Christ ML, LaPata RE. Uterine leiomyoma with skeletal muscle differentiation. Report of a case. Am J Clin Pathol 1991;96:344–7.
86. Ma KF, Chow LT. Sex cord-like pattern leiomyomatosis peritonealis disseminata: a hitherto undescribed feature. Histopathology 1992;21:389–91.
87. Irving JA, Carinelli S, Prat J. Uterine tumors resembling ovarian sex cord tumors are polyphenotypic neoplasms with true sex cord differentiation. Mod Pathol 2006;19:17–24.
88. Clement PB. The pathology of uterine smooth muscle tumors and mixed endometrial stromal-smooth muscle tumors: a selective review with emphasis on recent advances. Int J Gynecol Pathol 2000;19:39–55.
89. Mulvany NJ, Ostor AG, Ross I. Diffuse leiomyomatosis of the uterus. Histopathology 1995;27:175–9.
90. Clement PB. Pure mesenchymal tumors. In: Clement PB, Young RH, editors. Tumors and tumorlike lesions of the uterine corpus and cervix. New York: Churchill Livingstone; 1993. p. 265–328.
91. Gyure KA, Hart WR, Kennedy AW. Lymphangiomyomatosis of the uterus associated with tuberous sclerosis and malignant neoplasia of the female genital tract: a report of two cases. Int J Gynecol Pathol 1995;14:344–51.
92. Thomas EO, Gordon J, Smith-Thomas S, Cramer SF. Diffuse uterine leiomyomatosis with uterine rupture and benign metastatic lesions of the bone. Obstet Gynecol 2007;109:528–30.
93. Miranda-Guardiola F, Josa M, Valls VV, et al. A case of uterine leiomyomatosis extending into the right heart with an unusual echocardiographic appearance. Echocardiography 1997;14: 149–52.
94. Mulvany NJ, Slavin JL, Ostor AG, Fortune DW. Intravenous leiomyomatosis of the uterus: a clinicopathologic study of 22 cases. Int J Gynecol Pathol 1994;13:1–9.
95. Steinmetz OK, Bedard P, Prefontaine ME, et al. Uterine tumor in the heart: intravenous leiomyomatosis. Surgery 1996;119:226–9.
96. Topcuoglu MS, Yaliniz H, Poyrazoglu H, et al. Intravenous leiomyomatosis extending into the right ventricle after subtotal hysterectomy. Ann Thorac Surg 2004;78:330–2.
97. Uchida H, Hattori Y, Nakada K, Iida T. Successful one-stage radical removal of intravenous leiomyomatosis extending to the right ventricle. Obstet Gynecol 2004;103(5 Pt 2):1068–70.
98. Dal Cin P, Quade BJ, Neskey DM, et al. Intravenous leiomyomatosis is characterized by a der(14)t(12;14)(q15;q24). Genes Chromosomes Cancer 2003;36:205–6.
99. Quade BJ, Dal Cin P, Neskey DM, et al. Intravenous leiomyomatosis: molecular and cytogenetic analysis of a case. Mod Pathol 2002;15:351–6.
100. Nogales FF, Navarro N, Martinez de Victoria JM, et al. Uterine intravascular leiomyomatosis: an update and report of seven cases. Int J Gynecol Pathol 1987;6:331–9.
101. Ohmori T, Uraga N, Tabei R, et al. Intravenous leiomyomatosis: a case report emphasizing the vascular component. Histopathology 1988;13:470–2.
102. Clement PB, Young RH, Scully RE. Intravenous leiomyomatosis of the uterus. A clinicopathological analysis of 16 cases with unusual histologic features. Am J Surg Pathol 1988;12:932–45.
103. Lam PM, Lo KW, Yu MM, et al. Intravenous leiomyomatosis with atypical histologic features: a case report. Int J Gynecol Cancer 2003;13:83–7.
104. Coard KC, Fletcher HM. Leiomyosarcoma of the uterus with a florid intravascular component ('intravenous leiomyosarcomatosis'). Int J Gynecol Pathol 2002;21:182–5.
105. Kir G, Kir M, Gurbuz A, et al. Estrogen and progesterone expression of vessel walls with intravascular leiomyomatosis; discussion of histogenesis. Eur J Gynaecol Oncol 2004;25:362–6.
106. Lo KW, Lau TK. Intracardiac leiomyomatosis. Case report and literature review. Arch Gynecol Obstet 2001;264:209–10.
107. Parenti DJ, Morley TF, Giudice JC. Benign metastasizing leiomyoma. A case report and review of the literature. Respiration 1992;59:347–50.
108. Takemura G, Takatsu Y, Kaitani K, et al. Metastasizing uterine leiomyoma. A case with cardiac and pulmonary metastasis. Pathol Res Pract 1996;192:622–9.
109. Cohen DT, Oliva E, Hahn PF, et al. Uterine smooth-muscle tumors with unusual growth patterns: imaging with pathologic correlation. AJR Am J Roentgenol 2007;188:246–55.
110. Lee HJ, Choi J, Kim KR. Pulmonary benign metastasizing leiomyoma associated with intravenous leiomyomatosis of the uterus: clinical behavior and genomic changes supporting a transportation theory. Int J Gynecol Pathol 2008;27:340–5.
111. Crooks DM, Pacheco-Rodriguez G, DeCastro RM, et al. Molecular and genetic analysis of disseminated neoplastic cells in lymphangioleiomyomatosis. Proc Natl Acad Sci USA 2004;101:17462–7.
112. Goncharova EA, Goncharov DA, Spaits M, et al. Abnormal growth of smooth muscle-like cells in lymphangioleiomyomatosis: role for tumor suppressor TSC2. Am J Respir Cell Mol Biol 2006;34: 561–72.
113. Henske EP. Metastasis of benign tumor cells in tuberous sclerosis complex. Genes Chromosomes Cancer 2003;38:376–81.
114. Nucci MR, Dal Cin P, Drapkin R, et al. Unique cytogenetic profile in so-called benign metastasizing leiomyomata: evidence of a distinct clinicopathological entity. Mod Pathol 2003;16:202A.
115. Arif S, Ganesan R, Spooner D. Intravascular leiomyomatosis and benign metastasizing leiomyoma: an unusual case. Int J Gynecol Cancer 2006;16:1448–50.
116. Kayser K, Zink S, Schneider T, et al. Benign metastasizing leiomyoma of the uterus: documentation of clinical, immunohistochemical and lectin-histochemical data of ten cases. Virchows Arch 2000;437:284–92.
117. Tavassoli FA, Norris HJ. Peritoneal leiomyomatosis (leiomyomatosis peritonealis disseminata): a clinicopathologic study of 20 cases with ultrastructural observations. Int J Gynecol Pathol 1982;1: 59–74.
118. Quade BJ, McLachlin CM, Soto-Wright V, et al. Disseminated peritoneal leiomyomatosis. Clonality analysis by X chromosome inactivation and cytogenetics of a clinically benign smooth muscle proliferation. Am J Pathol 1997;150:2153–66.
119. Bekkers RL, Willemsen WN, Schijf CP, et al. Leiomyomatosis peritonealis disseminata: does malignant transformation occur? A literature review. Gynecol Oncol 1999;75:158–63.
120. Rubin SC, Wheeler JE, Mikuta JJ. Malignant leiomyomatosis peritonealis disseminata. Obstet Gynecol 1986;68:126–30.
121. D'Angelo E, Prat J. Uterine sarcomas: a review. Gynecol Oncol 2010;116:131–9.
122. Harlow BL, Weiss NS, Lofton S. The epidemiology of sarcomas of the uterus. J Natl Cancer Inst 1986;76:399–402.
123. Leibsohn S, d'Ablaing G, Mishell Jr DR, et al. Leiomyosarcoma in a series of hysterectomies performed for presumed uterine leiomyomas. Am J Obstet Gynecol 1990;162:968–74.
124. Brooks SE, Zhan M, Cote T, Baquet CR. Surveillance, epidemiology, and end results analysis of 2677 cases of uterine sarcoma 1989–1999. Gynecol Oncol 2004;93:204–8.
125. Perri T, Korach J, Sadetzki S, et al. Uterine leiomyosarcoma: does the primary surgical procedure matter? Int J Gynecol Cancer 2009;19:257–60.
126. Oliva E, Nielsen GP, Clement PB, et al. Epithelioid smooth muscle tumors of the uterus. A clinicopathologic analysis of 80 cases. Lab Invest 1997;76:107A.
127. King ME, Dickersin GR, Scully RE. Myxoid leiomyosarcoma of the uterus. A report of six cases. Am J Surg Pathol 1982;6:589–98.
128. Peacock G, Archer S. Myxoid leiomyosarcoma of the uterus: case report and review of the literature. Am J Obstet Gynecol 1989;160: 1515–18.
129. Kunzel KE, Mills NZ, Muderspach LI, d'Ablaing III G. Myxoid leiomyosarcoma of the uterus. Gynecol Oncol 1993;48:277–80.

130. Salm R, Evans DJ. Myxoid leiomyosarcoma. Histopathology 1985;9:159–69.
131. Taylor HB, Norris HJ. Mesenchymal tumors of the uterus. IV. Diagnosis and prognosis of leiomyosarcomas. Arch Pathol 1966;82:40–4.
132. Mayerhofer K, Obermair A, Windbichler G, et al. Leiomyosarcoma of the uterus: a clinicopathologic multicenter study of 71 cases. Gynecol Oncol 1999;74:196–201.
133. Atkins KA, Arronte N, Darus CJ, Rice LW. The use of p16 in enhancing the histologic classification of uterine smooth muscle tumors. Am J Surg Pathol 2008;32:98–102.
134. Bodner-Adler B, Bodner K, Czerwenka K, et al. Expression of p16 protein in patients with uterine smooth muscle tumors: an immunohistochemical analysis. Gynecol Oncol 2005;96:62–6.
135. Mittal K, Demopoulos RI. MIB-1 (Ki-67), p53, estrogen receptor, and progesterone receptor expression in uterine smooth muscle tumors. Hum Pathol 2001;32:984–7.
136. O'Neill CJ, McBride HA, Connolly LE, McCluggage WG. Uterine leiomyosarcomas are characterized by high p16, p53 and MIB1 expression in comparison with usual leiomyomas, leiomyoma variants and smooth muscle tumors of uncertain malignant potential. Histopathology 2007;50:851–8.
137. Jeffers MD, Farquharson MA, Richmond JA, McNicol AM. P53 immunoreactivity and mutation of the p53 gene in smooth muscle tumours of the uterine corpus. J Pathol 1995;177:65–70.
138. Akhan SE, Yavuz E, Tecer A, et al. The expression of Ki-67, p53, estrogen and progesterone receptors affecting survival in uterine leiomyosarcomas. A clinicopathologic study. Gynecol Oncol 2005;99:36–42.
139. D'Angelo E, Spagnoli LG, Prat J. Comparative clinicopathologic and immunohistochemical analysis of uterine sarcomas diagnosed using the World Health Organization classification system. Hum Pathol 2009;40:1571–85.
140. D'Angelo E, Espinosa I, Ali R, et al. Uterine leiomyosarcomas: tumor size, mitotic index, and biomarkers Ki67, and Bcl-2 identify two groups with different prognosis. Gynecol Oncol 2011;121:328–33.
141. Raspollini MR, Pinzani P, Simi L, et al. Uterine leiomyosarcomas express KIT protein but lack mutation(s) in exon 9 of c-KIT. Gynecol Oncol 2005;98:334–5.
142. Lehtonen HJ, Kiuru M, Ylisaukko-Oja SK, et al. Increased risk of cancer in patients with fumarate hydratase germline mutation. J Med Genet 2006;43:523–6.
143. Ylisaukko-oja SK, Kiuru M, Lehtonen HJ, et al. Analysis of fumarate hydratase mutations in a population-based series of early onset uterine leiomyosarcoma patients. Int J Cancer 2006;119:283–7.
144. Jeffers MD, Richmond JA, Macaulay EM. Overexpression of the c-myc proto-oncogene occurs frequently in uterine sarcomas. Mod Pathol 1995;8:701–4.
145. Hall KL, Teneriello MG, Taylor RR, et al. Analysis of Ki-ras, p53, and MDM2 genes in uterine leiomyomas and leiomyosarcomas. Gynecol Oncol 1997;65:330–5.
146. Trzyna W, McHugh M, McCue P, McHugh KM. Molecular determination of the malignant potential of smooth muscle neoplasms. Cancer 1997;80:211–17.
147. Dei Tos AP, Maestro R, Doglioni C, et al. Tumor suppressor genes and related molecules in leiomyosarcoma. Am J Pathol 1996;148:1037–45.
148. Hu J, Khanna V, Jones M, Surti U. Genomic alterations in uterine leiomyosarcomas: potential markers for clinical diagnosis and prognosis. Genes Chromosomes Cancer 2001;31:117–24.
149. Kawaguchi K, Oda Y, Saito T, et al. Mechanisms of inactivation of the p16INK4a gene in leiomyosarcoma of soft tissue: decreased p16 expression correlates with promoter methylation and poor prognosis. J Pathol 2003;201:487–95.
150. Chou CY, Huang SC, Tsai YC, et al. Uterine leiomyosarcoma has deregulated cell proliferation, but not increased microvessel density compared with uterine leiomyoma. Gynecol Oncol 1997;65:225–31.
151. Jeffers MD, Oakes SJ, Richmond JA, Macaulay EM. Proliferation, ploidy and prognosis in uterine smooth muscle tumours. Histopathology 1996;29:217–23.
152. Lennart K, Lennart B, Ulf S, Bernard T. Flow cytometric analysis of uterine sarcomas. Gynecol Oncol 1994;55(3 Pt 1):339–42.
153. Nola M, Babic D, Ilic J, et al. Prognostic parameters for survival of patients with malignant mesenchymal tumors of the uterus. Cancer 1996;78:2543–50.
154. Fletcher JA, Morton CC, Pavelka K, Lage JM. Chromosome aberrations in uterine smooth muscle tumors: potential diagnostic relevance of cytogenetic instability. Cancer Res 1990;50:4092–7.
155. Sandberg AA. Updates on the cytogenetics and molecular genetics of bone and soft tissue tumors: leiomyosarcoma. Cancer Genet Cytogenet 2005;161:1–19.
156. Quade BJ, Pinto AP, Howard DR, et al. Frequent loss of heterozygosity for chromosome 10 in uterine leiomyosarcoma in contrast to leiomyoma. Am J Pathol 1999;154:945–50.
157. Abeler VM, Royne O, Thoresen S, et al. Uterine sarcomas in Norway. A histopathological and prognostic survey of a total population from 1970 to 2000 including 419 patients. Histopathology 2009;54:355–64.
158. Major FJ, Blessing JA, Silverberg SG, et al. Prognostic factors in early-stage uterine sarcoma: a gynecologic oncology group study. Cancer 1993;71:1702–9.
159. Giuntoli 2nd RL, Gostout BS, DiMarco CS, et al. Diagnostic criteria for uterine smooth muscle tumors: leiomyoma variants associated with malignant behavior. J Reprod Med 2007;52:1001–10.
160. Koivisto-Korander R, Butzow R, Koivisto AM, Leminen A. Clinical outcome and prognostic factors in 100 cases of uterine sarcoma: experience in Helsinki University Central Hospital 1990–2001. Gynecol Oncol 2008;111:74–81.
161. Wang WL, Soslow R, Hensley M, et al. Histopathologic prognostic factors in stage I leiomyosarcoma of the uterus: a detailed analysis of 27 cases. Am J Surg Pathol 2011;35:522–9.
162. Denschlag D, Masoud I, Stanimir G, Gilbert L. Prognostic factors and outcome in women with uterine sarcoma. Eur J Surg Oncol 2007;33:91–5.
163. Larson B, Silfversward C, Nilsson B, et al. Prognostic factors in uterine leiomyosarcoma. Aclinical and histopathological study of 143 cases. The Radiumhemmet series 1936–1981. Acta Oncol 1990;29:185–91.
164. Nordal RR, Kristensen GB, Kaern J, et al. The prognostic significance of stage, tumor size, cellular atypia and DNA ploidy in uterine leiomyosarcoma. Acta Oncol 1995;34:797–802.
165. Kapp DS, Shin JY, Chan JK. Prognostic factors and survival in 1396 patients with uterine leiomyosarcomas: emphasis on impact of lymphadenectomy and oophorectomy. Cancer 2008;112:820–30.
166. Hensley ML, Blessing JA, Mannel R, Rose PG. Fixed-dose rate gemcitabine plus docetaxel as first-line therapy for metastatic uterine leiomyosarcoma: a Gynecologic Oncology Group phase II trial. Gynecol Oncol 2008;109:329–34.
167. Hensley ML, Ishill N, Soslow R, et al. Adjuvant gemcitabine plus docetaxel for completely resected stages I-IV high grade uterine leiomyosarcoma: results of a prospective study. Gynecol Oncol 2009;112:563–7.
168. Hardman MP, Roman JJ, Burnett AF, Santin AD. Metastatic uterine leiomyosarcoma regression using an aromatase inhibitor. Obstet Gynecol 2007;110:518–20.
169. Tavassoli FA, Devilee P, editors. Pathology and genetics of tumors of the breast and female genital organs. Lyon, France: International Agency for Research on Cancer; 2003.
170. Robboy SJ, Mehta K, Norris HJ. Malignant potential and pathology of leiomyomatous tumors of the uterus. Clin Consult Obstet Gynecol 1990;2:2–9.
171. Guntupalli SR, Ramirez PT, Anderson ML, et al. Uterine smooth muscle tumor of uncertain malignant potential: a retrospective analysis. Gynecol Oncol 2009;113:324–6.
172. Ip PP, Cheung AN, Clement PB. Uterine smooth muscle tumors of uncertain malignant potential (STUMP): a clinicopathologic analysis of 16 cases. Am J Surg Pathol 2009;33:992–1005.

Endometrial Stromal Tumors, Mixed Müllerian Tumors, Adenomyosis, Adenomyomas and Rare Sarcomas

Esther Oliva

CHAPTER OUTLINE

Endometrial Stromal Tumors	425
Introduction	425
Endometrial Stromal Nodule	425
Low-Grade Endometrial Stromal Sarcoma	427
High-Grade Endometrial Stromal Sarcoma	435
Undifferentiated Endometrial Sarcoma	435
Uterine Tumors Resembling Ovarian Sex Cord Tumors	436
Mixed Müllerian Tumors	438
Introduction	438
Müllerian Adenofibroma	438
Müllerian Adenosarcoma	439
Malignant Mixed Müllerian Tumor (Carcinosarcoma)	443
Adenomyosis	446
Adenomyomas	447
Endocervical- and Endometrioid-Type Adenomyomas	447
Atypical Polypoid Adenomyoma	449
PEComa	450
Other Rare Sarcomas	452
Rhabdomyosarcoma	452
Primitive Neuroectodermal Tumor (Ewing/Peripheral or Central Types)	453
Alveolar Soft Part Sarcoma	453

ENDOMETRIAL STROMAL TUMORS

INTRODUCTION

Even though endometrial stromal tumors represent the second most common category of mesenchymal tumors of the uterus, they are rare and account for less than 1% of all uterine tumors.[1] Endometrial stromal and related tumors are defined by the latest classification into the following four main categories based on resemblance to (or lack of) proliferative-type endometrial stroma: (1) endometrial stromal nodule, (2) low-grade endometrial stromal sarcoma, (3) high-grade endometrial stromal sarcoma and (4) undifferentiated endometrial sarcoma.[2]

ENDOMETRIAL STROMAL NODULE

Definition

This is a benign endometrial stromal tumor characterized by a well-delineated, expansile margin and composed of neoplastic cells that resemble proliferative phase endometrial stroma supported by a large number of small, thin-walled arteriolar vessels. Small irregularities in the form of finger-like projections or satellite islands ≤3 mm in maximum dimension and <3 in number are allowed.[2]

Clinical Features

Endometrial stromal nodule is the least common of all endometrial stromal tumors. Patients range widely in age (23–86 years) and they often present with abnormal vaginal/postmenopausal bleeding or enlarged uterus.[3,4] However, not infrequently, it is an incidental finding in patients who had a hysterectomy for 'leiomyomas.'

Gross Features

On gross examination, these tumors are centered in the endometrium forming polypoid masses that fill the uterine cavity but almost as frequently they are centered in the myometrium. They range in size from <1 to 22 cm; are well demarcated from the surrounding myometrium; and typically display a fleshy, homogeneous, yellow to tan cut surface (Figure 20.1). Cyst formation (more commonly centrally located) as well as areas of necrosis and/or hemorrhage can be encountered (Figure 20.1).[3,4] Rarely they may be predominantly cystic.[5]

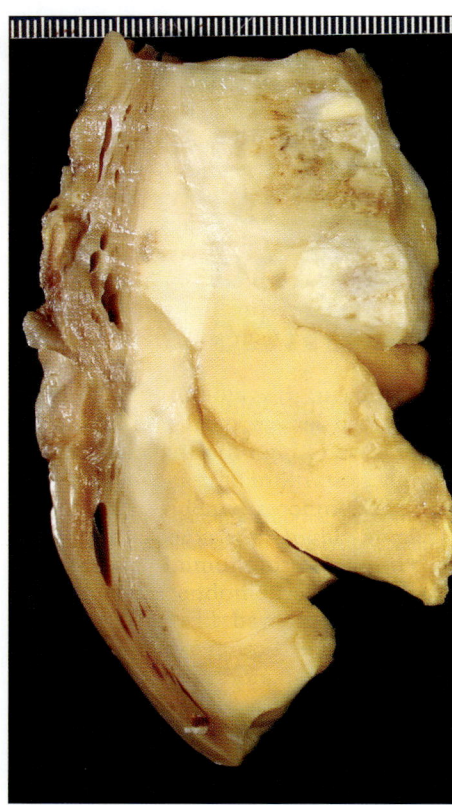

Figure 20.1 Endometrial stromal nodule. The tumor is well circumscribed from the adjacent myometrium and it has a tan to yellow cut surface with focal areas of necrosis and hemorrhage.

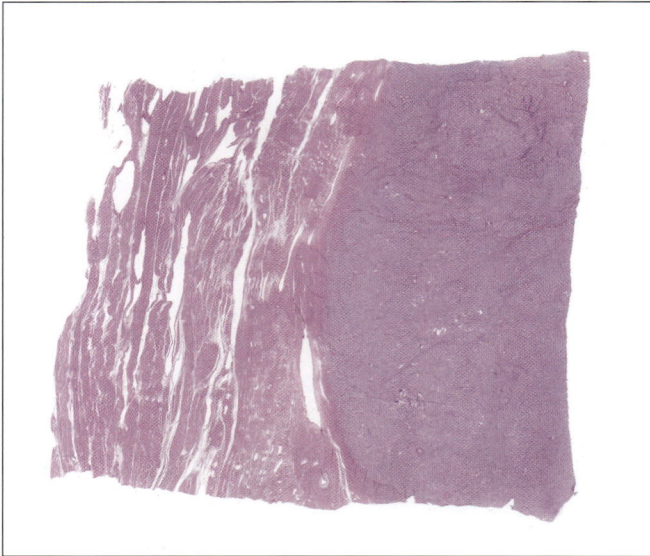

Figure 20.2 Endometrial stromal nodule. A smooth and well-circumscribed border with the surrounding myometrium is characteristic of this tumor.

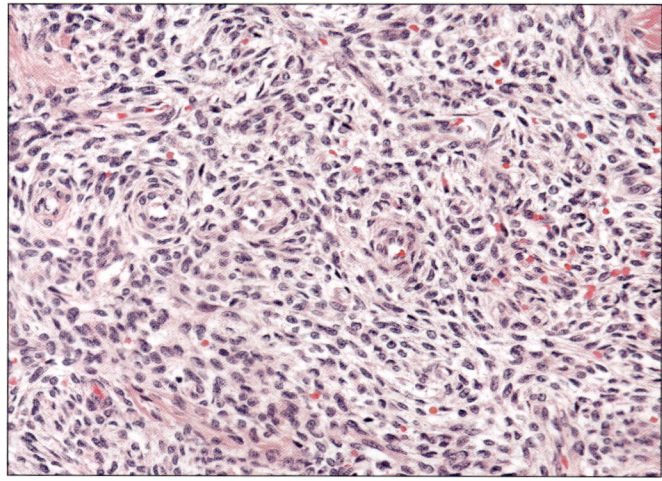

Figure 20.3 Endometrial stromal nodule. The tumor cells are small ('blue') with scant cytoplasm and oval to round nuclei that sometimes whorl around arterioles. The microscopic appearance overlaps with that of low-grade endometrial stromal sarcoma.

Microscopic Features

By definition these tumors should have a well-demarcated non-infiltrative margin with the surrounding myometrium (Figure 20.2). However, small irregularities in the form of finger-like projections or satellite islands ≤3 mm in maximum dimension and <3 in number are allowed.[3,6] The presence of lymphovascular invasion in a well-circumscribed endometrial stromal tumor excludes the diagnosis of endometrial stromal nodule.[2]

The tumor is composed of a diffuse proliferation of monotonous 'blue' cells that resemble proliferative phase endometrial stroma (Figure 20.3). Most of these tumors (if conventional morphology) are densely cellular. The neoplastic cells are small with scant cytoplasm and oval to round nuclei with small nucleoli (minimal cytologic atypia) and variable (sometimes brisk, up to 24/10 HPF) mitotic activity. No atypical mitoses are identified. They have a characteristic network of 'arteriole-like' vessels around which neoplastic cells often whorl, but this feature is only striking in less than one-third of tumors (Figure 20.3). Prominent hyalinization of the vessels as well as thin ectatic blood vessels can be seen. In contrast, large thick blood vessels are uncommon; and when present are typically seen close to the tumor–myometrium interface, probably representing entrapped pre-existent vessels. Another characteristic feature is the finding of collagen bands or plaques distributed randomly within the tumor (Figure 20.4). Foamy histiocytes single or in clusters may be present throughout. Infarct-type necrosis can be seen and may result in confluent hyalinization. Cysts, if present, often form secondary to necrosis or hemorrhage. They are lined by stromal cells that are often admixed with histiocytes and may be associated with cholesterol clefts.[3]

Differential Diagnosis

See following sections in endometrial stromal sarcomas.

Treatment and Prognosis

As endometrial stromal nodules are by definition benign, simple hysterectomy is the treatment of choice. However, a more conservative therapy may be considered in young patients who want to preserve fertility with close follow-up using a combination of ultrasound and hysteroscopy to monitor the growth of the tumor.

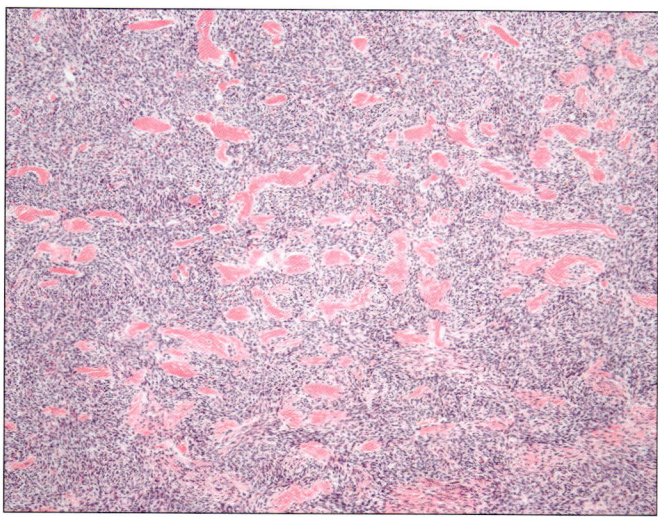

Figure 20.4 Endometrial stromal nodule. Multiple collagen bundles are interspersed among the neoplastic stromal cells.

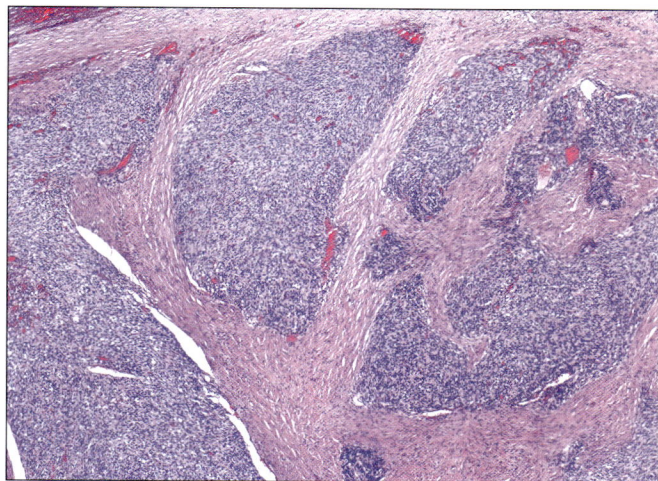

Figure 20.6 Low-grade endometrial stromal sarcoma. The tumor cells form irregular islands that infiltrate the myometrium without an associated desmoplastic response.

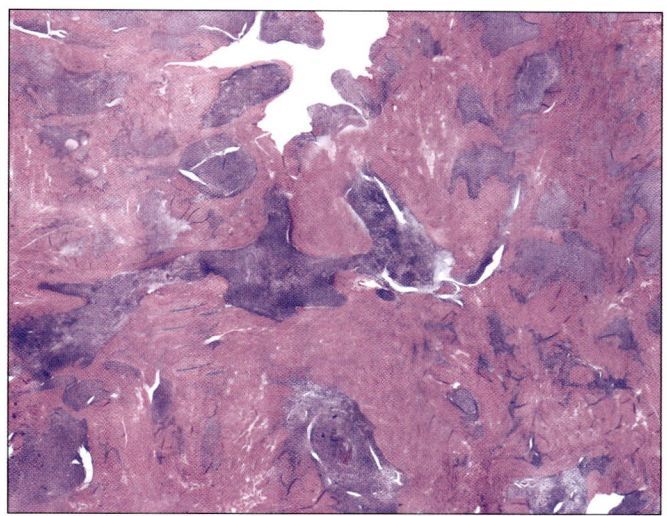

Figure 20.5 Low-grade endometrial stromal sarcoma. The tumor shows a diffuse permeative infiltrative growth.

LOW-GRADE ENDOMETRIAL STROMAL SARCOMA

Definition

Tumor composed of cells resembling those of proliferative phase endometrial stroma often associated with numerous arteriolar-like vessels that shows a permeative infiltrative growth ('tongue-like') into the myometrium with or without associated lymphovascular invasion.[2]

Clinical Features

Among uterine sarcomas, which constitute between 2% and 5% of all uterine malignancies, low-grade endometrial stromal sarcomas account for approximately 0.2–1% of all uterine malignancies and 6–20% of all uterine sarcomas, representing the second most common uterine sarcoma.[1]

These tumors tend to occur in premenopausal and perimenopausal women with a median age of 52 years (wide range) and do not have race predilection.[5,7] Most patients present with nonspecific signs or symptoms, including vaginal bleeding (most common), pelvic pain, and/or dysmenorrhea.[5]

Gross Features

Low-grade endometrial stromal sarcomas are typically poorly defined intracavitary and/or intramyometrial often confluent multinodular masses with a homogeneous soft tan to yellow or less commonly white cut surface. As occurs with endometrial stromal nodules, cyst formation as well as areas of necrosis and/or hemorrhage can be seen. However, in contrast to endometrial stromal nodules, intravascular (typically intravenous) worm-like plugs of tumor are variably present within the myometrium and para-uterine soft tissues (the latter easier to identify).[5,8–10] Of note, some low-grade endometrial stromal sarcomas display deceptively well-circumscribed borders due to very limited myometrial invasion that cannot be noticed on gross examination, closely mimicking the appearance of an endometrial stromal nodule. Thus, careful sampling of the tumor–myometrium interface is necessary in order to identify these areas and to establish a diagnosis of low-grade endometrial stromal sarcoma.[3]

Microscopic Features

Low-grade endometrial stromal sarcomas show an irregular interface with the myometrium with a tongue-like pattern of infiltration where irregularly shaped islands of tumor cells are unassociated with a stromal response (Figures 20.5 and 20.6). On high-power examination, the cytologic features are identical to those encountered in endometrial stromal nodules. Tumors are very cellular ('blue') and cells typically grow in sheets or vaguely storiform pattern; they have scant cytoplasm and uniform, oval to spindle-shaped nuclei with very small nucleolus (Figure 20.3). The neoplastic cells may focally whorl around small vessels

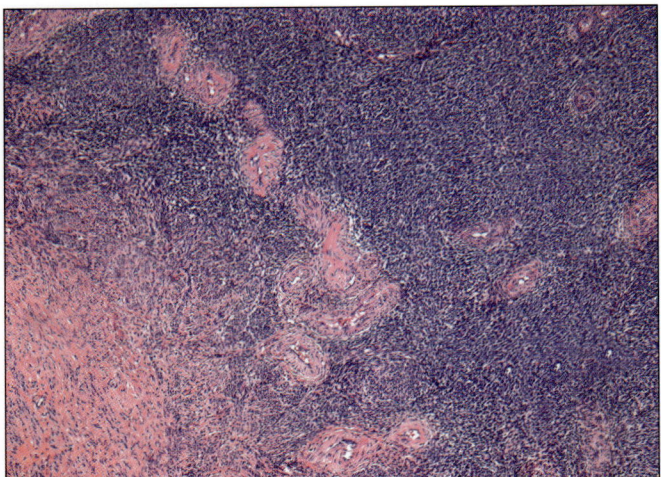

Figure 20.7 Low-grade endometrial stromal sarcoma. Thick blood vessels, most likely entrapped, are seen at the periphery of the tumor islands.

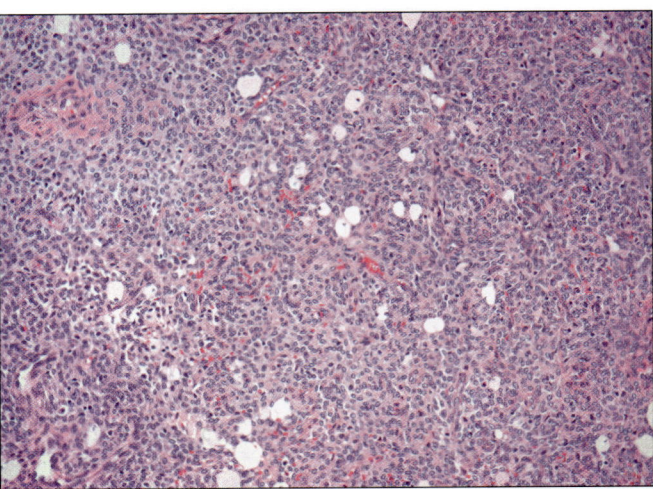

Figure 20.8 Low-grade endometrial stromal sarcoma. Stromal foam cells are interspersed between the neoplastic endometrial stromal cells. They may represent histiocytes, tumor cells, or both.

reminiscent of the arterioles seen in proliferative phase endometrium. By definition, significant degrees of nuclear atypia are absent and mitotic rate is usually <5/10 HPF but higher mitotic activity does not exclude this diagnosis. It is important to remember that tumors with typical morphology and characteristic tongue-like growth should be classified as low-grade endometrial stromal sarcoma regardless of their mitotic counts as the latter does not impact prognosis in this category of tumors. Arteriolar walls may be thickened due to hyalinization. Sometimes vessels may be thin and elongated, with a hemangiopericytoma-like morphology; however, thick blood vessels are uncommon and when present are located at the periphery of the tumor islands (Figure 20.7), likely being entrapped. Histiocytes (Figure 20.8), hyaline bands or plaques, and cholesterol clefts often next to areas of necrosis or cyst formation, as seen in endometrial stromal nodules, can also be noticed.[5,8–10]

ENDOMETRIAL STROMAL VARIANTS

Both endometrial stromal nodule and endometrial stromal sarcoma display the following types of differentiation (Table 20.1):

1. *Smooth muscle:* this type of differentiation has been reported in the literature based on morphologic, immunohistochemical, and ultrastructural studies.[5,11–16] As prognosis of these tumors relates to margin status of the endometrial stromal component, currently these tumors are defined as endometrial stromal neoplasms (nodule or sarcoma) in which the smooth muscle component accounts for >30% on H&E evaluation. On gross examination, the smooth muscle component may be seen as whitish and firm areas (if prominent) in contrast to the endometrial stromal component (soft and yellow-tan to light brown). On microscopic examination, smooth muscle differentiation can be seen as pale to 'pink' irregular islands of slightly epithelioid cells or much more characteristically as the so-called 'starburst' pattern present in a background of endometrial stromal neoplasia (Figure 20.9). The latter is characterized by a

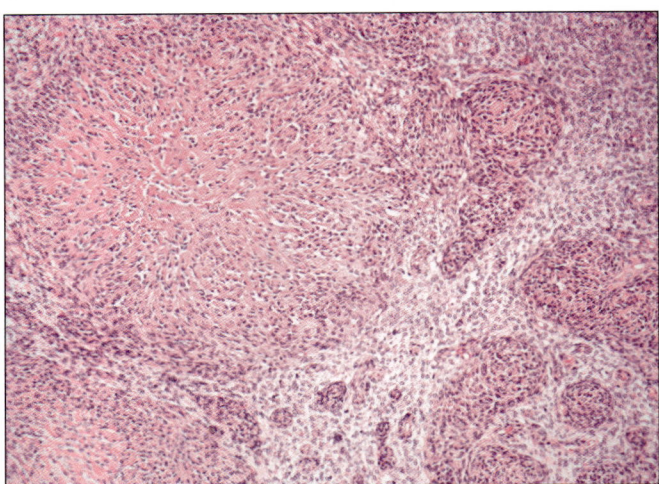

Figure 20.9 Low-grade endometrial stromal sarcoma with smooth muscle differentiation. A nodule of smooth muscle differentiation shows a central area of hyalinization with bands of collagen radiating toward the periphery where 'plump' cells are embedded (starburst pattern), which in turn form small fascicles of smooth muscle in a background of endometrial stromal neoplasia.

Table 20.1 Variant Features of Endometrial Stromal Tumors

1. Smooth muscle metaplasia
2. Myxoid and fibroblastic differentiation
3. Sex cord-like elements
4. Müllerian-type glands
5. Skeletal muscle differentiation
6. Epithelioid features
7. Rhabdoid appearance
8. Clear cytoplasm
9. Papillae/pseudopapillae
10. Adipose metaplasia
11. Bizarre nuclei
12. Osteoclast-type cells

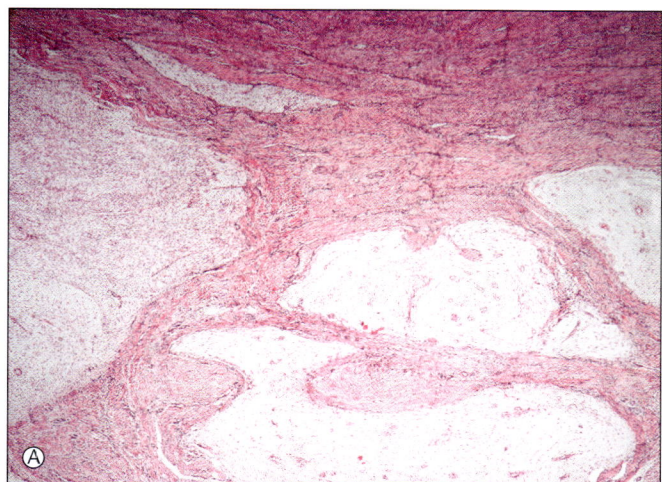

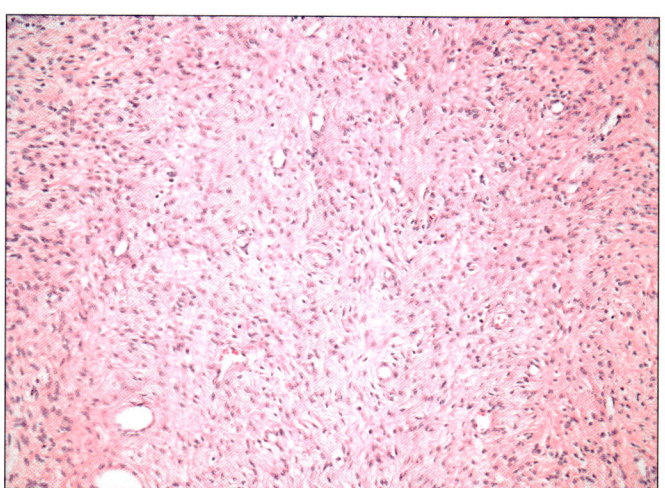

Figure 20.11 Endometrial stromal nodule with fibroblastic differentation. The tumor shows a prominent loose collagenous background.

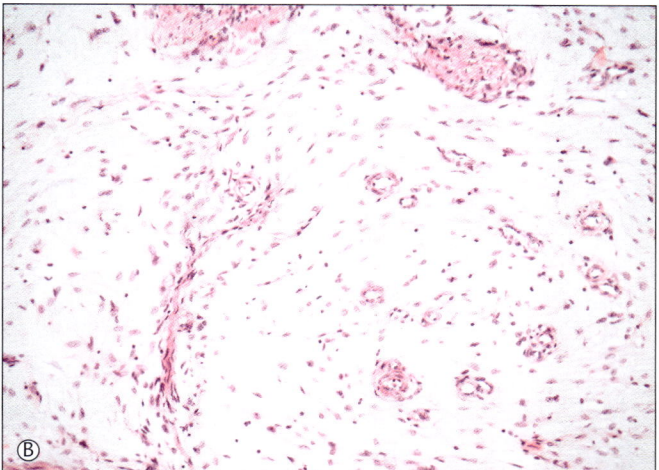

Figure 20.10 Low-grade endometrial stromal sarcoma with myxoid change. The tumor is strikingly hypocellular in contrast to conventional endometrial stromal sarcoma. However, it shows the typical 'tongue-like' pattern of infiltration **(A)** as well as the characteristic arterioles **(B)**.

central area of hyalinization from which collagen bands radiate toward the periphery and cells with an 'epithelioid' appearance are embedded in collagen fibers. These epithelioid cells form short and nonorganized fascicles of smooth muscle that in turn may transition into long and well-formed fascicles.[16] These starburst areas are often seen at the periphery of the tumor and they may also be present next to areas of 'sex cord-like' differentiation.[17] The smooth muscle cells are typically cytologically benign but rarely a malignant smooth muscle component has been reported.[16]

2. *Myxoid and fibroblastic*: these unusual types of differentiation are characterized either by prominent myxoid or by fibroblastic (loose collagen) background (Figures 20.10A and B, and 20.11) imparting a hypocellular appearance to the tumors in contrast to their typical hypercellular nature.[18,19] On gross examination, they can have a gelatinous (if myxoid) or firm and white (if fibroblastic) cut surface. However, other characteristic morphologic features of endometrial stromal neoplasia are present including the typical 'tongue' pattern of infiltration if low-grade sarcoma and arteriole-like vessels (Figure 20.10A and B). Cells are small with scant cytoplasm and oval to spindle shaped with minimal cytologic atypia and mitotic activity. Areas of conventional endometrial stromal neoplasm may be seen. Noteworthy, a fibroblastic component has been reported in approximately 50% of endometrial stromal tumors with *t(10;17)*, which are known to have a predominant high-grade round cell component and aggressive behavior (Figures 20.12 and 20.13).[20]

3. *Sex cord-like elements* have been reported with a variable frequency and extent in endometrial stromal tumors (up to 60%).[3,5,13,21–27] They consist of anastomosing cords, trabeculae, islands, small nests, tubules that may be retiform, or sheets of cells reminiscent of the patterns seen in granulosa and/or Sertoli cell tumors of the ovary (Figure 20.14). Cells typically show scant to abundant cytoplasm and round to oval nuclei, sometimes with grooves, indistinct or tiny nucleoli, and minimal mitotic activity. These sex cord-like elements are present within a background of typical endometrial stromal neoplasia or in a loose hypocellular background. Not infrequently they coexist with areas of smooth muscle differentiation, and in these instances both elements often merge imperceptibly with one another.[17]

4. *Glandular elements* may vary in number, but can be quite extensive. They can be seen in endometrial stromal nodules[4] but have been reported more frequently in endometrial stromal sarcomas.[15,28,29] Glands range from small and round (proliferative) to slightly irregular or cystically dilated (inactive). They have an endometrioid morphology, lined by cuboidal to columnar cells with eosinophilic and rarely clear cytoplasm and pseudostratified nuclei, which display a minimal degree of cytologic atypia in most cases (Figure 20.15).[4,15,28,29] Foci of grade I endometrioid carcinoma have been occasionally reported.[28]

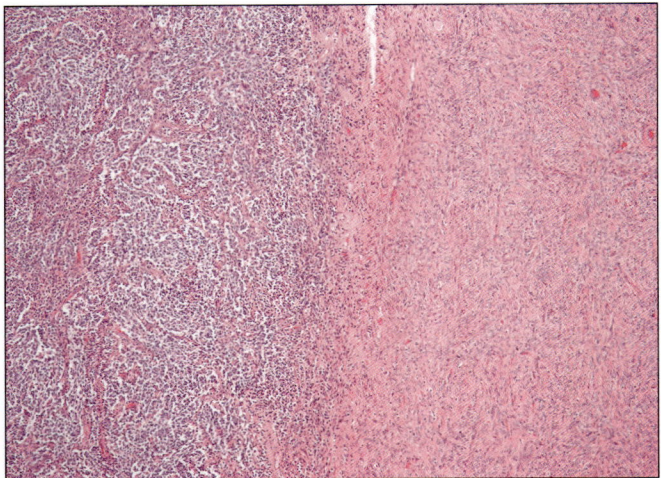

Figure 20.12 t(10;17) high-grade endometrial stromal sarcoma. Tumor cells with an epithelioid morphology (left) are juxtaposed to areas of endometrial stromal neoplasia with a fibroblastic appearance.

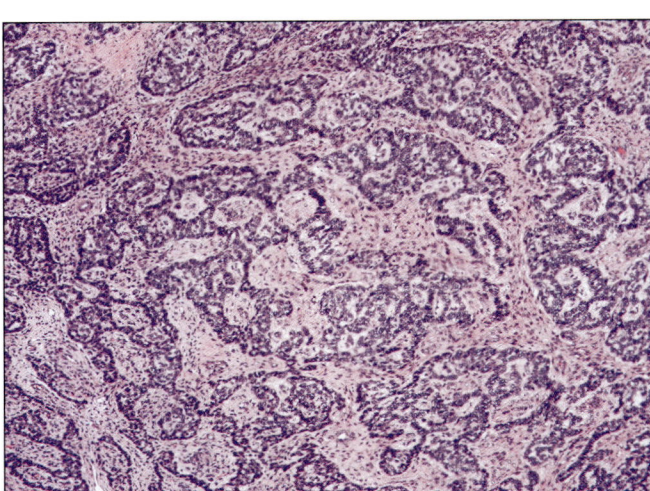

Figure 20.14 Low-grade endometrial stromal sarcoma with sex cord-like elements. Inter-anastomosing cords and trabeculae of 'epithelial-like' cells with architecture reminiscent of that of a granulosa cell tumor of the ovary are present in a background of neoplastic endometrial stromal cells.

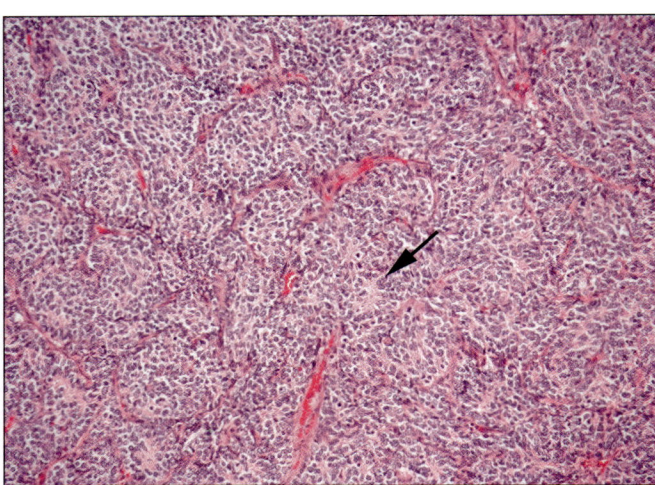

Figure 20.13 t(10;17) high-grade endometrial stromal sarcoma. The epithelioid areas are composed of cells with high-grade cytologic features and brisk mitotic activity. Pseudorosettes may be seen (arrow).

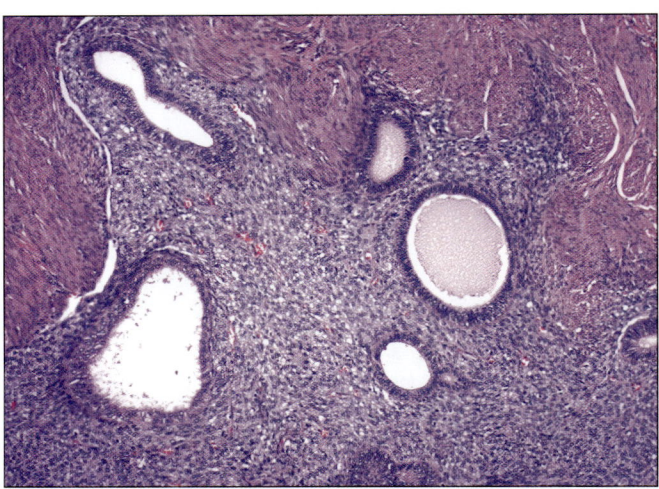

Figure 20.15 Low-grade endometrial stromal sarcoma with müllerian glandular elements. Benign endometrioid-type glands, with a slightly proliferative appearance, are present in an island of tumor.

5. *Skeletal muscle* may be seen as large cells with copious bright eosinophilic cytoplasm and abundant filament deposits typically wrapping around nuclei as well as cells having a strap-shaped morphology with cross striations. These cells are positive for myoglobin, myo-D1, and myogenin.[14,30]
6. *Epithelioid appearance* is defined as cells having abundant eosinophilic cytoplasm that confers an oval to polygonal appearance to the cells. This morphologic feature may be extensive within a given endometrial stromal tumor (up to 90% of cells).[3,31] Some of these cells may also have a granular quality of the cytoplasm (Figure 20.16).[31] Cells have bland cytologic features in contrast to the epithelioid cells seen in t(10;17) endometrial stromal tumors. This appearance has to be also distinguished from pseudodecidualization of neoplastic stromal cells that can occur in these tumors.
7. *Rhabdoid morphology* can be seen in endometrial stromal tumors more frequently in areas displaying sex cord-like differentiation. Cells characteristically have large eosinophilic hyaline cytoplasmic inclusions and eccentric vesicular nuclei often with prominent nucleoli.[25,26] By electron microscopy, abundant paranuclear deposits of intermediate filaments have been noted.[25]
8. *Cells with abundant clear cytoplasm* may rarely be seen,[32] adding to the differential diagnosis of uterine mesenchymal tumors with clear cells.
9. *True papillae and pseudopapillae* have been reported in endometrial stromal tumors, mostly endometrial

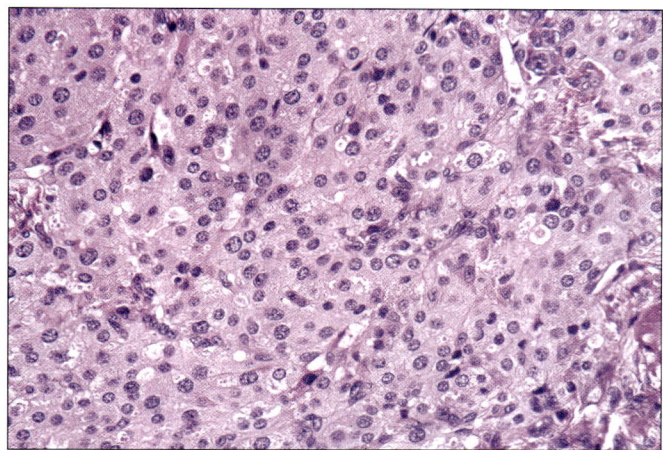

Figure 20.16 Low-grade endometrial stromal sarcoma with epithelioid cells. In contrast to the t(10;17) high-grade endometrial stromal sarcoma, the tumor cells have abundant eosinophilic granular cytoplasm and uniform round nuclei with no cytologic atypia.

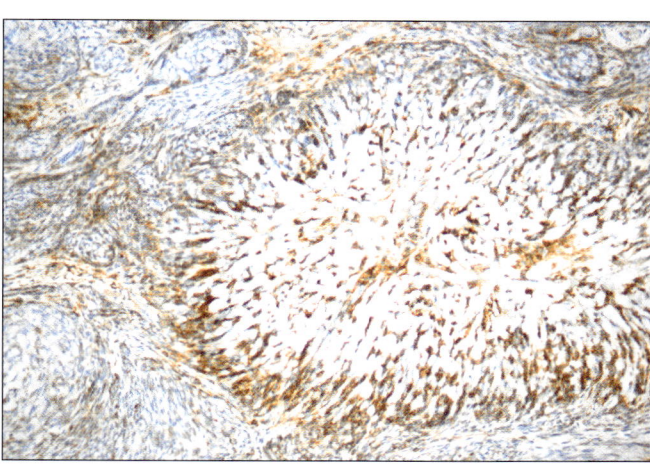

Figure 20.18 Low-grade endometrial stromal sarcoma with smooth muscle differentiation. Desmin immunoreaction highlights the smooth muscle component ('starburst') with minimal reaction of the background endometrial stroma.

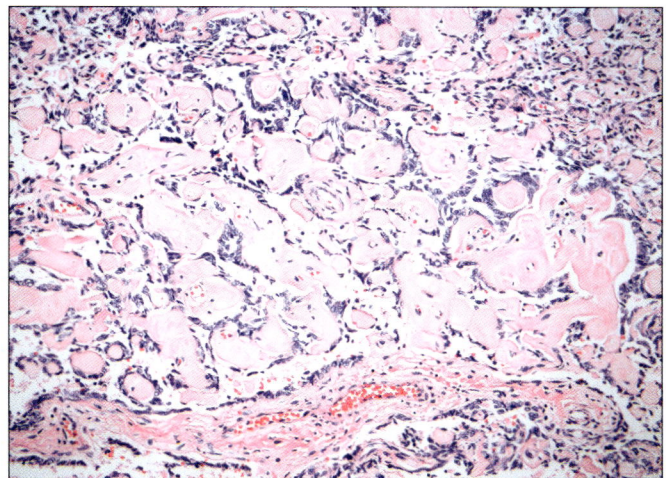

Figure 20.17 Low-grade endometrial stromal sarcoma with pseudopapillae. The tumor shows non-cohesive neoplastic endometrial stromal cells associated with abundant collagen imparting a pseudopapillary architecture.

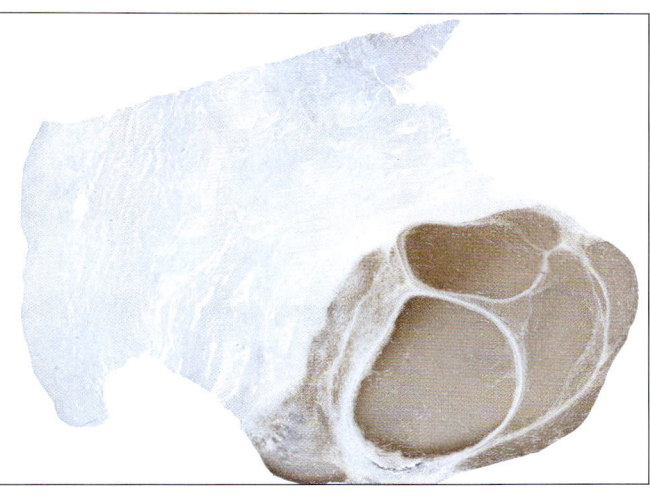

Figure 20.19 Low-grade endometrial stromal sarcoma. The infiltrating islands of tumor display diffuse and strong immunoreaction for CD10.

stromal sarcomas, either primary or metastatic, and may be a focal or diffuse finding. Papillae or pseudopapillae are typically small with angulated outlines and may have a glomeruloid appearance. They are lined by stromal cells, which are also present within the vascular cores associated with small vessels (Figure 20.17).[33]

10. *Mature adipose tissue* can occasionally be seen admixed with the neoplastic endometrial stromal cells.[30]
11. *Cells with bizarre nuclei* as noted more commonly in benign smooth muscle tumors (leiomyomas with bizarre nuclei) can rarely occur. They may be mononucleated or multinucleated and typically have nuclei with smudged chromatin and occasional intranuclear cytoplasmic inclusions.[30,31,34]
12. *Osteoclast-type cells* have also been reported in one endometrial stromal sarcoma.[35]

Immunohistochemical Features

Endometrial stromal tumors similar to normal endometrial stroma are surrounded by a network of reticulin fibers that can be highlighted by a reticulin stain. These tumors are also diffusely positive for vimentin, muscle-specific and smooth muscle actin, and often for keratins.[36,37] Areas of conventional endometrial stromal neoplasia show variable positivity (up to 30%) for desmin. Smooth muscle differentiation and sex cord-like elements are extensively positive for desmin and often for h-caldesmon, histone deacetylase (HDAC-8), and smooth muscle myosin (Figure 20.18).[11,13,18,37–40] CD10 is a very helpful marker in the diagnosis of endometrial stromal tumors as they typically display diffuse and strong immunoreactivity (Figure 20.19).[40,41] However, some tumors may only be weakly and focally positive or completely negative as typically occurs in t(10;17) endometrial stromal tumors[20]

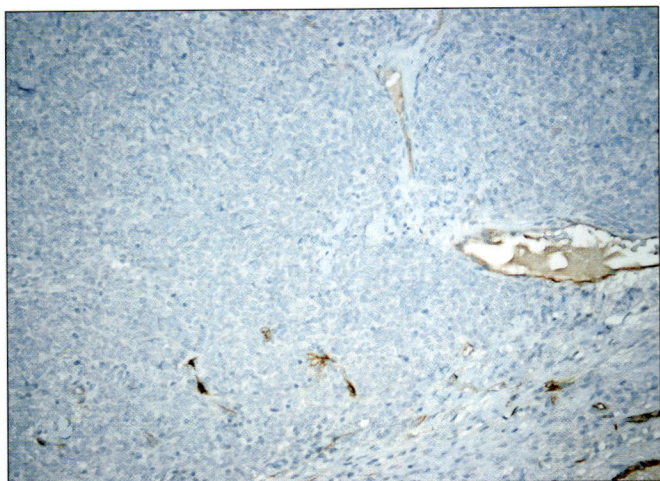

Figure 20.20 t(10;17) high-grade endometrial stromal sarcoma. CD10 staining is completely negative in the cytologically high-grade epithelioid component.

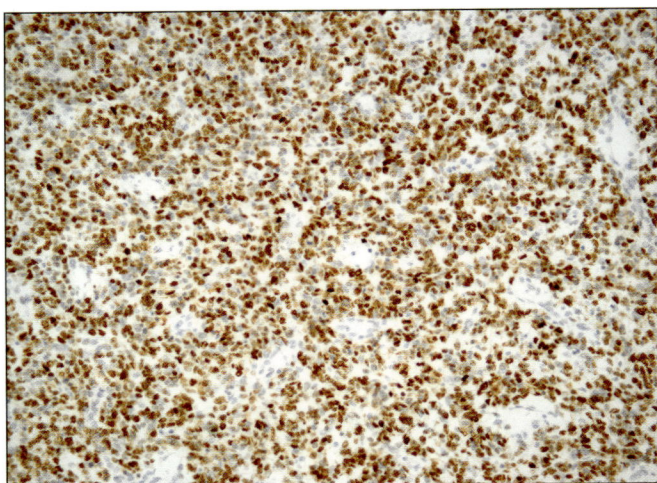

Figure 20.22 t(10;17) high-grade endometrial stromal sarcoma. The high-grade epithelioid areas are strongly and diffusely reactive for cyclin D1.

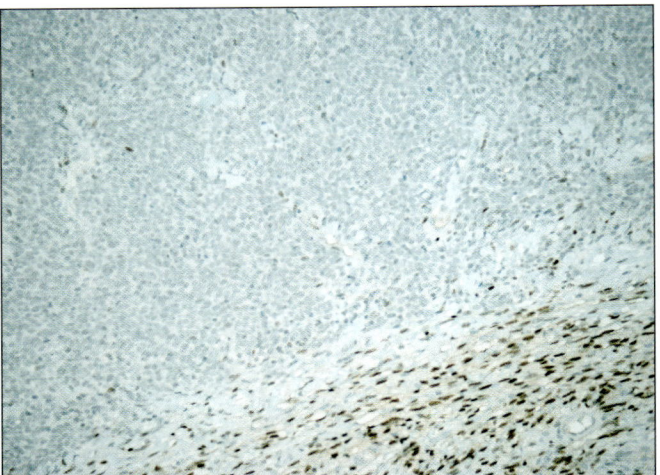

Figure 20.21 t(10;17) high-grade endometrial stromal sarcoma. The tumor cells are negative for ER in contrast to the adjacent fibroblastic component (ER positive).

(Figure 20.20) and undifferentiated endometrial sarcomas of pleomorphic type.[42] CD10 can also be positive in smooth muscle and sex cord-like areas.[40]

Endometrial stromal tumors express estrogen (ER) and progesterone (PR) receptors.[43,44] In contrast to normal endometrial stroma (ER-α and ER-β positive), endometrial stromal sarcoma cells typically express ER-α (involved in cellular proliferation) but not ER-β (involved in apoptosis). PR-A is overexpressed over PR-B in neoplastic endometrial stromal cells except in recurrences where PR-B expression is higher than PR-A.[45] The majority of endometrial stromal sarcomas with high-grade cytologic features, including endometrial stromal sarcomas with t(10;17) and undifferentiated endometrial sarcomas (especially if pleomorphic), are ER and PR negative (Figure 20.21).[20,45–48] Low-grade endometrial stromal sarcomas may also express androgen receptors with rare undifferentiated endometrial sarcomas being also positive.[49] Aromatase, which participates in extra-ovarian estrogen production, is expressed in endometrial stromal sarcomas, most frequently if high stage.[50]

WT1 is positive in non-neoplastic endometrial stroma as well as in endometrial stromal tumors.[51] Sex cord–stromal markers including inhibin, calretinin, CD99, and Melan-A (also known as Mart-1) can be positive in areas of epithelial (sex cord-like) differentiation.[21,24]

c-Kit has been reported to be positive in a small percentage of endometrial stromal tumors, but no mutation has been found.[52] It appears that c-kit may be more often positive in endometrial stromal sarcomas with high-grade cytologic features (especially if t(10;17)).

Nuclear β-catenin expression has been shown in up to 40% of low-grade endometrial stromal sarcomas[42] as well as in uniform undifferentiated endometrial sarcomas, the latter frequently associated with cyclin D1 expression and thought to be part of t(10;17) group of tumors.[42] p53 expression is typically absent in low-grade endometrial stromal sarcomas, but it has been reported in high-grade/undifferentiated endometrial sarcomas (more often if pleomorphic subtype, as expected).[48,53] Cyclin D1 is mostly expressed in endometrial stromal sarcomas with t(10;17)[54] (Figure 20.22), although rarely it has been detected in endometrial stromal nodules and low-grade endometrial stromal sarcomas, as well as uniform-type undifferentiated endometrial sarcomas.[42]

Differential Diagnosis

Among non-neoplastic processes, endometrial stromal tumors should be distinguished from *endometrial polyps* especially in curettage specimens if the polyp is fragmented and cellular and some fragments are only composed of endometrial stroma. In contrast to endometrial stromal tumors, stromal cells have an inactive 'compacted' appearance with unassociated mitotic activity. Even though small vessels reminiscent of the arterioles seen in endometrial stromal tumors may be present, large thick blood vessels are also found. Furthermore, some fragments may show inactive stromal cells admixed with endometrial glands.[55]

CHAPTER 20 — ENDOMETRIAL STROMAL TUMORS, MIXED MÜLLERIAN TUMORS, ADENOMYOSIS, ADENOMYOMAS   433

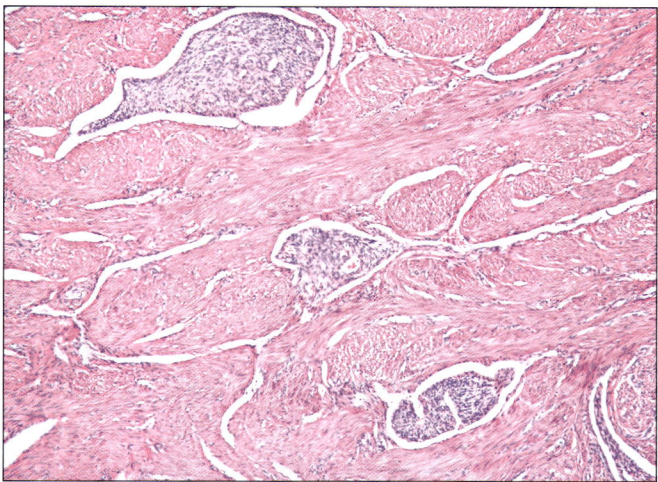

Figure 20.23 Gland-poor adenomyosis. Several islands of adenomyosis composed only of gland-free endometrial stroma are present within the myometrium. The stromal cells have an inactive and solid appearance.

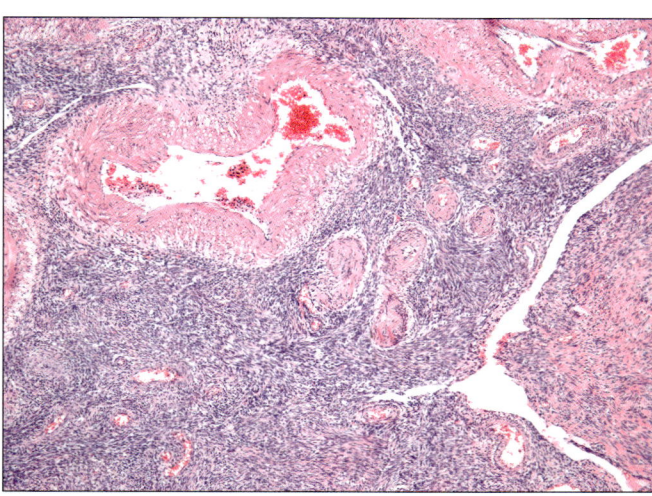

Figure 20.24 Highly cellular leiomyoma. The tumor has a vague fascicular architecture. Large and thick blood vessels as well as cleft-like spaces characteristic of this neoplasm are seen.

Gland-poor adenomyosis or intravascular adenomyosis (Figure 20.23) can be occasionally confused with an endometrial stromal sarcoma. Grossly these lesions do not form a mass but at most an irregular thickening or irregularity of the myometrial wall and typically represent an incidental finding. The islands of endometrial stroma have an inactive appearance without expansile borders in contrast to endometrial stromal sarcomas and areas of conventional adenomyosis are always identified.[56] However, endometrial stromal sarcomas may arise from adenomyotic foci as well as endometriosis.

A common pitfall is the misdiagnosis of a *highly cellular leiomyoma* as an endometrial stromal tumor, more frequently as a low-grade endometrial stromal sarcoma (Table 20.2). Highly cellular leiomyoma shares with the latter the following features: soft consistency and tan to yellow cut surface, dense cellularity ('blue'), striking vascularity, and irregular margins with the surrounding myometrium.[57] However, it also typically forms fascicles (easier to identify at its periphery), cells are spindled with elongated 'cigar-shaped' nuclei, and there is merging of the tumor cells with the surrounding myometrium. Small vessels can be found and may be misinterpreted as arterioles, but they do not show the morphology of typical arterioles seen in endometrial stromal tumors. Thick and large blood vessels and cleft-like spaces throughout the tumor are almost constant features of these tumors (Figure 20.24).[57] Some smooth muscle tumors may contain highly cellular areas alternating with conventional areas. If the latter are misinterpreted as myometrium, cellular areas may be diagnosed as endometrial stromal sarcoma. Gross evaluation as well as microscopic distinction of myometrium from neoplastic smooth muscle is key in rendering the correct diagnosis. Immunohistochemistry may be helpful in this differential diagnosis. As actins are positive in both categories of tumors they should not be used. CD10, although reported to be specific of endometrial stromal derivation, is often positive in highly cellular leiomyomas and thus should not be used in isolation. Muscle markers, including desmin, h-caldesmon, heavy chain myosin, and HDAC-8 are typically diffusely positive in smooth muscle tumors but can be positive in areas of conventional stromal neoplasia (desmin) and areas with smooth muscle or sex cord-like differentiation (desmin, h-caldesmon, heavy chain myosin).[19,38,40,58] Thus, using a panel of antibodies, which includes CD10, desmin, and h-caldesmon (or other specific smooth muscle markers), is most helpful in this differential diagnosis. It is also important to correlate positive areas with the corresponding morphologies of the

Table 20.2 Contrasting Features of Endometrial Stromal Tumors (ESTs) and Highly Cellular Leiomyomas (HCLs)

	EST	HCL
Yellow	Typical	Less common
Gross circumscription	Poor (if sarcoma)	Well demarcated
Microscopic circumscription	Poor (if sarcoma)	Limited interdigitation and merging with myometrium
Large thick blood vessels	Occasional (mostly at periphery)	Common (random)
Arterioles	Usual	Uncommon
Clefts	Rare	Common
Foamy histiocytes	Frequent	Rare
CD10 positivity	Diffuse and strong, in most	Up to 40% positive
Desmin positivity	Occasional (usual forms) Expected (if smooth muscle metaplasia)	Typical, diffuse
h-Caldesmon positivity	Negative (usual forms) Expected (if smooth muscle metaplasia)	Typical, diffuse

tumor. Oxytocin has also been used in the differential diagnosis of smooth muscle tumors and endometrial stromal tumors, the latter being typically negative.[59]

Cellular intravenous leiomyomatosis can enter in the differential diagnosis of endometrial stromal sarcomas due to their dense cellularity and intravascular growth especially if associated with a highly cellular leiomyoma. However, in most cases, the microscopic appearance of intravenous leiomyomatosis recapitulates that of typical leiomyomas showing a fascicular growth and large and thick blood vessels, as well as cleft-like spaces[60] and not infrequently a subendothelial proliferation of spindle cells may be seen 'colonizing' the walls of the veins.

Endometrial stromal tumors with myxoid differentiation should be distinguished from *myxoid smooth muscle tumors*, often leiomyosarcoma, as both tend to be hypocellular with a similar pattern of myometrial infiltration. However, extensive sampling should evidence a component of spindle or epithelioid leiomyosarcoma with highly atypical cells and brisk mitotic activity. Immunohistochemistry may be of limited utility as some endometrial stromal tumors with fibroblastic and/or myxoid background are positive for desmin[18] and positivity for muscle markers may be limited in myxoid smooth muscle tumors. If positive, p53 may favor a diagnosis of myxoid leiomyosarcoma as p53 positivity is restricted to undifferentiated endometrial sarcomas.[48,53]

Endometrial stromal tumors with sex cord-like differentiation should be distinguished from *uterine tumors resembling ovarian sex cord tumors* (*UTROSCTs*), as the latter lack any component of endometrial stromal neoplasia[22] (see the section Uterine tumors resembling ovarian sex cord tumors).

Endometrial stromal sarcomas with *t(10;17)* should be distinguished from *epithelioid leiomyosarcoma* and *epithelioid gastrointestinal stromal tumor secondarily involving the uterus* as all have epithelioid cells. Furthermore, *t(10;17)* endometrial stromal sarcomas are frequently CD10, ER, and PR negative and c-kit positive in the high-grade epithelioid areas,[20] creating a diagnostic challenge. As mentioned earlier, this morphologic variant of endometrial stromal sarcoma is associated with a low-grade fibroblastic component in 50% of cases, which, if present, may help to establish the correct diagnosis. These tumors are cyclin D1 positive while epithelioid leiomyosarcomas are typically desmin and caldesmon positive, often keratin and epithelial membrane antigen (EMA) positive,[40] and cyclin D1 negative.[54] Gastrointestinal stromal tumors present as one or multiple masses typically centered outside the uterus and they are positive for DOG-1 and to a lesser extent CD34 along with c-kit.[61]

Cytogenetics

t(7;17)(p15;q21) is the most common chromosomal translocation in endometrial stromal tumors resulting in the *JAZF1–SUZ12* gene fusion (Figure 20.25). It can be detected by cytogenetics, fluorescence *in situ* hybridization, or reverse transcriptase polymerase chain reaction (PCR). It has been reported in the majority of endometrial stromal nodules, approximately 50% of low-grade endometrial stromal sarcomas, and a minority of undifferentiated endometrial sarcomas, typically those classified as uniform type.[62–67] The presence of the *JAZF1–SUZ12* gene fusion in at least 50% of endometrial stromal nodules and in a significant, but smaller, subset of low-grade endometrial stromal sarcomas

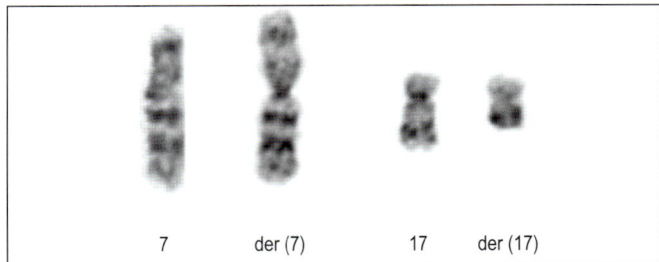

Figure 20.25 Low-grade endometrial stromal sarcoma. Karyotype analysis shows the common translocation involving chromosomes 7 and 17. (Courtesy of Paola Dal Cin.)

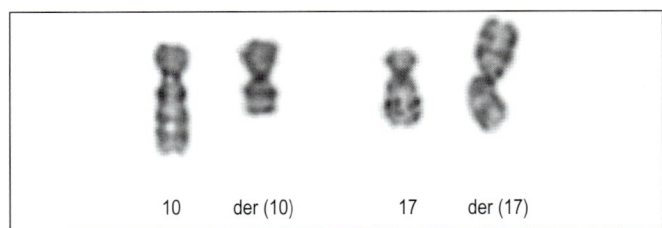

Figure 20.26 *t(10;17)* high-grade endometrial stromal sarcoma. *t(10;17)(q22;p13)* with genetic fusion between YWHAE and FAM22 occurs in a subset of high-grade endometrial stromal sarcomas that in 50% of cases has a concomitant low-grade fibromyxoid component. (Courtesy of Paola Dal Cin.)

suggests that *JAZF1–SUZ12* fusion represents an early event in the development of endometrial stromal tumors, and that additional events are necessary for tumor progression. The finding of identical translocations in occasional undifferentiated endometrial sarcomas and low-grade endometrial stromal sarcomas may indicate that at least some of the former tumors represent progression from low-grade tumors. The *JAZF1–SUZ12* cytogenetic abnormality has also been detected in morphologic variants of endometrial stromal tumors including those with smooth muscle, fibroblastic/myxoid, epithelioid, and sex cord-like differentiation, although to a lesser extent.[17,23,48,68,69] *t(6;17)(p21;p22)* and its variants represent the second most common cytogenetic abnormalities in endometrial stromal tumors.[66,70,71] A three-way *t(6p10q;10p)* has also been reported.[71] In general, it appears that there is no correlation between specific variant histologic subtypes and gene fusions among endometrial stromal tumors. However, recently, a *t(10;17)(q22;p13)* with genetic fusion between YWHAE and FAM22 (Figure 20.26)[66,72] has been reported in a subset of high-grade endometrial stromal sarcomas with a concomitant low-grade fibromyxoid component in 50% of cases. Also, *PHF1* genetic rearrangement has been found to occur more frequently in endometrial stromal sarcomas with sex cord differentiation than other morphologic variants.[73]

Treatment and Prognosis

Low-grade endometrial stromal sarcoma is a relatively indolent mesenchymal tumor with an overall 70–84% and 65–76% 5 and 10 year survival rate, respectively. Recurrences are common (in approximately half of patients), typically occurring years after the initial diagnosis. The most frequent sites include pelvis and abdomen but the tumor can also recur in lung and other locations.[10,74] Surgical–pathologic stage is the most powerful prognostic factor. It has been found that patients with tumors confined to the uterus (stage I or II) had an 89% 5 year disease-specific survival compared to 50% in patients with stage III or IV tumors.[7] Regarding the impact of stage, cytologic atypia, and mitotic activity in endometrial stromal sarcomas, by univariate analysis, brisk mitotic activity has correlated with poor outcome while cytologic atypia correlated with increased relapse although not with overall survival. However, by multivariate analysis, both parameters lost their predictive impact in stage I tumors in the largest study to date.[8] In a recent study, mitotic count and tumor cell necrosis were reported to be important prognostic factors in stage I endometrial stromal sarcomas and in conjunction could be used to stratify patients with low-grade endometrial stromal sarcomas into three prognostic categories.[75] Others, however, have found no association of tumor cell necrosis with prognosis.[8] Patients with endometrial stromal sarcomas are treated with radical hysterectomy and bilateral salpingo-oophorectomy to avoid secondary hormonal stimulation of the tumor. Younger patients who desire to preserve fertility can be treated with radiation, hormonal therapy, or aromatase inhibitors.[50] Gonadotropin-releasing hormone (GnRH) analogs can also be used as an adjunct as they reduce estrogen production in the ovaries.[75] Tumors with *t(10;17)* should be treated aggressively with a combination of radiation and chemotherapy as they do not respond to conventional treatment for low-grade endometrial stromal sarcoma.[20]

HIGH-GRADE ENDOMETRIAL STROMAL SARCOMA

Definition

This is malignant tumor of endometrial stromal derivation with high-grade, round-cell morphology sometimes associated with a low-grade spindle cell component that is most commonly fibromyxoid.[42] When unassociated with a low-grade component, these tumors should only be diagnosed after excluding other more common uterine sarcomas, including leiomyosarcoma, sarcomatous overgrowth in a müllerian adenosarcoma, malignant mixed müllerian tumor, or rhabdomyosarcoma.

Clinical Features

This is a rare tumor whose true frequency is unknown, as tumors previously considered undifferentiated uterine sarcoma may belong to this category. Patients range in age from 28–67 years (mean 50 years). Patients most often present with abnormal vaginal bleeding (menorrhagia or peri/postmenopausal bleeding) and can present with an enlarged uterus or a pelvic mass.

Gross Features

These tumors are often intracavitary polypoid or mural plaque-like masses. They typically range in size up to 9 cm (median 7.5 cm) and often show extrauterine extension at the time of diagnosis. They have a fleshy cut surface and are associated with extensive areas of necrosis and hemorrhage. They typically show destructive invasion of the myometrium in contrast to the permeative invasion of low-grade endometrial stromal sarcomas.

Microscopic Features

On low-power examination, these tumors may have the typical infiltrative growth and vasculature of its low-grade counterpart; however, there is usually confluent permeative and destructive growth, often with invasion into the outer half of the myometrium. There is a variable mixture of closely juxtaposed high-grade round cell (usually predominant) and low-grade spindle cell component. The round cell areas are hypercellular and the cells are arranged in vague to well defined nests and separated by a delicate capillary network. The round cells have modest amount of eosinophilic to granular cytoplasm, irregular nuclear contours and granular to often vesicular chromatin, with variably distinct nucleoli. Occasionally, the round cells are noncohesive imparting a pseudo-papillary/glandular appearance or have focal rhabdoid morphology. Occasionally, primitive neuroectodermal differentiation in the form of Flexner-Wintersteiner rosettes or Homer-Wright pseudo-rosettes may be seen (Figure 20.13). Mitotic activity is typically >10 per 10 HPF and is very striking. Necrosis is usually present. The spindle cell component often has fibromyxoid features. Lymphovascular invasion is typically present. Rarely, a high-grade sarcoma is seen in association with areas that have the appearance of conventional low-grade endometrial stromal sarcoma.

Immunohistochemistry and Somatic Genetics

The high-grade component of tumors with t(10;17) is CD10, ER and PR negative (Figures 20.20 and 20.21) but shows strong diffuse cyclin D1 positivity (>70% nuclei) (Figure 20.22); the low-grade spindle cell component is typically strongly and diffusely CD10, ER and PR positive and shows variable, heterogeneous cyclin D1 expression (<50%). The high-grade component is also typically c-Kit positive but DOG1 negative. High-grade endometrial stromal sarcoma typically harbours the *YWHAE-FAM22* genetic fusion as a result of t(10;17)(q22;p13).

Prognosis

In comparison to low-grade endometrial stromal sarcomas, patients have earlier and more frequent recurrences (often <1 year) and are more likely to die of disease. They appear to have a prognosis that is intermediate, between low-grade endometrial stromal sarcoma and undifferentiated uterine sarcoma.[20]

UNDIFFERENTIATED ENDOMETRIAL SARCOMA

Definition

This is a high-grade uterine sarcoma bearing no resemblance to proliferative-phase endometrium. Typically shows high-grade cytologic features without specific type of differentiation.[2]

Clinical Features

This tumor is rare. Patients are typically postmenopausal (mean age is 60 years). Approximately two-thirds of patients present with high-stage disease (stage III/IV). They typically have postmenopausal bleeding or signs/symptoms secondary to extra-uterine spread.

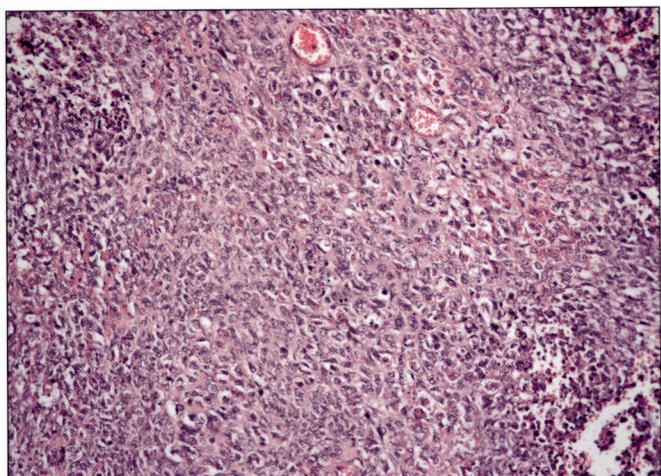

Figure 20.27 Undifferentiated endometrial sarcoma. The tumor cells grow in sheets, that display high-grade cytologic features and do not resemble endometrial stroma.

Gross Features

They are typically intraluminal polypoid masses, usually >10 cm, with a fleshy cut surface and areas of necrosis and/or haemorrhage.

Microscopic Features

On low-power magnification, margins are poorly defined with destructive invasion of the myometrium. The tumor cells are highly atypical, grow in sheets (Figure 20.27) or exhibit a storiform or herringbone patern. The cells can be polygonal or spindle and they show marked nuclear pleomorphism including multinucleated giant cells. Brisk mitotic activity including atypical forms is seen. The characteristic delicate vasculature reminiscent of spiral arterioles as well as the small uniform cells of the proliferative-type stroma are lacking. Lymphovascular invasion, necrosis, and hemorrhage are frequent. Rhabdoid morphology or myxoid background may be seen.

Immunohistochemistry and Somatic Genetics

These tumors are variably CD10 positive and typically ER and PR weakly positive or negative. Cyclin D1 can be diffusely positive but in those cases the tumors are also typically positive for CD10 (which excludes *YWHAE-FAM22* sarcomas). Focal smooth muscle actin, desmin, EMA or keratin positivity may be seen.[48]

These tumors can have complex chromosomal changes, including gains of 2q, 4q, 6q, 7p, 9q, 20q and losses of 3q, 10p, 14q.

Differential Diagnosis

As these tumors are poorly differentiated, extensive sampling is important in order to exclude other high-grade sarcomas (leiomyosarcoma or rhabdomyosarcoma), sarcomatous overgrowth in a müllerian adenosarcoma, or a malignant mixed müllerian tumor where the epithelial component is very limited and has only homologous sarcomatous elements. Leiomyosarcoma may have spindle or epithelioid cells and neoplastic cells with marked cytologic atypia. However, often they display well-developed fascicles and cigar-shaped nuclei. Immunohistochemical stains for smooth muscle markers are positive despite CD10, ER, and PR positivity. Spindle rhabdomyosarcoma is exceedingly rare. Cells are wavy with bright eosinophilic cytoplasm and may show cross striations. Muscle markers including myogenin and myo-D1 are typically positive.[76] Müllerian adenosarcoma with sarcomatous overgrowth as well as malignant mixed müllerian tumor may enter in the differential diagnosis if areas of conventional adenosarcoma or the carcinomatous component of a malignant mixed müllerian tumor have not been sampled.[77,78]

Prognosis and Treatment

Undifferentiated endometrial sarcomas are highly aggressive tumors that are associated with a dismal prognosis (<2 years).[48] Patients should be treated by radical hysterectomy and bilateral salpingo-oophorectomy and adjuvant radiation and/or chemotherapy.

UTERINE TUMORS RESEMBLING OVARIAN SEX CORD TUMORS

Definition

These uncommon neoplasms closely recapitulate the morphologic spectrum of sex cord–stromal tumors of the ovary, more frequently granulosa cell tumors.[79] Endometrial stromal tumors with any degree of sex cord-like (epithelial) differentiation were initially included under this category, with group A (stromal predominant) composed of tumors with some sex cord elements and group B having exclusively sex cord elements.[22] Currently only tumors composed of sex cord elements are diagnosed under this category.[55]

Clinical Features

These tumors are frequently seen in patients in their fourth to sixth decades who typically present with vaginal/postmenopausal bleeding or nonspecific symptoms and signs related to the growing uterine mass.[80]

Gross Features

They can be polypoid protruding into the endometrial cavity, intramyometrial, and rarely subserosal,[22] or centered in the cervix.[81] They range in size from microscopic to 15 (mean 6) cm[80] and are typically well circumscribed with a homogeneous yellow to tan or less frequently white to gray cut surface depending on the amount of intervening stroma. Areas of necrosis or hemorrhage are uncommon.

Microscopic Features

On low-power examination, these tumors are frequently but not always well circumscribed with a pushing border. Some tumors may have an infiltrative border where tumor cells are closely intermixed with fascicles of myometrium that may appear hyperplastic without associated stromal response.[55] On closer examination, uterine tumors resembling sex cord–stromal tumors are characterized by morphologic patterns that closely resemble those described in sex cord tumors of the ovary. Tumor cells are frequently arranged in cords (sometimes with plexiform pattern)

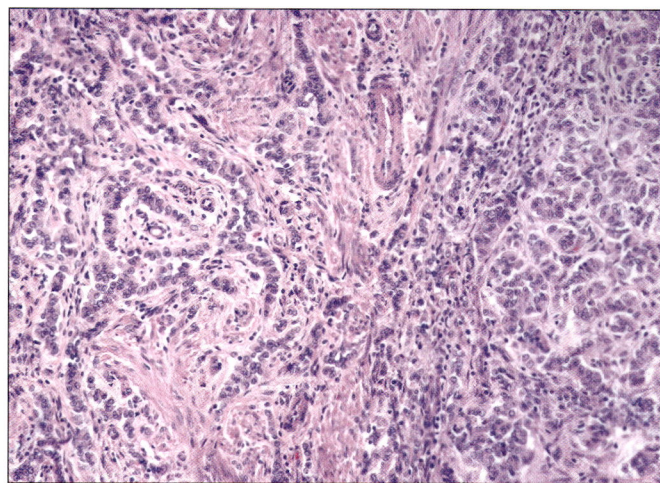

Figure 20.28 Uterine tumor resembling ovarian sex cord tumor. The neoplastic cells form cords, embedded in a collagenous stroma, which are reminiscent of an adult granulosa cell tumor.

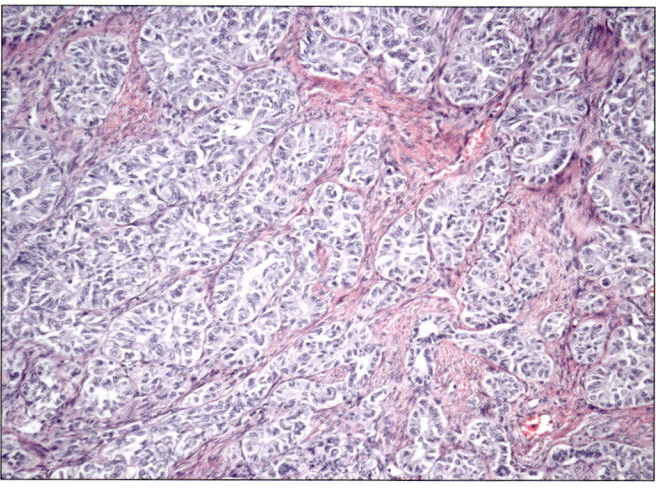

Figure 20.30 Uterine tumor resembling ovarian sex cord tumor. The neoplastic cells form tubular structures reminiscent of Sertoli cell tubules.

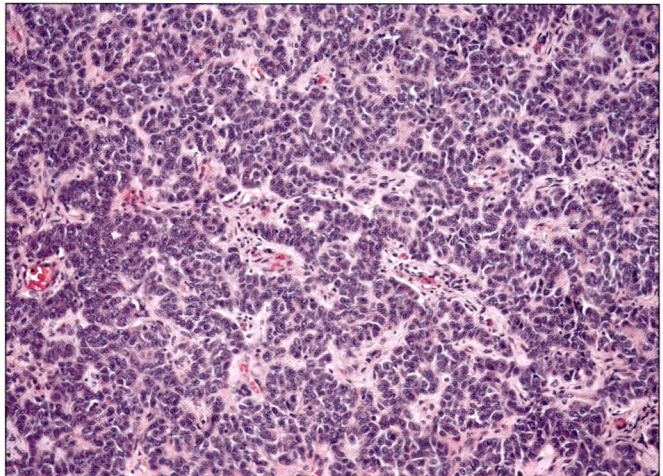

Figure 20.29 Uterine tumor resembling ovarian sex cord tumor. Closely packed interconnecting trabeculae composed of cells with 'epithelial' features are seen.

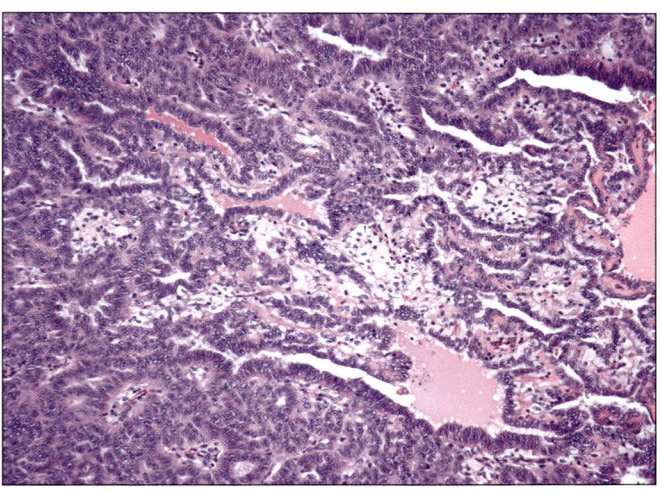

Figure 20.31 Uterine tumor resembling ovarian sex cord tumor. Less commonly, the tumor shows a retiform architecture similar to that seen in retiform Sertoli–Leydig cell tumors.

(Figure 20.28), anastomosing trabeculae (Figure 20.29), nests or irregularly shaped islands, and sheets reminiscent of granulosa cell tumor. However, hollow or solid tubules (Figure 20.30), some with a retiform architecture including small papillae with hyalinized cores reminiscent of Sertoli tubules seen in Sertoli–Leydig or Sertoli cell tumors, are also seen (Figure 20.31).[24,55,80,82] Rarely, cystic dilation of tubules, pseudopapillary architecture, Leydig-like or foam cells, and heterologous elements in the form of intestinal epithelium (as reported in ovarian Sertoli–Leydig cell tumor) can occur. Cells are usually small to medium sized with variable amounts of eosinophilic to pale sometimes vacuolated cytoplasm. Rarely rhabdoid morphology has been reported.[83] Nuclei are typically uniform with small but visible nucleoli and grooved nuclei may be seen. Mitotic figures are typically scant. The background stroma is frequently scarce with a loose fibroblastic appearance and no endometrial stromal component is present. Lymphovascular invasion is typically absent.[22]

Immunohistochemical Features

Uterine tumors resembling ovarian sex cord tumors are considered polyphenotypic as they often coexpress epithelial, smooth muscle, and sex cord markers. They are always vimentin positive and often express a variety of keratins (uncommonly CK7) (Figure 20.32A)[21,24,80,83,84] and to a much lesser extent EMA.[83,85] The tumor cells are often positive for smooth muscle markers including actin, desmin (Figure 20.32B), h-caldesmon, HDAC-8, and smooth muscle myosin heavy chain.[21,40,81,83–85] They also express calretinin, inhibin (Figure 20.32C), Melan-A, CD99, and WT1.[21,24,40,83,85] Inhibin also stains Leydig-like cells.[24] They are also variably positive for ER and PR[24,80,83,84,86] and can show focal CD10 and c-kit expression.[85]

Ultrastructural Features

These tumors show focal epithelial and variable sex cord-like differentiation but no definite smooth muscle differentiation, findings that overlap with those seen in sex–cord stromal tumors of the ovary.[87]

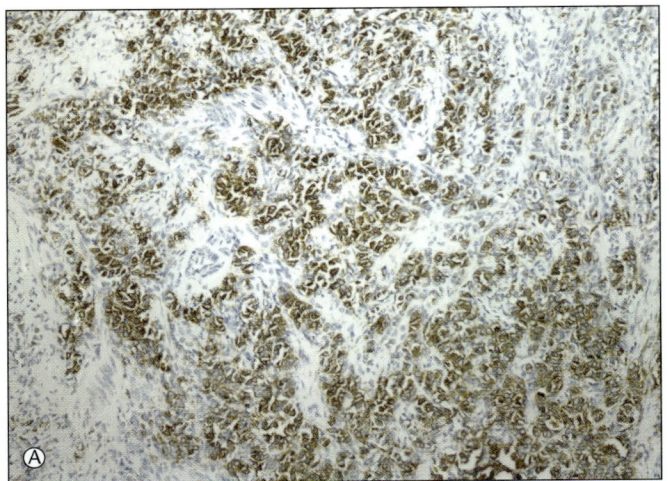
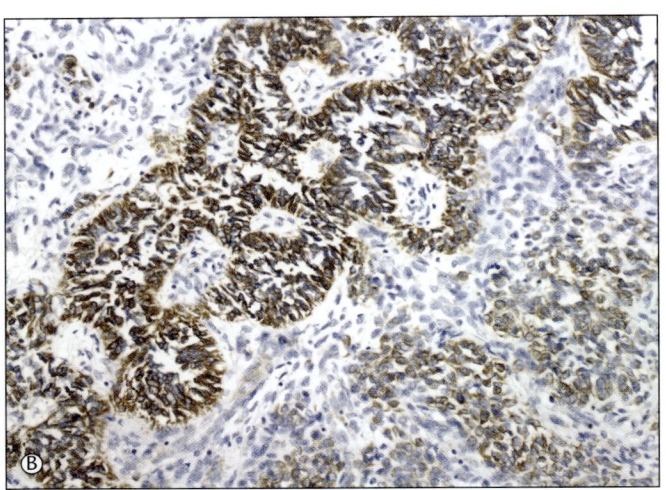
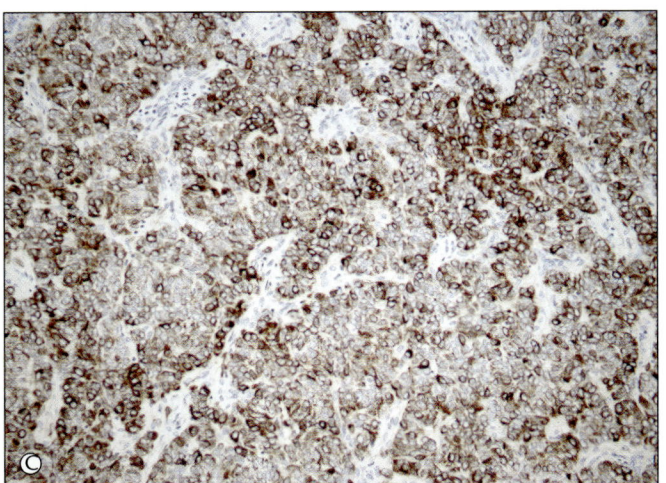

Figure 20.32 Uterine tumor resembling ovarian sex cord tumor. The tumor cells are often positive for AE1/AE3 **(A)** as well as desmin **(B)** and inhibin **(C)**.

Cytogenetics

Studies have shown that uterine tumors resembling ovarian sex cord–stromal tumors lack the *JAZF1–JJAZ1* gene fusion in contrast to endometrial stromal tumors with or without sex cord elements, suggesting an independent origin.[88]

Differential Diagnosis

The main differential diagnoses include endometrial stromal tumor with sex cord elements, endometrioid carcinoma including 'sertoliform' variant, and epithelioid smooth muscle tumors. Obviously, the presence of any endometrial stromal areas is diagnostic of endometrial stromal neoplasia. Furthermore, a diagnosis of uterine tumor resembling a sex cord ovarian tumor can only be made in a hysterectomy specimen where the specimen can be extensively sampled to exclude areas of endometrial stromal neoplasia.[55] Low-grade endometrioid carcinomas are by far more common than uterine tumors resembling ovarian sex cord tumors. They can be seen as thickening of the endometrium or irregularly infiltrating the myometrium and exhibit squamous, tubal, or mucinous metaplasia. However, some endometrioid carcinomas may have a sertoliform morphology and others may form cords and trabeculae associated with a hyalinized background,[89] while uterine tumors resembling sex cord tumors may have an endometrioid appearance especially if they show a retiform pattern. The finding of well-formed glands with squamous, tubal, or mucinous epithelium and negative staining for sex cord-like and smooth muscle markers supports a diagnosis of carcinoma. Epithelioid smooth muscle tumors may grow in sheets, cords, or nests and stain for smooth muscle markers, often for wide spectrum keratins as well as EMA but often are associated with a conventional spindle component and are negative for sex cord markers.[55] Other tumors that infrequently enter in the differential diagnosis include perivascular epithelial cell tumor (PEComa), malignant melanoma, or even metastatic lobular breast carcinoma.

Treatment and Prognosis

Uterine tumors resembling ovarian sex cord–stromal tumors are typically treated with hysterectomy as most are benign, although rare recurrences have been reported.[90,91] There are no well-established clinicopathologic criteria that can identify tumors with a more aggressive behavior.

MIXED MÜLLERIAN TUMORS

INTRODUCTION

This category of uterine tumors comprises müllerian adenosarcoma and malignant mixed müllerian tumor, and two other tumors that are either rare, müllerian adenofibroma, or likely nonexistent, carcinofibroma.

MÜLLERIAN ADENOFIBROMA

Definition

In contrast to its ovarian counterpart, müllerian adenofibroma of the uterus is exceedingly rare. It is defined as a biphasic neoplasm composed of benign epithelium and mesenchyme.[6]

Clinical Features

These tumors occur most often in perimenopausal or postmenopausal women but can be seen at a younger age.

Gross Features

They typically present as polypoid masses filling the endometrial cavity, but rarely may involve the lower uterine segment or cervix as occurs with müllerian adenosarcomas.[92] They have a spongy cut surface due to the presence of cysts that may be filled with mucoid or brown fluid. The cysts are surrounded by white firm tissue corresponding to the mesenchymal component.

Microscopic Features

The mesenchymal component may vary in cellularity from tumor to tumor but it is uniformly cellular within a given neoplasm. It is composed of cells with a fibroblastic or endometrial stromal morphology that lack cytologic atypia or mitotic activity but may show papillary growth.[92] Only one example showing a heterologous mesenchymal component, mature adipose tissue, has been reported (lipoadenofibroma).[93] The epithelial component most commonly resembles proliferative-phase endometrium, although mucinous, tubal, or hobnail cells may also be seen and the epithelium may be hyperplastic[90,94] but shows no cytologic atypia.[92]

Differential Diagnosis

The most important entity in the differential diagnosis is müllerian adenosarcoma. The presence of hypercellular periglandular stroma ('cuffing'), cytologic atypia, or mitotic activity in the stromal component should point toward the diagnosis of müllerian adenosarcoma. It has been shown that tumors with minimal cytologic atypia of the stromal component and <1 mitoses/10 HPF may be associated with an adverse outcome, challenging the concept of adenofibroma.[95] As periglandular cuffing may be very focal, hysterectomy is required to rule out the possibility of müllerian adenosarcoma. Thus, a diagnosis of müllerian adenofibroma should not be rendered in a curettage specimen or incomplete resection of the tumor.

Treatment and Prognosis

If correctly diagnosed, müllerian adenofibromas are benign tumors and have an excellent prognosis. However, some tumors initially diagnosed as adenofibromas have been associated with adverse outcome (multiple recurrences or even death of patients) and most likely represented adenosarcomas. Thus, extensive sampling is important in order to identify focal areas that fulfill the criteria of adenosarcoma.[95]

MÜLLERIAN ADENOSARCOMA

Definition

This biphasic müllerian uterine tumor is defined by the World Health Organization (WHO) as having benign epithelial and low-malignant homologous mesenchymal (sarcomatous) components,[6] with the latter responsible for their clinical behavior.

Clinical Features

They are uncommon neoplasms, representing between 5% and 10% of all uterine sarcomas.[73,96] The tumors are commonly located in the endometrium (approximately 90%) but may be centered in the myometrium, serosa, or cervix, and they have been reported to arise from adenomyosis, adenomyoma, or endometriosis.[97,98] Low-grade müllerian adenosarcomas typically occur in perimenopausal or postmenopausal women (average 58 years) but have been reported in a wide age range (14–90 years). Most patients present with vaginal bleeding, pelvic pain, a history of 'recurrent' endometrial polyps, or other nonspecific symptoms or signs.[92,99] Some patients have been reported to have a history of estrogen or tamoxifen use or prior radiation.[99,100]

Gross Features

Tumors may be large, ranging from 1 to 20 (mean 5–6.5) cm.[92,95,101] They frequently form a polypoid or less commonly a sessile mass that fills the endometrial cavity and may be seen protruding into the endocervical canal. Multifocality and diffuse growth have been reported. They are often well demarcated from the surrounding myometrium.[92] A leaf-like appearance may be noted. On sectioning, cysts alternate with solid white to tan to pink rubbery areas (Figure 20.33). The cysts may be filled with watery, mucoid, or brown fluid.[77,95] If there is sarcomatous overgrowth, it may be seen as soft, fleshy, white to gray areas (Figure 20.34) with associated foci of hemorrhage and/or necrosis.[101]

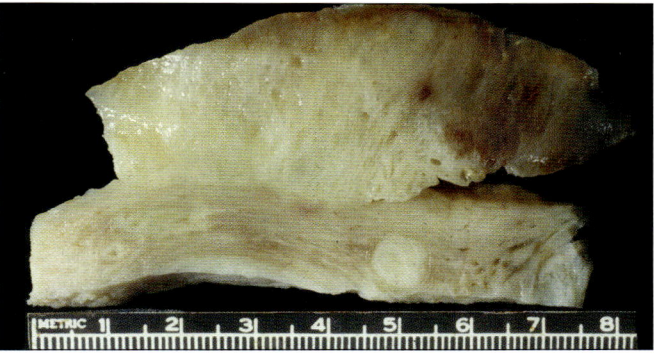

Figure 20.33 Müllerian adenosarcoma. The tumor is polypoid and has a spongy cut surface with solid white to tan areas punctuated by small cysts.

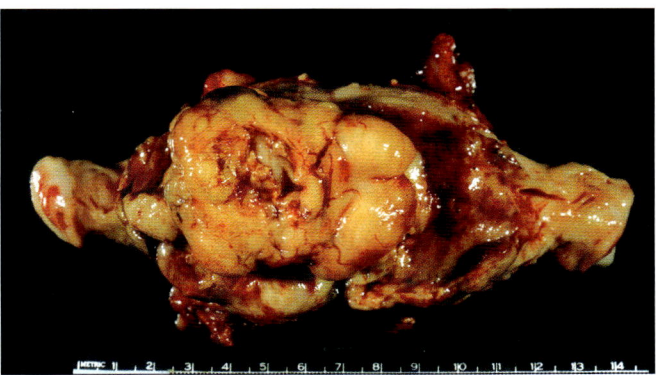

Figure 20.34 Müllerian adenosarcoma with sarcomatous overgrowth. A large polypoid mass with fleshy cut surface and focal hemorrhage is seen.

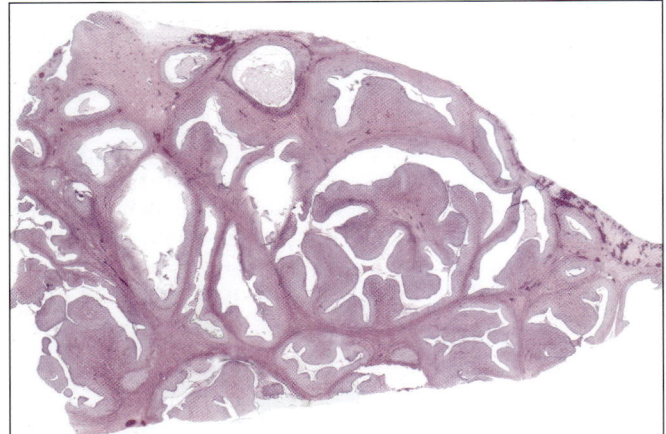

Figure 20.35 Müllerian adenosarcoma. The tumor shows a striking phyllodes architecture with numerous intraluminal polypoid projections.

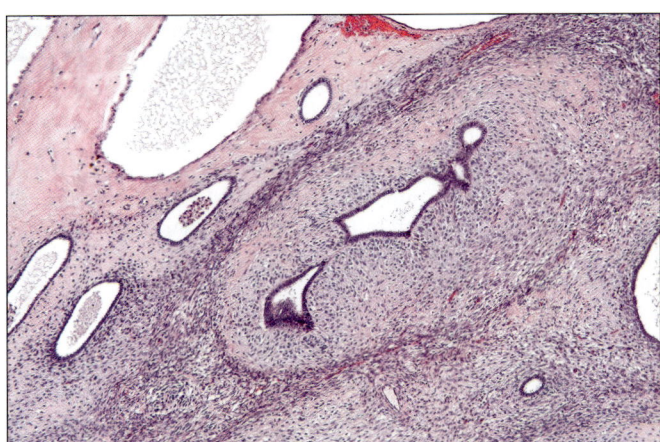

Figure 20.37 Müllerian adenosarcoma. Sometimes, the stroma around the glands is hypocellular due to collagen deposition.

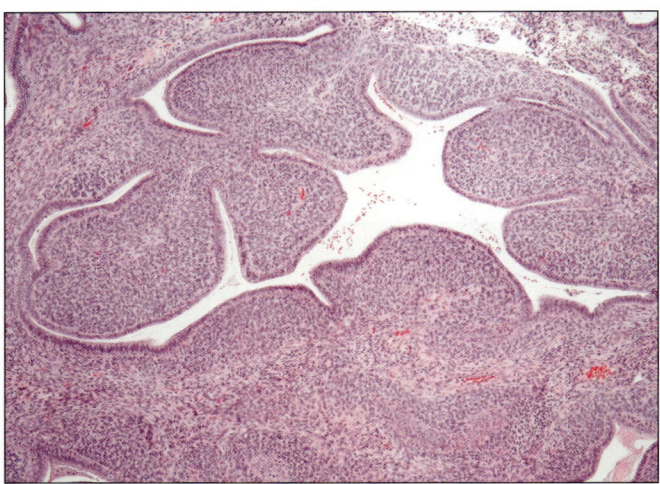

Figure 20.36 Müllerian adenosarcoma. Stromal condensation around glands is apparent.

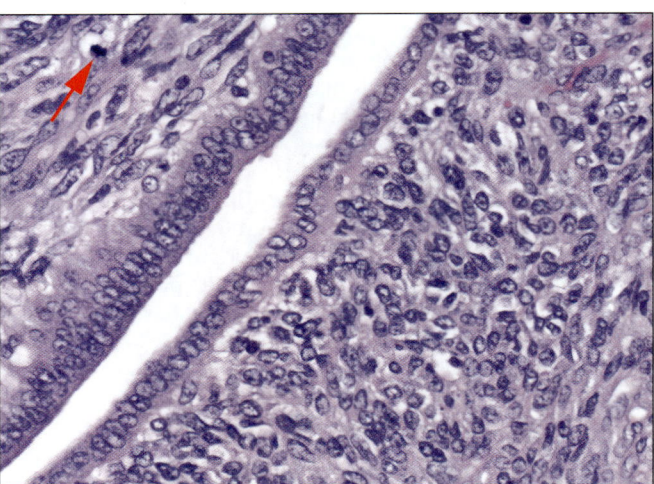

Figure 20.38 Müllerian adenosarcoma. The stromal cells around the glands are typically 'plump' with scant cytoplasm and enlarged nuclei and show scattered mitoses (arrow). The epithelium is typically endometrioid and lacks nuclear atypia.

Microscopic Features

On low-power examination, the tumors are commonly polypoid but may have prominent surface papillary projections and they are confined to the endometrium.[77,92] There is often a striking condensation (cuffing) of the cellular low-grade malignant stroma around müllerian glands, which may be small and round, cystically dilated, or display a phyllodes morphology with intraluminal polypoid projections of the stroma (Figures 20.35 and 20.36). However, rarely condensation may not be striking (Figure 20.37).[95] Increased stromal cellularity can also be seen under the surface epithelium. At higher magnification, the neoplastic cellular stroma resembles fibroblastic or endometrial stroma and is composed of cells with scant cytoplasm, enlarged vesicular nuclei with small nucleoli, and frequent mitoses when compared to the neoplastic stroma away from the glands (Figure 20.38). Even though a cut-off of 4 mitoses/10 HPF was used in the past to separate adenosarcoma from adenofibroma,[92] it was noted that tumors with characteristic but only focal periglandular cuffing and without prominent cellularity or atypia may be associated with lower mitotic counts and still recur.[77,95] Thus, in the most recent WHO classification, the mitotic threshold for the diagnosis of müllerian adenosarcoma is ≥1 mitoses/10 HPF,[6] but some do not require any mitotic activity if the tumor shows the typical low-power architecture. The stroma may show hyalinization, elastosis, edema, or myxoid change and multinucleated cells or foamy histiocytes may be seen.[77] The stromal component of müllerian adenosarcoma may show sex cord-like differentiation,[77,102] or smooth muscle metaplasia. The latter may be seen as closely apposed long intersecting fascicles of spindle or infrequently epithelioid cells often surrounding the stromal component but rarely in juxtaposition to the glands.[100,103] Less commonly fetal-type cartilage (most commonly if cervical) rhabdomyoblasts, mature adipocytic differentiation,[77,92,104] or areas of embryonal rhabdomyosarcoma or liposarcoma may be seen.[77] Rarely, cells with bizarre nuclei can occur. Glands are typically widely spaced within the tumor. They are lined by

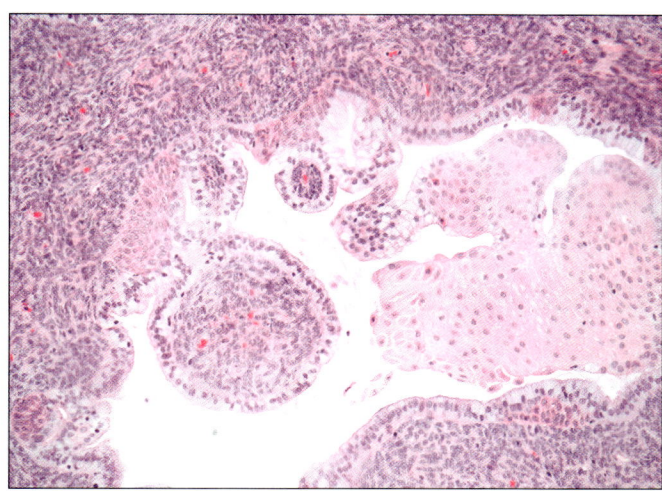

Figure 20.39 Müllerian adenosarcoma. The glands may be lined by endocervical-type or squamous epithelium. Notice the dense but uniform underlying stroma.

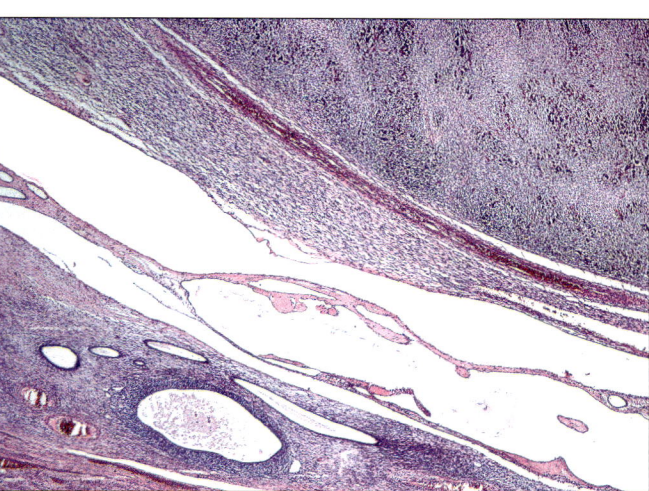

Figure 20.41 Müllerian adenosarcoma with sarcomatous overgrowth. Diffuse sarcomatous growth (upper right quadrant). Notice the presence of conventional adenosarcoma (bottom).

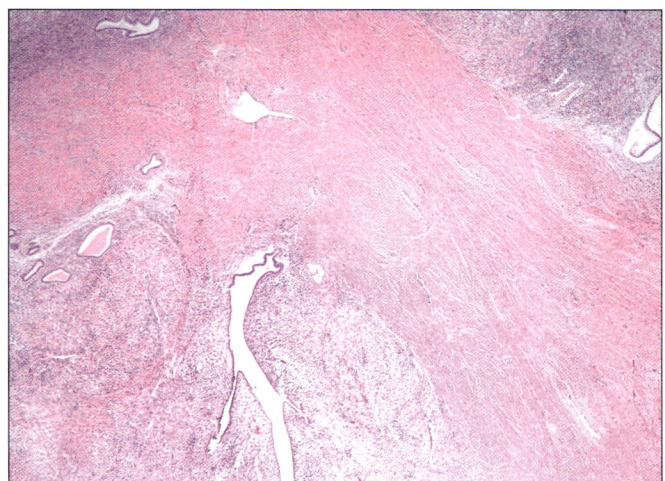

Figure 20.40 Müllerian adenosarcoma. Myometrial invasion is seen in less than 20% of cases and typically shows both mesenchymal and epithelial elements.

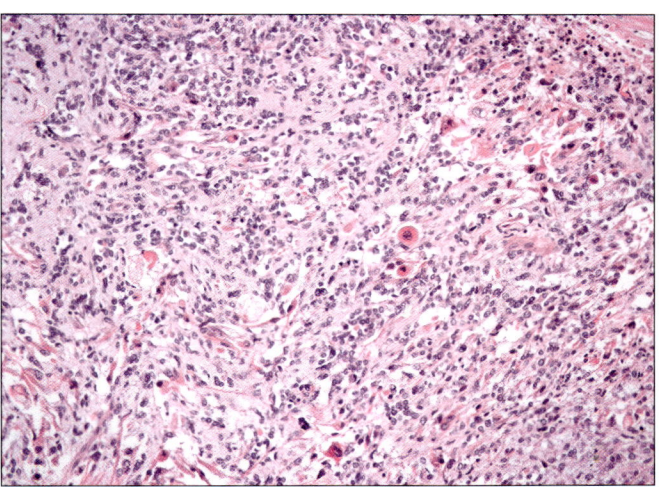

Figure 20.42 Müllerian adenosarcoma with sarcomatous overgrowth. Rhabdomyosarcoma is the most common type of heterologous sarcoma in sarcomatous overgrowth. Notice the presence of 'pink' rhabdomyoblasts.

endometrioid-type epithelium most often reminiscent of the proliferative phase, but endocervical mucinous, mature non-keratinizing squamous, or tubal epithelium may be seen (Figure 20.39). The cells are cuboidal or columnar, and they have round to oval nuclei with nucleoli and scattered mitotic figures more often if proliferative-type epithelium.[77,92] On rare occasions, glands may appear crowded (10%) and cytologic atypia may be marked (up to 30%), raising the diagnosis of focal atypical complex hyperplasia or even carcinoma arising in adenosarcoma.[77]

Morphologic features of prognostic importance are myometrial invasion (Figure 20.40) and sarcomatous overgrowth (Figure 20.41). If myometrial invasion (<20%), the 'invasive front' typically shows an infiltrative pattern and is composed of atypical stroma and glands.[77] Sarcomatous overgrowth is defined as the presence of sarcoma in >25% of the tumor, typically but not always high grade, most frequently as homologous poorly differentiated sarcoma or rhabdomyosarcoma if heterologous sarcoma (Figure 20.42).[101,105] Tumors with sarcomatous overgrowth more frequently show myometrial and vascular invasion compared than tumors without this feature.[95,101]

Immunohistochemical Features

The mesenchymal component of müllerian adenosarcomas expresses vimentin, CD10 (Figure 20.43A), WT1, ER and PR (Figure 20.43B), with variable expression of muscle markers (smooth muscle actin and desmin), androgen receptor, and keratins, closely resembling the immunohistochemical profile seen in endometrial stromal tumors.[95,106–109] There is low MIB1 expression and p53 is negative.[95,109] Stromal cells can also express CD34 as well as calretinin while c-kit

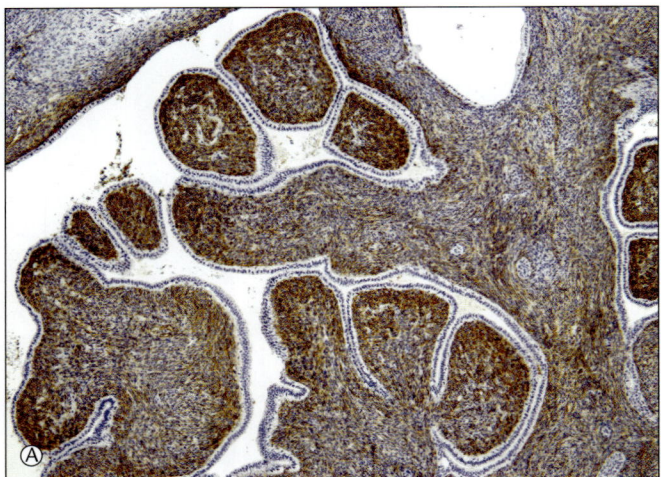

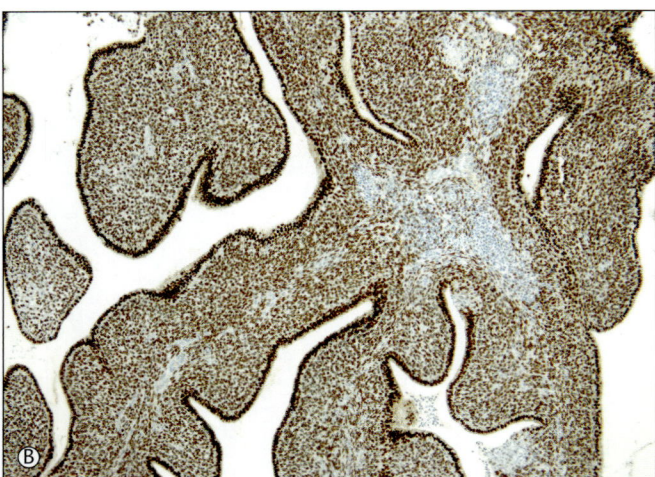

Figure 20.43 Müllerian adenosarcoma. The neoplastic stromal cells around the epithelial component typically react strongly for CD10 **(A)** and ER **(B)**. Notice that the epithelial cells are also ER positive.

	Adenomyoma	Adenofibroma/ Sarcoma
Intracavitary	Uncommon (except atypical polypoid adenomyoma)	Usual
Mural	Usual	Uncommon
Serosal	Occasional	Uncommon
Phyllodes-like	Rare	Typical
Papillary fronds	Rare	Common
Endometrial stroma	Non-neoplastic and scant (absent in atypical polypoid adenomyoma)	Neoplastic (mitoses usual in adenosarcoma)
Smooth muscle	Conspicuous (definitional)	Usually absent or inconspicuous

Table 20.3 Contrasting Features of Adenomyomas and Adenofibromas/Adenosarcomas

and inhibin if positive are typically weak and focal.[109] Areas with sex cord-like elements stain for calretinin, inhibin, Melan-A, and CD99, and areas of smooth muscle differentiation show strong and diffuse expression of smooth muscle markers. In contrast to the low-grade mesenchymal component, areas of sarcomatous overgrowth typically lose CD10, ER and PR expression and are associated with high MIB1 expression, while WT1 appears to be relatively preserved.[109] Recently, it has been shown that the Ki-67 labeling index in areas of periglandular cuffing is approximately 20% in contrast to <5% in stromal areas away from the epithelial component. The epithelial component typically expresses keratins as well as EMA, shows frequent ER and PR positivity, and rarely stains for CD10.[109]

Differential Diagnosis

The differential diagnosis of müllerian adenosarcoma includes non-neoplastic, benign, and malignant tumors, including cellular endometrial polyp, polypoid endometriosis, müllerian adenofibroma, adenomyoma, endometrial stromal tumors, carcinosarcoma, embryonal rhabdomyosarcoma (the latter mostly in the cervix), and pure high-grade sarcomas if sarcomatous overgrowth.

Cellular endometrial polyp in contrast to müllerian adenosarcoma is characterized by uniformly increased cellularity of the stroma lacking periglandular condensation, cytologic atypia, or mitotic activity. The presence of atypical multinucleated cells may also raise concern for adenosarcoma, but this finding in isolation lacks any significance.[110] It is not infrequent that some endometrial or endocervical polyps contain one or two glands surrounded by mildly hypercellular stroma with no cytologic atypia.

Polypoid endometriosis is composed of endometrial stroma and endometrial-type glands that may be cystically dilated; however, it lacks the typical periglandular stromal hypercellularity, intraglandular stromal papillae, or stromal cytologic atypia seen in müllerian adenosarcoma.[111]

Müllerian adenofibroma is an exceedingly rare biphasic tumor that lacks condensation of the neoplastic stroma around the glands, cytologic atypia, and mitotic activity.[95] This diagnosis should be made only after extensive sampling.

Adenomyomas are also in the differential diagnosis (Table 20.3) as they contain endometrial glands and stroma while müllerian adenosarcomas may have smooth muscle metaplasia.[100] However, adenomyomas are always grossly well circumscribed and the appearance of the predominant solid areas (smooth muscle) is identical to that of a leiomyoma.[112,113]

Atypical polypoid adenomyoma, in contrast to müllerian adenosarcoma, has a vague lobular architecture of the glandular component, with the lobules separated by benign (fibro-)muscular stroma, larger number of glands, as well as common squamous metaplasia (squamous morules). No low-grade malignant stroma is present.[114]

Endometrial stromal tumors, especially those with endometrioid-type glands, may be entertained in the differential diagnosis of müllerian adenosarcoma. However, glands in endometrial stromal tumors lack the periglandular stromal condensation. The neoplastic stroma permeates the myometrium with a 'tongue-like' pattern in contrast to the destructive infiltration seen in adenosarcoma. Furthermore, stroma in the invasive component of adenosarcoma is also higher grade than that seen in typical endometrial stromal sarcoma.[55] Immunohistochemistry is not helpful as it shows an overlapping profile in both tumor types.

Malignant mixed müllerian tumor (carcinosarcoma) enters in the differential diagnosis as some tumors may have a low-power architecture reminiscent of low-grade müllerian adenosarcoma.[115] However, stromal and epithelial components are typically high grade. Even though carcinoma may arise in an adenosarcoma, the malignant glandular elements are low grade and present in a background of low-grade sarcoma in contrast to carcinosarcomas that by definition are composed of high-grade malignant epithelium and stroma.[6]

Embryonal rhabdomyosarcoma often closely mimics the appearance of müllerian adenosarcoma at low-power magnification (more often in cervix) as both show a 'cambium layer' and 'collaring' of the malignant stroma around the glands and may have fetal-type cartilage. Müllerian adenosarcoma rarely contains rhabdomyoblasts.[77,116,117] Even though both are seen at a young age, rhabdomyosarcoma tends to occur in younger women and girls (mean 18 years).[116] Glands in rhabdomyosarcoma are not an integral part of the tumor (entrapped) and the malignant stroma away from the areas of subepithelial condensation is hypocellular, typically edematous, or myxoid alternating with small 'blue' aggregates of neoplastic cells. At higher magnification, the cells are hyperchromatic with brisk mitotic activity.[116,118]

Treatment and Prognosis

Patients are treated by total abdominal hysterectomy with bilateral salpingo-oophorectomy. If confined to the endometrium, adenosarcoma is frequently associated with a good outcome.[77,119] However, these tumors have a significant risk of recurrence, up to 26% in the largest series to date with approximately half of these patients dying from the disease (~10%).[77] Recurrences may be local (vagina, pelvis, or abdomen), or distant (bony metastases). In >50% of patients recurrences occur after 3 years of the initial diagnosis; thus, patients require long-term follow-up. Recurrences are composed of pure sarcoma (70%) or adenosarcoma and very rarely carcinosarcoma.[77,92] Myometrial invasion and sarcomatous overgrowth are the two most important prognostic factors in müllerian adenosarcoma.[77,92,105,120] In invasive tumors, the recurrence rate is estimated between 40% and 50%. If sarcomatous overgrowth is present, it is associated with a higher rate of myometrial and vascular invasion, and overall recurrence (70%), metastatic (40%), and death (60%) rates similar to other high-grade uterine sarcomas.[101]

MALIGNANT MIXED MÜLLERIAN TUMOR (CARCINOSARCOMA)

Definition

These tumors are defined as biphasic malignant neoplasms composed of high-grade epithelial and mesenchymal elements, which often are closely admixed but do not merge.[6]

Clinical Features

The incidence of malignant mixed müllerian tumors in the United States has been reported to be <1% of all gynecologic malignancies and 2–5% of all uterine malignancies.[78] They occur almost exclusively in postmenopausal women, most commonly Caucasian, but have been reported in premenopausal women including young girls.[121] Associated risk factors (obesity, exogenous estrogens, tamoxifen, and nulliparity) are similar to those reported in endometrial carcinoma.[122] Human papillomavirus (HPV) has been detected in patients with cervical tumors.[123] Up to 37% of women with malignant mixed müllerian tumors have a history of prior radiation and they tend to be younger patients. These tumors contain more often heterologous elements and they have more extensive disease at the time of diagnosis. Most women present with abnormal vaginal bleeding and an enlarged uterus and the serum CA125 level is often elevated.[90]

Gross Features

Most malignant mixed müllerian tumors arise in the uterine corpus and infrequently in the cervix. They typically form a bulky polypoid mass, ranging from 2 to 10 cm, that fills the uterine cavity (Figure 20.44); however, they may be seen as multiple polyps or plaques.[78] The cut surface is fleshy and white to gray and areas of hemorrhage and necrosis are common. Myometrial invasion is frequently seen commonly related to tumor size.[78]

Microscopic Features

These tumors are by definition biphasic on morphologic bases.[6] They are characterized by an intimate but haphazard admixture of carcinomatous and sarcomatous elements, although one of the components may predominate. In most carcinosarcomas, both components are high grade but, in rare instances, one or both may be low grade.[6] The carcinoma is usually serous (Figure 20.45) or endometrioid (with or without squamous metaplasia) and rarely may have clear cell, mucinous, squamous, or undifferentiated carcinoma components (including small cell carcinoma).[78,124] In up to 50% of these patients, endometrial hyperplasia or carcinoma (endometrioid or serous) is identified in the adjacent endometrium. In the cervix, the most common epithelial elements (exclusive or predominant) are represented by adenoid basal and keratinizing, nonkeratinizing, or basaloid squamous cell carcinoma (Figure 20.46), and much less

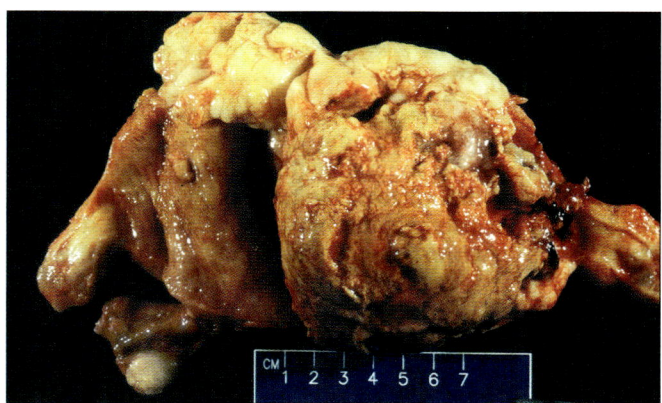

Figure 20.44 Malignant mixed müllerian tumor (carcinosarcoma). The bulky tumor fills the endometrial cavity and shows extensive necrosis and hemorrhage.

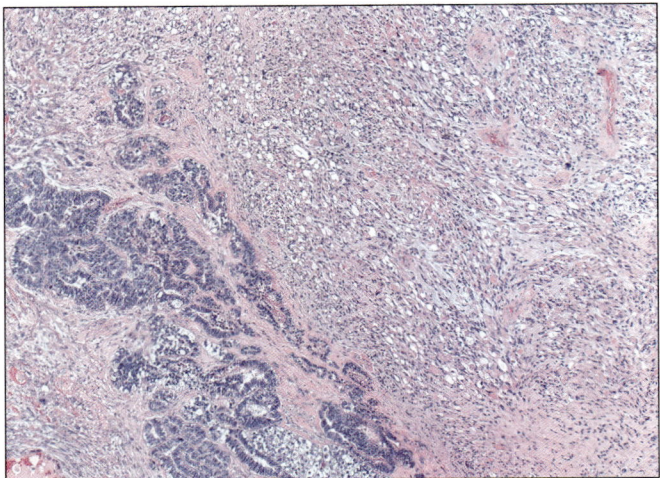

Figure 20.45 Malignant mixed müllerian tumor (carcinosarcoma). The tumor shows well-defined high-grade epithelial and mesenchymal components, the latter with numerous rhabdomyoblasts.

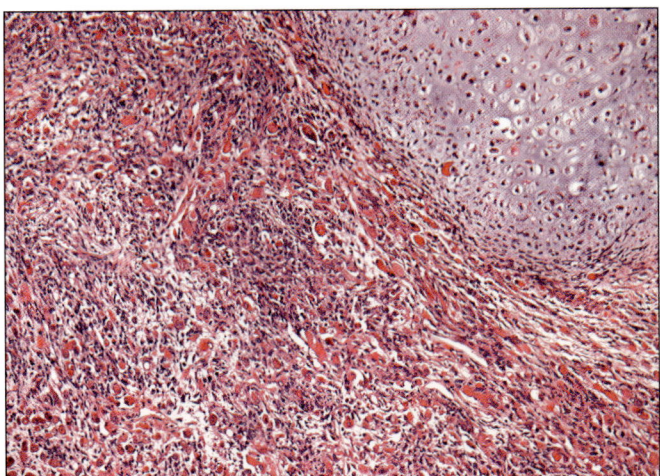

Figure 20.47 Malignant mixed müllerian tumor (carcinosarcoma). Rhabdomyosarcoma and chondrosarcoma are the most common heterologous elements. Both typically display high-grade nuclear features.

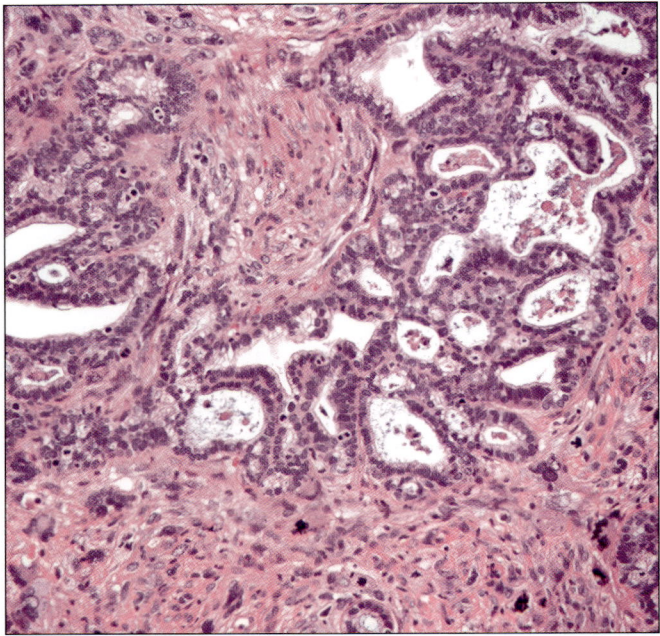

Figure 20.46 Malignant mixed müllerian tumor (carcinosarcoma) from endocervix. The epithelial component is neither endometrioid nor serous and appears lower grade. However, it is associated with high-grade homologous sarcoma (bottom).

often resemble adenoid cystic carcinoma or adenocarcinoma. It is typically associated with overlying squamous cell carcinoma *in situ*.[123] Rarely it may show neuroendocrine differentiation.[125] Homologous sarcomatous elements are more common than heterologous elements represented by high-grade sarcoma, NOS (undifferentiated endometrial sarcoma) (Figure 20.45), or rarely may resemble leiomyosarcoma or malignant fibrous histiocytoma.[78] Malignant heterologous mesenchymal elements may be seen in up to half of these tumors but their relative percentage varies depending on sampling and carefully identifying even small such foci. The most frequent heterologous components are rhabdomyosarcoma (typically also most extensive in amount), chondrosarcoma (Figure 20.47), and less often osteosarcoma or liposarcoma.[78,124] Rarely, neuroectodermal, melanocytic, yolk sac, and rhabdoid differentiation have been observed.[126–129] The finding of intracytoplasmic eosinophilic hyaline droplets is common (α-1-antitrypsin positive) but should not be confused with heterologous rhabdomyoblastic differentiation. Rare tumors may have adenosarcoma-like areas at low-power magnification, although when evaluated at higher power both stroma and glands are malignant.[115] Tumors arising in the uterine cervix usually show only a homologous sarcomatous component.[123] Deep myometrial invasion and lymphovascular invasion show more frequently the carcinomatous elements.[78]

Immunohistochemical Features

Both carcinomatous and sarcomatous elements are positive for keratins, vimentin, and often EMA.[123,130–133] Both express ER and PR, more frequently in the epithelial component, but to a lesser extent than carcinomas.[108,134] CD10 is positive, more commonly in the mesenchymal components.[108] The rhabdomyosarcomatous areas stain for desmin, myoglobin, myogenin, and myo-D1. Both carcinomatous and sarcomatous elements may show positivity for neuroendocrine markers including synaptophysin, neuron-specific enolase (NSE), and Leu-7. Expression of glial fibrillary acidic protein (GFAP) has been shown not only in areas of neuroectodermal differentiation but also in areas of homologous sarcoma. CD34 is more commonly expressed in the carcinomatous than sarcomatous component while c-kit may be expressed in the sarcomatous areas, but it is unassociated with mutations.[135,136] Both components are also typically p53, p16 (Figure 20.48),[124] and VEGF positive.[135] p53 mutations represent the most common genetic alteration.[137] Cervical tumors contain integrated HPV 16 by *in situ* hybridization in the carcinomatous and sarcomatous components.[123]

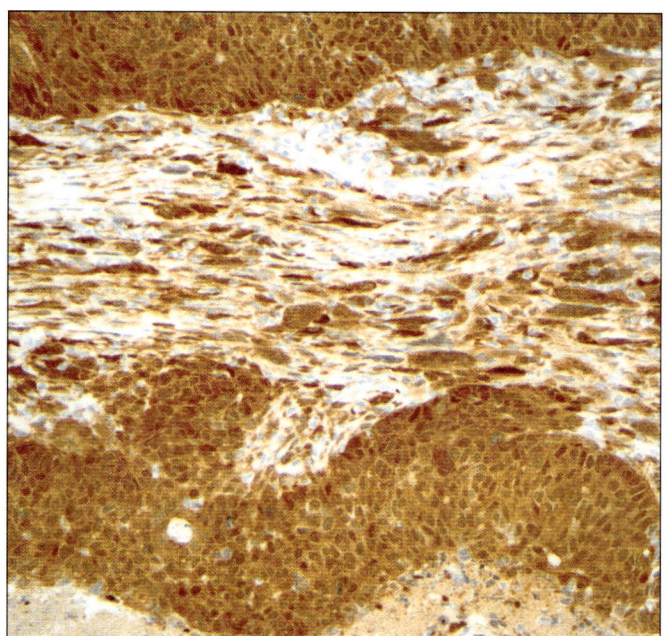

Figure 20.48 Malignant mixed müllerian tumor (carcinosarcoma) from endocervix. Both the squamous cell carcinoma and the homologous sarcoma components are strongly and diffusely reactive for p16.

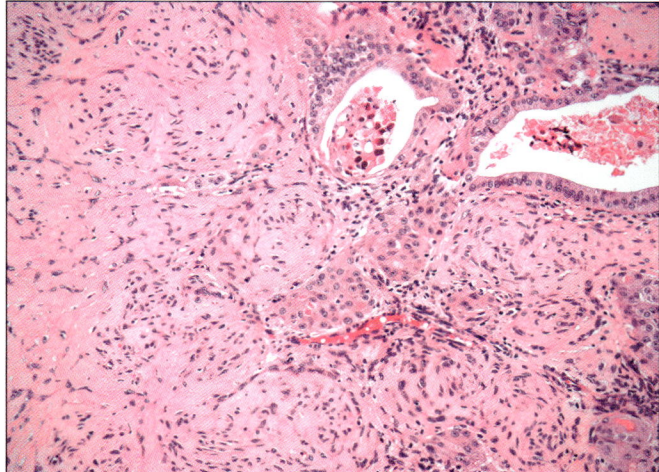

Figure 20.49 Endometrioid carcinoma with hyalinization, cording, and spindling. Well-formed endometrial glands merge with cords and spindle cells present within a hyalinized stroma. Although these tumors may be confused with malignant mixed müllerian tumor (carcinosarcoma), they are usually low grade and two distinct components cannot be delineated.

Histogenesis

Four main theories have been postulated to explain the histogenesis of these tumors: (1) the 'collision' theory suggests that the carcinomatous and sarcomatous components are independent tumors that have collided, (2) the 'combination' theory assumes that the two components arise from a common pluripotential cell, (3) the 'conversion' theory suggests that the sarcomatous component evolves from the carcinomatous component through metaplasia, and (4) the 'composition' theory postulates that the spindled component is a pseudosarcomatous stromal reaction to the carcinoma. The combination and conversion theories are most widely accepted. Molecular data have shown that most of these tumors are monoclonal in origin based on patterns of X chromosome inactivation, loss of heterozygosity, and p53 and K-ras mutations.[138–142] Recently it has been shown that carcinosarcomas undergo true epithelial–mesenchymal transition with loss of epithelial characteristics, including cadherin switching and acquisition of a mesenchymal phenotype, accompanied by expression and upregulation of all the E-cadherin repressors.[143] A small proportion of tumors may in fact represent true collision tumors.[144]

Differential Diagnosis

Carcinosarcomas should be distinguished from spindle, high-grade, and undifferentiated (or dedifferentiated) endometrioid carcinoma. Transition from typical to spindled cell areas as well as low-grade cytologic features of both components are typical features of spindle cell carcinoma (Figure 20.49). The absence of clear-cut sarcomatous areas and the presence of a better differentiated endometrioid component (on occasion) will favor a grade 3 endometrioid carcinoma. Undifferentiated carcinomas display noncohesive cells with a relatively monotonous appearance sometimes set in a myxoid background associated with a well-differentiated endometrioid carcinoma (dedifferentiated carcinoma). Although they may have rhabdoid cells, they lack well-defined sarcomatous areas.[145] Rarely endometrial carcinomas with heterologous elements may raise the differential diagnosis with carcinosarcoma. The most common heterologous element is mature bone (rarely fat or cartilage), which typically constitutes a very minor component of the tumor and has a benign appearance. Furthermore, the carcinoma is low grade and no homologous sarcoma is identified.[89] Some carcinosarcomas may have a low-power appearance that overlaps with that seen in müllerian adenosarcomas; however, the latter typically is composed of low-grade malignant stroma collaring around the epithelial elements that are typically benign or at most show low-grade malignant cytologic features.[99] Undifferentiated endometrial sarcomas and pure heterologous sarcomas may enter in the differential diagnosis when the carcinomatous elements represent a very minor component.

Treatment and Prognosis

Patients with carcinosarcoma should be treated by radical surgery including staging and chemoradiation as at the time of diagnosis metastases have been reported in ~30% of patients.[121] Five year survival rates range from 5% to 40% for patients with tumors of all stages.[121,134,146,147] Although approximately 50% of tumors are confined to the uterus at the time of diagnosis, overall survival rates range from 40% to 60% for patients with stage I and II tumors and most recurrences occur within the first 2 years. Clinical prognostic factors associated with survival in malignant mixed müllerian include age, race, performance, lymphadenectomy, and administration of radiation.[121] Among pathologic factors associated with outcome, stage is most important.[148–151]

446 PATHOLOGY OF THE FEMALE REPRODUCTIVE TRACT

These tumors appear to have a worse prognosis than endometrial serous and clear cell carcinomas. In stage I–II neoplasms, depth of myometrial invasion (40% have deep invasion) and lymphatic/vascular space involvement are significantly related to outcome.[151] The finding of clear cell or serous carcinoma is associated with a worse prognosis.[78] Within the sarcomatous component the presence of heterologous elements affects the overall prognosis in some studies including stage I tumors.[10,152] Extrauterine spread (stage III–IV) is reported in up to one-third of patients; carcinoma is the element more commonly found in metastases and the sarcomatous component or both elements are uncommon.[144] Most patients die from local pelvic recurrence rather that from metastatic disease.[96] Cervical malignant mixed müllerian tumors are more often confined to the uterus at initial diagnosis and may have a better prognosis than their uterine corpus counterparts.

ADENOMYOSIS

Definition

Adenomyosis is a non-neoplastic condition in which admixed endometrial stroma and glands are found within the body of the myometrium. It has been suggested that one medium-power field as the minimum distance from the junction (about 2–3 mm for a 10× objective) or alternatively involvement deeper than 25% of the myometrial thickness (2–3 mm in a 1 cm thick wall) is needed for this diagnosis.[153]

Clinical Features

Adenomyosis is seen mostly in women of late reproductive years and involves 5–70% of surgically removed uteri.[154] This wide frequency reflects differences in diagnostic stringency with its true prevalence around 20–25%.[155] Symptoms are nonspecific. Studies have also shown that parity is associated with an increased frequency of adenomyosis.[156] One study has shown that the incidence of adenomyosis among postmenopausal breast cancer patients treated with tamoxifen is three to four times higher than that of postmenopausal women not taking tamoxifen.[157] Using traditional clinical criteria, a correct diagnosis of adenomyosis is made in less than one-third of patients. The tendency to treat some gynecologic disorders, such as menorrhagia, by methods other than hysterectomy has led to a need for more precise methods, including magnetic resonance imaging (MRI), vaginal ultrasound, and myometrial needle biopsy in the diagnosis of adenomyosis as patients with deep adenomyosis respond poorly to endometrial ablation and other nonsurgical procedures.[158]

Pathogenesis

A number of factors play a role in the pathogenesis of adenomyosis and the mechanisms of its development. MRI has drawn attention to the most superficial specialized zone of myometrium, referred to as the 'junctional zone,'[159] which structurally and functionally differs from the outer myometrium. Abnormality of this zone, in which there is subendometrial smooth muscle hypertrophy with distortion of normal zonal architecture and loss of inner myometrial function, predisposes the secondary infiltration of the myometrium by endometrial elements.[159] Hormonal and immune factors also may play a role in the pathogenesis of adenomyosis.[160,161]

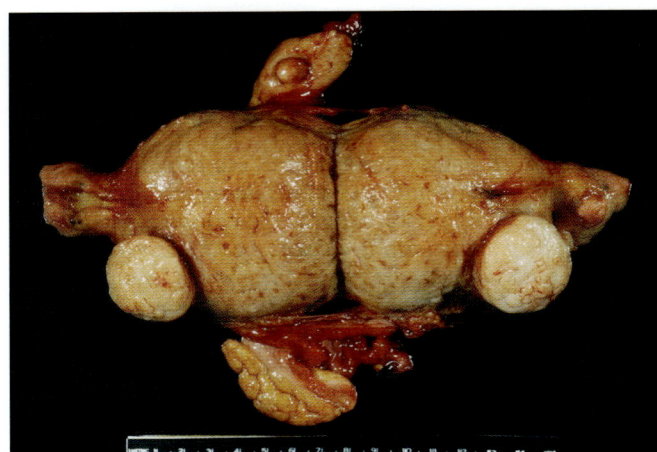

Figure 20.50 Adenomyosis. The uterine corpus is thickened and shows prominent trabeculation of the myometrium with multiple small foci of hemorrhage.

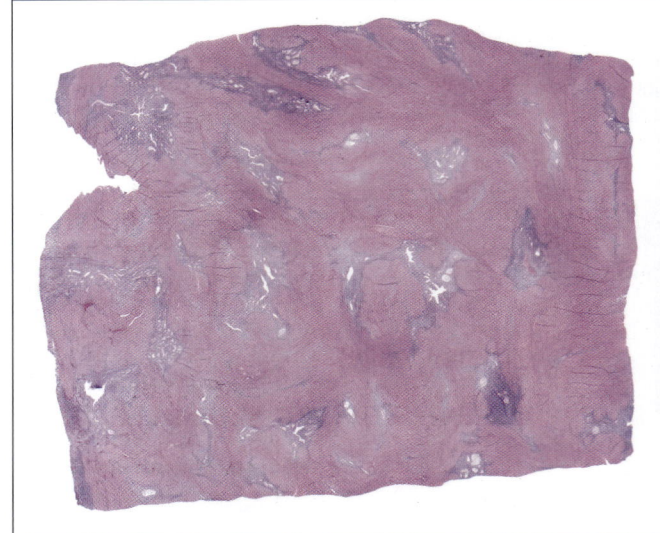

Figure 20.51 Adenomyosis. Numerous islands of endometrial glands and stroma are seen within the myometrium.

Gross Features

The uterus is often diffusely enlarged, affecting either one or both walls, and may show focal myometrial thickening or irregularity (if focal), or rarely may result in intramural masses that can grossly mimic a leiomyoma or the uterus may appear normal (if mild). Most of the grossly visible changes are secondary from the accompanying smooth muscle hypertrophy. Sectioning displays a prominent trabeculated cut surface with hypertrophic swirls of smooth muscle separating gray foci of endometrium that often appear as petechiae (Figure 20.50). Cystic spaces with blood may be seen.

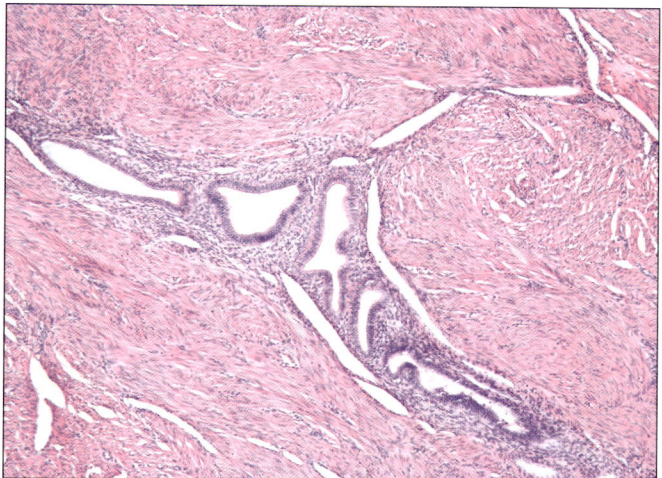

Figure 20.52 Adenomyosis. The endometrial glands and stroma have an inactive-to-atrophic appearance.

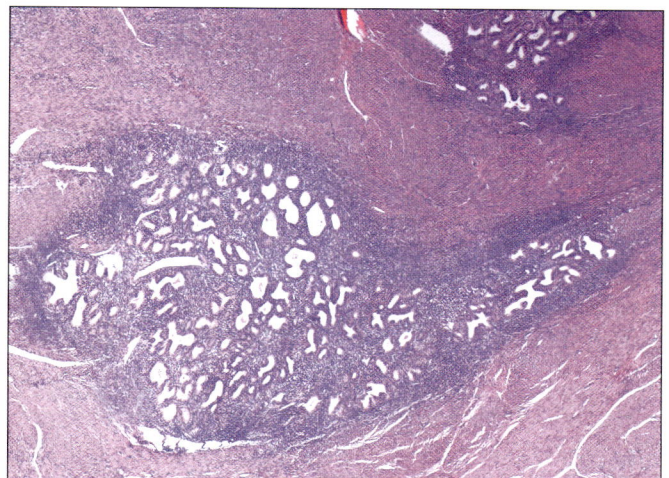

Figure 20.53 Adenomyosis involved by endometrial hyperplasia. Note the expansion of the adenomyotic focus secondary to the increased number of endometrial glands.

Microscopic Features

Typically islands of endometrial glands and stroma are seen deep within the myometrium (Figure 20.51), although rarely some islands may be composed of only endometrial stroma.[56] The outlines of the adenomyotic islands are characteristically angulated (Figure 20.52). The endometrial glands and stroma are usually inactive (compacted appearance) but occasionally secretory changes may be seen, and in pregnancy or with exogenous hormones, decidual change may occur. The surrounding myometrium is hypertrophied, often forming poorly defined nodules (Figure 20.52). Unusual changes such as glandular dilatation, epithelial metaplasias, and stromal fibrosis can occur and have been described in association with tamoxifen.[162] In some instances, adenomyotic foci can be found within vascular spaces.[56] It is important to remember that adenomyosis may be involved by hyperplasia or carcinoma (Figure 20.53).

Differential Diagnosis

In most instances the diagnosis of adenomyosis is straightforward. If gland poor or present within vascular spaces, it may be confused with a low-grade endometrial stromal sarcoma (see differential diagnosis for Low grade endometrial stromal sarcoma). It is important to recognize involvement of adenomyosis by endometrial carcinoma and distinguish it from small foci of myoinvasive carcinoma lacking associated stromal response that may mimic involvement of adenomyosis.[163,164] To establish the diagnosis of carcinoma within adenomyosis, a rim of benign endometrial stroma or a component of uninvolved adenomyosis within a particular island should be recognized so that there is a clear transition between both areas. This distinction is important as involvement of adenomyosis by an adenocarcinoma, even when deep in the myometrium, does not affect prognosis.[165–167] CD10 is not helpful in this differential diagnosis as stroma around neoplastic glands is also CD10 positive.[168] In these cases it is always important to evaluate the presence of adenomyotic foci not involved by carcinoma in the surrounding myometrium.

Treatment and Prognosis

Depending on associated symptoms, treatment may include hysterectomy to control severe symptoms.

ADENOMYOMAS

These are rare and frequently underdiagnosed benign biphasic tumors that are divided into three main categories: (1) endocervical-type adenomyoma, (2) endometrioid-type adenomyoma, and (3) atypical polypoid adenomyoma.

ENDOCERVICAL- AND ENDOMETRIOID-TYPE ADENOMYOMAS

Definition

These are biphasic tumors composed of either benign endocervical glands or endometrioid-type glands (the latter associated with variable amounts of endometrial stroma) and smooth muscle typically located in the endocervix (both) or corpus (endometrioid).[112]

Clinical Features

They occur more commonly in premenopausal women.[112,169] They may be asymptomatic and discovered incidentally during regular gynecologic examination, may present as a 'polyp' or 'fibroids' protruding through the external cervical os, or may result in abnormal bleeding or vaginal discharge, causing concern for malignancy.[112,113,169]

Gross Features

These tumors are frequently well circumscribed although unencapsulated and may be polypoid if submucosal and rarely multiple.[113] If in the corpus, they are most frequently submucosal.[112,169] They have a white to gray to slightly tan cut surface. The epithelial component may be seen as cysts while the mesenchymal areas have a firm consistency and a whorly cut surface.[113] Focal soft and gelatinous areas may be

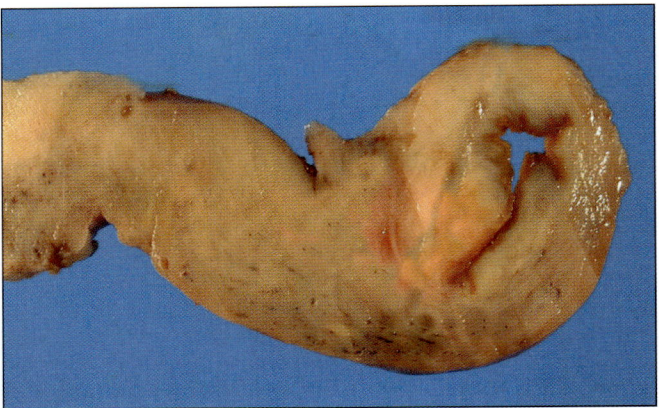

Figure 20.54 Endometrioid-type adenomyoma. The tumor is well circumscribed with a white to tan and whorly cut surface and a central hemorrhagic cyst.

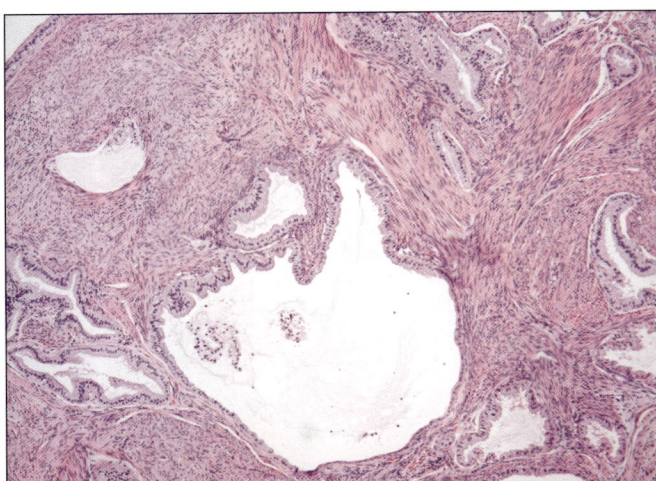

Figure 20.55 Endocervical-type adenomyoma. Irregularly shaped benign mucinous glands are admixed with mature smooth muscle.

detected (Figure 20.54).[112,169] Some tumors rarely may have a striking cystic cut surface.

Microscopic Features

At low-power magnification, adenomyomas show good circumscription. The epithelial component has irregularly shaped glands (scant or numerous but often not crowded), most frequently lined by either benign endocervical (Figure 20.55) or endometrioid-type epithelium (Figure 20.56). Endocervical cells have basal nucleus and abundant pale cytoplasm and may show tubal or tuboendometrioid metaplasia. Endometrioid cells show columnar cytoplasm and nuclear pseudostratification. Tubal, endocervical, or squamous epithelium may occasionally be seen in endometrioid-type adenomyomas. The smooth muscle component forms variably sized and shaped fascicles embedded in a collagenous background, but only has the appearance of a leiomyoma or its variants in endometrioid adenomyomas (Figure 20.56). Cells have bland cytologic features with eosinophilic cytoplasm and spindled 'cigar-shaped' nuclei. Bizarre nuclei may be seen. Mitotic activity is absent in both components.[113] Glands in endometrioid adenomyomas are surrounded by variable amounts of endometrial-type stroma (frequently weakly proliferative), which is typically less abundant than smooth muscle. Sex cord-like elements have been reported.[112] Areas of adenomyosis are commonly found in the vicinity of the tumors.[112,169]

Immunohistochemical Features

The endocervical epithelium shows luminal carcinoembryonic antigen (CEA) positivity, endometrioid glands show lateral positivity for vimentin while CD10 highlights the endometrial-type stroma and the smooth muscle component stains for muscle markers including smooth muscle actin, desmin and h-caldesmon.[113]

Differential Diagnosis

The most challenging differential diagnosis in endocervical adenomyoma is with adenoma malignum, especially in biopsy specimens. However, in the latter, glands often have complex outlines lined by cells with very abundant cytoplasm reminiscent of pyloric-type epithelium (HIK1083 and

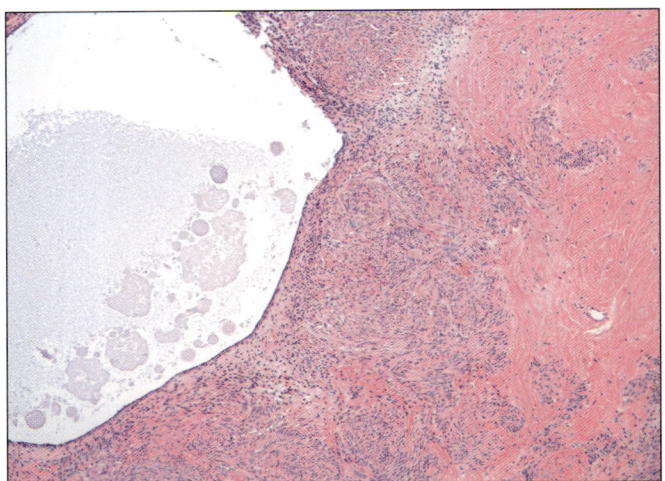

Figure 20.56 Endometrioid-type adenomyoma. A cystically dilated endometrioid gland is surrounded by a thin rim of endometrial stroma, which in turn is surrounded by benign smooth muscle that has the appearance of a leiomyoma.

cytoplasmic CEA positive), and at least focally display malignant cytologic features.[170] Adenoma malignum is associated with a diffuse thickening of the cervical wall and lymphovascular and perineural invasion, as well as conventional areas of adenocarcinoma.[170] Entities that should not be confused with endometrioid-type adenomyoma include atypical polypoid adenomyoma (see following section), endometrial polyp with smooth muscle metaplasia (smooth muscle only in stalk), leiomyoma with entrapped glands (glands only at the periphery),[112] adenomyosis, and rarely müllerian adenosarcoma or endometrial stromal tumor with smooth muscle differentiation (see differential diagnosis in these sections), or diffusely infiltrating endometrioid carcinoma.

Treatment and Prognosis

As these tumors are benign they are associated with an excellent outcome if completely removed by local excision or simple hysterectomy.[112,169,170]

ATYPICAL POLYPOID ADENOMYOMA

Definition

This is an unusual biphasic tumor of the uterus composed of endometrial-type glands and smooth muscle with a variable fibroblastic component.[171]

Clinical Features

It typically occurs in reproductive age women (mean 40 years),[114,172,173] but occurs a decade later if associated with myoinvasive carcinoma.[114] Patients often are nulliparous or have a history of infertility. It has been reported in patients with Turner syndrome. Patients present either with abnormal uterine bleeding, vaginal discharge, pelvic pain, or postcoital spotting.[114,172,173]

Gross Features

It is most commonly located in the lower uterine segment, forming a single polypoid lesion or infrequently multiple polyps.[114,174] They range from <0.5 to 6 (mean 2) cm[114] and often are well circumscribed with a lobulated or bosselated white to gray-tan, firm cut surface.[114,172,173] However, it is often fragmented (obtained by curettage) and only irregular pieces of firm and white to tan tissue may be seen.[114]

Microscopic Features

The tumor has a pushing border but the margin can be slightly irregular especially if associated with endometrial carcinoma.[114,173] Variable sized lobules of endometrial glands are embedded in a muscular or fibromuscular stroma (Figure 20.57). Glands are unevenly distributed within the lobules and may be closely packed and complex (Figure 20.58A). A three-tier system based on complexity of the glandular component has been advocated to convey its risk of recurrence.[114] Superficial myometrial invasion can be seen especially if there is complex glandular architecture. Glands are lined by endometrioid-type cells showing nuclear pseudostratification and variable cytologic atypia and mitoses (Figure 20.59). Squamous morules are common and may be associated with central necrosis (Figure 20.58B). Mucinous or ciliated metaplasia may also occur.[114,173] The stromal component is constituted by compact smooth muscle fascicles and less frequently by a fibroblastic/collagenous component,[114,173] and is cytologically bland although smooth muscle cells may be plump showing scattered mitoses (≤2/10 HPF).

Immunohistochemical Features

Endometrioid glands are vimentin, keratin, ER, and PR positive. Squamous morules often show extensive nuclear β-catenin expression that may also be present to a lesser extent in endometrial glands. The stromal component is

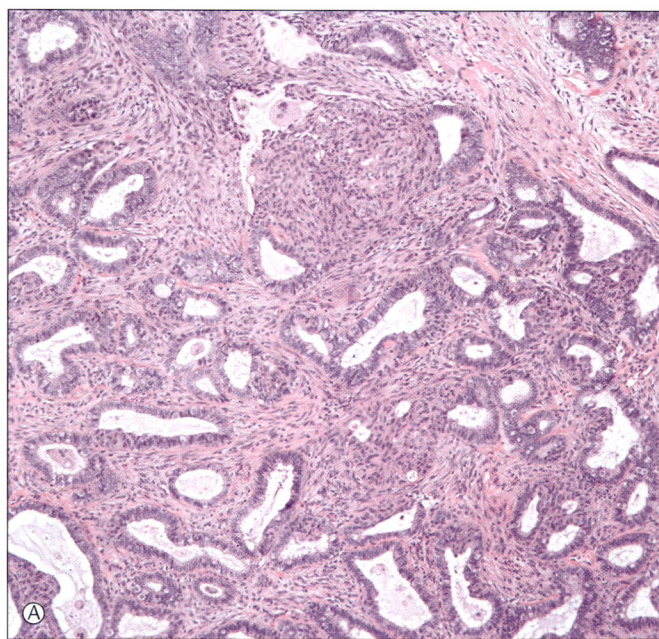

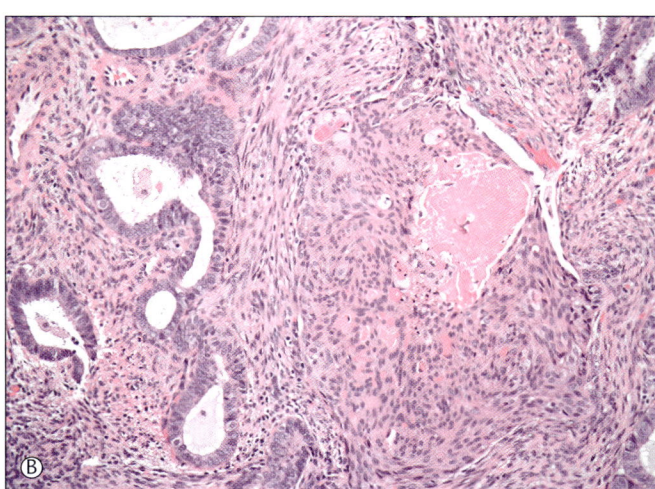

Figure 20.58 Atypical polypoid adenomyoma. The glandular elements appear closely packed but separated by muscular stroma. The glands are lined by endometrioid-type epithelium with squamous morular metaplasia **(A)**, which may be associated with central necrosis **(B)**.

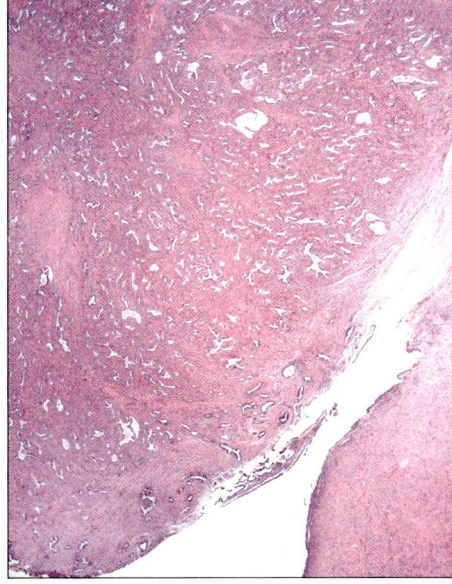

Figure 20.57 Atypical polypoid adenomyoma. At low power, the tumor has a vague lobulated architecture, with lobules being separated by fibromuscular stroma.

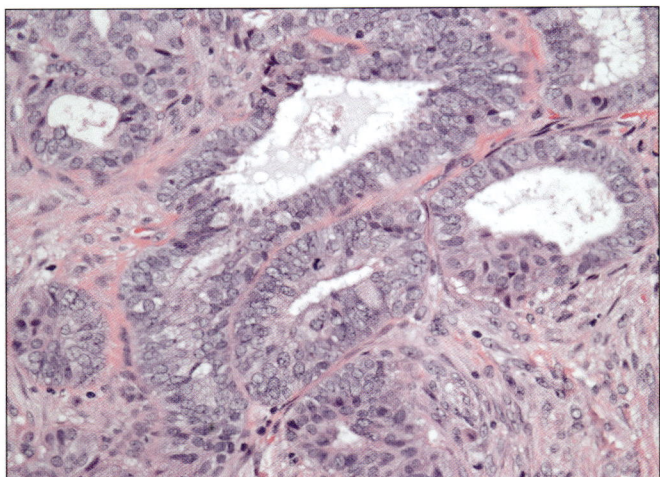

Figure 20.59 Atypical polypoid adenomyoma. The cells lining the glands show pseudostratification, nuclear atypia, and mitotic figures.

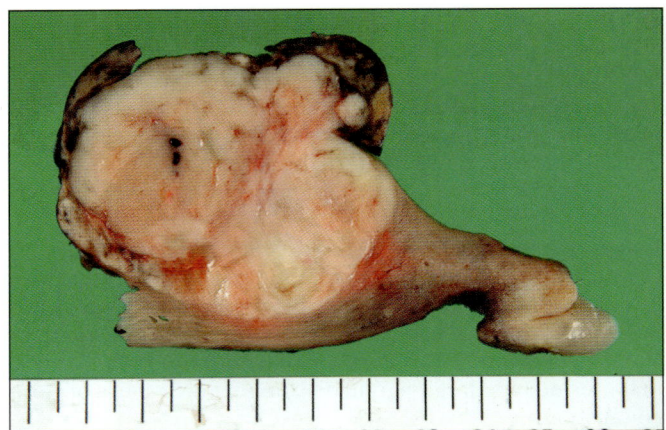

Figure 20.60 PEComa. A large mass appears protruding into the endometrial cavity. It shows a fleshy white to slightly yellow cut surface with areas of necrosis and hemorrhage.

extensively positive for smooth muscle markers (smooth muscle actin and desmin) if predominantly composed of smooth muscle with variable positivity for CD34, h-caldesmon, ER, and PR.[175,176]

Molecular Genetic Features

These tumors are associated with MLH1 hypermethylation (~40%) and microsatellite instability, molecular findings that overlap with those demonstrated in complex atypical hyperplasia and endometrioid carcinoma.[177]

Differential Diagnosis

Atypical polypoid adenomyoma should be distinguished from myoinvasive well-differentiated adenocarcinoma, endometrioid-type adenomyoma, and much less commonly low-grade müllerian adenosarcoma and malignant mixed müllerian tumor. Invasive adenocarcinoma, overall, lacks the lobular glandular architecture, squamous morular differentiation is much less common, and it is associated with desmoplastic stroma. CD10 may be useful in this differential diagnosis as it is expressed around invasive glands but not in the (fibro-) muscular stroma of atypical polypoid adenomyoma.[178] In endometrioid-type adenomyoma, the glandular component is typically scant, lacks a lobular architecture, any degree of cytologic atypia, and it is surrounded by varying amounts of endometrial-type stroma.[112,169] Müllerian adenosarcoma differs from atypical polypoid adenomyoma by its solid and cystic cut surface, phyllodes appearance, and low-grade malignant stromal component, that condensates around the glands without a lobular architecture.[99] Finally, the possibility of a malignant mixed müllerian tumor may be entertained but typically occurs in postmenopausal women and it is defined by the presence of high-grade epithelial and mesenchymal components.[6]

Treatment and Prognosis

Overall, atypical polypoid adenomyomas are associated with an excellent prognosis if completely excised. Patients may undergo local excision or hysterectomy and rarely are treated with hormonal therapy. However, there is a high rate of recurrence (up to 38%) if locally excised especially if there is an architecturally complex epithelial component bordering into adenocarcinoma while effects of hormonal therapy are limited.[114] It is important to state in the pathology report if non-neoplastic endometrium is present, as endometrial hyperplasia has been reported in approximately 6% of cases.[114,173] These lesions have also been associated with endometrioid carcinoma.

PEComa

Definition

The term PEComa encompasses a group of mesenchymal neoplasms composed of histologically and immunohistochemically distinctive perivascular epithelioid cells (PECs), which characteristically coexpress melanocytic and smooth muscle markers.[179] The uterus is the most common location within the female genital tract,[180–186] but they have been described in other locations.[183]

Clinical Features

These tumors occur in patients with a wide age range (25–75 years) and those with lymphangiomyomatosis are usually younger (mean 40 years). Some patients (more frequently with lymphangiomyomatosis) may harbor the tuberous sclerosis complex (*TSC1* or *TSC2* gene mutations).[187,188] Patients often present with abnormal vaginal or postmenopausal bleeding, less commonly with abdominal pain, and rarely hemoperitoneum, but it may be an incidental finding.[180–186]

Gross Features

PEComas are typically centered in the myometrium[180–186] and rarely are submucosal, subserosal, or cervical.[182,183,185] They are usually solitary but can be multiple,[186] ranging in size from <1 to 30 cm. They may have well-circumscribed borders or may infiltrate the myometrium.[181,186,189] The tumors often have a soft, fleshy, white to gray to yellow cut surface with variable areas of hemorrhage and necrosis (Figure 20.60).[181]

Microscopic Features

The tumor may have well-circumscribed margins although unencapsulated or may infiltrate the myometrium with a

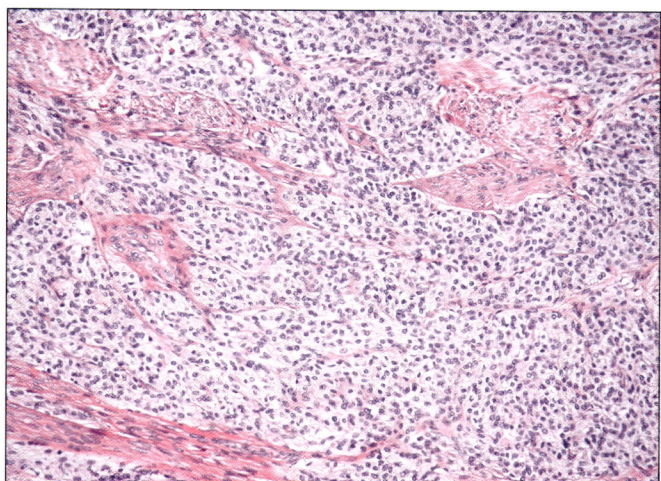

Figure 20.61 PEComa. The tumor shows closely packed nests of uniform cells with pale cytoplasm and round to oval nuclei.

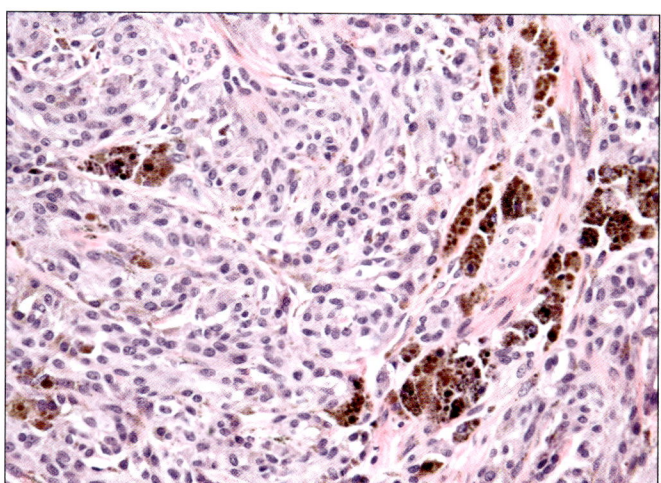

Figure 20.63 PEComa. The tumor cells are small with granular, pale cytoplasm and round to oval nuclei with small nucleoli. Notice the presence of abundant intracytoplasmic melanin pigment.

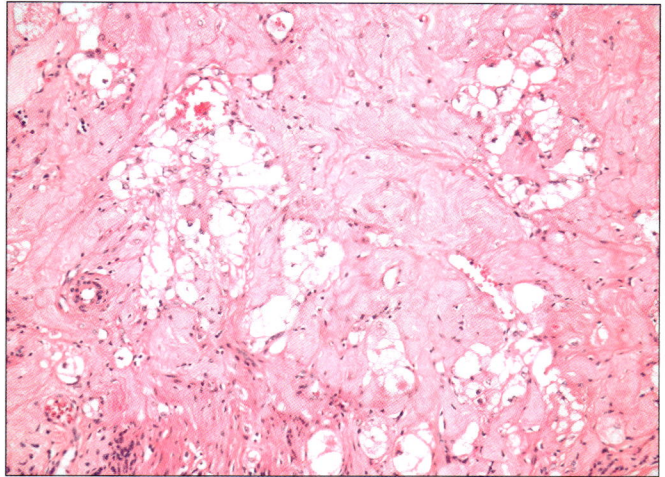

Figure 20.62 PEComa. Some tumors are extensively hyalinized and only scattered nests of tumor cells are seen (sclerosing variant).

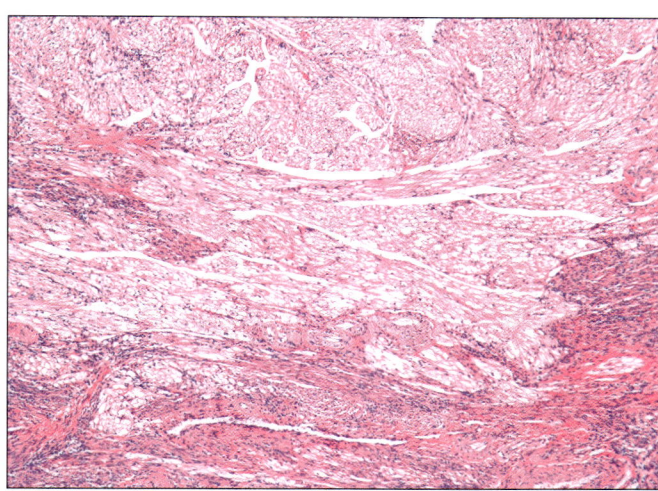

Figure 20.64 Lymphangioleiomyomatosis. Spindle to epithelioid cells form poorly demarcated fascicles and grow around lymphatics with slit-like shapes.

tongue-like or destructive growth.[181,186] The tumor cells are epithelioid or spindled and they grow in sheets, tight nests, or fascicles (Figure 20.61). Pseudoglandular and pseudopapillary growths have been reported.[181] They are associated with a striking delicate vascular network (reminiscent of sinusoidal vasculature of clear renal cell carcinoma) and cells are often arranged in a radial fashion around blood vessels.[183] Large, thick blood vessels can also be seen. Hyalinized plaques are present in between the neoplastic cells.[186] The tumors are usually moderately cellular, but if hyalinization is extensive they may appear hypocellular with scant nests or cords of epithelioid tumor cells (sclerosing PEComa) (Figure 20.62).[190] The epithelioid cells have abundant clear or eosinophilic/granular cytoplasm, and round to oval nuclei. Spindle cells typically form fascicles with pale eosinophilic cytoplasm and elongated nuclei with a wide range of cytologic atypia and mitotic activity (Figure 20.63). Focal intracytoplasmic melanin pigment may be seen (Figure 20.63). Nuclear pseudoinclusions, multinucleated tumor cells, some reminiscent of 'spider cells,' and sex cord-like features may be seen.[181,183,186] Necrosis may be encountered, and the latter as well as lymphovascular invasion are typically seen in malignant tumors.[180,181,183,186] PEComa in the uterus may be associated with lymphangioleiomyomatosis within the uterus, in lymph nodes, or other locations (Figure 20.64). The latter is characterized by a vague nodular proliferation of spindle to epithelioid cells, typically growing around dilated and irregularly shaped lymphatic spaces. The cells have overlapping cytologic features with PEComa cells.[188,191]

Immunohistochemical Features

PEComas are characterized by coexpression of melanocytic (HMB45, Melan-A, tyrosinase, micro-ophthalmia transcription factor, and less frequently S-100; Figure 20.65) and

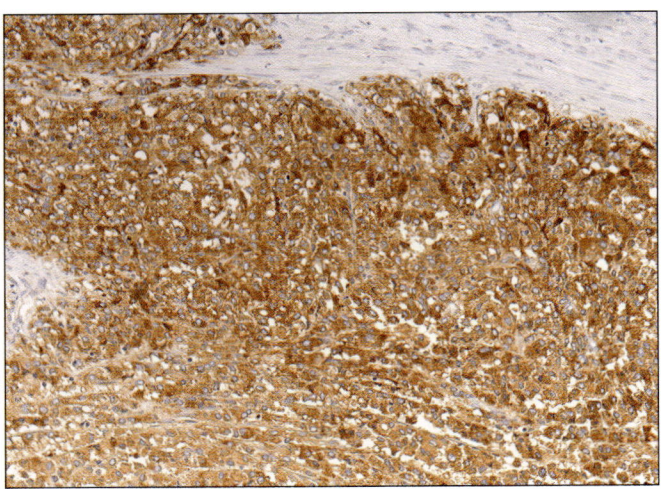

Figure 20.65 PEComa. The tumor cells react diffusely and strongly for HMB45.

smooth muscle markers (smooth muscle actin, muscle myosin, calponin, and to a lesser extent desmin (~30%) or caldesmon). Among melanocytic markers HMB45 and Melan-A are the most sensitive markers. In general, tumors that have a predominance of epithelioid cells tend to more strongly express melanocytic markers and the opposite occurs if the tumor has a predominant population of spindle cells. PEComas are frequently CD117 positive (no associated mutations). CD10 and TFE3 and rarely ER and PR can be positive while keratins (rarely focally positive), CD34, and WT1 and inhibin are negative. CD1a positivity has been reported, but results appear to be controversial.[192,193]

Histogenesis

Multiple origins have been proposed including melanocytic or neural crest,[194] smooth muscle,[186] pericytic, or from perivascular epithelioid cells.[180] In the uterus in particular, PEComas have been related to smooth muscle tumors by some investigators.[151,195,196] A study on comparative genomic hybridization has shown molecular evidence that PEComa is a distinctive neoplasm that often shows deletions on 16p in which the *TSC2* gene is located.[197]

Differential Diagnosis

Most common is the misinterpretation of a PEComa as a spindle and epithelioid smooth muscle tumor, an issue confounded by HMB45 positivity in some smooth muscle neoplasms.[196] Features that favor the latter include diffuse cytoplasmic eosinophilia, spindle cells with perinuclear vacuoles and cigar-shaped nuclei, absence of delicate vasculature, and radial arrangement of tumor cells around the vessels.[193] Even though HMB45 may be positive (may be explained by cross reaction), Melan-A and CD1a are typically negative.[192,193] As PEComa is positive for smooth markers, when confronted with this differential diagnosis it is important to add Melan-A in the diagnostic panel.[193] Gastrointestinal stromal tumors may secondarily involve the uterus and may have epithelioid and spindle cells and they are CD117 positive. However, they lack the delicate vasculature seen in PEComa, cells have eosinophilic fibrillar cytoplasm, and CD34 is negative.[183,198] Rarely, PEComas may be confused with clear cell carcinoma or alveolar soft part sarcoma. Even if PEComas may on occasion focally express keratin (anomalous expression), they never display diffuse and strong positivity, while carcinomas are negative for melanocytic markers. In contrast to PEComa, alveolar soft part sarcoma usually has more cytologic atypia including nucleolar prominence. Immunohistochemistry can also be helpful as these tumors do not express smooth muscle actin or melanocytic markers and they are TFE3 positive,[199] although PEComa may be focally positive for this marker.[183] Malignant melanoma may contain epithelioid and spindled cells as well as melanin pigment. Clinical history or finding an intraepithelial melanocytic component is crucial as both tumors show an overlapping immunohistochemical profile.

Treatment and Prognosis

Most PEComas are confined to the uterus, although extra-uterine disease has been reported in malignant tumors. Patients typically undergo total abdominal hysterectomy with or without adjuvant chemotherapy or radiation if the tumor is malignant.[181,183,186] Pathologic factors associated with adverse outcome ('high risk') include tumor size >5 cm, infiltrative growth, high-grade nuclear atypia, >1 mitoses/50 HPF, and necrosis. Approximately 70% of malignant PEComas have ≥2 of these features.[193,200] However, these pathologic features may be missing in some 'aggressive' PEComas, thus some investigators have suggested these tumors should be labeled as having uncertain malignant potential.[193]

OTHER RARE SARCOMAS

RHABDOMYOSARCOMA

These tumors are by far more common in the cervix than the corpus. The tree main subtypes include embryonal, pleomorphic, and alveolar (least common).[201] Pleomorphic rhabdomyosarcoma occurs in the corpus of perimenopausal and postmenopausal women while embryonal rhabdomyosarcoma is much less common in the corpus (reproductive age women) than in the cervix (girls and less frequently reproductive age women).[76,118,202,203] Patients typically present with abnormal vaginal/postmenopausal bleeding.

Gross Features

This tumor has typically a polypoid, sometimes grape-like configuration with a homogeneous fleshy and soft cut surface and common hemorrhage and necrosis.[76,118,203]

Microscopic Features

Pleomorphic rhabdomyosarcoma displays sheets of large atypical cells with abundant eosinophilic cytoplasm, large pleomorphic nuclei, and atypical mitoses (Figure 20.66).[118,202,203]

Immunohistochemical Features

Rhabdomyosarcomas are positive for muscle-specific actin, desmin, myogenin, and myo-D1, myf-4, myoglobin, and myosin but negative for smooth muscle actin. Rarely, they may express CD99, WT1, keratin, EMA or S-100.[76,203]

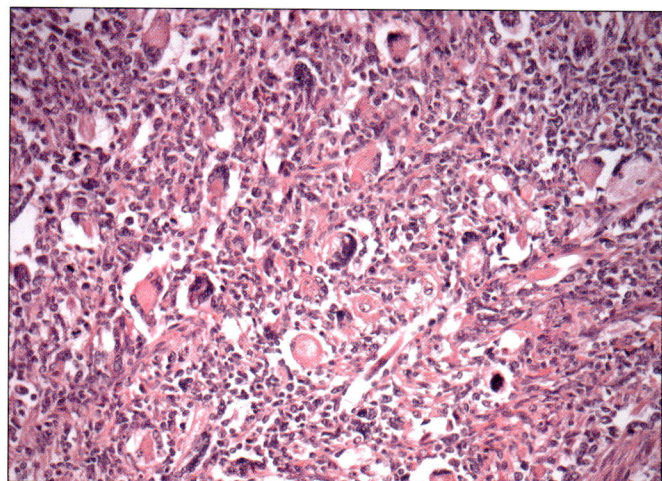

Figure 20.66 Pleomorphic rhabdomyosarcoma. There are numerous atypical rhabdomyoblasts with abundant eosinophilic cytoplasm.

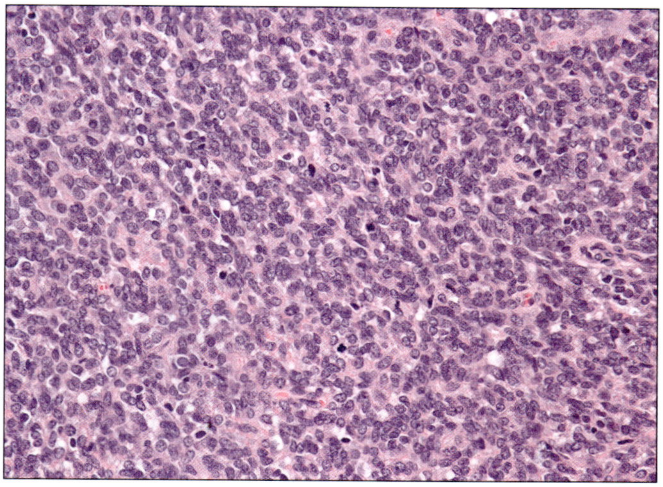

Figure 20.67 Primitive neuroectodermal tumor. The tumor cells grow in sheets. They are small with scant cytoplasm and show brisk mitotic activity.

Differential Diagnosis

Pleomorphic rhabdomyosarcoma should be distinguished from high-grade leiomyosarcoma, adenosarcoma with sarcomatous overgrowth, and carcinosarcoma. The main differential diagnosis of embryonal rhabdomyosarcoma is with müllerian adenosarcoma.

Treatment and Prognosis

Rhabdomyosarcomas are treated with a combination of surgery and chemotherapy, with or without radiotherapy. Age (adults worse), location (cervix better), histologic subtype (pleomorphic dismal prognosis), depth of invasion, and presence of metastasis at initial diagnosis are important prognostic factors.[118,203]

PRIMITIVE NEUROECTODERMAL TUMOR (EWING/PERIPHERAL OR CENTRAL TYPES)

These tumors rarely occur in the uterus of postmenopausal women and typically present with bleeding and a rapidly growing pelvic mass.[127,204] Tumor cells grow in sheets (Figure 20.67), but may form poorly defined lobules, nests, trabeculae, or cords. They are primitive 'blue,' uniform, small, and round, with scant cytoplasm and irregular hyperchromatic nuclei associated with high mitotic rate.[127,204] If of central type, they may show variable degrees of neuronal/neuroectodermal differentiation. Association with endometrioid endometrial carcinoma, adenosarcoma, carcinosarcoma, and rhabdomyosarcoma has been reported.[127] t(11;22)(q24;q12) present in peripheral primitive neuroectodermal tumor (PNET) is more helpful than immunohistochemistry in the differential diagnosis among PNET subtypes as both show similar profiles (vimentin, CD99, and FLI-1 positive). GFAP positivity points toward a central-type PNET. Neuroendocrine markers, neurofilaments, S-100, desmin, and GFAP show variable positivity, but cytokeratin is rarely positive.[127] Central PNET may show neurogenic differentiation by electron microscopy. The differential diagnosis includes cellular smooth muscle tumor and endometrial stromal tumors, two much more common neoplasms;

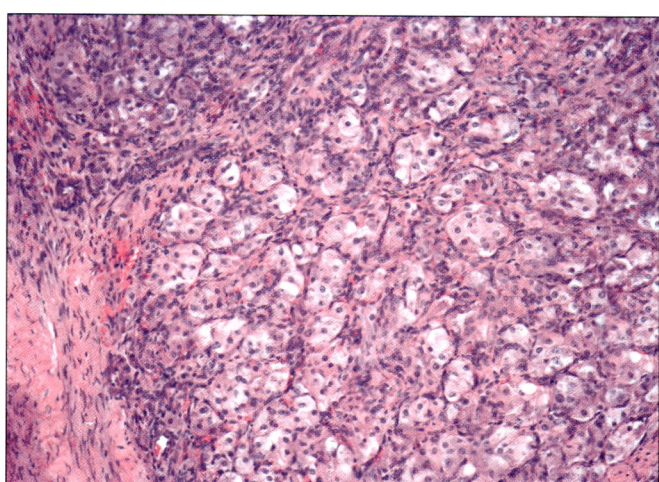

Figure 20.68 Alveolar soft part sarcoma. The tumor cells form small nests and have abundant pale granular cytoplasm and round nuclei with prominent nucleoli.

however, PNETs are typically CD10 and h-caldesmon negative. Rhabdomyosarcoma and lymphoma may also show overlapping histologic features with PNETs. Of note, CD99 and FLI-1 are sensitive but not specific markers of PNET, as rhabdomyosarcoma as well as lymphomas among other tumors have been reported to be positive for these markers.[205] Thus, it is most appropriate to use myogenin, myo-D1, or lymphoid markers in these scenarios. Patients are treated by surgery with or without adjuvant therapy; however, their overall survival is poor.[127]

ALVEOLAR SOFT PART SARCOMA

This soft-tissue neoplasm occurs more commonly in the cervix and lower uterine segment of adolescents and young women. Tumor cells typically have an alveolar or organoid growth separated by delicate fibrovascular septa (Figure 20.68). They display abundant eosinophilic

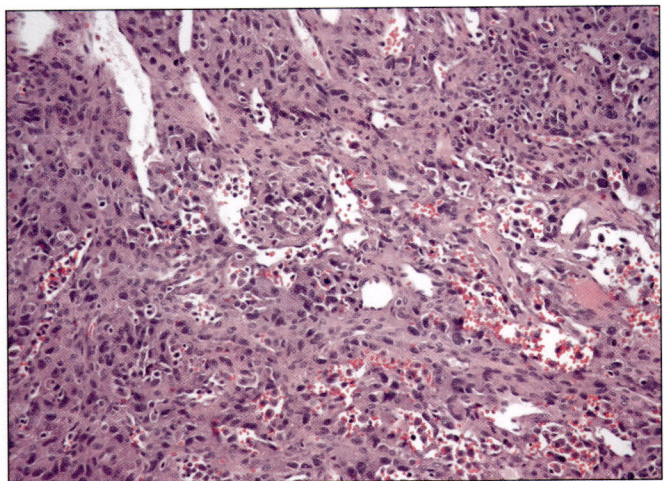

Figure 20.69 Angiosarcoma. There are irregular inter-anastomosing spaces that contain red blood cells and appear lined by tumor cells. The cells show abundant eosinophilic cytoplasm, atypical nuclei, and numerous mitoses.

granular, vacuolated, or clear cytoplasm that may contain periodic acid–Schiff-positive diastase-resistant granules or needle-shape crystals. Nuclei are uniformly large and vesicular with nucleoli and rare mitoses. TFE3 is typically strongly positive[199] while vimentin, smooth muscle markers (desmin, actin, and smooth muscle actin), and occasionally CD10, S-100, synaptophysin, NSE, myoglobin, and HMB45 are also positive. Cytogenetic studies reveal a *der(17)t(X;17)(p11.2;q25)*.[199,206] Patients are treated by surgery and they appear to have a better prognosis than their soft-tissue counterparts.

Other sarcomas occasionally reported in the uterus include *angiosarcoma* (may present as a hemorrhagic, ill-defined diffusely infiltrating mass or may simulate a leiomyoma with hemorrhage) (Figure 20.69),[207] malignant nerve sheath tumors,[208] *liposarcoma* (most likely arising from lipoleiomyoma),[209] *epithelioid sarcoma*,[210] *malignant rhabdoid tumor*,[211] *chondrosarcoma*,[212] and osteosarcoma.[213] Their histologic features are similar to their soft-tissue counterparts and they are associated with a very aggressive behavior.

REFERENCES

1. Harlow BL, Weiss NS, Lofton S. 1986 The epidemiology of sarcomas of the uterus. J Natl Cancer Inst 1986;76:399–402.
2. Hendrickson MR, Tavassoli F, Kempson RL, et al. Mesenchymal tumours and related lesions. In: Tavassoli F, Devilee P, editors. WHO classification of tumours. Pathology and genetics of tumors of breast and female genital organs. Lyon, France: IARC; 2003. p. 233–44.
3. Dionigi A, Oliva E, Clement PB, et al. Endometrial stromal nodules and endometrial stromal tumors with limited infiltration: a clinicopathologic study of 50 cases. Am J Surg Pathol 2002;26:567–81.
4. Tavassoli FA, Norris HJ. Mesenchymal tumours of the uterus. VII. A clinicopathological study of 60 endometrial stromal nodules. Histopathology 1981;5:1–10.
5. Fekete PS, Vellios F. The clinical and histologic spectrum of endometrial stromal neoplasms: a report of 41 cases. Int J Gynecol Pathol 1984;3:198–212.
6. McCluggage G, Haller U, Kurman RJ, et al. Mixed epithelial and mesenchymal tumors. In: Tavassoli F, Devilee P, editors. WHO classification of tumours. Pathology and genetics of tumours of the breast and female genital organs. Lyon, France: IARC Press; 2003. p. 245–9.
7. Chan JK, Kawar NM, Shin JY, et al. Endometrial stromal sarcoma: a population-based analysis. Br J Cancer 2008;99:1210–15.
8. Chang KL, Crabtree GS, Lim-Tan SK, et al. Primary uterine endometrial stromal neoplasms. A clinicopathologic study of 117 cases. Am J Surg Pathol 1990;14:415–38.
9. Hart WR, Yoonessi M. Endometrial stromatosis of the uterus. Obstet Gynecol 1977;49:393–403.
10. Norris HJ, Taylor HB. Mesenchymal tumors of the uterus. I. A clinical and pathological study of 53 endometrial stromal tumors. Cancer 1966;19:755–66.
11. Franquemont DW, Frierson Jr HF, Mills SE. An immunohistochemical study of normal endometrial stroma and endometrial stromal neoplasms. Evidence for smooth muscle differentiation. Am J Surg Pathol 1991;15:861–70.
12. Khalifa MA, Hansen CH, Moore Jr JL, et al. Endometrial stromal sarcoma with focal smooth muscle differentiation: recurrence after 17 years: a follow-up report with discussion of the nomenclature. Int J Gynecol Pathol 1996;15:171–6.
13. Lillemoe TJ, Perrone T, Norris HJ, et al. Myogenous phenotype of epithelial-like areas in endometrial stromal sarcomas. Arch Pathol Lab Med 1991;115:215–19.
14. Lloreta J, Prat J. Endometrial stromal nodule with smooth and skeletal muscle components simulating stromal sarcoma. Int J Gynecol Pathol 1992;11:293–8.
15. McCluggage WG, Cromie AJ, Bryson C, et al. Uterine endometrial stromal sarcoma with smooth muscle and glandular differentiation. J Clin Pathol 2001;54:481–3.
16. Oliva E, Clement PB, Young RH, et al. Mixed endometrial stromal and smooth muscle tumors of the uterus: a clinicopathologic study of 15 cases. Am J Surg Pathol 1998;22:997–1005.
17. Oliva E, de Leval L, Soslow RA, et al. High frequency of JAZF1-JJAZ1 gene fusion in endometrial stromal tumors with smooth muscle differentiation by interphase FISH detection. Am J Surg Pathol 2007;31:1277–84.
18. Oliva E, Young RH, Clement PB, et al. Myxoid and fibrous endometrial stromal tumors of the uterus: a report of 10 cases. Int J Gynecol Pathol 1999;18:310–19.
19. Yilmaz A, Rush DS, Soslow RA. Endometrial stromal sarcomas with unusual histologic features: a report of 24 primary and metastatic tumors emphasizing fibroblastic and smooth muscle differentiation. Am J Surg Pathol 2002;26:1142–50.
20. Lee CH, Marino-Enriquez A, Ou W, et al. The clinicopathologic features of YWHAE-FAM22 endometrial stromal sarcomas: a histologically high-grade and clinically aggressive tumor. Am J Surg Pathol 2012;36:641–53.
21. Baker RJ, Hildebrandt RH, Rouse RV, et al. Inhibin and CD99 (MIC2) expression in uterine stromal neoplasms with sex-cord-like elements. Hum Pathol 1999;30:671–9.
22. Clement PB, Scully RE. Uterine tumors resembling ovarian sex-cord tumors. A clinicopathologic analysis of fourteen cases. Am J Clin Pathol 1976;66:512–25.
23. Nucci MR, O'Connell JT, Huettner PC, et al. h-Caldesmon expression effectively distinguishes endometrial stromal tumors from uterine smooth muscle tumors. Am J Surg Pathol 2001;25:455–63.
24. Irving JA, Carinelli S, Prat J. Uterine tumors resembling ovarian sex cord tumors are polyphenotypic neoplasms with true sex cord differentiation. Mod Pathol 2006;19:17–24.
25. McCluggage WG, Date A, Bharucha H, et al. Endometrial stromal sarcoma with sex cord-like areas and focal rhabdoid differentiation. Histopathology 1996;29:369–74.
26. Rosty C, Genestie C, Blondon J, et al. [Endometrial stromal tumor associated with rhabdoid phenotype and and zones of 'sex cord-like' differentiation]. Ann Pathol 1988;18:133–6.
27. Zamecnik M, Michal M. Endometrial stromal nodule with retiform sex-cord-like differentiation. Pathol Res Pract 1998;194:449–53.
28. Clement PB, Scully RE. Endometrial stromal sarcomas of the uterus with extensive endometrioid glandular differentiation: a report of three cases that caused problems in differential diagnosis. Int J Gynecol Pathol 1992;11:163–73.
29. McCluggage WG, Ganesan R, Herrington CS. Endometrial stromal sarcomas with extensive endometrioid glandular differentiation: report of a series with emphasis on the potential for

misdiagnosis and discussion of the differential diagnosis. Histopathology 2009;54:365–73.
30. Baker PM, Moch H, Oliva E. Unusual morphologic features of endometrial stromal tumors: a report of 2 cases. Am J Surg Pathol 2005;29:1394–8.
31. Oliva E, Clement PB, Young RH. Epithelioid endometrial and endometrioid stromal tumors: a report of four cases emphasizing their distinction from epithelioid smooth muscle tumors and other oxyphilic uterine and extrauterine tumors. Int J Gynecol Pathol 2002;21:48–55.
32. Lifschitz-Mercer B, Czernobilsky B, Dgani R, et al. Immunocytochemical study of an endometrial diffuse clear cell stromal sarcoma and other endometrial stromal sarcomas. Cancer 1987;59:1494–9.
33. McCluggage WG, Young RH. Endometrial stromal sarcomas with true papillae and pseudopapillae. Int J Gynecol Pathol 2008;27:555–61.
34. Shah R, McCluggage WG. Symplastic atypia in neoplastic and non-neoplastic endometrial stroma: report of 3 cases with a review of atypical symplastic cells within the female genital tract. Int J Gynecol Pathol 2009;28:334–7.
35. Fadare O, McCalip B, Mariappan MR, et al. An endometrial stromal tumor with osteoclast-like giant cells. Ann Diagn Pathol 2005;9:160–5.
36. Aubry MC, Myers JL, Colby TV, et al. Endometrial stromal sarcoma metastatic to the lung: a detailed analysis of 16 patients. Am J Surg Pathol 2002;26:440–9.
37. Farhood AI, Abrams J. Immunohistochemistry of endometrial stromal sarcoma. Hum Pathol 1991;22:224–30.
38. de Leval L, Waltregny D, Boniver J, et al. Use of histone deacetylase 8 (HDAC8), a new marker of smooth muscle differentiation, in the classification of mesenchymal tumors of the uterus. Am J Surg Pathol 2006;30:319–27.
39. Devaney K, Tavassoli FA. Immunohistochemistry as a diagnostic aid in the interpretation of unusual mesenchymal tumors of the uterus. Mod Pathol 1991;4:225–31.
40. Oliva E, Young RH, Amin MB, et al. An immunohistochemical analysis of endometrial stromal and smooth muscle tumors of the uterus: a study of 54 cases emphasizing the importance of using a panel because of overlap in immunoreactivity for individual antibodies. Am J Surg Pathol 2002;26:403–12.
41. Chu PG, Arber DA, Weiss LM, et al. Utility of CD10 in distinguishing between endometrial stromal sarcoma and uterine smooth muscle tumors: an immunohistochemical comparison of 34 cases. Mod Pathol 2001;14:465–71.
42. Kurihara S, Oda Y, Ohishi Y, et al. Coincident expression of beta-catenin and cyclin D1 in endometrial stromal tumors and related high-grade sarcomas. Mod Pathol 2010;23:225–34.
43. Ioffe YJ, Li AJ, Walsh CS, et al. Hormone receptor expression in uterine sarcomas: prognostic and therapeutic roles. Gynecol Oncol 2009;115:466–71.
44. Kitaoka Y, Kitawaki J, Koshiba H, et al. Aromatase cytochrome P450 and estrogen and progesterone receptors in uterine sarcomas: correlation with clinical parameters. J Steroid Biochem Mol Biol 2004;88:183–9.
45. Balleine RL, Earls PJ, Webster LR, et al. Expression of progesterone receptor A and B isoforms in low-grade endometrial stromal sarcoma. Int J Gynecol Pathol 2004;23:138–44.
46. Bhargava R, Shia J, Hummer AJ, et al. Distinction of endometrial stromal sarcomas from 'hemangiopericytomatous' tumors using a panel of immunohistochemical stains. Mod Pathol 2005;18:40–7.
47. Jakate K, Azimi F, Ali RH, et al. Endometrial sarcomas: an immunohistochemical and JAZF1 re-arrangement study in low-grade and undifferentiated tumors. Mod Pathol 2013;26:95–105.
48. Kurihara S, Oda Y, Ohishi Y, et al. Endometrial stromal sarcomas and related high-grade sarcomas: immunohistochemical and molecular genetic study of 31 cases. Am J Surg Pathol 2008;32:1228–38.
49. Moinfar F, Regitnig P, Tabrizi AD, et al. Expression of androgen receptors in benign and malignant endometrial stromal neoplasms. Virchows Arch 2004;444:410–14.
50. Reich O, Regauer S. Aromatase expression in low-grade endometrial stromal sarcomas: an immunohistochemical study. Mod Pathol 2004;17:104–8.
51. Sumathi VP, Al-Hussaini M, Connolly LE, et al. Endometrial stromal neoplasms are immunoreactive with WT-1 antibody. Int J Gynecol Pathol 2004;23:241–7.
52. Rushing RS, Shajahan S, Chendil D, et al. Uterine sarcomas express KIT protein but lack mutation(s) in exon 11 or 17 of c-KIT. Gynecol Oncol 2003;91:9–14.
53. Jakate K, Azimi F, Ali RH, et al. Endometrial sarcomas: an immunohistochemical and JAZF1 re-arrangement study in low-grade and undifferentiated tumors. Mod Pathol 2013;26:95–105.
54. Lee CH, Ali RH, Rouzbahman M, et al. Cyclin D1 as a diagnostic immunomarker for endometrial stromal sarcoma with YWHAE-FAM22 rearrangement. Am J Surg Pathol 2012;36:1562–70.
55. Oliva E, Clement PB, Young RH. Endometrial stromal tumors: an update on a group of tumors with a protean phenotype. Adv Anat Pathol 2000;7:257–81.
56. Goldblum JR, Clement PB, Hart WR. Adenomyosis with sparse glands. A potential mimic of low-grade endometrial stromal sarcoma. Am J Clin Pathol 1995;103:218–23.
57. Oliva E, Young RH, Clement PB, et al. Cellular benign mesenchymal tumors of the uterus. A comparative morphologic and immunohistochemical analysis of 33 highly cellular leiomyomas and six endometrial stromal nodules, two frequently confused tumors. Am J Surg Pathol 1995;19:757–68.
58. Nucci MR, O'Connell JT, Huettner PC, et al. 2001 h-Caldesmon expression effectively distinguishes endometrial stromal tumors from uterine smooth muscle tumors. Am J Surg Pathol 1995;25:455–63.
59. Loddenkemper C, Mechsner S, Foss HD, et al. Use of oxytocin receptor expression in distinguishin g between uterine smooth muscle tumors and endometrial stromal sarcoma. Am J Surg Pathol 2003;27:1458–62.
60. Clement PB, Young RH, Scully RE. Intravenous leiomyomatosis of the uterus. A clinicopathological analysis of 16 cases with unusual histologic features. Am J Surg Pathol 1998;12:932–45.
61. Novelli M, Rossi S, Rodriguez-Justo M, et al. DOG1 and CD117 are the antibodies of choice in the diagnosis of gastrointestinal stromal tumours. Histopathology 2010;57:259–70.
62. Chiang S, Ali R, Melnyk N, et al. Frequency of known gene rearrangements in endometrial stromal tumors. Am J Surg Pathol 2011;35:1364–72.
63. Dal Cin P, Aly MS, De Wever I, et al. Endometrial stromal sarcoma t(7;17)(p15-21;q12-21) is a nonrandom chromosome change. Cancer Genet Cytogenet 1992;63:43–6.
64. Hennig Y, Caselitz J, Bartnitzke S, et al. A third case of a low-grade endometrial stromal sarcoma with a t(7;17)(p14 approximately 21;q11.2 approximately 21). Cancer Genet Cytogenet 1997;98:84–6.
65. Koontz JI, Soreng AL, Nucci M, et al. Frequent fusion of the JAZF1 and JJAZ1 genes in endometrial stromal tumors. Proc Natl Acad Sci USA 2001;98:6348–53.
66. Micci F, Walter CU, Teixeira MR, et al. Cytogenetic and molecular genetic analyses of endometrial stromal sarcoma: nonrandom involvement of chromosome arms 6p and 7p and confirmation of JAZF1/JJAZ1 gene fusion in t(7;17). Cancer Genet Cytogenet 2003;144:119–24.
67. Nucci MR, Harburger D, Koontz J, et al. Molecular analysis of the JAZF1-JJAZ1 gene fusion by RT-PCR and fluorescence in situ hybridization in endometrial stromal neoplasms. Am J Surg Pathol 2007;31:65–70.
68. Hrzenjak A, Moinfar F, Tavassoli FA, et al. JAZF1/JJAZ1 gene fusion in endometrial stromal sarcomas: molecular analysis by reverse transcriptase-polymerase chain reaction optimized for paraffin-embedded tissue. J Mol Diagn 2005;7:388–95.
69. Huang HY, Ladanyi M, Soslow RA. Molecular detection of JAZF1-JJAZ1 gene fusion in endometrial stromal neoplasms with classic and variant histology: evidence for genetic heterogeneity. Am J Surg Pathol 2004;28:224–32.
70. Hrynchak M, Horsman D, Salski C, et al. Complex karyotypic alterations in an endometrial stromal sarcoma. Cancer Genet Cytogenet 1994;77:45–9.
71. Micci F, Panagopoulos I, Bjerkehagen B, et al. Consistent rearrangement of chromosomal band 6p21 with generation of fusion genes JAZF1/PHF1 and EPC1/PHF1 in endometrial stromal sarcoma. Cancer Res 2006;66:107–12.
72. Regauer S, Emberger W, Reich O, et al. Cytogenetic analyses of two new cases of endometrial stromal sarcoma–non-random reciprocal translocation t(10;17)(q22;p13) correlates with fibrous ESS. Histopathology 2008;52:780–3.

73. D'Angelo E, Ali RH, Espinosa I, et al. 2012 Endometrial stromal sarcomas with sex cord differentiation are associated with PHF1 rearrangement. Am J Surg Pathol 2013;37:514–21.
74. Abeler VM, Royne O, Thoresen S, et al. Uterine sarcomas in Norway. A histopathological and prognostic survey of a total population from 1970 to 2000 including 419 patients. Histopathology 2009;54:355–64.
75. Reich O, Nogales FF, Regauer S. Gonadotropin-releasing hormone receptor expression in endometrial stromal sarcomas: an immunohistochemical study. Mod Pathol 2005;18:573–6.
76. McCluggage WG, Lioe TF, McClelland HR, et al. Rhabdomyosarcoma of the uterus: report of two cases, including one of the spindle cell variant. Int J Gynecol Cancer 2002;12:128–32.
77. Clement PB, Scully RE. Mullerian adenosarcomas of the uterus with sex cord-like elements. A clinicopathologic analysis of eight cases. Am J Clin Pathol 1989;91:664–72.
78. Silverberg SG, Major FJ, Blessing JA, et al. Carcinosarcoma (malignant mixed mesodermal tumor) of the uterus. A Gynecologic Oncology Group pathologic study of 203 cases. Int J Gynecol Pathol 1990;9:1–19.
79. Nogales F, Tavassoli FA. Sex cord-like, neuroectodermal and neuroendocrine tumours, lymphomas and leukaemias. In: Tavassoli FA, Devilee P, editors. WHO classifications of tumours. Pathology and genetics of tumours of the breast and female genital organs. Lyon, France: IARC; 2003.
80. Czernobilsky B, Mamet Y, David MB, et al. Uterine retiform sertoli-leydig cell tumor: report of a case providing additional evidence that uterine tumors resembling ovarian sex cord tumors have a histologic and immunohistochemical phenotype of genuine sex cord tumors. Int J Gynecol Pathol 2005;24:335–40.
81. Kabbani W, Deavers MT, Malpica A, et al. Uterine tumor resembling ovarian sex-cord tumor: report of a case mimicking cervical adenocarcinoma. Int J Gynecol Pathol 2003;22:297–302.
82. Nogales FF, Stolnicu S, Harilal KR, et al. Retiform uterine tumours resembling ovarian sex cord tumours. A comparative immunohistochemical study with retiform structures of the female genital tract. Histopathology 2009;54:471–7.
83. Hurrell DP, McCluggage WG. Uterine tumour resembling ovarian sex cord tumour is an immunohistochemically polyphenotypic neoplasm which exhibits coexpression of epithelial, myoid and sex cord markers. J Clin Pathol 2007;60:1148–54.
84. Krishnamurthy S, Jungbluth AA, Busam KJ, et al. Uterine tumors resembling ovarian sex-cord tumors have an immunophenotype consistent with true sex-cord differentiation. Am J Surg Pathol 1998;22(9):1078–82.
85. de Leval L, Lim GS, Waltregny D, et al. Diverse phenotypic profile of uterine tumors resembling ovarian sex cord tumors: an immunohistochemical study of 12 cases. Am J Surg Pathol 2010;34:1749–61.
86. Hauptmann S, Nadjari B, Kraus J, et al. Uterine tumor resembling ovarian sex-cord tumor–a case report and review of the literature. Virchows Arch 2001;439:97–101.
87. Gupta M, de Leval L, Selig M, et al. Uterine tumors resembling ovarian sex cord tumors: an ultrastructural analysis of 13 cases. Ultrastructural Pathol 2010;34:16–24.
88. Staats PN, Garcia JJ, Dias-Santagata DC, et al. Uterine tumors resembling ovarian sex cord tumors (UTROSCT) lack the JAZF1-JJAZ1 translocation frequently seen in endometrial stromal tumors. Am J Surg Pathol 2009;33:1206–12.
89. Murray SK, Clement PB, Young RH. Endometrioid carcinomas of the uterine corpus with sex cord-like formations, hyalinization, and other unusual morphologic features: a report of 31 cases of a neoplasm that may be confused with carcinosarcoma and other uterine neoplasms. Am J Surg Pathol 2005;29:157–66.
90. Clement PB, Scully RE. Uterine tumors with mixed epithelial and mesenchymal elements. Semin Diagn Pathol 1998;5:199–222.
91. O'Meara AC, Giger OT, Jurrer M, et al. Case report: recurrence of a uterine tumor resembling ovarian sex-cord tumor. Gynecol Oncol 2009;114:140–2.
92. Zaloudek CJ, Norris HJ. Adenofibroma and adenosarcoma of the uterus: a clinicopathologic study of 35 cases. Cancer 1981;48:354–66.
93. Horie Y, Ikawa S, Kadowaki K, et al. Lipoadenofibroma of the uterine corpus. Report of a new variant of adenofibroma (benign mullerian mixed tumor). Arch Pathol Lab Med 1995;119:274–6.
94. Miller KN, McClure SP. Papillary adenofibroma of the uterus. Report of a case involved by adenocarcinoma and review of the literature. Am J Clin Pathol 1992;97:806–9.
95. Gallardo A, Prat J. Mullerian adenosarcoma: a clinicopathologic and immunohistochemical study of 55 cases challenging the existence of adenofibroma. Am J Surg Pathol 2009;33:278–88.
96. Major FJ, Blessing JA, Silverberg SG, et al. Prognostic factors in early-stage uterine sarcoma. A Gynecologic Oncology Group study. Cancer 1993;71:1702–9.
97. Clarke BA, Mulligan AM, Irving JA, et al. Mullerian adenosarcomas with unusual growth patterns: staging issues. Int J Gynecol Pathol 2011;30:340–7.
98. Gollard R, Kosty M, Bordin G, et al. Two unusual presentations of mullerian adenosarcoma: case reports, literature review, and treatment considerations. Gynecol Oncol 1995;59:412–22.
99. Clement PB, Scully RE. Mullerian adenosarcoma of the uterus: a clinicopathologic analysis of 100 cases with a review of the literature. Hum Pathol 1990;21:363–81.
100. Clement PB, Oliva E, Young RH. Mullerian adenosarcoma of the uterine corpus associated with tamoxifen therapy: a report of six cases and a review of tamoxifen-associated endometrial lesions. Int J Gynecol Pathol 1996;15:222–9.
101. Clement PB. Mullerian adenosarcomas of the uterus with sarcomatous overgrowth. A clinicopathological analysis of 10 cases. Am J Surg Pathol 1989;13:28–38.
102. Hirschfield L, Kahn LB, Chen S, et al. Mullerian adenosarcoma with ovarian sex cord-like differentiation. A light- and electron-microscopic study. Cancer 1986;57:1197–200.
103. Fehmian C, Jones J, Kress Y, et al. Adenosarcoma of the uterus with extensive smooth muscle differentiation: ultrastructural study and review of the literature. Ultrastruct Pathol 1997;21:73–9.
104. Ramos P, Ruiz A, Carabias E, et al. Mullerian adenosarcoma of the cervix with heterologous elements: report of a case and review of the literature. Gynecol Oncol 2002;84:161–6.
105. Kaku T, Silverberg SG, Major FJ, et al. Adenosarcoma of the uterus: a Gynecologic Oncology Group clinicopathologic study of 31 cases. Int J Gynecol Pathol 1992;11:75–88.
106. Abeler VM, Nenodovic M. Diagnostic immunohistochemistry in uterine sarcomas: a study of 397 cases. Int J Gynecol Pathol 2011;30:236–43.
107. Amant F, Schurmans K, Steenkiste E, et al. Immunohistochemical determination of estrogen and progesterone receptor positivity in uterine adenosarcoma. Gynecol Oncol 2004;93:680–5.
108. Mikami Y, Hata S, Kiyokawa T, et al. Expression of CD10 in malignant mullerian mixed tumors and adenosarcomas: an immunohistochemical study. Mod Pathol 2002;15:923–30.
109. Soslow RA, Ali A, Oliva E. Mullerian adenosarcomas: an immunophenotypic analysis of 35 cases. Am J Surg Pathol 2008;32:1013–21.
110. Tai LH, Tavassoli FA. Endometrial polyps with atypical (bizarre) stromal cells. Am J Surg Pathol 2002;26:505–9.
111. Parker RL, Dadmanesh F, Young RH, et al. Polypoid endometriosis: a clinicopathologic analysis of 24 cases and a review of the literature. Am J Surg Pathol 2004;28:285–97.
112. Gilks CB, Clement PB, Hart WR, et al. Uterine adenomyomas excluding atypical polypoid adenomyomas and adenomyomas of endocervical type: a clinicopathologic study of 30 cases of an underemphasized lesion that may cause diagnostic problems with brief consideration of adenomyomas of other female genital tract sites. Int J Gynecol Pathol 2000;19:195–205.
113. Gilks CB, Young RH, Clement PB, et al. Adenomyomas of the uterine cervix of endocervical type: a report of ten cases of a benign cervical tumor that may be confused with adenoma malignum [corrected]. Mod Pathol 1996;9:220–4.
114. Longacre TA, Chung MH, Rouse RV, et al. Atypical polypoid adenomyofibromas (atypical polypoid adenomyomas) of the uterus. A clinicopathologic study of 55 cases. Am J Surg Pathol 1996;20:1–20.
115. Seidman JD, Chauhan S. Evaluation of the relationship between adenosarcoma and carcinosarcoma and a hypothesis of the histogenesis of uterine sarcomas. Int J Gynecol Pathol 2003;22:75–82.
116. Daya DA, Scully RE. Sarcoma botryoides of the uterine cervix in young women: a clinicopathological study of 13 cases. Gynecol Oncol 1988;29:290–304.
117. Dehner LP, Jarzembowski JA, Hill DA. Embryonal rhabdomyosarcoma of the uterine cervix: a report of 14 cases and a discussion of its unusual clinicopathological associations. Mod Pathol 2012;25:602–14.

118. Ferguson SE, Gerald W, Barakat RR, et al. Clinicopathologic features of rhabdomyosarcoma of gynecologic origin in adults. Am J Surg Pathol 2007;31:382–9.
119. Arend R, Bagaria M, Lewin SN, et al. Long-term outcome and natural history of uterine adenosarcomas. Gynecol Oncol 2010;119:305–8.
120. Verschraegen CF, Vasuratna A, Edwards C, et al. Clinicopathologic analysis of mullerian adenosarcoma: the M.D. Anderson Cancer Center experience. Oncol Rep 1998;5:939–44.
121. Garg G, Shah JP, Kumar S, et al. Ovarian and uterine carcinosarcomas: a comparative analysis of prognostic variables and survival outcomes. Int J Gynecol Cancer 2010;20:888–94.
122. Zelmanowicz A, Hildesheim A, Sherman ME, et al. Evidence for a common etiology for endometrial carcinomas and malignant mixed mullerian tumors. Gynecol Oncol 1998;69:253–7.
123. Grayson W, Taylor LF, Cooper K. Carcinosarcoma of the uterine cervix: a report of eight cases with immunohistochemical analysis and evaluation of human papillomavirus status. Am J Surg Pathol 2001;25:338–47.
124. Buza N, Tavassoli FA. Comparative analysis of P16 and P53 expression in uterine malignant mixed mullerian tumors. Int J Gynecol Pathol 2009;28:514–21.
125. Ribeiro-Silva A, Novello-Vilar A, Cunha-Mercante AM, et al. Malignant mixed Mullerian tumor of the uterine cervix with neuroendocrine differentiation. Int J Gynecol Cancer 2002;12:223–7.
126. Baschinsky DY, Niemann TH, Eaton LA, et al. Malignant mixed Mullerian tumor with rhabdoid features: a report of two cases and a review of the literature. Gynecol Oncol 1999;73:145–50.
127. Euscher ED, Deavers MT, Lopez-Terrada D, et al. Uterine tumors with neuroectodermal differentiation: a series of 17 cases and review of the literature. Am J Surg Pathol 2008;32:219–28.
128. Kajo K, Zubor P, Spacek J, et al. Carcinosarcoma of the uterus with melanocytic differentiation. Pathol Res Pract 2007;203:753–8.
129. Shokeir MO, Noel SM, Clement PB. Malignant mullerian mixed tumor of the uterus with a prominent alpha-fetoprotein-producing component of yolk sac tumor. Mod Pathol 1996;9:647–51.
130. Bitterman P, Chun B, Kurman RJ. The significance of epithelial differentiation in mixed mesodermal tumors of the uterus. A clinicopathologic and immunohistochemical study. Am J Surg Pathol 1990;14:317–28.
131. de Brito PA, Silverberg SG, Orenstein JM. Carcinosarcoma (malignant mixed mullerian (mesodermal) tumor) of the female genital tract: immunohistochemical and ultrastructural analysis of 28 cases. Hum Pathol 1993;24:132–42.
132. Costa MJ, Khan R, Judd R. Carcinoma (malignant mixed mullerian [mesodermal] tumor) of the uterus and ovary. Correlation of clinical, pathologic, and immunohistochemical features in 29 cases. Arch Pathol Lab Med 1991;115:583–90.
133. George E, Manivel JC, Dehner LP, et al. Malignant mixed mullerian tumors: an immunohistochemical study of 47 cases, with histogenetic considerations and clinical correlation. Hum Pathol 1991;22:215–23.
134. de Jong RA, Nijman HW, Wijbrandi TF, et al. Molecular markers and clinical behavior of uterine carcinosarcomas: focus on the epithelial tumor component. Mod Pathol 2011;24:1368–79.
135. Cimbaluk D, Rotmensch J, Scudiere J, et al. Uterine carcinosarcoma: immunohistochemical studies on tissue microarrays with focus on potential therapeutic targets. Gynecol Oncol 2007;105:138–44.
136. Winter 3rd WE, Seidman JD, Krivak TC, et al. Clinicopathological analysis of c-kit expression in carcinosarcomas and leiomyosarcomas of the uterine corpus. Gynecol Oncol 2003;91:3–8.
137. Lopez-Garcia MA, Palacios J. Pathologic and molecular features of uterine carcinosarcomas. Semin Diagn Pathol 2010;27:274–86.
138. Abeln EC, Smit VT, Wessels JW, et al. Molecular genetic evidence for the conversion hypothesis of the origin of malignant mixed mullerian tumours. J Pathol 1997;183:424–31.
139. Costa MJ, Vogelsan J, Young LJ. p53 gene mutation in female genital tract carcinosarcomas (malignant mixed mullerian tumors): a clinicopathologic study of 74 cases. Mod Pathol 1994;7:619–27.
140. Fujii H, Yoshida M, Gong ZX, et al. Frequent genetic heterogeneity in the clonal evolution of gynecological carcinosarcoma and its influence on phenotypic diversity. Cancer Res 2000;60:114–20.
141. Kounelis S, Jones MW, Papadaki H, et al. Carcinosarcomas (malignant mixed mullerian tumors) of the female genital tract: comparative molecular analysis of epithelial and mesenchymal components. Hum Pathol 1998;29:82–7.
142. Wada H, Enomoto T, Fujita M, et al. Molecular evidence that most but not all carcinosarcomas of the uterus are combination tumors. Cancer Res 1997;57:5379–85.
143. Castilla MA, Moreno-Bueno G, Romero-Perez L, et al. Micro-RNA signature of the epithelial-mesenchymal transition in endometrial carcinosarcoma. J Pathol 2011;223:72–80.
144. Sreenan JJ, Hart WR. Carcinosarcomas of the female genital tract. A pathologic study of 29 metastatic tumors: further evidence for the dominant role of the epithelial component and the conversion theory of histogenesis. Am J Surg Pathol 1995;19:666–74.
145. Tafe LJ, Garg K, Chew I, et al. Endometrial and ovarian carcinomas with undifferentiated components: clinically aggressive and frequently underrecognized neoplasms. Mod Pathol 2010;23:781–9.
146. Bodner-Adler B, Bodner K, Obermair A, et al. Prognostic parameters in carcinosarcomas of the uterus: a clinico-pathologic study. Anticancer Res 2001;21:3069–74.
147. Jonson AL, Bliss RL, Truskinovsky A, et al. Clinical features and outcomes of uterine and ovarian carcinosarcoma. Gynecol Oncol 2006;100:561–4.
148. Amant F, Cadron I, Fuso L, et al. Endometrial carcinosarcomas have a different prognosis and pattern of spread compared to high-risk epithelial endometrial cancer. Gynecol Oncol 2005;98:274–80.
149. Gagne E, Tetu B, Blondeau L, et al. Morphologic prognostic factors of malignant mixed mullerian tumor of the uterus: a clinicopathologic study of 58 cases. Mod Pathol 1989;2:433–8.
150. Iwasa Y, Haga H, Konishi I, et al. Prognostic factors in uterine carcinosarcoma: a clinicopathologic study of 25 patients. Cancer 1998;82:512–9.
151. Sartori E, Bazzurini L, Gadducci A, et al. Carcinosarcoma of the uterus: a clinicopathological multicenter CTF study. Gynecol Oncol 1997;67:70–5.
152. Ferguson SE, Tornos C, Hummer A, et al. Prognostic features of surgical stage I uterine carcinosarcoma. Am J Surg Pathol 2007;31:1653–61.
153. Parker WH. Etiology, symptomatology, and diagnosis of uterine myomas. Fertil Steril 2007;87:725–36.
154. Bergeron C, Amant F, Ferenczy A. Pathology and physiopathology of adenomyosis. Best Pract Res Clin Obstet Gynaecol 2006;20:511–21.
155. Parazzini F, Vercellini P, Panazza S, et al. Risk factors for adenomyosis. Hum Reprod 1997;12:1275–9.
156. Vercellini P, Parazzini F, Oldani S, et al. Adenomyosis at hysterectomy: a study on frequency distribution and patient characteristics. Hum Reprod 1995;10:1160–2.
157. Cohen I, Beyth Y, Tepper R, et al. Adenomyosis in postmenopausal breast cancer patients treated with tamoxifen: a new entity? Gynecol Oncol 1995;58:86–91.
158. McCausland AM, McCausland VM. Depth of endometrial penetration in adenomyosis helps determine outcome of rollerball ablation. Am J Obstet Gynecol 1996;174:1786–93; 1793–4.
159. Brosens JJ, de Souza NM, Barker FG. Uterine junctional zone: function and disease. Lancet 1995;346:558–60.
160. Ferenczy A. Pathophysiology of adenomyosis. Hum Reprod Update 1998;4:312–22.
161. Mori T, Singtripop T, Kawashima S. Animal model of uterine adenomyosis: is prolactin a potent inducer of adenomyosis in mice? Am J Obstet Gynecol 1991;165:232–4.
162. McCluggage WG, Desai V, Manek S. Tamoxifen-associated postmenopausal adenomyosis exhibits stromal fibrosis, glandular dilatation and epithelial metaplasias. Histopathology 2000;37:340–6.
163. Koshiyama M, Suzuki A, Ozawa M, et al. Adenocarcinomas arising from uterine adenomyosis: a report of four cases. Int J Gynecol Pathol 2002;21:239–45.
164. Mittal KR, Barwick KW. Diffusely infiltrating adenocarcinoma of the endometrium. A subtype with poor prognosis. Am J Surg Pathol 1988;12:754–8.
165. Ismiil N, Rasty G, Ghorab Z, et al. Adenomyosis involved by endometrial adenocarcinoma is a significant risk factor for deep myometrial invasion. Ann Diagn Pathol 2007;11:252–7.
166. Ismiil ND, Rasty G, Ghorab Z, et al. Adenomyosis is associated with myometrial invasion by FIGO 1 endometrial adenocarcinoma. Int J Gynecol Pathol 2007;26:278–83.

167. Mittal KR, Barwick KW. Endometrial adenocarcinoma involving adenomyosis without true myometrial invasion is characterized by frequent preceding estrogen therapy, low histologic grades, and excellent prognosis. Gynecol Oncol 1993;49:197–201.
168. Toki T, Shimizu M, Takagi Y, et al. CD10 is a marker for normal and neoplastic endometrial stromal cells. Int J Gynecol Pathol 2002;21:41–7.
169. Tahlan A, Nanda A, Mohan H. Uterine adenomyoma: a clinicopathologic review of 26 cases and a review of the literature. Int J Gynecol Pathol 2006;25:361–5.
170. Gilks CB, Young RH, Aguirre P, et al. Adenoma malignum (minimal deviation adenocarcinoma) of the uterine cervix. A clinicopathological and immunohistochemical analysis of 26 cases. Am J Surg Pathol 1989;13:717–29.
171. Mazur MT. Atypical polypoid adenomyomas of the endometrium. Am J Surg Pathol 1981;5:473–82.
172. Fukunaga M, Endo Y, Ushigome S, et al. Atypical polypoid adenomyomas of the uterus. Histopathology 1995;27:35–42.
173. Young RH, Treger T, Scully RE. Atypical polypoid adenomyoma of the uterus. A report of 27 cases. Am J Surg Pathol 1986;86:139–45.
174. Heatley MK. Atypical polypoid adenomyoma: a systematic review of the English literature. Histopathology 2006;48:609–10.
175. Horita A, Kurata A, Maeda D, et al. Immunohistochemical characteristics of atypical polypoid adenomyoma with special reference to h-caldesmon. Int J Gynecol Pathol 2011;30:64–70.
176. Soslow RA, Chung MH, Rouse RV, et al. Atypical polypoid adenomyofibroma (APA) versus well-differentiated endometrial carcinoma with prominent stromal matrix: an immunohistochemical study. Int J Gynecol Pathol 1996;15:209–16.
177. Ota S, Catasus L, Matias-Guiu X, et al. Molecular pathology of atypical polypoid adenomyoma of the uterus. Hum Pathol 2003;34:784–8.
178. Ohishi Y, Kaku T, Kobayashi H, et al. CD10 immunostaining distinguishes atypical polypoid adenomyofibroma (atypical polypoid adenomyoma) from endometrial carcinoma invading the myometrium. Hum Pathol 2008;39:1446–53.
179. Hornick JL, Fletcher CD. PEComa: what do we know so far? Histopathology 2006;48:75–82.
180. Bonetti F, Martignoni G, Colato C, et al. Abdominopelvic sarcoma of perivascular epithelioid cells. Report of four cases in young women, one with tuberous sclerosis. Mod Pathol 2001;14:563–8.
181. Bosincu L, Rocca PC, Martignoni G, et al. Perivascular epithelioid cell (PEC) tumors of the uterus: a clinicopathologic study of two cases with aggressive features. Mod Pathol 2005;18:1336–42.
182. Fadare O, Parkash V, Yilmaz Y, et al. Perivascular epithelioid cell tumor (PEComa) of the uterine cervix associated with intraabdominal 'PEComatosis': a clinicopathological study with comparative genomic hybridization analysis. World J Surg Oncol 2004;2:35.
183. Folpe AL, Mentzel T, Lehr HA, et al. Perivascular epithelioid cell neoplasms of soft tissue and gynecologic origin: a clinicopathologic study of 26 cases and review of the literature. Am J Surg Pathol 2005;29:1558–75.
184. Fukunaga M. Perivascular epithelioid cell tumor of the uterus: report of four cases. Int J Gynecol 2005;24:341–6.
185. Liang SX, Pearl M, Liu J, et al. 'Malignant' uterine perivascular epithelioid cell tumor, pelvic lymph node lymphangioleiomyomatosis, and gynecological pecomatosis in a patient with tuberous sclerosis: a case report and review of the literature. Int J Gynecol Pathol 2008;27:86–90.
186. Vang R, Kempson RL. Perivascular epithelioid cell tumor ('PEComa') of the uterus: a subset of HMB-45-positive epithelioid mesenchymal neoplasms with an uncertain relationship to pure smooth muscle tumors. Am J Surg Pathol 2002;26:1–13.
187. Cil AP, Haberal A, Hucumenoglu S, et al. Angiomyolipoma of the uterus associated with tuberous sclerosis: case report and review of the literature. Gynecol Oncol 2004;94:593–6.
188. Gyure KA, Hart WR, Kennedy AW. Lymphangiomyomatosis of the uterus associated with tuberous sclerosis and malignant neoplasia of the female genital tract: a report of two cases. Int J Gynecol Pathol 1995;14:344–51.
189. Clay MR, Gibson P, Lowell J, et al. Microscopic uterine lymphangioleiomyomatosis perivascular epithelioid cell neoplasm: a case report with the earliest manifestation of this enigmatic neoplasm. Int J Gynecol Pathol 2011;30:71–5.
190. Hornick JL, Fletcher CD. Sclerosing PEComa: clinicopathologic analysis of a distinctive variant with a predilection for the retroperitoneum. Am J Surg Pathol 2008;32:493–501.
191. Longacre TA, Hendrickson MR, Kapp DS, et al. Lymphangioleiomyomatosis of the uterus simulating high-stage endometrial stromal sarcoma. Gynecol Oncol 1996;63:404–10.
192. Fadare O, Liang SX. Epithelioid smooth muscle tumors of the uterus do not express CD1a: a potential immunohistochemical adjunct in their distinction from uterine perivascular epithelioid cell tumors. Ann Diagn Pathol 2008;12:401–5.
193. Folpe AL, Kwiatkowski DJ. Perivascular epithelioid cell neoplasms: pathology and pathogenesis. Hum Pathol 2010;41:1–15.
194. Fernandez-Flores A. Evidence on the neural crest origin of PEComas. Rom J Morphol Embryol 2011;52:7–13.
195. Silva EG, Deavers MT, Bodurka DC, et al. Uterine epithelioid leiomyosarcomas with clear cells: reactivity with HMB-45 and the concept of PEComa. Am J Surg Pathol 2004;28:244–9.
196. Simpson KW, Albores-Saavedra J. HMB-45 reactivity in conventional uterine leiomyosarcomas. Am J Surg Pathol 2007;31:95–8.
197. Pan CC, Jong YJ, Chai CY, et al. Comparative genomic hybridization study of perivascular epithelioid cell tumor: molecular genetic evidence of perivascular epithelioid cell tumor as a distinctive neoplasm. Hum Pathol 2006;37:606–12.
198. Hornick JL, Fletcher CD. 2002 Immunohistochemical staining for KIT (CD117) in soft tissue sarcomas is very limited in distribution. Am J Clin Pathol 2006;117:188–93.
199. Roma AA, Yang B, Senior ME, et al. TFE3 immunoreactivity in alveolar soft part sarcoma of the uterine cervix: case report. Int J Gynecol Pathol 2005;24:131–5.
200. Fadare O. Perivascular epithelioid cell tumor (PEComa) of the uterus: an outcome-based clinicopathologic analysis of 41 reported cases. Adv Anat Pathol 2008;15:63–75.
201. Fukunaga M. Pure alveolar rhabdomyosarcoma of the uterine corpus. Pathol Int 2011;61:377–81.
202. Fadare O, Bonvicino A, Martel M, et al. Pleomorphic rhabdomyosarcoma of the uterine corpus: a clinicopathologic study of 4 cases and a review of the literature. Int J Gynecol Pathol 2010;29:122–34.
203. Ordi J, Stamatakos MD, Tavassoli FA. Pure pleomorphic rhabdomyosarcomas of the uterus. Int J Gynecol Pathol 1997;16:369–77.
204. Daya D, Lukka H, Clement PB. Primitive neuroectodermal tumors of the uterus: a report of four cases. Hum Pathol 1992;23:1120–9.
205. McCluggage WG, Sumathi VP, Nucci MR, et al. Ewing family of tumours involving the vulva and vagina: report of a series of four cases. J Clin Pathol 2007;60:674–80.
206. Pang LJ, Chang B, Zou H, et al. Alveolar soft part sarcoma: a bimarker diagnostic strategy using TFE3 immunoassay and ASPL-TFE3 fusion transcripts in paraffin-embedded tumor tissues. Diagn Mol Pathol 2008;17:245–52.
207. Schammel DP, Tavassoli FA. Uterine angiosarcomas: a morphologic and immunohistochemical study of four cases. Am J Surg Pathol 1998;22:246–50.
208. Keel SB, Clement PB, Prat J, et al. Malignant schwannoma of the uterine cervix: a study of three cases. Int J Gynecol Pathol 1998;17:223–30.
209. McDonald AG, Dal Cin P, Ganguly A, et al. Liposarcoma arising in uterine lipoleiomyoma: a report of 3 cases and review of the literature. Am J Surg Pathol 2011;35:221–7.
210. Jeney H, Heller DS, Hameed M, et al. Epithelioid sarcoma of the uterine cervix. Gynecol Oncol 2003;89:536–9.
211. Hsueh S, Chang TC. Malignant rhabdoid tumor of the uterine corpus. Gynecol Oncol 1996;61:142–6.
212. Namizato CS, Muriel-Cueto P, Baez-Perez JM, et al. Chondrosarcoma of the uterus: case report and literature review. Arch Gynecol Obstet 2008;278:369–72.
213. Su M, Tokairin T, Nishikawa Y, et al. Primary osteosarcoma of the uterine corpus: case report and review of the literature. Pathol Int 2002;52:158–63.

Fallopian Tube 21

Elke A. Jarboe

CHAPTER OUTLINE

Introduction	459
Anatomy, Histology, and Function of the Fallopian Tube	459
Anatomy	459
Histology	460
Mucosal Epithelial Alterations	461
Function	462
Approach to Examining Tubal Specimens	462
Bilateral Tubal Ligation for Sterilization	462
Salpingectomy for Tubal Ectopic Gestation	463
Salpingectomy (with or without Oophorectomy and/or Hysterectomy)	463
Non-Neoplastic Lesions	463
Inflammation of the Fallopian Tubes	463
Infectious Salpingitis	464
Non-Granulomatous Salpingitis	464
Granulomatous Salpingitis	467
Salpingitis Isthmica Nodosa	469
Tubal Pregnancy	470
Cysts	472
Metaplasias and Rests	474
Torsion of the Fallopian Tube	475
Prolapse of the Fallopian Tube	476
Epithelial Proliferation Associated with Salpingitis	476
Tumors of the Fallopian Tube	477
Benign Tumors	477
Borderline Tumors	479
Malignant Tumors	479
Female Adnexal Tumor of Wolffian Origin	484

INTRODUCTION

As the fallopian tube is the intermediary between the ovary and the uterus, it is the seat of various interactions that culminate in a normally implanted pregnancy. Its multiple functions include conditioning of both gametes before fertilization, guiding their journeys before encounter, providing an appropriate chemical environment for fertilization, supplying nutriment to the fertilized ovum for its first few hours of life, and delivering it to the uterine cavity at the proper time for nidation. The exact processes by which these various mechanisms are accomplished are still rather poorly understood, partly because many of them vary significantly from species to species, so that the study of experimental animals does not always help to understand the situation in women. Recently, the fallopian tube has been implicated for its potential role in a more sinister pathologic process. A growing body of evidence strongly suggests that the distal fallopian tube is the site of origin for some proportion of high-grade pelvic serous cancers previously classified as primary ovarian or peritoneal malignancies. For a detailed discussion of this concept, see Chapter 25.

ANATOMY, HISTOLOGY, AND FUNCTION OF THE FALLOPIAN TUBE

ANATOMY

The fallopian tubes are derived from the müllerian ducts, which begin as invaginations of the celomic lining epithelium lateral to the cranial end of the mesonephric ducts at 5 weeks of intrauterine development. The lower ends fuse to the mesonephric ducts in the 7 week embryo, after which the mesonephric ducts undergo regression. The tube is 9–12 cm long *in vivo* but, being a muscular organ, its length can vary considerably. After fixation, it appears shorter, shrinking to a serpentine form. At the medial end, the tube is attached to the uterine cornu above and in front of the ovarian ligament, and above and behind the round ligament of the uterus. A sheet of pelvic peritoneum is folded over the tube, joining beneath it to form the mesosalpinx and then, beneath the mesovarium and ovarian ligament, to become the broad ligament. On the lateral wall of the pelvis, the tube arches backward over the ovary, its ostium facing the medial aspect of the latter.

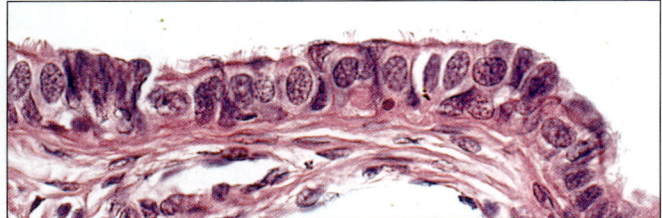

Figure 21.1 Normal tubal epithelium An admixture of secretory and ciliated cells constitute the majority of the cells.

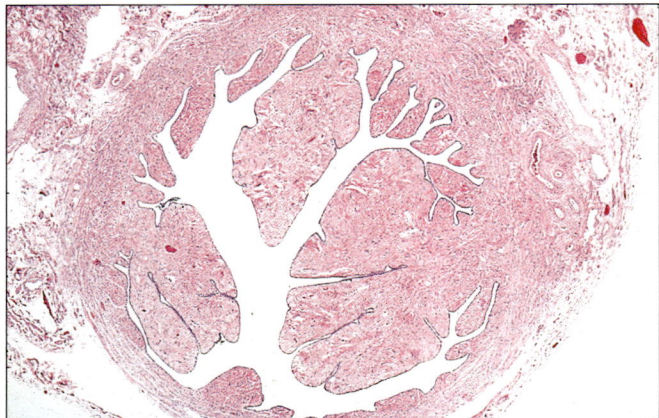

Figure 21.2 Atrophic tubal mucosa. The epithelium is thin and atrophic and the plical lamina propria is fibrotic.

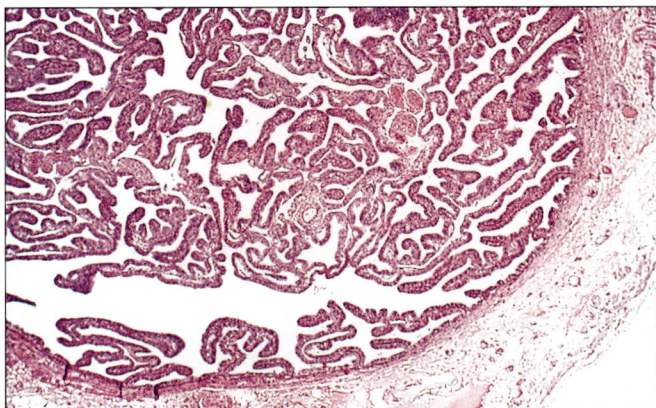

Figure 21.3 Normal ampulla. The mucosa forms a complex maze-like pattern of folds that branch but do not join.

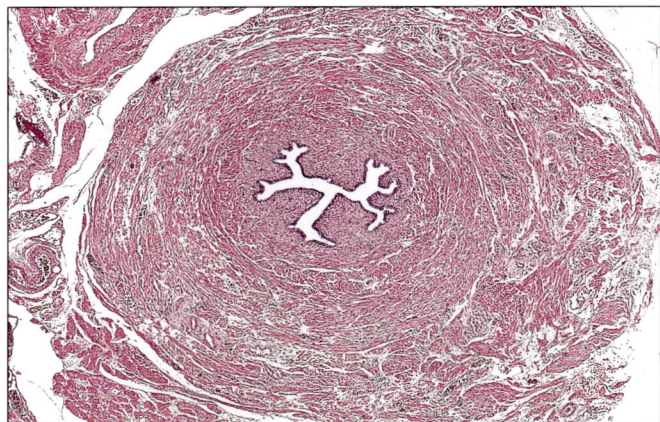

Figure 21.4 Normal isthmus. The lumen is narrow and stellate and the wall is thick.

The fallopian tube is divided into four zones, which, extending distally to proximally, are the infundibulum, the ampulla, the isthmus, and the interstitial (or intramural) portions. The infundibulum is the distal end of the tube and forms the funnel-like expansion opening onto the peritoneal cavity, about 1 cm in length and diameter that ends in a variable number of irregular, fringe-like extensions, the fimbriae. Proximal to the infundibulum and making up about half of the length of the tube is the ampullary portion. The ampulla is narrower than the infundibulum and runs a tortuous course. The isthmus, which is 2–3 cm in length, has a narrower lumen and more muscular wall than the ampulla. The interstitial portion of the tube has a lumen with a simple, stellate, or almost circular cross section. In this segment of the tube, the muscle of the tubal wall merges with that of the myometrium.

HISTOLOGY

The fallopian tube is composed of a mucosal lining, a muscular layer, and an outer serosa. The mucosa consists of nonstratified epithelium and a sparse underlying fibrovascular lamina propria. The epithelium (Figure 21.1) comprises three cell types: ciliated cells, secretory cells, and intercalated (or peg) cells. The ciliated cells have a centrally placed nucleus with a perinuclear halo, a prominent terminal bar, and definable surface cilia. The nuclei of the secretory cells vary in position, depending on the stage in the menstrual cycle. The intercalated cells are secretory cells that have discharged their secretions with the result that the cell walls are collapsed around the nucleus. The ciliated component is the most prominent near the fimbrial end of the tube and the secretory cells are more numerous in the isthmus than they are in the ampulla.

The tubal epithelium shows well-defined histologic alterations in response to cyclic hormonal variations, which affect the height of the epithelial cells, rather than the number of cilia, as happens in other primates. In the proliferative phase of the cycle the estrogen predominance results in epithelial cells with increasing height whereas in the progesterone-dominated secretory phase, the cell height may be as little as half that seen in the first half of the cycle. Similarly, the height of both epithelial cell types is low in pregnancy. Oral contraceptives produce a similar appearance to those of pregnancy; the epithelial cells are relatively flat and show a lack of secretory activity, features that doubtless play some part in the effectiveness of the medication. In the late postmenopausal state, the epithelium becomes thin and atrophic (Figure 21.2).

In cross section, at low-power magnification, the mucosa of the tubal ampulla (Figure 21.3) forms a complicated maze-like pattern of folds (the plicae) that branch but do not join. The epithelial surfaces of the plicae are apposed to one another so that even in the widest part of the tube the traversing ovum is not floating in a spacious lumen but is at all times nurtured by the ciliated and secretory epithelium with which it is in contact on all sides. These folds become less complex as the medial end of the tube is approached, becoming stellate in the isthmus (Figure 21.4) and forming an irregular, almost rounded, outline to the lumen in the interstitial part. In postmenopausal women, the plical stroma becomes fibrous and the plicae themselves club shaped, an appearance that may be mistaken for one sequela of infection, and the epithelium flattened.

The tubal musculature is arranged in a basket-weave fashion. This layer is thinnest at the tube's distal end and becomes progressively thicker as the cornu is approached. A subepithelial layer of mainly longitudinal muscle appears at the isthmus and continues along the interstitial portion. At this point, the spiral muscle becomes continuous with the myometrium.

MUCOSAL EPITHELIAL ALTERATIONS

SECRETORY CELL OUTGROWTHS AND p53 SIGNATURES

Expansions of morphologically unremarkable secretory cells, uninterrupted by ciliated cells, can occasionally be identified as discrete, linear foci in a background of the usual mixed ciliated and secretory cells populating the fallopian tube epithelium. Such expansions have been designated as secretory cell outgrowths (SCOUTs) when they comprise at least 30 or more secretory cells. The majority are associated with loss of expression of *PAX2*, a member of the pair box gene family, which is normally expressed in structures derived from the müllerian duct.[1] The related p53 signature is also composed of secretory cells, but with the incremental changes of acquired *p53* mutation, evidence of DNA damage, and relative predominance in the distal portion of the fallopian tube (Figure 21.5A and B).[2] Neither SCOUTs nor p53 signatures exhibit significant proliferative activity (Figure 21.5C). Both are currently interpreted as early clonal expansions short of neoplastic proliferation.

Both SCOUTs and p53 signatures are candidate early steps toward high grade serous tubal carcinoma, as discussed in Chapter 25. The reader is cautioned, however, that the prospective cancer risk of women with isolated SCOUTs and/or p53 signature is unknown, so neither is a diagnostic entity that should be invoked in clinical practice. Fallopian tubes from women with high-grade pelvic serous carcinoma harbor a significantly higher frequency of SCOUTs than those from women whose tubes were removed for a nonmalignant condition.[1] Tubes in which serous tubal intraepithelial carcinoma is present are more likely to contain p53 signatures than those without; in some cases, a p53 signature may be found in direct continuity with intraepithelial carcinoma. In a given case of pelvic serous carcinoma, shared *p53* mutations may be identified among p53 signatures, serous tubal intraepithelial carcinoma, and invasive tumor elsewhere in the pelvis.[2–5]

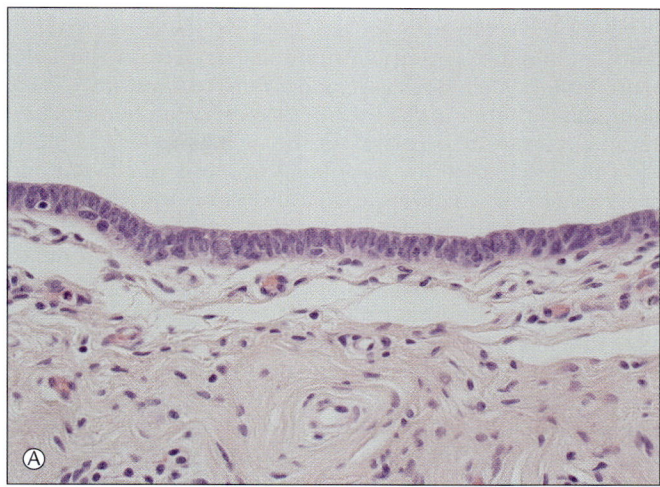

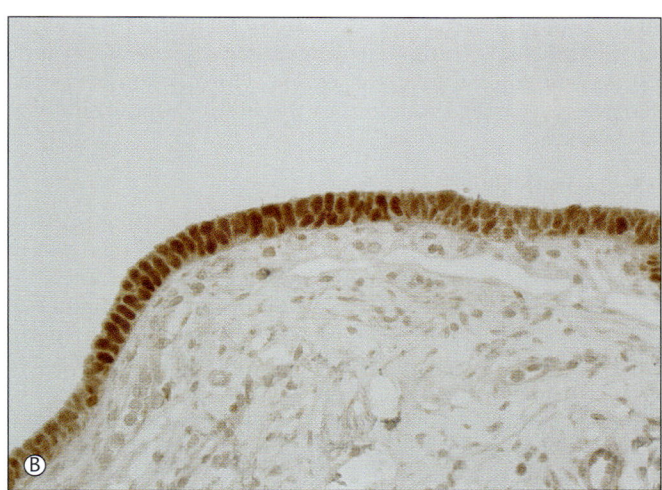

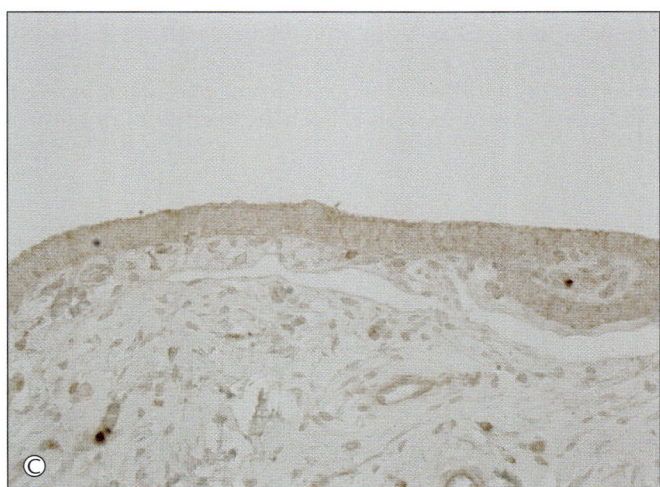

Figure 21.5 (A–C) The p53 signature is a histologically unremarkable stretch of tubal epithelium **(A)** that is associated with *p53* mutations, exhibiting strong nuclear staining for p53 **(B)** and has a low MIB1 index **(C)**.

OTHER MUCOSAL EPITHELIAL PROLIFERATIONS

Another notable pattern of epithelial growth in the fallopian tube, which does not appear to be associated with malignancy, either in the tube or elsewhere, is characterized by an apparent 'hyperplasia' of the normal mucosal epithelial cells. Such areas are populated by a mix of ciliated and secretory cells, which appear stratified or are arranged as small tufts. These areas may be focal or more diffuse. The cells themselves may exhibit some nuclear atypia, but not to the degree found in intraepithelial carcinoma. Mitotic activity is generally minimal (Figure 21.6). This mucosal alteration may be seen in the setting of pregnancy, but can be found in the tubes of non-pregnant women as well.

FUNCTION

The fallopian tube has three main functions in the reproductive process. First, it is responsible for transferring the ovum into its lumen when discharged from the ovary's rupturing follicle. Second, it provides an environment in which the sperm can fertilize the ovum. Third, it transfers the fertilized, cleaving embryo into the uterus after an interval of 3–4 days.

SPERM TRANSPORT

The mechanisms of sperm transport in the tube are not known. It is apparent that there is a rapid postcoital sperm movement along the whole genital tract and that, in different segments of the tract, including the tube, a number of 'storage compartments' are established from which sperm release occurs slowly. Although reduced sperm motility is a factor in male infertility, it is accepted that sperm do not have to be motile to be transported along the female genital tract. No information is known about the active part, if any, that the tube plays in sperm transport.

OVUM TRANSPORT

Ovum transport has been studied in detail, and the two essential elements are muscular activity and ciliary action. It would seem that these two mechanisms play a complementary role in ovum transport. Even so, each does not always appear necessary. Reproduction can take place when the muscular activity is paralyzed and ciliary action alone will carry the ovum across the ampullary part of the tube. The muscular contractions of the tubal wall are both phasic and tonic; it can undergo transient contractions as well as alter its basal tone. Contractile activity of the muscle takes place in coordinated waves. These result in peristaltic pulses along segments of the tube, although these are propagated only along random short lengths, with junctional pauses. Some claim that muscular activity is not essential for transport of the oocyte along its course.

The ciliary action in the tube is toward the uterus and is under the influence of many mediators. Physiologic levels of prostaglandins $F_{2\alpha}$, E_1, and E_2 stimulate the ciliary activity as do β-adrenergic agonists; the latter effect is potentiated by estrogen and progesterone. Recent data have shown that progesterone affects the tubal ciliary beat frequency.[6] Incubation with progesterone suppresses the beat frequency by 40–50% but estradiol has no effect. Cilia from the tubal ampulla beat significantly faster than those from fimbrial segments.

APPROACH TO EXAMINING TUBAL SPECIMENS

BILATERAL TUBAL LIGATION FOR STERILIZATION

Many methods are used, and the most popular is the Pomeroy operation and methods incorporating the use of clips or rings. The Pomeroy operation is an open procedure in which a loop of the tubal isthmus is pulled up and ligated with an absorbable suture followed by excision of the isolated loop. Histologic examination provides evidence that the operation has been carried out properly. Clips are also widely used. The clips are placed over the isthmus, where the tube is thinnest, so that the tubal lumen is completely occluded. Falope rings, made of Silastic, are placed over a loop of tube that is pulled up. The application of clips and rings is usually done as a laparoscopic procedure.

The most important aspect in the sectioning and preparation of the excised specimen for microscopic examination is that sufficient sections are made to show the complete cross section of the tube (Figure 21.7). An efficient method is to cut the fallopian tube into sections no more than 1–2 mm thick so that a single slide contains up to six sections. In this manner, even if some sections are embedded improperly or cut on a bias, at least a few should show the complete cross section, if in fact it is present. Any case where none of the pieces shows a complete cross section should be reported as incomplete (Figure 21.8). This can occur when the surgeon has removed arteries and fascia or only the tubal fimbriae. In these cases, it commonly happens that the clinician had difficulty definitively identifying the fallopian tube, even though this information was not transmitted to the pathologist. It is most important that an incomplete ligation be clearly reported in part for medicolegal consideration. The pathologist must be careful not to interpret a paratubal cyst as fallopian tube lumen; the latter has a much thicker wall with ample smooth muscle.

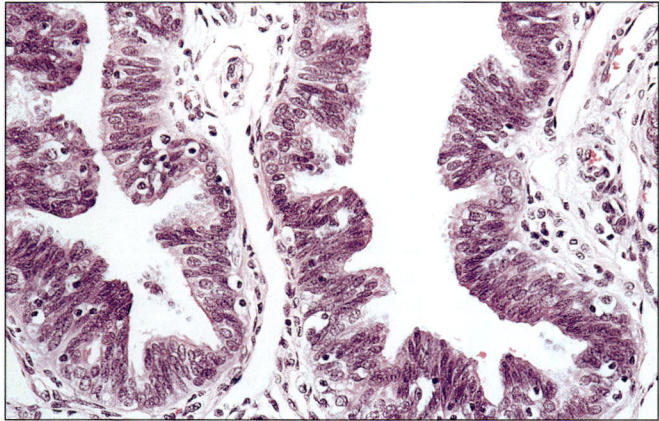

Figure 21.6 Mucosal epithelial proliferation. A prominent tufted appearance is present.

CHAPTER 21 — FALLOPIAN TUBE

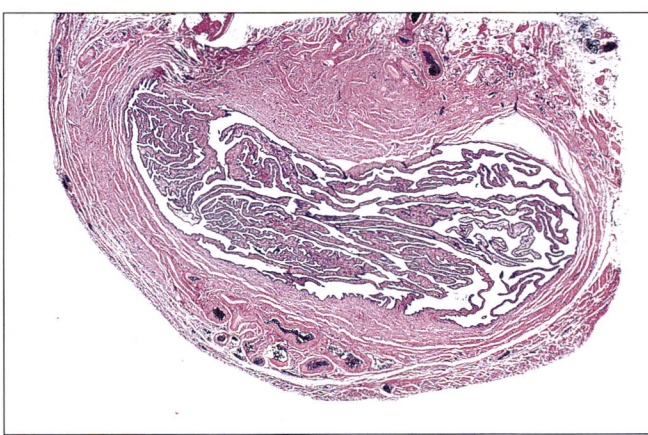

Figure 21.7 Sterilization procedure, complete transection. This section of the tube shows the complete circumference of muscular wall surrounding the mucosa, confirming complete transection of the tube.

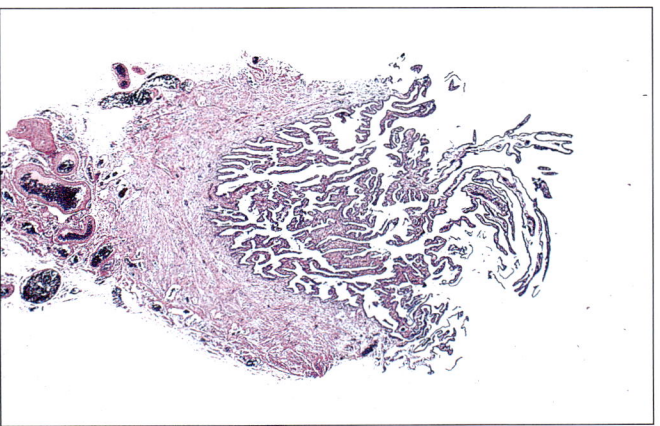

Figure 21.8 Sterilization procedure, incomplete transection. This is one of many sections from this sterilization procedure. Although tubal mucosa and muscular wall are present, the muscle does not surround the mucosa completely so that the transection cannot be confirmed as complete.

SALPINGECTOMY FOR TUBAL ECTOPIC GESTATION

Record the site and location of the gestation, if apparent. A rupture site, if present, should be described and sampled. If the ectopic pregnancy is not obvious, a focal enlargement or swelling should be sought. Blood distending the lumen should be documented. Blood clot should be examined carefully for gross evidence of chorionic villi. Multiple cross sections of the fallopian tube at the site of swelling and/or blood clot should be submitted for histopathologic review. Sections of fallopian tube adjacent to the site of swelling should also be sampled to look for evidence of prior salpingitis. Ectopic pregnancy removal by salpingostomy with preservation of the tube itself should be clearly conveyed in the report, as the patient is at risk for recurrence.

SALPINGECTOMY (WITH OR WITHOUT OOPHORECTOMY AND/OR HYSTERECTOMY)

THE SEE-FIM PROTOCOL

The majority of early serous carcinomas in the fallopian tube are detected microscopically rather than by gross examination, in the distal portion of the fallopian tube, in the fimbriae. Salpingectomy performed in high-risk patients, such as those undertaken prophylactically in *BRCA* mutant women, are a common setting for clinically and grossly occult disease. In an effort to facilitate a thorough examination of the distal fallopian tube a protocol for sectioning and extensively examining the fimbriated end (SEE-FIM) was developed (see also Chapter 35).[6] According to this protocol, the entire fallopian tube is first well fixed to prevent exfoliation of the mucosal epithelial cells. The fimbriae are then amputated from the proximal tube and sectioned longitudinally into multiple sections to permit maximum exposure of the fimbrial mucosa. The remainder of the tube is cross sectioned at 2–3 mm intervals and the entire tube is submitted for histopathologic review (Figure 21.9).

Indications for extensive tubal sampling are not yet clearly defined by clinical necessity, but should be considered in cases where it is desirable to maximize the likelihood of detecting early tubal cancer. Appropriate specimen types might include risk-reducing (prophylactic) salpingectomies; salpingectomies from women with a history of breast cancer; and salpingectomies in the setting of uterine, ovarian, or peritoneal disease. Some consensus is emerging from within the pathology community, with, for example, the Association of Directors of Anatomic and Surgical Pathology recommending an approach similar to SEE-FIM in prophylactically removed specimens, with an emphasis on longitudinal sectioning of the fimbriae.[7] This group also recommends sampling fimbriae as part of processing of routine tubal specimens.

Given that the distal fallopian tube is the site most likely to harbor occult tubal malignancy, the suggestion has been made by some authors to submit the entire fimbriae for histopathologic review even in cases in which tubes are removed for benign disease.[8] Currently, the incidence of occult carcinoma in the fallopian tube in the general population is unknown. However, with increasing attention focused on the distal tube, incidental tubal cancers are being discovered in cases otherwise unsuspected of harboring a malignancy.[8] A standard clinical response to incidentally discovered occult *in situ* tubal cancer has not yet been formulated, but there is a possibility for identification of individuals who may benefit from increased surveillance, or even early disease intervention.

NON-NEOPLASTIC LESIONS

INFLAMMATION OF THE FALLOPIAN TUBES

Inflammatory disease resulting from infection of the fallopian tubes and adjacent ovary is an increasing problem. The investigation and treatment of women with the disease is demanding more and more in the way of time and other resources. Identification of the disease early in its natural

PATHOLOGY OF THE FEMALE REPRODUCTIVE TRACT

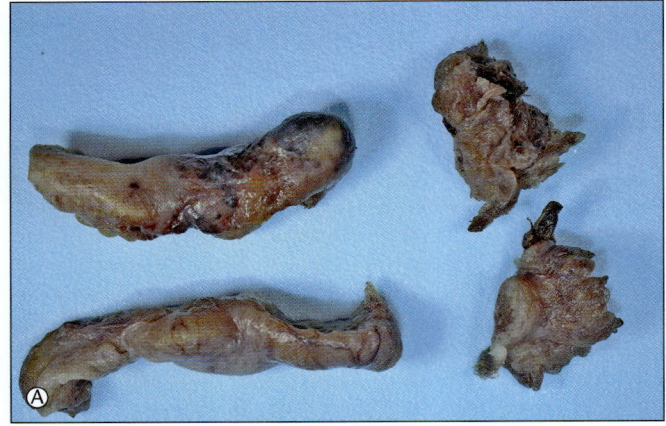

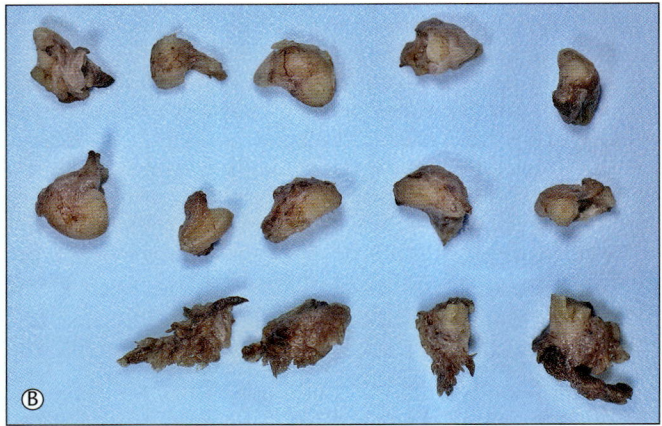

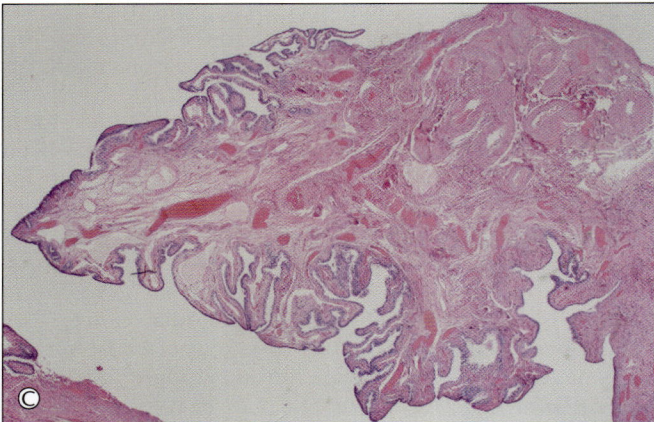

Figure 21.9 (A-C) The protocol for sectioning and extensively examining the fimbriated end (SEE-FIM protocol). Tubes are first fixed. The fimbriae are then amputated from the rest of the tube **(A)**, sectioned longitudinally into multiple sections **(B)**, and then submitted with the remainder of the tube, which has been cross sectioned at 2–3 mm intervals. Longitudinal sectioning permits maximum evaluation of the fimbrial mucosal epithelium (**C**, low-power magnification).

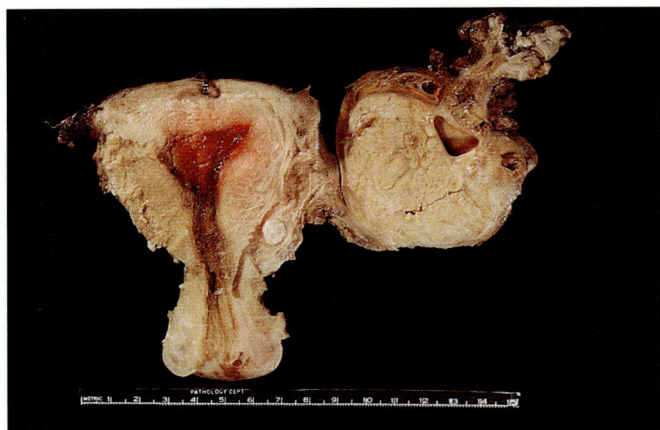

Figure 21.10 *Actinomyces* infection causing a tubo-ovarian abscess.

history is important to enable treatment to be effected before the damage becomes extensive and the consequent surgery destructive.

INFECTIOUS SALPINGITIS

Infectious salpingitis may be divided into the two major categories of non-granulomatous and granulomatous (or tuberculous) salpingitis.

NON-GRANULOMATOUS SALPINGITIS

Non-granulomatous salpingitis is predominantly a disease of young, sexually active women, and 70% of those with the disease are under the age of 25. Other factors that have an influence on the development of salpingitis include the method of contraception, induced abortion, and instrumentation of the cervix. Among the infectious organisms responsible for salpingitis, *Chlamydia trachomatis* and *Neisseria gonorrhoeae* remain of paramount importance and are responsible for ascending salpingitis.[9] Other causative microbial agents are the anaerobic bacteria (bacteroides, clostridia, and streptococci), *Mycoplasma hominis*, and *Ureaplasma urealyticum*, and miscellaneous organisms such as *Haemophilus influenzae* and group A streptococci. Bacterial vaginosis is a common concurrent disorder of women with acute salpingitis, and bacterial vaginosis microorganisms are commonly isolated from the upper genital tracts of patients with pelvic inflammatory disease.[9] Salpingitis caused by *Actinomyces israelii* is associated with the presence of an intrauterine contraceptive device, and may result in the development of a tubo-ovarian abscess (Figure 21.10). *Actinomyces*-like organisms can be identified in the pus (Figure 21.11). In practice, however, microbiologic investigations often show that the cultured material is already sterile by the time of the investigation, or else there is a combination of organisms.

The spread of etiologic organisms from the lower to the upper genital tract is canalicular, through the cervical canal and endometrial cavity and then into the fallopian tubes. Blockage of this route, either by cornual resection of the fallopian tubes or by sterilization, reduces the risk of salpingitis.[10] Salpingitis begins as a mucosal rather than a serosal infection.

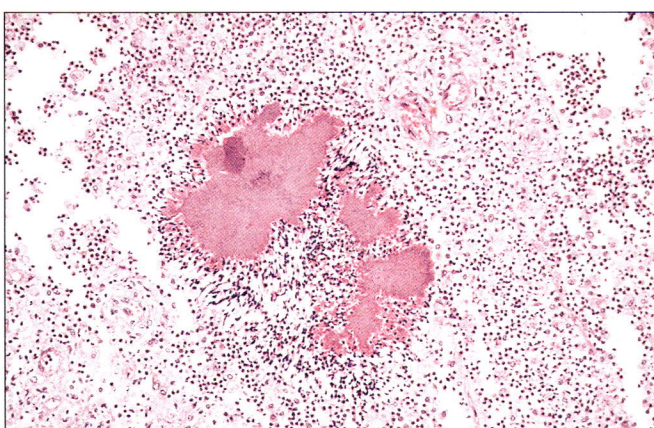

Figure 21.11 *Actinomyces*-like organisms in pus.

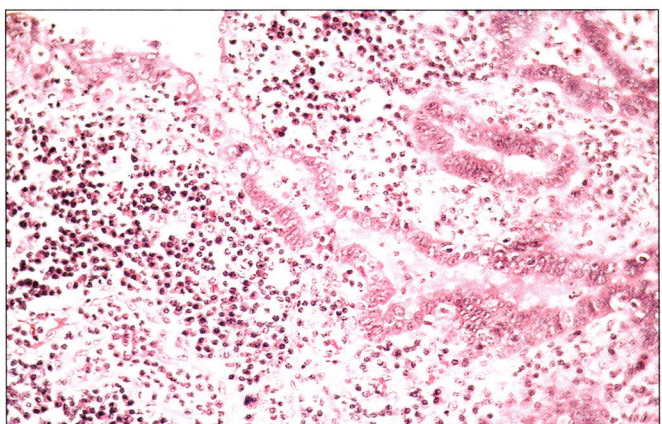

Figure 21.12 Acute salpingitis. The plicae are edematous and infiltrated by neutrophils.

Gross Features

In the acute phase of the disease, the tube is swollen, edematous, and congested. The acutely inflamed tube is rarely seen histologically, as treatment of the acute phase is medical rather than surgical.

In chronic salpingitis, the tube is thickened and congested, with adhesions on the surface, often binding the tube and ovary closely together. A pyosalpinx is a grossly enlarged tube, increased in both diameter and length, and containing pus. A hydrosalpinx characteristically shows a fusiform shape and is greatly enlarged with paper-thin walls. In both conditions, the fimbrial ends fuse, sealing the tube. Not uncommonly, the fimbriae cannot be identified.

Microscopic Features

The plicae are greatly swollen and densely infiltrated by neutrophils (Figure 21.12). The epithelial cells soon lose their cilia and the epithelium is shed in severe disease. The lumen contains pus (Figure 21.13). As the disease progresses to chronic salpingitis (Figures 21.14 and 21.15), the inflammatory infiltrate consists predominantly of plasma cells and then lymphocytes. The progression from acute to chronic non-granulomatous salpingitis may take several courses. If the fimbrial end of the tube remains patent, a chronic interstitial salpingitis may ensue, in which case the tube is thickened and the plicae fuse to form epithelial-lined cysts, which are the hallmark of chronic salpingitis. 'Follicular salpingitis' (Figure 21.16) rather confusingly refers to the epithelium-lined spaces rather than lymphoid collections. The inflammatory process may eventually become quiescent, leaving only the architectural sequelae of chronic salpingitis (Figure 21.17). Severe inflammation in the tube may spread to the adjacent ovary, resulting in a tubo-ovarian abscess (Figure 21.18). Occlusion of the fimbrial end of the tube prevents release of the tubal contents, so that a pyosalpinx may result (Figure 21.19). In pyosalpinx, the lumen is filled with pus (Figure 21.20) and the wall is thinned, although the attenuation is commonly less marked than in hydrosalpinx. Acute and chronic inflammatory cells infiltrate the plicae and wall. As the exudate is reabsorbed into the tubal wall concurrently with the quiescence of the inflammatory process, clear fluid replaces this pus and a

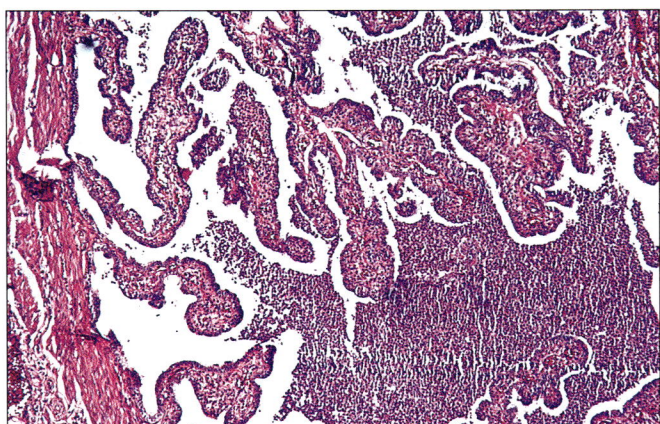

Figure 21.13 Acute salpingitis. The lumen is filled with pus and the plicae are engorged and inflamed.

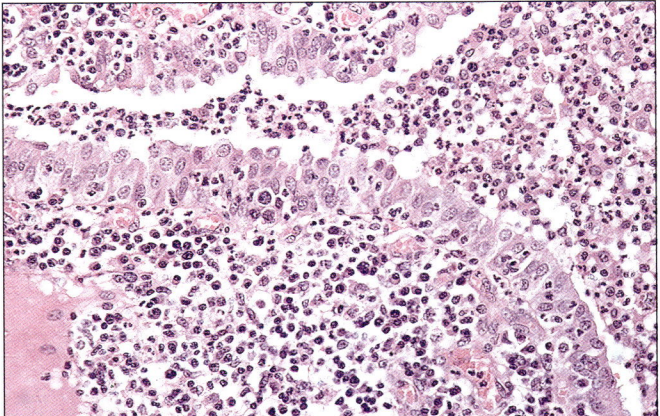

Figure 21.14 Chronic salpingitis. In this early stage of the disease, the plicae are infiltrated by plasma cells and lymphocytes and there is pus in the lumen. The epithelium is intact, although containing inflammatory cells.

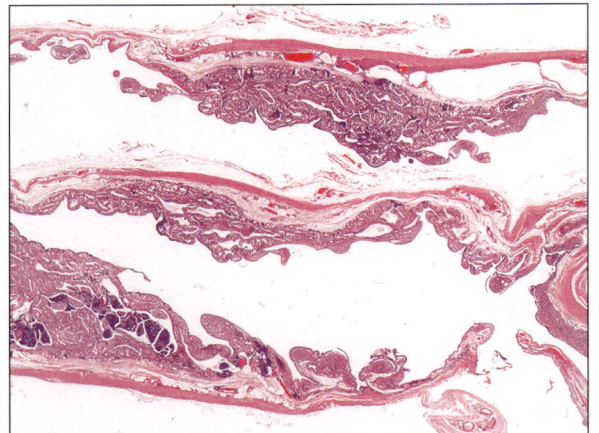

Figure 21.15 Chronic salpingitis. The infiltrate is now predominantly lymphocytic, with germinal centers.

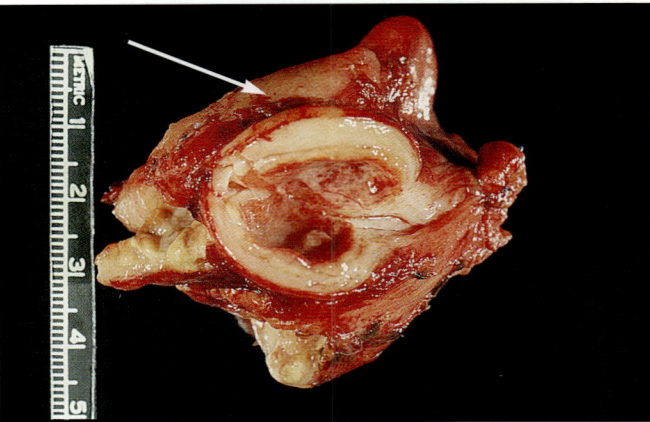

Figure 21.18 Tubo-ovarian abscess. The central mass is the ovary, which contains an abscess. Its cavity communicates with pus in the lumen of the tube (arrow).

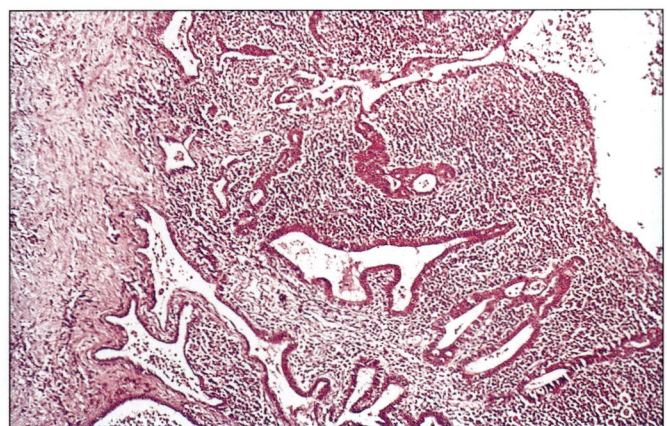

Figure 21.16 Chronic salpingitis. The plicae are partly fused, forming separate epithelium-lined spaces or 'follicles' separate from the central lumen ('follicular salpingitis'). Inflammation is still active.

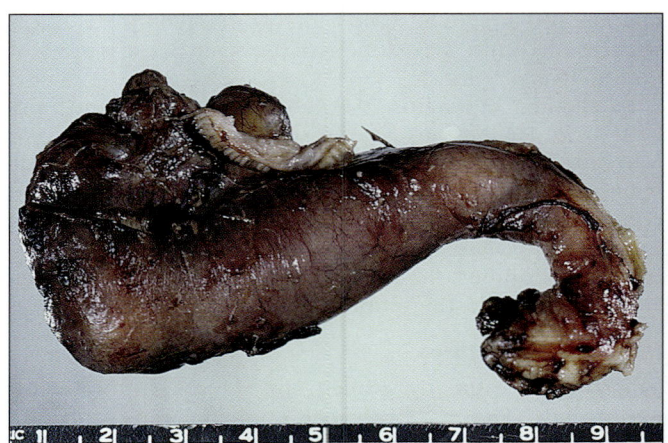

Figure 21.19 Pyosalpinx.

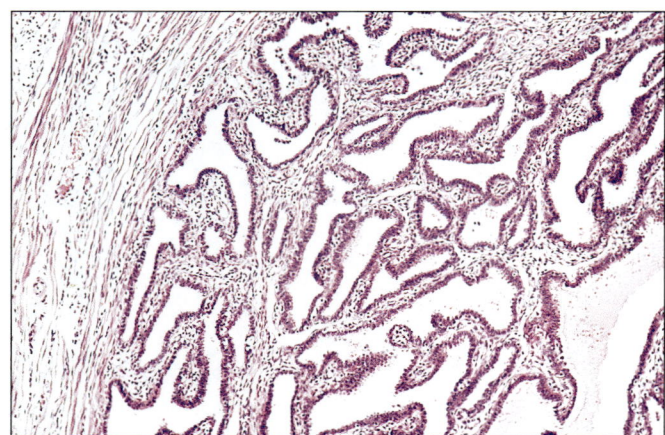

Figure 21.17 Chronic salpingitis, healed. The inflammation has subsided and is near absent, but the plicae remain fused by fibrosis.

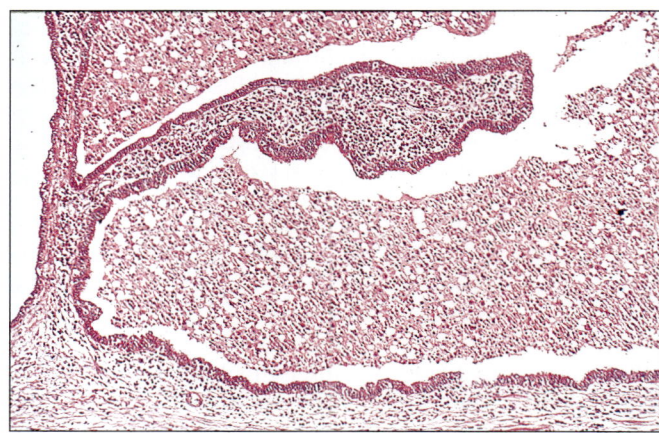

Figure 21.20 Pyosalpinx. The lumen contains pus.

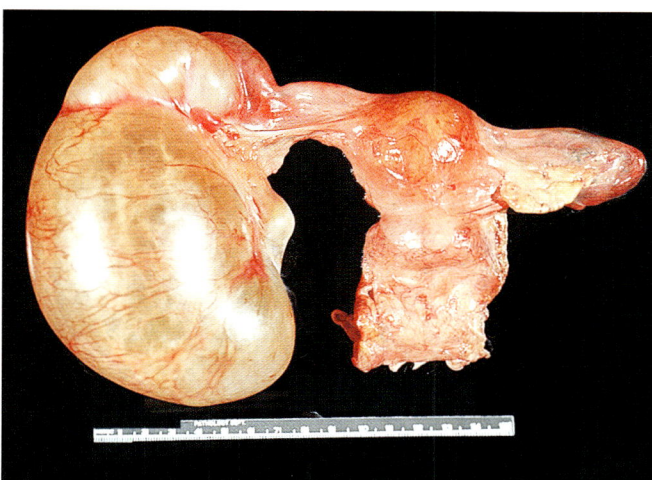

Figure 21.21 Hydrosalpinx.

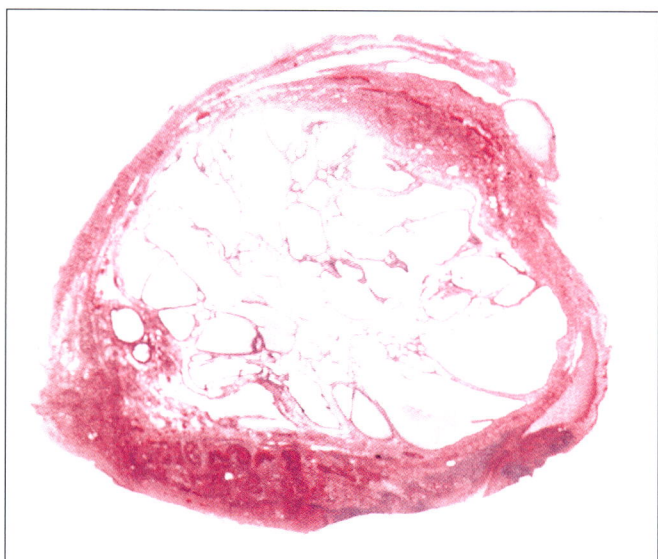

Figure 21.23 Hydrosalpinx follicularis.

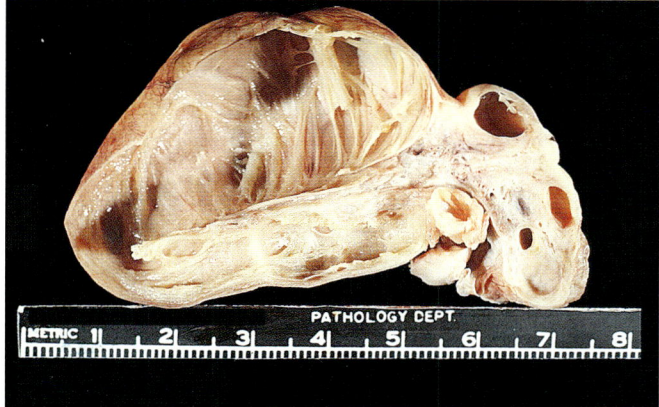

Figure 21.22 Hydrosalpinx. The convoluted shape (often called 'retort shaped') of the tube is seen on section.

hydrosalpinx results (Figures 21.21 and 21.22). In hydrosalpinx, the epithelium is generally thin and non-ciliated, although a few areas of morphologically normal cells may be seen. The wall of a hydrosalpinx is markedly thinned, with attenuation of smooth muscle and plicae. Usually, by this advanced stage in the disease process, there is little, if any, residual inflammatory infiltrate in the tissues of the wall. From a practical point of view, hydrosalpinx with tuboovarian adhesions is commonly misdiagnosed as ovarian 'serous cystadenoma' since it commonly presents as an adnexal mass. A careful microscopic examination identifying the muscular layer is diagnostic for hydrosalpinx. A small hydrosalpinx in which there is plical conglutination will have a 'honeycomb' cut surface and is termed a 'hydrosalpinx follicularis' (Figure 21.23). The relations among these inflammatory changes are shown in Figure 21.24.

The term 'pelvic inflammatory disease' (PID) implies chronic salpingitis with involvement of the surrounding structures, including ovary and parametrium. Adhesions are present on the surface of the tube, often spreading to involve the uterine serosa. PID typically has remissions and exacerbations and is difficult to eradicate. As a result of this cycle of events, in which acute salpingitis leads to chronic salpingitis, quiescence and then an exacerbation of the acute episode again, the histologic finding of acute and chronic salpingitis is commonplace. In these circumstances, the background architectural features of chronic salpingitis are seen, but the cellular infiltrate is predominantly of neutrophils, with pus in the lumen.

GRANULOMATOUS SALPINGITIS

Granulomatous salpingitis is nearly always tuberculous in origin. All age groups may be affected but the pattern of the disease has changed over the last few decades. Until the 1970s, tuberculosis of the female genital tract in the developed world affected mainly women of childbearing age but more recently the majority of cases are in postmenopausal women.[11] Whereas previously the main complaint of these women was infertility, tuberculosis accounting for about 40% of all cases of infertility,[12] the common symptoms are now pain and bleeding.[11] When tuberculosis affects the female genital tract, the tube is affected in nearly all cases and involvement of the endometrium is always secondary to it. The pelvic disease is, in turn, secondary to primary disease in the lungs or bowel, spreading to the tubes by hematogenous and lymphatic routes, respectively.

Gross Features

Tuberculous salpingitis is nearly always bilateral. The tube is thickened and congested and there are serosal adhesions. The fimbrial end of the tube is usually patent and the lumen may contain caseous debris (Figure 21.25). The wall is thickened and foci of caseation may be recognized within the tissue of the wall.

Microscopic Features

The hallmark of tuberculous salpingitis histologically is the epithelioid cell granuloma that is situated in the lamina

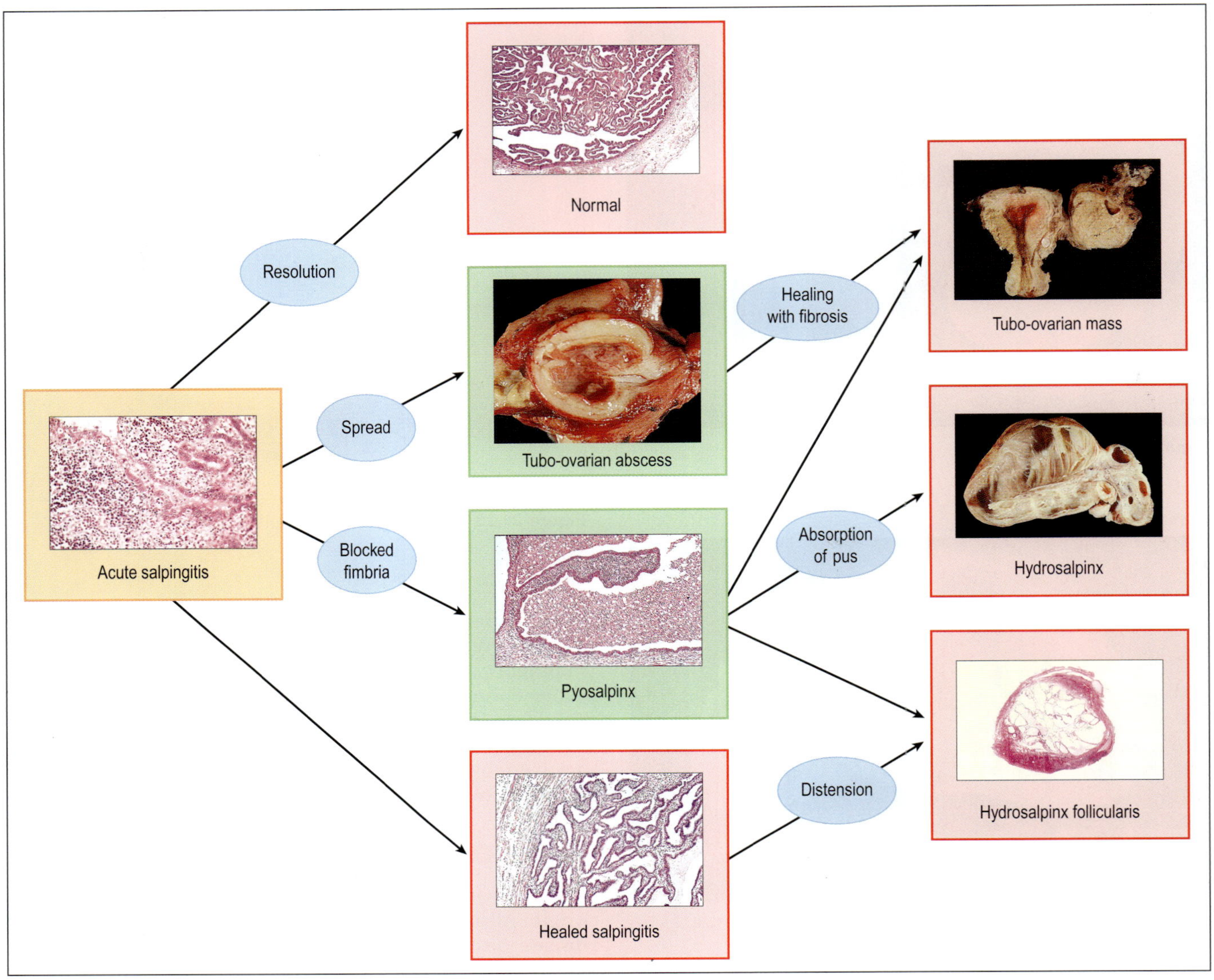

Figure 21.24 Relations among the appearances and stages of inflammation of the fallopian tube.

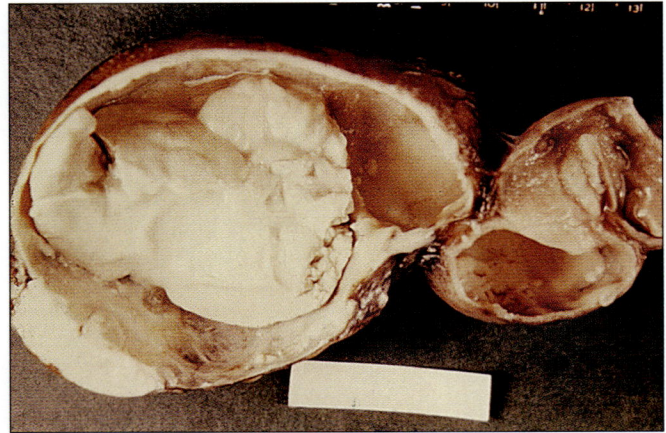

Figure 21.25 Tuberculous salpingitis. The wall is greatly distended and thinned and the lumen contains caseous material.

propria of the plicae (Figures 21.26 and 21.27) and, rarely, within the muscular wall. Caseation may or may not be present, but is more often seen in older women. A surrounding, dense lymphocytic infiltrate is found, both in the plical lamina propria and in the muscle, the latter is usually more conspicuous. A frequent finding is the presence of striking epithelial proliferation of the endosalpinx, a feature that may cause confusion with carcinoma (see later). Schaumann bodies are occasionally seen in tuberculous salpingitis (Figure 21.26). Although typically associated with sarcoidosis, these rounded, concentrically laminated calcified bodies may be seen in most forms of epithelioid cell granuloma. The histologic suggestion of tubal tuberculosis is confirmed if acid-fast bacilli are found in the sections, but this is achieved in only 1% of cases in which the culture proves positive. On a practical basis, staining is not useful. With the development of molecular pathology, polymerase chain reaction-based tuberculosis-specific bacilli DNA can be

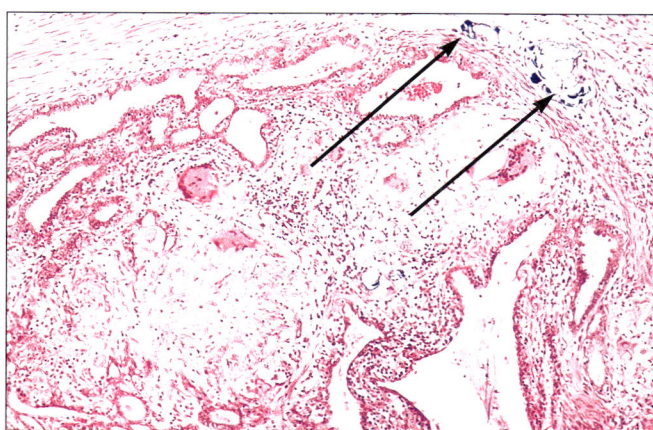

Figure 21.26 Tuberculous salpingitis. Epithelioid cell granulomas are present with giant cells. Schaumann bodies are also seen (arrows).

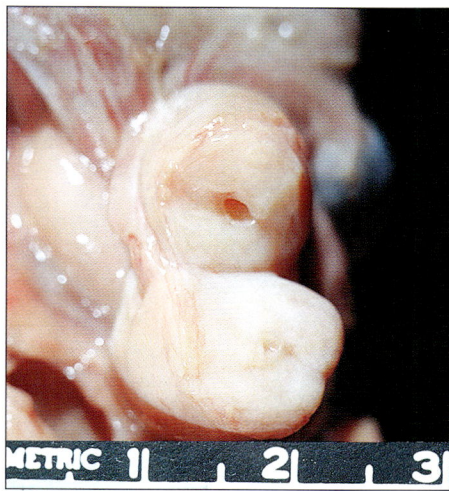

Figure 21.28 Salpingitis isthmica nodosa. The firm, round, isthmic nodule is bisected to demonstrate the central lumen.

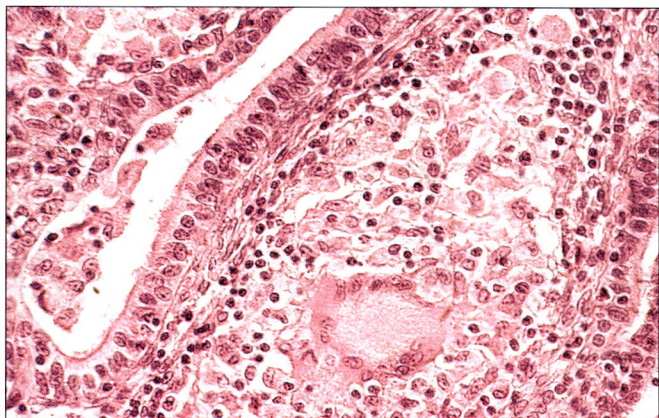

Figure 21.27 Tuberculous salpingitis.

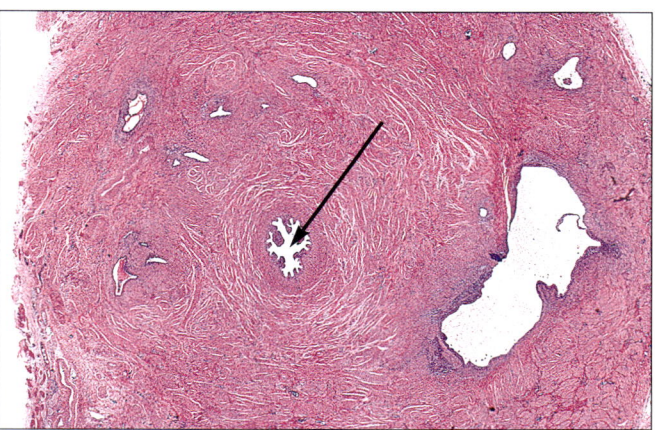

Figure 21.29 Salpingitis isthmica nodosa. The original lumen is still discernible near the center (arrow). The wall of the tube is greatly thickened by muscular hypertrophy and separate channels are present throughout the wall.

detected in 48 hours.[13] The differential diagnosis of tuberculous salpingitis in Europe is sarcoidosis, Crohn disease, and foreign-body granuloma. Worldwide, other conditions include schistosomiasis, blastomycosis, coccidioidomycosis, histoplasmosis, and enterobiasis. A positive tissue diagnosis of tuberculosis is often not possible and the decision to treat the patient must rest on the degree of clinical suspicion.

SALPINGITIS ISTHMICA NODOSA

Definition

An abnormality of the fallopian tube, salpingitis isthmica nodosa (SIN), occurs in 1% of Caucasian women and 10% of black women with a mean of 26 years. SIN consists of nodular swelling of the isthmic segment of the fallopian tube and is associated with diverticula of the lumen and smooth muscle proliferation. It has characteristic radiologic features and is significantly more common in women with ectopic pregnancy and infertility.

Pathology

SIN may be recognized grossly as a rounded, firm swelling, up to 2 cm in diameter, at the isthmic end of the tube (Figure 21.28), often merging with the cornual extremity of the uterus. The nodules are often bilateral and, occasionally, there may be more than one swelling on each tube. Most cases, however, cannot be detected macroscopically. The histologic appearances are striking and consist of a thickened wall due to hypertrophied musculature with epithelial-lined channels running between the muscle bundles and reaching close to the serosa (Figures 21.29 and 21.30). The epithelium lining these spaces is of normal, tubal type. The central lumen is always recognizable and the additional channels communicate with it and with each other, but not with the peritoneal cavity.

Histogenesis

The histogenesis of SIN remains unknown. Three potential mechanisms include:

1. The condition is postinflammatory.
2. The outcome results from 'mechanical' pressure, analogous to diverticular disease of the large bowel.
3. It is a developmental anomaly.

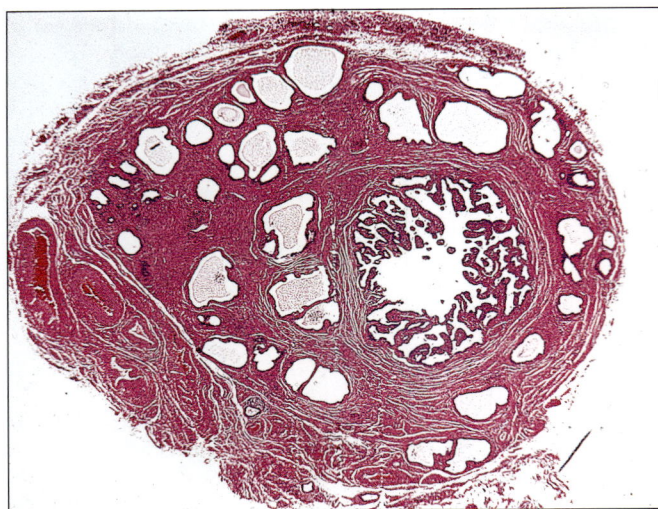

Figure 21.30 Salpingitis isthmica nodosa.

That SIN is the result of inflammatory changes is unlikely because of its low incidence compared with salpingitis, its position in the isthmus (inflammatory changes are more often in the ampulla), and the absence of fibrosis and of a cellular infiltrate. In favor of the mechanical theory is the finding of continuity between the original lumen and the peripheral channels, as well as the demonstration of small, direct outpouchings of epithelium into the muscle, which appear to initiate the process. The proposal that the condition reflects abnormal embryonic development could explain the findings.

Differential Diagnosis

SIN should be distinguished from endometriosis, chronic (infectious) salpingitis, and neoplasia. A diagnosis of endometriosis requires the presence of endometrial-type stroma surrounding the epithelial component, the latter consisting predominantly of non-ciliated, columnar cells, although areas of ciliation may be seen. Stroma is absent in SIN, the epithelium abutting directly onto the muscle. The distinction from chronic salpingitis is made by identifying smooth muscle bundles, which usually are prominent between the multiplicity of epithelial channels in SIN. In the inflammatory condition the channels are formed by fusion of the plicae with the result that fibrous tissue only, not muscle, intervenes between the diverticula. SIN is distinguished from carcinoma by the regular distribution of widely spread glands, lack of nuclear atypia, and the absence of a reactive stromal response.

TUBAL PREGNANCY

Etiology and Pathogenesis

Any factor that impairs the tube's ability to transport the fertilized ovum will predispose to tubal implantation of the ovum. Hence, congenital tubal abnormalities, failed tubal ligation, reconstructive tubal surgery, SIN, and, most importantly, postinflammatory tubal damage are all associated with an increased incidence of tubal pregnancies.[14]

The fertilized ovum may on occasion also implant in a normal tube. It has been argued that in these cases conception occurred during a cycle in which the non-implanted ovum was flushed back into the tube by a reflux of menstrual blood. Findings that support this hypothesis are that tubal gestation occurs only in humans and in primates that menstruate, and by the not uncommon finding that the tube with the pregnancy is on the side opposite to the corpus luteum of pregnancy. This latter phenomenon can also be due to transperitoneal or transuterine migration of the fertilized ovum into the contralateral tube where, due to its relatively advanced stage of development, it implants.

Natural History

Implantation occurs most commonly in the ampulla and may be plical, plicomural, or mural. It may also occur in the isthmus and interstitial portion. The earliest stages of pregnancy usually proceed in a manner that does not differ in any significant respect from the same process in an intrauterine site. The complications of tubal abortion, hemorrhage, or rupture soon supersede in all cases.

Tubal Abortion. A high proportion of tubal pregnancies abort at an early stage and may be expelled from the fimbrial end of the tube. This is invariably the case if implantation has been fimbrial or plical, simply because these sites offer insufficient tissue for adequate placentation, but it is also seen with mural implantation. There is often intramural and intraluminal hemorrhage and subsequent fetal death. Following abortion, degenerating chorionic villi may be retained in the tube as so-called 'chronic ectopic pregnancy' or they may be expelled via the uterus or be gradually absorbed. Hyalinized ghost villi may be identified in the tube as an incidental finding many months later.[15]

Tubal Hemorrhage. Although decidual change may be seen in the lamina propria of the fallopian tube during uterine or ectopic gestation, the change is focal and poorly developed. In normal pregnancy in the uterine body, decidualized endometrium acts as a buffer that constrains trophoblastic invasion. In the absence of this buffering zone in a tubal pregnancy, trophoblast infiltrates destructively into the vessels and muscle of the tube wall, resulting in hemorrhage and rupture. Even if there is no rupture, hemorrhage is invariably present at the time of presentation of a tubal ectopic pregnancy. Massive hemorrhage into the uterine wall may result if the implantation is interstitial.

Tubal Rupture. Tubal rupture complicates about 50% of cases of tubal pregnancy and appears to be due partly to the limited distensibility of the tube and partly to transmural trophoblastic invasion with penetration of the serosa. It is particularly likely to occur when the implantation is isthmic, because of this area's limited distensibility. Rupture is usually acute and is accompanied by intraperitoneal hemorrhage and the clinical features of an acute abdomen. Less commonly, there is a slow leakage of tubal contents and blood from the tube, which results in a gradually enlarging peritubal hematoma with dense adhesions between the tube and surrounding structures such as omentum and intestines. Occasionally, the ureters obstruct as a result of involvement in this peritubal mass. Although tubal rupture usually results in fetal death, the fetus occasionally retains sufficient attachment to its blood supply to maintain its viability. The trophoblast grows out through the rupture site and forms a secondary placental site in the abdomen or broad ligament. A secondary abdominal pregnancy of this type can occasionally proceed to term.

Pathology

Tubal Changes. The fallopian tube, as received by the pathologist after salpingectomy, can show a range of appearances that vary with the site of nidation, viability of the fetus, duration of pregnancy, and presence or absence of rupture. In typical cases the tube is focally or generally distended while the peritoneal surface is congested and sometimes inflamed (Figure 21.31). The fimbrial ostium can be occluded by blood clot or blood may be oozing from the ostium. If rupture has occurred, blood clot and placental tissue are sometimes seen protruding through the rupture site (Figure 21.32), and blood clot may envelop the tube. On opening the tube a complete amniotic sac and fetus is occasionally seen (Figures 21.33 and 21.34). More commonly, the lumen contains only fresh and old blood clot (Figure 21.35).

Histologic examination is usually required to confirm the diagnosis of tubal gestation (Figure 21.36). A critical aspect is determination of the tissue to be submitted for microscopic examination. In nearly all cases, tissue within the blood clot will contain chorionic villi. Occasionally, they will be attached to the tubal wall. The villi may appear fully normal, but more often show degenerative change such as fibrosis or hydropic swelling. Dysmorphic changes, associated with chromosomal anomalies or molar change (e.g., triploidy), are only rarely seen as these do not constitute the cause for the pregnancy loss. In some cases many sections of the blood clot have to be examined before placental villi are seen. In the rare case no residual villous tissue will be found, the only detectable abnormalities are the presence

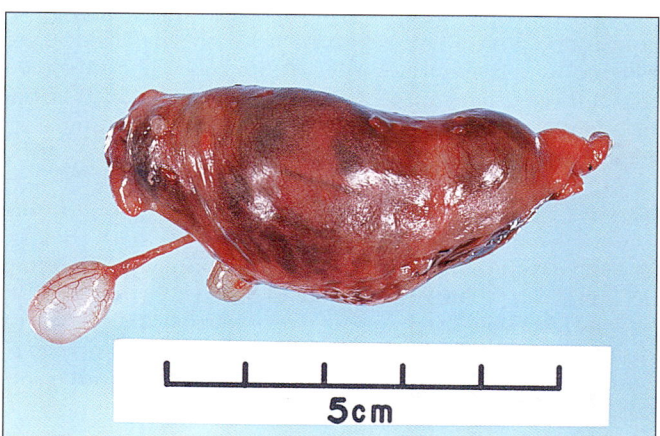

Figure 21.31 Tubal ectopic pregnancy.

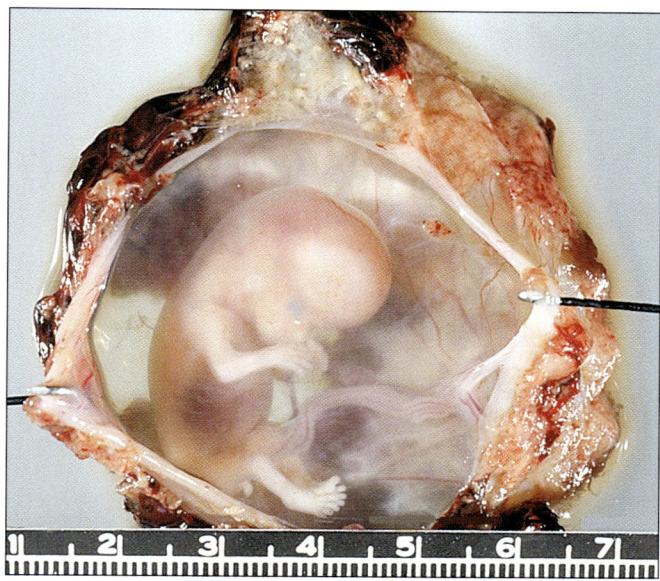

Figure 21.33 Tubal ectopic pregnancy. A fetus is present.

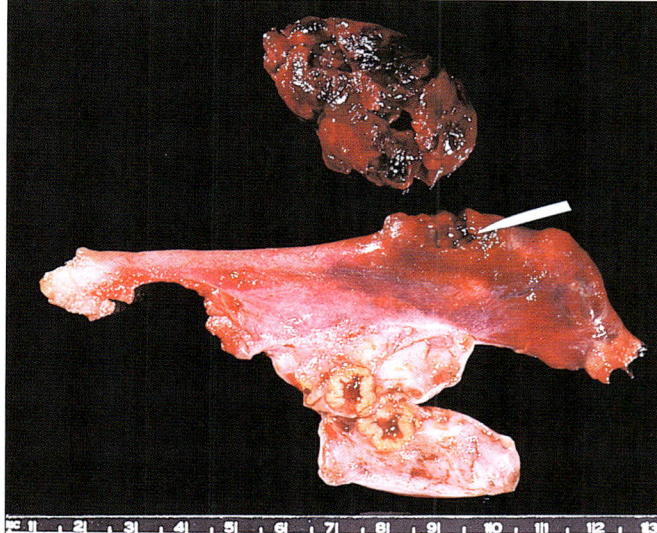

Figure 21.32 Ruptured tubal ectopic pregnancy (arrow).

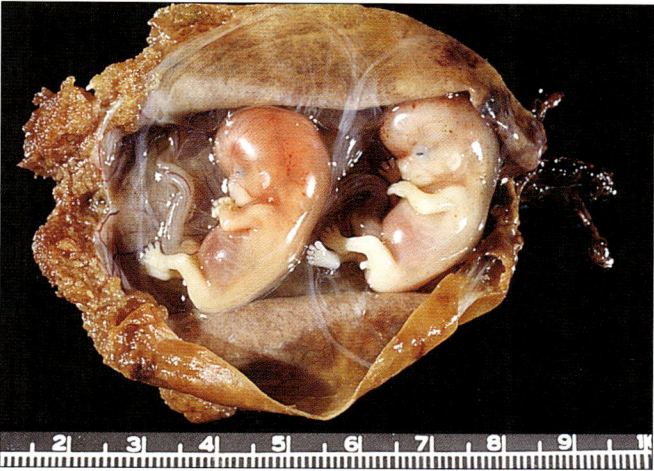

Figure 21.34 Tubal ectopic pregnancy. Twin fetuses are present.

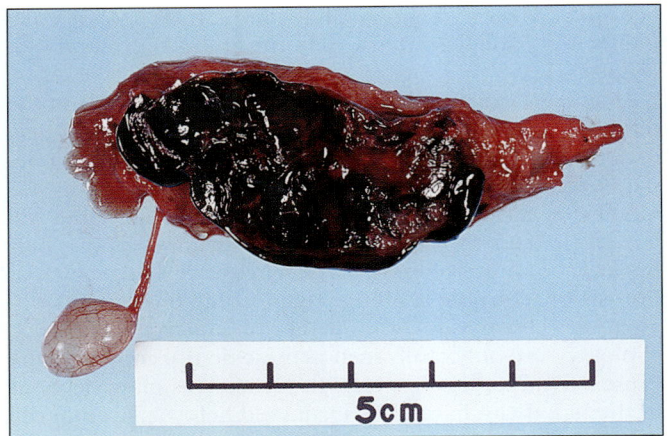

Figure 21.35 Tubal ectopic pregnancy. Sectioning shows only blood clot.

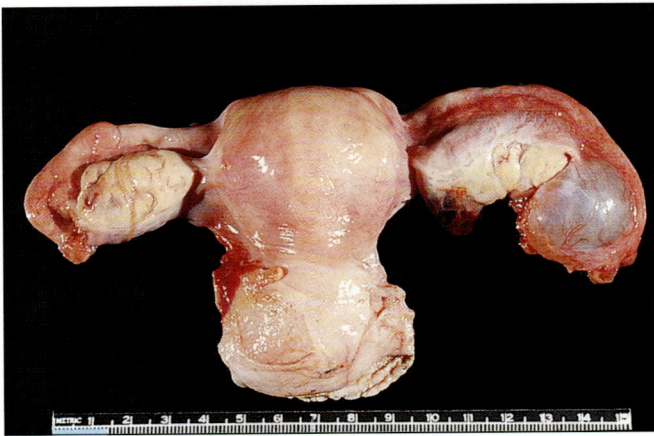

Figure 21.37 This paratubal cyst is thin walled and contains clear watery fluid.

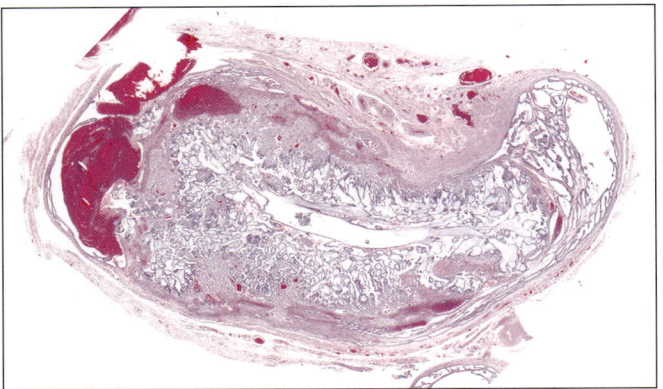

Figure 21.36 Tubal ectopic pregnancy, showing a virtually intact gestation sac. Chorionic villi are easily identifiable. A tiny fragment of embryo is present in the gestational sac itself. The fallopian tube parenchyma (right) shows evidence of old healed salpingitis with confluent plicae.

of inflammatory debris and nonspecific granulation tissue. Even in such circumstances, however, an implantation site can often be identified by the presence of extravillous trophoblastic cells that have infiltrated the tubal wall and invaded the vascular spaces. Curiously, tubal tissue more than a short distance from the region of the ectopic pregnancy may show no abnormality other than a minor degree of nonspecific inflammation. It is important to take a block from the fallopian tube medial to the implantation site to assess the presence or absence of pre-existing salpingitis, usually manifest as plical adhesions, as this offers not only some pointer as to a likely cause of the present ectopic, but is useful in the further management of the patient. Salpingitis is usually bilateral and a second ectopic in the contralateral tube is more likely in such patients (who frequently end up having some form of assisted conception).

Laparoscopic Salpingostomy. Although salpingectomy offers almost a 100% cure, laparoscopic methods are widely used that not only prevent maternal hemorrhage but also allow rapid recovery, preserve fertility, and reduce costs.[16]

Linear salpingostomy is now the standard laparoscopic operation when an ectopic pregnancy is unruptured but measures more than 4 cm by ultrasound. The products of conception are removed after an incision is made along the bulging antimesenteric border of the tube. The specimen the pathologist receives consists mainly of blood clot but frequently contains chorionic villi and trophoblastic fragments, enabling the diagnosis to be confirmed.

Uterine Changes. In tubal pregnancies the uterine endometrium undergoes decidual change to a degree similar to that found in an intrauterine pregnancy in about 45% of cases.[14] The endometrial glands are hypersecretory and an Arias-Stella change is seen focally in 60–70% of cases showing gestational changes. These appearances can, however, occur in any type of pregnancy and are not a specific feature of an ectopic gestation. In contrast to intrauterine pregnancies, curetted material shows little necrosis or inflammation. Indeed, this often is an important clue to the presence of an ectopic pregnancy. Depending on the time interval between fetal demise and curettage, the endometrium may show relatively poorly formed secretory changes and be inactive or even proliferative. In evaluating a curettage or biopsy specimen as part of a clinically suspected ectopic pregnancy, we have never personally encountered the situation where there was a documented pregnancy in the fallopian tube and chorionic villi were simultaneously found in the endometrial cavity. However, the pathologist must always be aware that villi are easily dislodged during tissue processing and may be artifactually introduced as contaminants from another case. Clues as to this possibility include position of the villi relative to other tissue fragments, lack of implantation site in the maternal tissues, and discordance between villous maturity and clinically suspected ectopic gestational age.

CYSTS

Cysts lying alongside the fallopian tube are referred to as paratubal cysts (Figure 21.37). They can be classified based on their origin as müllerian (paramesonephric), wolffian (mesonephric), or mesothelial. These subtypes are not

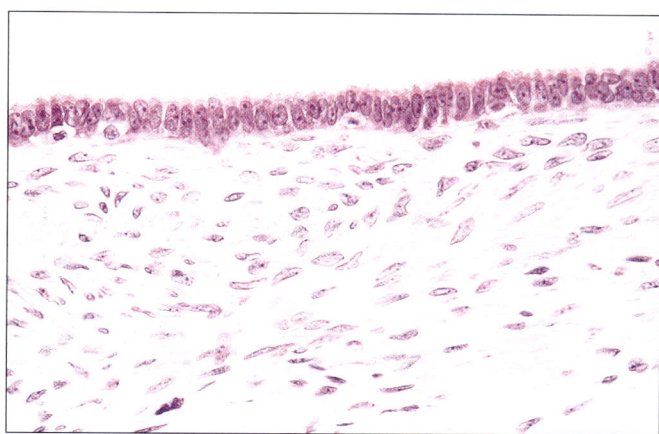

Figure 21.38 Broad ligament 'paratubal' cyst.

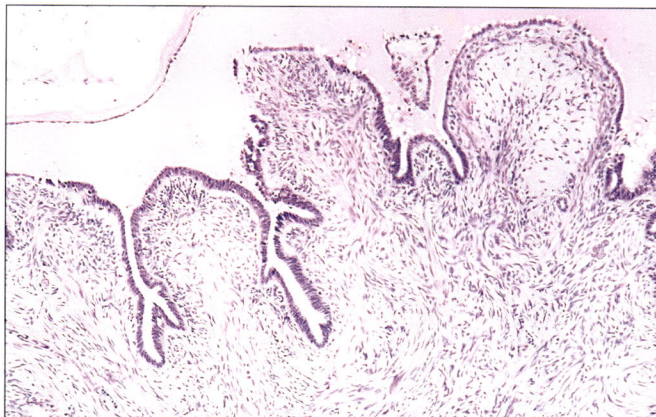

Figure 21.39 Paramesonephric (müllerian) cyst. Coarse, polypoid projections into the lumen may be seen.

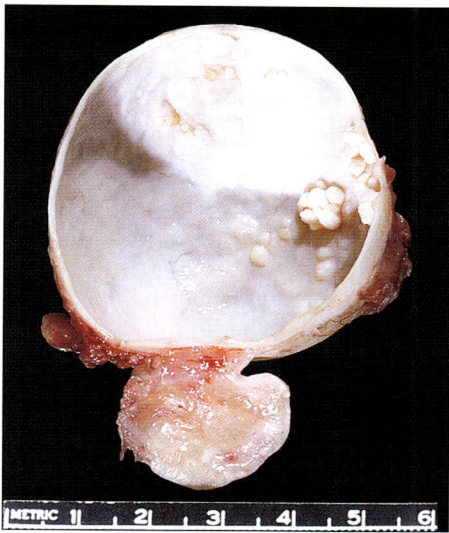

Figure 21.40 Paramesonephric (müllerian) cyst. A large cyst has papillary excrescences that arise from the internal surface.

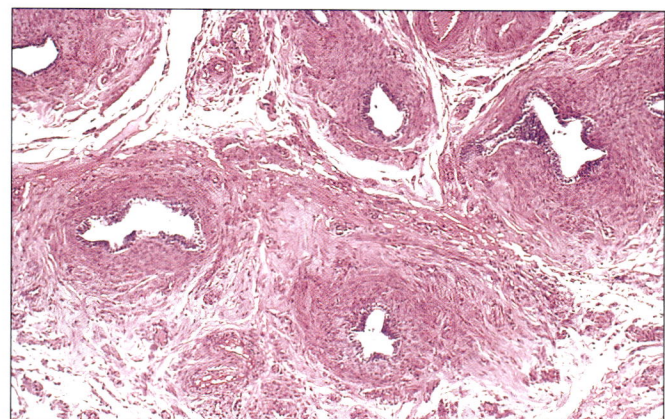

Figure 21.41 Mesonephric remnants.

always diagnostic at the time of presentation, because of either uncertain anatomic relationships or distortion of the wall and lining by dilation.

PARAMESONEPHRIC CYSTS

Paramesonephric cysts, when small, tend to be more laterally situated than those of mesonephric origin. The hydatid of Morgagni, usually seen as a cyst on a pedicle arising from the fimbria, is the most common example of a paramesonephric cyst. Others are found in close proximity to the tube or on its subserosal aspect. Paramesonephric cysts, often also termed 'broad ligament cysts,' are lined by a single layer of columnar cells that may be ciliated or non-ciliated (Figures 21.38 and 21.39). Smooth muscle is often present in their wall but is less prominent than in the mesonephric variety. Distinction between the two types of cyst is not always possible. Larger paramesonephric cysts may have papillary excrescences arising from the internal surface (Figure 21.40).

MESONEPHRIC CYSTS

The mesonephric remnants are the epoophoron and paroophoron, which continue as vestigial tubular structures between the tube and ovary (rete ovarii), passing medially toward the body of the uterus, to enter it at about the level of the internal cervical os and pass anterolaterally in the cervix as Gartner's duct. Non-neoplastic, noncystic mesonephric remnants are universally present between the tube and the ovary and are seen as a collection of thick-walled tubular structures lined by cuboidal epithelium with smooth muscle in their walls (Figure 21.41). These remnants may become cystic at any point along their course, so that mesonephric cysts may be found within the mesosalpinx and broad ligament or they may be pedunculated and situated just lateral to the ovary (Kobelt's cyst). Typically, the mesonephric cyst is lined by a single layer of epithelium that is of low columnar or cuboidal, non-ciliated type. Smooth muscle may be prominent in the wall of these cysts, often together with dense connective tissue and elastic fibers.

MESOTHELIAL INCLUSION CYSTS

Paratubal cysts lined by mesothelial cells can demonstrate a variety of morphologic appearances and exhibit a range of sizes. The cysts may be multilocular or unilocular, the latter of which are sometimes referred to as simple cysts. Their thin walls are composed of fibrous tissue. The lining cells are generally flattened or cuboidal and ciliated cells are absent. Transitional, or müllerian, metaplasia can also be observed within surface inclusion cysts.

METAPLASIAS AND RESTS

As in the cervix and endometrium, it is questionable whether the finding of a type of müllerian epithelium that is inappropriate to the site should strictly be referred to as 'metaplasia.' Nevertheless, the presence of mucinous epithelium and endometrial epithelium in the fallopian tube mucosa must be considered abnormal.

MUCINOUS METAPLASIA

This is an uncommon finding in which mucinous epithelium, exhibiting either an endocervical or gastrointestinal phenotype, replaces areas of tubal epithelium (Figure 21.42). Tubal mucinous metaplasia may occur in women with Peutz–Jeghers syndrome and has been reported in women with both ovarian and cervical mucinous tumors; this phenomenon may be associated with a mutation in the tumor suppressor gene *STK11*.[17] Tubal metaplasia in the setting of multifocal mucinous metaplasia and neoplasia of the female genital tract has also been described in women without Peutz–Jeghers syndrome.[18] The histogenesis of these multifocal mucinous lesions is unclear.

ENDOMETRIOSIS AND ENDOSALPINGIOSIS

Uterine endometrium is found in the interstitial and isthmic segments of the fallopian tube (Figure 21.43) in up to 25% and 10% of women, respectively. This change is identified both as an incidental finding in hysterectomy specimens and, more significantly, in cornual resections for infertility. The lesion represents a shift of the junction between endometrium and fallopian tube mucosa into the fallopian tube. It may be considered a normal morphologic variation even though it is often called 'endometriosis' or 'endometrial colonization.' This phenomenon, which may be related to the microenvironment adaptation, is often encountered in histologic examination of the tubal proximal stump, usually 1–4 years after tubal ligation. Endometrial colonization can also be caused by complete occlusion of the fallopian tube. It accounts for 15–20% of cases of infertility and may be associated with tubal pregnancy.[19]

Typical or serosal tubal endometriosis is most commonly associated with endometriosis elsewhere in the pelvis. In this condition, the myosalpinx and mucosa are not usually involved. In some cases of pelvic endometriosis, with or without tubal involvement, the plicae are expanded by masses of pseudoxanthoma cells, a lesion called pseudoxanthomatous salpingitis or pseudoxanthomatous salpingiosis.

Endosalpingiosis involving the tube and paratubal tissue is morphologically identical to that found elsewhere in the peritoneum. The glandular deposits of benign tubal epithelium can be found on the serosal surface of the tube and in the mesosalpinx. Not infrequently, psammoma bodies are present in association with the epithelium. Occasionally it is identified in women who also have endometriosis, suggesting a common etiology in some cases. A thorough discussion of both endometriosis and endosalpingiosis can be found in Chapter 22.

TRANSITIONAL METAPLASIA

Walthard rests are extremely common, small collections of transitional cells, rarely more than 1 mm in diameter, situated immediately beneath the tubal serosa (Figures 21.44 and 21.45). Grossly, Walthard rests are clear to tan-white soft nodules, usually less than 1 mm in diameter (Figure 21.46). The cells are of a rather nondescript type but some show longitudinal grooves in the nuclear membrane, resembling the appearance seen in Brenner tumor of the ovary. There is speculation that the cells of the Walthard rest and Brenner tumor arise in the same way, by transitional cell metaplasia of the serosal mesothelium. They may be solid or cystic. Walthard rests are of no significance whatsoever, apart from the importance of being recognized grossly for what they are and not mistaken clinically for pelvic tuberculosis, endometriosis, or disseminated tumor.

Compared with the very common transitional cell metaplasia of the serosa that Walthard rests represent, transitional cell metaplasia of the mucosa is extremely rare. It is likely that this is the same change that is described as 'reserve

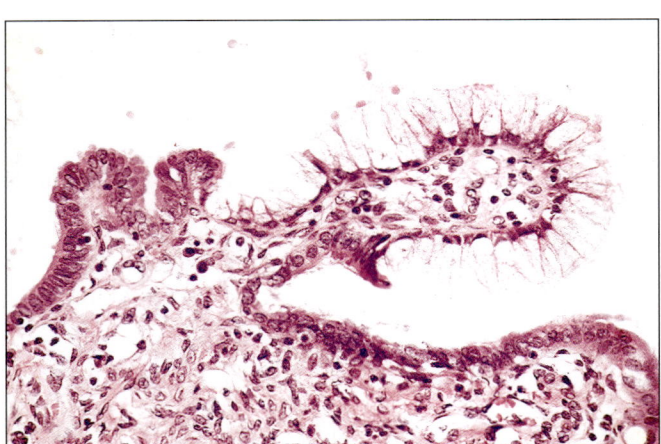

Figure 21.42 Mucinous metaplasia.

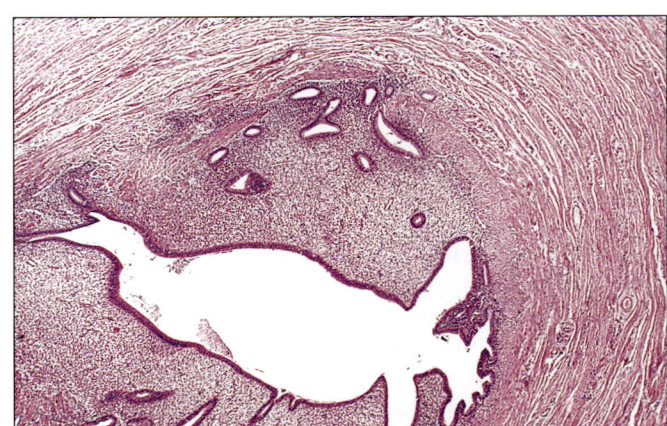

Figure 21.43 Endometrial replacement ('endometrialization or endometrial colonization'). Endometrial glands and stroma replace the tubal mucosa in the isthmus.

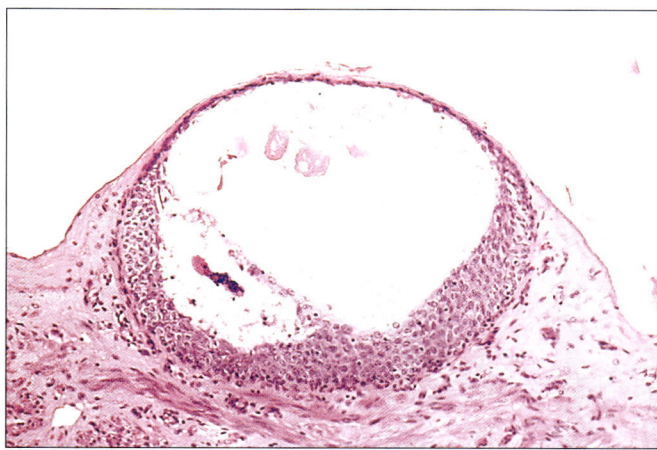

Figure 21.44 Walthard (urothelial differentiation) rest.

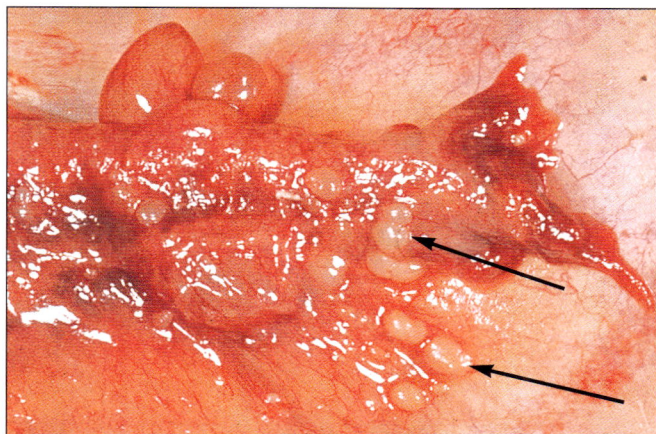

Figure 21.46 Walthard rests. Cystic Walthard rests (arrows) are present on the surface of the tube.

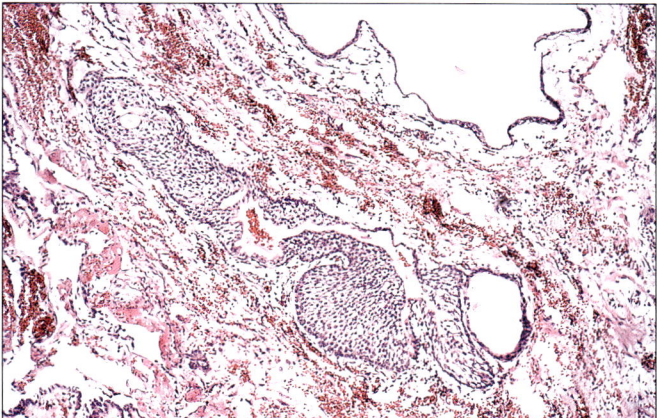

Figure 21.45 Walthard rest.

cell metaplasia' and may serve as a possible source of tubal transitional cell carcinomas.[20]

ADRENAL REST

An encapsulated collection of adrenal cortical cells is encountered as 1–3 mm yellow nodules in the broad ligament or mesosalpinx in as many as one-fourth of women (Figure 21.47). Also termed 'Marchand rest,' the heterotopic adrenal cells are identical to those of the adrenal cortex and are arranged in cords mimicking the zona fascicularis of the latter (Figure 21.48). Benign and malignant tumors may arise from them.

PSEUDODECIDUAL CHANGE (ECTOPIC DECIDUA)

The stromal cells of the fallopian tube lamina propria and subserosa readily undergo pseudodecidual change (Figure 21.49). It is seen in about one-third of salpingectomy specimens containing ectopic pregnancies, and in 5–8% of tubal segments excised for sterilization performed during cesarean section or in the immediate postpartum period.[19]

TORSION OF THE FALLOPIAN TUBE

The fallopian tube usually undergoes torsion with the ovary. Both become twisted together, often because the ovary is

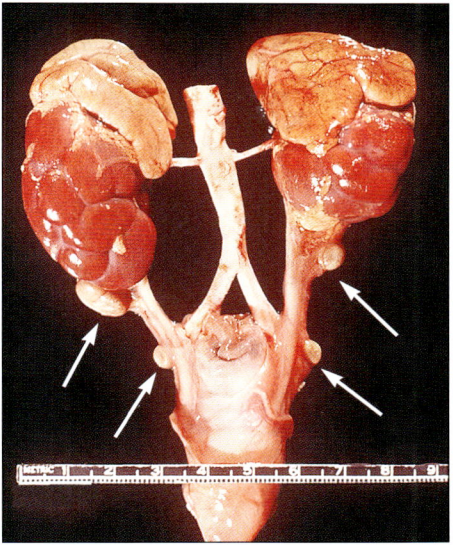

Figure 21.47 Adrenal rests. Although no longer related to the fallopian tubes, the adrenal rests (arrows) are clearly seen in these dissected organs from an infant.

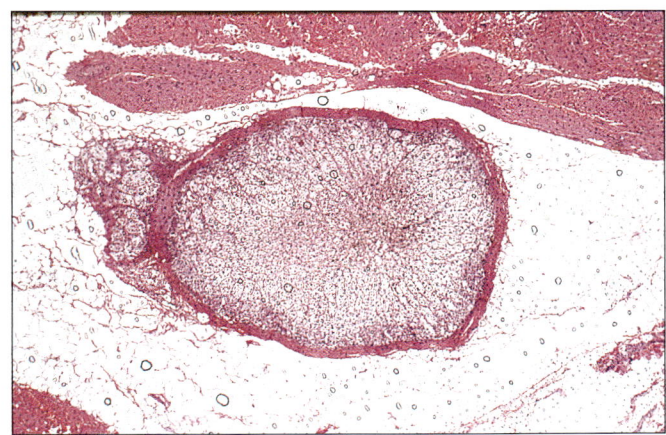

Figure 21.48 Adrenal rest.

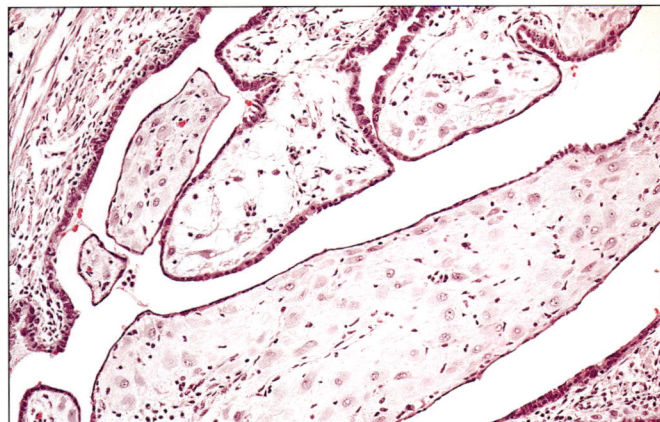

Figure 21.49 Pseudodecidual change.

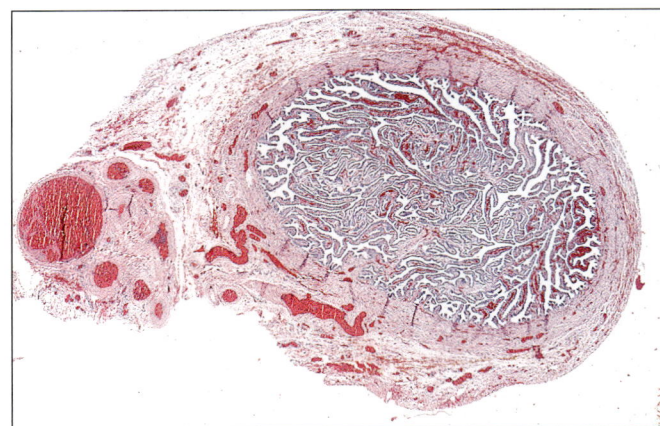

Figure 21.51 Torsion of the tube. At this early stage there is marked congestion. Infarction may follow.

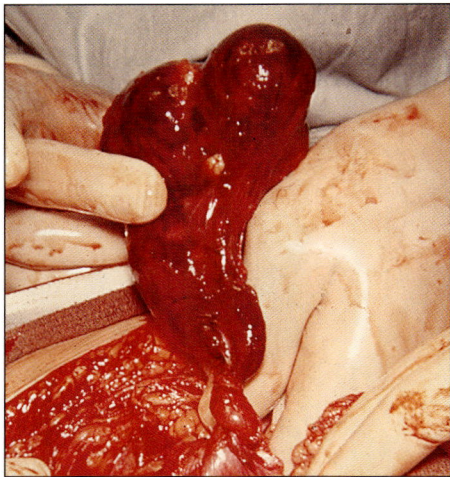

Figure 21.50 Torsion of the tube. A hydrosalpinx is present, an abnormality that precipitated twisting.

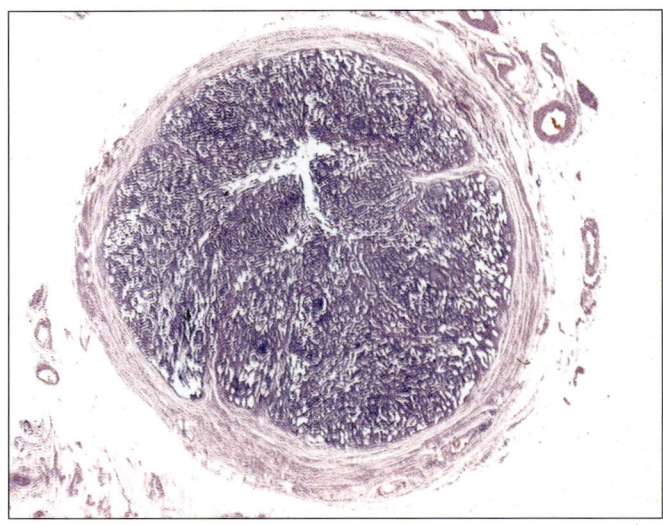

Figure 21.52 Epithelial proliferation associated with salpingitis. The diameter of the tube is greatly increased by what appears to be solid tissue.

enlarged. However, torsion may affect either organ independently and the tube is particularly at risk if it is diseased, as with a hydrosalpinx. The torsed tube is swollen and dark red-blue (Figure 21.50). Microscopy shows marked congestion initially (Figure 21.51), followed by infarction.

PROLAPSE OF THE FALLOPIAN TUBE

Tubal prolapse occurs occasionally after a hysterectomy, especially with vaginal hysterectomy. On clinical examination, a lesion simulating granulation tissue is seen at the vaginal apex. A misdiagnosis of papillary adenocarcinoma may happen if the tubal plicae and their lining of bland epithelium are not recognized (see Chapter 5).

EPITHELIAL PROLIFERATION ASSOCIATED WITH SALPINGITIS

Definition

Reactive hyperplasia of tubal epithelium is associated with salpingitis. It may be mistaken for carcinoma since the salpingitis may present as pseudocarcinomatous hyperplasia.[21]

Microscopic Features

This change results in the formation of multiple small glandular structures, often arranged in a highly complex pattern, amid inflamed, often edematous, tubal plicae (Figures 21.52–21.54). The complexity of the architectural pattern is compounded by the fusion of adjacent plicae, resulting in a striking back-to-back pseudoglandular pattern or a sieve-like pattern.[21] Epithelial stratification is often present and there may be loss of nuclear polarity. Nuclear atypia is of a mild to moderate degree only. Nucleoli are prominent in only half of the cases. Mitotic figures are rarely observed and these are normal. Moderate to marked chronic inflammatory changes are, of course, always present.

Reactive atypical hyperplasia may be distinguished from adenocarcinoma by the lack of solid epithelial areas, a feature nearly always seen in tubal carcinoma, the presence of only mild to moderate nuclear atypia and sparse, normal mitotic figures. Adenocarcinoma commonly shows moderate to severe atypia with prominent nucleoli and frequent mitotic figures.

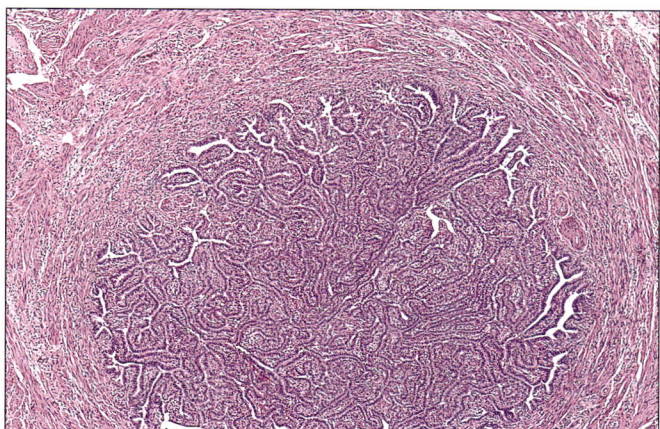

Figure 21.53 Epithelial proliferation associated with salpingitis.

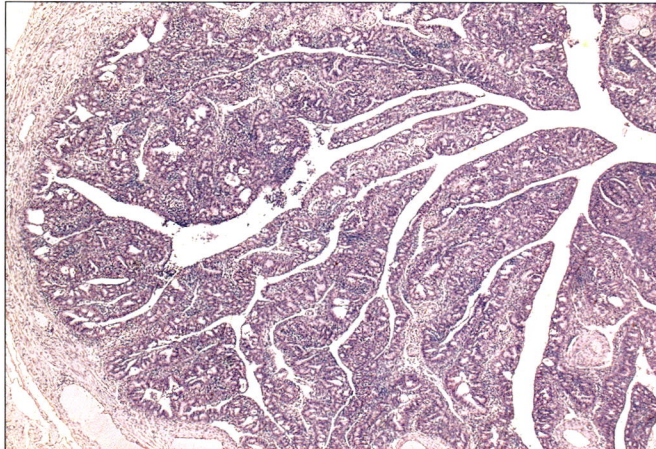

Figure 21.54 Epithelial proliferation associated with salpingitis. At higher power, the combination of inflammatory infiltrate and epithelial proliferation is apparent.

Table 21.1 Modified WHO Classification of Tumors of the Fallopian Tube

Epithelial tumors
  Benign
    Endometrioid polyp
    Papilloma
    Metaplastic papillary tumor
    Adenofibroma
    Cystadenoma
  Borderline
    Serous borderline tumor
    Endometrioid borderline tumor
    Mucinous borderline tumor
  Malignant
    Serous tubal intraepithelial carcinoma
    Serous adenocarcinoma
    Mucinous adenocarcinoma
    Endometrioid adenocarcinoma
    Clear cell adenocarcinoma
    Transitional cell carcinoma
    Squamous cell carcinoma
    Mixed carcinoma
    Undifferentiated carcinoma
Mixed epithelial–mesenchymal tumors, Malignant
  Adenosarcoma
  Carcinosarcoma
Soft-tissue tumors
  Benign
    Leiomyoma
    Others
  Malignant
    Leiomyosarcoma
    Others
Mesothelial tumors
  Solitary mesothelioma
  Adenomatoid tumor
Miscellaneous
  Wolffian adnexal tumor
Germ cell tumors
  Teratoma
    Mature
    Immature
    Others
Trophoblastic disease
  Hydatidiform mole
  Choriocarcinoma
Secondary tumors

TUMORS OF THE FALLOPIAN TUBE

Primary tubal neoplasms, most of which are malignant, are uncommonly diagnosed preoperatively. A modification of the World Health Organization (WHO) classification of fallopian tube tumors is shown in Table 21.1.[19]

BENIGN TUMORS

ADENOMATOID TUMOR

Definition

The adenomatoid tumor, also referred to as 'benign mesothelioma,' is the most common benign tumor of the fallopian tube but, nevertheless, is rare. It is always an incidental finding, usually in women who are in middle age or elderly, and is never symptomatic. Similar tumors are found in the uterus and ovary. Multiple small, slit-like or ovoid spaces lined by a single layer of flattened endothelial-like cells typify this condition.

Pathology

The adenomatoid tumor appears as a round or oval nodule, usually 1–3 cm in diameter, distending the tube (Figure 21.55). It is usually subserosal and in the outer wall, although it may be confined to the endosalpinx or spread throughout the wall. The neoplasm shows numerous slit-like, ovoid, and round spaces of various sizes, separated by bands of connective tissue (Figure 21.56). The spaces are lined by a single layer of low cuboidal or flattened cells with eosinophilic cytoplasm and oval nuclei (Figures 21.57–21.59). The tumor is not encapsulated and infiltrates the muscle of the tubal wall at its margins.

The main interest in these clinically unimportant tumors is in their histogenesis. Suggestions of their origin have

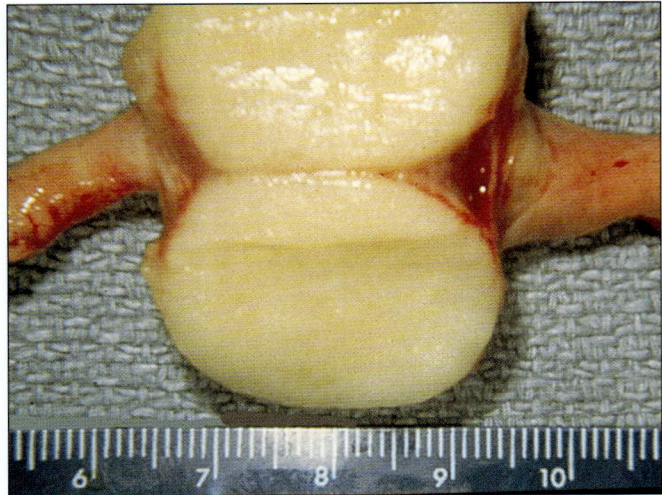

Figure 21.55 Adenomatoid tumor.

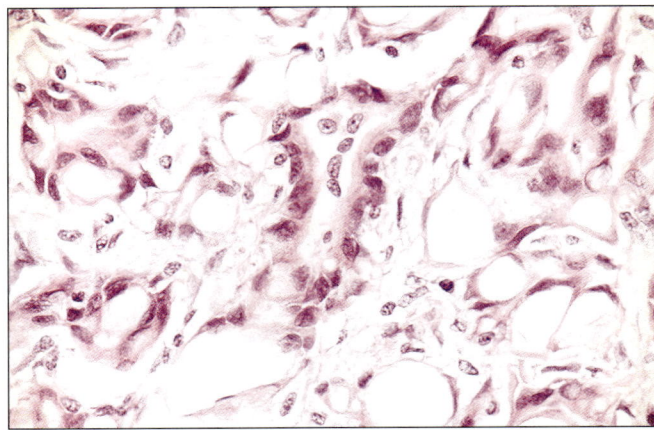

Figure 21.58 Adenomatoid tumor with variation in appearances.

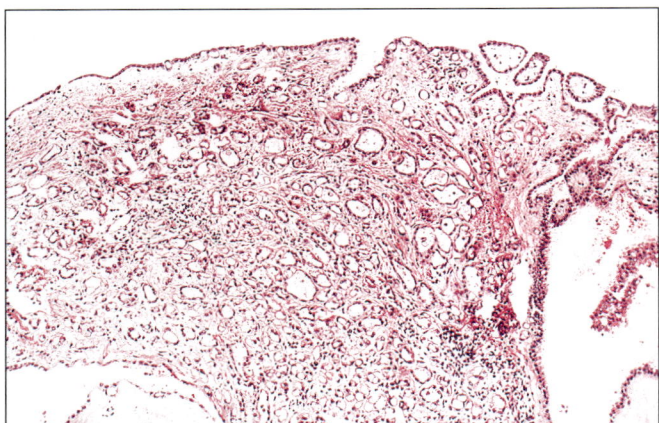

Figure 21.56 Adenomatoid tumor, which at low-power magnification discloses numerous slit-like, ovoid, and round spaces of various sizes, separated by bands of connective tissue.

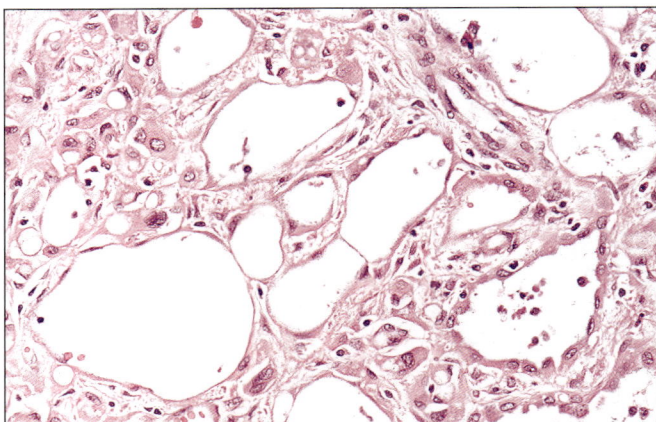

Figure 21.59 Adenomatoid tumor with lymphatic-like channels.

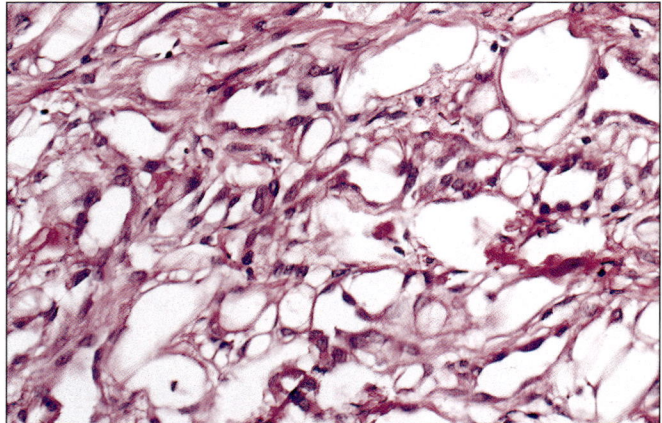

Figure 21.57 Adenomatoid tumor disclosing slit-like, ovoid, and round spaces of various sizes.

included mesonephric, vascular, lymphatic, müllerian, and mesothelial derivation. Electron microscopic and, more recently, immunohistochemical studies indicate that it is of mesothelial origin.

SEROUS CYSTADENOMA

These are occasionally found in the paratubal soft tissue and resemble their ovarian counterparts. They are distinguished from paratubal cysts by a thick, collagenous cyst wall. Cystadenoma can also be confused with hydrosalpinx; the latter is remarkable for the presence of smooth muscle in its wall.

ADENOFIBROMA

Once considered to be extremely rare, adenofibromas involving the fallopian tube have been recognized with greater frequency recently, due largely to the implementation of protocols that extensively sample the fimbriated end of the fallopian tube, where the overwhelming majority of tubal adenofibromas are located.[22] Most are present as microscopic foci; those forming larger masses are uncommon. Microscopically, they share features with ovarian adenofibromas, both morphologically and immunohistochemically, with the stromal component exhibiting positive staining for inhibin and CD10.[22]

LEIOMYOMAS

Leiomyomas are rare compared with the uterine variety and are usually small.[23]

OTHER BENIGN TUMORS

Of the rare benign tumors, about 50 mature cystic teratomas (dermoid cysts) have been reported, nearly all as incidental findings.[24] They resemble grossly and histologically the ovarian mature cystic teratoma and are thought to arise from misplaced germ cells, in this case extragonadal.

Rare examples of placental site nodule[25,26] and placental site trophoblastic tumor[27] have also been reported in the fallopian tube. Rarely, papillomas, ranging up to 3 cm in diameter, may occur in the tubal lumen.

Metaplastic papillary tumors are rare lesions that have been identified as incidental findings in tubal segments excised postpartum for sterilization.[19] They are composed of papillary nests of budding, proliferating cells with abundant eosinophilic cytoplasm (Figures 21.60 and 21.61). Rare mitotic figures may be seen. Whether these are genuine neoplastic lesions or the result of metaplasia and proliferation occurring during pregnancy is not known.

Very rare neoplasms include neurilemmoma, lipoma, chondroma, lymphangioma, ganglioneuroma, and hemangioma.[19]

BORDERLINE TUMORS

Compared with their ovarian counterparts, borderline tumors of the fallopian tube are uncommon, with limited experience about their clinical behavior. Most of the very limited number are serous and a very rare case is endometrioid.[28–30] Mucinous borderline tumors have been reported; when such cases are encountered, secondary spread to the tube from an undetected appendiceal mucinous tumor should always be excluded first.

The serous borderline tumor of the fallopian tube shows formation of papillary projections with focally prominent epithelial stratification and atypia. None has recurred, suggesting that these extremely uncommon tumors can be managed conservatively.[30]

MALIGNANT TUMORS

PRIMARY CARCINOMA OF THE FALLOPIAN TUBE

Definition

A malignant tumor arising from the epithelium of the fallopian tube mucosa.

General Features

Primary fallopian tube carcinoma has historically been considered to be a relatively uncommon neoplasm, with an estimated incidence of 0.41 per 100,000 (approximately 1/150, as common as ovarian cancer).[31] This assumption has been due, in part, to the stringent criteria classically used for ascribing a site of origin to the fallopian tube, including all of the following: the bulk of the tumor must be present in the tube; any tumor present in the ovary, peritoneum, or endometrium must be of smaller quantity than that in the tube; and early cancer should be identified in the tube. There is compelling and mounting evidence, however, to suggest that a significant proportion of cases of high-grade serous carcinoma classified as either ovarian or peritoneal in origin using conventional classification schemes have an origin in the distal fallopian tube. See Chapter 25 for a detailed discussion of this concept.

Clinical Features

The mean age of patients with fallopian tube carcinoma is about 60 years (age range, 26–86). Women who develop tubal carcinomas in the setting of a *BRCA* mutation present at a slightly younger mean age than those without.[32] Tubal carcinomas are uncommon in women under 40 years old.[33,34] Nulliparity, previous PID, and hormone replacement therapy may be associated with increased risk of developing tubal carcinoma, while oral contraceptive use may reduce the risk.[35,36] Early tubal carcinomas may be discovered in risk-reducing, prophylactic salpingectomies from women with *BRCA-1* or *BRCA-2* mutations, in specimens with coexisting high-grade serous carcinomas in other pelvic sites (ovary, peritoneum, uterus), and, very rarely, as incidental findings in specimens removed for non-malignant indications.

The correct diagnosis is rarely made preoperatively. The most common presenting signs and symptoms, including

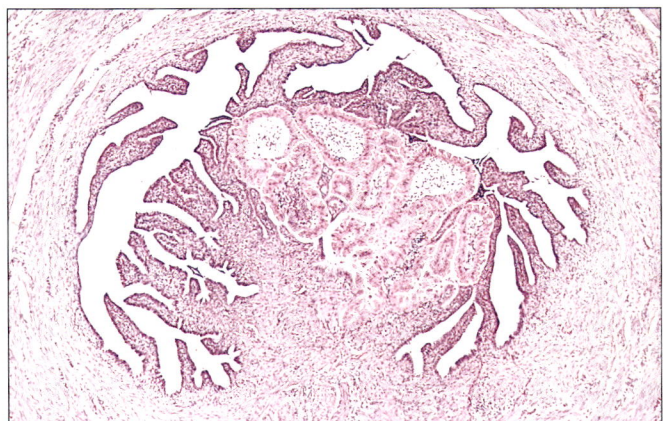

Figure 21.60 Metaplastic papillary lesion of pregnancy.

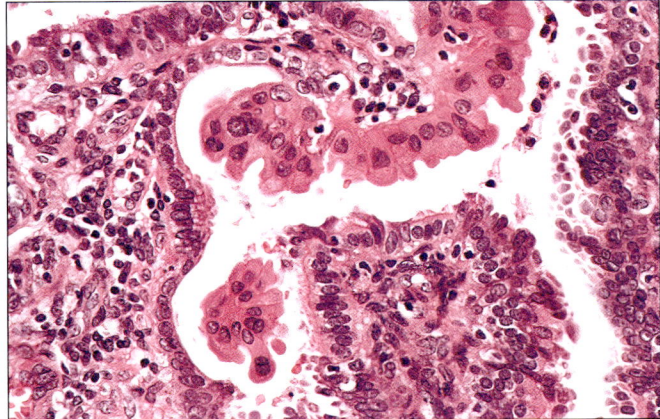

Figure 21.61 Metaplastic papillary lesion of pregnancy.

serosanguineous vaginal discharge, pain, and a palpable pelvic mass, are nonspecific and are seen in only a minority of women with the disease. 'Hydrops tubae profluens,' the classically described finding of colicky lower abdominal pain relieved by an intermittent serous, watery, vaginal discharge, occurs in fewer than 10% of patients.[32] Tumor may be identified in cervical cytology specimens or endometrial biopsies or curettages, but the findings are nonspecific for a tubal origin.

Gross Features

Tubal carcinoma can exhibit a variable gross appearance. The classic description is that of an enlarged, distended, tumor-filled tube with fused fimbriae, resembling a sausage or hydrosalpinx (Figure 21.62). The wall may or may not be thickened. In some cases, the tube is of overall normal size and shape, with grossly evident tumor present as friable nodules studding the fimbriae (Figure 21.63). Cases harboring only intraepithelial carcinoma will appear grossly unremarkable. About 20% of tubal carcinomas are bilateral.[37]

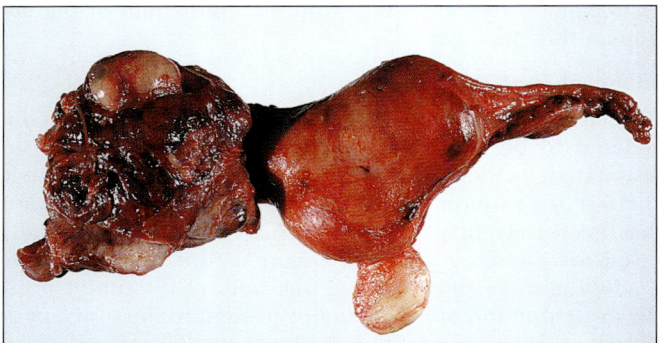

Figure 21.62 Serous carcinoma. The tube is enlarged, with solid, papillary, luminal growth.

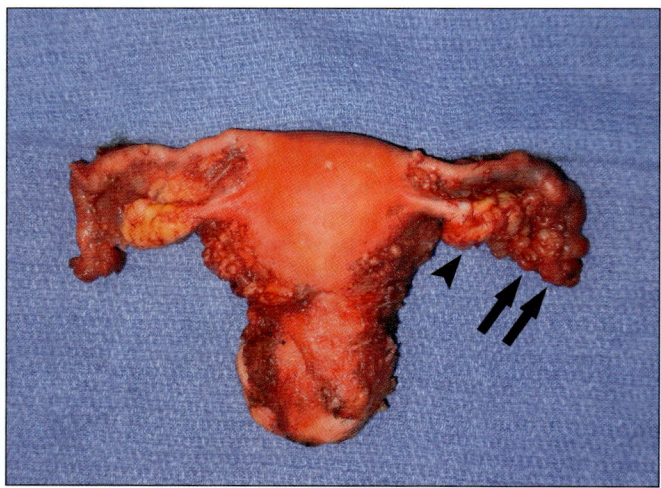

Figure 21.63 Primary fallopian tube carcinoma. The affected tube is of normal size and shape but is grossly remarkable for multiple nodules studding the fimbriae (arrows). A nodule of tumor is also present on the surface of the ovary (arrowhead).

Microscopic Features

Serous Tubal Intraepithelial Carcinomas. The majority of early noninvasive tubal carcinomas are found in the mucosal epithelium of the fimbriae, as serous tubal intraepithelial carcinomas (STICs). STICs exhibit the following microscopic features:

1. A *discrete population of epithelial cells replacing the normal mucosa*. Some STICs exhibit marked disorganized stratification with irregular fractures separating the cells (Figure 21.64A), while others are minimally stratified and 'thin' appearing (Figure 21.64B). The stratified STIC can generally be easily identified at low-power magnification, by virtue of its thickened, somewhat 'velvety' appearance relative to the adjacent non-neoplastic epithelium. Additionally, STICs often have an exfoliative appearance, with shedding of tumor cells from the surface, which may also be notable at low power (Figure 21.64A).
2. *Loss of cell polarity*. Even in the absence of stratification, the cells of a STIC almost always exhibit some loss of polarity.
3. *Increased nuclear to cytoplasmic ratio*.
4. *Often rounded nuclei with prominent nucleoli*.
5. *Absence of ciliated cells*.
6. *Usually stain positive for p53*. STICs are *p53* mutation-associated lesions; the majority exhibit strong, diffuse nuclear staining for p53 (Figure 21.64C). In a minority of STICs, staining for p53 is completely absent, which, in some cases, is due to a *p53* mutation with a resultant stop codon, yielding a truncated p53 protein, which is not detectable by immunohistochemical staining.[38]
7. *Increased rate of proliferation*. STICs have a high MIB1 index (approximately 70%) by immunohistochemical staining (Figure 21.64D).[5]

It is important to note that, while immunohistochemistry can be a useful diagnostic adjunct in supporting a morphologic impression of STIC, it should never be used as a substitute for the appropriate morphologic features. Additionally, when considering a diagnosis of STIC, they must be distinguished from lesser lesions of unknown clinical significance and diagnostic reproducibility. For example, the term 'tubal intraepithelial lesion in transition' (TILT) has been proposed for atypical foci of mitotically active p53-positive secretory cells, which exhibit features intermediate between p53 signatures and STICs.[5]

Benign Mimics. On occasion, foci of benign tubal epithelium can be identified that can raise suspicion for a neoplastic process. Tubal epithelium exhibiting architectural complexity with pseudostratification and occasional scattered atypical-appearing nuclei can be mistaken for neoplasia. In general, such a benign mimic will exhibit the presence of cilia diffusely, and overall polarity of the epithelium will be preserved. In especially challenging cases, immunostaining for p53 and MIB1 can serve as a useful diagnostic adjunct.

Serous Carcinoma. Serous carcinomas are the most common histologic type of epithelial tubal malignancy. Using classical criteria of a dominant tumor mass within the fallopian tube to assign a primary site, these are over half of

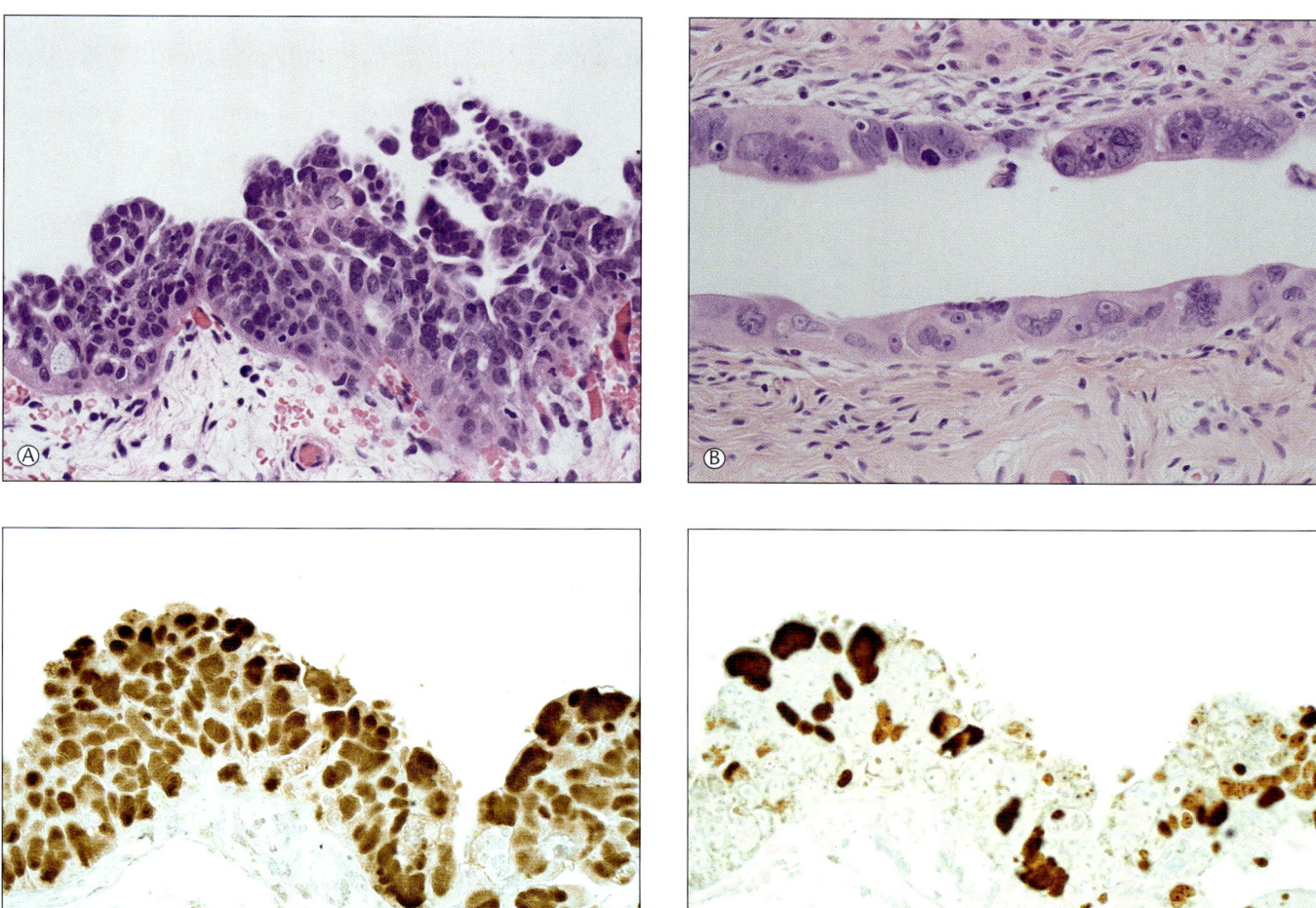

Figure 21.64 Serous tubal intraepithelial carcinoma. Some STICs are markedly stratified with fracture lines between cells; exfoliation of tumor cells from the surface is common **(A)**. Other STICs may be more thin, but still exhibit loss of cell polarity and atypical nuclei **(B)**. Most STICs stain strongly positive for p53 **(C)**, and have a high proliferative (MIB1-positive) index **(D)**.

all tubal carcinomas. This underestimates the true incidence, as new evidence suggests that grossly occult tubal serous carcinomas frequently present with a dominant metastatic ovarian mass, and thus have been considered primary ovarian tumors (see Chapter 25). As is true elsewhere in the pelvis, the majority of serous carcinomas involving the fallopian tube are high grade and demonstrate defects in the *p53* gene.[37] These poorly differentiated tumors are predominantly solid with usually at least focal areas of poorly formed papillae. Characteristic slit-like spaces are seen through solid sheets of tumor cells (Figure 21.65). The cells themselves have marked nuclear pleomorphism and a high mitotic rate with occasional structurally abnormal mitotic figures (Figures 21.66 and 21.67). Necrosis is common. STICs are frequently identified in association with high-grade serous carcinoma, and the presumed precursor lesion.[3] Low-grade serous tumors are rare in the fallopian tube. These are extensively papillary tumors with areas of stromal invasion. Papillae are lined by columnar to cuboidal cells, some of which may be ciliated, exhibiting generally mild cytologic atypia. Mitotic figures are typically infrequent (Figures 21.68 and 21.69). A transition from areas of borderline malignancy to carcinoma is common.

Endometrioid Carcinoma. About 12–25% of fallopian tube carcinomas are of endometrioid type.[37,39,40] Their pattern resembles that of endometrioid carcinomas in the uterus and ovary and is predominantly more glandular and less papillary than serous carcinomas. They are less likely to be bilateral than serous carcinomas.[40] A subtype of endometrioid carcinoma may resemble the female adnexal tumor of probable wolffian origin, and shows a mostly solid proliferation of small, oval to spindle cells punctured by small to cystic glands, many with luminal periodic acid–Schiff (PAS)-positive colloid-like secretions. Foci of typical endometrioid carcinoma are usually present but may be minor. These tumors usually are noninvasive.

Transitional Cell Carcinoma. Transitional cell carcinoma is the third most common histologic type of carcinoma found

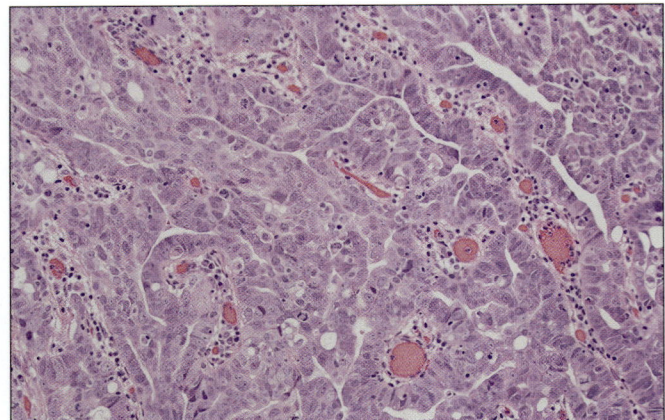

Figure 21.65 Serous carcinoma, high grade.

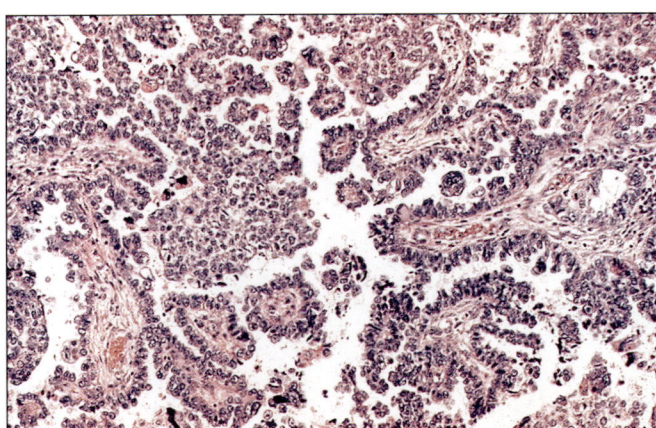

Figure 21.68 Low-grade serous carcinoma showing a typical papillary pattern.

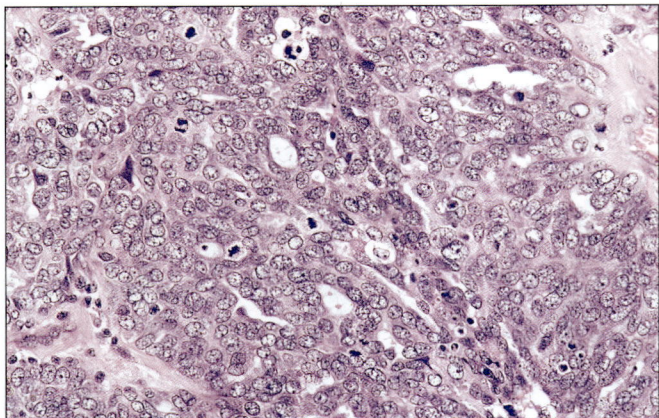

Figure 21.66 Serous carcinoma, high grade.

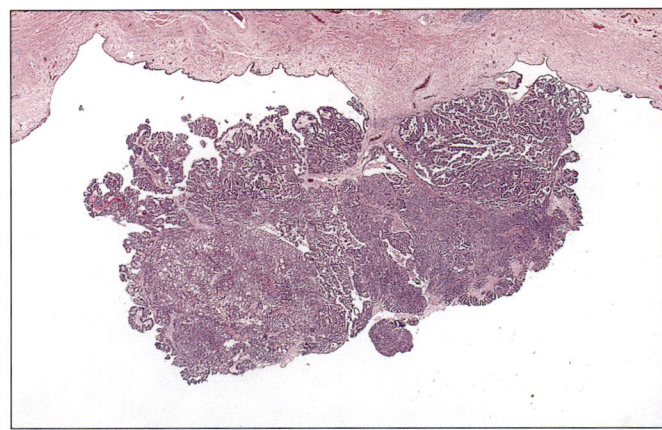

Figure 21.69 Serous carcinoma. The tumor is entirely mucosal and intraluminal.

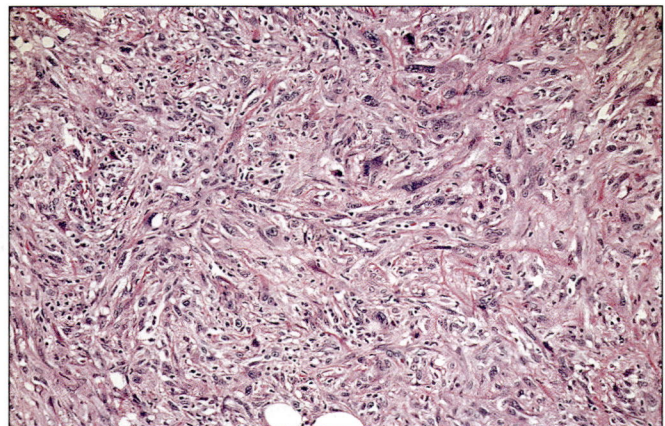

Figure 21.67 Serous carcinoma, high grade, invasive focus.

in the fallopian tube. One recent report found that 12% of tubal carcinomas were entirely of transitional cell type[37] while another found that as many as 57% of tubal carcinomas contained a transitional cell element.[41] These tumors are arranged as solid nests that show stratification. The cells have clear cytoplasm that may be slightly eosinophilic and some nuclei show nuclear grooves, the so-called 'coffee bean' appearance.[37] In our view, many such cases are more likely to be poorly differentiated serous carcinomas with a broad papillary or pseudopapillary growth pattern than a truly transitional cell type.

Clear Cell Carcinoma. Clear cell carcinoma of the fallopian tube is rare, constituting about 2% of tubal carcinomas.[37] The tumor has the same appearances as seen in the uterus and ovary. Solid zones of clear cells and papillary areas are present, together with a tubulocystic pattern with prominent hobnail cells.

Squamous Cell Carcinoma. Primary squamous cell carcinoma in the fallopian tube has been reported, but is rare.[42] Most cases are thought to represent transgenital spread of squamous intraepithelial lesions (SILs) from the cervix through the endometrium (Figures 21.70 and 21.71).[42]

Spread, Treatment, and Prognosis of Tubal Carcinoma

The current clinical staging system for carcinoma of the fallopian tube is shown in an abbreviated fashion in

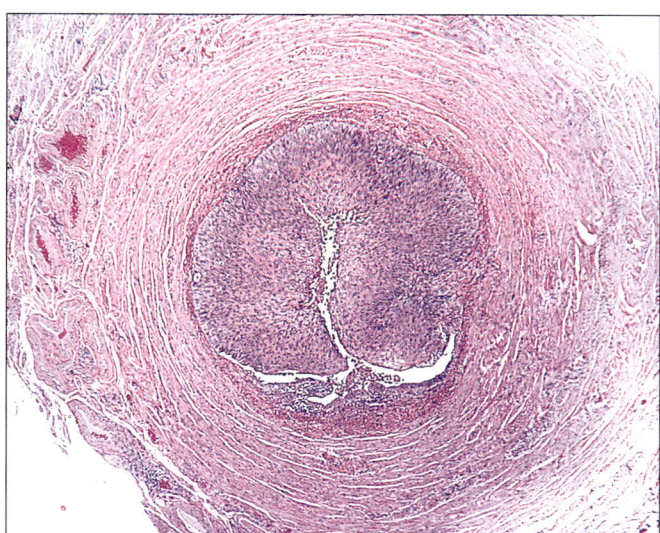

Figure 21.70 Cervical SIL, with transgenital spread to the tube lumen.

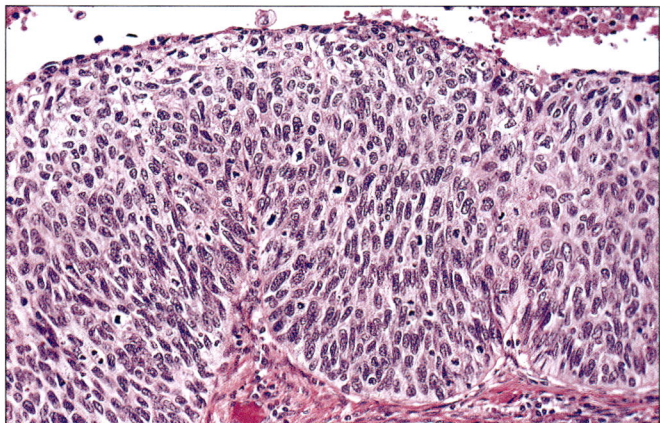

Figure 21.71 Cervical SIL, with transgenital spread to the tube lumen.

Appendix A. The spread of tubal carcinoma is generally similar to that of ovarian carcinoma. Transluminal spread into the peritoneal cavity with subsequent implantation on peritoneal surfaces is the predominant mode of spread, but direct involvement of adjacent organs, particularly ovary and uterus, is also important. Occasionally, spread may occur transluminally to involve endometrium and endocervix. Lymphatic spread from the fimbria is principally to the pelvic nodes, and to the para-aortic nodes from that portion of the tube near the uterus. In one small series, two of six patients with disease limited to the fallopian tube already had nodal metastases.[43,44]

Initial treatment is surgical, consisting of total hysterectomy with bilateral salpingo-oophorectomy and with staging procedures as for ovarian carcinoma. Postoperative radiation therapy is of some value but combination chemotherapy with cisplatin-containing agents, similar to that used for ovarian carcinoma, is most widely used.

Survival depends upon the extent of the disease at the time of diagnosis. The overall 5 year survival for stages I and II is about 50–60% and for stages III and IV is about 15–20%.[45,46] The overall 5 year survival for all stages is under 40%. Histologically high-grade lesions have the worst outcome but a better prognosis is associated with endometrioid type[37] and an inflammatory reaction around the tumor. The most important adverse prognostic factor remains advanced stage. Other adverse factors have included increasing age, vascular space invasion, and a high volume of residual tumor.

CARCINOSARCOMA

Definition

A rare mixed tumor composed of malignant glands and malignant mesenchyme, with an annual incidence of about 0.25 cases per million women.[47] Carcinosarcoma may be found anywhere along the female genital tract and, although much more common in the endometrium and ovary, about 70 cases of this tumor have been reported in the fallopian tube.

Clinical Features

The mean age at diagnosis is 59 years, with a range of 14–79 years. The majority of patients are postmenopausal although 17% are under 50 years old at diagnosis. Presentation is with nonspecific abdominal symptoms of pain or distension, often with vaginal spotting or bleeding. Physical examination usually reveals a pelvic mass, although initial evaluation may be normal.

Pathology

Carcinosarcomas of the tube are often relatively small when diagnosed. Larger tumors are difficult to distinguish from ovarian primaries. They appear grossly as polypoid growths filling the lumen of the tube, often with areas of hemorrhage and necrosis (Figure 21.72).

Microscopically, carcinosarcoma discloses a malignant epithelial element that may or may not have the pattern of an endometrioid adenocarcinoma, together with a mesenchymal element. As in the endometrium and ovary, the mesenchymal element may be homologous, containing elements indigenous to the endometrium, or heterologous, containing elements foreign to the endometrium, such a cartilage (Figure 21.73) or striated muscle.

Treatment and Prognosis

Recommended treatment is by surgery, followed by radiotherapy and/or chemotherapy. The prognosis is poor, the 5 year survival rate being about 15% and the mean survival only 16–20 months. Early stage disease is associated with a better prognosis,[48] and several long-term survivals are recorded.[47]

OTHER MALIGNANT TUMORS

Other rare malignant tumors that have been reported arising in the tube include leiomyosarcoma,[49] embryonal rhabdomyosarcoma,[50] immature teratoma,[51] and choriocarcinoma (Figure 21.74).[52]

TUMORS METASTATIC TO THE FALLOPIAN TUBE

Metastatic tumors from other gynecologic sites can spread to the fallopian tube, including rare transgenital spread of

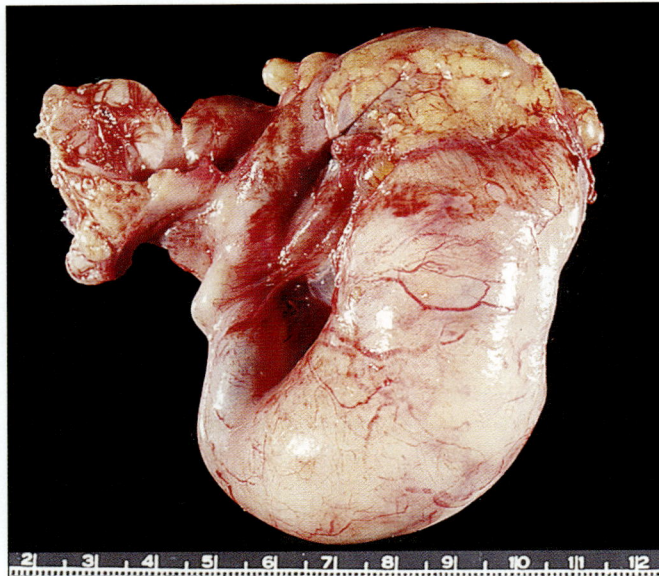

Figure 21.72 Carcinosarcoma.

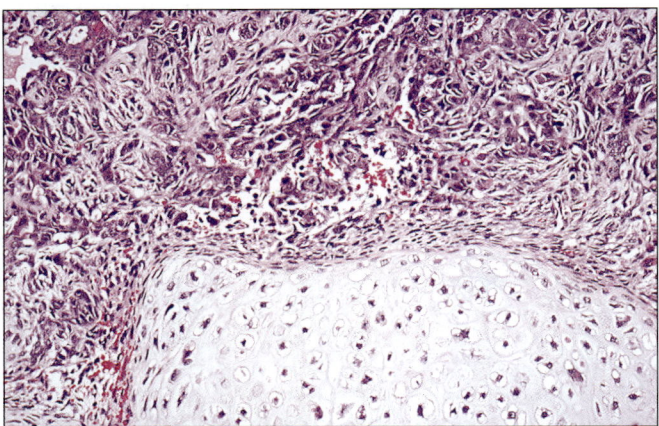

Figure 21.73 Carcinosarcoma. A heterologous tumor containing cartilage.

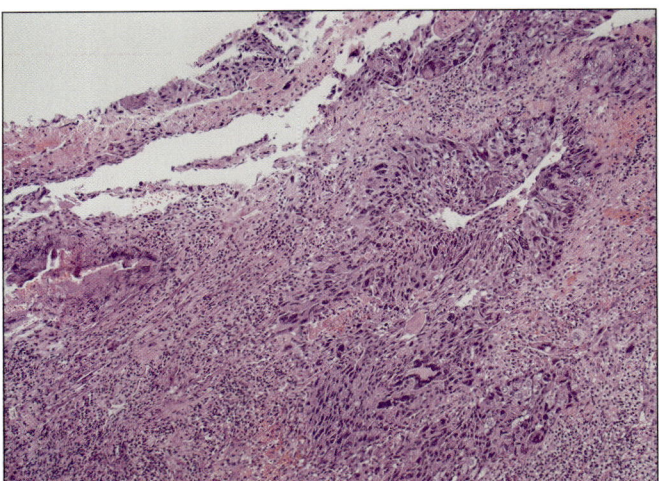

Figure 21.74 Tubal choriocarcinoma. Clinically, this case was presumed to be an ectopic tubal gestation.

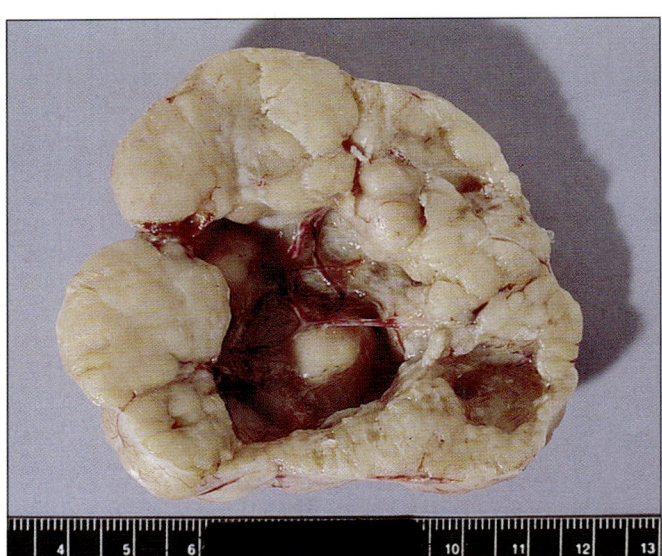

Figure 21.75 Adnexal tumor of probable wolffian origin.

cervical SILs as described above (Figures 21.70 and 21.71).[42] Tumors from non-gynecologic sites can spread to the fallopian tube, typically evident as deposits on the serosal surface of the tube or as tumor within lymphovascular spaces within the tube stroma.

FEMALE ADNEXAL TUMOR OF WOLFFIAN ORIGIN

Definition

A tumor of the broad ligament for which there is very strong evidence of a wolffian origin. About 40 cases have been reported.[19]

Clinical Features

The patients are 15–81 years of age. The tumors are asymptomatic and usually incidental findings, although a large tumor may present as a mass.

Gross Features

The tumors are unilateral, ranging from 0.5 to 18 cm in diameter, and are situated within the leaves of the broad ligament or pedunculated from it. Virtually all have bosselated, smooth outer surfaces. The cut surfaces (Figure 21.75) are gray-white to tan in color and rubbery to firm in consistency. Some are gritty, with focal areas of calcification that are sometimes sufficiently extensive to be seen on pelvic X-ray. Cystic areas are sometimes present.

Microscopic Features

Three main histologic patterns are described in these tumors:

- A sieve-like pattern (Figure 21.76), in which there are hollow tubules of varying size and shape, sometimes with cyst formation.
- Closely packed tubules, giving a dense, solid appearance (Figure 21.77). The tubules are winding, branching, and

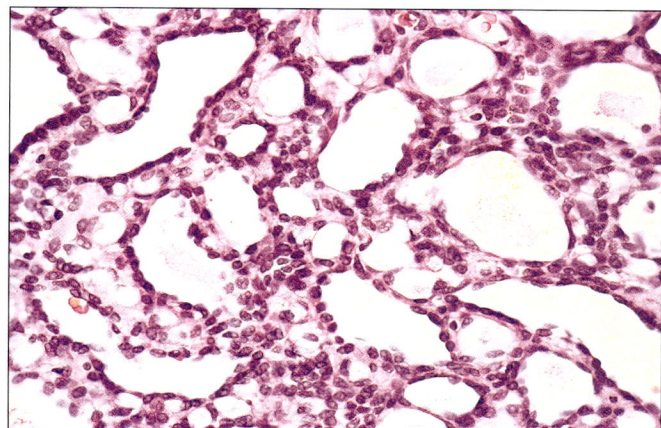

Figure 21.76 Adnexal tumor of probable wolffian origin. Solid areas between the cysts.

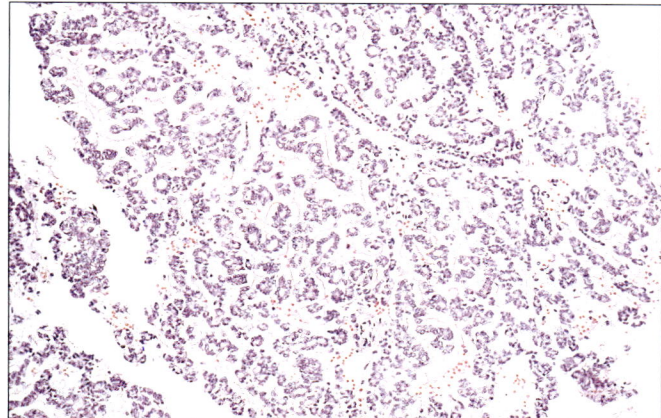

Figure 21.77 Adnexal tumor of probable wolffian origin. Closely packed tubules.

anastomosing, and are lined by cuboidal or columnar epithelial cells.
- Diffuse, solid sheets of cells.

The nuclei are round or oval and pale, with evenly dispersed chromatin. Most tumors have a low mitotic count. Some of those that behave in a malignant fashion contain pleomorphic nuclei and numerous mitotic figures, but not all clinically malignant tumors display these features.[19]

Origin

The tumors found in the broad ligament and mesosalpinx are considered by convention to be of wolffian origin because of their occurrence in the broad ligament, which is where wolffian remnants are located. Also, they do not resemble müllerian tumors by light microscopy, electron microscopy, or immunohistochemistry.[19] However, as the majority of female adnexal tumors of wolffian origin (FATWOs) share histologic features of sex cord–stromal tumors, particularly of Sertoli cell tumors or Sertoli–Leydig cell tumors, a possible extragonadal sex cord–stromal origin has been proposed.[53] It is difficult to study the tumor origin because of low incidence.

Differential Diagnosis

The differential diagnosis is sex cord–stromal tumors, particularly those containing Sertoli cells. No stromal cells of Leydig type have been demonstrated, nor has any patient shown hormonal manifestations. Inhibin reactivity is not helpful to differentiate FATWOs, Sertoli cell, or Sertoli–Leydig cell tumors as all of these tumors are consistently reactive.[53-55] In addition, although some areas of the tumors have a passing similarity to granulosa cell tumors, endometrioid adenocarcinomas, and clear cell carcinomas, these resemblances are only superficial and do not stand up to close scrutiny, although occasional confusion may occur.[56]

Prognosis

Five women have been reported with FATWOs that behaved in a malignant fashion.[33,34] All others have been benign, with follow-up ranging from a few months to 15 years.

REFERENCES

1. Chen EY, Mehra K, Mehrad M, et al. Secretory cell outgrowth, PAX2 and serous carcinogenesis in the fallopian tube. J Pathol 2010;222:110–6.
2. Lee Y, Miron A, Drapkin R, et al. A candidate precursor to serous carcinoma that originates in the distal tube. J Pathol 2007;211:26–35.
3. Kindelberger DW, Lee Y, Miron A, et al. Intraepithelial carcinoma of the fimbria and pelvic serous carcinoma: evidence for a causal relationship. Am J Surg Pathol 2007;31:161–9.
4. Carlson JW, Miron A, Jarboe EA, et al. Serous tubal intraepithelial carcinoma: its potential role in primary peritoneal serous carcinoma and serous cancer prevention. J Clin Oncol 2008;26:4160–5.
5. Jarboe E, Folkins A, Nucci MR, et al. Serous carcinogenesis in the fallopian tube: a descriptive classification. Int J Gynecol Pathol 2008;27:1–9.
6. Medeiros F, Muto MG, Lee Y, et al. The tubal fimbria is a preferred site for early adenocarcinoma in women with familial ovarian cancer syndrome. Am J Surg Pathol 2006;30:230–6.
7. Longacre TA, Oliva E, Soslow RA. Recommendations for the reporting of fallopian tube neoplasms. Virchows Arch 2007;450:25–9.
8. Semmel DR, Folkins AK, Hirsch MS, et al. Intercepting early pelvic serous carcinoma by routine pathological examination of the fimbria. Mod Pathol 2009;22:985–8.
9. Crossman SH. The challenge of pelvic inflammatory disease. Am Fam Physician 2006;73:859–64.
10. Abbuhl SB, Muskin EB, Shofer FS. Pelvic inflammatory disease in patients with bilateral tubal ligation. Am J Emerg Med 1997;15:271–4.
11. Honore LH. Pathology of the fallopian tube and broad ligament. In: Fox H, Wells M, editors. Haines and Taylor obstetrical and gynaecological pathology. 4th ed. New York: Churchill Livingstone; 1995. p. 623–71.
12. Parikh FR, Nadkarni SG, Kamat SA, et al. Genital tuberculosis—a major pelvic factor causing infertility in Indian women. Fertil Steril 1997;67:497–500.
13. Ortu S, Molicotti P, Sechi LA, et al. Rapid detection and identification of Mycobacterium tuberculosis by real time PCR and Bactec 960 MIGT. New Microbiol 2006;29:75–80.
14. Ramirez NC, Lawrence WD, Ginsburg KA. Ectopic pregnancy. A recent five-year study and review of the last 50 years' literature. J Reprod Med 1996;41:733–40.
15. Jacques SM, Qureshi F, Ramirez NC, et al. Retained trophoblastic tissue in Fallopian tubes: a consequence of unsuspected ectopic pregnancies. Int J Gynecol Pathol 1997;16:219–24.
16. Carson SA, Buster JE. Current concepts—ectopic pregnancy. N Engl J Med 1993;329:1174–81.
17. Kuragaki C, Enomoto T, Ueno Y, et al. Mutations in the STK11 gene characterize minimal deviation adenocarcinoma of the uterine cervix. Lab Invest 2003;83:35–45.

18. Mikami Y, Kiyokawa T, Sasajima Y, et al. Reappraisal of synchronous and multifocal mucinous lesions of the female genital tract: a close association with gastric metaplasia. Histopathology 2009;54:184–91.
19. Scully RE, Young RH, Clement RB. Tumors of the broad ligament and other uterine ligaments. Washington, DC: Armed Forces Institute of Pathology; 1998. p. 499–511.
20. Egan AJM, Russell P. Transitional (urothelial) cell metaplasia of the fallopian tube mucosa: morphological assessment of three cases. Int J Gynecol Pathol 1996;15:72–6.
21. Cheung AN, Young RH, Scully RE. Pseudocarcinomatous hyperplasia of the fallopian tube associated with salpingitis. A report of 14 cases. Am J Surg Pathol 1994;18:1125–30.
22. Bossuyt V, Medeiros F, Drapkin R, et al. Adenofibroma of the fimbria: a common entity that is indistinguishable from ovarian adenofibroma. Int J Gynecol Pathol 2008;27:390–7.
23. Schust D, Stovall DW. Leiomyomas of the fallopian tube. A case report. J Reprod Med 1993;38:741–2.
24. Kutteh WH, Albert T. Mature cystic teratoma of the fallopian tube associated with an ectopic pregnancy. Obstet Gynecol 1991;78:984–6.
25. Campello TR, Fittipaldi H, O'Valle F, et al. Extrauterine (tubal) placental site nodule. Histopathology 1998;32:562–5.
26. Nayar R, Snell J, Silverberg SG, et al. Placental site nodule occurring in a fallopian tube. Hum Pathol 1996;27:1243–5.
27. Su YN, Cheng WF, Chen CA, et al. Pregnancy with primary tubal placental site trophoblastic tumor: a case report and literature review. Gynecol Oncol 1999;73:322–5.
28. Alvarado-Cabrero I, Navani SS, Young RH, et al. Tumors of the fimbriated end of the fallopian tube: a clinicopathologic analysis of 20 cases, including nine carcinomas. Int J Gynecol Pathol 1997;16:189–96.
29. Krasevic M, Stankovic T, Petrovic O, et al. Serous borderline tumor of the fallopian tube presented as hematosalpinx: a case report. BMC Cancer 2005;5:129.
30. Zheng W, Wolf S, Kramer EE, et al. Borderline papillary serous tumor of the fallopian tube. Am J Surg Pathol 1996;20:30–5.
31. Stewart SL, Wike JM, Foster SL, et al. The incidence of primary fallopian tube cancer in the United States. Gynecol Oncol 2007;107:392–7.
32. Nordin AJ. Primary carcinoma of the fallopian tube: a 20-year literature review. Obstet Gynecol Surv 1994;49:349–61.
33. Brescia RJ, Cardoso de Almeida PC, Fuller Jr AF, et al. Female adnexal tumor of probable Wolffian origin with multiple recurrences over 16 years. Cancer 1985;56:1456–61.
34. Daya D. Malignant female adnexal tumor of probable Wolffian origin with review of the literature. Arch Pathol Lab Med 1994;118:310–12.
35. Hellstrom AC, Silfversward C, Nilsson B, et al. Carcinoma of the fallopian tube. A clinical and histopathological review: the Radiumhemmet series. Int J Gynecol Cancer 1994;4:395–400.
36. Vicus D, Finch A, Rosen B, et al. Risk factors for carcinoma of the fallopian tube in women with and without a germline BRCA mutation. Gynecol Oncol 2010;118:155–9.
37. Alvarado-Cabrero I, Young RH, Vamvakas EC, et al. Carcinoma of the fallopian tube: a clinicopathological study of 105 cases with observations on staging and prognostic factors. Gynecol Oncol 1999;72:367–79.
38. Jarboe EA, Miron A, Carlson JW, et al. Coexisting intraepithelial serous carcinomas of the endometrium and fallopian tube: frequency and potential significance. Int J Gynecol Pathol 2009;28:308–15.
39. Fujiwaki R, Takahashi K, Ryuko K, et al. Primary endometrioid carcinoma of the fallopian tube. Acta Obstet Gynecol Scand 1996;75:508–10.
40. Navani SS, Alvarado-Cabrero I, Young RH, et al. Endometrioid carcinoma of the fallopian tube: a clinicopathologic analysis of 26 cases. Gynecol Oncol 1996;63:371–8.
41. Uehira K, Hashimoto H, Tsuneyoshi M, et al. Transitional cell carcinoma pattern in primary carcinoma of the fallopian tube. Cancer 1993;72:2447–56.
42. Cheung ANY, So KF, Ngan HYS, et al. Primary squamous cell carcinoma of fallopian tube. Int J Gynecol Pathol 1994;13:92–5.
43. Cormio G, Lissoni A, Maneo A, et al. Lymph node involvement in primary carcinoma of the fallopian tube. Int J Gynecol Cancer 1996;6:405–9.
44. di Re E, Grosso G, Raspagliesi F, et al. Fallopian tube cancer. Incidence and role of lymphatic spread. Gynecol Oncol 1996;62:199–202.
45. Rauthe G, Vahrson HW, Burkhardt E. Primary cancer of the fallopian tube. Treatment and results of 37 cases. Eur J Gynaecol Oncol 1998;19:356–62.
46. Rosen AC, Ausch C, Hafner E, et al. A 15-year overview of management and prognosis in primary fallopian tube carcinoma. Austrian Cooperative Study Group for Fallopian Tube Carcinoma. Eur J Cancer 1998;34:1725–9.
47. Hellstrom AC, Auer G, Silfversward C, et al. Prognostic factors in malignant mixed müllerian tumor of the fallopian tube. Int J Gynecol Cancer 1996;6:467–72.
48. Ebert AD, Perez-Canto A, Schaller G, et al. Stage I primary malignant mixed müllerian tumor of the fallopian tube: report of a case with five-year survival after minimal surgery without adjuvant treatment. J Reprod Med 1998;43:598–600.
49. Ebert A, Goetze B, Herbst H, et al. Primary leiomyosarcoma of the fallopian tube. Ann Oncol 1995;6:618–9.
50. Buchwalter CL, Jenison EL, Fromm M, et al. Pure embryonal rhabdomyosarcoma of the fallopian tube. Gynecol Oncol 1997;67:95–101.
51. Li S, Zimmerman RL, LiVolsi VA. Mixed malignant germ cell tumor of the fallopian tube. Int J Gynecol Pathol 1999;18:183–5.
52. Muto MG, Lage JM, Berkowitz RS, et al. Gestational trophoblastic disease of the fallopian tube. J Reprod Med 1991;36:57–60.
53. Zheng W, Senturk BZ, Parkash V. Inhibin immunohistochemical staining: a practical approach for the surgical pathologist in the diagnoses of ovarian sex cord-stromal tumors. Adv Anat Pathol 2003;10:27–38.
54. Kommoss F, Oliva E, Bhan AK, et al. Inhibin expression in ovarian tumors and tumor-like lesions: an immunohistochemical study. Mod Pathol 1998;11:656–64.
55. McCluggage WG. Value of inhibin staining in gynecological pathology. Int J Gynecol Pathol 2001;20:79–85.
56. Fukunaga M, Bisceglia M, Dimitri L. Endometrioid carcinoma of the fallopian tube resembling a female adnexal tumor of probable wolffian origin. Adv Anat Pathol 2004;11:269–72.

Endometriosis 22

George L. Mutter

CHAPTER OUTLINE

Introduction	487	Considerations at Specific Anatomic Locations	498
Clinical Features of Endometriosis	487	Ovary	498
Distribution of Endometriosis	488	Peritoneal Surfaces	499
Epidemiology of Endometriosis	488	Fallopian Tube	499
Pathogenesis of Endometriosis	489	Cervix	499
Transplantation	489	Gastrointestinal Tract	500
Metaplastic Theory	490	Urinary Tract	500
Intrinsic Abnormalities of Endometriotic Tissue	490	Abdominal Wall	500
Local Feedback between Estrogen Production and Inflammation	490	Lymph Nodes	500
		Clinical Classification of Endometriosis	501
Altered Stromal–Epithelial Interaction	490	Infertility in Endometriosis	501
Etiologic Factors in Endometriosis	490	Endometriosis Presenting as a Benign Solid Tumor	501
Genetic Factors	490	Florid Endometriosis	501
Congenital Anatomic Abnormalities	491	Polypoid Endometriosis	502
Systemic Hormonal Factors	491	Malignancy in Endometriosis	502
Peritoneal Environment	491	Frequency and Types of Malignancies	503
Angiogenesis	491	Atypical Endometriosis and the Pathogenesis of Malignancy	504
Morphologic Features of Endometriosis	491		

INTRODUCTION

Endometriosis is the condition in which endometrial tissue, composed of both endometrial-type glandular epithelium and stroma, is found at sites outside the uterine cavity. In the past, adenomyosis and endometriosis were linked by a common terminology; the former was referred to as 'endometriosis interna' and the latter as 'endometriosis externa.' The two conditions are distinct,[1] however, with different symptoms and different epidemiologic and etiologic patterns: adenomyosis results from invagination of the basal endometrium lining the endometrial cavity into the uterine wall (see Chapter 20); endometriosis in most cases develops from endometrium that has implanted in the peritoneal cavity after retrograde transmission from the uterus through the fallopian tube.

CLINICAL FEATURES OF ENDOMETRIOSIS

Endometriosis is almost exclusively a disease of women in their reproductive years. It is currently the third leading cause of gynecologic hospitalization in the United States.[2] Its true incidence is unknown, although most reports estimate that it occurs in about 4–13% of all women of reproductive age,[3,4] 25–50% of infertile women,[5–7] 5–25% of those admitted for pelvic pain, 50% of teenagers with intractable dysmenorrhea,[3] and up to 7% of those admitted with pelvic masses. To determine the true incidence would require use of the most sensitive diagnostic test, laparoscopy, on a population of unselected premenopausal asymptomatic women. Clearly, such a prospective trial will never be performed.

The diagnosis is frequently made by laparoscopy in the late twenties or early thirties, and not infrequently in adolescence.[8] In the past, when diagnosis was based primarily on symptoms, patients tended to be older at the time of diagnosis. The condition has not been reported before puberty, which is not surprising, as the sex steroid hormones needed for endometrial growth are not sufficiently abundant. Endometriosis may also occur after menopause, mostly in postmenopausal women taking exogenous hormones.[9] In the minority who have not, other hormonal sources that are continuous and can sustain the process of endometriosis should be sought. One example is peripheral conversion of androgens in obese women.

Racial differences in the incidence of endometriosis, although once thought to be important, have not been confirmed in studies more adequately controlled for childbearing patterns and socioeconomic and other relevant factors.[10] Women with endometriosis are generally of lower parity than non-sufferers. The relationship between endometriosis and infertility is almost certainly a vicious cycle. The hormonal milieu in a woman who does not achieve pregnancy encourages the development of endometriosis. Once endometriosis develops, its presence contributes to the infertile state and the circle is established. Conversely, pregnancy often has a beneficial effect on the disease.

Most women with endometriosis present with secondary dysmenorrhea, dyspareunia, pelvic pain, or infertility. However, only about 5% have all four major symptoms. A small number of women with endometriosis develop a pelvic mass or, occasionally, ascites.[11] Many women with endometriosis are also asymptomatic. In one study two-fifths of the women in whom endometriosis was discovered during laparoscopic tubal ligation had no symptoms.[12]

The amount and character of the pain that the patient experiences correlate poorly with the actual extent of disease found.[13] Local microenvironment and physical effects seem to be more important factors than the anatomic location and extent of the endometriosis.[14] Production of cytokines and prostaglandins by the stromal cells of endometriosis has been suggested as a mechanism for stimulation of adjacent glands, and pain.[15] This is supported by studies showing that aromatase inhibitors such as letrozole, which diminish paracrine stromal production of estradiol and prostaglandins, can be effective in reducing the symptom of pain.[16]

DISTRIBUTION OF ENDOMETRIOSIS

The sites where endometriosis is most commonly found depend greatly on whether the diagnosis rests on clinical or histologic findings. In descending order of frequency, the two most frequent sites based on clinical findings alone are the uterosacral ligaments and ovaries (Table 22.1).[17] In most series, these two sites are each affected in over 60% of instances (due to multisite involvement). Most other sites are in the pelvis and include the pouch of Douglas, pelvic peritoneum, uterine surface, and fallopian tubes. The frequency of involvement ranges from 5% to 20%.

When tissue samples are selected from clinically suspicious areas, pathologic diagnosis is necessarily biased by clinical appearance. Additionally, endometriosis is a common incidental finding in bilateral salpingo-oophorectomy specimens (with or without hysterectomy) removed for unrelated reasons. Thus, in contrast to clinical series, the ovary is the principal tissue where the pathologist sees endometriosis (36% of specimens) (Table 22.2).[18] The fallopian tube, uterine serosa, and cul-de-sac each account for 6–14% of biopsy-proven specimens. The uterosacral ligaments are rarely biopsied, which explains why this site accounts for <2% of biopsy-proven endometriosis.

EPIDEMIOLOGY OF ENDOMETRIOSIS

Several risk factors have been identified that are associated with the development of endometriosis. Some evidence suggests that there may be a genetic basis to endometriosis as it occurs far more commonly in monozygotic than dizygotic twins.[19] The common features that appear to increase the risk of endometriosis relate to an increased exposure to

Table 22.1 Clinical Location of Endometrial Implants[17]

Location	Frequency (%)*
Uterosacral ligaments	63
Ovaries	
Superficial	56
Deep (endometrioma)	20
Ovarian fossae	33
Anterior vesicle pouch	22
Pouch of Douglas	19
Intestines	5
Fallopian tubes	5
Uterus	5

*Most individuals have multiple sites of involvement.

Table 22.2 Location of Endometriosis Based upon Biopsy Findings[18]

Location	Frequency (%)*
Ovary	36
Fallopian tube	14
Uterine serosa	12
Cul-de-sac	6
Cervix	3
Colon	3
Peritoneum	3
Appendix	2
Broad ligament	2
Pelvis	2
Uterosacral ligament	2
Vagina	2
Abdominal wall	1
Bladder	1
Fibrous tissue	1
Parametrium	1
Rectum	1
Small intestine	1
Other sites	7

*Based on 1323 biopsies and operative specimens.

menstruation, i.e., longer duration of flow or higher volumes of retrograde menstruation in states where estrogenic stimulation is maintained.[20,21] It is also frequent in women with cervical stenosis. The disease is more common where there is reduced parity, which reflects delayed childbearing, and is infrequent among multiparous women.[21] The risk is reduced for women using concurrent oral contraceptive medication, but not for such non-hormonal methods as intrauterine devices or diaphragms.[22] The risk increases after the use of the oral contraception medication is discontinued.

The occurrence of endometriosis relates also to increasing age, peaking at ages 40–44 years.[22] This may reflect increased numbers of menstrual cycles that have occurred before menopause has begun and the major source of estrogenic stimulation has ceased. Compared to women aged 25–29 years, the relative risk of endometriosis is 2.1 for women aged 30–34 years, 4.5 during the ages 35–39 years, and finally 6.1 for ages 40–44 years.

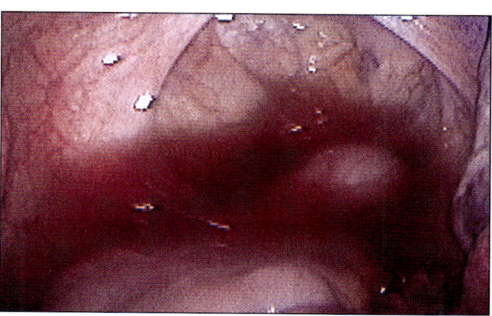

Figure 22.1 Blood in the pelvis from retrograde flow during menses.

PATHOGENESIS OF ENDOMETRIOSIS

Many theories have been proffered to explain the histogenesis of endometriosis. These are not necessarily mutually exclusive. The most widely discussed hypotheses include transplantation of endometrial fragments to ectopic sites, and metaplasia of the multipotential celomic peritoneum. The vast clinical experience and experimental studies in non-human primates favor an etiology that includes transplantation of exfoliated endometrial cells. Clonality studies of endometriotic cysts have shown that the epithelial component is monoclonal.[23,24] These results suggest that endometriotic cysts are outgrowths from a single cell of origin, consistent either with transformation of a single progenitor cell, or rare cells within transplanted tissue fragments capable of developing into endometriosis.

TRANSPLANTATION

The most easily understood, scientifically supported, and widely accepted mechanism is that, at menstruation, some of the menstrual products flow in a retrograde fashion through the lumen of the fallopian tubes into the pelvic peritoneal cavity.[25] The material drops to the pelvic floor and implants, in time regenerating into recognizable endometrium. This pathophysiology explains the most common sites of endometriosis. Abundant evidence indicates that menstrual retrograde flow does happen and, indeed, is a common phenomenon. Over 90% of women have blood in their pelvis at the time of menstruation, as identified by fluid examined at laparoscopy (Figure 22.1). Retrograde flow is, in itself, insufficient to cause endometriosis as only a small proportion will develop disease. Host inflammatory or immunologic factors may modify the outcome. Alternatively, sporadically acquired epigenetic or genetic changes within displaced endometrial tissues may alter the likelihood of successful implantation or persistence. Altered methylation of the *SF1* gene is one such possibility.[26]

The frequency with which endometriotic implants are found in the pelvic cavity both usually and under special conditions supports an origin from transplanted menstrual products. Studies have shown that the most frequent sites are where the menstrual products flow from the fimbrial ends of the tubes.[27] The uterine position is also of importance.[28] It is found significantly more commonly anteriorly in patients with severely anteflexed uteri. In contrast, when the uterus is retroflexed, anterior disease is uncommon. The more frequent finding of endometriosis in the left rather than the right ovary suggests that the endometrial retrograde flow is entrapped on entry by a shield formed in part by the sigmoid colon.

Further proof that menstrual material is viable has been obtained by collecting samples of menstrual products and injecting them subcutaneously into the anterior abdominal wall of animals. Excisional biopsy of the injection sites after several weeks showed lesions that resembled endometriosis in some subjects.[7]

Animal studies also support that menstrual products have the potential to implant and grow on a peritoneal surface. In baboons, a species with a high rate of spontaneous endometriosis, blood-stained peritoneal fluid was 10-fold more frequent (62% vs 6%) during menses than during non-menstrual phases.[29] Retrograde menstruation was also observed more frequently in animals that had spontaneously developed endometriosis than in animals that were free of disease and had a normal pelvis. Finally, the experimental intrapelvic injection of menstrual endometrium led to the development of endometriosis much more frequently than if normal secretory endometrium was injected.[30]

Several other routes of transplantation, i.e., vascular spread, lymphatic spread, and direct implantation, have been observed. All help explain the occurrence of disease at distant or unusual sites. Endometriosis in a location such as within the parenchyma of the lung is usually accepted as vascular spread. Fragments of endometrium may be seen in lymphatics in about 5% of women with endometriosis,[31,32] and occasionally in lymph nodes,[33] a phenomenon easiest explained by lymphatic spread. Finally, endometriosis in operative scars and in the cervix after cone biopsy or loop excision is easy to understand, as the endometrial tissue reaches the site by spillage at the time of operation and direct implantation.

The occurrence of endometriosis in young girls has been used as an argument that endometriosis arises by metaplasia, although, when occurring in young women, it is usually perimenarchal and accompanied by outflow obstruction caused by structural anomalies.[31]

METAPLASTIC THEORY

The metaplastic theory, for which there are scant data, proposes that endometriosis arises in the pelvis and elsewhere by endometrial metaplasia of the peritoneal serosa or serosa-like structures. The concept of the so-called 'secondary müllerian system'[34] attributes to the pelvic peritoneum the ability to differentiate, if appropriately stimulated, into any of the recognized types of müllerian epithelium.

One argument that proponents for both sides of the controversy have made concerns case reports of development of endometriosis in women who congenitally lack a uterus or do not menstruate.[35] One case, initially published as an example of endometriosis with an absent uterus, was later reported after new operative findings disclosed a functioning endometrium in a right rudimentary horn and retrograde menstruation through a fallopian tube with hematosalpinx.[36] In another instance, a 24-year-old woman with mosaic Turner syndrome was found to have endometrioma arising from the uterine serosa. However, as she had been receiving cyclic hormone-replacement therapy (HRT) for 5 years after laparoscopic gonadectomy and was having cyclic menstrual flow, it is likely that the endometriosis arose from retrograde menstruation.[37]

INTRINSIC ABNORMALITIES OF ENDOMETRIOTIC TISSUE

There are qualitative and quantitative differences between eutopic and ectopic endometrial tissues, which explain some aspects of lesion persistence and pain. The reader is referred to any of several excellent recent reviews for further details,[15,38] summarized in Figure 22.2 and the following sections.

LOCAL FEEDBACK BETWEEN ESTROGEN PRODUCTION AND INFLAMMATION

Aberrant expression of COX2 in endometriosis, which is normally present at only low levels in eutopic endometrium, leads to overproduction of the inflammatory mediator prostaglandin, PGE_2. In addition to the cascade of secondary inflammatory effects normally mediated by PGE_2, endometriotic tissues are defective in having a 'short circuit' between the normally independent inflammatory (Figure 22.2, red elements) and endocrine synthetic (Figure 22.2, blue elements) pathways. The inflammatory response provides positive feedback to the steroidogenic pathway of endometriotic tissues by abnormal activity of two genes: *SF1*, and aromatase. *SF1* is a nuclear receptor that positively regulates synthesis of androstenedione through a series of intermediaries. Epigenetic modification of the *SF1* promoter, by hypomethylation, is one possible mechanism of its overexpression in endometriotic tissues.[26] Androstenedione is not normally converted to estrogen in the endometrium, but, as endometriosis has high levels of aromatase, it is converted efficiently to estrone. Estrone has only low-level bioactivity in promoting proliferation of endometrial tissue, but can in turn be converted to the much more potent estradiol. Equilibrium between estrone and estradiol levels is disrupted in favor of the latter by specific inactivation of HSD17B2 in endometriosis. The resultant estradiol, produced locally as above, is locally proliferative and closes the connection between hormonal and inflammatory pathways through its positive feedback on COX2 activity.

ALTERED STROMAL–EPITHELIAL INTERACTION

The response of ectopic endometrial tissues to circulating steroid sex hormones is perturbed in a manner that confounds normal paracrine inhibition of glandular proliferation by stromal cells.[38] Normal endometrial stroma typically expresses progesterone receptors, enabling stromal cells to respond to circulating progesterone by paracrine secretion of retinoic acid. Upon exposure to locally secreted retinoic acid, the glandular cells convert estradiol to less active estrone, thereby mitigating the glandular mitogenic effects of estradiol. This paracrine mechanism of suppressing gland proliferation is compromised in endometriosis tissues, as the stromal (but not glandular) cells have reduced progesterone receptors.

ETIOLOGIC FACTORS IN ENDOMETRIOSIS

GENETIC FACTORS

Heritable factors are important in the development of endometriosis.[39–41] In an early study of women with histologically proven endometriosis, a surprisingly large proportion of their female relatives were similarly affected (6% of sisters, 8% of mothers, and 7% of first-degree female cousins). In contrast, only 1.0% of their husbands' sisters and 0.9% of their husbands' mothers were affected. Furthermore, those women with endometriosis whose first-degree relatives were affected were more likely to have a severe form of the disease than those women whose first-degree relatives were not affected. In another study comparing 515 cases with 149 control cases (women without endometriosis determined by laparoscopy performed during sterilization), endometriosis was found in 3.9% of mothers of cases but in only 0.7% of mothers of controls. It was also found in 4.8% of sisters of cases, but only 0.6% of sisters of controls. The relative risk of endometriosis in a first-degree relative was

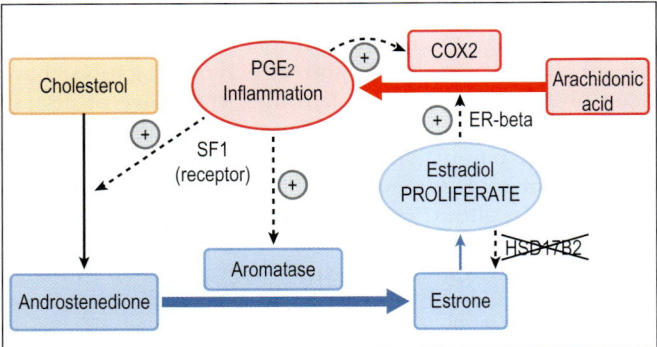

Figure 22.2 Unbroken cycle of inflammation and proliferation in endometriosis. The presence of aromatase (absent in eutopic endometrium) and abnormally high levels of COX2 in endometriotic tissues creates unchecked positive feedback loops for inflammation (red) and proliferation (blue). The cycle is augmented by additional changes not seen in native endometrium, including presence of *SF1* and deficiency of HSD17B2.[15]

7.2. The manifestations of endometriosis were far more severe in women with a positive family history than in those without (26% vs 12%).[42] Recent pilot surveys also suggest that there are high concordance rates for the presence of endometriosis in monozygotic but not dizygotic twins.[43,44] Large international collaborative projects are currently being undertaken to identify the multifactorial mode of inheritance.[45]

Endometriosis risk has been reported to be increased in women who carry specific pleomorphisms of vascular endothelial growth factor (*VEGF*), a gene that promotes angiogenesis.[46] A possible mechanism is enhanced *VEGF* biologic activity of the *VEGF* +936TC gene polymorphism, thereby facilitating implantation and growth of displaced endometrial tissues. The magnitude of increased risk is small, of the order of 1.18-fold.

CONGENITAL ANATOMIC ABNORMALITIES

Endometriosis in young girls does not occur much before the age of 11 years,[47] and when occurring in young women shortly after the onset of their menarche, is found associated with müllerian anomalies causing outflow tract obstruction.[31] On average, the elapsed time between the onset of menarche and the development of symptoms that require surgical intervention is 3 years if the woman has müllerian anomalies with outflow tract obstruction; it is nearly 7 years if outflow tract obstruction is present but the pelvic anatomy is normal.

SYSTEMIC HORMONAL FACTORS

Multiple lines of evidence support the importance of ovarian sex hormones in the genesis of endometriosis. Endometriosis is more common in women and primates where there are prolonged periods of unopposed estrogen exposure or in obese women who have higher levels of endogenous estrogen.[7] Conversely, it is much rarer in women who have decreased estrogen production during reproductive life. It often disappears after menopause or, when found on histologic examination, appears in an atrophic state. It may also regress with medical suppression, but reappears once ovarian activity resumes.[48] The relative contributions of circulating estrogen and progesterone are difficult to study independently, as they dynamically coexist in most women.

There are several emerging lines of evidence supporting a role for systemic and local progesterone effects in the development of endometriosis. Selective progesterone receptor modulators, which block the progesterone response through competitive interaction with the progesterone receptor, may be effective in treating endometriosis.[49] Larger prospective clinical trials of efficacy and demonstration of endometrial safety are needed before suitability for routine clinical use can be determined. As mentioned earlier, eutopic and ectopic endometrial tissues differ in their ability to respond to circulating progesterone, as the stroma of the former but not the latter contains progesterone receptors.

PERITONEAL ENVIRONMENT

The hormonal composition of the peritoneal environment is enriched by proximity of the ovaries, and local release of follicular fluid. Steroid hormone concentrations are exceedingly high in ovarian follicles, measuring 1000-fold higher than in plasma.[50] During the follicular phase, the concentration of estradiol in the peritoneal fluid increases progressively, rising after ovulation to a maximum of 40,000 pg/mL, which is a level 100 times that in the plasma. Progesterone levels both mirror and are higher than plasma levels. During the follicular phase, the levels in the peritoneal fluid are low (5–10 ng/mL), but jump abruptly after ovulation to 2000 ng/mL, decreasing slowly thereafter.

Endometriosis may be linked to abnormal immune function, a possible explanation for why only some women develop the disease even though retrograde menstruation is so common.[51] In addition to the hormonal milieu established by the ovary, peritoneal fluid contains multiple types of free-floating cells, including macrophages, mesothelial cells, leukocytes, lymphocytes, eosinophils, and mast cells. Macrophages are estimated to account for over 80% of the cells in normal women.[52] In women with endometriosis, there is a pronounced increase in the number of total leukocytes, including macrophages, helper T-lymphocytes, and natural killer cells, supporting the suggestion that active immunologic processes are occurring. Whether the changes observed are cause or effect remains unknown.

The differences that exist between superficial implants and those deeper (indicated in current classifications) may reflect the different local microenvironments to which each area of endometriosis is exposed. Peritoneal fluid factors would be expected to have a greater effect on superficial implants, whereas blood and ovarian hormonal factors regulate deep-seated endometriosis and cystic ovarian endometriosis.[50] Endometriotic tissue that has penetrated at least 5 mm beneath the peritoneal surface, and is therefore deep, correlates with more aggressive behavior as reflected by pelvic pain and infertility.[53]

ANGIOGENESIS

Under the transplantation theory, the retrograde endometrial flow must attach to and implant within the peritoneal cavity, and then establish and maintain an adequate blood supply. Growth of a new vascular bed is therefore critical if the endometriosis is to develop. A wide array of factors contribute to angiogenesis, and it has been suggested that basal activity of several polymorphic variants may alter the risk for endometriosis.[46,54]

Some evidence suggests that a key to angiogenic activity may lie in the contents of the peritoneal cavity rather than in the endometriotic explant itself.[55] Potent angiogenic growth factors are increased in the peritoneal fluid in patients with this disease. The activated peritoneal fluid macrophages and infiltrating macrophages are a rich source of this angiogenic growth factor.

MORPHOLOGIC FEATURES OF ENDOMETRIOSIS

In the most elemental terms, endometriosis can be diagnosed by finding both endometrial glands and stroma in the operative specimen. The appearances, however, can be protean and affected by topography, age of the lesion, and age of the patient. The laparoscopic appearances of the lesions are depicted in Figures 22.3–22.7.

Gross Features

The ages of the endometriotic deposits affect their gross appearances. The various colors reflect the deposit's functional states. Yellow-red surface stains, which reflect breakdown of blood products on the involved surfaces, often herald the presence of the earliest detectable lesions (Figure 22.3). Occasionally, early lesions will show vesicle formations (Figure 22.4), a state before the endometriotic foci begin to cycle and undergo tissue and blood breakdown. The red lesions also reflect an early form of the disease when the endometriosis is actively growing (Figure 22.5).[56] These red lesions evolve into the black (advanced) lesions in which some degree of bleeding has resolved (Figure 22.6). This is the most common form seen by the pathologist in operative specimens. Some lesions may be brown to slightly yellow-brown, which indicates the presence of hemosiderin. These lesions are also called 'café-au-lait spots.' The oldest (white) lesions, have fibrosis and scarring and often the color reflects the advanced degree of healing (Figure 22.7). Strangely, it is the white lesion where endometriosis is most easily confirmed histologically.[57] As lesions begin at different times, the various foci may differ from site to site. Seldom are endometriotic lesions solitary.

The changes seen laparoscopically are also seen macroscopically in the surgical specimen. In general, the first grossly recognizable lesions are blister-like blebs, some 2–3 mm in diameter, on the surface of the target organs. They are red and represent highly vascularized implants.[58] The tiny red lesions are the exclusive form of endometriosis found in 20% of adolescents with this disease. They have yet to show signs of repeated bleeding and scarring (fibrosis). Some investigators[59] believe that many of the red lesions should not be considered as endometriosis, assuming that virtually all women have retrograde menstruation and therefore some red lesions.

As the lesions advance in age, they enlarge, reaching a size of 3 mm to sometimes over 1 cm, sometimes singly or as a collection. As they go through repeated cycles, they become pigmented and blacker, largely from intraluminal debris, old blood, hemorrhagic stroma, hemosiderin-laden macrophages, and even some scarring. These lesions may be raised, bluish-red to bluish-black, and may resemble

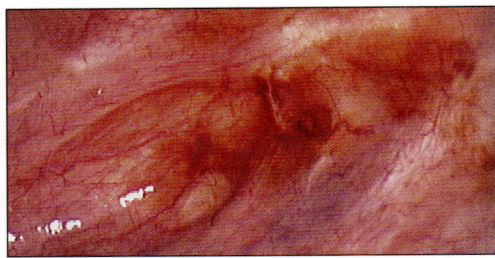

Figure 22.3 Yellow-red stain of endometriosis. This is the earliest manifestation of endometriosis seen laparoscopically.

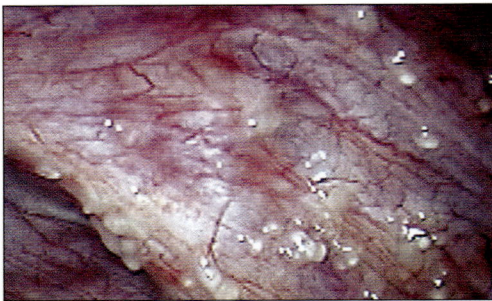

Figure 22.4 Vesicle formation in endometriosis on the broad ligament.

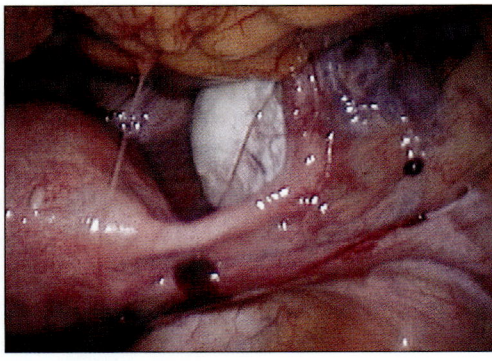

Figure 22.5 Red lesions on the broad ligament and ovary.

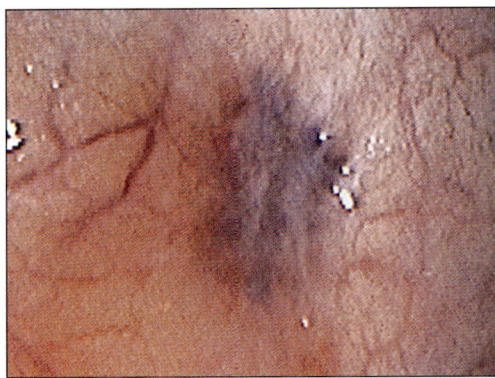

Figure 22.6 Black lesion in encometriosis with early scarring.

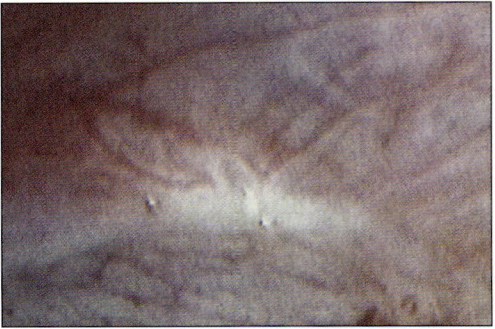

Figure 22.7 White lesion due to extensive fibrosis.

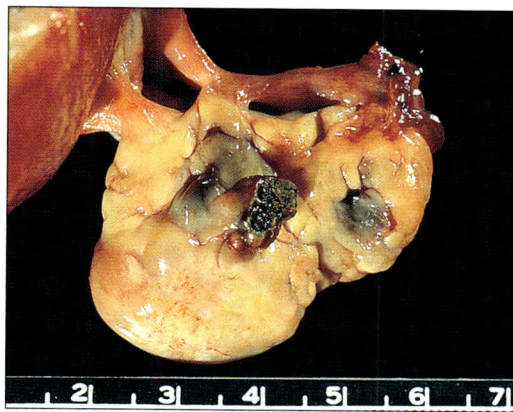

Figure 22.8 Black ('mulberry') lesion of endometriosis.

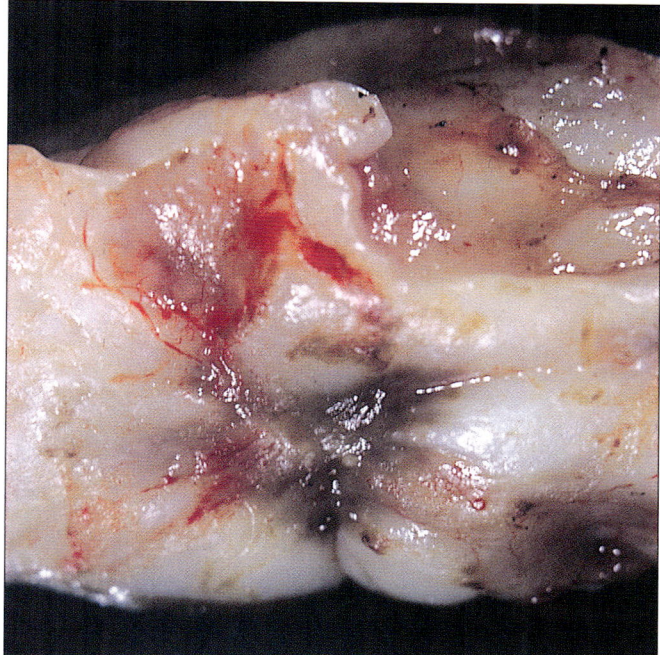

Figure 22.9 Scarred ('powder burn') lesion of endometriosis. The consequent extensive fibrosis has resulted in a puckered surface.

mulberries or blueberries (Figure 22.8). If they are more extensively fibrotic and scarred, they may also appear puckered ('powder burn') (Figure 22.9). Lesions that heal have undergone extensive fibrosis and scarring and are white. They have minimal stroma and are poorly vascularized. Black-and-white scarred lesions predominate in later years.

The disease site affects whether the endometriosis is serosal (including subserosal/subperitoneal) or whether it can be found deep within an organ (e.g., ovary). Implants of endometriosis grow poorly on the surface of the peritoneal mesothelium.[60] Rather, mesothelium quickly grows over the implant, encapsulating it as if it were a foreign body; such nodules appear to be located subperitoneally. In the ovary, these nodules enlarge during cyclical 'menstruation,' first appearing as small indentations into the cortex, and with time invaginating substantially into the ovarian substance. On cross section, these foci of developing endometriomas show the wall and base to actually consist of the ovarian cortex/serosa, the so-called 'inverted cortex' (Figure 22.10). Sometimes, the pearl-white appearance of the ovarian cortex is still recognizable. The tissue covering the endometrioma, i.e., the peritoneal cover, is an operculum consisting of fibrous tissue and mesothelium.

At some sites, the lesions may become grossly cystic, but the cysts generally do not become large, except in the ovary. In general, the cyst wall is rarely thicker than 2 mm, and the endometriotic tissue rarely more than 1.5 mm thick.[61] The term 'chocolate cyst' is often used to describe these cystic lesions (Figures 22.11 and 22.12). The term, though, can be misleading. It is purely descriptive, referring to the chocolate-colored contents. In fact, any hemorrhagic dysfunctional cyst can have the same appearance, be it from an old hemorrhagic corpus luteum, unruptured follicular cyst, or an endometrioid adenocarcinoma with extensive hemorrhage and necrosis.

In some cases, an organ involved with endometriosis may be greatly distorted by extensive fibrosis and scarring. Adhesions to surrounding structures are usually present and form an important basis of staging the severity of disease present.

Another feature that affects the appearance of the endometriosis is the age of the woman. A woman who is in her reproductive years will have the typical lesions, the microscopic appearances of which are as described below.

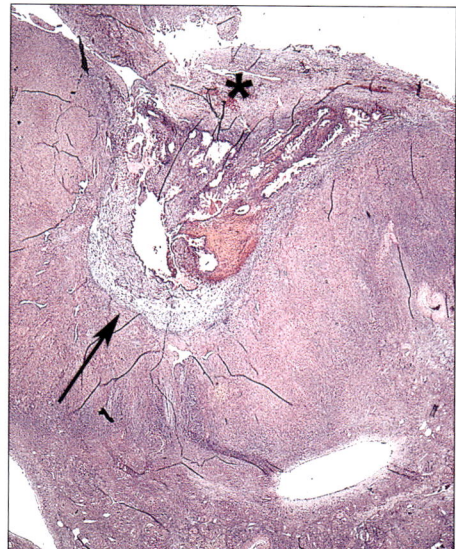

Figure 22.10 Inverted cortex of ovarian endometrioma. The inverted ovarian cortex lies at the base (arrow) of the endometrioma. A fibrous operculum (*) covers the upper surface of the endometrioma.

Women who are postmenopausal or who lack a source of estrogen stimulation will often have lesions marked by atrophy or near disappearance of either the epithelial or stromal component.

Microscopic Features

Endometriosis consists of endometrial glands surrounded by endometrial stroma, and both components must be

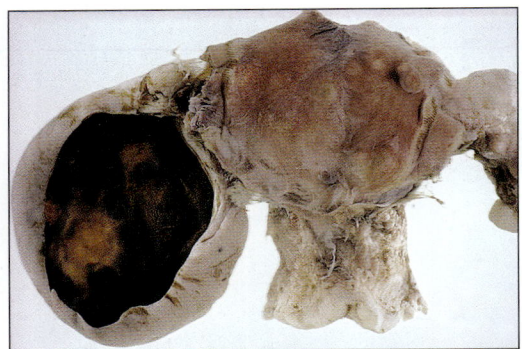

Figure 22.11 'Chocolate cyst' of the ovary. The endometrioma is large, and has displaced the ovary, which remains as a thickened aspect of the wall.

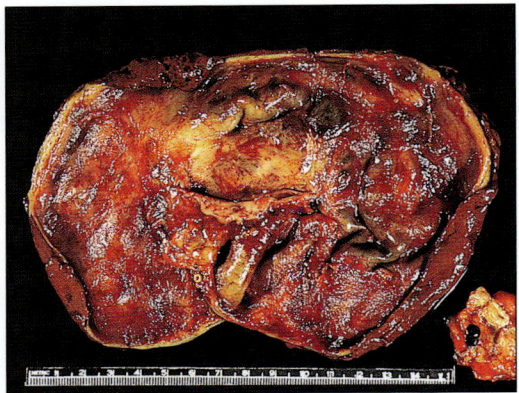

Figure 22.12 Large endometrioma, or 'chocolate cyst,' of ovary. The endometrioma has completely replaced the ovary.

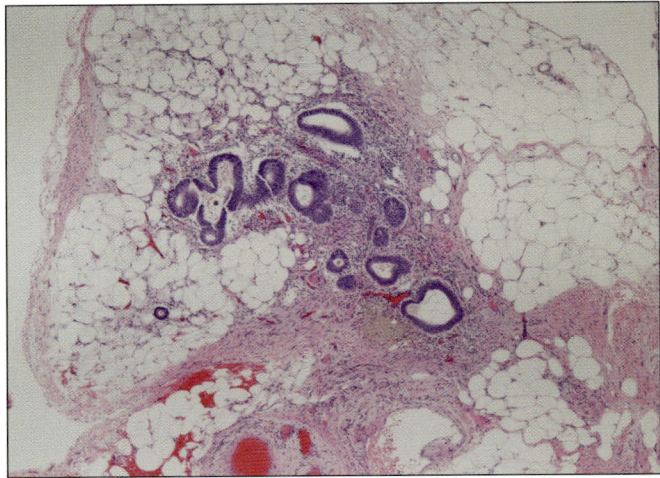

Figure 22.13 Endometriosis in the omentum. Disorganized glands resemble proliferative endometrial glands.

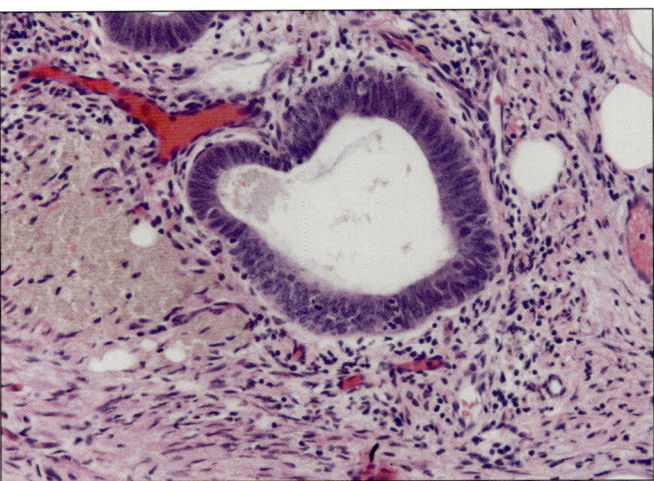

Figure 22.14 Endometriotic glands in the omentum surrounded by a cuff of cellular endometrial stroma and scattered hemosiderin.

definitively identified if errors in diagnosis are to be avoided. Hemorrhage and hemosiderin are often but not always present, and nonspecific as they are found in a wide variety of other conditions. On low-power magnification, the epithelium appears as a thin, dark layer that is sharply delineated from the underlying, paler stroma (Figure 22.13). The luminal surface of the epithelium may be slightly jagged and irregular. On high-power examination, the epithelium is one cell layer thick and has the appearance of an endometrial epithelium (Figure 22.14). The cells are usually tall and columnar with elongate cigar-shaped nuclei showing regular vertical orientation. The cytoplasm is eosinophilic and cilia are often identified. The glands usually appear to be relatively inactive, with only sparse mitoses, but florid proliferative and secretory activity may at times be observed.

Epithelial 'metaplasias' have been described in endometriosis, but in our experience are largely so common and interspersed that we consider them more of an intrinsic component than an abnormality.[62] Serous (tubal) metaplasia as alternating groups of ciliated and secretory cells is the most frequent (found in nearly half of cases) and may be either focal or widespread. Endometriotic lesions showing a prominent tubal metaplasia have been called 'endosalpingiosis,' a term we avoid as it is confusing. Clear cell metaplasia has been described in over a tenth of cases, but this can be difficult to distinguish from secretory changes, and particularly from the Arias-Stella reaction. Mucinous metaplasia is relatively rare and is usually focal. Squamous metaplasia has been reported to occur in long-standing endometriotic cysts.

The stroma generally resembles the normal stroma found in the endometrium, and consists of small spindle-shaped cells with inconspicuous cytoplasm. A delicate reticulin network that is much finer than that of native ovarian stroma supports the cells, as silver impregnation staining reveals. The presence of reticulin is also useful in some organs to distinguish between endometriosis and stroma that normally lacks reticulin investiture, e.g., cervix.[63] Various degrees of decidualized stromal cells may be seen if the endometriotic focus is cyclically functional. The cells may show a pseudodecidual response during the latter part of

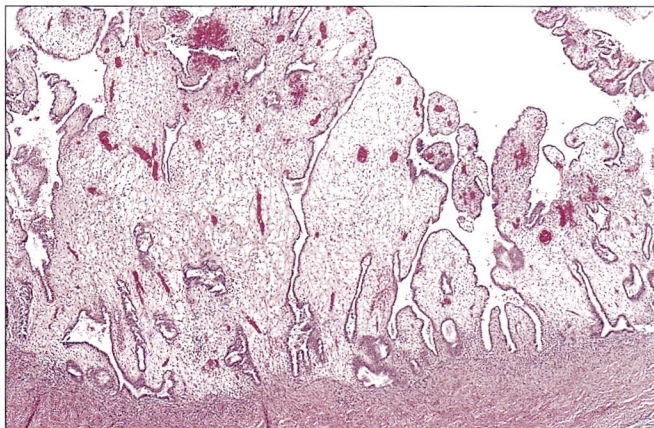

Figure 22.15 Pseudodecidual response of endometriosis to exogenous progestins.

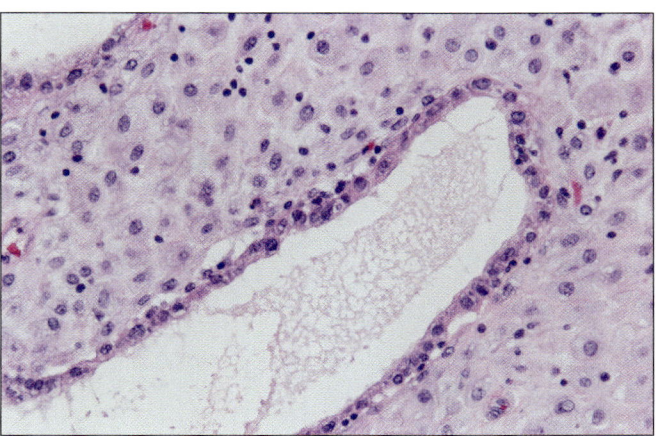

Figure 22.17 Pseudodecidual change in ovarian endometriosis of a woman 23 weeks pregnant. Detail.

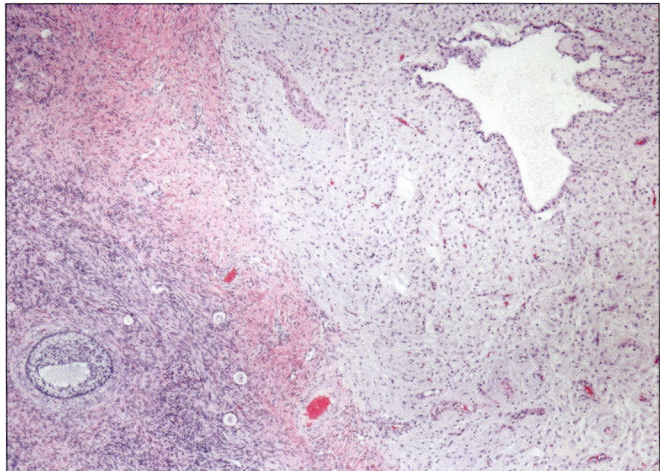

Figure 22.16 Pseudodecidual change in ovarian endometriosis of a woman 23 weeks pregnant.

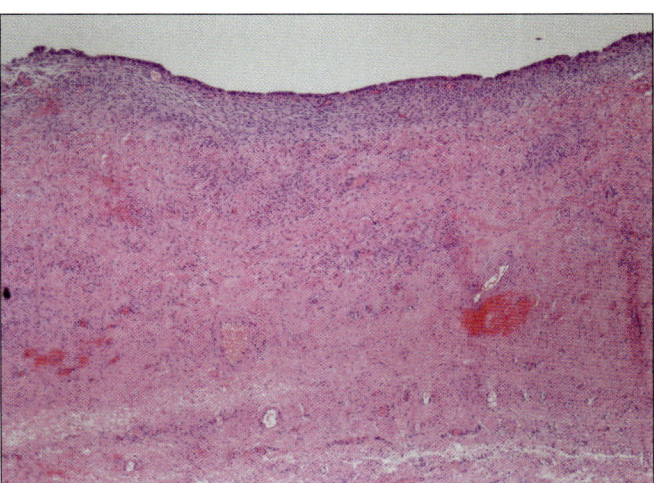

Figure 22.18 The lining epithelium and underlying cellular stroma is evident under low magnification in this ovarian endometrioma.

the menstrual cycle in association with exogenous administration of progestins (Figure 22.15) and during pregnancy (Figures 22.16 and 22.17).

A special form of endometriosis in which a central cystic space predominates is the endometrioma, which can present clinically as a mass (Figures 22.18 and 22.19). These may occur in any location, but most commonly in the ovary. A blood-filled space is lined by a flat simple epithelium and underlying stroma. Less commonly, partially (Figure 22.20) or well-formed glands (Figure 22.21) recapitulating normal endometrium are present. Expansion of the cystic space by blood or fluid can cause attenuation (Figure 22.18) or irritation (Figure 22.22) of the lining epithelium. Degenerative changes occur as described next.

Evidence of bleeding is initially seen as acute hemorrhage within the stroma or adjacent endometriotic tissues (Figures 22.23 and 22.24). In the case of endometriomas, breakdown of the epithelial lining can lead to bleeding into the lumen and disruption of the diagnostic lining (Figure 22.25).

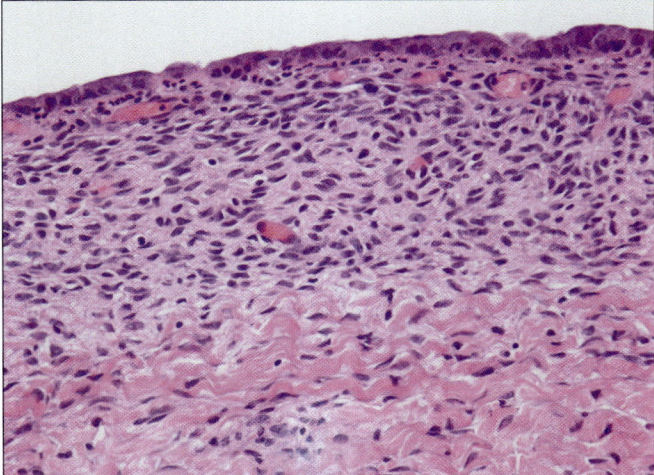

Figure 22.19 Endometriosis stromal cells have blunted nuclei and are randomly oriented compared with the adjacent ovarian stroma.

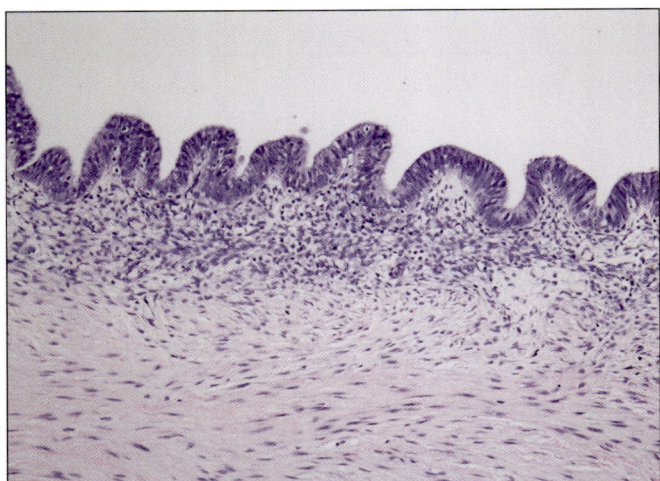

Figure 22.20 Lining of ovarian endometrioma with abortive gland formation.

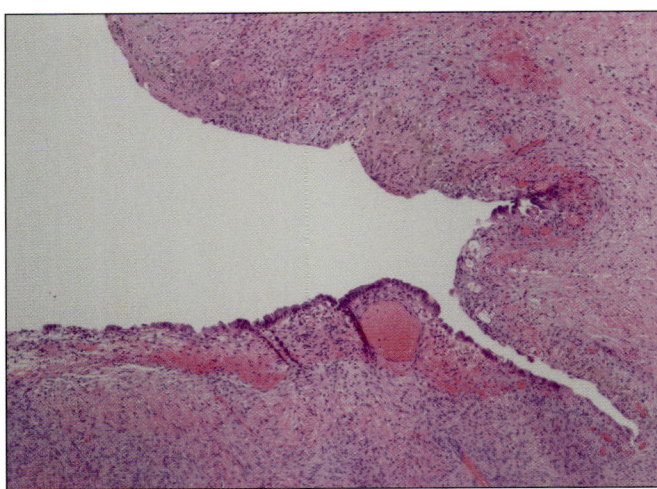

Figure 22.23 Partial erosion and reactive changes of the lining epithelium in an ovarian endometrioma. Hemosiderin-laden macrophases are in the wall.

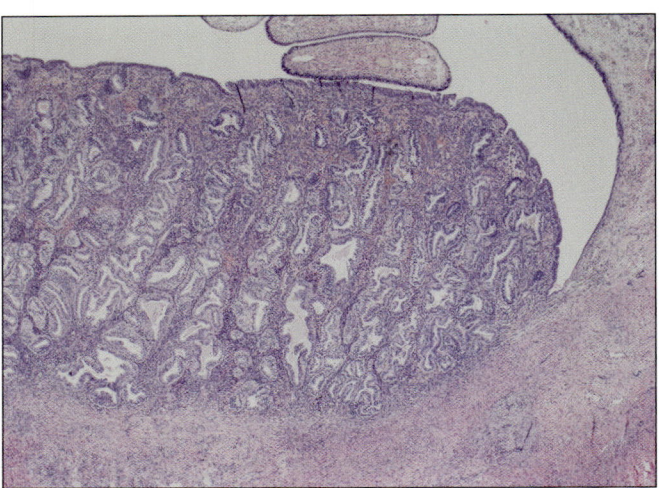

Figure 22.21 Florid endometriosis within an ovarian endometrioma. The exophytic component contains tubular glands and stroma recapitulating the structure of eutopic endometrium.

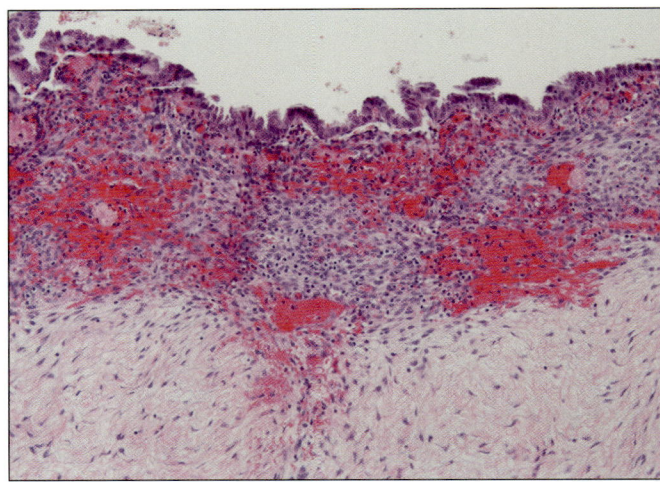

Figure 22.24 Acute hemorrhage is concentrated within the stroma of this ovarian endometrioma.

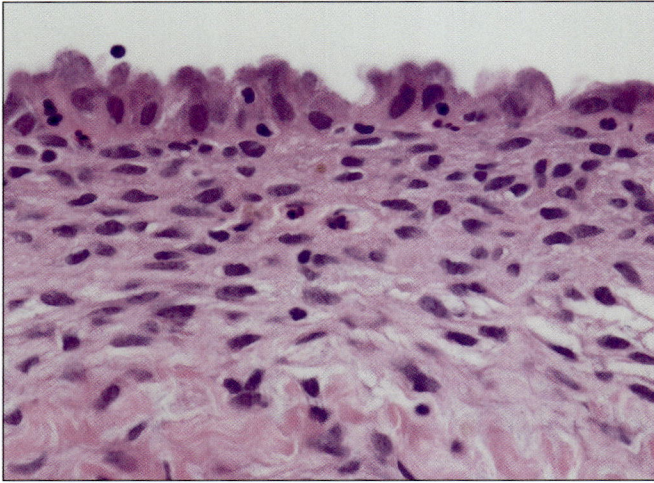

Figure 22.22 Mildly reactive surface lining of ovarian endometrioma.

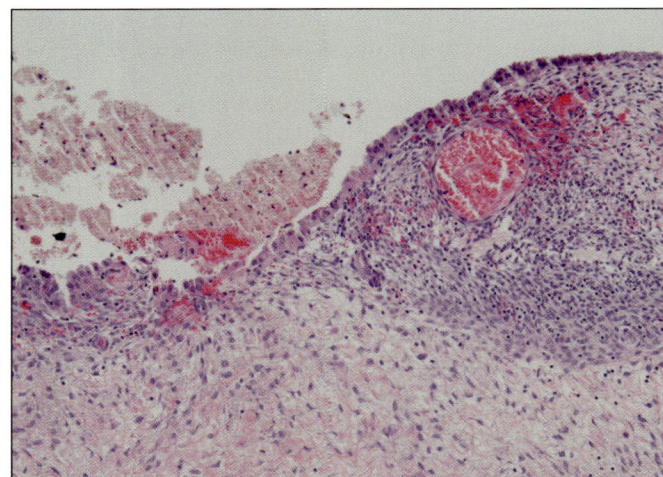

Figure 22.25 Re-epithelialized area (left) of an ovarian endometrioma that has lost most of its stroma by internal shedding.

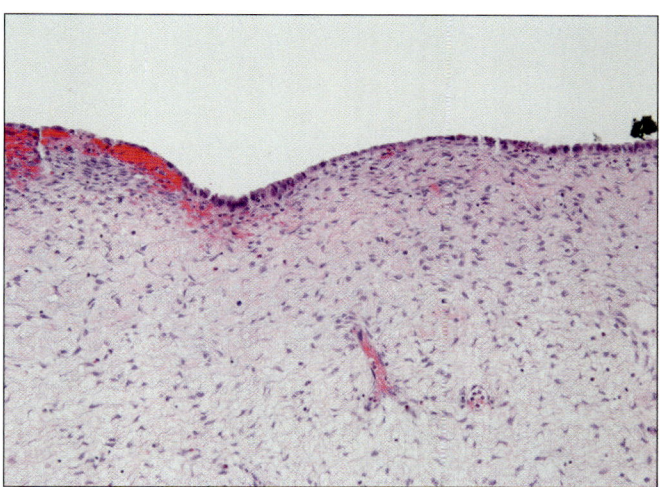

Figure 22.26 Stroma-poor region of endometrioma caused by re-epithelization of a previously shed lining.

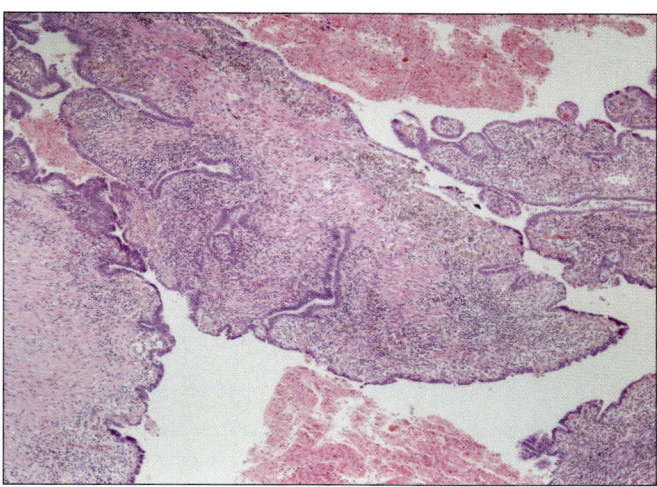

Figure 22.28 Blood in the lumen of the fallopian tube of a 50-year-old woman with an ovarian endometrioma. Plicae are blunted.

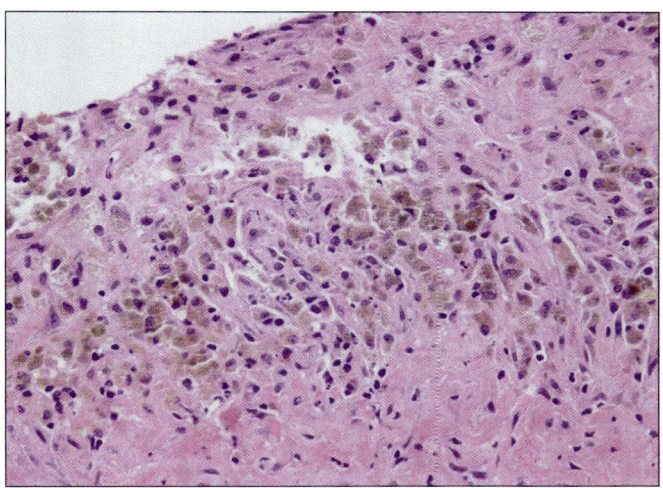

Figure 22.27 An eroded area of ovarian endometrioma where the lining has been replaced by a fibrinous exudate entrapping hemosiderin-laden macrophages. Diagnostic areas with epithelium and stroma were present elsewhere.

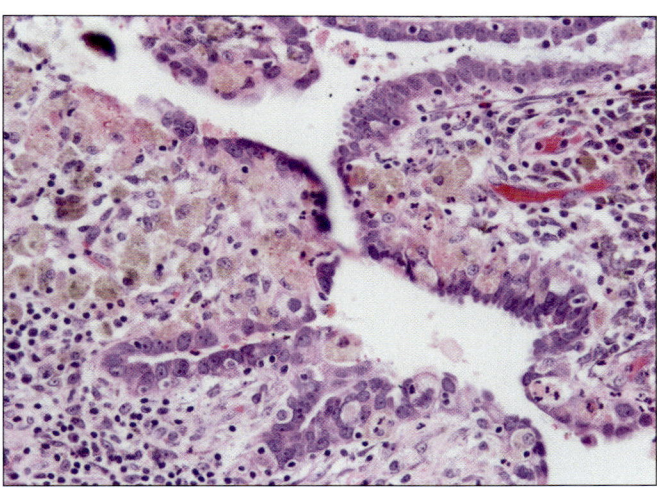

Figure 22.29 Hemosiderin-laden macrophages within stroma of tubal plicae. These changes are secondary to chronic bleeding from ovarian endometriosis.

Repair of eroded surfaces by re-epithelization can create a thin epithelial lining deficient in underlying endometrial stroma (Figure 22.26). In extreme cases, the entire lining and associated stroma is shed into the cyst, creating a pseudocyst lined by hemosiderin-laden macrophages entrapped in fibrin or fibrosis (Figure 22.27). These are no longer diagnostic of endometriosis, as a similar picture can be seen in any localized hemorrhage state such as created by ovarian functional cysts or pelvic inflammatory disease.

Blood sequestered within tissues degenerates to form hemosiderin pigment, which may be deposited directly within connective tissue or phagocytosed by macrophages (Figures 22.14 and 22.22). Hemosiderin-laden macrophages are a nonspecific end product of old bleeding from endometriosis or other causes. If fresh or old blood is directly released into the peritoneal cavity by rupture, it may enter the fallopian tube (Figure 22.28), causing irritation of the tubal lining and accumulation of hemosiderin-laden macrophages within tubal plicae (Figure 22.29).

The epithelial and stromal components may not always be satisfactorily identified, particularly when there has been extensive autolytic degeneration of an endometrioma lining as mentioned previously. In some cases of peritoneal surface endometriosis, multiple sections are necessary to disclose the characteristic findings. Particular attention should be paid when examining the slides to small crevice-like surface invaginations into the stroma (Figure 22.30). In one series of 77 patients with non-pigmented peritoneal lesions, 73 biopsy specimens showed both glands and stroma, 12 showed only endometrial-type stroma, and 10 had neither.[64] Except in the ovary, where hemorrhagic lesions other then endometriosis are common, a presumptive clinical diagnosis based on the laparoscopic findings is often possible.

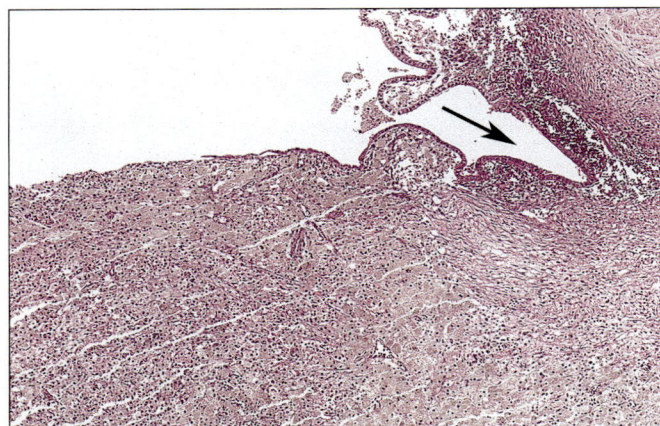

Figure 22.30 Endometriotic epithelium in a protected crevice. Occasionally, the epithelium from an endometrioma cannot be found except in an invagination where pressure atrophy is lacking (arrow), or during specimen preparation when the epithelium has not been wiped away. This shows epithelium around the protected crevice. In the extreme circumstance, only a dozen cells or so may be found in the crevice itself.

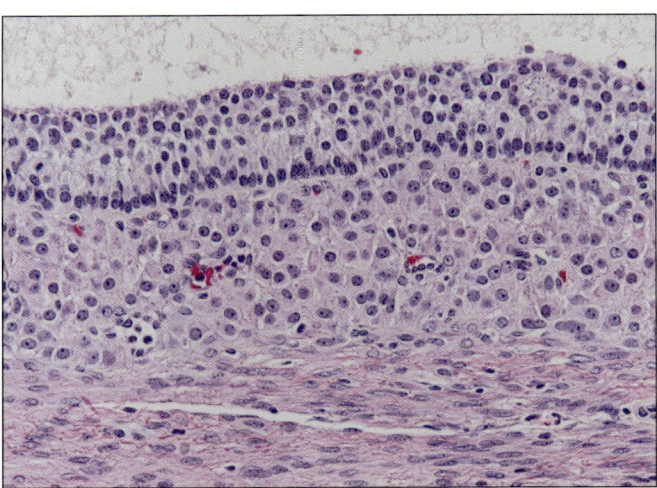

Figure 22.32 Granulosa layer in ovarian follicle. High-power magnification discloses stratified uniform small cells lacking the lining of a luminal epithelium seen in endometriosis.

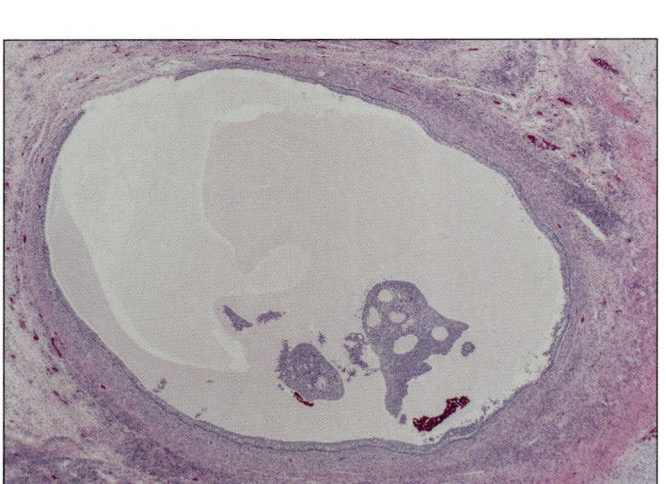

Figure 22.31 Graafian follicle of ovary. The granulosa layer is composed of uniform cells, thus lacking the lining layer of epithelium seen in endometriosis. When the cumulus oophorus (present here) is not in the plane of section they may be confused with an endometrioma.

Ovarian follicles may be confused with endometriosis. A normal follicle in the ovary that is in an advanced state of maturity may appear as a cystic structure surrounded by a hypercellular layer (Figure 22.31). An obvious cumulus oophorus may be lacking because of the plane of section. These can be distinguished from an endometrioma by the lack of a lining epithelium, and character of the stratified granulosa cells that line the follicle (Figure 22.32).

In postmenopausal women and women receiving selective estrogen response modulators, which are predominantly estrogen antagonists, foci of endometriosis in the peritoneal structures may be particularly difficult to identify and, when suspected, may be difficult to document conclusively. The lesions in this age group are typically atrophic and either the epithelial cells or sometimes the stromal cells are absent or, at most, debatably present. The stroma may also in part be fibrotic.

Endometriotic foci usually do not reflect the histologic appearances expected at the appropriate stages of the menstrual cycle. Indeed, they commonly lack cyclic changes. The morphologic appearance of tissue can provide some insight into which foci of endometriosis will be hormonally responsive. In general, the hormonal responsiveness of the implants reflects the quantity of stroma that surrounds the glands, its degree of vascularity, the degree of fibrosis, the presence of surface epithelium, characteristics of the glands themselves, and the presence of local stromal hemorrhage. Implants with greater amounts of fibrosis show progressively less hormonal responsiveness.[65]

CONSIDERATIONS AT SPECIFIC ANATOMIC LOCATIONS

The appearance and frequency of endometriosis varies somewhat by anatomic site. Furthermore, the differential diagnosis must always take into consideration the repertoire of diseases commonly seen at each location.

OVARY

Several conditions that are commonly misdiagnosed as endometriosis (or vice versa) have been described above. Corpus luteum cysts are the lesions most likely to be confused microscopically with chronic endometriotic cysts, since both have a ragged hemorrhagic internal surface. Microscopically, both are lined, at least focally, by fibrous tissue, and granulation tissue in which there are clusters of pale vacuolated cells. Endometrial glands and stroma are, of course, absent.

Ovarian serosal inclusion cysts are exceedingly common superficial cortical lesions. They are lined by cuboidal cells of surface epithelial type or by cells more typically identified as serous. The lesions are distinguished from small superficial endometriotic lesions by their lack of endometrial stroma, hemorrhage, or associated adhesions.

Mesothelial cysts are superficial lesions that do not impinge on the ovarian cortex. They are lined by cuboidal cells with small round nuclei that are readily distinguished from columnar endometrial cells with their cigar-shaped nuclei. Endometrial stroma is absent. They are usually the end result of inflammatory processes involving the ovarian capsular surface, so that adhesions and chronic inflammatory cells are often present.

Rete ovarii and parovarian vestigial remnants may superficially resemble endometriotic foci. The rete have a characteristic ramifying pattern and are surrounded by condensed ovarian, rather than endometriotic stroma lacking evidence of hemorrhage. Rete tubules are lined by cuboidal or columnar cells. Paramesonephric and mesonephric remnants are lined by tubal and cuboidal epithelium, respectively, with cuffs of smooth muscle.

Mature adult cystic teratomas should not cause confusion if there is an opportunity to examine the surgical specimen macroscopically or if multiple blocks have been sectioned. However, individual slides may show a cyst lining composed of macrophages, granulation tissue, and fibrous tissue—a picture also seen in endometriotic cysts. Close scrutiny should reveal the pathognomonic hair fragments or squamous cells.

PERITONEAL SURFACES

Endometriosis on the peritoneal surface, whether lining the abdominal wall or the serosal aspect of adnexal or other organs, often needs to be distinguished from benign müllerian inclusions arising in these locations or even small foci of serous borderline tumor metastatic from the ovary. The benign serous forms have been called 'endosalpingiosis' or 'benign müllerian inclusion cyst.' Quite commonly, the stroma that is present is miniscule in amount and has the appearance of reactive fibroblasts (Figure 22.33). In the absence of unequivocal endometrial-type stroma, endometriosis cannot be diagnosed. Implants of borderline tumors (see Chapters 25–27) lack endometrial stroma, but can be confused with endometriosis especially when accompanied by a reactive stromal response. Psammoma bodies are typical of reactive or proliferative serous lesions and less common in endometriosis. The diagnosis, however, should always be made on the appearance and context of the epithelium in question, rather than inferred by nonspecific changes such as psammoma bodies or hemorrhage.

In the peritoneal cavity, deciduosis and disseminated leiomyomas are manifestations of müllerian tissue present in the pregnant and the non-pregnant state, respectively. The subperitoneal foci of stroma decidualize and resemble the endometriotic lesions of pregnant women or patients receiving progesterone therapy. The absence of endometrial glands excludes endometriosis.

FALLOPIAN TUBE

Endometriosis of the fallopian tube has several patterns. A relatively uncommon, but highly distinctive form is the presence of endometrial tissue lining the tubal lumen itself, replacing the tubal mucosa ('endometrialization'). The

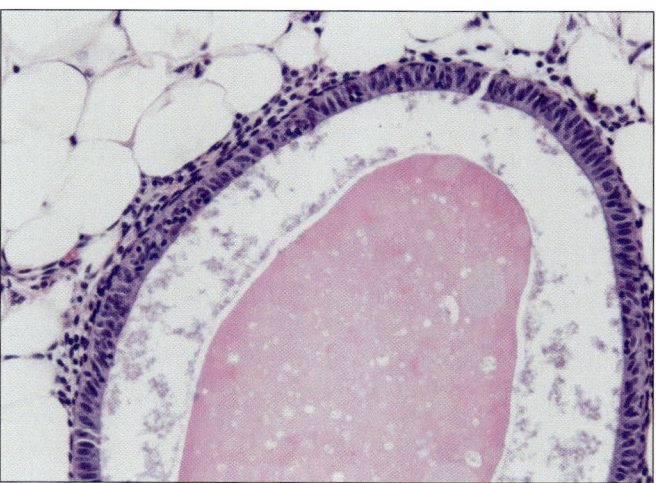

Figure 22.33 Serous müllerian inclusion in the omentum. There is a scant associated stroma that is not clearly endometrial in character, and present only focally. The differential diagnosis is endosalpingiosis versus endometriosis. This patient had foci of typical endometriosis elsewhere.

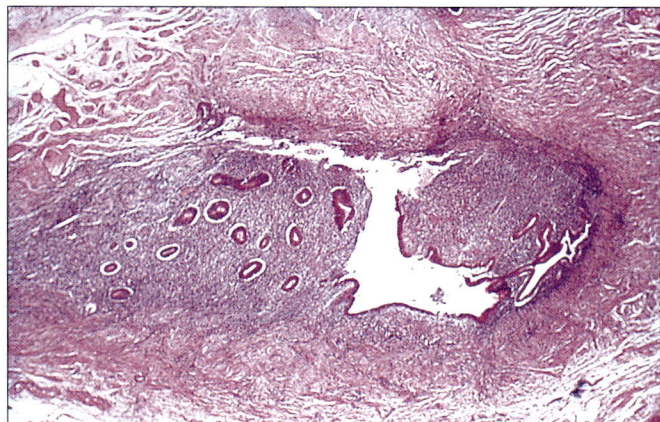

Figure 22.34 Endometriosis of fallopian tube lumen.

normal junction between endometrium and fallopian tube epithelium is usually situated at the inner end of the isthmic portion of the tube. Rather than finding the tubal plicae covered by ciliated epithelium, endometrial glands and stroma are present (Figure 22.34). This condition often produces complete blockage of the affected tube and is associated with infertility.

Sometimes, the endometriosis may be found in the wall, where it must be distinguished from salpingitis isthmica nodosum, a disease akin to adenomyosis of the uterine myometrium. The latter is usually localized to the tubal wall, often appears nodular due to reactive smooth muscle hyperplasia, and lacks unequivocal endometrial-type stroma. The two conditions may occur together.

CERVIX

Historically, endometriosis involving the cervix has been seen relatively infrequently (3% of biopsy and hysterectomy specimens). With the increased usage of loop electrosurgical excision and cone biopsy procedures, the frequency anecdotally has risen. When present in the endocervix, and especially if mitotically active, endometriosis can be mistaken for endocervical adenocarcinoma *in situ*. Characteristic stroma is most helpful in the distinction. Cervical implants may also represent transient adherence of endometrial cells shed during menses.

GASTROINTESTINAL TRACT

Extrapelvic endometriosis most commonly involves the gastrointestinal tract,[66] usually affecting those parts of the bowel that lie in proximity to the genital organs. It occurs in 5% of women with endometriosis. Symptoms, when present, depend on the site involved, and commonly are abdominal or rectal pain, or constipation.[67,68] Dysmenorrhea, dyspareunia, and infertility frequently accompany concomitant pelvic disease. Local symptoms reflect abnormal peristalsis or a distorted intestinal lumen. Constipation may occur with endometriosis in the distal colon, while patients with small intestinal lesions may have diarrhea or loose stools.

The gross appearance is usually that of a thickened bowel wall. At times, the endometriosis may simulate a colonic carcinoma if there is a circumferential stricture of the wall, but usually the endometriosis is distinctive in that there is prominent muscular hypertrophy. This thickened area of bowel wall is white and rubbery and sometimes discloses small, cystic spaces just visible to the naked eye (Figure 22.35). The wall also lacks the grittiness, scarring, and irregular tongues of invasive tumor seen with carcinomas. Usually, the mucosa is intact. Rectal bleeding, if present, is due to endometriotic tissue that swells during menstruation, resulting in mucosal tears.[69] Microscopically, typical foci of endometriosis are seen throughout the bowel wall (Figure 22.36), and sometimes may involve the submucosa. Occasionally, if endometriosis is not clinically evident and not present in the immediate zone of the biopsy, inflammatory bowel disease may be erroneously diagnosed.[70]

URINARY TRACT

The urinary tract is involved in 1.2% of women with endometriosis.[66] Of these, the bladder is most commonly affected (five-sixths of cases) and the disease is usually limited to the serosa. The wall, when involved, is usually thickened from fibrosis and muscular proliferation around the endometriotic foci. The ureter is affected less often (one-sixth of cases) and the kidney and urethra very rarely. Endometriosis can induce dramatic retroperitoneal fibrosis on occasion and, if the ureter is entrapped, represents an important cause of ureteric obstruction.[71]

ABDOMINAL WALL

Endometriosis in abdominal wall scars is seen most frequently following hysterotomy, a procedure that was a commonly used method of mid-trimester abortion in the early 1970s. The frequency with which endometriosis has been seen subsequently in the abdominal wall of women subjected to this operation emphasizes that endometrium has the potential to implant and proliferate when spilt into a wound. Although cesarean section is a common procedure, endometriosis is rarely a sequel. Endometriosis in the needle track has been reported following amniocentesis. It has also followed operations such as myomectomy or cesarean section that open the uterine cavity and thereby allow spillage of endometrium into the wound. Only rarely is it found in the scars of other operations, such as hysterectomy or appendectomy.

LYMPH NODES

Endometriosis is only occasionally found in lymph nodes (Figure 22.37), which is surprising given the prevalence of disease in the peritoneum and the occasional observation of endometrial cells in the myometrial lymphatics. When present in pericolic lymph nodes, it is easy to mistake the endometriosis for a metastatic adenocarcinoma of the intestines.[67] The presence in the lymph node of an endometrial-type epithelium that is associated with endometrial-type stroma should allow the diagnosis to be made with some

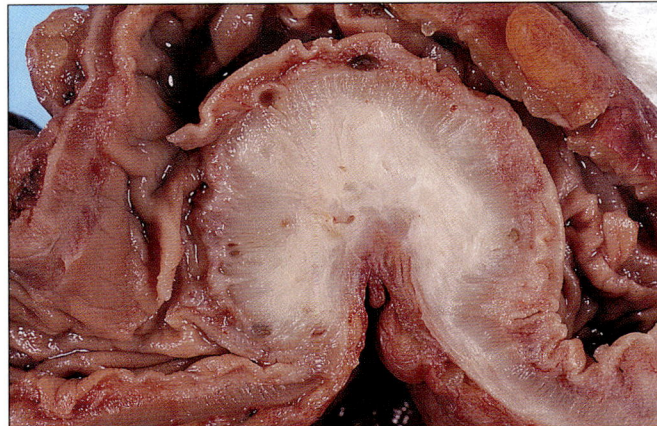

Figure 22.35 Endometriosis in colonic wall causing partial obstruction. Extensive fibrosis and muscle hypertrophy account for the white and tan-brown color, respectively.

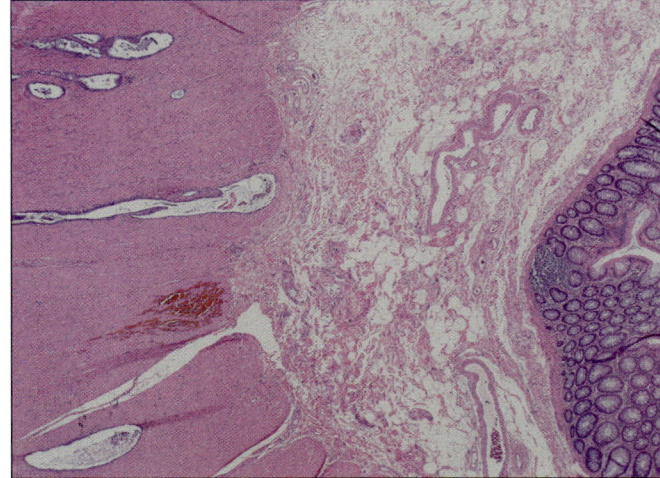

Figure 22.36 Deep endometriosis in the bowel wall.

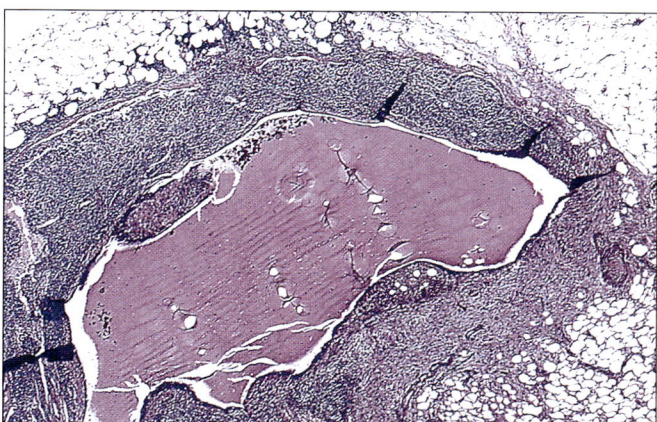

Figure 22.37 Endometriosis in colonic lymph node.

ease. Occasionally, the stroma may be decidualized, especially if the patient is pregnant or is taking progestational-type medication.

Far more commonly, pelvic or para-aortic lymph nodes may contain glands lined by a serous or endometrioid-type epithelium. In the absence of stroma, these glands may represent müllerian inclusion cysts (endosalpingiosis) or metastases from borderline serous tumors of the ovary.[72]

CLINICAL CLASSIFICATION OF ENDOMETRIOSIS

The schemes used to stage endometriosis by its severity and distribution have undergone substantial change since they were first introduced nearly 50 years ago. The various classifications began as descriptions of anatomic distribution of lesions, similar to contemporary systems for staging malignancies based on extent of disease. As this does not predict fertility outcomes very well on its own, measures of secondary damage (such as adhesions, organ distortion) and additional patient historical factors have been added to create composite scoring systems with improved predictive performance.

The anatomic staging scheme used most commonly today is the American Society for Reproductive Medicine (ASRM) criteria, revised in 1996.[73,74] The classification scheme is intended to be applied to symptomatic patients only, as there is no consensus regarding the need to stage asymptomatic patients. Scoring is based primarily on visual morphology at surgery (usually laparoscopy). Histologic confirmation is encouraged to improve accuracy, but is not a formal part of the system. The ASRM classification stratifies endometriosis by the extent of disease present and severity of disease found. It also assesses damage from the disease, namely pelvic adhesions. It has a weighted point score that assesses the extent of the endometriosis among organs and even within an organ, i.e., superficial (<1 mm) versus invasive (>5 mm) disease. It assesses the unilaterality of the disease, size of endometriomas, and type of adhesions (filmy vs dense). The cumulative scores result in a stage designation: stage 1 is minimal disease (1–5 points), stage 2 is mild disease (6–15 points), stage 3 is moderate disease (16–40 points), and stage 4 is extensive disease (>40 points). It has its limitations. Interobserver reproducibility is only fair to good,[75] and staging cut-offs are arbitrary.[76]

The 2010 Endometriosis Fertility Index (EFI) adds clinical historical parameters (age, fertility duration, prior pregnancies) and structural measures of adnexal function (distortion of ovaries and tubes) to the anatomic ASRM criteria, yielding a cumulative score that is linearly correlated with fertility outcome.[77] The EFI uses a four-tier scoring system of anatomic abnormalities of the ovary, fimbria, and tube, ordered sequentially by progressive impact on reproductive function. When combined with staged distribution of lesions using the ASRM system, and additional clinical background information, the prediction of fertility is improved over staging alone.[78] The EFI is reproducible and predictive of outcome, but clinical experience is limited due to its relatively recent vintage.[78]

INFERTILITY IN ENDOMETRIOSIS

Infertility and endometriosis go hand in hand.[77] Although precise figures of the relationship are difficult to determine, estimates are that about 30–50% of women with endometriosis suffer from infertility and 25–50% of infertile women have endometriosis.

The most obvious reasons for infertility would appear to be mechanical, resulting from functional changes caused by direct involvement of adnexal organs by endometriosis or its secondary effects. This is supported by the ability of clinical staging systems, such as the ASRM staging and EFI, mentioned previously, to predict fertility outcomes from this type of information.

There are many other factors that may contribute to reduced fertility in the patient with endometriosis.[74] These include systemic endocrine disorders caused by ovulatory dysfunction, poor oocyte quality, and regional effects of molecules elaborated by endometriotic implants. In the experimental situation, there is some evidence that the intraperitoneal inflammation itself rather than the implants is responsible for the reduced fecundity, comparable to the mechanism of contraception of the intrauterine device.

ENDOMETRIOSIS PRESENTING AS A BENIGN SOLID TUMOR

Endometriosis may present as a tumor mass when it grows as florid disease, or when it is the source of a stromal or glandular neoplasm that contributes to its bulk. The distinction between solid and cystic masses is somewhat arbitrary, as even the clinically solid lesions are actually multicystic, with interposed glands evident on microscopy. Solid masses of glandular endometriosis are less common than the endometrioma, which has a dominant cyst and the majority of its bulk contributed by its internal fluid contents.

FLORID ENDOMETRIOSIS

Endometriosis may grow as nodules or even large masses that microscopically show no more than broad expanses of admixed endometrial stroma and glands known as florid

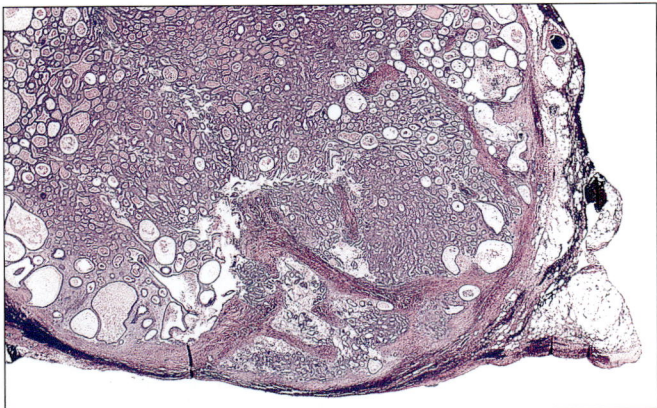

Figure 22.38 Florid endometriosis in omentum.

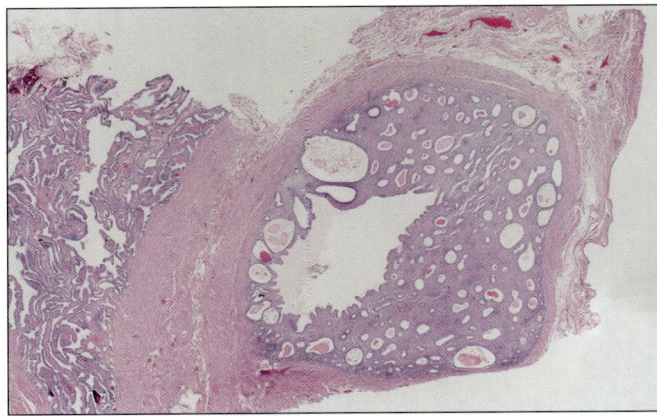

Figure 22.40 Polypoid endometriosis presenting as a mass adherent to the fallopian tube. The combination of tubulocystic glands and cellular stroma lacking hemorrhage is reminiscent of an endometrial polyp.

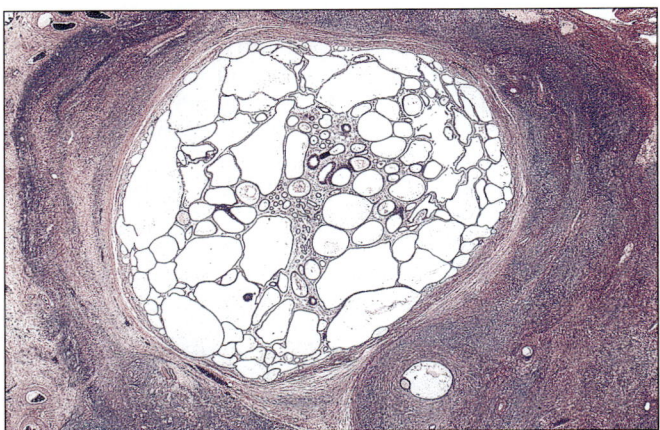

Figure 22.39 Florid endometriosis within ovary.

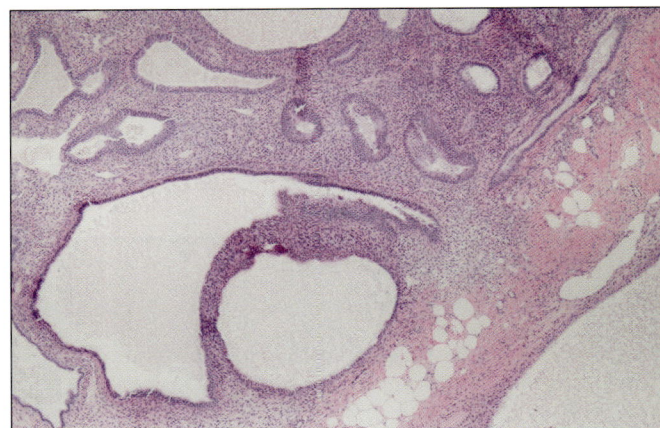

Figure 22.41 Detail of polypoid endometriosis showing fibrotic stroma.

endometriosis. These can be located in the pelvis (Figure 22.38), fat, or even located within organs (Figure 22.39). These are growth variants of endometriosis, sometimes referred to as an 'endometrial adenoma,' which otherwise have glandular and stromal components resembling that of usual endometriosis.

POLYPOID ENDOMETRIOSIS

Polypoid endometriosis is a distinctive solid lesion composed of endometrial stromal and glandular elements in which the stroma is fibrous, resembling that of endometrial polyps (Figures 22.40 and 22.41). Like endometrial polyps, blood vessels are prominent. It has a pathogenesis similar to that of endometrial polyps of the uterine cavity,[79] as both are clonal stromal neoplasms with secondary induction of müllerian-type epithelium. This is evident as clonal rearrangements of the *HMGA* gene found within the stromal, but not epithelial, cells of polypoid endometriosis.[80] A majority (18/24) are associated with endometriosis, and some occur within endometriomas (5/24), suggesting that they may originate from the stromal component of pre-existing endometriosis of the usual type.[81]

The site of involvement can be anywhere in the abdomen or pelvis, with a decreasing order of frequency in the colon, ovary, uterine serosa, cervical and/or vaginal mucosa, then other sites.[81] Bowel or ureteral obstruction, even vascular thrombosis, may result from impingement of adjacent structures. These clinical features, along with bulky solid growth, can easily be confused with a malignant process.[82,83] Polypoid endometriosis is a benign stromal neoplasm that can present with serious complications as described earlier, but it may undergo malignant transformation of its glandular or stromal components. It must be distinguished from müllerian adenosarcoma, which has periglandular condensations of mitotically active atypical stroma (Figures 22.42–22.44).

MALIGNANCY IN ENDOMETRIOSIS

For any number of reasons, the frequency of endometriosis transforming to cancer has been difficult to determine. Extensive sampling may be required to find a small focus of endometriosis adjacent to a malignant tumor or a cancer may destroy the endometriotic tissue from which it arose.

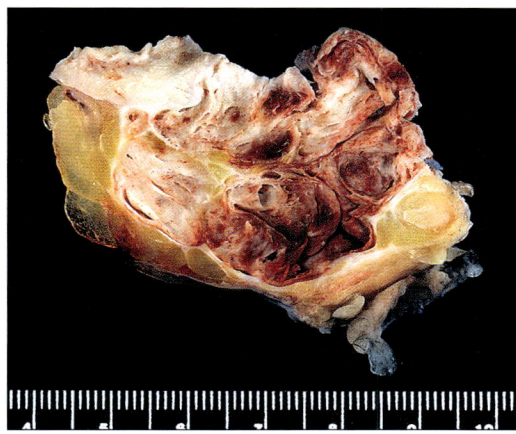

Figure 22.42 Adenosarcoma arising in omental endometriosis. The tumor, which was bloody and of a different texture, differed from the endometriosis spread throughout the abdominal cavity that was otherwise more rubbery and had evoked a fibrous stromal reaction.

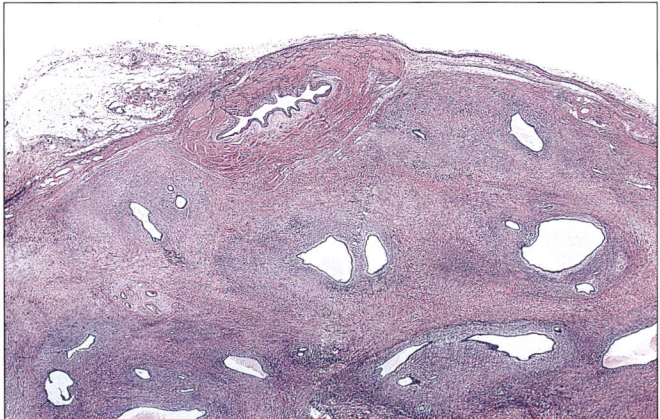

Figure 22.43 Extrapelvic adenosarcoma with periglandular cuffing.

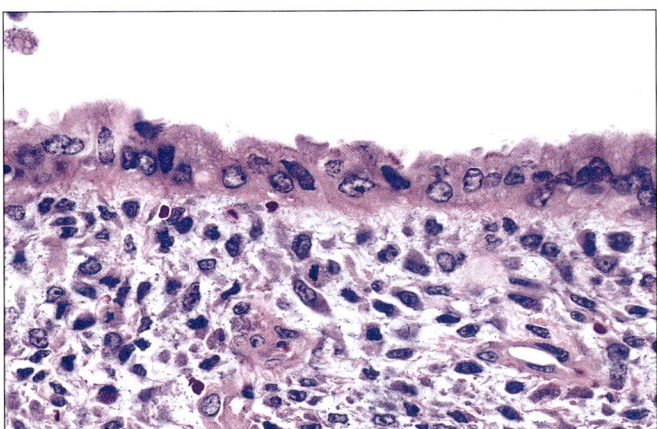

Figure 22.44 Adenosarcoma in the intestinal wall, high magnification. The epithelium shows cuboidal cells with atypical nuclei and copious eosinophilic cytoplasm.

Often, only the frequency of concomitant endometriosis has been recorded without a specific statement of how many cancers arose from the endometriotic tissue.

In general, the criteria for establishing an origin of malignancy from endometriosis include the following:

- Both cancer and benign endometrial tissue should be seen in the same organ.
- Both should have a continuous histologic relation to each other.
- The cancer must be shown to have arisen in this tissue and not invaded it from some other source.
- The tumor should be of a histologic type known to arise in the native endometrium.
- A gradual transition from benign to malignant epithelium is helpful, or at least documented atypia in the endometriosis adjacent to the malignant tumor.

These criteria are fulfilled in less than 10% of published cases. However, in nearly one-fourth of cases endometriosis can be identified in other parts of the affected organ (e.g., ovary), even though it is not in continuity with the tumor.

In recent years, conservation of clone-specific genetic changes has provided an accessible and objective means of establishing a direct lineage relationship between coexisting premalignant and malignant elements in a single patient.

FREQUENCY AND TYPES OF MALIGNANCIES

The ovary is by far the most common site where malignancy arises in association with endometriosis,[84,85] accounting for about 75% of such cases. However, tumor develops at virtually every site where endometriosis is found: cul-de-sac,[86] fallopian tube, groin, large bowel,[87] lymph node, omentum, pleura, rectovaginal septum,[88] scars,[89] ureter,[90] urinary bladder, vagina,[91,92] and vulva.[93]

The histologic types of malignancies that may arise from endometriosis is as diverse at that seen in the eutopic endometrium, and can include epithelial, stromal, or mixed neoplasms. Many are sufficiently rare that they are known primarily from case reports. This section will present the most commonly encountered forms of endometriosis-related malignancies, and readers are referred to relevant chapters on endometrial epithelial (Chapter 18) and uterine stromal (Chapter 20) tumors for the full repertoire of possibilities.

The frequency of malignant transformation is estimated at 1.1–3%.[18] The level of uncertainty relates to the sampling issues noted earlier. Among 1021 cases of endometriosis, malignancy was found in 56 (5.5%). However, only 11 (1.1%) were identified as arising within endometriosis with an additional 20 (1.9%) arising in the same organ but at some measurable distance from the microscopic endometriosis. The remaining 35 malignancies arose in patients with endometriosis, but in organs where no endometriosis was observed. In a report from a population-based study from a national cancer registry involving more than 20,000 women with endometriosis followed for a mean time of over 11 years, the relative risk of subsequently developing ovarian cancer was 1.9, rising to 4.2 among those subjects with a long-standing history of ovarian endometriosis.[94] The development of ovarian cancer was also raised in a second study with long-term follow-up.[95]

A recent meta-analysis of carcinoma risk elevation (odds ratio; OR) in patients with ovarian endometriosis found a statistically significant positive correlation with clear cell (OR = 3.05), and endometrioid (OR = 2.04) invasive adenocarcinomas.[96] Additionally, well-differentiated serous carcinomas have an elevated risk (OR = 2.11). As these are historical studies it is unclear how closely this 'well-differentiated' serous carcinoma in a three-grade system corresponds to more recent bimodal classification of serous cancers as low versus high grade based on nuclear cytology.[97] When data were adjusted and stratified from multiple studies, an association between endometriosis and serous borderline tumors lost statistical significance with an OR of 1.20.[97] Low-grade serous cancers of the ovary defined in this fashion have now been associated with borderline serous tumors undergoing malignant transformation by acquisition of KRAS mutations.[98]

Clear cell carcinoma (Figure 22.45) and endometrioid adenocarcinoma (Figure 22.46) account for roughly two-thirds of all endometriosis-associated cases.[18,99,100] While endometrioid adenocarcinoma is the more common of the two entities by a ratio between 1.3:1 to about 4:1,[101] women who have clear cell adenocarcinoma are often reported to have a much higher frequency of coexistent pelvic endometriosis. The rate of about 25–50% is much higher than for any other cell type, including endometrioid adenocarcinoma.[102,103] Mixtures of both endometrioid and clear cell adenocarcinoma are common.

Cancers of all other cell types arising in endometriosis are relatively uncommon. Endometriosis was found maximally in 8% of serous tumors in one study,[103] but in all other studies serous and all other cell types were present in under 5% of cases, regardless of whether it occurred in the ovary or extragonadally.[18,101,103] Endometrial-type stromal sarcoma (Figures 22.47 and 22.48), even though reported to be the second most common malignant neoplasm arising in extraovarian endometriosis, is nonetheless rare. The tumor we have seen with surprising frequency has been adenosarcoma arising in extrapelvic endometriosis (Figures 22.42 to 22.44), a lesion that can be distinguished from polypoid endometriosis (described previously) by the cuffing of glands with a condensation of cytologically atypical and mitotically active stromal cells.

ATYPICAL ENDOMETRIOSIS AND THE PATHOGENESIS OF MALIGNANCY

The molecular features of carcinoma arising from endometriosis correlate closely to those seen for carcinomas of similar histotype in the eutopic endometrium.[104] As with

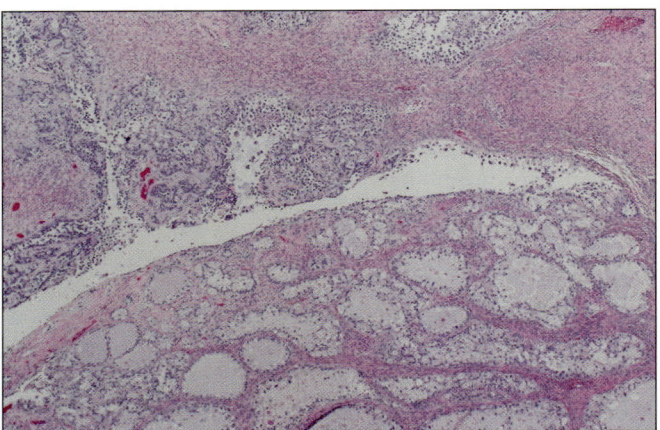

Figure 22.45 Clear cell adenocarcinoma of the ovary arising in association with atypical endometriosis (Figures 22.49 and 22.50).

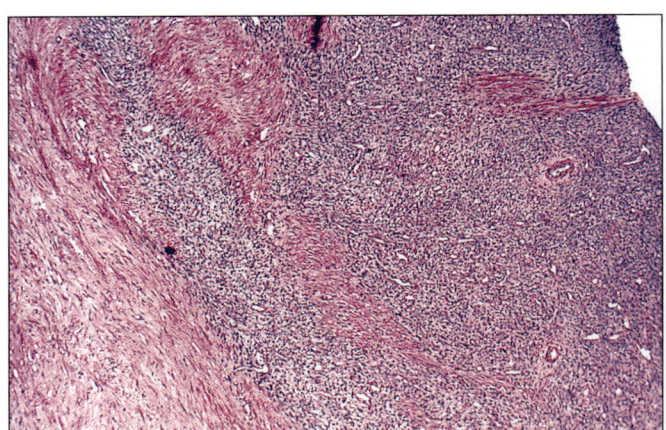

Figure 22.47 Stromal sarcoma arising in endometriosis.

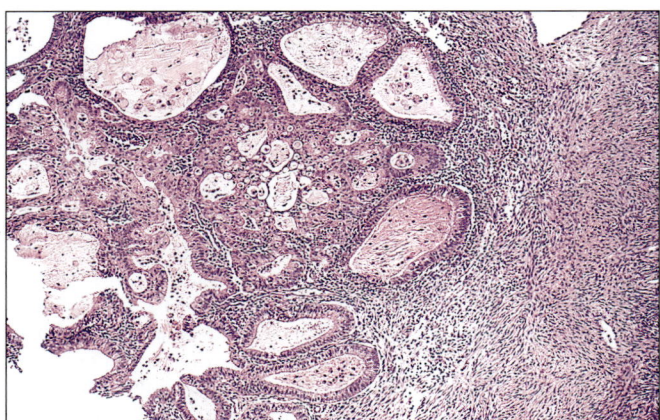

Figure 22.46 Endometrioid adenocarcinoma (cribriform) arising in atypical endometriosis.

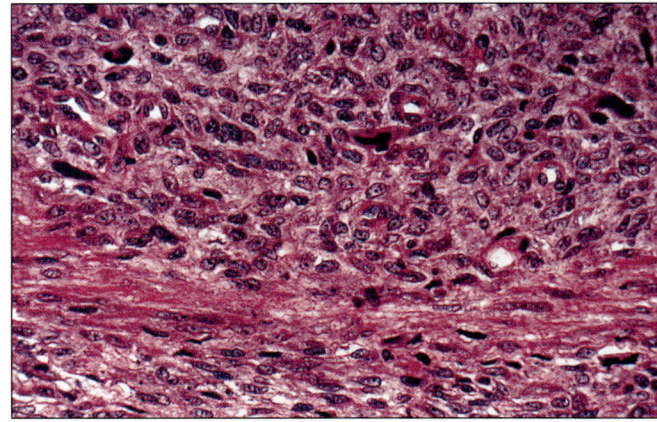

Figure 22.48 Stromal sarcoma with marked nuclear atypicality arising in endometriosis.

carcinoma arising in eutopic endometrium, the histologic appearance of premalignant changes intervening between benign endometriosis and carcinoma are pathway dependent. Generally these fall under the collective name of 'atypical endometriosis,' but those associated with clear cell carcinoma are somewhat different in appearance than those seen in endometrioid carcinomas. For purposes of simplifying the following discussion we divide these into 'atypical endometriosis, clear cell type,' and 'atypical endometriosis, endometrioid type.' In practice distinction between the two is not easy because of overlap, and a high degree of variation within each group. Often the clear cell versus endometrioid features of atypical endometriosis are not evident until it has progressed nearly all the way to malignancy. A further difficulty with the concept of atypical endometriosis is that some degree of cytologic atypia, exfoliation, and epithelial folding is common in degenerative areas of benign endometriosis. Caution must be exercised in its diagnosis and extrapolation of its clinical significance in the individual patient who does not already have an associated malignancy.

Atypical endometriosis, clear cell type, with characteristically atypical nuclei and vacuolated or foamy cytoplasm (Figures 22.49 and 22.50), is a precursor lesion to clear cell adenocarcinoma (Figures 22.45 and 22.51, same case as Figures 22.49 and 22.50). Atypical epithelium can be exfoliative and hobnail like, or flat. When arising from the flat surface of endometriomas, the atypical epithelium many not form discrete glands, and initially those glands that appear may be sparsely distributed. This is not always the case, and complex gland formation within exophytic epithelium or dense aggregates do occur. Lineage continuity between atypical endometriosis and adjacent clear cell carcinoma has been demonstrated at the molecular level, as identical PIK3CA mutations and loss of ARID1A protein[105] can be seen in endometriosis adjacent to clear cell carcinoma. Reliable diagnosis of this type of atypical endometriosis requires a high degree of nuclear pleomorphism and hyperchromasia, so as not to confuse it with reactive changes secondary to breakdown.

Atypical endometriosis, endometrioid type (Figures 22.52 and 22.53), is a lesion with features intermediate between endometriosis and endometrioid adenocarcinoma (Figure 22.54). It can resemble endometrial epithelial neoplasm of the eutopic endometrium (Chapter 17) in having prominent architectural features of increased gland density (Figure 22.55), and variable degrees of nuclear atypia (Figure 22.56). Endometrioid adenocarcinoma arising from endometriosis shows loss of function of PTEN (21%), KRAS (20%), β-catenin (25%), and PIK3CA (46%).[104]

ACKNOWLEDGMENT

The author would like to thank Dr. Stanley Robboy for his contributions carried forward from the previous edition of this chapter.

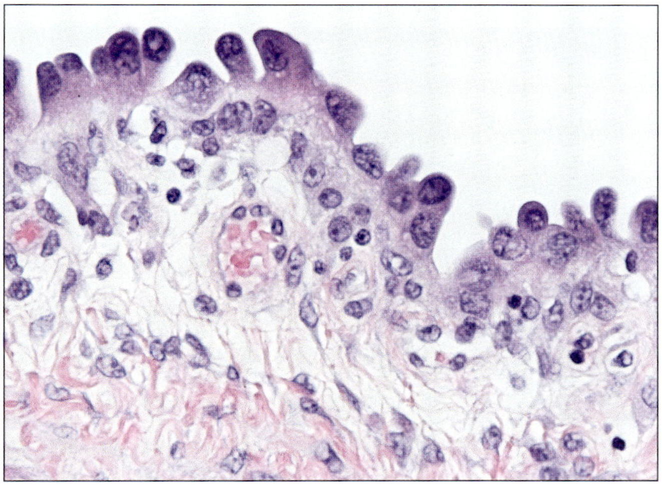

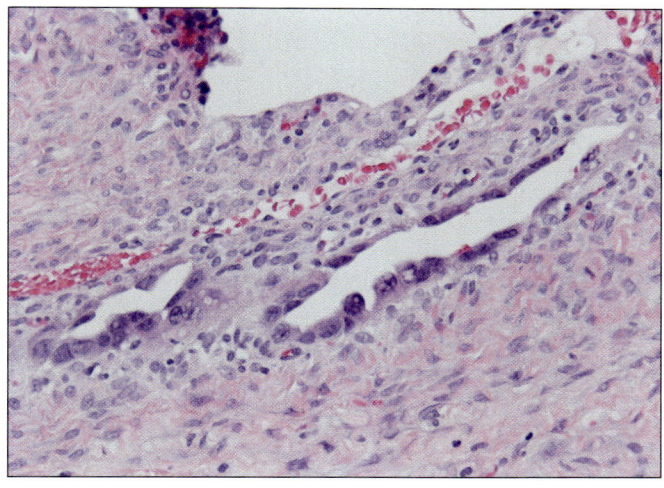

Figure 22.50 Atypical endometriosis, clear cell type, in ovary. Atypical glands are separated by stroma, and have not formed dense aggregates seen in the endometrioid type of atypical endometriosis.

Figure 22.49 Atypical endometriosis, clear cell type, in ovary. The epithelium is thin, but nuclei are irregularly enlarged with coarse chromatin. Note the lack of inflammatory reaction or erosion, which in addition to the hyperchromasia assist in distinction from reactive change.

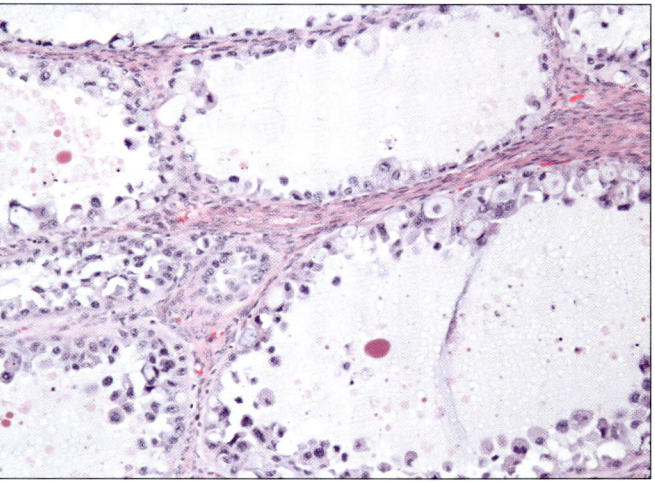

Figure 22.51 Clear cell adenocarcinoma of ovary, arising in association with endometriosis and atypical endometriosis.

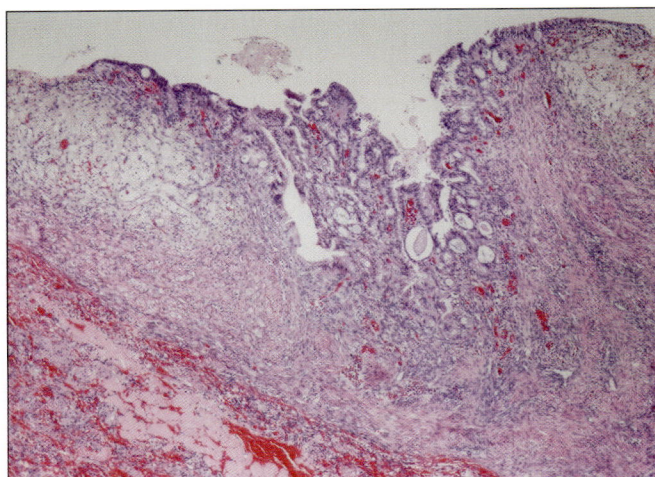

Figure 22.52 Atypical endometriosis, endometrioid type, in ovarian endometrioma. Lining epithelium is thickened, with a complex gland pattern.

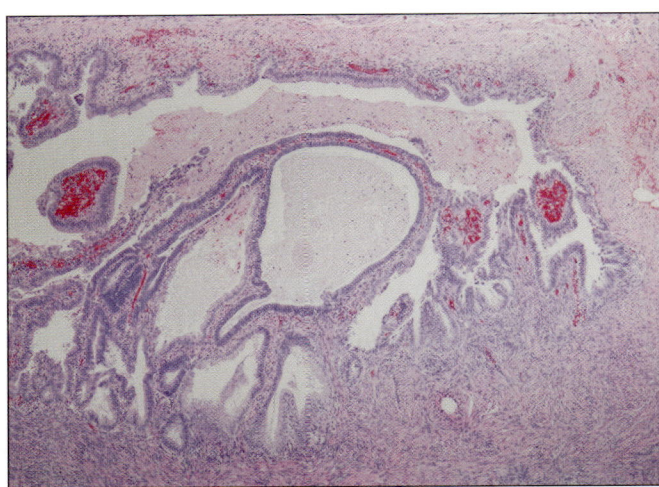

Figure 22.55 Atypical endometriosis, endometrioid type, in ovary. Glands are present at a high density, and demonstrate a variable cytology.

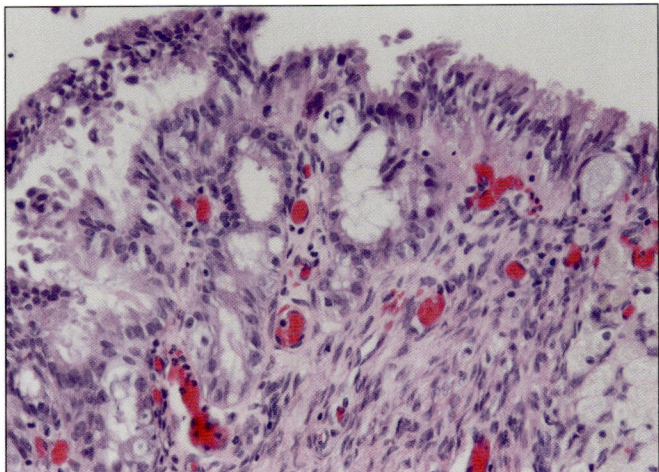

Figure 22.53 Atypical endometriosis, endometrioid type, in ovary. Cytologic atypia is moderate.

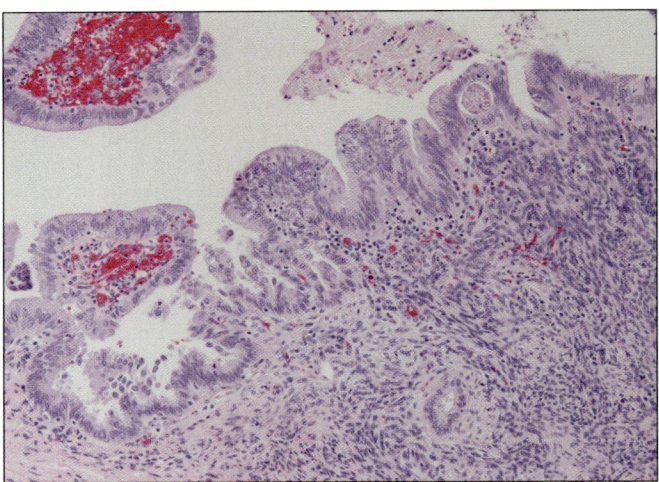

Figure 22.56 Detail of atypical endometriosis, endometrioid type, in ovary (Figure 22.55). Cytology is moderately atypical, and the convoluted epithelium forms glands off the surface.

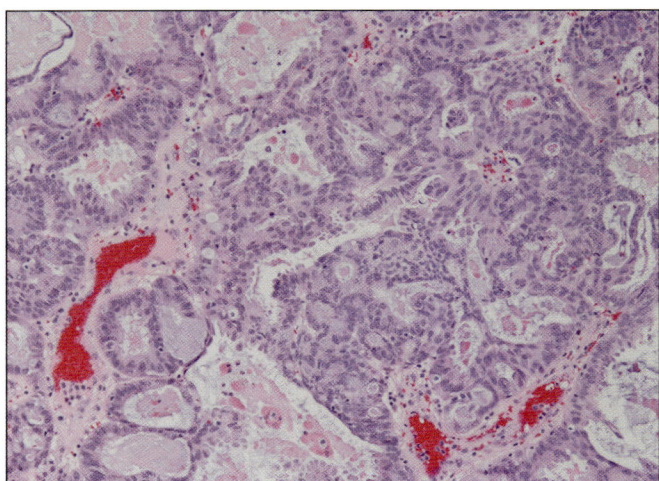

Figure 22.54 Endometrioid adenocarcinoma in ovary, arising from atypical endometriosis (Figures 22.52 and 22.53).

REFERENCES

1. Leyendecker G, Kunz G. [Endometriosis and adenomyosis]. Zentralbl Gynakol 2005;127:288–94.
2. McLeod BS, Retzloff MG. Epidemiology of endometriosis: an assessment of risk factors. Clin Obstet Gynecol 2010;53:389–96.
3. Cramer DW, Missmer SA. The epidemiology of endometriosis. In: Yoshinaga K, Parrott EC, editors. Endometriosis: emerging research and intervention strategies. New York: New York Academy of Sciences; 2002. p. 11–22.
4. Hompes PG, Mijatovic V. Endometriosis: the way forward. Gynecol Endocrinol 2007;23:5–12.
5. Allaire C. Endometriosis and infertility: a review. J Reprod Med 2006;51:164–8.
6. Giudice LC, Tazuke SI, Swiersz L. Status of current research on endometriosis. J Reprod Med 1998;43:252–62.
7. Osteen KG, Bruner KL, Eisenberg E. The disease endometriosis. In: Diamond MP, Osteen KG, editors. Endometrium and Endometriosis. Oxford: Blackwell Science; 1997. p. 20–4.
8. Coccia ME, Rizzello F, Comparetto C. Endometriosis and pain in an adolescent population. Proceedings of the World Meeting on Gynecologic Pelvic Pain and Endometriosis, Bolognia, Italy; 2006. p. 101–5.

9. Choi SW, Lee HN, Kang SJ, Kim HO. A case of cutaneous endometriosis developed in postmenopausal woman receiving hormonal replacement. J Am Acad Dermatol 1999;41:327–9.
10. Jacoby VL, Fujimoto VY, Giudice LC, et al. Racial and ethnic disparities in benign gynecologic conditions and associated surgeries. Am J Obstet Gynecol 2010;202:514–21.
11. Muneyyirci-Delale O, Neil G, Serur E, et al. Endometriosis with massive ascites. Gynecol Oncol 1998;69:42–6.
12. Balasch J, Creus M, Fabregues F, et al. Visible and non-visible endometriosis at laparoscopy in fertile and infertile women and in patients with chronic pelvic pain: a prospective study. Hum Reprod 1996;11:387–91.
13. Hurd WW. Criteria that indicate endometriosis is the cause of chronic pelvic pain. Obstet Gynecol 1998;92:1029–32.
14. Vercellini P. Endometriosis: what a pain it is. Semin Reprod Endocrinol 1997;15:251–61.
15. Bulun SE. Endometriosis. N Engl J Med 2009;360:268–79.
16. Abushahin F, Goldman KN, Barbieri E, et al. Aromatase inhibition for refractory endometriosis-related chronic pelvic pain. Fertil Steril 2011;96:939–42.
17. Shaw RW. An atlas of endometriosis. New York: Parthenon; 1993.
18. Stern RC, Dash R, Bentley RC, et al. Malignancy in endometriosis: frequency and comparison of ovarian and extraovarian types. Int J Gynecol Pathol 2001;20:133–9.
19. Treloar SA, O'Connor DT, O'Connor VM, Martin NG. Genetic influences on endometriosis in an Australian twin sample. sueT@qimr.edu.au. Fertil Steril 1999;71:701–10.
20. Eskenazi B, Warner ML. Epidemiology of endometriosis. Obstet Gynecol Clin North Am 1997;24:235–58.
21. Sangi-Haghpeykar H, Poindexter III AN. Epidemiology of endometriosis among parous women. Obstet Gynecol 1995;85:983–92.
22. Vessey MP, Villard-Mackintosh L, Painter R. Epidemiology of endometriosis in women attending family planning clinics. BMJ 1993;306:182–4.
23. Jimbo H, Hitomi Y, Yoshikawa H, et al. Evidence for monoclonal expansion of epithelial cells in ovarian endometrial cysts 24. Am J Pathol 1997;150:1173–8.
24. Nilbert M, Pejovic T, Mandahl N, et al. Monoclonal origin of endometriotic cysts. Int J Gynecol Cancer 1995;5:61–3.
25. D'Hooghe TM, Debrock S. Endometriosis, retrograde menstruation and peritoneal inflammation in women and in baboons. Hum Reprod Update 2002;8:84–8.
26. Bulun SE, Utsunomiya H, Lin Z, et al. Steroidogenic factor-1 and endometriosis. Mol Cell Endocrinol 2009;300:104–8.
27. Bricou A, Batt RE, Chapron C. Peritoneal fluid flow influences anatomical distribution of endometriotic lesions: why Sampson seems to be right. Eur J Obstet Gynecol Reprod Biol 2008;138:127–34.
28. Jenkins S, Olive DL, Haney AF. Endometriosis: pathogenetic implications of the anatomic distribution. Obstet Gynecol 1986;67:335–8.
29. D'Hooghe TM, Bambra CS, Raeymaekers BM, Koninckx PR. Increased incidence and recurrence of recent corpus luteum without ovulation stigma (luteinized unruptured follicle syndrome?) in baboons with endometriosis. J Soc Gynecol Investig 1996;3:140–4.
30. D'Hooghe TM. Clinical relevance of the baboon as a model for the study of endometriosis. Fertil Steril 1997;68:613–25.
31. Suginami H. A reappraisal of the coelomic metaplasia theory by reviewing endometriosis occurring in unusual sites and instances. Am J Obstet Gynecol 1991;165:214–18.
32. Ueki M. Histologic study of endometriosis and examination of lymphatic drainage in and from the uterus. Am J Obstet Gynecol 1991;165:201–9.
33. Abrao MS, Podgaec S, Dias Jr JA, et al. Deeply infiltrating endometriosis affecting the rectum and lymph nodes. Fertil Steril 2006;86:543–7.
34. Lauchlan SC. The secondary mullerian system revisited. Int J Gynecol Pathol 1994;13:73–9.
35. Oral E, Arici A. Pathogenesis of endometriosis. Obstet Gynecol Clin North Am 1997;24:219–33.
36. Acien P, Lloret M, Chehab H. Endometriosis in a patient with Rokitansky-Kuster-Hauser syndrome. Gynecol Obstet Invest 1988;25:70–2.
37. Tazuke SI, Milki AA. Endometrioma of uterine serosa in a woman with mosaic Turner's syndrome receiving hormone replacement therapy. Hum Reprod 2002;17:2977–80.
38. Kim JJ, Kurita T, Bulun SE. Progesterone action in endometrial cancer, endometriosis, uterine fibroids, and breast cancer. Endocr Rev 2013;34:130–62.
39. Ross HL, Bischoff FZ, Elias S. Genetics of endometriosis. In: Diamond MP, Osteen KG, editors. Endometrium and Endometriosis. Oxford: Blackwell Science; 1997. p. 70–4.
40. Vigano P, Somigliana E, Vignali M, et al. Genetics of endometriosis: current status and prospects. Front Biosci 2007;12:3247–55.
41. Wieser F, Wenzl R, Taylor RN, et al. Genetic basis of endometriosis. Gynakologie 2004;37:676–80.
42. Moen MH, Magnus P. The familial risk of endometriosis. Acta Obstet Gynecol Scand 1993;72:560–4.
43. Hadfield RM, Mardon HJ, Barlow DH, Kennedy SH. Endometriosis in monozygotic twins. Fertil Steril 1997;68:941–2.
44. Kennedy S. Is there a genetic basis to endometriosis? Semin Reprod Endocrinol 1997;15:309–18.
45. Kennedy S. The genetics of endometriosis. Eur J Obstet Gynecol Reprod Biol 1999;82:129–33.
46. Liang S, Huang Y, Fan Y. Vascular endothelial growth factor gene polymorphisms and endometriosis risk: a meta-analysis. Arch Gynecol Obstet 2012;286:139–46.
47. Emmert C, Romann D, Riedel HH. Endometriosis diagnosed by laparoscopy in adolescent girls. Arch Gynecol Obstet 1998;261:89–93.
48. Evers JL, Land JA, Dunselman GA, et al. 'The Flemish Giant,' reflections on the defense against endometriosis, inspired by Professor Emeritus Ivo A. Brosens. Eur J Obstet Gynecol Reprod Biol 1998;81:253–8.
49. Chabbert-Buffet N, Pintiaux A, Bouchard P. The imminent dawn of SPRMs in obstetrics and gynecology. Mol Cell Endocrinol 2012;358:232–43.
50. Koninckx PR, Kennedy SH, Barlow DH. Endometriotic disease: the role of peritoneal fluid. Hum Reprod Update 1998;4:741–51.
51. Dmowski WP, Braun DP. Immunologic aspects of endometriosis. In: Diamond MP, Osteen KG, editors. Endometrium and Endometriosis. Oxford: Blackwell Science; 1997. p. 174–81.
52. Dawood MY. Macrophages and macrophage-derived factors in normal reproductive tissues and endometriosis. In: Diamond MP, Osteen KG, editors. Endometrium and Endometriosis. Oxford: Blackwell Science; 1997. p. 146–51.
53. Brosens IA, Brosens JJ. Redefining endometriosis—Is deep endometriosis a progressive disease? Hum Reprod 2000;15:1–3.
54. Trovo de Marqui AB. Genetic polymorphisms and endometriosis: contribution of genes that regulate vascular function and tissue remodeling. Rev Assoc Med Bras 2012;58:620–32.
55. Smith SK. Angiogenesis. Semin Reprod Endocrinol 1997;15:221–7.
56. Donnez J, Van Langendonckt A, Casanas-Roux F, et al. Current thinking on the pathogenesis of endometriosis. Gynecol Obstet Invest 2002;54:52–62.
57. Stratton P, Winkel CA, Sinaii N, et al. Location, color, size, depth, and volume may predict endometriosis in lesions resected at surgery. Fertil Steril 2002;78:743–9.
58. Brosens IA. Endometriosis—a disease because it is characterized by bleeding. Am J Obstet Gynecol 1997;176:263–7.
59. Koninckx PR. Biases in the endometriosis literature. Illustrated by 20 years of endometriosis research in Leuven. Eur J Obstet Gynecol Reprod Biol 1998;81:259–71.
60. Brosens IA. Histologic appearances of endometriosis throughout the pelvis. In: Diamond MP, Osteen KG, editors. Endometrium and Endometriosis. Oxford: Blackwell Science; 1997. p. 27–35.
61. Muzii L, Bianchi A, Bellati F, et al. Histologic analysis of endometriomas: what the surgeon needs to know. Fertil Steril 2007;87:362–6.
62. Fukunaga M, Ushigome S. Epithelial metaplastic changes in ovarian endometriosis. Mod Pathol 1998;11:784–8.
63. Kim KR. Utility of trichrome and reticulin stains in the diagnosis of superficial endometriosis of the uterine cervix. Int J Gynecol Pathol 2001;20:173–6.
64. Jansen RP. Minimal endometriosis and reduced fecundability: prospective evidence from an artificial insemination by donor program. Fertil Steril 1986;46:141–3.
65. Metzger DA, Szpak CA, Haney AF. Histologic features associated with hormonal responsiveness of ectopic endometrium. Fertil Steril 1993;59:83–8.

66. Schwartz JL, Schwartz LB. Extrapelvic endometriosis. In: Diamond MP, Osteen KG, editors. Endometrium and Endometriosis. Oxford: Blackwell Science; 1997. p. 247–54.
67. Insabato L, Pettinato G. Endometriosis of the bowel with lymph node involvement. A report of three cases and review of the literature. Pathol Res Pract 1996;192:957–61.
68. Urbach DR, Reedijk M, Richard CS, Robboy SJ. Bowel resection for intestinal endometriosis. Dis Colon Rectum 1998;41:1158–64.
69. Case records of the Massachusetts general hospital. Weekly clinicopathological exercises. Case 28-1996. A 45-year old woman with abdominal pain and a polypoid mass in the colon. N Engl J Med 1996;335:807–12.
70. Langlois NE, Park KG, Keenan RA. Mucosal changes in the large bowel with endometriosis: a possible cause of misdiagnosis of colitis? Hum Pathol 1994;25:1030–4.
71. Henkel A, Christensen B, Schindler AE. Endometriosis: a clinically malignant disease. Eur J Obstet Gynecol Reprod Biol 1999;82:209–11.
72. Moore WF, Bentley RC, Berchuck A, Robboy SJ. Some mullerian inclusion cysts in lymph nodes may sometimes be metastases from serous borderline tumors of the ovary. Am J Surg Pathol 2000;24:710–18.
73. Canis M, Donnez JG, Guzick DS. Revised American Society for Reproductive Medicine classification of endometriosis: 1996. Fertil Steril 1997;67:817–21.
74. Practice Committee of the American Society for Reproductive Medicine. Endometriosis and infertility: a committee opinion. Fertil Steril 2012;98:591–8.
75. Rock JA, ZOLADEX Endometriosis Study Group. The revised American Fertility Society classification of endometriosis: Reproducibility of scoring. Fertil Steril 1995;63:1108–10.
76. Endometriosis and infertility: a committee opinion. Fertil Steril 2012;98:591–8.
77. Adamson GD, Pasta DJ. Endometriosis fertility index: the new, validated endometriosis staging system. Fertil Steril 2010;94:1609–15.
78. Kwek JW, H'ng MW, Chew SH, Tay EH. Florid polypoid endometriosis of the cervix with left ureteric obstruction: a mimic of cervical malignancy. Ultrasound Obstet Gynecol 2010;36:252–4.
79. Dal Cin P, Vanni R, Marras S, et al. Four cytogenetic subgroups can be identified in endometrial polyps. Cancer Res 1995;55:1565–8.
80. Medeiros F, Wang X, Araujo AR, et al. HMGA gene rearrangement is a recurrent somatic alteration in polypoid endometriosis. Hum Pathol 2012;43:1243–48.
81. Parker RL, Dadmanesh F, Young RH, Clement PB. Polypoid endometriosis—a clinicopathologic analysis of 24 cases and a review of the literature. Am J Surg Pathol 2004;28:285–97.
82. Dadhwal V, Deka D, Mathur S, et al. Vaginal polypoid endometriosis simulating neoplasia in a young woman. J Low Genit Tract Dis 2012;16:318–21.
83. Kwek JW, H'ng MW, Chew SH, Tay EH. Florid polypoid endometriosis of the cervix with left ureteric obstruction: a mimic of cervical malignancy. Ultrasound Obstet Gynecol 2010;36:252–4.
84. Ness RB. Endometriosis and ovarian cancer: thoughts on shared pathophysiology. Am J Obstet Gynecol 2003;189:280–94.
85. Van GT, Amant F, Neven P, et al. Endometriosis and the development of malignant tumours of the pelvis. A review of literature. Best Pract Res Clin Obstet Gynaecol 2004;18:349–71.
86. Kusaka M, Mikuni M, Nishiya M. A case of high-grade endometrial stromal sarcoma arising from endometriosis in the cul-de-sac. Int J Gynecol Cancer 2006;16:895–9.
87. Jones KD, Owen E, Berresford A, Sutton C. Endometrial adenocarcinoma arising from endometriosis of the rectosigmoid colon. Gynecol Oncol 2002;86:220–2.
88. Yazbeck C, Poncelet C, Chosidow D, Madelenat P. Primary adenocarcinoma arising from endometriosis of the rectovaginal septum: a case report. Int J Gynecol Cancer 2005;15:1203–5.
89. Chene G, Darcha C, Dechelotte P, et al. Malignant degeneration of perineal endometriosis in episiotomy scar, case report and review of the literature. Int J Gynecol Cancer 2007;17:709–14.
90. Salerno MG, Masciullo V, Naldini A, et al. Endometrioid adenocarcinoma with squamous differentiation arising from ureteral endometriosis in a patient with no history of gonadal endometriosis. Gynecol Oncol 2005;99:749–52.
91. Liu LT, Davidson S, Singh M. Mullerian adenosarcoma of vagina arising in persistent endometriosis: report of a case and review of the literature. Gynecol Oncol 2003;90:486–90.
92. Shah C, Pizer E, Veljovich DS, et al. Clear cell adenocarcinoma of the vagina in a patient with vaginal endometriosis. Gynecol Oncol 2006;103:1130–2.
93. Soliman NF, Hillard TC. Hormone replacement therapy in women with past history of endometriosis. Climacteric 2006;9:325–35.
94. Brinton LA, Gridley G, Persson I, et al. Cancer risk after a hospital discharge diagnosis of endometriosis. Am J Obstet Gynecol 1997;176:572–9.
95. Melin A, Sparen P, Persson I, Bergqvist A. Endometriosis and the risk of cancer with special emphasis on ovarian cancer. Hum Reprod 2006;21:1237–42.
96. Pearce CL, Templeman C, Rossing MA, et al. Association between endometriosis and risk of histological subtypes of ovarian cancer: a pooled analysis of case-control studies. Lancet Oncol 2012;13:385–94.
97. Malpica A, Deavers MT, Lu K, et al. Grading ovarian serous carcinoma using a two-tier system. Am J Surg Pathol 2004;28:496–504.
98. Kurman RJ, Shih I. Pathogenesis of ovarian cancer: lessons from morphology and molecular biology and their clinical implications. Int J Gynecol Pathol 2008;27:151–60.
99. Munkarah AR. Malignant transformation of endometriosis. In: Diamond MP, Osteen KG, editors. Endometrium and Endometriosis. Oxford: Blackwell Science; 1997. p. 42–6.
100. Toki T, Fujii S, Silverberg SG. A clinicopathologic study on the association of endometriosis and carcinoma of the ovary using a scoring system. Int J Gynecol Cancer 1996;6:68–75.
101. Vercellini P, Parazzini F, Bolis G, et al. Endometriosis and ovarian cancer. Am J Obstet Gynecol 1993;169:181–2.
102. Sainz de la CR, Eichhorn JH, Rice LW, et al. Histologic transformation of benign endometriosis to early epithelial ovarian cancer. Gynecol Oncol 1996;60:238–44.
103. Jimbo H, Yoshikawa H, Onda T, et al. Prevalence of ovarian endometriosis in epithelial ovarian cancer. Int J Gynaecol Obstet 1997;59:245–50.
104. Wei JJ, William J, Bulun S. Endometriosis and ovarian cancer: a review of clinical, pathologic, and molecular aspects. Int J Gynecol Pathol 2011;30:553–68.
105. Yamamoto S, Tsuda H, Takano M, et al. Loss of ARID1A protein expression occurs as an early event in ovarian clear-cell carcinoma development and frequently coexists with PIK3CA mutations. Mod Pathol 2012;25:615–24.

Normal Ovaries, Inflammatory and Non-Neoplastic Conditions

23

Ruthy Shaco-Levy, Stanley J. Robboy

CHAPTER OUTLINE

Anatomy, Histology, and Function	509
Anatomy	509
Histology	509
Physiology	510
Follicular Failure	**517**
Follicular Dysgenesis (Dysplasia)	517
Ovarian Failure	517
Hypogonadotropic Hypogonadism	522
Anomalies of Ovarian Development and Descent	**523**
Ectopic Ovarian Tissue	523
Dystopic Ovaries	523
Ovarian Agenesis	523
Splenogonadal Fusion	523
'Uterus-Like Mass' Replacing Ovary	523
Infectious Inflammatory Diseases	524
Bacterial Oophoritis	524
Viral Oophoritis	526
Parasitic Oophoritis	527
Fungal Oophoritis	529
Noninfectious Inflammatory Diseases	**529**
Sarcoidosis	529
Crohn Disease	529
Cortical Granulomas	530
Isolated Noninfectious Granulomas	530
Autoimmune Oophoritis	530
Necrotizing Arteritis	530
Giant Cell Arteritis	531
Polyarteritis Nodosa	531
Postpartum Ovarian Vein Thrombophlebitis	531

ANATOMY, HISTOLOGY, AND FUNCTION

ANATOMY

The ovaries are paired pelvic organs located close to the uterus, weighing 5–8 g and measure about $3.0 \times 2.0 \times 1.0$ cm in women of reproductive age. They normally shrink in size after menopause. The external surface is smooth until after puberty, when it increasingly convolutes in the normal course of maturation, rupture of the follicles, and repair.

Each ovary is attached along its hilar aspect to the broad ligament by a double fold of peritoneum, the mesovarium (Figure 23.1).[1] The ovarian ligament attaches the ovarian medial pole to the uterine cornu just below and behind the fallopian tube. The lateral pole of the ovary is attached to the pelvic wall by the suspensory ligament (infundibulopelvic ligament), a peritoneal fold containing the principal vascular supply and lymphatic drainage of the ovary. Veins from the left ovary drain into the left renal vein. Those of the right ovary drain into the right renal vein in 10% of women and directly into the inferior vena cava in 90%.[2]

The cut surface of the ovary consists of a narrow white outer cortex and a gray-pink medulla containing follicles and corpora albicantia that are often obvious macroscopically.

HISTOLOGY

The ovary is covered by a single layer of modified mesothelium originating from the celomic epithelium. This highly specialized mesothelial layer is continuous with the mesothelium of the peritoneal cavity at the ovarian hilus. Previously referred to as the 'germinal epithelium,' this layer is more appropriately designated as the 'surface epithelium.' The cells vary from columnar to cuboidal to flat (Figure 23.2). Immunohistochemically, the surface epithelial cells react for cytokeratin (CK)7, vimentin, Ber-EP4, N-cadherin, and calretinin,[3] but generally lack reactivity for CK20, desmin, and CA125. These cells are more active than the peritoneal mesothelial cells to which they are related and secrete or have receptors for inhibin, estrogen, progesterone, and androgens, as well as a range of growth factors and cytokines, such as epidermal growth factor, transforming growth factor-β (TGF-β), and tumor necrosis factor-α (TNF-α).[4] They form a delicate layer that is often partially denuded as a result of handling at surgery. The surface epithelium

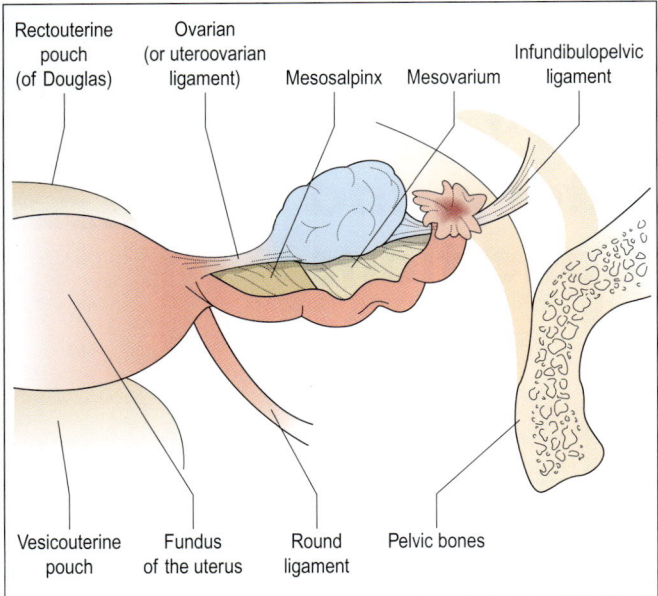

Figure 23.1 Ovarian ligaments. (Reproduced with permission from Prat, 2004.[1])

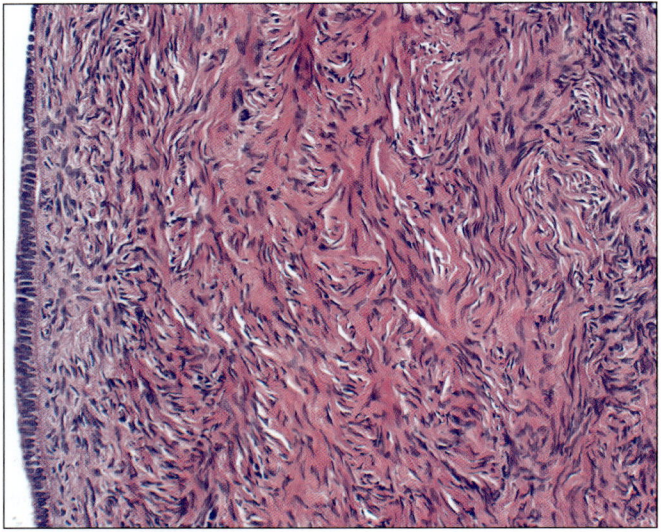

Figure 23.2 Cuboidal surface epithelial cells covering the ovary of a perimenopausal patient. They are separated from the underlying stroma by a distinct basement membrane.

often forms invaginations and inclusion cysts within the ovarian stroma. The ovarian surface epithelium is discussed further in relation to the histogenesis of epithelial tumors in both the ovary and the peritoneum (see Chapters 25 and 31, respectively).

Beneath the ovarian serosa lies the cortex, which is roughly divisible into an outer fibrous, relatively acellular collagenous zone, often termed the 'tunica albuginea,' and an inner, more cellular active cortex. The tunica albuginea is usually a well-defined layer in an active ovary, averaging about 0.3 mm as measured from the surface to the most superficially placed primordial follicle, but in some conditions, notably anovulatory states such as the polycystic ovary syndrome (see later), this outer cortical zone becomes an even more obvious 'capsule,' being wider and more densely collagenous. The underlying cellular part of the cortex contains the primordial, developing, and mature follicles. Its appearance varies considerably at different ages and, to some extent, during the menstrual cycle and pregnancy. The cortical stroma consists of uniform spindled cells arranged in bundles, often with a striking storiform pattern. From these cells derive the luteinized stromal cells and the theca cells that form the outer part of the follicle.

The central portion of the ovary is the medulla and, in young women, consists of active follicles and cellular stroma. The blood vessels, which enter at the hilum, are enmeshed in connective tissue generally poor in cells. As women approach middle age, the medulla fills with corpora albicantia and a meshwork of blood vessels with thick, hyalinized walls that render them more prominent than formerly. After menopause, the cortical stroma characteristically shrinks.

PHYSIOLOGY

OVARIAN DEVELOPMENT

The ovaries' two major functions are (1) release of mature ova at the time of ovulation and (2) the secretion of steroid hormones. Cyclic release of pituitary follicle-stimulating hormone (FSH) and luteinizing hormone (LH) control both functions. In turn, gonadotropin-releasing hormone (GnRH), which the hypothalamus secretes into the pituitary portal circulation, regulates the release of the two hormones. The ovarian steroid hormones stimulate the growth of the reproductive organs, foster the development of secondary sexual characteristics, and help maintain the implanted blastocyst. The production of these hormones depends upon the development and maturation of the follicles and the formation of the corpus luteum.

FOLLICULOGENESIS

The primordial germ cells arise from the yolk sac endoderm and migrate via the hindgut mesentery to the gonadal ridge, the migration commencing 3 weeks after fertilization.[5] At this stage the proliferating germ cells constitute the dominant growth, forming a finite complement of about six million ova by the sixth month of fetal life, to which there is no later addition. This proliferation is evident by the 8th week and is marked by the 13th week when the ovary consists largely of oogonial and oocytic clusters that taper proximally, with 'cords' only in the rete. Pregranulosa cells enclose individual germ cells to form primordial follicles (Figure 23.3A). At the primary oocyte stage, the cells are in the prophase of the first meiotic division and DNA synthesis resumes only in the event of fertilization. At birth, the ovary consists largely of scanty, loose stroma, enclosing primordial and maturing follicles and folded around stems of vascular connective tissue. The characteristic ovarian stroma develops during the first year. The total number of germ cells at birth exhibits a considerable variation around an approximate average of 500,000, already a significant loss from the second trimester maximum.

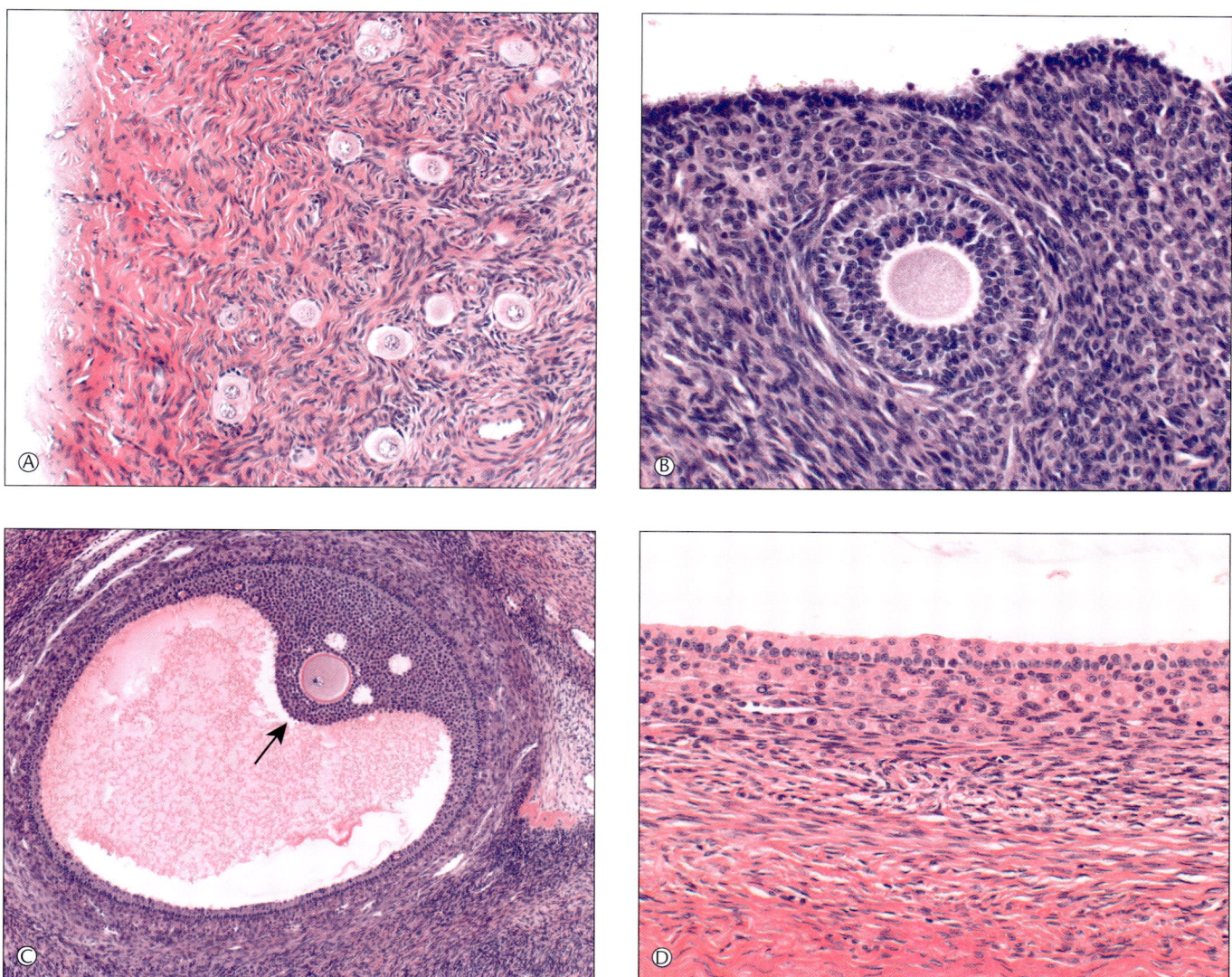

Figure 23.3 Preovulatory follicles. **(A)** Cellular superficial cortex containing a number of primordial follicles. An unusual variation is the presence of binovular follicles. **(B)** A late primary or preantral follicle with a prominent zona pellucida surrounding the ovum and an occasional Call–Exner body within the developing granulosa cell layer (above the ovum). The spindle-shaped cells of the emerging theca are apparent. A regressing cystic follicle forms the upper margin of the field. **(C)** Secondary or graafian follicle with an eccentric cumulus oophorus containing the oocyte (arrow). **(D)** Developing follicle showing the granulosa cell layer subtended by theca interna (plump cells) and theca externa (spindle cells) layers.

FOLLICULAR MATURATION

Follicular maturation begins in the third trimester of intrauterine life, becoming more frequent later. The development of a follicle at this stage of life is followed by its atresia. The number of maturing follicles becomes considerable in the first 2 years of postnatal life, falls to a low level at 4 years, and then increases again. At puberty individual follicles start to rupture and form corpora lutea, which then in turn regress.

Typically, a single dominant follicle develops, resulting in a single ovulation during each cycle. During the early follicular phase selection of a dominant follicle takes place. This complex process involves insulin-like growth factors and locally produced substances.[6–8] The early rise of FSH levels helps recruit the dominant follicle. The transient decrease in FSH during the midfollicular phase prevents development of subdominant follicles. The largest follicle has more granulosa cells and therefore more FSH receptors, enabling its continued growth despite the low FSH levels.[9] Moreover, the dominant follicle's granulosa cells are not only sensitized to FSH but at this stage express LH receptors and therefore respond directly to LH as well as FSH.[10,11]

Follicular maturation comprises enlargement of the ovum, formation of the zona pellucida around it, proliferation of the granulosa cells, and formation of a cavity among the latter. The enlarging follicle expands gradually. Several months are required for a new growing follicle to reach the preantral stage (0.15 mm), and an additional 70 days to reach a 2 mm size. It is likely that several hundred primordial follicles initiate growth each month, but only 20 or so become 'precursor' (preovulatory) follicles. From the time they enter the selectable stage during the late luteal phase, preovulatory follicles become sensitive to cyclic changes of FSH in terms of granulosa cell proliferation. From the mid-follicular phase, the preovulatory follicle synthesizes high quantities of estradiol, and, after the midcycle gonadotropin surge, very large amounts of progesterone. At this stage, the follicle is maximally responsive to gonadotropins, and especially to LH, which triggers granulosa wall dissociation and cumulus expansion as well as oocyte nuclear maturation. At this phase, the follicle is about 2–5 mm in diameter, with a fluid-filled antrum, more than one million granulosa cells, and a single oocyte. The other follicles undergo atresia at an early stage of development. Thus, as the follicle develops, its responsiveness to gonadotropins progressively increases under the control of local factors acting in an autocrine/paracrine fashion.[12] In addition to the critical endocrine signaling pathways between the hypothalamus, pituitary, and ovary, it is now evident that the proteins of the TGF-β superfamily secreted by the oocyte itself are important in influencing the microenvironment of the developing follicle.[13]

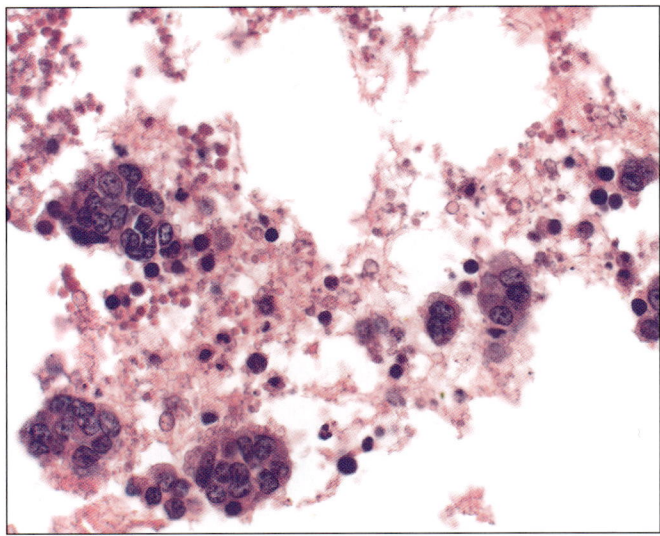

Figure 23.4 Shed granulosa cells from a mature preovulatory follicle.

Granulosa cell proliferation begins when the ovum starts to enlarge. The cells change from flat to cuboidal and then form several layers around the ovum (Figure 23.3B). Small periodic acid–Schiff (PAS)-positive droplets form between the granulosa cells and condense around the ovum to form small spaces. Enlargement or fusion of these spaces produces first an arcuate crevice and then a reniform cavity, the antrum (Figure 23.3C). The granulosa cells form a palisade at the periphery of the follicle and in turn are surrounded by a pale layer of specialized ovarian stroma, the theca interna. A basal lamina separates the granulosa cells from the cells of the theca interna. The theca externa is a poorly defined zone formed by the merging of the theca interna with the surrounding ovarian stroma (Figure 23.3D). Theca cells are fundamental for follicular growth, synthesizing all androgens required by the developing follicles for conversion into estrogens by the granulosa cells, and providing structural support of the growing follicle as it progresses through the developmental stages. Theca cells are likely recruited from surrounding stromal tissue by factors secreted from an activated primary follicle.[14] During maturation, the cytoplasm of the cells comprising the theca interna accumulates lipids, increases in amount, and becomes foamy or granular. In the dominant preovulatory follicle, the theca cell layer is well supplied with blood vessels but the granulosa cell layer remains avascular.

The follicular fluid is a modified transudate from the theca and adjacent vessels, which are believed to become more permeable because of locally released histamine. The same transudative process leads to the development of a loose-textured vascular shell around the outside of the follicle, the theca externa. As the antrum enlarges, the granulosa cell layer generally thins, but persists as a mound, the cumulus oophorus, around the ovum (Figure 23.3C). Granulosa cells aspirated from the developing follicle at this stage tend to be single or in small clusters with scanty amphophilic cytoplasm (Figure 23.4). Outside the cumulus the theca interna shows a corresponding thickening, the theca cone, which has a role in loosening the coherence of the tissues. The mature, preovulatory follicle is known as a graafian follicle. The final phase in follicular maturation is abrupt and largely mediated by the LH surge and a complex interaction of local cytokines.[15] It includes rapid accumulation of follicular fluid, loosening of the theca, and discharge of the fluid contents and ovum with the few attendant granulosa cells that form the corona radiata. The follicle then collapses, taking on a corrugated outline that becomes exaggerated as transformation into a corpus luteum advances. Bleeding into the thecal tissues may occur at about the time of ovulation but, as the granulosa is as yet avascular, there is normally no bleeding into the follicular cavity and peritoneum.

FORMATION OF THE CORPUS LUTEUM

The formation of the corpus luteum comprises two processes: (1) blood vessels grow into the collapsed granulosa cell layer from the theca, carrying theca cells with them (some bleeding now takes place into the cavity and, because of this, the corpus luteum of the current cycle appears bluish when seen through the surface of the ovary); and (2) the cells comprising the granulosa cell layer luteinize (Figure 23.5), the cells becoming strikingly large and pale, and readily distinguishable from the smaller and somewhat less pale luteinized theca cells ('theca–lutein cells'). Ultrastructural studies of the luteinized cells show abundant smooth endoplasmic reticulum with vesicular dilatations, mitochondria with tubular cristae, and numerous small lipid droplets, which are the familiar general features of the steroid-secreting cell.

When pregnancy occurs, the corpus luteum remains unchanged for about 50 days. It then doubles in size during the following 10 days and remains thus enlarged until about day 80, when it begins to shrink as the placenta takes over progesterone production. Hyaline bodies, about 10–20 μm in size, are found sparingly among the luteinized cells only in the corpus luteum of pregnancy (Figure 23.6A). Another

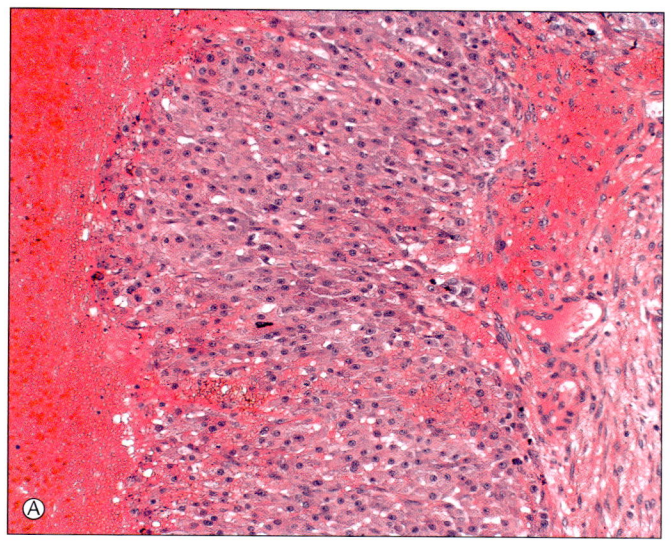
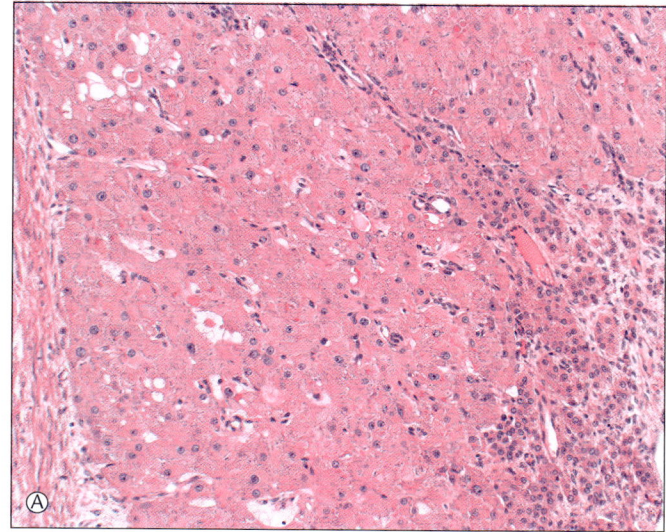
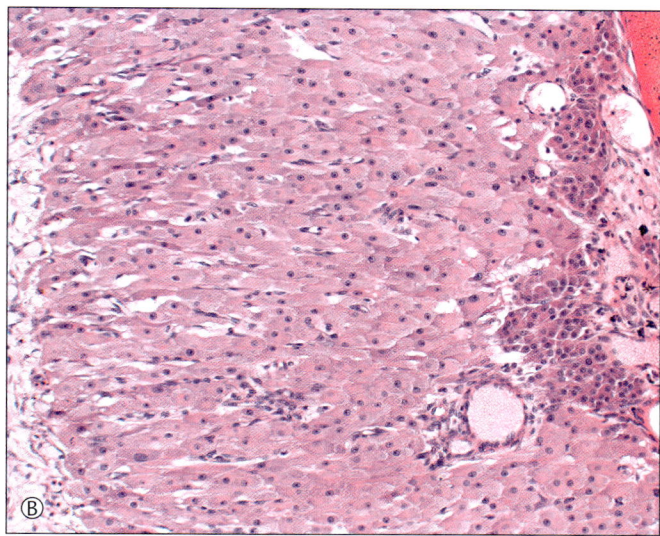
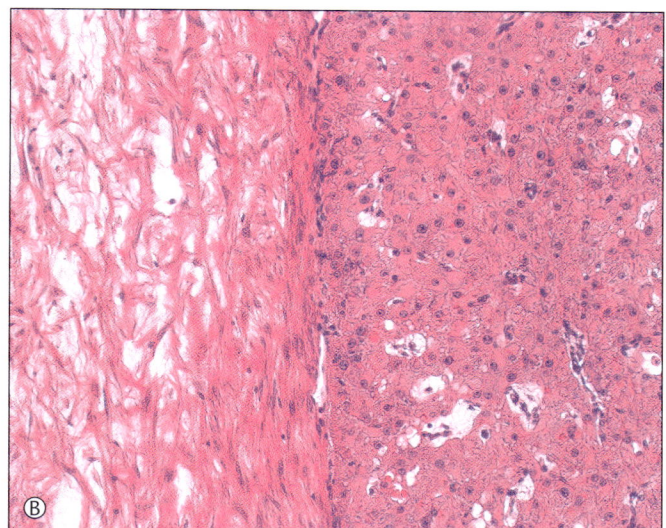

Figure 23.5 Corpus luteum. **(A)** Early corpus luteum with antrum to the left, granulosa lutein layer in the center, and poorly formed theca to the right but no vascularization of the granulosa. **(B)** Mature corpus luteum with vascularized granulosa and immature granulation tissue organizing the central coagulum (right).

Figure 23.6 Corpus luteum of pregnancy. **(A)** Established corpus luteum of pregnancy with organizing granulation tissue lining antrum to the right, granulosa lutein layer in the center, containing scattered hyaline bodies, and theca to the left. **(B)** Active corpus luteum of pregnancy with avascular collagenous connective tissue of many weeks' age.

histologic feature that, when present, distinguishes the corpus luteum of pregnancy from that of menstruation is the organization of the central coagulum to produce mature, avascular, collagenous connective tissue over a time period not available to the corpus luteum of menstruation prior to its programmed involution (Figure 23.6B).

INVOLUTION OF THE CORPUS LUTEUM

Unless stimulated by β-human chorionic gonadotropin (β-hCG), produced by the trophoblast of the fertilized zygote, the corpus luteum begins its programmed involution at about day 9, i.e., about day 23 of a normal 28 day cycle. The biologic mechanisms responsible for this physiologic destructive process of the corpus luteum (structural luteolysis) are complex and centered on apoptosis.[16,17] Hyaline and fatty changes appear to a variable extent in the luteinized granulosa cells (Figure 23.7A), together with an increase of acid phosphatase and PAS-positive intracellular material. This apoptotic change may occur acutely, with frank necrosis (Figure 23.7B). The average corpus luteum reaches about 1.5 cm in maximum size. It has shrunk only slightly by the end of the cycle, but then rapidly gets smaller. As it does so, its wavy lemon-yellow form becomes thinner and the color deepens to a darker yellow or orange. Eventually, the luteal pigment and the cells disappear. After several months, the corpus luteum completes its transformation into a much folded, collapsed shell of white, hyaline collagen, the corpus albicans (Figure 23.7C). Corpora albicantia persist in the medulla and are often conspicuous on the cut surface, particularly in later life. Regression of the corpus

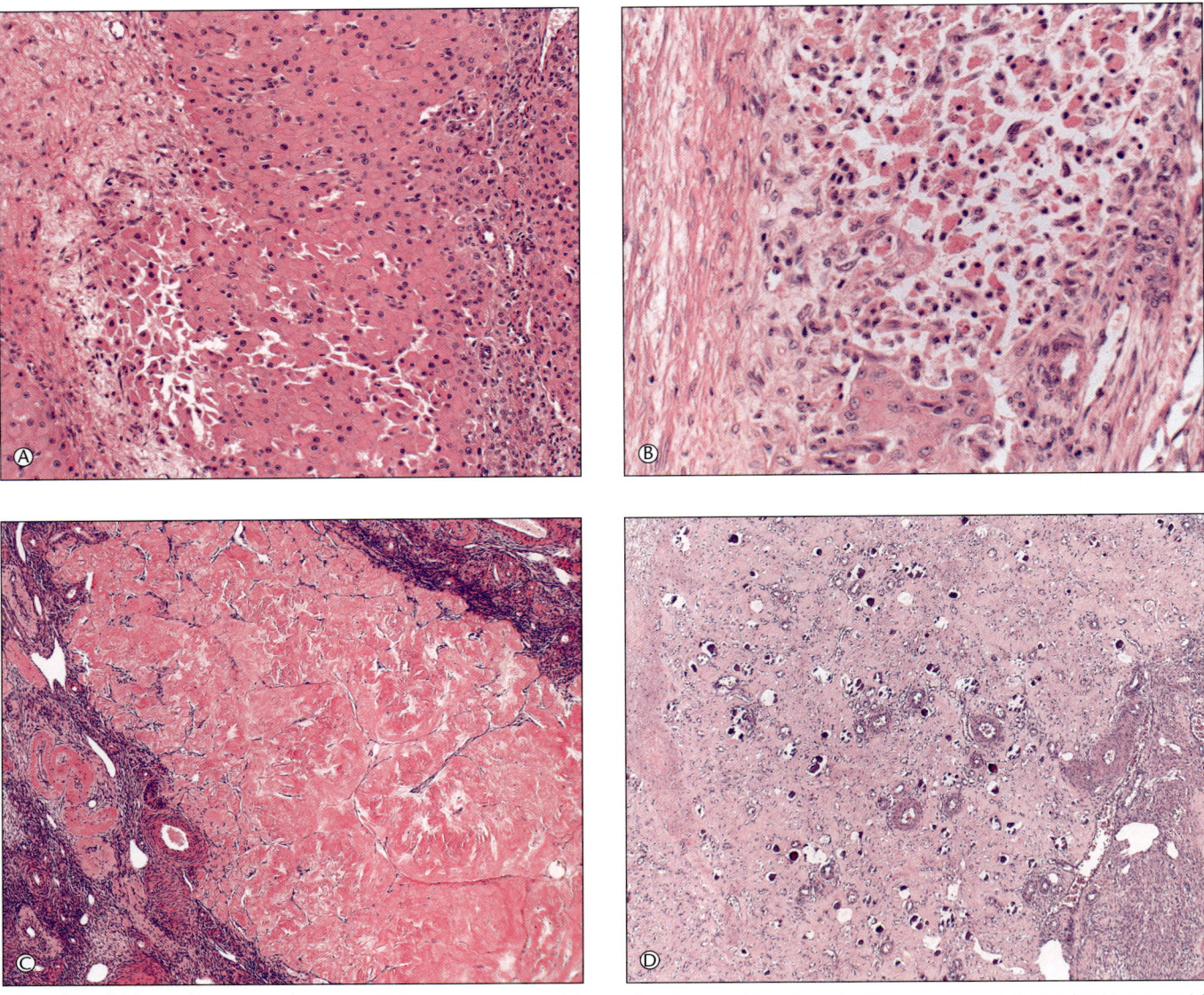

Figure 23.7 Regression of corpus luteum. **(A)** Regressing corpus luteum, showing considerable reduction in size of luteal cells (early apoptosis) and complete vascularization of the granulosa. **(B)** Hyperacute regression (diffuse apoptosis) of a corpus luteum, with frank necrosis. Surviving granulosa cells at the bottom. **(C)** Corpus albicans. **(D)** Regressed corpus luteum of pregnancy with prominent microcalcispherules.

luteum of pregnancy is occasionally accompanied by residual microcalcispherule formation (Figure 23.7D).

FOLLICULAR ATRESIA

During each cycle many follicles start to mature but usually only one ruptures to form a corpus luteum. Occasionally, two or three synchronous corpora lutea are found (one mechanism of multiple pregnancies). The follicles that do not complete maturation become atretic. In atretic antral follicles, granulosa cells stop proliferating and become apoptotic. Atresia may start at any stage during maturation and proceeds at rates varying from follicle to follicle and in different parts of the same follicle.[18,19] Atresia is triggered by a lack of some essential factors supporting follicular development. Specifically, terminal follicular development is strictly dependent upon gonadotropin supply (FSH, then LH in the final preovulatory stage). In addition, paracrine factors (growth factors, CKs, steroids, constituents of extracellular matrix) also play important roles in amplifying gonadotropin action in follicular cells.[20] The features of atresia include degeneration and shrinkage of the ovum; apoptosis of the granulosa cells or their transformation into connective tissue cells (Figure 23.8A); reversion of the cells of the theca interna to their original stromal form; invasion and obliteration of the shrinking cavity by stromal cells; and the formation of a hyalinized, collagenous membrane at the margin of the follicle. Eventually, the hyaline membrane alone persists to mark the site of the former follicle, which now appears as a compact white or gray nodule with a wavy outline, the corpus fibrosum (Figure 23.8B).

Macrophages laden with lipofuscin may accumulate around corpora albicantia and corpora fibrosa and may remain there for long periods. Care should be taken not to confuse degenerating luteinized cells containing lipofuscin and old hemorrhage with endometriosis.

CHAPTER 23 — NORMAL OVARIES, INFLAMMATORY AND NON-NEOPLASTIC CONDITIONS

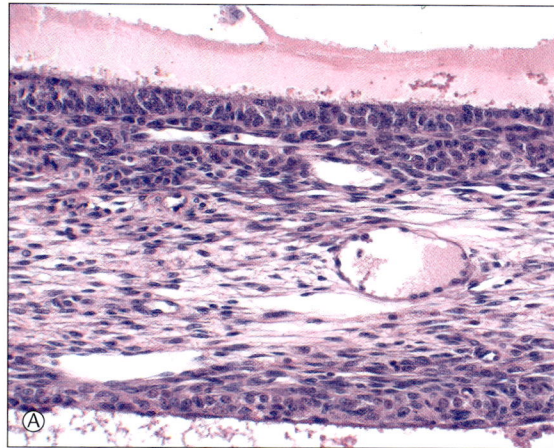

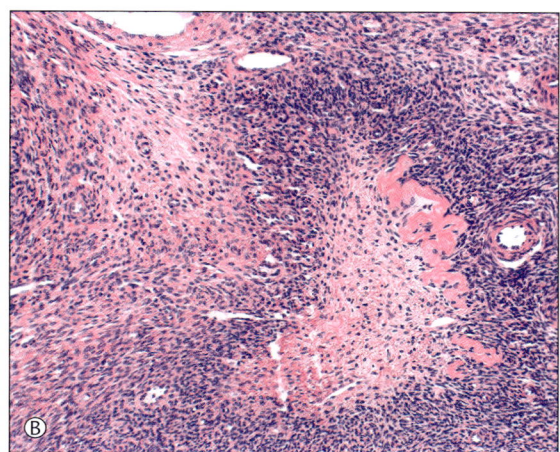

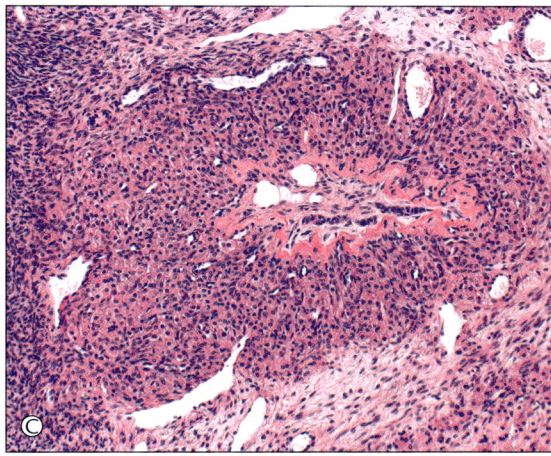

Figure 23.8 Follicular atresia. **(A)** Adjacent cystic follicles with early atresia in the lower follicle. The granulosa is degenerate and has been partly shed into the antrum. **(B)** Small follicle showing advanced atresia with typical festooned contour and fibroblastic tissue occupying the site of the original antrum. **(C)** Atretic follicle in early pregnancy displaying partial luteinization of the theca interna layer and central persistence of small cords of granulosa cells.

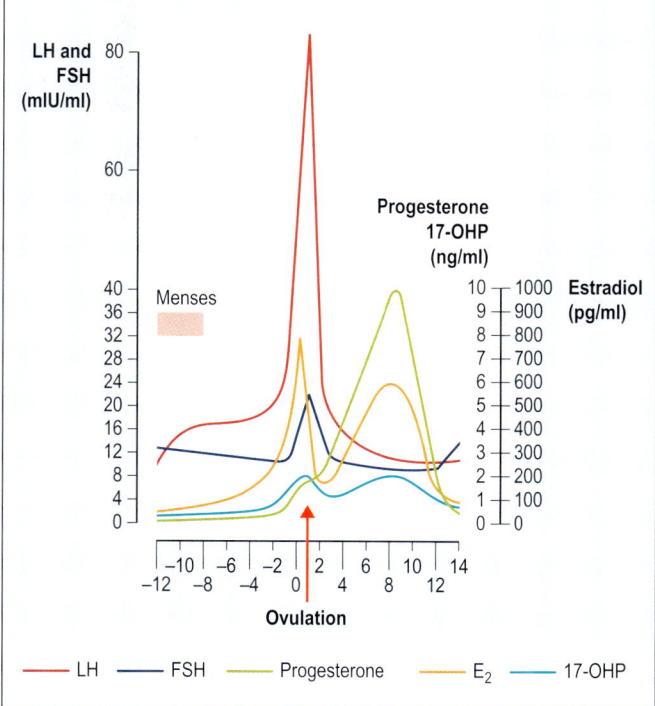

Figure 23.9 Normal menstrual cycle: plasma hormone levels. Ovulation occurs just after LH peak; 17-OHP, 17-α-hydroxyprogesterone. (Reproduced with permission from Prat, 2004.[1])

During pregnancy, follicle maturation and atresia diminish in the first 10 weeks. They then become more active and are associated with marked theca-cell luteinization (Figure 23.8C). The cellular stroma left after follicular atresia contributes to production of the cellular stroma that typifies the mature ovary and is absent at birth. Stroma formation depends largely on follicular activity and is depressed if follicles are lacking or inactive and increased if maturation and atresia are excessive, as in polycystic ovary syndrome. The medullary and juxtahilar stroma thus has a direct 'follicular' ancestry, which makes it easier to understand why the tumors that may rarely arise from it are similar to those that develop in the functioning cortical stroma, i.e., tumors of sex cord–stromal type.

THE HORMONAL BACKGROUND OF THE OVARIAN CYCLE

The normal menstrual (ovarian) cycle is depicted in Figure 23.9. Increasing levels of FSH stimulation are required for follicular growth.[21] Follicular antrum formation and antral expansion are absolutely dependent on pituitary FSH to which the larger follicles are more responsive. Early antral follicles (≤5 mm) develop normally even in infant ovaries but preovulatory (≥20 mm) growth depends on the adult FSH levels reached in ovulatory menstrual cycles and on the follicle capacity for estrogen synthesis. Follicular estrogens feeding back to the hypothalamic–pituitary axis control gonadotropin secretion, the secretion of FSH showing peaks on about days 4 and 14. Local interaction between estrogens and gonadotropins helps to coordinate preovulatory follicular maturation. Signaling by the gonadal paracrine activin and inhibin, which are members of the TGF-β superfamily, is crucial for follicular and oocyte development.[22,23] Immature antral follicles produce activin that enhances granulosa cell sensitivity and responsiveness to FSH, thus promoting follicular development, and simultaneously suppresses thecal androgen synthesis. Appropriate stimulation by FSH diverts the follicle to formation of inhibin, which suppresses the secretion of FSH and promotes androgen synthesis by LH-stimulated theca cells. Androgens in turn synergize with FSH to augment inhibin synthesis.

LH acts on specific receptors on theca cells to stimulate androgen production, with positive correlations between androgen receptor expression and follicular cell proliferation.[15] Furthermore, androgens are active through a conversion to estrogens in granulosa cells. The acute follicular enlargement leading to ovulation is associated with the peak of LH secretion on day 14 of the normal 28 day cycle, triggered by estrogen secreted by the dominant follicle. If pregnancy does not ensue, the corpus luteum's life span is maximally about 14 days. As mentioned previously, its degeneration begins by day 23 (day 9 postovulation). Its persistence during that time depends on the continuous low level of LH secretion, but on no other known luteotrophic stimulus. When pregnancy occurs, chorionic gonadotropin fosters maintenance of the corpus luteum.

All known steroidogenic sites in the ovary produce each of the main ovarian hormones from acetate by way of cholesterol. These include progesterone, androstenedione, testosterone, dihydroandrosterone, estradiol, and estrone 1, which are the main successive stages in cholesterol transformation. The exact roles of the granulosa cells and theca cells in the preovulatory follicle are difficult to study; the complex inter-relationships of the cells to each other are virtually impossible to reproduce *in vitro*. However, clearly the granulosa cells can synthesize pregnenolone and progesterone and convert androgens to estrogens by aromatization. Thecal tissue produces mainly androstenedione, with small amounts of estradiol. As the granulosa cell layer in the preovulatory follicle is avascular, the hormonal environment of these cells (and also that of the oocyte) is different from that of the blood. It is dependent, in part, upon the activity of the adjacent theca cells. Thus, the products of the granulosa cells must diffuse through at least some of the theca cell layer to reach the ovarian venous blood. While follicular fluid analysis gives only an indirect indication of the activity of both types of follicular cells, the dominant and therefore the most active preovulatory follicle in an ovary has the highest levels of estradiol in the fluid. This dominant follicle has the highest estrogen:androgen ratio in its secreted hormones of all the follicles and its granulosa cells have the highest capacity for androgen aromatization *in vitro*. Aromatase activity in the granulosa cells falls off shortly before ovulation, and synthesis of progesterone commences just prior to ovulation in response to the LH surge.

The levels of LH, FSH, and estradiol fall after ovulation, but there is sufficient LH to maintain the sensitive luteinized granulosa cells of the corpus luteum. Together the luteinized theca cells and luteinized granulosa cells of the corpus luteum produce both estradiol and its major product progesterone. Normal corpus luteum function depends on numerous regulatory factors, such as prostaglandins, oxytocin, steroids, growth factors, cytokines, and so forth.[24] The theca cells produce primarily estrogen and the luteinized granulosa cells produce mainly progesterone, which is reflected in the high plasma progesterone level during this phase of the cycle and the high pregnanediol excretion from the time of ovulation until the day or two preceding menstruation. Both hormones reach their peak in the midsecretory phase of the cycle, when estradiol levels are similar to those of the mid to late follicular phase. The stromal tissue produces mainly androstenedione, which has about one-tenth the androgenic activity of testosterone and is partly converted into the latter peripherally. The effects of these hormones on the pituitary are largely mediated through the hypothalamus. Secretion of FSH is inhibited by sufficient amounts of either estrogens or progesterone; the effect of estrogens on LH secretion is thought to be biphasic, and is stimulatory over a short length of time and inhibitory in the long term.

The ovaries are the primary source of androgens in the postmenopausal period when testosterone production in particular is maintained or even boosted, presumably due to increased stimulation of the ovarian stroma by LH.

THE OVARIAN HILUM AND ITS VICINITY

The rete ovarii consists of multiple intercommunicating channels lined by deeply staining, cuboidal to flattened epithelial cells exhibiting a characteristically angular, jagged-looking cross section (Figure 23.10). Nearer to the ovary the rete tubules are more rounded in outline and in this situation they often show traces of a muscle and connective tissue covering. The origin of the rete ovarii is disputed. It is generally considered as homologous with the straight seminiferous tubules of the testis. The relevant immunoprofile of the rete tubules includes strong reactivity for CD10[25] and non-reactivity for calretinin.[3]

Small groups of lutein-like cells are found in the mesovarium and in the ovarian hilum, often adjacent to nerves. These are the so-called 'ovarian hilar' (hilum or hilus) cells (Figure 23.11). They resemble the interstitial cells of the testis (Leydig cells) and contain lipofuscin pigment and

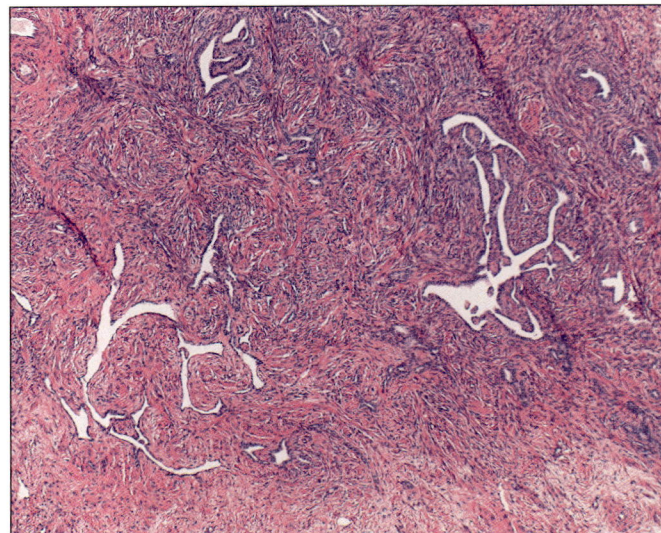

Figure 23.10 Normal rete ovarii, with jagged branching of slit-like epithelial-lined spaces.

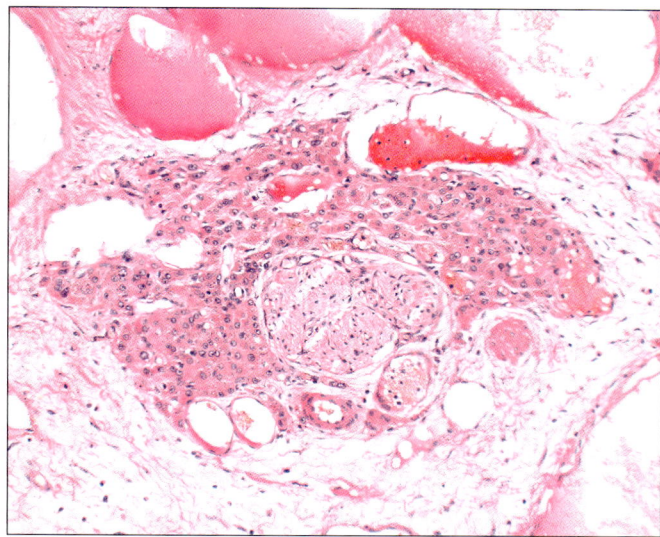

Figure 23.11 Hilus cells. Aggregate of hilus cells in close apposition to both autonomic nerve and dilated vascular spaces.

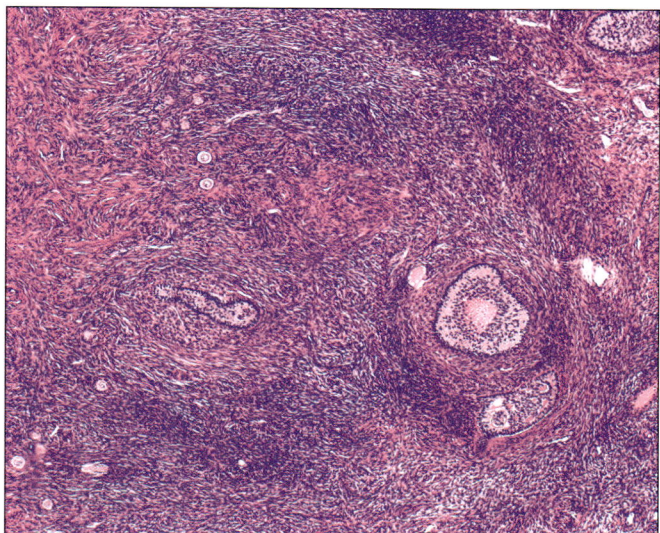

Figure 23.12 Dysplastic follicles in partial resistant ovary syndrome. Bizarre-shaped follicles with normal primordial follicles at top left.

Reinke crystals. They produce both androgens and estrogens and express α-inhibin and calretinin.[3]

FOLLICULAR FAILURE

FOLLICULAR DYSGENESIS (DYSPLASIA)

Definition

Dysplastic primary (preantral) and secondary (antral) follicles are occasionally encountered in otherwise normally functioning ovaries. The term 'follicular dysgenesis' has been applied to polyovular primordial follicles (i.e., containing two or more oocytes; see Figure 23.3A). However, we believe it is most appropriately applied to developing follicles that differ morphologically from normal by disorganized proliferated granulosa, frequently without an antrum despite the follicular size, and containing multiple Call–Exner bodies (Figure 23.12). Microscopically, these lesions have been likened to gonadoblastoma. They occur frequently (25%) in the ovaries of infants and young children. A similar morphologic pattern is seen in some cases of documented hypergonadotropic premature ovarian failure (POF) (Figures 23.12 and 23.13), but the relationship of the follicular changes to altered hypothalamic–pituitary–ovarian function remains unclear. Dysplastic follicles also occur in cases of autoimmune oophoritis and ovarian fibromatosis (see later).

Microscopic Features

The follicular outline is distorted with irregular extensions into the adjacent stroma (Figure 23.12). Sometimes follicular fragmentation produces small nests or cords of granulosa cells. Mitoses are reduced in these cells. Rarely, the cells contain cytoplasmic lipid. A prominent cuff of focally or partially luteinized theca interna cells surrounds about one-third of dysplastic follicles. Atresia of the dysplastic follicles is generally accompanied by persistent granulosa, a

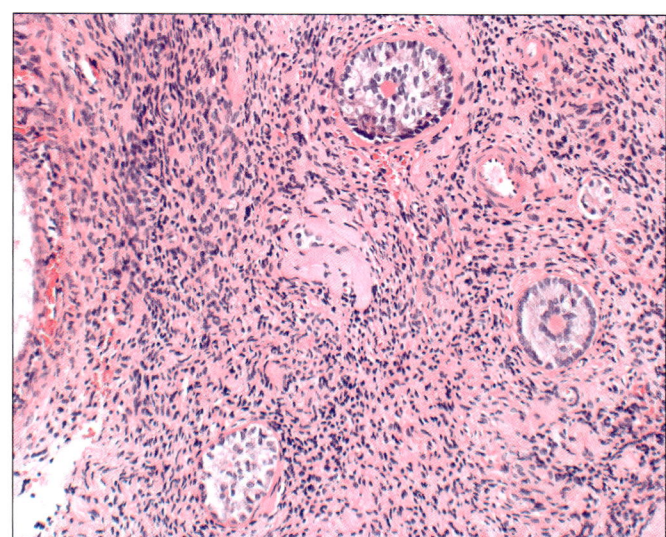

Figure 23.13 Dysplastic follicles in partial resistant ovary syndrome. Higher power of dysplastic follicles showing superficial resemblance to structures seen in SCTAT associated with the Peutz–Jeghers syndrome.

phenomenon only occasionally observed in normal ovaries. Occasional dysplastic follicles show convoluted and rounded deposits of hyaline PAS-positive material similar to, and continuous with, the basement membrane (glassy membrane) of the regressing follicles. These deposits are interposed between the cords of granulosa cells in a manner resembling sex cord tumors with annular tubules (SCTAT).

OVARIAN FAILURE

Definition

Failure of the ovary to ovulate or even to produce its steroids may result from multiple factors, ranging from never functioning or functioning abnormally from the start, or more commonly failing at some later time in life.

Ovarian failure may be associated with either elevated or depressed gonadotropin levels:

- *Hypergonadotropic hypogonadism* (primary ovarian failure) results from a congenital or acquired intrinsic ovarian defect, or failure of the ovaries to respond to pituitary gonadotropins despite the presence of follicles.
- *Hypogonadotropic hypogonadism* is due to failure of the pituitary gland to secrete gonadotropins (FSH and LH) in amounts sufficient to stimulate the ovaries.

Both primary ovarian failure and hypogonadotropic hypogonadism can present as primary or secondary amenorrhea. The median age at menopause in Western populations of women is approximately 51 years. While about 5% of women experience 'early' cessation of ovarian function at or prior to age 45, 1% of women experience POF, classically defined as 4–6 months of amenorrhea under the age of 40 years associated with menopausal levels of serum gonadotropins (FSH > 30U/I) and hypoestrogenism.[26] It represents a major cause of female infertility and renders remarkable impact on women's health due to premature osteoporosis, vaginal dryness, increased risk for cardiovascular disease, and shortened life span.[27–29] The human ovary is endowed at birth with a fixed number of primordial follicles, which steadily decreases throughout life due to atresia and recruitment for ovulation.[30] A causal relationship between follicular depletion and normal menopause clearly exists and there is a gradual acceleration toward follicular wastage, commencing more than a decade before cessation of menstrual activity. This suggests that follicle dynamics rather than neuroendocrine function determines the onset of menopause, both normal and premature.

POF is most commonly idiopathic,[27] but four broad etiologic categories are known:[31–33]

1. *Genetic.* Clear-cut X chromosome deletions or transpositions,[34–36] particularly those in the critical region, result in a truncated reproductive life span. Autosomal anomalies are less frequent causes.[37]
2. *Autoimmune.* POF may accompany any autoimmune polyglandular failure syndrome, most often in linkage with antithyroid and antiadrenal antibodies.[38,39]
3. *Iatrogenic.* Repeated ovarian surgery, uterine vascular embolization,[40] the underlying disease that led to surgery, or chemotherapy may trigger the failure.[41]
4. *Environmental.* Environmental toxins are difficult to pinpoint but, among others, industrial toxins[42,43] and galactose consumption[44] have been implicated.

Clinical Features

Ovarian failure affects approximately 1 in 10,000 women by age 20; 1 in 1000 women by age 30; 1 in 100 women by age 40.[45] Ovarian failure divides into two broad clinicopathologic subtypes: (1) premature follicular depletion, which has been recently termed primary ovarian insufficiency,[46] a state of irreversible ovarian failure due to depleted follicles (afollicular ovarian failure), and (2) the much rarer resistant ovary syndrome ('gonadotropin insensitivity syndrome'), in which primordial follicles are present but fail to respond appropriately to gonadotropin stimulation

Table 23.1 Ovarian Failure: Pathologic and Etiologic Classification

Afollicular (Premature Follicular Depletion, True Premature Menopause)

Exogenous (iatrogenic)
  Surgery
  Radiation
  Chemotherapeutic and other drugs
  Environmental toxins
Endogenous (spontaneous)
  Chromosomal, genetic, maldeveloped gonads
    Familial
    Galactosemia
    Mucopolysaccharidosis
    Blepharophimosis
    Malouf syndrome
    Perrault syndrome
    Roberts-SC phocomelia syndrome
  Autoimmune
  Infection (mumps, others)
  Hemorrhage
  Malignant infiltration
  Idiopathic

Follicular (Savage Syndrome, Gonadotropin-insensitivity Syndrome)

Idiopathic resistant ovary syndrome
Chronic (autoimmune) oophoritis
Galactosemia
Blepharophimosis

(follicular ovarian failure). This separation into afollicular and follicular forms is somewhat artificial, since many of the former are very likely end stages of various disorders. This distinction is nonetheless useful clinically, since premature follicular depletion signifies permanent loss of reproductive function.

Although ovarian biopsy, currently by minilaparoscopic techniques through a 2 mm port,[47] is not necessary for the diagnosis of ovarian failure, it is the best means to distinguish afollicular from follicular types and is therefore useful in counseling patients desiring pregnancy.[48] Recent research suggests that serum anti-müllerian hormone (AMH) levels can differentiate follicular from afollicular patients.[49,50] AMH is produced by the granulosa cells of early developing follicles, therefore serum AMH level is proportional to the number of small antral follicles; it is decreased with age and undetectable in the postmenopausal period.[51,52]

A combined pathologic and etiologic classification of ovarian failure is given in Table 23.1.

AFOLLICULAR OVARIAN FAILURE (PRIMARY OVARIAN INSUFFICIENCY, PREMATURE FOLLICULAR DEPLETION)

Etiology

Sometimes the cause of POF is obvious from the patient's history, e.g., bilateral oophorectomy, prior radiation, or chemotherapy. These exogenous or iatrogenic factors are discussed later.

In most cases, the etiology is unknown.[53] Genetic abnormalities more commonly present with primary rather than secondary amenorrhea, and include perturbations of the X chromosomes[27,34,36,45,46,54,55] as well as autosomal defects. Normal ovarian function requires two functioning X chromosomes.[28] The most obvious genetic cause of primary afollicular ovarian failure is Turner's syndrome, with complete or near complete loss of the second X chromosome.[28] Other well-documented causes of primary afollicular ovarian failure are mixed gonadal dysgenesis (Swyer syndrome; 46,XY), and so-called 'pure gonadal dysgenesis' (46,XX).[56] Additional reported associations include 47,XXX,[57] 48,XXXX,[58] 45,X/46,XX mosaicism,[59,60] structurally abnormal X chromosomes,[61] and balanced[62] and unbalanced[63] translocations of the X chromosome, including deletions of the distal portions of the Xq encompassing the fragile X locus.[64] The fragile X syndrome results from hypermethylation of the FMR1 gene causing the gene to be transcriptionally silenced. Recent reports of premutation-specific phenotypes unrelated to fragile X syndrome have shown up to 20-fold increased risks for POF among female carriers.[65,66]

About 10% of patients with POF have a family member with the same condition and a higher percentage if presenting during their teenage years. Some have a known specific genetic abnormality such as galactosemia. The mechanism of ovarian damage in galactosemia remains unknown, but appears to be independent of dietary management and most investigators favor a toxic effect of galactose or its metabolites on germ cells/follicular structures.[44,67,68] Ovarian failure occurs in females with the blepharophimosis, ptosis, and epicanthus inversus syndrome (BPES), a human disorder caused by mutations in the transcription factor gene *FOXL2* of chromosome 3 and shows facial dysmorphism,[69] and rarely in association with the Malouf syndrome,[70] Perrault syndrome,[71] Roberts-SC phocomelia syndrome,[72] noggin mutation,[73,74] cutis marmorata telangiectatica congenita syndrome,[75] Mulibrey nanism,[76,77] and specific types of leukodystrophy.[78]

The contribution of infections (including viral diseases) to POF is uncertain. Mumps oophoritis, although suspected clinically, has not been documented pathologically.

Although the etiology remains elusive in most cases with a normal 46,XX karyotype, ovarian autoimmune reaction occurs in 4–5% of women with ovarian insufficiency.[79] Clinical gonadal failure is found in both type I and type II autoimmune polyendocrine syndromes.[12,80] These include Addison's,[81] Grave's, and Hashimoto's diseases, rheumatoid arthritis,[82] myasthenia gravis,[83] diabetes mellitus,[84] pernicious anemia,[85] hypoparathyroidism,[85,86] and systemic lupus erythematosus,[87] ranging, in some studies, in up to 20–40% of patients with POF.

Further support lies in finding antiovarian antibodies in many POF patients (both with and without associated autoimmune disorders), and reports of response to corticosteroid therapy. Ovarian antibodies occur at a higher frequency in infertile women than in the general female population.[88] Antibodies in patients' sera have reacted against steroid-producing cells, gonadotropins and their receptors, corpus luteum, zona pellucida, and oocytes,[89] as well as producing a cytotoxic effect on granulosa cells in culture. Because of the association with other autoimmune diseases, investigation and close follow-up are recommended in such patients with POF.[79]

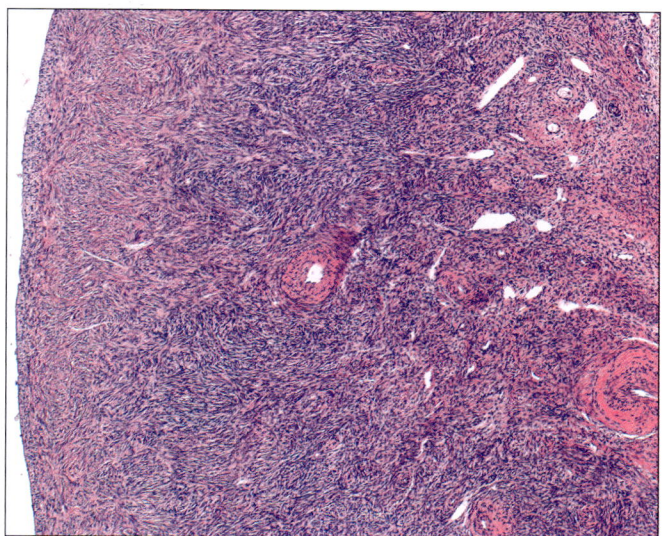

Figure 23.14 Premature follicular depletion. Dense cortical stroma devoid of primordial or developing follicles.

Some patients with premature follicular depletion have no etiologic factor that can be demonstrated clinically or histologically. Such unexplained cases may be due to an as yet undefined genetic defect resulting in congenitally small ovaries with reduced numbers of primordial follicles, or increased utilization of follicles or rapid follicular atresia.

Microscopic Features

The cortical stroma is dense and hypercellular and notable for a complete absence of primordial and antral follicles (Figure 23.14), although a rare primordial follicle does not exclude the diagnosis. Serosal epithelial inclusions are common, and care is needed to avoid confusing the smaller ones with primordial or preantral follicles. Atretic follicles (usually at corpus fibrosum stage) may be present, which indicates previous follicular activity. The deeper cortex and medulla often show evidence of previous ovulation, most commonly as corpora albicantia, but occasionally regressing corpora lutea. If there is no evidence of past or present follicular activity, nor any apparent corticomedullary differentiation, it may be difficult, especially in small laparoscopic biopsies, to confidently differentiate such an ovary from a streak (see above). Minor stromal changes may be present, such as small clusters of luteinized stromal cells or minor inflammatory foci that, in serial sections, exhibit no relationship to follicular remnants. It is reasonable to speculate that such infiltrates represent the end result of a chronic autoimmune oophoritis.

Treatment

Hormone replacement therapy remains the cornerstone of treatment, relieving menopausal symptoms and providing cardiovascular and bone protection.[90,91] The only solution presently available for the fertility problem is *in vitro* fertilization using donor oocytes.[27,92] Recent developments and sporadic success with physiologic estradiol/progesterone replacement cycles and cryopreservation of oocytes from unstimulated follicles[93] offer promise of alternatives to oocyte donation programs.

FOLLICULAR OVARIAN FAILURE. RESISTANT OVARY SYNDROME (SAVAGE SYNDROME, GONADOTROPIN-INSENSITIVITY SYNDROME)

Definition

Premature ovarian failure (POF) with continuous hypersecretion of pituitary gonadotropins, numerous morphologically normal ovarian primordial follicles, most with no evidence of development, and insensitivity of the ovaries to exogenous stimulation by human gonadotropins, even in massive doses. A rare follicle may reach the preantral stage and occasional follicles will reach the antral stage. In cases of secondary amenorrhea, stigmata of previous ovulation are usually present. Approximately 10% of cases of ovarian failure fall into this group.

Etiology

An established association exists in general between autoimmune disease and POF (see above), but this has not been specifically or widely extended to resistant ovary syndrome until studies reported a strong association between the latter and myasthenia gravis.[94] The key appears to be via blocking antibodies to the FSH receptor, analogous to the blocking antibodies of the acetylcholine receptor of myasthenia gravis. Some patients suffer from galactosemia or BPES and the overlap between afollicular and follicular variants of POF only adds uncertainty to etiology.

The history of apparently normal menstrual activity prior to the onset of symptoms and a resistance to exogenous gonadotropins suggests that the resistant ovary syndrome is usually an acquired disorder not related to any intrinsic abnormality of FSH. Since gonadotropin receptors are modulated by local estrogen production, an abnormality in estrogen metabolism may also be causative. Possibly, in the physiologic perimenopausal period, the last remaining follicles are relatively resistant to gonadotropin stimulation and that, by analogy, the picture of resistant ovary syndrome in women with POF may merely reflect a stage of premature perimenopause preceding total follicular depletion.

Microscopic Features

The cortical stroma appears uniformly dense and superficially sclerotic. Primordial follicles are variable in number and, as in normal ovaries, there is a tendency to clustering (Figure 23.15). Adequately sized biopsies and step-sectioning of these assume some importance in this context. Ova are histologically viable. In cases of partial ovarian resistance, i.e., those with some follicular development, dysplastic primary follicles are commonly observed. These are often enlarged and have rounded or irregular profiles outlined by thickened basement membranes. Call–Exner bodies may be numerous. Sometimes the granulosa cells are broken up by hyaline material forming small round nodules and ribbons in a pattern resembling that seen in SCTAT (see Chapter 28; Figure 23.13). Sometimes the hyaline material almost completely replaces the follicles. Morphologically similar follicles have been found in ovaries of stillborn fetuses, infants, and children, and have been most commonly identified in fetuses of 30–41 weeks' gestational age,

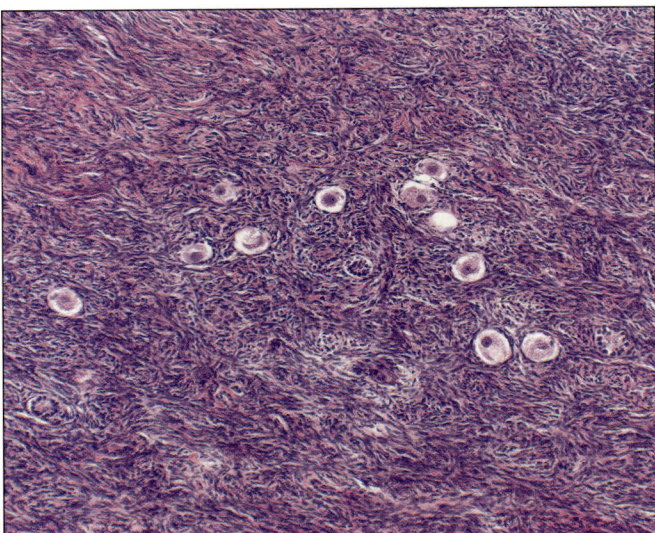

Figure 23.15 Resistant ovary syndrome in a patient with galactosemia. Cluster of primordial follicles in dense cortical stroma. No inflammatory infiltrate present.

a period when massive physiologic reduction of oocytes normally occurs. In occasional cases, oocytes are replaced by non-laminated granular basophilic material that may or may not be calcium. Rare early antral follicles may be present and evidence of previous ovulation, e.g., corpora albicantia, is not unexpected. Follicular atresia, when present, appears to be normal, with disappearance of the granulosa.

Behavior and Treatment

Ovarian resistance to gonadotropins may be relative rather than absolute. The process may be episodic, with known spontaneous remissions.[91,95,96] Thus, ovarian function and reproductive capacity are not necessarily irreversibly lost in such patients and, in fact, several reports note return of menses and, rarely, pregnancies following a diagnosis of resistant ovary syndrome. Estrogen therapy and high-dose gonadotropin therapy sometimes overcome the ovarian 'resistance.' In addition, high dosages of corticosteroids induced ovulation in POF patients with autoimmune phenomena.[39]

AUTOIMMUNE OOPHORITIS

Etiology

Some cases of POF may result from an abnormal self-recognition by the immune system. Between 10% and 30% of women with POF have a concurrent autoimmune disease, most commonly hypothyroidism, hyopoadrenalism, myasthenia gravis, systemic lupus erythematosus, rheumatoid arthritis, and Crohn disease. Autoimmune attack on the ovary might be general or partial and reversible, responsible for the fluctuating and variable courses.[97] Antiovarian autoantibodies (against steroid cells, gonadotropin receptors, and zona pellucida, as well as oocyte cytoplasm) are usually considered to be a suitable and independent marker of autoimmune ovarian disease, although their specificity and pathogenic role are questionable, as they are also often found in normal women.[31,98,99] Furthermore, the exact role

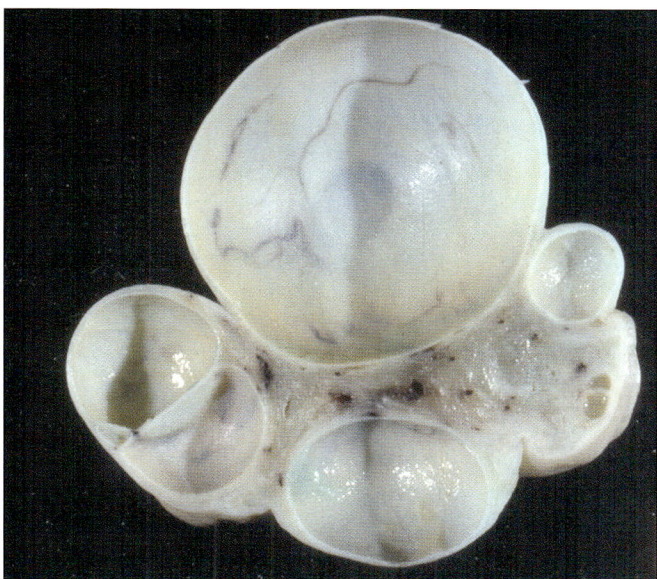

Figure 23.16 Autoimmune oophoritis displaying multiple large cystic follicles.

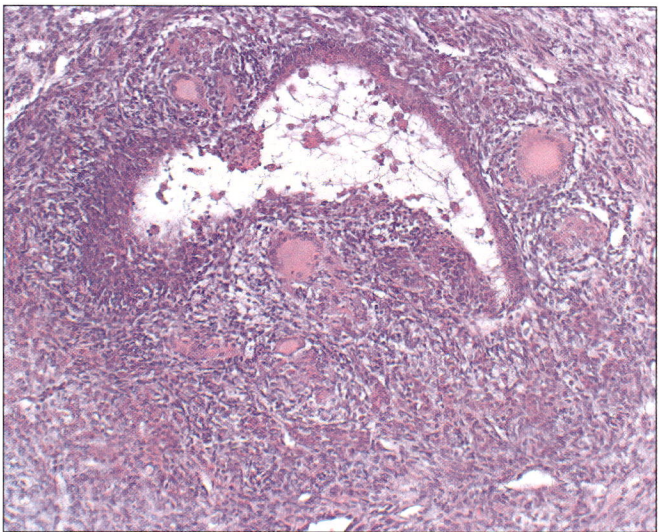

Figure 23.17 Chronic oophoritis in an 18-year-old woman with POF. Perifolliculitis which includes a well-formed sarcoid-like granuloma.

of cellular immunity and the efficiency of immunosuppressive therapy should be further clarified.

Gross Features

The ovaries are often of normal size, but many are greatly enlarged and even multicystic (Figure 23.16).

Microscopic Features

The characteristic sign of autoimmune oophoritis is follicles with an inflammatory infiltrate, usually as a mixture of B-cells (including plasma cells), T-cells (both CD4+ and CD8+), macrophages, and a few natural killer cells, sometimes with a granulomatous and eosinophilic reaction directed at follicular cells[100] (Figure 23.17). The infiltrate envelops the theca interna of developing follicles—the more advanced the follicles, the denser the inflammatory infiltrate and the greater the preponderance of plasma cells. The granulosa of affected follicles is only focally and sparsely infiltrated, but secondary degenerative features, such as hydropic change and apoptosis, may be observed. The follicular fluid contains few, if any, inflammatory cells (Figures 23.18 and 23.19). Primordial follicles are apparently entirely spared. With atresia of developing follicles, the inflammatory infiltrate subsides to some extent, though rarely completely (Figure 23.20). Dysplastic follicles may also be seen, similar to those described in the resistant ovary syndrome (see above). If ovulation occurs, both granulosa and theca–lutein layers of the corpora lutea are heavily infiltrated by lymphocytes and plasma cells[97] (Figure 23.21). The infiltrate occasionally is predominantly eosinophilic. Of note, in cases where POF is associated with adrenal autoimmunity, histologic examination almost always reveals the signs of autoimmune oophoritis. On the contrary, only a few patients whose POF is associated with non-adrenal immunity present with typical oophoritis. The rarity of inflammatory infiltrates in these patients does not exclude the possibility of an autoimmune mechanism. Follicular depletion might be the final

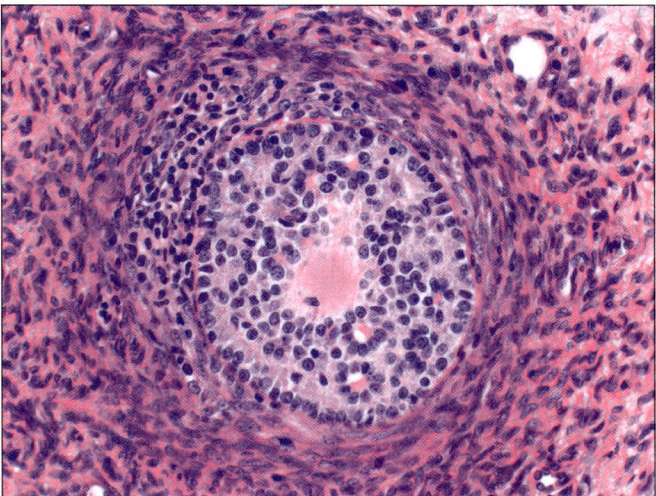

Figure 23.18 Chronic autoimmune oophoritis. Primary follicle with partial cuffing (left side) by an inflammatory infiltrate in the theca interna. Stroma elsewhere is not infiltrated.

stage of autoimmune process directed against ovarian structures.[97] The pathogenesis of autoimmune oophoritis is summarized in Figure 23.22. The cystic structures that are seen macroscopically are developing follicles or involuting corpora lutea, most likely due to elevated levels of pituitary gonadotropins. The intervening stroma is unremarkable.

Behavior and Treatment

Although uncommon, autoimmune oophoritis is important to recognize as it represents a definable, potentially treatable process that leads to POF and also indicates that the patient is at increased risk of having or developing other endocrine or non-endocrine autoimmune diseases (which may develop even several years after onset of amenorrhea).

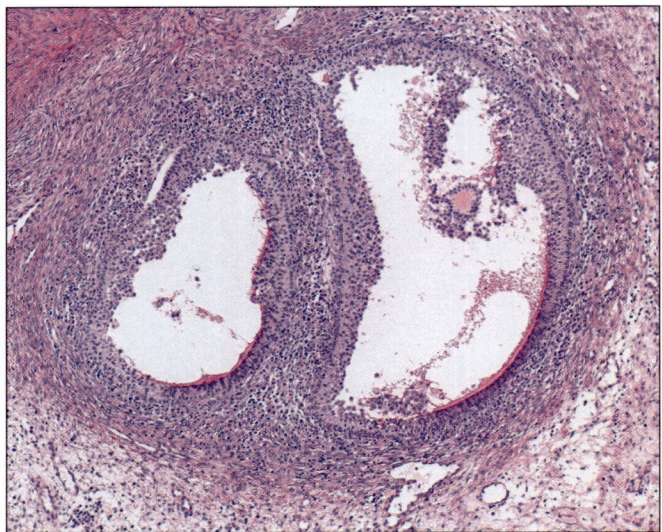

Figure 23.19 Chronic autoimmune oophoritis. Antral follicle with heavy chronic inflammatory infiltrate in the theca and lighter infiltrate in the granulosa that appears degenerate, especially in the region of the cumulus oophorus. Follicular fluid contains fibrin and a few inflammatory cells.

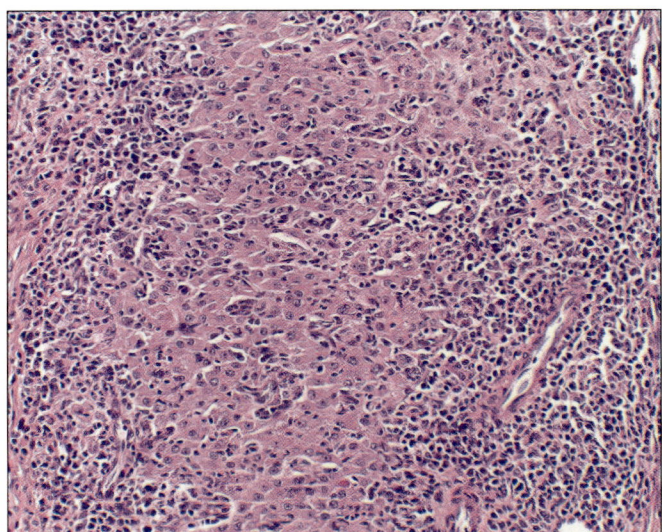

Figure 23.21 Autoimmune oophoritis in a 26-year-old woman with secondary infertility (same case as Figure 23.16). Heavy inflammatory infiltrate in the wall of a fresh corpus luteum with disruption of the granulosa cells.

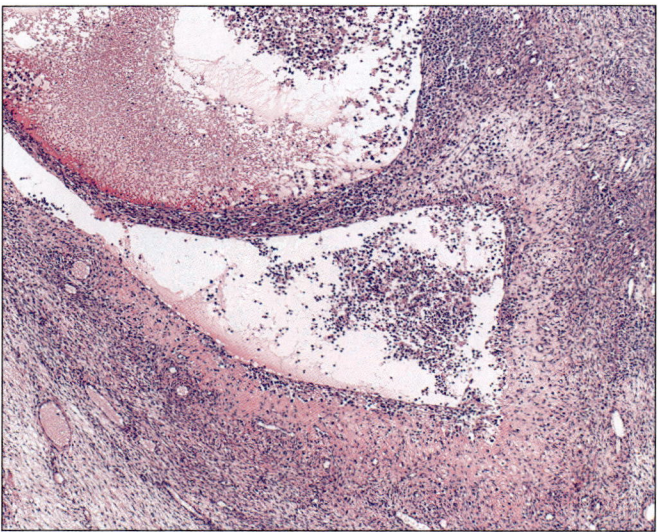

Figure 23.20 Chronic autoimmune oophoritis. Atretic follicle with diffuse lymphoplasmacytic infiltrate.

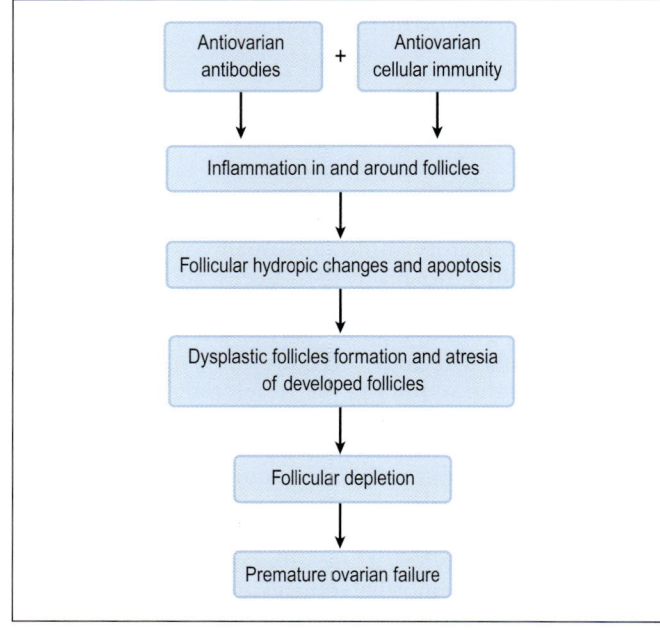

Figure 23.22 The stages in the pathogenesis of autoimmune oophoritis.

Antiadrenal antibodies may be useful predictors that adrenal failure may ensue. Management should be multidisciplinary, including hormone replacement therapy, immunosuppressive therapy in a selected population, and assisted conception techniques.[98] At present, no proven therapies are known that will improve follicular function for these women.[101]

HYPOGONADOTROPIC HYPOGONADISM

Etiology

This syndrome results from intrinsic disorders of the hypothalamus or hypophysis.[102,103] Acquired causes are more common and include tumors,[104] infections, granulomas, anorexia nervosa, radiation, surgery, and head trauma.

Congenital or hereditary causes include dysmorphic and polyglandular syndromes, isolated gonadotropin deficiency, and Kallmann syndrome (hypothalamic hypogonadism and anosmia).[105]

Microscopic Features

Primordial follicles are plentiful, but lack follicular development. If the onset of failure occurs after the menarche, corpora fibrosa or albicantia may be evident. The cortical

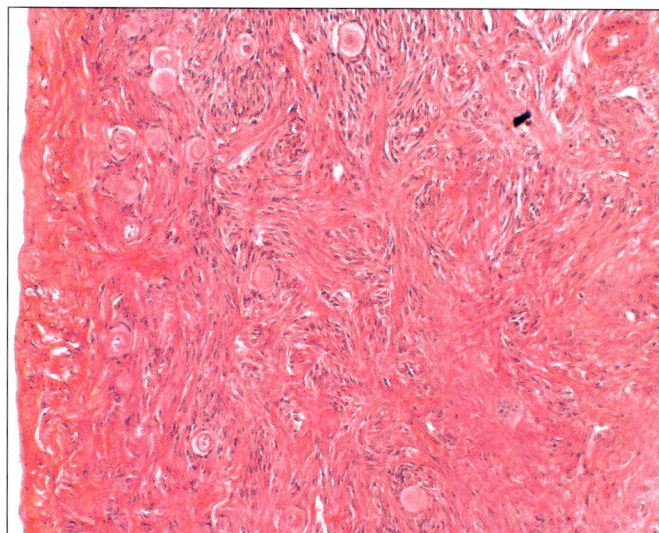

Figure 23.23 Hypogonadotropic hypogonadism. Dense cortical ovarian stroma with many primordial follicles. No evidence of current or past follicular activity.

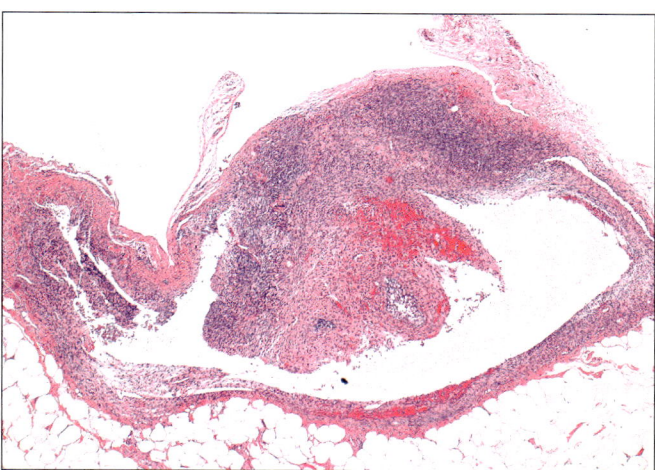

Figure 23.24 Ectopic ovary in a 32-year-old woman occurring in the omentum. No history of previous pelvic or abdominal surgery.

and medullary stroma is unremarkable and there is no inflammation. To this extent the picture may be indistinguishable from the resistant ovary syndrome (Figure 23.23).

ANOMALIES OF OVARIAN DEVELOPMENT AND DESCENT

ECTOPIC OVARIAN TISSUE

Anomalous ovarian development and descent are rarely encountered. Ectopic ovarian tissue may occur in the presence or less commonly in the absence of normally sited ovaries. As many as 36% of ectopic ovaries have been associated with other congenital malformations of the genitourinary system (such as unicornuate or bicornuate uterus, vaginal aplasia, agenesis of the kidney and ureter, bladder diverticulum, etc).[106]

Ectopic ovarian tissue may be located at some distance from the eutopic ovary, in the pelvis (in relation to the uterus, bladder, or pelvic wall) and abdomen (retroperitoneum, omentum, mesentery of the colon, kidney)[107] (Figure 23.24). It may be single or multiple and range from a few millimeters to the dimensions of a normal ovary. It may contain grossly visible follicular structures. The vast majority are incidental findings at autopsy, laparoscopy, or surgery.[108] The documented sites of ectopic ovarian tissue may possibly explain the origin of ovarian-type tumors in extraovarian sites such as the broad ligament and retroperitoneum. Exceptionally rare cases of documented pathology in ectopic ovarian tissue have been reported.[109-111] The additional ovarian tissue possesses functional potential, accounting for persistent menstruation after bilateral oophorectomy. Ectopic ovarian tissue is more commonly seen as small nodules up to 1 cm across, situated near a normally placed ovary, either within or suspended from the broad ligament.[106] It is considered as postsurgical or postinflammatory implants, which are mostly solitary and rarely display pathology.[111]

DYSTOPIC OVARIES

One or both ovaries, structurally and functionally normal, may be found in abnormal positions due to aberrant descent into the pelvis.[112] They have been identified as high as the lower pole of the kidney, close to their embryologic site of origin, within the retroperitoneal tissues, and as low as the inguinal canal. In some instances, malposition (dystopia) or maldescent of the ovaries is associated with ipsilateral anomalies of the müllerian duct derivatives.[113] In some patients, displacement may be due to torsion, detachment, and parasitic attachment to the omentum or other intraperitoneal structures.

OVARIAN AGENESIS

Confusion exists concerning the terms 'agenesis' and 'dysgenesis' and many reports in the early literature undoubtedly were examples of streak gonads rather than true agenesis.

Rarely, one ovary may be absent in an otherwise normal woman.[114] Associated findings include agenesis or malformation of the ipsilateral fallopian tube,[115] uterus, round ligament, kidney and ureter, alone or in combination.[113] However, most reported cases of absent ovaries probably result from antenatal torsion of an otherwise normal fallopian tube and ovary with necrosis and resorption of the adnexal structures.

SPLENOGONADAL FUSION

In this rare congenital anomaly splenic tissue is abnormally associated with the gonads or mesonephric remnants.[116] Many of these patients have severe congenital malformations of the extremities.[117]

'UTERUS-LIKE MASS' REPLACING OVARY

In this rare condition the ovary[118] or adjacent broad ligament[119] is replaced by a uterus-like mass with a central cavity lined by endometrial tissue and surrounded by a thick, smooth muscle wall. This lesion is most likely a congenital malformation of müllerian duct origin, an interpretation supported by the presence of congenital abnormalities of the urinary tract in several reported cases.

INFECTIOUS INFLAMMATORY DISEASES

BACTERIAL OOPHORITIS

PELVIC INFLAMMATORY DISEASE

Definition

Most examples of acute and chronic suppurative oophoritis are associated with pelvic inflammatory disease (PID), a generic term for infection of the female genital organs. PID usually begins as ascending, often recurrent, infection of the genital tract that tends to localize in the fallopian tubes but may also involve adjacent structures such as the peritoneum and ovaries.

Etiology

Gonococci and chlamydiae are the bacteria most commonly isolated. Once tissue damage has occurred, secondary bacterial invaders, chiefly anaerobic, may replace the initial organisms. Acute salpingitis results in the production of inflammatory exudate, including fibrin, from the tubal serosa and ostia, leading to adhesions to adjacent pelvic and sometimes abdominal organs.

Isolated ovarian abscesses, unassociated with salpingitis, are unusual. Almost all cases display a predisposing factor such as a recent gynecologic operation, childbirth, or use of an intrauterine contraceptive device (IUD). *Escherichia coli* and *Bacteroides* spp. are the most common organisms isolated. As opposed to the insidious development of ovarian abscesses in association with PID, isolated abscesses have an acute presentation, usually with abdominal pain. Rupture is likely if surgical treatment is not prompt. Acute peritonitis and pelvic abscess are expected sequelae.

The presence of an IUD increases the risk of developing PID compared with non-users, and especially predisposes to unusual organisms such as *Actinomyces* spp. (see later). Oophoritis may complicate other pelvic and abdominal infections such as diverticulitis and appendicitis.

Secondary infection of pre-existing cysts is a recognized clinical risk. One percent of mature cystic teratomas are said to become infected, usually by coliforms. Endometriotic cysts are also prone to secondary suppurative inflammation.

Gross Features

The ovaries usually resist the invasion of pathogenic bacteria, and their involvement in PID is often limited to a peri-oophoritis, even in the presence of tubo-ovarian inflammatory masses. However, recurrent or severe PID may result in ovarian parenchymal involvement, initially as an acute diffuse oophoritis. Abscess formation, usually in continuity with a pyosalpinx (tubo-ovarian abscess), sometimes follows and this may result in permanent loss of ovarian parenchyma. In chronic PID there may be an increase in cystic follicles and follicular or corpus luteum cysts, but chronic PID does not influence growth of follicles or their ability to ovulate. An outer layer of dense fibrous tissue is usually present.

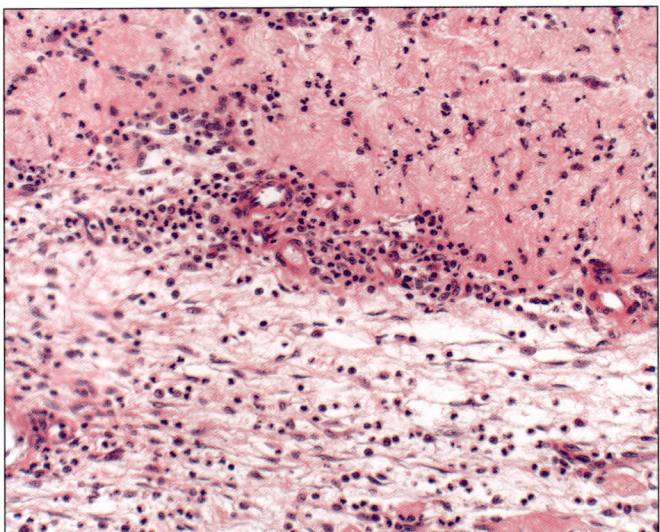

Figure 23.25 Acute suppurative oophoritis. Edematous parenchyma with diffuse neutrophilic infiltrate that even involves a corpus fibrosum (top).

Microscopic Features

Acute diffuse oophoritis shows neutrophil infiltration, edema, vascular dilatation, and focal hemorrhage. Follicular structures may be involved (Figure 23.25). Abscesses display central accumulations of necrotic debris or cavities lined by granulation tissue admixed with inflammatory cells (Figure 23.26). Large, foamy, lipid-laden macrophages may be conspicuous if there has been extensive hemorrhage and necrosis. Hemosiderin and lipofuscin (ceroid) pigment may also be demonstrable.

Acute peri-oophoritis exhibits neutrophil infiltration and fibrin exudation. Groups of peritoneal macrophages adhere to the serosal surfaces. The exudate becomes organized by the ingrowth of proliferating fibroblasts and capillaries, i.e., granulation tissue. Concurrent with this reparative process is a proliferation of mesothelial cells, which may be quite exuberant. Peri-oophoritis resolves but leaves behind adhesions, scattered lymphocytes, and sometimes psammoma bodies as residua of the inflammatory process.

Chronic diffuse oophoritis is rarely observed in patients with PID (Figure 23.27). Focal lymphocytic infiltrates are associated with autoimmune oophoritis.

In most cases of suppurative oophoritis, the fallopian tubes are also inflamed. However, in cases of isolated ovarian abscess, endosalpingitis is absent, although there may be tubal edema and perisalpingitis.

XANTHOGRANULOMATOUS OOPHORITIS

This is a rare variant of chronic oophoritis. Some patients have a history of PID.[120] *Bacteroides* spp. have been isolated in some cases. Predisposing factors include antibiotic treatment, cervical stenosis, and endometriosis. No association with malignancy or radiotherapy has been reported.

Macroscopically, xanthogranulomatous oophoritis usually forms a yellow, well-circumscribed mass (4–8 cm in diameter), with hemorrhage, necrosis, and abscess formation.

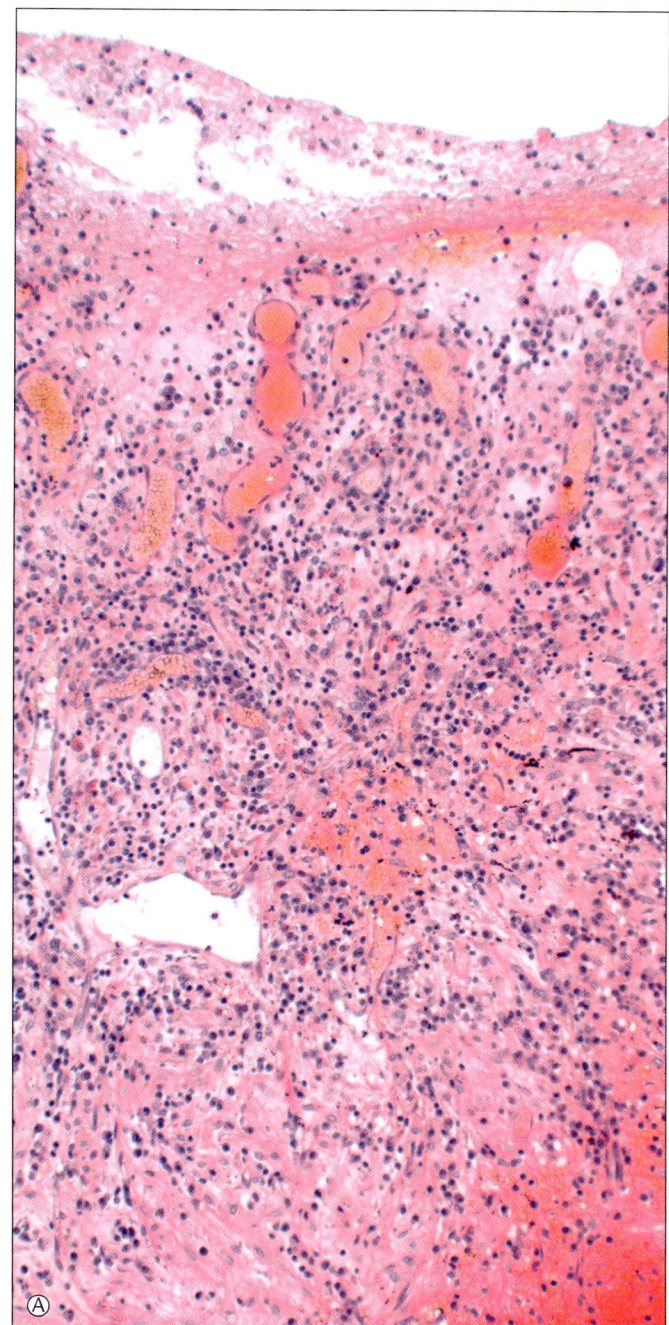

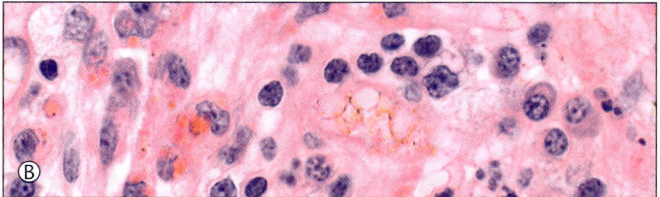

Figure 23.26 Ovarian abscess (chronic phase). **(A)** Thick fibrous wall with shaggy lining. Heavy infiltrate of chronic inflammatory cells. **(B)** Detail of cellular infiltrate: plasma cells, lymphocytes, and foamy macrophages.

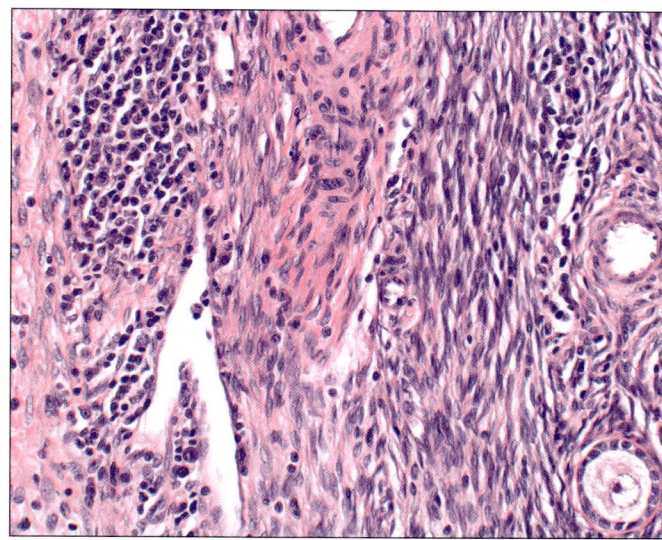

Figure 23.27 Chronic lymphoplasmacytic oophoritis. Patchy infiltrate adjacent to a resolving abscess.

Stigmata of PID are generally present elsewhere. Microscopically, sheets of foamy macrophages dominate the picture, interspersed with non-vacuolated, sometimes multi-nucleated histiocytes and other inflammatory cells. The foamy cells contain lipid as well as PAS-positive cytoplasmic granules (lysosomes). Hemosiderin deposition and fibroblastic proliferation are usually present.

MALACOPLAKIA

This chronic inflammatory process rarely involves the female genital tract of postmenopausal women,[121] and is more often identified in the renal pelvis and bladder. The lower genital tract (especially the vagina) is more commonly affected than the ovaries (see Chapter 7).

ACTINOMYCOSIS

Etiology

Pelvic actinomycosis is rare and in older reports was almost always secondary to ileocecal disease.[122] Although actinomycotic PID, associated with IUD use, has been recognized since the 1920s, the popularity of the new generation IUDs in the 1960s was followed by a spate of reports, which continues. There appears to be a correlation with prolonged IUD usage, although actinomycosis may present even after removal of the IUD,[123] and rare reports have been unassociated with IUD use.[124] The organism is readily identified in cervicovaginal smears of 8–30% of IUD users, but only rarely, and in small numbers, in non-users. Up to 25% of those with positive smears develop clinical PID (not necessarily due to actinomycosis).

Culture of the organisms is successful in less than one-third of the histologically confirmed cases but other anaerobic bacteria are isolated from the abscesses in most cases. Almost all patients with actinomycotic PID have an actinomycotic endometritis. Uterine curettings and tissue adherent to a removed IUD can also be used for histologic examination and culture.

Gross Features

Adnexal involvement is frequently unilateral and forms a large distorted tubo-ovarian mass, which may mimic pelvic malignancy at laparotomy.[125] Sectioning shows multiple shaggy abscesses containing purulent blood-stained material separated by dense fibrous scar tissue (Figure 23.28). Sulfur granules may be evident macroscopically.

Microscopic Features

The actinomycotic colonies are located in the center of abscesses and are surrounded by polymorphs and necrotic debris (Figure 23.29). Occasional multinucleated histiocytes are in close proximity to the colonies. Foamy histiocytes are often conspicuous in the adjacent granulation tissue. Plasma cells and lymphocytes are more obvious in the peripheral zone of fibrous tissue. The colonies consist of branching filaments; the central denser portion is hematoxylinophilic, but the peripheral radiating clubs are eosinophilic. The organisms are Gram positive and acid fast with certain modified stains (Putt stain) but not in solutions where full-strength acids are used (traditional Ziehl–Neelsen stain). With these stains, the organism can often be seen as a central core through the length of the club.

TUBERCULOSIS

Etiology

Although most genital tuberculosis (TB) is blood-borne from a pulmonary focus, fewer than half the patients have a history of TB or an abnormal chest X-ray. Within the pelvis, tubercle bacilli preferentially lodge in the fallopian tubes, from which direct spread to the ovaries may occur. Less commonly, the infection spreads via lymphatics from a tuberculous focus in the urinary or gastrointestinal tracts. Overall, the incidence of genital TB is low with the ovaries involved in 13–63% of such patients, and tuberculous endometritis is its most common manifestation[126] (Figure 23.30). The ovaries may also be involved incidentally in tuberculous peritonitis (see Table 23.2 for a differential diagnosis of tuberculoid granulomas and Chapter 31 for further details). Genital TB is strongly associated with infertility.

VIRAL OOPHORITIS

MUMPS

Transient acute oophoritis may occur during the course of mumps infection in adult women. While orchitis is a well-known and common manifestation of mumps infection in males, the occurrence of oophoritis in infected females is less well recognized and is said to be less frequent, of the

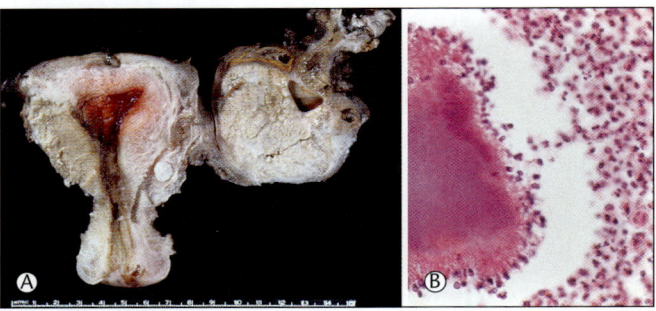

Figure 23.28 Actinomycosis. **(A)** The ovary is replaced by a mass of grayish-white nodular tissue. **(B)** A sulfur granule surrounded by polymorphonuclear leukocytes is seen on the right. (Reproduced with permission from Prat, 2004.[1])

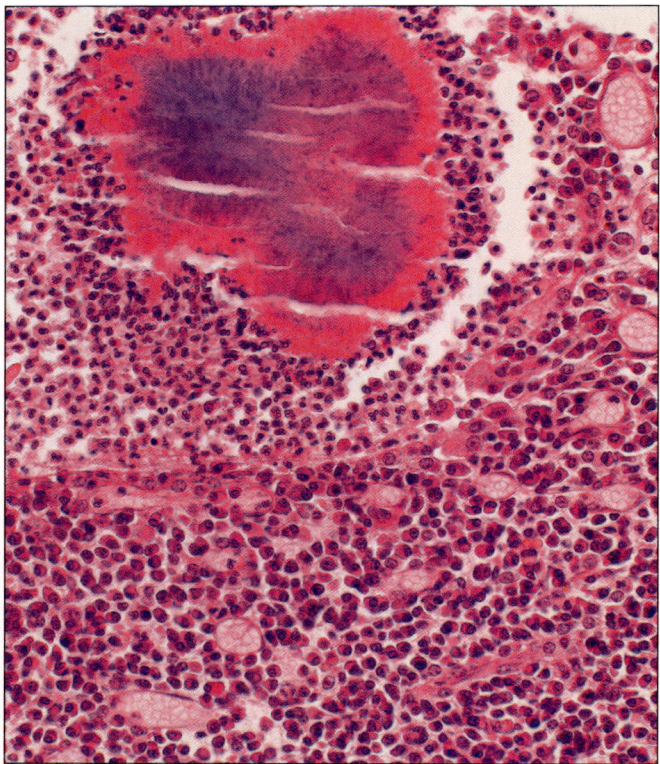

Figure 23.29 Ovarian actinomycosis. Detail of cellular infiltrate composed of lymphocytes, plasma cells, neutrophils (adjacent to a 'sulfur granule').

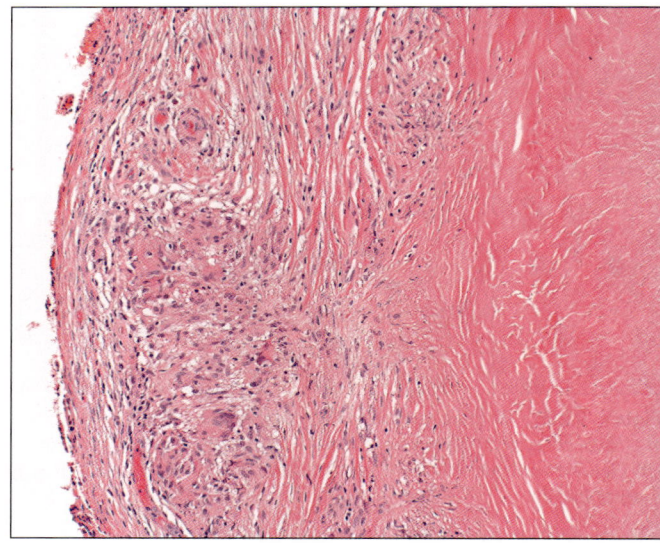

Figure 23.30 Microbiologically confirmed peritoneal TB involving the ovarian cortex.

Table 23.2 Oophoritis: Differential Diagnosis by Tissue Reaction[a]

Acute or Chronic Suppuration

Acute diffuse oophoritis associated with PID
Ovarian abscess associated with PID
Isolated ovarian abscess
Actinomycosis
Foreign body
Coccidioidomycosis, blastomycosis
Schistosomiasis[b]

Acute Serositis (without Parenchymal Inflammation)

Ruptured tubal ectopic gestation
Generalized peritonitis
Peritoneal carcinomatosis

Eosinophilic Infiltration

Foreign-body reactions, especially starch[c]
Enterobiasis[c]
Schistosomiasis[c]
Autoimmune oophoritis[b]
Isolated noninfectious granulomatous oophoritis[b]

Lymphoplasmacytic Infiltration

Autoimmune oophoritis
Resolving phases of suppurative oophoritis
CMV oophoritis

Foreign-body Granulomas

Exogenous substances, e.g., sutures, talc, starch, radiographic media, parasites, intestinal contents
Endogenous substances, e.g., contents of mature cystic teratomas, keratin from uterine adenoacanthomas, cauterized tissue

Sarcoidal Granulomas

Sarcoidosis
Crohn disease
Foreign-body reactions, especially starch[c]
'Cortical granulomas'
Autoimmune oophoritis[b]

Necrotizing Granulomas

Tuberculosis[c]
Foreign-body reactions, especially starch[b,c] and radiographic media[b,c]
Enterobiasis[c]
Coccidioidomycosis, blastomycosis
Isolated noninfectious granulomatous oophoritis
Schistosomiasis[b]

[a]Note that an etiologic agent may be associated with more than one type of reaction.
[b]Rare feature of the condition.
[c]Predominantly serosal lesions.

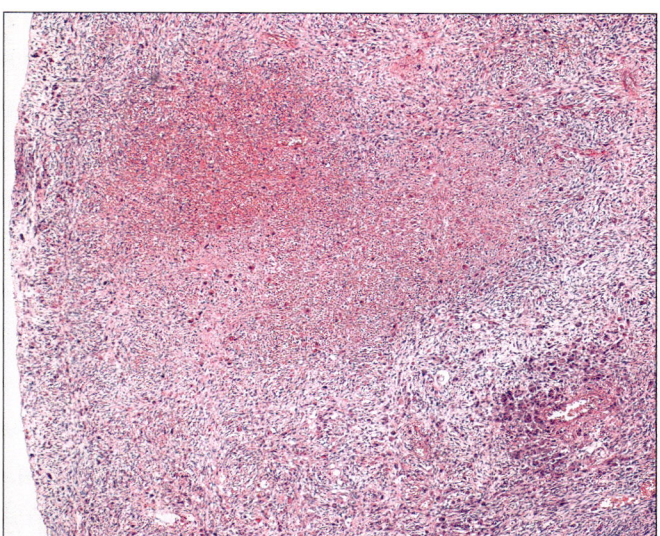

Figure 23.31 Cytomegalovirus oophoritis from an immunosuppressed 37-year-old woman. Wedge-shaped cortical infarct.

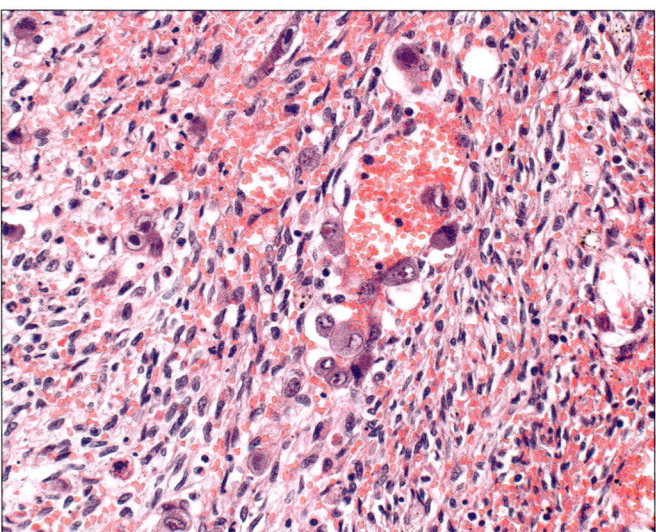

Figure 23.32 Detail of Figure 23.31. Infected endothelial and stromal cells with intranuclear and intracytoplasmic inclusions.

It often presents as a mass lesion, and typically shows extensive cortical coagulative necrosis with areas of hemorrhage, associated with a mixed inflammatory infiltrate (Figure 23.31). Within and bordering the necrotic area are sheets and clusters of enlarged virally infected stromal and endothelial cells with abundant amphophilic cytoplasm, large intranuclear inclusions, and variable intracytoplasmic inclusions (Figure 23.32). A chronic inflammatory cell infiltrate is present in the surrounding viable parenchyma.

PARASITIC OOPHORITIS

SCHISTOSOMIASIS (BILHARZIASIS)

Etiology

Schistosomiasis, although prevalent in large parts of the world, rarely affects the ovary.[132] It represents so-called

order of 5%.[127] There are no reports in the literature of the histologic features of mumps oophoritis.

CYTOMEGALOVIRUS

Cytomegalovirus (CMV) oophoritis is rare, and is reported only in immunocompromised patients,[128–130] usually as part of a disseminated infection.[131]

ectopic disease, i.e., not related directly to the life cycle of the organism. Worms preferentially lodge in the mesenteric and portal (*Schistosoma mansoni* and *S. japonicum*) or vesical veins (*S. haematobium*) but may access the genital tract via venous anastomoses such as those between mesenteric and ovarian veins. It is usually an incidental finding, although some patients with upper genital tract infections have symptoms suggestive of PID, and some develop serious complications such as ectopic pregnancy and infertility. The genital tract is involved more frequently by *S. haematobium* than with *S. mansoni* infection. *S. haematobium* predominantly involves the lower genital tract, while *S. mansoni* has a predilection for tubes and ovaries.

Microscopic Features

If the schistosomal infection is merely an incidental finding, the ovaries are likely to be of normal size. Small white nodules appear on their surfaces and often elsewhere on the pelvic peritoneum as well simulating metastatic carcinoma. In patients clinically affected, the ovaries may be three times their normal size; rarely in the form of ovarian pseudotumor.[132] They display necrosis, abscesses, tuboovarian adhesions, and adhesions to other pelvic structures in most cases.

Living worms and dead ova usually provoke little tissue reaction (Figure 23.33), but dead worms and living ova incite a granulomatous reaction when they enter the tissues. Ova are more commonly identified than worms. The cellular infiltrate consists of epithelioid cells, foreign-body giant cells, lymphocytes, plasma cells, and eosinophils. Some granulomas appear tuberculoid. Sometimes the cellular reaction to freshly laid ova is predominantly eosinophilic, with formation of abscesses. The Splendore–Hoeppli phenomenon (radiating eosinophilic deposits around ova) may also be observed. The peripheral zone of the granulomas consists of fibrous tissue that gradually increases in amount and may replace entire lesions. Dead ova frequently calcify and are found within the ovarian parenchyma and, more often, within veins of the outer uterine wall or broad ligament.

Schistosomal ova can be readily differentiated from each other in histologic preparations if spines are visible in the plane of section. The ova are 80–160 μm long and 30–90 μm wide. *S. haematobium* and *S. mansoni* are elongate. *S. haematobium* has a terminal spine while that of *S. mansoni* is lateral. *S. japonicum* is round to ovoid and has a lateral spine that is less prominent than that of *S. mansoni* (Figure 23.34).

ENTEROBIASIS

Etiology

Extraintestinal enterobiasis, caused by *Enterobius* (*Oxyuris*) *vermicularis* (pinworm, threadworm), is rare, and usually involves women with inflammatory or granulomatous lesions in the genital tract or the pelvic peritoneum. Parasites gain entry to the peritoneal cavity by ascending the genital tract after migrating to the introitus from the anus. Once in the

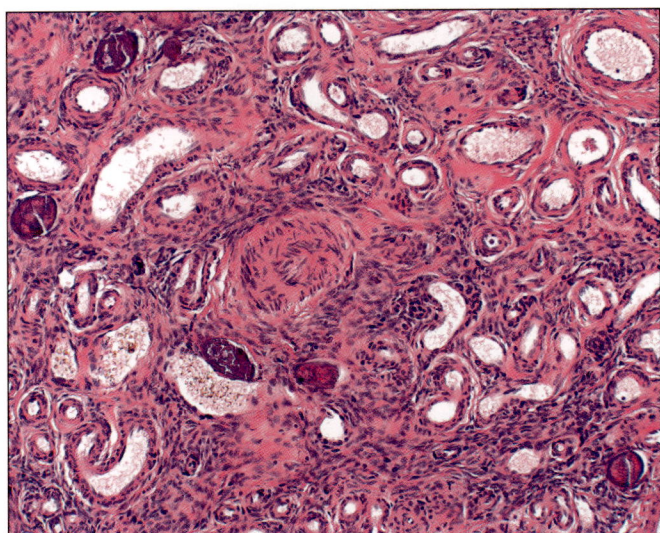

Figure 23.33 Ovarian medulla containing degenerate, calcified, schistosomal ova. Note the complete absence of an inflammatory reaction.

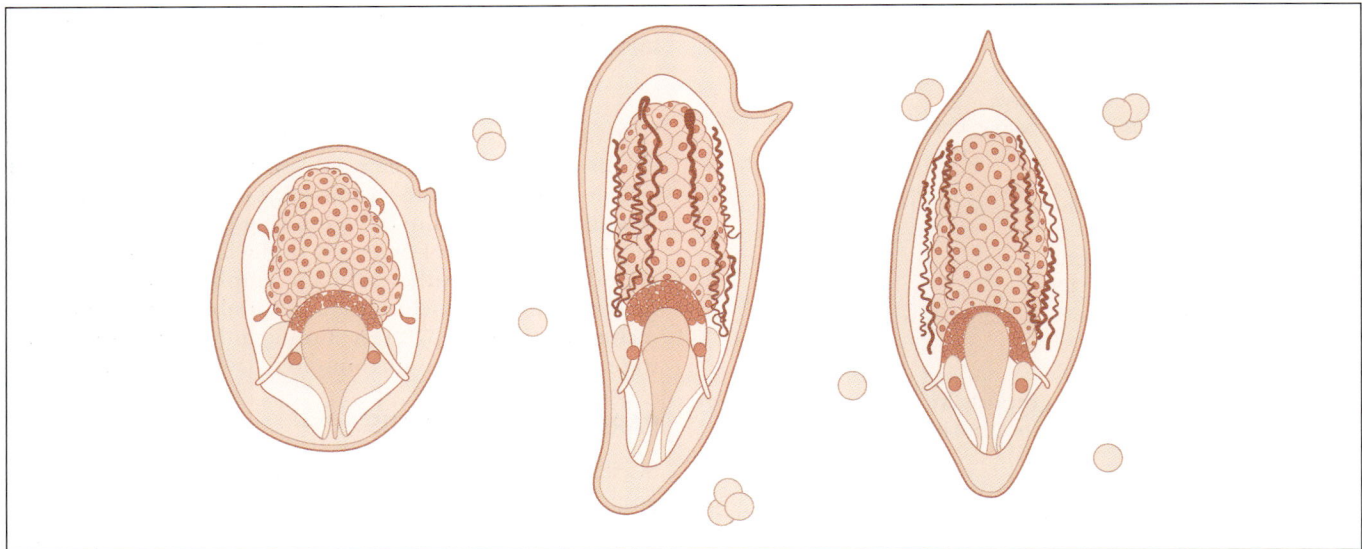

Figure 23.34 Parasitic ova. From left to right: *S. japonicum, S. mansoni, S. haematobium*. Circles represent the size of red blood cells.

peritoneal cavity the worms die and their ova are released, inciting an inflammatory reaction. Although mostly asymptomatic or causing minor clinical problems, they may lead to severe infectious complications. *E. vermicularis* may occasionally cause generalized peritonitis and tubo-ovarian abscess formation with necrotizing epithelioid granulomas that may mimic malignancy.[133]

Pathology

Macroscopically, ovarian granulomas are soft yellow-brown serosal nodules, up to 1 cm in diameter, sometimes associated with adhesions. Larger lesions may show central softening.

Microscopically, the granulomatous inflammation centers on the ova, which are oval (up to 60 μm long and 30 μm wide) with double-contoured smooth shells, flattened on one side, in which embryonic structures may be identified. Degenerate worms are rarely identified. Ova (and worms) lie within necrotic debris that contains numerous eosinophils. Beyond this is a zone of granulation tissue that includes epithelioid histiocytes and lymphocytes. The granulomas show peripheral fibrosis. The ova and, indeed, entire granulomas may calcify.

The finding of large necrotizing pelvic granulomas, particularly if associated with an eosinophilic infiltrate, should prompt a search for a possible causative parasite. Processing additional tissue and cutting step sections foster the identification. *Enterobius* ova can be distinguished from those of *Schistosoma* by their smaller size and lack of spines (Figure 23.34).

ECHINOCOCCOSIS

Echinococcosis or hydatid disease is an endemic parasitic disease in many countries, caused most commonly by the larval stage of the *Echinococcus granulosus*. In humans the most common site of echinococcal cysts is the liver followed by the lungs, but they can be located in any part of the body. Genital involvement is rare, occurring in but 0.1–0.3% of infected females, with the ovary the most common location. Ovarian involvement is generally secondary to peritoneal spread of daughter cysts due to rupture of a liver hydatid cyst. Such ovarian involvement may present clinically and on ultrasound as an ovarian cystic mass.[134,135]

Hydatid cysts measure up to 16 cm in diameter and show the characteristic triple-layered wall consisting of innermost germinal epithelium (with its brood capsules and scolices), hyaline-laminated membrane, and outermost adventitial fibrous tissue (of host origin). A calcified cyst wall, a very useful radiologic sign, is usually associated with regression of the cyst following death of the parasite.

FUNGAL OOPHORITIS

COCCIDIOIDOMYCOSIS

Etiology

This fungal disease is endemic in certain semi-arid areas of North, Central, and South America and is caused by *Coccidioides immitis*. Genital infection is rare, even in cases of disseminated fatal coccidioidomycosis, which generally occur in immunosuppressed patients. As in TB, genital involvement usually results from blood-borne spread of organisms from a pulmonary lesion that is generally radiologically inactive or apparently healed. Pelvic coccidioidomycosis is usually associated with peritonitis.

Pathology

In cases with adnexal involvement the fallopian tubes and ovaries show dense serosal adhesions and multiple small white nodules on the serosal surfaces. In addition, the ovaries may contain abscess cavities.

The inflammatory reaction is either tuberculoid granulomatous, which may progress to caseation and cavitation, or suppurative with microabscess formation. The fungal elements are seen in tissues as spherules (sporangia) measuring 20–200 μm in diameter that have thin doubly refractile walls. The enclosed endospores, 2–3 μm in diameter, are released into the tissues upon rupture of the spherules. A rapid diagnosis of pelvic coccidioidomycosis is fostered by identifying the spherules in wet preparations of peritoneal fluid or purulent exudates.

BLASTOMYCOSIS

Genital tract involvement in North American blastomycosis is rare and results from venereal transmission or hematogenous spread from a pulmonary lesion. The tissue reaction to the fungus resembles that seen in coccidioidomycosis, i.e., either suppurative or tuberculoid granulomatous inflammation. The budding, thick-walled yeast bodies, 8–20 μm diameter, are readily found in sections.

NONINFECTIOUS INFLAMMATORY DISEASES

SARCOIDOSIS

Etiology

Sarcoidosis rarely involves the female genital tract, even in the active stage of the disease when granulomas may be widely disseminated throughout the body. The uterus is more often affected than the adnexa. Most patients have current or recent evidence of pulmonary sarcoidosis.[136] The serum CA125 is sometimes elevated.

Microscopic Features

Ovarian granulomas are distributed at random through the cortex, medulla, and hilus. As in extragenital sites, the discrete noncaseating granulomas are composed of epithelioid histiocytes with small numbers of giant cells of Langhans or foreign-body type, sometimes containing crystalloid inclusions. A diagnosis of ovarian sarcoidosis in the absence of systemic disease should be made with great caution since the histologic changes alone are not pathognomonic (Table 3.2; Figure 23.35). TB and mycoses, especially if endemic in the patient's locality, should be excluded by the appropriate special stains and preferably culture. The sections should be screened with the aid of polarizing filters for foreign bodies, particularly starch granules and parasitic elements.

CROHN DISEASE

Crohn disease has a tendency to form fistulas and may involve contiguous organs. Ovarian involvement is the result of direct extension of the inflammatory process from the

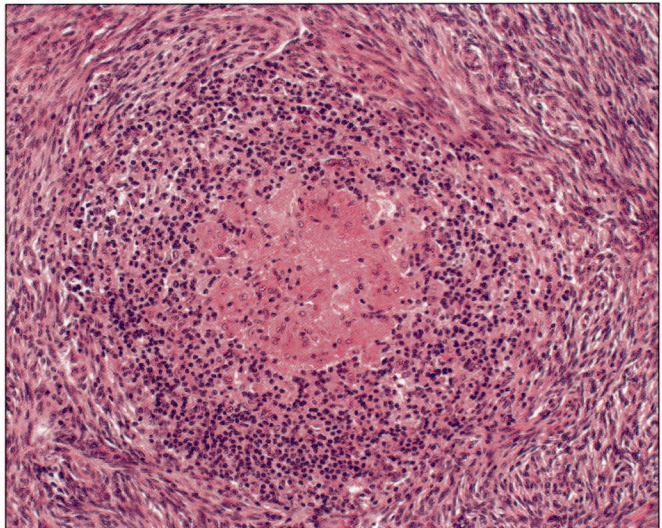

Figure 23.35 Sarcoidosis. Typical sarcoidal granuloma in ovarian cortex, an incidental finding in a postmenopausal woman with known clinical sarcoidosis. No microorganisms or foreign bodies could be identified.

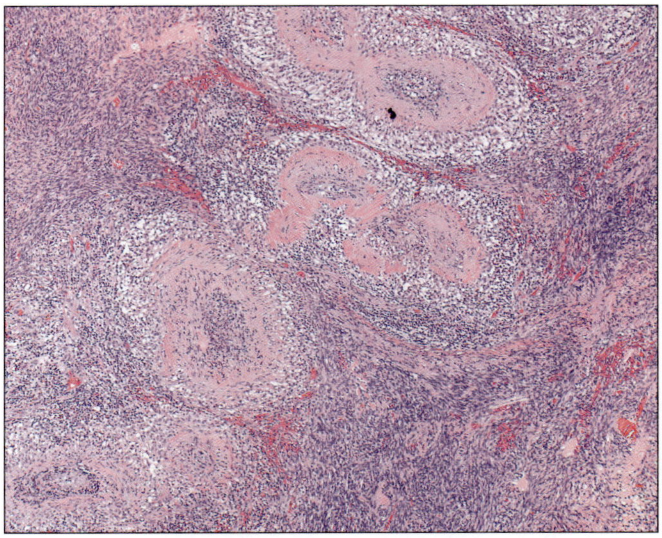

Figure 23.36 Isolated necrotizing arteritis. Incidental finding in an ovary which also contained a small, benign transitional cell tumor. No evidence of systemic vasculitis.

adherent segment of intestine.[137] The right ovary, by virtue of its proximity to the terminal ileum, is more commonly affected, but the left ovary is also occasionally involved. Crohn disease may also cause ovarian vein thrombosis with consequent ovarian pain and enlargement.[138]

Ovarian granulomas may be restricted to the serosa and superficial cortex, or widely distributed in the parenchyma. They are sarcoidal in type and set in a background of lymphocytic infiltration. A more destructive combined suppurative and granulomatous reaction occurs also in association with an ileo-ovarian 'fistula.' The ipsilateral fallopian tube is generally involved as well. Differential diagnosis is not problematic once the clinical and surgical details are available. However, prudence dictates that other infective causes of granulomatous oophoritis, such as actinomycosis or TB (Table 3.2), which may also be associated with ileocecal disease, be excluded.

CORTICAL GRANULOMAS

Cortical granulomas are a frequent incidental microscopic finding. They are more common in postmenopausal women but can be seen in premenopausal women as well. They are well circumscribed, 100–500 μm in diameter, and consist of loose ovarian stroma containing small numbers of lymphocytes and epithelioid cells (which may represent either luteinized stromal cells or macrophages), multinucleated giant cells, and occasional anisotropic fat crystals. The lesions are well vascularized but eventually become fibrotic and hyalinized.

ISOLATED NONINFECTIOUS GRANULOMAS

Isolated noninfectious granulomas typically occur in premenopausal women without evidence of systemic granulomatous disease or of genital tract infection of potentially granulomatous type. In most patients the granulomas are incidental findings and there is a history of previous surgery (in the preceding several months or years) involving the now affected ovary, suggesting that the granulomas may possibly be a reaction to traumatized tissues.

The granulomas are multiple and may be bilateral. They are small, with an acellular hyaline core bordered by palisading histiocytes and peripheral fibrosis. The lesions resemble the necrobiotic rheumatoid-like granulomas that may be found in the cervix following cone biopsy or loop excision of the transformation zone.

AUTOIMMUNE OOPHORITIS

See discussion in the previous section Ovarian Failure.

NECROTIZING ARTERITIS

Etiology

A small proportion of patients with necrotizing arteritis suffer from a systemic connective tissue disorder such as lupus erythematosus, while others give a history of drug therapy, especially penicillin, suggesting an allergic basis to the lesion. In the majority, however, no underlying cause can be identified and these appear to be cases of idiopathic, isolated, visceral necrotizing vasculitis. Further investigation and follow-up of asymptomatic patients with uterine and adnexal involvement are usually unrewarding in uncovering systemic disease.[139]

Microscopic Features

Medium-sized arteries and arterioles are affected (Figure 23.36). The most striking feature is fibrinoid necrosis of the media with some associated disruption of the internal elastic lamina. Fibrin is often seen in the lumen, but thrombosis and tissue infarction do not occur. An inflammatory infiltrate, chiefly lymphocytic, permeates the vessel wall and adventitia. Neutrophils and eosinophils, but not giant cells, may be present in small numbers. If eosinophils are prominent, polyarteritis nodosa should be considered (see later).

GIANT CELL ARTERITIS

Giant cell arteritis of the female genital tract is a rare usually asymptomatic finding in elderly women, and is occasionally associated with temporal arteritis. It may occur as an isolated finding or as part of generalized giant cell arteritis.[140] The patients may present with fatigue, fever, weight loss, anemia, and sometimes pelvic mass. The clinical significance of this disorder is uncertain. It may be associated with later development of giant cell arteritis elsewhere in the body. Symptomatic patients treated with prednisone often show improvement.

Microscopic Features

Small- to medium-sized arteries display random segmental involvement. Intimal edema and fibrosis narrow the lumen. The media is expanded by a granulomatous inflammatory infiltrate consisting of lymphocytes and histiocytes, some epithelioid and multinucleated giant cells. There is destruction of elastic fibers, especially in the internal elastic lamina. Inflammatory cells, mainly lymphocytes, extend into the intima and adventitia. Eosinophils are conspicuous by their absence. Fibrinoid necrosis and thromboses are rarely seen.

POLYARTERITIS NODOSA

Polyarteritis nodosa is a systemic necrotizing vasculitis that affects numerous organs. The female genital tract, including the ovaries, rarely may be involved in polyarteritis nodosa.[141,142] Arguably, the 'localized' form involving only the ovaries should be classified as polyarteritis nodosa or isolated necrotizing arteritis (see previous section).

Microscopic Features

Medium-sized and small arteries are affected. They show fibrinoid necrosis and an acute, predominantly eosinophilic, inflammatory infiltrate (Figure 23.37). Older lesions show lymphocytes and plasma cells. Thromboses, when developing, may result in infarction of distal tissues.

POSTPARTUM OVARIAN VEIN THROMBOPHLEBITIS

Etiology

The pathologist rarely encounters postpartum ovarian vein thrombophlebitis and thrombosis, a potentially life-threatening condition, because standard management does not include oophorectomy.[143] The condition complicates about 1 in 1000 deliveries. It is part of the spectrum of pelvic thrombophlebitis, but selective involvement of the ovarian veins makes the condition clinically distinct from non-puerperal cases in which the uterine and iliac veins are predominantly affected. Some consider the condition to be infective, with the primary source the placental bed. Postpartum hypercoagulability, together with dilatation and stasis, potentiate thrombosis in the inflamed veins. Peculiarities in ovarian venous blood flow postpartum (antegrade on the right but retrograde on the left) result in preferential spread of infection to the right side. The right side is involved in 90% of unilateral cases and 14% of all cases are bilateral. Ultrasound and computer-assisted tomographic scanning help to confirm the diagnosis. Management is with antibiotics and anticoagulation.

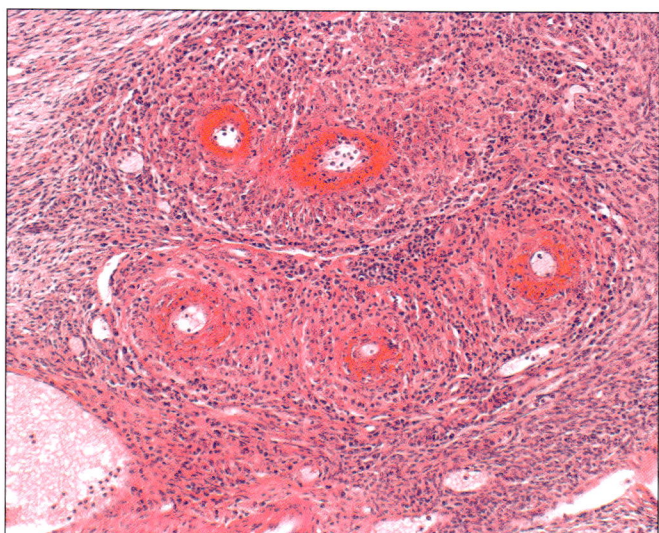

Figure 23.37 Acute necrotizing arteritis in a patient with systemic evidence of polyarteritis nodosa.

Microscopic Features

At laparotomy, the thrombosed ovarian veins are markedly enlarged (up to 10 mm in diameter), tortuous, tense, and firm; thrombus sometimes extends into the ovaries. The inferior vena cava, left renal vein, or both may be involved in continuity. The ovaries and fallopian tubes are dark and congested, but their viability is not usually compromised and infarction rarely occurs. The ovarian veins, if available for histologic examination, show thrombophlebitis.

REFERENCES

1. Prat J. Pathology of the ovary. Saunders: Philadelphia; 2004.
2. Koc Z, Ulusan S, Oguzkurt L. Right ovarian vein drainage variant: is there a relationship with pelvic varices? Eur J Radiol 2006;59:465–71.
3. Cao QJ, Jones JG, Li M. Expression of calretinin in human ovary, testis, and ovarian sex cord-stromal tumors. Int J Gynecol Pathol 2001;20:346–52.
4. Auersperg N, Ota T, Mitchell GW. Early events in ovarian epithelial carcinogenesis: progress and problems in experimental approaches. Int J Gynecol Cancer 2002;12:691–703.
5. Russell P, Farnsworth A. Surgical pathology of the ovaries. 2nd ed. New York: Churchill Livingstone; 1997.
6. Kwintkiewicz J, Giudice LC. The interplay of insulin-like growth factors, gonadotropins, and endocrine disruptors in ovarian follicular development and function. Semin Reprod Med 2009;27:43–51.
7. Messinis IE, Messini CI, Dafopoulos K. The role of gonadotropins in the follicular phase. Ann N Y Acad Sci 2010;1205:5–11.
8. Sirotkin AV. Transcription factors and ovarian functions. J Cell Physiol 2010;225:20–6.
9. Sharif K, Afnan M. Ovarian function and ovulation induction. In: Shaw RW, Soutter WP, Stanton SL, editors. Gynaecology. 2nd ed. New York: Churchill Livingstone; 1997. p. 223–36.

10. Hillier SG. Current concepts of the roles of follicle stimulating hormone and luteinizing hormone in folliculogenesis. Hum Reprod 1994;9:188–91.
11. Zeleznik AJ, Hillier SG. The role of gonadotropins in the selection of the preovulatory follicle. Clin Obstet Gynecol 1984;27:927–40.
12. Arif S, Varela-Calvino R, Conway GS, Peakman M. 3 beta hydroxysteroid dehydrogenase autoantibodies in patients with idiopathic premature ovarian failure target N- and C-terminal epitopes. J Clin Endocrinol Metab 2001;86:5892–7.
13. Juengel JL, McNatty KP. The role of proteins of the transforming growth factor-beta superfamily in the intraovarian regulation of follicular development. Hum Reprod Update 2005;11:143–60.
14. Young JM, McNeilly AS. Theca: the forgotten cell of the ovarian follicle. Reproduction 2010;140:489–504.
15. Hugues JN, Cedrin-Durnerin I. Role of luteinizing hormone in follicular and corpus luteum physiology. Gynecol Obstet Fertil 2000;28:738–44.
16. Carambula SF, Pru JK, Lynch MP, et al. Prostaglandin F2alpha- and FAS-activating antibody-induced regression of the corpus luteum involves caspase-8 and is defective in caspase-3 deficient mice. Reprod Biol Endocrinol 2003;1:15.
17. Sugino N, Okuda K. Species-related differences in the mechanism of apoptosis during structural luteolysis. J Reprod Dev 2007;53:977–86.
18. Gougeon A. Human ovarian follicular development: from activation of resting follicles to preovulatory maturation. Ann Endocrinol (Paris) 2010;71:132–43.
19. Gougeon A. Regulation of ovarian follicular development in primates: facts and hypotheses. Endocr Rev 1996;17:121–55.47.
20. Monniaux D, Huet C, Pisselet C, et al. [Mechanism, regulation, and manipulations of follicular atresia]. Contracept Fertil Sex 1998;26(7–8):528–35.
21. Meduri G, Bachelot A, Cocca MP, et al. Molecular pathology of the FSH receptor: new insights into FSH physiology. Mol Cell Endocrinol 2008;282:130–42.
22. Eldar-Geva T, Spitz IM, Groome NP, et al. Follistatin and activin A serum concentrations in obese and non-obese patients with polycystic ovary syndrome. Hum Reprod 2001;16:2552–6.
23. Hillier SG. Paracrine support of ovarian stimulation. Mol Hum Reprod 2009;15:843–50.
24. Del Vecchio RP. The role of steroidogenic and nonsteroidogenic luteal cell interactions in regulating progesterone production. Semin Reprod Endocrinol 1997;15:409–20.
25. Ordi J, Romagosa C, Tavassoli FA, et al. CD10 expression in epithelial tissues and tumors of the gynecologic tract: a useful marker in the diagnosis of mesonephric, trophoblastic, and clear cell tumors. Am J Surg Pathol 2003;27:178–86.
26. Persani L, Rossetti R, Cacciatore C. Genes involved in human premature ovarian failure. J Mol Endocrinol 2010;45:257–79.
27. Maclaran K, Horner E, Panay N. Premature ovarian failure: long-term sequelae. Menopause Int 2010;16:38–41.
28. Santoro N. Mechanisms of premature ovarian failure. Ann Endocrinol (Paris) 2003;64:87–92.
29. Skillern A, Rajkovic A. Recent developments in identifying genetic determinants of premature ovarian failure. Sex Dev 2008;2:228–43.
30. Gougeon A. The biological aspects of risks of infertility due to age: the female side. Rev Epidemiol Sante Publique 2005;53:2S37–45.
31. Goswami D, Conway GS. Premature ovarian failure. Hum Reprod Update 2005;11:391–410.
32. Mahmoud MS, Merhi ZO, Yelian FD. Mechanisms of premature ovarian failure: reappraisal and overview. J Reprod Med 2007;52:623–9
33. Santoro N. Research on the mechanisms of premature ovarian failure. J Soc Gynecol Investig 2001;8(1 Suppl Proceedings):S10–2.
34. Fassnacht W, Mempel A, Strowitzki T, Vogt PH. Premature ovarian failure (POF) syndrome: towards the molecular clinical analysis of its genetic complexity. Curr Med Chem 2006;13:1397–410.
35. Layman LC. Genetic causes of human infertility. Endocrinol Metab Clin North Am 2003;32:549–72.
36. Rizzolio F, Bione S, Sala C, et al. Chromosomal rearrangements in Xq and premature ovarian failure: mapping of 25 new cases and review of the literature. Hum Reprod 2006;21:1477–83.
37. Simpson JL, Rajkovic A. Ovarian differentiation and gonadal failure. Am J Med Genet 1999;89:186–200.
38. Chernyshov VP, Radysh TV, Gura IV, et al. Immune disorders in women with premature ovarian failure in initial period. Am J Reprod Immunol 2001;46:220–5.
39. Hoek A, Schoemaker J, Drexhage HA. Premature ovarian failure and ovarian autoimmunity. Endocr Rev 1997;18:107–34.
40. Kovacs P, Stangel JJ, Santoro NF, Lieman H. Successful pregnancy after transient ovarian failure following treatment of symptomatic leiomyomata. Fertil Steril 2002;77:1292–5.
41. Chen WY, Manson JE. Premature ovarian failure in cancer survivors: new insights, looming concerns. J Natl Cancer Inst 2006;98(13):880–1.
42. Matikainen T, Perez GI, Jurisicova A, et al. Aromatic hydrocarbon receptor-driven Bax gene expression is required for premature ovarian failure caused by biohazardous environmental chemicals. Nat Genet 2001;28:355–60.
43. Miller KP, Borgeest C, Greenfeld C, et al. In utero effects of chemicals on reproductive tissues in females. Toxicol Appl Pharmacol 2004;198:111–31.
44. Forges T, Monnier-Barbarino P, Leheup B, Jouvet P. Pathophysiology of impaired ovarian function in galactosaemia. Hum Reprod Update 2006;12:573–84.
45. Persani L, Rossetti R, Cacciatore C, Bonomi M. Primary ovarian insufficiency: X chromosome defects and autoimmunity. J Autoimmun 2009;33:35–41.
46. Welt CK. Primary ovarian insufficiency: a more accurate term for premature ovarian failure. Clin Endocrinol 2008;68:499–509.
47. Pellicano M, Zullo F, Cappiello F, et al. Minilaparoscopic ovarian biopsy performed under conscious sedation in women with premature ovarian failure. J Reprod Med 2000;45:817–22.
48. Abe N, Takeuchi H, Kikuchi I, Kinoshita K. Effectiveness of microlaparoscopy in the diagnosis of premature ovarian failure. J Obstet Gynaecol Res 2006;32:224–9.
49. La Marca A, Pati M, Orvieto R, et al. Serum anti-mullerian hormone levels in women with secondary amenorrhea. Fertil Steril 2006;85:1547–9.
50. Meduri G, Massin N, Guibourdenche J, et al. Serum anti-Mullerian hormone expression in women with premature ovarian failure. Hum Reprod 2007;22:117–23.
51. Hansen KR, Hodnett GM, Knowlton N, Craig LB. Correlation of ovarian reserve tests with histologically determined primordial follicle number. Fertil Steril 2011;95:170–5.
52. LaMarca A, Broekmans FJ, Volpe A, et al. Anti-Mullerian hormone (AMH): what do we still need to know? Hum Reprod 2009;24:2264–75.
53. Nippita TA, Baber RJ. Premature ovarian failure: a review. Climacteric 2007;10:11–22.
54. Davison RM, Fox M, Conway GS. Mapping of the POF1 locus and identification of putative genes for premature ovarian failure. Mol Hum Reprod 2000;6:314–8.
55. Zinn AR. The X chromosome and the ovary. J Soc Gynecol Investig 2001;8(1 Suppl Proceedings):S34–6.
56. Hisama FM, Zemel S, Cherniske EM, et al. 46,XX gonadal dysgenesis, short stature, and recurrent metabolic acidosis in two sisters. Am J Med Genet 2001;98:121–4.
57. Holland CM. 47,XXX in an adolescent with premature ovarian failure and autoimmune disease. J Pediatr Adolesc Gynecol 2001;14:77–80.
58. Rooman RP, Van Driessche K, Du Caju MV. Growth and ovarian function in girls with 48,XXXX karyotype—patient report and review of the literature. J Pediatr Endocrinol Metab 2002;15:1051–5.
59. Devi AS, Metzger DA, Luciano AA, Benn PA. 45,X/46,XX mosaicism in patients with idiopathic premature ovarian failure. Fertil Steril 1998;70:89–93.
60. Diao FY, Xu M, Liu JY. [Analysis of X chromosome mosaicism in patients with premature ovarian failure by fluorescent in-situ hybridization]. Zhonghua Fu Chan Ke Za Zhi 2003;38:20–3.
61. Leppig KA, Disteche CM. Ring X and other structural X chromosome abnormalities: X inactivation and phenotype. Semin Reprod Med 2001;19:147–57.
62. Banerjee N, Kriplani A, Takkar D, Kucheria K. Balanced X; 22 translocation in a patient with premature ovarian failure. Acta Genet Med Gemellol (Roma) 1997;46:241–4.
63. Ashraf M, Jayawickrama NS, Bowen-Simpkins P. Premature ovarian failure due to an unbalanced translocation on the X chromosome. BJOG 2001;108:230–2.

64. Bussani C, Papi L, Sestini R, et al. Premature ovarian failure and fragile X premutation: a study on 45 women. Eur J Obstet Gynecol Reprod Biol 2004;112:189–91.
65. Allen EG, He W, Yadav-Shah M, Sherman SL. A study of the distributional characteristics of FMR1 transcript levels in 238 individuals. Hum Genet 2004;114:439–47.
66. Mila M, Mallolas J. [Fragile X syndrome: premature ovarian failure. Preimplantation and preconception genetic diagnosis]. Rev Neurol 2001;33 Suppl 1:S20–3.
67. Gubbels CS, Land JA, Rubio-Gozalbo ME. Fertility and impact of pregnancies on the mother and child in classic galactosemia. Obstet Gynecol Surv 2008;63:334–43.
68. Rubio-Gozalbo ME, Gubbels CS, Bakker JA, et al. Gonadal function in male and female patients with classic galactosemia. Hum Reprod Update 2010;16:177–88.
69. Loffler KA, Zarkower D, Koopman P. Etiology of ovarian failure in blepharophimosis ptosis epicanthus inversus syndrome: FOXL2 is a conserved, early-acting gene in vertebrate ovarian development. Endocrinology 2003;144:3237–43.
70. Narahara K, Kamada M, Takahashi Y, et al. Case of ovarian dysgenesis and dilated cardiomyopathy supports existence of Malouf syndrome. Am J Med Genet 1992;44:369–73.
71. Bellassoued M, Mnif M, Marouene H, et al. [Perrault's syndrome: two cases]. Ann Endocrinol (Paris) 2001;62:534–7.
72. De Ravel TJ, Fryns JP, Van Driessche J, Vermeesch JR. Complex chromosome re-arrangement 45,X,t(Y;9) in a girl with sex reversal and mental retardation. Am J Med Genet 2004;124A:259–62.
73. Di Pasquale E, Beck-Peccoz P, Persani L. Hypergonadotropic ovarian failure associated with an inherited mutation of human bone morphogenetic protein-15 (BMP15) gene. Am J Hum Genet 2004;75:106–11.
74. Kosaki K, Sato S, Hasegawa T, et al. Premature ovarian failure in a female with proximal symphalangism and Noggin mutation. Fertil Steril 2004;81:1137–9.
75. Sills ES, Harmon KE, Tucker MJ. First reported convergence of premature ovarian failure and cutis marmorata telangiectatica congenita. Fertil Steril 2002;78:1314–6.
76. Karlberg N, Jalanko H, Perheentupa J, Lipsanen-Nyman M. Mulibrey nanism: clinical features and diagnostic criteria. J Med Genet 2004;41:92–8.
77. Karlberg S, Tiitinen A, Lipsanen-Nyman M. Failure of sexual maturation in Mulibrey nanism. N Engl J Med 2004;351(24):2559–60.
78. Schiffmann R, van der Knaap MS. The latest on leukodystrophies. Curr Opin Neurol 2004;17:187–92.
79. LaMarca A, Brozzetti A, Sighinolfi G, et al. Primary ovarian insufficiency: autoimmune causes. Curr Opinion Obstet Gynecol 2010;22:277–82.
80. Falorni A, Laureti S, Santeusanio F. Autoantibodies in autoimmune polyendocrine syndrome type II. Endocrinol Metab Clin North Am 2002;31:369–89, vii.
81. Dal Pra C, Chen S, Furmaniak J, et al. Autoantibodies to steroidogenic enzymes in patients with premature ovarian failure with and without Addison's disease. Eur J Endocrinol 2003;148:565–70.
82. Cutolo M, Sulli A, Pizzorni C, et al. Hypothalamic–pituitary–adrenocortical and gonadal functions in rheumatoid arthritis. Ann N Y Acad Sci 2003;992:107–17.
83. Ryan MM, Jones Jr HR. Myasthenia gravis and premature ovarian failure. Muscle Nerve 2004;30:231–3.
84. Dorman JS, Steenkiste AR, Foley TP, et al. Menopause in type 1 diabetic women: is it premature? Diabetes 2001;50:1857–62.
85. Maclaren N, Chen QY, Kukreja A, et al. Autoimmune hypogonadism as part of an autoimmune polyglandular syndrome. J Soc Gynecol Investig 2001;8(1 Suppl Proceedings):S52–4.
86. Myhre AG, Halonen M, Eskelin P, et al. Autoimmune polyendocrine syndrome type 1 (APS I) in Norway. Clin Endocrinol (Oxf) 2001;54:211–7.
87. Medeiros MM, Silveira VA, Menezes AP, Carvalho RC. Risk factors for ovarian failure in patients with systemic lupus erythematosus. Braz J Med Biol Res 2001;34:1561–8.
88. Tuohy VK, Altuntas CZ. Autoimmunity and premature ovarian failure. Curr Opin Obstet Gynecol 2007;19:366–9.
89. Forges T, Monnier-Barbarino P, Faure GC, Bene MC. Autoimmunity and antigenic targets in ovarian pathology. Hum Reprod Update 2004;10:163–75.
90. Fernandes AM, Arruda Mde S, Bedone AJ. Twin gestation two years after the diagnosis of premature ovarian failure in a woman on hormone replacement therapy. A case report. J Reprod Med 2002;47:504–6.
91. Nelson LM. Primary ovarian insufficiency. N Engl J Med 2009;360:606–14.
92. Anasti JN. Premature ovarian failure: an update. Fertil Steril 1998;70:1–15.
93. Hovatta O. Cryopreservation and culture of human primordial and primary ovarian follicles. Mol Cell Endocrinol 2000;169(1–2):95–7.
94. Chiauzzi VA, Bussmann L, Calvo JC, et al. Circulating immunoglobulins that inhibit the binding of follicle-stimulating hormone to its receptor: a putative diagnostic role in resistant ovary syndrome? Clin Endocrinol (Oxf) 2004;61:46–54.
95. Aslam MF, Gilmour K, McCune GS. Spontaneous pregnancies in patients with resistant ovary syndrome while on HRT. J Obstet Gynaecol 2004;24:573–4.
96. Mueller A, Berkholz A, Dittrich R, Wildt L. Spontaneous normalization of ovarian function and pregnancy in a patient with resistant ovary syndrome. Eur J Obstet Gynecol Reprod Biol 2003;111:210–3.
97. Dragojevic-Dikic S, Marisavljevic D, Mitrovic A, et al. An immunological insight into premature ovarian failure (POF). Autoimmun Rev 2010;9:771–4.
98. Kalu E, Panay N. Spontaneous premature ovarian failure: management challenges. Gynecol Endocrinol 2008;24:273–9.
99. Ramos-Casals M, Trejo O, Garcia-Carrasco M, et al. Triple association between hepatitis C virus infection, systemic autoimmune diseases, and B cell lymphoma. J Rheumatol 2004;31:495–9.
100. Lewis J. Eosinophilic perifolliculitis: a variant of autoimmune oophoritis? Int J Gynecol Pathol 1993;12:360–4.
101. Nelson LM, Bakalov VK. Mechanisms of follicular dysfunction in 46,XX spontaneous premature ovarian failure. Endocrinol Metab Clin North Am 2003;32:613–37.
102. Meysing AU, Kanasaki H, Bedecarrats GY, et al. GNRHR mutations in a woman with idiopathic hypogonadotropic hypogonadism highlight the differential sensitivity of luteinizing hormone and follicle-stimulating hormone to gonadotropin-releasing hormone. J Clin Endocrinol Metab 2004;89:3189–98.
103. Timmreck LS, Reindollar RH. Contemporary issues in primary amenorrhea. Obstet Gynecol Clin North Am 2003;30:287–302.
104. Trimarchi CP, Russo P. Cyclic estrogen-progestin hormone therapy as a new therapeutic approach in the treatment of functional alterations of the hypothalamus–pituitary–ovary axis: case reports. Endocr Res 2002;28:155–60.
105. Hoffman B, Bradshaw KD. Delayed puberty and amenorrhea. Semin Reprod Med 2003;21:353–62.
106. Vendeland LL, Shehadeh L. Incidental finding of an accessory ovary in a 16-year-old at laparoscopy. A case report. J Reprod Med 2000;45:435–8.
107. Hartigan K, Pecha B, Rao G. Intrarenal supernumerary ovary excised with partial nephrectomy. Urology 2006;67:424 e11–2.
108. Litos MG, Furara S, Chin K. Supernumerary ovary: a case report and literature review. J Obstet Gynaecol 2003;23:325–7.
109. Kamiyama K, Moromizato H, Toma T, et al. Two cases of supernumerary ovary: one with large fibroma with Meig's syndrome and the other with endometriosis and cystic change. Pathol Res Pract 2001;197:847–51.
110. Kuga T, Esato K, Takeda K, et al. A supernumerary ovary of the omentum with cystic change: report of two cases and review of the literature. Pathol Int 1999;49:566–70.
111. Sharatz SM, Trevino TA, Rodriguez L, West JH. Giant serous cystadenoma arising from an accessory ovary in a morbidly obese 11-year-old girl: a case report. J Med Case Rep 2008;2:7–10.
112. Trinidad C, Tardaguila F, Fernandez GC, et al. Ovarian maldescent. Eur Radiol 2004;14:805–8.
113. Kaya H, Sezik M, Ozkaya O, Kose SA. Mayer–Rokitansky–Kuster–Hauser syndrome associated with unilateral gonadal agenesis. A case report. J Reprod Med 2003;48:902–4.
114. Mylonas I, Hansch S, Markmann S, et al. Unilateral ovarian agenesis: report of three cases and review of the literature. Arch Gynecol Obstet 2003;268:57–60.
115. Dueck A, Poenaru D, Jamieson MA, Kamal IK. Unilateral ovarian agenesis and fallopian tube maldescent. Pediatr Surg Int 2001;17(2–3):228–9.

116. Cualing H, Wang G, Noffsinger A, Fenoglio-Preiser C. Heterotopic ovarian splenoma: report of a first case. Arch Pathol Lab Med 2001;125:1483–5.
117. Bonneau D, Roume J, Gonzalez M, et al. Splenogonadal fusion limb defect syndrome: report of five new cases and review. Am J Med Genet 1999;86:347–58.
118. Mitra S, Nicol A, Scott GI. Uterus-like mass of the ovary. J Obstet Gynaecol 1997;17:94–5.
119. Ahmed AA, Swan RW, Owen A, et al. Uterus-like mass arising in the broad ligament: a metaplasia or mullerian duct anomaly? Int J Gynecol Pathol 1997;16:279–81.
120. Gray Y, Libbey P. Xanthogranulomatous salpingitis and oophoritis: a case report and review of the literature. Arch Pathol Lab Med 2001;125:260–3.
121. Chou SC, Wang JS, Tseng HH. Malacoplakia of the ovary, fallopian tube and uterus: a case associated with diabetes mellitus. Pathol Int 2002;52:789–93.
122. Benkiran L, Gamra L, Lamalmi N, et al. [Pelvic actinomycosis simulating adnexal malignant tumor]. Med Trop (Mars) 2002;62:73–6.
123. Dunn TS, Cothren C, Klein L, Krammer T. Pelvic actinomycosis: a case report. J Reprod Med 2006;51:435–7.
124. Burlando SC, Paz LA, De Feo LG, et al. [Ovarian abscess due to Actinomyces sp. in absence of an intrauterine contraceptive device]. Medicina (B Aires) 2001;61(5 Pt 1):577–80.
125. Dogan NU, Salman MC, Gultekin M, et al. Bilateral actinomyces abscesses mimicking pelvic malignancy. Int J Gynaecol Obstet 2006;94:58–9.
126. Jahromi BN, Parsanezhad ME, Ghane-Shirazi R. Female genital tuberculosis and infertility. Int J Gynecol Obstet 2001;75:269–72.
127. Hviid A, Rubin S, Muhlemann K. Mumps. Lancet 2008;371:932–44.
128. Manfredi R, Alampi G, Talo S, et al. Silent oophoritis due to cytomegalovirus in a patient with advanced HIV disease. Int J STD AIDS 2000;11:410–2.
129. Nieto Y, Ross M, Gianani R, et al. Post-mortem incidental finding of cytomegalovirus oophoritis after an allogeneic stem cell transplant. Bone Marrow Transplant 1999;23:1323–4.
130. Ortiz-Rey JA, Touza F, Perez-Valcarcel J, Perez-Villanueva J. [Oophoritis due to cytomegalovirus in a female AIDS patient]. Med Clin (Barc) 1997;108:357–8.
131. Yu J, Solano FX, Seethala RR. Bilateral cytomegalovirus (CMV) oophoritis mimicking widely metastatic carcinoma: a case report and review of the literature. Diagn Pathol 2007;2:50–4.
132. Batista TP, Romao de Andrade JJ, Magnata de Fonte Filho LA. Schistosoma mansoni: an unusual cause of ovarian pseudotumor. Arch Gynecol Obstet 2010;281:141–3.
133. Craggs B, De Waele E, De Vogelaere K, et al. Enterobius vermicularis infection with tuboovarian abscess and peritonitis occurring during pregnancy. Surg Infections 2009;10:545–7.
134. Tampakoudis P, Assimakopoulos E, Zafrakas M, et al. Pelvic echinococcus mimicking multicystic ovary. Ultrasound Obstet Gynecol 2003;22:196–8.
135. Yuksel M, Demirpolat G, Sever A, et al. Hydatid disease involving some rare locations in the body: a pictorial assay. Korean J Radiol 2007;8:531–40.
136. Parveen AS, Elliott H, Howells R. Sarcoidosis of the ovary. J Obstet Gynaecol 2004;24:465.
137. Monneuse O, Pilleul F, Gruner L, et al. MRI evaluation in a rare case of Crohn's disease complicated by abscess of the ovary. Gastroenterol Clin Biol 2006;30:153–4.
138. Marcovici I, Goldberg E. Ovarian vein thrombosis associated with Crohn's disease: a case report. Am J Obstet Gynecol 2000;182:743–4.
139. Pilch H, Schaffer U, Gunzel S, et al. (A)symptomatic necrotizing arteritis of the female genital tract. Eur J Obstet Gynecol Reprod Biol 2000;91:191–6.
140. Bell DA, Mondschein M, Scully RE. Giant cell arteritis of the female genital tract. A report of three cases. Am J Surg Pathol 1986;10:696–701.
141. Herve F, Heron F, Levesque H, Marie I. Ascites as the first manifestation of polyarteritis nodosa. Scand J Gastroenterol 2006;41:493–5.
142. Kaya E, Utas C, Balkanli S, et al. Isolated ovarian polyarteritis nodosa. Acta Obstet Gynecol Scand 1994;73:736–8.
143. Kominiarek MA, Hibbard JU. Postpartum ovarian vein thrombosis: an update. Obstet Gynecol Surv 2006;61:337–42.

Non-Neoplastic and Tumor-Like Conditions of the Ovary

Emanuela F. Veras, Jennifer H. Crow, Stanley J. Robboy

CHAPTER OUTLINE

Dysfunctional Cysts	535
Cysts Derived from Preovulatory Follicles (Follicular Cysts)	536
Corpus Luteum Cysts	538
Corpus Albicans Cysts	539
Simple (Unclassified) Cysts	540
Tumor-Like Lesions Associated with Pregnancy	540
Luteomas of Pregnancy (Nodular Theca–Lutein Hyperplasia of Pregnancy)	540
Multiple Theca–Lutein Cysts (Hyperreactio Luteinalis)	542
Solitary Luteinized Follicular Cysts of Pregnancy and Puerperium	542
Leydig (Hilus) Cell Hyperplasia	543
Deciduosis (Ectopic Decidua)	543
Ovarian Granulosa Cell Proliferations of Pregnancy	544
Ovarian Pregnancy	544
Primary Ovarian Trophoblastic Disease	545
Other Ovarian Lesions	546
Reactive Stromal Tumor-Like Lesions	546
Polycystic Ovary Syndrome	546
Stromal Hyperplasia and Hyperthecosis	548
Leydig (Hilus) Cell Hyperplasia	551
Massive Ovarian Edema and Fibromatosis	552
Sequelae of Surgery or Trauma	556
Ovarian Remnant Syndrome (Residual or Remnant Ovary Syndrome)	556
Ovarian 'Drilling' for Polycystic Ovary Syndrome	557
Splenosis (Autotransplantantion of Splenic Tissue)	557
Iatrogenic Disorders of the Ovaries	558
Radiotherapy Damage	558
Chemotherapeutic and Immunosuppressive Drugs	558
Oral Contraceptives	558
Progesterone	559
Danazol	559
(GnRH) Analogs	559
Ovulation-Induction Agents	559
Tamoxifen	560
Ovarian Hemorrhage and Adnexal Torsion	560
Ovarian Hemorrhage	560
Adnexal Torsion	560
Müllerianosis and Reactive Mesothelial Lesions	561

DYSFUNCTIONAL CYSTS

Definitions

Dysfunctional ovarian cysts derive from the follicular apparatus either before or after ovulation (Table 24.1). They may result from or cause disordered hypothalamic–pituitary–ovarian function. Although not always functional in the sense of producing steroid hormones, the cysts all have or have had the potential to do so at some stage in their development.

Ultrasound examination is used widely in the diagnosis and surveillance of these cysts, which achieve clinical importance if they exceed 3 cm in premenopausal and early postmenopausal women or 1 cm in late postmenopausal women, and if they do not disappear on repeat scanning. Most disappear spontaneously within 2–3 weeks. Cyst aspiration is not recommended, as the cysts often recur and the sensitivity for the detection of malignancy is low.

'Polycystic ovaries' is a term that should be reserved for the abnormal ovaries found in association with functional hyperandrogenism (the Stein–Leventhal and related

Table 24.1	Classification of Dysfunctional Ovarian Cysts

Cysts derived from preovulatory follicles
    Follicular cyst—unluteinized
    Follicular cyst—luteinized
        Granulosa lutein cyst
        Theca–lutein cyst
    Follicular cyst—atretic
Cysts derived from corpus luteum
    Cystic corpus luteum
    Corpus luteum cyst
    Corpus albicans cyst
Simple cysts

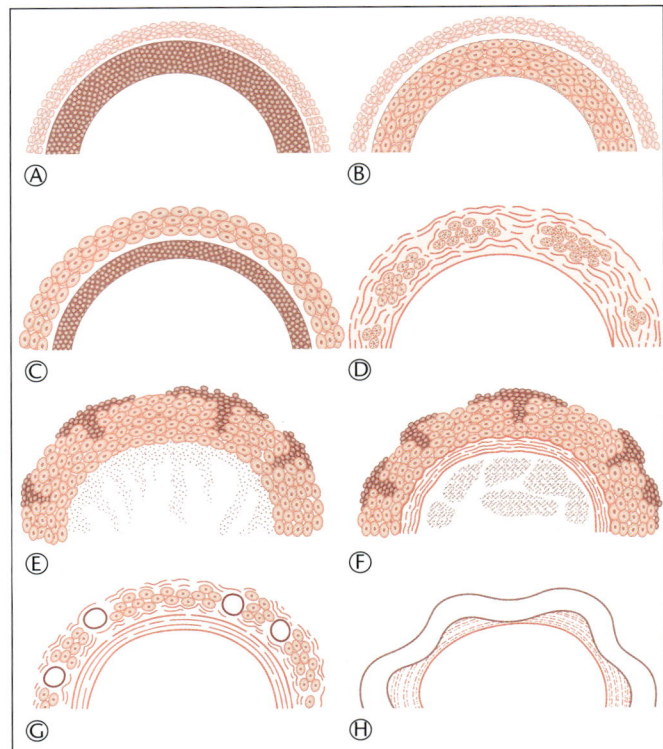

Figure 24.1 Comparative morphology of dysfunctional cysts. **(A)** Unluteinized follicular cyst. **(B)** Granulosa lutein cyst. **(C)** Theca–lutein cyst. **(D)** Involuting follicular cyst. **(E)** Cystic corpus luteum. **(F)** Corpus luteum cyst (early). **(G)** Corpus luteum cyst (late). **(H)** Corpus albicans cyst.

clinical syndromes; see later). The ovaries commonly have thick white capsules, and display multiple cystic follicles and small, luteinized follicular cysts of atretic type, absence of stigmata of recent ovulation, and occur with a characteristic disturbance of hypothalamic–pituitary function. Ovaries displaying several cysts, but otherwise not fitting into this category, should be called 'multicystic' to avoid confusion.

Corpus luteum cysts also derive from the follicular apparatus but show evidence of prior ovulation, which distinguishes them from follicular cysts. Ovulation is indicated by convolution of the cyst lining (which results from collapse of the follicle) with the characteristic invaginations of theca–lutein (paralutein) cells into the inner zone of granulosa lutein cells. A layer of fibrous tissue lining the inner surface of the cyst, resulting from organization of the corpus luteum hematoma, also indicates that ovulation has occurred.

Features distinguishing the various types of cysts derived from the follicular apparatus appear diagrammatically in Figure 24.1.

CYSTS DERIVED FROM PREOVULATORY FOLLICLES (FOLLICULAR CYSTS)

Etiology

The etiology of follicular cysts (by definition ≥3.0 cm) is not always obvious but in most cases reflects disordered function of the pituitary–ovarian axis. Pathologic cystic change may develop either in the follicular growth phase or during atresia. Unluteinized follicular cysts (Figure 24.1A), which produce predominantly estradiol, result from excessive ovarian stimulation (either by endogenous follicle-stimulating hormone (FSH) or by ovulation-induction agents) or an abnormal response to normal stimulation.

Granulosa lutein cysts are follicular cysts with predominantly luteinized granulosa cells (which are internal to the basal lamina; see Figure 24.1B). Like corpora lutea, the granulosa cells secrete progesterone. An unknown proportion of granulosa lutein cysts results from failure of follicular rupture at the expected time of ovulation and is the basis of the luteinized unruptured follicle syndrome, which occurs more frequently in infertile than in normal fertile women.[1]

Theca–lutein cysts are follicular cysts with luteinization predominantly of the theca interna (which is external to the basal lamina; see Figure 24.1C). Androstenedione is the characteristic steroid product. These cysts develop when there is prolonged exposure to luteinizing hormone (LH) or beta human chorionic gonadotropin (β-hCG), either endogenous, such as in polycystic ovary syndrome (PCOS; see later) or hyperreactio luteinalis syndrome of pregnancy (multiple theca–lutein cysts), or exogenous, as in the ovarian hyperstimulation syndrome. Atretic follicular cysts can also elaborate androstenedione.

Clinical Features

Ovarian cysts in the fetus are more frequent than were once thought, with an estimated incidence of about one in 2500 births. They are usually diagnosed in the third trimester by ultrasound or magnetic resonance imaging (MRI).[2] A cyst size below 4–5 cm usually carries a low risk of torsion, whereas larger cysts have a high risk, and therefore may warrant decompression. However, the criteria and recommendations for therapy vary widely.[2–4] Since torsion can lead to ovarian loss and thus impact future fertility, the goal of intervention is to preserve fertility.[2,6] Therapeutic intervention is usually prompted by acute torsion in the newborn or persistent cysts exceeding 5 cm in diameter in children older than 6 months of age.

In prepubertal girls, follicular cysts form a significant proportion of ovarian lesions that come to surgical intervention. Common clinical presentations are pain, vomiting, diarrhea, and constipation, sometimes precipitated by ovarian torsion. A less common but well-recognized association is with isosexual pseudoprecocity, either idiopathic or associated with hypothyroidism or the McCune–Albright syndrome (polyostotic fibrous dysplasia, cutaneous melanin pigmentation, and endocrine organ hyperactivity).[7,8]

During the reproductive years, unluteinized follicular cysts may produce sufficient estradiol to cause irregular or prolonged (dysfunctional) uterine bleeding. The endometrium in such cases may show disordered proliferative phase changes or hyperplasia. Granulosa lutein cysts secrete progesterone, but rarely in sufficient amounts to disturb the menstrual cycle. Atretic cysts, if numerous (as in the PCOS), may synthesize sufficient androstenedione to produce hirsutism or virilization. Observation shows that most regress spontaneously over a few cycles and that therapy with contraceptive agents does not accelerate this process.[9,10] Persistence should raise the suspicion of neoplasia.

During pregnancy, pre-existing follicular cysts may become luteinized. New cysts rarely develop but a notable exception is the hyperreactio luteinalis syndrome (multiple theca–lutein cysts). Large solitary luteinized follicular cysts may present as adnexal masses in the third to fourth months of pregnancy or postpartum, or are incidental findings at cesarean section.

Symptomatic follicular cysts are rare after menopause, although some sporadic follicular activity (generally without ovulation) continues in the early years.

Gross Features

These are usually single and 3–10 cm in diameter. Solitary luteinized follicle cysts of pregnancy and puerperium have a median diameter of 25 cm. They are smooth lined and contain clear proteinaceous fluid or altered blood.

Microscopic Features

Unluteinized follicular cysts show the microscopic features of physiologic growing cystic follicles, with well-preserved granulosa and theca layers separated by a basal lamina (Figure 24.2). However the cumulus oophorus and oocyte are no longer present. The lining may be somewhat attenuated secondary to dilatation. There is no trace of the festooned pattern of a corpus luteum. During involution the lining is often incomplete and later appears as small clusters of lutein cells in the compressed ovarian stroma, which becomes progressively fibrotic. As involution continues, distinguishing features become increasingly difficult to identify and definitive diagnosis may not be possible (Figure 24.3); in this situation the cyst is better designated 'simple' (see later).

Cytologically, unluteinized follicular cysts contain numerous granulosa cells that have been shed into the fluid and reflect the normal lining. The cells are arranged singly and in tight clusters. The clusters may be irregular in shape, some with papillary configurations. Granulosa cells contain round to oval nuclei and a small rim of distinct cytoplasm. The chromatin is coarsely granular. Nuclear grooves are occasionally seen. Mitoses may be identified. The cells are uniform with negligible variation from cell to cell. Degenerative changes may be present.

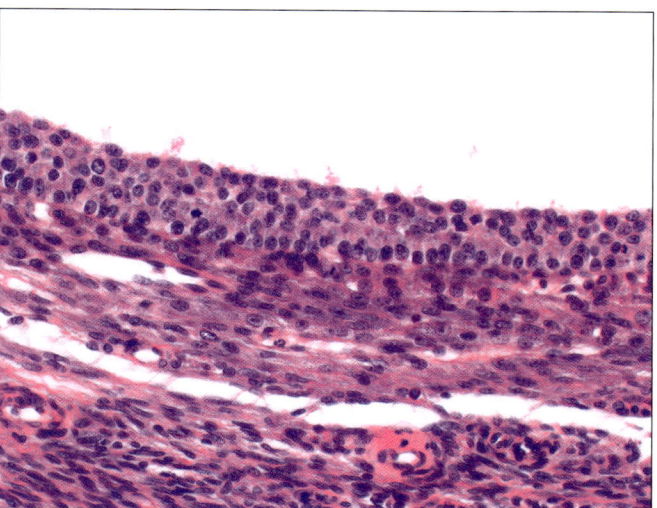

Figure 24.2 Unluteinized follicular cyst. About four layers of uniform small granulosa cells are present above the basal lamina.

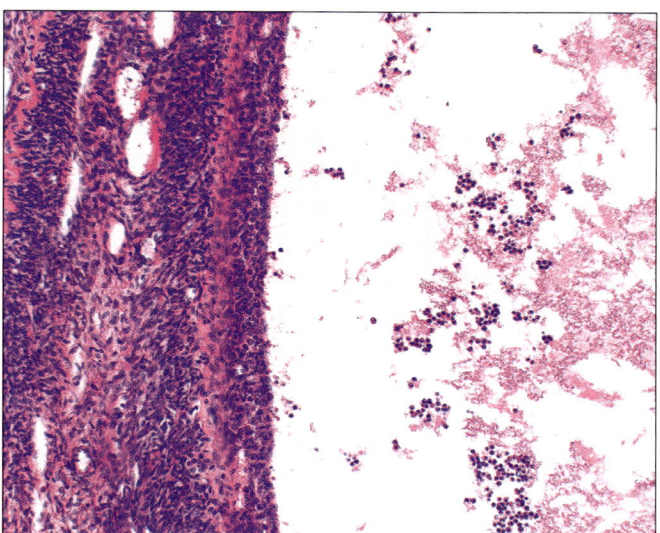

Figure 24.3 Involuting follicular cyst. Smooth internal contour and inapparent lining cells of follicular origin. Shed granulosa cells in the lumen are a useful guide to diagnosis.

Luteinized follicular cysts show the general features of unluteinized follicular cysts as described above, but in addition some of the cells in the cyst wall are luteinized. The granulosa (granulosa lutein cyst; see Figure 24.4) or theca layer (theca–lutein cyst; see Figures 24.5 and 24.6), or occasionally both, luteinize, although the cyst is classified according to the layer predominantly affected. Luteinization appears as enlarged cells with increased eosinophilic or finely vacuolated cytoplasm. The changes are similar to those in a corpus luteum.

Cytologically, luteinized follicular cysts contain single and/or clusters of luteinized granulosa cells with round to oval nuclei, coarse chromatin, and small prominent nucleoli. Cell cytoplasm is ample and foamy. Mitotic figures may be found. The cells lack pleomorphism. Degenerative

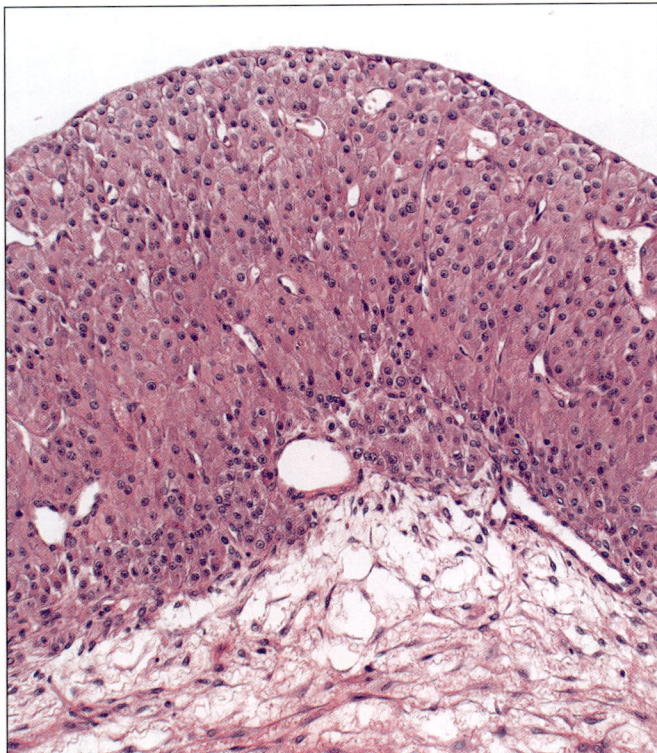

Figure 24.4 Granulosa lutein cyst lined by large eosinophilic cells. The thecal layer is relatively inconspicuous.

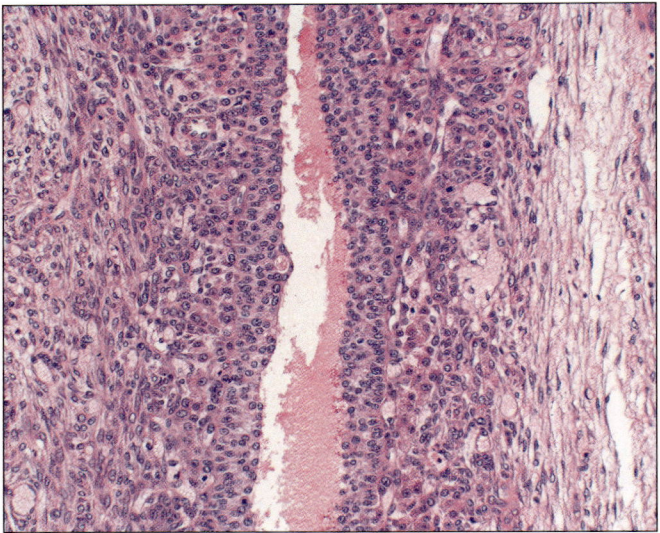

Figure 24.5 Theca–lutein cyst. Thick lining of small granulosa cells with large luteinized theca cells beneath basal lamina (from patient with PCOS).

changes may be present in single cells with obvious nuclear pyknosis.

Atretic follicular cysts are lined by ovarian stroma in which there are small clusters of luteinized theca cells. They may be indistinguishable from involuting follicular cysts of other types.

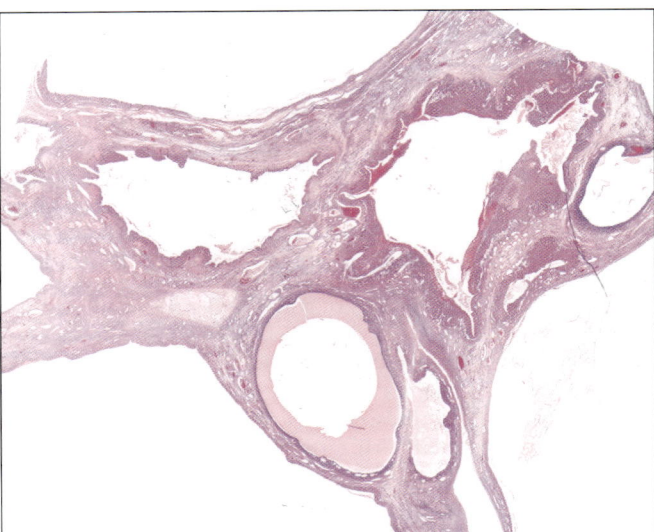

Figure 24.6 Multiple theca–lutein cysts in pregnancy. Ribbons of luteinized cells line cysts.

Differential Diagnosis

Cysts derived from a corpus luteum can be distinguished from luteinized follicular cysts by their retention, partially or focally, of their convoluted lining with invaginations of paralutein cells, and by their innermost lining of fibrous tissue (the result of organization of the central coagulum). In addition a well-defined vascular zone may be evident.

Cystic granulosa cell tumors may be difficult to distinguish from follicular cysts. They are often considerably larger and always unilateral. The neoplastic cells lining the cysts may show prominent luteinization and may display mitotic activity. Although most granulosa cell tumors are estrogenic, 15–30% of the cystic variants are clinically androgenic, a feature not associated with follicular cysts except in the specific clinical situations mentioned above.

CORPUS LUTEUM CYSTS

Etiology

These are cysts derived from corpora lutea of menstruation or pregnancy that result from excessive central hemorrhage. Small physiologic hemorrhages occur 2–4 days after ovulation during the stage when the corpus luteum vascularizes. They usually organize rapidly, but if the hemorrhage is excessive and the corpus luteum becomes overdistended with blood, involution is likely to be delayed.

Clinical Features

Most are asymptomatic. In some non-pregnant women, this delayed involution (sometimes called 'persistent corpus luteum') and its continuing production of progesterone may result in minor menstrual disturbances (so-called 'irregular shedding').

Gross Features

Corpora lutea of menstruation rarely exceed 3 cm (average size 2 cm) but may do so if there is an unusually large

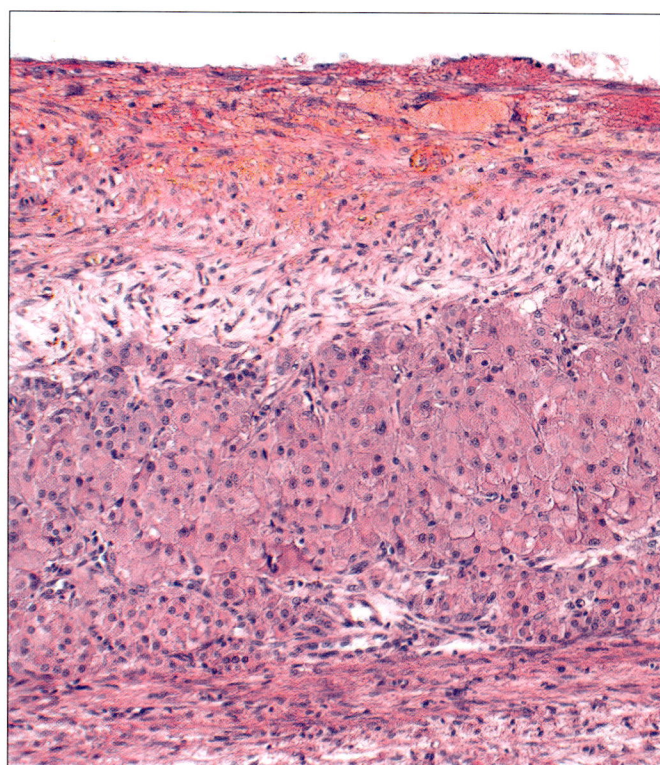

Figure 24.7 Early corpus luteum cyst. Organizing hematoma at top and thin zone of involuting vacuolated luteinized cells below.

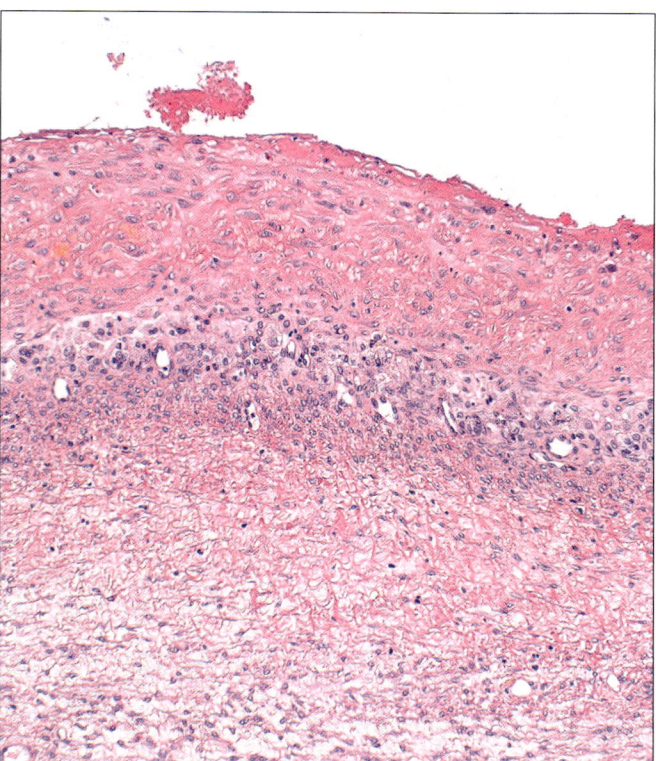

Figure 24.8 Late corpus luteum cyst. Inner zone of fibrous tissue with involuting vacuolated luteinized cells beneath.

fluid-filled central cavity. Cystic corpora lutea of pregnancy often exceed 5 cm and may exceed 10 cm in diameter. They are not infrequently identified on routine ultrasound examination in early pregnancy. They contain clear fluid or altered blood. Rupture may be evident. They are generally smooth lined with an incomplete band of yellow tissue in the wall.

Microscopic Features

Cystic corpora lutea display the same features as their non-cystic counterparts. The distension leads to some attenuation of the convolutions but without loss of distinctive cell layers. The fibrous tissue lining contains mature collagen demonstrable with a trichrome connective tissue stain. Peripheral clusters of small paralutein (theca–lutein) cells may still be seen between larger groups of granulosa lutein cells (Figure 24.7). The granulosa and theca–lutein cells are smaller than those seen in a fresh corpus luteum. The nuclei are small, hyperchromatic, and lack mitotic activity, while the cytoplasm is usually finely vesicular. With progressive involution, fewer and smaller islands of lutein cells are found within the increasingly fibrotic wall, but a well-defined zone of small blood vessels remains to mark the phase of vascularization (Figure 24.8).

Cytologically, corpus luteum cysts contain numerous fully luteinized granulosa cells singly and in clusters and mixed with fresh blood and scattered hemosiderin-laden macrophages. Unlike those from follicular cysts, these cells are large and polyhedral in shape with eccentric, round nuclei. Hemorrhagic corpus luteum cysts may be identified by these features as well as the presence of abundant fibrin and some fibroblasts in the smear background. Regressing corpora lutea may contain large luteinized cells, as well as numerous macrophages with yellow hematoidin pigment.

Differential Diagnosis

Luteinized follicular cysts appear macroscopically like corpus luteum cysts but are less likely to be hemorrhagic. The microscopic distinction hinges around evidence of ovulation as indicated earlier. Follicular cysts generally lack the zone of vascularization. Some long-standing cysts may be very difficult to classify.

Endometriotic cysts may be impossible to distinguish macroscopically from corpus luteum cysts but should be suspected if there is evidence of endometriosis elsewhere. Microscopic identification of endometrial glands or stroma within the cyst confirms the diagnosis.

CORPUS ALBICANS CYSTS

The corpus albicans is typically a small, solid, hyalinized fibrous scar, but occasionally has a central cavity containing clear fluid. The cysts are rarely more than 1 cm in diameter, and develop after corpora lutea involute. The mechanism of fluid retention or accumulation is not known.

Microscopically, the cyst wall consists of a convoluted ribbon-like band of hyalinized acellular fibrous tissue, usually with an innermost lining of looser fibrous connective tissue with a smoother outline. The cysts are nonfunctional and are too small to produce symptomatic adnexal masses.

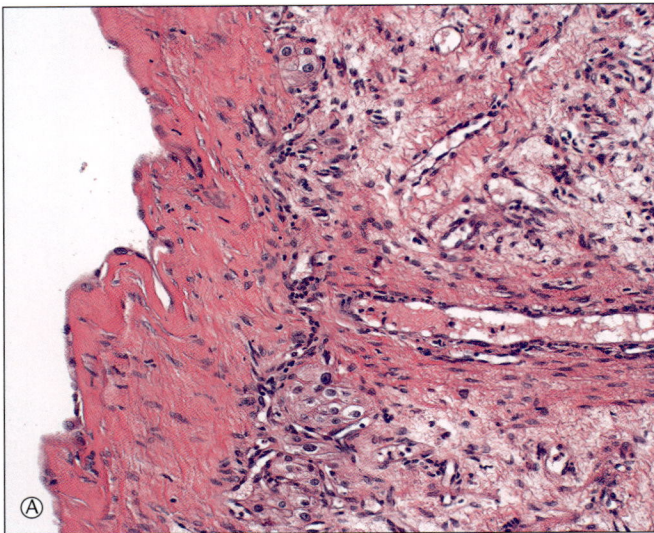 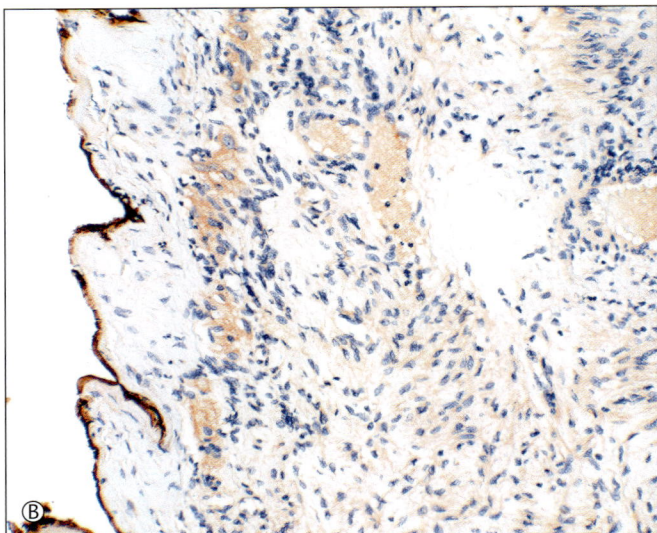

Figure 24.9 Simple cyst. **(A)** A dense fibrous tissue wall is lined by barely perceptible 'epithelial' cells. Occasional lutein-like cells beneath this fibrous layer suggest origin from the follicular apparatus. **(B)** Persistent α-inhibin reactivity in the lining cells (as well as the lutein-like cells in the wall) support this interpretation.

SIMPLE (UNCLASSIFIED) CYSTS

Definition

These are ovarian cysts or cyst-like structures that lack identifiable linings. Some produce symptomatic adnexal masses but most are incidental findings. The cysts are usually less than 10 cm in diameter, solitary, and have a smooth internal surface and a variable content of clear fluid or altered blood. Most are of follicular origin, although some arise as epithelial cysts.

Microscopic Features

The lining usually consists only of a narrow band of dense fibrous tissue or compressed ovarian stroma. There may be occasional small clusters of involuting lutein cells in the cyst wall, suggesting an origin from the follicular apparatus. Sometimes there is a complete or partial lining of apparent epithelial cells that are too attenuated for their origin to be identified (Figure 24.9A) but, even here, persistent reactivity for α-inhibin may be present (Figure 24.9B). Some cysts undoubtedly represent epithelial cystomas. Some are lined by granulation tissue or organizing hematoma. Such lesions may be endometriotic in origin but lack overall the necessary diagnostic features. There is probably no benefit in precisely categorizing 'simple' cysts. All are benign and most are non-neoplastic.

TUMOR-LIKE LESIONS ASSOCIATED WITH PREGNANCY

Non-neoplastic ovarian lesions encountered exclusively in pregnancy or the puerperium involute spontaneously after the pregnancy ends and radical surgery is clearly inappropriate treatment. Other ovarian enlargements not necessarily exclusive to pregnancy are also seen, e.g., corpus luteum, endometriotic, and paraovarian cysts.

LUTEOMAS OF PREGNANCY (NODULAR THECA–LUTEIN HYPERPLASIA OF PREGNANCY)

Definition

These are multinodular, often multicentric or bilateral, tumor-like masses of lutein cells that develop during an otherwise normal pregnancy (presenting usually in the third trimester) and involute in the puerperium. They represent the extreme example of nodular theca–lutein hyperplasia of pregnancy.

Clinical Features

About one-fourth of patients become hirsute or virilized. Approximately 80% of cases occur in black women. Rarely, female fetuses display masculinizing signs at birth.

Etiology

The lesions most likely arise from the lutein cells found during pregnancy as isolated groups in the stroma or in the walls of atretic follicles. Some patients have a history suggestive of PCOS. β-hCG is necessary for the development of luteomas, but is unlikely to be the only etiologic factor since the lesions are not associated with trophoblastic disease or with early pregnancy, when β-hCG levels are at their highest. Morphologic and clinical similarities exist between luteomas and multiple theca–lutein cysts (hyperreactio luteinalis), and it is possible that they are related forms of theca–lutein cell hyperplasia. Unlike luteomas, hyperreactio luteinalis is associated with conditions of pathologic β-hCG elevation, multiple gestations, and abnormal pregnancy states.

Gross Features

Luteomas are usually 6–12 cm in diameter but may exceed 20 cm. They are circumscribed, multinodular solid masses with a soft gray-brown to tan cut surface. Small cystic spaces may be present. Those removed in the puerperium may be softer and paler or even frankly necrotic.

Microscopic Features

Luteomas display sheets of large eosinophilic cells that are broken up into groups by numerous delicate blood vessels. An organoid pattern (Figure 24.10) is common. A trabecular arrangement is less frequently seen. The cell size is intermediate between that of granulosa and theca–lutein cells. The reticulin pattern of fibers around groups rather than individual cells is also intermediate between the abundant pericellular distribution of reticulin fibers in the theca interna and the paucity of fibers in the granulosa layer. Follicular spaces containing colloid-like material may be present but the intracellular hyaline droplets ('colloid bodies') typical of corpora lutea of pregnancy are rare. The cytoplasm is eosinophilic and sometimes finely vacuolated but contains little stainable lipid. The round central nuclei have a prominent nucleolus and abundant euchromatin. There may be mild nuclear pleomorphism and some mitotic figures (<3 per 10 HPF) (Figure 24.10). The remainder of the ovary shows the physiologic changes of pregnancy but small theca–lutein cysts may be evident as well. Early involutional changes include nuclear pyknosis and increased cytoplasmic vacuolization. Eventually the luteoma is reduced to sheets of necrotic cells (Figure 24.11). Even at this late stage, the typical reticulin pattern may still be useful diagnostically.

Differential Diagnosis

Non-cystic aggregates of large lutein-like cells include a plethora of entities in the differential diagnosis, some neoplastic, some not (Figure 24.12). The clinical context and gross features of the lesions all contribute to their separation.

Nodular stromal hyperthecosis may occur in pregnancy. The ovaries are uniformly enlarged and display multiple microscopic nodules of spindle-shaped luteinized stromal cells, arranged in bundles rather than nests. Reticulin fibers invest individual cells that have pale or finely vacuolated cytoplasm containing abundant lipid.

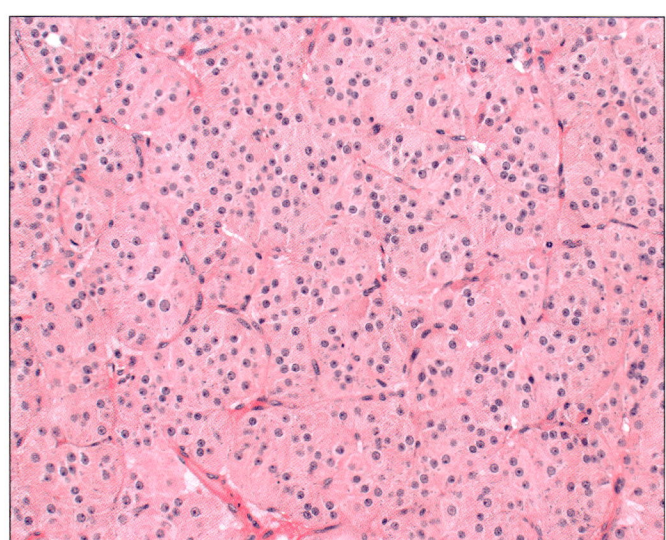

Figure 24.10 Luteoma of pregnancy. Distinctly organoid pattern with cell groups separated by delicate vessels. Note mild nuclear variation.

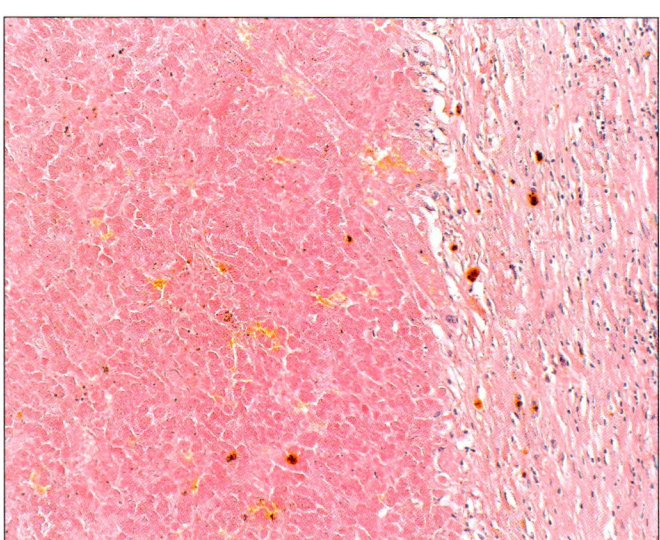

Figure 24.11 Luteoma of pregnancy. Involuted luteoma 5 months postpartum; sheets of ghost cells with some organization (granulation tissue) at margin.

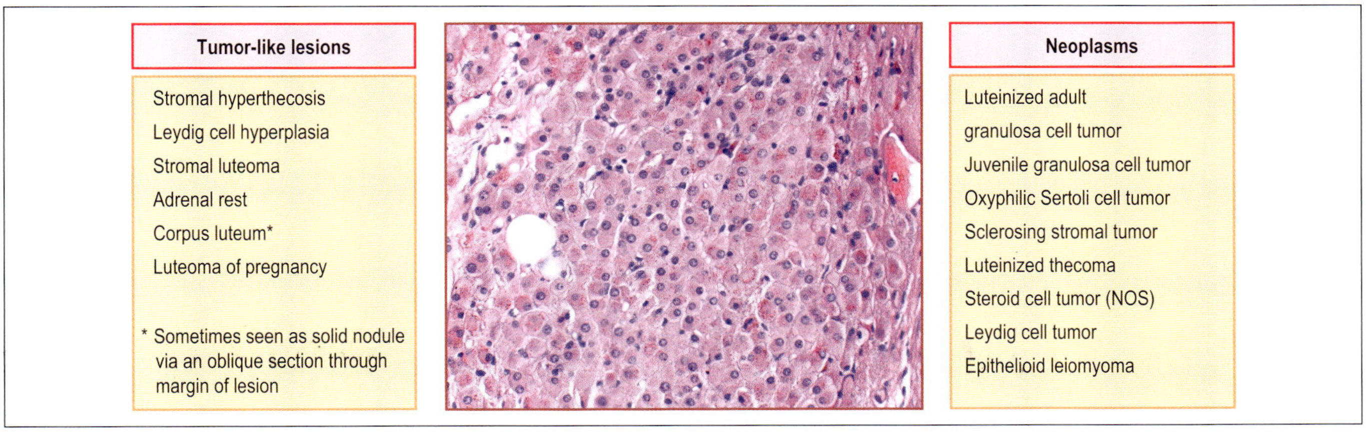

Tumor-like lesions	Neoplasms
Stromal hyperthecosis	Luteinized adult granulosa cell tumor
Leydig cell hyperplasia	Juvenile granulosa cell tumor
Stromal luteoma	Oxyphilic Sertoli cell tumor
Adrenal rest	Sclerosing stromal tumor
Corpus luteum*	Luteinized thecoma
Luteoma of pregnancy	Steroid cell tumor (NOS)
	Leydig cell tumor
	Epithelioid leiomyoma

* Sometimes seen as solid nodule via an oblique section through margin of lesion

Figure 24.12 Non-cystic aggregates of lutein-like cells: differential diagnosis.

Table 24.2 Steroid Cell Tumor versus Pregnancy Luteoma: Differential Diagnosis

	Steroid Cell Tumor	Pregnancy Luteoma
Clinical		
Mean age:	47 years	26 years
Relationship to pregnancy	None	Diagnosed at or near term or in puerperium
Racial tendency	None	80% in black women
Laterality	Almost always unilateral	Often bilateral and multicentric
Endocrine features	75% of women virilized	25% develop hirsutism during pregnancy; female newborn sometimes with hermaphroditic signs
Histologic		
Intracellular lipid	Abundant	Relatively little or none
Necrosis	If present, only focal puerperium	Diffuse acute regressive changes if removed postpartum
Adjacent uninvolved ovary	No pregnancy changes	Pregnancy changes (deciduosis, hyperthecosis)

Steroid cell tumors are almost always unilateral (excepting for stromal luteomas) and sometimes arise in the ovarian hilus. They are solid, lobulated tumors composed of eosinophilic or finely vacuolated cells arranged in a diffuse or, less commonly, a trabecular pattern—not dissimilar to that of luteomas. Reticulin surrounds single cells or small groups. Mitotic activity is variable but rarely as prominent as in luteomas of pregnancy. The most helpful distinguishing microscopic features are the abundant stainable intracytoplasmic lipids in all steroid cell tumors and the presence of crystalloids of Reinke in Leydig cell tumors (Table 24.2).

Thecomas are usually unilateral. They may be focally luteinized in pregnancy and resemble luteomas. However, the basic spindle shape of the cells is still evident. Sclerosing stromal tumors, closely related to thecomas, display a striking lobulated pattern that is due to bands of edematous immature or mature collagenous stroma (absent in luteomas). Within the lobules is abundant pericellular reticulin as seen in thecomas. Another helpful distinguishing feature is the mixed population of spindle and polyhedral eosinophilic cells (mostly the latter). Granulosa cell tumors are rare in pregnancy but, when they occur, are usually of the juvenile type, which may closely resemble luteomas.

MULTIPLE THECA–LUTEIN CYSTS (HYPERREACTIO LUTEINALIS)

Etiology and Clinical Features

While theca–lutein cysts (luteinized follicular cysts) occur at any age and in many different clinical situations, multiple bilateral theca–lutein cysts are classically associated with molar pregnancies or choriocarcinoma, occurring in 25% of such cases. They also occur with Rh isoimmunization, nonimmune hydrops, chronic renal failure,[11] multiple pregnancies,[12] and even apparently normal singleton pregnancies.[13,14] Rarely, a similar clinicopathologic picture results from ovarian hyperstimulation, provoked by ovulation-induction agents (see later), a condition occasionally associated with clinical evidence of hyperglycemia or virilization.[15] Although multiple bilateral theca–lutein cysts are usually associated with abnormally elevated β-hCG levels, additional factors may be necessary for their genesis. The cysts may persist into, or appear first, in the puerperium when β-hCG levels have fallen. In the latter situation the cysts probably initially developed during pregnancy under the influence of β-hCG but were then maintained by the FSH and LH levels that rose soon after parturition if lactation was not established. The condition almost always regresses within a few weeks after parturition. For this reason surgery during pregnancy, which is often required for diagnostic purposes or management of acute abdomen or shock, should be as conservative as possible. Intraoperative frozen-section examination of an incisional ovarian biopsy may obviate unnecessarily extensive surgery based on the erroneous presumption of malignant disease.

Gross and Microscopic Features

Both ovaries are involved and measure up to 15 cm across. Sectioning shows multiple cysts 1–4 cm in diameter that contain yellowish fluid or blood, separated by edematous stroma (Figure 24.13). The follicular cysts show hyperplasia and prominent luteinization of the theca interna layer; the granulosa is often luteinized as well (Figures 24.6 and 24.14). The edematous stroma may also contain large clusters of luteinized stromal cells.

Differential Diagnosis

Solitary luteinized follicular cysts of pregnancy and the puerperium (see later) are large, unilateral, and unilocular. Hemorrhage and edema are usually absent. There is no distinct separation of granulosa and theca layers. Cystic ovarian neoplasms, while also in the differential diagnosis, can be easily distinguished from hyperreactio luteinalis by microscopic examination.

SOLITARY LUTEINIZED FOLLICULAR CYSTS OF PREGNANCY AND PUERPERIUM

Definition

A large, distinctive follicular cyst of the ovary may occur during pregnancy.[16,17] Such cysts present as adnexal masses in the third to fourth months of pregnancy or postpartum, or are incidental findings at cesarean section. The involved ovaries exhibit large (average diameter 25 cm), unilocular, thin-walled cysts (Figure 24.15), which contain clear or mucoid fluid. The pathogenesis is unknown, but β-hCG stimulation is probably important.

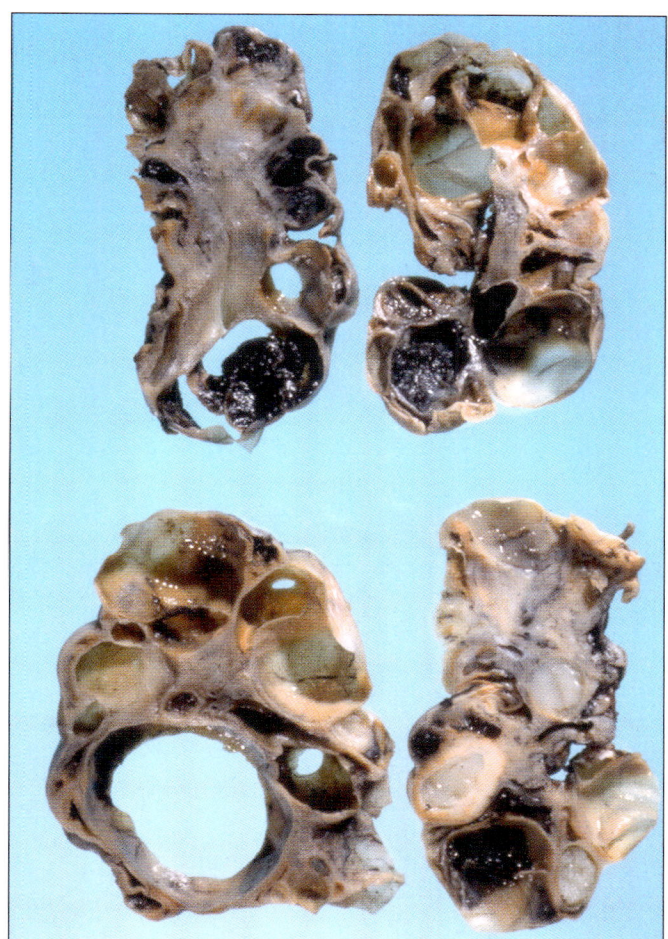

Figure 24.13 Multiple theca–lutein cysts in pregnancy. Multiple cysts and intervening hemorrhagic edematous stroma.

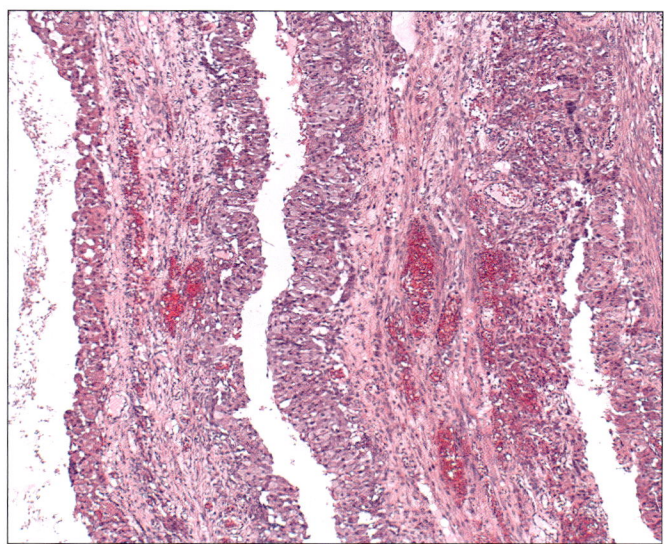

Figure 24.14 Hyperreactio luteinalis. Detail of Figure 24.6. Luteinization of both theca and granulosa with some early necrosis (cytoplasmic eosinophilia) of the lining (at top).

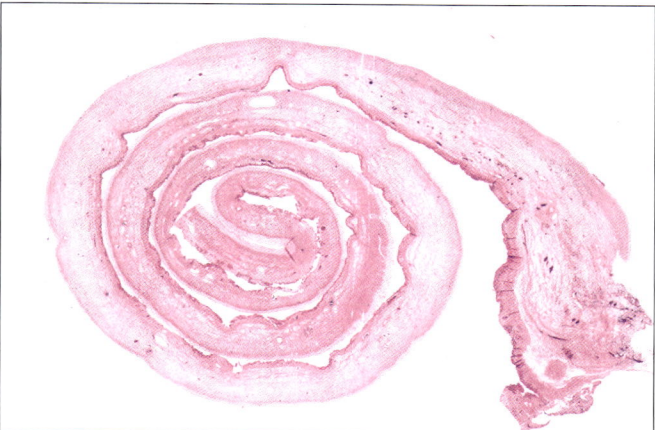

Figure 24.15 Solitary 23 cm luteinized follicular cyst ('jam roll' preparation). Removed 2 months postpartum following torsion.

Microscopic Features

Microscopically, a single layer or multiple layers of large luteinized cells line the cysts, with only a sparse reticulin network. Similar cells are sometimes also present in the fibrous wall of the cysts but these cells are not obviously thecal in type, i.e., there is no clear definition of the granulosa and theca elements of the cyst wall usually seen in cysts of follicular origin. A striking feature is the focal presence of large, pleomorphic and hyperchromatic nuclei in the luteinized cells (Figure 24.16). This feature, together with the remarkably large cyst size and lack of recognizable separation of lining cells into granulosa and theca layers, distinguish this entity morphologically from the follicular cysts of non-pregnant women. Mitotic figures are lacking.

LEYDIG (HILUS) CELL HYPERPLASIA

This condition has a close association with pregnancy. It is asymptomatic, but may be found incidentally in ovaries biopsied or excised for indications such as tumor. For greater detail, see the following sections.

DECIDUOSIS (ECTOPIC DECIDUA)

Etiology

Deciduosis (extrauterine decidual change or ectopic decidua) is a quasi-physiologic process that arises in the subcelomic mesenchyme as a result of the progesterone stimulus of pregnancy. It is thus an expression of müllerianosis. It can be identified, if carefully sought, in the cortex or surface of most ovaries from term or near-term pregnancies. It is found with greater difficulty in the first and second trimesters. Deciduosis also develops on the peritoneal surfaces of other pelvic and abdominal structures and may be exaggerated in patients with trophoblastic disease. This decidual change is also regularly observed in the stroma of ovarian endometriotic deposits during pregnancy.

Gross and Microscopic Features

Deciduosis appears as serosal macules 1–5 mm across, which are flat or slightly raised in contour. Decidual foci consist of superficial discrete collections of cells cytologically similar

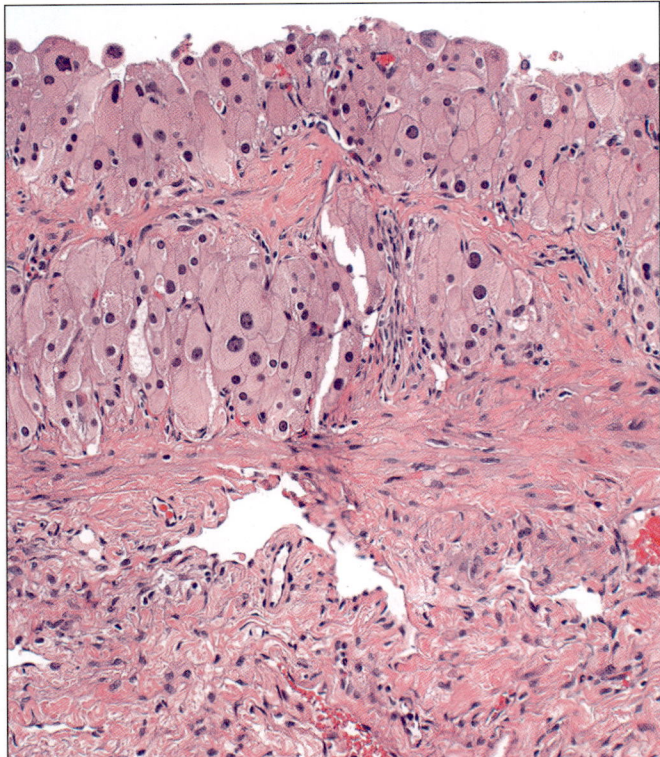

Figure 24.16 Theca–lutein cyst. Detail of cyst wall showing luteinized cells with pleomorphic hyperchromatic nuclei (same case as Figure 24.25).

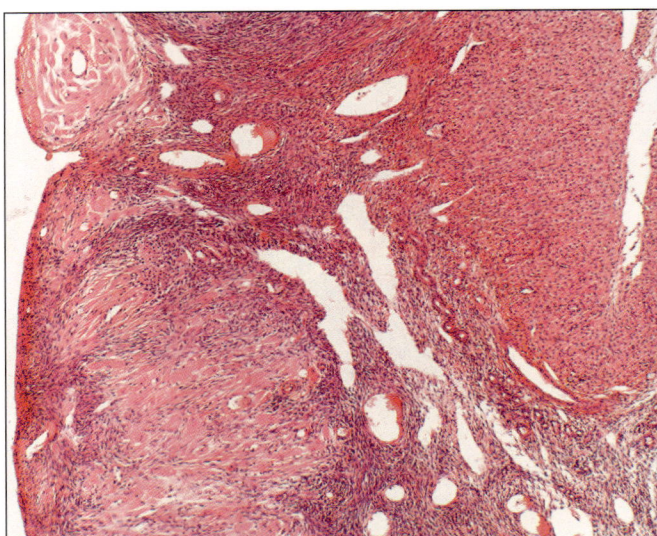

Figure 24.17 Ovarian deciduosis. Subserosal plaque, with central capillary, plus clustered decidual cells in adjacent cortex. Note stromal luteinization below.

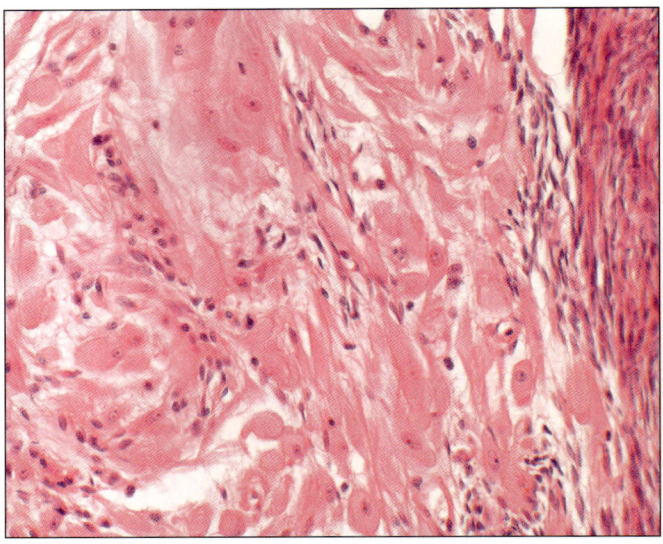

Figure 24.18 Detail of deciduosis (same case as Figure 24.17). Decidual cells showing abundant cytoplasm, round to oval nuclei with prominent nucleoli. Occasional lymphocytes present.

to the decidual cells of gestational endometrium, i.e., distinct cell margins, abundant, slightly eosinophilic, finely granular cytoplasm, and central, small, round pale nuclei with conspicuous nucleoli. Capillaries are prominent and the decidual cells sometimes appear to sheathe them. A sprinkling of lymphocytes may be present (Figures 24.17 and 24.18). Most commonly the foci are nodular or plaque-like but some lie just beneath the serosal surface and are surrounded by edematous stroma. Decidual foci may become confluent.

OVARIAN GRANULOSA CELL PROLIFERATIONS OF PREGNANCY

Definition
Proliferations of granulosa cells occur rarely as incidental findings in pregnant women. The lesions are usually multiple and are present within atretic follicles.[18]

Microscopic Features
The arrangement of the granulosa cells mimics similar patterns seen with granulosa cell tumors, i.e., solid, microfollicular, trabecular, or insular (Figure 24.19). Usually, the granulosa cells contain scanty cytoplasm and grooved nuclei resembling the cells of the adult-type granulosa cell tumor. Less commonly, the cells are luteinized with non-grooved nuclei of variable size, or sertoliform with vacuolated cytoplasm suggestive of lipid.

OVARIAN PREGNANCY

Definition
Definitive diagnosis of ovarian pregnancy requires proof of ovarian nidation and exclusion of tubal nidation with secondary ovarian involvement, and the following criteria are applicable:

- The tube must be intact and clearly separate from the ovary.
- The fetal sac should occupy the normal position of the ovary and be connected to the uterus by the utero-ovarian ligament.

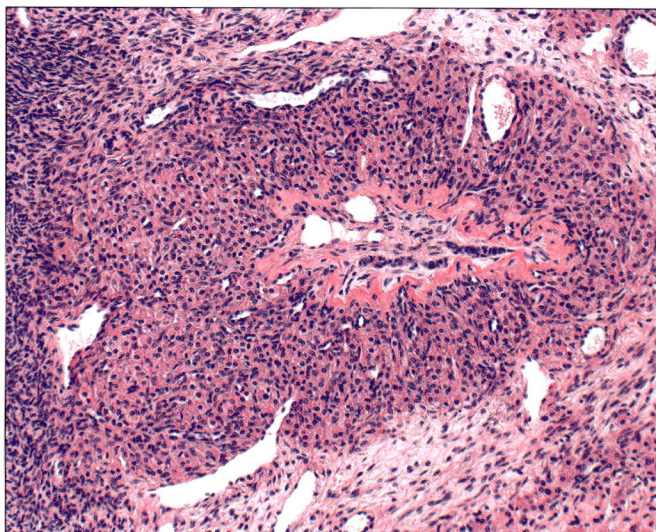

Figure 24.19 Re-emergence of granulosa cells within an atretic follicular remnant in pregnancy. Small trabecular arrangements are seen centrally. The residual perifollicular theca cells are luteinized as are scattered stromal cells nearby.

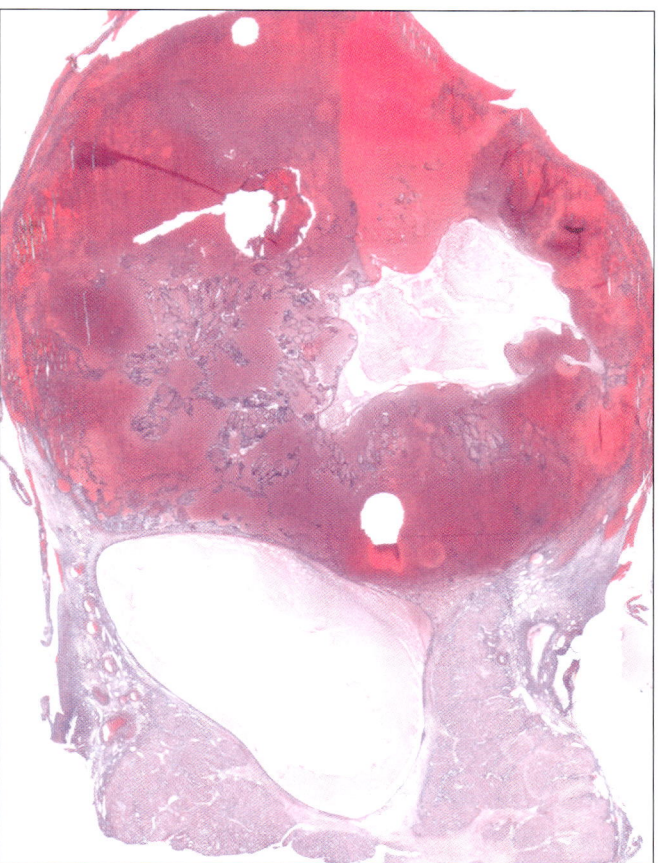

Figure 24.20 Ectopic ovarian pregnancy. Chorionic vesicle and immature villi surrounded by blood clot. Corpus luteum at bottom.

- Definite ovarian tissue must be present in the sac wall. These criteria obviously become more difficult to establish in more advanced gestations. In these cases confirmation of ovarian pregnancy requires the demonstration of ovarian tissue at several places in the fetal sac wall.
- The serum β-hCG should fall to non-pregnant levels upon removal of the ovarian lesion.

Etiology

Ovarian nidation occurs about once in every 10,000 pregnancies and accounts for 0.5–3% of ectopic gestations.[19–21] Exceptionally rarely, the ovarian nidation may be multiple,[22] or occur with a synchronous intrauterine pregnancy.[23,24] A strong relationship exists between ovarian ectopic pregnancies and use of intrauterine contraceptive devices, but the nature of this relationship remains unclear.[20] In marked contrast to patients with tubal ectopics, patients with ovarian pregnancies are highly fertile and have a lower than average incidence of pelvic inflammatory disease and endometriosis. The pathogenesis is best explained by chance fertilization of an unexpectedly mature ovum within the fimbriae, or on the ovarian surface, and subsequent implantation in the ovarian parenchyma. Intrafollicular implantation and development of the conceptus within the corpus luteum itself is considered highly unlikely. This is not only because the ovum would not have completed its first meiotic division and matured to the point of being able to accept fertilization, but also because of the inhospitable environment in the hemorrhagic corpus luteum. Ovarian endometriosis is thought to play no role in local nidation.

Microscopic Features

Histologic examination is necessary to confirm that trophoblastic tissue is present in juxtaposition to unequivocal ovarian structures. A corpus luteum of pregnancy can often be identified close to the hemorrhagic implantation site (Figures 24.20 and 24.21). Deciduosis and other pregnancy-associated alterations may be noted in the adjacent parenchyma. If a partial rather than a complete oophorectomy has been performed, it may be difficult to confirm the diagnosis solely by pathologic examination of the material submitted.

PRIMARY OVARIAN TROPHOBLASTIC DISEASE

Ovarian hydatidiform mole is an extremely rare lesion that develops subsequent to ovarian pregnancy. The ovary is grossly enlarged and replaced by an encapsulated hemorrhagic mass of vesicles. Confirmation of primary ovarian origin requires exclusion of extension from a molar pregnancy arising within the uterus or fallopian tube, as well as demonstration that the molar tissue is intraovarian. Gestational choriocarcinoma in the ovary may be either metastatic from the uterus or a primary tumor developing subsequent to ovarian pregnancy.[25,26] Exclusion of the former beyond reasonable doubt is implicit in confirming the latter possibility, something that is extraordinarily difficult to do. A useful term might be 'choriocarcinoma occurring solely in the ovary' rather than forcing a particular case into the primary or metastatic category. Ovarian choriocarcinoma can also coexist with an apparently normal uterine gestation, further confounding the issue. The morphology of choriocarcinoma and the problems in diagnosis

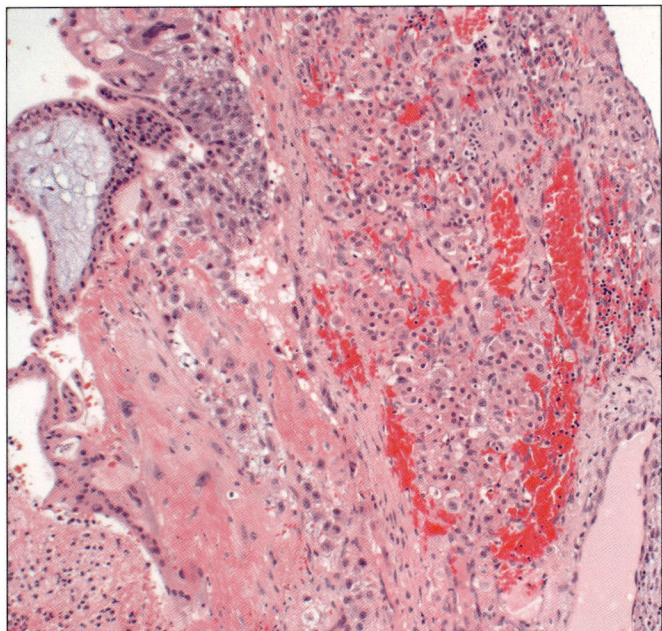

Figure 24.21 Ectopic ovarian pregnancy. Note immature villi and villous trophoblast to the left and scattered extravillous trophoblastic cells infiltrating the granulosa lutein cells of the corpus luteum to the right.

Table 24.3 Primary Ovarian Tumors Diagnosed or Removed during Pregnancy*

Surface Epithelial Stromal Tumors	
Serous	
Benign	13
Proliferating	1
Mucinous	
Benign	24
Proliferating	1
Malignant	1
Sex Cord–Stromal Tumors	
Thecoma	1
Sclerosing stromal tumor	1
Fibroma	1
Germ Cell Tumors (Teratomas)	
Immature	1
Mature (Dermoid cysts)	67
Monodermal (struma)	2
Total	133

*There were 119,157 live births at King George V Hospital from 1950 to 1975.

of non-gestational choriocarcinoma (germ cell tumor)[27] are discussed in Chapter 29.

OTHER OVARIAN LESIONS

TORSION

Approximately 10–20% of neoplastic and non-neoplastic ovaries torse during pregnancy,[28] which may be due to physiologic dislocation of the ovaries in pregnancy and to the softening and edema of the pelvic tissues, especially ligaments. Torsion involves all forms of cysts and neoplasms that occur during the reproductive years (see later) and rarely may even involve a primary ovarian pregnancy itself.[29]

DISSEMINATED PERITONEAL LEIOMYOMATOSIS

Disseminated peritoneal leiomyomatosis displays innumerable nodules, 2–3 mm in diameter, scattered throughout the peritoneal cavity but particularly conspicuous in the pelvis and omentum. Ovarian involvement occurs in 25% of cases. The nodules are superficial, discrete, and well circumscribed and composed of whorled smooth muscle, similar to the familiar uterine leiomyomas, but may also contain some fibroblasts and decidual cells. The condition usually presents in association with pregnancy or use of the oral contraceptive pill. Resolution may be spontaneous after parturition but can also be accelerated by progesterone.

OVARIAN NEOPLASMS

The true incidence of ovarian neoplasms in pregnancy is difficult to assess from the literature and to a greater extent depends on the method of diagnosis (clinical or surgical) and whether non-neoplastic lesions are included.[30–32] A reasonable figure based on multiple series is one tumor per 1000 live births, of which 2–5% are malignant (contrasted with 20% of ovarian tumors in general) (Table 24.3).

REACTIVE STROMAL TUMOR-LIKE LESIONS

POLYCYSTIC OVARY SYNDROME

Definition

Polycystic ovary syndrome (PCOS), also called Stein–Leventhal syndrome, is the prototypic form of chronic hyperandrogenic oligo- or anovulation. It is a common heterogeneous metabolic disorder that is often familial, and affects at least 10% of infertility cases in reproductive age women. By definition, the syndrome is unassociated with any underlying adrenal or pituitary disorders or ovarian tumors. It may manifest with hyperinsulinemia, hyperlipidemia, diabetes mellitus, and cardiac disease, as well as the better recognized hyperandrogenism, hirsutism, infertility, and chronic anovulation. This definition is essentially clinical, which means that the finding of enlarged ovaries with numerous follicle cysts by echography or gross inspection is not an essential diagnostic requirement.

Presenting features are to some extent age dependent, from precocious puberty in childhood, through hirsutism and menstrual irregularities in teenagers, infertility and glucose intolerance in adulthood, to frank diabetes and cardiovascular disease in older patients.

The term 'polycystic ovaries,' as some use it, applies to many (possibly up to 25%) asymptomatic women with

Table 24.4 Criteria for Diagnosing Polycystic Ovary Syndrome (PCOS) and Related Disorders

Criteria of the U.S. National Institutes of Health

PCOS

- Presence of menstrual abnormalities and anovulation
- Presence of clinical and/or biochemical hyperandrogenemia
- Absence of hyperprolactinemia or thyroid disease
- Absence of late onset congenital adrenal hyperplasia
- Absence of Cushing's syndrome

Polycystic Ovaries

- Presence of polycystic ovaries on ultrasound examination
- Absence of menstrual or cosmetic symptoms
- Absence of biochemical hyperandrogenemia

Idiopathic Hirsutism

- Presence of excess hair growth
- Absence of biochemical hyperandrogenemia

Proposed Criteria (European Society of Human Reproduction and Embryology and American Society of Reproductive Medicine)*

PCOS is diagnosed if any two of the following are present:
- Presence of polycystic ovaries on ultrasound examination
- Clinical or biochemical hyperandrogenism
- Menstrual dysfunction with anovulation

*Symposium on PCOS, Rotterdam, The Netherlands, May 1, 2003.

---

typical ultrasound features.[33] The term 'polycystic ovary syndrome' generally is reserved for those women who have morphologic features of polycystic ovaries associated with typical clinical symptoms of oligo- or anovulation, as well as biochemical signs of hyperandrogenism. Indeed some recent publications exclude polycystic ovaries as a key diagnostic criterion for PCOS (Table 24.4). Polycystic ovaries may simply reflect the pathology of that subset of women who seem to ovulate best when thin, unlike their 'normal' counterparts who need a certain amount of body fat to ovulate regularly and would thus become amenorrheic when pathologically thin. Some believe that 'polyfollicular' should replace the term 'polycystic' and that 'functional hyperandrogenism' should replace 'PCOS.'[34]

Etiology

The disorder is probably the most common hormonal abnormality in women of reproductive age and certainly is a leading cause of infertility. In young women, precocious puberty and hyperinsulinemia are early manifestations of PCOS. It is frequently associated with insulin resistance and type 2 diabetes, possibly on the basis of pancreatic β-cell dysfunction,[35] and management with insulin sensitizers such as metformin is currently popular for the induction of ovulation.[36] Obesity exacerbates the insulin resistance and favors the progression from impaired glucose tolerance to clinical diabetes in these patients.[37] Whether obesity is a cause or an effect of PCOS is unclear, but the latter is more likely.

Insulin also, in turn, signals the body to release testosterone, with somatic as well as skin and hair manifestations. Skin symptoms, such as acne or hirsutism, are not only determined by serum androgen levels but also by the activity of the skin's hormone receptors and the activity of enzymes such as 5-α reductase. Women who exhibit amenorrhea, hirsutism, and enlarged polycystic ovaries represent the severe end of the disease spectrum.

A distinct familial clustering of women with PCOS suggests that heredity factors are also etiologically important. Candidate genes for PCOS include those related to androgenic pathways and metabolic associations of the syndrome. More recently, genes encoding inflammatory cytokines have been identified as target genes for PCOS. Evidence is mounting for a susceptibility gene that maps near D19S884 on chromosome19p13.3.[38] Nevertheless, despite much detailed investigation, no one gene seems to play a pivotal role in the genesis of PCOS. It remains probable that PCOS is the final outcome of different, interrelated, genetic anomalies that influence each other and perpetuate the syndrome.[39]

Investigational Profile

Nearly all patients with PCOS have at least subtle laboratory abnormalities. Often, they are at the upper limits of 'normal,' showing only a tendency, rather than a discrete abnormality. By contrast, serious pathology may be more evident by a marked elevation, or suppression of a single test.

Many have sustained high LH levels due to an increase in LH pulse size and frequency. These high LH levels (usually above 20 IU/L) result in excessive theca cell growth and consequent androgen production. Among women with PCOS, this subgroup with high serum LH levels is at highest risk for infertility and miscarriage.[40] Most patients have normal or slightly lower levels of FSH, and an LH/FSH ratio greater than 2. Provided the LH level is not lower than 8 IU/L, this may be used to suggest the diagnosis in women with clinical features of PCOS.

Hyperinsulinemia or abnormalities of the insulin-like growth factor axis are frequently found. Although the women are often obese, their hyperinsulinemia appears independent of their obesity. Insulin inhibits sex hormone-binding globulin production and stimulates ovarian androgen production.[41] Most have demonstrable androgen excess with raised levels of total testosterone (usually 2.4–4.2 nmol/L), androstenedione (usually 10.5–17.5 nmol/L), DHEA, and DHEA sulfate (about 40% of women with PCOS will have at least one of these androgens elevated). Obese and anovulatory women with PCOS usually have low levels of sex hormone-binding globulin resulting in high free testosterone levels. The presence or absence of hirsutism depends on whether these androgens are converted peripherally by 5-α reductase to the more potent androgen dihydrotestosterone and 3-α-diol-G, as reflected by increased levels of 3-α-diol-G.

About 20% of women with PCOS also have mildly elevated levels of prolactin (20–30ng/ml), possibly related to increased pulsatility of gonadotropin-releasing hormone (GnRH) or to a relative dopamine deficiency or to both.

The most consistent ultrasound feature is more than 10 peripherally placed symmetrical small follicles (2–8 mm in diameter; the so-called 'string of pearls') in association with increased stroma and often an ovarian volume exceeding 12 cm^3. Sometimes the ovary is virtually filled with small cysts. In other cases, it is heterogeneously dense with barely detectable microcystic changes (some women with characteristic clinical features of PCOS have normal-sized ovaries). Note, any hyperandrogenic state may manifest these appearances. Diffusely enlarged ovaries without a discrete mass on ultrasound, in the absence of adrenal findings, are consistent with the diagnosis of stromal hyperthecosis, which is probably a less common variant in the PCOS spectrum.

Gross Features

Both ovaries are ovoid or globular and usually symmetrically enlarged to twice their normal size or more with a thickened glistening white capsule. The cut surfaces typically show a somewhat thickened capsule with a linear subcapsular aggregation of multiple small follicles up to about 8 mm in diameter and containing clear fluid, and an absence of stigmata of previous ovulation (Figure 24.22).

Microscopic Features

The tunica albuginea is usually thickened, often threefold but occasionally up to 10-fold, with accentuated, layered interlacing bundles of fibrocollagenous connective tissue (Figure 24.23). This finding is not specific for PCOS and is found in many anovulatory states. Primordial follicles are present in appropriate or slightly reduced numbers and there are many cystic follicles at about the 4–8 mm stage of development (Figure 24.22). The relatively uniform size of the cystic follicles is a typical feature of PCOS. Follicular atresia is prominent. Apart from aberrant follicular development, theca cell hyperplasia occurs in all cases. The theca interna layer is often two to three times thicker than normal. The theca cells may be larger than normal with more obvious eosinophilic cytoplasm or appear frankly luteinized. The granulosa of these follicles is either indistinguishable from normal or exhibits early regressive changes with disaggregation and lack of mitotic activity.

Differential Diagnosis

The morphologic changes described previously are found in other clinical settings such as 92% of women with idiopathic hirsutism, 87% of women with oligomenorrhea, 82% of women with congenital adrenal hyperplasia, and in almost 25% of 'normal women.' They should, therefore, be regarded as typical but not diagnostic of PCOS. Using pelvic ultrasound, the main characteristic feature of polycystic ovaries is the presence of more than 10 peripheral small follicles in association with increased stroma. Clinically also, late onset congenital adrenal hyperplasia and other virilizing disorders may mimic polycystic ovaries.

For the pathologist, other conditions that may resemble PCOS include the ovarian hyperstimulation syndrome, the swollen ovary syndrome, and hyperreactio luteinalis with multiple theca–lutein cysts and prominence of luteinized stromal cells in enlarged ovaries. The clinical context of this latter condition associated with a pregnancy episode or trophoblastic disease hardly lends itself to ready confusion.

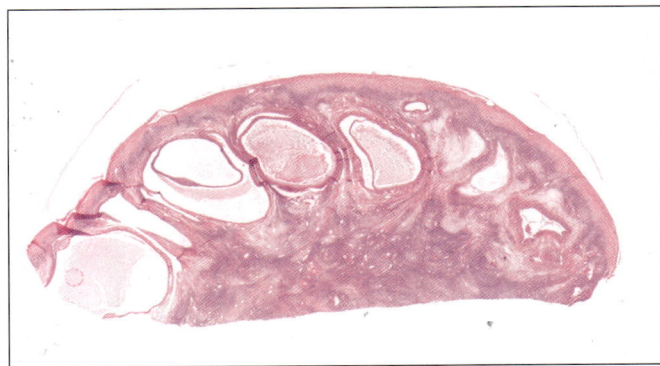

Figure 24.22 PCOS. Whole-mount showing thickened capsule and numerous antral follicles. No stigmata of ovulation are seen.

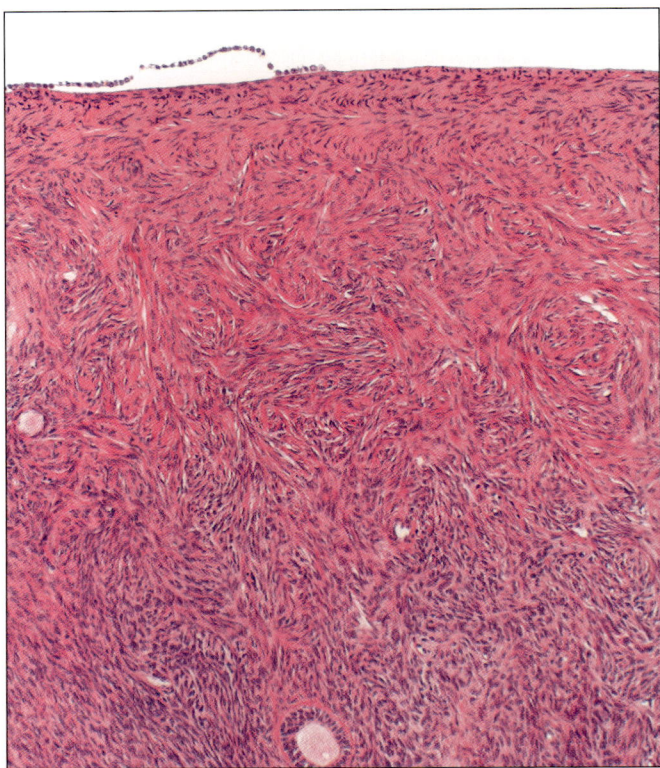

Figure 24.23 Low power of thickened and somewhat fibrotic tunica delimited by the serosa and subjacent primordial and primary follicles.

STROMAL HYPERPLASIA AND HYPERTHECOSIS

Definitions and Clinical Features

Stromal hyperplasia is the exaggerated presence of the cortical stroma that is characteristically ovarian. Mild hyperplasia of the cortical and medullary stroma is found in the ovaries of about one-third of perimenopausal and postmenopausal women. It is nearly always diffusely bilateral. As the apparent severity of the changes does not correlate well with clinical symptoms, some suggest that the term 'stromal hyperplasia' should be reserved for definite and florid cases. Minimum criteria should be an obliterated normal distinction between cortex and medulla or at least some nodularity to the proliferating stroma. Most women are older and many are postmenopausal. Clinical symptoms result from excess androgen (androstenedione) production by the hyperplastic stroma,[42,43] with or without dominant peripheral aromatization to estrone.[44]

Hyperthecosis is the presence of luteinized cells of thecal origin located in the stroma distant from the follicles. They may be single or in groups and may be clustered or scattered diffusely. It regularly occurs in association with ovarian stromal hyperplasia on the one hand and merges imperceptibly with the PCOS on the other. Like stromal hyperplasia, it may on occasion be asymptomatic, but is more usually accompanied by marked defeminization and virilization[45] and only occasionally by estrogenic signs. Although isolated luteinized stromal cells are common in postmenopausal ovaries, clinical hyperthecosis occurs mostly in women of reproductive age and may rarely present as virilization in pregnancy that ameliorates spontaneously after delivery, or as endometrial hyperplasia. These changes are also seen in association with endometrial hyperplasias and cancer.

Gross Features

Both ovaries are enlarged, up to twice the normal size. The capsule is thickened and the cut surface is uniformly pale yellow to fawn in color, often with blurring of the division into cortex and medulla (Figure 24.24). In severe cases, nodularity will be present.

Microscopic Features

Stromal hyperplasia shows a variable but marked proliferation of plump but otherwise undistinguished spindled stromal cells, each invested by reticulin fibrils, recapitulating the storiform swathes and whorls of normal ovarian stroma (Figure 24.25). The medulla is most affected by this proliferation and the usually obvious corticomedullary interface may be obliterated. Stromal hyperplasia may be entirely diffuse (Figure 24.26), but rather more commonly exhibits a focal or widespread nodular pattern, particularly in the cortex. Fat stains usually reveal widespread intracytoplasmic lipid. Small foci of hyalinization are quite frequently encountered in the superficial cortex.

Stromal hyperthecosis is typified by isolated or aggregated lutein-like cells throughout each ovary. These cells generally are more numerous in the medulla (Figure 24.27) than the cortex (Figure 24.28), and they are large and polyhedral with abundant eosinophilic granular or finely vacuolated cytoplasm and rounded central nuclei, each with a single, small to sometimes prominent nucleolus (Figure 24.27). Focal regression is sometimes seen with hyalinization and a mild lymphohistiocytic infiltrate (Figure 24.29). A continuum exists between such diffuse cases and those in which the lutein cells form multiple discrete small nodules (see Figure 24.30; nodular stromal hyperthecosis). The cortex frequently contains small cystic follicles, each with a prominent luteinized theca interna layer. Stigmata of recent ovulation are absent, but follicular atresia is sometimes increased.

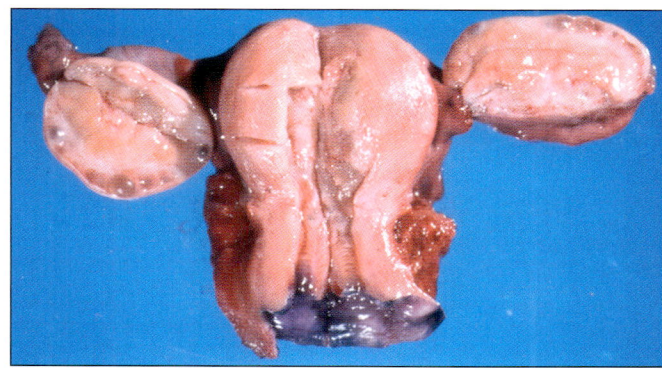

Figure 24.24 Cortical stromal hyperplasia. Extrafascial hysterectomy for endometrial carcinoma (note tumor in right fundus). Ovaries are uniformly enlarged and the soft, fawn cut surface shows blurring of usual distinction between cortex and medulla.

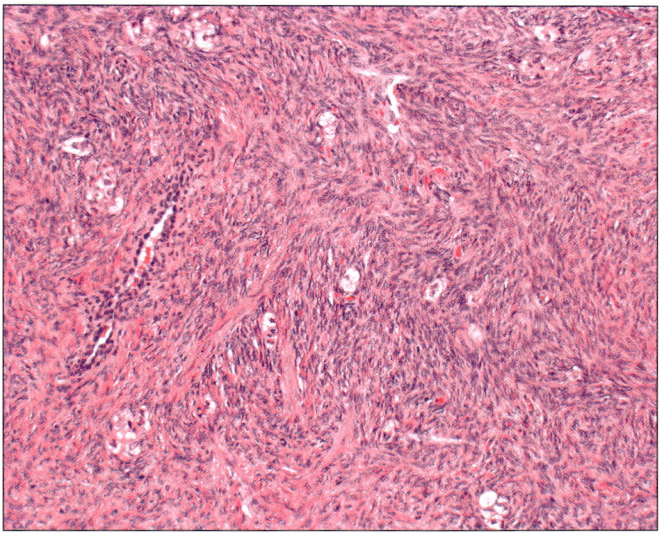

Figure 24.25 Cortical stromal hyperplasia. Characterized by swirls and bands of small spindle cells, more cellular but otherwise indistinguishable from normal ovarian cortex. It is a moot point as to how prominent isolated luteinized cells with foamy cytoplasm can be without reclassifying a lesion as hyperthecosis (see Figure 24.41).

Differential Diagnosis

In occasional cases, one or more nodules become dominant, suggesting a neoplasm graced by a specific name, such as stromal luteoma. In accord with similar pathologic processes in other endocrine glands (e.g., thyroid, parathyroid), the diagnosis of stromal luteoma should be made with caution in the presence of multiple hyperplastic nodules of theca-like cells, and the term is best reserved for those lipid cell tumors of stromal origin that arise in the absence of such diffuse or nodular ovarian stromal hyperplasia or hyperthecosis. These tumor-like nodules are composed entirely of large rounded lutein cells (Figure 24.31), and average about 1 cm in diameter. Reinke crystalloids are absent, distinguishing them from Leydig cell tumors of stromal (or non-hilar) origin. Paradoxically, Leydig cell hyperplasia and Leydig cell tumors may also occur in association with hyperthecosis. The spindled non-luteinized theca-like cells of partly luteinized

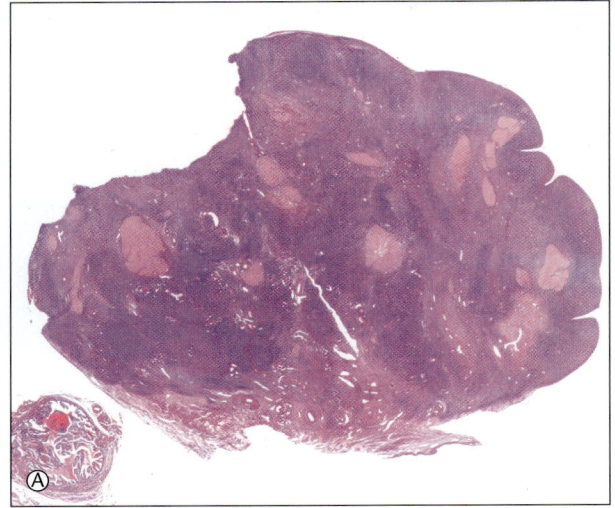

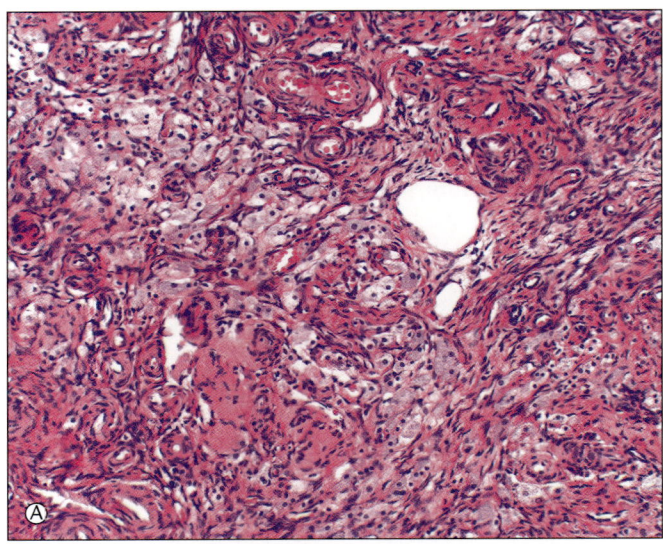

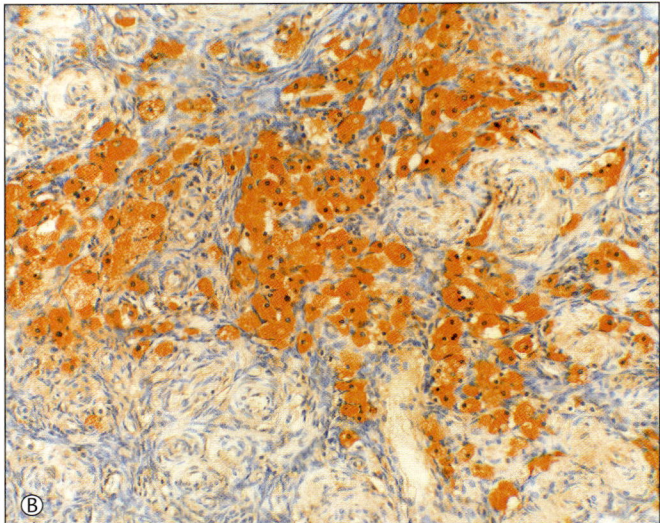

Figure 24.27 Stromal hyperthecosis. Medullary clusters of luteinized stromal cells. **(A)** H&E, **(B)** immunostain for estradiol.

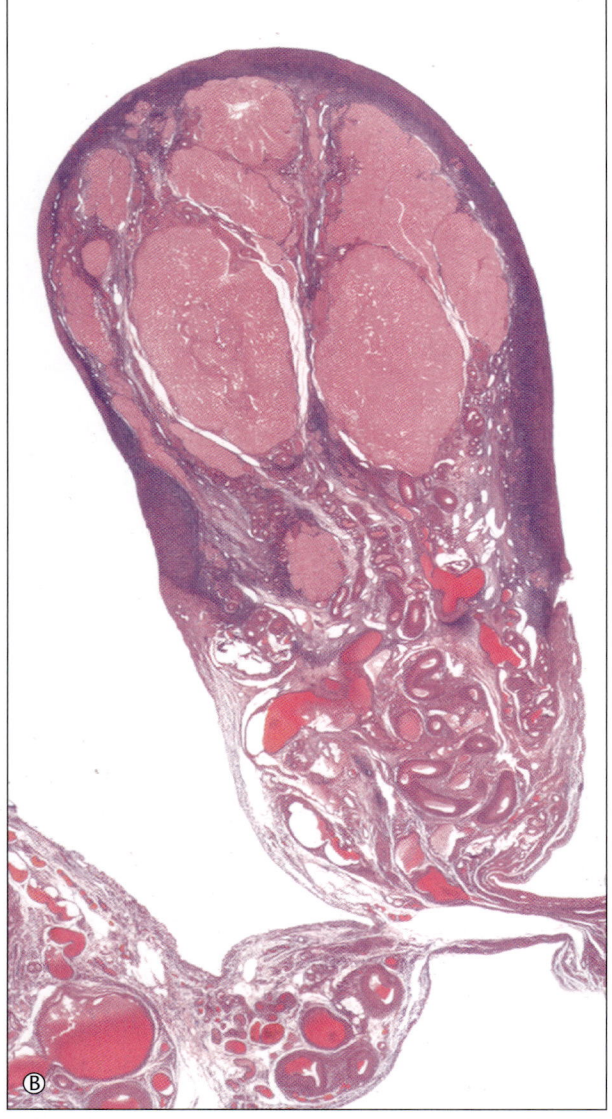

Figure 24.26 **(A)** Section of diffusely hyperplastic postmenopausal ovary. Note obliteration of normal corticomedullary junction. **(B)** Normal postmenopausal ovary for comparison.

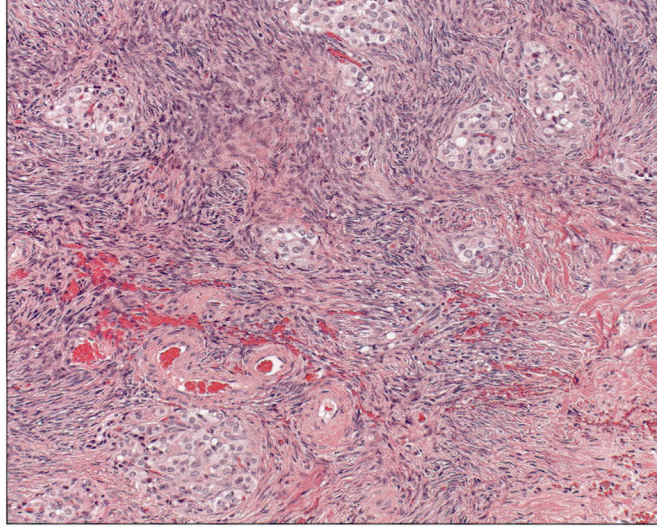

Figure 24.28 Stromal hyperthecosis. Discrete clusters of luteinized stromal cells in hyperplastic cortical stroma.

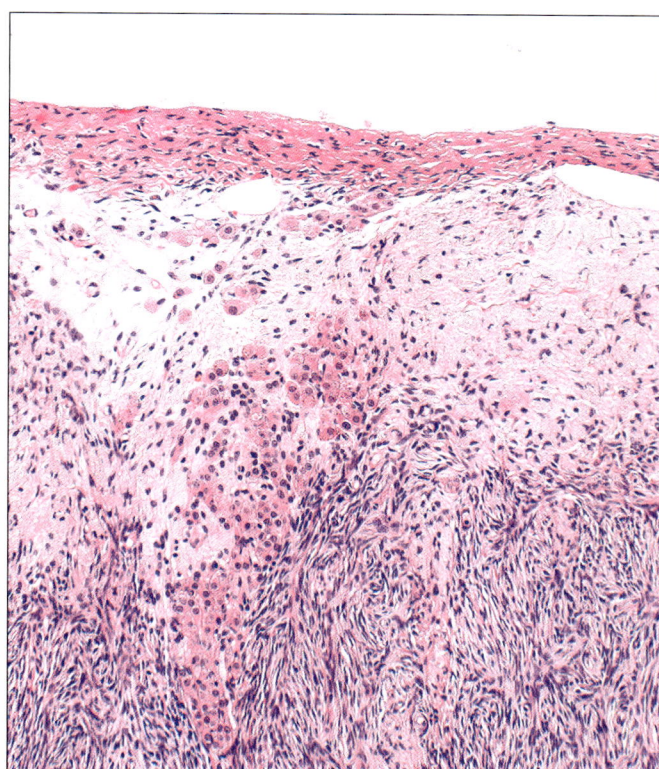

Figure 24.29 Hyperthecosis. A small collection of residual luteinized stromal cells is noted, while the remainder of the focus has undergone hyalinization.

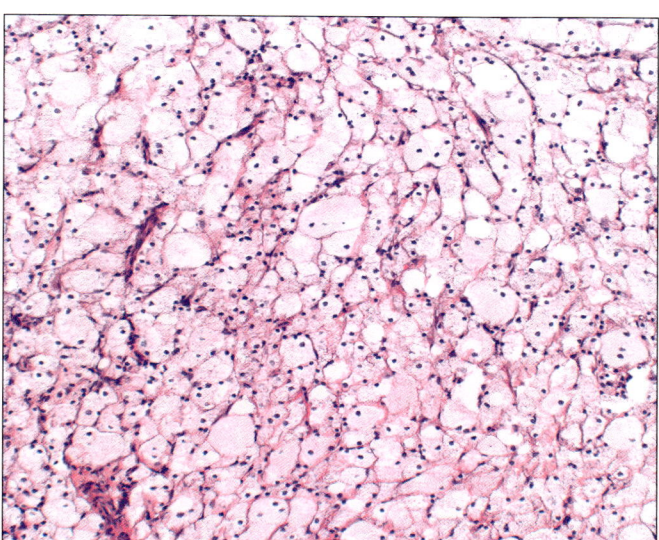

Figure 24.31 Stromal luteoma. Large vacuolated lutein cells from a solitary 9 mm nodule.

LEYDIG (HILUS) CELL HYPERPLASIA

Definition

Leydig cells are rounded to polygonal cells with central nuclei and eosinophilic cytoplasm that are infrequently observed in routine sections of the ovaries unless specifically sought, despite their documented presence in at least 80% of cases. Their casual observation, therefore, usually indicates some degree of hyperplasia.

Etiology

Prominent Leydig cells are most regularly seen in response to raised gonadotropin levels during pregnancy or at menopause. Occasionally the pregnancy-associated Leydig cell hyperplasia is severe, sufficient to produce visible mitotic activity in these cells (an otherwise extremely rare occurrence). In non-pregnant women, Leydig cell hyperplasia most frequently occurs against a background of stromal hyperplasia and hyperthecosis.

Clinical Features

Leydig cell hyperplasia is generally of a mild degree and unassociated with clinical endocrine disturbance. Although the endocrine profile is neither consistent nor specific for Leydig cell hyperplasia, there may be increased serum testosterone levels.

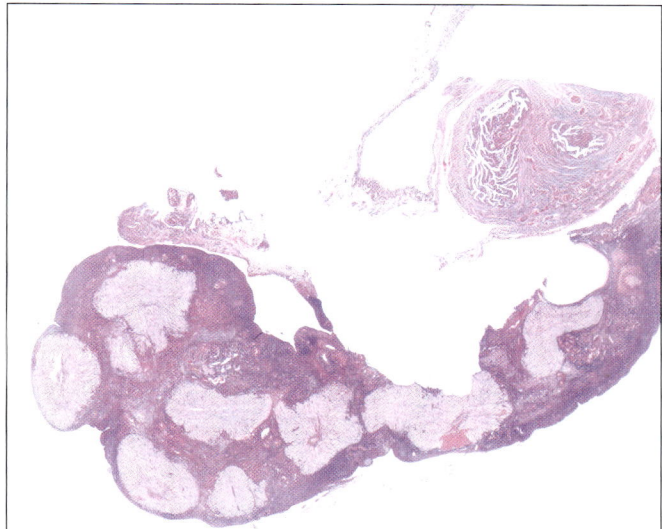

Figure 24.30 Nodular stromal hyperthecosis from a virilized woman. Multiple discrete nodules of large pale lutein cells against a background of stromal hyperplasia.

thecomas are also absent, as are the perivascular hyaline plaques typical of thecomas.

Behavior and Treatment

Virilizing hyperthecosis, unlike PCOS, tends not to respond to clomiphene treatment, but a measure of success has been achieved with the use of GnRH agonists.[46]

Microscopic Features

The hyperplasia appears as clusters and nodules of typical rounded or polygonal Leydig cells with moderately sized, vesicular, central nuclei and eosinophilic, granular to finely vacuolated cytoplasm (Figure 24.32). Yellow-brown intracytoplasmic lipochrome (lipofuscin) pigment is often focally observed, and Reinke crystalloids are sometimes found in occasional cells although they may be sparse. Nuclear pleomorphism is not common, although bizarre hyperchromatic nuclei may be encountered in the hyperplastic Leydig cells of postmenopausal women.

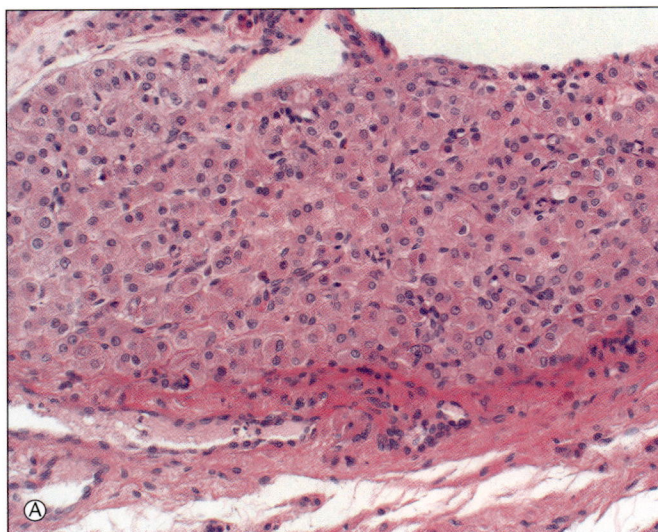

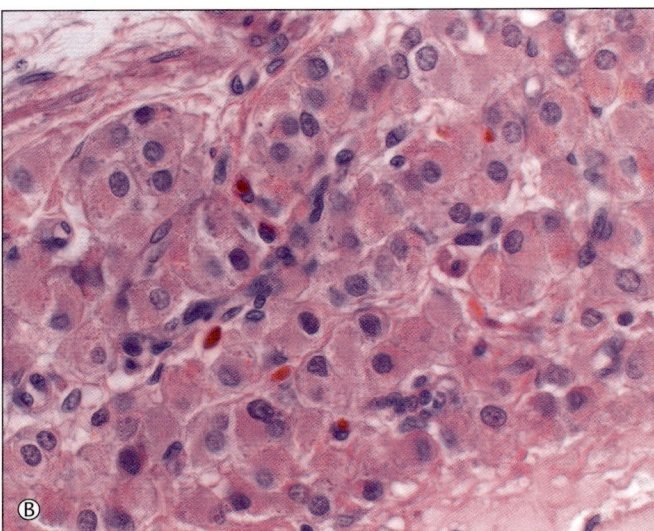

Figure 24.32 Leydig cell hyperplasia. **(A)** Large nodule of typical polygonal Leydig cells associated with a number of small vessels. **(B)** Leydig cells with uniform, rounded, central, vesicular nuclei and eosinophilic, slightly granular cytoplasm containing abundant cytochrome pigment and occasional refractile Reinke crystals.

The nodules or clusters of Leydig cells vary greatly from area to area and, although most prominent in the ovarian hilus, may extend into the mesovarium. Small capillary vessels are identifiable among the Leydig cells, and nonmyelinated nerves can be disclosed in apposition to many of the cell clusters (Figure 24.33). Cells immunostain strongly for α-inhibin and calretinin.

Leydig cells (with typical Reinke crystalloids) may also be found in hyperplastic and neoplastic conditions. Non-neoplastic stromal Leydig cells may be seen in simple stromal hyperplasias or stromal proliferations reactive to metastatic carcinomas or primary epithelial ovarian neoplasms. Rarely, typical Leydig cells are noted in benign ovarian stromal tumors, the so-called 'stromal–Leydig cell tumors' and 'pure Leydig cell tumors of non-hilar type.' Unlike Leydig cell tumors of hilus cell origin, these lesions

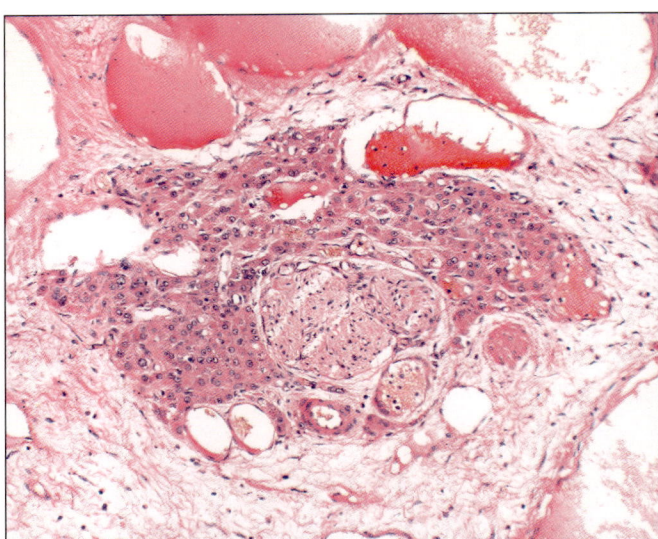

Figure 24.33 Leydig cell hyperplasia. Small nodule of Leydig cells adjacent to a number of small vessels and sheathing a small nerve.

are characteristically multinodular, bilateral, and found in ovaries with stromal hyperplasia and hyperthecosis.

MASSIVE OVARIAN EDEMA AND FIBROMATOSIS

MASSIVE OVARIAN EDEMA

Definition
This rare tumor-like entity exhibits gross enlargement of one or both ovaries by an accumulation of edema fluid in the stroma that separates normal follicular structures.

Etiology
Massive ovarian edema is thought to result from partial or intermittent torsion of an otherwise normal ovary (observed at operation in one-half of cases), compromising venous and lymphatic drainage but not causing ischemic necrosis.[47–49]

Clinical Features
Most examples occur in women in their second and third decades, but sometimes also in prepubertal girls.[48–52] These women present with acute abdominal pain and/or a palpable adnexal mass, and less commonly with menstrual disturbances. Masculinization of varying degrees is sometimes present, clinically suggestive of the PCOS in some cases, a pathologic condition that may coexist with massive ovarian edema.[53] Possibly, both the edema and the abnormal hormone production result from a local para-endocrine factor.

Gross and Microscopic Features
The enlarged ovary may be up to 35 cm in diameter (averaging 11 cm) with a soft pearly external surface. The cut surface is almost featureless and myxoid, from which regularly exudes protein-rich edema fluid (Figure 24.34). The typical histologic features are diffuse edema of the medulla and inner cortex with relative sparing of the superficial cortex and tunica albuginea, which are often thick and fibrotic. Cystic follicles beneath the tunica (Figure 24.35) and other normal cortical and medullary structures such as

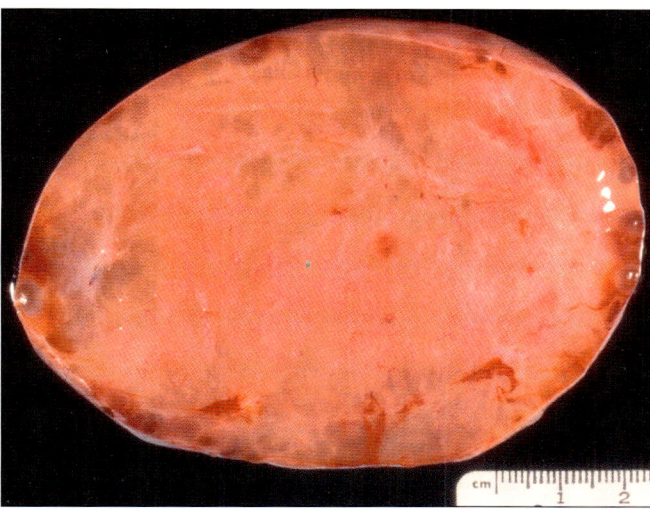

Figure 24.34 Massive ovarian edema. Featureless cut surface of an ovary with massive edema. Follicles are apparent beneath the capsule.

corpora albicantia are normal if seen, but separated by loose myxoid tissue. Small fields of normal-appearing ovarian stroma may be present in less edematous areas. The marked edema widely separates stellate stromal cells and scanty intervening collagen (Figure 24.36), making vascular and lymphatic channels abnormally prominent. There may be some congestion and foci of red cell extravasation. Small numbers of lymphocytes, mast cells, and macrophages may be observed rarely. Focal necrosis is uncommon. Over 40% of examples show isolated or clustered luteinized stromal cells, and are thought to be the source of excess steroid hormone production in those patients presenting with virilization. The luteinization is usually confined to edematous areas, but may be seen also in the contralateral edematous or non-edematous ovary. It appears to be related directly to the duration of symptoms.

Differential Diagnosis

Other ovarian lesions that may show marked focal or generalized edema include ovarian fibromas and fibrothecomas. The relation between massive ovarian edema and fibromatosis is yet to be settled but is more likely to represent disparate responses to the same pathologic stimulus rather than one (fibromatosis) being a precursor of the other (massive edema). Sclerosing stromal tumors tend to compress the surrounding normal ovarian tissue and have a pseudolobular pattern with focal hyalinization. Metastatic carcinomas and malignant lymphomas may be sufficiently edematous as to grossly resemble massive ovarian edema. This applies particularly to Krukenberg tumors, in which the diagnostic signet-ring cells may be quite sparse indeed. In cases of patchy edema and focal condensation of plump cortical stromal cells, either a stain for mucin, such as with Alcian blue, or an immunostain for cytokeratin is helpful to identify the metastatic signet-ring cells.

Behavior and Treatment

Unilateral salpingo-oophorectomy has been the traditional surgical procedure for massive ovarian edema, largely

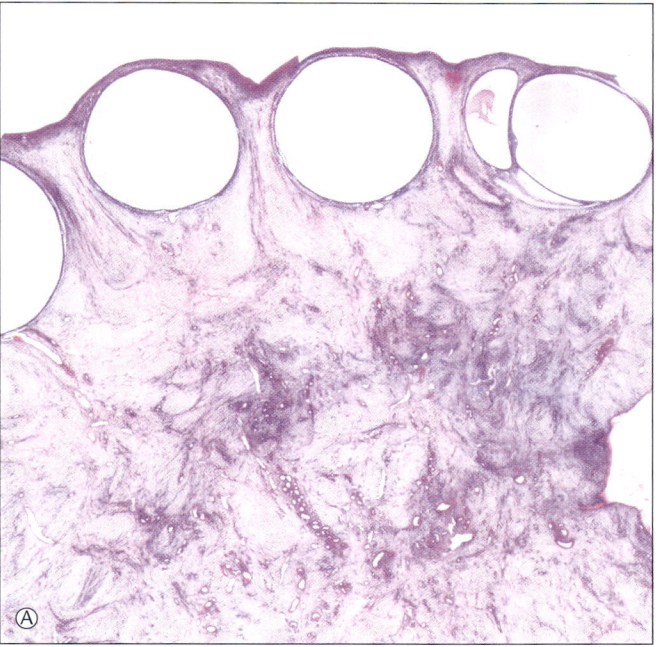

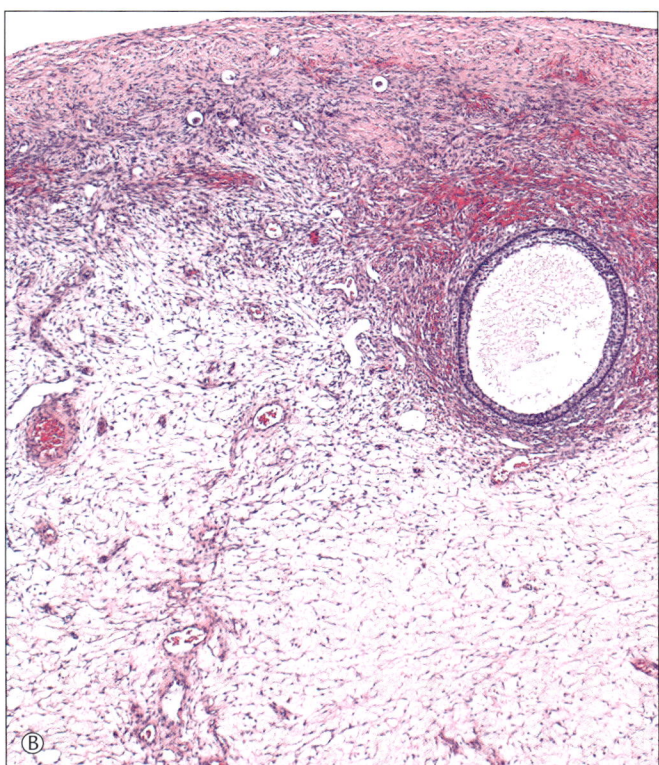

Figure 24.35 Massive ovarian edema. **(A)** Edema maximal in the deeper cortex and medulla, with relative sparing of the superficial cortex. **(B)** Higher power showing preservation of follicular structures in the superficial cortex.

driven by a failure to consider the diagnosis preoperatively, or when faced, at laparotomy, with a unilateral solid ovarian 'mass.' It is mostly unilateral and, usually, exclusion of an underlying neoplastic process that may have predisposed to the partial torsion in an individual case requires microscopic examination of the enlarged ovary. The young age of the patients, a small but significant risk of bilaterality or of 'recurrence' in the contralateral ovary,[54,55] and the consequent importance of retention of reproductive capacity, however, suggest a more conservative approach. Preoperative ultrasound or MRI may be helpful.[56–58] An intraoperative frozen section examination of a large wedge biopsy of the affected ovary to exclude underlying neoplasia and to confirm viability of the edematous ovary can be followed by surgical tethering of the ovary to the uterus or side wall of the pelvis.[59] An alternative conservative approach has involved use of oral contraceptive agents.

FIBROMATOSIS

Definition

The term was first applied to a tumor-like condition of unknown cause showing florid overgrowth of collagen-producing spindle cells that enveloped normal follicular structures and led to thickening of the superficial cortex.

Etiology

The strong clinical overlap with massive edema—young age, clinical manifestations of menstrual irregularities, abdominal pain and less commonly virilization, and finding of torsion in some cases at operation—as well as transitional appearances between the two entities suggest a common pathogenesis. We believe that they represent different ends of a single pathologic spectrum. At the 'immature' or acute end, the usually large ovarian masses are either 'acellular' lesions (typical massive ovarian edema; see above) or, rarely, highly cellular fibroblastic tumor-like lesions reported variously as 'thecomas,' 'secondary massive edema,' 'sarcoma-like ovarian nodules,' 'malignant luteinized thecoma,' 'fibromatosis,'[60]

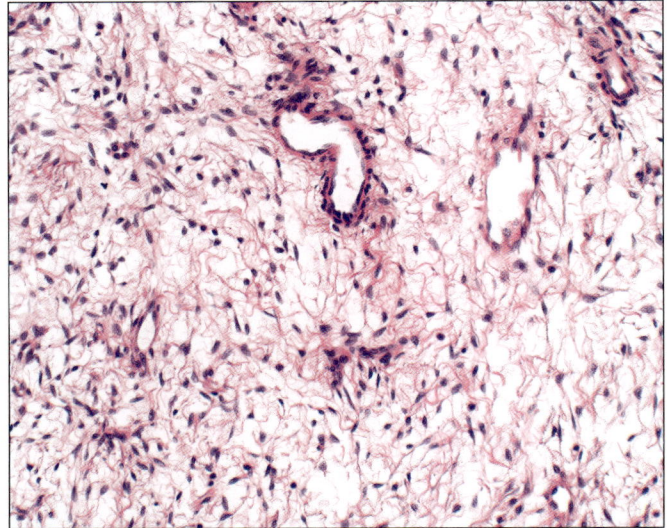

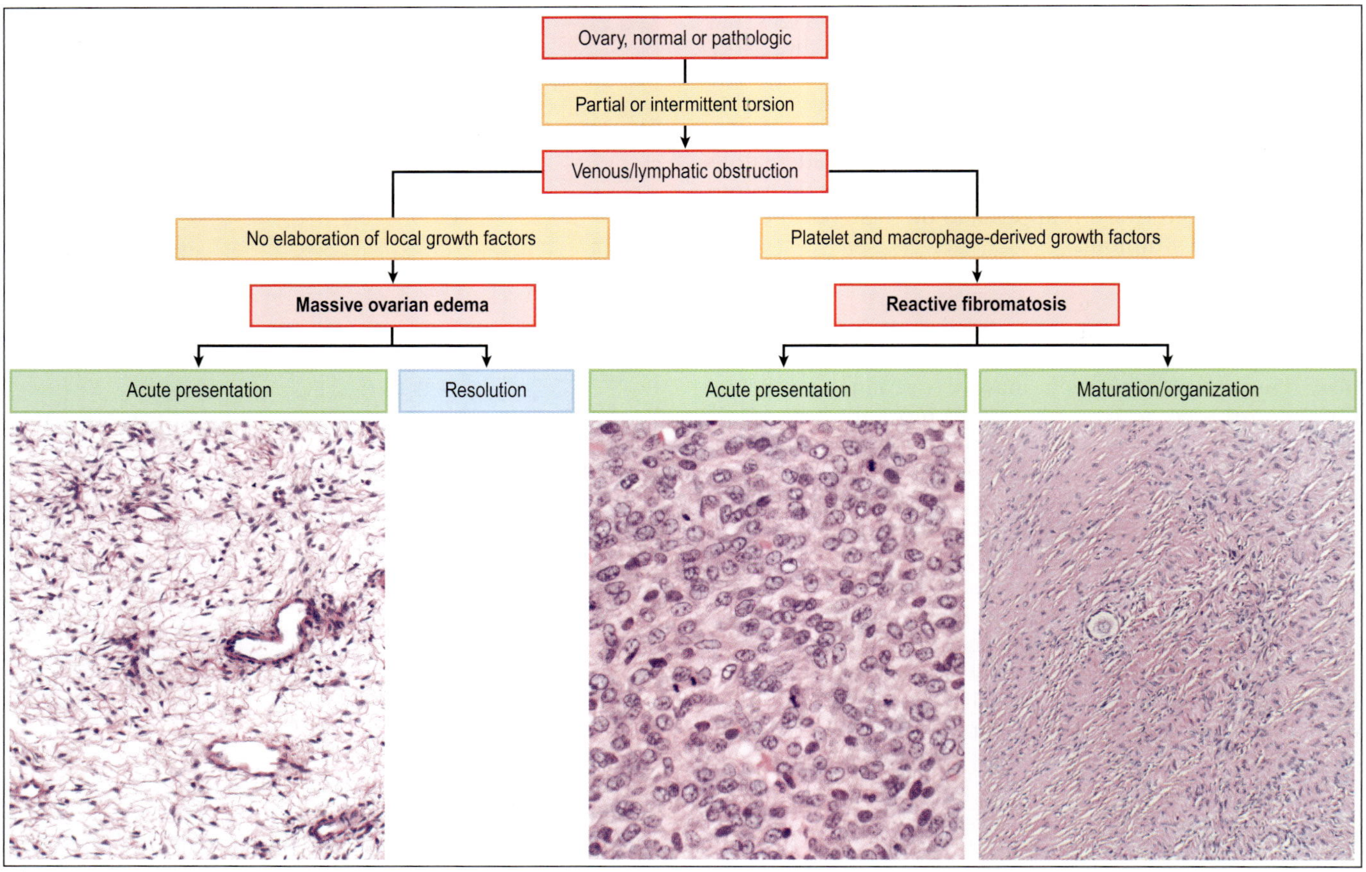

Figure 24.36 Massive ovarian edema. Stellate stromal cells widely separated by gross interstitial edema. Same case as Figure 24.35a.

Figure 24.37 Ovarian fibromatosis and massive edema. Notional relationships within this group of pathologic entities.

and 'luteinized thecoma with sclerosing peritonitis.'[61] The characteristics of this combined group are the following:

- Young age (mean age 24 years, range 4–76 years)
- Abdominal pain and swelling associated with pelvic masses and ascites/pleural effusions in many cases
- Frequent association between abdominal fibromatosis/sclerosing peritonitis and ovarian fibromatosis/massive ovarian edema
- Occasional exposure to antiepileptic drugs or to β-adrenergic blocking agents (particularly in patients under 10 years of age).

Although the underlying mechanism for ovarian fibromatosis is unknown, speculation is that local tissue injury, e.g., surgery, incomplete or intermittent ovarian torsion, stimulates platelets and macrophages to secrete locally acting growth factors that in turn induce massive fibroblastic proliferation and/or edema. Possibly, patients who present in the acute phase exhibit either massive ovarian edema or florid mitotically active 'immature' fibromatosis with/without associated peritoneal pathology, and those who present in a subacute or resolving phase exhibit the better documented 'mature' form of acellular sclerotic fibromatosis (Figure 24.37).

Gross Features

The ovaries are enlarged but sometimes only marginally so. The cut surface of the 'mature' forms is densely sclerotic and pale. The immature or cellular variants are usually large solid masses, averaging about 15 cm in diameter with fibrinous adhesions on the external surface, with tan-white and smooth cut surfaces, frequently focally hemorrhagic.

Microscopic Features

The mature variant of fibromatosis exhibits collagen-producing spindle cells that proliferate around and between normal follicles and produce a thickened fibrotic cortex. The proliferative process varies from densely acellular bands of collagen to intersecting bundles of spindle cells with a storiform pattern resembling ovarian cortex. Minor foci of uninvolved cortex and edema may be present (Figure 24.38), as may rare luteinized cells in the fibromatous zones or adjacent normal cortex. Microscopic foci of sex-cord differentiation may appear as isolated epithelial-like structures, or may be aggregated around areas of hypercellularity, suggesting development from old follicular remnants.

Immature ovarian fibromatosis shows densely cellular swathes and intersecting bundles of spindle-shaped fibroblasts or myofibroblasts (Figure 24.39). Areas of apparent maturation of the myofibroblastic stroma suggest a transition from immature fibromatosis toward more typical examples of fibromatosis (Figure 24.38). In most instances, this process totally obliterates the normal architecture of the ovary, but in ovaries that are only slightly enlarged it may be confined to the cortex. The proliferating myofibroblastic cells, which are immunoreactive for vimentin and smooth muscle actin, have scanty cytoplasm and round to oval, vesicular, but remarkably bland nuclei. Nucleoli are small or inapparent. Mitoses are numerous, regularly exceeding 20 mitotic figures/10 HPF; but atypical mitoses are not seen (Figure 24.40). Reticulin stains show a fine pericellular

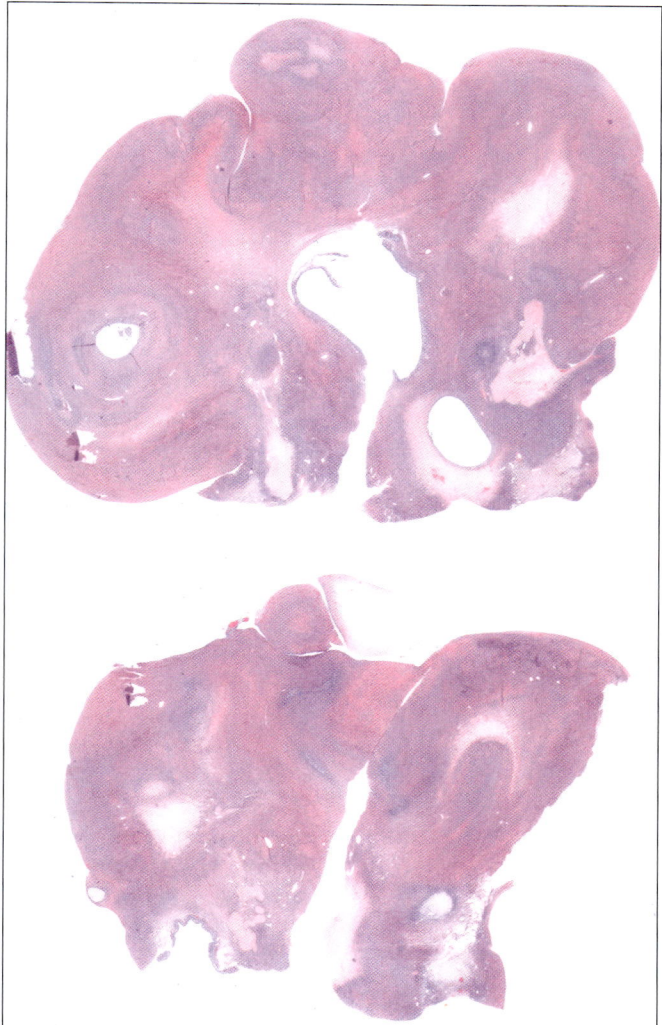

Figure 24.38 Low-power survey of ovarian fibromatosis. Irregular replacement by dense sclerotic fibrous tissue is seen with focal edema, entrapped follicular remnants and small areas of uninvolved cortex.

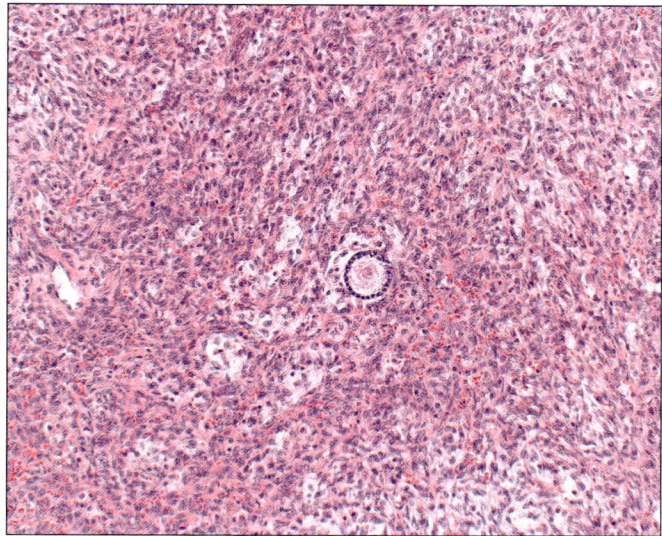

Figure 24.39 Immature fibromatosis. Plump spindle-shaped myofibroblastic cells enveloping residual primordial follicle.

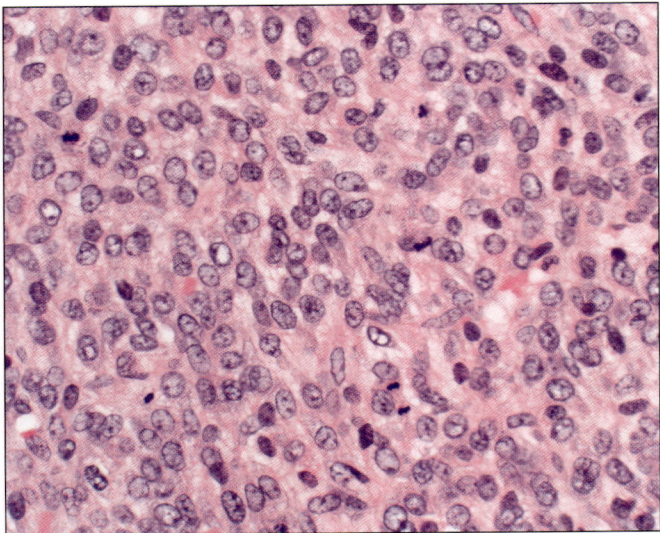

Figure 24.40 Immature fibromatosis. Higher power of proliferating myofibroblastic cells seen in Figure 24.39. Note bland oval nuclei, but numerous mitoses.

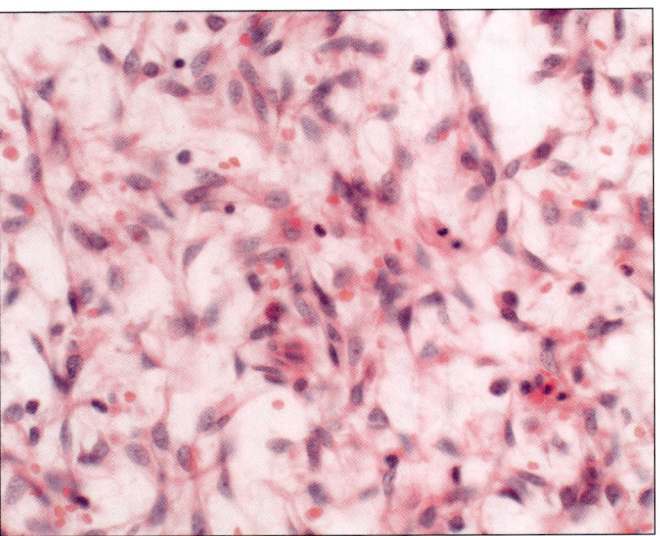

Figure 24.41 Immature fibromatosis. Intercellular edema imparts a 'tissue culture' appearance to proliferating mesenchymal cells, and a morphologic pattern that overlaps that of massive ovarian edema.

meshwork of fibrils. Hemorrhage is seen focally but no necrosis.

This architectural pattern merges into areas more typical of massive ovarian edema with conspicuous intercellular edema fluid, microcyst formation, dilated lymphatics and sinusoidal blood vessels, and interstitial hemorrhages. At the interfaces, the proliferating fibroblasts assume a 'tissue-culture' appearance (Figure 24.41).

Scattered in both the cellular fibroblastic and edematous areas are single or nested lutein-like cells. These cells exhibit small to moderate amounts of eosinophilic cytoplasm and rounded central nuclei, often with an obvious central nucleolus. Cells intermediate between the lutein-like cells and fibroblasts are seen.

Another important morphologic feature, reported occasionally, is entrapped follicular structures, crucial because (as with massive ovarian edema) it represents strong evidence that the process is not neoplastic. These are usually unremarkable primordial follicles (Figure 24.39), but may be 'dysplastic' (see above).

Differential Diagnosis

Stromal hyperthecosis (see above), like many cases of immature fibromatosis, is commonly bilateral and occurs in young women. It is not associated, however, with ascites or an acute presentation, does not cause massive enlargement of the ovaries, does not obliterate ovarian architecture, and is not associated with either collagen production or proliferating mitotically active fibroblastic cells.

Luteinized thecomas, the neoplasms that most closely resemble immature fibromatosis, may occur in young women, but with vanishing rarity under the age of 20 years. In contrast, one-half of patients with fibromatosis in which the ovary shows florid proliferative features are younger than 20 years of age. Some are under age 10 years. Most luteinized thecomas are estrogenic (>50%), unilateral (>90%), and unassociated with ascites or peritoneal pathology while fibromatosis is hormonally inactive or occasionally androgenic, commonly bilateral, and may present in association with similar fibroblastic peritoneal lesions. Histologically, luteinized thecomas are not edematous and do not incorporate native ovarian follicles.

SEQUELAE OF SURGERY OR TRAUMA

OVARIAN REMNANT SYNDROME (RESIDUAL OR REMNANT OVARY SYNDROME)

Definition

This condition exists if a patient who has had a 'total bilateral oophorectomy' later develops a palpable mass or experiences pelvic pain or other symptoms referable to ovarian tissue that has been left behind.[62]

Etiology

Residual ovarian tissue should not be confused with accessory or supernumerary ovaries (see above). The incomplete oophorectomy is usually the consequence of difficult surgical dissection secondary to adhesions caused by endometriosis or pelvic inflammatory disease, which often has been complicated further by previous surgery.

Clinical Features

Pelvic masses and pelvic pain are the most common presenting symptoms.[62] In a premenopausal patient, climacteric symptoms fail to develop and, if the uterus has been left behind, continuing cyclic vaginal bleeding may occur. Clinical suspicions in these patients is confirmed if the serum FSH and LH remain within the premenopausal range. Hormonal therapy may help alleviate symptoms, but surgery is the definitive treatment.

Pathology

At re-exploration, ovarian remnants may be found attached by usually dense adhesions to any of the residual pelvic

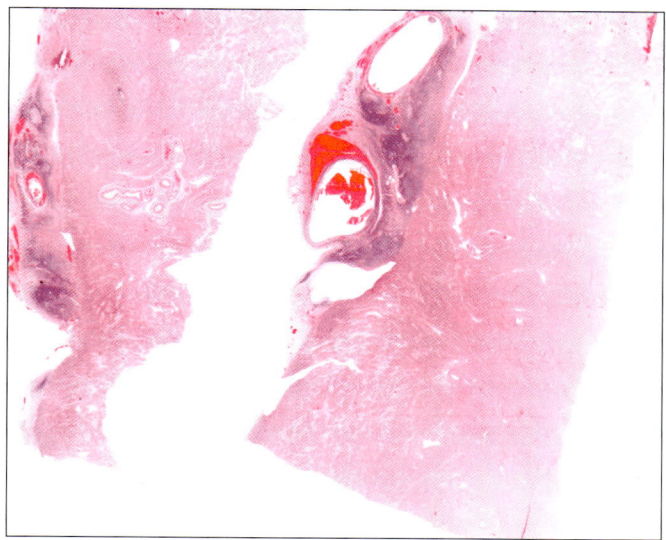

Figure 24.42 Ovarian remnant. An island of identifiable ovarian cortical tissue containing developing follicles, densely adherent to the uterine wall.

structures, including the uterus (Figure 24.42), or pelvic wall. Remnants may also show incidental endometriotic or dysfunctional cysts, but most display only normal functional ovarian parenchyma.[62] Obstruction or compression of the ureter, the colon, or bladder may occur.[63] Rare cases of adenocarcinoma developing in a remnant have been also reported.[64]

OVARIAN 'DRILLING' FOR POLYCYSTIC OVARY SYNDROME

One form of surgical therapy, for patients resistant to medical management of PCOS, is so-called laparoscopic 'drilling.'[65] This has largely replaced the older forms of corticomedullary stromal reduction such as wedge resection[66] and produces a peculiar pattern of tissue necrosis (Figure 24.43). Although pathognomonic and instantly identifiable with prior experience, this appearance would be utterly mysterious to the pathologist without relevant clinical information.

SPLENOSIS (AUTOTRANSPLANTANTION OF SPLENIC TISSUE)

Etiology

Splenosis is sometimes a complication of trauma, usually a motor vehicle accident, which has resulted in splenic rupture necessitating splenectomy, or rupture of a diseased spleen.[67] Nodules of splenic tissue, usually less than 1 cm in diameter, are randomly distributed in the peritoneal cavity and may be found adherent to the ovaries (Figure 24.44). Splenosis is generally asymptomatic but may cause abdominal or pelvic pain simulating endometriosis, or produce intestinal obstruction due to the development of adhesions. The gynecologic surgeon may encounter splenosis as an incidental finding or mistakenly interpret the widespread fleshy reddish-brown or purplish peritoneal nodules as endometriotic deposits.

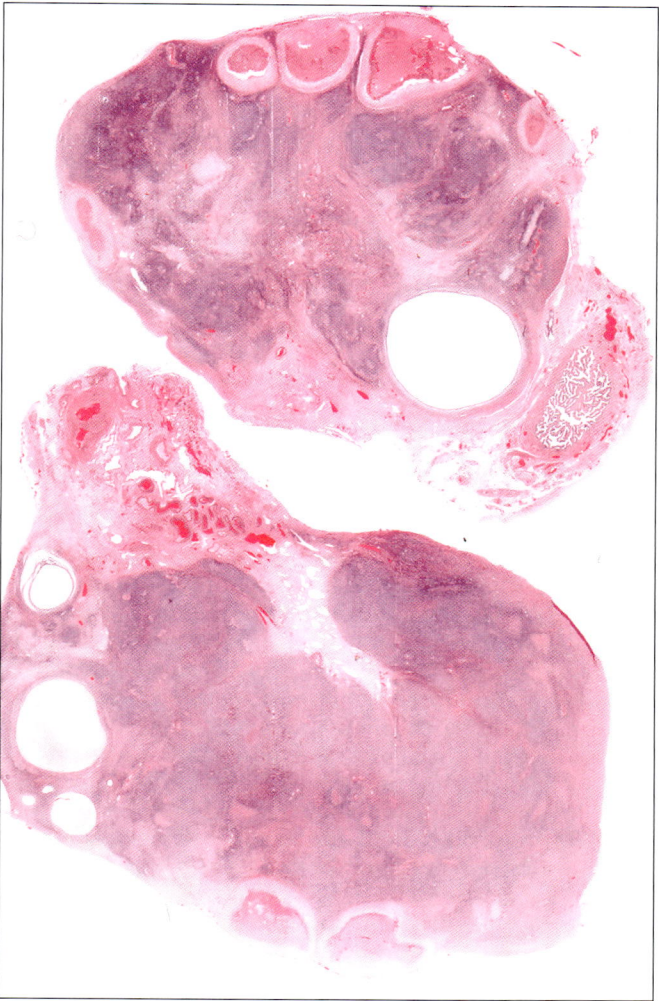

Figure 24.43 Ovarian drilling. A distinct pattern of acute focal tissue necrosis induced by laparoscopic diathermy to the ovarian cortex and superficial medulla of an ovary in a patient with PCOS.

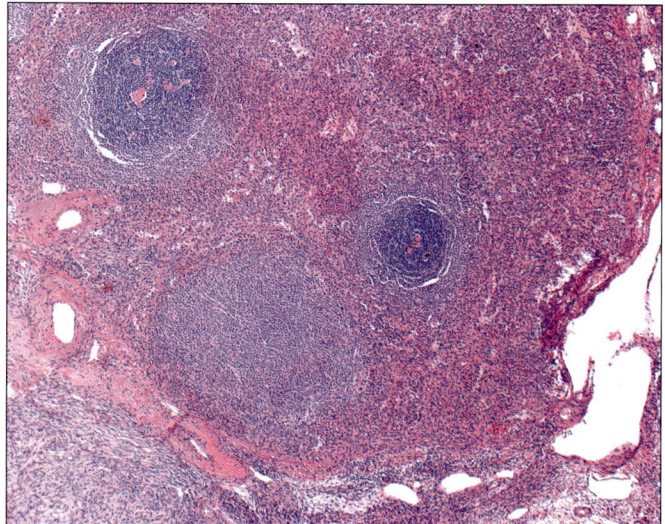

Figure 24.44 Ovarian splenosis. Ovarian splenotic nodules thought to represent endometriosis at laparotomy, in a 28-year-old woman with infertility. History of motor vehicle accident followed by splenectomy 17 years previously. Note ovarian cortical stroma at top left.

Microscopic Features

The implants are encased by fibrous tissue that simulates a splenic capsule, but lack smooth muscle and elastic fibers. Larger nodules usually show all the histologic components of normally sited splenic parenchyma (Figure 24.44) but, in smaller lesions, red pulp only may be evident.

IATROGENIC DISORDERS OF THE OVARIES

RADIOTHERAPY DAMAGE

Etiology

The ovaries may be exposed to external high-dose ionizing radiation for various reasons, most commonly for the treatment of malignant disease, either in children or adults. In the past, radiotherapy was used to induce an artificial menopause and to treat some non-malignant conditions such as endometriosis. Apart from achieving the desired radiotherapeutic effect on tumor growth, the most important issue at stake for young patients undergoing treatment for malignant disease is that of subsequent fertility. In contrast to gametogenesis in males, proliferation of oogonia ceases *in utero* and the number of oocytes is then fixed and cannot be replenished. Destruction of these germ cells *in utero* may lead to ovarian dysgenesis and postnatally to premature ovarian failure. The mitotically active oogonia are much more sensitive to radiation than oocytes that are in a resting phase (prophase of their first meiotic division) until just before ovulation. Ovarian follicles also vary in their sensitivity. Actively growing follicles are most vulnerable, possibly because their rapidly proliferating granulosa cells are radiosensitive, and their destruction may lead to death of the oocyte that they invest. The effects of radiation vary with the age of the patient (younger patients are generally more tolerant), the dose, the extent of the radiation field, and the use of concurrent chemotherapy.[68–70] Damage to the ovary may manifest during treatment as acute ovarian failure, or years later as premature menopause. Lead shielding and oophoropexy have been partially successful in protecting fertility. Cryopreservation of eggs prior to treatment is an emerging option, as freezing technology has improved.[71]

Microscopic Features

The first observable light-microscopic change in radiated oocytes is nuclear pyknosis. Condensed chromatin and a damaged nuclear envelope are evident ultrastructurally. The cytoplasmic damage that follows is manifest as eosinophilia. Granulosa cells exhibit pyknosis and karyolysis very soon after a radiation insult and, if a sufficient number of these cells are destroyed and regeneration is inadequate, the oocyte will die and the follicle will undergo atresia. Granulosa lutein cells show cytoplasmic vacuolation. The chronic effect on the follicular apparatus is decreased follicular activity, demonstrated by a progressive reduction in the numbers of growing and involuting follicles and corpora lutea, culminating in primordial follicle depletion.

The acute and chronic radiation effects in the non-specialized ovarian structures are similar to those documented more often in other organs. Stromal edema and fibrin exudation progress to stromal hyalinization, fibrosis,

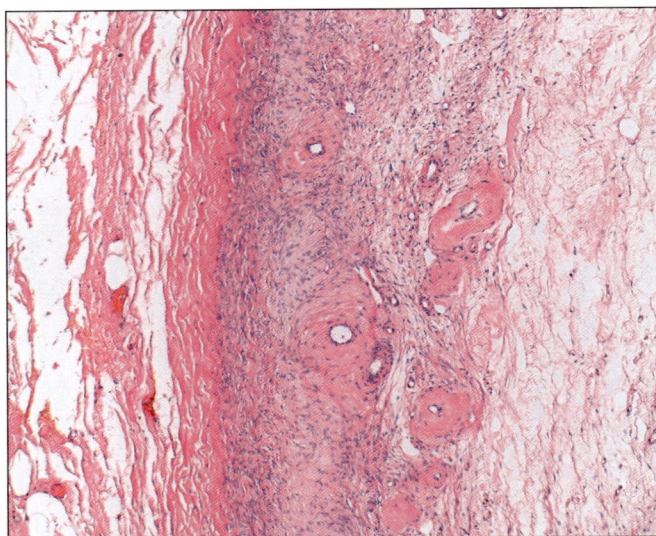

Figure 24.45 Chronic radiation damage. Dense peri-ovarian adhesions are subtended by atrophic, hyalinized cortex displaying vessels with hyalinized media and some fibrinoid change.

and capsular adhesions (Figure 24.45). Vascular changes are most conspicuous in arteries, which show fibrinoid necrosis, thrombosis, hyalinized media, foam cell accumulation, and myointimal proliferation. However, damage to the microvasculature is considered to be the prime mediator of delayed radiation injury, particularly ischemic necrosis and fibrosis.

CHEMOTHERAPEUTIC AND IMMUNOSUPPRESSIVE DRUGS

Etiology

From limited morphologic studies, antineoplastic drugs have a similar general effect on the ovary to ionizing radiation; namely, death of selected cells, especially those that are proliferating at the time of the insult. Individual drugs have a variable ovarian toxicity, and factors that influence the response of patients to radiotherapy also operate with respect to chemotherapy.[72,73] Adult women are more likely to develop temporary or permanent amenorrhea due to oocyte destruction than prepubertal children treated for cancer with cytotoxic agents alone, due to the low level of ovarian follicular activity before puberty. Attempts to simulate a quiescent state, and thus mitigate the damaging effect of chemotherapy in adults, have been made by giving oral contraceptives during therapy.

Microscopic Features

Biopsies show capsular thickening, peri-oophoritis, stromal fibrohyalinization, necrotizing vasculitis, hemorrhage, and disintegrating follicles.

ORAL CONTRACEPTIVES

Etiology

Combined estrogen–progestogen contraceptive pills inhibit ovulation chiefly by suppressing the release of pituitary gonadotropins, and in particular by suppressing the LH surge or disrupting the endometrial cycle.[74]

Microscopic Features

Morphologic effects on the ovaries depend on the type of preparation administered. High-dose formulas suppress all functional activity, and the ovaries shrink to postmenopausal size. Follicular growth is inhibited, no corpora lutea are formed, and the ovarian stroma becomes dense and fibrous. The basement membrane around primordial follicles thickens but oocytes are unaffected. After several months of therapy, corpora albicantia may be the only evidence of previous follicular activity. With low-dose preparations, there may be continuing folliculogenesis, including the development of mature (Graafian) follicles. Ovulation is still inhibited; the follicles undergo atresia, and corpora lutea do not form. Randomized controlled trials indicate that modern oral contraceptives are unlikely to prevent the development of functional cysts or to hasten their disappearance.[74]

Differential Diagnosis

Although practical problems in differential diagnosis are unlikely to arise, similar morphologic ovarian changes that correlate with functional arrest are also seen in women with (see above) hypogonadotropic hypogonadism, resistant ovary syndrome, and prolonged hyperprolactinemia.

PROGESTERONE

Etiology

Short-term high-dose progesterone therapy is used to manage various gynecologic disorders, including endometriosis and abnormal uterine bleeding, especially due to anovulation. Low-dose progestins are used in the contraceptive 'mini-pill.'

Microscopic Features

High-dose progesterone suppresses follicular activity and ovulation can be inhibited. Foci of deciduosis may occur in the ovarian cortex and beneath the pelvic peritoneum (Figure 24.46). Ovarian (and extraovarian) endometriotic lesions may exhibit a progestogenic effect similar to that more commonly encountered in the endometrium. The endometriotic glands are small, poorly developed and relatively inactive, while the stroma shows a decidual reaction. Low-dose progestins do not cause such conspicuous morphologic alterations. Follicular activity usually continues, and ovulation, with formation of a normal corpus luteum, occurs in about 40% of cases. There is defective ovulation in a further 30%. Follicular cysts have been noted occasionally.

DANAZOL

Etiology

This is an isoxazol derivative of a synthetic steroid 17-α ethinyltestosterone, used in the treatment of endometriosis, dysfunctional uterine bleeding, benign breast disease, and angioedema, and causes profound ovarian suppression and inhibits ovulation. It has a complex action, interfering with cyclical FSH and LH production, directly inhibiting

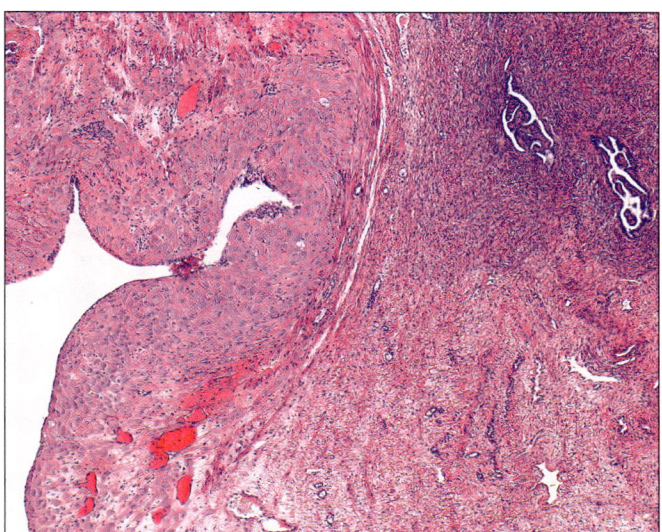

Figure 24.46 Pseudodeciduosis beneath the mesothelium of the ovarian hilus. From a woman recently treated with progesterone.

follicular development and steroidogenesis, and also having a weak androgenic effect.

Microscopic Features

The ovaries become small and follicular activity is arrested. Endometriotic lesions shrink and may be difficult to identify, even microscopically. The endometriotic glands become very small and are lined by atrophic cuboidal cells. The endometriotic stroma is compact and similarly inactive, and may be difficult to differentiate from cortical stroma.

(GnRH) ANALOGS

The most widely studied GnRH analog is goserelin. It acts on the hypothalamic–pituitary axis to suppress ovarian function, decreasing LH and estradiol levels to postmenopausal values. By virtue of its mode of action, goserelin causes the ovaries to become small and follicular activity ceases. Unlike tamoxifen (see later), there is no estrogen agonist-like effect.[75,76]

OVULATION-INDUCTION AGENTS

Ovulation-induction agents, especially clomiphene citrate, pulsatile GnRH therapy, and human menopausal gonadotropins, produce an iatrogenic form of hyperreactio luteinalis (see above) known as the 'ovarian hyperstimulation syndrome' (OHSS). This complication develops only after β-hCG is given at the time of ovulation, and is particularly prone to occur in women with the PCOS. Pathology is localized to the ovaries at the time the condition is triggered. The syndrome is unpredictable and potentially life-threatening when organs different from the ovaries become involved, causing ascites, hydrothorax, or coagulation disturbances resulting in thromboembolic phenomena. The different clinical and laboratory findings are the basis for classifications of mild, moderate, and severe OHSS.[77]

Pathology

In severe cases the ovaries become massively enlarged and pathologic examination shows changes identical to multiple theca–lutein cysts as well as one or more corpora lutea.

TAMOXIFEN

Tamoxifen is increasingly used as adjuvant therapy in premenopausal women with breast cancer. The hormonal effects of tamoxifen in premenopausal women are associated with increased levels of estradiol and progesterone whereas FSH and LH remain normal or increase slightly. Tamoxifen is structurally similar to clomiphene and is equivalent for induction of ovulation. The elevated serum levels of estrogen and progesterone may result from maturation of multiple ovarian follicles. There is no evidence that tamoxifen exposure is associated with an increase in benign or malignant primary ovarian neoplasms[78] or metastatic ovarian neoplasms. Further study is necessary to better define any association between tamoxifen and endometriosis.

Microscopic Features

Multiple and single ovarian follicular cysts have been reported in premenopausal women treated with tamoxifen. but it is debatable whether their incidence is increased. Necrosis and torsion are recognized but rare complications.

OVARIAN HEMORRHAGE AND ADNEXAL TORSION

OVARIAN HEMORRHAGE

Etiology

Small hemorrhages are common in normally functioning ovaries. The well-vascularized theca interna of developing follicles is prone to hemorrhage but usually only a small intrafollicular or perifollicular hematoma is formed. Slight bleeding occurs with follicular rupture at ovulation. Bleeding also occurs regularly in the vascularization stage of the corpus luteum. This is usually slight but, if excessive, may lead to the formation of a corpus luteum cyst (see later).

On occasion, profuse hemorrhage from the previous sources (mostly corpora lutea) causes ovarian rupture and bleeding into the peritoneal cavity. Hemoperitoneum from a corpus luteum may occur at any time during the reproductive years, but the risk is increased during pregnancy and in coagulopathic[79,80] and thrombocytopenic patients.[81] Rupture occurs most often on day 20–26 of the menstrual cycle, and two-thirds of cases involve the right ovary.

Microscopic Features

Pathologic examination of the excised tissues (oophorectomy, wedge excision, or cystectomy) will readily identify the source of the bleeding, except when extensive interstitial hemorrhage has obscured morphologic detail. In these cases, the operative findings and clinical features should provide a presumptive diagnosis. Sometimes examination of the blood clot evacuated from the peritoneal cavity may yield diagnostic material such as groups of lutein cells (Figure 24.47).

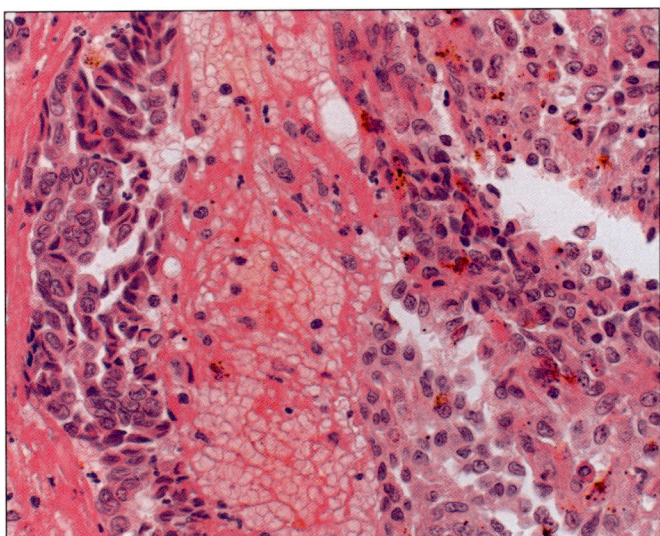

Figure 24.47 Peritoneal blood clot, containing granulosa cells, retrieved at laparotomy from a young woman with a ruptured follicular cyst.

ADNEXAL TORSION

Etiology

Torsion involving the ovary may occur in isolation or together with the fallopian tube. It is an uncommon but not rare gynecologic occurrence.[82] It presents most frequently during the reproductive years, but about 25% of cases involve children and, of these, a significant minority occurs in neonates and infants less than 8 months of age. Otherwise unexplained absence of an ovary has been attributed to subclinical torsion and consequent 'autoamputation' occurring in childhood or, perhaps, even *in utero*. Massive ovarian edema may be a variation on the theme; the clinicopathologic differences are dictated by the degree and speed of torsion and the stage at which the condition is diagnosed.

The tube and ovary usually undergo torsion as a single unit, rotating around the broad ligament as an axis. Less commonly, the ovary twists alone, around the mesovarium and even more rarely the tube alone undergoes torsion.[83] The right side is more commonly affected, and the left ovary is less freely mobile because of the presence of the sigmoid colon.

In adults, most cases are secondary to pathologic ovarian enlargements. Ovaries, once exceeding a diameter of 6 cm, are lifted out of the pelvic confines and become more freely mobile. A wide range of cystic and neoplastic diseases have been identified in twisted ovaries, the most common lesions being cystic teratomas (Figure 24.48) or cystadenomas. There is an increased risk of torsion of normal fallopian tube and ovary in pregnancy because of increased ovarian mobility within the abdomen during this period, most usually in the first half of pregnancy.[29,84] Torsion also occurs in association with ovarian hyperstimulation syndrome (see above).[85]

In children, torsion of apparently normal ovaries accounts for approximately one-third of cases, and occasionally may be bilateral.[86,87]

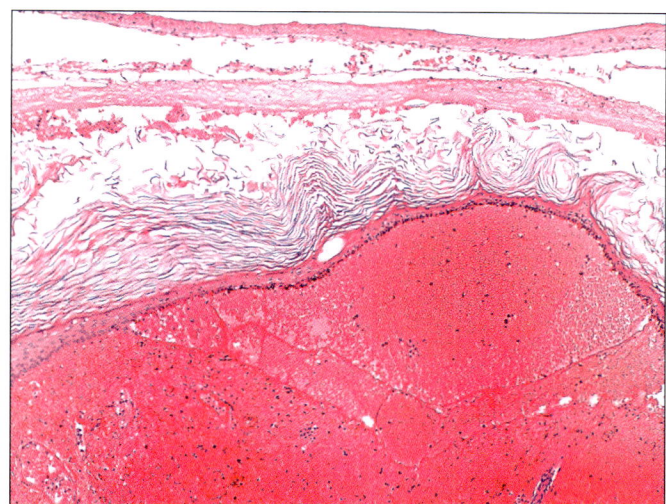

Figure 24.48 Torsion due to benign tumor. Diffuse hemorrhage into the wall of a mature cystic teratoma with surviving squamous lining at top.

Microscopic Features

Microscopy confirms hemorrhage, edema, and ischemic change and, often, frank necrosis. Normal structures may be difficult to identify. Multiple blocks of more solid or apparently viable areas, especially cyst walls, should be examined to determine the nature of any underlying pathologic condition and to exclude the possibility of a malignant neoplasm (Figure 24.48). We have found that staining for reticulin fibers, which regularly survive prolonged *in vivo* infarction, is particularly helpful in giving a 'skeletal' picture of the underlying vascular, stromal, and epithelial architecture long after all cellular detail is lost or obscured by hemorrhage. Complex cystic or papillary patterns are suspicious of underlying neoplasms and may even give the experienced observer hints of histologic type. Organoid structures may represent the infarcted tissues of a dermoid cyst. The accompanying fallopian tube if torsed may show similar ischemic changes and, less frequently, the apparent cause of adnexal torsion, such as a hydrosalpinx.

MÜLLERIANOSIS AND REACTIVE MESOTHELIAL LESIONS

'Müllerianosis' is a generic term applied to that group of epithelial and mesenchymal 'metaplasias' and proliferations that are frequent in the female peritoneal cavity, commonly around the pelvic viscera and especially the ovaries. In many ways, they exhibit the same morphologic features as their cellular analogs lining or forming the müllerian duct derivatives, such as endosalpinx (the fallopian tube mucosal lining), endometrium, smooth muscle, and so forth.

The epithelial metaplasias that fall loosely into this group of lesions would, therefore, include 'endosalpingiosis' and 'endocervicosis.' Extension by common usage rather than rational argument might also include transitional cell metaplasia as occurs in Walthard cell rests. The mesenchymal or stromal lesions in this group include 'deciduosis' (regularly encountered in pregnant patients) and 'disseminated peritoneal leiomyomatosis.' Mixed lesions would include endometriosis. Nonspecific peritoneal inclusions and proliferations are to one side of this morphologic spectrum but, clearly, are to be considered in their pathogenesis.

REFERENCES

1. Qublan H, Amarin Z, Nawasreh M, et al. Luteinized unruptured follicle syndrome: incidence and recurrence rate in infertile women with unexplained infertility undergoing intrauterine insemination. Hum Reprod (Oxford) 2006;21(8):2110–13.
2. Kuroiwa M, Hatakeyama SI, Suzuki N, et al. Neonatal ovarian cysts: management with reference to magnetic resonance imaging. Asian J Surg 2004;27(1):43–8.
3. Galinier P, Carfagna L, Juricic M, et al. Fetal ovarian cysts management and ovarian prognosis: a report of 82 cases. J Pediatr Surg 2008;43(11):2004.
4. Shimada T, Miura K, Gotoh H, et al. Management of prenatal ovarian cysts. Early Hum Dev 2008;84(6):417–20.
5. Slodki M, Janiak K, Respondek-Liberska M, et al. Assessment of the usefulness of ultrasound screening in fetal ovarian cysts. Ginekol Polska 2008;79(2):120–5.
6. Mittermayer C, Blaicher W, Grassauer D, et al. Fetal ovarian cysts: development and neonatal outcome. Ultraschall Med 2003;24(1):21–6.
7. de Sanctis C, Lala R, Matarazzo P, et al. Pubertal development in patients with McCune-Albright syndrome or pseudohypoparathyroidism. J Pediatr Endocrinol Metab 2003;16(Suppl 2):293–6.
8. Lytras A, Tolis G. Reproductive disturbances in multiple neuroendocrine tumor syndromes. Endocr Relat Cancer 2009;16(4):1125–38.
9. Grimes DA, Jones LB, Lopez LM, Schulz KF. Oral contraceptives for functional ovarian cysts. Cochrane Database Syst Rev 2006(4):CD006134.
10. Grimes DA, Jones LB, Lopez LM, Schulz KF. Oral contraceptives for functional ovarian cysts. Cochrane Database Syst Rev (Online) 2009;(2)(2):CD006134.
11. Coccia ME, Pasquini L, Comparetto C, Scarselli G. Hyperreactio luteinalis in a woman with high-risk factors. A case report. J Reprod Med 2003;48(2):127–9.
12. Tanaka Y, Yanagihara T, Ueta M, et al. Naturally conceived twin pregnancy with hyperreactio luteinalis, causing hyperandrogenism and maternal virilization. Acta Obstet Gynecol Scand 2001;80(3):277–8.
13. Csapo Z, Szabo I, Toth M, et al. Hyperreactio luteinalis in a normal singleton pregnancy. A case report. J Reprod Med 1999;44(1):53–6.
14. Le Vaillant C, Tremouilhac C, Boog G. [Luteinized cystic ovarian hyperplasia during a normal pregnancy]. J Gynecol Obstet Biol Reprod (Paris) 2003;32(4):368–74.
15. Sherer DM, Dalloul M, Khoury-Collado F, et al. Hyperreactio luteinalis presenting with marked hyper-glycemia and bilateral multicystic adnexal masses at 21 weeks gestation. Am J Perinatol 2006;23(2):85–8.
16. Haddad A, Mulvany N, Billson V, Arnstein M. Solitary luteinized follicle cyst of pregnancy—Report of a case with cytologic findings. Acta Cytol 2000;44(3):454–8.
17. Wang XY, Vinta MK, Myers S, Fan F. Solitary luteinized follicle cyst of pregnancy and puerperium. Pathol Res Pract 2006;202(6):471–3.
18. Satyanarayana S, Bohre JK. Ovarian granulosa cell 'tumorlet' and mature follicles with ectopic decidua in pregnancy—a case report. Indian J Pathol Microbiol 2001;44(2):149–50.
19. Ercal T, Cinar O, Mumcu A, et al. Ovarian pregnancy; relationship to an intrauterine device. Aust N Z J Obstet Gynaecol 1997;37(3):362–4.
20. Raziel A, Schachter M, Mordechai E, et al. Ovarian pregnancy—a 12-year experience of 19 cases in one institution. Eur J Obstet Gynecol Reprod Biol 2004;114(1):92–6.
21. Raziel A, Mordechai E, Schachter M, et al. A comparison of the incidence, presentation, and management of ovarian pregnancies

22. Knight JA, Marrett LD. Parental occupational exposure and the risk of testicular cancer in Ontario. J Occup Environ Med 1997;39(4):333–8.
23. Melilli GA, Avantario C, Farnelli C, et al. Combined intrauterine and ovarian pregnancy after in vitro fertilization and embryo transfer: a case report. Clin Exp Obstet Gynecol 2001;28(2):100–1.
24. Selo-Ojeme DO, GoodFellow CF. Simultaneous intrauterine and ovarian pregnancy following treatment with clomiphene citrate. Arch Gynecol Obstet 2002;266(4):232–4.
25. Danihel L, Losch A, Kainz C, et al. Bilateral primary leiomyoma of the ovary. Wien Klin Wochenschr 1995;107(14):436–8.
26. Namba A, Nakagawa S, Nakamura N, et al. Ovarian choriocarcinoma arising from partial mole as evidenced by deoxyribonucleic acid microsatellite analysis. Obstet Gynecol 2003;102(5 Pt 1):991–4.
27. Balat O, Kutlar I, Ozkur A, et al. Primary pure ovarian choriocarcinoma mimicking ectopic pregnancy: a report of fulminant progression. Tumori 2004;90(1):136–8.
28. Born C, Wirth S, Stabler A, Reiser M. Diagnosis of adnexal torsion in the third trimester of pregnancy: a case report. Abdom Imaging 2004;29(1):123–7.
29. Pan HS, Huang LW, Lee CY, et al. Ovarian pregnancy torsion. Arch Gynecol Obstet 2004;270(2):119–21.
30. Bromley B, Benacerraf B. Adnexal masses during pregnancy: accuracy of sonographic diagnosis and outcome. J Ultrasound Med 1997;16(7):447–52.
31. Pitynski K, Basta A, Szczudrawa A, Oplawski M. [Ovarian tumors in pregnancy in the material of the Department of Gynecology and Oncology Collegium Medicum of Jagiellonian University in Cracow]. Ginekol Pol 2002;73(4):371–5.
32. Sayedur Rahman M, Al-Sibai MH, Rahman J, et al. Ovarian carcinoma associated with pregnancy. A review of 9 cases. Acta Obstet Gynecol Scand 2002;81(3):260–4.
33. Koivunen R, Laatikainen T, Tomas C, et al. The prevalence of polycystic ovaries in healthy women. Acta Obstet Gynecol Scand 1999;78(2):137–41.
34. Geisthovel F. A comment on the European Society of Human Reproduction and Embryology/American Society for Reproductive Medicine consensus of the polycystic ovarian syndrome. Reprod Biomed Online 2003;7(6):602–5.
35. Pelusi B, Gambineri A, Pasquali R. Type 2 diabetes and the polycystic ovary syndrome. Minerva Ginecol 2004;56(1):41–51.
36. Fleming R. The use of insulin sensitising agents in ovulation induction in women with polycystic ovary syndrome. Hormones (Athens) 2006;5(3):171–8.
37. Salehi M, Bravo-Vera R, Sheikh A, et al. Pathogenesis of polycystic ovary syndrome: What is the role of obesity? Metab Clin Exp 2004;53(3):358–76.
38. Strauss 3rd JF. Some new thoughts on the pathophysiology and genetics of polycystic ovary syndrome. Ann N Y Acad Sci 2003;997:42–8.
39. Fratantonio E, Vicari E, Pafumi C, Calogero AE. Genetics of polycystic ovarian syndrome. Reprod Biomed Online 2005;10(6):713–20.
40. Homburg R. Adverse effects of luteinizing hormone on fertility: fact or fantasy. Baillieres Clin Obstet Gynaecol 1998;12(4):555–63.
41. Sabuncu T, Harma M, Harma M, et al. Sibutramine has a positive effect on clinical and metabolic parameters in obese patients with polycystic ovary syndrome. Fertil Steril 2003;80(5):1199–204.
42. Leong S, Trivedi AN. A case of ovarian stromal hyperplasia causing hirsutism in a post-menopausal woman. Aust N Z J Obstet Gynaecol 2001;41(1):102–3.
43. Sluijmer AV, Heineman MJ, Koudstaal J, et al. Relationship between ovarian production of estrone, estradiol, testosterone, and androstenedione and the ovarian degree of stromal hyperplasia in postmenopausal women. Menopause 1998;5(4):207–10.
44. Jongen VH, Hollema H, van der Zee AG, et al. Ovarian stromal hyperplasia and ovarian vein steroid levels in relation to endometrioid endometrial cancer. BJOG 2003;110(7):690–5.
45. Manieri C, Di Bisceglie C, Fornengo R, et al. Postmenopausal virilization in a woman with gonadotropin dependent ovarian hyperthecosis. J Endocrinol Invest 1998;21(2):128–32.
46. Krug E, Berga SL. Postmenopausal hyperthecosis: functional dysregulation of androgenesis in climacteric ovary. Obstet Gynecol 2002;99(5 Pt 2):893–7.
47. Carvalho JP, Diegoli MS, Carvalho FM, Diegoli CA. Adnexal torsion following gonadotropin-releasing hormone analog therapy: a case report. Rev Hosp Clin Fac Med Sao Paulo 2004;59(3):128–30.
48. Friedrich M, Ertan AK, Axt-Fliedner R, et al. Unilateral massive ovarian edema (MOE): a case report. Clin Exp Obstet Gynecol 2002;29(1):65–6.
49. Mohan H, Mohan P, Bal A, Tahlan A. Massive ovarian oedema: report of two cases. Arch Gynecol Obstet 2004;270(3):199–200.
50. Kanumakala S, Warne GL, Stokes KB, et al. Massive ovarian edema causing early puberty. J Pediatr Endocrinol Metab 2002;15(6):861–4.
51. Natarajan A, Wales JK, Marven SS, Wright NP. Precocious puberty secondary to massive ovarian oedema in a 6-month-old girl. Eur J Endocrinol 2004;150(2):119–23.
52. Nogales FF, MartinSances L, MendozaGarcia E, et al. Massive ovarian oedema. Histopathology 1996;28(3):229–34.
53. Guvenal T, Cetin A, Tasyurt A. Unilateral massive ovarian edema and polycystic ovaries. A case report. Eur J Obstet Gynecol Reprod Biol 2001;97(2):258–9.
54. de la Cruz SI, Llanos Arriaga V, Narro Tristan H, et al. [Bilateral ovary massive edema. Unusual gynecologic pathology. Report of 2 cases]. Ginecol Obstet Mex 2001;69:72–6.
55. Valenzuela P, Dominguez P. Bilateral massive edema of the ovary. Zentralbl Gynakol 1999;121(5):258–9.
56. Tanaka T, Umesaki N, Ogita S. Camptothecin and mitomycin combination chemotherapy on ovarian clear cell carcinoma with multiple systemic metastases. Eur J Gynaecol Oncol 2000;21(4):377–9.
57. Umesaki N, Tanaka T, Miyama M, Kawamura N. Sonographic characteristics of massive ovarian edema. Ultrasound Obstet Gynecol 2000;16(5):479–81.
58. Umesaki N, Tanaka T, Miyama M, et al. Successful preoperative diagnosis of massive ovarian edema aided by comparative imaging study using magnetic resonance and ultrasound. Eur J Obstet Gynecol Reprod Biol 2000;89(1):97–9.
59. Kocak M, Caliskan E, Haberal A. Laparoscopic conservation of the ovaries in cases with massive ovarian oedema. Gynecol Obstet Invest 2002;53(2):129–32.
60. Scurry J, Allen D, Dobson P. Ovarian fibromatosis, ascites and omental fibrosis. Histopathology 1996;28(1):81–4.
61. Clement PB, Young RH, Hanna W, Scully RE. Sclerosing peritonitis associated with luteinized thecomas of the ovary. A clinicopathological analysis of six cases. Am J Surg Pathol 1994;18(1):1–13.
62. Magtibay PM, Nyholm JL, Hernandez JL, Podratz KC. Ovarian remnant syndrome. Am J Obstet Gynecol 2005;193(6):2062–6.
63. Terzibachian JJ, Gay C, Bertrand V, et al. Value of ureteral catheterization in laparoscopy. Gynecol Obstet Fertil 2001;29(6):427–32.
64. Donnez O, Squifflet J, Marbaix E, et al. Primary ovarian adenocarcinoma developing in ovarian remnant tissue ten years after laparoscopic hysterectomy and bilateral salpingo-oophorectomy for endometriosis. J Min Inv Gyncol 2007;14(6):752–7.
65. Farquhar C, Lilford R, Marjoribanks J, Vanderkerchove P. Laparoscopic drilling by diathermy or laser for ovulation induction in anovulatory polycystic ovary syndrome. Chichester, UK: John Wiley; 2007.
66. Balen A. Surgical treatment of polycystic ovary syndrome. Best Pract Res Clin Endocrinol Metab 2006;20(2):271–80.
67. Vydianath B, Gurumurthy M, Crocker J. Solitary ovarian splenosis. J Clin Pathol 2005;58(11):1224–5.
68. Green DM, Sklar CA, Boice JD, et al. Ovarian failure and reproductive outcomes after childhood cancer treatment: Results from the Childhood Cancer Survivor Study. J Clin Oncol 2009;27(14):2374.
69. Gross E, Champetier C, Pointreau Y, et al. Tolérance à l'irradiation des tissus sains: les ovaires. Cancer/Radiothérapie 2010;14(4–5):373.
70. Wo JY, Viswanathan AN. Impact of radiotherapy on fertility, pregnancy, and neonatal outcomes in female cancer patients. Int J Radiat Oncol Biol Phys 2009;73(5):1304–12.
71. Technology PCotASfRMaSfAR. Ovarian tissue and oocyte cryopreservation. Fertil Steril 2008;90(5, Suppl 1):S241.
72. Meirow D, Nugent D. The effects of radiotherapy and chemotherapy on female reproduction. Hum Reprod Update 2001;7(6):535–43.
73. Stroud JS, Mutch D, Rader J, et al. Effects of cancer treatment on ovarian function. Fertil Steril 2009;92(2):417–27.

74. Group ECW. Ovarian and endometrial function during hormonal contraception. Hum Reprod (Oxford) 2001;16(7):1527.
75. Goel S, Sharma R, Hamilton A, Beith J. LHRH agonists for adjuvant therapy of early breast cancer in premenopausal women. Chichester, UK: John Wiley; 2009.
76. Jonat W. Luteinizing hormone-releasing hormone analogues—the rationale for adjuvant use in premenopausal women with early breast cancer. Br J Cancer 1998;78(Suppl 4):5–8.
77. Golan A, Weissman A. A modern classification of OHSS. Reprod BioMed Online 2009;19(1):28.
78. McGonigle KF, Vasilev SA, Odom-Maryon T, Simpson JF. Ovarian histopathology in breast cancer patients receiving tamoxifen. Gynecol Oncol 1999;73(3):402–6.
79. Castellino G, Cuadrado MJ, Godfrey T, et al. Characteristics of patients with antiphospholipid syndrome with major bleeding after oral anticoagulant treatment. Ann Rheum Dis 2001;60(5):527–30.
80. Cretel E, Cacoub P, Huong DL, et al. Massive ovarian haemorrhage complicating oral anticoagulation in the antiphospholipid syndrome: a report of three cases. Lupus 1999;8(6):482–5.
81. Castro-Lizano N, Calleja C, Galindo-Rodriguez G, Avina-Zubieta JA. Ovarian haemorrhage, rupture and haemoperitoneum secondary to thrombocytopenia in a patient with SLE. Lupus 2003;12(8):648–50.
82. Huchon C, Fauconnier A. Adnexal torsion: a literature review. Eur J Obstet Gynecol Reprod Biol 2010;150(1):8–12.
83. Antoniou N, Varras M, Akrivis C, et al. Isolated torsion of the fallopian tube: a case report and review of the literature. Clin Exp Obstet Gynecol 2004;31(3):235–8.
84. Prefumo F, Ciravolo G. Adnexal torsion in late pregnancy. Arch Gynecol Obstet 2009;280(3):473–4.
85. Bellver J, Escudero E, Pellicer A. Bilateral partial oophorectomy in the management of severe ovarian hyperstimulation syndrome (OHSS): ovarian mutilating surgery is not an option in the management of severe OHSS. Hum Reprod (Oxford) 2003;18(7):1363.
86. Abes M, Sarihan H. Oophoropexy in children with ovarian torsion. Eur J Pediatr Surg 2004;14(3):168–71.
87. Beaunoyer M, Chapdelaine J, Bouchard S, Ouimet A. Asynchronous bilateral ovarian torsion. J Pediatr Surg 2004;39(5):746–9.

25 Ovarian Epithelial-Stromal Tumors. Serous Tumors

Jaime Prat, Elke Jarboe

CHAPTER OUTLINE

Epithelial/Stromal Tumors	564	Serous Borderline Tumors of the Peritoneum	579
Borderline Tumors	565	**Serous Carcinomas**	**580**
Carcinomas	565	Low-grade Serous Carcinomas	580
Benign and Borderline Serous Tumors	565	High-grade Serous Carcinomas	582
Benign Serous Tumors	565		
Serous Borderline Tumors	567		
Serous Borderline Tumors in Lymph Nodes	578		

EPITHELIAL/STROMAL TUMORS

The tumors in this category account for approximately two-thirds of all ovarian tumors and for about 90% of all ovarian cancers in the Western world.[1,2] Epithelial ovarian tumors are heterogeneous neoplasms that are primarily classified according to cell type into serous, mucinous, endometrioid, clear cell, transitional, and squamous cell tumors.[1–3] However, benign counterparts of these cells are not found in the normal ovary and their neoplastic occurrence has long been attributed to müllerian 'neometaplasia' of the ovarian surface epithelium (mesothelium), which derives from the celomic epithelium. Specifically, since the celomic epithelium gives rise to the müllerian ducts, it was proposed that, as the surface epithelium becomes malignant, it would acquire the morphologic features of the müllerian duct epithelium; i.e., serous (fallopian tube-like), endometrioid (endometrium-like), and mucinous (endocervical-like). This aberrant differentiation constitutes the basis for ovarian tumor classification. However, even if an origin from the surface epithelium cannot be excluded, there is now compelling evidence that a number of tumors thought to be primary ovarian cancers actually originate in other pelvic organs and involve the ovary secondarily. In fact, it has been discovered that high-grade serous carcinomas (HGSCs) may arise from precursor epithelial lesions in the distal fimbriated end of the fallopian tube,[4–10] whereas endometrioid and clear cell carcinomas originate from ovarian endometriosis.[11,12] The relative importance of the fallopian tube mucosa compared with the ovarian surface epithelium (mesothelium) in the genesis of high-grade serous ovarian cancers is still a subject of debate. On the other hand, it can be argued that tumors arising in endometriosis are ultimately of endometrial origin. Thus, in some cases, the term ovarian cancer may not be accurate, and it has been suggested that it should be replaced with the terms pelvic or peritoneal cancer. However, given the confusion that might follow in the literature, we think it best to keep the term ovarian cancer until the various possible origins of these diseases are known better.

Some epithelial ovarian tumors, particularly those in the serous category, may be exophytic, intracystic (endophytic), or both. The presence of exophytic growth is indicated by the word 'surface,' which is added to the designation, i.e., 'serous surface papillary adenocarcinoma.' In contrast, cystic tumors with intracystic growth are variably called 'serous adenocarcinoma' or described by the prefix *cyst-* before their name, i.e., 'serous cystadenocarcinoma.' Most surface epithelial–stromal neoplasms are predominantly epithelial, with only a minor component derived from the ovarian stroma. When gland-forming tumors have a predominant stromal component, the terms 'adenofibroma' and 'cystadenofibroma' (if grossly visible cysts are present) are used.

However, the subdivision of epithelial–stromal tumors that is most important from a clinical viewpoint is their classification into benign, borderline, and carcinoma forms, because it generally correlates with prognosis. This is done according to the amount of tumor cell proliferation, the degree of nuclear atypia, and the presence or absence of stromal invasion.[1,2]

BORDERLINE TUMORS

Borderline tumors (also designated as tumors of low malignant potential) show histologic and cytologic features that are intermediate between those of clearly benign and clearly malignant tumors of the same cell type(s). They exhibit epithelial proliferation greater than that seen in their benign counterparts but an absence of *destructive invasion* of the stroma or confluent growth, and are associated with a much better prognosis, stage for stage, than that of ovarian carcinomas.[2,3,13] Even in the absence of invasiveness within the ovary, borderline tumors of the serous type can either implant on peritoneal surfaces or be associated with independent foci of primary serous peritoneal neoplasia, and, rarely, invasion of the underlying tissues occurs in both circumstances.[14–21] Exceptionally, tumors of borderline malignancy spread via lymphatics and blood vessels. In addition, a small number of these tumors are combined with or transform over time into obviously invasive carcinomas.[15,19,21] Although favorable in the majority of cases, the biologic behavior of the borderline tumors differs from that of the obviously benign tumors of the same cell type(s). Therefore, the designation 'tumors of borderline malignancy' should be kept. Alternative terms such as *proliferating*, *atypical*, and *atypical proliferative*[22] are misleading because they do not imply the malignant potential of a small but significant number of these tumors and discourage complete surgical staging and follow-up of the patients.[1–3,13,19] Subdivision of the borderline group into benign and malignant, based on the presence of micropapillary architecture, is artificial since tumors with or without micropapillary pattern may rarely be associated with invasive peritoneal implants and poor outcome. Although the word 'borderline' may suggest uncertainty, it accurately describes the ambiguous histologic and biologic features of these neoplasms and remains the most appropriate term. Accordingly, it has been recommended by the World Health Organization (WHO) for the last four decades.[3]

The distinction between borderline tumors and carcinomas is one of the most common problems in ovarian tumor pathology, yet the literature on borderline tumors is confusing, particularly with regard to their diagnostic features and treatment. Although the WHO[3] has recommended the presence or absence of 'obvious invasion' of the stroma, most practitioners do not require obvious stromal invasion for the diagnosis of carcinoma if the epithelial cells are malignant cytologically. To promote terminology agreement, the WHO has proposed such tumors be classified as borderline *with intraepithelial carcinoma*. The extent of the carcinomatous epithelium should be noted in the pathology report.[1–3]

CARCINOMAS

Malignant epithelial tumors (carcinomas) are the most common ovarian cancers, accounting for 90% of cases.[2,3] Although traditionally referred to as a single entity, ovarian cancer is not a homogeneous disease but rather a group of diseases, each with different morphology and biologic behavior. Currently, based on histopathology, immunohistochemistry, and molecular genetic analysis, at least five main types of ovarian carcinomas are identified: HGSCs (70%), endometrioid carcinomas (10%), clear cell carcinomas (10%), mucinous carcinomas (3%), and low-grade serous carcinomas (LGSCs; <5%).[23,24] These tumors account for 98% of ovarian carcinomas, can be reproducibly diagnosed by light microscopy, and are inherently different diseases, as indicated by differences in epidemiologic and genetic risk factors, precursor lesions, patterns of spread, molecular events during oncogenesis, response to chemotherapy, and prognosis. The fact that one tumor type (HGSCs) accounts for over two-thirds of cases does not justify classifying ovarian carcinomas into only two pathogenetic types, lumping together the other four (endometrioid, clear cell, mucinous, and LGSCs) as 'type I carcinomas.'[25] In fact, the latter tumors are clinically, morphologically, and molecularly distinct diseases that individually bear resemblance neither to HGSCs nor to each other. Thus, classifying ovarian carcinomas into only two pathogenetic types ('types I and II')[25] appears to be artificial and simplistic.

BENIGN AND BORDERLINE SEROUS TUMORS

Serous tumors in both their benign and borderline forms show ciliated epithelial cells and other cell types resembling those of the fallopian tube. Although the less differentiated tumors lose the cytologic features of tubal epithelium, they usually exhibit distinctive patterns of growth, including fine and complex papillary structures with prominent cellular budding and glands with irregular slit-like lumens and solid sheets. Psammoma bodies and larger calcific deposits are usually found. Serous tumors, whether benign, borderline, or malignant, tend to be uniform throughout a given specimen, usually lacking the admixtures of these three subtypes so common in mucinous tumors. The Systematized Nomenclature of Medicine (SNOMED) classification of serous tumors is as follows:

- Benign serous tumors
  - Serous adenofibroma, cystadenofibroma
  - Serous surface papilloma
  - Serous cystadenoma
  - Serous papillary cystadenoma
- Serous borderline tumor
- Serous carcinoma
- Epidemiology.

In the Western world, serous tumors account for 30–40% of all ovarian tumors. Of these, approximately 70% are benign, 5–10% borderline, and 20–25% carcinomas.[1] Borderline and invasive serous tumors together account for about 30% of the non-benign ovarian tumors.

BENIGN SEROUS TUMORS

Clinical Features

Benign serous tumors may occur at any age but are most common during the fifth decade. Usually, the tumors are asymptomatic and discovered incidentally during ultrasound investigation of another gynecologic disorder.

Macroscopic Features

Benign serous tumors are usually endophytic (cystadenomas), but may be exophytic (surface papillomas) or both.

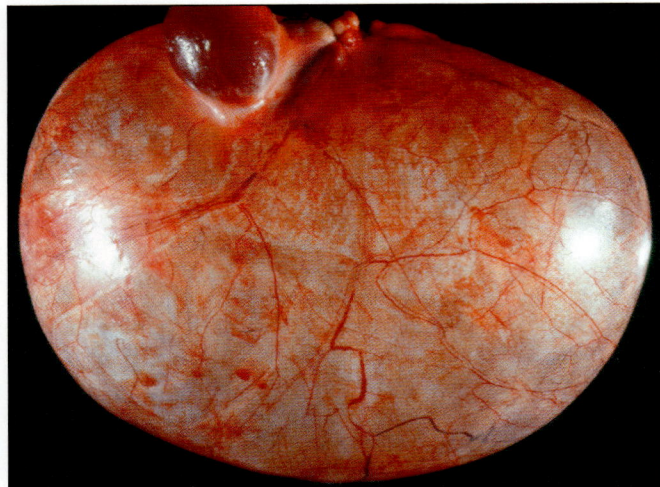

Figure 25.1 Serous cystadenoma. Unilocular thin-walled cyst.

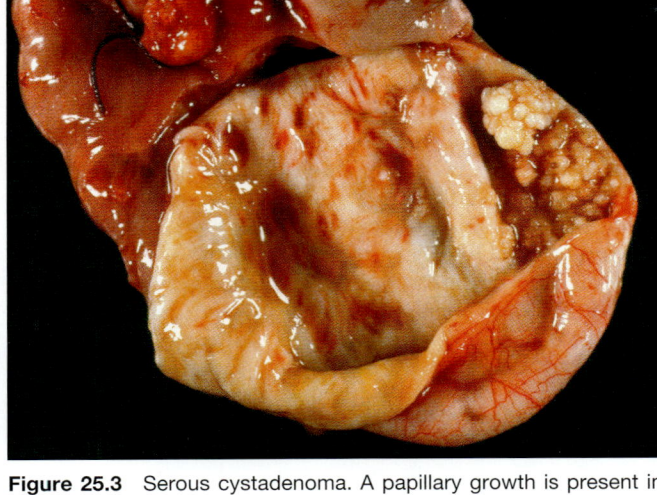

Figure 25.3 Serous cystadenoma. A papillary growth is present in the lumen of the cyst.

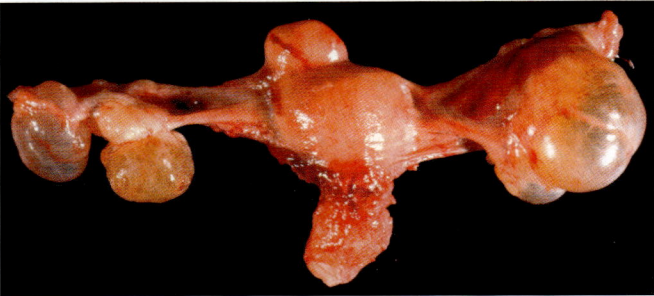

Figure 25.2 Serous cystadenoma, bilateral.

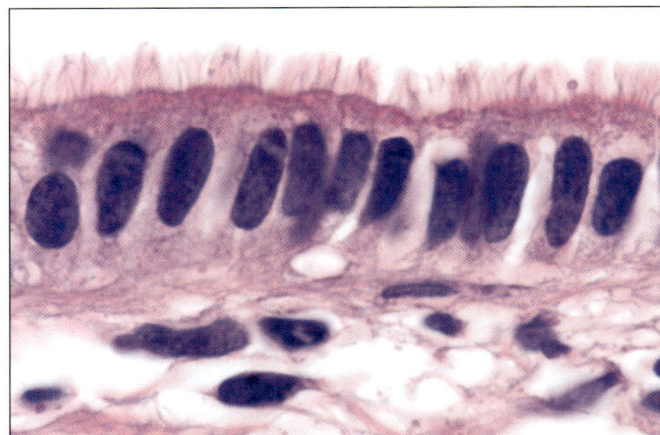

Figure 25.4 Serous cystadenoma. Ciliated epithelium similar to that of the fallopian tube.

Serous cystadenomas are usually unilocular (Figure 25.1) but may be multilocular, and have thin-walled cyst(s) (Figure 25.2) filled with watery or occasionally thin mucinous fluid. They average about 10 cm in size. Customarily, a benign serous tumor is diagnosed only if the lesion is >1 cm in diameter. The cyst(s) may have a smooth inner surface or have polypoid excrescences (Figure 25.3), which are firm if their stroma is fibrous and soft if it is edematous. Serous cystadenomas are bilateral in approximately 10–20% of cases (Figure 25.2).

Serous surface papillomas appear as polypoid excrescences on the outer surface of the ovary. The surface tumors are often accompanied by underlying cystic components. Serous adenofibromas are hard, white, predominantly fibromatous tumors with small glands or cysts that contain clear fluid. When bilateral, their firm consistency may suggest the diagnosis of cancer.

Microscopic Features

The cysts and polypoid excrescences of benign serous tumors are typically lined by pseudostratified epithelium similar to that of the fallopian tube, which is frequently ciliated (Figure 25.4). Tumors lined entirely by nonciliated cuboidal or columnar epithelium that resembles ovarian surface epithelium are also generally included in the serous

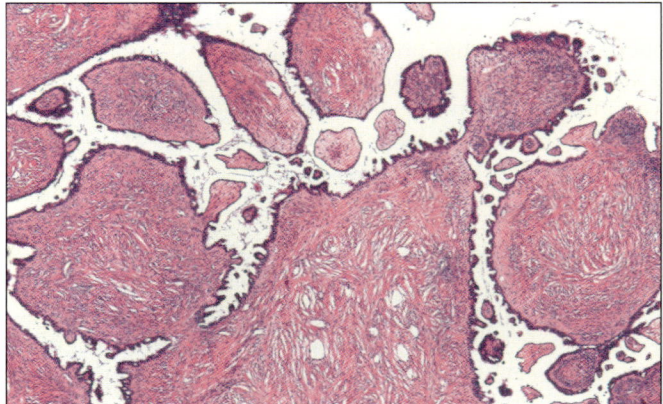

Figure 25.5 Serous papillary cystadenoma. The polypoid excrescences are composed predominantly of dense fibrous tissue.

category despite their indifferent appearance. The epithelial cells of benign serous tumors may secrete mucin, but, when it is present, it is usually confined to the lumens of cysts and apical portion of the cytoplasm of the epithelial cells. Mitoses are rare. There is no nuclear atypia. Psammoma bodies are infrequent (10%). Papillae when found are composed almost entirely of stroma (Figure 25.5), which may be collagenous or markedly edematous. In adenofibromas and cystadenofibromas, glands and cysts are scattered within a predominantly fibromatous stroma. Otherwise typical benign cystic or surface serous tumors containing minor foci (<10%) consistent with borderline neoplasia (cell stratification and nuclear atypia) are kept in the benign category for clinical purposes.[1]

Differential Diagnosis

Serous cystadenomas may be confused with rare examples of cystic struma ovarii (Chapter 29), but the latter exhibits at least minor foci of identifiable thyroid follicles in the cyst's outer wall. Rare rete cystadenomas may simulate serous cystadenomas but, in addition to their hilar location, often show a thick layer of smooth muscle and are lined by cells lacking cilia. Common peritoneal cysts, lined by mesothelial cells, often mimic serous cystadenomas. Serous surface papillary adenofibromas should be distinguished from the common small surface stromal proliferations sometimes seen in adult women. The latter lesions are typically multifocal, have a simple cuboidal epithelial lining, and do not form a mass lesion.

SEROUS BORDERLINE TUMORS

Clinical Features

Serous borderline tumors (SBTs) account for one-fourth to one-third of the non-benign serous tumors.[26,27] They are most common in the fourth and fifth decades, with an average patient age of 42 years.[21] Although often asymptomatic, the tumor may sometimes present with abdominal enlargement and pain due to rupture or torsion. Approximately 70% are confined to one or both ovaries (stage I) at the time of diagnosis; the remaining tumors have spread within the pelvis (stage II) or upper abdomen (stage III). Only rare cases have extended beyond the abdomen (stage IV) at the time of presentation.[19,27] One-third of the stage I tumors are bilateral.[27]

Macroscopic Features

Serous borderline tumors have one or more cysts that are lined by polypoid excrescences and closely packed finer papillae (endophytic growth) (Figure 25.6). The cysts contain thick mucinous fluid, which does not necessarily indicate the mucinous nature of the tumor. The polypoid excrescences contain fibrous or edematous stroma. Serous borderline cystadenofibromas are firm, white, fibromatous tumors with a cystic component of variable size. In almost 50% of SBTs the papillary growth covers the outer surface of the ovary (serous surface papillary borderline tumor).[28] Frequently, both exophytic and endophytic papillary components are present (Figure 25.7). The typical gross features of serous carcinomas, such as friability, hemorrhage, and necrosis, are not seen in SBTs.

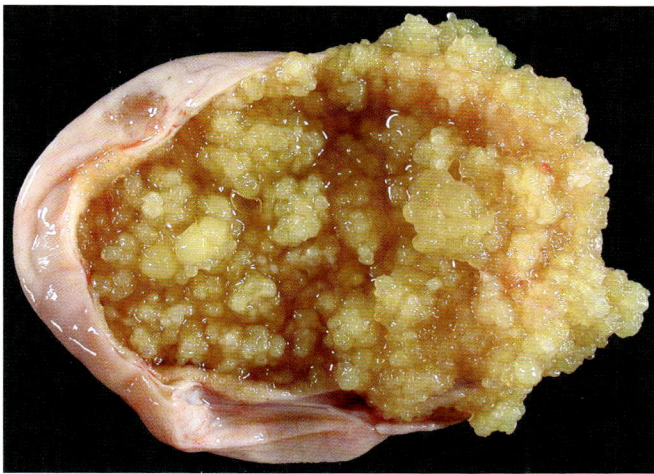

Figure 25.6 Serous borderline tumor. Intracystic growth of soft papillary excrescences. (Courtesy of Dr. Jeronimo Forteza, Santiago, Spain.)

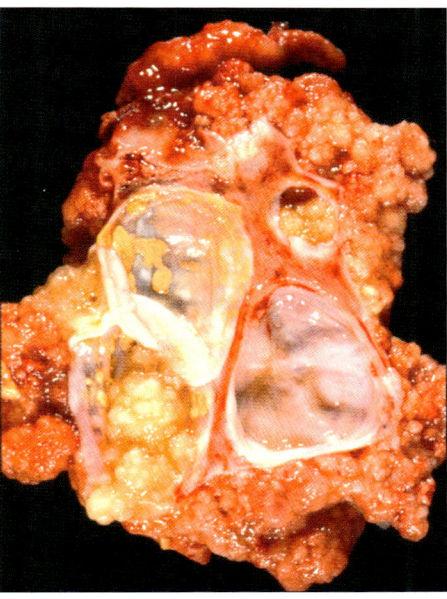

Figure 25.7 Serous borderline tumor. The external surface is covered by confluent polypoid excrescences and closely packed small papillae (exophytic growth). The sectioned surface shows a solid and cystic tumor with intracystic papillary growth.

Microscopic Features

SBTs show stromal polypoid excrescences, glands, and papillae lined by stratified cuboidal to columnar epithelial cells and ciliated cells resembling those of the fallopian tube (Figures 25.8–25.11). Larger hobnail cells with ample eosinophilic cytoplasm (Figure 25.12) and mesothelial-like cells may also be present. Eosinophilic cells are increased when microinvasion has occurred. The lining epithelial cells show mild to moderate nuclear atypia (rarely severe) and mitoses are rare; therefore, the histologic pattern usually differs from that of carcinoma *in situ* of other organs. Psammoma bodies are found in about one-fourth of cases. The three most important diagnostic features are (1) arborizing papillae that form increasingly smaller branches

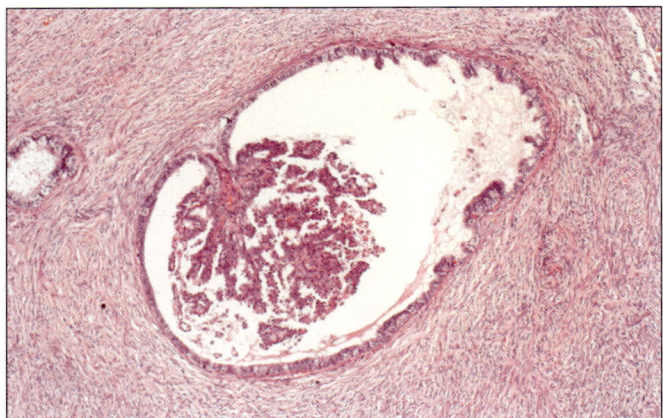

Figure 25.8 Small serous borderline tumor arising within a surface epithelial inclusion cyst.

ending in clusters of epithelial cells that appear to be detached from the stroma (hierarchical pattern of branching), (2) varying degree of nuclear atypia, and (3) absence of 'frank' stromal invasion or solid sheets of tumor with a cribriform pattern.[1]

Several changes within SBTs may result in overdiagnosis of carcinoma. The pathologist's main problems while dealing with SBTs are listed below.

- Pseudoinvasion
- Self-implantation
- Mesothelial cell hyperplasia
- Micropapillary pattern
- Microinvasion
- Peritoneal implants
- SBT in lymph nodes
- SBT of the peritoneum.

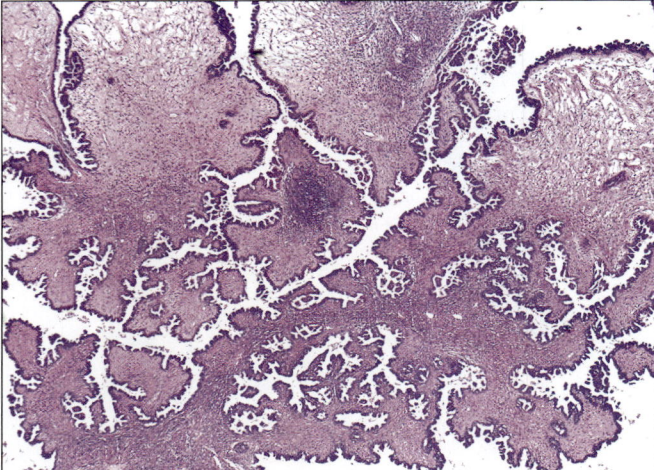

Figure 25.9 Serous borderline tumor, typical pattern. The epithelial papillae show hierarchical and complex branching without stromal invasion. Some papillae have fibroedematous stalks.

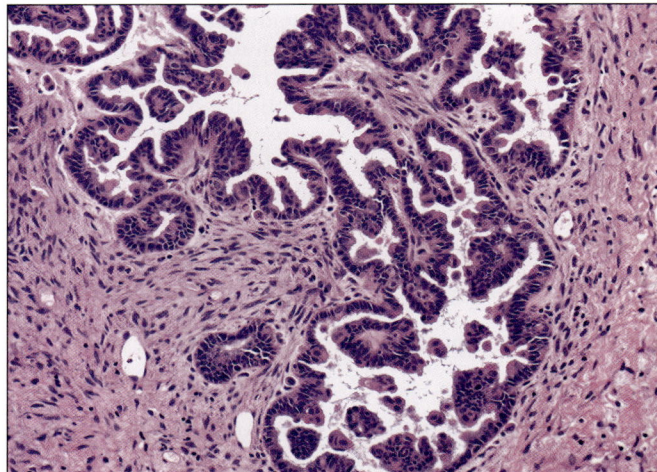

Figure 25.11 Serous borderline tumor, typical pattern. The papillae are lined by stratified cuboidal-to-columnar epithelial cells with hyperchromatic slightly atypical nuclei.

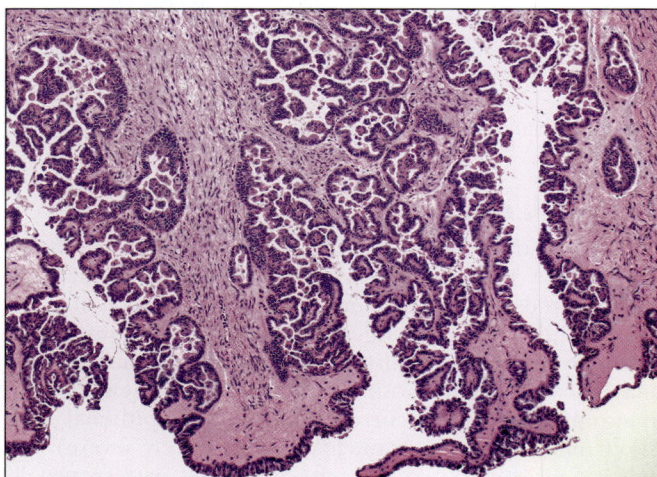

Figure 25.10 Serous borderline tumor, typical pattern. Orderly penetration of the stroma by glands and microcysts with papillae, without stromal reaction. Detachment of small cell nests from the stratified lining epithelium.

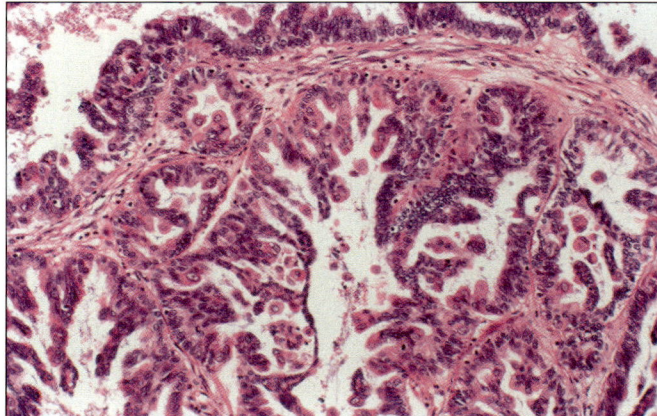

Figure 25.12 Serous borderline tumor. The lining cells are stratified with cellular budding and show moderate atypia. Larger hobnail cells with abundant eosinophilic cytoplasm are seen.

PSEUDOINVASION, AUTOIMPLANTS, AND MESOTHELIAL CELL HYPERPLASIA

Serous borderline tumors often show a relatively complex proliferation of glands and papillae (Figure 25.10). The glands often invaginate into the stroma and, particularly when sectioned tangentially, may appear as if they have invaded the stroma. This *pseudoinvasion* differs, however, from the destructive stromal invasion of a carcinoma. The stroma about the pseudoinvasion is similar to the stroma elsewhere and the glands have an orderly distribution. In carcinoma, it forms a desmoplastic stroma typically and the neoplastic glands have a more disorderly arrangement. Exceptionally, an SBT implants on itself and may exhibit focal desmoplastic stroma. *Autoimplants* are sharply circumscribed desmoplastic plaques usually on the outer surface but occasionally on the inner (cystic) surface of the tumor, resembling noninvasive desmoplastic implants on extraovarian peritoneum (Figure 25.13).[29] Although the term *autoimplant* suggests that this lesion might arise by detachment of exophytic SBT and subsequent reattachment to itself, occurrence of this phenomenon has not been confirmed. Autoimplants seem to lack clinical significance. Sometimes, SBTs are partly covered by fibrous adhesions associated with *mesothelial hyperplasia*, which may be erroneously interpreted as surface borderline tumor or even carcinoma. The mesothelial cells, however, lack nuclear atypia and are typically arranged in a linear fashion (Figure 25.14).

MICROPAPILLARY PATTERN

Rarely, SBTs show an exuberant micropapillary (or focal cribriform) proliferation without destructive stromal invasion (Figure 25.15).[19] There is a filigree pattern of highly complex micropapillae growing in a nonhierarchical fashion from fibrous stalks (Figure 25.16) composed of stratified nonciliated cuboidal cells with high nuclear to cytoplasmic ratio. Nuclear atypia is only mild with occasional higher grade nuclei present (Figure 25.17). Mitotic figures are rare and no abnormal forms are seen.[30] In contrast to the typical SBT, which usually shows variable degrees of cell proliferation and nuclear atypia, the micropapillary or cribriform SBT (Figure 25.18) exhibits a homogeneous and marked degree of cell proliferation and uniform mild nuclear atypia

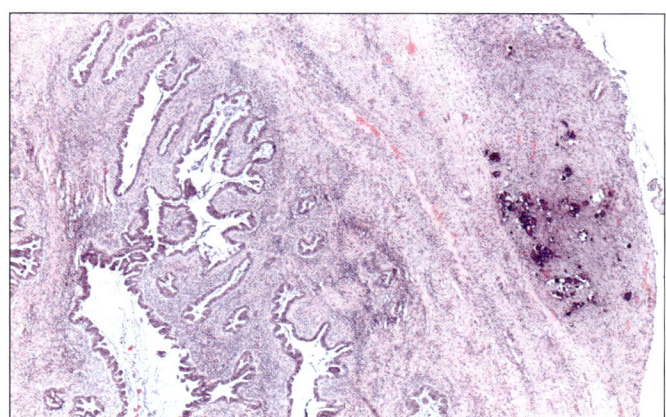

Figure 25.13 Serous borderline tumor with autoimplantation. The upper right corner of the figure shows desmoplastic tissue with numerous psammoma bodies creating an image similar to that of a desmoplastic peritoneal implant. Note the sharp demarcation with the ovarian stroma.

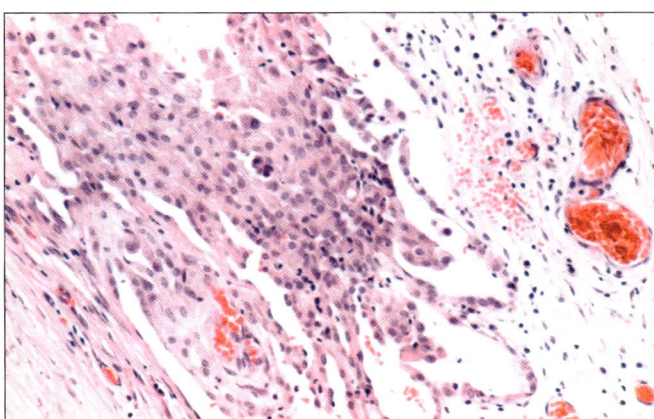

Figure 25.14 Mesothelial hyperplasia on the surface of an seous borderline tumor. The mesothelial cells lack nuclear atypia and are typically arranged in a linear fashion.

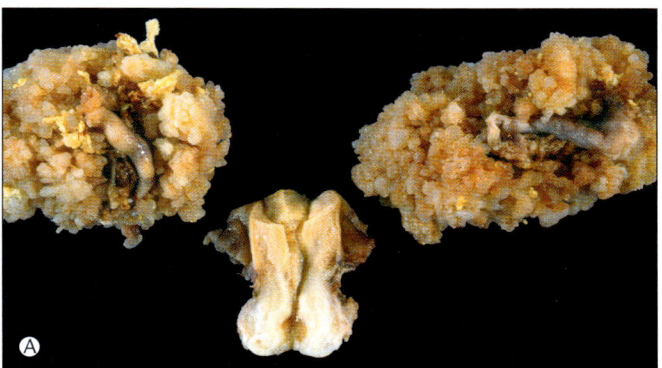

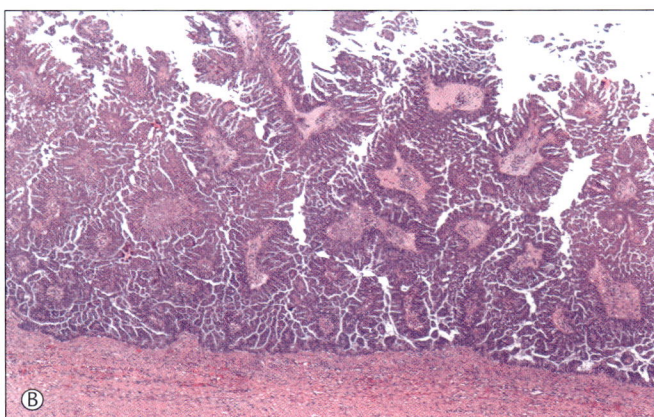

Figure 25.15 **(A)** Bilateral serous borderline tumor (SBT) with micropapillary proliferation. Both tumors show prominent exophytic papillary growth.[19] (Reproduced with permission of Lippincott Williams & Wilkins.) **(B)** SBT with micropapillary pattern. The highly complex micropapillae grow in a nonhierarchical fashion from fibrovascular stalks. Stromal invasion is not present.

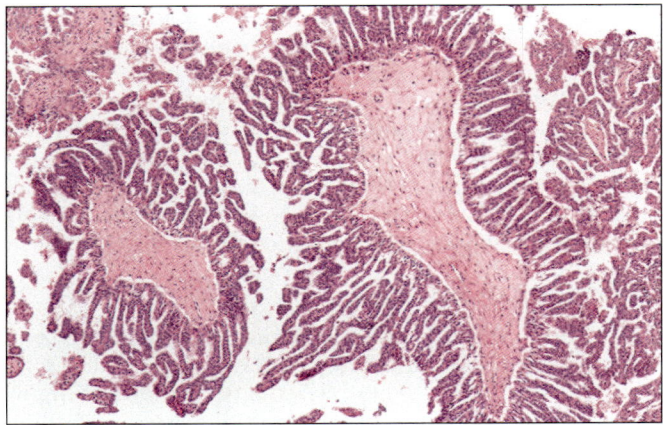

Figure 25.16 Serous borderline tumor with micropapillary pattern ('Medusa head-like appearance'). Filigree network of small micropapillae, at least five times as long as wide, arising directly from papillary stalks.

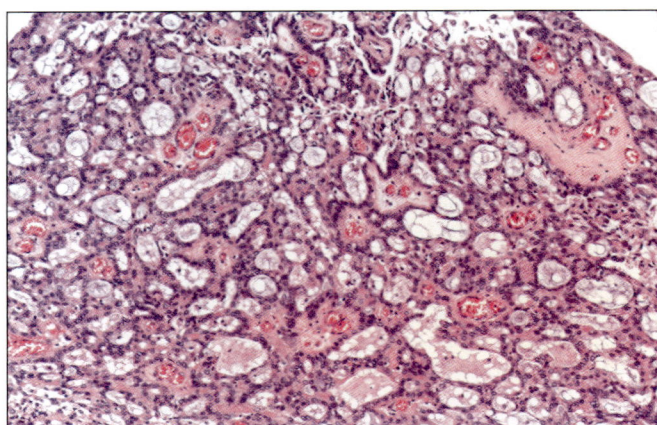

Figure 25.18 Serous borderline tumor with cribriform architecture.

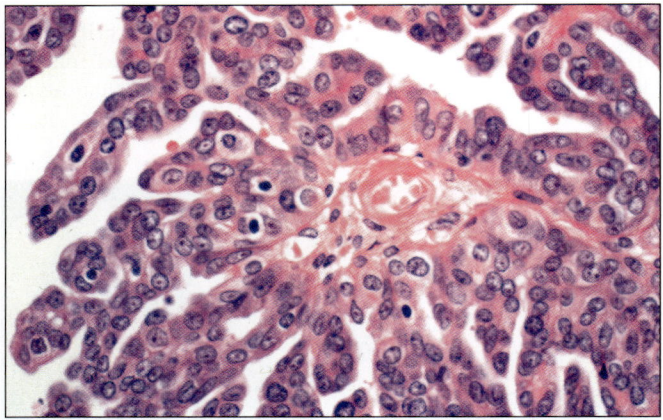

Figure 25.17 Serous borderline tumor with micropapillary pattern. Nuclear atypia is uniform and only moderate (grade 2).

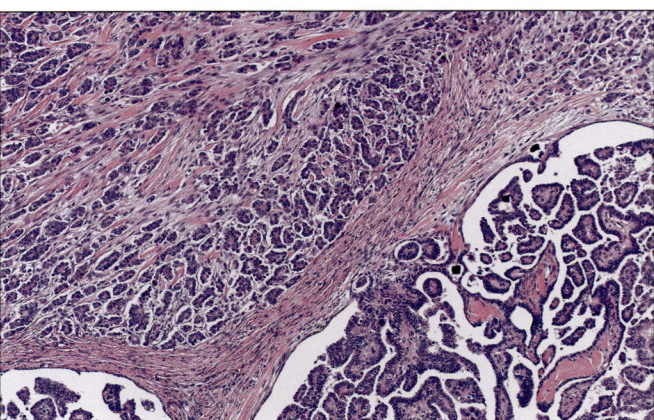

Figure 25.19 Low-grade serous micropapillary carcinoma (upper left) adjacent to serous borderline tumor with micropapillary pattern (lower right). Note the presence of destructive stromal invasion (larger than 10 mm^2).

(Figure 25.17). Most micropapillary tumors contain areas of typical SBT, indicating the former's probable origin.[30] When the micropapillary architecture exceeds 5 mm in greatest dimension, it has been recommended to segregate these tumors from the less proliferative SBTs, claiming that they are likely to progress to invasive carcinoma, particularly as invasive peritoneal implants.[30] Subsequently, it was required that the 'micropapillae' should be five times as long as wide (Figure 25.16).[31]

It has been shown that bilaterality, ovarian surface growth, and advanced stage (noninvasive implants) are more common features of micropapillary SBTs than of typical SBTs, but a strong association of the former tumors with invasive implants and poor outcome has been inconsistent. Although in four studies[21,31–33] micropapillary SBTs were more frequently associated with invasive implants, micropapillary architecture did not have a significant adverse effect on survival when controlled for implant type. Stage II–III micropapillary SBTs with noninvasive peritoneal implants had the same favorable prognosis as typical SBTs (Table 25.1);[16,19,21,30–34] thus, from a prognostic viewpoint, micropapillary SBTs are closer to typical SBTs than to carcinomas. However, although largely noninvasive, serous tumors with prominent micropapillary architecture may contain areas of frank stromal invasion (Figure 25.19); therefore, extensive sampling is indicated in these cases.

The micropapillary pattern (Figures 25.16 and 25.17), almost always associated with typical SBT, most likely represents a degree of epithelial proliferation intermediate between SBT and LGSCs. By analogy with cervical neoplasia, the difference between typical SBT and micropapillary SBT is like between cervical intraepithelial neoplasia (CIN) 2 and CIN 3. Although the micropapillary pattern in combination with other clinical and pathologic features (i.e., advanced stage, invasive implants, and microinvasion) may be associated with increased risk of disease progression, taken individually, micropapillarity is not a specific predictor of adverse prognosis.[21,33,34] Almost all patients dying of recurrent tumor had invasive peritoneal implants, which are the key feature associated with a poor prognosis.

Table 25.1 Literature Comparison: Advanced Stage Serous Borderline Tumors with Micropapillary Pattern[16,19,21,30–34]

	Burks et al.[30]	Seidman and Kurman[16]	Eichhorn et al.[31]	Prat and de Nictolis[19]	Longacre et al.[21]	Park et al.[33]	Avril et al.[34]
Total cases	10	11	19	13	23	33	2
Cases with invasive implants	6[b]	10[b]	3	1	5	5	0
Chemotherapy[a]	8/10 (80%)	5/9 (56%)	5/17 (29%)	9/12 (75%)	—	10/33 (30%)	1
5 year follow-up	5	10	10	9	23	—	2
Alive, no tumor	0	3	6	8	17	29	2
Alive, recurrent tumor in contralateral oophorectomy	0	0	2	1	0	3	0
Alive, progressive residual/recurrent tumor	2[b]	3[b]	0	1[c]	0	0	0
Died of tumor	2	4	2	0	5	1	0
Died of unrelated causes	1	0	0	0	1	0	0
Follow-up <5 years	5	1	5	3	0	—	0
Lost to follow-up	0	0	3	1	0	0	0
Recent cases	0	0	1	0	0	0	0

[a]Number of patients/number of patients with postoperative treatment information (%).
[b]Including 'implants with micropapillary' pattern but without recognizable invasion of underlying tissue.
[c]Patient died of tumor subsequent to her report.

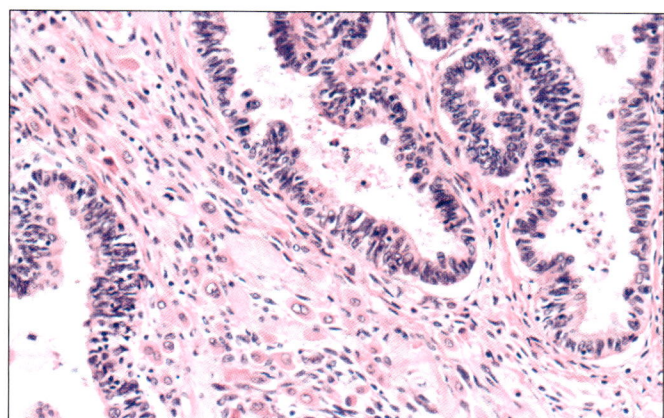

Figure 25.20 Serous borderline tumor with microinvasion. Stromal microinvasion by single epithelial cells and small clusters of such cells with abundant eosinophilic cytoplasm.

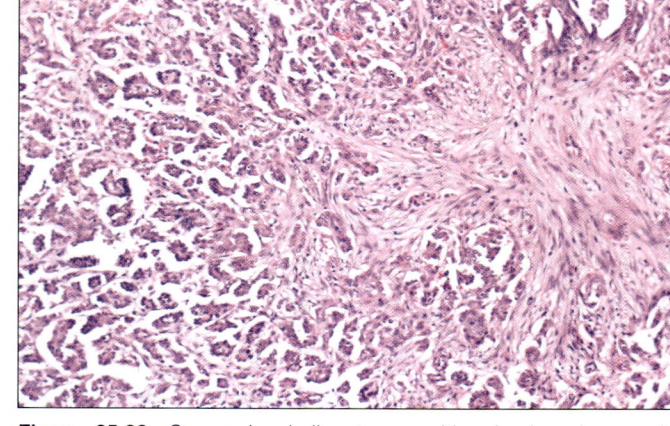

Figure 25.22 Serous borderline tumor with microinvasive carcinoma (2 mm). Destructive invasion of the stroma by malignant-appearing cells and desmoplastic response.

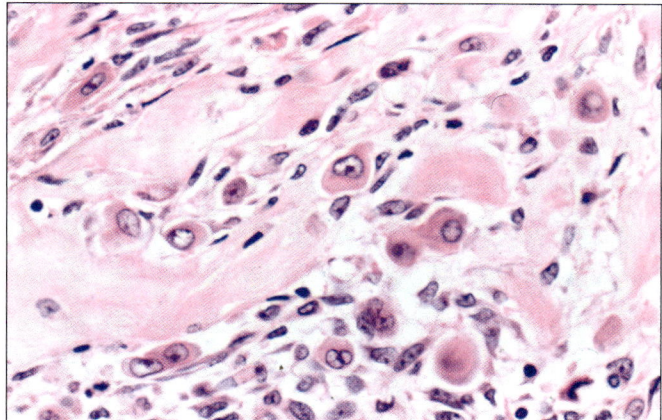

Figure 25.21 Serous borderline tumor with microinvasion. The invasive cells show ample eosinophilic cytoplasm and vesicular nuclei with prominent nucleoli.

MICROINVASION

Approximately 10% of otherwise typical SBTs contain one or more discrete foci of stromal microinvasion,[15,19,21,35–38] which are made up of single epithelial cells or small clusters of such cells with abundant eosinophilic cytoplasm (Figures 25.20 and 25.21). Often, the cell nests appear surrounded by clefts that separate the epithelium from the stroma (Figures 25.22 and 25.23). These microscopic foci (arbitrarily defined as not exceeding 10 mm^2 in area, or 3 mm maximum linear dimension) are typically unassociated with a significant stromal reaction and are easily overlooked on routinely stained sections.[1] Cytokeratin (CK) stains help to visualize the invasive epithelial cells (Figure 25.24). Occasionally, foci of lymphatic invasion may be present.[36] Several patients with these tumors have been pregnant at the time of diagnosis.[38]

Table 25.2 Literature Comparison: Serous Borderline Tumors with Microinvasion[15,19,35–38]

	Tavassoli[35]	Bell and Scully[36]	Nayar et al.[37]	Kennedy and Hart[15]	Prat and de Nictolis[19]	McKenney et al.[38]
Total cases	18	21	7	4	20	60
Advanced stage	6	2	—	1	9	26
Invasive implants/distant metastasis	1	1	0	0	1	2
Lymph node metastasis	1	1	0	0	2	7
Chemotherapy	4	3	—	3	4	9
Radiotherapy	1	0	—	0	1	4
5 year follow-up (or until death)	5	—	6	3	11	—
Alive, no tumor	4	—	6	3	9	41
Alive, progressive residual/recurrent tumor	0	1	0	0	1	2
Died of tumor	1	0	0	0	1*	7
Follow-up <5 years	13	—	1	1	5	—
Lost to follow-up	0	4	0	0	4	10

*Incomplete surgical staging.

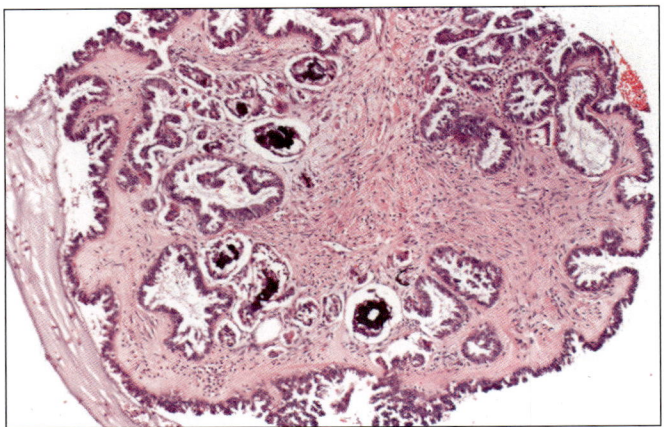

Figure 25.23 Serous borderline tumor with microinvasion. The stroma contains numerous small papillae and clusters of tumor cells surrounded by clefts.

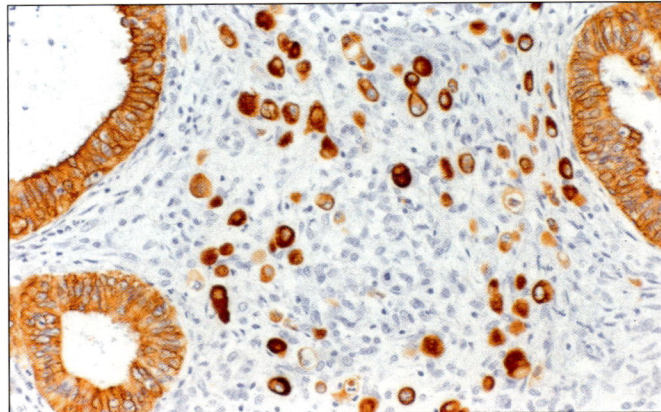

Figure 25.24 Serous borderline tumor with microinvasion. The invasive cells show a strong cytokeratin immunoreaction.

SBTs with microinvasion are associated with a higher frequency of bilaterality, exophytic ovarian surface growth, and advanced stage than typical SBTs lacking microinvasion, yet the rate of invasive implants is similar in both tumor groups.[19] At least five studies[15,19,35–37] (Table 25.2)[15,19,35–38] have confirmed that SBTs with or without microinvasion have a similar prognosis. However, two recent reports[21,38] suggested that microinvasion may represent a risk factor for disease progression that is independent of stage and implant status. SBTs with microinvasion (Figures 25.20 and 25.21) should be distinguished from SBTs with *microinvasive carcinoma*. The latter shows 'destructive' invasion of the stroma by malignant-appearing cells and desmoplastic response (Figure 25.22).[39] The lesion resembles an invasive peritoneal implant or LGSC. Lymphatic invasion is common and can be demonstrated by D2-40 immunoreaction.[40]

Immunohistochemistry

SBTs show positive immunoreaction for CK7, epithelial membrane antigen (EMA), and OC-125. WT1 is weakly positive. Some cases show focal positivity for CK20. Most cases express estrogen and progesterone receptors (ERs/PRs). p53 is usually negative but can be focally positive; however, focal nuclear reaction for p53 does not correlate with *TP53* mutations.[41]

PERITONEAL IMPLANTS

One controversial aspect of SBTs is their association in ~30–40% of cases with peritoneal implants.[14–21] Implants are found more frequently in patients with tumors that have an exophytic component than in those that do not.[28] They rarely present as bulky disease (Figure 25.25), and, in most cases, are either microscopic or small macroscopic (≤1–2 cm) lesions. Their histologic appearance may vary greatly, ranging from foci of benign glandular epithelium resembling endosalpingiosis, to noninvasive papillae, plaques, or nodules of borderline epithelium and stroma, to invasive implants resembling an LGSC.[14] Endosalpingiosis, typified by glands, cysts, and occasionally papillae with psammoma bodies, is a benign peritoneal lesion frequently associated with ovarian SBTs (Figure 25.26). It may rarely be the substrate for the development of peritoneal SBTs or carcinomas, but its presence should not change the stage of a synchronous ovarian SBT.

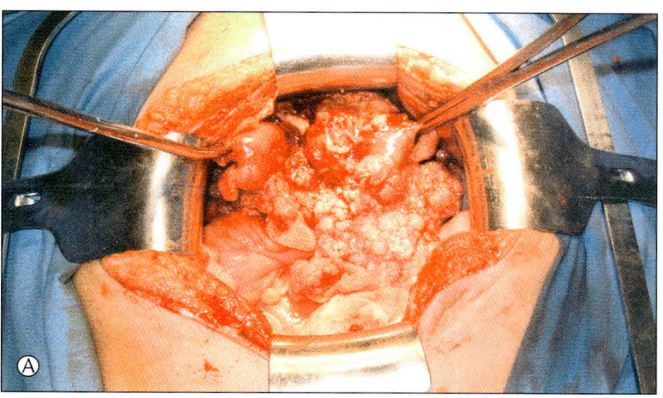 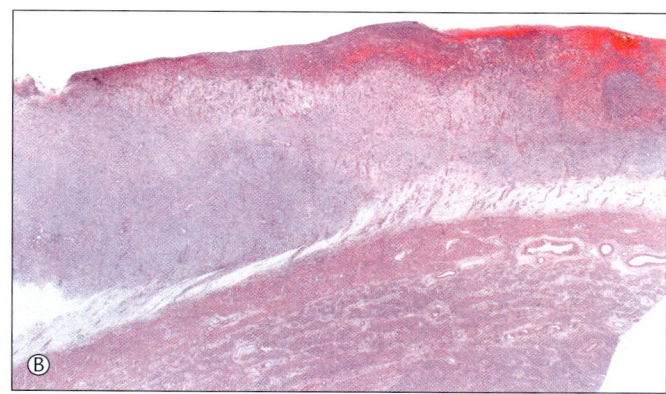
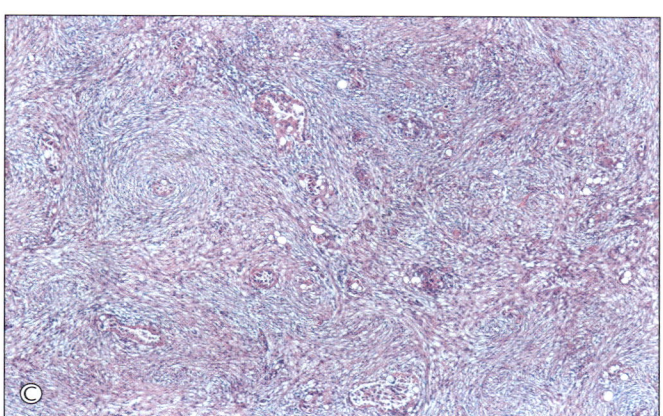 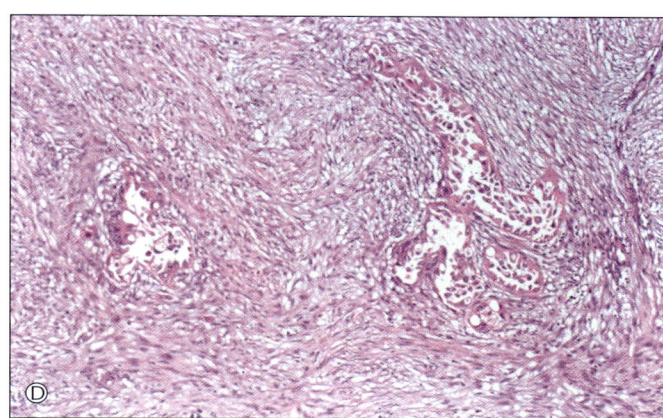

Figure 25.25 **(A)** Serous borderline tumor (SBT) with noninvasive implants. At laparotomy, the uterus was covered by a soft grayish white and hemorrhagic mass (400 g). (Courtesy of Dr. Isidre Boguna, Barcelona, Spain.) **(B)** Noninvasive desmoplastic implant of SBT. The implant appears plastered upon the uterine serosa without invading the underlying myometrium. The surface of the implant shows hemorrhage and necrosis. **(C)** Noninvasive desmoplastic implant of SBT. The implant is largely composed of a fibroblastic proliferation which surpasses quantitatively the glandular epithelial component. **(D)** Noninvasive desmoplastic implant of SBT. Two epithelial glands containing hobnail cells with moderately atypical nuclei are surrounded by dense fibroblastic stroma.

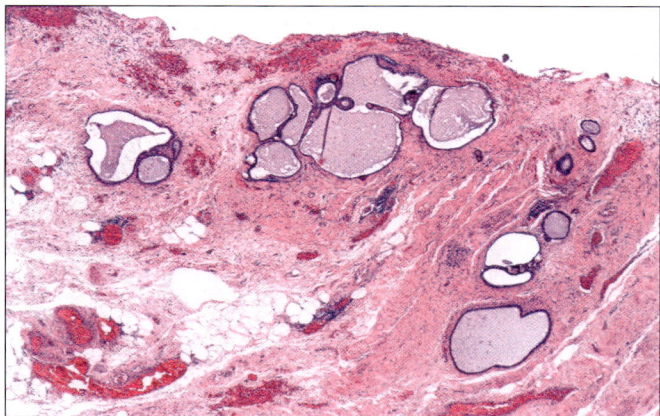

Figure 25.26 Endosalpingiosis. Glands lined by flattened tubal-like epithelium lay in the parametrium.

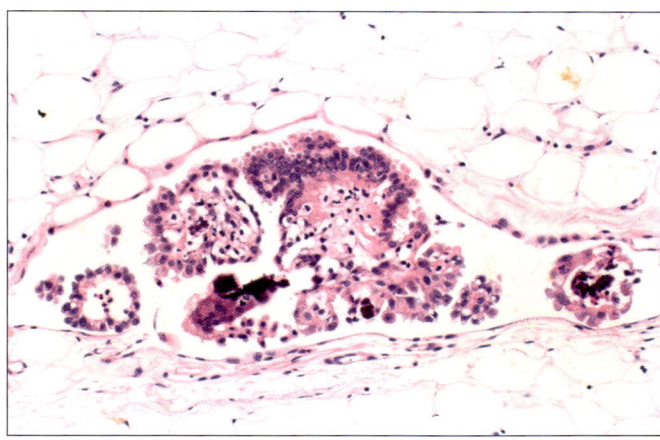

Figure 25.27 Noninvasive epithelial implant of serous borderline tumor within a smoothly contoured invagination of the omental fat. The epithelial proliferation contains calcifications and resembles that of the primary ovarian tumor.

The peritoneal implants of SBTs have been classified histologically into *noninvasive* and *invasive* types with the former further subdivided into *epithelial* and *desmoplastic* subtypes.[14] The *epithelial* subtype of noninvasive implants shows papillary proliferations of atypical epithelial cells resembling those of the ovarian SBT (Figure 25.27); they are typically present on the surface of the peritoneum (Figure 25.28)[19] or in smoothly contoured subperitoneal invaginations and exhibit little or no stromal reaction.[14] In contrast, the *desmoplastic* subtype of noninvasive implant is largely composed

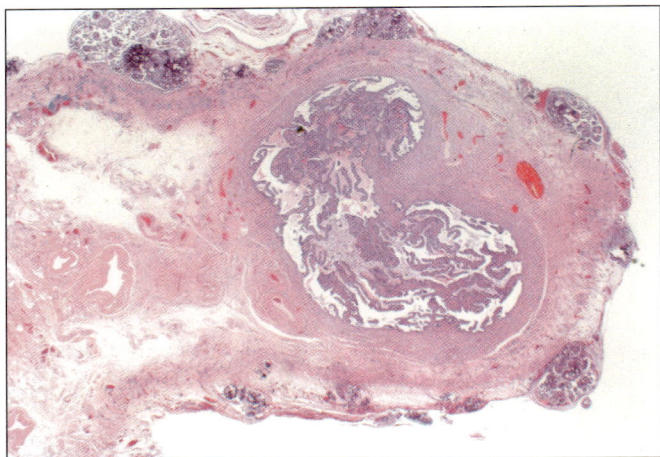

Figure 25.28 Numerous noninvasive epithelial implants of serous borderline tumor on the serosa of the fallopian tube.[19] (Reproduced with permission of Lippincott Williams & Wilkins.)

of a stromal proliferation, which is plastered upon serosal surfaces or invaginations between lobules of omental fat (Figures 25.25B–D, 25.29,[13] and 25.30[43]). The stromal reaction surpasses quantitatively the epithelial component of the implant. In late lesions, small glands and papillae lined by atypical serous cells as well as psammoma bodies are entrapped by dense fibroblastic tissue that is often infiltrated by acute and chronic inflammatory cells. Early implants show necrosis with surface fibrin deposition and hemorrhage (Figure 25.30[34]).[14] *Invasive* implants, which represent approximately 12% of the cases,[14,19–21,31] manifest a disorderly infiltration of normal tissues, such as the omentum; in contrast to the well-defined limits of the desmoplastic implants, the invasive implants exhibit irregular borders (Figure 25.31). They usually show a greater epithelial cell population (Figure 25.32[19]) and resemble histologically a low-grade serous adenocarcinoma (Figure 25.33[42]); marked cytologic atypia may be present.[14] Implants should be sampled extensively since noninvasive and

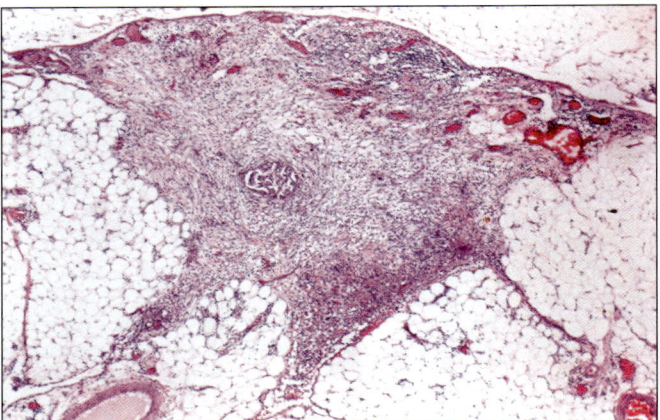

Figure 25.29 Noninvasive desmoplastic implant of serous borderline tumor. The implant invaginates between adjacent lobules of omental fat. Scattered nests of tumor cells are present within a loose fibroblastic stroma.[13] (Reproduced with permission of Lippincott Williams & Wilkins.)

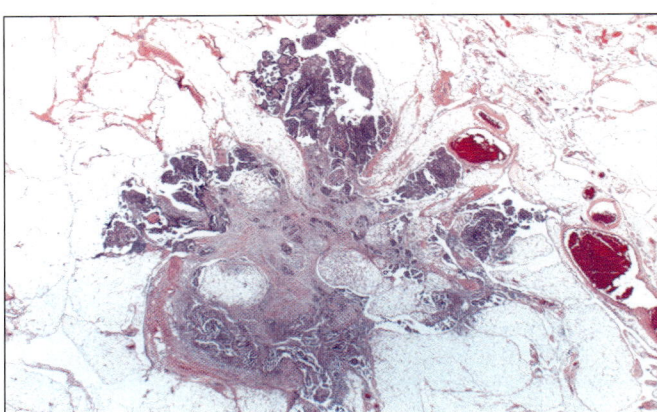

Figure 25.31 Invasive omental implant of serous borderline tumor. The implant is composed predominantly of epithelial cells which invade the adipose tissue in an irregular fashion.

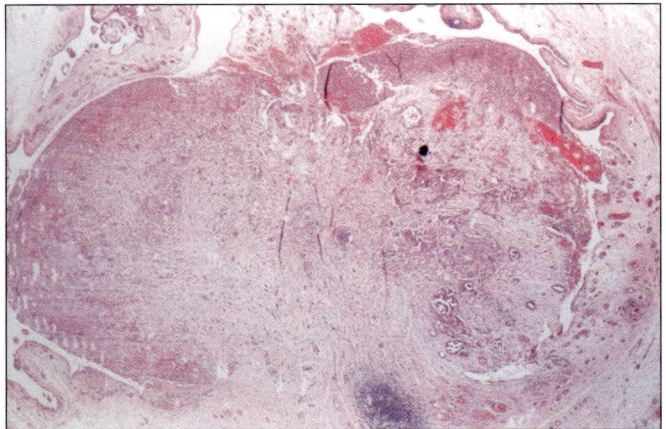

Figure 25.30 Noninvasive desmoplastic implant of serous borderline tumor. The sharply circumscribed nodule is composed predominantly of granulation tissue-like stroma and contains only scattered nests of tumor cells. Foci of hemorrhage and necrosis are seen at the periphery.[42] (Reproduced with permission of Lippincott Williams & Wilkins.)

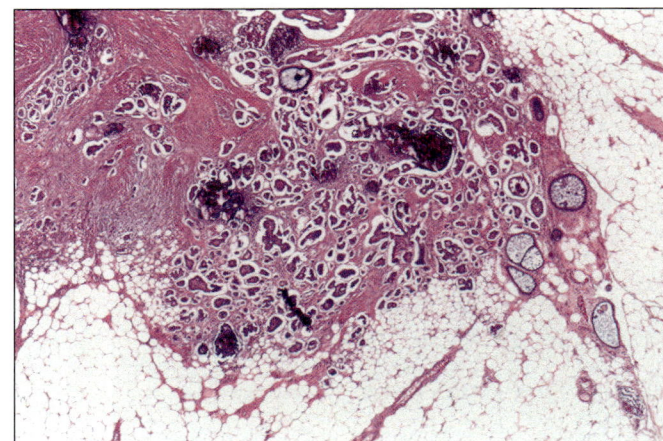

Figure 25.32 Invasive omental implant of serous borderline tumor. The tumor glands and papillae appear disorderly distributed within a desmoplastic ('collagenized') stroma and many of them are surrounded by clefts.[19] (Reproduced with permission of Lippincott Williams & Wilkins.)

invasive implants may coexist. Also, some implants of serous carcinomas may be noninvasive and simulate the desmoplastic noninvasive implants of SBTs. The former implants, however, usually contain highly atypical epithelial cells.

At least 11 studies of SBTs with peritoneal implants (Table 25.3)[14–19,21,31,33,34,42–44] have clearly demonstrated that separation of the implants into invasive and noninvasive subtypes carries important prognostic implications. The rare tumors that were fatal were mostly those with invasive peritoneal implants.

Despite the poor prognosis associated with invasive implants when they actually invade the underlying tissues, their diagnostic criteria remain problematic. Truly invasive implants are rare lesions; i.e., from a population exceeding 3 million people, only six patients with stage III SBTs with invasive implants were encountered during a 17 year period.[20] Some investigators, however, have reported higher rates of invasive implants (up to 35% in one series) but a lack of correlation between their presence and adverse prognosis.[17] Such a discrepancy could be explained by the inclusion of desmoplastic noninvasive implants in the category of invasive implants.

Although the use of more liberal histologic criteria (i.e., solid epithelial nests surrounded by clefts and micropapillary architecture) increased the proportion of invasive implants in a recently reported series to more than 50%,[44] association with death due to progressive disease was less significant than by three other groups using more stringent diagnostic rules.[19,20,31] In fact, one of the latter studies confirmed that solid epithelial nests surrounded by clefts and micropapillary architecture are found more often in invasive than noninvasive implants;[19] in that series, obvious destructive invasion was the only feature of the peritoneal implants specifically associated with poor outcome.[19] As stated earlier, the presence of epithelial cell clusters surrounded by clefts or halos is a characteristic feature of stromal microinvasion (which is associated with a favorable prognosis; Figure 25.23). In contrast, an abundant epithelial component (Figures 25.31 and 25.32[19]), whether micropapillary or not, favors the diagnosis of invasion. Noninvasive desmoplastic implants typically contain an excess of granulation tissue-like stroma and minimal epithelial component in the form of small cellular nests or glands (Figures 25.25B–D, 25.29,[13] and 25.30[42]).[14] The finding of single isolated cells in the stroma is not enough histologic evidence to diagnose the implant as invasive; such isolated cells can also be found in approximately one-third of the noninvasive desmoplastic implants.[44]

The characteristic features of noninvasive epithelial implants, noninvasive desmoplastic implants, and invasive implants can be summarized as follows.

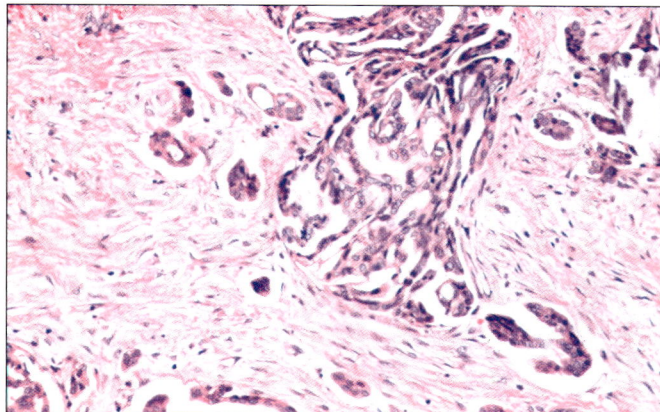

Figure 25.33 Invasive omental implant of serous borderline tumor. The tumor resembles an LGSC. The intervening stroma appears desmoplastic.[42] (Reproduced with permission of Lippincott Williams & Wilkins.)

Table 25.3 Death from Tumor among Patients with Ovarian Serous Borderline Tumors Associated with Peritoneal Implants (Literature Review, 1984–2011)[14–19,21,31,33,34,42–44]

	Noninvasive Implants	Invasive Implants
McCaughey et al.[43]	2/13	4/5
Bell DA et al.[14]	3/50	5/6[a]
de Nictolis et al.[42]	0/10	4/9
Kennedy and Hart[15]	1/25[b]	0/1[c]
Seidman and Kurman[16]	1/51	2/3
Gershenson et al.[17,18]	6/73	6/39
Eichhorn et al.[31]	0/30	2/3
Bell KA et al.[44]	2/29[d]	6/31[e]
Prat and de Nictolis.[19]	0/34	3/6[f]
Longacre et al.[21]	2/85	5/14[g]
Park et al.[33]	0/14	1/5
Avril et al.[34]	0/8	0/0
Total	17/422	38/122

[a] One patient died of tumor subsequent to her report.
[b] Transformation into serous carcinoma.
[c] Follow-up 23 months.
[d] One patient was alive with progressive disease (AWPD).
[e] Thirteen patients were AWPD.
[f] The other three patients were AWPD.
[g] One patient was AWPD and one died of leukemia but had persistent tumor.

Noninvasive Epithelial Implants

- Papillary proliferations resembling ovarian SBT
- On peritoneal surface or in smoothly contoured invaginations
- Well-defined margins
- Little or no stromal reaction
- Psammoma bodies

Noninvasive Desmoplastic Implants

- Stromal proliferation plastered on serosal surfaces or between lobules of omental fat
- Well-defined margins
- Excess of granulation tissue-like stroma (>50%) and minimal epithelial component
- Hemorrhage, necrosis (early changes), fibrosis, and calcification (late changes)

Invasive Implants

- Disorderly distributed glands destructively invading normal tissue
- Poorly defined irregular margins

- Abundant epithelial component
- Dense collagenous stroma without significant inflammation
- Resemble LGSCs
- Aneuploidy

Because the ovarian and peritoneal lesions found in stage II–III SBTs may have various histologic appearances, and as the extraovarian peritoneal mesothelium has the potential to give rise to müllerian epithelial lesions, i.e., endosalpingiosis and serous neoplasms, some investigators have postulated that some of the peritoneal implants associated with ovarian SBTs represent independent foci of primary peritoneal neoplasia rather than true implants.[45] Others, however, favor the 'implantation' explanation based on the fact that two-thirds of SBTs with an exophytic component are associated with implants (in contrast to less than 5% of those that are exclusively endophytic).[28]

Immunohistochemical studies have shown that invasive implants show loss of calretinin-positive mesothelial cells and CD34-positive fibroblasts, which are preserved in noninvasive implants. Smooth muscle actin-positive myofibroblasts are present in both invasive and noninvasive implants.[46]

Somatic Genetics

Recent molecular genetic studies indicate that SBTs and HGSCs represent separate pathogenetic entities. SBTs with and without micropapillary pattern frequently display B-RAF/K-RAS mutations but rarely mutant TP53. In contrast, B-RAF/K-RAS mutations are rare in HGSCs, but TP53 mutations occur in approximately 60% of cases (see later).[47,48] B-RAF/K-RAS mutations also occur in the epithelium of cystadenomas adjacent to SBTs, suggesting that they precede the development of the latter tumors.[49] K-RAS mutations are also present in the glandular inclusions (endosalpingiosis) in the peritoneum and lymph nodes of patients with ovarian SBT.[50] RNA expression profiles of ovarian serous tumors have disclosed that the mitogenic MAP kinase pathway is activated in SBTs; however, activation of downstream genes involved in extracellular matrix degradation is absent, suggesting an uncoupling of both events.[51] Gene expression profiling has also shown prominent expression of wild p53, cyclin-dependent kinase inhibitor p21, and other p53-modulated genes in SBTs, suggesting that this signaling pathway may play an important role in the distinct phenotype associated with this tumor.[52] Although the profiles for invasive LGSCs did not contain the enhanced p53 signaling activity observed in SBTs, the former tumors were aligned with the SBTs instead of HGSCs.[52] These findings provide additional proof that typical SBTs, SBTs with micropapillary pattern, and invasive LGSCs are closely related neoplasms and different from usual HGSCs. The rare invasive LGSCs with micropapillary pattern (Figure 25.19; which also have B-RAF/K-RAS mutations) probably represent SBTs with infiltrative stromal invasion greater than microinvasion.

Clonality studies have examined whether multiple, synchronous, or metachronous SBTs (found at different sites in the abdominal cavity) arise as a result of spread from a single ovarian site, or whether such deposits are polyclonal representing independent primary tumors. Two studies based on X chromosome inactivation analysis support a multifocal origin of bilateral and advanced SBTs.[53,54] However, tumor-related changes may interfere with X chromosome inactivation and this method poorly assesses clonality. In contrast, loss of heterozygosity (LOH) is an irreversible genetic event acquired during tumorigenesis. Its weakness, however, is that the absence of informative markers and the failure to detect LOH underestimates the frequency of clonality.

Recently, clonality of invasive and noninvasive peritoneal implants and lymph node deposits has been investigated by genome-wide allelotyping and B-RAF/K-RAS mutation analysis in 10 patients using 23 microsatellite markers. Concordant LOH for 1–5 microsatellite markers was found in all five informative cases in all tumor sites. In addition, identical K-RAS and B-RAF mutations were detected in four and two cases, respectively (Figure 25.34[55]). These findings strongly support the metastatic nature of noninvasive and invasive peritoneal implants and lymph node deposits.

Histogenesis

Ovarian SBTs have traditionally been thought to arise from the ovarian surface epithelium (mesothelium), from the müllerian epithelium within the ovary (surface epithelial inclusion cysts), or from endosalpingiosis. Recently, however, and based on the more frequent finding of papillary tubal hyperplasia[56] and secretory cell outgrowths lacking PAX2 expression[57] in the fallopian tubes of patients with SBTs compared to controls, a direct origin from the tubal epithelium with secondary ovarian involvement has been suggested.

Differential Diagnosis

SBTs are only rarely confused with other neoplasms. Their distinction from LGSCs has already been discussed. SBTs differ from endocervical-like (müllerian) mucinous borderline tumors by the lack of both intracellular mucin and a neutrophilic infiltrate (see later). SBTs may also occur as a component of mixed müllerian borderline tumors. Retiform Sertoli–Leydig cell tumors (Chapter 28) can have areas indistinguishable from SBTs on routine staining, but occur in a younger age group, have other distinctive features such as long ribbons of sex cord-type cells, and other patterns of Sertoli–Leydig cell tumors. These tumors, like most sex cord tumors, are often reactive for α-inhibin.

Biologic Behavior

The overall outcome of SBTs is extremely favorable. For patients with stage I tumors, the risk of recurrence or the development of a second SBT has been estimated to be only 5–10%.[15,19,21] The tumors rarely recur beyond 10 years.

Most SBTs maintain their microscopic features and indolent clinical behavior, and usually do not progress over the years to frankly invasive carcinoma.[15] However, rare cases of late recurrence in the form of carcinoma have been described.[58] In a more recent study, progression of SBT to LGSC occurred in 6–7% of patients late in the course of the disease and was associated with poor prognosis. Almost 80% occurred in patients without prior history of invasive implants.[21] Of eight cases of SBT with malignant behavior, all had ovarian surface involvement, three exhibited focal stromal invasion greater than microinvasion, and only two were SBT with micropapillary pattern.[59] Although exceptional, malignant transformation of SBT to HGSC may also occur early[60] or following multiple recurrences[19] (Figure 25.35).

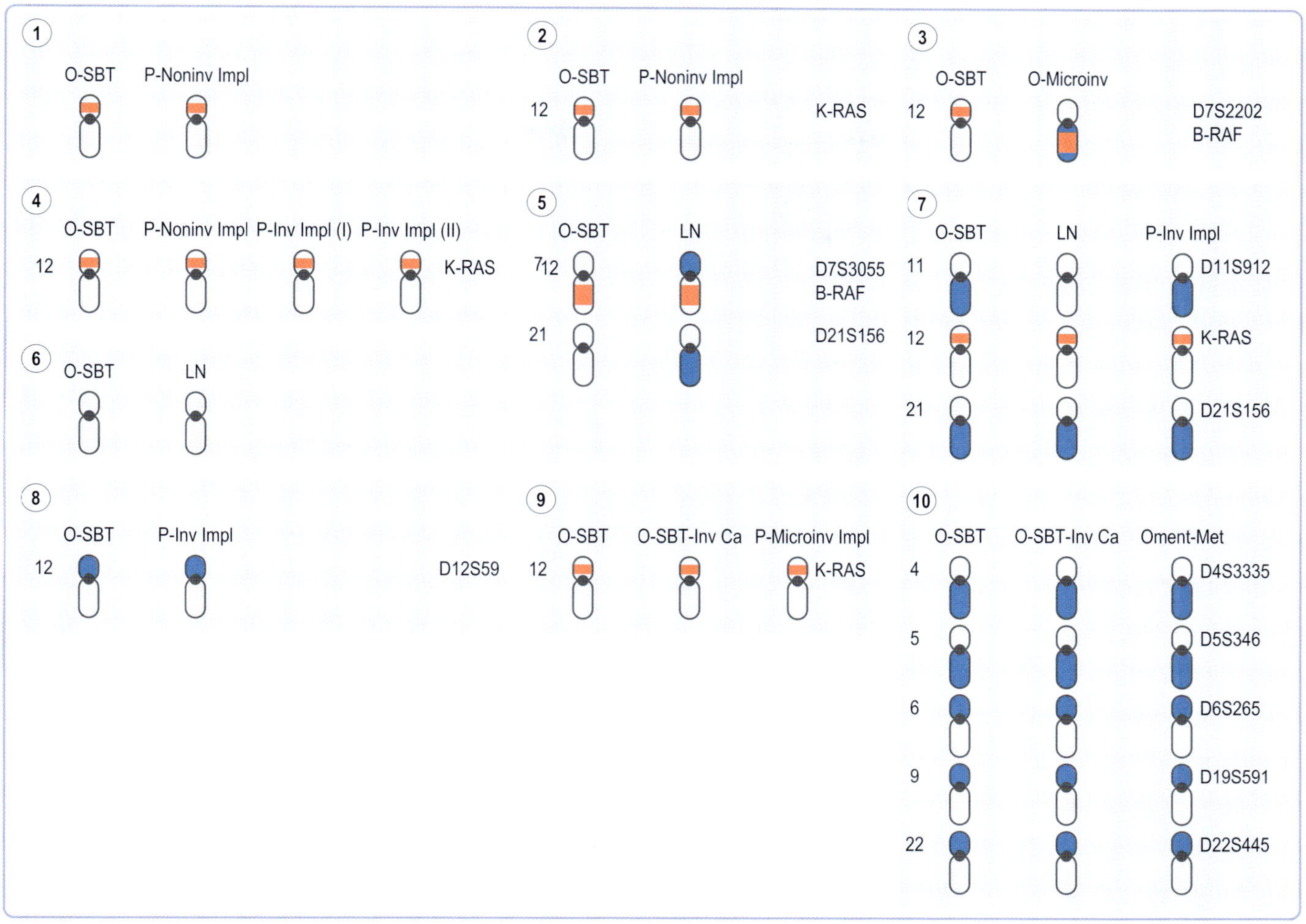

Figure 25.34 Clonal analysis of 10 serous borderline tumors (SBT) with peritoneal implants and/or lymph node involvement. O-SBT, ovarian SBT; P-Noninv Impl, noninvasive peritoneal implant; O-Microinv, ovarian SBT with focus of microinvasion too small to warrant the diagnosis of serous carcinoma; P-Inv Impl, invasive peritoneal implant; LN, SBT with lymph node involvement; O-SBT-Inv Ca, ovarian SBT with invasive foci allowing the diagnosis of LGSC; P-Microinv Impl, noninvasive peritoneal implant with foci of microinvasion; Oment-Met, omental metastasis of serous carcinoma. LOH is indicated in blue; *B-RAF/K-RAS* mutation is indicated in red; microsatellite markers for which the LOH was found are indicated on the right. Chromosome numbers where LOH and mutations were found are on the left.[55] (Reproduced with permission of John Wiley & Son, Ltd.)

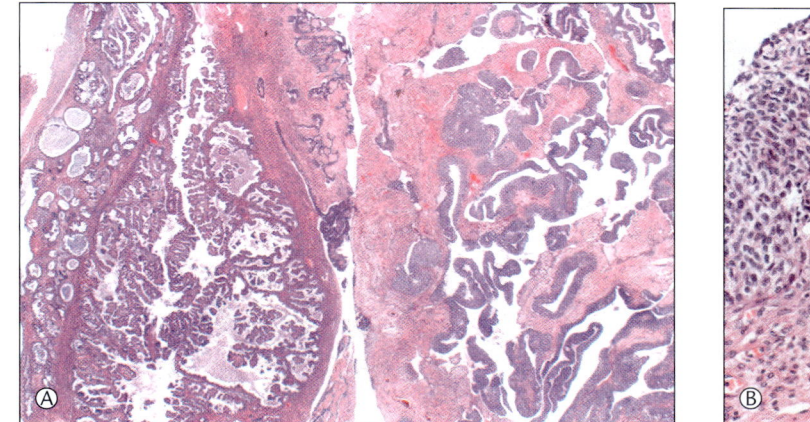
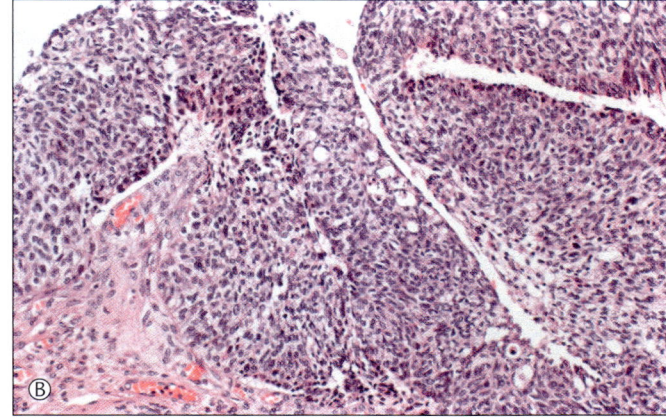

Figure 25.35 **(A)** Serous borderline tumor (SBT) with malignant transformation. The sixth recurrent pelvic tumor shows a component of TCC (right), which had not been identified in previous specimens. The patient had 12 recurrent tumors resected over a period of 11 years. **(B)** SBT with malignant transformation. Higher magnification of the TCC.

Although exophytic SBTs are more often associated with synchronous peritoneal implants than intracystic SBTs, the presence of ovarian surface involvement does not necessarily predict progression of disease.[15,28] As previously stated, most fatal SBTs have had invasive implants.[14–19,21,31,42–44]

SEROUS BORDERLINE TUMORS IN LYMPH NODES

At staging surgery, the frequency of lymph node involvement in patients with ovarian SBTs varies from 20% to 30%.[21,61–63] However, this high rate of regional lymph node 'metastasis' may be artificial. On the other hand, most studies with clinical follow-up data indicate that lymph node status is not an independent prognostic factor for patient survival.

Glandular inclusions lined by benign serous epithelium (endosalpingiosis or müllerian inclusion cysts) are encountered in pelvic and para-aortic lymph nodes in approximately half of patients with SBTs in whom lymph nodes are examined but in only 10% of women who undergo lymphadenectomies for other reasons (Figure 25.36). Thus, it is not surprising that proliferative lesions, including SBTs and even LGSCs, develop occasionally from these glandular inclusions. When this occurs in a patient with an ovarian SBT, distinction between primary nodal and metastatic tumor can be difficult.

If the SBT in the nodes is a focal finding, confined to the parenchyma or capsule of the lymph node, and appears associated with numerous benign inclusions, it is logical to interpret the nodal proliferation in these cases as independent SBT arising from endosalpingiosis.[1,64,65] In other cases, there is involvement of vascular sinuses at the periphery of the node (Figure 25.37), suggesting metastatic spread to the node. Molecular genetic investigations have shown identical K-RAS mutations in ovarian SBTs and nodal endosalpingiosis, suggesting that some glandular inclusions may represent bland-appearing forms of metastatic SBT.[50,66]

Whether the lymph node involvement represents synchronous neoplasia or true metastatic SBT does not change the favorable prognosis of these patients and should not influence their treatment. A recent report, however, has suggested that nodular epithelial aggregates (Figure 25.38; 1–8 mm) often accompanied by desmoplastic stromal reaction (Figure 25.39) and micropapillary architecture tend to be associated with decreased disease-free survival.[63] Rarely, SBTs involve extra-abdominal lymph nodes, including cervical lymph nodes, and simulate metastatic carcinoma from thyroid, breast, or lung.[19,67] In these cases, positive immunoreactions for markers of müllerian differentiation, such as WT1, CK7, and PAX8, and negative reactions for TTF-1, CK20, and GCDFP-15 may be helpful.

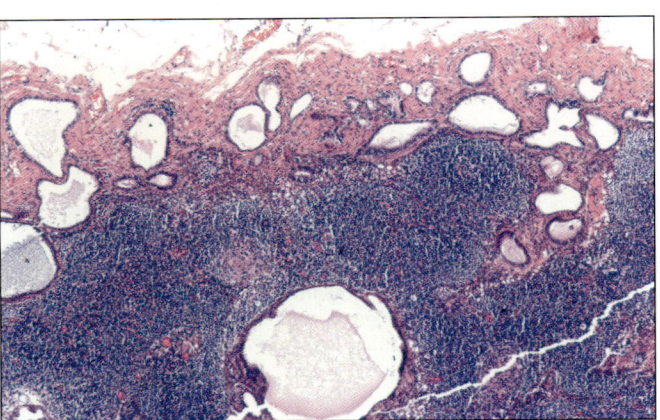

Figure 25.36 Benign müllerian inclusion glands in a pelvic lymph node.

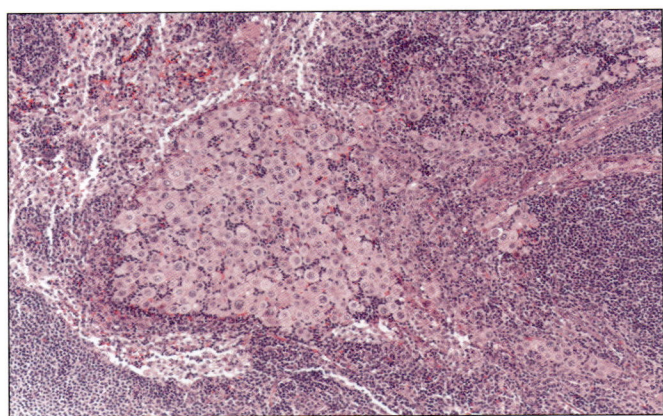

Figure 25.38 Serous borderline tumor. Lymph node involvement by nodular epithelial aggregates.

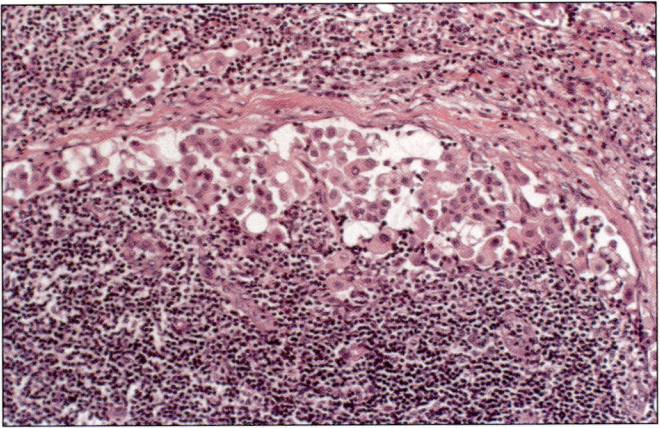

Figure 25.37 Serous borderline tumor. Lymph node involvement. Tumor cell clusters fill up a sinus.

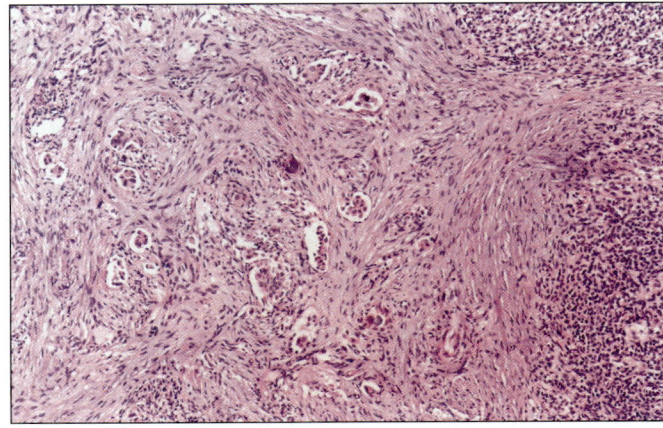

Figure 25.39 Serous borderline tumor. Lymph node involvement showing desmoplastic stromal reaction.

Lymph node involvement by SBT associated with endosalpingiosis should be distinguished from metastatic LGSC, which typically shows numerous papillae packing the sinuses and replacing extensively the nodal tissue in a haphazard fashion. But, even in these cases, the possibility of primary nodal LGSC arising independently of the ovarian tumor (Figure 25.40) cannot be easily excluded.[19]

Another nodal lesion that may cause confusion in identifying metastatic tumor is CK-positive mesothelial cells, singly or in groups, occupying either the subcapsular sinuses or the lymph node parenchyma.[68,69] This phenomenon is due to marked proliferation of mesothelial cells as a result of peritoneal involvement by tumor; the mesothelial cells are subsequently filtered ('deportation') from the peritoneal fluid by regional lymph nodes.[68] Immunostaining with a panel of antibodies may be of help. The most useful marker is Ber-Ep4, which reacts with serous tumors but not with mesothelioma. In contrast, calretinin, CK5, and thrombomodulin all react with mesothelioma but not with serous carcinomas.[70]

SEROUS BORDERLINE TUMORS OF THE PERITONEUM

Tumors histologically identical to SBTs may arise as primary neoplasms of the peritoneum with minimal or no ovarian surface involvement.[71,72] The ages of the patients range from 16 to 67 (mean 32) years. Infertility and abdominal pain are the most frequent presenting symptoms but one-third of the lesions are incidental findings at laparotomy performed for other various reasons.[71] At operation, the peritoneal lesions may be focal or diffuse. They typically appear as fibrous adhesions or granular lesions of the peritoneal surfaces (up to 6 mm in diameter) and may be mistaken for peritoneal carcinomatosis. They are found mainly in the pelvic peritoneum, but can involve the upper abdominal peritoneum including omentum.[71] In these patients, the ovaries are typically of normal size, and frequently exhibit adhesions and focal granularity similar to that seen in the extraovarian peritoneum. Microscopically, the tumors may resemble either the epithelial or desmoplastic subtypes of noninvasive implants of ovarian SBTs. Psammoma bodies are prominent (Figures 25.41 and 25.42).[71] Endosalpingiosis and chronic salpingitis are common associated findings in these patients.[71]

The standard treatment is total abdominal hysterectomy and bilateral salpingo-oophorectomy (TAH-BSO) and omentectomy. Younger patients who desire to maintain fertility may be treated conservatively.[72] The prognosis is excellent, although, rarely, invasive LGSC of the peritoneum may develop and occasional death due to tumor may occur.[71]

Treatment

Surgery is the cornerstone of treatment for patients with SBTs. In menopausal and postmenopausal women and in those who have completed their childbearing, the standard treatment is TAH-BSO. Abdominal exploration, careful staging, and removal of all grossly identifiable tumors should be done. In young women with unilateral tumors and normal-appearing contralateral ovaries who wish to preserve their reproductive capacity, unilateral oophorectomy, or even an ovarian cystectomy, can be safely performed.[15,73,74] Although a staging procedure for SBTs is often thought to be too radical, comprehensive surgical staging is

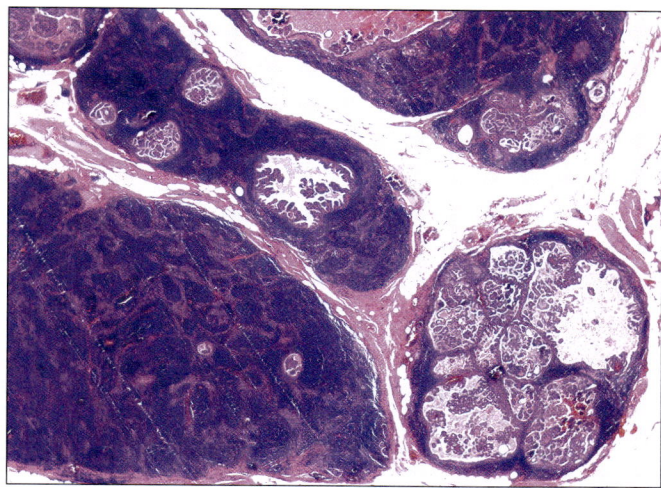

Figure 25.40 Nodal serous borderline tumor and low-grade serous carcinoma probably arising from nodal endosalpingiosis. The patient had bilateral ovarian SBTs resected 10 years earlier.

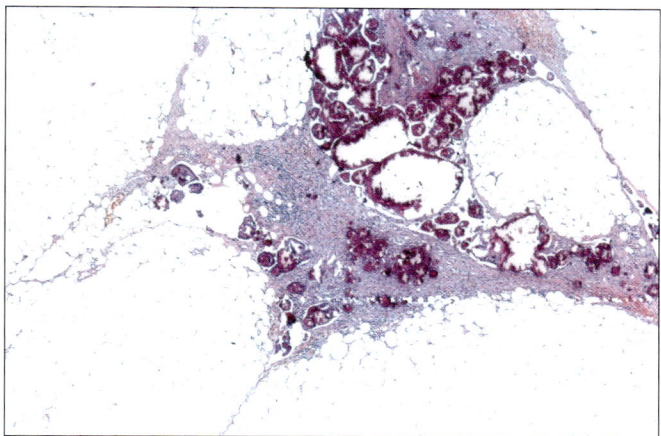

Figure 25.41 Serous borderline tumor of the peritoneum. The tumor is well circumscribed and resembles a noninvasive desmoplastic implant. Psammoma bodies and larger calcific deposits are seen.

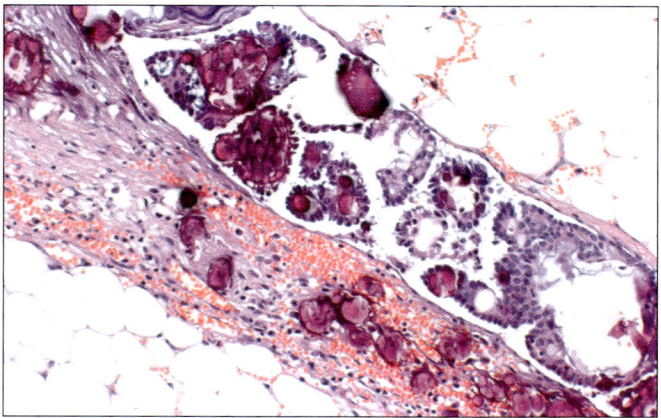

Figure 25.42 Serous borderline tumor of the peritoneum. The tumor extends between lobules of adipose tissue. The ovaries were free of tumor.

recommended in patients with apparent stage I SBTs to exclude the presence of peritoneal implants.[75] Between 16% and 30% of patients with stage I and 75% with stage II have been upgraded to stage III after a restaging operation.[75] Follow-up examination is mandatory. After the patient's family is complete, hysterectomy with residual salpingo-oophorectomy has been advocated, but its value has been questioned.[76] If a similar tumor develops in the contralateral ovary (5–10% of the cases), the patient can be successfully treated in most cases by reoperation alone.[15,19] For patients with advanced stage SBTs, postoperative treatment has varied from no additional therapy to various forms of chemotherapy and radiation therapy. The literature presents no clear evidence that adjuvant therapy alters the course of the disease and, unfortunately, many patients have died as a result of adverse complications of such treatments.[15] The current treatment approach is to recommend postoperative chemotherapy (carboplatin plus paclitaxel) to those patients with invasive peritoneal implants, or noninvasive implants with macroscopic residual disease.[15,77] For patients with recurrent SBTs, secondary cytoreductive surgery and optimal resection has been associated with high overall survival.[78]

Prognosis

Survival of patients with SBTs is much higher than that of serous carcinomas (see below). According to the most recent "annual" report (2003) of the International Federation of Gynecology and Obstetrics (FIGO),[79] the 5 year survival rates for patients with disease that is stages I–IIIb are roughly between 88% and >95% and about 60% for disease that is stage IIIC or IV. Estimates of 20 year survival are about 80%. Other than the adverse effect of invasive implants, there is no agreement in the literature as to which prognostic factors are important.[33] Although positive peritoneal cytology is predictive for survival in cases of ovarian carcinoma, this is not the case in SBTs.[80] According to most investigators, SBTs with micropapillary pattern or SBTs with microinvasion have a prognosis similar to that of tumors lacking these features. Likewise, focal lymph node involvement has not demonstrated any effect on survival. The vast majority of SBTs display a diploid DNA histogram. Aneuploid SBTs are thought to be associated with poorer prognosis.[80]

SEROUS CARCINOMAS

It is now accepted that low-grade serous carcinoma (LGSC) and high-grade serous carcinoma (HGSC) are fundamentally different tumor types and, consequently, different diseases.[81] LGSCs are associated, in most cases, with a serous borderline component, carry *K-RAS* and *B-RAF* mutations, and are unrelated to *TP53* mutations and *BRCA* abnormalities.[41,82] In contrast, HGSCs are not associated with SBTs and typically exhibit *TP53* mutations and *BRCA* abnormalities. However, recent investigations suggest that both types of serous carcinoma may originate from tubal epithelium either in the fallopian tube or in the ovary.[4–10,56,57]

LOW-GRADE SEROUS CARCINOMAS

Low-grade serous carcinomas are uncommon and account for less than 5% of all cases of ovarian carcinoma.[83] Grossly,

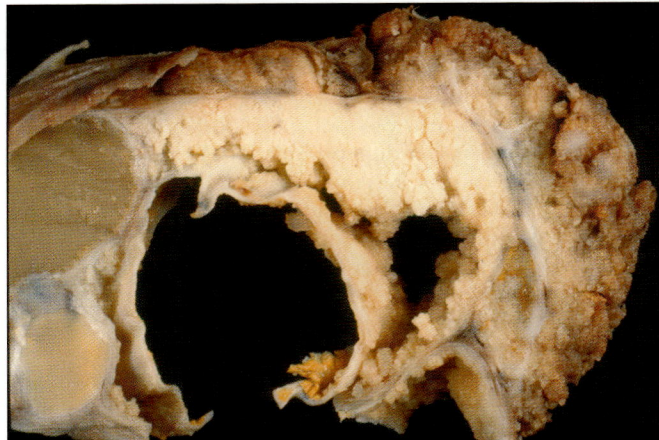

Figure 25.43 Low-grade serous carcinoma. The solid and cystic neoplasm resembles an SBT. It shows confluent papillae within the cysts and lacks hemorrhage and necrosis.

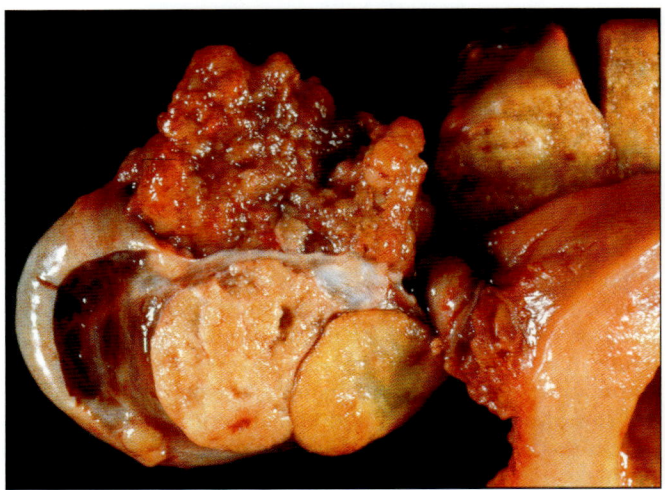

Figure 25.44 Low-grade serous carcinoma. Solid and cystic tumor (bottom) with an exophytic borderline component (top).

they resemble SBTs exhibiting cystic and papillary growth with little if any necrosis (Figure 25.43). These tumors frequently show a noninvasive serous borderline component (Figure 25.44; with or without micropapillary pattern) as they likely represent progression of SBTs beyond microinvasion. Whereas the presence of small foci of LGSC in an ovarian borderline tumor is associated with an excellent prognosis, patients with advanced stage disease fare less favorably. Nevertheless, the disease usually follows a relatively indolent course.

Microscopic Features

Microscopically, LGSCs show small papillae of tumor cells with small and uniform nuclei (grade 1) within variable amounts of hyalinized stroma, which often contains psammoma bodies (Figures 25.45 and 25.46). Mitotic figures are rare. Uniformity of the nuclei is the principal criterion for distinguishing between LGSC and HGSC, with <3-fold variability. This distinction has been shown to be highly reproducible.[84] Tumors showing nuclei of intermediate size often have *TP53* mutations and should be classified as HGSC.[85] LGSCs rarely progress to high-grade tumors.

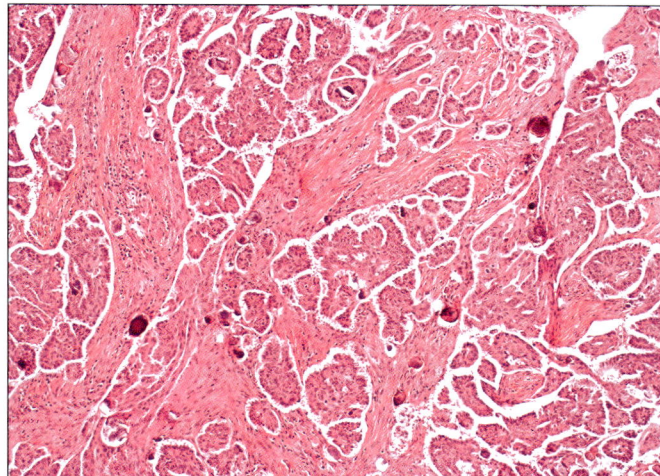

Figure 25.45 Low-grade serous carcinoma. The papillary tumor shows epithelial cells with small and uniform nuclei (grade 1). The stroma appears hyalinized and contains psammoma bodies.

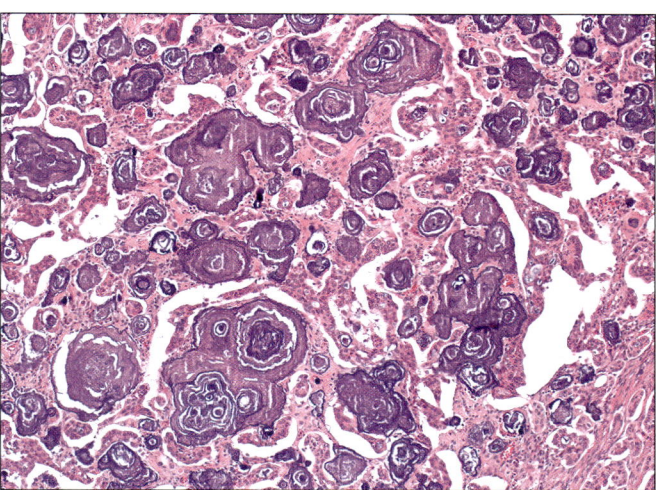

Figure 25.47 Serous psammocarcinoma. The invasive and well-differentiated epithelial component is partly covered by psammoma bodies.

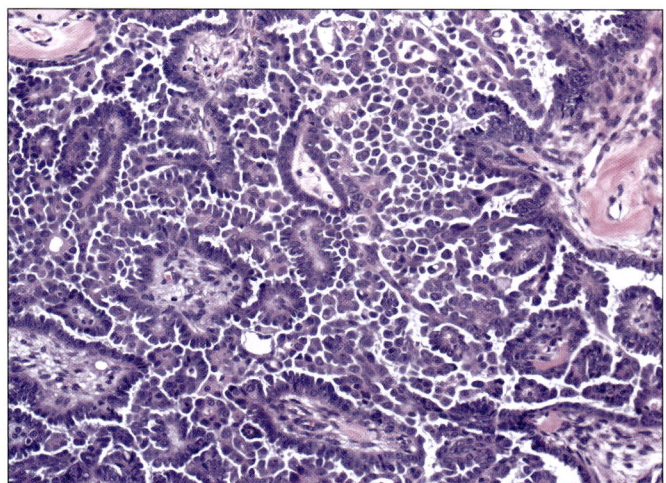

Figure 25.46 Low-grade serous carcinoma. The tumor cells are rounded with scant cytoplasm and mild or moderately atypical nuclei. Mitotic figures are rare.

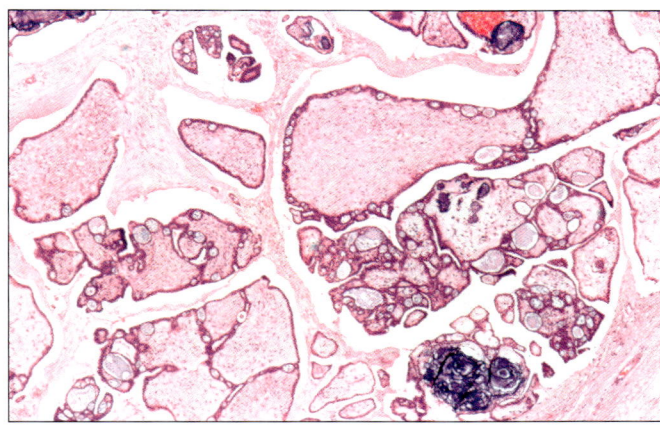

Figure 25.48 Low-grade serous papillary adenocarcinoma,. Broad papillae lined by tumor cells appear in non-lymphatic spaces within fibrous stroma.

Psammocarcinoma is a very rare form of LGSC with a favorable prognosis.[86] This tumor, which behaves clinically more like an SBT than a serous carcinoma, differs in its microscopic features from the former by infiltrating the ovarian stroma (Figure 25.47). Four criteria recommended for the diagnosis of psammocarcinoma include: (1) invasion of the ovarian stroma (or, in extraovarian sites, invasion of any intraperitoneal tissue); (2) only mild to moderate nuclear atypia; (3) epithelial nests <15 cells in their largest dimension; and (4) the presence of psammoma bodies in at least 75% of papillae or nests.[86] Although all 18 reported tumors were stage III at presentation, there has been only one death, turning out a survival rate of 94%.

A rare variant of well-differentiated serous carcinoma consists of broad papillae lined by tumor cells lying in non-lymphatic spaces within fibrous stroma (Figure 25.48); the spaces probably result from secretion of serous fluid by the neoplastic cells.[1]

Immunohistochemistry and Somatic Genetics

The biomarker expression profile of LGSCs is similar to that of their high-grade counterparts (see later). Only p53 is usually negative and Ki-67 immunoreaction differs significantly between the two tumor types, with a median Ki-67 labeling index of 2.5% in LGSCs versus 22.4% in HGSCs.[87] B-RAF or K-RAS mutations are present in LGSCs (38% and 19%, respectively).[82,88] LGSCs do not show chromosomal instability and lack the complex genetic abnormalities seen in HGSCs. LGSCs are not associated with BRCA germline mutations.

Differential Diagnosis

With regard to the distinction between LGSC and SBT, micropapillarity, by itself, is not sufficient to warrant a diagnosis of carcinoma in the absence of invasion. If there are invasive foci measuring <10 mm^2, the tumor is considered to be borderline with microinvasion.[39] Tumors with larger invasive components are classified as LGSC. Histopathologically, invasive peritoneal implants and LGSC are identical lesions, which are only distinguished by the timing of the disease and the volume of the tumor. Whereas invasive implants are early superficial lesions of microscopic or small macroscopic size (≤1–2 cm), LGSC frequently presents as bulky disease.[89] Although the independent peritoneal origin of the invasive implants associated with ovarian SBT cannot be completely excluded, we have recently demonstrated identical *B-RAF* and *K-RAS* mutations as well as identical LOH in a series of ovarian SBTs, peritoneal implants, and lymph node deposits. Such findings support a monoclonal origin of these tumors and the secondary nature of the implants.[55]

Treatment

The response rate to conventional therapy for LGSCs is difficult to determine because this tumor type has only recently been recognized and existing data may reflect case series that include some cases of HGSC. Data from a series of patients with SBTs who experienced a recurrence as carcinoma, indicate that, in most cases, LGSCs do not respond to conventional ovarian carcinoma chemotherapy.[90] Although data are limited, cytoreduction seems to be more effective.[78]

HIGH-GRADE SEROUS CARCINOMAS

Clinical Features

High-grade serous carcinoma is the most common type of ovarian cancer and accounts for approximately 70% of ovarian carcinomas.[23] The average age of patients is 56 years (ranging from 45 to 65 years). Although most patients have symptoms, these are often subtle and easily confused with those of benign conditions of the gastrointestinal and urinary tracts. Accordingly, about 80% of patients present with advanced stage disease, and tumors confined to the ovary at diagnosis are distinctly uncommon (<5%). The most important risk factor is a strong family history of ovarian or breast cancer, which is present in only 10–15% of patients (see the section Genetic susceptibility).[91] In fact, most patients with a history of breast cancer who present later with an adnexal or pelvic mass are found to have independent HGSCs of the ovary, fallopian tube, or peritoneum and not breast cancer recurrence.[92,93]

Tumor dissemination can occur by local extension throughout the abdominopelvic peritoneum, and through lymphatics to the retroperitoneal pelvic, para-aortic, and mesenteric lymph nodes. Ascites may occur in all stages, but becomes more evident when the tumor involves the upper abdomen (stage III). Metastatic disease is commonly found in the omentum. The most common extra-abdominal site of disease is the pleural space. Less frequently, distant metastases occur, through the bloodstream, in the parenchyma of the liver, spleen, lungs, and other organs. Advanced intra-abdominal tumor is often associated with signs of intestinal obstruction, including nausea, vomiting, and abdominal pain. Ultrasound, MRI and CT have no clearly established role in preoperative tumor staging. Laparotomy and surgical exploration of the abdominal cavity remain the standard approach for staging.

In 10–20% of patients with advanced stage HGSC, the ovaries are of normal size or minimally enlarged, or exhibit

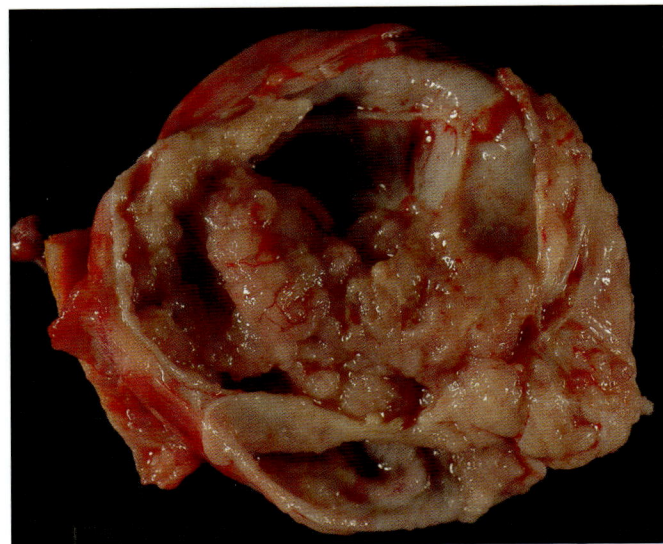

Figure 25.49 High-grade serous carcinoma. The tumor is cystic and solid. The cysts contain closely packed papillae, which appear more confluent than those of an SBT. There are foci of necrosis and hemorrhage.

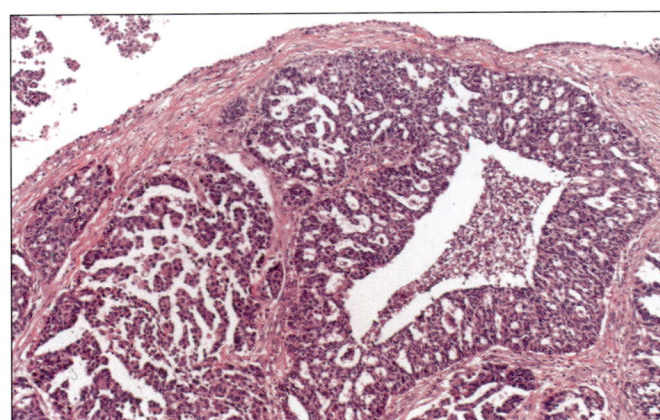

Figure 25.50 High-grade serous carcinoma. Small cellular papillae without fibrous cores and solid areas with slit-like spaces.

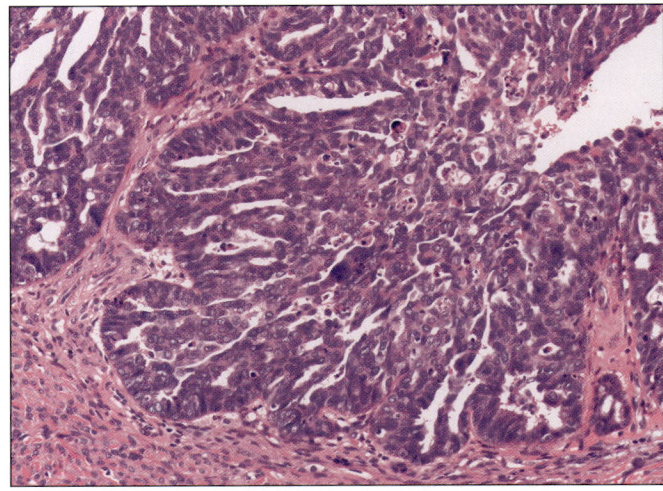

Figure 25.51 High-grade serous carcinoma. The slit-like spaces tend to be uniform in size and oriented radially.

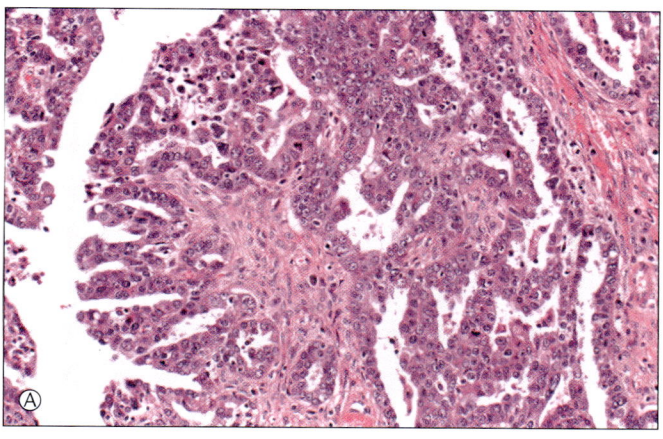

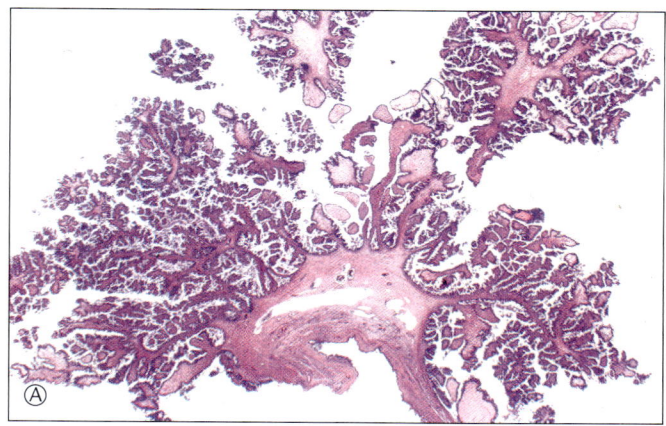

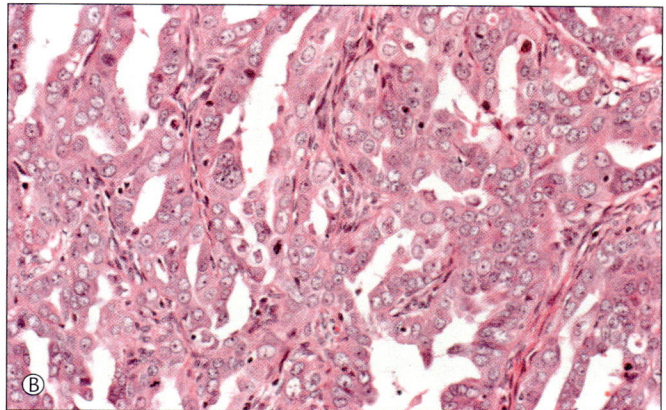

Figure 25.52 High-grade serous carcinoma. **(A)** Closely packed papillae lacking fibrous cores. **(B)** Marked nuclear atypia, prominent nucleoli and mitoses.

Figure 25.53 **(A)** High-grade serous carcinoma (HGSC) resembling a serous borderline tumor. Hierarchical and complex branching without obvious stromal invasion. **(B)** HGSC. The tumor cells show marked nuclear atypia and high mitotic activity.

mainly surface involvement. These findings warrant a diagnosis of primary peritoneal HGSC (see the section Differential diagnosis below and Chapter 31).

Macroscopic Features

Serous carcinomas range in size from microscopic to over 20 cm in diameter and are bilateral in two-thirds of all cases (one-third of stage I cases).[1] Rare serous carcinomas appear as closely packed soft surface papillae, requiring microscopic examination for their distinction from SBTs. The papillae tend to be softer and more confluent than those of SBTs (Figure 25.49). Poorly differentiated tumors are predominantly solid, multinodular masses with necrosis and hemorrhage. Omental metastases usually are firm tumor masses with grayish white cut surfaces. Grossly normal omentum contains microscopic tumor in 20% of cases.

Microscopic Features

High-grade serous carcinomas show papillary and solid growth with slit-like glandular lumens and severe nuclear atypia (Figures 25.50–25.55). The papillae are irregularly branching and highly cellular with little or no stromal support (Figure 25.50). The slit-like spaces tend to be uniform in size and oriented radially (Figure 25.51). The tumor cells are typically of intermediate size, with scattered bizarre mononuclear giant cells exhibiting prominent nucleoli (Figure 25.52). In contrast to LGSCs, these tumors show >3-fold variation in nuclear size (Figure 25.55). Although nuclear features are the chief criterion for distinguishing between HGSC and LGSC, the mitotic activity can be used in cases with equivocal degrees of nuclear pleomorphism; mitotic activity greater than 12/10 HPFs favors a diagnosis of HGSC.[23,81] In these tumors, mitotic activity is often several times this diagnostic threshold and is associated with abundant apoptotic bodies. Abnormal mitoses are common (Figure 25.55). Necrosis and hemorrhage are usually prominent. Psammoma bodies are often present in varying numbers (30%). Serous carcinomas tend to be uniform throughout. Rarely do high- and low-grade forms coexist.

High-grade and predominantly solid carcinomas showing serous differentiation, even in a minority of the tumor, should be classified as HGSC (rather than mixed serous/undifferentiated); to date, no underlying molecular differences between these tumors and pure HGSC have been detected.[94] HGSCs may contain various other cell types as a minor component (<10%), but do not influence the outcome. For example, they may contain clear cells, but the characteristic architectural features of clear cell carcinoma are absent. Rare serous carcinomas undergo focal squamous differentiation.

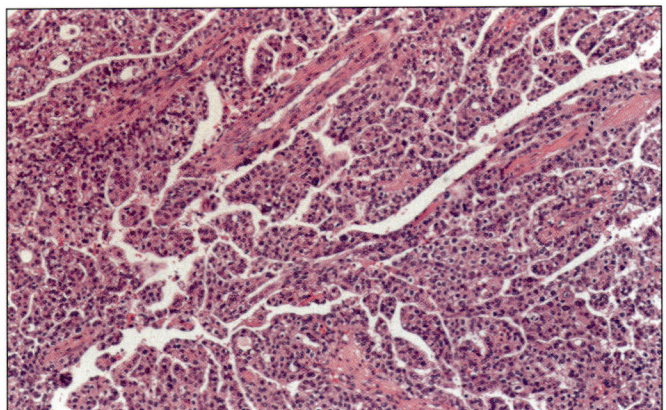

Figure 25.54 High-grade serous carcinoma resembling a mesothelioma. The tumor cells are predominantly small and uniform but a few bizarre mononuclear giant cells are seen.

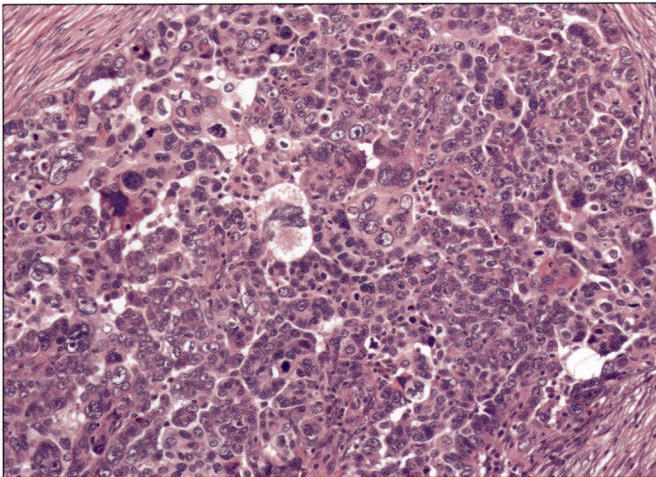

Figure 25.55 High-grade serous carcinoma. Marked nuclear pleomorphism and high mitotic activity.

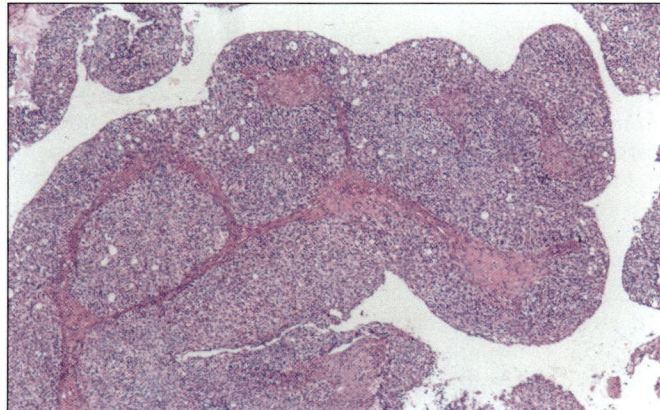

Figure 25.56 Transitional-like carcinoma (TCC). Multilayered papilla with smooth luminal borders protruding into an empty space.

Ovarian transitional cell carcinoma (TCC), not associated with a benign or borderline Brenner component, differs clinically and pathologically from malignant Brenner tumor (see Chapter 27) and is now classified as a morphologic variant of HGSCs, i.e., transitional-like adenocarcinoma. The tumor shows thick, blunt, undulating papillae of transitional cell differentiation (Figure 25.56) in contrast with the papillae of typical HGSCs, which are generally thinner. The bands of epithelium are multilayered, have a relative uniform width of at least a dozen cells, and typically contain microspaces (87%).[95] It is now believed that ovarian TCC represents an HGSC with morphologic features of transitional cell differentiation rather than being a distinct tumor type. This view is supported by the frequent coexistence of TCC foci within otherwise conventional HGSC[95] as well as their similar immunoprofile and genetic alterations.[96,97]

Immunohistochemistry

HGSCs show cytoplasmic immunoreactivity for CK7 but not for CK20. They are also reactive for CAM5.2, AE1/AE3, EMA, B72.3, Ber-Ep4, Leu-M1, and CA125 (90%), but not for calretinin, CK5, and other mesothelial markers. α-Inhibin, a marker of sex cord stromal tumors, may be rarely reactive. TTF-1, a marker for lung and thyroid carcinomas, is focally or weakly positive (nuclear reactivity) in 25–35% of serous carcinomas, but occasionally can be diffusely positive.[98,99] CD99 is often positive.

Most HGSCs immunoreact for p53, BRCA1, WT1, and p16. They also exhibit a high proliferation index as indicated by an increased nuclear expression of Ki-67. Only strong and diffuse p53 and p16 reactions should be considered positive. Nuclear WT1 reaction occurs in approximately 80% of cases of HGSC and LGSC but in less than 5% of ovarian carcinomas of other types.[87,100,101] ER is expressed in approximately two-thirds of cases of HGSC and is also expressed in LGSCs and endometrioid carcinomas but is negative in almost all clear cell carcinomas and mucinous carcinomas.[101] WT1-positive tumors are more often high-stage, high-grade, bcl-2 positive, and have a higher proliferation index based on increased nuclear staining for Ki-67, as compared to WT1-negative tumors.[102]

Genetic Susceptibility

Women with germline mutations in *BRCA1* or *BRCA2* have a 30–70% risk of developing ovarian cancer by the age of 70, mainly HGSC.[103] *BRCA1* and *BRCA2* are essential components of the homologous recombination DNA system required to repair DNA double-strand breaks (DSBs).[104] Like *TP53* mutations, *BRCA* inactivation seems to be a consistent genetic alteration of HGSC. Besides germline mutation, inactivation of the *BRCA* pathway may result from somatic mutation in either *BRCA1* or *BRCA2*,[105] or promoter hypermethylation in *BRCA1*.[106]

Histogenesis and Genetic Profile

The traditional view that HGSCs arise from the ovarian surface epithelium or epithelial inclusion cysts has been recently challenged by the identification, in women with *BRCA1* or *BRCA2* germline mutations, of serous tubal intraepithelial carcinoma (STIC) in the distal fimbriated end of the fallopian tube as the probable precursor of advanced HGSC.[4-8] Cytologically, the cells of STIC show secretory differentiation[8] and resemble those of HGSC. They lack cilia and show nuclear enlargement, hyperchromasia, loss of polarity, prominent nucleoli, and mitotic figures. STIC shows immunohistochemical evidence of double-stranded DNA damage, as indicated by nuclear staining for γ-H2AX.[10] Like HGSC, STIC diffusely and strongly expresses p53 and the Ki-67 proliferation index is usually markedly elevated (mean labeling index, 72%; range, 40–95%).[10] p16 and WT1 may also be expressed. Furthermore, the finding of identical *TP53* mutations in both STIC and concomitant tumors classified as ovarian in origin[7] indicates a clonal relationship between them and suggests that the distal fallopian tube (fimbria) is an important site for the initiation of HGSC. Nevertheless, implantation of tubal-type epithelium into the ovary (endosalpingiosis) or mesothelial surface invaginations (inclusion cysts) may explain the origin of those HGSCs lacking STIC. In such cases the primary tumor would appear to originate from the ovary. Currently, the relative proportion of HGSCs of ovarian and tubal derivation is unknown mainly because the growth of tumor in advanced stage cancers conceals the primary site. However, extensive examination of the fallopian tubes from 55 consecutive cases of HGSC (ovarian, tubal, or pelvic) revealed involvement of the endosalpinx in 70% and STIC in approximately 50% of the cases.[7]

The discovery of STICs in risk-reducing salpingo-oophorectomy (RRSO) specimens from women with known *BRCA* mutations and/or a strong family history of ovarian cancer has resulted in extensive research into the role of the fallopian tube in pelvic serous carcinogenesis.[4-10] Early studies revealed small foci of strongly p53-immunoreactive cells in largely histologically normal fallopian tube epithelium.[8] These foci, which predominate in the distal portion of the fallopian tube, have been designated 'p53 signatures.' Like STIC, p53 signatures are composed exclusively of secretory cells (at least 12 consecutive immunoreactive cells), and the majority exhibit evidence of DNA damage by immunoreaction for γ-H2AX.[8-10] They are more frequent and multifocal in tubes with STIC and, in some cases, can be identified in direct continuity with STIC. About 57% of p53 signatures contain *TP53* mutations;[8] however, Ki-67 proliferation index is low (mean, 3%). p53 signatures probably represent early clonal expansion short of neoplastic proliferation[107] and, surprisingly, are found in both women with and those without *BRCA1* or *BRCA2* mutations at the same frequency (10–38% vs 17–33%, respectively); should BRCA loss have caused p53 signature foci, one would expect a much higher frequency in women with germline mutations in *BRCA1* or *BRCA2*, but this does not occur.[8] Thus, *TP53* mutation is an early event in the genesis of HGSC, occurring in p53 signature foci and leading to STIC in the distal fallopian tube. *BRCA1* mutation also occurs early in the development of STIC but after *TP53* mutation.[107] It is possible that germline mutations of *BRCA1* act as a promoter for the development of STIC.[9]

A morphologic continuum of epithelial changes taking place in the distal fallopian tube has been described.[10] The transition is as follows: normal fallopian tube epithelium, overexpression of p53, STIC, and, finally, invasive serous carcinoma. Clonality of the precursor cells in both the so-called p53 signature and STICs are the strongest support for the fimbriated end of the fallopian tube as a site of origin for HGSC.[6] Concentration of *TP53* mutant lesions in the distal fallopian tube suggests a vulnerability of these cells to DNA damage. In fact, the secretory cells of the tubal epithelium have a limited ability to repair DNA DSBs, as shown by the persistence of γ-H2AX-immunoreactive foci after DNA damage.[108] This might explain why this tissue seems to be especially sensitive to inactivating *BRCA* mutations.

The protocol for sectioning and extensively examining the fimbriated end (SEE-FIM protocol) was developed for processing RRSO (see Chapter 21).[6] According to this protocol, the entire tube is initially fixed for at least 4 hours to prevent denuding of the mucosal epithelial cells. Then, the fimbriated end is amputated from the proximal tube and sectioned longitudinally into multiple (at least four) sections and the entire tube is submitted for histologic review. With more extensive sectioning of these specimens, an increased rate of detection of early cancer (up to 17%) can be obtained.[109]

Although a significant number of HGSCs may not arise from the ovary, and the term 'ovarian cancer' would not be histogenetically precise in every case, ovarian involvement is the rule in almost all cases. Furthermore, in view of the rarity of HGSC associated with tubal tumor masses, it seems unlikely that all HGSCs originate in the fallopian tube. Thus, as indicated previously, the term HGSC of the ovary should be kept until the different origins of the ovarian tumors are better understood. Terms like 'müllerian' or 'pelvic' would create confusion for patients, physicians, and medical investigators.[110]

Pathogenetic Model

Similar to the now well-recognized adenoma–carcinoma sequence in colorectal cancer pathogenesis, it was thought for many years that progression of ovarian epithelial–stromal tumors occurs from benign cystadenomas to borderline tumors, to well-differentiated carcinomas, and ultimately to poorly differentiated carcinomas. This was assumed without taking the five major histologic types into account. Nevertheless, since HGSCs represent the majority of ovarian carcinomas, most reports on molecular pathology of ovarian carcinoma in the older literature refer mainly to HGSC. However, as indicated earlier, HGSC and LGSC are essentially two different diseases. In fact, whereas the benign–borderline–malignant sequence seems to apply quite well to LGSC, the sequence of genetic alterations in HGSC is substantially different.

A pathogenetic model that includes the stages of initiation and progression of HGSC taking into account biomarkers of early tumorigenesis has recently been described (Figure 25.57[107]). This model, essential for effective screening and treatment, proposes as primary events early p53 loss followed by BRCA loss, leading to deficiency in homologous recombination repair (HRR) of DSBs, which triggers chromosomal instability (genetic chaos) and widespread copy number changes.[107,111,112] Secondary and tertiary events then cause global changes in gene expression followed by mutations to facilitate tumor evolution. Once chromosomal instability is set up by mutation in *TP53* and *BRCA* inactivation, gene copy number is the major determinant of progression of HGSC.[107]

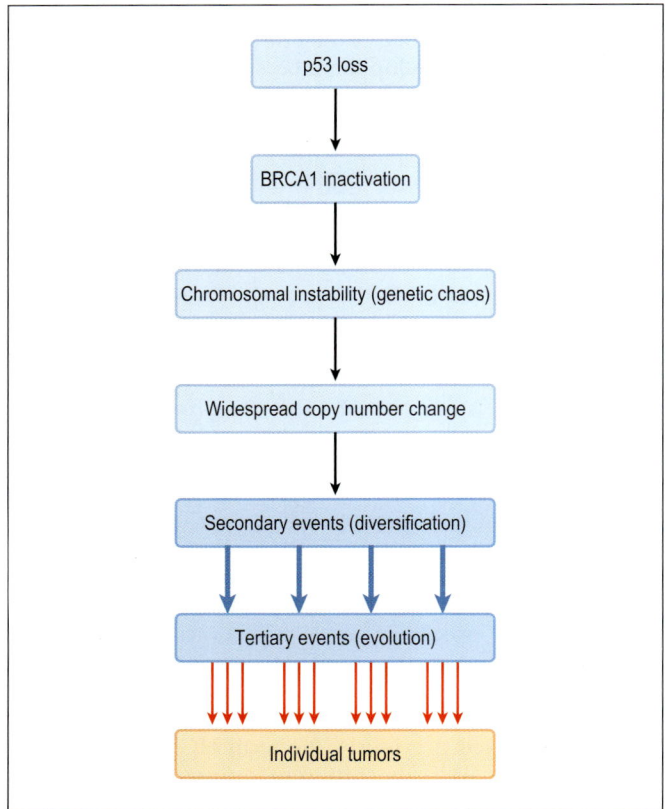

Figure 25.57 Initiation and progression of HGSC of the ovary. This model proposes that the sequence of primary events were as follows: early p53 loss followed by BRCA loss, leading to deficiency in HRR of DSBs, which triggers chromosomal instability (genetic chaos) and widespread copy number changes. Copy number change can be a driver of molecular subtype specification and results in global changes in gene expression. Subsequent mutations facilitate tumor progression. (Modified from Bowtell.[107])

Differential Diagnosis

Approximately 10–20% of patients with advanced stage HGSC have normal sized or slightly enlarged ovaries with exclusively surface involvement. These tumors are classified as primary peritoneal serous carcinomas and should be distinguished from ovarian serous carcinomas. According to the Gynecologic Oncology Group, the following are required to meet the criteria for primary peritoneal carcinoma: (1) both ovaries must be normal in size or enlarged by a benign process; (2) the involvement in the extraovarian peritoneum must be greater than on the surface of either ovary; and (3) the ovarian tumor involvement must be either nonexistent, confined to ovarian surface epithelium without stromal invasion, or involving the cortical stroma with tumor size less than 5×5 mm.[113] From a clinical viewpoint, the distinction is not critical because the prognosis and treatment are similar.

Although HGSC is the most common papillary carcinoma of the ovary, other carcinomas, particularly endometrioid, and clear cell carcinomas may be papillary as well, and enter the differential diagnosis. The papillae in endometrioid carcinomas are typically larger and villous, as in uterine villoglandular carcinomas. Squamous differentiation and adenofibromatous growth are common in endometrioid carcinomas but rare in serous carcinomas. Endometrioid carcinomas are more likely low-grade carcinomas associated with coexistent adenocarcinoma of the uterine corpus (in 15–20% of cases)[114] and with endometriosis in the ovaries or elsewhere in the pelvis (about 30%) than their serous counterparts. In fact, most high-grade non-papillary adenocarcinomas would be currently classified as HGSCs.[115]

Diffuse and strong immunoreaction for WT1, p53, and p16 favor an HGSC, while the opposite immunoprofile is more common in endometrioid carcinoma. Nuclear reaction for β-catenin may be found in endometrioid carcinoma but not in HGSC. The papillae in clear cell carcinomas are lined by hobnail or clear cells and typically have hyalinized cores; other distinctive features of clear cell carcinoma are almost always present. Hobnail cells may be seen in otherwise typical serous carcinomas but are almost always present in small foci. A further useful marker is the presence of occasional bizarre mononuclear giant cells (Figure 25.54) among sheets of small uniform cells. These may be the only feature suggestive of serous neoplasia in otherwise undifferentiated carcinomas. A useful immunohistochemical panel for this distinction is HNF-1β, WT1, and ER. The most common immunoprofiles are HNF-1β–, WT1+, and ER+ in HGSC and HNF-1β+, WT1–, and ER– in clear cell carcinoma.[101]

Some HGSCs contain cells with abundant eosinophilic cytoplasm and may mimic malignant mesotheliomas (see Chapter 30) but are usually distinguished by their intraovarian location, distinctive glandular pattern, and nuclear features. The typical tubular and papillary patterns of mesotheliomas differ from the more disorderly patterns of serous carcinomas. Malignant mesothelioma cells are typically less pleomorphic than those of serous carcinoma and their papillae are less cellular. Psammoma bodies are much less common in mesotheliomas then in HGSCs. The most useful immunohistochemical markers are the Ber-Ep4-defined surface glycoprotein, which is positive in HGSC but negative in mesothelioma, and calretinin, CK5/6, and thrombomodulin, all three of which are positive in mesothelioma but negative in serous carcinomas.[70,116] Additionally, lack of reactivity for carcinoembryonic antigen, B72.3, Leu-M1, ER, PR, and CA125 favor a diagnosis of mesothelioma over carcinoma[116] (see Chapter 30).

Primary serous carcinoma of the ovary must be distinguished from metastatic serous carcinoma of the fallopian tube and endometrium. In cases exhibiting myometrial vascular invasion, bilateral and surface ovarian involvement, and tumor present in the ovarian hilus within vascular spaces, the diagnosis of secondary involvement by the endometrial carcinoma is obvious. In other cases, the ovarian tumor is either, an independent primary neoplasm, or the only primary tumor that has spread to the endometrium (see Chapter 27). WT1 can be useful, as peritoneal serous carcinomas are positive like their ovarian counterparts, whereas endometrial serous carcinomas are usually negative or weakly positive.

Patients with a history of breast cancer, particularly *BRCA1* or *BRCA2* mutation carriers, who present with an adnexal or pelvic mass, are more likely to have independent ovarian or tubal HGSC than metastases from the breast cancer by a 3:1 ratio.[92,93] Occasionally, however, metastatic poorly differentiated carcinoma from the breast may closely simulate serous carcinoma both microscopically and in its pattern of spread within the abdomen. In such cases, comparison of both tumors in terms of their grades, patterns, and cell types facilitates the diagnosis. The 'single-file' infiltrative patterns typical of lobular breast carcinomas are rarely seen in serous carcinomas. Demonstration of intracellular mucin is also useful. Immunohistochemistry may rarely be helpful in difficult cases. Reactivity for GCDFP-15 favors metastatic breast carcinoma whereas WT1, PAX8, and CA125 reactivity favors primary ovarian carcinoma; however, a panel of markers is recommended as no currently available individual marker is entirely specific for breast or ovarian carcinomas.

Treatment and Prognosis

The initial treatment includes abdominal exploration, meticulous staging, and resection of all grossly identifiable disease (bulk resection).[117] FIGO stage is the strongest predictor of outcome in ovarian cancer. The most recent version of the FIGO staging for cancer of the ovary, fallopian tube, and peritoneum (Rome, 2012) is shown in Appendix A. Whereas complete staging would be sufficient surgical treatment for tumors in stages I and II, patients with advanced disease require cytoreductive surgery. Stage I ovarian cancer is confined to the ovaries and, as indicated above, less than 5% of HGSCs are stage I tumors. Tumor rupture, ovarian surface involvement by tumor cells, or presence of malignant cells in peritoneal washings or ascitic fluid, warrant a stage IC. However, several recent studies have questioned the worse prognosis of stage IC tumors compared to stage I carcinomas. Currently, it is unclear whether upstaging based on dense adhesions of an apparent stage I tumor is justified.[118-120]

Less than 10% of HGSCs are found in stage II; i.e., extension or metastasis to extraovarian/extratubal pelvic organs or tissues. Stage II includes examples of direct extension to the tubes/ovaries and pelvic sidewall, as well as pelvic peritoneal metastases. Thus, it includes resectable and curable tumors that have extended to adjacent organs, and tumors that have seeded the pelvic peritoneum and are associated with poor prognosis. Noteworthy, the sigmoid colon is within the pelvis, and, therefore, sigmoid involvement equals stage II.

HGSC most commonly presents in stage III and the vast majority of these are stage IIIC. These tumors typically spread along the abdominopelvic peritoneum involving the omentum, serosa of the small and large bowel, mesentery, paracolic gutters, diaphragm, and peritoneal surfaces of the liver and spleen. Ascites is found in almost all cases and positive lymph nodes are found in a high number of patients who undergo node sampling or lymphadenectomy and in almost 80% of advanced stage tumors.

The new FIGO staging includes a revision of the stage III patients. Allotment to stage IIIA1 is based on spread to the retroperitoneal lymph nodes without intraperitoneal dissemination, because an analysis of these patients indicates that their survival is significantly better than those who have intraperitoneal dissemination.[121,122] Nodal metastasis without peritoneal metastasis is relatively uncommon (about 9% of cases).[122] The majority of these have positive para-aortic nodes. Isolated positive pelvic nodes with negative para-aortic nodes is very uncommon (0-3%).[123]

Volume of residual disease is an important prognostic factor in most studies, but this applies only to stages IIIC and IV. The parameter that defines optimal cytoreduction is residual disease less than 1 cm.[124] Stage IV is defined as distant metastasis and includes patients with parenchymal liver metastases and extra-abdominal metastases; 12-21% of patients present in stage IV.[79]

Stage I serous carcinoma is treated by TAH-BSO. Unilateral salpingo-oophorectomy can be alternatively done on young women who desire preservation of fertility. Close follow-up is essential in those cases; residual adnexa and uterus may be removed after childbearing is completed. Postoperatively, patients with HGSC receive combination chemotherapy. The chemotherapeutic agents most commonly used for epithelial ovarian cancers are platinum compounds (cisplatin and carboplatin), alkylating agents, and taxol. Intraperitoneal chemotherapy has not been universally accepted for at least three reasons: toxic effects, intraperitoneal treatment delivery issues, and complications (e.g., intraperitoneal adhesions, infections).[125] Neoadjuvant chemotherapy followed by debulking surgery produces similar outcomes to primary debulking followed by chemotherapy in stages IIIC and IV disease.[125]

The most promising targets in clinical trials are angiogenesis and homologous recombination deficiency. Increased production of vascular endothelial growth factor (VEGF), frequently observed in hypoxia or inflammation, results in increased endothelial cell proliferation and decreased apoptosis.[126] The humanized monoclonal anti-VEGF antibody bevacizumab has shown promising anti-tumor activity alone and in combination with cytotoxic chemotherapy. Treatment with poly (ADP-ribose) polymerase (PARP) inhibitors relies upon the inherent defect in homologous recombination that occurs in BRCA-deficient tumors by inhibiting the alternative DNA repair pathway involving base excision repair. PARP inhibitors have been shown to have activity in epithelial ovarian, fallopian tube, and primary peritoneal cancer in phase I and II clinical trials.

The rates of long-term survival (>10 years) in patients with early stage disease (stage I or II) are 80-95%. In contrast, 75% of patients present with advanced disease (stage III or IV) and have low long-term survival rates (10-30%).[127]

REFERENCES

1. Scully RE, Young RH, Clement PB. Tumors of the ovary, maldeveloped gonads, fallopian tube, and broad ligament. In: Rosai J, Sobin LH, editors. Atlas of tumor pathology. 3rd ed, vol. 23. Washington, DC: Armed Forces Institute of Pathology; 1998.
2. Prat J. Pathology of the ovary. Philadelphia: Saunders; 2004. p. 83-109.
3. Lee KR, Tavassoli FA, Prat J, et al. Tumours of the ovary and peritoneum: surface epithelial-stromal tumours. In: Tavassoli FA, Devilee P, editors. World Health Organization classification of tumours. Pathology and genetics of tumours of the breast and female genital organs. Lyon, France: IARC Press; 2003. p. 117-45.
4. Piek JM, van Diest PJ, Zweemer RP, et al. Dysplastic changes in prophylactically removed fallopian tubes of women predisposed to developing ovarian cancer. J Pathol 2001;195:451-6.
5. Piek JM, van Diest PJ, Zweemer RP, et al. Tubal ligation and risk of ovarian cancer. Lancet 2001;358:844.
6. Medeiros F, Muto MG, Lee Y, et al. The tubal fimbria is a preferred site for early adenocarcinoma in women with familial ovarian cancer syndrome. Am J Surg Pathol 2006;30:230-6.

7. Kindelberger DW, Lee Y, Miron A, et al. Intraepithelial carcinoma of the fimbria and pelvic serous carcinoma: evidence for a causal relationship. Am J Surg Pathol 2007;31:161–9.
8. Lee Y, Miron A, Drapkin R, et al. A candidate precursor to serous carcinoma that originates in the distal fallopian tube. J Pathol 2007;211:26–35.
9. Folkins AK, Jarboe EA, Saleemuddin A, et al. A candidate precursor to pelvic serous cancer (p53 signature) and its prevalence in ovaries and fallopian tubes from women with BRCA mutations. Gynecol Oncol 2008;109:168–73.
10. Jarboe E, Folkins A, Nucci MR, et al. Serous carcinogenesis in the fallopian tube: a descriptive classification. Int J Gynecol Pathol 2008;27:1–9.
11. Obata K, Morland SJ, Watson RH, et al. Frequent PTEN/MMAC mutations in endometrioid but not serous or mucinous epithelial ovarian tumors. Cancer Res 1998;58:2095–7.
12. Sato N, Tsunoda H, Nishida M, et al. Loss of heterozygosity on 10q23.3 and mutation of the tumor suppressor gene PTEN in benign endometrial cyst of the ovary: possible sequence progression from benign endometrial cyst to endometrioid carcinoma and clear cell carcinoma of the ovary. Cancer Res 2000;60:7052–6.
13. Prat J. Ovarian tumors of borderline malignancy (tumors of low malignant potential): a critical appraisal. Adv Anat Pathol 1999;6:247–74.
14. Bell DA, Weinstock MA, Scully RE. Peritoneal implants of ovarian serous borderline tumors. Histologic features and prognosis. Cancer 1988;62:2212–22.
15. Kennedy AW, Hart WR. Ovarian papillary serous tumors of low malignant potential (serous borderline tumors). A long term follow-up study, including patients with microinvasion, lymph node metastasis, and transformation to invasive serous carcinoma. Cancer 1996;78:278–86.
16. Seidman JD, Kurman RJ. Subclassification of serous borderline tumors of the ovary into benign and malignant types. A clinicopathologic study of 65 advanced stage cases. Am J Surg Pathol 1996;20:1331–45.
17. Gershenson DM, Silva EG, Levy L, et al. Ovarian serous borderline tumors with invasive peritoneal implants. Cancer 1998;82:1096–103.
18. Gershenson DM, Silva EG, Tortolero-Luna G, et al. Serous borderline tumors of the ovary with noninvasive peritoneal implants. Cancer 1998;83:2157–63.
19. Prat J, de Nictolis M. Serous borderline tumors of the ovary. A long-term follow-up study of 137 cases, including 18 with micropapillary pattern and 20 with microinvasion. Am J Surg Pathol 2002;26:1111–28.
20. Gilks CB, Alkushi A, Yue JJ, et al. Advanced-stage serous borderline tumors of the ovary: a clinicopathological study of 49 cases. Int J Gynecol Pathol 2003;22:29–36.
21. Longacre TA, McKenney JK, Tazelaar HD, et al. Ovarian serous tumors of low malignant potential (borderline tumors). Outcome-based study of 276 patients with long-term (≥5-year) follow-up. Am J Surg Pathol 2005;29:707–23.
22. Seidman JD, Kurman RJ. Ovarian serous borderline tumors: a critical review of the literature with emphasis on prognostic factors. Hum Pathol 2000;31:539–57.
23. Gilks CB, Prat J. Ovarian carcinoma pathology and genetics: recent advances. Hum Pathol 2009;40:1213–23.
24. Prat J. Ovarian carcinomas: five distinct diseases with different origins, genetic alterations, and clinicopathological features. Virchows Arch 2012;460:237–49.
25. Kurman RJ, Shih IM. The origin and pathogenesis of epithelial ovarian cancer: a proposed unifying theory. Am J Surg Pathol 2010;34:433–43.
26. Koonings PP, Campbell K, Mishell Jr DR, Grimes DA. Relative frequency of primary ovarian neoplasms: a ten year reviews. Obstet Gynecol 1989;74:921–26.
27. Pettersson F. Annual report of the results of treatment in gynecological cancer. Stockholm, Sweden: International Federation of Gynecology and Obstetrics; 1991.
28. Segal GH, Hart WR. Ovarian serous tumors of low malignant potential (serous borderline tumors). The relationship of exophytic surface tumor to peritoneal 'implants.' Am J Surg Pathol 1992;16:577–83.
29. Rollins SE, Young RH, Bell DA. Autoimplants in serous borderline tumors of the ovary: a clinicopathologic study of 30 cases of a process to be distinguished from serous adenocarcinoma. Am J Surg Pathol 2006;30:457–62.
30. Burks RT, Sherman ME, Kurman RJ. Micropapillary serous carcinoma of the ovary. A distinctive low-grade carcinoma related to serous borderline tumors. Am J Surg Pathol 1996;20:1319–30.
31. Eichhorn JH, Bell DA, Young RH, Scully RE. Ovarian serous borderline tumors with micropapillary and cribriform patterns: A study of 40 cases and comparison with 44 cases without these patterns. Am J Surg Pathol 1999;23:397–409.
32. Deavers MT, Gershenson DM, Tortolero-Luna G, et al. Micropapillary and cribriform patterns in ovarian serous tumors of low malignant potential. A study of 99 advanced stage cases. Am J Surg Pathol 2002;26:1129–41.
33. Park JY, Kim DY, Kim JH, et al. Micropapillary pattern in serous borderline ovarian tumors: does it matter? Gynecol Oncol 2011;123:511–16.
34. Avril S, Hahn E, Specht K, et al. Histopathologic features of ovarian borderline tumors are not predictive of clinical outcome. Gynecol Oncol 2012;127:516–24.
35. Tavassoli FA. Serous tumor of low malignant potential with early stromal invasion (serous LMP with microinvasion). Mod Pathol 1988;1:407–13.
36. Bell DA, Scully RE. Ovarian serous borderline tumors with stromal microinvasion: a report of 21 cases. Hum Pathol 1990;21:397–403.
37. Nayar R, Siriaunkgul S, Robbins KM, et al. Microinvasion in low malignant potential tumors of the ovary. Hum Pathol 1996;27:521–7.
38. McKenney JK, Balzer BL, Longacre TA. Patterns of stromal invasion in ovarian serous tumors of low malignant potential (borderline tumors): a reevaluation of the concept of stromal microinvasion. Am J Surg Pathol 2006;30:1209–21.
39. Bell DA, Longacre TA, Prat J, et al. Serous borderline (low malignant potential, atypical proliferative) ovarian tumors. Workshop perspectives. Hum Pathol 2004;35:934–48.
40. Sangoi AR, McKenney JK, Dadras SS, et al. Lymphatic vascular invasion in ovarian serous tumors of low malignant potential with stromal microinvasion: a case control study. Am J Surg Pathol 2008;32:261–8.
41. Singer G, Stöhr R, Cope L, et al. Patterns of p53 mutations separate ovarian serous borderline tumors and low- and high-grade carcinomas and provide support for a new model of ovarian carcinogenesis. A mutational analysis with immunohistochemical correlation. Am J Surg Pathol 2005;29:218–24.
42. de Nictolis M, Montironi R, Tommasoni S, et al. Serous borderline tumors of the ovary: a clinicopathologic, immunohistochemical and quantitative study of 44 cases. Cancer 1992;70:152–60.
43. McCaughey WTE, Kirk ME, Lester W, Dardick I. Peritoneal epithelial lesions associated with proliferative serous tumors of ovary. Histopathology 1984;8:195–208.
44. Bell KA, Smith Sehdev AE, Kurman RJ. Refined diagnostic criteria for implants associated with ovarian atypical proliferative serous tumors (borderline) and micropapillary serous carcinomas. Am J Surg Pathol 2001;25:419–32.
45. Russell P. Borderline epithelial tumours of the ovary: a conceptual dilemma. Clin Obstet Gynecol 1984;11:259–77.
46. Lee ES, Leong AS-Y, Kim Y-S, et al. Calretinin, CD34 and alpha-smooth muscle actin in the identification of peritoneal invasive implants of serous borderline tumors of the ovary. Mod Pathol 2006;19:364–72.
47. Caduff RF, Svoboda-Newman SM, Ferguson AW, et al. Comparison of mutations of Ki-ras and p53 immunoreactivity in borderline and malignant epithelial ovarian tumors. Am J Surg Pathol 1999;23:323–8.
48. Singer G, Kurman RJ, Chang H-W, et al. Diverse tumorigenic pathways in ovarian serous carcinoma. Am J Pathol 2002;160:1223–8.
49. Ho CL, Kurman RJ, Dehari R, et al. Mutations of BRAF and RAS precede the development of ovarian serous borderline tumors. Cancer Res 2004;64:6915–18.
50. Alvarez AA, Moore WF, Robboy SJ, et al. K-ras mutations in mullerian inclusion cysts associated with serous borderline tumors of the ovary. Gynecol Oncol 2001;80:201–6.

51. Sieben NLG, Oosting J, Flanagan AM, et al. Differential gene expression in ovarian tumors reveals Dusp-4 and serpina-5 as key regulators for benign behavior of serous borderline tumors. J Clin Oncol 2005;23:7257–64.
52. Bonome T, Lee JY, Park DC, et al. Expression profiling of serous low malignant potential, low-grade, and high-grade tumors of the ovary. Cancer Res 2005;65:10602–12.
53. Gu J, Roth LM, Younger C, et al. Molecular evidence for the independent origin of extra-ovarian papillary serous tumors of low malignant potential. J Natl Cancer Inst 2001;93:1147–52.
54. Lu KH, Bell DA, Welch WR, et al. Evidence for the multifocal origin of bilateral and advanced human serous borderline ovarian tumors. Cancer Res 1998;58:2328–30.
55. Sieben NLG, Roemen GMJM, Oosting J, et al. Clonal analysis favours a monoclonal origin for serous borderline tumors with peritoneal implants. J Pathol 2006;210:405–11.
56. Kurman RJ, Vang R, Junge J, et al. Papillary tubal hyperplasia: the putative precursor of ovarian atypical proliferative (borderline) serous tumors, noninvasive implants, and endosalpingiosis. Am J Surg Pathol 2011;35:1605–14.
57. Laury AR, Ning G, Quick CM, et al. Fallopian tube correlates of serous borderline tumors. Am J Surg Pathol 2011; 35:1759–65.
58. Silva EG, Tornos C, Zhuang Z, et al. Tumor recurrence in stage I ovarian serous neoplasms of low malignant potential. Int J Gynecol Pathol 1998;17:1–6.
59. Lee KR, Castrillon DH, Nucci MR. Pathologic findings in eight cases of ovarian serous borderline tumors, three with foci of serous carcinoma, that preceded death or morbidity from invasive carcinoma. Int J Gynecol Pathol 2001;20:329–34.
60. Parker RL, Clement PB, Chercover DJ, et al. Early recurrence of ovarian serous borderline tumor as high-grade carcinoma: a report of two cases. Int J Gynecol Pathol 2004;23:265–72.
61. Leake JF, Rader JS, Woodruff JD, Rosenshein NB. Retroperitoneal lymphatic involvement with epithelial ovarian tumors of low malignant potential. Gynecol Oncol 1991;42:124–30.
62. Tan LK, Flynn SD, Carcangiu ML. Ovarian serous borderline tumors with lymph node involvement. Clinicopathologic and DNA content study of seven cases and review of the literature. Am J Surg Pathol 1994;18:904–12.
63. McKenney JK, Balzer BL, Longacre TA. Lymph node involvement in ovarian serous tumors of low malignant potential (borderline tumors): pathology, prognosis, and proposed classification. Am J Surg Pathol 2006;30:614–24.
64. Djordjevic B, Malpica A. Lymph node involvement in ovarian serous tumors of low malignant potential: with lymph node involvement: a clinicopathologic study of thirty-six cases. Am J Surg Pathol 2010;34:1–9.
65. Djordjevic B, Clement-Kruzel S, Atkinson NE, Malpica A. Nodal endosalpingiosis in ovarian serous tumors of low malignant potential with lymph node involvement: a case for a precursor lesion. Am J Surg Pathol 2010;34:1442–8.
66. Moore WF, Bentley RC, Berchuck A, Robboy SJ. Some mullerian inclusion cysts in lymph nodes and peritoneum are metastases from serous borderline tumors of the ovary. Am J Surg Pathol 2000;24:710–18.
67. Djordjevic B, Malpica A. Ovarian serous tumors of low malignant potential with nodal low-grade serous carcinoma. Am J Surg Pathol 2012;36:955–63.
68. Clement PB, Young RH, Oliva E, et al. Hyperplastic mesothelial cells within abdominal lymph nodes: mimic of metastatic ovarian carcinoma and serous borderline tumor—a report of two cases associated with ovarian neoplasms. Mod Pathol 1996;9:879–86.
69. Argani P, Rosai J. Hyperplastic mesothelial cells in lymph nodes: report of six cases of a benign process that can simulate metastatic involvement by mesothelioma or carcinoma. Hum Pathol 1998;29:339–46.
70. McCluggage WG. Immunohistochemical and functional biomarkers of value in female genital tract lesions. Int J Gynecol Pathol 2006;25:101–20.
71. Bell DA, Scully RE. Serous borderline tumors of the peritoneum. Am J Surg Pathol 1990;14:230–9.
72. Biscotti CV, Hart WR. Peritoneal serous papillomatosis of low malignant potential (serous borderline tumors of the peritoneum). A clinicopathologic study of 17 cases. Am J Surg Pathol 1992;16:467–75.
73. Barnhill DR, Kurman RJ, Brady MF, et al. Preliminary analysis of the behavior of stage I ovarian serous tumors of low malignant potential: a Gynecologic Oncology Group study. J Clin Oncol 1995;13:2752–6.
74. Lim-Tan SK, Cajigas HE, Scully RE. Ovarian cystectomy for serous borderline tumors: a follow-up study of 35 cases. Obstet Gynecol 1988;72:775–81.
75. Lin PS, Gershenson DM, Bevers MW, et al. The current status of surgical staging of ovarian serous borderline tumors. Cancer 1999;85:905–11.
76. Papadimitriou DS, Martin-Hirsch P, Kitchener HC, et al. Recurrent borderline tumors after conservative treatment management in women wishing to retain their fertility. Eur J Gynecol Oncol 1999;20:94–7.
77. Gershenson DM. Contemporary treatment of borderline ovarian tumors. Cancer Invest 1999;17:206–10.
78. Bristow RE, Gossett DR, Shook DR, et al. Recurrent micropapillary serous ovarian carcinoma: the role of secondary cytoreductive surgery. Cancer 2002;95:791–800.
79. Heintz AP, Odicino F, Maisonneuve P, et al. Carcinoma of the ovary. Int J Gynecol Obstet 2003;83S:133–66.
80. Zuna RE, Behrens A. Peritoneal washing cytology in gynecologic cancers. J Natl Cancer Inst 1996;88:980–7.
81. Malpica A, Deavers MT, Lu K, et al. Grading ovarian serous carcinoma using a two-tier system. Am J Surg Pathol 2004;28:496–504.
82. Singer G, Oldt 3rd R, Cohen Y, et al. Mutations in BRAF and KRAS characterize the development of low-grade ovarian serous carcinoma. J Natl Cancer Inst 2003;95:484–6.
83. Gershenson DM, Sun CC, Lu KH, et al. Clinical behavior of stage II–IV low-grade serous carcinoma of the ovary. Obstet Gynecol 2006;108:361–8.
84. Malpica A, Deavers MT, Tornos C, et al. Inter-observer and intraobserver variability of a two-tier system for grading ovarian serous carcinoma. Am J Surg Pathol 2007;31:1203–8.
85. Ayhan A, Kurman RJ, Yemelyanova A, et al. Defining the cut-point between low- and high-grade ovarian serous carcinomas: a clinicopathologic and molecular genetic analysis. Am J Surg Pathol 2009;33:1220–4.
86. Gilks CB, Bell DA, Scully RE. Serous psammocarcinoma of the ovary and peritoneum. Int J Gynecol Pathol 1990;9:110–21.
87. Köbel M, Kalloger SE, Boyd N, et al. Ovarian carcinoma subtypes are different diseases: implications for biomarker studies. PLoS Med 2008;5:e232.
88. Jones S, Wang T-L, Kurman RJ, et al. Low-grade serous carcinomas of the ovary contain very few point mutations. J Pathol 2012; 226:413–20.
89. Shvartsman HS, Sun CC, Bodurka CC, et al. Comparison of the clinical behavior of newly diagnosed stages II–IV low-grade serous carcinoma of the ovary with that of serous ovarian tumors of low malignant potential that recur as low grade serous carcinoma. Gynecol Oncol 2007;105:625–9.
90. Crispens MA, Bodurka D, Deavers M, et al. Response and survival in patients with progressive or recurrent serous ovarian tumors of low malignant potential. Obstet Gynecol 2002;99:3–10.
91. Prat J, Ribe A, Gallardo A. Hereditary ovarian cancer. Hum Pathol 2005;36:861–70.
92. Curtin JP, Barakat RR, Hoskins WJ. Ovarian disease in women with breast cancer. Obstet Gynecol 1994;84:449–52.
93. Garg R, Zahurak ML, Trimble EL, et al. Abdominal carcinomatosis in women with a history of breast cancer. Gynecol Oncol 2005;99:65–70.
94. Gilks CB, Ionescu DN, Kalloger SE, et al. Tumor cell type can be reproducibly diagnosed and is of independent prognostic significance in patients with maximally debulked ovarian carcinoma. Hum Pathol 2008;39:1239–51.
95. Eichhorn JH, Young RH. Transitional cell carcinoma of the ovary: a morphologic study of 100 cases with emphasis on differential diagnosis. Am J Surg Pathol 2004;28:453–63.
96. Cuatrecasas M, Catasus L, Palacios J, Prat J. Transitional cell tumors of the ovary: a comparative clinicopathologic, immunohistochemical, and molecular genetic analysis of Brenner tumors and transitional cell carcinomas. Am J Surg Pathol 2009;33:556–7.
97. Ali RH, Seidman JD, Luk M, et al. Transitional cell carcinoma of the ovary is related to high-grade serous carcinoma and is distinct

from malignant Brenner tumor. Int J Gynecol Pathol 2012;31:499–506.
98. Baker PM, Oliva E. Immunohistochemistry as a tool in the differential diagnosis of ovarian tumors: an update. Int J Gynecol Pathol 2005;24:39–55.
99. Kubba LA, McCluggage WG, Liu J, et al. Thyroid transcription factor-1 expression in ovarian epithelial neoplasms. Mod Pathol 2008;21:485–90.
100. Al-Hussaini M, Stockman A, Foster H, McCluggage WG. WT-1 assists in distinguishing ovarian from uterine serous carcinoma and in distinguishing between serous and endometrioid ovarian carcinoma. Histopathology 2004;44:109–15.
101. Köbel M, Kalloger SE, Carrick J, et al. A limited panel of immunomarkers can reliably distinguish between clear cell and high-grade serous carcinoma of the ovary. Am J Surg Pathol 2009;33:14–21.
102. Yamamoto S, Tsuda H, Kita T, et al. Clinicopathological significance of WT1 expression in ovarian cancer: a possible accelerator of tumor progression in serous adenocarcinoma. Virchows Arch 2007;451:27–35.
103. Risch HA, McLaughlin JR, Cole DE, et al. Population BRCA1 and BRCA2 mutation frequencies and cancer penetrances: a kin-cohort study in Ontario, Canada. J Natl Cancer Inst 2006;98:1694–706.
104. Venkitaraman AR. Linking the cellular functions of BRCA genes to cancer pathogenesis and treatment. Annu Rev Pathol 2009;4:461–87.
105. Geisler JP, Hatterman-Zogg MA, Rathe JA, Buller RE. Frequency of BRCA1 dysfunction in ovarian cancer. J Natl Cancer Inst 2002;94:61–7.
106. Esteller M, Silva JM, Dominguez G, et al. Promoter hypermethylation is a cause of BRCA1 inactivation in sporadic breast and ovarian tumors. J Natl Cancer Inst 2000;92:564–9.
107. Bowtell DD. The genesis and evolution of high-grade serous ovarian cancer. Nat Rev Cancer 2010;10:803–8.
108. Levanon K, Ng V, Piao HY, et al. Primary ex vivo cultures of human fallopian tube epithelium as a model for serous ovarian carcinogenesis. Oncogene 2010;29:1103–13.
109. Powell CB, Kenley E, Chen LM, et al. Risk reducing salpingo-oophorectomy in BRCA mutation carriers: role of serial sectioning in the detection of occult malignancy. J Clin Oncol 2005;23:127–32.
110. Vaughan S, Coward JI, Bast Jr RC, et al. Rethinking ovarian cancer: recommendations for improving outcomes. Nat Rev Cancer 2011;11:719–25.
111. Pothuri B, Leitao MM, Levine DA, et al. Genetic analysis of the early natural history of epithelial ovarian carcinoma. PLoS One 2010;5:e10358.
112. Norquist BM, Garcia RL, Allison KH, et al. The molecular pathogenesis of hereditary ovarian carcinoma: alterations in the tubal epithelium of women with BRCA1 and BRCA2 mutations. Cancer 2010;116:5261–71.
113. Schorge JO, Muto MG, Lee SJ, et al. BRCA1-related papillary serous carcinoma of the peritoneum has a unique molecular pathogenesis. Cancer Res 2000;60:1361–4.
114. Irving JA, Catasus L, Gallardo A, et al. Synchronous endometrioid carcinomas of the uterine corpus and ovary: Alterations in the beta-catenin (CTNNB1) pathway are associated with independent primary tumors and favorable prognosis. Hum Pathol 2005;36:605–19.
115. Kobel M, Kalloger SE, Baker PM, et al. Diagnosis of ovarian carcinoma cell type is highly reproducible: a transcanadian study. Am J Surg Pathol 2010;34:984–93.
116. Yaziji H, Gown AM. Immunohistochemical analysis of gynecologic tumors. Int J Gynecol Pathol 2001; 20:64–78.
117. Cannistra SA. Cancer of the ovary. N Engl J Med 2004;351:2519–29.
118. Chan JK, Tian C, Monk B, et al. Prognostic factors for high-risk early-stage epithelial ovarian cancer: a Gynecologic Oncology Group study. Cancer 2008;112:2202–10.
119. Leitao MM, Boyd J, Hummer A, et al. Clinicopathologic analysis of early-stage sporadic ovarian carcinoma. Am J Surg Pathol 2004;28:147–59.
120. Obermair A, Fuller A, Lopez-Varela E, et al. A new prognostic model for FIGO stage I epithelial ovarian cancer. Gynecol Oncol 2007;104:607–11.
121. Onda T, Yoshikawa H, Yasugi T, et al. Patients with ovarian carcinoma upstaged to stage III after systematic lymphadenectomy have similar survival to stage I/II patients and superior survival to other stage III patients. Cancer 1998;83:1555–60.
122. Cliby WA, Aletti GD, Wilson TO, et al. Is it justified to classify patients to stage IIIC epithelial ovarian cancer based on nodal involvement only? Gynecol Oncol 2006;103:797–801.
123. Harter P, Gnauert K, Hils R, et al. Pattern and clinical predictors of lymph node metastases in epithelial ovarian cancer. Int J Gynecol Cancer 2007;17:1238–44.
124. Bristow RE, Tomacruz RS, Armstrong DK, et al. Survival effect of maximal cytoreductive surgery for advanced ovarian carcinoma during the platinum era: a meta-analysis. J Clin Oncol 2002;20:1248–59.
125. Hennessy BT, Coleman RL, Markman M. Ovarian cancer. Lancet 2009;374:1371–82.
126. Ferrara N, Gerber HP, LeCouter J. The biology of VEGF and its receptors. Nat Med 2003;9:669–76.
127. McGuire WP, Hoskins WJ, Brady MF, et al. Cyclophosphamide and cisplatin compared with paclitaxel and cisplatin in patients with stage III and stage IV ovarian cancer. N Engl J Med 1996;334:1–6.

Ovarian Mucinous Tumors

26

Jaime Prat

CHAPTER OUTLINE

General Features	591	Mucinous Cystic Tumors Associated with Pseudomyxoma Peritonei	598
Benign Mucinous Tumors	592	Mucinous Adenocarcinomas	600
Mucinous Borderline Tumors	593	Mural Nodules	604
Mucinous Borderline Tumors, Endocervical-Like	593		
Mucinous Borderline Tumors, Gastrointestinal Type	595		

GENERAL FEATURES

Mucinous tumors show cysts and glands lined by epithelial cells containing intracytoplasmic mucin. The tumor cells may resemble those of the endocervix, gastric pylorus, or intestine. They are typically diastase resistant PAS positive, and mucicarmine positive. Mucinous tumors account for 10–15% of all primary ovarian tumors.[1] Approximately 80% are benign and the remainder are borderline tumors, non-invasive carcinomas, and invasive carcinomas.[1] Although they generally occur in older women (mean ages 51–54 years), mucinous borderline tumors and carcinomas are more common in the first two decades than their serous counterparts.[2] Mucinous tumors, especially the borderline tumors, tend to be the largest of all ovarian tumors. Many of them are 15–30 cm in diameter and weigh up to 4000 g or more.[2]

Mucinous ovarian tumors are difficult to interpret. Over the past 40 years, their classification has changed considerably as a result of the following: (1) the separation of mucinous borderline tumors from mucinous carcinomas, (2) the recognition of mucinous borderline tumors *with intraepithelial carcinoma* (IEC), (3) the evidence that most ovarian mucinous cystic tumors associated with pseudomyxoma peritonei are low-grade appendiceal mucinous neoplasms that involve the ovary secondarily, and (4) the increasing recognition of metastatic adenocarcinomas of intestinal and pancreatic origin that closely resemble primary ovarian mucinous tumors.

Although mucinous ovarian tumors are currently classified as surface epithelial tumors, their origin is unclear in most cases. Some mucinous tumors are of germ cell origin (monodermal teratomas), but neometaplasia of the ovarian surface epithelium is an alternative explanation for their development.[2] In fact, transitions between mucinous tumors and serous and endometrioid tumors are occasionally seen. Also, serous and endometrioid tumors may secrete mucin from the apical pole of the epithelial cells, resulting in abundant intracystic mucus, but are not generally intracytoplasmic. Mucinous tumors may be associated with dermoid cysts (3–5%), Brenner tumors, and mucinous tumors of other organs such as the uterine cervix and appendix.[2] In patients with the Peutz–Jeghers syndrome, well-differentiated mucinous ovarian tumors may be accompanied by minimal deviation adenocarcinomas ('adenoma malignum') of the cervix. Occasionally, mucinous cystic ovarian tumors may develop from heterologous gastrointestinal elements in a Sertoli–Leydig cell tumor.

Mucinous ovarian tumors are among the most common non-endocrine neoplasms presenting hormonal manifestations. Most times, the endocrine symptoms are due to the secretion of steroid hormones, which the ovarian stroma adjacent to the tumor produces.[2,3] The serum level of inhibin (a hormone produced by ovarian granulosa and lutein cells that inhibits the secretion of follicle-stimulating hormone by the anterior pituitary gland) is considered to be a tumor marker for mucinous borderline tumors and carcinomas, possibly due to the reactive luteinized cells that develop in the adjacent stroma.[4] Less frequently, patients present with Zollinger–Ellison syndrome, secondary to gastrin secretion by neuroendocrine cells in the gastrointestinal mucinous epithelium, and rarely, the carcinoid syndrome (see Chapter 29). CA125, carcinoembryonic antigen (CEA), and CA19-9 are often elevated in mucinous carcinomas.

Ovarian mucinous tumors are subdivided into benign, borderline, and malignant categories depending on their degree of cell proliferation, nuclear atypia, and the presence or absence of stromal invasion. In contrast to serous tumors, which are characteristically homogeneous in their degree of differentiation, mucinous tumors often are heterogeneous. Benign-appearing, borderline, and invasive patterns may coexist within an individual neoplasm; also, not infrequently, the degree of malignancy of the carcinomatous component varies from noninvasive to invasive and from well-differentiated to poorly differentiated or even undifferentiated (anaplastic) carcinoma. Such morphologic continuum suggests that tumor progression occurs from cystadenoma and borderline tumor to noninvasive, microinvasive, and invasive carcinoma. This hypothesis is supported by studies of *K-RAS* mutations, which are common in mucinous ovarian tumors and represent an early event in mucinous ovarian tumorigenesis. Mucinous borderline tumors have a higher frequency of *K-RAS* mutations than that of mucinous cystadenomas, but lower than mucinous carcinomas.[5–9] Using microdissection, the same *K-RAS* mutation has been detected in benign-appearing, borderline, and malignant areas of the same tumor.[5] From a practical viewpoint, the prognostic evaluation of mucinous ovarian tumors other than benign cystadenomas is difficult because of their typical large size, and the great variation in the degree of differentiation of individual tumors. Extensive sampling is important, especially of areas that appear nodular or solid.

BENIGN MUCINOUS TUMORS

Clinical Profile

Benign mucinous cystadenomas constitute approximately 80% of ovarian mucinous tumors. They occur most frequently during the third to sixth decades, although may also be encountered in younger women. This age distribution accounts for their frequent occurrence during pregnancy.

Macroscopic Features

Mucinous cystadenomas are often large (mean size, 10 cm), unilateral, multilocular, but sometimes unilocular cystic tumors containing mucoid material. The outer cyst wall is often thick with a smooth or bosselated surface. The rare mucinous cystadenofibromas and adenofibromas are partly to almost completely solid with small cysts (Figure 26.1). Benign mucinous tumors are typically unilateral in 95% of cases.

Microscopic Features

Mucinous cystadenomas are composed of glands and cysts lined by a single layer of columnar cells with abundant intracellular mucin. Cellular stratification is minimal, and nuclei are basally located with only mild atypia (Figure 26.2).[10] If epithelial proliferation resembling a borderline mucinous tumor is present, this feature must be limited to <10% of the epithelial volume for the tumor to qualify as a cystadenoma.[11] Papillae are unusual except in rare cases of mucinous cystadenomas of endocervical type, which are conspicuously papillary. Goblet cells, neuroendocrine cells, and, rarely, Paneth cells may be encountered in mucinous cystadenomas of gastrointestinal type. However, gastric foveolar-type epithelium or intestinal epithelium with goblet cells is found more often in mucinous borderline tumors and carcinomas. Reactive nuclear atypia and mitotic activity can be seen in peripheral crypt-like structures. The stroma is fibrocollagenous and exhibits variable cellularity. Occasionally, marked prominence of the stroma occurs between glands, giving rise to patterns of adenofibroma (Figure 26.3). Stromal cellularity may be increased in the vicinity of the epithelium where lutein-like cells are seen in 25% of cases. Rare benign tumors may show definite Leydig cells (with crystals) in the adjacent stroma. Smooth muscle may develop sometimes in the stroma running parallel to the cyst linings.

Rupture of mucinous glands and cysts is common, resulting in extravasation of mucin into the stroma, and often a marked inflammatory response. Such a finding must be distinguished from large pools of dissecting mucin (pseudomyxoma ovarii), which is a characteristic feature of mucinous ovarian tumors associated with pseudomyxoma peritonei (see later). In about 5% of mucinous cystadenomas, the mucin in the stroma typically elicits a histiocytic and foreign body giant cell response (mucin granuloma) (Figure 26.4). Extruded neoplastic epithelium from an adjacent ruptured gland, particularly if accompanied by a mucin

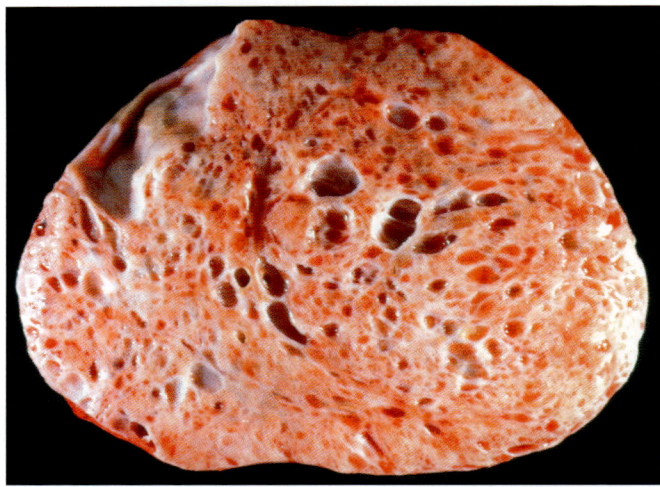

Figure 26.1 Mucinous cystadenofibroma. The sectioned surface appears partly solid with numerous small cysts.

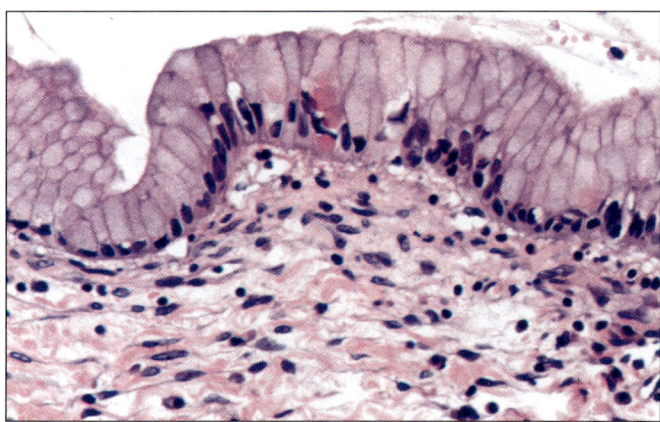

Figure 26.2 Mucinous cystadenoma. The cytoplasms appear full of mucin and the nuclei are small and basal.

granuloma, should be distinguished from stromal microinvasion (see later). Mucinous cystadenomas and adenofibromas are benign but can recur if incompletely excised. Tumor rupture is not associated with recurrence.

Mucinous cystadenomas are associated with dermoid cysts in 5% of cases[2] and with Brenner tumors in 18%.[12] Accordingly, it has been suggested that mucinous tumors of intestinal type may be of germ cell origin or arise from Brenner tumors.

MUCINOUS BORDERLINE TUMORS

Mucinous borderline tumors (MBTs) exhibit an epithelial proliferation of mucinous-type cells greater than that seen in their benign counterparts, but without destructive stromal invasion. The proliferative areas must constitute greater than 10% of the epithelial volume of the tumor.[11] In the Western world, MBTs are less common than serous borderline tumors (SBTs). Of the 20% of primary mucinous tumors that are not cystadenomas, MBTs outnumber the invasive carcinomas.[13] MBTs have been subclassified into two different clinicopathologic forms: the most common form is composed of gastrointestinal-type epithelium and is designated MBT of *gastrointestinal type*. A second and less common variant of MBT contains endocervical-type epithelium and has been named MBT *endocervical-like* (Figure 26.5).[14]

MUCINOUS BORDERLINE TUMORS, ENDOCERVICAL-LIKE

Endocervical MBTs,[14] also designated as müllerian MBTs, account for 10–15% of MBTs. About 140 cases have been reported.[14-17] These tumors differ in many respects from intestinal MBTs, as shown in Table 26.1. The average age of the patients with endocervical MBTs is 40 years, with a range of 15–84 years.[14-17] An association with endometriosis is frequent (35–50%).[16] At the time of diagnosis, most tumors are confined to the ovary and approximately 20% have spread to the peritoneum or regional lymph nodes.[14]

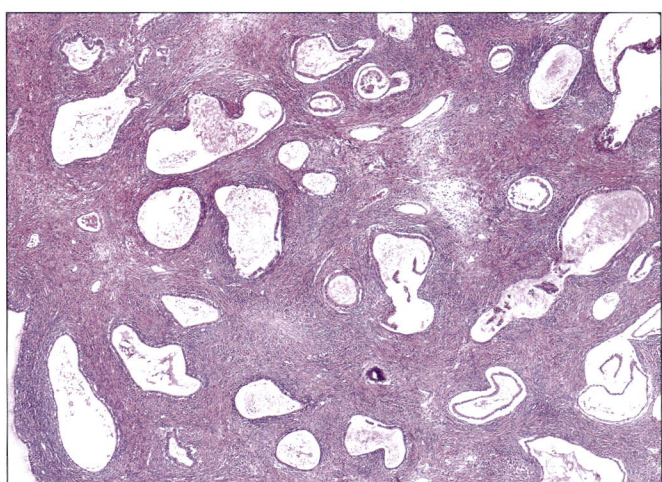

Figure 26.3 Mucinous cystadenofibroma. Benign mucinous cystic glands lay in dense fibrous stroma.

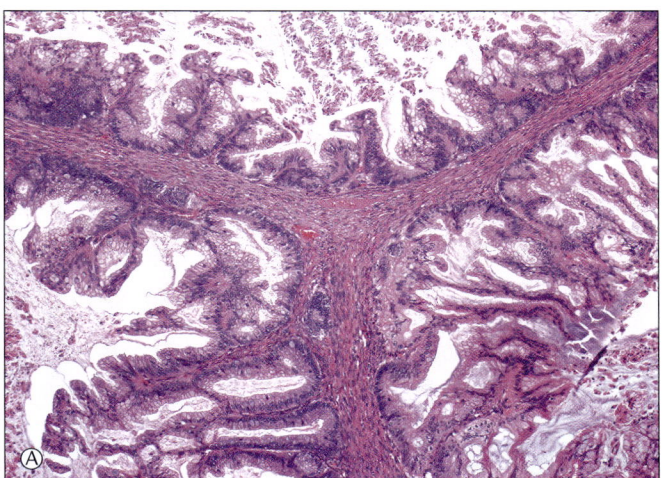

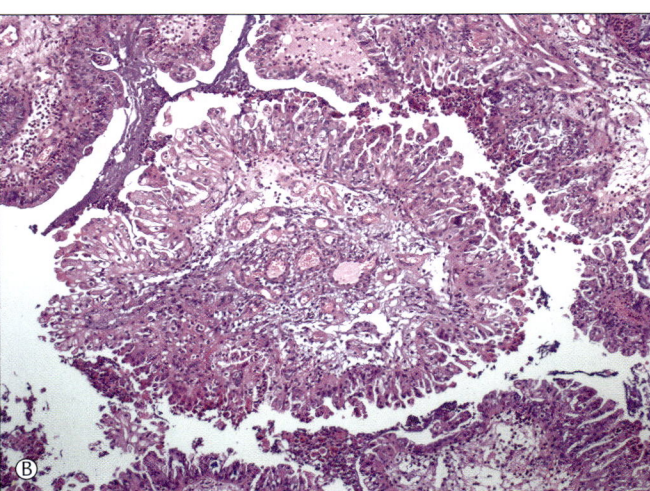

Figure 26.5 Mucinous borderline tumors. **(A)** The gastrointestinal-type tumor resembles a colonic polyp and contains goblet cells. **(B)** The endocervical-like (müllerian type) tumor shows mucinous epithelial cells resembling endocervical epithelium (upper left) and indifferent cells. None of the tumors shows stromal invasion.

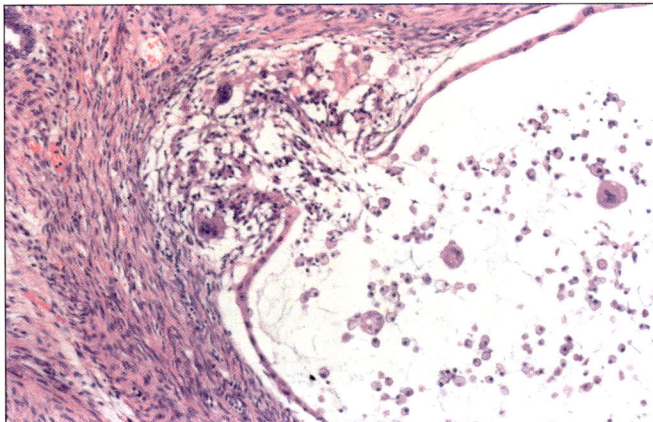

Figure 26.4 Mucinous cystadenofibroma. Ruptured gland with mucin granuloma.

Table 26.1 Mucinous Borderline Tumors[14]		
	Endocervical-like MBT (%)	Intestinal-type MBT (%)
Frequency	15	85
Average age (years)	34	41
Bilaterality	40	6
Diameter (cm)	8	19
Multilocular	20	72
Goblet cells	0	100
Grimelius +ve cell	3	86
Acute inflammation	100	0
Endometriosis	30	6
Stage II–III	24	10
Impl +/or LN Mets	20	0
Pseudomyxoma P	0	17

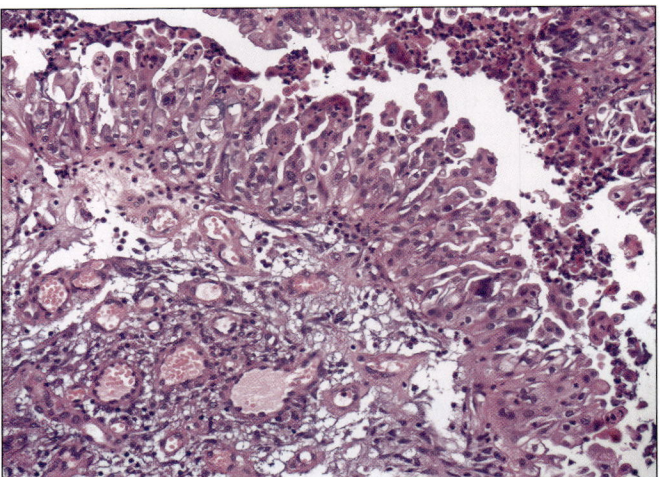

Figure 26.7 Mucinous borderline tumor, endocervical-like (müllerian type). Mucinous and indifferent cells with eosinophilic cytoplasm and tufting. A neutrophil infiltration is seen.

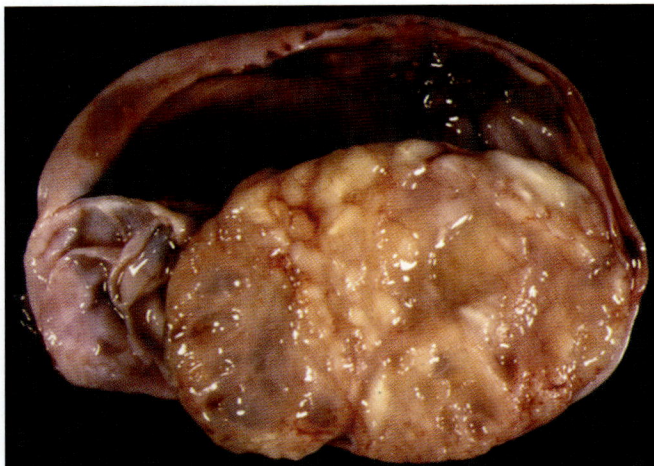

Figure 26.6 Mucinous borderline tumor, endocervical-like (müllerian type). The sectioned surface shows a solid mucinous nodule arising in an endometriotic cyst.

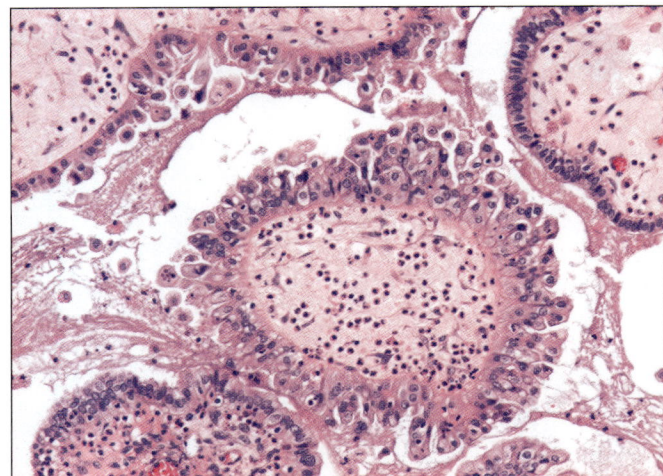

Figure 26.8 Mucinous borderline tumor, endocervical-like (müllerian type). Stratification with cellular budding is evident. Neutrophils are seen in the stroma and epithelium. (Reproduced with permission of Lippincott Williams & Wilkins.)

No association with pseudomyxoma peritonei has been described.

Macroscopic Features

The tumors average 8–10 cm in diameter, with a range from 2 to 36 cm. About 80% are unilocular or contain three or fewer locules. Most of them show grossly visible intracystic papillae (Figure 26.6). From 12% to 40% are bilateral at presentation[14–17] and the contralateral ovary is subsequently involved by an endocervical-type MBT in an additional 7% of cases.[14]

Microscopic Features

The tumors contain complex papillae architecturally similar to those of SBTs. The epithelial lining is composed of columnar, mucin-containing cells that resemble endocervical cells as well as indifferent polygonal cells with abundant eosinophilic cytoplasm that are usually located at the tips of papillae (Figure 26.7).[14] The nuclei exhibit mild to focally severe atypia. Mitotic figures are infrequent. No destructive invasion of the stroma is observed. Nuclear stratification in the absence of recognizable stromal invasion cannot be used as a diagnostic criterion of carcinoma in endocervical-type MBTs as the polygonal eosinophilic cells may be stratified up to 20 or more in height (Figure 26.8).[14] Rare tumors exhibit foci of micropapillary growth similar to the micropapillary pattern seen in SBTs.[15] Other epithelial cells of müllerian type may be present, including ciliated serous cells, endometrioid cells, and squamous epithelium.[18,19] From 30% to 50% of the tumors show a transition from mucinous neoplasia to endometriosis.[14,16,18] No areas of intestinal differentiation are usually seen. Typically, polymorphonuclear leukocytes infiltrate the stroma of the papillae, the neoplastic epithelium, and the intraluminal mucin in almost all cases (Figure 26.9).

Endocervical-type MBTs with intraepithelial carcinoma have been described.[15–17] Morphologic features of the intraepithelial carcinoma include foci showing a cribriform pattern of growth and stroma-free cellular papillae, or nuclear features of malignancy (Figure 26.10). In most cases, the

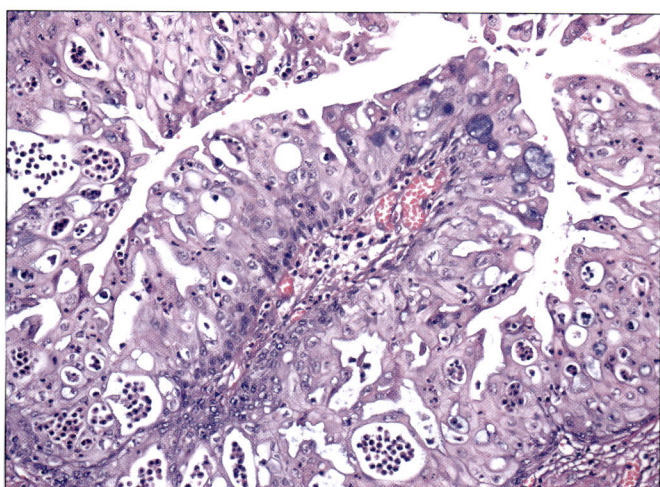

Figure 26.9 Mucinous borderline tumor, endocervical-like (müllerian type). Cellular stratification and prominent intraepithelial neutrophil infiltration.

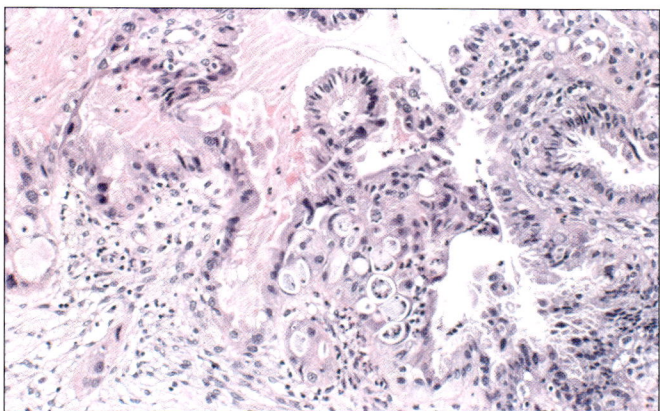

Figure 26.10 Mucinous endocervical-like borderline tumor with IEC and microinvasion. The lining epithelium shows cell stratification, cribriform pattern, and marked nuclear atypia. A nest of invasive cells is seen at the lower left corner.

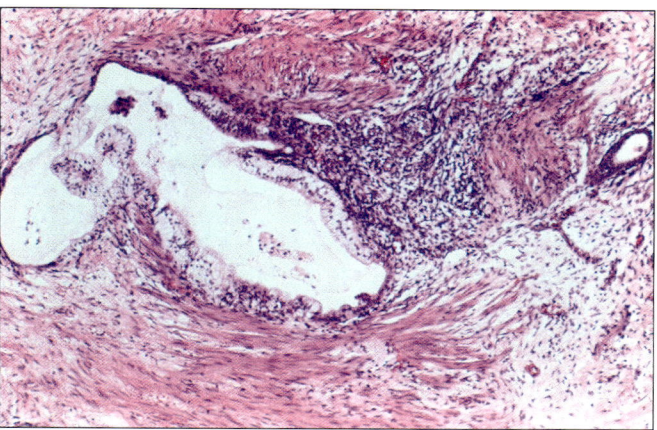

Figure 26.11 Isolated peritoneal implant of mucinous endocervical-like borderline tumor.

intraepithelial carcinoma in endocervical-type MBT consists of multiple foci usually measuring less than 1 or 2 mm in linear dimension. Classification of these tumors as intraepithelial carcinoma seems justified by the mean 7 year disease-free follow-up interval for 10 patients with this diagnosis.[15-17] Since few cases have been reported and the follow-up intervals were relatively short, the favorable behavior of these tumors needs confirmation by additional investigations.

Microinvasion has been described in 24 endocervical-type MBTs (19%) from five different series.[15-17,20,21] The microinvasive foci ranged from <2 to 5 mm in greatest diameter, and were similar to those found more commonly in SBTs (Figure 26.10). Twelve patients with prolonged follow-up were without evidence of disease at an average of 8 years.[15-17,20,21]

Endocervical-type MBTs may be associated with pelvic or abdominal implants (3–20%), which are characteristically discrete and contain mucinous glands in a fibrous stroma (desmoplastic implants) (Figure 26.11).[14,16] In some cases the peritoneal implants may arise from independent foci of endometriosis. Some implants may appear invasive.

Immunohistochemistry and Somatic Genetics

Endocervical MBTs frequently express cytokeratin 7 (CK7; 100%), estrogen receptor (ER; 100%), progesterone receptor (PR; 67%), CA125 (92%), and mesothelin (83%). Expression of WT1 is rare (8%) and, in contrast to gastrointestinal MBTs, immunoreactivity for CK20 and CDX2 is absent.[22-24] Therefore, the gastrointestinal and endocervical types of MBTs are immunophenotypically distinctive tumors. Whereas the former express markers of intestinal-type differentiation (CK20 and CDX2), the latter show expression of müllerian-type markers (ER, PR, CA125, and mesothelin). The müllerian immunoprofile of endocervical MBTs, as well as their frequent association with endometriosis, supports the concept that this subtype of mucinous tumors is closely related to endometrioid tumors and justifies the designation 'müllerian.' Designating this tumor partially as 'seromucinous' is incomplete, and ignores the common presence of other müllerian components such as endometrioid or squamous elements.[19] Furthermore, the recent finding in these tumors of loss of expression or mutation of *ARID1A*, which occurs in most endometriosis-associated ovarian tumors but not in pure serous tumors, favors the term müllerian over seromucinous.[25]

Treatment and Prognosis

Stage I endocervical-type MBTs are generally treated like SBTs (see Chapter 25). If the contralateral normal-appearing ovary is conserved, the patient should be followed closely for possible development of a similar tumor in it. The prognosis of endocervical-type MBT is excellent and approximates that of SBTs. Recent studies report that foci of IEC or microinvasion do not influence the prognosis.[15-17] No deaths from these tumors have been well documented, although most reported follow-up has been under 5 years.[14-16,26-28] There is no evidence that chemotherapy is necessary or helpful, even for patients with higher stage disease.[2,14]

MUCINOUS BORDERLINE TUMORS, GASTROINTESTINAL TYPE

These tumors account for 85% of MBTs and occur most frequently in the fourth to seventh decades (average age, 52 years).[2,26-34] About 80–90% are stage I and only 5% are bilateral.[2,26–34] Of note, metastatic mucinous tumors in the ovary often mimic primary ovarian mucinous neoplasms, particularly adenocarcinomas of the pancreas and large intestine (see Chapter 30).[35] Microscopically, the metastatic tumor may appear deceptively 'benign,' 'borderline,' or malignant. It has been established that most, if not all, ovarian mucinous tumors associated with pseudomyxoma peritonei are secondary tumors, frequently low-grade appendiceal mucinous neoplasms (see later).[36] Bilaterality is exceptional in stage I ovarian mucinous tumors; therefore, tumor involvement of both ovaries should raise the suspicion of metastatic carcinoma.

Macroscopic Features

On gross examination, the tumors average 19 cm in diameter, are usually cystic and multilocular, and contain mucinous fluid (Figure 26.12). Papillae and polypoid excrescences may line the cysts. MBTs of gastrointestinal type cannot be distinguished grossly from mucinous cystadenomas and cystadenocarcinomas. These tumors should be sampled extensively, particularly the solid portions, since variable degrees of epithelial proliferation and nuclear atypia (from benign to borderline, and to carcinoma) coexist frequently within an individual neoplasm.

Microscopic Features

Microscopically, MBTs of gastrointestinal type consist of cysts and glands lined by atypical epithelium of gastric pyloric type. The cysts may contain papillae that are typically thin and branching (Figure 26.13). The lining epithelium almost always contains goblet cells and may have argyrophil cells and occasional Paneth cells. The epithelial cells are usually stratified to two or three layers, nuclear atypia is mild to moderate, and mitotic figures vary from few to numerous. High-grade nuclear features are absent and stromal invasion is not seen (Figure 26.14). The overall appearance resembles that of a hyperplastic or adenomatous colonic polyp. Most tumors also

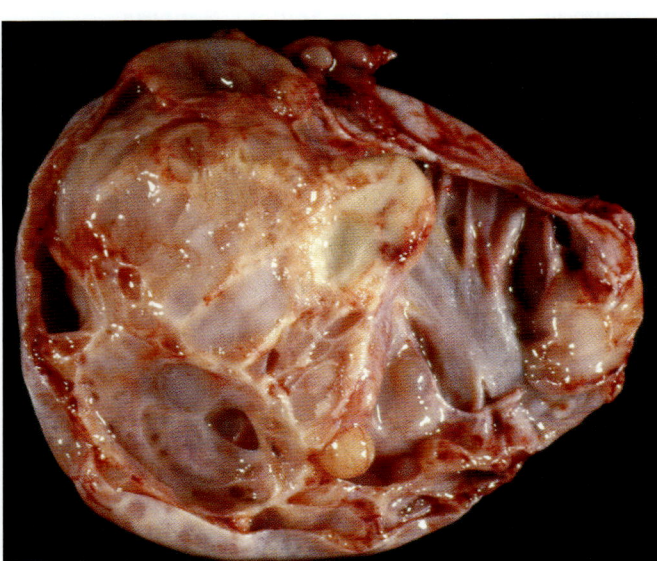

Figure 26.12 Mucinous cystic borderline tumor of intestinal type. The sectioned surface shows a multiloculated cystic tumor with largely smooth cyst walls.

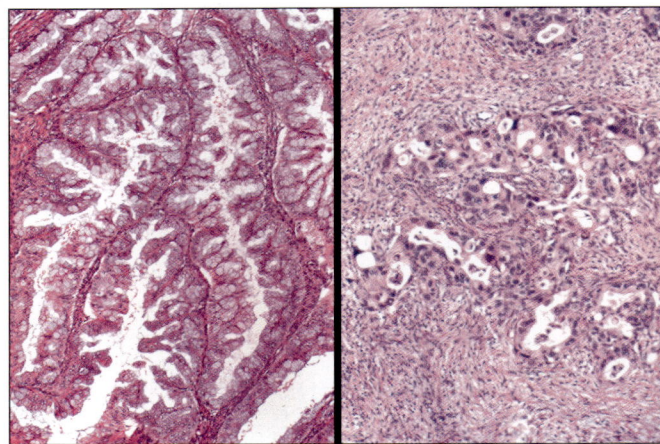

Figure 26.14 Mucinous borderline tumor (left) and mucinous carcinoma (right). The borderline tumor shows branching papillae with minimal stromal support, stratification into two or three cell layers, and mild nuclear atypia without stromal invasion. In contrast, the carcinoma exhibits severe nuclear atypia and obvious stromal invasion.

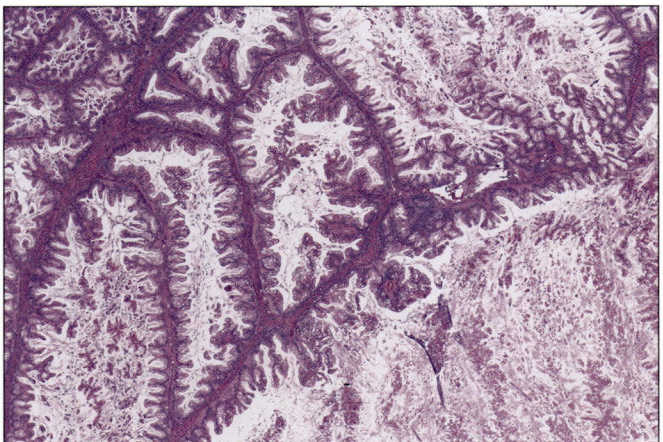

Figure 26.13 Mucinous cystic borderline tumors of intestinal type. Intraglandular proliferation of mucinous epithelium with filiform branching papillae. There is no stromal invasion.

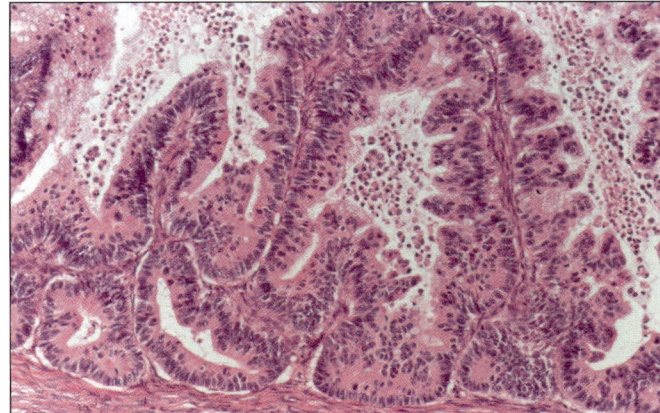

Figure 26.15 Mucinous borderline tumor with IEC. There is cell proliferation with glandular architectural complexity. The glands are lined by high-grade malignant nuclei with mitotic figures.

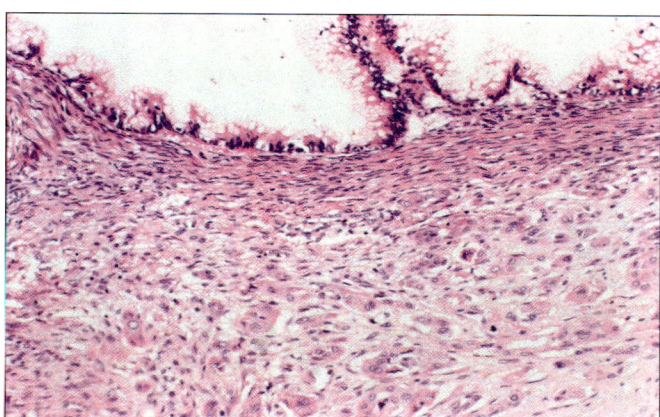

Figure 26.16 Mucinous borderline tumor with microinvasion. Stromal microinvasion by single epithelial cells and small clusters of such cells with abundant eosinophilic cytoplasm and minimal nuclear atypia.

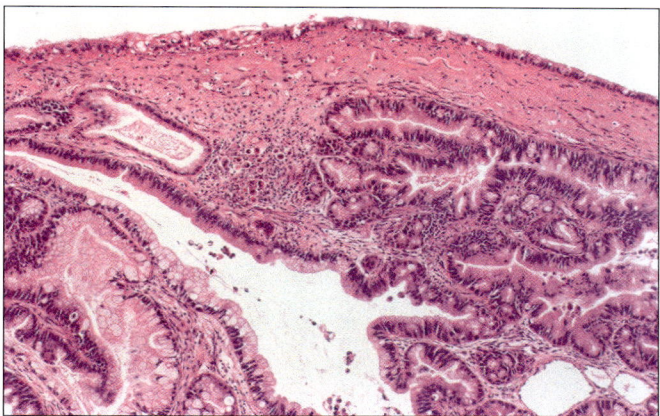

Figure 26.17 Mucinous borderline tumor with intraepithelial and microinvasive carcinoma. Stromal microinvasion by single epithelial cells with severe nuclear atypia (center left).

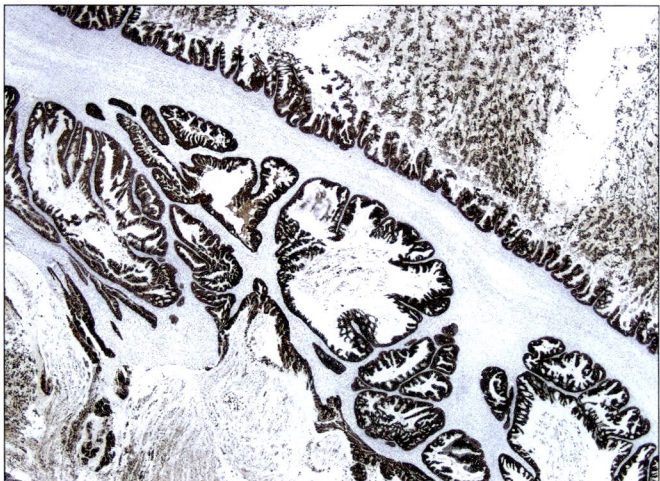

Figure 26.18 Mucinous borderline tumor intestinal type. Immunoreaction for CK7.

contain foci of benign mucinous epithelium, which resembles endocervical or gastric epithelium. Occasionally, pools of extravasated mucin dissect into the stroma and may be associated with a histiocytic and foreign-body–giant-cell reaction (mucin granuloma) or may lack an inflammatory cell response (pseudomyxoma ovarii). Focal necrosis and acute inflammation are not uncommon.

Noninvasive MBTs of gastrointestinal type may exhibit areas of epithelial cell proliferation of four or more layers, scattered foci of cribriform or stroma-free papillary architecture, and moderate (grade 2) or severe atypical (grade 3) nuclei (Figure 26.15). Whether tumors with such areas should be classified as noninvasive carcinomas or as borderline tumors has remained controversial for many years.[13] Numerous studies,[26–34] however, have shown that these tumors are almost always clinically benign, and we recommend classifying them as mucinous borderline tumors *with intraepithelial carcinoma*.[2,37] Currently, the preferred and exclusive criterion for this diagnosis is marked nuclear atypia (grade 3); neither a cribriform pattern nor epithelial stratification of greater than three cell layers qualify.[34,38] No minimum quantity of malignant-appearing epithelium is required for inclusion into this histologic category. The upper limit, however, merges imperceptibly with invasive carcinoma with an expansile growth pattern (see later) and has been arbitrarily established as 10 mm^2. Because of their *in situ* malignant change, MBT with IEC requires more extensive sampling than pure intestinal-type MBTs to exclude stromal invasion. Cell pseudostratification and cribriform-like pattern caused by tangential sectioning characteristically lacks high-grade nuclear atypia and should not be interpreted as IEC.[13]

Ten per cent of intestinal-type MBTs contain one or more foci of stromal microinvasion (also arbitrarily defined as not exceeding 10 mm^2). Individual microinvasive foci usually are <1 or 2 mm in greatest dimension. Their histologic appearances vary from small nests of tumor cells admixed with extracellular mucin in a normal ovarian stroma to irregular glands associated with a fibroblastic or edematous stroma, or tiny nests or isolated tumor cells within clear spaces. On the basis of less than 100 reported cases,[20,21,30–34] the presence of these foci does not alter the favorable prognosis of intestinal-type MBT. Nevertheless, MBT with stromal microinvasion should be distinguished from microinvasive carcinoma. Whereas the microinvasive component and the adjacent glands of the former tumors exhibit only low-grade (borderline) nuclear atypia (Figure 26.16), the cells of microinvasive carcinomas usually contain grade 3 nuclei (Figure 26.17).[13,32,38] Recently, a case of MBT with intraepithelial and microinvasive carcinoma associated with aggressive behavior has been reported.[39] Stromal microinvasion may be difficult to distinguish from extruded neoplastic epithelium from an adjacent ruptured gland, particularly if accompanied by a mucin granuloma (Figure 26.4). Cytokeratin immunostaining reveals that mucin granulomas contain tumor cells more often than suspected on H&E.[33]

Immunohistochemistry and Somatic Genetics

The immunophenotype of gastrointestinal MBT differs from that of endocervical MBT. Both types of MBTs are reactive for CK7 (Figure 26.18), but only the gastrointestinal type immunoreacts for CK20 and CDX2.[22] CK20 immunoreaction is usually focal and less extensive than CK7 expression. PAX8 is variably positive and ER and PR are negative. *K-RAS* mutations are present in 29–73% of cases.[5–8,40]

Treatment and Prognosis

Stage I intestinal-type MBTs are treated similarly to SBTs. In a young woman who wishes to preserve her reproductive function, unilateral oophorectomy can be safely performed. Prolonged follow-up is recommended to exclude development of a similar tumor in the contralateral ovary. When performing a consultation in the operating room (frozen section), the pathologist should be mindful that additional postoperative sampling may disclose a carcinomatous component in the permanent sections. Following this message, the surgeon is more likely to undertake appropriate staging. If there is gross evidence of pseudomyxoma peritonei or the patient has bilateral ovarian tumors, removal of the appendix as well as exploration of the abdomen for a possible source of metastasis is recommended.

According to the International Federation of Gynecologists and Obstetricians (FIGO) annual report,[41] MBTs are confined to one or both ovaries (stage I) in 82% of cases, stage II in 6%, stage III in 10%, and stage IV in 2%. However, almost all stage II–III intestinal MBTs are associated with pseudomyxoma peritonei. After excluding this group of patients in which the ovarian tumor is virtually always secondary (metastatic) from a primary appendiceal tumor (see later), it has been questioned whether the noninvasive intestinal-type MBTs have any malignant potential as the 5 year survival nears 100% in these women. Moreover, some investigators have proposed abandoning the borderline denomination for these tumors and replacing it with 'atypical proliferative mucinous tumors.'[30] Others,[31,32] however, believe that the term 'borderline' should be retained because it better reflects the view that these tumors represent intermediate stages of mucinous tumorigenesis and may be accompanied by intraepithelial and frankly invasive carcinomas.

Overall survival for MBTs with IEC is 95% with most recent studies showing 100% survival. In a recent report, 6 of 144 patients (4.2%) had tumor recurrence. Risk factors for recurrence included FIGO stage ≥IC, microinvasion, age less than 45 years, and IEC. The amount of IEC was also associated with risk of recurrence.[34] The recurrence rate for mucinous tumors with microinvasive carcinoma is 5% and the tumor-related death rate is less than 5% with adverse behavior limited to FIGO stage ≥IC tumors.[33]

In advanced stage intestinal-type MBTs not associated with pseudomyxoma peritonei, the metastases appear as invasive peritoneal implants and the prognosis is similar to that of ovarian mucinous carcinomas with metastases. In these cases, it is likely that areas of invasion within the ovarian tumor were not sampled.[13,31,32]

MUCINOUS CYSTIC TUMORS ASSOCIATED WITH PSEUDOMYXOMA PERITONEI

Pseudomyxoma peritonei is a clinical term for localized or widespread intraperitoneal deposits of extracellular mucin ('gelatinous ascites') caused by rupture or leakage of an intra-abdominal tumor, usually a low-grade (adenomatous) mucinous tumor of the appendix and, less frequently, a metastatic appendiceal or colonic mucinous adenocarcinoma.[36,42–44] The mucinous deposits result from MUC2-expressing goblet cells, which secrete large quantities of extracellular mucin in a ratio of mucin:cells exceeding 10:1.[45] The gelatinous material should be thoroughly sampled and examined microscopically. The mucus may be acellular or may contain mucinous epithelial cells (Figure 26.19). The degree of atypia (described as low grade or high grade) of the tumor cells present in the mucinous deposits should be indicated in the report, as well as whether the mucin dissects into tissues with a fibrous response or is merely on the surface. Patients in whom the tumor cells appear low grade usually have a more favorable clinical course than those where the tumor appears cytologically malignant (peritoneal carcinomatosis).[31,46] Nevertheless, the former tumors may lead to significant morbidity and mortality (10 year survival rate of 45%).[44,47]

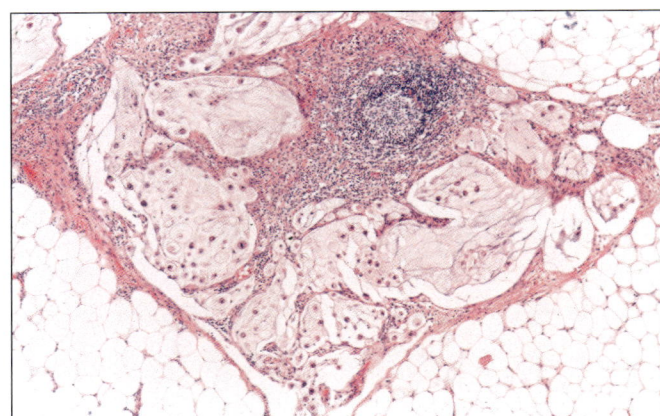

Figure 26.19 Pseudomyxoma peritonei associated with mucinous tumors of the appendix and ovaries. Note the presence of tumor cells floating in pools of mucin dissecting through the fat.

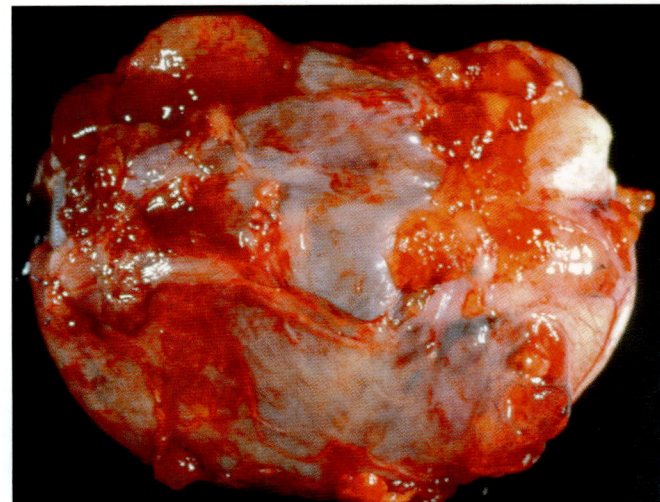

Figure 26.20 Cystic ovarian tumor secondary to low-grade mucinous tumor of the appendix associated with pseudomyxoma peritonei. Note the presence of mucin deposits on the surface of the cyst.

Historically, pseudomyxoma peritonei was thought to be the typical pattern of spread of a ruptured primary mucinous tumor of the ovary, usually a borderline tumor of gastrointestinal type. However, we now know that ruptured primary ovarian mucinous tumors are not associated with the subsequent development of pseudomyxoma peritonei.[13,31] In fact, patients with the latter condition often have ovarian tumors that are usually bilateral or right sided and multicystic. They develop secondarily after incorporation of peritoneal mucin and tumor cells into the ovaries. Typically, there is ovarian surface involvement and/or pools of mucin dissecting through the ovarian stroma (pseudomyxoma ovarii) (Figures 26.20–26.22), which are rare findings in primary mucinous ovarian tumors. The tumor cysts are lined by unusually tall mucinous epithelium of intestinal type with slightly atypical nuclei (see Chapter 30).[36] The secondary ovarian tumors are easily mistaken for primary mucinous borderline tumors (Figure 26.23).

The appendiceal tumors may be small and rupture sites can be sealed after evacuation of mucus and retraction of the appendiceal wall (Figures 26.24 and 26.25).[36] In patients with pseudomyxoma peritonei, the appendix should be excised and examined entirely for a primary low-grade tumor that is often undetected by the surgeon.[46,47]

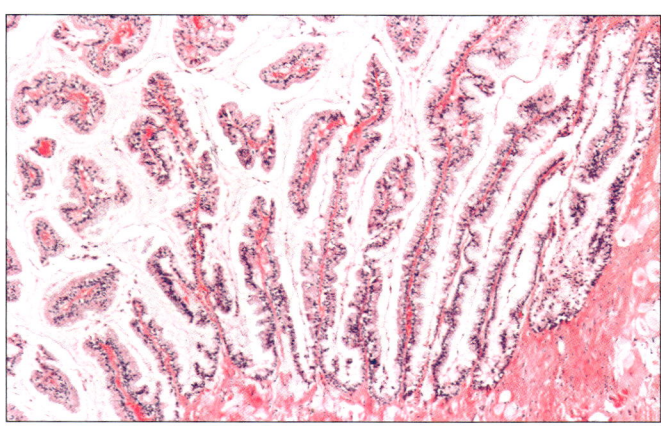

Figure 26.23 Low-grade mucinous appendiceal tumor associated with pseudomyxoma peritonei and involving the ovary. The tumor resembles a mucinous borderline tumor of the ovary. (Reproduced with permission of Lippincott Williams & Wilkins.)

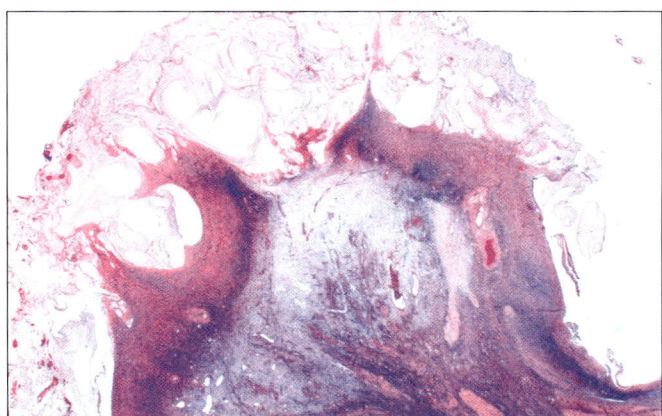

Figure 26.21 Low-grade mucinous appendiceal tumor associated with pseudomyxoma peritonei involving the surface of the ovary.

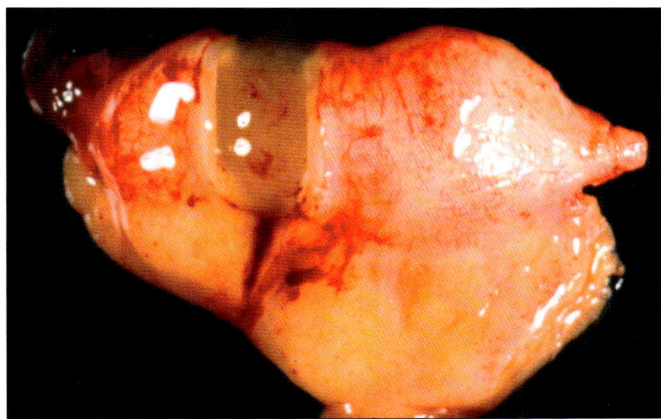

Figure 26.24 Mucinous appendiceal tumor (mucocele) associated with pseudomyxoma peritonei and bilateral ovarian mucinous tumors.

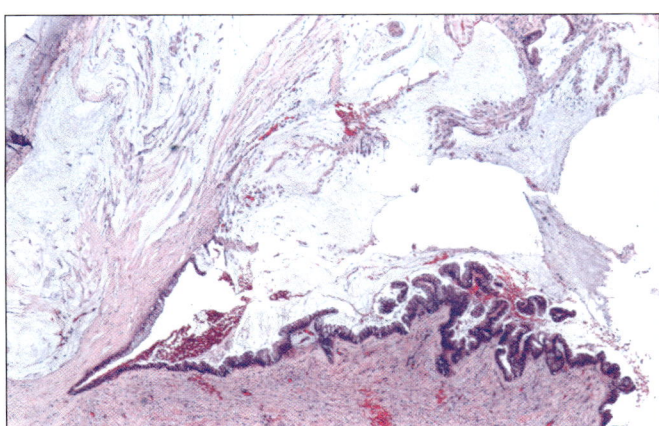

Figure 26.22 Low-grade mucinous appendiceal tumor associated with pseudomyxoma peritonei involving the ovary. Pools of mucin dissecting through the ovarian stroma (pseudomyxoma ovarii).

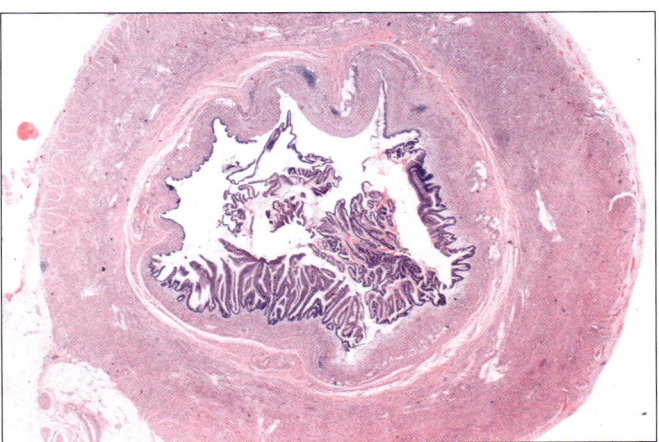

Figure 26.25 Low-grade mucinous appendiceal tumor associated with pseudomyxoma peritonei and bilateral ovarian mucinous tumors. (Reproduced with permission of Lippincott Williams & Wilkins.)

In patients with sychronous mucinous tumors of the appendix and ovaries, molecular genetic analyses support the conclusion that the appendiceal tumor is the primary neoplasm. The concordance of K-RAS mutational pattern in both tumors in each patient[48,49] suggest that they are not separate neoplasms, but originate from the same clone which, in the light of the clinicopathologic data, is most likely of appendiceal origin.

While there is general agreement today that most tumors associated with pseudomyxoma peritonei arise in the appendix,[31,36,42–44] it is still open to question whether some of these neoplasms are ovarian in origin. One explanation, albeit rare, is an origin in a mature ovarian teratoma where the appendix is proven to be normal.[31,36,50–54] In most reported cases, the mucinous tumors were of borderline malignancy and not reactive for CK7. Reactivity for CK20 supported their gastrointestinal-type teratomatous origin.[31,50–54]

Prognosis and Treatment

Patients with pseudomyxoma peritonei containing epithelial cells that are benign or low-grade malignant usually have a protracted clinical course. The 10 and 15 year survival rates are 63% and 59%, respectively. In contrast, when the mucinous epithelial cells appear malignant (peritoneal carcinomatosis) the clinical course is more aggressive, and ~90% of patients died within 3 years. In patients with pseudomyxoma peritonei from appendiceal origin, cytoreductive surgery and hyperthermic intraperitoneal chemotherapy may achieve long-term survival.[55]

MUCINOUS ADENOCARCINOMAS

Over the past 40 years, the number of mucinous ovarian tumors diagnosed as primary carcinomas has been largely reduced due to the following: (1) the separation of mucinous borderline tumors from mucinous carcinomas; (2) the classification of most ovarian mucinous cystic tumors associated with pseudomyxoma peritonei as secondary neoplasms from the appendix; and (3) the recognition of metastatic adenocarcinomas, mainly of intestinal, pancreatic, and biliary tract origin, which mimic primary ovarian mucinous tumors (Figure 26.26). In the first modern study, only 22 (3%) of 688 primary mucinous tumors confined to the ovary at diagnosis were obviously invasive carcinomas.[56] In a consecutive series of 124 ovarian carcinomas from a single institution, only three (2.4%) were mucinous carcinomas.[57] Thus, the reported frequency of 15% for mucinous adenocarcinomas primary in the ovary may be overestimated, and most contemporary studies have been based on a relatively small number of cases.[29–32,57]

Macroscopic Features

Mucinous carcinomas are usually large (8–40 cm; mean 16–19 cm in greatest dimension),[58] unilateral, multilocular or unilocular cystic masses containing mucinous fluid (Figure 26.27). They often exhibit papillary and solid areas that may be soft and mucoid or firm, hemorrhagic, and necrotic. Extensive sampling of mucinous ovarian tumors, especially the more solid areas, is critical, as benign, borderline, and malignant components may coexist within a single specimen and the malignant areas may involve only a small portion of the tumor. The tumors are bilateral in only 5% of cases. Bilateral mucinous carcinomas or unilateral carcinomas under 10 cm in greatest dimension should raise the suspicion of metastases.

Microscopic Features

Over 80% of invasive mucinous carcinomas show components of mucinous borderline tumor of intestinal type or mucinous cystadenoma, or both, suggesting a progression from benign to borderline, and from borderline to

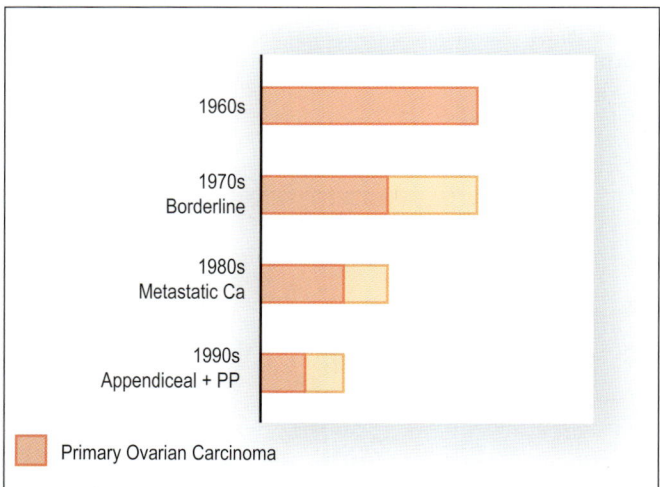

Figure 26.26 Mucinous tumors of the ovary. Over the last 40 years, the percentage of primary mucinous carcinomas (Ca) of the ovary has been largely reduced because of the introduction of the borderline category of tumors (1970s); the realization that metastatic adenocarcinomas, particularly of the large intestine and pancreas, can simulate primary ovarian tumors (1980s); and, last, the finding that most mucinous ovarian tumors associated with 'pseudomyxoma peritonei' (PP) are secondary neoplasms, often from the appendix.

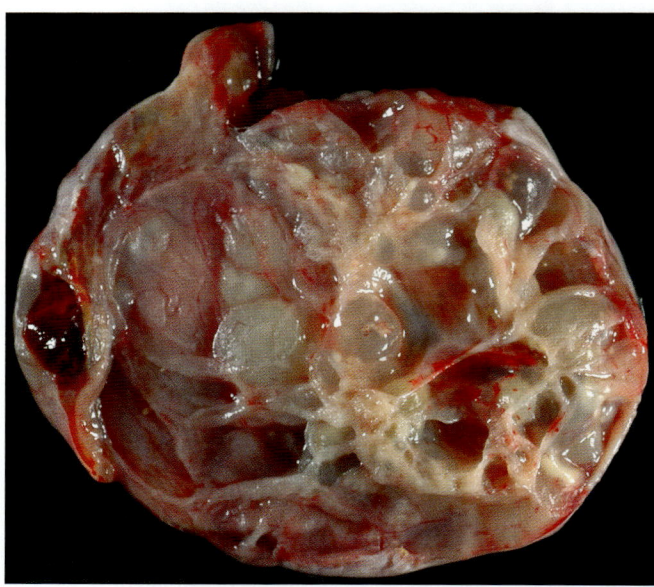

Figure 26.27 Mucinous cystadenocarcinoma. The sectioned surface shows a multiloculated tumor.

malignant mucinous neoplasia. The remaining 20% of carcinomas appear exclusively malignant. According to their pattern of invasion, mucinous carcinomas are divided into two categories: (1) an *expansile* type without demonstrable destructive stromal invasion, but exhibiting back-to-back or complex malignant glands without or with minimal intervening stroma and exceeding 10 mm^2 in area (>3 mm in each of two linear dimensions) (Figures 26.28–26.30) and (2) an *infiltrative* type, showing obvious stromal invasion in the form of glands, cell clusters, or individual cells, disorderly infiltrating the stroma and frequently associated with a desmoplastic stromal reaction (Figure 26.31).[31] Stromal invasion must exceed 10 mm^2 in area in order to be classified as carcinoma; otherwise a diagnosis of microinvasive carcinoma is warranted. An infiltrative pattern, particularly in the setting of bilateral ovarian involvement, should raise suspicion for metastatic mucinous carcinoma. The expansile pattern of growth has also been referred to as the 'noninvasive,' 'intraglandular,'[58] or 'confluent glandular'[30] pattern. Both patterns may coexist in a single tumor.

Rare mucinous carcinomas of the endocervical-like or mixed müllerian type have been described;[15,59] three cases were associated with endometriosis and one with an endocervical-type MBT of the contralateral ovary.[59] In our experience, such cases are indistinguishable from endometrioid carcinoma.[16]

Immunohistochemistry

Although selected immunostains help to distinguish primary from secondary ovarian tumors, immunohistochemistry is considerably less useful when the ovarian neoplasm is of mucinous type. Most ovarian mucinous borderline tumors

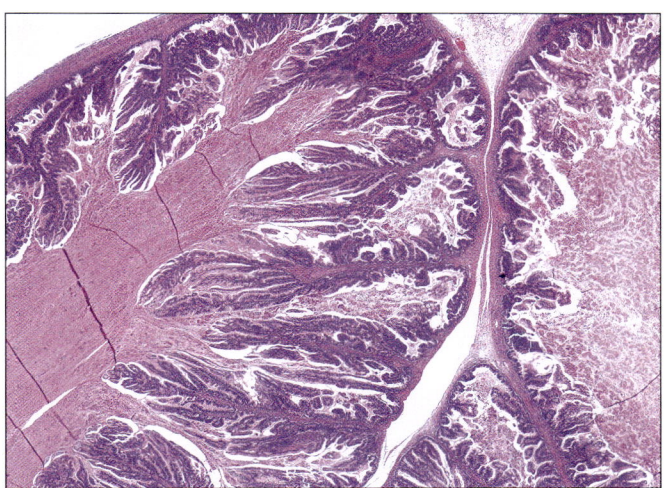

Figure 26.28 Mucinous carcinoma with expansile invasion. Confluent, complex glandular proliferation without obvious stromal invasion.

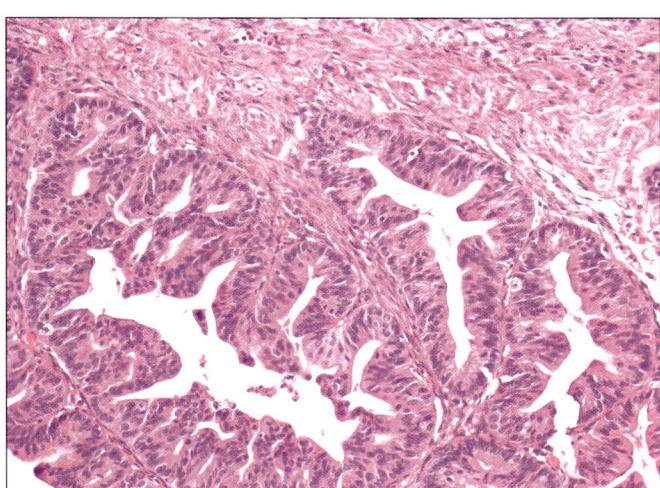

Figure 26.30 Mucinous carcinoma with expansile invasion. Papillary glands lined by cells with grade 2 or 3 malignant nuclei. Mitotic figures are seen.

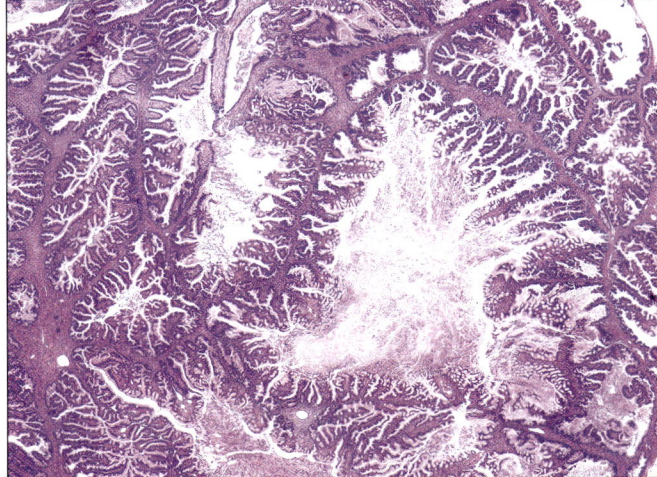

Figure 26.29 Mucinous carcinoma with expansile invasion. Closely packed (back-to-back) malignant glands with little to no stromal support. Stromal invasion is not obvious.

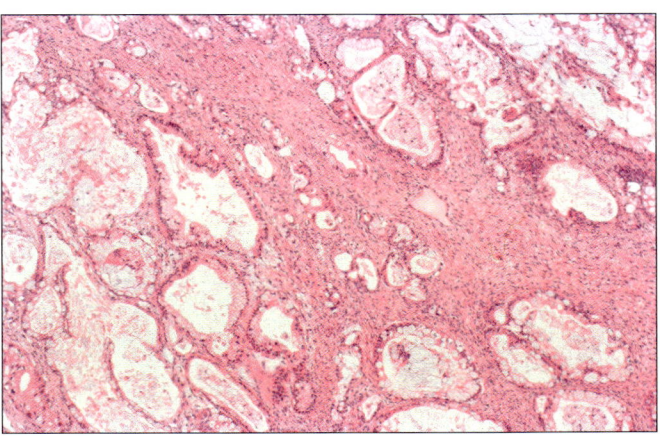

Figure 26.31 Mucinous carcinoma with infiltrative invasion. Mucinous glands infiltrate a desmoplastic stroma.

and carcinomas are of intestinal type and, therefore, their immunophenotype frequently overlaps with that of metastatic gastrointestinal tumors. Cytokeratin immunostains are the most commonly used.[60] Primary ovarian mucinous tumors are almost always (up to 80%) immunoreactive for CK7 whereas colorectal adenocarcinomas are usually CK7 negative.[61] However, CK7 is usually positive in metastatic carcinomas of the pancreas, notorious for masquerading as primary ovarian tumors, and it is also focally expressed by many other carcinomas, including those of stomach, gallbladder, small bowel, appendix, lung, breast, thyroid, uterus, and bladder.[62–64] Ovarian mucinous borderline tumors and carcinomas are immunoreactive for CK20 in 65% and 75% of cases, respectively, but the reaction is typically weak and focal.[60,63,64] In contrast, colorectal adenocarcinomas are diffusely and strongly reactive for CK20.[61,64,65] Therefore, a CK7-negative/CK20-positive immunoprofile suggests metastatic adenocarcinoma.[60,64] Although the vast majority of colorectal adenocarcinomas express CK20, poorly differentiated and right-sided tumors can be CK20 negative.[61] Thus, immunostains for CK7 and CK20 should be interpreted with caution, always in the light of all clinical information, and with the understanding that no tumor shows absolute consistency in its staining with these markers.

Other immunohistochemical stains have greater overlap in their expressions and should not be used individually in this differential diagnosis. Ovarian mucinous tumors can express CDX2 (nuclear staining);[22] exhibit focal expression of p16; and are negative for ER, PR, and CA125.[66,67] Loss of Dpc4 immunoreactivity occurs in almost 50% of metastatic carcinomas of the pancreas, whereas most primary ovarian mucinous carcinomas are focally or diffusely positive.[64] Human papillomavirus (HPV) DNA assessment may be helpful for distinguishing mucinous adenocarcinoma of the cervix metastatic to the ovary from a primary ovarian mucinous carcinoma. p16 expression is also a reliable surrogate marker for HPV.[67]

Mucinous tumors arising in association with mature cystic teratomas, often showing pseudomyxoma ovarii, may have a lower intestinal tract CK7–/CK20+ immunoprofile, which may suggest a metastatic tumor from the lower intestinal tract.[54]

Differential Diagnosis

The most important differential diagnosis of mucinous ovarian carcinoma is with metastatic mucinous carcinoma that may present clinically as a primary ovarian tumor. Most of these originate in the large intestine, appendix, pancreas, biliary tract, stomach, or cervix (see Chapter 30).[35,36,61,64,68,69] Common features that favor a primary mucinous carcinoma are an expansile pattern of invasion and a complex papillary architecture; a borderline or benign-appearing component is commonly found.[68] Features favoring a metastatic mucinous carcinoma are bilaterality, small size (<10 cm), a multinodular growth pattern, ovarian surface involvement by epithelial cells (surface implants), hilar involvement, signet-ring cell component, vascular space invasion, and presence of extraovarian disease.[68] The finding of abundant extracellular mucin (pseudomyxoma ovarii) should always raise the suspicion of metastatic carcinoma. Most primary mucinous carcinomas of the ovary are unilateral and stage I.[30–32,58] Nevertheless, metastatic mucinous adenocarcinomas, particularly colorectal carcinomas, may be large (≥10 cm) and unilateral in approximately 40% of cases.[70,71]

Well-differentiated endometrioid carcinomas containing foci of benign-appearing endocervical-like cells are best interpreted as endometrioid adenocarcinomas, grade 1, with areas of mucinous metaplasia. Some endometrioid adenocarcinomas secrete large amounts of mucin into the lumens of their glands and cysts, but the mucin is present only in the glycocalyx of the tumor cells. These tumors are considered to be mucin-rich endometrioid carcinomas rather than mucinous carcinomas.[2]

Sertoli–Leydig cell tumors with heterologous mucinous elements may appear on gross examination as mucinous cystic tumors. The problem may be accentuated if a mucinous tumor is producing androgens and virilizing the patient because of its luteinized stroma. Microscopically, there is Sertoli–Leydig cell tumor, typically of the intermediate type with abundant sex-cord-like structures, between the cyst locules, rather than stroma or lutein cells. Other heterologous elements such as carcinoid or mesenchymal tissues (skeletal muscle or cartilage) may be present also in heterologous Sertoli–Leydig cell tumors to aid in the differential diagnosis.[2]

Somatic Genetics

As indicated above, tumor heterogeneity is common and probably reflects tumor progression (Figures 26.32 and 26.33). In the sequence of malignant transformation from benign and borderline mucinous tumors to infiltrative carcinoma, intraepithelial (noninvasive) carcinomas and carcinomas with purely expansile (not obvious) invasion represent transitional stages of mucinous carcinogenesis.[31,32] Molecular studies support this hypothesis of genetic alterations in mucinous tumors.[5,7] An increasing frequency of codon 12/13 *K-RAS* mutations in benign, borderline, and carcinomatous mucinous ovarian tumors favors the viewpoint that *K-RAS* mutational activation is an early event in mucinous ovarian tumorigenesis (Figures 26.34 and 26.35).[5,7] *K-RAS* mutations have been reported in 44% of mucinous carcinomas and 79% of mucinous borderline tumors. Overexpression/amplification of *HER2* has been

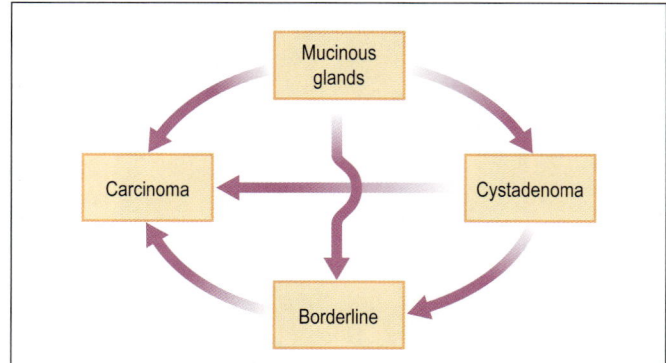

Figure 26.32 Mucinous carcinomas: histogenesis. In contrast to serous carcinomas, which typically show morphologic uniformity, malignant mucinous intestinal tumors frequently exhibit a morphologic transition from benign, to borderline, and to carcinoma.

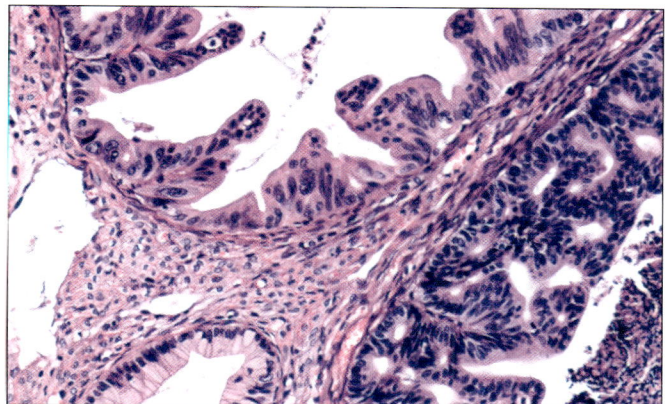

Figure 26.33 Mucinous tumor of intestinal type. Three neoplastic components appear next to each other: benign (bottom left), borderline with marked proliferation and nuclear atypia (top), and carcinoma with cribriform pattern and central necrosis (bottom right). (Reproduced with permission of Lippincott Williams & Wilkins.)

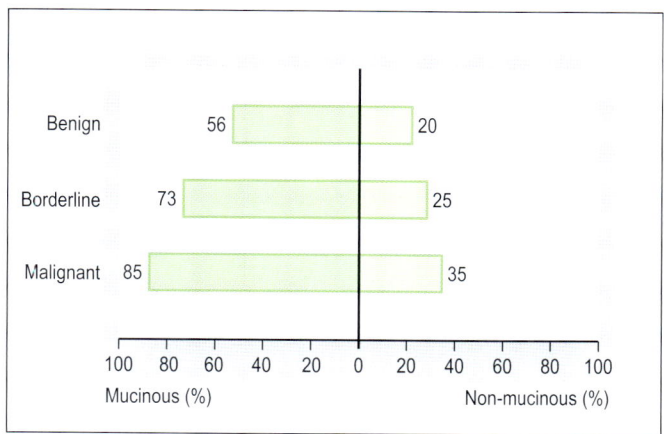

Figure 26.34 *K-RAS* investigation in two large series of mucinous and non-mucinous epithelial ovarian tumors. *K-RAS* mutations were encountered more frequently in mucinous (68%) than in non-mucinous (30%) tumors. They occurred in benign, borderline, and fully malignant tumors, but their presence increased significantly with the degree of malignancy.[5]

found in 19% of mucinous carcinomas and 6% of mucinous borderline tumors. *K-RAS* mutations were near mutually exclusive of *HER2* amplification. In mucinous carcinomas, either *HER2* amplification/overexpression or *K-RAS* mutation was associated with decreased risk of recurrence or death when compared to cases with neither feature.[72]

Treatment and Prognosis

Treatment of mucinous carcinomas is similar to that of serous carcinomas (see earlier). FIGO stage is the single most important prognostic factor, and stage I carcinomas have an excellent prognosis. However, the prognosis in cases with extraovarian spread is poor.[28,30–32,58] According to the FIGO annual report,[41] mucinous carcinomas are confined to one or both ovaries in 49% of the cases, are stage II in 11%, stage III in 29%, and stage IV in 10%. The 5 year survival for patients with stage I mucinous carcinomas is 83%; stage II, 55%; stage III, 21%; and stage IV, 9%.[41] After excluding cases of metastatic tumor from non-ovarian sites and cases of pseudomyxoma peritonei of intestinal origin, more than 80% of mucinous carcinomas are stage I (confined to ovary) at the time of diagnosis.[31,32,58]

Advanced stage mucinous carcinoma of the ovary is very rare and is associated with poor overall survival (14 months).[73] Survival for advanced stage mucinous neoplasms is inferior to that of serous carcinomas.[74] Most patients with extraovarian disease at presentation die of disease.[73]

Prognosis within and across FIGO stage also reflects specifics of histologic features. Infiltrative stromal invasion is biologically more aggressive than expansile invasion. Among 59 cases of invasive carcinoma in two recent series,[31,32] all 20 cases with expansile invasion were stage I and no patient experienced recurrent disease. Of the 25 infiltrative carcinomas with follow-up data, only 9 of 13 patients with stage I disease and 1 of 12 with higher stage disease (stage IIA) had favorable outcomes. Furthermore, in contrast to previous reports,[30,31,58] one series[32] showed that high nuclear grade (grade 3) was predictive of behavior independent of the surgical stage (Table 26.2).

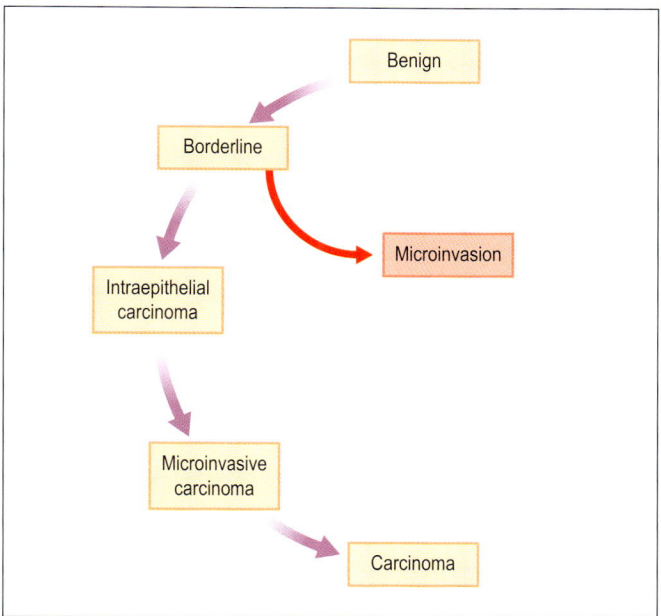

Figure 26.35 Progression of mucinous tumors.

Table 26.2	Stage I Mucinous Carcinomas: Prognosis[32]	
Favorable	**Unfavorable**	
Expansile	Infiltrative	($p = 0.005$)
Nuclear G1–2	Nuclear G3	($p = 0.021$)
Intact	Ruptured	

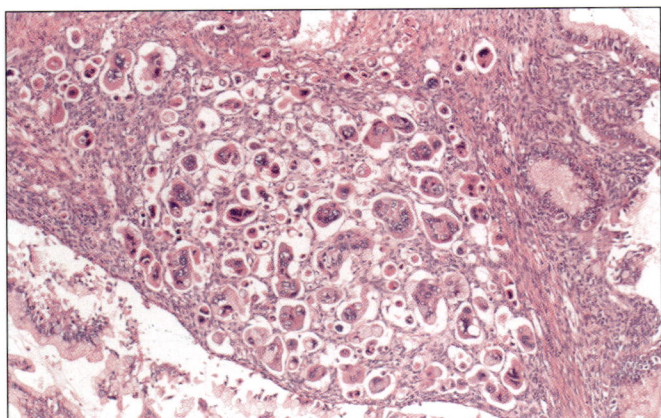

Figure 26.36 Invasive mucinous carcinoma. Small focus (1.3 mm^2) of invasion. Notice the presence of highly malignant (nuclear grade 3) carcinomatous cells. This stage IIIB ruptured cystic tumor showed a predominant borderline component but contained several foci of invasive carcinoma, the largest 10.2 mm^2 in area.

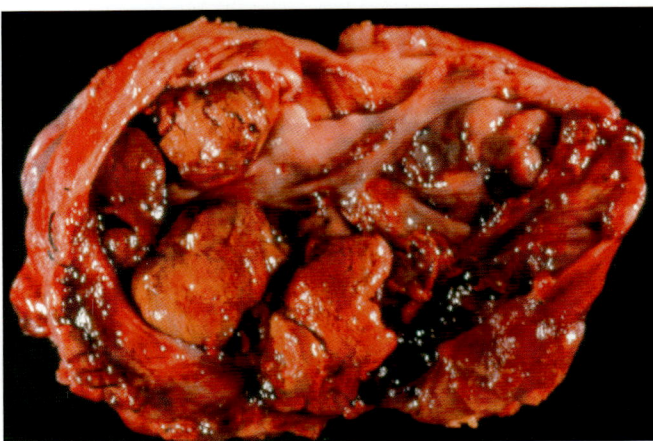

Figure 26.37 Sarcoma-like mural nodules in a mucinous cystic tumor. Four red to brown nodules protrude into the lumen of the cyst.

The combination of extensive and infiltrative stromal invasion, high nuclear grade, and tumor rupture should be considered a strong predictor of recurrence for stage I mucinous carcinomas.[32]

Foci of stromal invasion <10 mm^2 have been designated 'microinvasive,' and cases with this finding have had a favorable outcome.[20,21,27,28,31,32] However, experience with these tumors is still scarce, and occasional carcinomas with stromal invasion barely beyond the limit accepted for microinvasion have produced metastases (Figure 26.36).[32,75]

MURAL NODULES

Mucinous cystic tumors of the ovary, whether benign, borderline, or malignant, may contain one or more mural nodules that differ notably in their microscopic features from those of the underlying mucinous neoplasm. The nodules have been classified into three major subtypes: sarcoma-like mural nodules, nodules of anaplastic carcinoma, and sarcoma.[76] Mixed nodules have also been described.

Sarcoma-like mural nodules occur predominantly in middle-aged women (mean age, 39 years) as red-brown nodules (0.6–6 cm in diameter) (Figure 26.37) that appear sharply demarcated from the adjacent mucinous epithelium (Figures 26.38 and 26.39). The nodules are almost always multiple. They are associated with mucinous carcinoma in about half the cases and with benign and MBTs in the remainder (Figure 26.40). They exhibit a heterogeneous cell population with numerous multinucleated cells of the epulis type, atypical spindle cells, and inflammatory cells (Figure 26.41). In some nodules the predominant elements are spindle-shaped cells of moderate size containing hyperchromatic nuclei and pleomorphic mononucleated or binucleated giant cells. The mitotic index in the most cellular areas is 5–10/10 HPF. Sarcoma-like mural nodules usually coexpress vimentin (strong/diffuse) and cytokeratin (focal/weak).[76] All cases described have had a benign clinical course.[76]

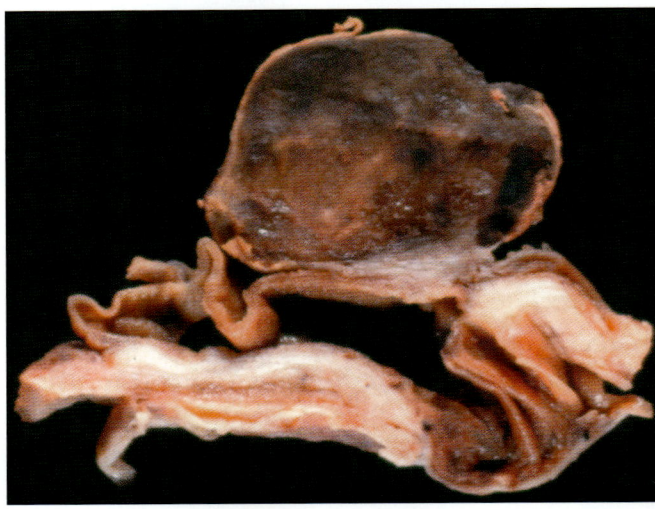

Figure 26.38 Sarcoma-like mural nodules in a mucinous cystic tumor. The sectioned surface shows a hemorrhagic nodule which appears well circumscribed. (Reproduced with permission of Lippincott Williams & Wilkins.)

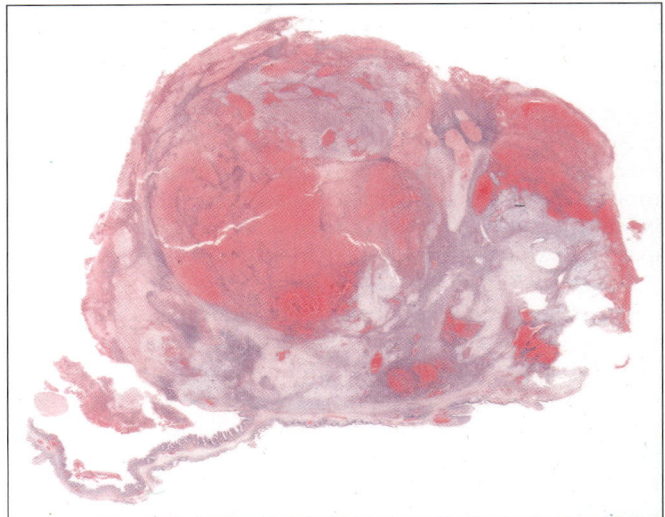

Figure 26.39 Sarcoma-like mural nodule in a mucinous cystic tumor. The nodule shows extensive hemorrhage and is well demarcated from the mucinous epithelial component (bottom).

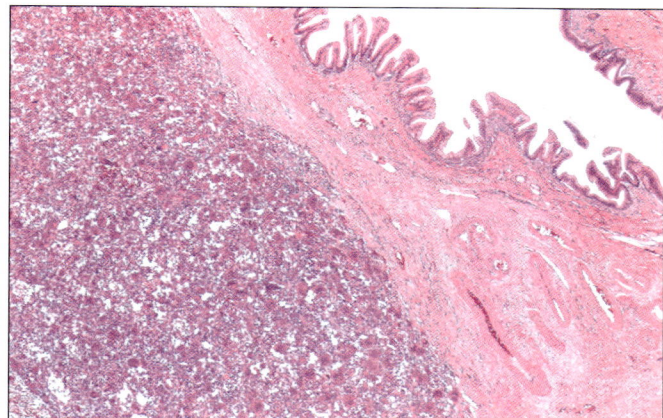

Figure 26.40 Sarcoma-like nodule in the wall of a mucinous cystic tumor. The nodule exhibits a heterogeneous cell population with numerous multinucleated cells of the epulis type. (Reproduced with permission of Lippincott Williams & Wilkins.)

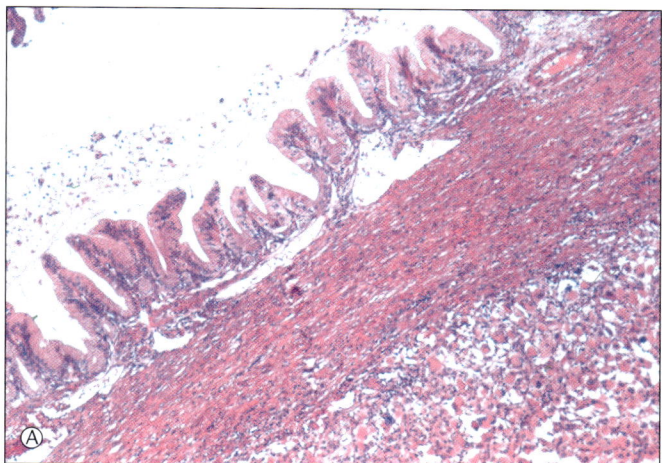

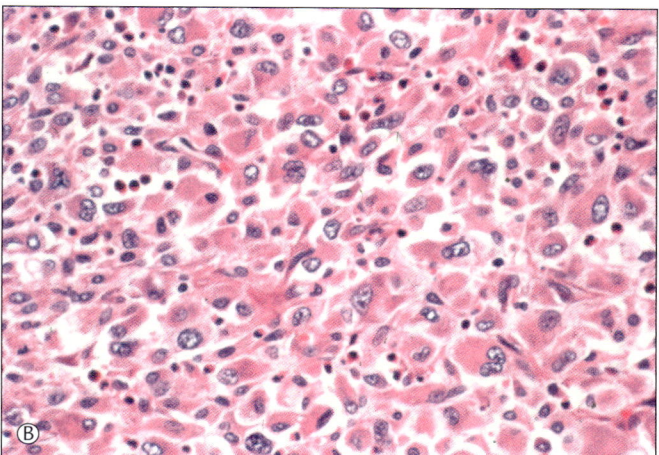

Figure 26.42 Anaplastic carcinoma in mucinous cystic tumor. The epithelial lining of the cyst appears of borderline malignancy (A). The undifferentiated component is characterized by a diffuse arrangement of cells with abundant eosinophilic cytoplasm and grade 3 nuclei (B).

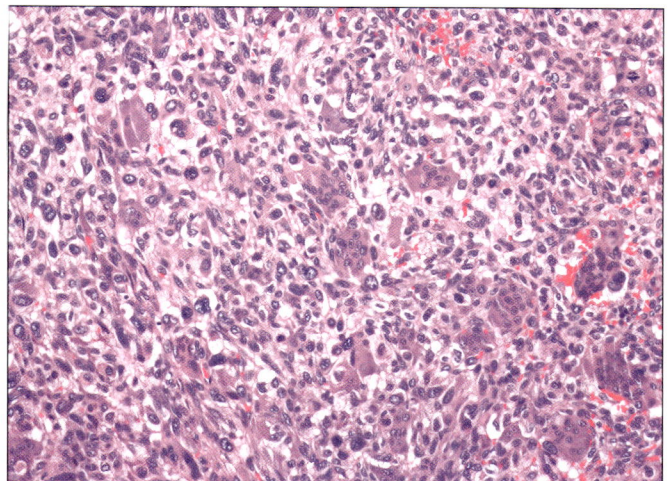

Figure 26.41 Sarcoma-like mural nodule in a mucinous cystic tumor. The cells of the nodule include osteoclast-like giant cells and smaller mononuclear cells with marked nuclear atypia.

The nodules of anaplastic carcinoma may show: (1) large rhabdoid cells with abundant eosinophilic cytoplasm, eccentric nuclei, and one or more prominent nucleoli (Figure 26.42); (2) sarcomatoid spindle cells often exhibiting a herringbone pattern; or (3) pleomorphic cells.[77] The size of the anaplastic nodules ranges from microscopic to about 10 cm and they may be single or multiple. Frequently, there is invasion of the surrounding tissue and, occasionally, lymphovascular space invasion.[77] In contrast to sarcoma-like mural nodules, the tumor cells react strongly for cytokeratin (Figure 26.43). Although initially thought to carry an invariably unfavorable prognosis, recent data indicate that these nodules when found within unruptured stage I mucinous cystic tumors may be associated with a favorable prognosis.[32,77]

Various types of true sarcomatous nodules have been reported, such as fibrosarcoma, rhabdomyosarcoma, and

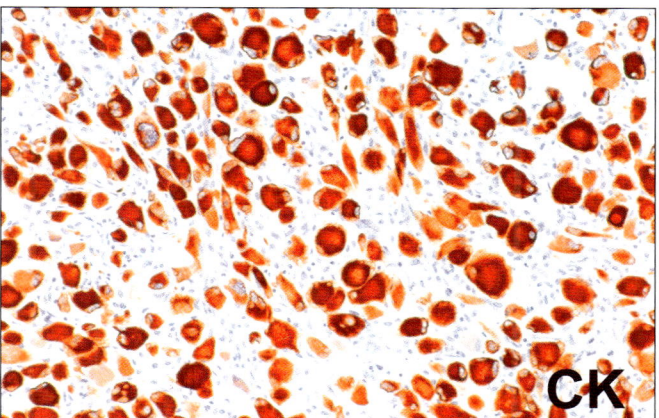

Figure 26.43 Anaplastic carcinoma in mucinous cystic tumor. Strongly positive cytokeratin immunoreaction.

undifferentiated sarcoma. These tumors carry a poor prognosis.

Mural nodules of different types may be present in the same neoplasm and individual nodules may exhibit mixed morphologic features. Negative immunoreaction for cytokeratins does not rule out anaplastic carcinoma, as the anaplastic cells may have lost cytokeratin expression. In one report, the diagnosis of carcinoma was supported by strong p53 immunostaining, which highlighted the nests of carcinomatous cells within the reactive component.[78]

REFERENCES

1. Koonings PP, Campbell K, Mishell Jr DR, Grimes DA. Relative frequency of primary ovarian neoplasms: a ten year reviews. Obstet Gynecol 1989;74:921–6.
2. Scully RE, Young RH, Clement PB. Tumors of the ovary, maldeveloped gonads, fallopian tube, and broad ligament. In: Rosai J, Sobin LH, editors. Atlas of tumor pathology. 3rd ed. vol. 23. Washington, DC: Armed Forces Institute of Pathology; 1998.
3. Matias-Guiu X, Prat J. Ovarian tumors with functioning stroma: an immunohistochemical study with hCG mono and polyclonal antibodies. Cancer 1990;65:2001–5.
4. Healy DL, Burger HG, Mamers P, et al. Elevated serum inhibin concentrations in postmenopausal women with ovarian tumors. N Engl J Med 1993;329:1539–42.
5. Cuatrecasas M, Villanueva A, Matias-Guiu X, Prat J. K-ras mutations in mucinous ovarian tumors: a clinicopathologic and molecular study of 95 cases. Cancer 1997;79:1581–6.
6. Ichikawa Y, Nishida M, Suzuki H, et al. Mutation of K-ras protooncogene is associated with histological subtypes in human mucinous ovarian tumors. Cancer Res 1994;54:33–5.
7. Mandai M, Konishi I, Kuroda H, et al. Heterogeneous distribution of K-ras-mutated epithelia in mucinous ovarian tumors with special reference to histopathology. Hum Pathol 1998;28:34–40.
8. Mok SC, Bell DA, Knapp RC, et al. Mutation of K-ras protooncogene in human ovarian epithelial tumors of borderline malignancy. Cancer Res 1993;53:1489–92.
9. Gemignani ML, Schlaerth AC, Bogomolniy F, et al. Role of KRAS and BRAF gene mutations in mucinous ovarian carcinoma. Gynecol Oncol 2003;90:378–81.
10. Bell DA. Mucinous adenofibromas of the ovary. A report of 10 cases. Am J Surg Pathol 1991;15:227–32.
11. Ronnett BM, Kajdacsy-Balla A, Gilks CB, et al. Mucinous borderline ovarian tumors: points of general agreement and persistent controversies regarding nomenclature, diagnostic criteria, and behavior. Hum Pathol 2004;35:949–60.
12. Seidman JD, Khedmati F. Exploring the histogenesis of ovarian mucinous and transitional cell (Brenner) tumors: a study of 120 tumors. Arch Pathol Lab Med 2008;132:1753–60.
13. Hart WR. Mucinous tumors of the ovary: A review. Int J Gynecol Pathol 2005;24:4–25.
14. Rutgers JL, Scully RE. Ovarian müllerian mucinous papillary cystadenomas of borderline malignancy. A clinicopathologic analysis. Cancer 1988;61:340–8.
15. Shappell HW, Riopel MA, Smith Sehdev AE, et al. Diagnostic criteria and behavior of ovarian seromucinous (endocervical-type mucinous and mixed cell-type) tumors: atypical proliferative (borderline) tumors, intraepithelial, microinvasive, and invasive carcinomas. Am J Surg Pathol 2002;26:1529–41.
16. Rodriguez IM, Irving JA, Prat J. Endocervical-like mucinous tumors of the ovary. A clinicopathological analysis of 31 cases. Am J Surg Pathol 2004;28:1311–18.
17. Dubé V, Roy M, Plante M, et al. Mucinous ovarian tumors of Mullerian-type: an analysis of 17 cases including borderline tumors and intraepithelial, microinvasive, and invasive carcinomas. Int J Gynecol Pathol 2005;24:138–46.
18. Rutgers JL, Scully RE. Ovarian mixed-epithelial papillary cystadenomas of borderline malignancy of müllerian type. A clinicopathologic analysis. Cancer 1988;61:546–54.
19. Nagai Y, Kishimoto T, Nikaido T, et al. Squamous predominance in mixed-epithelial papillary cystadenomas of borderline malignancy of mullerian type arising in endometriotic cysts: a study of four cases. Am J Surg Pathol 2003;27:242–7.
20. Nayar R, Siriaunkgul S, Robbins KM, et al. Microinvasion in low malignant potential tumors of the ovary. Hum Pathol 1996;27:521–7.
21. Khunamornpong S, Russell P, Dalrymple JC. Proliferating (LMP) mucinous tumors of the ovaries with microinvasion: morphologic assessment of 13 cases. Int J Gynecol Pathol 1999;18:238–46.
22. Vang R, Gown AM, Barry TS, et al. Ovarian atypical proliferative (borderline) mucinous tumors: gastrointestinal and seromucinous (endocervical-like) types are immunophenotypically distinctive. Int J Gynecol Pathol 2006;25:83–9.
23. Lin X, Lindner JL, Silverman JF, Liu Y. Intestinal type and endocervical-like ovarian mucinous neoplasms are immunophenotypically distinct entities. Appl Immunohistochem Mol Morphol 2008;16:453–8.
24. Yasunaga M, Ohishi Y, Oda Y, et al. Immunohistochemical characterization of mullerian mucinous borderline tumors: possible histogenetic link with serous borderline tumors and low-grade endometrioid tumors. Hum Pathol 2009;40:965–74.
25. Wu CH, Mao TL, Vang R, et al. Endocervical-type mucinous borderline tumors are related to endometrioid tumors based on mutation and loss of expression of ARID1A. Int J Gynecol Pathol 2012;31:297–303.
26. Guerrieri C, Hogberg T, Wingren S, et al. Mucinous borderline and malignant tumors of the ovary. A clinicopathologic and DNA ploidy study of 92 cases. Cancer 1994;74:2329–40.
27. Siriaunkgul S, Robbins KM, McGowan L, Silverberg SG. Ovarian mucinous tumors of low malignant potential: a clinicopathologic study of 54 tumors of intestinal and müllerian type. Int J Gynecol Pathol 1995;14:198–208.
28. Nomura K, Aizawa S. Clinicopathologic and mucin histochemical analyses of 90 cases of ovarian mucinous borderline tumors of intestinal and mullerian types. Pathol Int 1996;46:575–80.
29. De Nictolis M, Montironi R, Tommasoni S, et al. Benign, borderline and well-differentiated malignant intestinal mucinous tumors of the ovary: a clinicopathologic, histochemical, immunohistochemical and nuclear quantitative study of 57 cases. Int J Gynecol Pathol 1994;13:10–21.
30. Riopel MA, Ronnett BM, Kurman RJ. Evaluation of diagnostic criteria and behavior of ovarian intestinal-type mucinous tumors. Atypical proliferative (borderline) tumors and intraepithelial, microinvasive, invasive and metastatic carcinomas. Am J Surg Pathol 1999;23:617–35.
31. Lee KR, Scully RE. Mucinous tumors of the ovary. A clinicopathologic study of 196 borderline tumors (of intestinal type) and carcinomas, including an evaluation of 11 cases with 'pseudomyxoma peritonei.' Am J Surg Pathol 2000;24:1447–64.
32. Rodriguez IM, Prat J. Mucinous tumors of the ovary. A clinicopathologic analysis of 75 borderline tumors (of intestinal type) and carcinomas. Am J Surg Pathol 2002;26:139–52.
33. Kim K-R, Lee H-I, Lee S-K, et al. Is stromal microinvasion in primary mucinous ovarian tumors with 'mucin granuloma' true invasion? Am J Surg Pathol 2007;31:546–54.
34. Khunamornpong S, Settakorn J, Sukpan K, et al. Mucinous tumor of low malignant potential ('borderline' or 'atypical proliferative' tumor) of the ovary: a study of 171 cases with the assessment of intraepithelial carcinoma and microinvasion. Int J Gynecol Pathol 2011;30:218–30.
35. Young RH, Hart WR. Metastases from carcinomas of the pancreas simulating primary mucinous tumors of the ovary: a report of seven cases. Am J Surg Pathol 1989;13:748–56.
36. Young RH, Gilks CB, Scully RE. Mucinous tumors of the appendix associated with mucinous tumors of the ovary and pseudomyxoma peritonei. A clinicopathological analysis of 22 cases supporting an origin in the appendix. Am J Surg Pathol 1991;15:415–29.
37. Lee KR, Tavassoli FA, Prat J, et al. Tumours of the ovary and peritoneum: surface epithelial-stromal tumours. In: Tavassoli FA, Devilee P, editors. World Health Organization classification of tumours. Pathology and genetics of tumours of the breast and female genital organs. Lyons, France: IARC Press; 2003.
38. Ronnett BM, Kajdacsy-Balla A, Gilks CB, et al. Mucinous borderline ovarian tumors: points of general agreement and persistent con-

troversies regarding nomenclature, diagnostic criteria, and behavior. Hum Pathol 2004;35:949–60.
39. Ludwick C, Gilks CB, Miller D, et al. Aggressive behavior of stage I ovarian mucinous tumors lacking extensive infiltrative invasion: a report of four cases and review of the literature. Int J Gynecol Pathol 2005;24:205–17.
40. Garrett AP, Lee KR, Colitti CR, et al. k-ras mutation may be an early event in mucinous ovarian tumorigenesis. Int J Gynecol Pathol 2001;20:244–51.
41. Pettersson F. Annual report of the results of treatment in gynecological cancer. Stockholm, Sweden: International Federation of Gynecology and Obstetrics; 1991.
42. Prayson RA, Hart WR, Petras RE. Pseudomyxoma peritonei. A clinicopathologic study of 19 cases with emphasis on site of origin and nature of associated ovarian tumors. Am J Surg Pathol 1994;18:591–603.
43. Ronnett BM, Kurman RJ, Zahn CM, et al. Pseudomyxoma peritonei in women: a clinicopathologic analysis of 30 cases with emphasis on site of origin, prognosis, and relationship to ovarian mucinous tumors of low malignant potential. Hum Pathol 1995;26:509–24.
44. Misdraji J, Yantiss RK, Graeme-Cook FM, et al. Appendiceal mucinous neoplasms. A clinicopathologic analysis of 107 cases. Am J Surg Pathol 2003;27:1089–103.
45. O'Connell JT, Tomlinson JS, Roberts AA, et al. Pseudomyxoma peritonei is a disease of MUC2-expressing goblet cells. Am J Pathol 2002;161:551–64.
46. Ronnett BM, Yan H, Kurman RJ, et al. Patients with pseudomyxoma peritonei associated with disseminated peritoneal adenomucinosis have a significantly more favorable prognosis than patients with peritoneal mucinous carcinomatosis. Cancer 2001;92:85–91.
47. Bradley RF, Stewart JH, Russell GB, et al. Pseudomyxoma peritonei of appendiceal origin: a clinicopathologic analysis of 101 patients uniformly treated at a single institution, with literature review. Am J Surg Pathol 2006;30:551–9.
48. Cuatrecasas M, Matias-Guiu X, Prat J. Synchronous mucinous tumors of the appendix and the ovary associated with pseudomyxoma peritonei: A clinicopathologic study of six cases with comparative analysis of c-Ki-ras mutations. Am J Surg Pathol 1996;20:739–46.
49. Szych C, Staebler A, Connolly DC, et al. Molecular genetic evidence supporting the clonality and appendiceal origin of Pseudomyxoma peritonei in women. Am J Pathol 1999;154:1849–55.
50. Ronnett BM, Seidman JD. Mucinous tumors arising in ovarian mature cystic teratomas: Relationship to the clinical syndrome of pseudomyxoma peritonei. Am J Surg Pathol 2003;27:650–7.
51. Pranesh N, Menasce LP, Wilson MS, O'Dwyer ST. Pseudomyxoma peritonei: unusual origin from an ovarian mature cystic teratoma. J Clin Pathol 2005;58:1115–17.
52. Marquette S, Amant F, Vergote I, Moerman P. Pseudomyxoma peritonei associated with a mucinous ovarian tumor arising from a mature cystic teratoma. A case report. Int J Gynecol Pathol 2006;25:340–3.
53. Vang R, Gown AM, Zhao C, et al. Ovarian mucinous tumors associated with mature cystic teratomas: morphologic and immunohistochemical analysis identifies a subset of potential teratomatous origin that shares features of lower gastrointestinal tract mucinous tumors more commonly encountered as secondary tumors in the ovary. Am J Surg Pathol 2007;31:854–69.
54. McKenney JK, Soslow RA, Longacre TA. Ovarian mature teratomas with mucinous epithelial neoplasms: morphologic heterogeneity and association with pseudomyxoma peritonei. Am J Surg Pathol 2008;32:645–55.
55. Chua TC, Moran BJ, Sugarbaker PH, et al. Early- and long-term outcome data of patients with pseudomyxoma peritonei from appendiceal origin treated by a strategy of cytoreductive surgery and hyperthermic intraperitoneal chemotherapy. J Clin Oncol 2012;30:2449–56.
56. Hart WR, Norris HJ. Borderline and malignant mucinous tumors of the ovary. Histologic criteria and clinical behavior. Cancer 1973;31:1031–45.
57. Seidman JD, Kurman RJ, Ronnett BM. Primary and metastatic mucinous adenocarcinomas in the ovaries. Incidence in routine practice with a new approach to improve intraoperative diagnosis. Am J Surg Pathol 2003;27:985–93.
58. Hoerl HD, Hart WR. Primary ovarian mucinous cystadenocarcinomas. A clinicopathologic study of 49 cases with long term follow-up. Am J Surg Pathol 1998;22:1449–62.
59. Lee KR, Nucci MR. Ovarian mucinous and mixed epithelial carcinomas of mullerian (endocervical-like) type: a clinicopathologic analysis of four cases of an uncommon variant associated with endometriosis. Int J Gynecol Pathol 2003;22:42–51.
60. Vang R, Gown AM, Barry TS, et al. Cytokeratins 7 and 20 in primary and secondary mucinous tumors of the ovary: analysis of coordinate immunohistochemical expression profiles and staining distribution in 179 cases. Am J Surg Pathol 2006;30:1130–9.
61. Park SY, Kim HS, Hong EK, Kim WH. Expression of cytokeratins 7 and 20 in primary carcinomas of the stomach and colorectum and their value in the differential diagnosis of metastatic carcinomas to the ovary. Hum Pathol 2002;33:1078–85.
62. Soslow RA, Rouse RV, Hendrickson MR, et al. Transitional cell neoplasms of the ovary and urinary bladder: A comparative immunohistochemical analysis. Int J Gynecol Pathol 1996;15:257–65.
63. Chu PG, Weiss LM. Keratin expression in human tissues and neoplasms. Histopathology 2002;40:403–39.
64. Ji H, Isacson C, Seidman J, et al. Cytokeratins 7 and 20, Dpc4, and MUC5AC in the distinction of metastatic mucinous carcinomas in the ovary from primary ovarian mucinous tumors: Dpc4 assists in identifying metastatic pancreatic carcinomas. Int J Gynecol Pathol 2002;21:391–400.
65. Lee MJ, Lee HS, Kim WH, et al. Expression of mucins and cytokeratins in primary carcinomas of the digestive system. Mod Pathol 2003;16:403–10.
66. Vang R, Gown AM, Barry TS, et al. Immunohistochemistry for estrogen and progesterone receptors in the distinction of primary and metastatic mucinous tumors in the ovary: an analysis of 124 cases. Mod Pathol 2006;19:97–105.
67. Vang R, Gown AM, Farinola M, et al. p16 expression in primary ovarian mucinous and endometrioid tumors and metastatic adenocarcinomas in the ovary: utility for identification of metastatic HPV related endocervical adenocarcinomas. Am J Surg Pathol 2007;31:653–63.
68. Lee KR, Young RH. The distinction between primary and metastatic mucinous carcinomas of the ovary: gross and histologic findings in 50 cases. Am J Surg Pathol 2003;27:281–92.
69. Elishaev E, Gilks CB, Miller D, et al. Synchronous and metachronous endocervical and ovarian neoplasms: evidence supporting interpretation of the ovarian neoplasms as metastatic endocervical adenocarcinomas simulating primary ovarian surface epithelial neoplasms. Am J Surg Pathol 2005;29:281–94.
70. Khunamornpong S, Suprasert P, Pojchamarnwiputh S, et al. Primary and metastatic mucinous adenocarcinomas of the ovary: Evaluation of the diagnostic approach using tumor size and laterality. Gynecol Oncol 2006;101:152–7.
71. Yemelyanova AV, Vang R, Judson K, et al. Distinction of primary and metastatic mucinous tumors involving the ovary: analysis of size and laterality data by primary site with reevaluation of an algorithm for tumor classification. Am J Surg Pathol 2008;32:128–38.
72. Anglesio MS, Kommoss S, Tolcher MC, et al. Molecular characterization of mucinous ovarian tumours supports a stratified treatment approach with HER2 targeting in 19% of carcinomas. J Pathol 2013;229:111–20.
73. Zaino RJ, Brady MF, Lele SM, et al. Advanced stage mucinous adenocarcinoma of the ovary is both rare and highly lethal: a Gynecologic Oncology Group study. Cancer 2011;117:554–62.
74. Schiavone MB, Herzog TJ, Lewin SN, et al. Natural history and outcome of mucinous carcinoma of the ovary. Am J Obstet Gynecol 2011;205:480.e1–8.
75. Nomura K, Aizawa S. Noninvasive, microinvasive, and invasive mucinous carcinomas of the ovary. A clinicopathologic analysis of 40 cases. Cancer 2000;89:1541–6.
76. Bagué S, Rodríguez IM, Prat J. Sarcoma-like mural nodules in mucinous cystic tumors of the ovary revisited: A clinicopathologic analysis of 10 additional cases. Am J Surg Pathol 2002;26:1467–76.
77. Provenza C, Young RH, Prat J. Anaplastic carcinoma in mucinous ovarian tumors: a clinicopathologic study of 34 cases emphasizing the crucial impact of stage on prognosis, their histologic spectrum, and overlap with sarcoma-like mural nodules. Am J Surg Pathol 2008;32:383–9.
78. Nakamura E, Shimizu M, Mikami Y, et al. Ovarian mucinous cystadenocarcinoma with malignant mural nodules. Pathol Int 1998;48:645–8.

27 Ovarian Endometrioid, Clear Cell, Transitional, and Mixed Epithelial–Stromal Tumors

Jaime Prat

CHAPTER OUTLINE

Endometrioid Tumors	608
Epithelial Tumors	609
Mixed Tumors (Tumors with a Sarcomatous Component)	618
Tumors of Smooth Muscle	623
Clear Cell Tumors	624
Benign Clear Cell Tumors	625
Borderline Clear Cell Tumors	625
Clear Cell Adenocarcinomas	626
Transitional Cell Tumors	629
Benign Brenner Tumor	629
Borderline and Malignant Brenner Tumors	630
Squamous Cell Lesions	633
Epidermoid (Squamous Cell) Cysts	633
Squamous Cell Carcinomas	633
Mixed Epithelial Tumors	633
Undifferentiated Carcinomas	634
Miscellaneous and Unclassified Tumors	635
Small Cell Undifferentiated Carcinoma, Hypercalcemic Type	635
Small Cell Carcinoma, Pulmonary Type	636
Undifferentiated Carcinoma of Non-Small Cell (Neuroendocrine) Type	636
Cysts and Adenomas of the Rete Ovarii	636
Adenomatoid Tumors	636
Hepatoid Carcinomas	637
Female Adnexal Tumors of Wolffian Origin	637

ENDOMETRIOID TUMORS

Endometrioid tumors of the ovary resemble those encountered more frequently in the endometrium.[1,2] They include endometrioid carcinomas, endometrioid stromal sarcomas, adenosarcomas, and malignant mesodermal mixed tumors (carcinosarcomas). Endometrioid carcinomas are the most common. Although an origin from endometriosis can be demonstrated in some cases, it is not required for the diagnosis (almost all müllerian tumors can originate from endometriosis).[1,2] Recent molecular genetic studies, however, suggest that most endometrioid *cancers* are caused by the malignant transformation of endometriosis and do not derive from the ovarian surface epithelium.[3–6]

The epithelial cells of endometrioid tumors resemble those of proliferative endometrium. Diastase–periodic acid–Schiff (PAS) and mucicarmine staining reveal some extracellular mucin plus staining of the luminal glycocalyx. Ten percent of tumors contain argyrophil cells of neuroendocrine type. Secretory changes similar to those seen in postovulatory endometrium are frequently seen in well-differentiated tumors and squamous elements are common. Most ovarian endometrioid carcinomas are moderately or well-differentiated tumors with a predominantly glandular or papillary architecture. Presently, the poorly differentiated carcinomas tend to be classified as high-grade serous carcinomas, suggesting that high-grade endometrioid carcinoma is not a distinct tumor type.[7] The Systematized Nomenclature of Medicine (SNOMED) classification of endometrioid tumors is as follows:

Adenofibroma
  Cystadenofibroma
Cystadenoma
Endometrioid borderline tumor
Endometrioid adenocarcinoma
  Not otherwise specified
  Malignant adenofibroma
  Variant with squamous differentiation
  Ciliated variant
  Oxyphilic variant

Secretory variant
Sertoliform variant
Malignant mesodermal (müllerian) mixed tumor (carcinosarcoma)
Adenosarcoma
Endometrioid stromal
Undifferentiated sarcoma

EPITHELIAL TUMORS

Clinical Features

Endometrioid epithelial tumors represent 2–4% of all ovarian tumors.[2] Benign endometrioid tumors (mostly adenofibromas) are rare and account for <1% of benign ovarian tumors. Only 2–3% of borderline ovarian tumors are endometrioid. Endometrioid carcinomas account for 10–15% of ovarian carcinomas, representing the second most common form of ovarian epithelial malignancy;[2] however, when strict criteria are used (i.e., close resemblance to uterine endometrioid carcinoma and reclassification of nonspecific high-grade carcinomas as serous carcinomas), the frequency falls to <10%.

Benign, borderline, and malignant endometrioid epithelial tumors occur most commonly in women in the perimenopausal or postmenopausal age groups, with mean ages of 56, 51, and 56 years, respectively.[2] Most patients with borderline endometrioid tumors have endometriosis (63%) and concomitant endometrial hyperplasia/carcinoma is common (39%).[8] Similarly, about 40% of the endometrioid carcinomas are associated with documented ipsilateral ovarian or pelvic endometriosis.[2,9] Patients whose tumors are accompanied by endometriosis are 5–10 years younger on average than patients without associated ovarian endometriosis.[2,10,11] Endometriosis-related ovarian carcinomas are more frequently low grade and low stage and have a more favorable prognosis than carcinomas unrelated to endometriosis.[12] Endometrioid carcinomas are confined to the ovaries and adjacent pelvic structures in 70% of cases. They are bilateral in 28% of all cases and in 13% of those in International Federation of Gynecologists and Obstetricians (FIGO) stages I–II.

Endometrioid carcinoma of the ovary is associated in 15–20% of cases with carcinoma of the endometrium.[2,13] The favorable outcome in those cases in which the tumor is limited to both organs suggests that these are mostly independent primary tumors arising as a result of a müllerian field effect or due to implantation of endometrial stem cells carrying genetic abnormalities.[13–15] The criteria for distinguishing ovarian metastasis, uterine metastasis, and independent primary tumors of both organs are presented in the following sections.

Like most ovarian carcinomas, many endometrioid carcinomas are asymptomatic. Some present as a pelvic mass with or without pain, and may be associated with endocrine symptoms secondary to steroid hormone secretion by the specialized ovarian stroma.[16] Serum CA125 is elevated in over 80% of the cases.[17]

Pathogenesis

The frequent association of ovarian endometrioid carcinomas with endometriosis, endometrial carcinoma, or both, suggests that some ovarian endometrioid carcinomas may

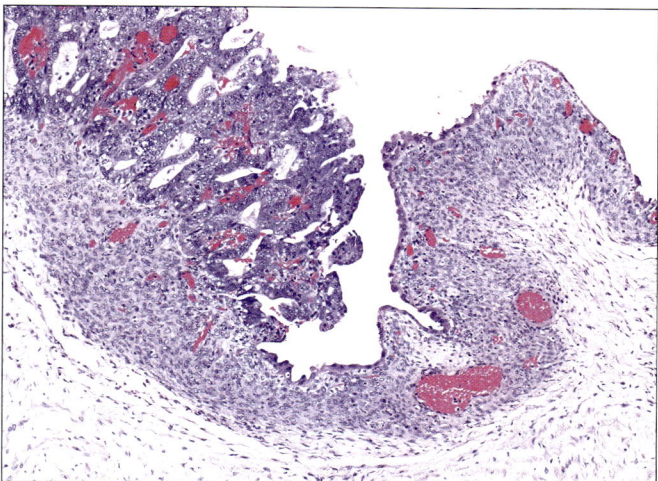

Figure 27.1 Endometrioid adenocarcinoma arising from endometriosis.

have the same risk factors for their development as endometrial carcinomas. Up to 42% of the endometrioid carcinomas are associated with ipsilateral ovarian or pelvic endometriosis,[10] an entity in which the entire spectrum of endometrial hyperplasia can be seen[18] (see Chapter 22). Several epidemiologic studies have shown that ovarian endometriosis is associated with an increased risk of developing ovarian endometrioid and clear cell carcinomas (CCCs)[9,12,19,20] and a direct transition from ovarian atypical endometriosis to carcinomas has been described in 15–32% of cases[11] (Figure 27.1). Atypical ipsilateral endometriosis occurs in up to 23% of endometrioid carcinomas and may have a role in the process of transformation to malignancy.[11,18] Occasionally, however, the lining epithelium of endometriotic cysts shows large cells with abundant eosinophilic cytoplasm and large, hyperchromatic, smudgy nuclei. This cytologic change is often seen in the absence of carcinoma and its malignant potential is unknown.[21]

In cases of ovarian endometrioid carcinoma associated with endometriosis, common genetic alterations have been encountered in the adjacent endometriosis, atypical endometriosis, and adenocarcinoma.[4] In mice harboring K-RAS mutations that result in the development of benign lesions reminiscent of endometriosis, deletion of PTEN leads to the induction of invasive endometrioid carcinoma.[22] Recently, AT-rich interactive domain 1A (ARID1A) gene mutations have been discovered in endometrioid carcinomas and CCCs as well as in adjacent endometriosis.[23] These findings indicate that inactivation of tumor suppressor genes such as PTEN or ARID1A may represent early events in the malignant transformation of endometriosis.[6]

BENIGN ENDOMETRIOID TUMORS

Most benign endometrioid tumors are unilateral endometrioid adenofibromas. These rare tumors have a mean size of about 10 cm in diameter, and about one-sixth are bilateral. The external surface is smooth and the cut surface is firm and densely fibrous displaying variably sized cystic spaces. The cysts contain clear or yellowish fluid. Occasionally, the tumors are predominantly cystic.

The rare endometrioid cystadenomas are similar to endometriotic cysts but lack endometrial stroma, hemosiderin-laden macrophages, and a myofibroblastic wall. Nevertheless, their frequent merging with endometriotic cysts suggests that a pure endometrioid cystadenoma may not even exist. Adenofibromas have non-mucinous glands lying within an abundant fibromatous stroma. Tall columnar epithelium resembles that of proliferative endometrium, with basophilic to deeply eosinophilic cytoplasm and elongate nuclei with relatively coarse chromatin and small but obvious nucleoli, or inactive endometrium with uniform dark nuclei and scanty cytoplasm. Mitoses are rarely seen. Squamous differentiation in the form of morules is a common finding.[1,2]

BORDERLINE ENDOMETRIOID TUMORS

Pathologic Features

Borderline endometrioid tumors may appear as either multilocular cystadenofibromas similar to benign tumors or cystic tumors with solid but friable mural nodules.

There is no agreement on the criteria for the diagnosis of borderline endometrioid tumors. Most are adenofibromatous and show crowded endometrial-like glands and cystic spaces embedded in stroma that varies from ovarian to hyaline or collagenous (Figure 27.2). The second most common pattern is villoglandular or papillary with an atypical cell lining similar to atypical hyperplasia of the endometrium also in a fibromatous background. By World Health Organization (WHO) criteria, these tumors exhibit glands or cysts lined by atypical or cytologically malignant endometrioid-type cells without obvious stromal invasion (Figure 27.3).[1] Mitoses range up to 4 mitotic figures per 10 HPF but are rarely atypical. Squamous metaplasia, present in one-third to one-half of cases, may be occasionally both florid (Figure 27.4) and keratinizing. It may give rise to a foreign body giant cell reaction. Stromal luteinization occasionally occurs. An uncommon stromal change is focal metaplastic benign bone formation. When the epithelial component is carcinomatous the term borderline endometrioid tumor with *intraepithelial carcinoma* is used and the tumor is graded 1–3 (Figure 27.3). Microinvasion is arbitrarily defined as the presence of one or more foci of epithelial cells haphazardly infiltrating the stroma, 10 mm^2 or less in area.[2] Tumors exhibiting confluent glandular growth (5 mm or more in maximum diameter) and destructive stromal invasion greater than microinvasion are diagnosed as invasive carcinomas. Cytologic atypia and microinvasion do not appear to affect the favorable prognosis of borderline endometrioid tumors and conservative treatment, i.e., unilateral salpingo-oophorectomy, appears to be curative. However, only 134 cases have been reported and clinical follow-up data are limited.[8,24]

Immunohistochemistry and Somatic Genetics

The immunohistochemical profile of borderline endometrioid tumors resembles that of endometrioid carcinomas (see later). In both, β-catenin gene mutation appears to be an early event in tumorigenesis.[25] In a study of eight borderline endometrioid tumors, a strong nuclear β-catenin immunoreaction (in both, the glandular and squamous components) was obtained in all cases, and seven (90%)

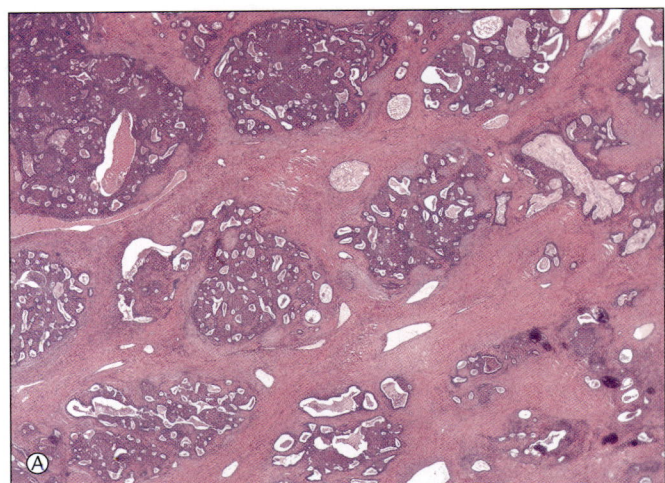
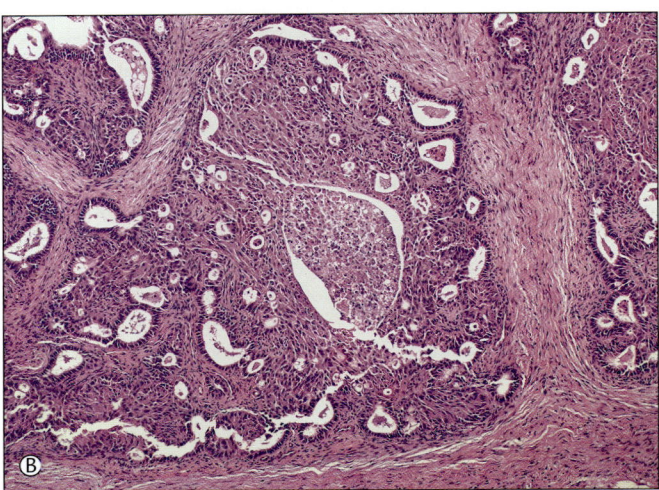

Figure 27.2 Borderline endometrioid adenofibroma. **(A)** Crowded endometrial-like glands and cystic spaces are embedded in dense fibrous stroma. **(B)** The squamous differentiation confirms the endometrioid nature of the tumor.

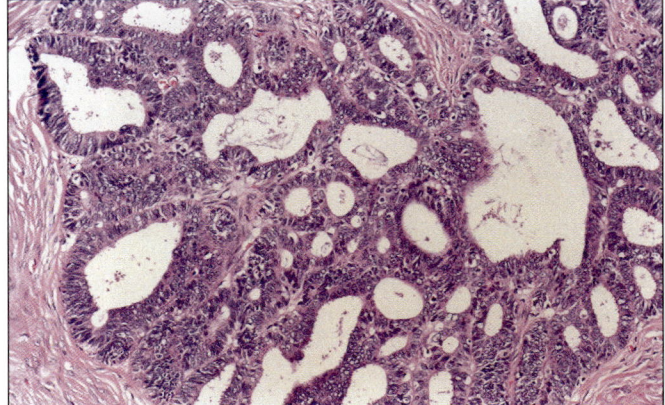

Figure 27.3 Borderline endometrioid adenofibroma with well-differentiated (grade 1) intraepithelial carcinoma. Island of crowded glands with cribriform pattern and moderate nuclear atypia without obvious stromal invasion.

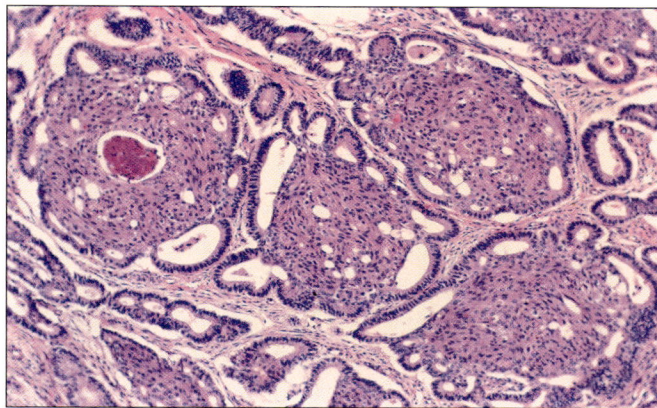

Figure 27.4 Borderline endometrioid adenofibroma. Endometrioid glands are partly replaced by squamous morules with occasional central necrosis. (Reproduced with permission of Lippincott Williams & Wilkins.)

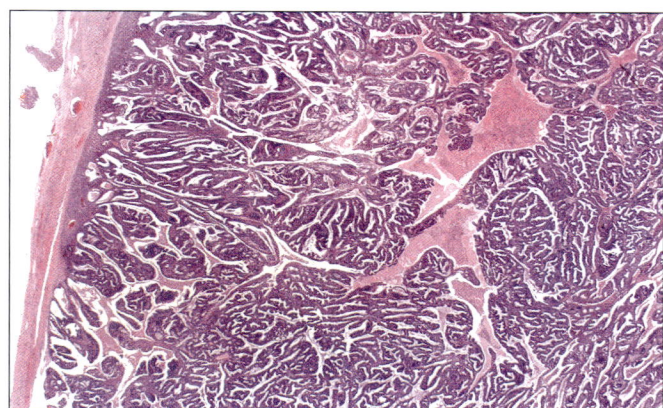

Figure 27.6 Well-differentiated endometrioid adenocarcinoma (grade 1). The tumor shows a villoglandular pattern.

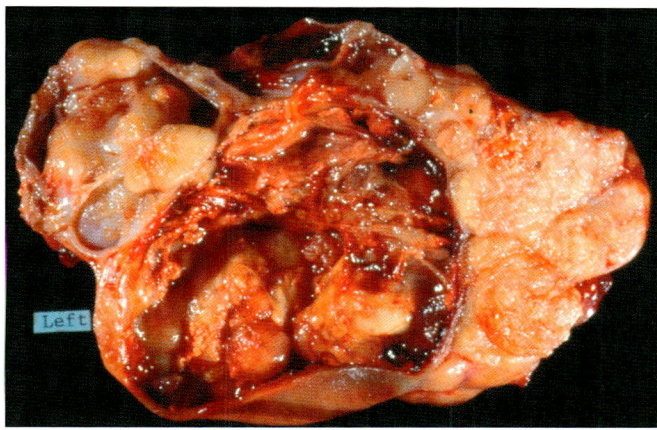

Figure 27.5 Endometrioid adenocarcinoma arising from an endometriotic cyst. The polypoid tumor protrudes from the inner surface of the sectioned cyst and has extended through the capsule.

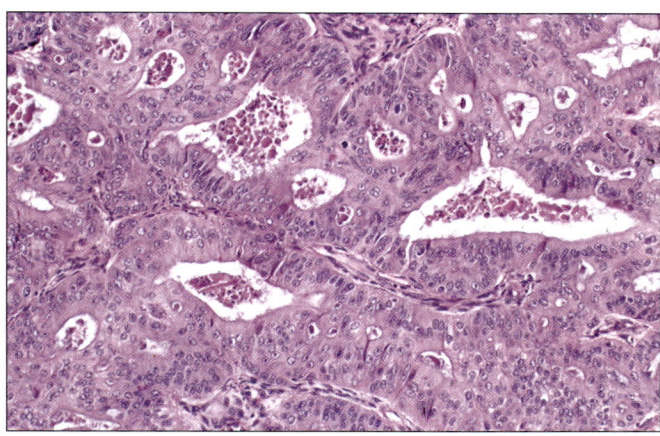

Figure 27.7 Endometrioid adenocarcinoma. The crowded neoplastic glands are lined by stratified non-mucin-containing epithelium. Nuclear atypia is moderate.

had β-catenin gene (*CTNNB1*) mutations. Only one tumor had a *PTEN* mutation. Neither *K-RAS* mutations nor microsatellite instability were encountered.

ENDOMETRIOID CARCINOMAS

Macroscopic Features

Endometrioid carcinomas are predominantly cystic, measuring 12–20 cm in diameter, with usually smooth outer surfaces. The cut surfaces reveal friable soft masses or papillae partly filling cystic spaces that may contain blood-stained fluid. Rarely, they are completely solid, exhibiting hemorrhage or necrosis. Mucus may sometimes fill the cystic spaces. The tumor, if it has arisen in an endometriotic cyst, tends to be a polypoid nodule projecting into the lumen of a thick-walled blood-filled cyst (Figure 27.5).

Microscopic Features

Ovarian endometrioid carcinomas closely resemble endometrioid carcinomas of the uterine corpus. Most tumors show confluent glandular proliferation or 'expansile invasion.'[26] There is back-to-back arrangement of the glands with reduction of the stroma, glandular branching, cribriform pattern, and complex papillary proliferation (Figure 27.6). Less frequently, the tumors exhibit destructive infiltrative growth characterized by obvious stromal invasion in the form of glands, cell clusters, or individual cells, disorderly infiltrating the stroma and frequently associated with a desmoplastic or inflammatory stromal reaction.[26]

Most endometrioid carcinomas are well differentiated— particularly those arising from endometriotic cysts—and show round, oval, or tubular glands lined by stratified non-mucin-containing epithelium (Figure 27.7). Mitoses range up to about 5 per 10 HPF. Cribriform or villoglandular patterns may be present (Figure 27.8). The broad blunt papillae with obvious connective tissue cores differ from the usually fine micropapillae of serous carcinomas. Squamous differentiation occurs in 30–50% of the cases, often in the form of morules (cytologically benign-appearing squamous cells) (Figure 27.9).[2] Occasionally, the squamous elements appear malignant and are then intimately admixed with or

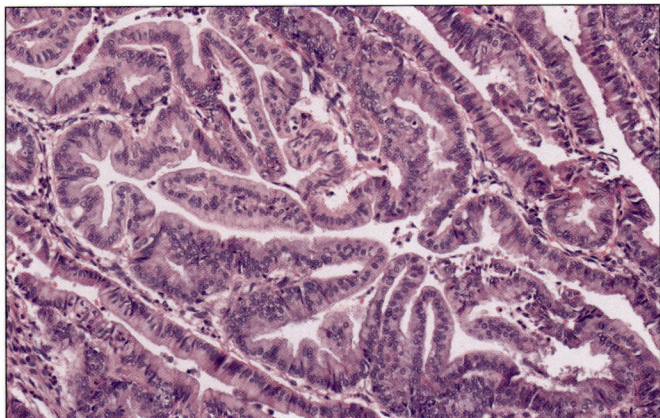

Figure 27.8 Well-differentiated endometrioid adenocarcinoma with villoglandular architecture.

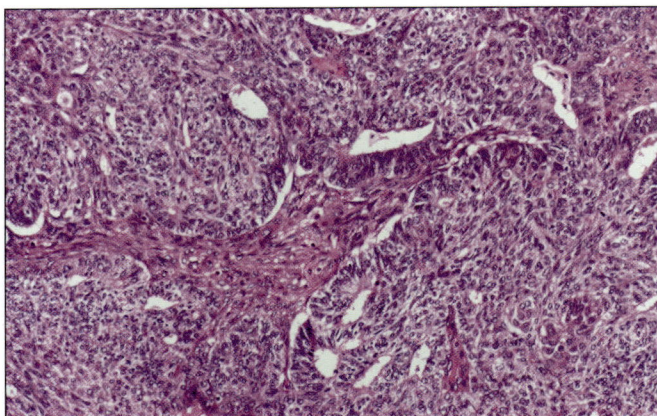

Figure 27.10 Endometrioid adenocarcinoma with spindle-shaped epithelial cells. The spindle-shaped cells merge almost imperceptibly with the glandular epithelium (abortive squamous differentiation).

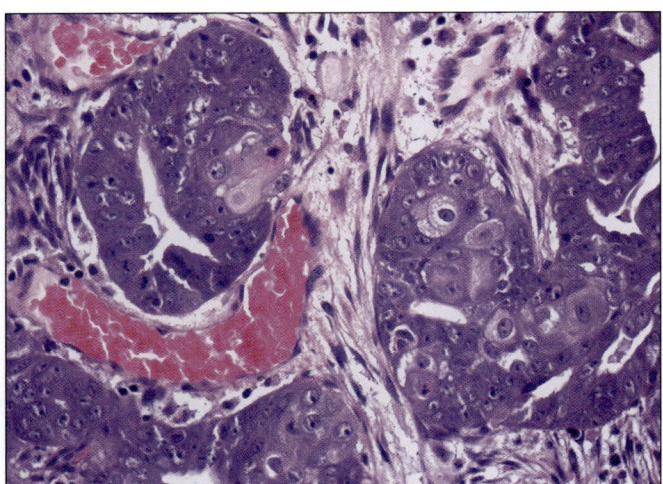

Figure 27.9 Moderately differentiated endometrioid adenocarcinoma with squamous differentiation.

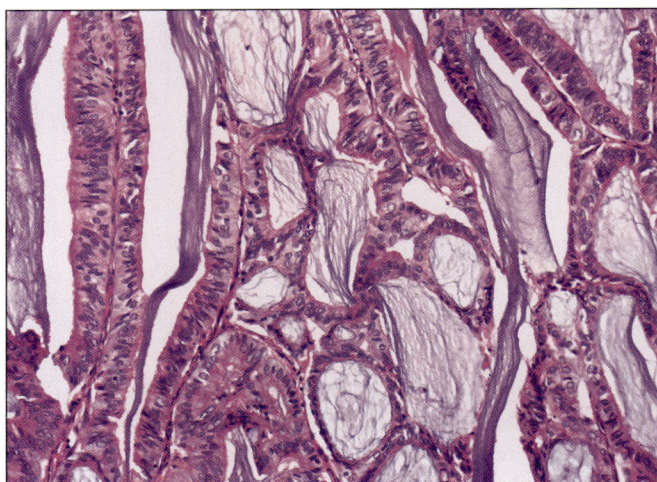

Figure 27.11 Endometrioid adenocarcinoma, mucin-rich form. The glands are filled with mucin.

separated from the glandular component. The current designation 'endometrioid carcinoma with squamous differentiation' is generally preferable to the adenoacanthoma or adenosquamous carcinoma, even though the latter terms in many cases more succinctly convey the degree of histologic differentiation of the squamous epithelium.[1,2] Aggregates of spindle-shaped epithelial cells are an occasional finding in endometrioid carcinoma (Figure 27.10).[27] Rarely, the spindle cell nests undergo a transition to clearly recognizable squamous cells, suggesting that the former may represent abortive squamous differentiation.[27] Some well-differentiated endometrioid carcinomas, almost always with a squamous component, may have a prominent fibrous stroma (malignant adenofibromas). Stromal invasion in such tumors is difficult to document and inferred only by the extent and complexity of the glandular component and the presence of a desmoplastic stroma.

Rare examples of mucin-rich (Figure 27.11), secretory, ciliated cell, and oxyphilic types have been described.[28,29] In the mucin-rich variant, glandular lumens and apex of the cell cytoplasm are occupied by mucin.[30] Minor foci of mucinous epithelium are present in some endometrioid carcinomas and should not lead to the diagnosis of mucinous carcinoma. The secretory type contains vacuolated cells with supranuclear and/or subnuclear vacuoles resembling those of an early secretory endometrium.[2] Hobnail cells are not seen. The oxyphilic variant has a prominent component of large polygonal tumor cells with abundant eosinophilic cytoplasm and round central nuclei with prominent nucleoli.[29]

Occasional tumors contain solid areas punctuated by tubular or round glands or small rosette-like glands (microglandular pattern) simulating an adult granulosa cell tumor.[31] Unlike the Call–Exner bodies found in granulosa cell tumors, the microglands in endometrioid carcinomas contain intraluminal mucin. The nuclei of endometrioid carcinomas are usually round and hyperchromatic, whereas those of granulosa cell tumors are round, oval, or angular, pale, and grooved[31] (see Chapter 28). Rare

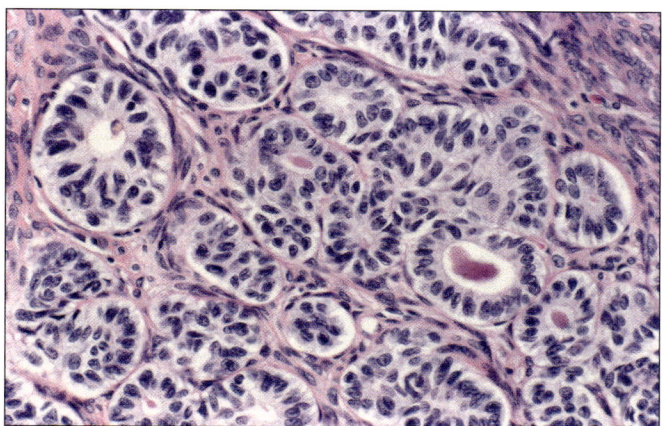

Figure 27.12 Endometrioid adenocarcinoma resembling a Sertoli cell tumor. Tubular glands lined by cells with oval nuclei and clear cytoplasms, resembling the tubules of a Sertoli cell tumor.

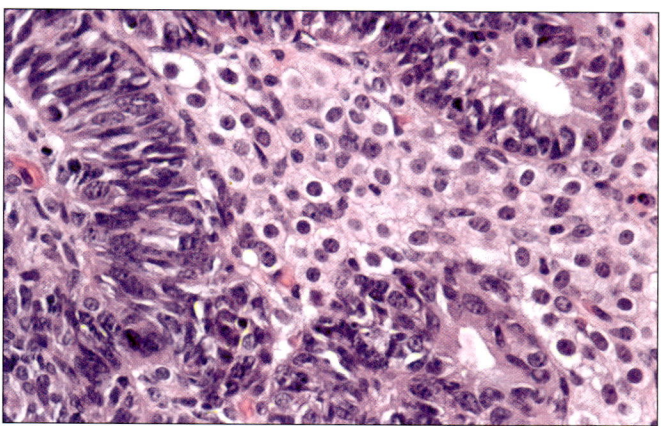

Figure 27.14 Endometrioid adenocarcinoma resembling a Sertoli–Leydig cell tumor. The tubular glands contain high-grade nuclei. The luteinized ovarian stromal cells resemble Leydig cells.

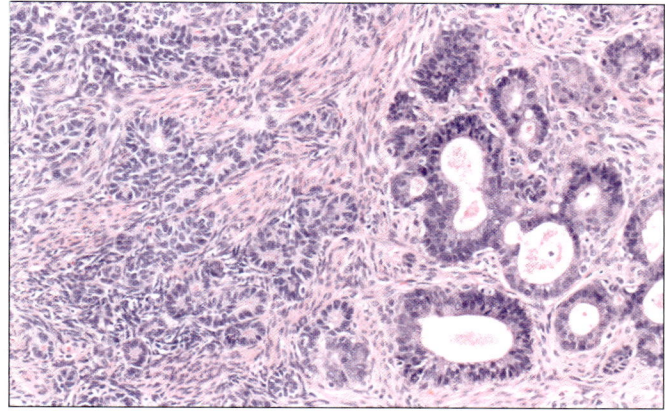

Figure 27.13 Endometrioid adenocarcinoma resembling a Sertoli cell tumor. The small tubular glands, resembling the tubules of a Sertoli cell tumor (left), appear adjacent to typical glands of endometrioid carcinoma (right).

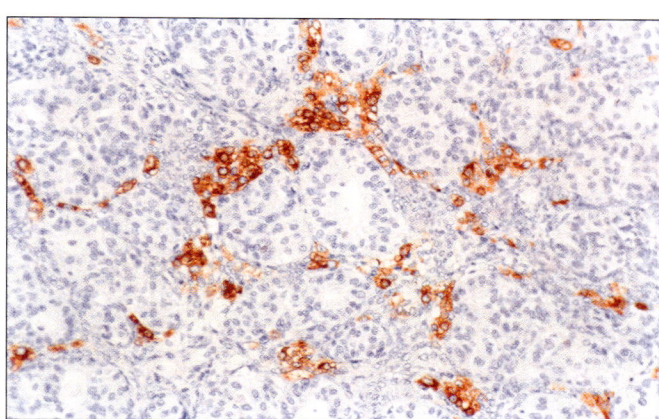

Figure 27.15 Endometrioid adenocarcinoma resembling a Sertoli–Leydig cell tumor. Immunoreaction for α-inhibin is positive in the luteinized stromal cells and negative in the epithelial cells.

cases of endometrioid carcinomas of the ovary show focal to extensive areas resembling Sertoli and Sertoli–Leydig cell tumors (Figures 27.12 and 27.13).[31-33] They contain small, well-differentiated hollow tubules, solid tubules or, rarely, thin cords resembling sex cords. Furthermore, the stroma may appear cellular and fibrous, resembling the spindle cell component of stromal tumors. When the stroma is luteinized (Figure 27.14), this variant (designated as 'endometrioid carcinoma resembling sex cord–stromal tumor' or 'sertoliform endometrioid carcinoma') may be mistaken for a Sertoli–Leydig cell tumor, particularly if the patient is virilized. However, typical glands of endometrioid carcinoma and squamous differentiation are each present in 75% of the tumors, facilitating their recognition as an endometrioid carcinoma.[31] Furthermore, immunostains for α-inhibin (Figure 27.15) and calretinin show reactivity in the luteinized stromal cells and Sertoli cells but not in the cells of endometrioid carcinoma.[34] At surgery, most of these tumors are confined to the ovary (FIGO stage I).

Rarely, endometrioid carcinomas may exhibit an adenoid basal or adenoid cystic-like component[35] (Figure 27.16). Recently, endometrioid carcinomas with transitional cell-like differentiation have been reported.[36] More rarely, endometrioid carcinomas may contain yolk sac tumor elements. These tumors are often large and have an unfavorable prognosis.[37,38] Immunoreactions for α-fetoprotein (AFP) and glypican-3 are strongly positive in the yolk sac tumor component.

Most well-differentiated endometrioid adenocarcinomas contain areas of endometriosis, endometrioid adenofibroma, or borderline endometrioid tumor.[26,39]

Poorly differentiated endometrioid carcinomas are rare and have a predominantly solid pattern with focal microglandular areas. Mitotic activity is high (up to 5 or more mitoses per HPF) and squamous or secretory change infrequent. Hemorrhage and/or necrosis are prominent. However, most high-grade carcinomas with these features would be currently classified as serous carcinomas.[40]

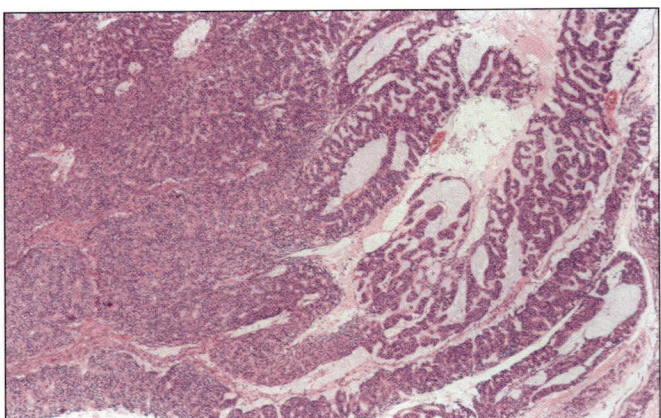

Figure 27.16 Adenoid cystic-like component in endometrioid carcinoma.

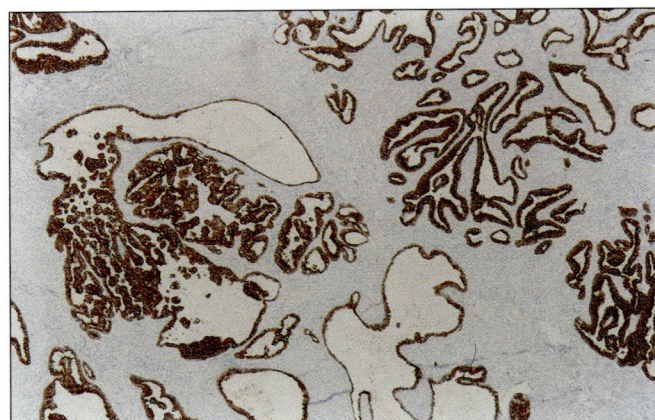

Figure 27.17 Endometrioid adenocarcinoma. Positive immunoreaction for CK7.

Sometimes, ovarian carcinomas with a predominantly endometrioid component are mixed with other epithelial types such as clear cell and serous carcinoma. A mixed epithelial tumor is diagnosed when 10% or more of a second or third type of epithelium is present.[1]

About 10% of endometrioid carcinomas contain argyrophilic cells of neuroendocrine type. Occasionally, bone metaplasia can be found.

Immunohistochemistry

Endometrioid carcinomas react strongly with epithelial markers including cytoplasmic immunoreaction for cytokeratins (CK7, 97%; CK20, 13% positive) (Figure 27.17) and membranous reaction for epithelial membrane antigen (EMA). The rate of immunoreactivity for other markers is as follows: vimentin, 31%; B72.3, 86%; OC-125, 76%; and carcinoembryonic antigen (CEA), 30%. Estrogen receptors (ERs) and progesterone receptors (PRs) are positive in the majority of cases.[41] WT1 and p16 are usually negative[42,43] but WT1 can be positive in 17–29%[44–47] and focal p16 immunoreactivity can occur in up to half of cases.[44] BRCA1 protein is usually positive (nuclear reaction).[48] Inhibin is usually negative,[34,49] but calretinin is strongly positive in 10%, and weakly positive in an additional 10–25%.[45,50] CD99 is often positive. PTEN expression is negative in well-differentiated carcinomas; however, PTEN immunoreaction is unreliable.[51] Most tumors with microsatellite instability, approximately 10–15% of ovarian endometrioid adenocarcinomas,[52] show negative immunoreaction for hMLH1 and hMSH2 proteins.[53] Strong and diffuse immunoreactivity for p53 should raise the differential diagnosis of high-grade serous carcinoma.

Grading

Grading of endometrioid carcinoma of the ovary uses the same criteria as for endometrial adenocarcinoma[54] (see Chapter 18). Grade I tumors are glandular or papillary neoplasms exhibiting <5% of solid tumor growth (Figure 27.6). Grade II tumors show 5–50% solid growth, and grade III tumors show >50% solid tumor growth (Figure 27.18). Areas of squamous or spindle cell differentiation are not counted as solid growth. When the nuclei are highly atypical and the

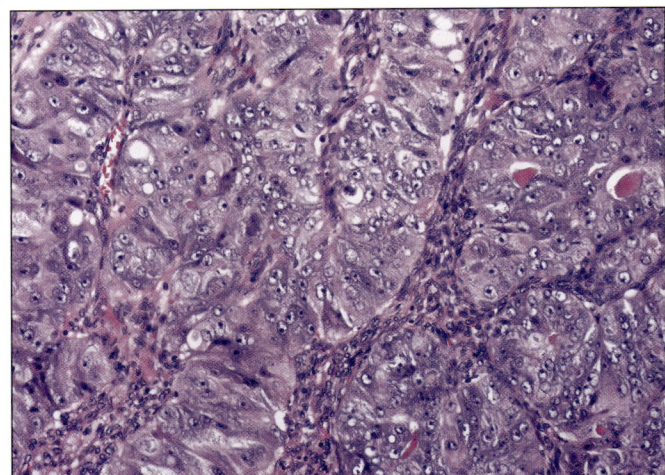

Figure 27.18 Endometrioid carcinoma. Predominantly solid tumor with grade 3 nuclei.

architectural glandular pattern is grade I or II, the overall tumor grade is increased by one. Most ovarian endometrioid carcinomas are well differentiated, and show low-grade nuclei. Thus, nuclear grade is the best discriminator.

Spread and Metastasis

Stage I carcinomas are bilateral in 17% of the cases. The stage distribution of endometrioid carcinomas differs from that of serous carcinomas. According to the FIGO annual report, 31% of the tumors are stage I, 20% stage II, 38% stage III, and 11% stage IV.[55] However, in a review of 874 cases from 19 series, 43% of the tumors were stage I.[24]

Genetic Susceptibility

Most endometrioid carcinomas occur sporadically but occasional cases develop in families with germline mutations in DNA mismatch repair genes, mainly MSH-2 and MLH-1 (Muir–Torre syndrome).[56] This syndrome, a variant of the hereditary nonpolyposis colorectal cancer (HNPCC) syndrome, reflects an inherited autosomal dominant susceptibility to develop cutaneous and visceral neoplasms.[57]

Somatic Genetics

The molecular genetic alterations of well-differentiated ovarian endometrioid carcinomas are similar to those of their uterine counterparts. Compared with uterine endometrioid carcinomas, the ovarian tumors have similar frequency of β-catenin abnormalities but a lower rate of microsatellite instability and *PTEN* alterations.[52] β-catenin protein, encoded by the *CTNNB1* gene located in 3p21, maintains cell polarity by interacting with E-cadherin at the cell membrane. In the cytoplasm, free β-catenin interacts with the adenomatous polyposis coli (APC) protein and may function as a transcription factor. The APC protein downregulates β-catenin by cooperating with the glycogen synthase kinase 3-β (GSK-3-β), inducing phosphorylation of the serine–threonine residues coded in exon 3 of the *CTNNB1* gene and its degradation through the ubiquitin–proteasome pathway. *CTNNB1* activating mutations alter recognition sequences and inhibit phosphorylation, resulting in cytoplasmic and nuclear accumulation of β-catenin, signal transduction, and transcriptional activation through the LEF/Tcf pathway. Increased β-catenin expression caused by *CTNNB1* or *APC* mutations results in uncontrolled activation of target genes such as matrix metalloproteinase-7 (*MMP-7*) and cyclin D1 (*CD1*). Activating mutations of the *CTNNB1* gene occur in 38–50% of ovarian endometrioid carcinomas (Figure 27.19)[52,58,59] and nuclear β-catenin immunoreaction is seen in the tumor cells in over 80% of these cases. Endometrioid carcinomas with *CTNNB1* mutations often show squamous differentiation, and are low-grade and early stage tumors associated with good prognosis.[52,60]

The tumor suppressor gene *PTEN* is located in chromosome 10q23.3, a genomic region undergoing loss of heterozygosity (LOH) in a wide variety of human cancers. *PTEN* encodes a lipid phosphatase that antagonizes the PI3K/AKT pathway by dephosphorylating PIP_3, the product of PI3K. PI3K is a heterodimer enzyme consisting of a catalytic subunit (p110) and a regulatory subunit (p85). The *PIK3CA* gene, located on chromosome 3q26.32, codes for the p110 catalytic subunit of PI3K. Decreased *PTEN* activity causes activation of the PI3K/AKT pathway and expression of several genes involved in suppression of apoptosis and cell cycle progression. *PTEN* may be inactivated by several mechanisms such as mutation, LOH at 10q23, and promoter hypermethylation. Loss of function of the two alleles is needed for *PTEN* inactivation and, usually, mutation and LOH coexist. *PTEN* is mutated in approximately 20% of endometrioid ovarian tumors (Figure 27.20) and in 46% of those with 10q23 LOH.[5,52] *PTEN* mutations occur between exons 3 and 8. The majority of endometrioid carcinomas with *PTEN* mutations are well-differentiated and stage I tumors, suggesting that *PTEN* inactivation is an early event in this subset of ovarian tumors.[5,52,60] The finding of 10q23 LOH and *PTEN* mutations in endometriotic cysts that are adjacent to endometrioid carcinomas with similar genetic alterations provides additional evidence for the precursor role of endometriosis in ovarian carcinogenesis.[6]

PIK3CA mutations, mainly clustered in exons 9 and 20, have been identified in up to 20% of ovarian endometrioid carcinomas but in only 2% of serous carcinomas.[61] In some tumors, *PIK3CA* and *PTEN* mutations co-occur and an additive effect on the PI3K pathway has been suggested.[62] In both the ovary and the endometrium, PIK3CA mutations are associated with adverse prognostic parameters.[63]

Microsatellites are repetitive DNA sequences usually one to five nucleotides in length. Microsatellite instability refers to alterations in the DNA of tumor cells in which the number of sequence repeats in these microsatellites differs from the number of repeats at the same locus in DNA from the patient's normal cells. Microsatellite instability has been found in 12–20% of ovarian endometrioid carcinomas.[52,58,64] Cancer patients from HNPCC kindreds have an inherited germline mutation either in MLH-1, MSH-2, MSH-6, or in PMS-2 ('first hit') and carcinoma develops after the instauration of a deletion or mutation in the contralateral allele ('second hit').[65] In contrast, in sporadic tumors, MLH-1 inactivation by promoter hypermethylation is the main cause of mismatch repair deficiency leading to accumulation of myriads of mutations in coding and non-coding DNA sequences (Figure 27.21).[52,58,64] Short-tandem repeats are particularly susceptible to mismatch repair alterations; however, most occur in non-coding DNA sequences and subtle mutations (insertions or deletions) do not result in

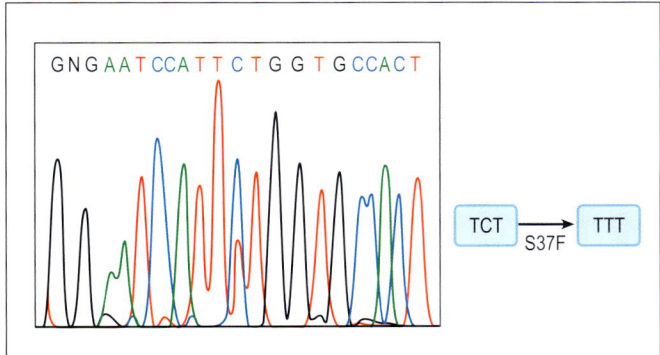

Figure 27.19 Endometrioid adenocarcinoma. DNA sequencing of exon 3 of the β-catenin (*CTNNB1*) gene discloses a TCT to TTT point mutation at codon 37 (S37F).

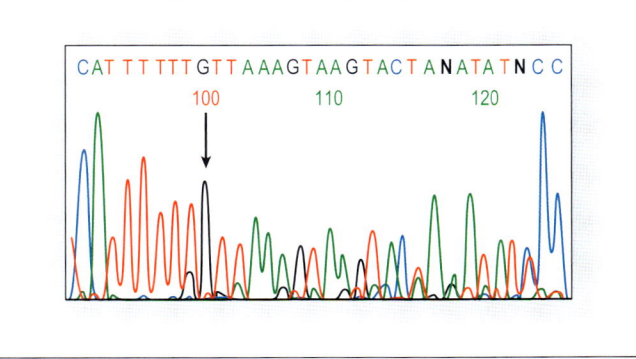

Figure 27.20 Endometrioid adenocarcinoma. Partial representative nucleotide sequencing of antisense strand around the (A) 6 tract in exon 8 of *PTEN*. Sequence analysis of polymerase chain reaction (PCR) product of tumor DNA showed the deletion of one nucleotide in the poly-A tract.[13] (Reproduced with permission from Irving et al.[13])

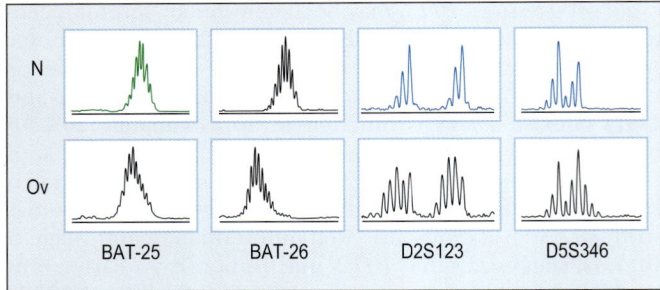

Figure 27.21 Endometrioid adenocarcinoma. Microsatellite instability for the loci BAT-25, BAT-26, D2S123, and D5S346 (capillary electrophoresis).

the production of abnormal proteins. However, some mononucleotide repeats are located within the coding sequence of important genes such as *BAX, IGFIIR, hMSH3, hMSH6, MBD4, CHK-1,* or caspase-5, which may be potential targets during tumor progression in ovarian endometrioid carcinomas with microsatellite instability.[64]

Inactivating mutations of *ARID1A*, which encodes a subunit of the SWI/SNF chromatin remodeling complex, have been found in 30% of endometrioid carcinomas.[23] The mutations are typically frameshift or nonsense mutations that result in loss of protein expression. p53 mutations have been reported in up to 60% of endometrioid carcinomas arising in the ovary, most often in high-grade tumors. However, recent studies indicate that many ovarian tumors previously diagnosed as high-grade endometrioid carcinomas lack the characteristic mutations of low-grade endometrioid carcinoma and have gene expression profiles indistinguishable from high-grade serous carcinomas.

Differential Diagnosis

The distinction of endometrioid tumors from mucinous neoplasms has been discussed in Chapter 26.

1. *High-grade serous carcinoma.* As indicated above, most ovarian endometrioid adenocarcinomas are low-grade carcinomas that exhibit rounded glands and broad papillae lacking the slit-like spaces typical of high-grade serous carcinomas. Furthermore, not infrequently they show squamous differentiation and an adenofibroma component. In contrast to high-grade serous carcinoma, ovarian endometrioid adenocarcinomas usually fail to react for WT1, are only focally immunoreactive for p16, and show positive PR and vimentin immunoreaction. Nuclear reaction for β-catenin is frequently positive whereas p53 is usually negative.
2. *Endometrioid adenofibroma versus Brenner tumor.* Both tumors exhibit a prominent fibrous stromal component. Endometrioid tumors generally have an epithelial component in the form of glands with lumens, whereas in Brenner tumors the epithelial component typically consists of branching nests and trabeculae of transitional cells; a glandular component, if present in the Brenner tumor, is frequently mucinous. Nuclear grooves, characteristic of the transitional cells of Brenner tumors, are not found in squamous morules.
3. *Endometrioid adenocarcinoma, secretory type, versus clear cell adenocarcinoma.* The secretory form of endometrioid adenocarcinoma displays glands lined by well-differentiated cells with basal and supranuclear vacuoles. The tubulocystic pattern of CCC exhibits glands lined by hobnail cells with high-grade nuclei. In addition CCC, unlike secretory carcinoma, usually contains areas where the tumor is composed of sheets of tumor cells with clear cytoplasm.
4. *Ovarian tumor of wolffian origin.* The glands of endometrioid carcinoma commonly contain intraluminal mucin, which is absent in wolffian tumors. Wolffian tumors are reactive for CD10 but rarely reactive for EMA and B72.3.[2]
5. *Yolk sac tumor (glandular variant).* Typically occurs in young women, shows other more common patterns, and exhibits reactivity for AFP and glypican-3 (see Chapter 29). Occasionally, yolk sac differentiation is encountered in endometrioid carcinomas.[38]
6. *Granulosa cell tumor (insular, trabecular, or microfollicular).* In contrast to Call–Exner bodies, endometrioid carcinomas contain microglands with intraluminal mucin. Also, the nuclei of endometrioid carcinomas are usually round and hyperchromatic, whereas those of granulosa cell tumors are round, oval, or angular, pale and grooved.[31] Carcinomas are reactive for EMA, whereas granulosa cell tumors are reactive for FOXL2, α-inhibin, and calretinin.
7. *Sertoli–stromal cell tumors.* Most occur at an average age of 25 years and are usually unilateral (bilaterality, 2%). Endometrioid carcinomas are bilateral in about 28% of the cases. Typical endometrioid glands (Figure 27.13) with intraluminal mucin and squamous differentiation are each found in three-fourths of tumors resembling Sertoli–stromal cell tumors.[31] α-Inhibin and calretinin are positive in Sertoli cells.[34,49]
8. *Identical patterns of endometrioid carcinoma involving both the ovary and uterine corpus (independent primaries vs metastatic tumors).* This problem is discussed later. The good prognosis in cases in which the tumor is limited to both organs provides strong evidence that the neoplasms are independent primaries in most of such cases.[13,14] According to FIGO, the primary site of the tumor should be determined by its initial clinical manifestations.[55]
9. *Metastatic colonic adenocarcinoma.* This differential diagnosis is covered more fully in Chapter 30. Bilaterality, 'dirty' necrosis, amputated glands, desmoplastic stroma, vascular invasion, and 'too high grade' nuclei, all favor metastatic carcinoma. In addition, metastatic colonic carcinoma is usually reactive for CK20, CEA, and CDX-2, whereas endometrioid carcinoma is reactive for CK7 (Figure 27.17).

Treatment and Prognosis

The treatment of endometrioid carcinomas is similar to that of ovarian cancers in general. The 5 year survival rate of patients with stage I carcinoma is 78%, stage II 63%, stage III 24%, and stage IV 6%.[55] Patients with grade I and II tumors have a higher survival rate than those with grade III tumors. Peritoneal foreign body granulomas to keratin found in cases of endometrioid carcinoma with squamous

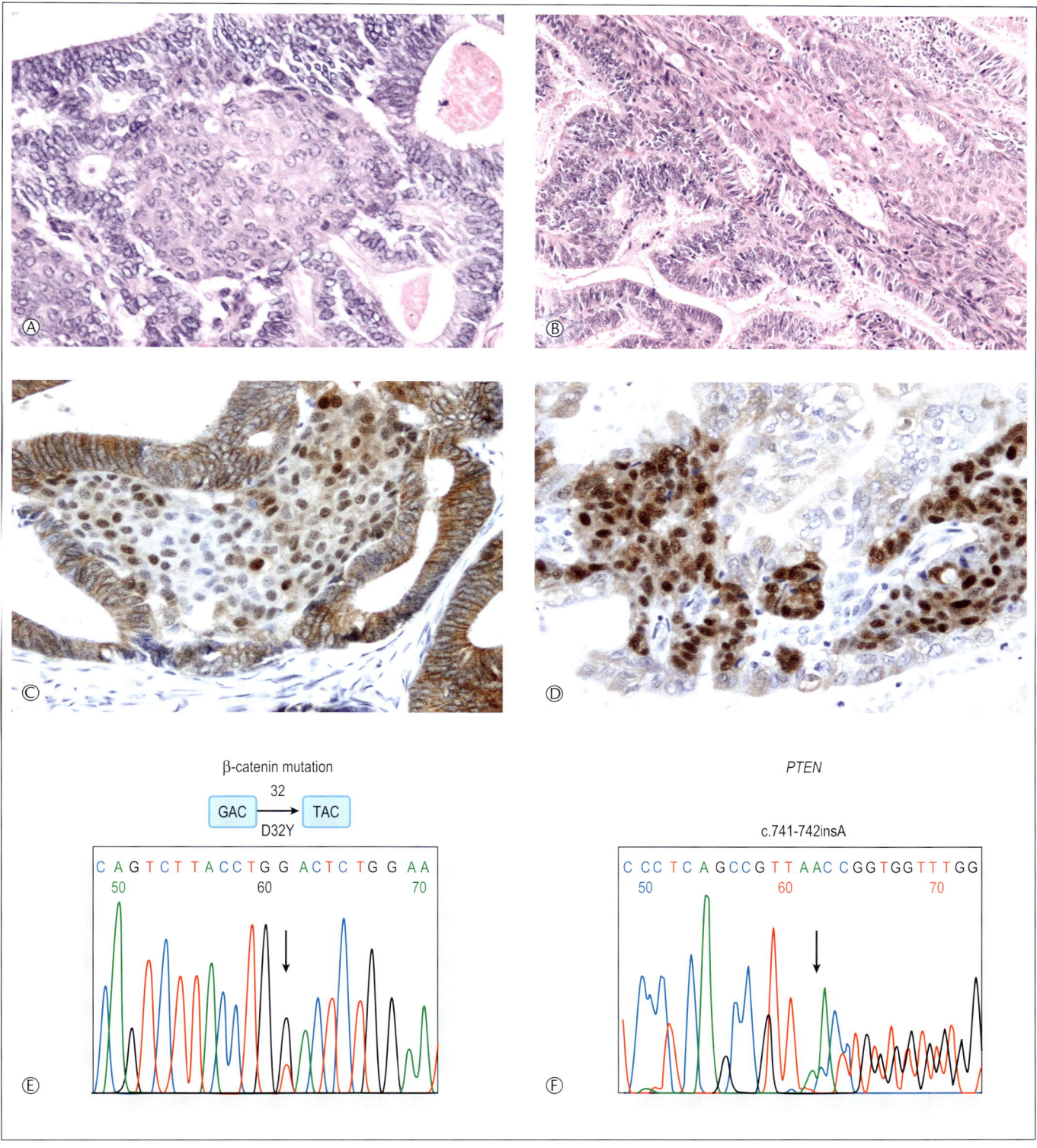

Figure 27.22 Synchronous, independent primary endometrioid carcinomas of the uterus (left) and ovary (right). Both tumors are grade 1 with squamous differentiation as shown in **(A)** (uterus) and **(B)** (ovary). Nuclear accumulation of β-catenin is most prominent in squamous morules (**C,** uterus; **D,** ovary). Sequence analysis of exon 3 of *CTNNB1* reveals an identical GAC → TAC point mutation (D32Y) in both uterine and ovarian tumors **(E)**. Sequencing histogram of *PTEN* frameshift mutation **(F)**. An identical bp insertion in exon 7 was detected in both tumors.[13] (Reproduced with permission from Irving et al.[13])

differentiation do not seem to affect the prognosis adversely in the absence of viable-appearing tumor cells.[2] Endometrioid carcinomas with a mixed clear cell, serous, or undifferentiated carcinoma component are reported to have a worse prognosis.[67]

SIMULTANEOUS ENDOMETRIOID CARCINOMAS OF THE OVARY AND ENDOMETRIUM

Simultaneous carcinomas of the ovary and uterine corpus, usually detected as synchronous and less frequently as metachronous tumors, occur in 15–20% of ovarian tumors and in approximately 5% of uterine tumors.[1] Both tumors are of endometrioid type in the majority of cases. Accurate diagnosis, as independent primary tumors or metastases, has important prognostic implications and is necessary for appropriate staging and treatment. Independent primary low-grade endometrioid carcinomas limited to the endometrium and ovary are associated with favorable outcome and require no additional treatment other than oophorectomy and hysterectomy. In contrast, metastatic tumors usually carry an adverse prognosis and adjuvant therapy is indicated.

Assessment of conventional pathologic features including tumor size, histologic type, and grade; pattern of tumor growth; vascular invasion; and coexisting atypical hyperplasia or endometriosis allows the distinction in most cases.[1] For example, in cases of low-grade endometrial carcinomas associated with hyperplasia and minimal or no myometrial invasion, the ovarian tumor can safely be regarded as primary, particularly if it shows endometriosis, adenofibroma, or a borderline tumor component. In contrast, bilaterality and multinodular growth, as well as vascular space and tubal invasion, are characteristic features of ovarian metastases. In patients with simultaneous carcinomas, however, the 5 year survival is 70–92%, and the median survival is 10 years or longer;[68,69] thus, follow-up favors two independent adenocarcinomas since most patients survive without recurrence.[14,70,71]

Occasionally, the differential diagnosis can be difficult or impossible as the tumors may show overlapping features.[1] Even if patient follow-up is the single most conclusive factor in such cases, ancillary techniques may help to establish the correct diagnosis.[13,70,72] Most of the strategies have relied upon the presence or absence of clonal genetic alterations in the ovarian and endometrial adenocarcinomas to identify metastatic or independent primary tumors, respectively. It must be emphasized that the results of these analyses should always be interpreted in the light of the clinicopathologic findings.[72–75] Also, it should be kept in mind that independent primary carcinomas may show identical gene mutations (Figure 27.22), reflecting induction of the same genetic abnormalities by a common carcinogenic agent acting in two separate sites of a single anatomic region. Alternatively, the genetic profiles of metastatic carcinomas may differ from those of their corresponding primary tumors as a result of tumor progression. In other words, the genetic profile can be identical in independent tumors and different in metastatic carcinomas.[73,75]

A recent study has revealed a frequency of molecular alterations in both independent and metastatic tumors, including *MI* and *PTEN* mutations, which is higher than that observed in single sporadic tumors. Nuclear immunoreactivities for β-catenin and *CTNNB1* mutations were restricted to independent uterine and ovarian tumors and were absent in metastatic tumors (Figure 27.23). These findings correlated with the clinical outcome.[13]

MIXED TUMORS (TUMORS WITH A SARCOMATOUS COMPONENT)

These tumors, which are uncommon in the ovary, occur more frequently in the uterus and, rarely, in the pelvic and abdominal peritoneum or the omentum. They show malignant mesenchymal cells admixed with benign or malignant epithelial elements.

MALIGNANT MESODERMAL MIXED TUMORS (CARCINOSARCOMAS)

These tumors are composed of high-grade carcinoma of different müllerian types and sarcoma. The latter component may be homologous (tissue types native to the müllerian tract, i.e., endometrial stroma, fibrous tissue, and smooth muscle) or heterologous (foreign tissue, such as skeletal muscle, adipose tissue, cartilage, and bone). Any of these various components may be widespread or limited to small foci.[1] Approximately one-third fall into the homologous group. Occasionally, these complex neoplasms arise in ovarian endometriosis.

General Features

Malignant mesodermal (müllerian) mixed tumors (MMMTs) account for 2% of all ovarian cancers. They occur in the sixth to eighth decades, and are rare before the age of 40 years.[2] Recent immunohistochemical and molecular genetic studies[76–78] support a clonal origin of both tumor components (epithelial and mesenchymal-like elements) and, accordingly, a proposal to designate these tumors 'undifferentiated or metaplastic carcinoma' has been made.[79] However, preserving the currently accepted term MMMT, which indicates the type(s) of neoplastic differentiation, is recommended because of the unique clinicopathologic features of this tumor.

Macroscopic Features

The tumors are bilateral in one-third of the cases.[2] They are usually large (15–20 cm mean diameter), friable, solid and/or cystic with areas of necrosis and hemorrhage (Figure 27.24). Occasionally, bone or cartilage can be palpated.

Microscopic Features

Most tumors display a complex admixture of epithelial and malignant stromal elements and transitions are uncommon. The epithelial component is most frequently high-grade serous (Figure 27.25), endometrioid, or undifferentiated carcinoma. Occasionally, squamous, mucinous, or clear cell carcinoma is found. If the epithelium is mucinous, care should be taken to distinguish such tumors from mucinous cystic tumors with mural nodules (see Chapter 26). The sarcomatous elements are usually hypercellular sheets of small hyperchromatic round to spindle-shaped cells with a high mitotic rate and lacking apparent differentiation. In the homologous type, the sarcoma component resembles fibrosarcoma, malignant fibrous histiocytoma, or high-grade endometrial stromal sarcoma. The heterologous tumor most

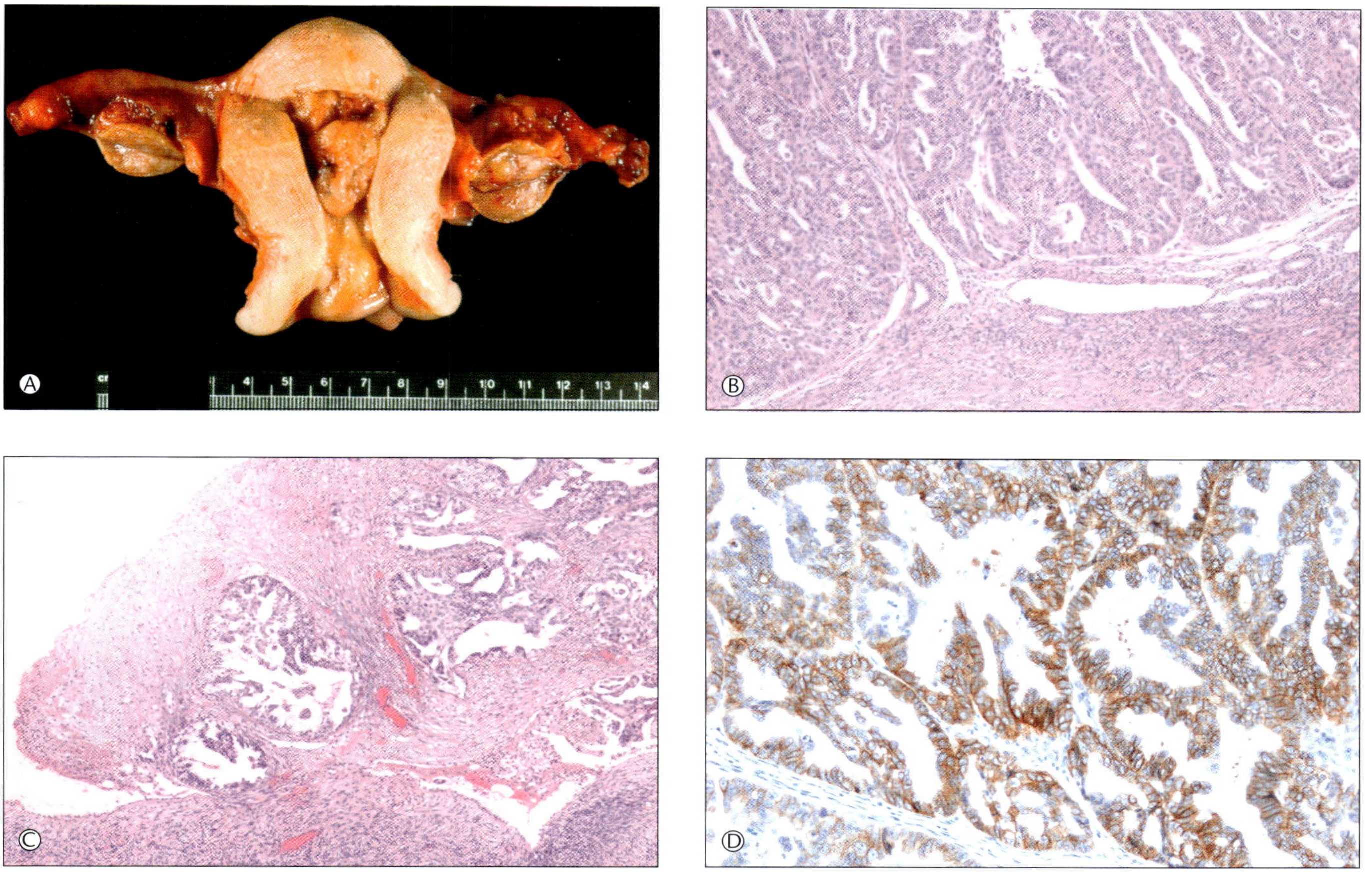

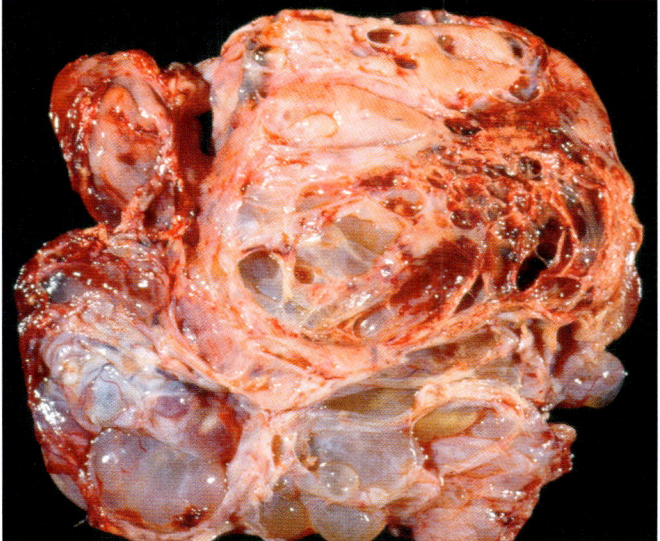

Figure 27.23 Primary endometrioid carcinoma of the uterine corpus with bilateral ovarian metastases. **(A)** Polypoid tumor filling the endometrial cavity, with surface involvement of both ovaries. **(B)** The uterine tumor is a minimally invasive (<1 mm) grade 3 endometrioid carcinoma. **(C)** The ovarian surfaces are extensively involved by metastatic grade 3 endometrioid carcinoma. **(D)** Membranous pattern of β-catenin immunoreactivity is observed in the uterine tumor (shown) as well as both ovaries and omental metastases.[13] (Reproduced with permission from Irving et al.[13])

Figure 27.24 Malignant mesodermal mixed tumor (carcinosarcoma). The sectioned surface reveals a solid and cystic tumor with areas of hemorrhage.

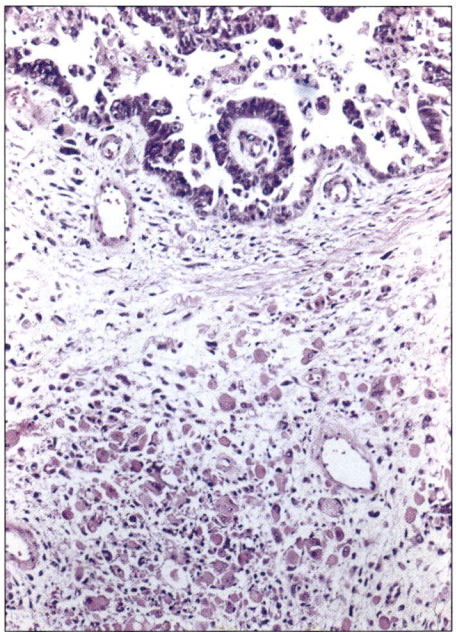

Figure 27.25 Malignant mesodermal mixed tumor, heterologous. The epithelial component is high-grade serous carcinoma (top). There is a rhabdomyosarcoma component (bottom).

often contains chondrosarcoma, rhabdomyosarcoma (Figure 27.25), or both. Rarely, osteosarcoma or liposarcoma is present. PAS-positive, diastase-resistant hyaline bodies are common in the sarcoma component. Glial, neuronal, and trophoblastic differentiation may be encountered.

Immunohistochemistry

As a general rule, reactivity for EMA and cytokeratins (AE1/AE3 and CAM5.2) but not for vimentin helps distinguish poorly differentiated carcinoma from sarcoma. However, in MMMTs, the sarcomatous component may also react for cytokeratins and EMA[7] and reactivity with vimentin in not uncommon in the epithelial component. The presence of heterologous components may be confirmed by immunohistochemistry including desmin, myogenin, and myoD1 for rhabdomyosarcoma or S-100 for chondrosarcoma. Reactivity with chromogranin, neural specific enolase, and synaptophysin is found in one-sixth of the cases.

Histogenesis

MMMTs are of epithelial cell origin and molecular studies favor a monoclonal origin by showing concordant *TP53* abnormalities within the carcinoma and sarcoma component.[76,77,80] Further indirect evidence supporting the epithelial origin is that MMMTs may present as recurrence of high-grade serous carcinomas,[81] and that the metastatic pattern of MMMTs is also similar to that of high-grade serous carcinomas.

Somatic Genetics

MMMTs are probably monoclonal as the histologically different components share similar allelic losses and retentions.[76–78] A cell line developed from an MMMT has expressed both epithelial and mesenchymal antigens.[82] Tumor progression (clonal evolution) could explain the heterogeneous pattern of LOH in either the carcinoma or sarcoma components of the neoplasm.[77]

Differential Diagnosis

1. *MMMT versus immature teratoma.* Immature teratoma occurs predominantly in children and adolescents and typically contains elements derived from all three germ layers. Neuroectodermal tissue, which is rarely found in MMMT, is almost always the predominant malignant component. In addition, the malignant epithelial component of immature teratoma has an embryonal appearance and the cartilaginous component resembles fetal cartilage with uniform nuclei, in contrast to the cartilage found in MMMT in which the cells are bizarre and appear clearly malignant (chondrosarcoma) (see Chapter 29).
2. *MMMT versus poorly differentiated Sertoli–Leydig cell tumor with heterologous elements.* The latter tumor nearly always occurs in young women, many of whom present because of virilization. Usually, some area is better differentiated and readily diagnosable as Sertoli–Leydig tumors. Reactivity for α-inhibin and calretinin (Sertoli–Leydig) and EMA (in MMMT) also facilitates the diagnosis (see Chapter 28).
3. *MMMT versus endometrioid stromal sarcomas with sex cord-like differentiation.* The latter tumors are better differentiated than MMMTs and often exhibit sex cord differentiation (see later).
4. *MMMT versus sarcoma-like mural nodules in mucinous cystic tumor.* The mural nodules may be reactive, composed of anaplastic carcinoma, or truly sarcomatous (see Chapter 26).

Tumor Spread and Prognosis

Over 75% of MMMTs have spread beyond the ovary at the time of diagnosis, 60% being stage III and 10% stage IV.[1] The metastases commonly contain both carcinomatous and sarcomatous components. The prognosis is very poor. After cytoreductive surgery and platinum-based chemotherapy, the overall 5 year survival is under 30%. Only 25% of patients survive 2 years (median survival, 10 months).[1]

MÜLLERIAN ADENOSARCOMAS

Ovarian adenosarcomas are usually unilateral and predominantly solid tumors containing numerous small cysts. Over 50 cases have been reported.[83,84] They occur in older women (mean age, 54 years) and have a much worse prognosis than their more common uterine counterparts; 50% die within 5 years.

Microscopically, the tumors exhibit both a malignant stromal and a glandular component. The glandular epithelium, which is usually of endometrioid type (Figure 27.26), appears benign or less frequently atypical. The stroma resembles a cellular fibroma, low-grade fibrosarcoma, or low-grade endometrial stromal sarcoma. Typically, it is most cellular adjacent to the glands forming cuffs around them ('periglandular cuffing'). The glands become cystic and polypoid projections of stroma into the lumens (phyllodes-like pattern) are often present. Mitoses in the stromal cells range from 2 to <40 per 10 HPF.[83] Heterologous elements, sex cord-like structures, and sarcomatous overgrowth are occasionally found.

Adenosarcomas should be distinguished from adenofibromas, polypoid endometriosis, sex cord–stromal tumors, and endometrial stromal sarcomas.

Adenosarcoma of the ovary is a far more aggressive tumor than its counterpart in the endometrium. About half will have spread beyond the ovary by the time of diagnosis. Treatment is primarily surgical, although radiation therapy and chemotherapy have also been used. For stage I cancer,

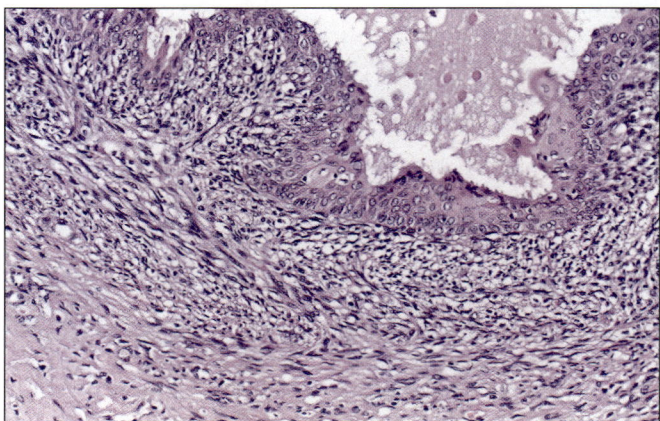

Figure 27.26 Adenosarcoma. Squamous differentiation and cuff of cellular stroma.

tumor rupture and high-grade and sarcomatous overgrowth are associated with a higher rate of recurrence.[83]

ENDOMETRIOID STROMAL SARCOMAS

These tumors consist of cells resembling the stromal cells of normal proliferative endometrium. They may derive from foci of ovarian endometriosis (coexistent endometriosis is present in almost half the cases), from foci of gland-free endometrial stroma in the ovary (stromal endometriosis) or, possibly, may arise directly from the ovarian stromal cells following metaplasia into endometrial stromal-type cells.[66]

Clinical Features

Endometrioid stromal sarcoma (ESS) of the ovary is not a common tumor and <60 cases have been reported to date.[66,85] The patients were 11–76 years of age. The majority of tumors occurred during the fifth and sixth decades. The presenting symptoms, which were nonspecific, were related to the presence of a pelvic mass. In one of the larger series,[66] the tumor was, at the time of operation, confined to the ovary in only one-sixth of patients; it involved other pelvic structures or had spread into the abdomen in over one-third for each group and had metastasized to the lungs in the remainder. About 30% of the patients had a similar tumor in the uterus, for which reason a metastasis to the ovary was strongly considered in some.[66]

Macroscopic Features

The tumors generally are up to 15 cm in diameter and unilateral in 75% of cases.[66] They are predominantly solid, though foci of cystic change are present in over half. On section they usually have a yellow-white homogeneous appearance (Figure 27.27), with foci of necrosis relatively uncommon.

Microscopic Features

Histologically, ovarian ESSs, like their more common uterine counterparts, exhibit sheets of uniform cells resembling the stromal cells of normal proliferative endometrium (Figure 27.28). In contrast to the uterine tumors, fibromatous areas are frequently present (Figure 27.29).[66] An important diagnostic feature is the presence of a prominent network of small arterioles (Figure 27.30), closely resembling the spiral vessels seen in normal late secretory endometrium. This network is most clearly seen in reticulin-stained sections.[66] The tumor cells are small and oval to spindle shaped, and usually have scanty cytoplasm. The intravascular growth characteristic of uterine ESSs of low-grade malignancy is not seen within the ovarian tumors but is typically present when the neoplasm extends beyond the ovary.[66] The tumor cells may contain abundant intracellular lipid and, although usually growing in uniform sheets, can, like similar uterine tumors, show an epithelial or sex cord-like pattern. In almost half the cases, endometriosis is identified adjacent to the tumor (Figure 27.31), or a few glands of endometrioid type are found within it.[66]

Immunohistochemistry and Somatic Genetics

ESSs immunoreact for vimentin and CD10. Muscle-associated proteins and low molecular weight cytokeratins

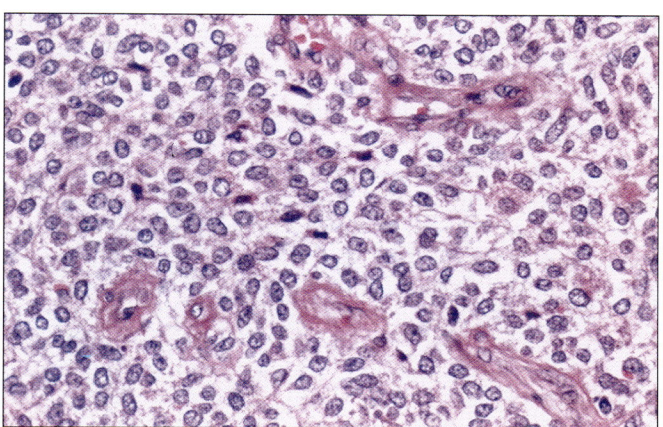

Figure 27.28 Endometrioid stromal sarcoma, low grade. The tumor consists of a monotonous collection of small cells resembling endometrial stromal cells. Note the presence of small arterioles resembling the spiral arterioles of the normal late secretory endometrium.

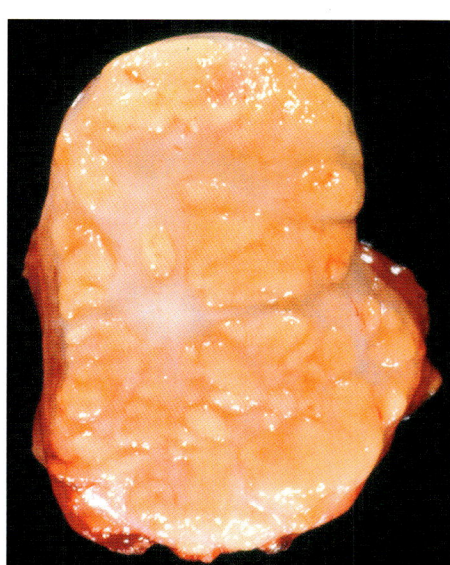

Figure 27.27 Endometrioid stromal sarcoma. The sectioned surface of the tumor is solid and multinodular.

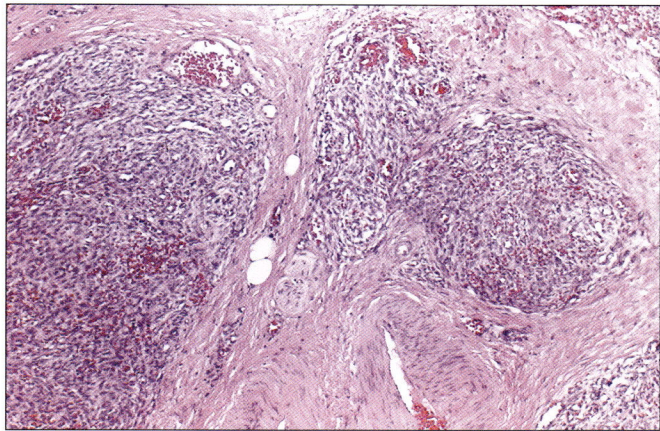

Figure 27.29 Endometrioid stromal sarcoma, low grade. Cellular nodules intersected by dense fibrous bands.

are only focally expressed. Calretinin and α-inhibin are not expressed. Approximately half of the reported extrauterine ESSs have similar genetic alterations to their uterine counterparts, including fusions of *JAZF1–JJAZ1(SUZ12)*, *EPC1-PHF1*, and *PHF1* rearrangement.[86] No ovarian ESSs exhibiting the novel genetic fusion *YWHAE–FAM22* resulting from translocation t(10;17) (q22,p13), as seen in the corresponding uterine tumors, has been described.[87]

Differential Diagnosis

The cytologic features and the presence of a rich vascular network allow for the differentiation of ESS from other types of ovarian sarcoma. An adenosarcoma may, however, be mimicked if endometriotic glands are trapped within the tumor. Nevertheless, the focal presence of the glands, as opposed to their uniform distribution throughout an adenosarcoma, together with the absence of any stromal condensation around the glands (periglandular cuffing), usually indicates the correct diagnosis. A sex cord-like pattern, if a prominent feature of an ESS, may lead to confusion with a granulosa cell tumor; the epithelial-like cells, however, lack the nuclear features of granulosa cells. Furthermore, granulosa cell tumors lack the individual cellular investment by reticulin fibrils so characteristic of ESS. The usual advanced stage and the frequent bilaterality of ESS argue against a diagnosis of any tumor in the sex cord–stromal category. A lack of reactivity for FOXL2, calretinin, and/or α-inhibin also helps to identify the tumor as a stromal sarcoma.[88–90]

Nearly one-third of ovarian ESSs are associated with a prior, synchronous, or subsequent uterine ESS.[66] When the uterine lesions precede the ovarian neoplasms by many years, the tumors most likely represent independent primary neoplasms of each organ. In synchronous cases, however, it may be impossible to exclude metastasis from one organ to the other, especially if other pelvic structures are involved. Some[85] regard the tumor as an ovarian primary only if both the tumor is confined to the ovary and the uterus has been shown to be disease free on pathologic examination. Others[2] accept ovarian endometriosis also as evidence of an ovarian origin. Obviously, it is important to review any prior hysterectomy specimen in a patient with an ovarian ESS. If the uterus has not been removed at the time of operation, it is more than a remote possibility that a uterine ESS may have been left behind or will subsequently develop.[2]

Tumors that lack endometrial stromal differentiation and are composed of pleomorphic mesenchymal cells with highly atypical nuclei and prominent nucleoli should be diagnosed as undifferentiated ovarian sarcoma.[85]

Prognosis

Ovarian ESSs behave similarly to uterine ESSs with nuclear atypia and mitotic activity of prognostic significance. Tumors without nuclear atypia and showing <10 mitoses per 10 HPF are associated with a good prognosis, even if there is extrauterine spread. In the largest series reported,[66] only 10% of patients whose neoplasms lacked nuclear atypia and contained <10 mitoses per 10 HPF died of their disease. While patients with extraovarian spread survived over the short term, longer term follow-up studies indicate that the disease may nonetheless be fatal even after 10 years.[2] The prognosis of tumors exhibiting nuclear atypia and containing more than 10 mitoses per 10 HPF (Figure 27.32) was comparable to that of other ovarian sarcomas, and three-fourths of women die within 4 years.[66]

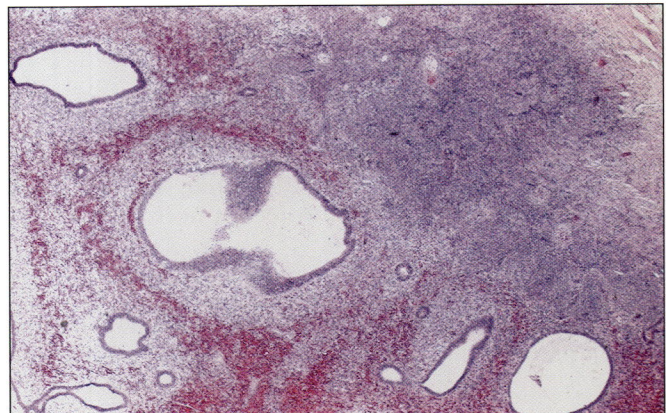

Figure 27.31 Endometrioid stromal sarcoma, low grade, arising from endometriosis.

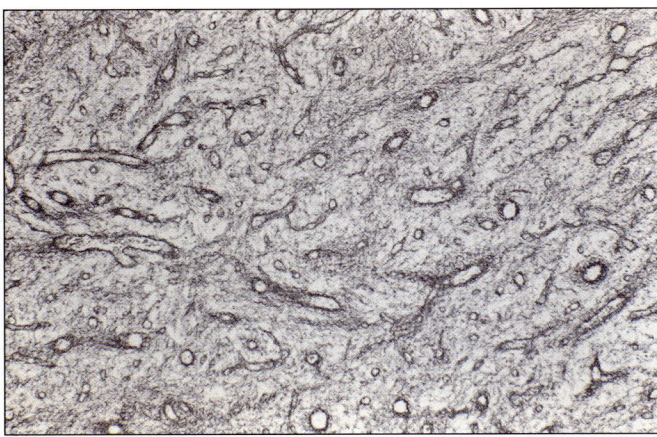

Figure 27.30 Endometrioid stromal sarcoma, low grade. Reticulin staining discloses a prominent vascular pattern.

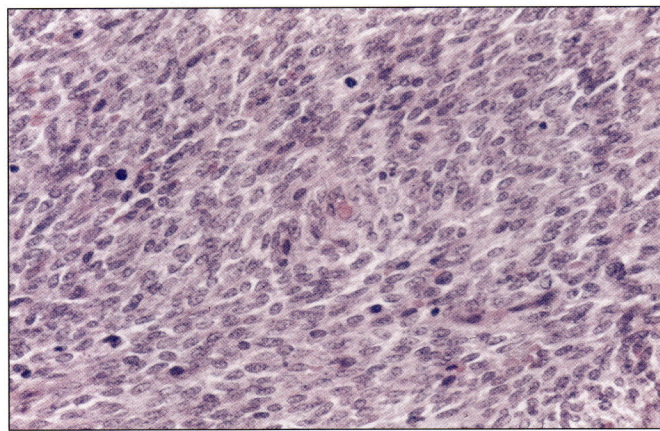

Figure 27.32 Endometrioid stromal sarcoma, high grade. There is nuclear atypia and several mitotic figures are seen.

Treatment

The primary treatment of ovarian ESS is surgical. In menopausal or postmenopausal patients, hysterectomy with bilateral salpingo-oophorectomy is the treatment of choice. Because of the high frequency of bilateral ovarian involvement and the possibility of synchronous or subsequent uterine ESS, a similar approach may be optimal even for younger women. Both progesterone and radiotherapy have been used for residual or recurrent disease. Tumors of low-grade malignancy (<10 mitoses per 10 HPF) typically run an indolent course and patients with untreated residual disease may remain free of symptoms for many years.

TUMORS OF SMOOTH MUSCLE

LEIOMYOMAS

Ovarian leiomyomas are rare.[91] The mean age at presentation is 43 years, but they have been encountered in females as young as age 3 and as old as 103 years. Most are asymptomatic but about one-third complained of nonspecific pelvic mass symptoms such as abdominal pain or swelling. Rarely, torsion occurs. Ascites has developed in a few patients.

The tumors are usually unilateral, and range in size from 1 to 24 cm in diameter. Although lacking a true capsule, leiomyomas tend to be sharply circumscribed, which helps distinguish them from the far more common ovarian fibromas, which are solid and firm and on section have a white, gray, or brown cut surface. Leiomyomas have a whorled or multinodular structure and although commonly solid may show areas of myxoid or pseudocystic change. Foci of hemorrhage, necrosis, or calcification are common.

Histologically, the ovarian leiomyoma has the typical features of that associated with the uterus, i.e., interlacing bundles of smooth muscle fibers, sometimes admixed with collagenous septa. The muscle cells have elongated blunt-ended or cigar-shaped nuclei. Occasional multinucleated giant cells may be present, but there is otherwise no pleomorphism. Mitotic figures are either absent or extremely sparse. Like the uterine counterpart, cellular and mitotically active ovarian leiomyomas exist.[91] Both lack significant nuclear atypia. Mitotically active ovarian leiomyomas may contain up to 15 mitoses per 10 HPF, but should not have atypical mitotic figures. Leiomyomas with extensive hyalinization and epithelioid cells may be confused with sex cord–stromal tumors (see Chapter 28) and those exhibiting myxoid change may resemble yolk sac tumors (see Chapter 29).[91] Immunostains for desmin, α-inhibin, calretinin, and AFP may facilitate the diagnosis.

The histogenesis of ovarian leiomyomas is uncertain. Possible origins are from the smooth muscle fibers of the ovarian ligaments, ovarian blood vessels, or smooth muscle fibers of the cortical stroma.

Ovarian leiomyomas, including those considered as cellular or 'mitotically active,' are benign and can be treated conservatively. Criteria for distinguishing between benign and malignant smooth muscle tumors of the ovary are similar to those used for uterine smooth muscle tumors. Moderate to severe nuclear atypia, tumor cell necrosis, and infiltrative margins correlated with malignant behavior.[91] Cytologically atypical leiomyomas with <5 mitoses per 10 HPF that lack tumor cell necrosis may be considered atypical leiomyomas (of 'uncertain malignant potential').[91] A mitotic count of >5 mitoses per 10 HPF in a cytologically atypical ovarian smooth muscle tumor should be regarded as an adverse sign especially if any other adverse histologic features are present.

LEIOMYOSARCOMAS

Ovarian leiomyosarcomas are extremely uncommon and <50 examples have been reported.[91] The tumors usually occur in elderly women (mean age, 58 years). The presenting symptoms are abdominal pain or an awareness of an abdominal mass. The tumors are almost always unilateral and are generally large with a mean of 14 cm; some are as large as 30 cm.[91] Grossly the tumors have a nodular outer surface and on section most are predominantly solid, often with extensive hemorrhage and necrosis. The cut surface tends to be gray-white and usually has a more fleshy texture than that of a leiomyoma. The histologic appearances are variable and range from very well-differentiated tumors (Figure 27.33) that resemble atypical leiomyomas to highly pleomorphic sarcomas (Figure 27.34) with only few areas of a recognizably smooth muscle nature. As in the uterus, the diagnosis rests on the presence of at least two of the following three

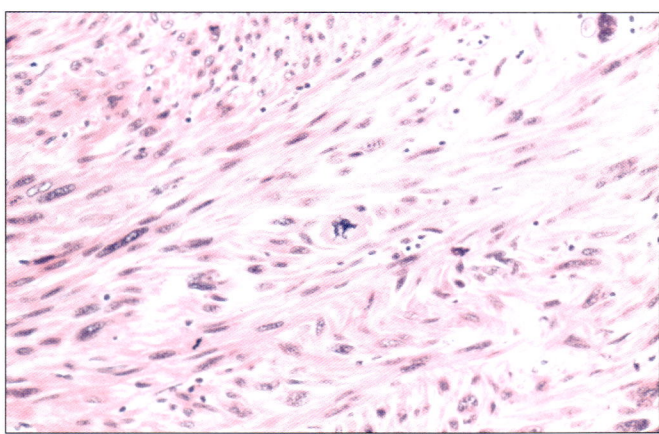

Figure 27.33 Well-differentiated ovarian leiomyosarcoma. Interlacing fascicles of smooth muscle fibers. An atypical mitotic figure is present.

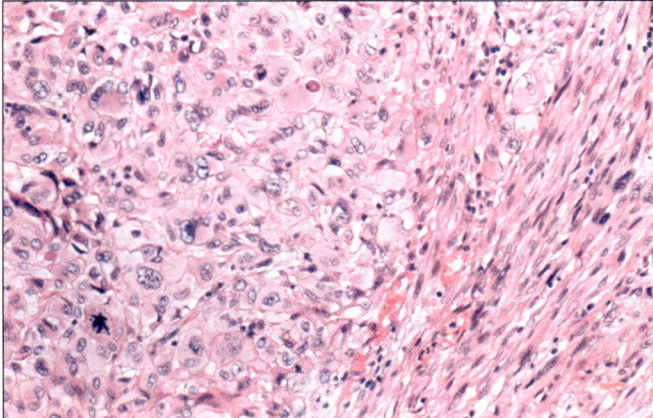

Figure 27.34 Epithelioid leiomyosarcoma. Typical leiomyosarcoma is seen to the right and epithelioid cells with abundant eosinophilic cytoplasm on the left. An atypical mitotic figure is seen.

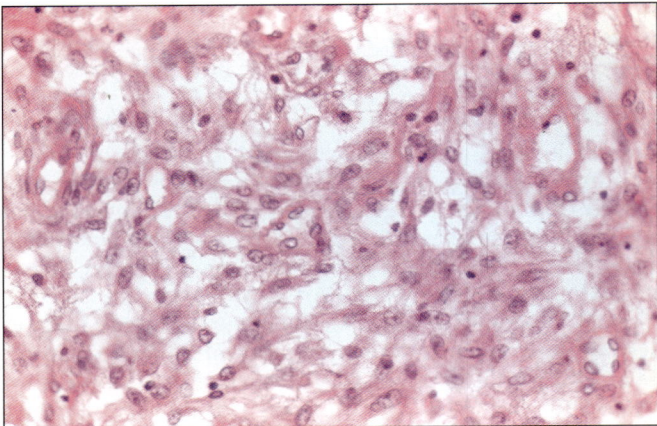

Figure 27.35 Myxoid leiomyosarcoma. Loose reticular meshwork of elongated cells without significant atypicality or mitotic activity.

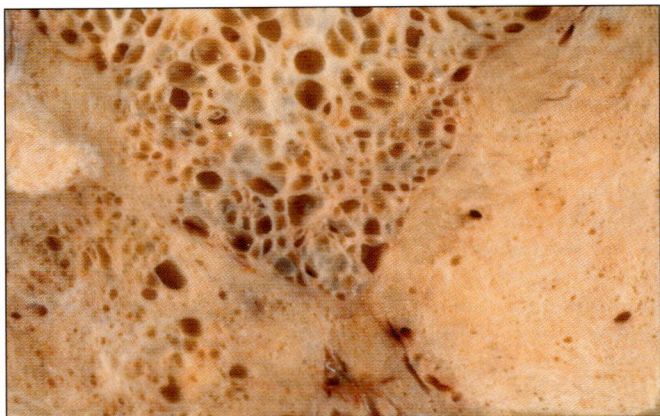

Figure 27.36 Borderline clear cell adenofibroma. The sectioned surface shows numerous small cysts (parvilocular cystoma).

histologic features: moderate or severe cytologic atypia, a mitotic count of ≥10 mitoses per 10 HPF, and geographic tumor cell necrosis. The mitotic count may range from 4 to 25 mitoses per 10 HPF and atypical mitoses are frequently seen. However, in the absence of tumor cell necrosis, a mitotic count of ≥5 mitotic figures/10 HPF in a cytologically atypical ovarian tumor warrants a diagnosis of leiomyosarcoma.[91]

Ovarian leiomyosarcomas are aggressive neoplasms and have commonly spread beyond the ovary at the time of initial diagnosis. The treatment of choice is probably radical surgery although radiotherapy or chemotherapy may prolong survival in some instances. Approximately 70% of patients develop recurrent disease at a mean of 20 months and 62% died of tumor within a year.[91]

MYXOID LEIOMYOSARCOMA

Myxoid leiomyosarcoma of the ovary is an extremely rare tumor.[91] Unlike the usual leiomyosarcoma, the myxoid variants are large gelatinous masses sowing cystic change, necrosis, and hemorrhage. Microscopically, the tumors exhibit a reticular meshwork of elongated cells surrounded by abundant basophilic myxoid material (Figure 27.35). The differential diagnosis includes massive edema, ovarian myxoma, yolk sac tumor (see Chapter 29), and a myxoid sarcomatous component of MMMT (see previously). Positive immunoreactions for smooth muscle markers may be helpful in establishing the nature of the tissue and hence the diagnosis. Due to the decreased cellular density the myxoid change causes, mitotic counts are usually low and therefore deceptive. Clinical stage seems to be the most reliable prognostic indicator, but, unfortunately, this feature is of no use if the tumor is stage Ia. Like its uterine counterpart, myxoid leiomyosarcoma of the ovary is highly aggressive, with most patients dying within 2 years of diagnosis.[91]

CLEAR CELL TUMORS

General Features

Ovarian clear cell tumors are composed of the following types of epithelial cells: clear cells (containing glycogen) similar to those of renal cell carcinoma; 'hobnail' cells (with large nuclei that protrude from the apparent cytoplasmic limits into a lumen) that line cysts and tubules; and less frequently flat, cuboidal, oxyphilic, or mucin-containing signet-ring cells.

Benign clear cell tumors are exceptional, and the borderline forms account for <1% of ovarian borderline tumors.[2] Most clear cell tumors of the ovary are carcinomas and represent approximately 10% of ovarian carcinomas in the Western world. Most are diagnosed during the fifth to seventh decades.[92] Among ovarian cancers, clear cell carcinomas CCCs have the highest association with ovarian and pelvic endometriosis, paraendocrine hypercalcemia (2–10%),[92–94] and venous thromboembolism (20–45%);[95] it has also been related to Lynch syndrome.[96–98] CCC occurs not only in the ovary, but also in the endometrium, fallopian tube, cervix, and vagina.

CCC was initially considered to arise from mesonephric remnants, and the designations 'mesonephroma' and 'mesonephric carcinoma' were used. However, it is now accepted that these tumors are of müllerian origin.[2] Most occur along the course of müllerian duct derivatives or within the ovary, which is involved by endometriosis, commonly associated with CCC (up to 50% of cases). CCC also arises from müllerian-derived vaginal adenosis in girls and young women exposed prenatally to diethylstilbestrol.[2] Last, CCC recapitulates the hypersecretory endometrium of pregnancy (Arias-Stella change).[2] The SNOMED classification is as follows:

- Clear cell cystadenoma
- Clear cell cystadenofibroma
- Clear cell tumor of borderline malignancy
- Clear cell adenofibroma of borderline malignancy
- Clear cell adenocarcinoma

Macroscopic Features

Benign or borderline clear cell adenofibromas have a nonspecific gross appearance and an average diameter of about 10–12 cm.[2] Occasionally, the cystic glands may be so extensive as to render the tumor's sectioned surface as sponge like (parvilocular cystoma) (Figure 27.36). CCCs range up to 30 cm in diameter with a mean of 15 cm. They may be

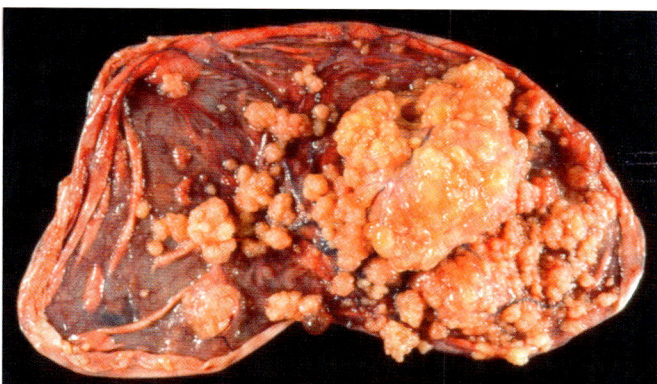

Figure 27.37 CCC. The predominantly cystic tumor contains multiple yellow-brown polypoid masses that protrude into the lumen of the cyst.

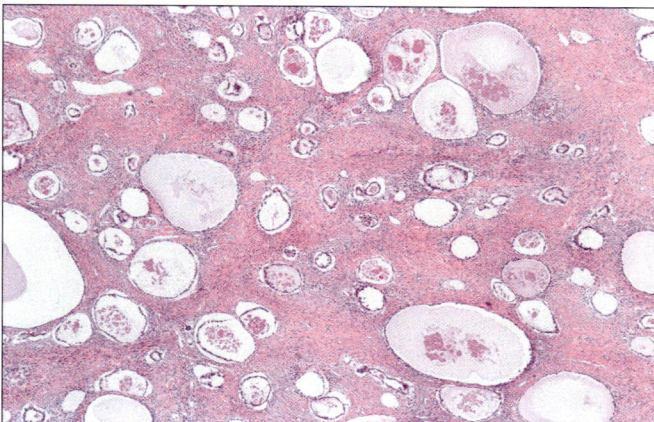

Figure 27.39 Borderline clear cell adenofibroma with microinvasion. Cystic glands lined by flat and hobnail cells lie in an abundant fibromatous stroma.

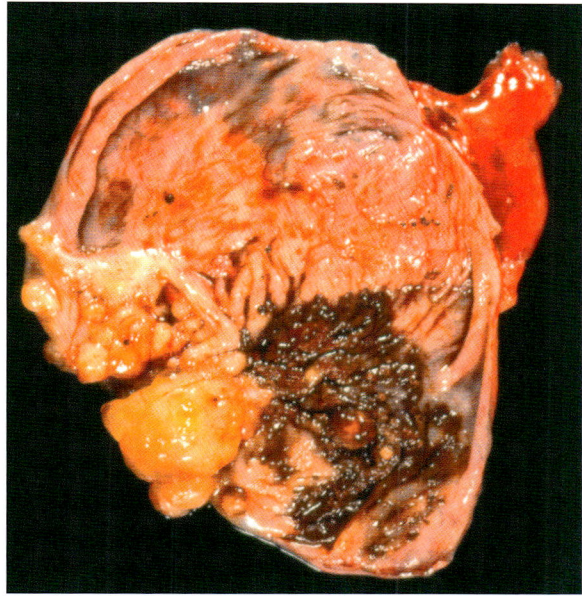

Figure 27.38 Clear cell adenocarcinoma arising in endometriotic cyst. The polypoid yellow tumor protrudes into the lumen of a unilocular endometriotic (chocolate) cyst.

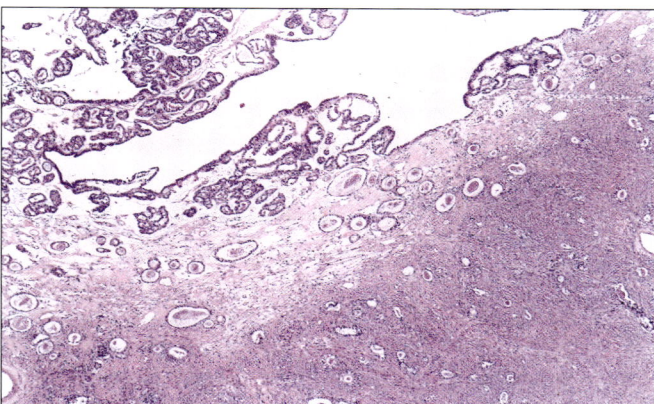

Figure 27.40 Clear cell adenocarcinoma in borderline adenofibroma. The invasive carcinoma, composed of oxyphilic cells, appears in the upper left corner of the figure.

predominantly solid but are more often predominantly cystic (unilocular or multilocular) containing one or more white, yellow, or brown polypoid masses that protrude into the lumens (Figure 27.37).[1,2,92] The polypoid solid tissue may represent carcinoma or an adenofibromatous component, from which some CCCs arise. The cyst lumens contain serous or mucinous fluid or chocolate-colored material when the tumor has arisen in an endometriotic cyst (Figure 27.38). Benign and borderline clear cell tumors are almost always unilateral; stage I carcinomas are bilateral in 4% of the cases.[55] Compared to other cell types, CCC is more likely to be stage IC due to a higher risk of tumor rupture.[99,100]

BENIGN CLEAR CELL TUMORS

Nearly all benign clear cell tumors are adenofibromas. The tubular glands are lined by a single layer of hobnail cells, clear cells, or less commonly 'indifferent' cuboidal cells. The nuclei are regular in size and shape. Cellular atypia, if present, is only mild and focal. Solid sheets of clear cells and luminal tufting are absent. Mitoses are rarely encountered. The intervening stroma is compact and fibrocollagenous, and is often more cellular adjacent to the epithelial elements. The diagnosis should only be made after thorough sampling to exclude a malignant component.

BORDERLINE CLEAR CELL TUMORS

Borderline clear cell tumors (Figure 27.39) show atypical epithelium without invasion (one or more foci each under 10 mm^2 do not alter the designation).[1,2] Nuclear atypia, epithelial budding, and mitoses (up to 3 per 10 HPF) are present. True papillae are rarely seen. Before a diagnosis of a benign or a borderline clear cell adenofibroma is rendered, the specimen should be extensively sampled for occult CCC in as much as these tumor subtypes occur far more often in the company of CCC than in pure form (Figure 27.40).[2]

CLEAR CELL ADENOCARCINOMAS

CCCs exhibit a variety of patterns and cell types that are often admixed.[2] The most common patterns are tubulocystic (Figure 27.41) and papillary (Figure 27.42). A predominantly solid pattern is less frequent (Figure 27.43). The papillae are often complex. Rarely, CCC has a reticular pattern, simulating a yolk sac tumor.

The most common cell types are the clear and the hobnail cells. Clear cells are clustered in solid nests or masses (Figure 27.43) whereas hobnail cells line lumens and papillae (Figures 27.41 and 27.42). Clear cells are rounded or polyhedral, have distinct cell borders, and contain eccentric rounded nuclei with prominent nucleoli. The hobnail cells contain bulbous dark nuclei that protrude into lumens beyond their apparent cytoplasmic limits (Figure 27.44). Less common cell types are flattened cells (that line deceptively benign-looking cysts), cuboidal cells, oxyphilic cells with abundant eosinophilic cytoplasm (Figure 27.45),[2] and

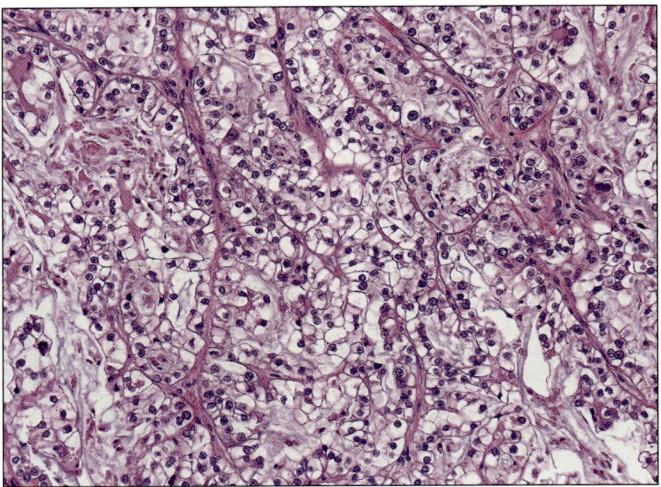

Figure 27.43 Clear cell adenocarcinoma. The tumor has a solid pattern. The clear cells are polyhedral and have eccentric hyperchromatic nuclei.

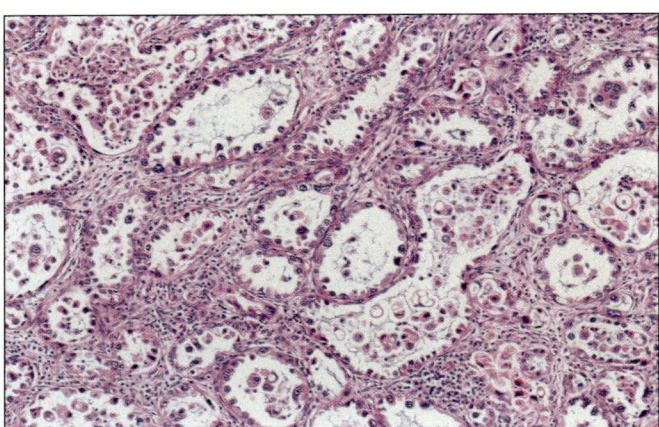

Figure 27.41 Clear cell adenocarcinoma with tubulocystic pattern. The cysts are lined by markedly atypical hobnail cells.

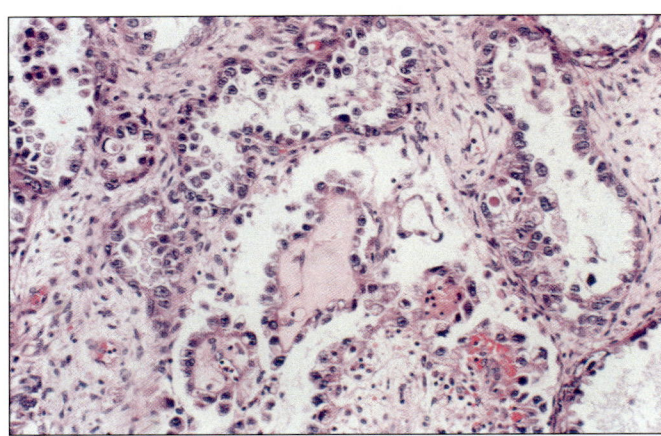

Figure 27.44 Clear cell adenocarcinoma with tubulocystic and papillary features. Occasional signet-ring cells are present.

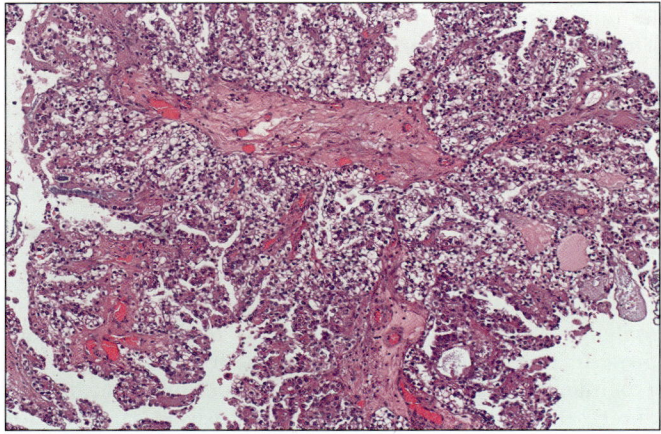

Figure 27.42 Clear cell adenocarcinoma. The tumor shows a papillary pattern. The papillae, lined by clear cells and hobnail cells, have hyalinized cores.

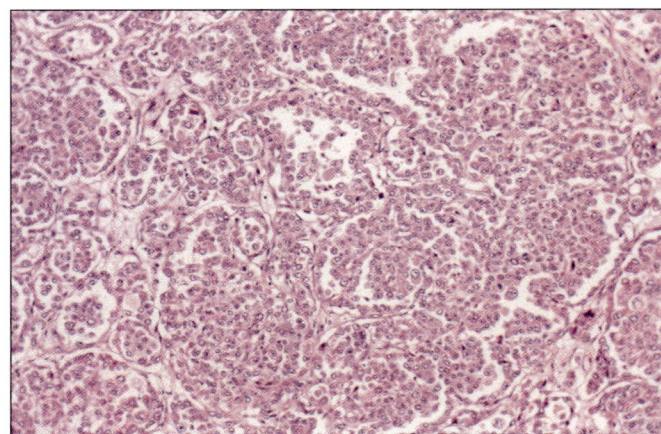

Figure 27.45 Clear cell adenocarcinoma oxyphilic type. The tumor cells have abundant eosinophilic cytoplasm and form solid aggregates.

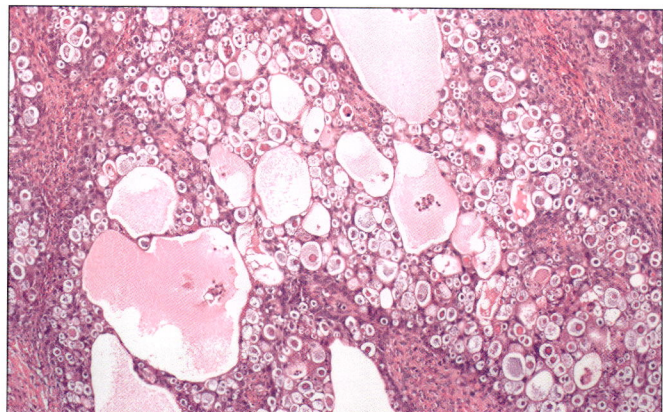

Figure 27.46 Clear cell adenocarcinoma with small cystic glands and signet-ring cells. The glands contain inspissated eosinophilic secretion.

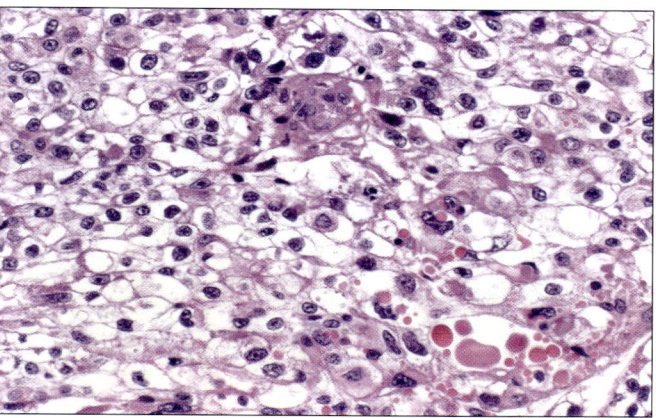

Figure 27.48 Clear cell adenocarcinoma. Numerous intracytoplasmic hyaline globules are seen on the lower right corner.

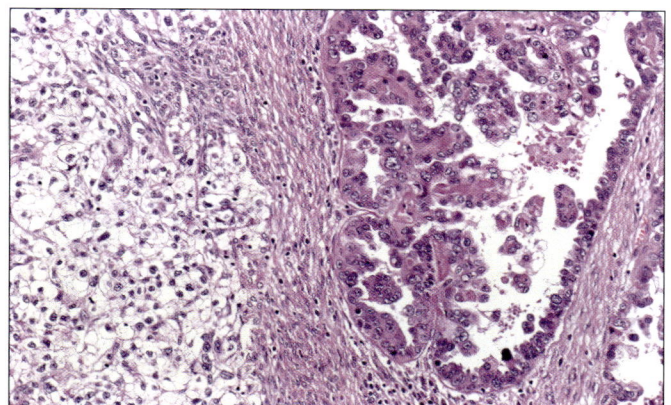

Figure 27.47 Clear cell adenocarcinoma. Mixed papillary and solid patterns.

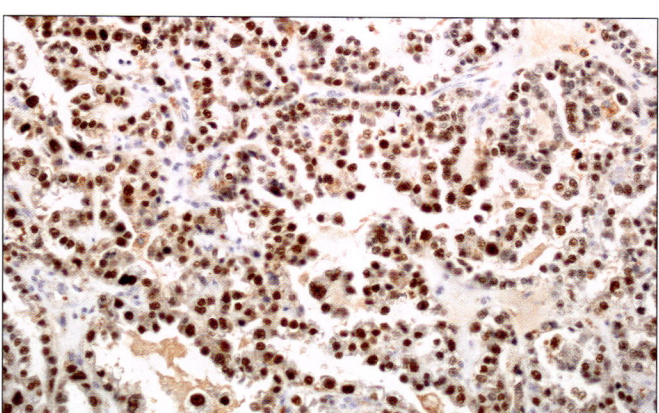

Figure 27.49 Clear cell adenocarcinoma. Strong nuclear immunoreaction for HNF-1β.

signet-ring cells containing mucin, typically in the form of inspissated eosinophilic material in the center of the vacuole (bull's eye appearance) (Figure 27.46). Rarely, the latter cells predominate in CCC. The various patterns are often admixed (Figure 27.47). Mitoses are less frequent than in other types of ovarian carcinomas and usually number <2 mitoses per 10 HPF. Indeed, a mitotic rate of 6 or greater per 10 HPF is regarded as an adverse prognostic variable.[101]

The clear cells contain glycogen. Except in the mucin-containing signet-ring cells, mucinous secretion (PAS–diastase resistant), if present, is found in the lumens and along the cytoplasmic apex of the lining cells.

The presence of clear cells alone is not sufficient for a diagnosis of CCC because cells with clear cytoplasm can be seen in high-grade serous carcinoma and endometrioid carcinoma.[102,103] Three characteristic microscopic features help in the diagnosis of CCC: (1) multiple complex papillae, (2) densely hyaline basement membrane material or mucoid stroma expanding the cores of the papillae,[2] and (3) hyaline bodies, which are present in approximately 25% of cases (Figure 27.48). The spherule-like mucoid stroma and hyalinized stroma represent different phases of the stromal remodeling process.[104,105] In exceptional cases, extensive amounts of basement membrane material, which characteristically stains for type IV collagen and laminin, occupy the stroma. CCC is occasionally admixed with endometrioid carcinoma, to which it is closely related.

Immunohistochemistry

CCCs react strongly and diffusely for epithelial markers including keratins, specifically CAM5.2, CK7, EMA, Leu M1, and B72.3. Immunoreactions for CA125 are positive in 50% of cases and for vimentin in about 50%. AFP, CK20, p53, CD10, and CEA are usually negative.[42,102,106,107] WT1 is positive in 10% and thyroid transcription factor (TTF) in <20%.[102,106,108,109] ER and PR are negative.[102] The hyalinized stroma is immunoreactive for laminin and type IV collagen.[110] CCCs are usually positive for hepatocyte nuclear factor-1β (HNF-1β) in >90% of cases (Figure 27.49).[110–112]

HNF-1β is upregulated in ovarian clear cell tumors, including benign, borderline tumors, and carcinomas.[110] This transcription factor facilitates glycogen synthesis and is expressed in mid-to-late secretory and gestational endometrium (Arias-Stella reaction),[110] atypical and inflammatory endometriosis, and CCC.[110] HNF-1β regulates several specific genes of CCC, including dipeptidyl peptidase IV (glycogen synthesis), osteopontin (progesterone-regulated endometrial secretory protein), angiotensin-converting enzyme 2 (ferritin induction, iron deposition, antiapoptosis), annexin 4 (paclitaxel resistance), and UGT1A1 (detoxification).[113] Thus, HNF-1β appears to play an important role in the pathogenesis and behavior of CCC.

Somatic Genetics

CCCs lack the *BRCA* abnormalities, chromosomal instability, or complex karyotypes of high-grade serous carcinoma.[114] Recently, it has been found that nearly half the CCCs (46–57%) carry *ARID1A* mutations and lack BAF250 protein. In two cases, *ARID1A* mutations and loss of BAF250a expression were found in the tumor and adjacent endometriosis but not in distant endometriosis. This finding suggests that *ARID1A* inactivation occurs early during malignant transformation of endometriosis.[23] *PIK3CA*-activating mutations occur in 33% and *PTEN*-inactivating mutations in 8%.[61,115,116] Most *PIK3CA*-activating mutations (71%) occur in *ARID1A*-deficient carcinomas.[117] These results suggest that loss of ARID1A-associated protein occurs as a very early event, similar to *PIK3CA* mutation, and loss of *ARID1A* can cooperate with *PIK3CA* mutations during oncogenesis. Mutations in *K-RAS* and *TP53* are present in some CCCs but their frequency is very low.

Genetic Susceptibility

CCC is associated with Lynch syndrome (most commonly with germline mutations in MSH2),[96–98] but not with hereditary ovarian–breast cancer syndrome (*BRCA1* or *BRCA2* mutations).

Differential Diagnosis

1. *High-grade serous carcinoma.* The papillae of CCC are more delicate and the stroma is more frequently hyalinized than in serous carcinoma. CCC usually shows lower mitotic rate. Conversely, serous carcinomas not infrequently contain focal areas with clear cells; in the absence of the typical papillary and tubulocystic architecture of CCC, these should not be diagnosed as CCC. A useful panel for this distinction is HNF-1β, WT1, and ER. The most common immunoprofiles are HNF-1β–, WT1+, and ER+ in high-grade serous carcinoma and HNF-1β+, WT1–, and ER– in CCC.[112]
2. *Dysgerminoma.* A CCC may simulate a dysgerminoma when it has a diffuse pattern composed entirely of clear cells (Figure 27.43). The dysgerminoma cell is rounded with flattened edges in contrast to the polyhedral cell of CCC; and the nuclei of dysgerminoma, unlike those of the CCC, are central and contain one to several prominent nucleoli. Lymphocytes are almost always seen in dysgerminoma, especially in fibrous septa, but are lacking in CCC. Granulomas are also often seen in dysgerminoma, but rarely, if ever, in CCC. Immunoreactions for placental-like alkaline phosphatase (PLAP), CD117, D2-40 (podoplanin), and LIN28, as well as nuclear transcription factors SALL 4 and OCT-4 are positive in dysgerminoma but not in CCC.[118,119] On the contrary, CCCs show strong diffuse reactivity for cytokeratins (dot-like/focal in dysgerminoma) and EMA, as expected in an epithelial tumor. Finally, the older age of patients with CCC would be unusual in germ cell tumors.
3. *Yolk sac tumor.* CCCs may display a loose, edematous appearance simulating the reticular pattern of a yolk sac tumor; both tumors may be papillary and contain hyaline bodies. The nuclei in yolk sac tumors, however, almost always appear more primitive than in CCC and their papillae may occasionally contain a central vessel (Schiller–Duval body) and lack a hyalinized eosinophilic core. The presence of other types of germ cell neoplasia within the neoplasm excludes a diagnosis of CCC. Of note, hyaline bodies are seen in one-fourth of CCCs as well as commonly in yolk sac tumors. AFP is demonstrable in almost all yolk sac tumors but in only 10% of CCCs. SALL4 and LIN28 are much better than AFP and glypican-3 for distinguishing yolk sac tumor from CCC.[118–120]
3. *Juvenile granulosa cell tumor.* The young age of the patient, the associated estrogenic symptoms, α-inhibin reactivity, and the presence of more typical tumor patterns facilitate the diagnosis.
4. *Krukenberg tumor.* Rare cases of CCC that are predominantly composed of mucin-containing signet-ring cells (Figure 27.46) may be difficult to distinguish from a Krukenberg tumor. However, Krukenberg tumors occur in patients who are known to have a primary mucinous carcinoma elsewhere, and are bilateral in 80% of the cases. Additional sections usually show the typical microscopic features of CCC, i.e., hyalinized papillae, hobnail cells, and tubulocystic pattern.
5. *Metastatic renal cell carcinoma.* The very rare metastatic renal cell carcinoma may be indistinguishable from the rare primary ovarian CCC, which is composed exclusively of clear cells (Figure 27.43). In most cases of ovarian CCC, however, the additional presence of other patterns (e.g., tubulocystic) and cell types and conspicuous extracellular luminal mucin permits microscopic differentiation. In contrast, renal cell carcinomas may show a sarcomatoid pattern and are typically CK7 negative and CD10 positive; the opposite pattern for CCC of the ovary.[107,121] Moreover, papillary renal cell carcinoma type II (eosinophilic) immunoreacts for racemase (milk fat protein) whereas CCC does not. Clinical data, including radiologic studies, may be necessary in some cases to exclude metastatic renal cell carcinoma.
6. *Steroid cell tumor/hepatoid yolk sac tumor/hepatoid carcinoma.* CCCs composed predominantly or exclusively of oxyphil cells (Figure 27.45) may closely resemble steroid cell tumors or other ovarian tumors exhibiting abundant eosinophilic cytoplasm such as the hepatoid yolk sac tumor and hepatoid carcinoma. However, typical foci of CCC are usually present in the oxyphilic variant of the tumor. In addition, the nuclei in oxyphilic CCC are typically eccentric in contrast to the central nuclei of steroid cell tumors. The degree of cytologic atypia in CCC generally exceeds that of steroid cell tumors. The hepatoid yolk sac tumor generally occurs in young females and, in addition, often contains other foci of more typical yolk

sac neoplasia. The hepatoid carcinoma occurs in an age group that is generally similar to that of CCC but lacks the typical foci of CCC usually present in the oxyphilic form of the tumor. In contrast to oxyphilic CCC, the hepatoid yolk sac tumor and hepatoid carcinoma are reactive for AFP.

7. *Arias-Stella change.* The glands of CCC resemble the hypersecretory glands of the Arias-Stella phenomenon, which occasionally may be encountered in ovarian endometriosis associated with either intrauterine or extrauterine pregnancy or trophoblastic disease. The Arias-Stella phenomenon usually involves a focus of closely packed glands. The epithelial cells exhibit marked nuclear pleomorphism and hyperchromatism, but, of importance, the nuclear material has a smudged appearance. The cytoplasm is vacuolated and clear or may be densely eosinophilic. Unlike CCC, the Arias-Stella phenomenon is associated with decidua and typically shows nuclear polyploidy. CCC develops predominantly in postmenopausal women, and usually contains near diploid or aneuploid nuclear DNA.

Tumor Spread and Staging

Patients with CCC present as stage I disease in 35–60% of cases, stage II in 10–22%,[122] stage III in 29%, and stage IV in 9%.[55]

Treatment and Prognosis

Treatment is similar to that applied to other ovarian carcinomas. Most patients with clear cell borderline tumors, including those with microinvasion, have a favorable prognosis. CCC is currently considered as an unfavorable histologic type with a worse prognosis in advanced stages than other malignant epithelial–stromal tumors, and a poor response to platinum-based chemotherapy.[93,123] The prognosis of CCC resembles that of undifferentiated carcinomas.[123] The 5 year survival rate for patients with stage I carcinomas is 69%; stage II, 55%; stage III, 14%; and stage IV, 4%.[1]

Recently, it has been suggested that CCC with an adenofibromatous component may represent a distinct subgroup of CCC that is associated with more favorable prognosis than CCC without an adenofibromatous component (5 year survival 78.8% vs 49.3%).[124,125] In contrast, other investigators claimed that, compared to cystic CCC, adenofibromatous CCCs are diagnosed more often in advanced stages (stages II–IV) and are associated with less favorable outcome (5 year survival 77% vs 37%).[126]

TRANSITIONAL CELL TUMORS

Ovarian tumors that contain epithelial cells histologically resembling those of the urothelium are grouped in the transitional cell category of tumors. This group of neoplasms constitutes 1–2% of all ovarian tumors and includes: (1) benign Brenner tumors, exhibiting a prominent stromal component and transitional cell nests, and (2) borderline (noninvasive) and malignant (invasive) Brenner tumors, both of which are associated with a benign Brenner tumor component.

Transitional cell carcinomas (TCCs), not associated with a benign or borderline Brenner component, differ clinically from malignant Brenner tumors and are now classified as variants of high-grade serous carcinomas.

- Brenner tumor
- Borderline Brenner tumor
- Malignant Brenner tumor

Histogenesis

Transitional cell tumors appear to derive directly from the ovarian surface epithelium that undergoes metaplasia to form urothelial-like epithelium. Although transitional cell differentiation in the form of Walthard nests occurs frequently in the pelvic peritoneum (perisalpinx and ovarian hilus), it represents the least common type of ovarian surface epithelial differentiation.[2] Walthard nests and small Brenner tumors have been found to arise occasionally from the rete ovarii, which is also of celomic or mesonephric derivation.[2] In rare cases, Brenner nests lie adjacent to or within a dermoid cyst, a struma ovarii, or a carcinoid tumor, suggesting a possible germ cell origin for at least some cases.[2] The similarity of Walthard nests and transitional cell tumors to urothelium is evident at both histologic and ultrastructural levels. However, the cytokeratin immunohistochemical profile of the ovarian transitional cell tumors, parallels that of müllerian (negative CK20) rather than urothelial (positive CK20) tumors.[127,128] CK7, CEA, EMA, and CA19-9 may be expressed by both ovarian and urinary tract neoplasms. Urothelial markers such as uroplakin III (Uro-III) and thrombomodulin are consistently positive in Brenner tumors but rarely positive in TCC of the ovary.[127,129] Additionally, the ovarian tumors are CA125 positive. These findings, along with a frequent mixture of other müllerian epithelial elements (mucinous, serous) in the tumors, have prompted grouping of transitional cell tumors with the other 'epithelial–stromal tumors.'

BENIGN BRENNER TUMOR

Clinical Features

Benign Brenner tumors represent <5% of benign epithelial–stromal tumors.[1] They are found in women of both reproductive and postmenopausal years, usually between the ages of 30 and 60 years.[2] Most are asymptomatic and are typically found incidentally in ovaries removed for some other reason. Brenner tumors with functioning stroma are associated with endocrine symptoms of estrogenic or androgenic type.

Macroscopic Features

Approximately half of the benign Brenner tumors are grossly visible. Many are under 2 cm in size and only a few exceed 10 cm in diameter. Less than 10% are bilateral. The sectioned surface of the typical Brenner tumor shows a nodular, sharply circumscribed (but unencapsulated), and lobulated fibrous mass that has a brownish tinge (Figure 27.50). Small cysts are common, and a rare tumor is predominantly cystic. Focal calcification may be seen. About one-fourth exhibit a cystic component, but this usually represents mixed (mucinous) epithelial differentiation.

Microscopic Features

Benign Brenner tumors show round to oval nests or trabeculae of mature transitional cells within a prominent

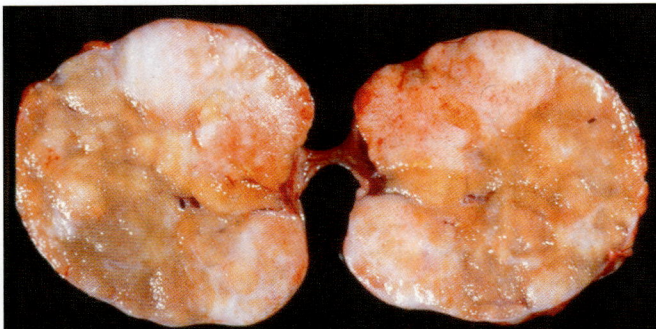

Figure 27.50 Brenner tumor. On section, the tumor appears solid, yellowish-brown and multinodular. The gray areas correspond to the fibromatous stroma.

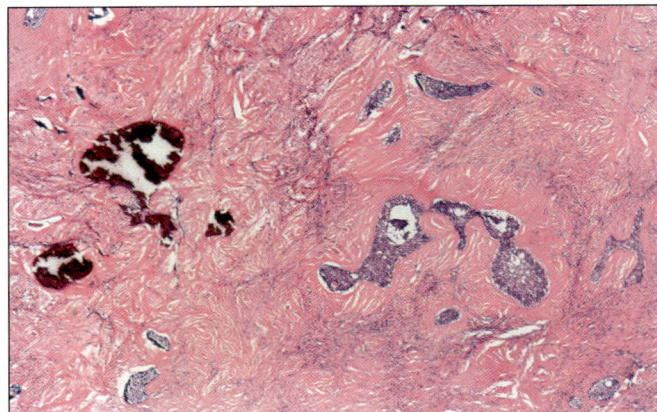

Figure 27.51 Brenner tumor. Several nests of transitional cells lie in a fibromatous stroma, which shows focal calcification.

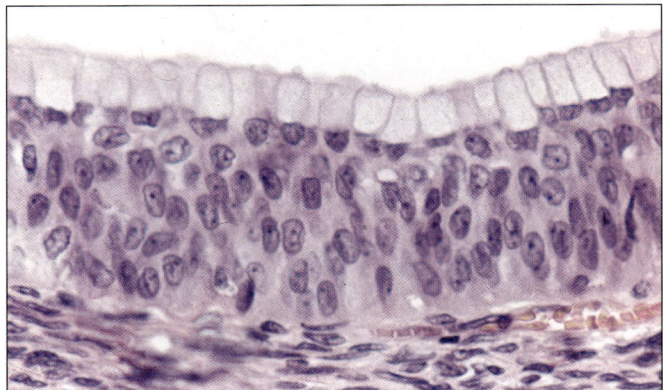

Figure 27.52 Brenner tumor. Cavitated nest of transitional cells lined by mucinous columnar epithelium.

fibromatous stroma (Figure 27.51). The apparent islands are in reality branches of a tree-like structure that in cortical tumors is in continuity with the ovarian surface epithelium. The epithelial cells are round to polygonal with distinct cell membranes and eosinophilic to clear cytoplasm. The oval nuclei have fine, evenly dispersed chromatin, obvious nucleoli, and often longitudinal grooving (so-called 'coffee-bean' appearance). This last feature is not always prominent and, moreover, it is nonspecific. It can be found in other ovarian tumors such as the adult granulosa cell tumor. Epithelial atypia is rare, as are mitoses (<1 per 10 HPF). The nests may be solid or have a central cavity containing densely eosinophilic, mucin-positive material. The lumina may be lined by mucinous (Figure 27.52), sometimes ciliated serous, or indifferent epithelium. Occasionally, squamous differentiation is found within the Brenner nests. Often the cell nests become cystic and these microcysts (containing eosinophilic debris or mucin) are mostly lined by otherwise unremarkable transitional cells. Cystic change may be more prominent, to the point of having macroscopically visible cysts forming a significant portion of the tumor. Typical transitional cell epithelium commonly lines these cysts but, sometimes, it is a mucinous epithelium that gives rise to one-sided overgrowth. The extreme of this spectrum is for a small nodule of transitional cell tumor to be found in the wall of an otherwise typical benign mucinous cystadenoma (see section Mixed Epithelial Tumors).

The Brenner epithelial nests are scattered throughout a stromal component that has the microscopic features of an ovarian fibroma or more rarely a thecoma, and may contain luteinized cells. There is much variation in cellularity, which is inversely proportional to collagen formation and hyalinization, the latter most often prominent around, or in juxtaposition to, epithelial nests. Dystrophic spiculate calcification is frequently present in such sites (Figure 27.51). New bone formation and marked stromal edema may occur.

Immunohistochemistry and Somatic Genetics

As evidence of some urothelial differentiation, benign Brenner tumors express Uro-III and thrombomodulin in three-fourths of cases, but they do not immunoreact for CK20.[127–129,131,134] They express CK7, S-100P, and GATA3. One-third of the tumors contain intracytoplasmic neuroendocrine granules, which are reactive for serotonin, but not for peptide hormones. *K-RAS* mutations at codon 12 have been identified in three of five benign Brenner tumors in one study.[133] This finding supports the hypothesis that, in ovarian tumors, *K-RAS* mutations are genetic events closely related to the mucinous phenotype.

BORDERLINE AND MALIGNANT BRENNER TUMORS

Clinical Features

Only 5% of Brenner tumors are borderline or malignant and, unlike their benign counterparts, the great majority occur in women over 50 years of age.[1,2] The patients present with an abdominal mass or pain. Some may have abnormal vaginal bleeding. Most tumors are confined to the ovary at the time of diagnosis. While borderline tumors are almost always unilateral, 10% of malignant Brenner tumors are bilateral.[2]

Macroscopic Features

Borderline Brenner tumors are typically large with a median size of 16–20 cm. Although they are usually cystic and unilocular or multilocular, with papillomatous masses

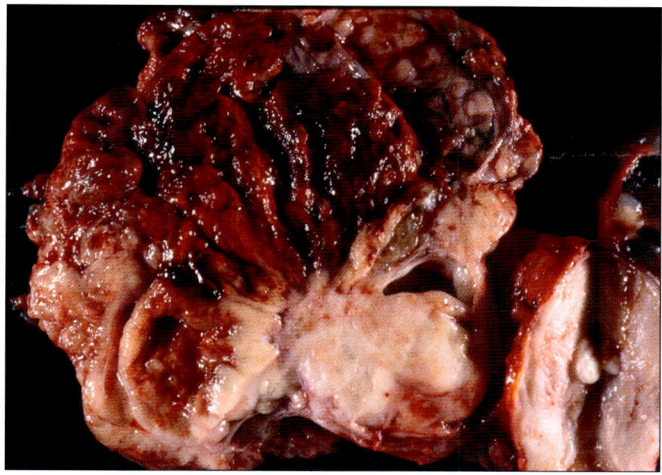

Figure 27.53 Malignant Brenner tumor. Large, solid and cystic polypoid tumor. A fibroma-like component (benign Brenner tumor) is seen at the bottom.

protruding into one or more of the locules, occasional tumors are solid. Malignant Brenner tumors may be solid or cystic with mural nodules; they have no distinctive features except that, in contrast to TCCs, they may exhibit a benign Brenner tumor component, which may be fibromatous and calcified (Figure 27.53).[1,2]

Microscopic Features

Microscopically, the polyps of the borderline tumors resemble urothelial papillary neoplasms (Figure 27.54) and exhibit the same spectrum of architectural and cytologic features. By definition, there is no stromal invasion. A benign Brenner tumor component is typically present (Figure 27.55) but may be small and easily overlooked. The mitotic rate is highly variable and focal necrosis is common. Mucinous metaplasia may be extensive. The criteria for the diagnosis of borderline and frankly malignant Brenner tumors and the designations used for these neoplasms are somewhat controversial. Since there are no reported cases of borderline tumors of any grade that have spread beyond

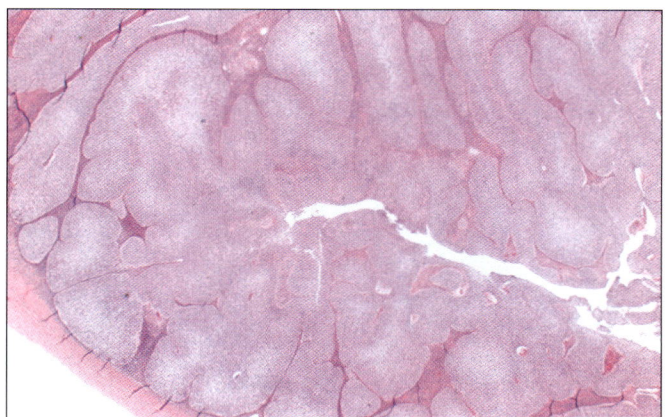

Figure 27.54 Borderline Brenner tumor. Confluent papillae lined by transitional cells protrude into a cystic space.

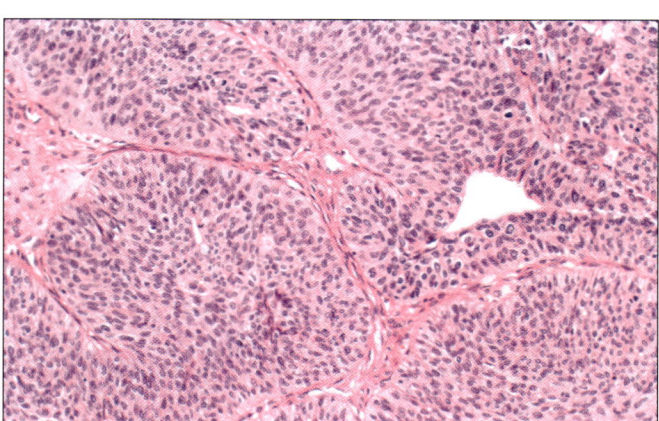

Figure 27.56 Malignant Brenner tumor. Large, closely packed, solid aggregates of transitional cells.

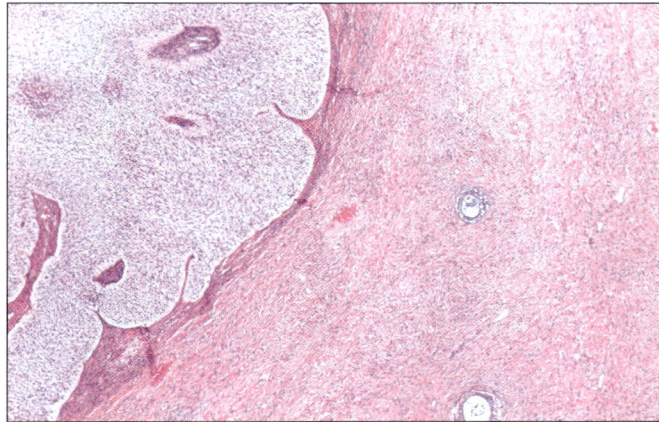

Figure 27.55 Borderline Brenner tumor. Two benign Brenner nests with central cavities lie in the adjacent fibromatous stroma.

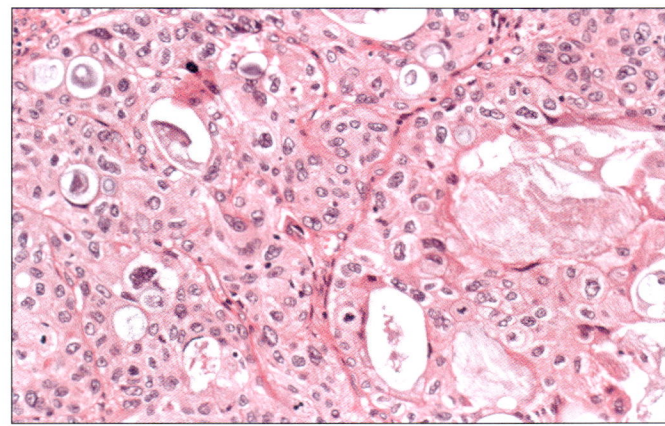

Figure 27.57 Malignant Brenner tumor. The irregular masses of TCC contain many small pools filled with mucin.

the ovary or have followed an aggressive behavior, some investigators have designated these tumors as 'proliferating' rather than borderline. Others, however, designate those resembling grade 2 or 3 TCC of the urinary tract as borderline 'with intraepithelial carcinoma.'[2] The finding of severe atypia should suggest further sampling in order to exclude the presence of an invasive component.

Malignant Brenner tumors are usually suspected on sectioning when solid cancerous masses are found. Microscopically, invasive transitional or squamous cell carcinoma (Figures 27.56 and 27.57), alone or mixed with each other, are evident together with a benign or borderline Brenner component (Figure 27.58).[1,2] Cysts are lined by multilayered epithelium featuring hyperchromatic and pleomorphic nuclei and prominent mitotic activity. With the exception of a few reported cases in which cellular atypia has been described as mild, the malignancy of the tumor cells is usually quite obvious. Discrete nests of carcinoma cells may undergo central necrosis producing a 'comedo carcinoma' pattern and occasional bizarre tumor giant cells are seen. However, as in other malignant epithelial adenofibromas, the demonstration of unequivocal stromal invasion is subjective and may necessitate extensive sampling. Irregularity, branching, and confluent epithelial nests; depletion of stroma by crowded epithelial masses; and desmoplastic stromal reactions are useful diagnostic features. Mucinous elements and, more rarely, mucinous adenocarcinoma may coexist with the transitional component. Occasionally, a prominent signet-ring mucinous component may be found (Figure 27.59).

Immunohistochemistry

The immunoprofile resembles that of benign Brenner tumors (see earlier) with a variable pattern of antigen expression in the invasive component. Borderline Brenner tumors are immunoreactive for p63, epidermal growth factor receptor (EGFR), RAS, GATA3, and CEA; and may be usually positive for S-100, uroplakin, and thrombomodulin. Rb, cyclin D1, p16, p53, and CK20 are usually weak or negative. Like their benign counterparts, malignant Brenner tumors express CK7 (Figure 27.60) but not CK20; however, urothelial markers such as uroplakin and thrombomodulin have been demonstrated in some cases.[127,134] The tumors react for cell proliferation markers, such as EGFR, cyclin D1, and *K-RAS* but, in contrast to transitional-like carcinoma of high-grade serous type, do not react for WT1, ER, p16, and p53.[135,136]

Genetic Profile

PIK3CA mutations (exon 9) have been demonstrated in a case of malignant Brenner tumor.[135] It has been suggested that malignant Brenner tumors are low-grade carcinomas with activation of the PI3K/AKT pathway through EGFR; however, EGFR amplification was not encountered in the reported case.[135] The genetic profile differs from that of transitional-like carcinoma of high-grade serous type, in which p53 mutations result in chromosomal instability, a feature of high-grade carcinomas.[135]

Differential Diagnosis

In the absence of a benign or proliferating transitional cell component, the distinction between malignant Brenner

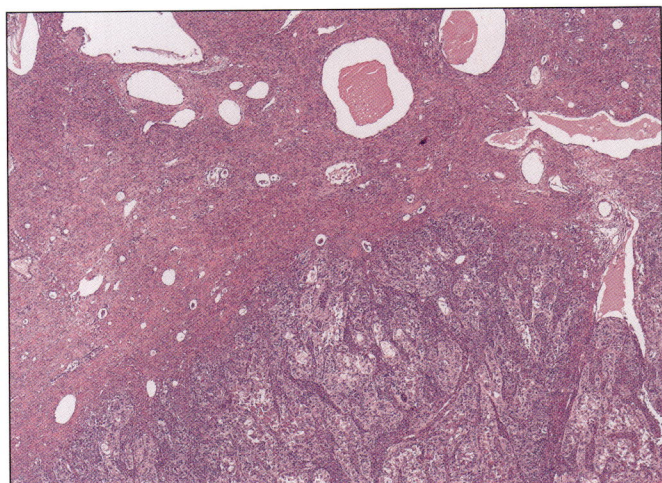

Figure 27.58 Malignant Brenner tumor. Several cavitated nests of benign Brenner component are seen in the vicinity of the invasive carcinoma.

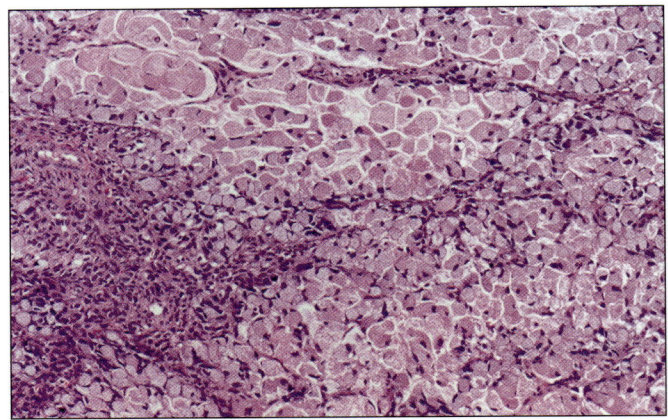

Figure 27.59 Malignant Brenner tumor with a prominent signet-ring mucinous epithelial component.

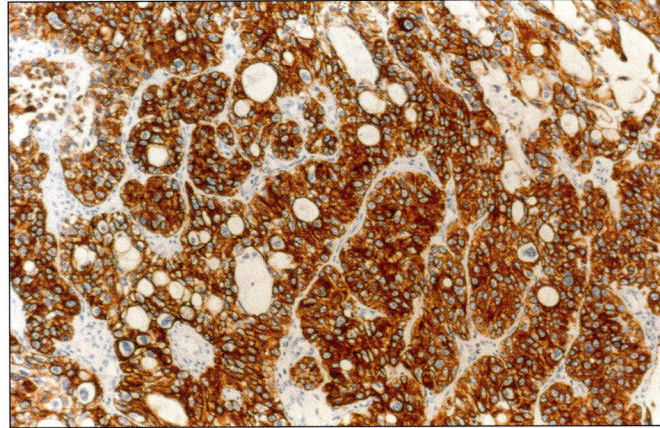

Figure 27.60 Malignant Brenner tumor. Positive immunoreaction for CK7.

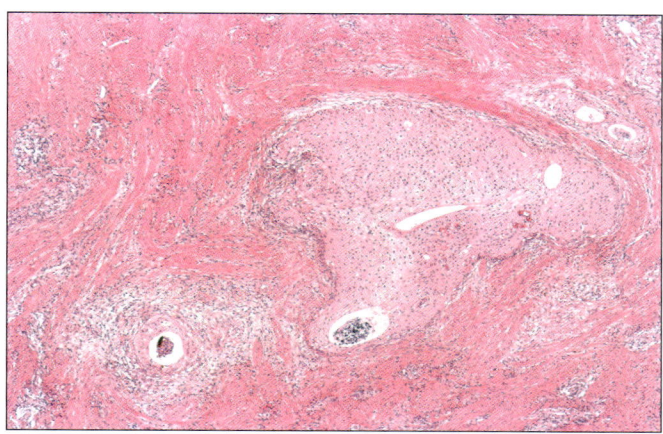

Figure 27.61 Recurrent borderline Brenner tumor. Myometrial invasion by partly cavitated masses of transitional tumor cells.

tumors and other poorly differentiated ovarian carcinomas may be difficult. Identification of a mucin-secreting adenocarcinoma component, if present, would strongly favor malignant Brenner tumor, while origin from or juxtaposition to an endometriotic cyst would favor a tumor of endometrioid type. Differentiating between TCC primary in the ovary and metastases to the ovaries from the urinary tract often requires clinical information.

Treatment and Prognosis

Borderline Brenner tumors can be treated by conservative surgery when they occur in young women. Malignant Brenner tumors are treated like other epithelial cancers. Of more than 50 reported borderline Brenner tumors, only one case is known to have spread beyond the ovary after incomplete laparoscopic resection[2,135] (Figure 27.61). Most malignant Brenner tumors are stage I and have an excellent prognosis (88% 5 year survival). About one-fifth, however, present with extraovarian spread and behave similarly to other ovarian cancers.[137]

SQUAMOUS CELL LESIONS

EPIDERMOID (SQUAMOUS CELL) CYSTS

These rare lesions are usually incidental findings. Epidermoid cysts not associated with teratomatous elements may originate from the surface epithelium of the ovary or from the rete ovarii. They are lined by keratinizing squamous epithelium and contain a creamy material that is usually seen on gross examination. Multiple sections are required to rule out a dermoid cyst.

SQUAMOUS CELL CARCINOMAS

Ovarian squamous cell carcinomas may have several histogenetic origins. Most seem to be of germ cell origin, as they arise from the walls of dermoid cysts. Less frequently, they occur in association with endometriosis, as a component of a malignant Brenner tumor, or in pure form where they are considered to be of epithelial–stromal origin.[138] Rare cases are associated with squamous cell carcinoma of the cervix (*in situ*, or invasive), raising the question of their metastatic nature.[139,140] The finding of a benign epithelial lesion, such as endometriosis, mucinous cystadenoma, Brenner tumor, or epidermoid cysts within the same ovary, suggests a primary epithelial neoplasm. The presence of these associated lesions may have prognostic implications, as pure squamous cell carcinomas generally behave more aggressively than those arising in endometriosis. Also, a malignant squamous cell component can be extensive in ovarian carcinomas of other types, particularly endometrioid carcinomas and malignant Brenner tumors. Most ovarian squamous cell carcinomas have spread beyond the ovary at the time of presentation, and the prognosis is poor.[138]

MIXED EPITHELIAL TUMORS

Most ovarian epithelial–stromal tumors are pure and easily classified into one of the five major categories (i.e., high-grade serous, low-grade serous, mucinous, endometrioid, and clear cell carcinomas). In some cases, however, two or more histologic types reside within the same tumor, or the tumor type cannot be identified by available criteria. Sampling of the tumor should be extensive enough to include all different components. Using WHO convention, mixed epithelial ovarian tumors are those in which the minor components are grossly recognizable, or account for at least 10% of the tumor on microscopical examination.[1] Mixed epithelial tumors represent <4% of epithelial–stromal tumors. Endometrioid tumors with squamous differentiation and neuroendocrine tumors associated with an epithelial–stromal tumor are excluded from this definition. The SNOMED classification of Mixed Epithelial Tumors is as follows:

- Benign mixed epithelial tumor
- Borderline mixed epithelial tumor
- Malignant mixed epithelial tumor

The association of different types of epithelial–stromal tumors is not surprising in view of their common müllerian derivation. Almost all combinations of mixed epithelial tumors have been described. Among the best known are Brenner tumor with a mucinous cystic component, endocervical-like mucinous (seromucinous) cystadenoma of borderline malignancy exhibiting other epithelial cell types of müllerian derivation,[2] endometrioid carcinoma admixed with CCC,[67] endometrioid carcinoma with a serous or undifferentiated component, and transitional-like carcinoma of high-grade serous type with another type of carcinoma. In fact, transitional cell-like differentiation is commonly found in endometrioid and serous carcinomas.

Whereas in benign and borderline tumors the mixture of different cell types is not prognostically relevant, the presence of a high-grade serous or undifferentiated component in a carcinoma has long been known to have a negative effect on prognosis, particularly for stage III and IV tumors. The 5 year survival rate for stage III tumors falls from 63% to 8%.[67] Prognostic data regarding transitional cell differentiation in carcinomas are still controversial and, similarly, there is no statistical evidence that mixed endometrioid and CCCs behave differently from either of the two pure types.

UNDIFFERENTIATED CARCINOMAS

Undifferentiated carcinomas lack significant differentiation, or contain only minor (<5%) areas of differentiation.[1,2] They account for <5% of ovarian carcinomas. Most of these tumors are currently classified as high-grade serous carcinomas. The SNOMED term is Undifferentiated carcinoma.

Clinical Features

The patients generally are older (mean, 54 years) with a range of ages from 39 to 72 years. The clinical presentation resembles that of other ovarian cancers: abdominal pain, swelling, weight loss, and urinary or intestinal symptoms. At laparotomy, 90% of the tumors show extraovarian spread, and half are stage III (Figure 27.62).[1,2]

Pathologic Features

Undifferentiated carcinomas are bilateral in 15% of cases (Figure 27.63). They are predominantly solid with extensive hemorrhage and necrosis. Surface adhesions and capsular rupture are common. Microscopically, they show a uniform population of large- to medium-sized cells arranged in solid groups with high-grade nuclei and numerous mitotic figures (Figure 27.64). Foci of high-grade serous or transitional-like carcinoma of high-grade serous type may be present. If tumors with undifferentiated areas are classified based on the areas showing a recognizable growth pattern, they usually will end up classified as high-grade serous carcinomas. As noted previously, most tumors considered in the past to be mixed high-grade serous/endometrioid, high-grade serous/clear cell, or high-grade serous/transitional cell are, based on molecular studies, better classified as high-grade serous carcinomas. Rare undifferentiated carcinomas are of small cell hypercalcemic type or show neuroendocrine features (see later).[141,142] Undifferentiated carcinomas may occasionally exhibit focal choriocarcinoma with chorionic gonadotropin (hCG) secretion.[143]

Immunohistochemistry

Undifferentiated carcinoma is reactive for EMA, CAM5.2, CK7, B72.3, and CEA (20%); and unreactive for CK20 and vimentin. CA125 is usually positive (80%).[144]

Differential Diagnosis

Undifferentiated carcinomas may be confused with diffuse granulosa cell tumors of the adult type, which have much better prognosis, and with transitional-like carcinoma of high-grade serous type. Most granulosa cell tumors have low-grade nuclei and lack both high mitotic activity and abnormal mitotic figures so characteristic of undifferentiated carcinomas. Moreover, granulosa cell tumors fail to react with EMA but typically react with vimentin, α-inhibin, and FOXL2. Undifferentiated carcinomas of small cell type show the same immunoprofile as the large cell type.[145] Estrogenic and androgenic endocrine manifestations so commonly associated with granulosa cell tumors are not seen in patients with undifferentiated carcinomas. The distinction between undifferentiated and transitional-like carcinoma of high-grade serous type is discussed in Chapter 25.

Undifferentiated carcinomas not otherwise specified (NOS) should also be distinguished from poorly differentiated ovarian tumors of other types, particularly the small cell carcinoma with hypercalcemia (see later), which typically occurs in the first three decades of life, neuroendocrine carcinomas (see later), and lymphomas. Rarely, undifferentiated carcinomas from other organs metastasize to the ovary (Chapter 30).

Prognosis

The 5 year survival rate of patients with undifferentiated carcinoma ranges from 17% (stage III) to 68% (stage I).

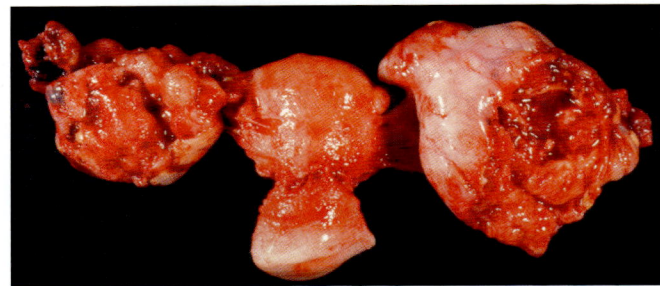

Figure 27.63 Undifferentiated carcinoma, bilateral. Predominantly solid tumors, which have extended through the capsule.

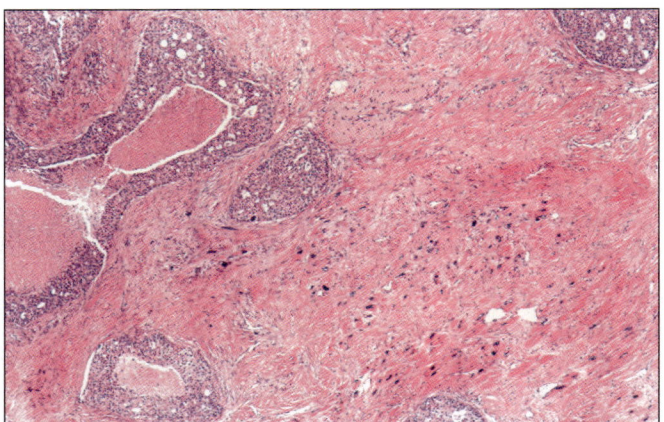

Figure 27.62 Metastatic undifferentiated carcinoma to the right undersurface of the diaphragm.

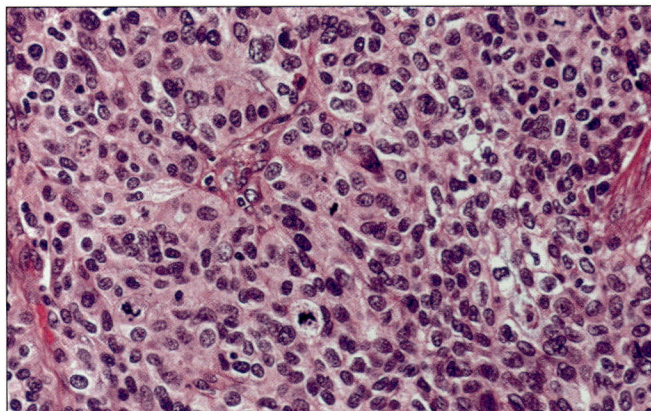

Figure 27.64 Undifferentiated carcinoma. The tumor cells have atypical nuclei with abnormal mitoses and moderate amount of cytoplasm.

MISCELLANEOUS AND UNCLASSIFIED TUMORS

SMALL CELL UNDIFFERENTIATED CARCINOMA, HYPERCALCEMIC TYPE

Clinical Features

This tumor is the most common form of undifferentiated carcinoma of the ovary in females under 40 years of age and has been associated with hypercalcemia in 66% of the cases in which the calcium level has been measured.[146] The mechanism by which hypercalcemia develops, and spontaneously regresses after the tumor is resected, is unknown. Serum parathormone (PTH) levels have been normal in several cases and attempts to demonstrate PTH within the tumor cells have been unsuccessful. However, PTH-related peptide (PTHRP) has been elevated in the serum[95] or detected by immunohistochemistry in some cases.[147] Binding of PTHRP to a receptor common for PTH and PTHRP would explain that tumor secretion of PTHRP may produce the biochemical features of hyperparathyroidism. The tumor is occasionally familial.[146] Most patients present with abdominal swelling and pain related to the tumor. Even though the neoplasm is almost always unilateral, half will already be extraovarian at the time of laparotomy.[146]

Pathologic Features

Grossly, the small cell carcinoma of hypercalcemic type is usually large (15–20 cm) and predominantly solid, resembling a lymphoma or dysgerminoma because of its cream-colored and uniform cut surface. Hemorrhage, necrosis, and cystic degeneration are common. Two patterns are found microscopically.[146] The more common shows tumor cells that are small, closely packed, and frequently arranged in diffuse sheets (Figures 27.65 and 27.66) and cords resembling a lymphoma or a juvenile granulosa cell tumor. Follicle-like structures lined by tumor cells are present in 80% of the cases (Figure 27.67). These spaces typically contain eosinophilic fluid, but sometimes it is basophilic. The nuclei may display a single prominent nucleolus and mitoses are numerous. The second form consists of larger cells exhibiting epithelioid or rhabdoid features (Figure 27.68), such as abundant eosinophilic cytoplasm and prominent nucleoli. Mixed patterns often occur. The tumor stroma may be edematous or myxoid. Interestingly, mucinous glands, atypical mucinous cells, or signet-ring cells are present in 10% of the tumors.[146]

Immunohistochemistry, DNA Cytometry, and Ultrastructure

The tumor cells are diploid[148] and typically reactive for cytokeratins (CAM5.2) (Figure 27.69), EMA, and also vimentin, but unreactive for α-inhibin.[30] It is variable for WT1, neuron-specific enolase, chromogranin, parathyroid hormone, and parathyroid hormone-related protein.[30,147] Immunohistochemistry is useful in order to exclude lymphoma, primitive neuroectodermal tumor, metastatic melanoma, and desmoplastic small round cell tumor. Ultrastructural analysis shows the tumor to be of epithelial appearance with small desmosomes and tight junctions. The cytoplasm contains dilated granular endoplasmic reticulum with amorphous material. Some neurosecretory granules have been found.[146]

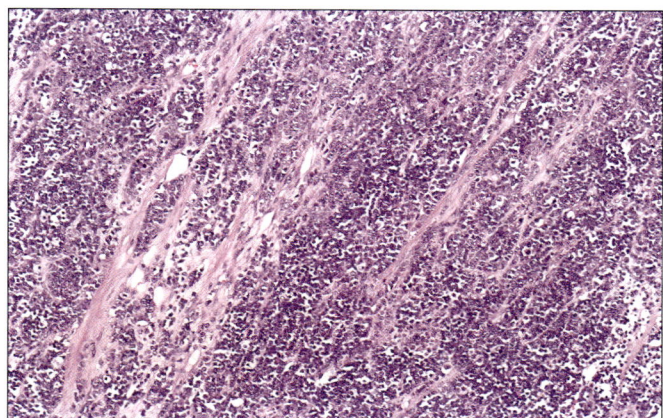

Figure 27.65 Small cell carcinoma, hypercalcemic type. The tumor cells grow in nests. The stroma appears fibrous and focally hyalinized.

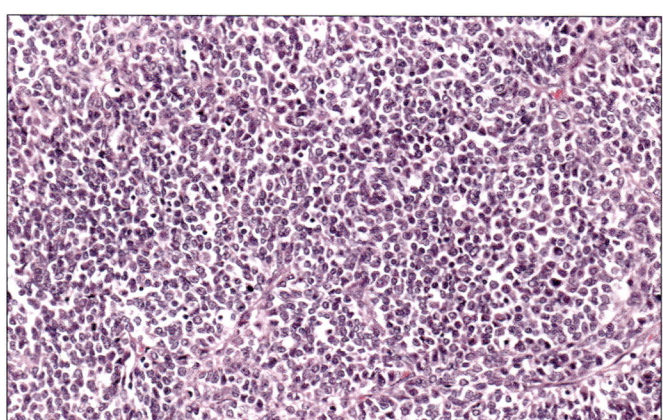

Figure 27.66 Small cell carcinoma, hypercalcemic type. Closely packed epithelial cells exhibiting hyperchromatic nuclei and scanty cytoplasm.

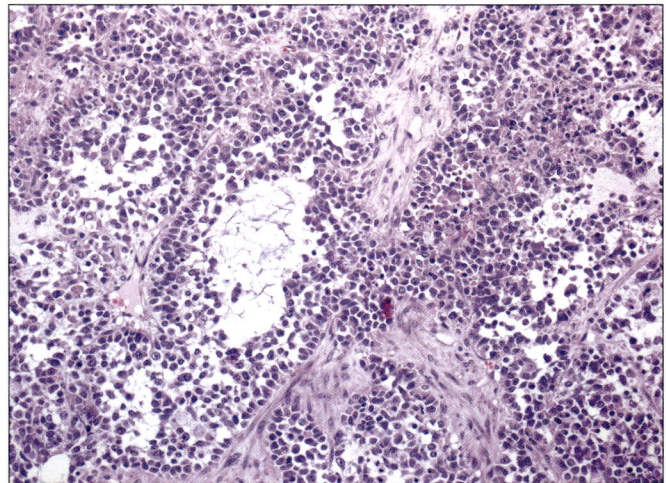

Figure 27.67 Small cell carcinoma, hypercalcemic type. Follicle-like structures.

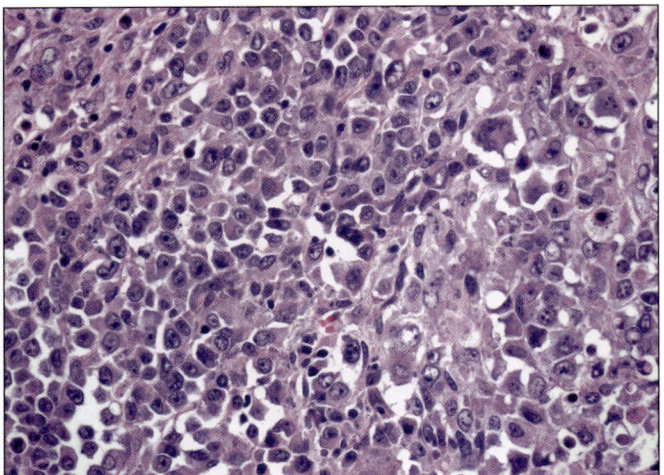

Figure 27.68 Small cell carcinoma, hypercalcemic type. Large cells with abundant eosinophilic cytoplasm and round clear nuclei with prominent nucleoli appear admixed with smaller cells.

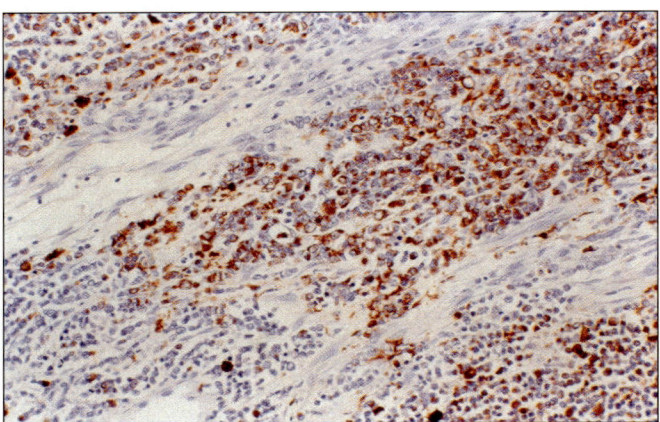

Figure 27.69 Small cell carcinoma, hypercalcemic type. Cytokeratin immunoreaction.

The tumor is thought to be epithelial but the specific cell type is unknown.

Genetic Profile

In a recent study of 21 cases, neither *TP53* (exons 5–8) nor *K-RAS* (exon 2, codons 12 and 13) mutations were identified.[149]

Differential Diagnosis

Small cell carcinomas are most often misinterpreted as granulosa cell tumors of either the adult or juvenile type. These differential diagnoses are discussed in Chapter 28. The absence of membrane immunostaining for MIC2 protein (CD99) distinguishes small cell carcinomas from primitive neuroectodermal tumors. Small cell carcinomas can also be confused with malignant lymphomas and sometimes with metastatic malignant melanoma and metastatic alveolar rhabdomyosarcoma. Clinicopathologic features and immunohistochemistry usually clarify these differential diagnoses.

Prognosis

The prognosis is poor even for stage I tumors, with only one-third of patients surviving 5 years. Most patients with higher stage tumors will die of disease within 2 years.[146]

SMALL CELL CARCINOMA, PULMONARY TYPE

These highly malignant tumors are histologically similar to small cell carcinomas of the lung and should be distinguished from metastases of the latter. Patients are generally older than those with small cell carcinomas of the hypercalcemic type and most of them present with high-stage disease.[142] Microscopically, most cells have scanty cytoplasm, nuclei with stippled chromatin, and inconspicuous nucleoli, which are typically molded by adjacent nuclei. Immunohistochemical study of nine cases revealed immunoreaction for cytokeratin in six, EMA in five, and chromogranin in two. All nine tumors were vimentin negative. Perinuclear dot-like reaction for CK20 and variable TTF-1 expression have also been found.[150] Although the histogenesis of these tumors is unclear, the concurrence of some with endometrioid carcinoma or its variants, or with Brenner tumors, suggests a surface epithelial derivation. Most tumors are aneuploid.[142]

UNDIFFERENTIATED CARCINOMA OF NON-SMALL CELL (NEUROENDOCRINE) TYPE

These tumors, which are highly malignant and occur in older women (average age of 60 years), are recognized because of their trabecular and insular growth pattern. The tumor cells are of medium to large size and contain large nuclei, which may exhibit central macronucleoli. Each of the eight reported cases was admixed with surface epithelial tumors (seven mucinous and one endometrioid). The diagnosis is established by the presence of argyrophilic granules and reactivity for cytokeratins, chromogranin and synaptophysin, serotonin, and neuron-specific enolase. The associated surface epithelial components confirm the primary nature of the tumor.[141,151]

CYSTS AND ADENOMAS OF THE RETE OVARII

Rete ovarii tubules may become dilated to form cysts. These are usually only small hilar lesions but larger cysts, up to 12 cm in diameter, also occur. Some have been associated with virilization in postmenopausal women. The cysts are lined by non-ciliated cuboidal or, less commonly, ciliated columnar epithelium, and their fibrous walls exhibit bundles of smooth muscle and often peripheral Leydig cell hyperplasia. The epithelial lining may undergo squamous metaplasia, representing one possible origin of ovarian epidermoid cysts (see earlier). Adenomas disclose cords and tubules lined by cells similar to those seen in the normal rete.

ADENOMATOID TUMORS

Adenomatoid tumors are considered benign mesotheliomas. These tumors are more frequently encountered, as incidental findings, subserosally in the uterus and fallopian tubes. They may also occur rarely in the hilar region where they form well-circumscribed white to yellow nodules

1–1.5 cm in diameter. The cut surface shows a honeycomb pattern of small cystic spaces. Microscopically, vascular-like spaces are lined by flattened or cuboidal cells, in turn surrounded by stroma. The tumor cells have eosinophilic or vacuolated cytoplasm that is Alcian blue positive at pH 2.5; this reaction, including the nonspecific stromal staining, can be eliminated by prior incubation with hyaluronidase. Adenomatoid tumors are reactive for low molecular weight cytokeratin, WT1, calretinin, and D2-40 but not for ER, PR, and Ber-EP4.

HEPATOID CARCINOMAS

This rare subtype of ovarian carcinoma resembles hepatocellular carcinoma (Figure 27.70) and gastric hepatoid carcinoma, and shows reactivity for AFP, albumin, and α-1-antitrypsin.[152] Most patients are postmenopausal and, by the time of diagnosis, most tumor will have spread beyond the ovary.[152] Sheets, trabeculae, and cords of cells with moderate to large amounts of eosinophilic cytoplasm and round to oval central nuclei are characteristic. Hyaline bodies may be numerous. These tumors are commonly admixed with serous, or less frequently with mucinous or endometrioid, carcinomas, strongly suggesting a surface epithelial origin.[132,152,153]

Hepatoid carcinoma must be distinguished from the rare hepatocellular carcinoma metastatic to the ovary and other ovarian tumors that have cells with abundant eosinophilic cytoplasm, particularly the hepatoid yolk sac tumor (see Chapter 29), steroid cell tumors (see Chapter 28), and oxyphilic CCCs (see earlier). Clinicopathologic features must be considered in making the distinction between hepatoid carcinoma and metastatic hepatocellular carcinoma. A hepatic mass suggestive of a primary neoplasm is strong evidence in favor of metastasis to the ovary.

The presence of bile pigment cannot be considered diagnostic of hepatic origin as it is found sometimes in hepatoid carcinomas arising at other sites. Hepatoid yolk sac tumor almost always develops in young women and usually shows additional typical patterns of yolk sac/germ cell neoplasia. Steroid cell tumors are often associated with endocrine manifestations and generally are not reactive for AFP. Similarly, hepatoid carcinoma is unreactive for α-inhibin.

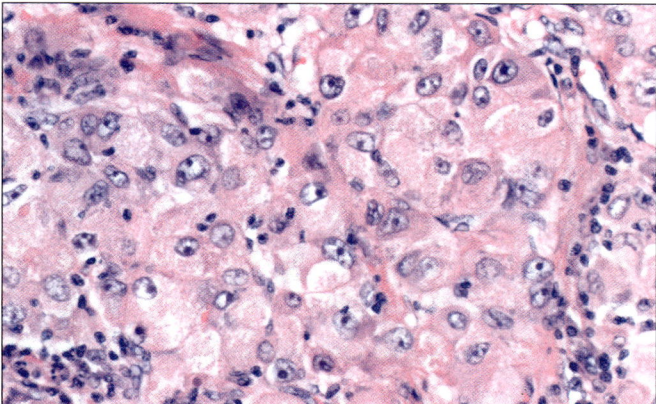

Figure 27.70 Hepatoid carcinoma. The polygonal tumor cells have abundant eosinophilic cytoplasm and round nuclei with prominent nucleoli.

Hepatoid carcinoma of the ovary is a highly malignant tumor.[152,153] Most patients present with disseminated tumor and die of the disease within a few years of diagnosis.

FEMALE ADNEXAL TUMORS OF WOLFFIAN ORIGIN

These unilateral and almost always benign tumors mimic serous or endometrioid neoplasms and Sertoli cell tumors. Unlike the latter tumors, they typically occur in the broad ligament, the mesosalpinx (see Chapter 21), or in the ovarian hilus, but when larger in size they may be misinterpreted as ovarian tumors. They arise from mesonephric (wolffian) remnants.[154,155] Grossly, the tumors appear solid and gray, tan, or yellow. They range from 2 to 20 cm (average 12 cm) in diameter.[154,155] Microscopically, the picture is that of a diffuse tubular, trabecular, or microcystic (sieve-like) growth of small- to medium-sized epithelial cells with variable quantities of fibrous stroma. The tubal lumens and sieve-like spaces usually contain eosinophilic, colloid-like material. Nuclear atypia is mild and mitotic figures are rare. The tumor cells do not contain mucin but occasionally may contain glycogen. They are immunoreactive for pan-cytokeratin, CD10, and vimentin, but they are EMA negative.[156] Calretinin, low molecular weight cytokeratin (CAM5.2), and androgen receptor are often positive but sometimes may be negative. Tumors occasionally express CK7 and α-inhibin is almost always positive.[157] CK20 is typically negative. Only rare malignant examples characterized by nuclear pleomorphism, high mitotic index, and vascular invasion have been reported.[155]

REFERENCES

1. Lee KR, Tavassoli FA, Prat J, et al. Tumours of the ovary and peritoneum: Surface epithelial-stromal tumours. In: Tavassoli FA, Devilee P, editors. World Health Organization classification of tumours. Pathology and genetics of tumours of the breast and female genital organs. Lyons, France: IARC; 2003.
2. Scully RE, Young RH, Clement PB. Tumors of the ovary, maldeveloped gonads, fallopian tube, and broad ligament. In: Atlas of tumor pathology, third series. Fascicle 23. Washington, DC: Armed Forces Institute of Pathology; 1998. p. 153–64.
3. Jiang X, Hitchcock A, Bryan EJ, et al. Microsatellite analysis of endometriosis reveals loss of heterozygosity at candidate ovarian tumor suppressor gene loci. Cancer Res 1996;56:3534–9.
4. Jiang X, Morland SJ, Hitchcock A, et al. Allelotyping of endometriosis with adjacent ovarian carcinoma reveals evidence of a common lineage. Cancer Res 1998;58:1707–12.
5. Obata K, Morland SJ, Watson RH, et al. Frequent PTEN/MMAC mutations in endometrioid but not serous or mucinous epithelial ovarian tumors. Cancer Res 1998;58:2095–7.
6. Sato N, Tsunoda H, Nishida M, et al. Loss of heterozygosity on 10q23.3 and mutation of the tumor suppressor gene PTEN in benign endometrial cyst of the ovary: possible sequence progression from benign endometrial cyst to endometrioid carcinoma and clear cell carcinoma of the ovary. Cancer Res 2000;60:7052–6.
7. Tothill RW, Tinker AV, George J, et al. Australian Ovarian Cancer Study Group, Gertig D, DeFazio A, Bowtell D. Novel molecular subtypes of serous and endometrioid ovarian cancer linked to clinical outcome. Clin Cancer Res 2008;14:5198–208.
8. Roth LM, Emerson RE, Ulbright TM. Ovarian endometrioid tumors of low malignant potential: a clinicopathologic study of 30 cases with comparison to well-differentiated endometrioid adenocarcinoma. Am J Surg Pathol 2003;27:1253–9.
9. Erzen M, Rakar S, Klancnik B, Syrjanen K. Endometriosis-associated ovarian carcinoma (EAOC): an entity distinct from

9. other ovarian carcinomas as suggested by a nested case-control study. Gynecol Oncol 2001;83:100–8.
10. McMeekin DS, Burger RA, Manetta A, et al. Endometrioid adenocarcinoma of the ovary and its relationship to endometriosis. Gynecol Oncol 1995;59:81–6.
11. Sainz de la Cuesta R, Eichhorn JH, Rice LW, et al. Histologic transformation of benign endometriosis to early epithelial ovarian cancer. Gynecol Oncol 1996;60:238–44.
12. Brinton LA, Gridley G, Persson I, Bergqvist A. Cancer risk after a hospital discharge diagnosis of endometriosis. Am J Obstet Gynecol 1997;176:572–9.
13. Irving JA, Catasus L, Gallardo A, et al. Synchronous endometrioid carcinomas of the uterine corpus and ovary: alterations in the beta-catenin (CTNNB1) pathway are associated with independent primary tumors and favorable prognosis. Hum Pathol 2005;36:605–19.
14. Falkenberry SS, Steinhoff MM, Gordinier M, et al. Synchronous endometrioid tumors of the ovary and endometrium. A clinicopathologic study of 22 cases. J Reprod Med 1996;41:713–18.
15. Fujii H, Matsumoto T, Yoshida M, et al. Genetics of synchronous uterine and ovarian endometrioid carcinoma: combined analyses of loss of heterozygosity, PTEN mutation, and microsatellite instability. Hum Pathol 2002;33:421–8.
16. Matias-Guiu X, Prat J. Ovarian tumors with functioning stroma. An immunohistochemical study of 100 cases with human chorionic gonadotropin monoclonal and polyclonal antibodies. Cancer 1990;65:2001–5.
17. Leake J, Woolas RP, Daniel J, et al. Immunocytochemical and serological expression of CA 125: a clinicopathological study of 40 malignant ovarian epithelial tumours. Histopathology 1994;24:57–64.
18. Fukunaga M, Nomura K, Ishikawa E, Ushigome S. Ovarian atypical endometriosis: its close association with malignant epithelial tumors. Histopathology 1997;30:249–55.
19. Borgfeldt C, Andolf E. Cancer risk after hospital discharge diagnosis of benign ovarian cysts and endometriosis. Acta Obstet Gynecol Scand 2004;83:395–400.
20. Stern RC, Dash R, Bentley RC, et al. Malignancy in endometriosis: frequency and comparison of ovarian and extraovarian types. Int J Gynecol Pathol 2001;20:133–9.
21. Seidman JD. Prognostic importance of hyperplasia and atypia in endometriosis. Int J Gynecol Pathol 1996;15:1–9.
22. Dinulescu DM, Ince TA, Quade BJ, et al. Role of K-RAS and PTEN in the development of mouse models of endometriosis and endometrioid ovarian cancer. Nat Med 2005;11:63–70.
23. Wiegand KC, Shah SP, Al-Agha OM, et al. ARID1A mutations in endometriosis-associated ovarian carcinomas. N Engl J Med 2010;363:1532–43.
24. Bell KA, Kurman RJ. A clinicopathologic analysis of atypical proliferative (borderline) tumors and well-differentiated endometrioid adenocarcinomas of the ovary. Am J Surg Pathol 2000;24:1465–79.
25. Oliva E, Sarrio D, Brachtel EF, et al. High frequency of beta-catenin mutations in borderline endometrioid tumors of the ovary. J Pathol 2006;208:708–13.
26. Chen S, Leitao MM, Tornos C, et al. Invasion patterns in stage I endometrioid and mucinous ovarian carcinomas: a clinicopathologic analysis emphasizing favorable outcomes in carcinomas without destructive stromal invasion and the occasional malignant course of carcinomas with limited destructive stromal invasion. Mod Pathol 2005;18:903–11.
27. Tornos C, Silva EG, Ordonez NG, et al. Endometrioid carcinoma of the ovary with a prominent spindle-cell component, a source of diagnostic confusion. A report of 14 cases. Am J Surg Pathol 1995;19:1343–53.
28. Eichhorn JH, Scully RE. Endometrioid ciliated-cell tumors of the ovary: a report of five cases. Int J Gynecol Pathol 1996;15:248–56.
29. Pitman MB, Young RH, Clement PB, et al. Endometrioid carcinoma of the ovary and endometrium, oxyphilic cell type: a report of nine cases. Int J Gynecol Pathol 1994;13:290–301.
30. Aguirre P, Thor AD, Scully RE. Ovarian small cell carcinoma: histogenetic considerations based on immunohistochemical and other findings. Am J Clin Pathol 1989;92:140–9.
31. Young RH, Prat J, Scully RE. Ovarian endometrioid carcinomas resembling sex cord-stromal tumors. A clinicopathologic analysis of 13 cases. Am J Surg Pathol 1982;6:513–22.
32. Ordi J, Schammel DP, Rasekh L, Tavassoli FA. Sertoliform endometrioid carcinomas of the ovary: a clinicopathologic and immunohistochemical study of 13 cases. Mod Pathol 1999;12:933–40.
33. Roth LM, Liban E, Czernobilsky B. Ovarian endometrioid tumors mimicking Sertoli and Sertoli-Leydig cell tumors. Sertoliform variant of endometrioid carcinoma. Cancer 1982;50:1322–31.
34. Matias-Guiu X, Pons C, Prat J. Mullerian inhibiting substance, alpha-inhibin, and CD99 expression in sex cord-stromal tumors and endometrioid ovarian carcinomas resembling sex cord-stromal tumors. Hum Pathol 1998;29:840–5.
35. Eichhorn JH, Scully RE. 'Adenoid cystic' and basaloid carcinomas of the ovary: evidence for a surface epithelial lineage. A report of 12 cases. Mod Pathol 1995;8:731–40.
36. Karnezis AN, Aysal A, Zaloudek CJ, Rabban JT. Transitional cell-like morphology in ovarian endometrioid carcinoma. Morphologic, immunohistochemical, and behavioral features distinguishing it from high-grade serous carcinoma. Am J Surg Pathol 2013;37:24–37.
37. Rutgers JL, Young RH, Scully RE. Ovarian yolk sac tumor arising from an endometrioid carcinoma. Hum Pathol 1987;18:1296–9.
38. Nogales FF, Bergeron C, Carvia RE, et al. Ovarian endometrioid tumors with yolk sac tumor component, an unusual form of ovarian neoplasm. Analysis of six cases. Am J Surg Pathol 1996;20:1056–66.
39. Yemelyanova AV, Cosin JA, Bidus MA. Pathology of stage I versus stage III ovarian carcinoma with implications for pathogenesis and screening. Int J Gynecol Cancer 2008;18:465–9.
40. Köbel M, Kalloger SE, Baker PM, et al. Diagnosis of ovarian carcinoma cell type is highly reproducible: a transcanadian study. Am J Surg Pathol 2010;34:984–93.
41. Lee P, Rosen DG, Zhu C, et al. Expression of progesterone receptor is a favorable prognostic marker in ovarian cancer. Gynecol Oncol 2005;96:671–7.
42. McCluggage WG. Immunohistochemical and functional biomarkers of value in female genital tract lesions. Int J Gynecol Pathol 2006;25:101–20.
43. O'Neill CJ, Deavers MT, Malpica A, et al. An immunohistochemical comparison between low-grade and high-grade ovarian serous carcinomas: significantly higher expression of p53, MIB1, BCL2, HER-2/neu, and C-KIT in high grade neoplasms. Am J Surg Pathol 2005;29:1034–41.
44. Vang R, Gown AM, Farinola M, et al. p16 expression in primary ovarian mucinous and endometrioid tumors and metastatic adenocarcinomas in the ovary: utility for identification of metastatic HPV related endocervical adenocarcinomas. Am J Surg Pathol 2007;31:653–66.
45. Cathro HP, Stoler MH. The utility of calretinin, inhibin and WT1 immunohistochemical staining in the differential diagnosis of ovarian tumors. Hum Pathol 2005;36:195–201.
46. Zhao C, Bratthauer GL, Barner R, et al. Comparative analysis of alternative and traditional immunohistochemical markers for the distinction of ovarian Sertoli cell tumor from endometrioid tumors and carcinoid tumor: a study of 160 cases. Am J Surg Pathol 2007;31:255–66.
47. Zhao C, Bratthauer GL, Barner R, et al. Diagnostic utility of WT1 immunostaining in ovarian Sertoli cell tumor. Am J Surg Pathol 2007;31:1378–86.
48. Thrall M, Gallion HH, Kryscio R, et al. BRCA1 expression in a large series of sporadic ovarian carcinomas: a Gynecologic Oncology Group study. Int J Gynecol Cancer 2006;16(Suppl. 1):166–71.
49. Aguirre P, Thor AD, Scully RE. Ovarian endometrioid carcinomas resembling sex cord-stromal tumors. An immunohistochemical study. Int J Gynecol Pathol 1989;8:364–73.
50. Lugli A, Forster Y, Haas P, et al. Calretinin expression in human normal and neoplastic tissues: a tissue microarray analysis on 5233 tissue samples. Hum Pathol 2003;34:994–1000.
51. Gomes CP, Andrade LA. PTEN and p53 expression in primary ovarian carcinomas: immunohistochemical study and discussion of pathogenetic mechanisms. Int J Gynecol Cancer 2006;16(Suppl. 1):254–8.
52. Catasús L, Bussaglia E, Rodríguez IM, et al. Molecular genetic alterations in endometrioid carcinomas of the ovary: Similar frequency of beta-catenin abnormalities but lower rate of microsatellite instability and PTEN alterations than in uterine endometrioid carcinomas. Hum Pathol 2004;35:1360–8.

53. Liu J, Albarracin CT, Chang K-H, et al. Microsatellite instability and expression of hMLH1 and hMSH2 proteins in ovarian endometrioid cancer. Mod Pathol 2004;17:75–80.
54. Zaino RJ, Kurman RJ, Diana KL, Morrow CP. The utility of the revised International Federation of Gynecology and Obstetrics histologic grading of endometrial adenocarcinoma using a defined nuclear grading system: a Gynecologic Oncology Group study. Cancer 1995;75:81–6.
55. Pettersson F. Annual report of the results of treatment in gynecological cancer. Stockholm, Sweden: International Federation of Gynecology and Obstetrics; 1991.
56. Machín P, Catasus L, Pons C, et al. Microsatellite instability and immunostaining for MSH-2 and MLH-1 in cutaneous and internal tumors from patients with the Muir-Torre syndrome. J Cutan Pathol 2002;29:415–20.
57. Southey MC, Young M-A, Whitty J, et al. Molecular pathologic analysis enhances the diagnosis and management of Muir-Torre syndrome and gives insight into its underlying molecular pathogenesis. Am J Surg Pathol 2001;25:936–41.
58. Moreno-Bueno G, Gamallo C, Perez-Gallego L, et al. Beta-catenin expression pattern, beta-catenin gene mutations, and microsatellite instability in endometrioid ovarian carcinomas and synchronous endometrial carcinomas. Diagn Mol Pathol 2001;10:116–22.
59. Palacios J, Gamallo C. Mutations in the beta-catenin gene (CTNNB1) in endometrioid ovarian carcinomas. Cancer Res 1998;58:1344–7.
60. Gamallo C, Palacios J, Moreno G, et al. Beta-catenin expression pattern in stage I and II ovarian carcinomas: relationship with beta-catenin gene mutations, clinicopathological features, and clinical outcome. Am J Pathol 1999;155:527–36.
61. Campbell IG, Russell SE, Choong DY, et al. Mutation of the PIK3CA gene in ovarian and breast cancer. Cancer Res 2004;64:7678–81.
62. Oda K, Stokoe D, Taketani Y, et al. High frequency of coexistent mutations of PIK3CA and PTEN genes in endometrial carcinoma. Cancer Res 2005;65:10669–73.
63. Catasus L, Gallardo A, Cuatrecasas M, Prat J. PIK3CA mutations in the kinase domain (exon 20) of uterine endometrial adenocarcinomas are associated with adverse prognostic parameters. Mod Pathol 2008;21:131–9.
64. Gras E, Catasus Ll, Arguelles R, et al. Microsatellite instability, MLH-1 promoter hypermethylation, and frameshift mutations at coding mononucleotide repeat microsatellites in ovarian tumors. Cancer 2001;92:2829–36.
65. Lynch HT, Casey MJ, Snyder CL, et al. Hereditary ovarian carcinoma: heterogeneity, molecular genetics, pathology, and management. Mol Oncol 2009;3:97–137.
66. Young RH, Prat J, Scully RE. Endometrioid stromal sarcomas of the ovary: a clinicopathologic analysis of 23 cases. Cancer 1984;53:1143–55.
67. Tornos C, Silva EG, Khorana SM, Burke TW. High-stage endometrioid carcinoma of the ovary. Prognostic significance of pure versus mixed histologic types. Am J Surg Pathol 1994;18:687–93.
68. Soliman PT, Slomovitz BM, Broaddus RR, et al. Synchronous primary cancers of the endometrium and ovary: a single institution review of 84 cases. Gynecol Oncol 2004;94:456–62.
69. Storey DJ, Rush R, Stewart M, et al. Endometrioid epithelial ovarian cancer: 20 years of prospectively collected data from a single center. Cancer 2008;112:2211–20.
70. Prat J, Matias-Guiu X, Barreto J. Simultaneous carcinoma involving the endometrium and the ovary. A clinicopathologic, immunohistochemical, and DNA flow cytometric study of 18 cases. Cancer 1991;68:2455–9.
71. Pearl ML, Johnston CM, Frank TS, Roberts JA. Synchronous dual primary ovarian and endometrial carcinomas. Int J Gynaecol Obstet 1993;43:305–12.
72. Fujita M, Enomoto T, Wada H, et al. Application of clonal analysis. Differential diagnosis for synchronous primary ovarian and endometrial cancers and metastatic cancer. Am J Clin Pathol 1996;105:350–9.
73. Emmert-Buck MR, Chuaqui R, Zhuang Z, et al. Molecular analysis of synchronous uterine and ovarian endometrioid tumors. Int J Gynecol Pathol 1997;16:143–8.
74. Shenson DL, Gallion HH, Powell DE, Pieretti M. Loss of heterozygosity and genomic instability in synchronous endometrioid tumors of the ovary and endometrium. Cancer 1995;76:650–7.
75. Matias-Guiu X, Lagarda H, Catasus LI, et al. Clonality analysis in synchronous or metachronous tumors of the female genital tract. Int J Gynecol Pathol 2002;21:205–11.
76. Abeln EC, Smit VT, Wessels JW, et al. Molecular genetic evidence for the conversion hypothesis of the origin of malignant mixed mullerian tumours. J Pathol 1997;183:424–31.
77. Fujii H, Yoshida M, Gong ZX, et al. Frequent genetic heterogeneity in the clonal evolution of gynecological carcinosarcoma and its influence on phenotypic diversity. Cancer Res 2000;60:114–20.
78. Thompson L, Chang B, Barsky SH. Monoclonal origins of malignant mixed tumors (carcinosarcomas). Evidence for a divergent histogenesis. Am J Surg Pathol 1996;20:277–85.
79. McCluggage WG. Uterine carcinosarcomas (malignant mixed Mullerian tumors) are metaplastic carcinomas. Int J Gynecol Cancer 2002;12:687–90.
80. Jin Z, Ogata S, Tamura G, et al. Carcinosarcomas (malignant mullerian mixed tumors) of the uterus and ovary: a genetic study with special reference to histogenesis. Int J Gynecol Pathol 2003;22:368–73.
81. Gallardo A, Matias-Guiu X, Lagarda H, et al. Malignant mullerian mixed tumor arising from ovarian serous carcinoma: a clinicopathologic and molecular study of two cases. Int J Gynecol Pathol 2002;21:268–72.
82. Becker JL, Papenhausen PR, Widen RH. Cytogenetic, morphologic and oncogene analysis of a cell line derived from a heterologous mixed mullerian tumor of the ovary. In Vitro Cell Dev Biol Anim 1997;33:325–31.
83. Eichhorn JH, Young RH, Clement PB, Scully RE. Mesodermal (Müllerian) adenosarcoma of the ovary: a clinicopathologic analysis of 40 cases and review of the literature. Am J Surg Pathol 2002;26:1243–58.
84. Gallardo A, Prat J. Mullerian adenosarcoma: a clinicopathologic and immunohistochemical study of 55 cases challenging the existence of adenofibroma. Am J Surg Pathol 2009;33:278–88.
85. Chang KL, Crabtree GS, Lim Tan SK, et al. Primary extrauterine endometrial stromal neoplasms: a clinicopathologic study of 20 cases and a review of the literature. Int J Gynecol Pathol 1993;12:282–96.
86. Nucci MR, Harburger D, Koontz J, et al. Molecular analysis of the JAZF1-JJAZ1 gene fusion by RT-PCR and fluorescence in situ hybridization in endometrial stromal neoplasms. Am J Surg Pathol 2007;31:65–70.
87. Lee CH, Marino-Enriquez A, Ou W, et al. The clinicopathologic features of YWHAE-FAM22 endometrial stromal sarcomas: a histologically high-grade and clinically aggressive tumor. Am J Surg Pathol 2012;36:641–53.
88. Deavers MT, Malpica A, Liu J, et al. Ovarian sex cord-stromal tumors: an immunohistochemical study including a comparison of calretinin and inhibin. Mod Pathol 2003;16:584–90.
89. Zheng W, Sung CJ, Hanna I, et al. Alpha and beta subunits of inhibin/activin as sex cord-stromal differentiation markers. Int J Gynecol Pathol 1997;16:263–71.
90. Al-Agha OM, Huwait HF, Chow C, et al. FOXL2 is a sensitive and specific marker for sex cord-stromal tumors of the ovary. Am J Surg Pathol 2011;35:484–94.
91. Lerwill MF, Sung R, Oliva E, et al. Smooth muscle tumors of the ovary. A clinicopathologic study of 54 cases emphasizing prognostic criteria, histologic variants, and differential diagnosis. Am J Clin Pathol 2004;28:1436–51.
92. Komiyama S, Aoki D, Tominaga E, et al. Prognosis of Japanese patients with ovarian clear cell carcinoma associated with pelvic endometriosis: clinicopathologic evaluation. Gynecol Oncol 1999;72:342–6.
93. Pather S, Quinn MA. Clear cell cancer of the ovary—is it chemosensitive? Int J Gynecol Cancer 2004;15:432–7.
94. Tan DSP, Kaye S. Ovarian clear cell adenocarcinoma: a continuing enigma. J Clin Pathol 2007;60:355–60.
95. Tsunematsu R, Saito T, Iguchi H, et al. Hypercalcemia due to parathyroid hormone-related protein produced by primary ovarian clear cell adenocarcinoma: case report. Gynecol Oncol 2000;76:218–22.
96. Lu F, Gilks CB, Mulligan AM, et al. Prevalence of loss of expression of DNA mismatch repair proteins in primary epithelial ovarian tumors. Int J Gynecol Pathol 2012;31:524–31.

97. Ketabi Z, Bartuma K, Bernstein I, et al. Ovarian cancer linked to Lynch syndrome typically presents as early-onset, non-serous epithelial tumors. Gynecol Oncol 2011;121:462–5.
98. Cai KQ, Albarracin CT, Rosen D, et al. Microsatellite instability and alteration of the expression of hMLH1 and hMSH2 in ovarian clear cell carcinoma. Hum Pathol 2004;35:552–9.
99. Mizuno M, Kikkawa F, Shibata K, et al. Long-term prognosis of stage I ovarian carcinoma: prognostic importance of intraoperative rupture. Oncology 2003;65:29–36.
100. Takano M, Kikuchi Y, Yaegashi N, et al. Clear cell carcinoma of the ovary: a retrospective multicentre experience of 254 patients with complete surgical staging. Br J Cancer 2006;94:1369–74.
101. Kennedy AW, Biscotti CV, Hart WR, Tuason LJ. Histologic correlates of progression-free interval and survival in ovarian clear cell adenocarcinoma. Gynecol Oncol 1993;50:334–8.
102. Han G, Gilks CB, Leung S, et al. Mixed ovarian epithelial carcinomas with clear cell and serous components are variants of high-grade serous carcinoma: an interobserver correlative and immunohistochemical study of 32 cases. Am J Surg Pathol 2008;32:955–64.
103. Silva EG, Young RH. Endometrioid neoplasms with clear cells: a report of 21 cases in which the alteration is not of typical secretory type. Am J Surg Pathol 2007;31:1203–8.
104. Kato N, Takeda J, Fukase M, Motoyama T. Alternate mucoid and hyalinized stroma in clear cell carcinoma of the ovary: manifestation of serial stromal remodeling. Mod Pathol 2010;23:881–8.
105. Kato N, Takeda J, Fukase M, Motoyama T. Hyalinized stroma in clear cell carcinoma of the ovary: how is it formed? Hum Pathol 2012;43:2041–6.
106. Baker PM, Oliva E. Immunohistochemistry as a tool in the differential diagnosis of ovarian tumors: an update. Int J Gynecol Pathol 2005;24:39–55.
107. Cameron RI, Ashe P, O'Rourke DM, et al. A panel of immunohistochemical stains assists in the distinction between ovarian and renal clear cell carcinoma. Int J Gynecol Pathol 2003;22:272–6.
108. Acs G, Pasha T, Zhang PJ. WT1 is differentially expressed in serous, endometrioid, clear cell, and mucinous carcinomas of the peritoneum, fallopian tube, ovary, and endometrium. Int J Gynecol Pathol 2004;23:110–18.
109. Howell NR, Zheng W, Cheng L, et al. Carcinomas of ovary and lung with clear cell features: can immunohistochemistry help in differential diagnosis? Int J Gynecol Pathol 2007;26:134–40.
110. Kato N, Sasou S, Motoyama T. Expression of hepatocyte nuclear factor-1beta (HNF-1beta) in clear cell tumors and endometriosis of the ovary. Mod Pathol 2006;19:83–9.
111. Köbel M, Kalloger SE, Boyd N, et al. Ovarian carcinoma subtypes are different diseases: implications for biomarker studies. PLoS Med 2008;5:e232.
112. Köbel M, Kalloger SE, Carrick J, et al. A limited panel of immunomarkers can reliably distinguish between clear cell and high-grade serous carcinoma of the ovary. Am J Surg Pathol 2009;33:14–21.
113. Kobayashi H, Yamada Y, Kanayama S, et al. The role of hepatocyte nuclear factor-1beta in the pathogenesis of clear cell carcinoma of the ovary. Int J Gynecol Cancer 2009;19:471–9.
114. Press JZ, De Luca A, Boyd N, et al. Ovarian carcinomas with genetic and epigenetic BRCA1 loss have distinct molecular abnormalities. BMC Cancer 2008;8:17.
115. Kuo KT, Mao TL, Jones S, et al. Frequent activating mutations of PIK3CA in ovarian clear cell carcinoma. Am J Pathol 2009;174:1597–601.
116. Yamamoto S, Tsuda H, Takano M, et al. PIK3CA mutation is an early event in the development of endometriosis-associated ovarian clear cell adenocarcinoma. J Pathol 2011;225:189–94.
117. Yamamoto S, Tsuda H, Takano M, et al. Loss of ARID1A protein expression occurs as an early event in ovarian clear-cell carcinoma development and frequently coexists with PIK3CA mutations. Mod Pathol 2012;25:615–24.
118. Cao D, Guo S, Allan RW, et al. SALL4 is a novel sensitive and specific marker of ovarian primitive germ cell tumors and is particularly useful in distinguishing yolk sac tumor from clear cell carcinoma. Am J Surg Pathol 2009;33:894–904.
119. Xue D, Peng Y, Wang F, et al. RNA-binding protein LIN28 is a sensitive marker of ovarian primitive germ cell tumours. Histopathology 2011;59:452–9
120. Nogales FF, Preda O, Nicolae A. Yolk sac tumours revisited. A review of their many faces and names. Histopathology 2012;60:1023–33.
121. Ohta Y, Suzuki T, Shiokawa A, et al. Expression of CD10 and cytokeratins in variant and renal clear cell carcinoma. Int J Gynecol Pathol 2005;24:239–45.
122. Pectasides D, Fountzilas G, Aravantinos G, et al. Advanced stage clear-cell epithelial ovarian cancer: the Hellenic Cooperative Oncology Group experience. Gynecol Oncol 2006;102:285–91.
123. Goff BA, Sainz de la Cuesta R, Muntz HG, et al. Clear cell carcinoma of the ovary: a distinct histologic type with poor prognosis and resistance to platinum-based chemotherapy in stage III disease. Gynecol Oncol 1996;60:412–17.
124. Yamamoto S, Tsuda H, Yoshikawa T, et al. Clear cell adenocarcinoma associated with clear cell adenofibromatous components: a subgroup of ovarian clear cell adenocarcinoma with distinct clinicopathologic characteristics. Am J Surg Pathol 2007;31:999–1006.
125. Yamamoto S, Tsuda H, Takano M, et al. Clear-cell adenofibroma can be a clonal precursor for clear-cell adenocarcinoma of the ovary: a possible alternative clear-cell carcinogenic pathway. J Pathol 2008;216:103–10.
126. Veras E, Mao T-L, Ayhan A, et al. Cystic and adenofibromatous clear cell carcinomas of the ovary: distinctive tumors that differ in their pathogenesis and behavior: a clinicopathologic analysis of 122 cases. Am J Surg Pathol 2009;33:844–53.
127. Logani S, Oliva E, Amin MB, et al. Immunoprofile of ovarian tumors with putative transitional cell (urothelial) differentiation using novel urothelial markers: histogenetic and diagnostic implications. Am J Surg Pathol 2003;27:1434–41.
128. Soslow RA, Rouse RV, Hendrickson MR, et al. Transitional cell neoplasms of the ovary and urinary bladder: a comparative immunohistochemical analysis. Int J Gynecol Pathol 1996;15:257–65.
129. Ogawa K, Johansson SL, Cohen SM. Immunohistochemical analysis of uroplakins, urothelial specific proteins, in ovarian Brenner tumors, normal tissues, and benign and neoplastic lesions of the female genital tract. Am J Pathol 1999;155:1047–50.
130. Ordonez NG. Role of immunohistochemistry in distinguishing epithelial peritoneal mesotheliomas from peritoneal and ovarian serous carcinomas. Am J Surg Pathol 1998;22:1203–14.
131. Ordonez NG. Transitional cell carcinomas of the ovary and bladder are immunophenotypically different. Histopathology 2000;36:433–8.
132. Scurry JP, Brown RW, Jobling T. Combined ovarian serous papillary and hepatoid carcinoma. Gynecol Oncol 1996;63:138–42.
133. Cuatrecasas M, Erill N, Musulen E, et al. K-RAS mutations in non-mucinous ovarian epithelial tumors: A molecular analysis and clinicopathological study of 144 patients. Cancer 1998;82:1088–95.
134. Riedel I, Czernobilsky B, Lifschitz-Mercer B, et al. Brenner tumors but not transitional cell carcinomas of the ovary show urothelial differentiation: immunohistochemical staining of urothelial markers, including cytokeratins and uroplakins. Virchows Arch 2001;438:181–91.
135. Cuatrecasas M, Catasus L, Palacios J, Prat J. Transitional cell tumors of the ovary: a comparative clinicopathologic, immunohistochemical, and molecular genetic analysis of Brenner tumors and transitional cell carcinomas. Am J Surg Pathol 2009;33:556–67.
136. Ali RH, Seidman JD, Luk M, et al. Transitional cell carcinoma of the ovary is related to high-grade serous carcinoma and is distinct from malignant Brenner tumor. Int J Gynecol Pathol 2012;31:499–506.
137. Austin RM, Norris HJ. Malignant Brenner tumor and transitional cell carcinoma of the ovary: a comparison. Int J Gynecol Pathol 1987;6:29–39.
138. Pins MR, Young RH, Daly WJ, Scully RE. Primary squamous cell carcinoma of the ovary. A report of 37 cases. Am J Surg Pathol 1996;20:823–33.
139. Mai KT, Yazdi HM, Bertrand MA, et al. Bilateral primary ovarian squamous cell carcinoma associated with human papillomavirus infection and vulvar and cervical intraepithelial neoplasia. Am J Surg Pathol 1996;20:767–72.
140. Sworn MJ, Jones H, Letchworth AT, et al. Squamous intraepithelial neoplasia in an ovarian cyst, cervical intraepithelial neoplasia and human papillomavirus. Hum Pathol 1995;26:344–7.
141. Eichhorn JH, Lawrence WD, Young RH, Scully RE. Ovarian neuroendocrine carcinomas of non small cell type associated with surface epithelial adenocarcinomas. A study of five cases

and a review of the literature. Int J Gynecol Pathol 1996;15: 303–14.
142. Eichhorn JH, Young RH, Scully RE. Primary ovarian small cell carcinoma of pulmonary type. A clinicopathologic, immunohistologic, and flow cytometric analysis of 11 cases. Am J Surg Pathol 1992;16:926–38.
143. Oliva E, Andrada E, Pezzica E, Prat J. Ovarian carcinomas with choriocarcinomatous differentiation. Cancer 1993;72:2441–6.
144. Kuwashima Y, Takayama S. Immunohistochemical characterization of undifferentiated carcinomas of the ovary. J Cancer Res Clin 1994;120:672–7.
145. Riopel MA, Perlman EJ, Seidman JD, et al. Inhibin and epithelial membrane antigen immunohistochemistry assist in the diagnosis of sex cord-stromal tumors and provide clues to the histogenesis of hypercalcemic small cell carcinomas. Int J Gynecol Pathol 1998;17:46–53.
146. Young RH, Oliva E, Scully RE. Small cell carcinoma of the ovary, hypercalcemic type. A clinicopathologic analysis of 150 cases. Am J Surg Pathol 1994;18:1102–16.
147. Matias-Guiu X, Prat J, Young RH, et al. Human parathyroid hormone-related protein in ovarian small cell carcinoma. An immunohistochemical study. Cancer 1994;73:1878–81.
148. Eichhorn JH, Bell DA, Young RH, et al. DNA content and proliferative activity in ovarian small cell carcinomas of the hypercalcemic type. Implications for diagnosis, prognosis and histogenesis. Am J Clin Pathol 1992;98:579–86.
149. D'Angelo E, Rivera C, Canet B, et al. Small cell carcinoma hypercalcemic type: consistent clinicopathologic features and lack of molecular markers. Mod Pathol 2012;25S–264A.
150. Carlson JW, Nucci MR, Brodsky J, et al. Biomarker-assisted diagnosis of ovarian, cervical and pulmonary small cell carcinomas: the role of TTF-1, WT-1 and HPV analysis. Histopathology 2007;51:305–12.
151. Veras E, Deavers MT, Silva EG, et al. Ovarian nonsmall cell neuroendocrine carcinoma: a clinicopathologic and immunohistochemical study of 11 cases. Am J Surg Pathol 2007;31:774–82.
152. Ishikura H, Scully RE. Hepatoid carcinoma of the ovary. A newly described tumor. Cancer 1987;60:2775–84.
153. Tochigi N, Kishimoto T, Supriatna Y, et al. Hepatoid carcinoma of the ovary: a report of three cases admixed with common surface epithelial carcinoma. Int J Gynecol Pathol 2003;22:266–71.
154. Kariminejad MH, Scully RE. Female adnexal tumor of probable Wolffian origin: a distinctive pathologic entity. Cancer 1973;31:671–7.
155. Young RH, Scully RE. Ovarian tumors of probable Wolffian origin: a report of 11 cases. Am J Surg Pathol 1983;7:125–36.
156. Rahilly MA, Williams ARW, Krausz T, al Nafussi A. Female adnexal tumor of probable Wolffian origin: a clinicopathologic and immunohistochemical study of three cases. Histopathology 1995;26:69–74.
157. Kommoss F, Oliva E, Bahn AK, et al. Inhibin expression in ovarian tumors and tumor-like lesions: an immunohistochemical study. Mod Pathol 1998;11:656–64.

28 Ovarian Sex Cord–Stromal and Steroid Cell Tumors

Jaime Prat

CHAPTER OUTLINE

General Features	642	Steroid Cell Tumors	662
Granulosa Cell Tumors	643	Stromal Luteoma	662
Adult Granulosa Cell Tumor	643	Leydig Cell Tumor	663
Juvenile Granulosa Cell Tumor	647	Steroid Cell Tumor, Adrenal Cortical Type	664
Thecoma	650	Steroid Cell Tumor (NOS)	664
Typical Form	650	Endocrine Syndromes Associated With Ovarian Tumors	665
Luteinized Thecoma	651	Ovarian Tumors with Functioning Stroma	665
Fibroma	652	Hypercalcemia	666
Cellular Fibroma	653	Hyperthyroidism	666
Fibrosarcoma	654	Carcinoid Syndrome	666
Sclerosing Stromal Tumor	654	Zollinger–Ellison Syndrome	666
Signet-Ring Stromal Tumor	655	Hyperprolactinemia	667
Microcystic Stromal Tumor	655	Cushing Syndrome	667
Sertoli–Stromal Cell Tumors	656	Hypoglycemia	667
Sertoli Cell Tumors	656	Hyperaldosteronism	667
Sertoli-Leydig Cell Tumors	656		
Sex Cord Tumor With Annular Tubules	661		
Gynandroblastoma	661		

GENERAL FEATURES

Sex cord–stromal tumors account for approximately 8% of all ovarian tumors and are the most common functioning tumors associated with endocrine manifestations.[1] These tumors contain granulosa cells, theca cells (and their luteinized derivatives), Sertoli cells, Leydig cells, and fibroblasts of gonadal stromal origin, either separately or in combination and exhibiting varying degrees of differentiation.[1]

Sex cord–stromal tumors arise from ovarian cells specialized in steroid hormone production. The designation *sex cord–stromal* tumors (which is favored by the World Health Organization (WHO) over *gonadal stromal* tumors) simply reflects the uncertainty about the origin of the gonadal sex cords;[2] it is still unclear whether they derive from the celomic epithelium (sex cords) or the gonadal mesenchyme (stroma). Sex cords are identified in the developing testis by the fifth week of embryonic life but are not found in the developing ovary where nests of pregranulosa cells (of apparent stromal origin) enveloping the germ cells are evident later in embryonic life.[1] Some authors do not accept the term 'sex cords' to describe progenitors of granulosa cells. However, the hyphenated term (sex cord–stroma) acknowledges that this category of ovarian tumors may be composed of sex cord derivatives (granulosa and Sertoli cells) that appear as *epithelial* elements, stromal derivatives (theca, lutein, and Leydig cell) that have the appearance of *mesenchymal* (gonadal stromal) cells, or derivatives of both precursors.[1,2]

Tumors composed of ovarian cell types are usually estrogenic, whereas those composed of cells of testicular type are androgenic, but tumors in either group may be nonfunctioning; rarely, tumors made up of female elements are androgenic, and tumors composed of Sertoli and Leydig cells are associated with estrogenic manifestations. Therefore, there is not always a strict correlation between the morphology of the tumor cells and the type of hormone they secrete.[2]

Because of the great diversity of histologic patterns, evaluation of sex cord–stromal tumors requires awareness of the patient's age and clinical history, thorough sampling of the tumor, and immunohistochemical validation. The most helpful markers currently available are α-inhibin, calretinin, and epithelial membrane antigen (EMA). The first two are typically positive in sex cord–stromal tumors and the third is typically negative.[3–5] Recently, a likely 'driver' point mutation of the *FOXL2* gene has been identified in the vast majority of adult granulosa cell tumors (97%) but only rarely in juvenile granulosa cell tumors (10%).[6] FOXL2, together with α-inhibin and calretinin, forms an immunomarker panel that will result in positive immunoreaction in essentially all cases of sex cord–stromal tumors.[7]

The distribution of the various sex cord–stromal tumors at the Massachusetts General Hospital over a 25 year period was as follows: tumors in the thecoma–fibroma group (87%), GCTs (12%), Sertoli–Leydig cell tumors (SLCTs) (0.05%), and unclassified (0.05%).[1] Most clinically malignant sex cord–stromal tumors are GCTs.

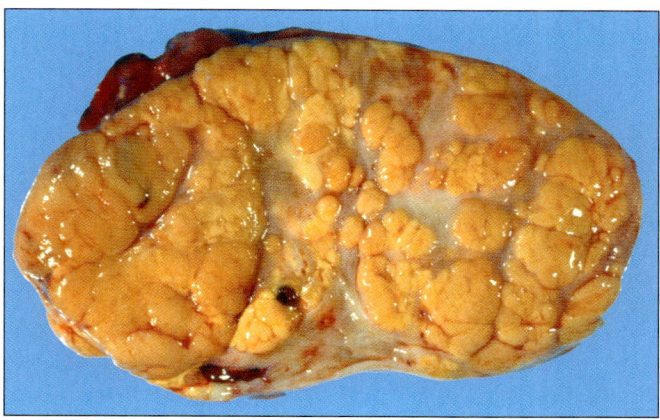

Figure 28.1 Adult granulosa cell tumor. The section surface is solid, lobulated, and yellow.

GRANULOSA CELL TUMORS

Granulosa cell tumors (GCTs) comprise two different clinicopathologic subtypes: adult and juvenile.[1,2] The *adult* form occurs more often in middle-aged and postmenopausal women and characteristically contains microfollicles and uniform cells with scanty cytoplasm and pale, grooved nuclei; in contrast, the *juvenile* subtype occurs mainly in children and younger women, and typically shows large rudimentary follicles and cells with moderate to abundant cytoplasm and darker nuclei usually without grooves.[1,2]

ADULT GRANULOSA CELL TUMOR

Clinical Features

Adult granulosa cell tumors (AGCTs) account for 1–2% of all ovarian tumors and 95% of all GCTs. They occur mainly in menopausal and postmenopausal women of about 50–55 years of age and are the most common ovarian tumors associated with estrogenic symptoms (75% of cases).[1, 8–12]

Functioning AGCTs (which are typically estrogenic tumors) may be associated with various clinical syndromes depending upon the age of the patient: women in the reproductive age group usually present with irregular and excessive uterine bleeding (*metropathia hemorrhagica*), but *amenorrhea*, lasting from months to years, may precede the abnormal bleeding, or may be the only endocrine symptom.[1] In postmenopausal women, the most common symptom is *postmenopausal bleeding* secondary to breakdown of endometrial hyperplasia or carcinoma. Occasionally, swelling, tenderness, and discharge from the breasts are prominent. Vaginal cytology typically shows increased maturation of squamous epithelial cells. Most of the clinical symptoms are related to the continuous estrogen stimulation of the endometrium: luteinizing hormone (LH) secretion from the anterior pituitary stops; ovulation does not occur, and progesterone is not secreted; the estrogenic stimulation of

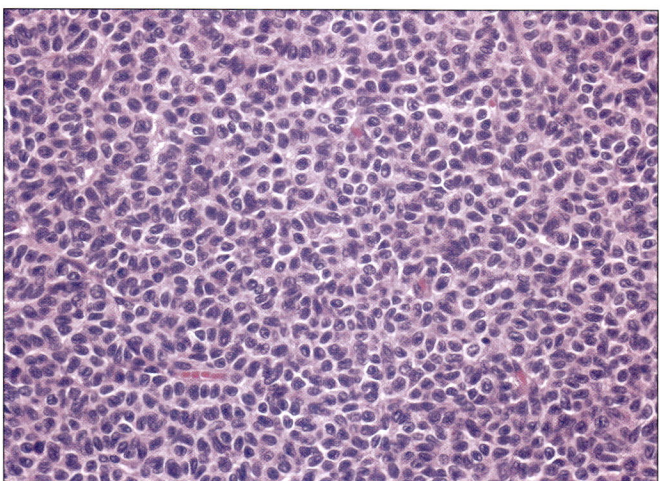

Figure 28.2 Adult granulosa cell tumor. Diffuse pattern. The regular-sized nuclei appear in a disorderly arrangement.

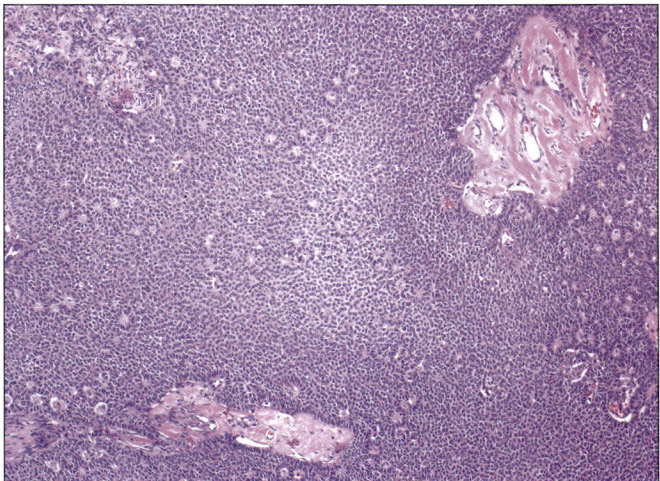

Figure 28.3 Adult granulosa cell tumor. Microfollicular pattern. Numerous Call–Exner bodies are seen.

the endometrium results in endometrial hyperplasia (usually simple but occasionally complex atypical hyperplasia). Endometrial carcinoma occurs in approximately 5% of cases[1] and is almost always a grade 1 endometrioid adenocarcinoma, which never metastasizes and almost never causes the death of the patient. Rare cases of AGCT appear before puberty and are associated with *isosexual pseudoprecocity*, due to estrogen production by the ovarian tumor. Although AGCTs are mostly estrogenic, very rare cases, usually large thin-walled cystic tumors, are associated with *androgenic* manifestations.[13]

In addition to endocrine symptoms, patients with AGCTs have signs and symptoms related to a pelvic mass such as abdominal pain and swelling; the tumor is palpable on pelvic examination in almost 90% of cases. Approximately 10% of patients present with acute abdominal symptoms due to rupture of the tumor with hemoperitoneum.[1] AGCTs are confined to the ovary (International Federation of Gynecology and Obstetrics stage I) in 60–90% of cases.[9–11,14] Extraovarian spread occurs to the peritoneum and omentum and occasionally to the liver or lungs.[15] Lymph node metastases are uncommon.

Macroscopic Features

The tumors are unilateral in over 95% of cases. About 10–15% are ruptured. The average diameter is 12 cm but their size ranges from microscopic to very large masses. They are cystic and solid and the cysts characteristically contain blood clots. The solid component varies from yellow (Figure 28.1) to white depending upon the amount of lipid-containing cells, and from soft to firm depending on the quantity of granulosa cells and stromal cells.

Microscopic Features

Histologically, there is a proliferation of granulosa cells often with a stromal component of theca cells, fibroblasts, or both. The granulosa cells grow in a wide variety of patterns, which are commonly admixed and lack prognostic significance. The most common pattern is the diffuse pattern in which the tumor cells grow in sheets with no organized structure (Figure 28.2). More characteristic but less common (30–50%) is the microfollicular pattern, which shows numerous rosette-like structures that simulate the Call–Exner bodies of the Graafian follicle (Figures 28.3 and 28.4). These small spaces contain eosinophilic debris or hyalinized basement membrane material and are surrounded by a circular row of typical granulosa cells. The cells contain scanty cytoplasm and pale, angular, or oval, often grooved, nuclei arranged haphazardly in relation to one another and to the follicles (Figure 28.4). The macrofollicular pattern is uncommon and shows cysts lined by well-differentiated granulosa cells and underlying theca cells (Figures 28.5). In totally cystic tumors, the cells lining the cysts may so closely mimic those of non-neoplastic ovarian follicles that distinction on a purely histologic basis is difficult. Tumor cells grow in anastomosing bands in the trabecular pattern, in undulating ribbons and cords in the gyriform, or in a watered-silk pattern (Figure 28.6), and in circumscribed nests and islands in the insular pattern (Figure 28.7). Some tumors may exhibit a diffuse sarcomatoid pattern characterized by somewhat spindle-shaped cells. Whatever the histologic pattern may be, the best

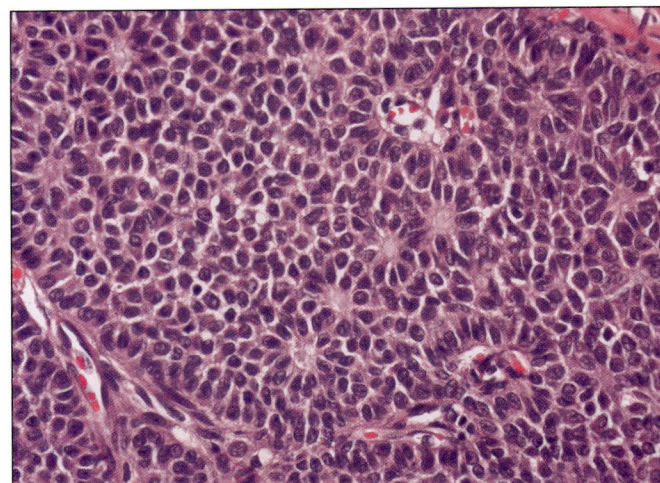

Figure 28.4 Adult granulosa cell tumor. Microfollicular pattern. Numerous Call-Exner bodies containing degenerated material are surrounded by granulosa cells with grooved nuclei.

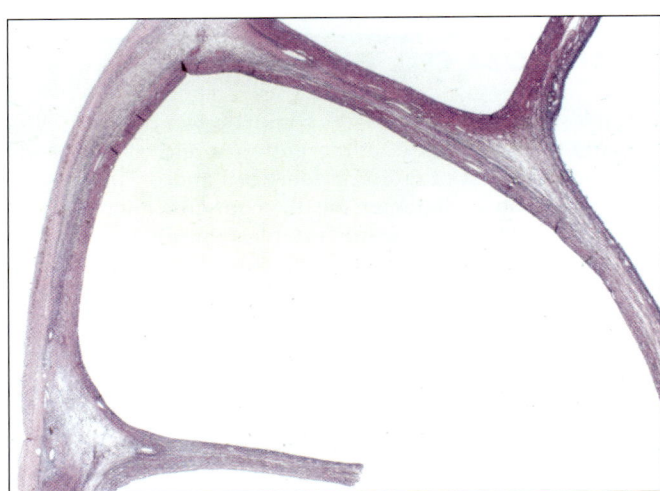

Figure 28.5 Adult granulosa cell tumor. Macrofollicular pattern. The large cystic cavities resemble follicle cysts.

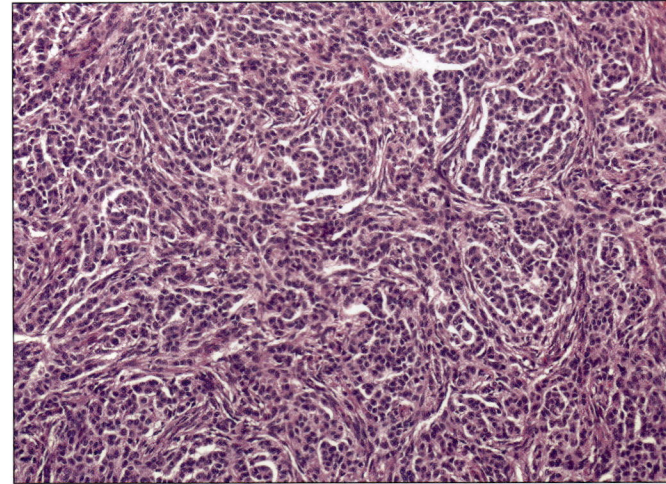

Figure 28.6 Adult granulosa cell tumor. Gyriform pattern.

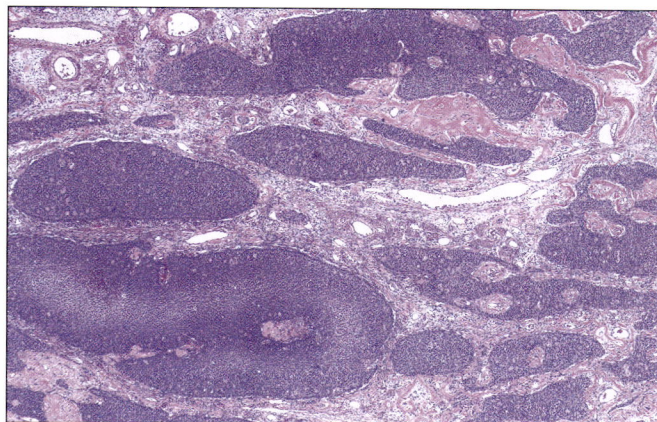

Figure 28.7 Adult granulosa cell tumor. Insular and microfollicular patterns. The tumor cells grow in well-defined islands containing Call–Exner bodies.

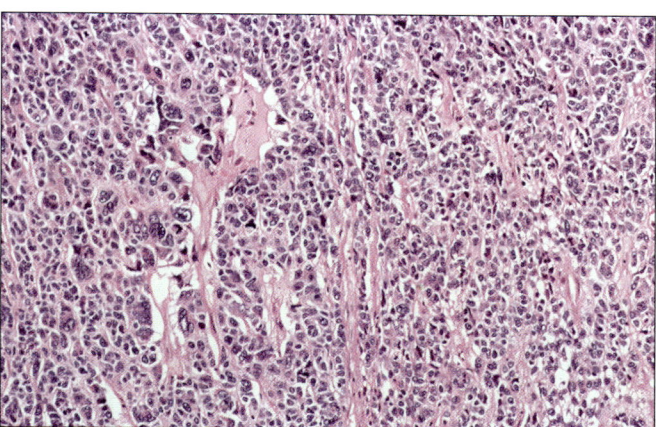

Figure 28.9 Adult granulosa cell tumor with bizarre nuclei. Large, hyperchromatic nuclei, including multinucleated forms, are present.

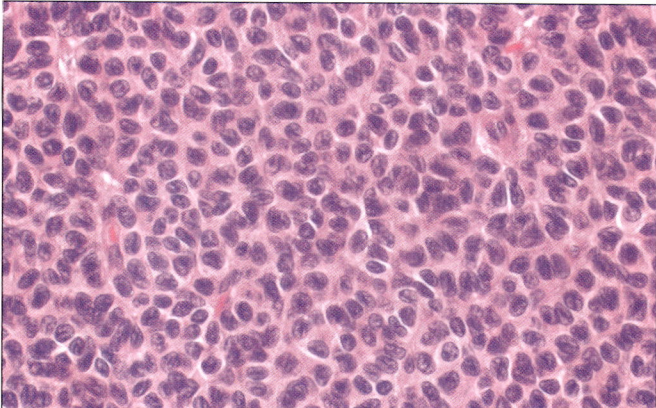

Figure 28.8 Adult granulosa cell tumor. The tumor cells have pale angular nuclei, many of which are grooved.

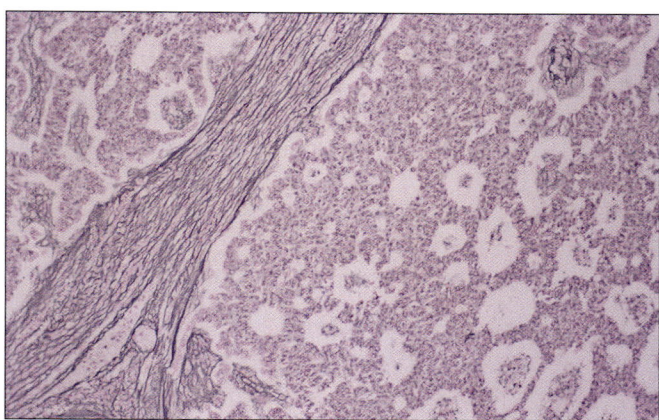

Figure 28.10 Adult granulosa cell tumor. A reticulin stain shows fibrils in the theca cell component and their absence in the granulosa cell compartment.

morphologic markers of the AGCT are (1) the presence of Call–Exner bodies (microfollicular) (Figure 28.4) and (2) the cell nuclei, which appear uniform and haphazardly oriented to one another and are oval, round, and angular and pale, often grooved, and lack significant pleomorphism (Figure 28.8).

Approximately 2% of AGCTs contain scattered cells with bizarre, large, hyperchromatic nuclei (Figure 28.9).[1] The mitotic activity in AGCTs varies, but is usually low; most tumors have 1–2 mitoses per 10 HPF. The presence of numerous mitoses, particularly abnormal forms, should raise the suspicion of poorly differentiated carcinoma.

The stromal component of AGCTs varies from fibromatous to thecomatous (granulosa–theca cell tumor) and it is best enhanced by the reticulin stains (Figure 28.10). In contrast to theca cells and fibroblasts, which are individually invested by fibrils, the granulosa cell component of the tumor contains few fibrils.[1] Occasional GCTs with hepatocellular differentiation have been reported.[16,17] In contrast to lutein or Leydig cells, the hepatic-type cells are negative for inhibin.[17]

Immunohistochemistry

α-Inhibin (Figure 28.11), calretinin, and FOXL2 (Figure 28.12) are the most important positive immunoreactions.[7] Calretinin is a more sensitive but less specific marker than α-inhibin.[18,19] Steroidogenic factor-1 (SF-1), WT1, and CD56 are also positive.[19,20] Almost all GCTs are vimentin positive. Monoclonal antibodies against low molecular weight cytokeratins (CK) 8 and 18 (CAM5.2, AE1/3) stain 30–60% of the tumors.[3,21] Most GCTs are immunoreactive for smooth muscle actin but negative for desmin.[21] Positive nuclear or cytoplasmic stain for S-100 protein has been reported in 50% of the tumors.[3,21] There is membrane staining for CD99 (MIC2 gene product) in 70% of GCTs.[22] Positive reaction for müllerian-inhibiting substance (MIS) has also been reported.[23] The most significant negative immunoreactions are for EMA and CK7, which are almost always absent in GCTs.[3,21]

Genetic Profile

Over 80% of the GCTs are diploid. Cytogenetic abnormalities have been detected by comparative genomic hybridization and fluorescence *in situ* hybridization (FISH) and

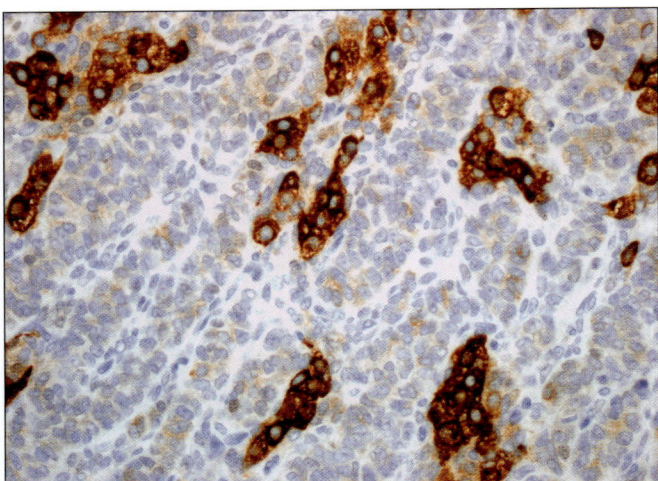

Figure 28.11 Luteinized adult granulosa cell tumor. The tumor cells are immunoreactive for α-inhibin, particularly the luteinized stromal cells.

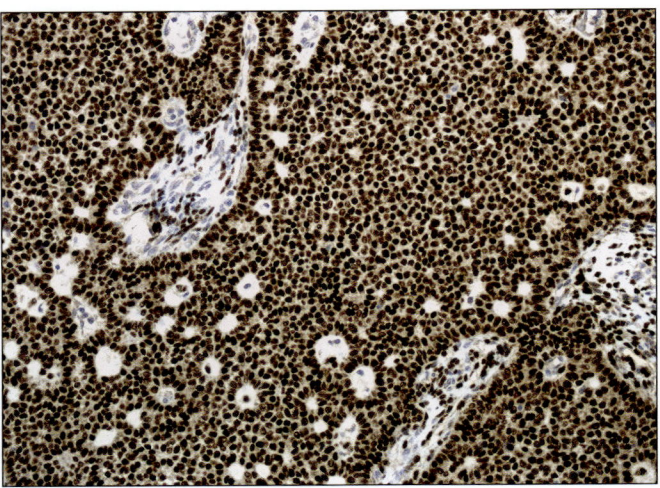

Figure 28.12 Adult granulosa cell tumor. The tumor cells are immunoreactive for FOXL2.

Table 28.1	Differentiation between AGCT and Undifferentiated Carcinoma	
	AGCT	**Undifferentiated Carcinoma**
Bilaterality	5%	15%
Stage	I	III
Nuclei	Paled, grooved, uniform	Hyperchromatic, pleomorphic
Prognosis	Favorable	Poor

include trisomy 12 and 14 and monosomy 22.[24,25] Over 90% of GCTs contain a missense point mutation 402 C→G (C134W) in the *FOXL2* gene at 3q22.3, presumably an early event in tumorigenesis.[6]

Differential Diagnosis

1. *Undifferentiated carcinoma versus diffuse AGCT.* The typical nuclear features of AGCT (Figure 28.8) differ from those of undifferentiated carcinoma, namely nuclear hyperchromatism, pleomorphism, and atypical mitotic activity; carcinomas are often associated with higher stage and adverse clinical course. In difficult cases, positive immunostains for α-inhibin, calretinin, and vimentin and lack of staining for EMA favor the diagnosis of AGCT. FOXL2 immunoreaction is helpful (see Chapter 25, and Table 28.1).[3,7,26,27]

2. *Small cell carcinoma of hypercalcemic type versus diffuse AGCT.* The small cell carcinoma is often found in advanced stage and has an aggressive clinical course; it is associated with hypercalcemia in two-thirds of patients, lacks estrogenic symptoms, and contains hyperchromatic nuclei and numerous mitoses. Immunohistochemical staining may facilitate the diagnosis (see Chapter 27).

3. *Endometrioid stromal sarcoma (primary or metastatic from the uterus) versus diffuse AGCT.* The stromal sarcoma lacks endocrine symptoms and is frequently bilateral; microscopically, it shows numerous small arterioles, individual investment of tumor cells by reticulin fibers, and tongue-like pattern of infiltration mainly outside the ovary. Positive immunoreactions for α-inhibin, calretinin, and FOXL2 and negative CD10 staining support the diagnosis of AGCT (see Chapter 27).

4. *Thecoma and cellular fibroma versus diffuse AGCT.* The distinction may be aided by reticulin stains.

5. *Large solitary luteinized follicle cyst of pregnancy and puerperium versus unilocular cystic AGCT.* Patients with the former lesion have a history of recent pregnancy. The follicle cyst shows large luteinized cells with large bizarre nuclei. In contrast, the unilocular cystic AGCT is lined by non-luteinized cells with typical granulosa cell nuclei (see Chapter 24).

6. *Endometrioid carcinoma (well differentiated and microglandular, resembling a sex cord–stromal tumor; sertoliform carcinoma) versus microfollicular, trabecular, or insular AGCT.* Foci of typical endometrioid carcinoma with mucin-secreting glands are usually found in the former; also, carcinomatous (atypical) nuclei with numerous and often abnormal mitoses are seen. Squamous differentiation and adenofibromatous (müllerian) features are common. In carcinomas, α-inhibin and calretinin immunostains are negative (but positive in luteinized stromal cells), whereas cytokeratins and EMA are strongly positive (see Chapter 27).[23,26]

7. *Insular carcinoid tumor versus microfollicular AGCT.* The different nuclear features, calcification of acini of carcinoid tumors, and neuroendocrine markers should facilitate the differential diagnosis (see Chapter 29).

8. *Sex cord tumor with annular tubules (SCTAT) versus microfollicular AGCT.* The former tumor shows larger hyaline deposits than Call–Exner bodies as well as ring-shaped tubules; in cases associated with the Peutz–Jeghers syndrome (PJS) the SCTATs are small, multiple, and bilateral.

9. *Gonadoblastoma versus insular or microfollicular AGCT.* Background of intersexual condition, presence of germ cells, and larger hyaline deposits than Call–Exner bodies all favor gonadoblastoma (see Chapter 29).

10. *Metastatic melanoma versus GCT.* Histologic features of melanoma, melanin pigment, positive S-100, and

HMB-45 and negative α-inhibin and calretinin all favor the former diagnosis (see Chapter 30).

11. *Metastatic breast carcinoma (particularly of lobular type) versus diffuse AGCT*. Bilaterality, history of breast cancer, presence of intracellular mucin, negative α-inhibin, positive EMA, and GCDFP-15 are all features of metastatic breast cancer (see Chapter 30).

Spread and Metastasis

All AGCTs are potentially malignant and capable of extending beyond the ovary, or recurring after apparently complete removal. Spread occurs mainly within the pelvis and lower abdomen; although rare, distant metastases have been reported in many locations.[15] Most recurrences appear within 5 years but they can be detected many years postoperatively (occasionally after 20 or 30 years).[1]

Treatment and Prognosis

In menopausal or postmenopausal women, the optimal treatment is bilateral salpingo-oophorectomy with total hysterectomy. It is reasonable to conserve the opposite ovary and uterus of a young woman with an AGCT confined to one ovary. The recurrence rate is 10–15% for stage IA tumors and 20–30% overall. Recurrence is usually fatal, but reoperation, radiotherapy, and chemotherapy (similar to that used in malignant germ cell tumors) can be helpful.[28]

The 10 year survival varies from 60% to 90%.[8–12] Patients with stage I tumors have much better prognosis than those with higher stage tumors (86% vs 49% 10 year survival).[9] The most consistent indicator of aggressive behavior has been the presence of metastases or invasion of structures outside the ovary at the time of diagnosis.[9,12] Also unfavorable but less significant factors are large tumor size (>6 cm in diameter)[11] and tumor rupture.[9] There is no correlation between the microscopic pattern and the clinical outcome. Flow cytometric results regarding DNA ploidy are contradictory.[29]

JUVENILE GRANULOSA CELL TUMOR

Clinical Features

Juvenile granulosa cell tumors (JGCTs) account for only 5% of GCTs and have been so designated because they usually occur in women less than 30 years of age, half of them in the first decade of life.[1,30] These tumors differ histologically from the more common AGCTs and contain cells that appear less mature; they are often mistaken for other neoplasms, usually malignant germ cell tumors.

JGCTs occurring before puberty are associated in 80% of cases with isosexual pseudoprecocity, due to estrogen production by the ovarian tumor.[30] They account for 10% of cases of sexual precocity. The large majority of cases (90%) of sexual precocity are central (idiopathic or constitutional), and result from premature release of gonadotropins by the hypothalamus (anterior pituitary gland) with no detectable organic lesion. In these cases (true precocity) ovulation occurs and there is a possibility of pregnancy. This does not occur in the cases of pseudoprecocity secondary to estrogen production by a functioning ovarian tumor. The GCTs that occur before puberty are almost always palpable on pelvic or rectal examination.[1,30] Noteworthy, other ovarian tumors (of non-endocrine type) secreting human chorionic gonadotropin (hCG) can also be associated with isosexual pseudoprecocity in young females.[1] In adult women, however, the most common symptom of the JGCT is uterine bleeding as a result of endometrial hyperplasia.[1,30]

In the largest series reported,[30] which included 125 JGCTs, 44% occurred in the first decade, 34% in the second decade, 18% in the third decade, and only 3% after the age of 30 years. Eighty-two percent of the tumors encountered before the age of normal puberty were associated with isosexual pseudoprecocity. Eight cases of JGCTs that developed in patients with Ollier disease (multiple enchondromatosis),[31] and three with Maffuci syndrome (Ollier disease with hemangiomas) have been reported, indicating that the JGCT is a rare component of these disorders.[30] At operation, JGCTs are almost always unilateral (98%) and more than 95% of them are confined to the ovary (stage I). Extraovarian spread is found in only 2% of patients, mostly confined to the pelvis.[30]

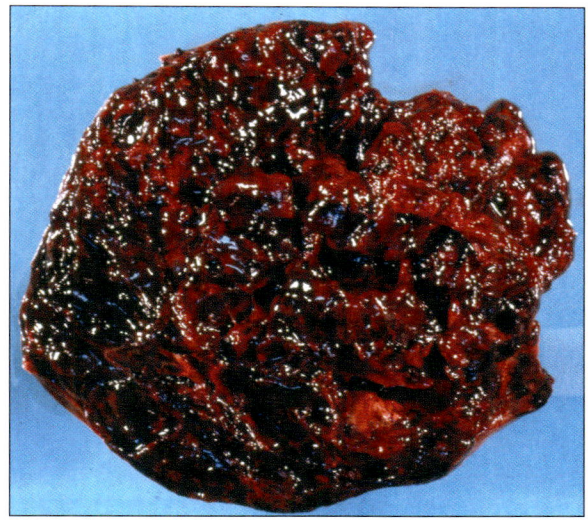

Figure 28.13 Juvenile granulosa cell tumor. The section surface is solid and cystic with extensive hemorrhage.

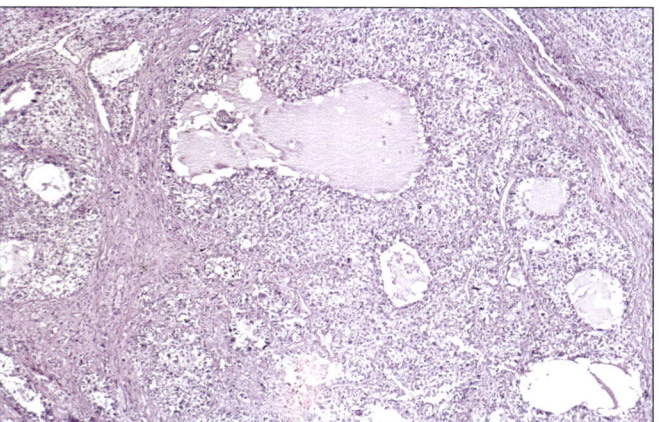

Figure 28.14 Juvenile granulosa cell tumor. Numerous oval to round follicles containing eosinophilic fluid.

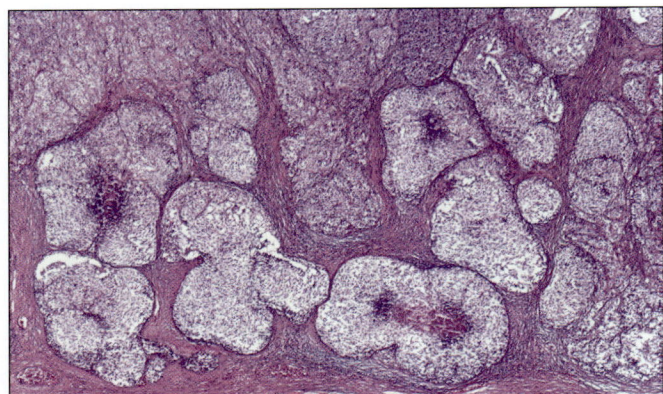

Figure 28.15 Juvenile granulosa cell tumor. The tumor cells form solid nodules, some of which exhibit central necrosis.

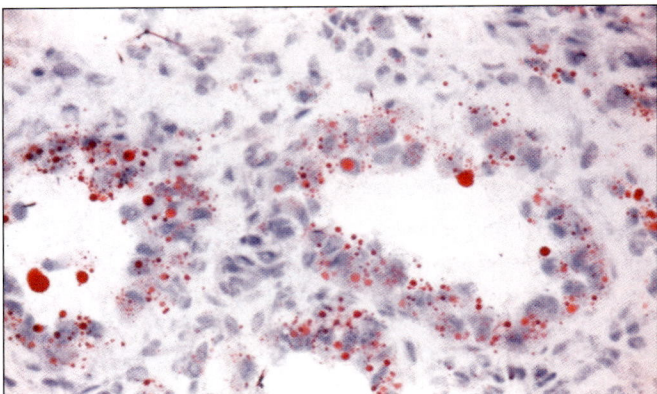

Figure 28.17 Juvenile granulosa cell tumor. Positive fat (ORO) stain.

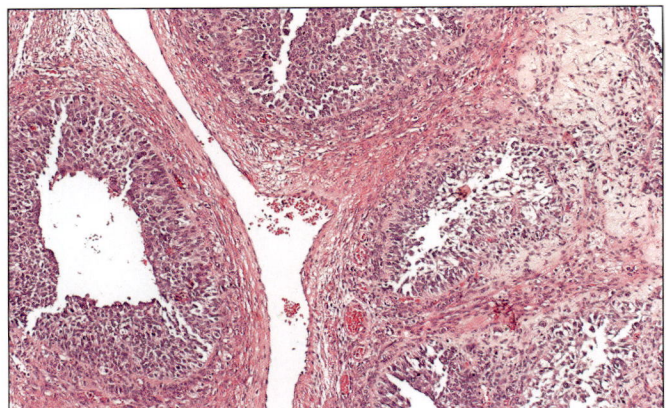

Figure 28.16 Juvenile granulosa cell tumor. Well-defined follicles of varying sizes separated by fibrovascular tissue.

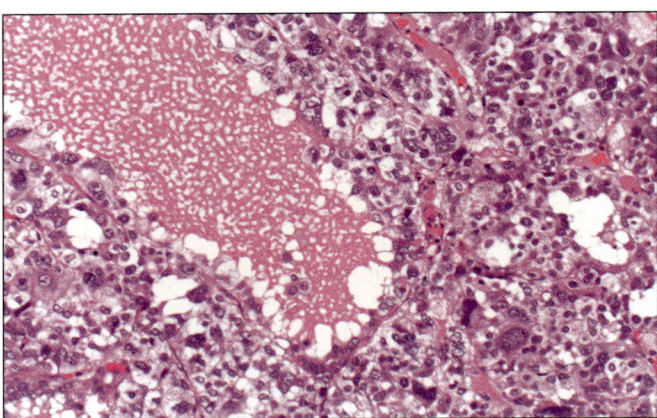

Figure 28.18 Juvenile granulosa cell tumor. A follicle is surrounded by cells with large bizarre nuclei.

Macroscopic Features

The tumors range from 3 to 32 cm (average 12.5) in diameter and appear similar to the AGCT. They are usually either uniformly solid or partly solid containing cysts that are often filled with blood (Figure 28.13); less commonly the tumors are composed predominantly of one or more thin-walled cysts. The neoplastic tissue is gray or yellow and occasionally large areas of necrosis or hemorrhage suggest a highly malignant tumor.[1,30]

Microscopic Features

Microscopic examination shows diffuse sheets or nodules of neoplastic granulosa cells, which may be solid but more often are punctured by follicular spaces (Figure 28.14). Generally the follicles do not reach the large size of those encountered in the macrofollicular form of the AGCT; although they vary in size and shape, they are usually round to oval (Figures 28.15 and 28.16). The lumens typically contain eosinophilic or basophilic material that stains with mucicarmine in about two-thirds of cases. Papillae lined by granulosa cells grow into the cystic spaces in some tumors.[32] Theca cells may be present in varying amounts and occasionally the granulosa and theca cells are arranged in a disorderly fashion; in such cases reticulin stains may help to differentiate them, with fibrils investing the theca cells individually, but the granulosa cells only in groups. Fat stains (ORO) are positive (Figure 28.17).

The cytologic features of the JGCT also differ from those of the AGCT. The nuclei of both the granulosa and theca cells appear less mature in the former than the latter, showing hyperchromatism (Figure 28.18) and often considerable mitoses, which may be atypical; nuclear atypia varies from minimal to severe and nuclear grooves are absent. Rare cases of anaplastic JGCT exhibit a sheet-like growth with striking nuclear atypia resembling undifferentiated carcinoma. Another cytologic feature of these tumors is luteinization of both granulosa and theca cells (Figure 28.19) with fat stains typically showing abundant intracytoplasmic lipid in the two cell types.

Immunohistochemistry and Genetic Profile

Like the adult variant, JGCTs show immunoreaction for inhibin (Figure 28.20), calretinin, MIS, FOXL2, and SF-1.[7,20] There is strong membrane reaction for CD99 (Figure 28.21) and CD56.[22] The tumor cells are vimentin positive and react for low molecular weight cytokeratin in 25–50% of cases.[21] EMA is usually negative, as is typical of sex cord–stromal tumors, but sometimes may be focally positive.[33] Trisomy 12 has been demonstrated in many cases by FISH.[34]

The *FOXL2* (C402G) mutation that is present in AGCTs is absent in JGCTs.[6,35]

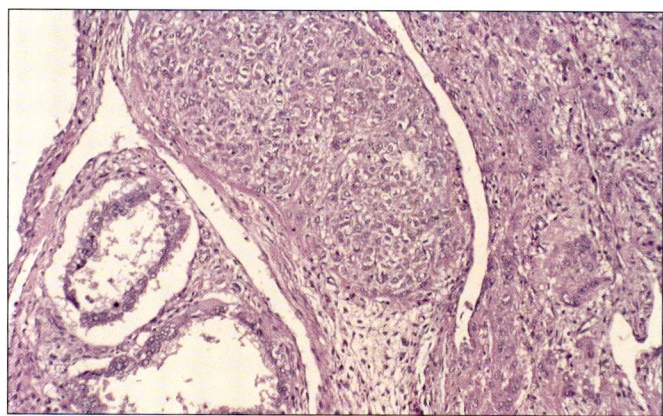

Figure 28.19 Juvenile granulosa cell tumor. Nests of luteinized granulosa and theca cells with pale eosinophilic cytoplasm.

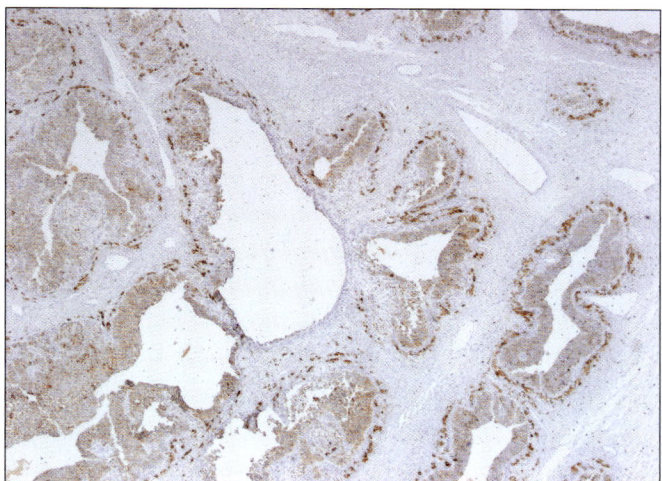

Figure 28.20 Juvenile granulosa cell tumor. The tumor cells are immunoreactive for α-inhibin, particularly the theca cells that surround rudimentary follicles.

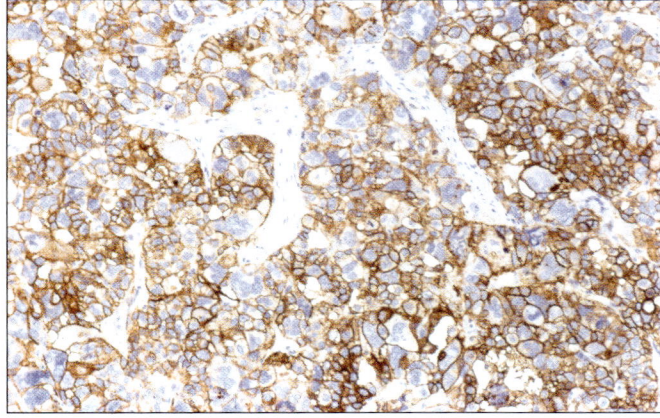

Figure 28.21 Juvenile granulosa cell tumor. The immunostaining for CD99 shows a characteristic membranous pattern.

Table 28.2 Differentiation between JGCT and Small Cell Carcinoma

JGCT	Small Cell Carcinoma
Rarely malignant	Highly malignant
No ↑ Ca^{2+}	↑ Ca^{2+} frequent
Estrogenic	Never estrogenic
Follicles + + +	Follicles +
Thecomatous stroma	Nonspecific stroma
Abundant cytoplasm	Scanty cytoplasm

Differential Diagnosis

1. *Adult granulosa cell tumor.* There are regular follicles, Call–Exner bodies, nuclear features (nuclear grooves), and lack of luteinization (except in pregnancy).
2. *Malignant germ cell tumor (yolk sac tumor, embryonal carcinoma).* Although the nuclei of JGCTs may occasionally appear severely atypical, they do not look as uniformly malignant (embryonal) as those of a primitive germ cell tumor. The latter lacks the typical follicular pattern and shows positive immunoreactions for hCG, α-fetoprotein, and cytokeratins, as well as nuclear transcription factors SALL4, LIN28, and OCT-4 or glypican-3 (see Chapter 29).
3. *Thecoma.* The patients are older and there is absence of follicles, predominance of theca cells, mild nuclear atypia, and characteristic reticulin stain.
4. *Clear cell or undifferentiated carcinoma.* Symptoms include older age of the patient, carcinomatous cells throughout the specimen, and negative α-inhibin in almost all cases.
5. *Small cell carcinoma of hypercalcemic type.* There is a lack of estrogenic symptoms, hypercalcemia, predominance of small cells (although it may contain large, rhabdoid-appearing cells focally), absence of the luteinized theca cell component, and higher mitotic rate. There are also negative α-inhibin and calretinin, and positive cytokeratin stains (see Chapter 27 and Table 28.2).
6. *Metastatic malignant melanoma.* It is rare in young patients; there is a clinical history of melanoma, bilaterality, positive S-100 protein, and HMB-45 stains (Melan-A immunostaining can be positive in sex cord–stromal tumors; see Chapter 30).

Prognosis

Although the JGCT usually appears histologically more malignant than the AGCT, the follow-up data in four series of cases indicate a high cure rate.[30,36–38] The stage of the tumor correlates best with prognosis. In the largest series reported, only 2 of 80 stage I tumors with follow-up information were clinically malignant. Both patients had stage IC tumors. All three stage II tumors were fatal.[30] Contrary to the AGCT, almost all recurrences of the JGCT appear within 3 years postoperatively. The clinically malignant tumors were on average larger than those with a favorable outcome (20 vs 12 cm).[30] Even if the *FOXL2* (C402G) mutation, which is consistently present in AGCTs, is absent in JGCTs, patients with the latter tumors and higher FOXL2 protein expression had worse overall survival and disease-free survival than those with negative or weakly immunoreactive tumors.[35] Neither DNA ploidy nor the S-phase fraction are predictive of the outcome. Some patients with advanced or recurrent disease respond to platinum-based combination chemotherapy.[39]

THECOMA

Thecomas are stromal tumors composed of lipid-containing cells resembling theca cells, lutein cells, and fibroblasts. These tumors can be divided into *typical* and *luteinized* variants.[1]

TYPICAL FORM

General Features

Typical thecomas are one-third as common as GCTs.[1] They occur in older patients than those with GCTs (mean age, 59 years) and are estrogenic in almost all cases.[1,40] About 60% of the patients present with uterine bleeding and 21% have an endometrial carcinoma.[40]

Macroscopic Features

Like GCTs, thecomas are unilateral in 97% of cases.[1] Grossly, they are typically solid yellow masses (Figure 28.22) of about 7 cm in diameter. Cystic change and calcification may occur.

Microscopic Features

Typical thecomas are composed of sheets of round to spindle cells with ill-defined pale cytoplasm, often vacuolated and lipid-rich, alternating with collagen-producing fibroblasts (Figure 28.23). The nuclei vary from round to spindle shape and typically lacks atypia and mitoses. A fibromatous component often intersects sheets of theca-like cells. Hyaline plaques or even large zones of hyalinization may be present. Foci of calcification may also be found. Extensively calcified thecomas occasionally occur, especially in young women.[41] Typical thecomas may also contain scattered 'sex cord elements.'[1] Contrary to GCTs, reticulin fibrils typically invest individual thecoma cells (Figure 28.24).

Rarely, mild nuclear atypia or even bizarre nuclei are seen in otherwise typical tumors, but severe atypia, high mitotic activity, and malignant behavior are extremely rare. Most of the tumors reported as 'malignant thecomas' probably represent examples of fibrosarcomas or diffuse GCTs.[1]

Immunohistochemistry and Cytogenetics

Thecomas are immunoreactive for vimentin, inhibin, calretinin, and other sex cord markers. Immunoreactions for cytokeratin are negative.[18,26] Trisomy 12 can often be identified in thecomas.[34]

Differential Diagnosis

Thecomas and fibromas have overlapping features. They are essentially similar neoplasms, and typical thecomas are most frequently functioning tumors and contain lipid-rich cells that immunoreact for α-inhibin. Fat stains, however, are not helpful in distinguishing between thecomas and fibromas because otherwise typical-appearing fibromas can contain abundant lipid and some thecomas contain very little. The

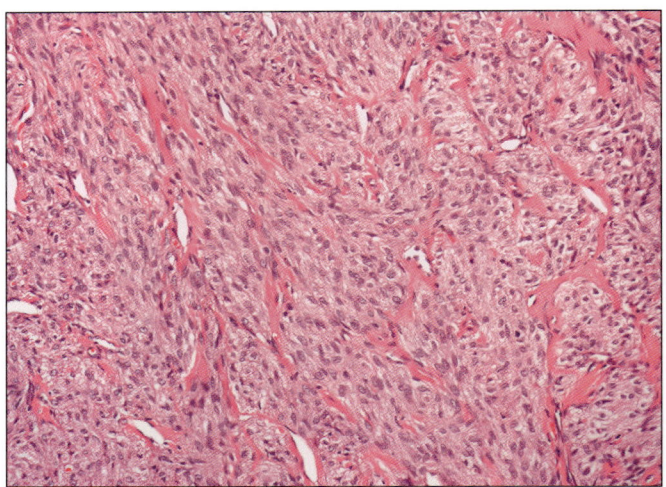

Figure 28.23 Thecoma. The tumor cells are vacuolated.

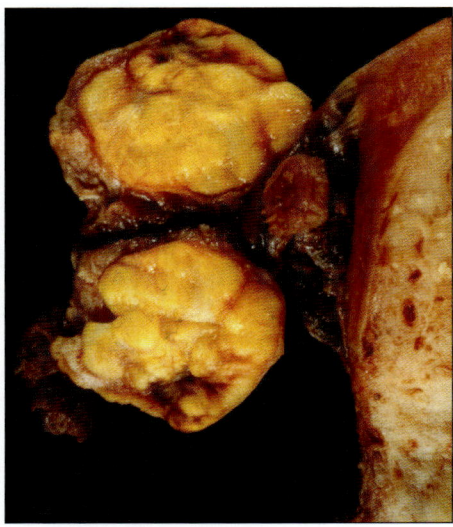

Figure 28.22 Thecoma. The sectioned surface is lobulated and yellow.

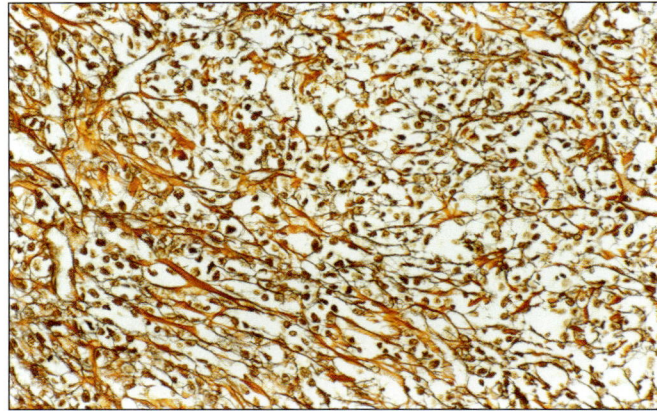

Figure 28.24 Thecoma, reticulin stain. Individual tumor cells appear invested by fibrils.

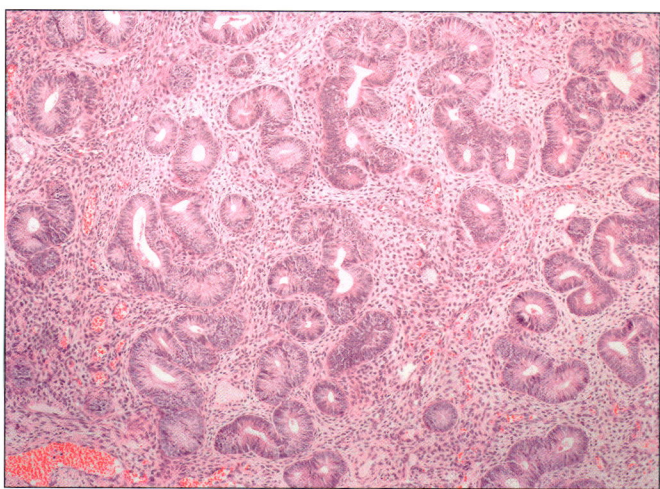

Figure 28.25 Endometrial hyperplasia without atypia from a 65-year-old patient with thecoma (see also Figures 28.22 and 28.23).

term 'thecoma' should be reserved for stromal tumors either containing moderate to large amounts of cytoplasmic lipid or associated with clinical or laboratory evidence of steroid hormone secretion. In contrast, fibromas are nonfunctioning tumors composed almost exclusively of spindle cells producing collagen and containing only small amounts of cytoplasmic lipid. Tumors with intermediate features are classified as 'tumors in the thecoma–fibroma group.'

Treatment and Prognosis

Typical thecomas are almost invariably benign and surgical excision is the appropriate treatment. In cases associated with endometrial hyperplasia (Figure 28.25) or carcinoma, hysterectomy and bilateral salpingo-oophorectomy is the standard treatment.

LUTEINIZED THECOMA

General Features

Luteinized thecomas occur in a younger age group than typical thecomas. Although they are most common in postmenopausal women, 30% develop in women under 30 years of age.[42] Approximately half of them are estrogenic, 40% nonfunctioning, and 10% androgenic.[42] A rare variant of the luteinized thecoma is that associated with sclerosing peritonitis, which may be complicated by intestinal obstruction and can be fatal.[43,44] Like luteinized thecomas of the usual type, these tumors occur mainly in young patients who present with abdominal swelling and ascites. The cause of the sclerosing peritonitis is unknown.

Macroscopic Features

Except for the lesions associated with sclerosing peritonitis, the gross features of luteinized thecomas are similar to those of typical thecomas. The former lesions are often bilateral ranging from normal-sized or slightly enlarged ovaries with a striking cerebriform appearance (Figure 28.26) to large tumors up to 31 cm in diameter.[43] On section, there is prominent cortical edema and cystic change. The lack of a discrete mass in some cases suggests that they may

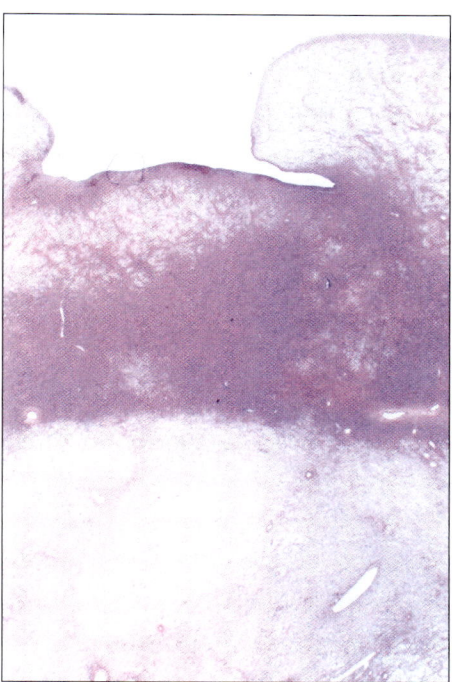

Figure 28.26 Luteinized thecoma in a patient with sclerosing peritonitis. The ovarian surface (top) shows a polypoid contour. There is striking edema.

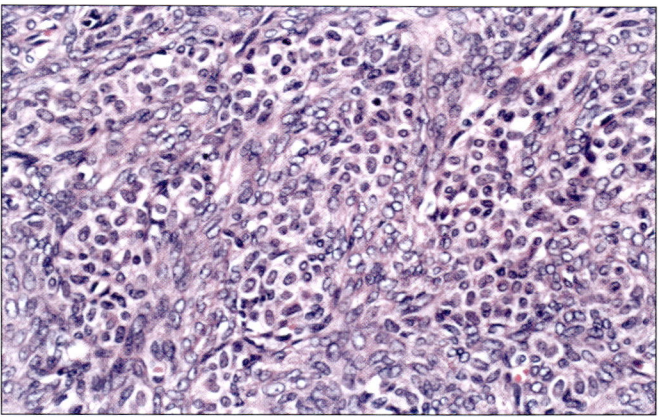

Figure 28.27 Luteinized thecoma in a patient with sclerosing peritonitis. Clusters of luteinized cells are admixed with spindle cells.

represent a hyperplastic rather than neoplastic process. The sclerosing peritonitis involves the omentum, peritoneum, and intestinal serosa. There is fibroblastic proliferation, collagen, and inflammation with fibrin deposition.

Microscopic Features

Luteinized thecomas have the appearance of a fibroma or a typical thecoma but contain sharply defined lutein (steroid-type) cells, singly or forming nests (Figures 28.27 and 28.28) or masses. These cells are polyhedral or rounded cells with abundant eosinophilic cytoplasm and central, round nuclei with single prominent nucleoli.[1,42,45,46] Occasionally, the steroid-type cells contain crystals of Reinke and these rare tumors, which may cause virilization, have been designated 'stromal–Leydig cell tumors.'[42] The variant associated with

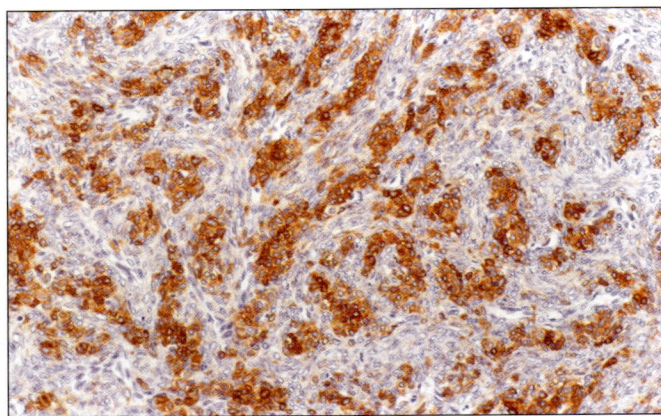

Figure 28.28 Luteinized thecoma in a patient with sclerosing peritonitis. The luteinized cells immunoreact for α-inhibin.

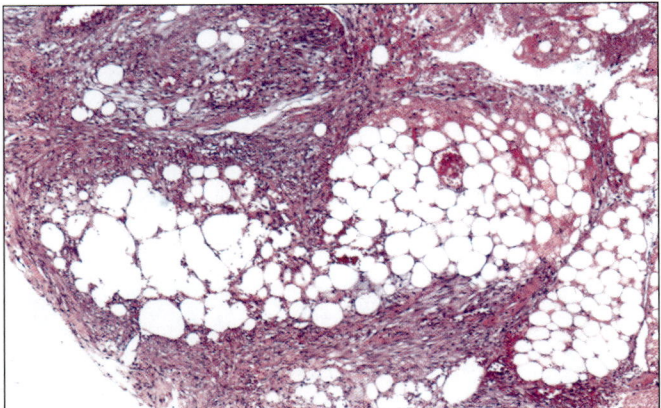

Figure 28.29 Sclerosing peritonitis in a patient with luteinized thecoma. The fat lobules are surrounded by cellular fibromatous tissue.

sclerosing peritonitis (Figure 28.29) is characterized by a dense proliferation of spindle cells admixed with lutein cells. There is minimal nuclear atypia but mitotic figures may be numerous (up to 40 per 10 HPF). In some cases there is diffuse edema with microcystic change.[43]

Genetic Profile

Loss of heterozygosity (LOH) at 9q22.3 (*PTCH* gene) but not 19p13.3 (*STK11* gene) has been reported in luteinized thecomas.[47]

Differential Diagnosis

Extensively luteinized thecomas may be confused with steroid cell tumors,[45] but the different clinical and pathologic features of both tumors help to distinguish them. The fibromatous component of steroid tumors usually represents <10% of the tumor.[1] Luteinized thecomas may also be confused with stromal hyperthecosis, but the latter is always bilateral and characterized microscopically by nests of lutein cells on a background of normal stromal cells. In contrast, luteinized thecomas are rarely bilateral (except for those associated with sclerosing peritonitis) and contain large collagen-producing spindle cells and theca-like cells. The striking luteinization of thecomas in pregnant patients can create confusion with pregnancy luteomas. The latter, however, are multiple in half of the cases, contain no lipid, and lack fibromatous features.[42]

Luteinized thecomas associated with sclerosing peritonitis can be confused with various non-neoplastic and neoplastic lesions. The prominent nodular surface in some cases, or the marked ovarian enlargement in others, serves to distinguish these thecomas from stromal hyperthecosis. Furthermore, the stromal cells in hyperthecosis lack the mitotic activity often found in luteinized thecomas. Massive edema and fibromatosis are hypocellular and associated with either diffuse edema or extensive collagen deposition. Immunohistochemical stains (positive calretinin and α-inhibin (Figure 28.28) and negative EMA and cytokeratin reactions) may help to distinguish these rare lesions from metastatic lobular carcinoma of the breast, particularly in bilateral cases.

Treatment and Prognosis

The treatment of luteinized thecomas of the usual type is similar to that of typical thecomas. Exceptionally, mitotically active luteinized thecomas with nuclear atypia metastasize.[42] The criteria for separating benign and malignant luteinized thecomas are similar to those used for distinguishing between cellular fibromas and fibrosarcomas[48,49] (see later). Luteinized thecomas associated with sclerosing peritonitis are treated adequately by excision of the ovarian tumors and abdominal surgery, including lysis of adhesions, omentectomy, and bowel resection. None of the reported tumors have spread beyond the ovary, but three patients died of complications from their peritoneal disease.[43]

FIBROMA

Although fibromas can arise from nonspecific ovarian tissues, there is a continuous histologic spectrum between thecomas and fibromas and most fibromas are considered sex cord–stromal tumors developing from the specialized ovarian stroma.

General Features

Fibromas account for about 4% of all ovarian tumors.[1,50] They occur in women of all ages, but are most common between 50 and 60 years. Although most of them are asymptomatic, some patients may develop abdominal pain, abdominal enlargement, or urinary disturbances.[50] In about 5% of cases there is an acute onset of abdominal pain because of torsion of the neoplasm. Although steroid hormone production is exceptional, the fibroma is occasionally accompanied by two unusual clinical syndromes: Meigs syndrome[51] and the basal cell nevus (Gorlin) syndrome.[52] The former, which is found in only 1–2% of cases, is defined as ascites and pleural effusion accompanying a fibrous ovarian tumor and disappearing after the resection of the tumor.[51] When a fibroma is associated with Meigs syndrome and elevated CA125 levels, the clinical picture is very similar to that of an ovarian carcinoma and it may be only after laparotomy and surgical staging that the final diagnosis is established.[53]

Ascites alone is associated with 15–30% of ovarian fibromas over 10 cm in diameter.

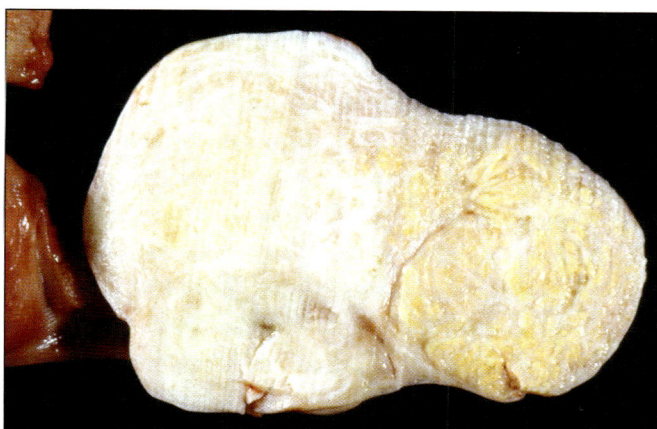

Figure 28.30 Fibroma. The sectioned surface is grayish yellow and solid.

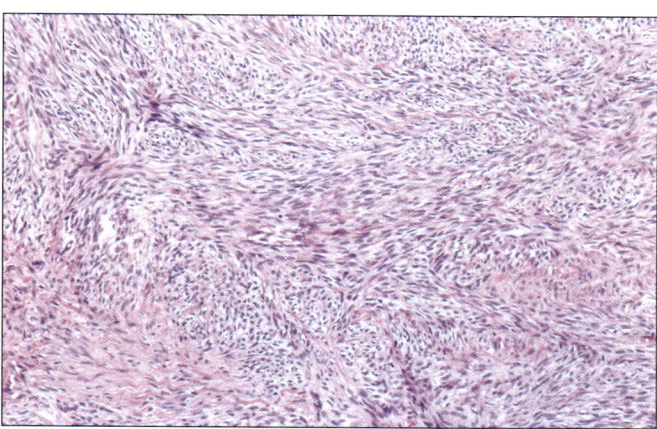

Figure 28.31 Fibroma. The spindle cells are arranged in intersecting bundles.

Ovarian fibromas occur in a high proportion of young women with the basal cell nevus syndrome and in these patients the fibromas are almost always bilateral, multiple, and calcified.[52]

Macroscopic Features

Fibromas are bilateral in about 8% of cases and have an average diameter of 6 cm.[1,50] They have a smooth, lobulated outer surface and on section appear as uniformly white or grayish white solid tissue (Figure 28.30); sometimes, however, the cut surface has a whorled appearance. Fibromas are cystic in about 20% of cases and calcification is not uncommon and is sometimes massive. Rarely, a fibroma may show ossification.[1,50]

Microscopic Features

Fibromas are formed of interlacing bundles of spindle cells resembling fibroblasts (Figure 28.31), which often show a 'feathertail' pattern. Nuclear palisading is sometimes seen and occasionally a storiform pattern, similar to that of fibrous histiocytomas, is present. Although the cellularity varies, it is usually not marked; when striking the tumor is classified as a cellular fibroma (see later). The tumor cells are small and have narrow ovoid nuclei. Cytologic atypia and mitotic activity are usually absent. The cell cytoplasm may contain small amounts of lipid. Occasionally, it contains eosinophilic hyaline globules. Sharply delineated hyaline plaques are sometimes present and a more diffuse hyalinization is not uncommon; many fibromas show a variable degree of intercellular edema or myxoid change. Occasional fibromas contain scattered foci of sex cord elements (Figure 28.32). Ovarian fibromas immunoreact for calretinin (95–100%) and α-inhibin (15–70%).[18]

Differential Diagnosis

Fibromas should be distinguished from thecomas (see previously), sclerosing stromal tumors (SSTs; see later), and non-neoplastic lesions such as massive edema and fibromatosis. Usually, in the last two conditions, there is preservation of follicles, corpora lutea, and corpora albicantia, whereas fibromas almost always displace these structures.

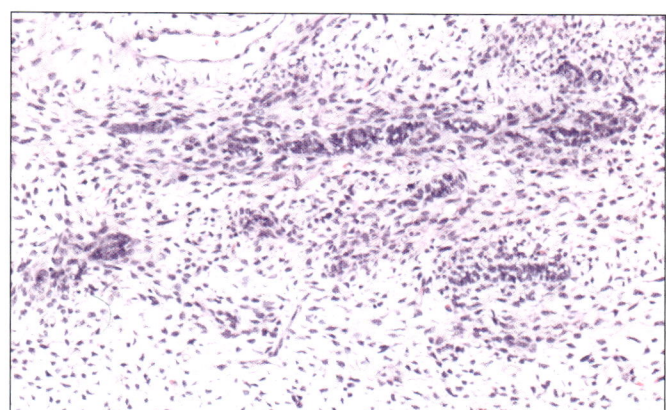

Figure 28.32 Fibroma with scattered sex cord elements.

Krukenberg, Brenner, and carcinoid tumors may resemble fibromas on gross examination, but their characteristic epithelial components facilitate the correct diagnosis on microscopic examination.

Treatment and Prognosis

Fibromas are benign and oophorectomy will result in rapid resolution of any ascites or hydrothorax that may be present. Exceptionally, benign fibromas seed implants onto the peritoneum; if both these and the ovarian tumor appear histologically benign the prognosis is excellent and the peritoneal nodules should not be taken as evidence of malignancy.

CELLULAR FIBROMA

Approximately 10% of ovarian fibromas are densely cellular (almost as much as a diffuse GCT) and have been descriptively named 'cellular fibromas.'[48] The clinical features of these tumors are similar to those of typical fibromas. Grossly, however, cellular fibromas are larger (average size, 12 cm) and softer than the usual ovarian fibromas and their sectioned surfaces, which are solid (Figure 28.33), may exhibit hemorrhage and necrosis.

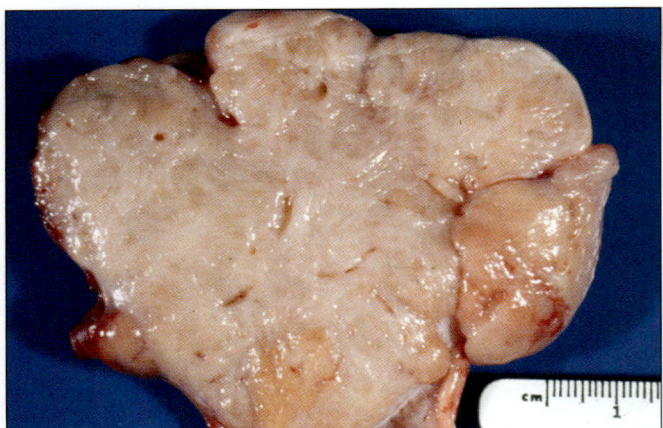

Figure 28.33 Cellular fibroma. The sectioned surface has a fleshy appearance which differs from that of a typical fibroma.[48] (Reproduced with permission of John Wiley and Sons; Prat J, Scully RE. Cellular fibromas and fibrosarcomas of the ovary. A comparative clinicopathologic analysis of seventeen cases. Cancer 1981;47:2663–2670)

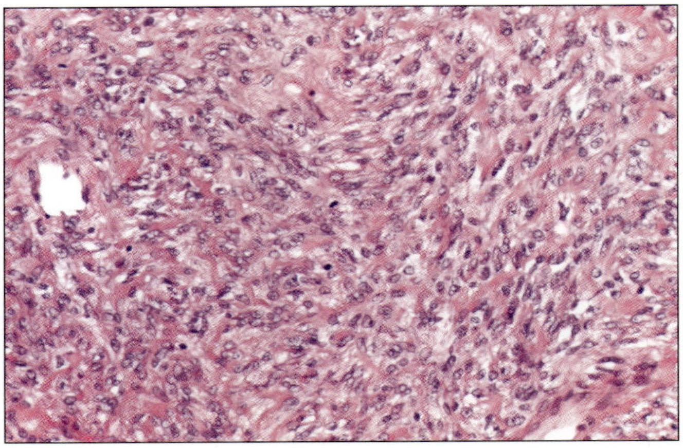

Figure 28.34 Cellular fibroma. The tumor is cellular but lacks significant atypia. A mitotic figure is seen. The patient died of recurrent tumor.

Microscopically, cellular fibromas are composed largely of densely cellular tissue with a few areas of hypocellular fibrous tissue. The cells are spindle shaped and arranged in intersecting bundles or in a storiform pattern. They have ill-defined cytoplasmic borders and round to oval hyperchromatic nuclei. The nuclei are slightly or moderately atypical, and between 1 and 3 mitotic figures per 10 HPF are present (Figure 28.34). Higher mitotic rates are still compatible with cellular fibroma ('mitotically active cellular fibroma') provided there is no appreciable cytologic atypia.[48,49] A gain of trisomy 12 cells has been demonstrated by FISH in eight of these tumors.[54]

Because of the typically benign course and infrequent bilaterality of cellular fibromas, they can justifiably be treated by unilateral salpingo-oophorectomy in a young woman who wants to retain her fertility. If the tumor is adherent it should be removed as completely as is technically feasible. Patients with ruptured tumors should be followed carefully because of the possibility of intra-abdominal recurrence.[48]

FIBROSARCOMA

Pure fibrosarcomas are among the most common form of ovarian sarcoma.[1] They are often found in older women (average, 58 years) and are almost always unilateral and large masses (average size, 17 cm).[48] On gross examination, they are soft and lobulated and completely replace the ovary. Sectioning typically shows solid, grayish white to tan tissue that often has areas of hemorrhage and necrosis.

Microscopically, the tumors are densely cellular, and the spindle-shaped cells are arranged in a herringbone or storiform pattern. The tumor cells have indistinct borders, eosinophilic cytoplasm, and hyperchromatic nuclei with prominent nucleoli. There is a moderate to marked degree of pleomorphism and the number of mitotic figures ranges from 4 to 25 per 10 HPF (Figure 28.35).[48] Mitotic activity (particularly normal mitotic figures) in excess of 4 per 10 HPF in the absence of moderate to severe atypia does not signify a fibrosarcoma. In such cases, a diagnosis of mitotically active cellular fibroma is made.[48,49]

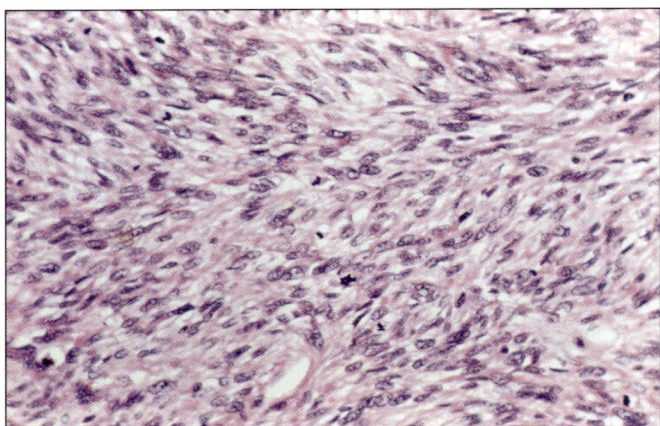

Figure 28.35 Fibrosarcoma. The tumor shows moderate nuclear atypia and several mitoses including abnormal forms.

The MIB1 labeling index and the proliferative index (percentage of cells in S + G2 + M phases) are higher in fibrosarcomas than in cellular fibromas of the ovary. Trisomy 12 and trisomy 8 have been reported in an ovarian fibrosarcoma.[54] Fibrosarcomas are highly aggressive neoplasms associated with poor prognosis.

SCLEROSING STROMAL TUMOR

This rare form of stromal tumor differs clinically from fibromas and thecomas in its age distribution. Approximately 80% of these tumors occur in patients who are less than 30 years old (average age 27 years).[55,56] In contrast, only about 10% of fibromas and thecomas develop during that age period. Most patients present with nonspecific symptoms related to a unilateral adnexal mass. Unlike typical thecomas, sclerosing stromal tumors (SSTs) are usually

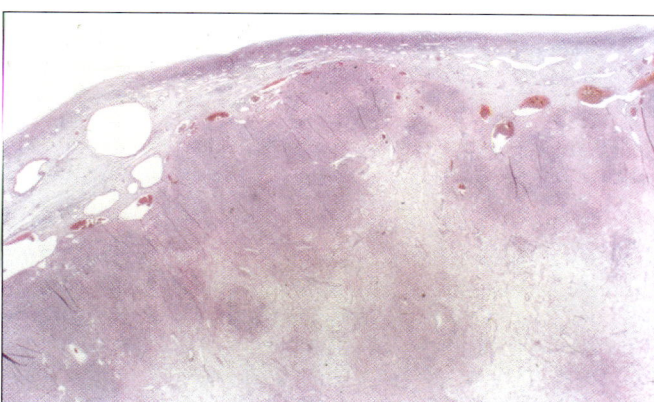

Figure 28.36 Slerosing stromal tumor. Cellular pseudolobules appear separated by edematous fibrous tissue.

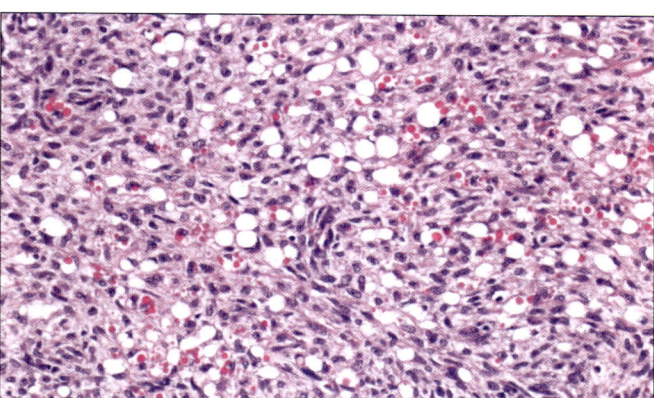

Figure 28.38 Signet-ring stromal tumor. Numerous vacuolated cells with eccentric nuclei are admixed with spindle-shaped cells. Note the presence of hyaline bodies.

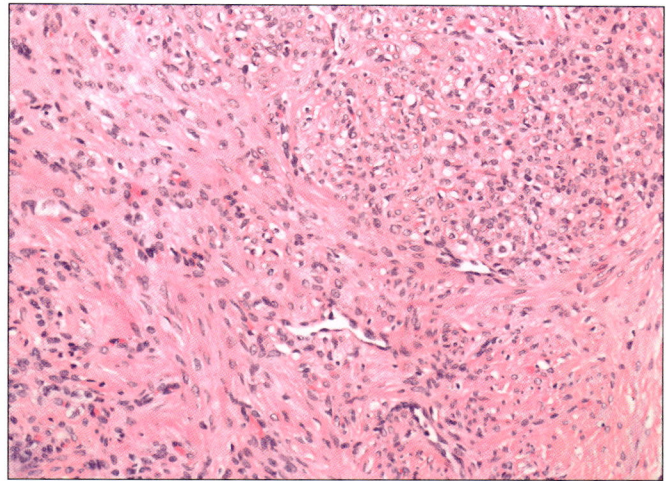

Figure 28.37 Slerosing stromal tumor. Spindle-shaped fibroblasts are admixed with rounded vacuolated cells. Note the presence of thin-walled blood vessels.

nonfunctioning, and if hormonally active, are usually androgenic, most frequently during pregnancy.[57]

Grossly, the tumors are predominantly solid masses (average diameter, 10 cm) with yellow areas, edema, and cyst formation. The microscopic features of the SST are distinctive. Low-power microscopic examination typically shows ill-defined cellular pseudolobules separated by edematous fibrous tissue (Figure 28.36). The nodules contain two types of cells: spindle cells producing collagen and round to oval degenerated lutein cells (Figure 28.37). The latter have a vacuolated cytoplasm and contain lipid. Mitotic activity is low. A network of thin-walled blood vessels, 'hemangiopericytoma-like,' is usually present within the nodules.

Immunohistochemical expression of vimentin, inhibin, calretinin, α-glutathione S-transferase, and CD34 has been demonstrated in SSTs.[58] Smooth muscle actin and muscle-specific actin and desmin are usually positive.[56] Immunoreactions for vascular permeability factor/vascular endothelial growth factor (VPF/VEGF) and its receptor, fms-like tyrosine kinase 1 (flt-1), have also been detected in the lutein cells and small- to medium-sized blood vessels, respectively.[59] These findings explain the prominent vasculature and edema characteristic of SSTs. Trisomy 12 has also been identified.[59,60]

The typical microscopic features of SSTs serve to distinguish them from fibromas and thecomas. Rarely, the vacuolated cells in SST can simulate the signet-ring cells of a Krukenberg tumor. The vacuoles in SST, however, contain lipid instead of mucin and immunostains for cytokeratin are negative. All reported cases of SST have been benign.

SIGNET-RING STROMAL TUMOR

This rare neoplasm occurs in adults and is nonfunctioning. Only eight cases have been reported.[61–64] The clinical and macroscopic features are similar to those of ovarian fibromas. Microscopically, spindle cells are diffusely distributed and merge almost imperceptibly with rounded cells containing eccentric nuclei and single large vacuoles resembling signet-ring cells (Figure 28.38). Hyaline bodies are frequently present. Stains for lipid and mucin are negative. Ultrastructural studies have revealed that in some cases the vacuoles result from diffuse edema of the cytoplasmic matrix, in other cases from swelling of mitochondria, and in still others from cytoplasmic pseudoinclusions of edematous extracellular matrix.[62,63] The main differential diagnosis is Krukenberg tumor, but negative mucin, EMA, and cytokeratin stains exclude that diagnosis.[64] The signet-ring stromal tumor lacks the pseudolobulation, lipid-rich cells, and prominent vascularity of the SST. Inhibin has been negative in all cases tested.

MICROCYSTIC STROMAL TUMOR

This benign stromal tumor shows a characteristic microcystic pattern.[65] In the only reported series of 16 cases, all patients were adults (mean 45 years) and the tumors were nonfunctioning, confined to the ovary (stage I), and had a mean size of 10 cm. They were cystic or solid and cystic. On microscopic examination, the appearance varies according to the relative prominence of the three fundamental components: microcysts, solid cellular regions, and fibrous stroma. These regions are punctuated by small cysts that anastomose with each other, giving a distinctive appearance (Figure 28.39). The neoplastic cells contain granular eosinophilic cytoplasm and round to oval nuclei with small nucleoli (Figure 28.40). Mitotic figures are rare. The tumors are typically negative for inhibin but positive for CD10. About one-third of the tumors examined to date have been cytokeratin positive but they have been EMA negative. The tumors show WT1 nuclear immunoreactivity and nuclear staining of β-catenin.[66] Mutation analysis in two cases revealed the presence of an identical point mutation, c.98C>G, in exon 3 of *CTNNB1* (β-catenin).[66] This finding suggests that dysregulation of the Wnt/β-catenin pathway plays an important role in the pathogenesis of this ovarian stromal tumor.

SERTOLI–STROMAL CELL TUMORS

SERTOLI CELL TUMORS

These uncommon tumors are composed of hollow or solid tubules intersected by stroma with only rare or no Leydig cells.[1,67–69] They account for 4% of Sertoli–stromal cell tumors. They may occur at any age but are most common in women with an average age of 30 years. Sertoli cell tumors are usually nonfunctioning but may be estrogenic or rarely androgenic. Lipid-rich Sertoli cell tumors are associated with isosexual pseudoprecocity,[1] and oxyphil Sertoli cell tumors with the Peutz–Jeghers syndrome (PJS).[70] The endometrium may be hyperplastic. A decidual reaction caused by progestins produced by the tumor is occasionally seen.[71] One tumor was malignant with distant metastases.[68]

Sertoli cell tumors are unilateral and stage I.[67–69] They average 9 cm in diameter and appear solid, lobulated, and yellow-brown. Microscopically, the tumors exhibit a prominent tubular architecture. The tubules are surrounded by a basement membrane that may coalesce to form hyalinized areas. Hollow tubules are lined by columnar to cuboidal cells with pale or eosinophilic cytoplasm (Figure 28.41). Other patterns include trabecular, diffuse, alveolar, pseudopapillary, and retiform. Spindle cells may be prominent. The Sertoli cells show mild nuclear atypia and very few mitoses. Bizarre nuclei may be rarely found. Vimentin, WT1,[72] SF-1,[73] cytokeratins, inhibin (Figure 28.42), calretinin, and CD99 are usually positive. EMA is negative.

Endometrioid carcinomas may resemble Sertoli cell tumors ('sertoliform' variant).[74,75] Struma ovarii and primary or metastatic carcinoid tumours may also mimic Sertoli cell tumors. The possibility that a sertoliform tumor could be a Sertoli cell adenoma in a phenotypic female with androgen insensitivity syndrome should also be considered.

SERTOLI-LEYDIG CELL TUMORS

Clinical Features

Sertoli-Leydig cell tumors (SLCTs) are rare and account for less than 0.5% of all ovarian tumors;[1] they occur in all age

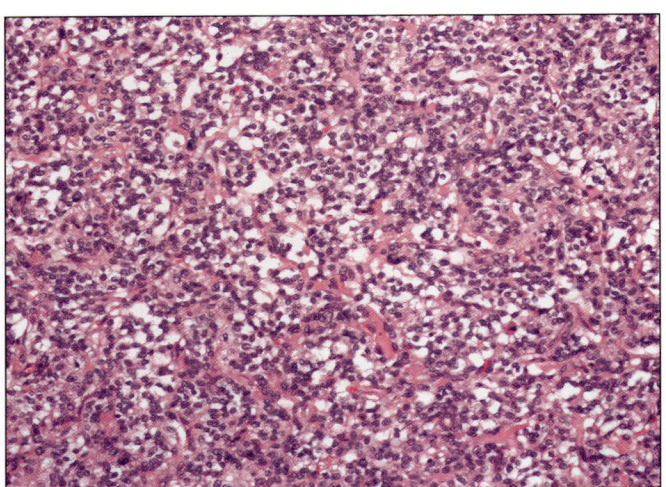

Figure 28.39 Microcystic stromal tumor.

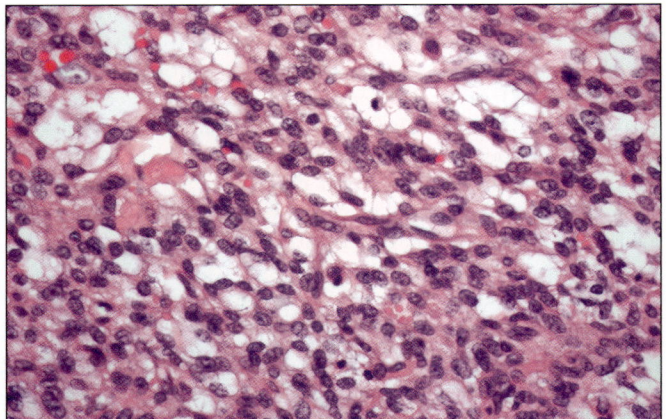

Figure 28.40 Microcystic stromal tumor. The small cysts anastomose with each other, giving a distinctive appearance.

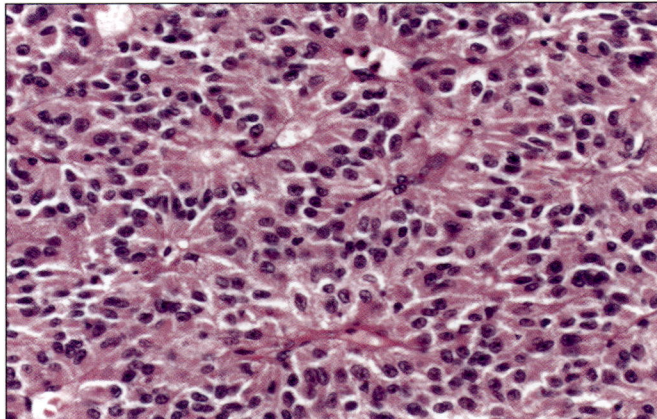

Figure 28.41 Sertoli cell tumor. The almost solid tubules are lined by cuboidal to columnar cells with eosinophilic cytoplasm. No mitotic activity is seen.

groups but they peak during reproductive years (average age, 25 years).[76–79] Tumors developing in patients with a germline *DICER-1* mutation occur at a younger median age of 13 years.[80] SLCTs are unilateral in over 98% of cases. They produce androgens and masculinize the patients in 40–60% of cases, but many tumors are nonfunctioning and some even have estrogenic effects.[77,79] Testosterone and a variety of androgenic precursors may be secreted in variable proportions. Androgenic manifestations include amenorrhea, hirsutism, breast atrophy, enlargement of the clitoris, and hoarseness. In contrast to virilizing adrenal tumors, urinary 17-ketosteroid values are usually normal or only slightly raised. About 20% of cases are associated with elevated serum levels of α-fetoprotein.[81] Patients may present with abdominal pain, ascites, or tumor rupture. SLCTs are stage IA in about 80% of cases.[76–79] Only 2–3% of tumors have spread beyond the ovary, usually within the pelvis and rarely into the upper abdomen. Poorly differentiated tumors more often are ruptured and present at a more advanced stage than tumors of intermediate differentiation. Well-differentiated tumors are almost always stage IA.

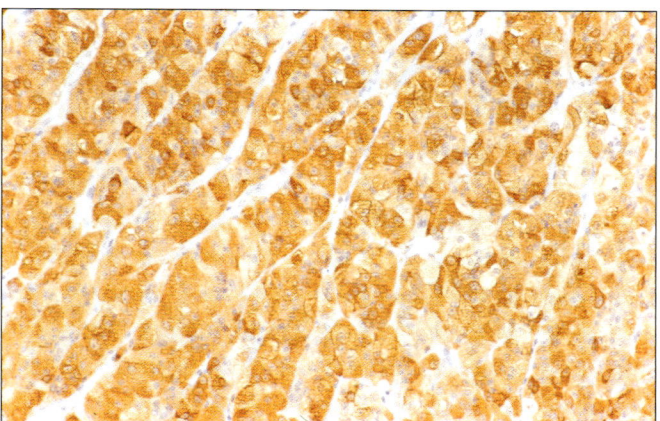

Figure 28.42 Sertoli cell tumor. Immunoreaction for α-inhibin.

Macroscopic Features

The tumors vary in their gross appearance from solid, lobulated, yellow masses (Figure 28.43) to unilocular or multilocular cysts containing blood. Their average diameter is 13 cm.[76–79] Poorly differentiated tumors including those containing mesenchymal heterologous elements are often large, hemorrhagic, and necrotic.[82] Retiform tumors and those with mucinous heterologous elements tend to be cystic or predominantly cystic and may contain numerous papillae (Figure 28.44).[83–86]

Microscopic Features

Unlike granulosa cell tumors, Sertoli-Leydig cell tumors have a wide variety of microscopic patterns that correlate with prognosis. Five histologic subtypes are distinguished: well differentiated, of intermediate differentiation, and poorly differentiated. Additionally, the last two categories may contain heterologous elements, a retiform component, or both.

1. Well-differentiated tumors form hollow or solid tubules composed of cuboidal to columnar Sertoli cells, separated by a fibrous stroma, and admixed with nests of large round Leydig cells. The histologic appearance resembles that of the fetal testis (Figure 28.45) or even the tubular glands of a well-differentiated endometrioid adenocarcinoma. The nuclei are round and lack atypia and mitotic activity. Crystals of Reinke can be seen in some of the Leydig cells in 20% of cases.[87]
2. Tumors of intermediate differentiation contain cellular lobules of immature gonadal stromal cells separated by edematous stroma (Figures 28.46 and 28.47). The hyperchromatic spindle-shaped cells merge with cords and tubules of atypical Sertoli cells (Figure 28.48). The immature Sertoli cells contain small, round, oval, or angular nuclei; the abortive tubules resemble early sex cords of the embryonic testis (Figure 28.47).[76–78] In tumors of intermediate differentiation, mitotic figures average 5 per 10 HPF. Rarely, bizarre nuclei may be seen. Leydig cells are found in clusters at the periphery of the cellular

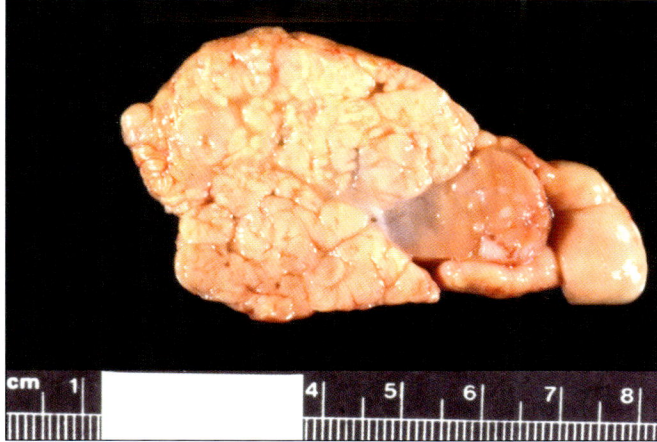

Figure 28.43 Sertoli-Leydig cell tumor. The sectioned surface is lobulated and gray-yellow.

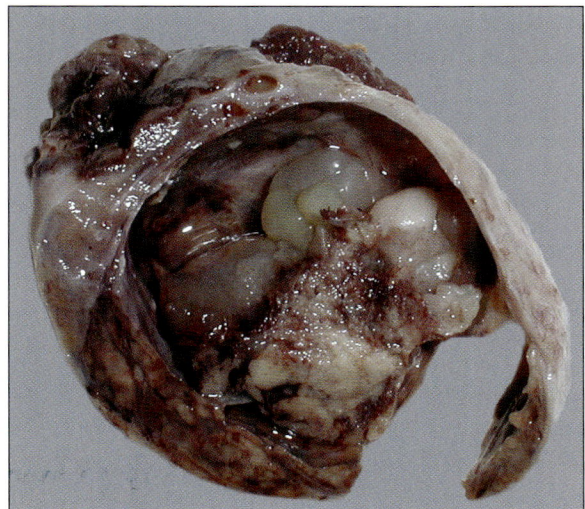

Figure 28.44 Sertoli-Leydig cell tumor, retiform type. Opened cystic tumor. The lumen of the cyst is partly filled with edematous polypoid structures. (Courtesy of Dr. Giuseppe Nuciforo, Catania, Italy).

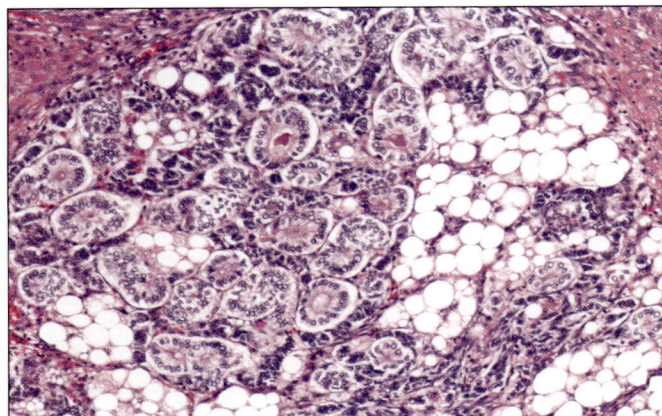

Figure 28.45 Well-differentiated Sertoli-Leydig cell tumor from a 29-year-old woman with virilization. The hollow tubules are lined by mature Sertoli cells. The intervening stroma contains numerous Leydig cells exhibiting large cytoplasmic vacuoles that were filled with lipid.

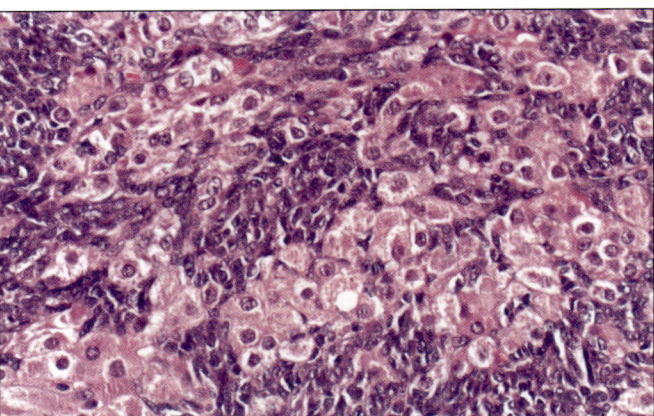

Figure 28.47 Sertoli-Leydig cell tumor of intermediate differentiation. The Sertoli cells have oval and angular nuclei whereas those of the Leydig cells are round and contain prominent nucleoli.

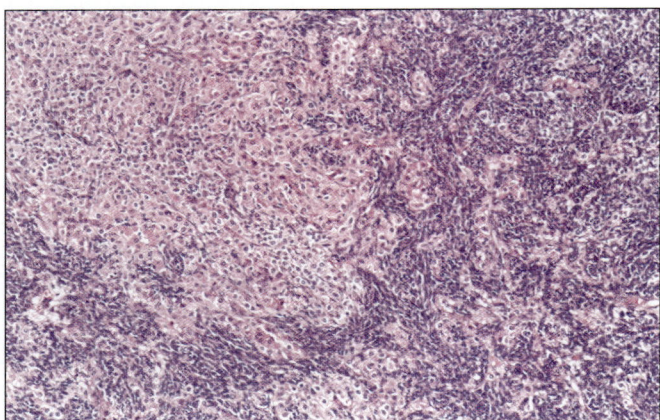

Figure 28.46 Sertoli-Leydig cell tumor of intermediate differentiation. Masses and clusters of Leydig cells with abundant eosinophilic cytoplasm separate aggregates of smaller Sertoli cells with scanty cytoplasm.

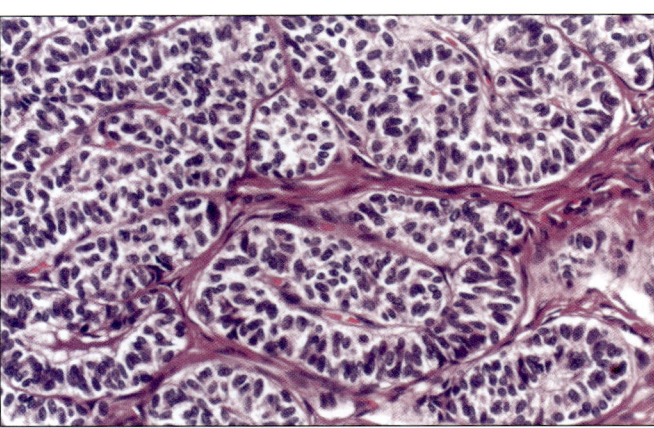

Figure 28.48 Sertoli-Leydig cell tumor of intermediate differentiation. Solid tubules of well-differentiated Sertoli cells resembling those of the fetal testis.

lobules or admixed with other elements. They may be vacuolated, contain lipofuscin, or rarely have Reinke crystals. The Leydig cells lack nuclear atypia and mitotic activity.

3. Poorly differentiated or *sarcomatoid* SLCTs are composed of spindle cells with vague trabecular arrangement resembling a fibrosarcoma (Figure 28.49). Leydig cells may or may not be present. Mitotic figures are usually numerous with a mean of over 20 per 10 HPF.[77,78]
4. Fifteen percent of SLCTs show areas of slit-like spaces that mimic the rete of the ovary or testis (Figure 28.50); they have been designated *retiform* SLCTs.[83] They occur on average about a decade earlier than other SLCTs, are less often virilizing, and are frequently papillary simulating epithelial–stromal tumors, particularly serous borderline tumors, and yolk sac tumors.[83–85] The papillae often contain hyalinized cores. Some tumors show a multicystic pattern with sieve-like spaces lined by flattened cells. Approximately 30% of poorly differentiated LSCTs have retiform elements.

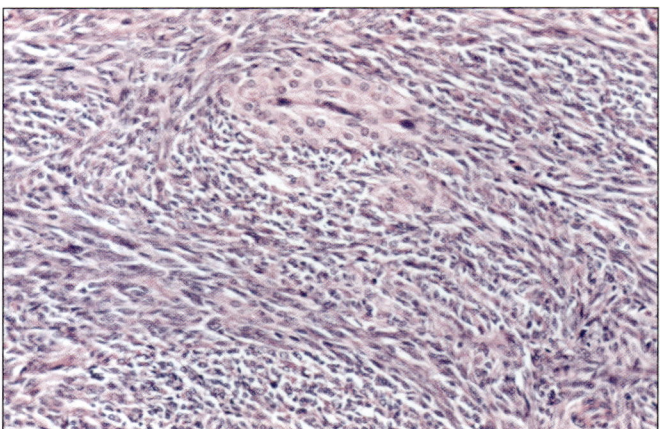

Figure 28.49 Sertoli-Leydig cell tumor, poorly differentiated ('sarcomatoid'). The tumor cells are spindle shaped and resemble those of a sarcoma. A nest of Leydig cells is seen.

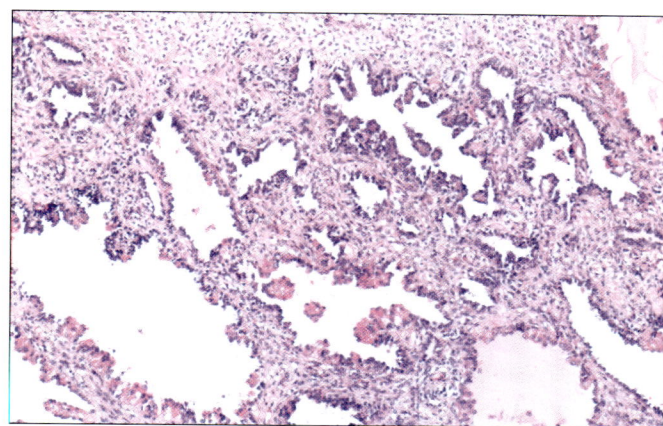

Figure 28.50 Sertoli-Leydig cell tumor, retiform. The tumor shows a papillary architecture. The papillae are partly covered by hyaline bodies.

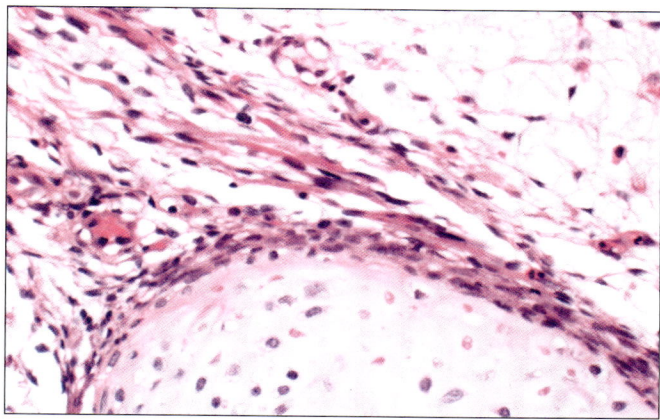

Figure 28.52 Sertoli-Leydig cell tumor with heterologous elements. Island of fetal-type cartilage (bottom) and bundles of rhabdomyoblasts.

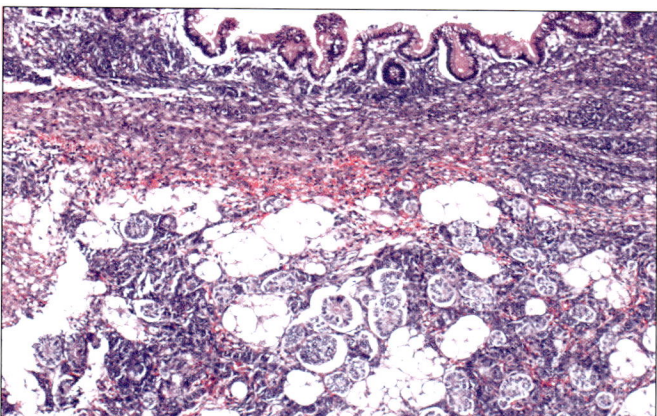

Figure 28.51 Well-differentiated Sertoli-Leydig cell tumor with heterologous elements. Well-differentiated gastrointestinal mucinous epithelium containing goblet cells (top).

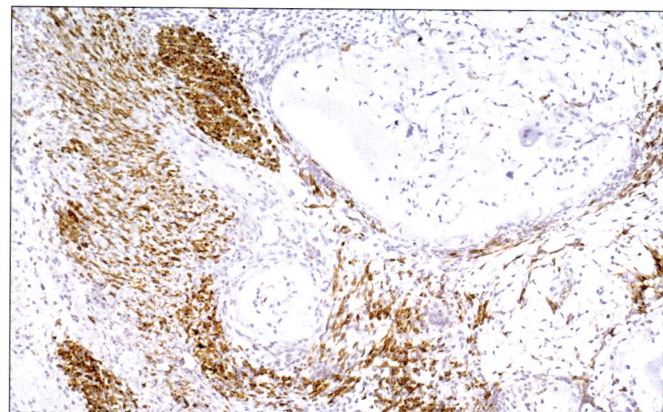

Figure 28.53 Sertoli-Leydig cell tumor with heterologous elements. The rhabdomyoblasts immunoreact for desmin. Unstained mucinous glands are also seen.

5. Twenty percent of the tumors contain *heterologous elements* such as neoplastic mucinous glands (Figure 28.51), cartilage, and skeletal muscle (Figure 28.52).[82,86] Glands and cysts are lined by well-differentiated mucinous epithelium of gastrointestinal type containing goblet cells, argentaffin cells, and Paneth cells; the mucinous epithelium may appear benign, borderline, or of low-grade malignancy. Focal insular carcinoid may be present.[86] Mesenchymal heterologous elements are found in only 5% of all SLCTs and include areas of fetal cartilage, embryonal rhabdomyosarcoma (Figures 28.52 and 28.53), or both.[82] Hepatic tissue has been found in 56% of the tumors with retiform differentiation (Figure 28.54).[88,89] One recurrent heterologous tumor contained neuroblastoma.[82]

SLCTs are divided into well-differentiated, intermediate, and poorly differentiated forms based on the degree of tubular differentiation of the Sertoli cell component and the quantity of spindle cell gonadal stroma. Both Sertoli cell elements and Leydig cells are seen less frequently in the poorly differentiated tumors. Heterologous elements and/or a retiform pattern may be seen in all but the well-differentiated variant. Unlike the theca cells in GCTs, the Leydig cell component is an integral part of the neoplastic process at least in some cases.

Immunohistochemistry

SLCTs are immunoreactive for vimentin, cytokeratins, inhibin (Figure 28.55), calretinin, progesterone receptor, androgen receptor, CD56, SF-1, and WT1. The intensity of expression differs between sex cord and stromal components. SLCTs react for FOXL2 in approximately half of cases.[7] DICER1 immunoreaction is strong in Sertoli cells and weak in Leydig cells.[80] Leydig cells in SLCTs do not react for FOX L2, WT1, and CD99, but express Melan-A.[20]

Genetic Susceptibility

Mutations in *DICER1*, a gene encoding an RNase III endoribonuclease, are found in 60% of SLCTs. Germline mutations have been identified in families affected by pleuropulmonary blastoma in childhood, multinodular goiter, and SLCTs.[80,90,91]

Differential Diagnosis

1. Sertoli cell tumors and hamartomas occur in the abdominal testes of patients with the *androgen-insensitivity syndrome*. Such patients have normal female habitus,

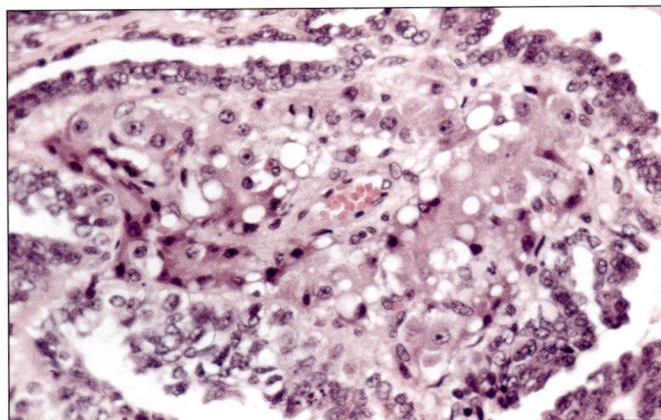

Figure 28.54 Retiform Sertoli-Leydig cell tumor with heterologous elements. A central aggregate of hepatocytes is seen.

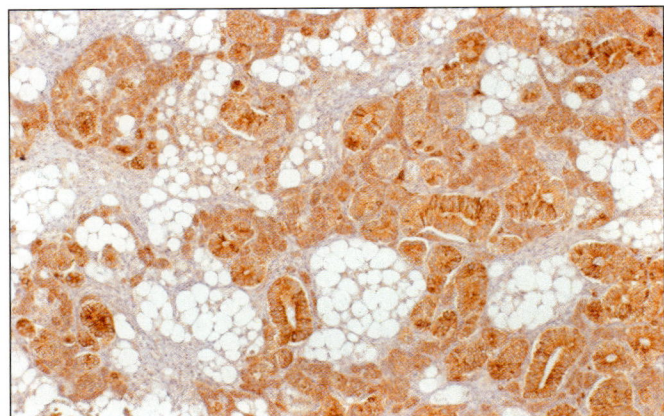

Figure 28.55 Sertoli-Leydig cell tumor, well differentiated. Immunoreaction for α-inhibin.

Table 28.3	Survival Rates for SLCTs
Differentiation	**% Survival**
Well differentiated	100
Of intermediate differentiation	89
Poorly differentiated	41
With intestinal heterologous elements	97
Poorly differentiated with mesenchymal heterologous elements	12.5

absence of pubic or axillary hair, primary amenorrhea, no uterus, and 46,XY karyotype.

Most SLCTs immunoreact for α-inhibin and calretinin. Positive results should facilitate the differential diagnosis with the following tumors:

2. *Endometrioid carcinomas resembling sex cord–stromal tumor.* Endometrioid carcinomas show mucin secretion, areas of squamous differentiation (nests of cells, morules, and keratinizing foci), and an adenofibromatous component (see Chapter 27).
3. *Endometrioid stromal sarcomas with sex cord-like differentiation* (see Chapter 27).
4. *Krukenberg tumors with tubular pattern and stromal luteinization.* Krukenberg tumors are bilateral in most cases and contain markedly atypical cells, including signet-ring cells that contain mucin. Other general features of metastatic tumors will be present (see Chapter 30).
5. *Carcinoid tumors of the trabecular type* may be confused with SLCTs of intermediate differentiation. The ribbons of the carcinoid tumor are much longer and more evenly distributed than the sex cord structures of the latter tumors. The stroma of the carcinoid tumors is less cellular and more fibromatous than that of SLCTs and does not contain Leydig cells. Primary carcinoid tumors are associated with teratomatous elements in about 70% of cases (see Chapter 29), and metastatic carcinoids are usually bilateral and are frequently accompanied by peritoneal metastases (see Chapter 30).
6. *Struma ovarii* with solid tubular pattern may be difficult to distinguish from an SLCT. The finding of true thyroid follicles, calcium oxalate crystals, and positive immunostaining for thyroglobulin facilitate the correct diagnosis (see Chapter 29).
7. *Ependymoma*, primary or metastatic, may be confused with an SLCT. The finding of perivascular pseudorosettes composed of cells with fibrillary cytoplasmic processes and the positive glial fibrillary acidic protein immunoreactivity are helpful (see Chapter 29).
8. *Female adnexal tumors of wolffian origin* are rarely associated with endocrine symptoms (see Chapter 27)
9. *Teratoma.* SLCTs with heterologous elements may be misdiagnosed as teratomas. However, gonadal teratomas do not contain gonadal cell types and SLCTs do not contain ectodermal elements (except in a single reported case of neuroblastoma; see Chapter 29).[82]
10. *Malignant mesodermal mixed tumors (MMMTs).* Heterologous SLCTs containing cartilage or skeletal muscle may be erroneously interpreted as MMMTs. Nevertheless, the latter usually occur in postmenopausal patients and the cartilage component appears histologically malignant (chondrosarcoma; see Chapter 27).
11. Retiform SLCTs may be confused with *yolk sac tumors* because of the young age of the patient and the presence of a papillary architecture. The former, however, are accompanied by androgenic symptoms in 25% of cases and do not contain the primitive germ cells of yolk sac tumors. α-fetoprotein and glypican-3 immunoreactions are also helpful in this differential diagnosis (see Chapter 29).

Treatment and Prognosis

In young women, the treatment of choice is unilateral salpingo-oophorectomy. In those patients with virilizing SLCTs, normal menses return in about 4 weeks following removal of the tumor.[79] Radical surgery and chemotherapy are indicated for tumors at an advanced stage. In contrast to GCTs, which often recur many years postoperatively, SLCTs tend to recur earlier, within 1–2 years (Table 28.3).[77,78,82]

Almost all SLCTs are benign, with the rare malignant cases falling into the category of poorly differentiated tumors (60%) and those with mesenchymal heterologous elements.[82] Not enough cases of retiform SLCT have been reported to establish its prognosis, but it appears to be worse than that of SLCTs in general.[84,85] Malignant behavior takes the form of intra-abdominal spread, ordinarily without distant metastases.[77,78,82]

SEX CORD TUMOR WITH ANNULAR TUBULES

This tumor has distinctive morphologic features, which are intermediate between granulosa cell and Sertoli cell tumor.[92,93] One-third of cases are associated with the Peutz–Jeghers syndrome (PJS) (mucocutaneous pigmentation, gastrointestinal hamartomatous polyps, rarely well-differentiated adenocarcinoma of the uterine cervix, and carcinomas of colon, pancreas, or breast) and have been found in patients of an average age of 27 years (Figure 28.56).[92,93] The ovarian lesions are often incidental operative findings.[93] In patients without the syndrome (average age, 34 years), the tumors often form unilateral palpable masses and are estrogenic in about half of the cases.[93] In both cases, the tumors are composed of simple and complex ring-shaped tubules containing central hyaline nodules of basement membrane material (Figure 28.57).[92,93] The cells lining the tubules have an antipodal arrangement with the nuclei located at opposite ends of the cells. Nuclear atypia and mitotic figures are rare. In patients with the PJS, multiple bilateral tumorlets are scattered within the ovarian stroma and calcification of the tubules is common (60%; Figure 28.58).[92]

Sex cord tumor with annular tubules (SCTAT) show positive immunoreaction for vimentin, inhibin, calretinin, FOXL2, SF-1, WT1, and CD56.[18] There is positive reaction for cytokeratin but not for EMA. Germline-inactivating mutations of the PJS gene (*STK11/LKB1*) at chromosome 19p13.3 have been found in most PJS patients; however, somatic mutations have not been encountered in sporadic tumors.[94] In sporadic sex cord–stromal tumors, LOH at 19p13.3 apparently targets a gene different from *STK11* and may play a role in their pathogenesis, especially in tumors containing sex cord derivatives.[95] LOH at the 19p13.3 region has also been found in three of eight well-differentiated adenocarcinomas of the cervix.

SCTATs associated with PJS have a favorable clinical course. About 20% of the SCTATs unassociated with PJS have been clinically malignant.[93] Features associated with aggressive behavior include large size and invasive appearance, marked nuclear atypia, and high mitotic activity. The tumors spread via lymphatics. Recurrences are often late. Treatment is primarily surgical. MIS, α-inhibin, and progesterone are useful serum tumor markers.[1]

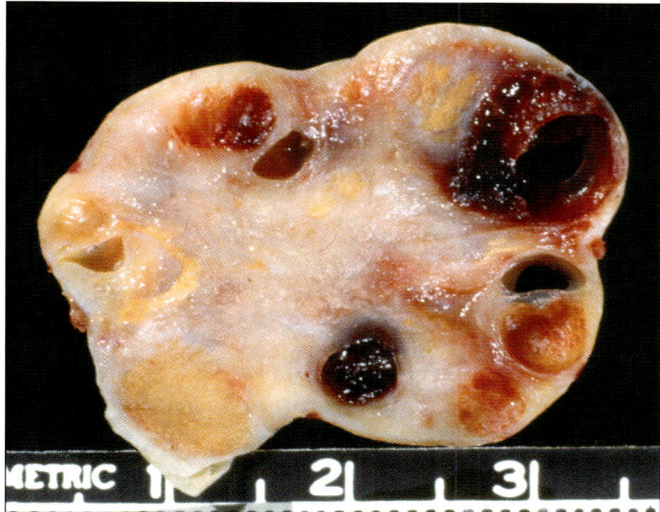

Figure 28.56 Sex cord tumor with annular tubules. Section of ovary from a woman with Peutz–Jeghers syndrome. Several small yellow-pale nodules are seen.

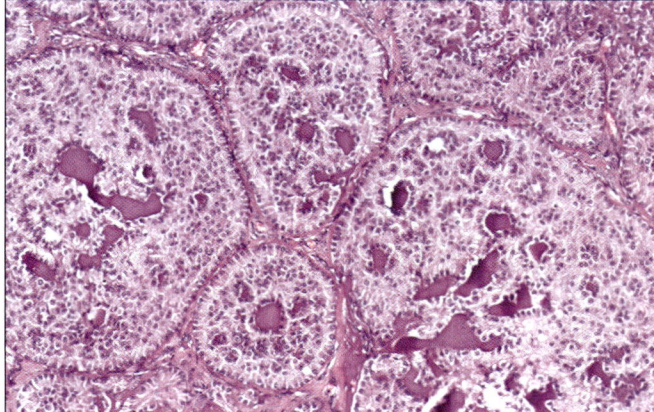

Figure 28.57 Sex cord tumor with annular tubules. Complex annular tubules encircling numerous hyaline masses. Nuclei are arranged in antipodal manner at the periphery of the nests and around the hyaline mass.

GYNANDROBLASTOMA

Rarely, a sex cord–stromal tumor may include both granulosa–theca cell and Sertoli–Leydig cell components. The minor component should account for at least 10% of the tumor. Most of these tumors have been benign. Those with hormonal function have produced androgens.

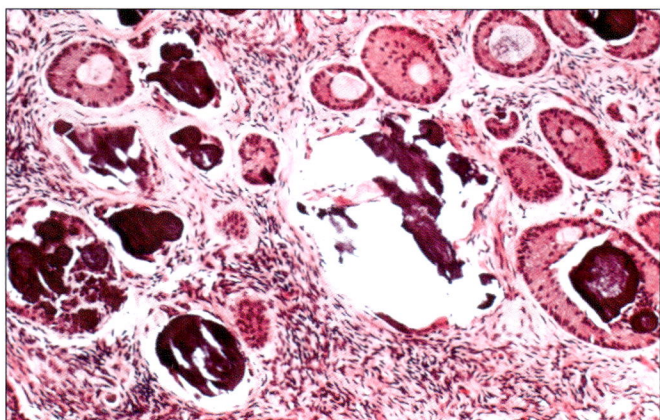

Figure 28.58 Sex cord tumor with annular tubules. Calcification of the tubules.

STEROID CELL TUMORS

The term steroid cell tumors refers to a group of ovarian neoplasms composed of cells resembling steroid hormone-secreting cells (lutein cells, Leydig cells, or adrenal cortical cells). Although these tumors have been previously designated as lipid (lipoid) cell tumors, up to one-fourth of them contain little or no lipid.[1,2] Consequently, the more appropriate and accurate term steroid cell tumors has been proposed for these neoplasms because it reflects both the cytologic features of the tumor cells and their capacity to secrete steroid hormones (Figure 28.59).[1,2] Steroid tumors have been subdivided into four different subtypes: stromal luteomas, Leydig cell tumors, adrenal cortical-type tumors, and steroid cell tumors NOS (not otherwise specified) (Table 28.4).[1,2] These neoplasms are uncommon and represent only approximately 0.1% of all ovarian tumors;[1,2] nevertheless, they are clinically remarkable lesions, which are often associated with hyperestrogenism or masculinization (Table 28.5).[96] All steroid cell tumors are immunoreactive for α-inhibin.

STROMAL LUTEOMA

Stromal luteoma is a benign and small steroid cell tumor usually found within the ovarian stroma and presumably arising from it.[1,97,98] The stromal origin of this tumor is supported by the finding of lutein cells in cases of stromal hyperthecosis, a non-neoplastic lesion associated with the neoplasm in over 90% of the cases (in the ipsilateral or contralateral ovary).[97,98] In fact, in some cases of stromal hyperthecosis, nests of lutein cells may appear as nodules (nodular hyperthecosis).[1] The stromal luteoma accounts for 20% of all steroid cell tumors, and 80% of them occur in postmenopausal women (mean age, 58 years).[97,98] The tumor appears as a unilateral, well-circumscribed, solid, reddish yellow nodule, less than 3 cm in diameter (Figure 28.60). Microscopically, it is composed of lutein cells with relatively little lipid (Figure 28.61) and abundant lipochrome pigment. The nuclei are round and contain prominent nucleoli. Mitotic figures are uncommon. The

Table 28.4 Steroid Cell Tumors

1. Stromal luteoma
2. Leydig cell tumor
   a. Hilus
   b. Non-hilus
3. Adrenal cortical type
4. NOS

Table 28.5 Steroid Cell Tumors (Clinical Features)[96]

Clinical Manifestations	Stromal Luteoma	Hilus C+	Hilus C−	Steroid Cell Tumor (NOS)
Androgenic (%)	12	83	33	52
Estrogenic (%)	60	0	44	8
Cushing syndrome (%)	0	0	0	6
Nonfunctioning (%)	20	17	23	27

C+, with Reinke crystals; C−, without Reinke crystals.

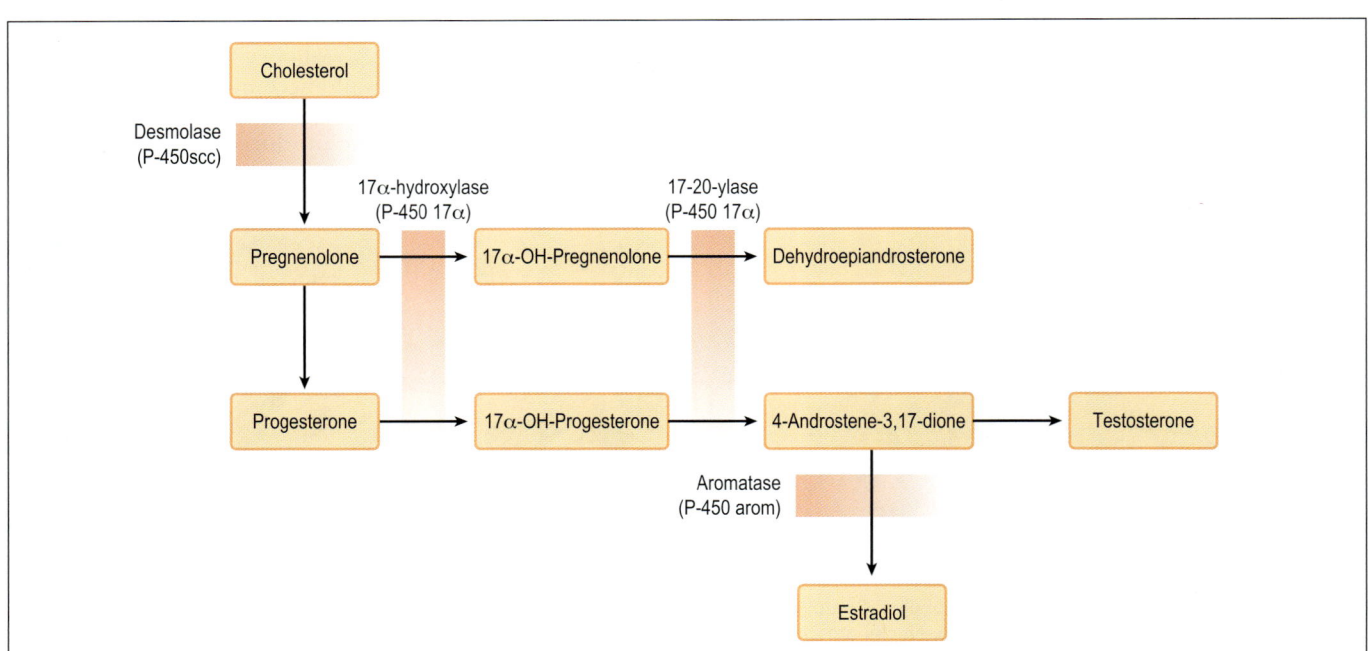

Figure 28.59 Ovarian steroidogenic pathway.

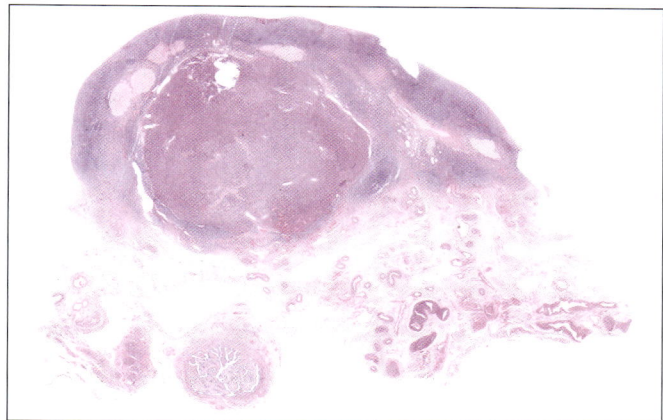

Figure 28.60 Stromal luteoma. The tumor is surrounded by a rim of ovarian parenchyma. A section of the fallopian tube is seen at the bottom.

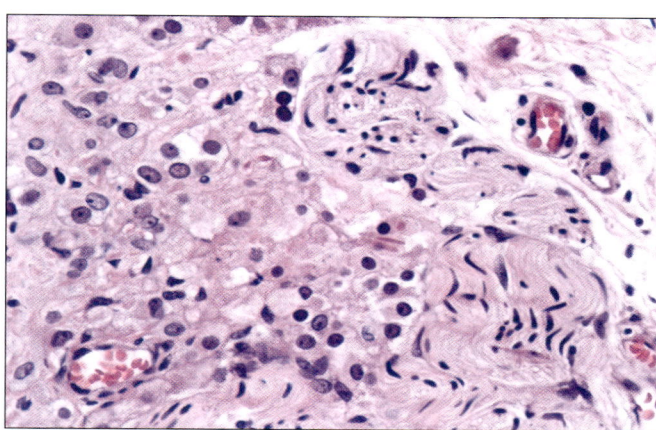

Figure 28.62 Hilus cells. Reinke crystals are seen in the center of the field. A strand of a nerve is present in the right side of the figure.

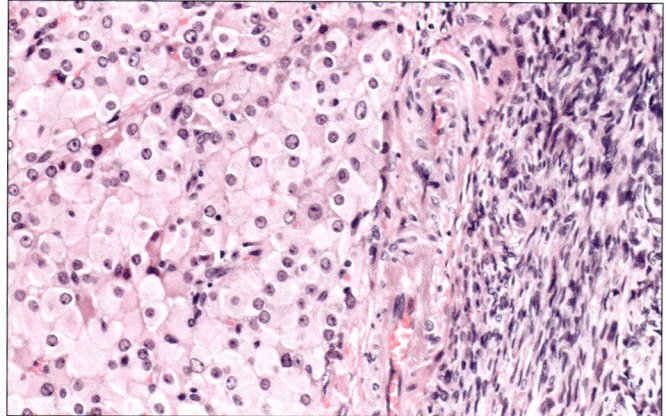

Figure 28.61 Stromal luteoma. The tumor is sharply demarcated from the ovarian stroma. The tumor cells are polygonal and contain little lipid.

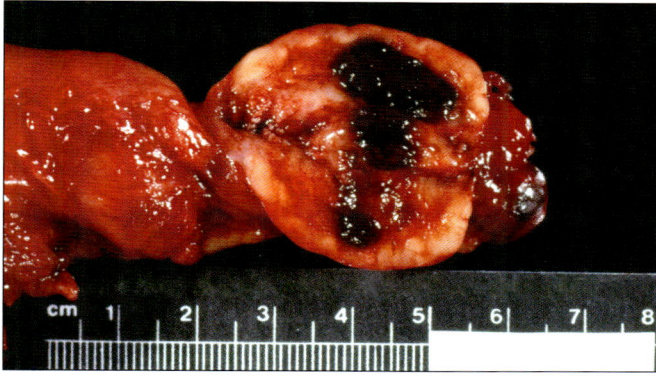

Figure 28.63 Leydig cell tumor. The cut surfaces of the bisected ovary show a dark-brown mass.

tumor cells are arranged in a vague organoid pattern. In some cases, the artifactual formation of irregular spaces with hemorrhage can lead to an erroneous diagnosis of vascular tumor. In contrast to the other types of steroid cell tumor, stromal luteoma is commonly associated with hyperestrogenism (60%), although some rare cases have been androgenic (12%).[97–99]

LEYDIG CELL TUMOR

Leydig cell tumors derive from Leydig cells, which are normally located in the ovarian hilus and contain crystals of Reinke in their cytoplasm on either light microscopy (Figure 28.62) or electron microscopy.[96] Accordingly, the vast majority of reported tumors have been located in the hilus and have been thought to arise from hyperplastic hilus (Leydig) cells; they have been designated *hilus cell tumors*. Less frequently, Leydig cell tumors develop within the ovarian stroma, far from the hilus, and then are described as Leydig cell tumors (non-hilar type).[1,96]

Leydig cell tumors, which represent 15% of steroid cell tumors, usually occur in postmenopausal women (mean age, 58 years), and are associated with hirsutism or virilization in 80% of cases.[1,96] They secrete predominantly testosterone and, therefore, the urinary 17-ketosteroid levels are often normal or only slightly elevated.[1,96] Grossly, the tumors appear as small dark or reddish brown to yellow nodules; most of them are less than 5 cm in diameter (Figure 28.63). Microscopically, they are composed of polygonal cells arranged in nests. In some cases, Leydig cell tumors may contain cells with nuclear pseudoinclusions or marked nuclear pleomorphism (so-called *endocrine atypia*) (Figure 28.64). These pleomorphic tumors often exhibit Reinke crystals and lipochrome pigment. Leydig cell tumors with crystals are more frequently associated with virilization than Leydig cell tumors without crystals. When crystals are not found, the diagnosis of Leydig cell tumor is favored by its hilar location, the finding of hilus cell hyperplasia around non-medullated nerves, fibrinoid necrosis of vessel walls, and nuclear clustering with nucleus-free zones.[1,96] Immunostains for α-inhibin are strongly positive. Practically all reported cases of hilus cell tumor have been benign.[1,96]

Mutations of LH receptor gene have been associated with the development of testicular Leydig cell tumors.[100]

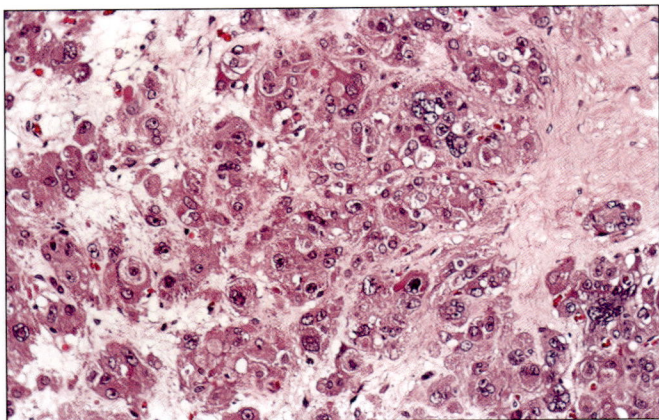

Figure 28.64 Leydig cell tumor. The polygonal cells have abundant eosinophilic cytoplasm and are arranged in nests. Some of them contain bizarre nuclei.

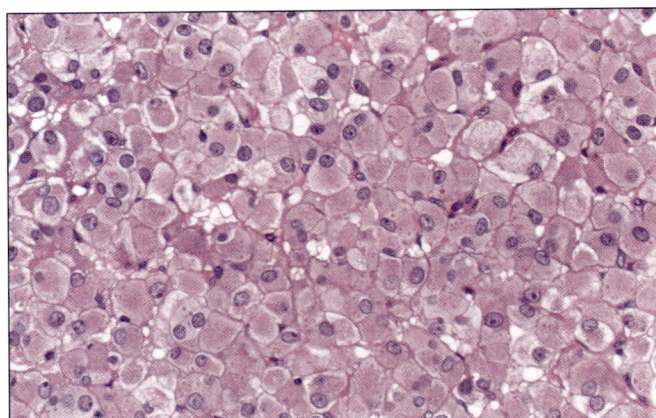

Figure 28.65 Steroid cell tumor NOS. The tumor cells are polygonal and have abundant eosinophilic cytoplasm and small round nuclei.

STEROID CELL TUMOR, ADRENAL CORTICAL TYPE

The morphologic similarity between steroid cell tumors and adrenal cortical tumors suggests that some of the former neoplasms may arise from adrenal cortical rests.[1] These rests are extremely rare within the ovary, but they can be encountered in the mesovarium (broad ligament) in approximately 25% of women. In rare patients with steroid cell tumors, the responses of elevated levels of urinary 17-ketosteroids and 17-hydroxycorticosteroids to ACTH stimulation and dexamethasone suppression have been more concordant with an adrenal cortical tumor than one of ovarian type. Furthermore, the occasional association of such tumors with the adrenogenital syndrome or Cushing's syndrome also supports their adrenal cortical nature.[1] α-Inhibin immunostaining helps in the differential diagnosis.

STEROID CELL TUMOR (NOS)

Steroid cell tumors NOS comprise a heterogeneous group of neoplasms that probably includes large stromal luteomas or Leydig cell tumors; however, since they lack Reinke crystals and their topographic origin is no longer evident, they cannot be classified accordingly.[1,101] They represent 60% of steroid cell tumors.[1] In one series, the clinically malignant tumors accounted for 28% of cases.[101] The tumors may occur at any age, but characteristically at a younger age (mean, 43 years) than the other types of steroid cell tumors.[1,101] They are associated with hirsutism or virilization in approximately 50% of cases, but may be estrogenic in 10% of cases. Four tumors have produced cortisol and caused Cushing's syndrome and one has secreted aldosterone.[1,102]

Steroid cell tumors NOS are almost always unilateral. Bilaterality has been reported in only 6% of cases.[96] Their size ranges from 1.2 to 45 cm with the malignant tumors having the largest diameters.[101] The neoplasms may show different gross and microscopic features. Some of them are brown while others are yellow. Some tumors are composed of polygonal-shaped eosinophilic cells (Figure 28.65) whereas others show cells with clear cytoplasm containing abundant lipid (Figure 28.66). These tumors are positive for inhibin, calretinin, and Melan-A, a marker that can help in

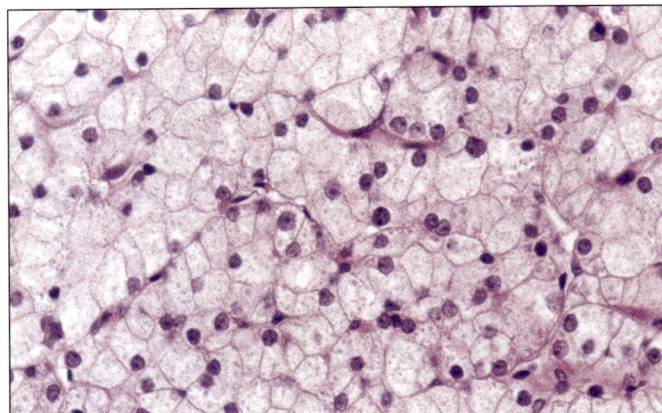

Figure 28.66 Steroid cell tumor NOS. The tumor cells have abundant pale (lipid-rich) cytoplasm.

the distinction from other sex cord–stromal tumors;[103] they are negative for FOXL2.

Differential Diagnosis

Steroid cell tumors, particularly those in the NOS category, may be confused with the tumors and tumor-like conditions contained in the following list. Positive immunohistochemical reactions for inhibin, calretinin, and SF-1 should exclude tumors in the differential diagnosis except for those in the sex cord–stromal category. However, steroid cell tumors are positive for Melan-A[103] and negative for FOXL2.

1. *Granulosa cell tumors and thecomas with marked luteinization.* The presence of non-luteinized areas with some composed of spindle cells, the characteristic nuclear features, and the reticulin stains facilitate the correct diagnosis (See Figure 28.11).
2. *Clear cell carcinoma (oxyphilic type).* These tumors have glycogen-rich cytoplasm and excentric nuclei. Also, other patterns of clear cell carcinoma such as tubulocystic, papillary, and glandular are not found in steroid cell tumors.
3. *Hepatoid yolk sac tumors and hepatoid carcinomas.* Both tumors have epithelial cells, which may form glands. Immunoreaction for α-fetoprotein is characteristic.

4. *Struma ovarii (oxyphilic type).* The presence of true thyroid follicles, an association with other teratomatous elements, and immunostaining for thyroglobulin should help in establishing the correct diagnosis.
5. *Paraganglioma and pheochromocytoma (primary or metastatic).* Along with the clinical features, staining for chromogranin and the finding of dense core granules by ultrastructural examination permit the distinction of these tumors from steroid cell tumors.
6. *Melanomas (primary or metastatic)* have higher nuclear atypicality than steroid cell tumors. Nevertheless, the melanin granules of the former may be confused with the lipochrome pigment of the latter. Immunoreaction for S-100 protein and HMB-45 may be helpful in some cases.
7. *Metastatic carcinomas from kidney, adrenal cortex, and liver.* Clinical, radiologic, and immunohistochemical findings may facilitate the correct diagnosis.
8. *Pregnancy luteomas* resemble lipid-poor steroid cell tumor and are frequently virilizing (see Chapter 24). However, about half of the pregnancy luteomas are multiple and approximately one-third are bilateral. Nuclear atypia is absent but mitoses may be numerous. Steroid cell tumors with mitotic activity usually exhibit marked nuclear atypia.

Treatment and Prognosis

As with other types of endocrine tumor, it may be impossible to predict whether these tumors will have a malignant behavior on the basis of the clinicopathologic features. Nevertheless, some clinical and pathologic findings should be taken into account when considering the possibility of malignancy. Age of presentation is a good indicator of malignant behavior; the vast majority of malignant tumors occur in women older than 51 years.[101] Other features to be considered are (1) 2 or more mitoses per 10 HPF, (2) grade 2 or 3 nuclear atypia, (3) diameter of 7 cm or greater, (4) hemorrhage, and (5) necrosis.[101] Approximately 40% of the tumors show clinical signs of malignancy. In a young patient with a stage IA tumor, unilateral salpingo-oophorectomy is the standard treatment. Follow-up by measurement of hormone levels is important. In older patients with low-stage tumors, hysterectomy with bilateral salpingo-oophorectomy is advised. For advanced-stage tumors, bulk removal is recommended.[101]

ENDOCRINE SYNDROMES ASSOCIATED WITH OVARIAN TUMORS

Ovarian tumors with obvious endocrine manifestations represent <5% of all ovarian neoplasms, and malignant 'functioning' ovarian tumors <10% of all ovarian cancers.[1,2] Nevertheless, the frequency of functioning ovarian tumors at a subclinical level is probably much higher according to various laboratory data. For example, it has been reported that over one-third of the cases of ovarian cancer in postmenopausal women are associated with abnormal cornification in vaginal smears, suggesting an increased estrogen level.[104] Furthermore, approximately half of the postmenopausal women with common epithelial tumors (which are usually considered to be nonfunctioning) have elevated urinary estrogen and/or pregnandiol levels.[105]

OVARIAN TUMORS WITH FUNCTIONING STROMA

In 1958, Morris and Scully[106] defined ovarian tumors with functioning stroma (OTFS) as tumors, other than sex cord–stromal or steroid cell neoplasms, whose stroma is consistent with steroid hormone secretion and are associated with estrogenic, androgenic, or progestogenic manifestations. In these tumors the neoplastic cells are not primarily responsible for steroid hormone production, but by growing within the ovarian stroma stimulate its cells or the adjacent hilus cells, which subsequently produce estrogens, androgens, progesterone, or combinations of these hormones. The mechanism by which this stimulation occurs is not well known. Possibly, secretion of hCG or hCG-like substance by the tumor cells is the triggering factor.[107] This phenomenon appears to be unique in the ovary among all endocrine glands. Almost all types of ovarian tumors (benign or malignant and primary or metastatic) can exhibit a functioning stroma, but the frequency of such association varies considerably depending upon the histologic type. It is found most frequently in mucinous (Figure 28.67) and endometrioid tumors and metastatic carcinomas from the gastrointestinal tract.[108]

From a microscopical viewpoint, OTFS can be separated into two categories: the more common forms in which the stroma of the tumor is condensed or luteinized; and the less frequent tumors in which the peripheral stromal (Figure 28.68) or hilus cells become activated.[109,110] Urinary estrogen levels have been correlated with the degree of stromal activation.[108] In the same study, 40 of 80 (50%) postmenopausal women with benign and malignant surface epithelium stromal tumors or metastatic carcinomas to the ovaries had

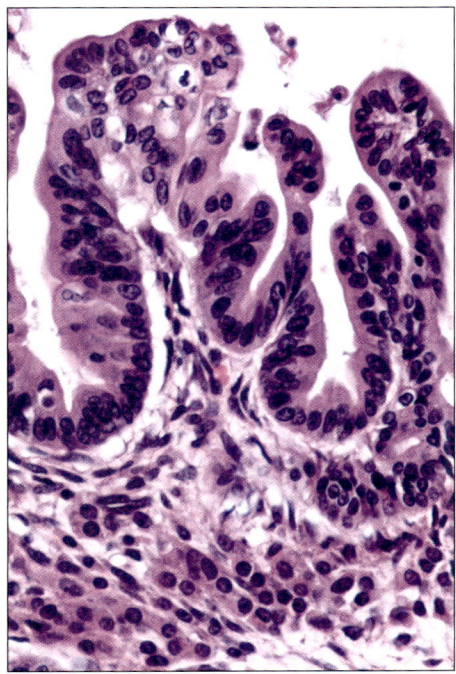

Figure 28.67 Mucinous borderline tumor with luteinization of stroma. Nests of lutein cells are seen below the neoplastic mucinous epithelium.

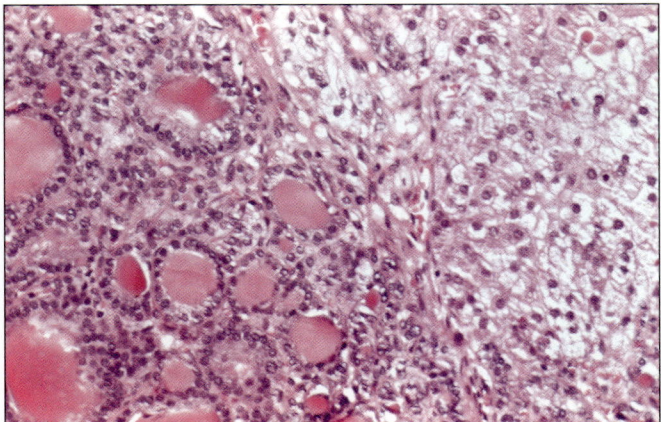

Figure 28.68 Struma ovarii with peripheral development of lutein cells. The lutein cells (right) are vacuolated. This tumor was associated with elevated estrogen levels and endometrial hyperplasia.

elevated urinary estrogen levels; 73% of these patients had activation of the ovarian stroma and 68% had a proliferative or hyperplastic endometrium. In these patients, the finding of mitoses in the fallopian tube epithelium is also indicative of estrogenic stimulation. Rare OTFS have been associated with progestational changes resulting in a decidual reaction or Arias-Stella change in the endometrium.[111]

From a pathogenetic viewpoint, OTFS may fall into three groups: (1) tumors that contain syncytiotrophoblastic cells, such as undifferentiated carcinoma, embryonal carcinoma, choriocarcinoma, and about 5% of dysgerminomas; (2) those in which the tumor occurs during pregnancy and the high hCG level of the pregnant state is the cause of stromal activation (virilizing Krukenberg tumors and mucinous cystic tumors are the most common OTFS that are diagnosed during pregnancy); and (3) tumors that do not contain trophoblastic cells and do not occur during pregnancy. In the third group, by far the most common, the explanation for the stromal change is less clear.

The possible explanations include: (1) the mechanical effect of the tumor, which expands and compresses the adjacent stroma as it does the enlarging follicle, would stimulate the development of theca-like cells; (2) the tumor would induce proliferation of the adjacent ovarian stroma with subsequent increase of mitotic activity in the stromal cells (apparently postmitotic cells are most receptive to stimulation by hLH, whose plasma levels are characteristically high in postmenopausal women); or (3) the ectopic production of hCG or hCG-like substances by the tumor cells.

In a study of 100 non-selected primary and metastatic ovarian tumors for investigating the frequency of stromal activation and its possible relation to hCG or hCG-like secretion by tumor cells,[107] stromal luteinization was present in 13 cases and stromal condensation in 16. The tumors most commonly associated with activation of the ovarian stroma were mucinous tumors (11 cases) and metastatic gastrointestinal adenocarcinomas (six cases). Two polyclonal and four monoclonal antibodies were used. A correlation between hCG production by the tumor cells, determined by immunohistochemistry, and activation (condensation or luteinization) of the ovarian stroma was encountered.

Immunoreaction for hCG was more frequently found in tumors with morphologically active stroma than in those with an inactive stroma.[107] These results indicate that hCG or hCG-like substances may play a role in activating the stroma of both primary and metastatic ovarian tumors.

It is known that ovarian carcinoma cells may secrete abnormal amounts of steroid hormones. As these cells or their neighbor stromal cells may also have aromatase activity, it is possible that steroid interconversions occur and result in endocrine manifestations.

HYPERCALCEMIA

Paraendocrine hypercalcemia is often associated with malignant tumors from different organs. Approximately 50 ovarian tumors accompanied by hypercalcemia have been reported. In these cases, no recognizable clinical manifestations have been described. The two types of ovarian tumor that are most frequently associated with elevated serum calcium levels are the small cell carcinoma (the so-called hypercalcemic type) and the clear cell carcinoma. Rare examples of dysgerminoma, serous tumors, or squamous cell carcinomas arising from pre-existing dermoid cysts have also been reported in association with hypercalcemia.

The small cell carcinoma, which is associated with hypercalcemia in two-thirds of cases, was first described in 1982[112] (see Chapter 27). Several substances including osteoblast activating factor, prostaglandins, vitamin D-like substance, parathormone (PTH), and PTH-related peptide have been considered as potential responsible agents for the hypercalcemia. Attempts to demonstrate PTH immunostaining in these ovarian tumors have been unsuccessful in most cases.[113] Immunostaining for PTH-related peptide has been described in five of seven cases of small cell carcinoma of the ovary, suggesting that PTH-related peptide is the responsible substance for the hypercalcemia associated with these ovarian tumors.[114]

HYPERTHYROIDISM

Rare strumal carcinoids have been accompanied by evidence of hypersecretion of thyroid hormone in the form of postoperative thyroid storm or hypothyroidism.[115] In cases of struma ovarii, biochemically documented thyroid hyperfunction has rarely been documented.

CARCINOID SYNDROME

Of the three main types of carcinoid tumors of the ovary—insular, trabecular, and strumal—33% of the insular tumors and a single case of strumal carcinoid have been accompanied by the carcinoid syndrome.[115,116] In these cases, the syndrome occurs in the absence of hepatic or other metastases since the secreted hormones enter the systemic circulation directly, bypassing the portal venous system and avoiding hepatic inactivation. The syndrome has been cured by removal of the ovarian tumor.

ZOLLINGER–ELLISON SYNDROME

Mucinous ovarian tumors contain endocrine cells in their glandular epithelium in over 30% of the cases.[117] A wide variety of peptide hormones have been demonstrated in these cells by immunohistochemistry. Eleven mucinous tumors of the ovary have produced the Zollinger–Ellison syndrome.[118] Gastrin-containing cells were identified by immunohistochemistry in 10 of the cases. The patients had elevated serum gastrin levels that disappeared after removal of the tumors.

HYPERPROLACTINEMIA

Two cases of ovarian dermoid cyst containing prolactinomas of 2.5 cm and 1 mm each have been reported.[119,120] The patients, aged 41 and 25 years, respectively, presented with amenorrhea and hyperprolactinemia.

CUSHING SYNDROME

Five cases of typical Cushing syndrome have been caused by cortisol production by steroid cell tumors.[102] Four tumors occurred in adults, had spread beyond the ovary at the time of presentation, and were eventually fatal. The fifth tumor developed in a 2-year-old girl who presented with the syndrome and isosexual precocity, both of which regressed postoperatively. This tumor probably originated from adrenal cortical rests.

Other ovarian tumors have rarely been associated with Cushing syndrome through either ectopic production of ACTH or anterior pituitary tissue (which had given rise to an ACTH-producing adenoma) within a dermoid cyst.

HYPOGLYCEMIA

Six ovarian tumors associated with hypoglycemia have been reported. They have included a dysgerminoma, a fibroma, a malignant schwannoma, a strumal carcinoid tumor, and a carcinoid tumor with a mixed insular and trabecular pattern.[121]

HYPERALDOSTERONISM

Twelve cases of hypertension due to hormone secretion by an ovarian tumor have been reported.[122,123] In eight cases, the hypertension was associated with a renin-secreting tumor and secondary hyperaldosteronism. In three cases, an aldosterone-secreting ovarian tumor resulted in primary hyperaldosteronism and low or normal plasma renin levels. In four cases the tumor also produced steroid hormones. Eight tumors were sex cord–stromal tumors, two were steroid cell tumors, one was a mucinous adenocarcinoma, and one was a leiomyosarcoma. One of the sex cord–stromal tumors occurred in a patient with Gorlin syndrome (see earlier) and another developed in a woman with Peutz–Jeghers syndrome (see earlier). Three tumors were clinically malignant and two were fatal. Immunoreaction for renin or prorenin was detected in five of the sex cord–stromal tumors and the leiomyosarcoma.

REFERENCES

1. Scully RE, Young RH, Clement PB. Sex cord-stromal tumors. In: Tumors of the ovary, maldeveloped gonads, fallopian tube, and broad ligament. Atlas of tumor pathology, 3rd series. Fascicle 23. Washington DC: Armed Forces Institute of Pathology; 1998. p. 169–238.
2. Prat J. Pathology of the ovary. Philadelphia: Saunders; 2004. p. 197–249.
3. Aguirre P, Thor AD, Scully RE. Ovarian endometrioid carcinomas resembling sex cord-stromal tumors: an immunohistochemical study. Int J Gynecol Pathol 1989;8:364–73.
4. Baker PM, Oliva E. Immunohistochemistry as a tool in the differential diagnosis of ovarian tumors: an update. Int J Gynecol Pathol 2004;24:39–55.
5. McCluggage WG. Immunohistochemical markers as a diagnostic aid in ovarian pathology. Diagn Histopathol 2008;14:335–51.
6. Shah SP, Kobel M, Senz J, et al. Mutation of FOXL2 in granulosa-cell tumors of the ovary. N Engl J Med 2009;360:2719–29.
7. Al-Agha OM, Huwait HF, Chow C, et al. FOXL2 is a sensitive and specific marker for sex cord-stromal tumors of the ovary. Am J Surg Pathol 2011;35:484–94.
8. Bjorkholm E, Pettersson F. Granulosa-cell and theca-cell tumors. The clinical picture and long term outcome for the Radiumhemmet series. Acta Obstet Gynecol Scand 1980;59:361–5.
9. Bjorkholm E, Silversward C. Prognostic factors in granulosa cell tumors. Gynecol Oncol 1981;11:261–74.
10. Evans AT, Gaffey TA, Malkasian Jr GD, Annegers JF. Clinicopathologic review of 118 granulosa and 82 theca cell tumors. Obstet Gynecol 1980;55:231–7.
11. Fox H, Agrawal K, Langley FA. A clinicopathological study of 92 cases of granulosa cell tumor of the ovary with special reference to the factors influencing prognosis. Cancer 1975;35:231–41.
12. Stenwig JT, Hazekamp JT, Beecham JB. Granulosa cell tumors of the ovary. A clinicopathological study of 118 cases with long-term follow-up. Gynecol Oncol 1979;7:136–52.
13. Nakashima N, Young RH, Scully RE. Androgenic granulosa cell tumors of the ovary. A clinicopathological analysis of seventeen cases and review of the literature. Arch Pathol Lab Med 1984;108:786–91.
14. Lauszus FF, Petersen AC, Greisen J, Jakobsen A. Granulosa cell tumor of the ovary: a population-based study of 37 women with stage I disease. Gynecol Oncol 2001;81:456–60.
15. Thrall MM, Paley P, Pizer E, et al. Patterns of spread and recurrence of sex cord-stromal tumors of the ovary. Gynecol Oncol 2011;122:242–5.
16. Nogales FF, Concha A, Plata C, Ruiz-Avila I. Granulosa cell tumor of the ovary with diffuse true hepatic cell differentiation simulating stromal luteinization. Am J Surg Pathol 1993;17:85–90.
17. Ahmed E, Young RH, Scully RE. Adult granulosa cell tumor of the ovary with foci of hepatic cell differentiation. A report of four cases and comparison with two cases of granulosa cell tumor with Leydig cells. Am J Surg Pathol 1999;23:1089–93.
18. Deavers MT, Malpica A, Liu J, et al. Ovarian sex cord-stromal tumors: an immunohistochemical study including a comparison of calretinin and inhibin. Mod Pathol 2003;16:584–90.
19. Cathro HP, Stoler MH. The utility of calretinin, inhibin, and WT1 immunohistochemical staining in the differential diagnosis of ovarian tumors. Hum Pathol 2005;36:195–201.
20. Zhao C, Vinh TN, McManus K, et al. Identification of the most sensitive and robust immunohistochemical markers in different categories of ovarian sex cord-stromal tumors. Am J Surg Pathol 2009;33:354–66.
21. Costa MJ, DeRose PB, Roth LM, et al. Immunohistochemical phenotype of ovarian granulosa cell tumors: absence of epithelial membrane antigen has diagnostic value. Hum Pathol 1994;25:60–6.
22. Loo KT, Leung AKF, Chan JKC. Immunohistochemical staining of ovarian granulosa cell tumours with MIC2 antibodies. Histopathology 1995;27:388–90.
23. Matias Guiu X, Pons C, Prat J. Müllerian inhibiting substance, alpha-inhibin, and CD99 expression in sex cord-stromal tumors and endometrioid ovarian carcinomas resembling sex cord-stromal tumors. Hum Pathol 1998;29:840–5.
24. Lin YS, Eng HL, Jan YJ, et al. Molecular cytogenetics of ovarian granulosa cell tumors by comparative genomic hybridization. Gynecol Oncol 2005;97:68–73.
25. Geiersbach KB, Jarboe EA, Jahromi MS, et al. FOXL2 mutation and large-scale genomic imbalances in adult granulosa cell tumors of the ovary. Cancer Genet 2011;204:596–602.

26. Kommoss F, Oliva E, Bhan AK, et al. Inhibin expression in ovarian tumors and tumor-like lesions: an immunohistochemical study. Mod Pathol 1998;11:656–64.
27. Riopel MA, Perlman EJ, Seidman JD, et al. Inhibin and epithelial membrane antigen immunohistochemistry assist in the diagnosis of sex cord-stromal tumors and provide clues to the histogenesis of hypercalcemic small cell carcinomas. Int J Gynecol Pathol 1998;17:46–53.
28. Schwartz PE, Smith JP. Treatment of ovarian stromal tumors. Am J Obstet Gynecol 1976;125:402–11.
29. Evans MP, Webb MJ, Gaffey TA, et al. DNA ploidy of ovarian granulosa cell tumors. Lack of correlation between DNA index or proliferative index and outcome in 10 patients. Cancer 1995;75:2295–8.
30. Young RH, Dickersin GR, Scully RE. Juvenile granulosa cell tumor of the ovary. A clinicopathologic analysis of 125 cases. Am J Surg Pathol 1984;8:575–96.
31. Velasco-Oses A, Alonso-Alvaro A, Blanco-Pozo A, Nogales Jr FF. Ollier's disease associated with ovarian juvenile granulosa cell tumor. Cancer 1988;62:222–5.
32. Irving JA, Young RH. Granulosa cell tumors of the ovary with a pseudopapillary pattern: a study of 14 cases of an unusual morphologic variant emphasizing their distinction from transitional cell neoplasms and other papillary ovarian tumors. Am J Surg Pathol 2008;32:581–6.
33. McCluggage WG. Immunoreactivity of ovarian juvenile granulosa cell tumours with epithelial membrane antigen. Histopathology 2005;46:235–6.
34. Shashi V, Golden WL, von Kap Herr C, et al. Interphase fluorescence in situ hybridization for trisomy 12 on archival ovarian sex cord-stromal tumors. Gynecol Oncol 1994;55:349–54.
35. D'Angelo E, Mozos A, Nakayama D, et al. Prognostic significance of FOXL2 mutation and mRNA expression in adult and juvenile granulosa cell tumors of the ovary. Mod Pathol 2011;24:1360–7.
36. Lack EE, Perez-Atayde AR, Murthy AS, et al. Granulosa theca cell tumors in premenarchal girls. A clinical and pathologic study of ten cases. Cancer 1981;48:1846–54.
37. Zaloudek C, Norris HJ. Granulosa tumors of the ovary in children. A clinical and pathologic study of 32 cases. Am J Surg Pathol 1982;6:503–12.
38. Calaminus C, Wessalowski R, Harms D, Gobel U. Juvenile granulosa cell tumors of the ovary in children and adolescents: results from 33 patients registered in a prospective cooperative study. Gynecol Oncol 1997;65:447–52.
39. Schneider DT, Calaminus G, Wessalowski R, et al. Therapy of advanced ovarian juvenile granulosa cell tumors. Klin Padiatr 2002;214:173–8.
40. Bjorkholm E, Silversward C. Theca cell tumors. Clinical features and prognosis. Acta Radiol Oncol 1980;19:241–4.
41. Young RH, Clement PB, Scully RE. Calcified thecomas in young women. A report of four cases. Int J Gynecol Pathol 1988;7:343–50.
42. Zhang J, Young RH, Arseneau J, Scully RE. Ovarian stromal tumors containing lutein or Leydig cells (luteinized thecomas and stromal Leyding cell tumors). A clinicopathological analysis of fifty cases. Int J Gynecol Pathol 1982;1:270–85.
43. Clement PB, Young RH, Hanna W, Scully RE. Sclerosing peritonitis associated with luteinized thecomas of the ovary. A clinicopathological analysis of six cases. Am J Surg Pathol 1994;18:1–13.
44. Staats PN, McCluggage WG, Clement PB, Young RH. Luteinized thecomas (thecomatosis) of the type typically associated with sclerosing peritonitis: a clinical, histopathologic, and immunohistochemical analysis of 27 cases. Am J Surg Pathol 2008;32:1273–90.
45. Hughesdon PE. Lipid cell thecomas of the ovary. Histopathology 1983;7:681–92.
46. Roth LM, Sternberg WH. Partly luteinized theca cell tumor of the ovary. Cancer 1983;51:1697–704.
47. Tsuji T, Catasus L, Prat J. Is loss of heterozygosity at 9q22.3 (PTCH gene) and 19p13.3 (STK11 gene) involved in the pathogenesis of ovarian stromal tumors? Hum Pathol 2005;36:792–6.
48. Prat J, Scully RE. Cellular fibromas and fibrosarcoma of the ovary: a comparative clinicopathologic analysis of seventeen cases. Cancer 1981;47:2663–70.
49. Irving JA, Alkushi A, Young RH, Clement PB. Cellular Fibromas of the ovary: a study of 75 cases including 40 mitotically active tumors emphasizing their distinction from fibrosarcoma. Am J Surg Pathol 2006;30:928–38.
50. Dockerty MB, Masson JV. Ovarian fibromas: a clinical and pathologic study of two hundred and eighty three cases. Am J Obstet Gynecol 1944;47:741–52.
51. Meigs JV. Fibroma of the ovary with ascites and hydrothorax. Meigs' syndrome. Am J Obstet Gynecol 1954;67:962–87.
52. Gorlin RJ. Nevoid basal-cell carcinoma syndrome. Medicine (Baltim) 1987;66:98–113.
53. Domingo P, Montiel JA, Monill JM, Prat J. Pseudo-Meigs syndrome with elevated CA125 levels. Arch Intern Med 1998;158:1378–9.
54. Tsuji T, Kawauchi S, Utsunomiya T, et al. Fibrosarcoma versus cellular fibroma of the ovary: A comparative study of their proliferative activity and chromosome aberrations using MIB-1 immunostaining, DNA flow cytometry, and fluorescence in situ hybridization. Am J Surg Pathol 1997;21:52–9.
55. Chalvardjian A, Scully RE. Sclerosing stromal tumors of the ovary. Cancer 1973;31:664–70.
56. Zekioglu O, Ozdemir N, Terek C, et al. Clinicopathological and immunohistochemical analysis of sclerosing stromal tumours of the ovary. Arch Gynecol Obstet 2010;282:671–6.
57. Cashell AW, Cohen ML. Masculinizing sclerosing stromal tumor of the ovary during pregnancy. Gynecol Oncol 1991;43:281–5.
58. Tiltman AJ, Haffajee Z. Sclerosing stromal tumors, thecomas, and fibromas of the ovary: an immunohistochemical profile. Int J Gynecol Pathol 1999;18:254–8.
59. Kawauchi S, Tsuji T, Kaku T, et al. Sclerosing stromal tumor of the ovary: a clinicopathologic, immunohistochemical, ultrastructural, and cytogenetic analysis with special reference to its vasculature. Am J Surg Pathol 1998;22:83–92.
60. Moulla A, Giakoustidis D, Leontsini M. Sclerosing stromal tumors of the ovary: a clinicopathologic, immunohistochemical and cytogenetic analysis of three cases. Eur J Gynaecol Oncol 2004;25:257–60.
61. Ramzy I. Signet-ring stromal tumor of ovary. Histochemical, light, and electron microscopic study. Cancer 1976;38:166–72.
62. Suárez A, Palacios J, Burgos E, Gamallo C. Signet-ring stromal tumor of the ovary: a histochemical, immunohistochemical and ultrastructural study. Virchows Arch A 1993;422:333–6.
63. Dickersin GR, Young RH, Scully RE. Signet-ring stromal and related tumors of the ovary. Ultrastructural Pathol 1995;19:401–19.
64. Vang R, Bagué S, Tavassoli FA, Prat J. Signet ring stromal tumor of the ovary: clinicopathologic analysis with comparison to Krukenberg tumor. Int J Gynecol Pathol 2003;23:45–51.
65. Irving JA, Young RH. Microcystic stromal tumor of the ovary: report of 16 cases of a hitherto uncharacterized distinctive ovarian neoplasm. Am J Surg Pathol 2009;33:367–75.
66. Maeda D, Shibahara J, Sakuma T, et al. β-catenin (CTNNB1) S33C mutation in ovarian microcystic stromal tumors. Am J Surg Pathol 2011;35:1429–40.
67. Tavassoli FA, Norris HJ. Sertoli tumors of the ovary. A clinicopathologic study of 28 cases with ultrastructural observations. Cancer 1980;46:2281–97.
68. Young RH, Scully RE. Ovarian Sertoli cell tumors. A report of ten cases. Int J Gynecol Pathol 1984;2:349–63.
69. Oliva EA, Alvarez T, Young RH. Sertoli cell tumors of the ovary. A clinicopathological and immunohistochemical study of 54 cases. Am J Surg Pathol 2005;29:143–56.
70. Ferry J, Young RE, Engel G, Scully RE. Oxyphil Sertoli cell tumor of the ovary: a report of three cases, two in patients with the Peutz-Jeghers syndrome. Int J Gynecol Pathol 1994;13:259–66.
71. Tracy SL, Askin FB, Reddick RL, et al. Progesterone secreting Sertoli cell tumor of the ovary. Gynecol Oncol 1985;22:85–96.
72. Zhao C, Bratthauer GL, Barner R, Vang R. Diagnostic Utility of WT1 immunostaining in ovarian Sertoli cell tumor. Am J Surg Pathol 2007;31:1378–86.
73. Zhao C, Barner R, Vinh TN, et al. SF-1 is a diagnostically useful immunohistochemical marker and comparable to other sex cord-stromal tumor markers for the differential diagnosis of ovarian Sertoli cell tumor. Int J Gynecol Pathol 2008;27:507–14.
74. Young RH, Prat J, Scully RE. Ovarian endometrioid carcinomas resembling sex cord-stromal tumors. A clinicopathologic analysis of 13 cases. Am J Surg Pathol 1982;6:513–22.
75. Ordi J, Schammel DP, Rasekh L, Tavassoli FA. Sertoliform endometrioid carcinomas of the ovary: a clinicopathologic and immunohistochemical study of 13 cases. Mod Pathol 1999;12:933–40.

76. Roth LM, Anderson MC, Govan AD, et al. Sertoli-Leydig cell tumors. A clinicopathologic study of 34 cases. Cancer 1981;48: 187–97.
77. Zaloudek C, Norris HJ. Sertoli-Leydig tumors of the ovary. A clinico-pathologic study of 64 intermediate and poorly differentiated neoplasms. Am J Surg Pathol 1984;8:405–18.
78. Young RH, Scully RE. Ovarian Sertoli-Leydig cell tumors. A clinicopathological analysis of 207 cases. Am J Surg Pathol 1985;9: 543–69.
79. Gui T, Cao D, Shen K, et al. A clinicopathological analysis of 40 cases of ovarian Sertoli-Leydig cell tumors. Gynecol Oncol 2012;127:384–9.
80. Rio Frio T, Bahubeshi A, Kanellopoulou C, et al. *DICER1* mutations in familial multinodular goiter with and without ovarian Sertoli-Leydig cell tumors. JAMA 2011;305:68–77.
81. Gagnon S, Tetu B, Silva EG, McCaughey WTE. Frequency of alpha-fetoprotein production by Sertoli-Leydig cell tumors of the ovary: an immunohistochemical study of eight cases. Mod Pathol 1989;2:63–7.
82. Prat J, Young RH, Scully RE. Ovarian Sertoli-Leydig cell tumors with heterologous elements. II. Cartilage and skeletal muscle: A clinicopathologic analysis of twelve cases. Cancer 1982;50: 2465–75.
83. Young RH, Scully RE. Ovarian Sertoli-Leydig cell tumors with retiform pattern: a problem in histopathologic diagnosis. Am J Surg Pathol 1983;77:755–71.
84. Roth LM, Slayton RE, Brady LW, et al. Retiform differentiation in ovarian Sertoli–Leydig cell tumors. A clinicopathologic study of six cases from a gynecologic oncology group study. Cancer 1985;55:1093–8.
85. Mooney EE, Nogales FF, Bergeron C, Tavassoli FA. Retiform Sertoli-Leydig cell tumors: clinical, morphological and immunohistochemical findings. Histopathology 2002;41:110–17.
86. Young RH, Prat J, Scully RE. Ovarian Sertoli–Leydig cell tumors with heterologous elements. I. Gastrointestinal epithelium and carcinoid: a clinicopathologic analysis of thirty-six cases. Cancer 1982;50:2448–56.
87. Young RH, Scully RE. Well-differentiated ovarian Sertoli-Leydig cell tumors. A clinicopathological analysis of 23 cases. Int J Gynecol Pathol 1984;3:277–90.
88. Young RH, Pérez-Atayde AR, Scully RE. Ovarian Sertoli-Leydig cell tumor with retiform and heterologous components. Report of a case with hepatocytic differentiation and elevated serum alpha-fetoprotein. Am J Surg Pathol 1984;8:709–18.
89. Mooney EE, Nogales FF, Tavassoli FA. Hepatocytic differentiation in retiform Sertoli-Leydig cell tumors: distinguishing a heterologous element from Leydig cells. Hum Pathol 1999;30:611–17.
90. Heravi-Moussavi A, Anglesio MS, Cheng SW, et al. Recurrent somatic DICER1 mutations in nonepithelial ovarian cancers. N Engl J Med 2012;366:234–42.
91. Schultz KA, Pacheco MC, Yang J, et al. Ovarian sex cord-stromal tumors, pleuropulmonary blastoma and DICER1 mutations: a report from the International Pleuropulmonary Blastoma Registry. Gynecol Oncol 2011;122:246–50.
92. Scully RE. Sex cord tumor with annular tubules. A distinctive ovarian tumor of the Peutz-Jeghers syndrome. Cancer 1970;25:1107–21.
93. Young RH, Welch WR, Dickersin GR, Scully RE. Ovarian sex cord tumor with annular tubules: review of 74 cases including 27 with Peutz–Jeghers syndrome and 4 with adenoma malignum of the cervix. Cancer 1982;50:1384–402.
94. Connolly DC, Katabuchi H, Cliby WA, Cho KR. Somatic mutations in the STK11/LKB1 gene are uncommon in rare gynecological tumor types associated with Peutz-Jegher's syndrome. Am J Pathol 2000;156:339–45.
95. Kato N, Romero M, Catasus L, Prat J. STK11/LKB1 Peutz-Jegher's gene is not involved in the pathogenesis of sporadic sex cord-stromal tumors although LOH at 19p13.3 indicates another gene alterations in these tumors. Hum Pathol 2004;35:1101–4.
96. Paraskevas M, Scully RE. Hilus cell tumor of the ovary. A clinicopathological analysis of 12 Reinke crystal-positive and 9 crystal-negative cases. Int J Gynecol Pathol 1989;8:299–310.
97. Scully RE. Stromal luteoma of the ovary. A distinctive type of lipoid-cell tumor. Cancer 1964;17:769–78.
98. Hayes MC, Scully RE. Stromal luteoma of the ovary: a clinicopathologic analysis of 25 cases. Am J Surg Pathol 1987;6:313–21.
99. Chico A, Garcia JL, Matias-Guiu X, et al. A gonadotropin dependent stromal luteoma: a rare cause of post-menopausal virilization. Clin Endocrinol 1995;43:645–9.
100. Liu G, Duranteau L, Carel JC, et al. Leydig-cell tumor caused by an activating mutation of the gene encoding the luteinizing hormone receptor. N Engl J Med 1999;341:1731–6.
101. Hayes MC, Scully RE. Ovarian steroid cell tumor (not otherwise specified): a clinicopathological analysis of 63 cases. Am J Surg Pathol 1987;11:835–45.
102. Young RH, Scully RE. Ovarian steroid cell tumors associated with Cushing's syndrome. A report of three cases. Int J Gynecol Pathol 1987;6:40–8.
103. Jones MW, Harri R, Dabbs DJ, Carter GJ. Immunohistochemical profile of steroid cell tumor of the ovary: a study of 14 cases and a review of the literature. Int J Gynecol Pathol. 2010;29: 315–20.
104. Rubin DK, Frost JK. The cytologic detection of ovarian cancer. Acta Cytol 1963;7:191–5.
105. Rome RM, Laverty CR, Brown JB. Ovarian tumours in postmenopausal women. Clinicopathological features and hormonal studies. J Obstet Gynecol Br Commonw 1973;80:984–91.
106. Morris JM, Scully RE. Tumors with 'functioning' stroma. In: Endocrine pathology of the ovary. St. Louis, MO: Mosby; 1958. p. 131.
107. Matias-Guiu X, Prat J. Ovarian tumors with functioning stroma. An immunohistochemical study of 100 cases with human chorionic gonadotropin monoclonal and polyclonal antibodies. Cancer 1990;65:2001–5.
108. Rome RM, Fortune DW, Quinn MA, Brown JB. Functioning ovarian tumors in postmenopausal women. Obstet Gynecol 1981;57:705–10.
109. Scully RE. Ovarian tumors with functioning stroma. In: Fox H, editor. Haines and Taylor obstetrical and gynaecological pathology, vol. 2. 4th ed. Edinburgh: Churchill Livingstone; 1995.
110. Rutgers JL, Scully RE. Functioning ovarian tumors with peripheral steroid cell proliferation: a report of twenty-four cases. Int J Gynecol Pathol 1986;5:319–37.
111. Zaloudek CJ, Tavassoli FA, Norris HJ. Dysgerminoma with syncytiotrophoblastic giant cells. A histologically and clinically distinctive subtype of dysgerminoma. Am J Surg Pathol 1981;5:361–7.
112. Dickersin GR, Kline IW, Scully RE. Small cell carcinoma of the ovary with hypercalcemia: a report of eleven cases. Cancer 1982;49:188–97.
113. Aguirre P, Thor AD, Scully RE. Ovarian small cell carcinoma. Histogenetic considerations based on immunohistochemical and other findings. Am J Clin Pathol 1989;92:140–9.
114. Matias-Guiu X, Prat J, Young RH, et al. Human parathyroid hormone-related protein in ovarian small cell carcinoma. Cancer 1994;73:1878–81.
115. Robboy SJ, Scully RE. Strumal carcinoid of the ovary: an analysis of 50 cases of a distinctive tumor composed of thyroid tissue and carcinoid. Cancer 1980;46:2019–34.
116. Robboy SJ, Norris HJ, Scully RE. Insular carcinoid primary in the ovary: a clinicopathologic analysis of 48 cases. Cancer 1975;36: 404–18.
117. Aguirre P, Scully RE, Dayal Y, DeLellis RA. Mucinous tumors of the ovary with argyrophil cells. An immunohistochemical analysis. Am J Surg Pathol 1984;8:345–56.
118. Boixeda D, Roman AL, Pascasio JM, et al. Zollinger–Ellison syndrome due to gastrin-secreting ovarian cystadenocarcinoma. Case report. Acta Chir Scand 1990;156:409–10.
119. Kallenberg GA, Pesce CM, Norman B, et al. Ectopic hyperprolactinemia resulting from an ovarian teratoma. JAMA 1990;263: 2472–4.
120. Palmer PE, Bogojavlensky S, Bhan AK, Scully RE. Prolactinoma in wall of ovarian dermoid cyst with hyperprolactinemia. Obstet Gynecol 1990;75:540–3.
121. Ashton MA. Strumal carcinoid of the ovary associated with hyperinsulinemic hypoglycemia and cutaneous melanosis. Histopathology 1995;27:463–7.
122. Anderson PW, d'Ablaing G, Penny R, et al. Secretion of prorenin by a virilizing ovarian tumor. Gynecol Oncol 1992;45:58–61.
123. Fox R, Eckford S, Hirschowitz L, et al. Refractory gestational hypertension due to a renin-secreting ovarian fibrothecoma associated with Gorlin's syndrome. Br J Obstet Gynaecol 1994;101: 1015–17.

29 Ovarian Germ Cell Tumors

Jaime Prat

CHAPTER OUTLINE

General Features	670	Immature Teratomas	681
Dysgerminoma	671	Monodermal Teratomas	683
Yolk Sac Tumor (Primitive Endodermal Tumor)	674	Carcinoma in Dermoid Cysts	688
		Mixed Malignant Germ Cell Tumors	688
Embryonal Carcinoma	678	Mixed Germ Cell Sex Cord-Stromal Tumor	688
Polyembryoma	678		
Nongestational Choriocarcinoma	679	Gonadoblastoma	688
Teratomas	679		
Mature Teratomas	679		

GENERAL FEATURES

Germ cell tumors arise from primordial germ cells and account for approximately 30% of all ovarian tumors. Over 95% of them are benign dermoid cysts (mature cystic teratomas) and the remaining 5% are malignant. Malignant germ cell tumors (MGCTs) represent approximately 3% of all ovarian cancers in Western countries and about 20% in Asian and African populations, where surface epithelial cancers are much less common.[1]

Germ cell tumors replicate in a distorted form various stages of normal embryogenesis and, like the embryo, are capable of developing complex and highly differentiated tissues.[2] The malignant potential of ovarian germ cell tumors is inversely related to their degree of differentiation. Some traditional views on the histogenesis of germ cell tumors have been recently challenged. Although germ cell tumors of the ovary are morphologically similar to testicular germ cell tumors, they may not necessarily have an identical origin.[3] Testicular germ cell tumors originate from primitive germ cells with a malignant character, whereas ovarian germ cell tumors have a parthenogenetic origin from postmeiotic or meiotic cells.[4] For this reason, embryonal carcinoma (EC) occurs more frequently in the testis than the ovary. Nevertheless, an unknown percentage of MGCTs developing in phenotypic females may, in fact, represent testicular germ cell tumors (seminomas, ECs, mixed germ cell tumors), as they may have originated from the malignant germ cell component of gonadoblastomas present in dysgenetic gonads of patients with an unrecognized Y chromosome-containing genotype.[5] Rarely, germ cell tumors may arise from pre-existing somatic neoplasms of the female genital tract.[6–9] In these cases, the teratoid tumors derive most likely from a pluripotent stem cell population of somatic neoplasms. Recent evidence suggests that germinomas may not be end-stage tumors, as traditionally believed, but some of them could be precursors to germ cell neoplasms capable of further differentiation.[10–15] The occasional morphologic overlap between the primitive or immature forms of germ cell tumors, such as germinoma, EC, and yolk sac tumor (YST), supports the view that these tumors constitute a closely related group of neoplasms capable of embryonic or extraembryonic differentiation.[10,16] The new concepts of tumor histogenesis have been represented in a tridimensional tetrahedron model of inter-relationships between the different components (Figure 29.1). Nevertheless, the most popular histogenetic scheme[17] (shown in Figure 29.2) forms the basis for the current World Health Organization (WHO) classification of ovarian germ cell tumors (Table 29.1).[18]

MGCTs generally occur in younger women (75% in women under 30 years) and account for two-thirds of ovarian cancers in the first two decades.[1,19] The tumors are usually large (median size is 16 cm). Bilateral tumors are rare except dysgerminomas (10–20% bilaterality). Abdominal enlargement and pelvic pain are the most common presenting symptoms. Teenagers who present with abdominal masses and who have never menstruated should be evaluated for the possibility of a gonadoblastoma that has undergone malignant progression. Preoperative karyotyping can be helpful to identify underlying chromosomal abnormalities. Human chorionic gonadotropin (hCG) and α-fetoprotein (AFP) levels are useful markers in the diagnosis and in monitoring the postoperative course of these

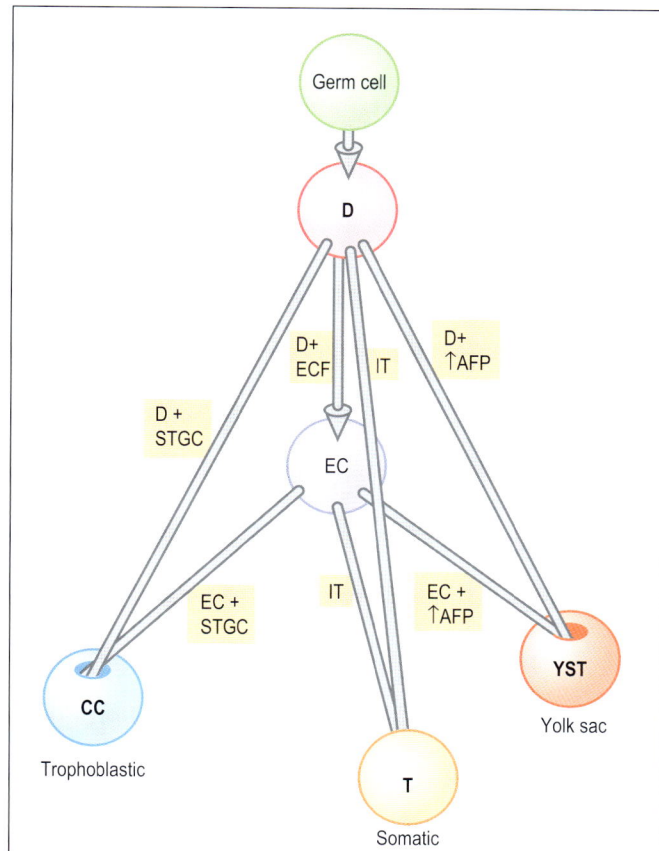

Figure 29.1 Tetrahedron model of germ cell histogenesis. D, dysgerminoma; D+ECF, dysgerminoma with early carcinomatous features; EC, embryonal carcinoma; D+STGC, dysgerminoma with syncytiotrophoblastic giant cells; D+↑AFP, dysgerminoma with elevated α-fetoprotein; IT, immature teratoma; EC+STGC, embryonal carcinoma with syncytiotrophoblastic giant cells; EC+↑AFP, embryonal carcinoma with elevated α-fetoprotein; CC, choriocarcinoma; T, mature teratoma; YST, yolk sac tumor.[11] (Modified with permission of Taylor & Francis.)

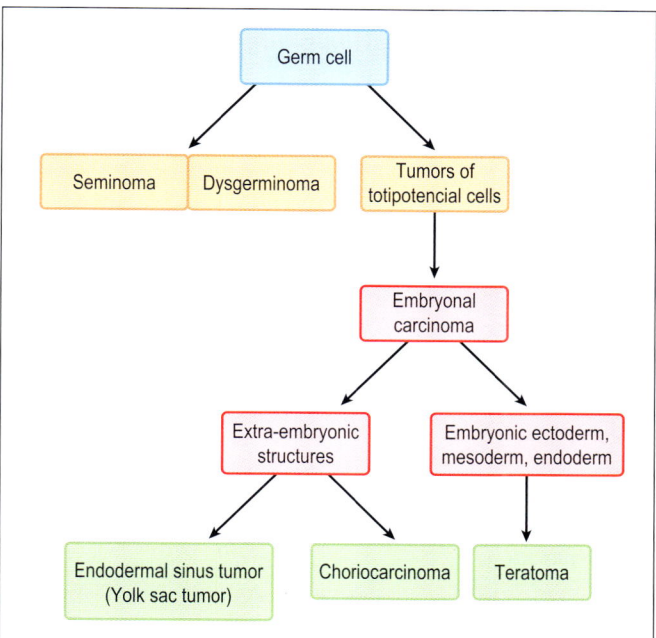

Figure 29.2 Germ cell tumors. Traditional histogenetic scheme.[17] (Data from Teilum G. Special tumors of the ovary and testis. Comparative pathology and histological identification. JB Lippincott, Philadelphia, 1976: p. 68)

patients. Moreover, recent stem cell research has provided several highly diagnostic pluripotency markers, including transcription factors and cytoplasmic/membranous proteins that are sequentially expressed in MGCTs according to their differentiation stage.[20,21]

MGCTs are now frequently cured by fertility-sparing surgery and combination chemotherapy including bleomycin, etoposide, and cisplatin.[22] For patients with advanced stage disease, maximum cytoreductive surgery appears to be beneficial. About 60–75% of women have stage I disease and 25–30% have stage III disease. For patients with early stage disease, cure rates approach 100%. For those with advanced stage disease, cure rates are reportedly at least 75%.[22]

The relative frequencies of the various types of MGCTs are shown in Table 29.2. Most MGCTs occur in a pure form, but approximately 15% of cases contain two or more types. The prognosis of patients with a mixed MGCT usually reflects that of its most malignant component. Therefore, it is important to sample these tumors extensively, particularly areas with different gross appearance. One section per every centimeter in tumor diameter is recommended. Most

MGCTs are composed of primitive tissues (i.e., dysgerminoma, YST); less frequently, malignant neoplasms of the adult type arise in dermoid cysts, usually in older patients.

DYSGERMINOMA

Clinical Features

Dysgerminoma is one of the most common MGCTs of the ovary, but it accounts for only 1–2% of all ovarian cancers. They occur almost exclusively in children and young women. The average patient age is 22 years.[23] Most patients present with a rapidly growing abdominal mass that often causes lower abdominal pain or pressure and may simulate pregnancy. Premenarchal patients with a pelvic mass should have their karyotype determined, as approximately 5% of dysgerminomas arise from gonadoblastomas in phenotypic females with abnormal gonads. These patients have pure gonadal dysgenesis (46,XY, bilateral streak gonads) or mixed gonadal dysgenesis (45,X/46,XY, unilateral streak gonad, contralateral testis). The estimated risk of malignancy is 28% by the age of 20 years for the former patients and 19% risk by the same age for the latter. Therefore, prophylactic removal of the gonads is recommended in both groups of patients at an early age.[1] Almost all patients with dysgerminoma have elevated serum levels of lactic dehydrogenase (1 and 2 fractions) at presentation.[24] In rare cases (3–5%), dysgerminomas may produce hCG and these patients may present with endocrine symptoms that are characteristically estrogenic (menstrual irregularities, isosexual pseudoprecocity, pseudopregnancy), but rarely androgenic.[25] Serum levels of CA125, placental-like alkaline phosphatase (PLAP), and neuron-specific enolase (NSE) have been elevated in some cases. Paraneoplastic hypercalcemia has been described in

Table 29.1 WHO Histologic Classification of Ovarian Germ Cell Tumors

Dysgerminoma
   Variant–syncytiotrophoblast cells

Yolk Sac Tumor (Primitive Endodermal Tumor)
   Polyvesicular vitelline tumor
   Hepatoid
   Glandular
      Intestinal
      Endometrioid-like
   Parietal

Embryonal Carcinoma

Polyembryoma

Nongestational Choriocarcinoma

Teratomas
   Immature
   Mature (adult)
      Solid
      Cystic
      With secondary tumor
      Fetiform (homunculus)
   Monodermal
      Struma ovarii
      Carcinoid tumor
         Insular
         Trabecular
         Strumal carcinoid tumor
         Mucinous carcinoid tumor
      Neuroectodermal tumors
      Sebaceous tumors
      Others

Mixed Germ Cell Tumors

Gonadoblastoma
   With MGCTs

Mixed Germ Cell Sex Cord–Stromal Tumor

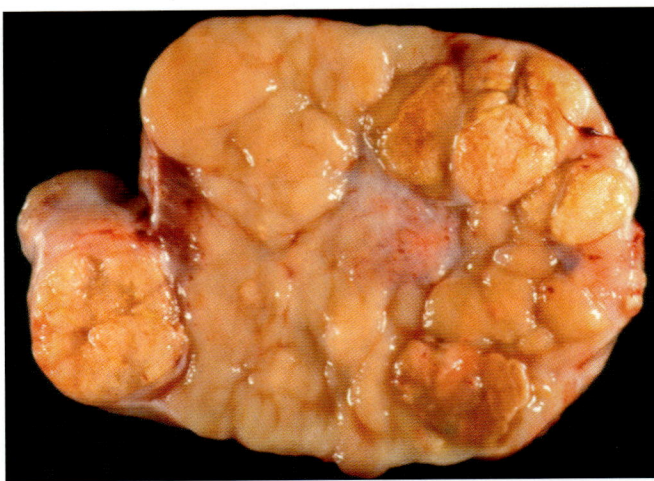

Figure 29.3 Dysgerminoma. The sectioned surface appears solid, yellowish white, and lobulated. Note the absence of significant hemorrhage and necrosis.

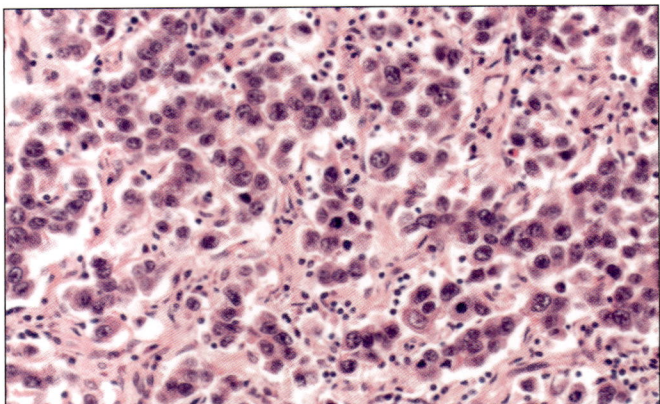

Figure 29.4 Dysgerminoma. The tumor cells are distributed in nests separated by delicate fibrous septa. The stroma contains numerous lymphocytes.

Table 29.2 Approximate Frequency of MGCTs of the Ovary

• Dysgerminoma	33%
• YST	10%
• EC	—
• Polyembryoma	—
• Choriocarcinoma	<1%
• Teratoma	
• Immature	36%
• Malignancy in dermoid cyst	5%
• Monodermal	—
• Mixed	15%

Macroscopic Features

Dysgerminomas are characteristically solid, and are well-encapsulated tumors with an average diameter of 15 cm. On section, they are lobulated, soft, and fleshy, and may appear gray-white or light tan (Figure 29.3). Areas of coagulative necrosis and hemorrhage typically associated with cystic change may be seen. Such areas should be sampled to rule out the presence of other types of MGCT. The presence of calcification suggests an underlying gonadoblastoma. Dysgerminoma is the only MGCT that has a significant rate of bilaterality. Gross involvement of the contralateral ovary is seen in 10% of cases, and in another 10% microscopic foci of tumor are found.[1]

Microscopic Features

The microscopic appearance of dysgerminoma is identical to that of testicular seminoma and extragonadal germinoma. It is composed of a monotonous population of rounded cells resembling primordial germ cells in a predominantly diffuse or insular arrangement. The cells may also grow as trabeculae, cords, or small nests (Figure 29.4).

some patients.[26] One tumor occurred in a patient with a germline *BRCA1* mutation.[27] About two-thirds of dysgerminomas are stage IA at diagnosis; higher stage tumors involve the contralateral ovary (20%), pelvic and para-aortic lymph nodes, and/or the pelvic and abdominal peritoneum.

Lack of intercellular cohesion may result in the formation of pseudoglandular spaces. The tumor cells are polygonal, with discrete cell membranes and abundant eosinophilic to clear, glycogen-rich, cytoplasm. The nuclei are large, central, and rounded, and they contain one or a few prominent nucleoli. Mitotic figures are often numerous. Aggregates of tumor cells are usually separated by thin fibrous septa almost always infiltrated by T-lymphocytes.[28] In some tumors, lymphocytes are abundant and may form follicles with germinal centers. In approximately 20% of the cases, epithelioid sarcoid-like granulomas with multinucleated giant cells are present (Figure 29.5).[1] About 5% of dysgerminomas contain syncytiotrophoblastic giant cells (SGCs) in the absence of any other non-germinomatous differentiation.[25] Such tumors, which have the same prognosis as dysgerminomas in which SGCs are absent, should be sampled extensively to rule out foci of choriocarcinoma or EC. The SGCs have a perivascular location, are immunoreactive for human chorionic gonadotropin (hCG)(Figure 29.6), and are often associated with stromal luteinization. The luteinized stromal cells, which may be admixed with the tumor cells or located at the periphery of the neoplasm,[29] are probably responsible for the estrogenic or androgenic symptoms that are found in some patients.

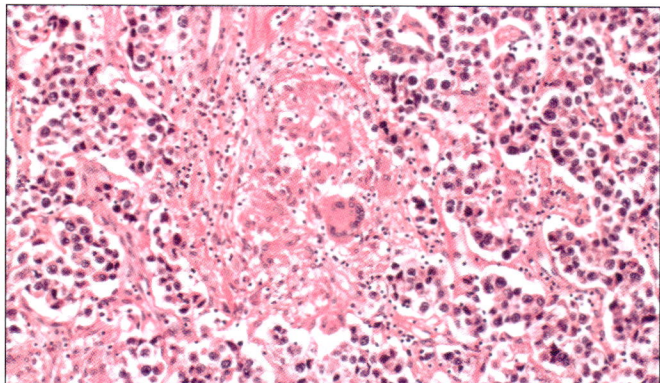

Figure 29.5 Dysgerminoma. A sarcoid-like granuloma is present.

Immunohistochemistry

Dysgerminoma cells show cytoplasmic and membranous immunoreaction for vimentin, PLAP, CD117 (*c-kit*), and D2-40 (podoplanin); the membranous reaction is characteristic of dysgerminoma.[30,31] There is nuclear immunoreaction for the stem cell/primitive germ cell nuclear transcription factors OCT3/4, NANOG, and SALL4[31–33] (Table 29.3). OCT3/4 is expressed very early during embryogenesis and has an essential role in blastocyst differentiation. However, when the female germ cells enter meiosis the expression of OCT3/4 is downregulated. OCT3/4 regularly shows positivity in dysgerminoma (Figure 29.7) but can also be expressed in EC and in some immature neural elements of ovarian teratoma.

SALL4 can also show positivity in EC, YST, and primitive areas of immature teratoma (IT).[33] Dysgerminomas may exhibit limited cytoplasmic dot- or rim-like staining for cytokeratin (Figure 29.8) but epithelial membrane antigen

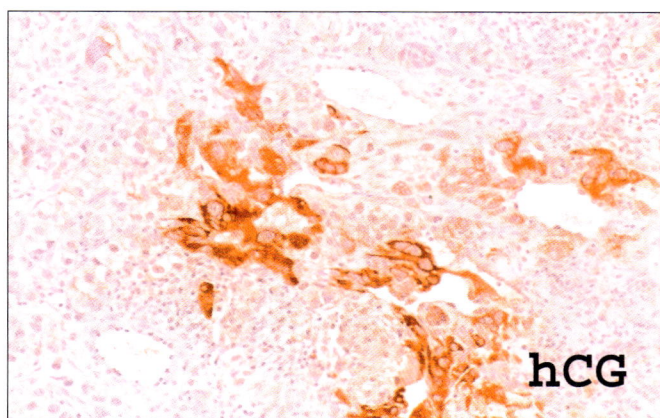

Figure 29.6 Dysgerminoma with syncytiotrophoblastic giant cells. Positive immunostain for hCG.

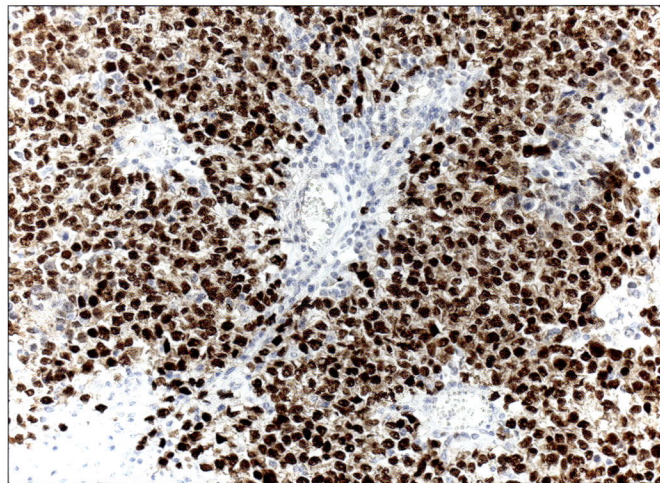

Figure 29.7 Dysgerminoma. OCT3/4-positive nuclear immunoreaction recognizes germ cells in poorly fixed specimen. (Courtesy of Dr. Francisco Nogales.)

Table 29.3 Immunohistochemical Markers for Ovarian Germ Cell Tumors

Marker	GB	DYS	EC	YST	IT	Choriocarcinoma
PLAP	+	+	±	±	±	±
SALL4	+	+	+	+	±	±
LIN28	+	+	+	+	±	±
OCT3/4	+	+	+	−	−	−
SOX2	−	−	+	−	+	−
D2-40	+	+	−	−	−	±
CD30	−	−	+	−	−	−
AFP	−	−	−	+	±	−
Glypican-3	−	−	−	+	±	±
β-hCG	−	−	−	−	−	+

GB, gonadoblastoma; DYS, dysgerminoma; EC, embryonal carcinoma; IT, immature teratoma; and YST, yolk sac tumor.

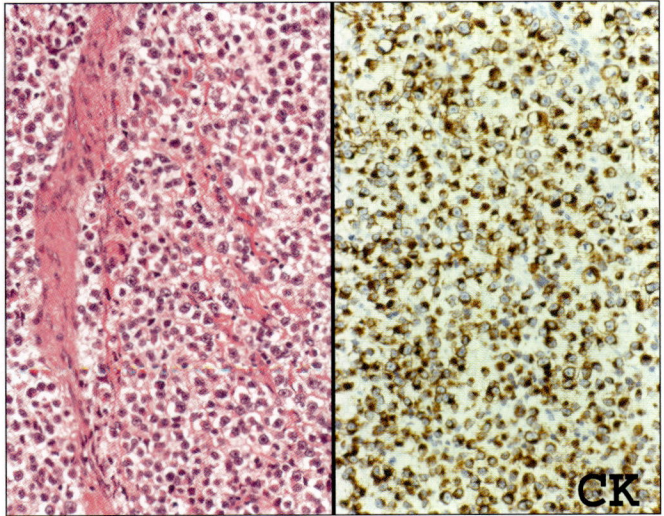

Figure 29.8 Dysgerminoma. Positive 'dot-like' immunostain for cytokeratin.

(EMA) is negative. The SGCs that are found in a small percentage of dysgerminomas exhibit positive cytoplasmic staining for hCG (Figure 29.6).

Somatic Genetics

Dysgerminomas, like seminomas, show by comparative genomic hybridization frequent (75%) chromosome 12p gain, usually in the form of an isochromosome 12p.[34] The *c-kit* gene encodes a tyrosine kinase receptor (KIT), which is required in normal spermatogenesis and is expressed in seminomas and dysgerminomas. *c-kit* point mutations localized to exon 17, codon 816 (Asp>Val), involving the phosphotransferase domain, have been identified in 25–50% of ovarian dysgerminomas.[35-37] The mutations are in exon 17, not in the exon 11 location, which confers susceptibility to imatinib therapy.

Genetic Susceptibility

Dysgerminoma is the most common malignant gonadal tumor in patients with gonadal dysgenesis and a Y chromosome. In these cases, the dysgerminoma typically arises in a gonadoblastoma.

Differential Diagnosis

Dysgerminoma should be distinguished from the solid type of YST, EC, clear cell carcinoma, and large cell lymphoma. The solid YST is almost always associated with other more typical patterns that are not seen in dysgerminomas. YSTs exhibit greater nuclear variation, contain hyaline bodies, immunoreact for AFP and glypican-3, and lack the lymphocytic infiltrate of dysgerminomas. Moreover, in contrast to dysgerminoma, YSTs fail to react for D2-40 and OCT3/4. The extremely rare EC shows larger cells with more ample nuclei that are more hyperchromatic and irregular than those of dysgerminoma. ECs are CD30 and cytokeratin positive, almost always contain SGCs, and lack the stromal infiltrate of lymphocytes. The distinction of dysgerminoma from clear cell carcinoma is discussed in Chapter 27. Large cell lymphomas may resemble dysgerminomas both grossly and microscopically. Lymphomas, however, are bilateral in approximately one-half of the cases, and simultaneous involvement of the ipsilateral tube occurs in 25% of them[38] (see Chapter 30). Careful attention to the nuclear features and immunostains for PLAP, D2-40, SALL4, and lymphoid markers facilitate the correct diagnosis. Poorly fixed dysgerminomas may occasionally be misdiagnosed as poorly differentiated carcinomas, as the cellular features of the former tumors are lost.

Treatment and Prognosis

The treatment of patients with dysgerminoma is primarily surgical, including the resection of the ovarian tumor and complete surgical staging. Given that the tumor mainly affects young females, for whom preservation of fertility is important, unilateral adnexectomy with frequent patient follow-up (every 2–3 months for the first 2–3 years) is the treatment of choice. This conservative approach is currently used in young patients even in the presence of metastasis.[39] Therefore, biopsy of an apparently normal contralateral ovary is not recommended as it increases the risk of infertility. Dysgerminoma is highly sensitive to chemotherapy, which is usually reserved for the treatment of recurrent disease.[23,40] Although these tumors are equally sensitive to radiotherapy, its use has been discontinued in an effort to preserve patient fertility, and cisplatin-based chemotherapy is currently preferred.[22] In young patients whose karyotype analysis reveals a Y chromosome, both ovaries should be removed.[1] When the patient's fertility is not a factor, hysterectomy with bilateral salpingo-oophorectomy is recommended; chemotherapy is subsequently administered in the case of higher stage tumors.[22] Postoperative work-up includes the serum markers AFP and hCG, chest X-ray, and abdominopelvic CT or MRI. Recurrence in the retained contralateral ovary can occur in 5–15% of cases over the next 2 years.[1] About 75% of the recurrences occur within the first postoperative year, and the most common sites are the peritoneal cavity and the retroperitoneal lymph nodes.[1]

Patients with dysgerminoma have an excellent prognosis. The 5 year survival rate is greater than 95% for patients with stage IA tumor, and 85% for those with advanced stage or recurrent tumor.[22] Features associated with recurrence include a tumor diameter greater than 10 cm, and age younger than 20 years.[41] Although the designation 'anaplastic dysgerminoma' has been applied to tumors with numerous mitoses, there is no evidence that such tumors are associated with a worse prognosis, and therefore this term is not recommended. Most dysgerminomas are nondiploid and ploidy is not a useful prognostic factor.[42]

YOLK SAC TUMOR (PRIMITIVE ENDODERMAL TUMOR)

Clinical Features

Yolk sac tumors (YSTs) (also referred to as *primitive endodermal tumors*) account for approximately 10% of MGCTs and are almost as common as dysgerminoma in patients under the age of 20 years.[1] They occur at a median age of 18 years and are rare over the age of 40 years.[1,43–45] Patients most frequently present with abdominal pain and a large, rapidly growing, pelvic mass. Rupture or torsion of the tumor occurs in about 10% of patients. YSTs consistently produce

AFP, which can be demonstrated in the patient's serum, usually at a level greater than 1000 ng/ml. This substance, which is normally produced in the yolk sac of the developing embryo, may serve as a tumor marker in monitoring the patient during and after therapy. Lower serum levels of AFP may be encountered in other tumors that also occur in young females such as IT and Sertoli–Leydig cell tumors (SLCTs). CA125 and carcinoembryonic antigen (CEA) are also elevated in 100% and 10% of YSTs, respectively. Rare examples of YST have occurred in older patients in association with mucinous or endometrioid tumors; in such cases, a somatic cell rather than a germ cell origin is almost certain.[6,8,9]

Yolk sac tumor is a highly malignant neoplasm. At laparotomy, evidence of extraovarian spread has been reported in 30–70% of cases.[44,45] In an older study,[46] subclinical metastases were present in 84% of cases regarded as 'stage I' tumors, which most likely reflects incomplete staging. When the tumor spreads beyond the ovary, it involves the omentum and peritoneum, the para-aortic lymph nodes, and the liver.

Macroscopic Features

Yolk sac tumors are large, well-encapsulated masses, with an average diameter of 15 cm. The external surface is usually smooth and glistening. The sectioned surface is characteristically solid and cystic and shows soft, gray to yellow tissue with extensive areas of hemorrhage and necrosis (Figure 29.9). When a polyvesicular vitelline component is present, the tumor shows a microcystic appearance.[1] Although YSTs are bilateral in less than 5% of patients, the contralateral ovary may contain a dermoid cyst in about 10% of cases.[1]

Microscopic Features

Although YSTs often exhibit a wide variety of microscopic patterns, most tumors have a reticular architecture reflecting extraembryonic differentiation.[46,47] They are composed of a network of irregular spaces lined by primitive epithelial cells with glycogen-rich, clear cytoplasm, and large, hyperchromatic nuclei with prominent nucleoli; mitotic figures are numerous (Figure 29.10). The most characteristic feature is the presence of isolated papillary projections with a central blood vessel and peripheral sleeve of embryonic epithelial cells (Schiller–Duval bodies; Figure 29.11). Cross sections of this structure once were erroneously compared with immature glomeruli (Schiller's mesonephroma).[48] In fact, they closely resemble invaginations of yolk sac endoderm, as seen best in the rat placenta, forming the endodermal sinuses of Duval.[46] Nevertheless, Schiller–Duval bodies are present in only 20% of cases.[47] The term 'endodermal sinus tumor' is misleading, since the endodermal sinus is neither a structure present in human embryogenesis nor a constant feature of these neoplasms. Accordingly, the designation primitive endodermal tumor has recently been proposed.[49] Another distinctive feature is the presence of brightly eosinophilic, periodic acid–Schiff (PAS)-positive, diastase-resistant hyaline globules (Figure 29.10). Occasionally, multiple small vesicles with eccentric constrictions resembling the yolk sac vesicle of the normal embryo are present, and the tumor is designated a polyvesicular vitelline tumor (Figure 29.12).[46,50,51] This pattern recapitulates the subdivision of the primary yolk sac vesicle into a large component lined by flat cells (vestigial primary yolk sac) and a

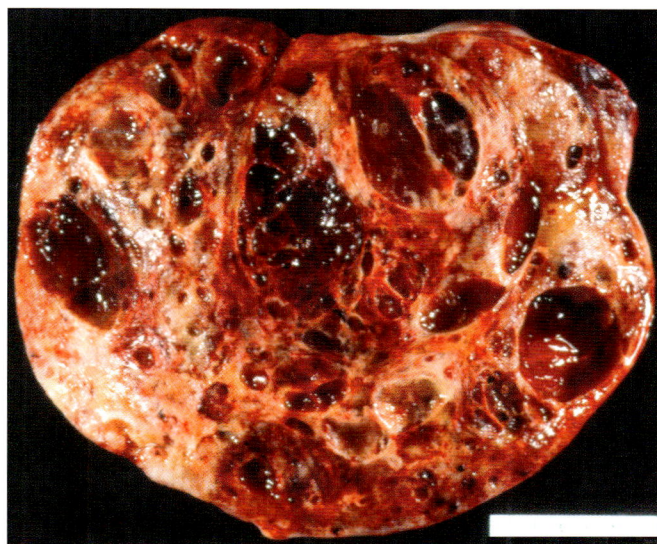

Figure 29.9 Yolk sac tumor. Solid and cystic tumor with extensive hemorrhage, necrosis, and gelatinous degeneration.

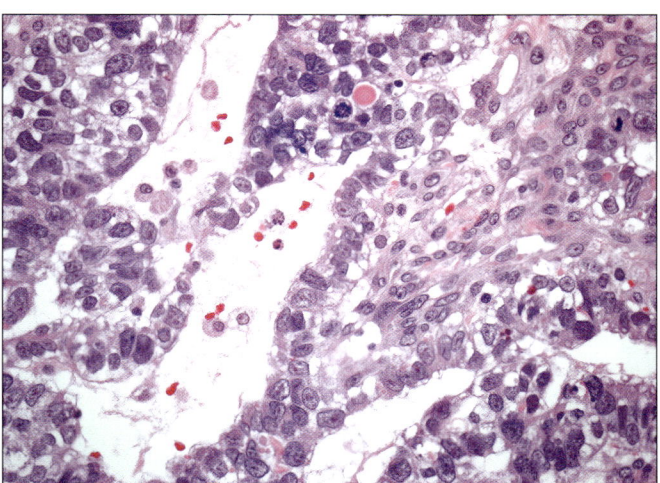

Figure 29.10 Yolk sac tumor. Reticular pattern. Irregular spaces lined by primitive epithelial cells with glycogen-rich, clear cytoplasm, and large, hyperchromatic nuclei with prominent nucleoli. A hyaline body is present (upper center). Mitotic figures are seen.

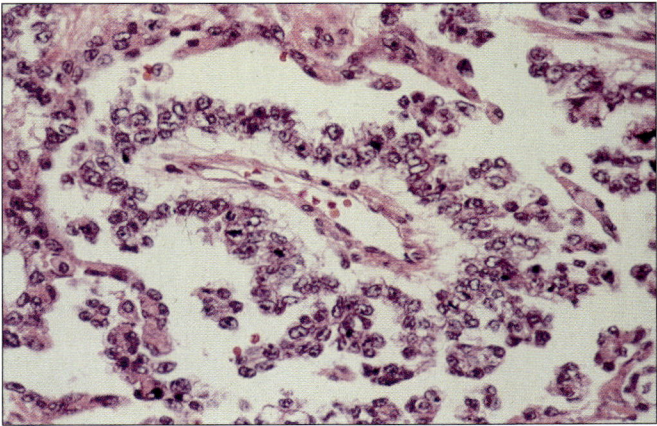

Figure 29.11 Yolk sac tumor. Schiller–Duval (glomeruloid) body. Central blood vessel and peripheral sleeve of embryonic epithelial cells.

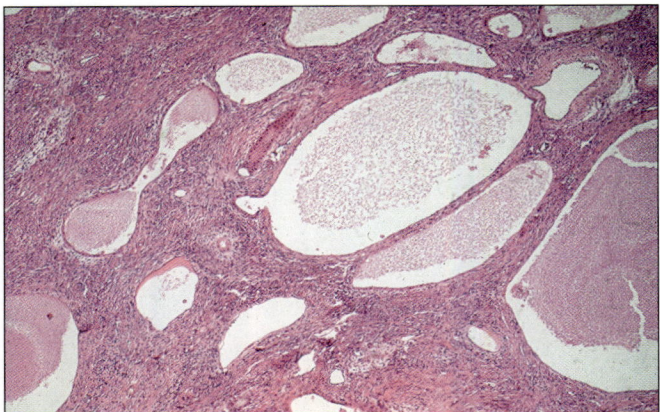

Figure 29.12 Yolk sac tumor, polyvesicular vitelline variant. The vesicles are lined by flattened epithelial cells and some of them exhibit eccentric constrictions.

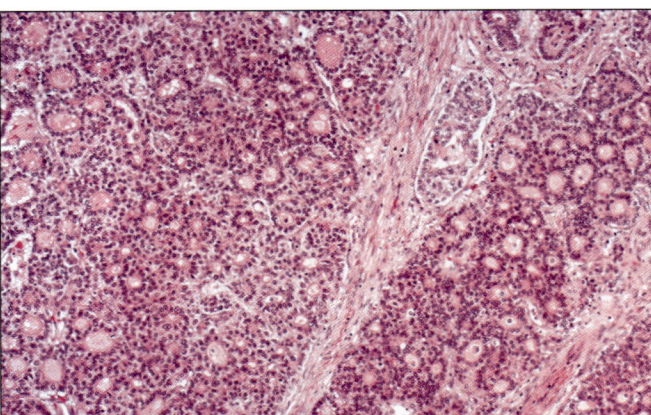

Figure 29.14 Yolk sac tumor, glandular variant, intestinal type. The tumor shows a cribriform pattern.

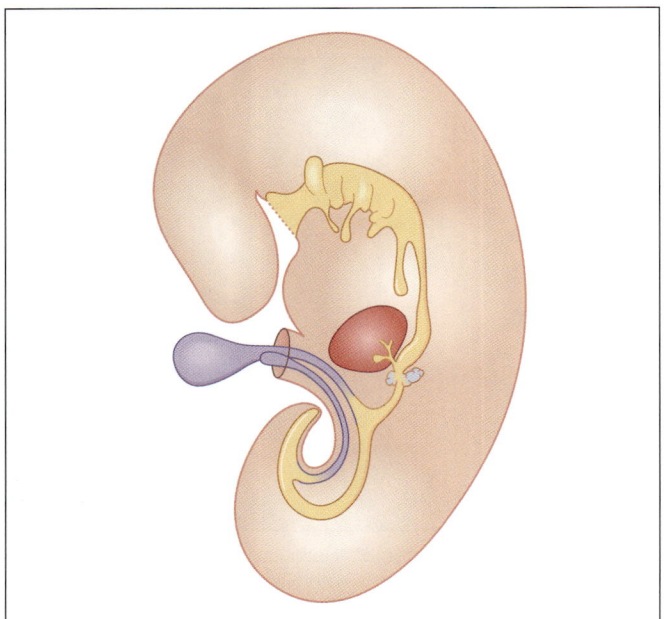

Figure 29.13 Diagram of a median longitudinal section through a 10 mm human embryo (about 6 weeks old). The primitive yolk sac (blue) is in continuity with the midgut. The rudiment of the liver and biliary tract appears attached to the ventral wall of the foregut. (Modified from Prat J, Pathology of the ovary. Saunders, Philadelphia, 2004. With permission.)

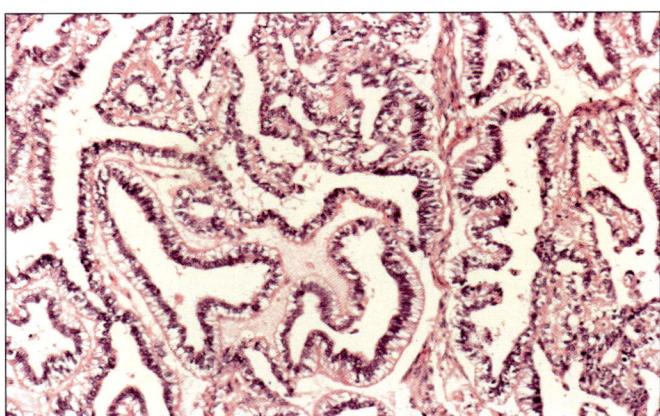

Figure 29.15 Yolk sac tumor, endometrioid-like glandular variant. The tumor glands resemble those of the secretory endometrium.

smaller component lined by taller epithelium that simulates the forerunner of the primitive gut and its appendages (secondary yolk sac vesicle) in normal embryogenesis (Figure 29.13). Like the normal yolk sac vesicle, the neoplastic yolk sac may give rise to tumors of embryonal type. These tumors recapitulate primitive gut (glandular YST) and primitive liver (hepatoid YST).[52–56]

Endodermal-type glands may be found in approximately 50% of YSTs, often admixed with reticular and polyvesicular vitelline components.[1] In some tumors, a glandular pattern predominates, and may appear as rounded cribriform aggregates of primitive epithelial cells ('intestinal' variant; Figure 29.14),[52] or glands of 'endometrioid' type, which can be mistaken for typical or secretory endometrioid adenocarcinoma (endometrioid-like variant; Figure 29.15);[53] foci of carcinoid tumor have been described in one of the latter tumors.[57] Occasionally, the mature intestinal component may give rise to a mucinous carcinoma.[58]

Although small foci of hepatoid differentiation are found in 16–48% of YSTs,[55,56] neoplasms with a predominant hepatoid component are infrequent.[54,59] These tumors are characterized by compact masses of large polyhedral cells with abundant eosinophilic cytoplasm, and round central nuclei with prominent single nucleoli, separated by thin fibrous bands, resembling hepatocellular carcinoma (Figure 29.16). Hyaline bodies are usually numerous. In some cases, glandular spaces containing mucin are present. Ultrastructural examination of hepatoid YSTs reveals features similar to hepatocellular carcinoma.[54] A 'parietal' differentiation characterized by small extracellular accumulations of basement membrane material has been described in over 90% of YSTs.[55] Rarely, YSTs may contain SGCs.

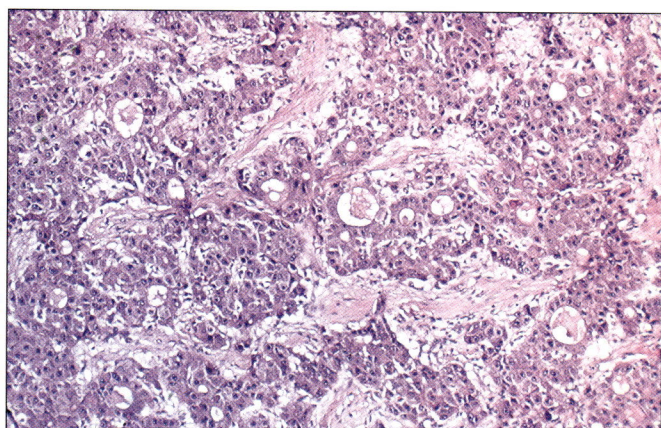

Figure 29.16 Yolk sac tumor, hepatoid variant. The tumor is composed of compact masses and nests of large polyhedral cells with abundant eosinophilic cytoplasm separated by a fibrous stroma. Note the striking resemblance to a hepatocellular carcinoma.

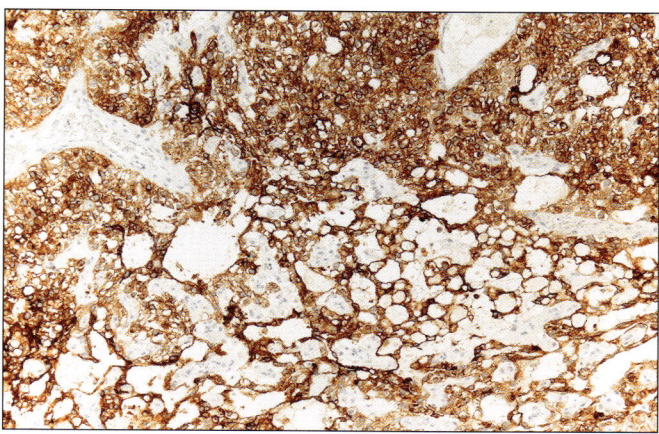

Figure 29.18 Yolk sac tumor. Glypican-3 immunoreaction delineates a clean microcystic pattern. (Courtesy of Dr. Francisco Nogales.)

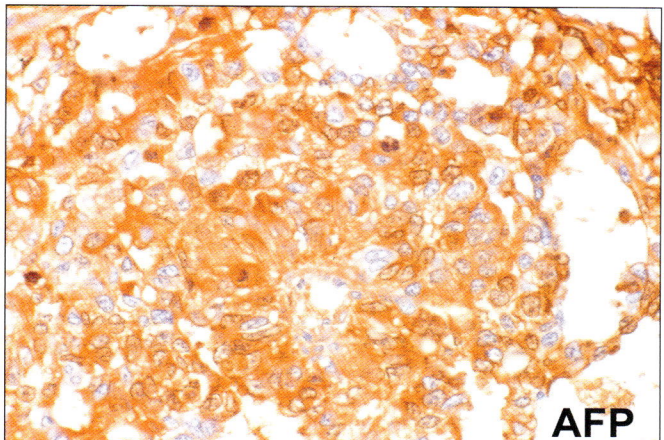

Figure 29.17 Yolk sac tumor. Schiller–Duval body exhibiting a strong immunoreaction for AFP.

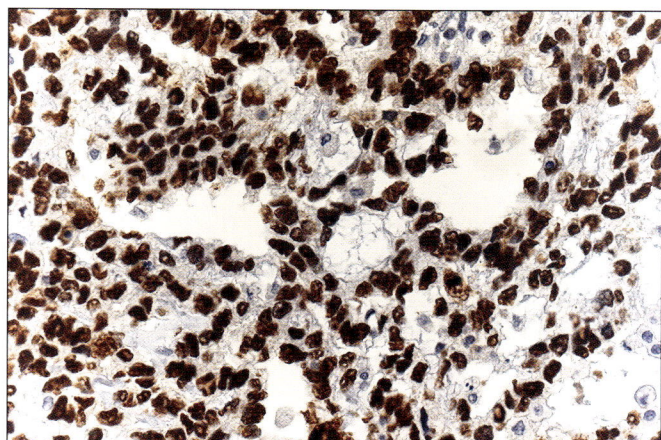

Figure 29.19 Yolk sac tumor. SALL4 nuclear immunoreaction in epithelial and in some mesenchymal cells. (Courtesy of Dr. Francisco Nogales.)

The loose stromal component of YST recapitulates the extraembryonic mesenchyme (magma reticulare),[46] and may be the site of origin of the sarcomas that develop in some patients after chemotherapy.[60,61]

Immunohistochemistry

Similar to the primitive gut (secondary yolk sac) and its appendages, YSTs are immunoreactive for AFP (Figure 29.17), glypican-3 (Figure 29.18), SALL4 (Figure 29.19), villin, CDX2, and hepatocyte paraffin antigen 1.[33] AFP is expressed often focally either as granular cytoplasmic deposits or delineating intracellular canaliculi. Glypican-3 immunoreaction is usually stronger than that of AFP;[62] however, it is not as specific since it is expressed by other germ cell tumors and clear cell carcinoma.[63] Nuclear transcription factor SALL4 is regularly expressed in both epithelium and mesenchyme[32] and there is cytoplasmic reactivity of RNA-binding protein LIN28.[64] Villin is also constantly expressed in membranes and cytoplasms of epithelial cells.

The different endodermal elements may be immunoreactive for their corresponding tissue markers, i.e., hepatic components for hepatocyte paraffin antigen 1,[65] intestinal elements for CDX2,[49] and foregut-derived epithelia for thyroid transcription factor 1.[33] However, YSTs are negative for OCT4, SOX2, D2-40, and CD30 (Table 29.3). Combined expression of AFP, glypican-3, villin, SALL4, or LIN28 makes an ideal panel for confirming the diagnosis.[49]

Differential Diagnosis

Because of their various microscopic patterns, YSTs can be confused with many other ovarian tumors, both primary and metastatic. The most common problems in differential diagnosis include clear cell carcinoma and endometrioid adenocarcinoma (see Chapter 27), the retiform variant of SLCT (see Chapter 28), and hepatoid carcinoma (see Chapter 27). YSTs should also be distinguished from other germ cell tumors such as dysgerminoma and the very rare EC. These differential diagnoses are discussed under those headings.

Treatment and Prognosis

The treatment of YST includes surgical exploration, unilateral salpingo-oophorectomy, and frozen section for diagnosis.[22,44] Although gross metastases should be removed, a thorough surgical staging is not necessary because all patients need chemotherapy.[44] Prior to combination chemotherapy, the prognosis for patients with YSTs was dismal despite apparently adequate surgery. In one large study of patients treated prior to 1975 the 3 year survival was only 13%.[47] The development of the vincristine, dactinomycin, and cyclophosphamide (VAC) combination chemotherapy dramatically changed the outlook for patients with YSTs. Currently, cisplatin-based chemotherapy provides still better results. Survival rates have approached 100% for patients with stage I tumors, and 75% for patients with higher stage tumors.[22] Serum AFP can be used to monitor the response to treatment and to detect tumor recurrence. Adverse prognostic factors include tumor stage II or higher, gross residual tumor after surgery, and ascitic fluid of more than 100 ml.[45] The good long-term outcome in two polyvesicular-vitelline tumor (PVVT) cases supports prior evidence that this form of YST may be more indolent than the conventional forms of the tumor.[51]

EMBRYONAL CARCINOMA

Embryonal carcinoma (EC) is a very rare ovarian tumor that is morphologically identical to EC of the testis. For many years, it was confused with YST, which it resembles.[66] From a histogenetic viewpoint, EC has been considered a pluripotent stem cell tumor capable of differentiating along different pathways.[67] The patients are young (median age, 12 years), present with an abdominal mass, and consistently have a positive pregnancy test as a result of hCG production by the tumor.[66] Premenarchal patients have endocrine manifestations in about half of the cases; usually, they include isosexual pseudoprecocity, irregular bleeding, amenorrhea, or hirsutism. Laparotomy reveals peritoneal spread in 40% of cases.[66] Grossly, ECs are large (17 cm), unilateral tumors that exhibit solid and variegated cut surfaces. Foci of hemorrhage and necrosis are common. Histologically, ovarian EC resembles testicular Embryonal carcinoma; it is composed of large primitive cells distributed in solid masses, often exhibiting central necrosis, gland-like spaces, and papillae. The nuclei are round and vesicular. Mitotic figures, including atypical forms, are numerous. Hyaline globules are usually present. SGCs immunoreactive for hCG are almost always present (Figure 29.20).

Embryonal carcinoma is most often found in the ovary as a component of a mixed germ cell tumor. The tumor cells are immunoreactive for cytokeratin, PLAP, CD30, NSE, AFP, and hCG. The last two substances can be used as tumor markers. Nuclear transcription factors OCT3/4 and SALL4 are positive and SOX2 is variably positive.[31,32,68] Immunoreaction for EMA is negative. Most ECs contain an isochromosome, i12p. EC should be distinguished from other MGCTs (dysgerminoma, YST), juvenile granulosa cell tumor (JGCT), and undifferentiated carcinomas in the surface-epithelial category. In contrast to EC, the last two tumors rarely produce AFP and usually lack SGCs. Unilateral

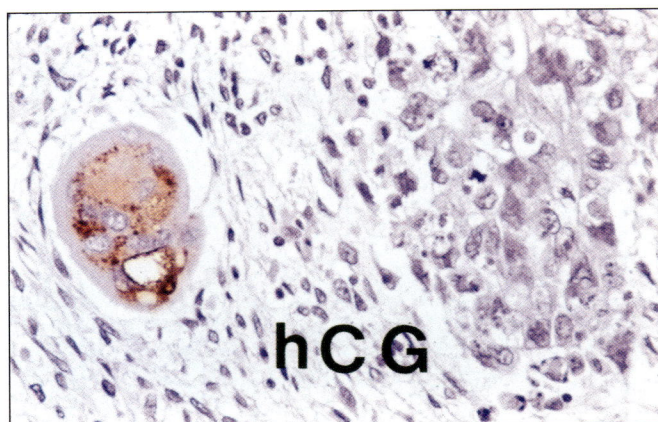

Figure 29.20 Embryonal carcinoma. A syncytiotrophoblastic giant cell shows positive immunostaining for hCG.

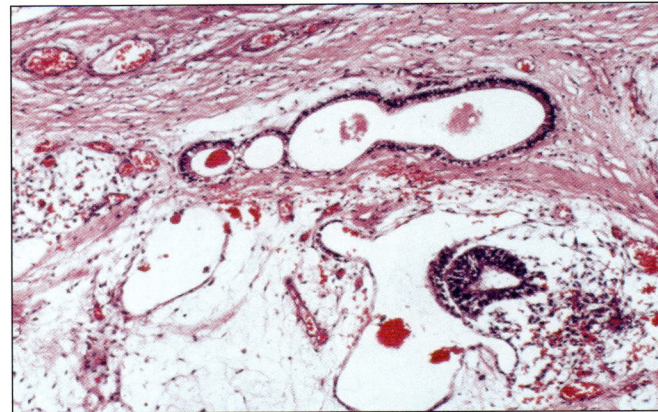

Figure 29.21 Polyembryoma. Embryoid body with embryonic disc (dark) and yolk sac vesicle. The yolk sac shows an eccentric constriction (secondary yolk sac) lined by a thicker epithelium. Enteric differentiation is seen (top).

salpingo-oophorectomy is the recommended surgical procedure. Although these tumors are highly malignant, cisplatin-based combination chemotherapy has resulted in some long-term survivors.

POLYEMBRYOMA

Rare cases of MGCT contain large numbers of embryoid bodies in various stages of development, typically distributed in a primitive mesenchymal stroma.[69–72] Only 15 ovarian polyembryomas have been reported in the English literature, most of them found as components of mixed germ cell tumors in children or young women.[72] Serum levels of AFP and hCG may be elevated. Grossly, polyembryomas are unilateral large tumors with a microcystic cut surface. Microscopically, the embryoid bodies resemble perfect or imperfect early embryos and contain germ discs, yolk sacs, amniotic cavities, chorionic elements, and extraembryonic mesenchyme in an edematous stroma (Figure 29.21). Well-differentiated enteric glands and mature or immature hepatic tissue, which may secrete bile, are found in some cases. The yolk sac components of the embryoid bodies and the nests of liver cells are immunoreactive for AFP. The behavior of polyembryomas is similar to that of other MGCTs. Conservative surgery and combination chemotherapy is the recommended treatment.

NONGESTATIONAL CHORIOCARCINOMA

Pure nongestational choriocarcinoma of the ovary is an exceedingly rare and highly malignant tumor that develops before puberty. It accounts for less than 1% of MGCTs.[1] More frequently, choriocarcinoma is seen as a component of a mixed MGCT[73] (only 45 pure cases have been reported).[74] Clinically, these patients present with abdominal enlargement and pain and, occasionally, there is hemoperitoneum simulating a tubal pregnancy.[75] The pregnancy test is positive and the elevated serum level of hCG may lead to isosexual pseudoprecocity in children or menstrual abnormalities in older patients.[75] Serum β-hCG levels range from hundreds to more than 2,000,000 mIU/ml.[74] Grossly, choriocarcinomas are large (4–25 cm), hemorrhagic, and friable tumors. Microscopically, much of the tumor is hemorrhagic and necrotic. The viable areas show cytotrophoblastic and syncytiotrophoblastic cells arranged in a plexiform pattern (Figure 29.22). The former cells are mononucleated with vesicular nuclei, abundant clear cytoplasm, and well-defined borders; the syncytiotrophoblastic cells have abundant vacuolated basophilic or amphophilic cytoplasm and several dark nuclei. In some tumors, the plexiform pattern may not be apparent.[1] Intermediate trophoblastic cells are present in some cases. Vascular invasion is frequent. The syncytiotrophoblastic cells are immunoreactive for hCG, cytokeratins, human placental lactogen, PLAP, EMA, CD10, CEA, α-inhibin, and GLP-3.

The clinical symptoms and histologic picture of germ cell-derived choriocarcinomas are similar to those of gestational choriocarcinoma; however, the remarkable response to chemotherapy (methotrexate or actinomycin D) associated with the latter tumors does not occur.[76] Although gestational choriocarcinomas of the ovary are almost invariably metastatic from uterine or tubal choriocarcinomas, they may occasionally follow an ovarian pregnancy.[1,75] The finding of a corpus luteum of pregnancy may be of help in establishing the gestational nature of the tumor. Similarly, the presence of a paternal component by DNA analysis or HLA typing is characteristic of gestational choriocarcinomas.[77–79] Rare cases of poorly differentiated carcinomas with choriocarcinomatous differentiation and hCG secretion have been reported.[8,80] Unilateral salpingo-oophorectomy followed by combination chemotherapy has resulted in cures or prolonged remissions.

TERATOMAS

Teratomas are germ cell tumors composed of an array of tissues derived from two or three embryonic layers (ectoderm, mesoderm, and endoderm) in any combination. The great majority of teratomas are benign cystic tumors that contain mature elements and are designated mature cystic teratomas or dermoid cysts. The presence of any immature tissue warrants a diagnosis of IT, which is a potentially malignant neoplasm. Nevertheless, typical dermoid cysts containing very small foci of immature tissue have a benign behavior and should not be reported as grade 1 IT.[81] Rarely, teratomas may be predominantly or exclusively composed of endodermal or ectodermal tissues (monodermal teratomas).[1] The pathogenesis of teratomas has always excited speculation because of their exotic composition. Cytogenetic analysis, using chromosome-banding techniques, has revealed that ovarian teratomas are parthenogenetic tumors that develop from a single germ cell after its first meiotic division.[82] Also, genetic analysis of mature ovarian teratomas has demonstrated genotypic differences between homozygous teratomatous tissue and heterozygous host tissue.[83]

MATURE TERATOMAS

Clinical Features

Mature teratomas, usually dermoid cysts, represent the most common ovarian neoplasms, accounting for 27–44% of all primary ovarian tumors and over two-thirds of all ovarian tumors in patients under 15 years of age.[1,84] Most patients are between 20 and 40 years, but the tumors occur at all ages. Although they usually occur in pure form, dermoid cysts are found grossly within 26% of ITs and in the ovary contralateral to a MGCT in about 5–10% of cases.[1,81] Most patients with mature teratomas present the typical signs and symptoms of benign ovarian tumors, but approximately 25% are asymptomatic and the tumors are discovered on routine examination. Radiologically, dermoid cysts are characterized by central areas of very low density enclosed by a ring of increased capsular density.[85] Calcified tissues including bone and teeth may be present and facilitate the radiologic diagnosis. Dermoid cysts may undergo torsion or rupture, with acute abdominal symptoms, or hemoperitoneum. Leakage of the cyst contents into the abdominal cavity results in granulomatous peritonitis, which may mimic tuberculosis or metastatic carcinoma.[86] Peritoneal melanosis may also occur. Autoimmune hemolytic anemia has been reported in some cases. Mature solid teratomas may occasionally produce mature peritoneal glial implants (grade 0), which have an excellent prognosis.[87]

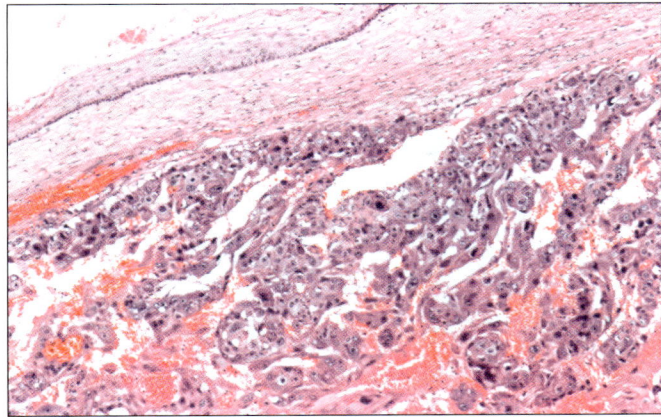

Figure 29.22 Choriocarcinoma arising in a dermoid cyst.

Although mature teratomas are benign tumors, malignant transformation may occur in approximately 1–2% of cases, usually in postmenopausal women (mean age, 51–62 years). Almost any component may become malignant, but squamous cell carcinoma accounts for 80% of the cases.[1,88]

Macroscopic Features

Mature teratomas are almost always cystic tumors and are bilateral in approximately 15% of cases. They range in size from 0.5 to 40 cm (average 15 cm) and have a smooth grayish white external surface. On section, a unilocular or, less frequently, a multilocular cyst lined by skin appears filled with sebaceous material and hair (Figure 29.23). The cyst contents are liquid at body temperature but they solidify at room temperature. A solid nodule composed of fat tissue with teeth or bone usually protrudes into the cyst lumen (Rokitansky's protuberance). Dermoid cysts may contain a great variety of mature somatic tissues that may be seen grossly, such as brain tissue, bone, cartilage, adipose tissue, mucinous cysts, and thyroid. In rare cases, partially developed organs may be identified. Rarely, mature teratomas are completely solid and differ grossly from ITs by the absence of hemorrhagic and necrotic areas.[89] Twenty-two cases of a rare type of mature solid teratoma resembling a malformed human fetus have been reported. This form of teratoma has been designated homunculus or fetiform teratoma.[90] Dermoid cysts that are unusually large and adherent to surrounding structures or that contain mural nodules, or extensive necrosis and hemorrhage, are suspicious of harboring a secondary malignant tumor.[1]

Microscopic Features

Mature teratomas are composed of adult and sometimes fetal-type tissue derived from two or three embryonic layers. Ectodermal elements predominate in almost all cases, particularly epidermis (Figure 29.24), pilosebaceous structures, teeth, sweat glands, and neural tissue (usually glia).[1] In mature solid teratomas, well-differentiated glia may constitute the predominant component. Other ectodermal derivatives, such as cerebrum, cerebellum, choroid plexus, and retina, may also be found. The common presence of cranially derived tissues in one study suggests that the type of differentiation in mature cystic teratomas parallels anterior embryonic plate development.[91] Frequent endodermal elements include respiratory and gastrointestinal structures and thyroid tissue. The most common mesodermal derivatives are smooth or striated muscle, adipose tissue, bone, teeth, and cartilage. Less frequently, adrenal, pituitary, pancreatic, renal, thymic, mammary, or prostatic tissue are encountered.[92] Although mitotic figures are rare, they may be seen in recognizable fetal tissues.[1] The various tissues exhibit an organoid arrangement; for instance, cartilage, mucinous glands, and respiratory epithelium may appear together as in normal bronchus. Rarely, a florid benign vascular proliferation may be found in association with glial tissue and can be misinterpreted as an immature component.[93]

Benign tumors, such as carcinoid, struma, adrenal adenoma, prolactinoma, glomus tumor, sebaceous adenomas, and nevus, may develop within a dermoid cyst.[1,94–97] Six mucinous–intestinal tumors associated with pseudomyxoma peritonei arose in ovarian dermoid cysts.[98,99] The great majority of secondary cancers are invasive or, rarely, *in situ* squamous cell carcinomas (see later). Sebaceous carcinomas, sarcomas, and melanomas are occasionally seen.[1,100]

Treatment and Prognosis

Dermoid cysts are treated conservatively, particularly in children and young women. Ovarian cystectomy is adequate treatment. With the exception of rare cases in which a secondary malignant tumor develops, dermoid cysts are benign tumors even if they contain microscopic foci of immature neural tissue.[81] Similarly, mature solid teratomas, including those associated with mature implants, have a favorable clinical course.[87] Patients with squamous cell carcinoma that has disseminated beyond the ovary typically have a poor prognosis.[88]

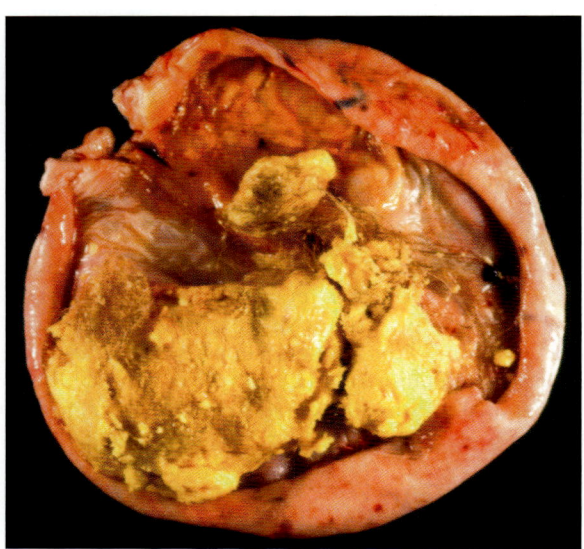

Figure 29.23 Dermoid cyst (mature cystic teratoma). The cyst contains sebaceous material and hairs.

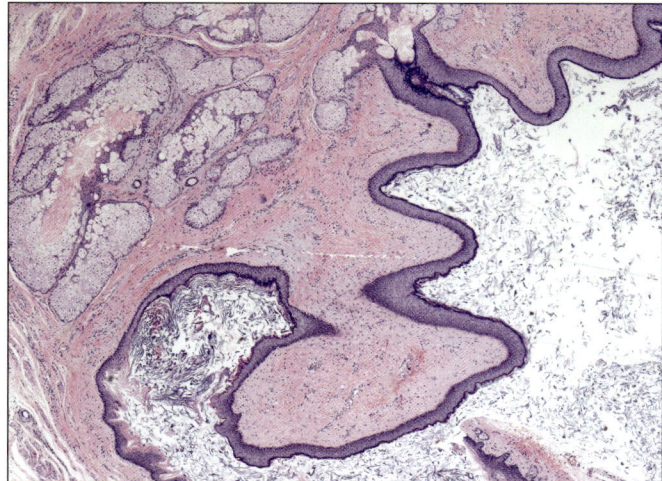

Figure 29.24 Dermoid cyst (mature cystic teratoma). Squamous epithelium and sebaceous glands.

IMMATURE TERATOMAS

Clinical Features

Immature teratomas (ITs) are probably the most common MGCTs of the ovary, representing about 36% of such tumors and 1% of ovarian cancers in general.[101-105] Only 3% of ovarian teratomas are immature. They occur predominantly in children and young women, at a median age of 18 years, who have a palpable abdominal mass and complain of pelvic or abdominal pain. In rare cases, ITs are preceded by ipsilateral dermoid cysts that have been removed some years previously.[81] Serum AFP can be elevated in patients with pure IT but levels only rarely exceed 1000 ng/ml. Higher levels almost always indicate the presence of a YST component.[106] Other tumor markers include hCG, NSE, CEA, and CA125. Extraovarian spread, usually in the form of peritoneal implants and less frequently as lymph node metastases, is found in one-third of patients at the time of surgery.[87,102-105] Ruptured or adherent tumors are most commonly associated with peritoneal implants.[87]

Macroscopic Features

Immature teratomas are typically large (mean size, 18 cm), encapsulated tumors that are ruptured in nearly 50% of cases.[102] On section, they are predominantly solid, but small cysts containing mucin or blood are often seen (Figure 29.25). The solid areas, which usually correspond to neural tissue, are soft, fleshy, and gray to pink and frequently show hemorrhage and necrosis. Foci of bone and cartilage may be present. Grossly visible dermoid cysts are found in 26% of cases.[81] The tumor is almost always unilateral, but the contralateral ovary contains a dermoid cyst in about 10% of patients.[1]

Microscopic Features

Most tumors contain a mixture of mature and immature embryonal elements. The embryonic-type tissue varies from microscopic foci to large amounts and is composed predominantly of neuroepithelial rosettes (Figure 29.26) and tubules admixed with areas of hypercellular glia with numerous mitoses. The neuroepithelial rosettes are lined by crowded cells (Figure 29.27) and may be pigmented. Islands of immature cartilage, bone, skeletal muscle, and glandular structures are distributed through a myxoid stroma. Embryonal endodermal elements, such as hepatic tissue and intestinal-type epithelium, may also be found.[56] The presence of these elements in grade 3 ITs (see later) with markedly elevated serum AFP levels should alert the pathologist to perform a diligent search for a YST component. In childhood ITs, such a component may develop as well-differentiated glandular or hepatoid YST.[106] Two cases of ITs composed predominantly of endodermal elements without neural component have been described (Figure 29.28).[107] Rarely, immature renal tissue,[108] SGCs, and yolk sac-like tissue may be found.[102,109] Vascular proliferation occurs in relationship with neural tissues.[93]

The relative amount of primitive neuroepithelial tissue is an important factor in grading and determining the prognosis of ITs.[89] Grading is performed by a subjective,

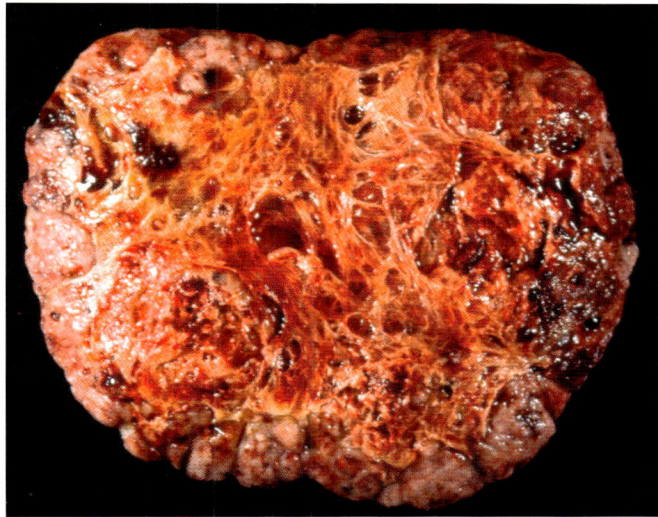

Figure 29.25 Immature teratoma. The sectioned surface is predominantly solid but also shows numerous small cysts containing bloody fluid.

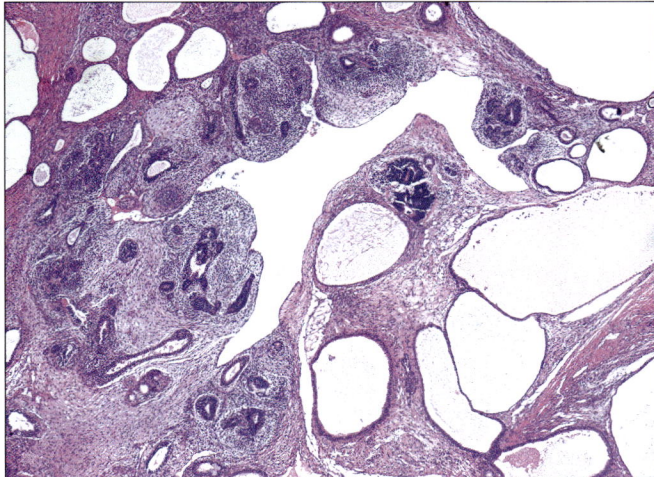

Figure 29.26 Immature teratoma. The tumor shows both immature neuroepithelial and mesenchymal elements.

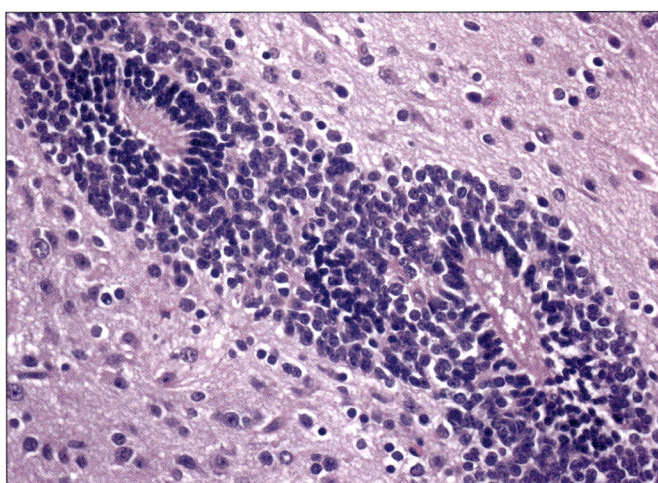

Figure 29.27 Immature teratoma. Glial tissue with neuroepithelial tubules.

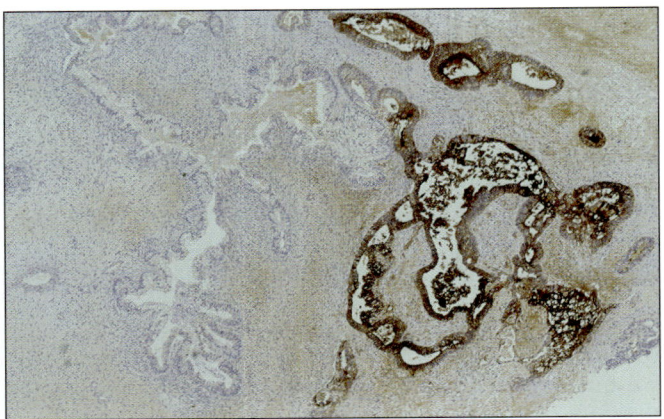

Figure 29.28 Immature endodermal teratoma. The tumor is exclusively composed of endodermal elements without neural component. The intestinal-like glands show positive AFP immunoreaction.

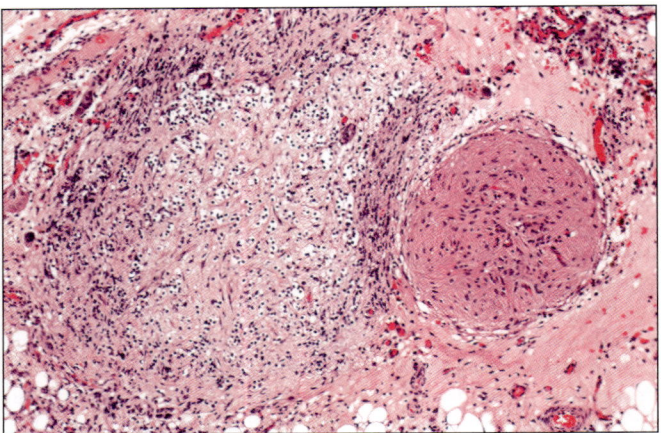

Figure 29.29 Peritoneal implant of immature teratoma. The implant is partly composed of immature glial tissue (left).

Table 29.4 Grading of Ovarian Immature Teratomas[102]

Immature Teratoma: Histologic Grade		
(Immature Neural Tissue)		
G1	Rare foci	<1 LPF/slide
G2	Moderate	>1, <4 LPF/slide
G3	Abundant	>4 LPF/slide

semiquantitative analysis of the relative amount and atypicality of the immature neural tissue (neuroepithelial tubules and neural blastema) present in the tumor. Grade 1 has been applied to tumors with rare foci of immature neural tissue that occupy less than one low-power field (LPF) (40×) in any slide, grade 2 to tumors with moderate amounts of immature neural tissue occupying more than 1 but less than 4 LPF in any slide, and grade 3 to tumors with immature neural tissue occupying 4 or more LPFs in any slide (Table 29.4).[102] The grading system is also applied to peritoneal implants (Figure 29.29) and lymph node metastases. A two-grade system (low grade and high grade), which combines grades 2 and 3, has been proposed but has not been formally adopted.[109] ITs as well as mature solid teratomas may be associated with mature (grade 0) peritoneal implants (so-called peritoneal gliomatosis).[87] The pathogenesis of this phenomenon is unclear and both, direct seeding of immature cells from the primary tumor with subsequent differentiation in the peritoneum[87] and peritoneal metaplasia[110] from stem cells have been proposed. In some cases, the glial implants appear admixed with endometriosis.[111] As mature and immature implants may coexist, generous sampling of the peritoneal lesions is recommended.[1] The pelvic and para-aortic lymph nodes may also contain similar glial tissue.[112]

Immunohistochemistry

SALL4 is positive in both intestinal and neural immature tissues.[63] SOX2, however, identifies more specifically immature neural areas, highlighting them, and is helpful for grading of immature teratoma.[33] Glypican-3 may also exhibit a patchy neuroepithelium immunoreaction. The neuroectodermal tissues are also immunoreactive for several neural markers, including glial fibrillary acidic protein (GFAP), NSE, S-100 protein, neurofilament protein, synaptophysin, and nerve growth factor receptor. The intestinal-type glands and hepatic tissue stain strongly for AFP.[56] SGCs stain positively for hCG.

Somatic Genetics

Immature teratomas seem to originate from premeiotic germ cells.[113] By comparative genomic hybridization, ITs exhibit fewer DNA changes than other ovarian germ cell tumors. No gain of 12p or i(12p) has been identified.[114] Grades 1–2 ITs are diploid in 90% of cases, whereas most grade 3 tumors are aneuploid.[115]

Differential Diagnosis

Immature teratoma is distinguished from mature solid teratoma by the presence of immature embryonal tissue. The finding of fetal cartilage and mitotically active cerebrum or cerebellum does not justify the diagnosis of immature teratoma.[89] Typical dermoid cysts may contain minor foci of immature neural tissue.[81] Malignancy arising in a dermoid cyst occurs most commonly in postmenopausal patients. In contrast to IT, only one element, usually squamous epithelium, is malignant (see later). IT is a frequent component of mixed MGCTs; therefore, the presence of other primitive elements such as dysgerminoma or YST should be excluded by generous sampling. In primitive mixed tumors occurring in children and adolescents, the YST components may be of the glandular (enteric) or hepatoid type and, thus, difficult to distinguish from the embryonal or fetal gastrointestinal glands or hepatocytes that can be found in pure ITs.[106] The additional presence of extraembryonal patterns (reticular or polyvesicular vitelline patterns) of YST, as well as the typically elevated serum levels of AFP, facilitate the differential diagnosis.[106] The differential diagnosis between immature teratomas and malignant mixed müllerian tumor with heterologous elements and primitive neuroectodermal tumors is discussed in Chapter 27 and in the following sections, respectively.

Treatment and Prognosis

In a young patient whose tumor appears localized to a single ovary (stage IA), a unilateral salpingo-oophorectomy and surgical staging should be done. If preservation of fertility is not an issue, or the contralateral ovary or uterus is involved, a total abdominal hysterectomy and bilateral salpingo-oophorectomy should be carried out. Any peritoneal lesions should be sampled carefully and submitted for histologic evaluation. The primary prognostic factor in patients with immature teratoma is the tumor grade. Patients with stage IA, grade 1 tumors or those with exclusively mature (grade 0) glial implants have an excellent prognosis and are treated by surgery alone. Patients with grade 2 or 3, stage IA, or those with immature implants should receive combination chemotherapy.[103–105] The VAC regimen has been replaced by platinum-containing regimens such as cisplatin, etoposide, and bleomycin (BEP). In patients with no residual tumor after surgery, the survival rate is 90–100%.[103,116] Prognosis is less favorable for patients with residual gross tumor or recurrent IT. Following chemotherapy, high-grade implants typically disappear, or are replaced by mature, necrotic, or fibrotic tissue.[87] Mature implants may continue to grow ('growing teratoma syndrome') and may require reoperation. However, on rare occasions, gliomatosis peritonei can induce a florid vascular proliferation that may result in peritoneal hemorrhage and shock.[117] Rare cases of glioblastoma multiforme arising from peritoneal gliomatosis have been described.[118] Cytogenetically abnormal or aneuploid ITs may be associated with a worse prognosis than karyotypically normal or diploid tumors.[119]

According to a report from the Pediatric Oncology Group, surgery alone is curative in children and adolescents with IT of any grade, and chemotherapy should only be used for cases with tumor recurrence.[106] In such cases, the presence of a YST component rather than the grade of the IT component is the only valid predictor of recurrence.[106]

MONODERMAL TERATOMAS

STRUMA OVARII

Clinical Features

Over 20% of dermoid cysts may contain thyroid tissue on microscopic examination, but the term struma ovarii is only applied to teratomas composed either exclusively or predominantly of such tissue. Struma ovarii is the most common form of monodermal teratoma accounting for 3% of all ovarian teratomas.[120] Most patients are in their fifth decade.[120] Along with a palpable abdominal mass, patients may present with ascites and hydrothorax ('pseudo-Meigs' syndrome'), cervical thyroid enlargement, and hyperthyroidism with high pelvic iodine uptake.[121]

Macroscopic Features

Most tumors are unilateral and range from 0.5 to 10 cm in diameter. On section, the thyroid tissue appears solid, gelatinous, and typically brown or green-brown (Figure 29.30). Usually, struma occurs in a pure form; less frequently, it is associated with a dermoid cyst or is a component of strumal carcinoid. Occasionally, strumas are found in the wall of mucinous cystadenomas or are admixed with Brenner tumor.[122] Some cases of struma ovarii appear as unilocular

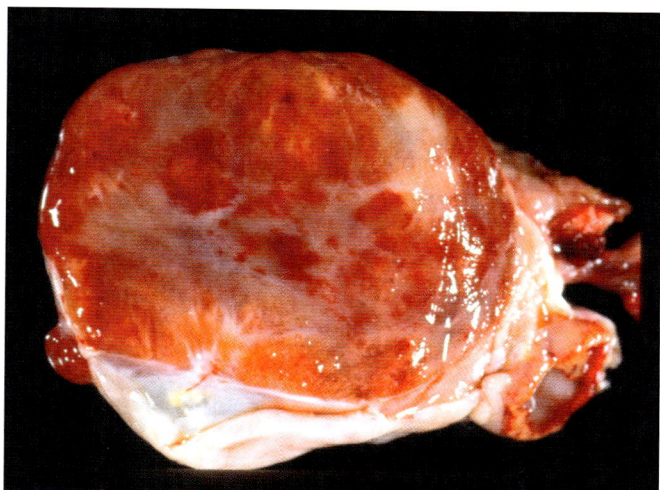

Figure 29.30 Struma ovarii. The sectioned surface is solid and red to brown.

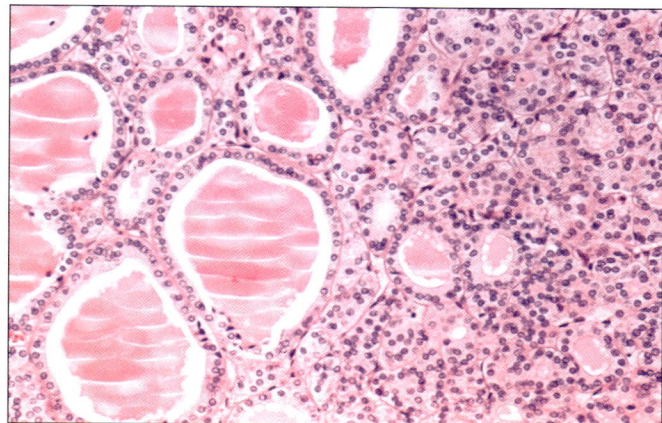

Figure 29.31 Struma ovarii. The tumor resembles a thyroid adenoma with mixed macrofollicular and microfollicular pattern.

or multilocular cysts containing brown to green gelatinous fluid.[123] Rarely, the contralateral ovary contains a dermoid cyst or even another struma.

Microscopic Features

Struma ovarii may appear as normal thyroid tissue or an adenoma of the macrofollicular, microfollicular, embryonal, or mixed type (Figure 29.31). Clear cell, oxyphilic, and solid tubular forms of thyroid adenoma also occur.[124] Under polarized light, birefringent calcium oxalate crystals are often found within the colloid, which is immunoreactive for thyroglobulin. Tumor cells also show immunohistochemical expression of TTF-1. They exhibit only mild nuclear atypia and mitotic figures are rare. In cystic strumas, thyroidal differentiation may not be readily apparent. The thin fibrous septa are lined by flat to cuboidal nonspecific epithelial cells and the characteristic thyroid follicles may be sparse in the cyst wall.[123]

The criteria for malignant change in struma ovarii have not been uniformly established. Malignant strumas are rare, and most of them are characterized by a papillary architecture (or a follicular pattern with occasional papillae) and the presence of cells with overlapping ground-glass nuclei.[125] Follicular carcinomas are difficult to diagnose since struma has no true capsule but is surrounded only by stroma, and capsular invasion cannot be a criterion for malignancy;[126] also, true vascular invasion is exceedingly rare and has not proved to be a valid prognostic parameter.[125,126] Poorly differentiated carcinomas are rare.[125]

Differential Diagnosis

Cystic struma is often mistaken for a serous or mucinous cystic tumor; however, the green to brown color of the cyst contents and, microscopically, the focal presence of thyroid follicles on the cyst wall, and the occasional association with other teratomatous elements in the struma permit its identification.[123] Cysts closely resembling thyroid follicles may be found in endometrioid carcinomas, clear cell carcinomas, Sertoli-Leydig cell tumors (SLCTs), and pregnancy luteomas, but other typical morphologic features in such tumors almost always facilitate their distinction. A predominant microfollicular pattern may be misinterpreted as the Call–Exner bodies of a granulosa cell tumor (GCT). Oxyphilic strumas may be mistaken for other oxyphilic tumors, such as steroid cell tumors, and strumas with a solid tubular pattern may simulate Sertoli cell tumors. In these cases, the finding of true thyroid follicles and calcium oxalate crystals and immunoreactivity for thyroglobulin and TTF-1 confirms the diagnosis of struma.[124] The rare case of ovarian metastasis from carcinoma of the thyroid gland is usually diagnosed after obtaining additional clinical data.

Treatment and Prognosis

Benign struma ovarii is treated by oophorectomy. Patients with malignant struma should be treated by oophorectomy and removal of as much extraovarian tumor as technically feasible. In some of these patients, extraovarian disease has been treated successfully with ^{132}I.[127]

Most cases of struma have been clinically benign. Although in the older literature 5–10% of strumas have been considered malignant, only a few cases have been associated with metastasis or recurrence. In the remaining cases, the diagnosis of malignancy has been based exclusively on microscopic criteria, and some tumors originally thought to be malignant are now interpreted as benign strumal carcinoids.[128] Clinically malignant struma ovarii can develop from histologically malignant strumas, adenomas of various types, or even benign thyroid tissue. In fact, ovarian tumors with subtle atypical nuclear features, which are suggestive of but not diagnostic for the follicular variant of papillary thyroid carcinoma, still can metastasize.[129] No single histologic feature can reliably predict a malignant behavior, but ascites, larger tumor size (over 12 cm), ovarian surface invasion, and extensive adhesions favor a malignant clinical behavior.[125,130] Rare cases of benign-appearing struma implants on the peritoneum (so-called peritoneal strumosis) have been associated with indolent clinical course and prolonged survival.[131] These cases have also been designated 'highly differentiated follicular carcinomas.'[132] In the largest series reported of malignant struma ovarii, the overall survival rate was 89% at 10 years and 84% at 25 years, indicating the need for routine long-term follow-up.[125]

CARCINOIDS

Clinical Features

Ovarian carcinoids are the second most common monodermal teratomas. They may occur in pure form (15%) or, more often, combined with other teratomatous elements (85%) such as a dermoid cyst or a struma ovarii (strumal carcinoid).[128] They may also be a component of a mucinous cystic tumor or a Brenner tumor. The pure carcinoids are divided into insular, trabecular, and mucinous types, and resemble carcinoids of the gastrointestinal tract.[133–135] Although ovarian carcinoids may occur at any age, most patients are perimenopausal or postmenopausal women who present with nonspecific symptoms, such as abdominal enlargement and pain. The carcinoid syndrome (facial flushing, diarrhea, bronchospasm, hypertension, and edema secondary to carcinoid heart disease) has been described in 30% of cases of insular carcinoid, and less often in trabecular (13%) and strumal (3.2%) carcinoids.[136,137] It typically disappears after removal of the tumor.[133] Patients with the syndrome usually have tumors larger than 7 cm in diameter. Other clinical findings include chronic constipation, hypoglycemia, and hyperthyroidism associated with strumal carcinoids. Occasionally, androgenic or estrogenic symptoms related to stromal luteinization or peripheral steroid cell proliferation may develop.[1]

Gross Features

Although ovarian carcinoids are unilateral tumors, the contralateral ovary contains a dermoid cyst, a mucinous tumor, or a Brenner tumor in 15% of cases.[1] Carcinoid tumors are firm, yellow-tan, and predominantly solid tumors. Exclusively cystic tumors are rare. Occasionally, the carcinoid may form a nodule that protrudes into the lumen of a dermoid cyst (Figure 29.32) or a mucinous cystic tumor,[138] or be admixed with a Brenner tumor or struma (strumal carcinoid). In some cases, the carcinoid and struma can be separately recognized on gross examination.

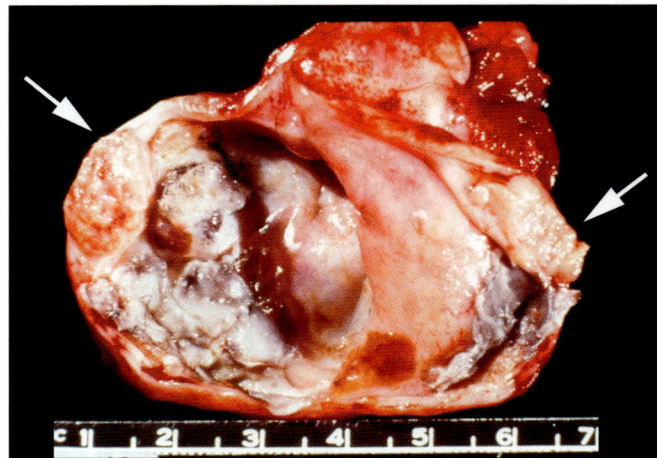

Figure 29.32 Ovarian carcinoid tumor (arrows) in the wall of a dermoid cyst.

CHAPTER 29 — OVARIAN GERM CELL TUMORS   685

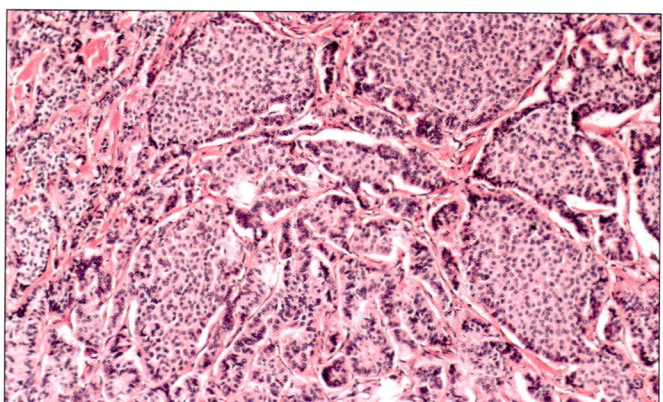

Figure 29.33 Insular carcinoid. Cellular nests containing small round acini are separated by fibrous stroma.

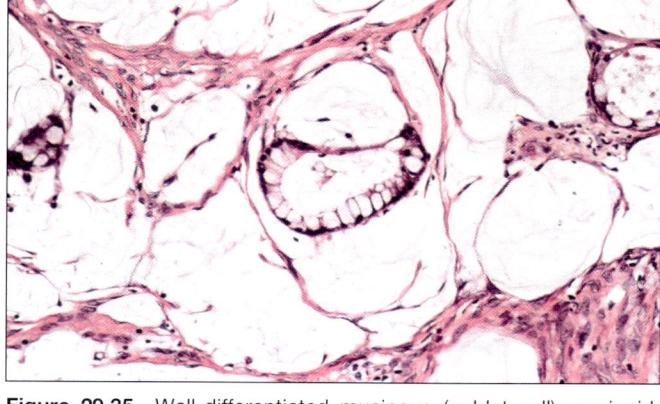

Figure 29.35 Well-differentiated mucinous (goblet cell) carcinoid. Nests composed of cuboidal to columnar goblet cells lie in pools of mucin.

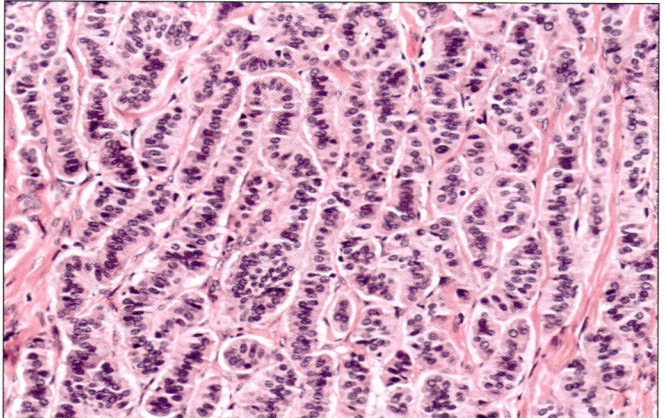

Figure 29.34 Trabecular carcinoid.

Microscopic Features

All ovarian carcinoids are composed, at least in part, of round to cuboidal neuroendocrine cells that have uniform round nuclei, coarse chromatin granules, and small nucleoli. Mitotic figures are rare. The cytoplasm is characteristically abundant and varies from clear to eosinophilic. Four histologic types of carcinoid tumor may be found in the ovary. The insular type is the most common, accounting for 26–53% of cases.[133,136,137] It resembles midgut carcinoid and is characterized by cellular nests or islands separated by a fibromatous stroma (Figure 29.33). The cellular islands often show small tubular acini lined by columnar cells, particularly at their periphery. The acinar lumens contain eosinophilic secretion, which may be calcified. The peripheral cells of the islands and the acinar cells contain red-brown argentaffin granules. Respiratory or gastrointestinal epithelium may also be present.

Trabecular carcinoids account for 23–29% of cases.[136,137] They are characterized by wavy, parallel cords, ribbons, or trabeculae of cells separated by fibrous stroma and resemble hindgut or foregut carcinoids (Figure 29.34).[134] The cords are composed of columnar cells with oblong nuclei oriented perpendicular to the axis of the cord. Typically, intracytoplasmic argyrophilic granules are found at both poles of the nucleus. Associated teratomatous elements are almost always present.

Mucinous (goblet cell) carcinoids constitute only 1.5% of cases and resemble goblet cell carcinoids arising in the appendix.[135,137] Unlike the appendiceal tumors, however, the ovarian mucinous carcinoids are often associated with other neoplastic elements. In fact, they are thought to develop from appendiceal tissue within a teratoma. The mucinous carcinoids have been subdivided into three groups: well differentiated, atypical, and carcinomatous.[135] In the well-differentiated tumors, small nests or glands composed of goblet cells and cuboidal to columnar cells may be floating within pools of mucin that appear surrounded by a fibrous stroma (Figure 29.35). The nuclei are uniform, small, and round to oval. The neuroendocrine nature of the tumor cells is usually confirmed by immunohistochemistry. Atypical tumors show crowded glands or a cribriform pattern. Tumors with a carcinomatous component contain islands and large masses of tumor cells, crowded glands, and isolated signet-ring cells. These tumors show severe nuclear atypia and numerous mitoses. Combinations of the three histologic subtypes may occur.

Strumal carcinoid is the second most common type and accounts for 26–44% of cases. It is characterized by coexistence of carcinoid and thyroid tissue.[128,136,137] The two components may be contiguous (Figure 29.36) or, more often, intimately admixed; either component may predominate. The carcinoid is trabecular in approximately half of the cases. The thyroid component resembles normal thyroid tissue or follicular adenoma. In areas of intimate mixture, the carcinoid cells characteristically replace the original lining cells of the thyroid follicles (Figure 29.37). Consequently, neuroendocrine granules are found not only within the cells of the trabecular carcinoid, but also within those lining the colloid-filled spaces.[128,139] Mucinous glands and cysts or even a mucinous carcinoma component may be present in about 40% of cases.[140]

Immunohistochemical Findings

Carcinoids are immunoreactive to neuroendocrine markers such as chromogranin (Figure 29.38), synaptophysin, and Leu-7.[141] They are often positive for CDX2. Additionally,

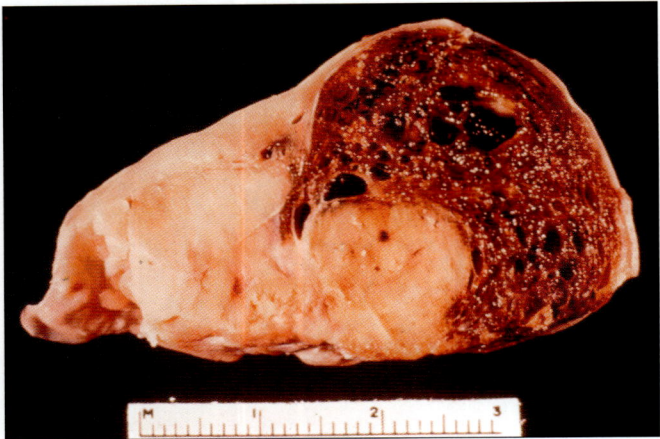

Figure 29.36 Strumal carcinoid. The brown strumal component (right) is predominantly cystic and appears sharply demarcated from the solid white carcinoid tissue (left). (Reproduced with permision of J.B. Lippincott Company.)

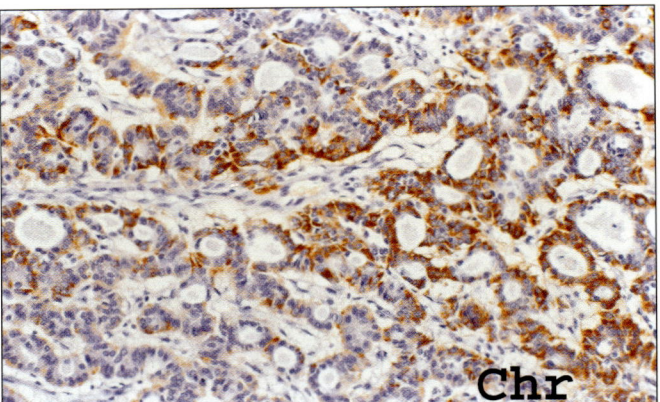

Figure 29.38 Carcinoid tumor. Positive immunostain for chromogranin.

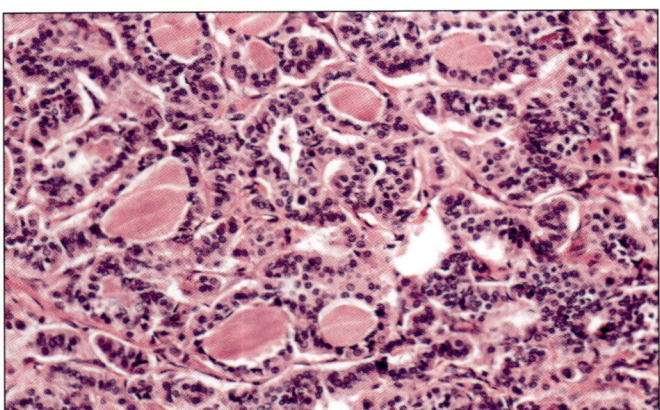

Figure 29.37 Strumal carcinoid. The tumor is characterized by an admixture of thyroid follicles and trabeculae of carcinoid cells. The carcinoid cells typically replace the original lining cells of the thyroid follicles.

various peptide hormones can be detected in about 25% of cases, including serotonin, gastrin, pancreatic polypeptide, vasoactive intestinal peptide, insulin, glucagon, substance P, peptide YY, neurotensin, β-endorphin, ACTH, and somatostatin.[142] Insular and trabecular carcinoids are CK7 positive and CK20 negative. In contrast, mucinous (goblet cell) carcinoids show a CK7(−)/CK20 diffuse profile.[143] In strumal carcinoids, thyroglobulin, TTF-1, and CK7 are usually expressed in the strumal component but not in the carcinoid component.[139,140,144] Calcitonin and amyloid may be present in rare examples of these tumors,[128] but immunostains for CEA are negative.

Differential Diagnosis

In the absence of other teratomatous elements, primary ovarian carcinoid may be difficult to distinguish from metastatic carcinoma. Along with a clinical history of carcinoid tumor in the gastrointestinal tract, lung, or elsewhere, evidence favoring metastasis includes bilaterality, multinodularity, peritoneal metastases, and persistence of the carcinoid syndrome or elevated 5-hydroxyindolacetic acid levels in the urine after removal of the ovarian tumor.[145] For mucinous (goblet cell) carcinoid, a metastatic appendiceal carcinoma with goblet cell carcinoid-like and signet-ring cell features must be excluded.[146] These findings are also helpful in distinguishing ovarian mucinous carcinoid with signet-ring cells from Krukenberg tumor.

Ovarian carcinoids can be confused with other primary ovarian tumors, particularly Brenner tumor, GCT, and Sertoli or SLCT. In contrast to the cells of carcinoid tumors, those of Brenner tumors have a characteristic urothelial appearance with grooved nuclei. Furthermore, unlike the carcinoid islands, Brenner nests often contain glands lined by mucinous cells. The granulosa cells surrounding a Call–Exner body lack the eosinophilic cytoplasm and typically have pale, grooved, haphazardly oriented nuclei instead of the round, coarsely stippled nuclei of carcinoid cells. The sex cords in SLCTs of intermediate differentiation are less uniform, and more sparsely distributed than the elongated ribbons of trabecular carcinoid. The presence of other distinctive patterns of SLCT usually facilitates the diagnosis. Immunohistochemical staining for neuroendocrine, thyroid, and sex cord–stromal (α-inhibin) markers can be helpful in difficult cases.

Treatment and Prognosis

Ovarian carcinoids are tumors of low malignant potential and less than 5% are complicated by metastasis and death. Most tumors occur in perimenopausal women and, therefore, the standard treatment is hysterectomy and bilateral salpingo-oophorectomy. Unilateral adnexectomy is adequate treatment for young women. Ovarian trabecular carcinoids do not metastasize and are associated with good prognosis. Strumal carcinoid typically follows a benign course and is only rarely associated with metastases.[128,139] Most of the malignant tumors have been of the insular or mucinous (carcinomatous) type.[135] A few patients have died of progressive carcinoid heart disease.

NEUROECTODERMAL-TYPE TUMORS

Sixty-five neuroectodermal tumors, similar to neoplasms of the central nervous system (CNS), have been described in the ovary.[147–153] They included well-differentiated tumors, mainly ependymomas (Figure 29.39), but also astrocytomas and oligodendrogliomas; primitive tumors resembling medulloblastoma, medulloepithelioma, central neurocytoma, and neuroblastoma (Figure 29.40A–D); and anaplastic neoplasms resembling glioblastoma multiforme. Most patients were in their twenties to thirties (range, 6–69 years) and presented with abdominal/pelvic pain, abdominal mass, and fullness.[147,151] All tumors but one were unilateral.[154] The primitive and anaplastic tumors are typically large (average 14 cm, range 4–29 cm), had a malignant gross appearance, and often extended beyond the ovary.

Given their association with teratomas, most neuroectodermal-type tumors are thought to be of germ cell origin. Tumors not associated with teratomas (particularly ependymomas and primitive neuroectodermal tumors; PNETs) may result from neometaplasia occurring in müllerian-related tissues.[155] In the largest series reported, all oligodendrogliomas and most astrocytomas were associated with teratomas but only 1 of 19 ependymomas was so.[147,152,153] Also, most primitive tumors (except PNETs) and all glioblastoma multiforme were associated with teratomas.[147,151] But even if most cases are essentially germ cell tumors, they should be classified separately from grade 2–3 ITs in which the neuroectodermal elements do not resemble tumors of the CNS.[147] Whereas the IT with predominant neuroectodermal differentiation is easily recognized because of the presence of many other teratomatous elements, the pure or almost pure neuroectodermal-type

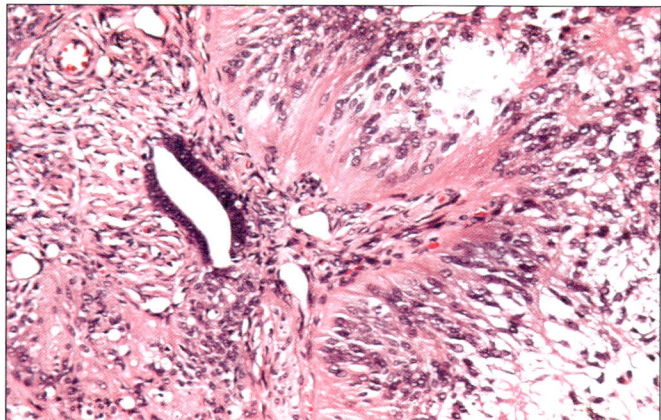

Figure 29.39 Ependymoma. Cells with fibrillary cytoplasmic processes form perivascular pseudorosettes.

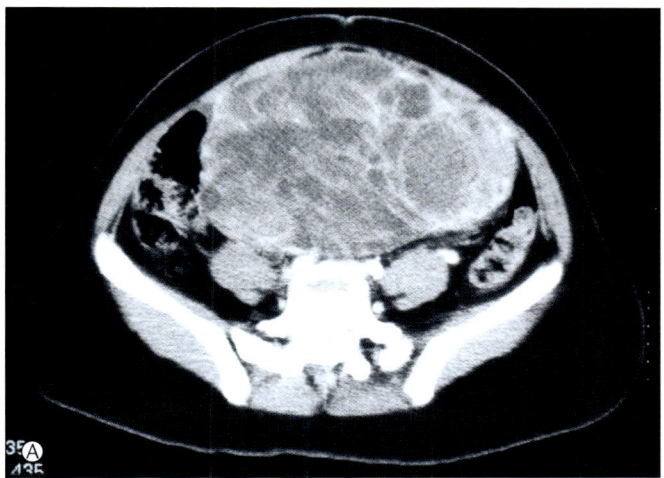
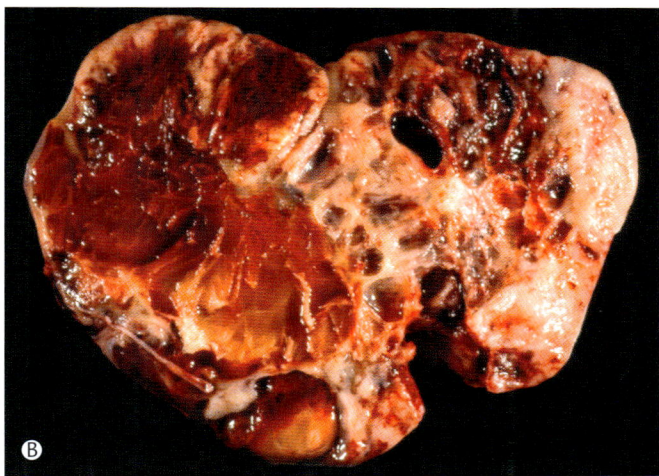
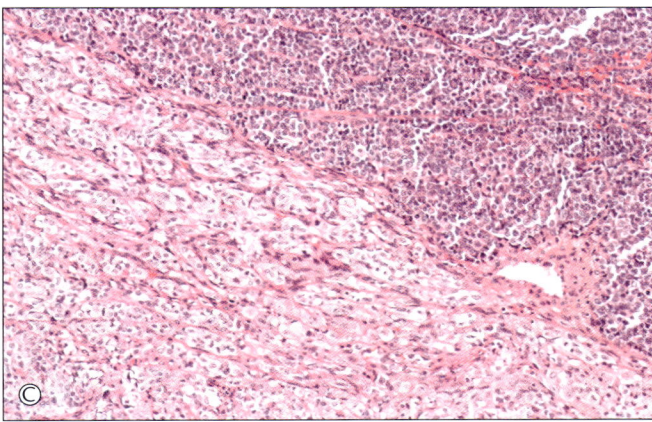
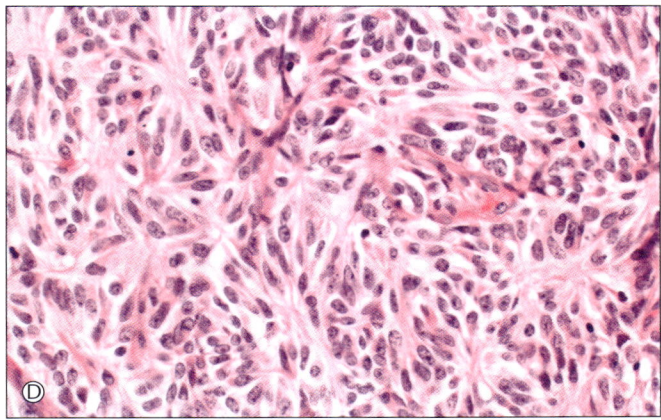

Figure 29.40 Primitive neuroectodermal tumor (PNET). **(A)** CT scan shows a solid abdominal mass, 18 cm in greatest diameter. **(B)** The sectioned surface of the tumor is solid and cystic with extensive hemorrhage and necrosis. **(C)** Typical biphasic pattern composed of large (lower left) and small (upper right) cells. **(D)** Homer–Wright rosettes.

tumor is frequently confused with other types of ovarian tumors such as granulosa cell tumor, small cell carcinoma of the hypercalcemic type, and endometrioid carcinoma. Extensive sampling and immunohistochemical stains for glial fibrillary acidic protein (GFAP) and MIC2 protein (CD99) facilitate the correct diagnosis. Ovarian ependymomas are more likely to express various cytokeratins, and estrogen receptor and progesterone receptor than their CNS counterparts.[156] The EWS/FLI-1 chimeric transcript, secondary to t(11;22)(q24;q12) chromosomal translocation, characteristic of the PNET family, has been identified by reverse transcription polymerase chain reaction in a case of ovarian neuroectodermal tumor.[157] Clinical stage is the most important prognostic factor. However, ovarian ependymomas are associated with good prognosis even in an advanced stage.[148,150] In contrast, the primitive and anaplastic tumors have a poor outcome.[147]

CARCINOMA IN DERMOID CYSTS

SQUAMOUS CELL CARCINOMA

Malignant change occurs in 1–2% of dermoid cysts. Any component may be involved, but squamous cell carcinomas account for 80% of cases. Nonepithelial malignant tumors are exceedingly rare.[158] The tumors occur at an average age of about 55 years.[158–160] Presentation varies from an ordinary dermoid cyst to obvious ovarian cancer. In patients 45 years or older, a diameter larger than 10 cm and elevated CEA and squamous cell carcinoma antigen levels are suspicious of malignancy and imaging may be confirmatory.[159]

Average size is about 14 cm.[159] Tumors are solid or solid and cystic with a polypoid mass showing areas of necrosis. A thickened wall is characteristic. Microscopically, the tumors show papillary, nodular, and infiltrative features.[88] Almost all squamous cell carcinomas arise from respiratory or gastrointestinal-type epithelium rather than skin and may show transmural extension and local invasion (Figure 29.41).[161] Unlike squamous cell carcinomas associated with other ovarian tumors that are more frequently bilateral, carcinomas arising in dermoid cyst are typically unilateral.[88]

Outcome is highly dependent on stage and tumors confined to the ovary have a favorable outcome. The overall 5 year survival is 15–52% for all stages[161] and 75.7% for stage I tumors.

ADENOCARCINOMA

Adenocarcinoma is the second most common malignancy arising in dermoid cysts, accounting for 7% of cases.[162] Most tumors arise from gastrointestinal and respiratory type epithelium.[59,163] Rarely, carcinomas of sweat glands, sebaceous glands, salivary glands, mammary glands,[164,165] and carcinosarcoma[166] may occur. Patients' ages range from 17 to 66 years (mean, 39 years) and preoperative elevated serum level of CEA and CA19.9 and imaging are helpful for the preoperative diagnosis.[167]

Mucinous tumors arising in dermoid cysts show a wide morphologic spectrum, including benign, malignant, and low-grade tumors resembling mucinous appendiceal tumors; some may show goblet cells, signet-ring cells, and carcinoid-like morphology.[143,168] Pseudomyxoma ovarii is common and in some cases is associated with pseudomyxoma peritonei. Immunohistochemical stains for CK7 and CK20 are of limited value in the differential diagnosis with a secondary tumor. Search of teratomatous elements in the ovarian mass and careful examination of the intestines, in particular appendix and rectum, are important for establishing the correct diagnosis.

The main prognostic parameters are stage and grade. Mucinous borderline tumors confined to the ovary have a favorable prognosis. Also, patients with adenocarcinomas limited to the ovary may have a favorable outcome.[169]

MIXED MALIGNANT GERM CELL TUMORS

In ~10–20% of malignant germ cell tumors (MGCTs) of the ovary, particularly of a primitive nature, a combination of two or more neoplastic types is found.[73] The proportion of each tumor type parallels the incidence of germ cell tumors and influences prognosis. Although any combination is possible, dysgerminoma and YST is the most common; immature teratoma is the third most common component; and EC, choriocarcinoma, and polyembryoma are less frequently encountered.[73] In fact, the latter tumors are rarely found in the ovary in a pure form, but rather as components of mixed MGCTs. Mixed MGCTs may secrete either AFP or hCG, or both, or neither, depending on their components. A panel of immunomarkers including OCT3/4, CD30, and glypican-3 is useful for characterizing the tumor component. Proper identification of the various components requires careful gross examination and extensive sampling of the tumor. Contemporary results indicate that tumor stage is the only significant prognostic factor in patients treated with combination chemotherapy.[170]

MIXED GERM CELL SEX CORD–STROMAL TUMOR

GONADOBLASTOMA

Gonadoblastoma is a rare *in situ* form of MGCT consisting of a mixture of immature sex-cord cells and germ cells that arises almost exclusively in dysgenetic gonads. It occurs

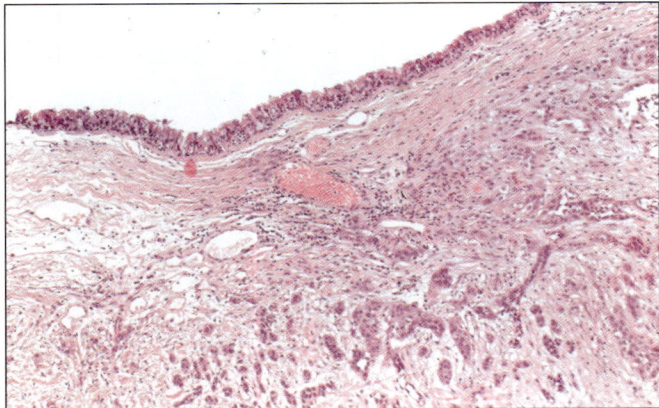

Figure 29.41 Squamous cell carcinoma arising in a dermoid cyst. Invasive squamous cell carcinoma underlies respiratory epithelium lining the cyst.

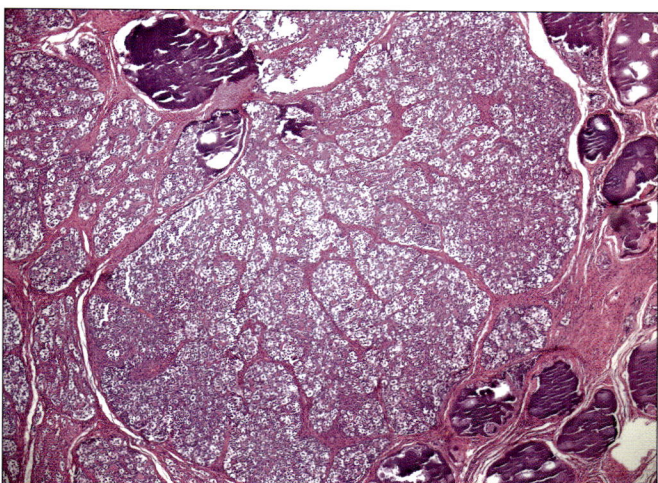

Figure 29.42 Gonadoblastoma. Cellular nests surrounded by connective tissue stroma. Foci of calcification are seen.

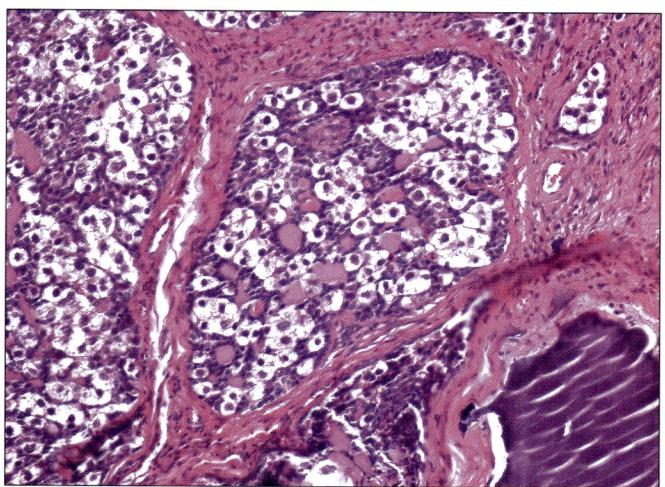

Figure 29.43 Gonadoblastoma. A nest composed of large germ cells admixed with smaller sex cord derivatives. Numerous rounded pink hyaline bodies are surrounded by the smaller cells.

Table 29.5 Gonadoblastoma (Phenotype and Karyotype)

Female—MGD	90%
Male	10%
Y chromosome	95%
• 46,XY	Most frequent
• 45,X/46,XY	1%
• Mosaic with Y	
46,XX/45,X0	5%

mainly in young patients, often before the age of 20 years.[171] Most patients are virilized phenotypic females, but nearly all of them are genotypic males, i.e., have a Y chromosome. The underlying gonadal abnormality is almost always 46,XY pure gonadal dysgenesis or mixed gonadal dysgenesis, which is frequently associated with a 45,X/46,XY karyotype (Table 29.5). A gene that increases susceptibility to gonadoblastoma in patients with dysgenetic gonads has been identified in the long arm of the Y chromosome (GBY region). This gene (*TSPY1*) encodes the testis-specific protein 1, which is thought to have a role in cell cycle regulation.[172] Rare patients are phenotypic men with varying degrees of feminization.

Grossly, the tumor varies in appearance, from soft and fleshy to firm and completely calcified, depending upon the presence or absence of an associated MGCT, calcification, or both. Whereas pure gonadoblastomas are typically less than 8 cm in size, those with an MGCT are usually larger.[1] Gonadoblastomas may arise from indeterminate gonads (60%), dysgenetic testes (20%), or streak gonads (20%);[1] the tumors are bilateral in more than 40% of cases.[1]

Microscopically, the tumor contains both immature germ cells and sex cord–stromal cells, which resemble granulosa or Sertoli cells, arranged in small islands (Figure 29.42) and intermixed with rounded pink hyaline bodies (basement membrane-type material) (Figure 29.43). Leydig cells or lutein cells are distributed through the intervening stroma in two-thirds of the cases and are responsible for the endocrine manifestations.[171] Calcification may be extensive and detected by X-rays. Overgrowth by an MGCT occurs in approximately half the cases.[1] The malignant tumor is a germinoma in 80% of cases, and less frequently yolk sac tumor (YST), embryonal carcinoma (EC) choriocarcinoma, or IT.[1] MGCTs associated with gonadoblastoma are usually diploid.

The germ cells in gonadoblastoma have the same immunophenotype as dysgerminoma cells. They show positive membrane and cytoplasmic reactivity for placental alkaline phosphatase (Figure 29.44), CD117 (*c-kit*), and D2-40 (podoplanin), and they exhibit nuclear reactivity for OCT3/4 and SALL4.[32,173] Cytoplasmic and membrane immunoreaction for TSPY is present in the germ cells.[174]

The sex cord–stromal cells show positive cytoplasmic reaction for inhibin (Figure 29.45), vimentin, and cytokeratin, and nuclear staining for WT1 and FOXL2, but they lack reactivity for SOX9.[175] This suggests a closer relationship to granulosa cells than to Sertoli cells. The hyaline material in the tumor cell nests is PAS positive and reacts with anti-laminin antibodies. Luteinized cells in the stroma around the gonadoblastoma nests react strongly for inhibin and calretinin.

Gonadoblastoma should be distinguished from pure dysgerminoma and sex cord tumor with annular tubules (SCTAT). In a patient with dysgenetic gonads and a Y chromosome, the finding of calcification within a dysgerminoma should raise the question of its origin in gonadoblastoma. Although SCTAT resembles gonadoblastoma, it lacks a germ cell component.[1] Other mixed germ cell sex cord–stromal tumors that lack the characteristic pattern of gonadoblastoma and develop in children with apparently normal gonads and a normal karyotype have been described.[176] Pure gonadoblastoma is benign unless it is overgrown by an MGCT; however, because of the frequency of this event, it is regarded as an '*in situ*' form of MGCT and treated by gonadectomy.[1]

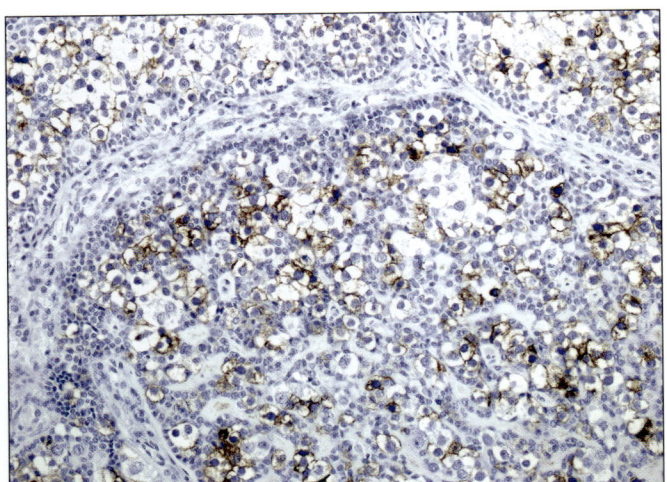

Figure 29.44 Gonadoblastoma. The germ cells immunoreact for PLAP.

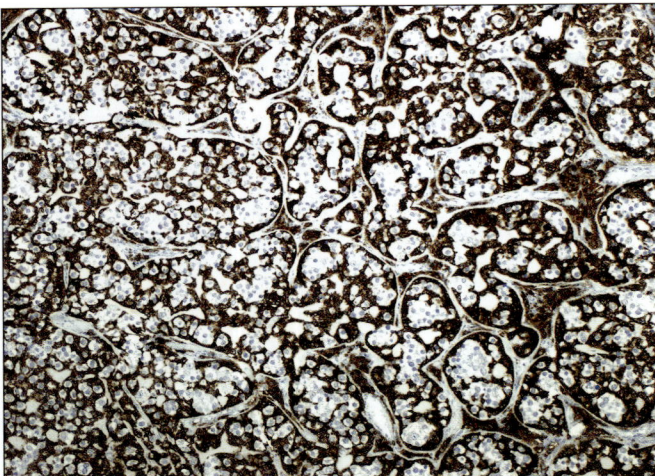

Figure 29.45 Gonadoblastoma. The sex cord–stromal elements show immunoreactivity for inhibin.

REFERENCES

1. Scully RE, Young RH, Clement PB. Tumors of the ovary, maldeveloped gonads, fallopian tube, and broad ligament. In: Atlas of tumor pathology, 3rd series. Fascicle 23. Washington, DC: Armed Forces Institute of Pathology; 1998. p. 239–312.
2. Pierce GB. Teratocarcinoma: a model for developmental concept of cancer. In: Moscona AA, Monroy A, editors. Current topics in developmental biology, vol. 2. New York: Academic Press; 1967. p. 223–46.
3. Damjanov I. Pathobiology of human germ cell neoplasia. Recent Results Cancer Res 1991;123:1–19.
4. Ulbright TM. Germ cell tumors of the gonads: a selective review emphasizing problems in differential diagnosis, newly appreciated, and controversial issues. Mod Pathol 2005;18(Suppl 2): S61–79.
5. Oosterhuis JW, Stoop H, Honecker F, Looijenga LH. Why human extragonadal germ cell tumours occur in the midline of the body: old concepts, new perspectives [discussion in Int J Androl 2007; 30(4):263–4]. Int J Androl 2007;30:256–63.
6. Rutgers JL, Young RH, Scully RE. Ovarian yolk sac tumor arising from endometrioid carcinoma. Hum Pathol 1987;18:1296–9.
7. Mazur MT, Talbot Jr WH, Talerman A. Endodermal sinus tumor and mucinous cystadenofibroma of the ovary. Occurrence in an 82 year old woman. Cancer 1988;62:2011–15.
8. Oliva E, Andrada E, Pezzica E, Prat J. Ovarian carcinomas with choriocarcinomatous differentiation. Cancer 1993;72:2441–6.
9. Nogales FF, Bergeron C, Carvia RE, et al. Ovarian endometrioid tumors with yolk sac tumor component, an unusual form of ovarian neoplasm. Analysis of six cases. Am J Surg Pathol 1996;20:1056–66.
10. Walt H, Arrenbrecht S, Delozier-Blanchet CD, et al. A human testicular germ cell tumor with borderline histology between seminoma and embryonal carcinoma secreted beta HCG and AFP only as a xenograft. Cancer 1986;58:139–46.
11. Srigley JR, Mackay B, Toth P, Ayala A. The ultrastructure and histogenesis of male germ cell neoplasia with emphasis on seminoma with early carcinomatous features. Ultrastruct Pathol 1988;12:67–86.
12. Damjanov I. Is seminoma a relative or a precursor of embryonal carcinoma? Lab Invest 1989;60:1–3.
13. Oosterhuis JW, Castedo SMMJ, Dejong B, et al. Ploidy of primary germ cell tumors of the testis; pathogenesis and clinical relevance. Lab Invest 1989;60:14–21.
14. Czaja JT, Ulbright TM. Evidence for the transformation of seminoma to yolk sac tumor, with histogenetic considerations. Am J Clin Pathol 1992;97:468–77.
15. Parkash V, Carcangiu ML. Transformation of ovarian dysgerminoma to yolk sac tumor: evidence for a histogenetic continuum. Mod Pathol 1995;8:881–7.
16. Cardoso de Almeida PC, Scully RE. Diffuse embryoma of the testis. A distinctive form of mixed germ cell tumor. Am J Surg Pathol 1983;7:633–42.
17. Teilum G. Special tumors of ovary and testis and related extragonadal lesions. Comparative pathology and histological identification. Philadelphia: JB Lippincott; 1976.
18. Prat J, Cao D, Carinelli S, et al. Tumours of the ovary: Germ cell tumours. In Kurman RJ, Carcangiu ML, Herrington S, Young RH, editors. World Health Organization (WHO) classification of tumours of female reproductive organs. 4th ed. Lyons, France: IARC Press; 2014.
19. Prat J. Pathology of the ovary. Philadelphia: Saunders; 2004. p. 251–81.
20. Tapia N, Arauzo-Bravo MJ, Ko K, Scholer HR. Concise review: challenging the pluripotency of human testis-derived ESC-like cells. Stem Cells 2011;29(8):1165–9.
21. Wang Z, Oron E, Nelson B, et al. Distinct lineage specification roles for NANOG, OCT4, and SOX2 in human embryonic stem cells. Cell Stem Cell 2012;10:440–54.
22. Gershenson DM. Management of ovarian germ cell tumors. J Clin Oncol 2007;25:2938–43.
23. Vicus D, Beiner ME, Klachook S, et al. Pure dysgerminoma of the ovary 35 years on: a single institutional experience. Gynecol Oncol 2010;17:23–6.
24. Pressley RH, Muntz HG, Falkenberry S, Rice LW. Serum lactic dehydrogenase as a tumor marker in dysgerminoma. Gynecol Oncol 1992;44:281–3.
25. Zaloudek CJ, Tavassoli FA, Norris HJ. Dysgerminoma with syncytiotrophoblastic giant cells. A histologically and clinically distinctive subtype of dysgerminoma. Am J Surg Pathol 1981;5:361–7.
26. Radhakrishnan S, Haq S, Lofts F, et al. Ovarian dysgerminoma associated with hypercalcemia. Br J Obstet Gynaecol 2001;108: 1302–4.
27. Werness BA, Ramus SJ, Whittemore AS, et al. Primary ovarian dysgerminoma in a patient with a germline BRCA1 mutation. Int J Gynecol Pathol 2000;19:390–4.
28. Dietl J, Horny HPI, Ruck P, Kaiserling E. Dysgerminoma of the ovary: an immunohistochemical study of tumor infiltrating lymphoreticular cells and tumor cells. Cancer 1993;71:2562–8.
29. Rutgers JL, Scully RE. Functioning ovarian tumors with peripheral steroid cell proliferation: a report of twenty-four cases. Int J Gynecol Pathol 1986;5:319–37.
30. Sever M, Jones TD, Roth LM, et al. Expression of CD117 (c-kit) receptor in dysgerminoma of the ovary: diagnostic and therapeutic implications. Mod Pathol 2005;18:1411–16.
31. Chang MC, Vargas SO, Hornick JL, et al. Embryonic stem cell transcription factors and D2-40 (podoplanin) as diagnostic immunohistochemical markers in ovarian germ cell tumors. Int J Gynecol Pathol 2009;28:347–55.

32. Cao D, Guo S, Allan RW, et al. SALL4 is a novel sensitive and specific marker of ovarian primitive germ cell tumors and is particularly useful in distinguishing yolk sac tumor from clear cell carcinoma. Am J Surg Pathol 2009;33:894–904.
33. Nogales FF, Dulcey I, Preda O. Issues in gynecologic pathology. Germ cell tumors of the ovary. An update. Arch Pathol Lab Med 2013;137:104–12.
34. Cossu-Rocca P, Zhang S, Roth LM, et al. Chromosome 12p abnormalities in dysgerminoma of the ovary: a FISH analysis. Mod Pathol 2006;19:611–15.
35. Hoei-Hansen CE, Kraggerud SM, Abeler VM, et al. Ovarian dysgerminomas are characterised by frequent KIT mutations and abundant expression of pluripotency markers. Mol Cancer 2007;6:12.
36. Cheng L, Roth LM, Zhang S, et al. KIT gene mutation and amplification in dysgerminoma of the ovary. Cancer 2011;117:2096–103.
37. Hersmus R, Stoop H, van de Geijn GJ, et al. Prevalence of c-KIT mutations in gonadoblastoma and dysgerminomas of patients with disorders of sex development (DSD) and ovarian dysgerminomas. PLoS One 2012;7:e43952.
38. Osborne BM, Robboy SJ. Lymphomas or leukemia presenting as ovarian tumors. An analysis of 42 cases. Cancer 1983;52:1933–43.
39. Zhang R, Sun YC, Zhang GY, et al. Treatment of malignant ovarian germ cell tumors and preservation of fertility. Eur J Gynaecol Oncol 2012;33:489–92.
40. Mangili G, Sigismondi C, Lorusso D, et al. Is surgical restaging indicated in apparent stage IA pure ovarian dysgerminoma? The MITO group retrospective experience. Gynecol Oncol 2011;121:280–4.
41. Gershenson DM, Copeland JL, Del Junco G, et al. Second-look laparotomy in the management of malignant germ cell tumors of the ovary. Obstet Gynecol 1986;67:789–94.
42. Palmquist MB, Webb MJ, Lieber MM, et al. DNA ploidy of ovarian dysgerminomas: correlation with clinical outcome. Gynecol Oncol 1992;44:13–16.
43. Fujita M, Inoue M, Tanizawa O, et al. Retrospective review of 41 patients with endodermal sinus tumor of the ovary. Int J Gynecol Cancer 1993;3:329–35.
44. Gershenson DM, Del Junco G, Herson J, Rutledge FN. Endodermal sinus tumor of the ovary: the M.D. Anderson experience. Obstet Gynecol 1983;61:194–202.
45. Kawai M, Kano T, Furuhashi Y, et al. Prognostic factors in yolk sac tumors of the ovary. A clinicopathologic analysis of 29 cases. Cancer 1991;67:184–92.
46. Teilum G. Endodermal sinus tumor of the ovary and testis. Comparative morphogenesis of the so-called mesonephroma ovarii (Schiller) and extraembryonic (yolk sac-allantoic) structures of the rat's placenta. Cancer 1959;12:1092–105.
47. Kurman RJ, Norris HJ. Endodermal sinus tumor of the ovary: a clinicopathologic analysis of 71 cases. Cancer 1976;38:2404–19.
48. Schiller W. Mesonephroma ovarii. Am J Cancer 1939;35:1–21.
49. Nogales FF, Preda O, Nicolae A. Yolk sac tumours revisited: a review of their many faces and names. Histopathology 2012;60:1023–33.
50. Nogales Jr FF, Matilla A, Nogales O, Galera-Davidson HL. Yolk sac tumors with pure and mixed polyvesicular vitelline patterns. Hum Pathol 1978;9:553–66.
51. Young RH, Ulbright TM, Policarpio-Nicolas ML. Yolk sac tumor with a prominent polyvesicular vitelline pattern: a report of three cases. Am J Surg Pathol 2013;37:393–8.
52. Cohen MB, Friend DS, Molnar JJ, Talerman A. Gonadal endodermal sinus (yolk sac) tumor with pure intestinal differentiation: a new histologic type. Pathol Res Pract 1987;182:609–16.
53. Clement PB, Young RH, Scully RE. Endometrioid-like yolk sac tumor of the ovary. A clinicopathological analysis of eight cases. Am J Surg Pathol 1987;11:767–78.
54. Prat J, Bhan AK, Dickersin GR, et al. Hepatoid yolk sac tumor of the ovary (endodermal sinus tumor with hepatoid differentiation). A light microscopical, ultrastructural and immunohistochemical study of seven cases. Cancer 1982;50:2355–68.
55. Ulbright TM, Roth LM, Brodhecker CA. Yolk sac differentiation in germ cell tumors. A morphologic study of 50 cases with emphasis on hepatic, enteric, and parietal yolk sac features. Am J Surg Pathol 1986;10:151–64.
56. Nakashima N, Fukatsu T, Nagasaki T, et al. The frequency and histology of hepatic tissue in germ cell tumors. Am J Surg Pathol 1987;11:682–92.
57. Dickersin GR, Oliva E, Young RH. Endometrioid-like variant of ovarian yolk sac tumor with foci of carcinoid: an ultrastructural study. Ultrastruct Pathol 1995;19:421–9.
58. Nogales FF, Buritica C, Regauer S, Gonzalez T. Mucinous carcinoid as an unusual manifestation of endodermal differentiation in ovarian yolk sac tumors. Am J Surg Pathol 2005;29:1247–51.
59. Devouassoux-Shisheboran M, Schammel DP, Tavassoli FA. Ovarian hepatoid yolk sac tumours: morphological, immunohistochemical and ultrastructural features. Histopathology 1999;34:462–9.
60. Michael H, Ulbright TM, Brodhecker CA. The pluripotential nature of the mesenchyme-like component of yolk sac tumor. Arch Pathol Lab Med 1989;113:1115–19.
61. Ulbright TM, Loehrer PJ, Roth LM, et al. The development of non-germ cell malignancies within germ cell tumors. A clinicopathologic study of 11 cases. Cancer 1984;54:1824–33.
62. Zynger DL, Everton MJ, Dimov ND, et al. Expression of glypican 3 in ovarian and extragonadal germ cell tumors. Am J Clin Pathol 2008;130:224–30.
63. Rabban JT, Zaloudek CJ. A practical approach to immunohistochemical diagnosis of ovarian germ cell tumours and sex cord-stromal tumours. Histopathology 2013;62:71–88.
64. Xue D, Peng Y, Wang F, et al. RNA-binding protein LIN28 is a sensitive marker of ovarian primitive germ cell tumours. Histopathology 2011;59:452–9.
65. Pitman MB, Triratanachat S, Young RH, Oliva E. Hepatocyte paraffin 1 antibody does not distinguish primary ovarian tumors with hepatoid differentiation from metastatic hepatocellular carcinoma. Int J Gynecol Pathol 2004;23:58–64.
66. Kurman RJ, Norris HJ. Embryonal carcinoma of the ovary. A clinicopathologic entity distinct from endodermal sinus tumor resembling embryonal carcinoma of the adult testis. Cancer 1976;38:2420–33.
67. Kleinsmith LJ, Pierce Jr GB. Multipotentiality of single embryonal carcinoma cells. Cancer Res 1964;24:1544–51.
68. Cheng L, Zhang S, Talerman A, Roth LM. Morphologic, immunohistochemical, and fluorescence in situ hybridization study of ovarian embryonal carcinoma with comparison to solid variant of yolk sac tumor and immature teratoma. Hum Pathol 2010;41:716–23.
69. Takeda A, Ishizuka T, Goto T, et al. Polyembryoma of ovary producing alpha-fetoprotein and HCG: immunoperoxidase and electron microscopic study. Cancer 1982;14:1878–89.
70. Nakashima N, Murakami S, Fukatsu T, et al. Characteristics of 'embryoid body' in human gonadal germ cell tumors. Hum Pathol 1988;19:1144–54.
71. Prat J, Matías-Guiu X, Scully RE. Hepatic yolk sac differentiation in an ovarian polyembryoma. Surg Pathol 1989;2:147–50.
72. Jondle DM, Shahin MS, Sorosky J, Benda JA. Ovarian mixed germ cell tumor with predominance of polyembryoma. A case report with literature review. Int J Gynecol Pathol 2002;21:78–81.
73. Kurman RJ, Norris HJ. Malignant mixed germ cell tumor of the ovary. A clinical and pathologic analysis of 30 cases. Obstet Gynecol 1976;48:579–89.
74. Lv L, Yang K, Wu H, et al. Pure choriocarcinoma of the ovary: a case report. J Gynecol Oncol 2011;22:135–9.
75. Axe SR, Klein VR, Woodruff JD. Choriocarcinoma of the ovary. Obstet Gynecol 1985;66:111–14.
76. Jacobs AJ, Newland JR, Green RK. Pure choriocarcinoma of the ovary. Obstet Gynecol Surv 1982;37:603–9.
77. Grover V, Grover RK, Usha R, et al. Primary pure choriocarcinoma of the ovary. Gynecol Obstet Invest 1990;30:61–3.
78. Fisher RA, Newlands ES, Jeffreys AJ, et al. Gestational and non-gestational trophoblastic tumors distinguished by DNA analysis. Cancer 1992;69:839–45.
79. Shigematsu T, Kamura T, Arima T, et al. DNA polymorphism analysis of a pure non-gestational choriocarcinoma of the ovary: case report. Eur J Gynaecol Oncol 2000;21:153–4.
80. Hafezi-Bakhtiari S, Morava-Protzner I, Burnell MJ, et al. Choriocarcinoma arising in a serous carcinoma of ovary: an example of histopathology driving treatment. J Obstet Gynaecol Can 2010;32:698–702.
81. Yanai-Inbar I, Scully RE. Relations of ovarian dermoid cysts and immature teratomas: an analysis of 350 cases of immature

82. Linder D, McCaw BK, Hecht F. Parthenogenic origin of benign ovarian teratomas. N Engl J Med 1975;292:63–6.
83. Vortmeyer AO, Devouassoux-Shisheboran M, Li G, et al. Microdissection-based analysis of mature ovarian teratoma. Am J Pathol 1999;154:987–91.
84. Koonings PP, Campbell K, Mishell Jr DR, Grimes DA. Relative frequency of primary ovarian neoplasms: a 10-year review. Obstet Gynecol 1989;74:921–6.
85. Zakin D. Radiologic diagnosis of dermoid cysts in the ovary. Obstet Gynecol Surv 1976;31:165–84.
86. Comerci Jr JT, Licciardi F, Bergh PA, et al. Mature cystic teratoma: a clinicopathologic evaluation of 517 cases and review of the literature. Obstet Gynecol 1994;84:22–8.
87. Robboy SJ, Scully RE. Ovarian teratoma with glial implants on the peritoneum. An analysis of 12 cases. Hum Pathol 1970;1:643–53.
88. Pins MR, Young RH, Daly WJ, Scully RE. Primary squamous cell carcinoma of the ovary. Report of 37 cases. Am J Surg Pathol 1996;20:823–33.
89. Thurlbeck WM, Scully RE. Solid teratoma of the ovary. A clinicopathological analysis of 9 cases. Cancer 1960;13:804–11.
90. Abbott TM, Hermann Jr WJ, Scully RE. Ovarian fetiform teratoma (homunculus) in a 9-year-old girl. Int J Gynecol Pathol 1984;2:392–402.
91. Chen E, Fletcher CD, Nucci MR. Meningothelial proliferations in mature cystic teratoma of the ovary: evidence for the common presence of cranially derived tissues paralleling anterior embryonic plate development. An analysis of 25 consecutive cases. Am J Surg Pathol 2010;34:1014–18.
92. Halabi M, Oliva E, Mazal PR, et al. Prostatic tissue in mature cystic teratoma of the ovary: a report of four cases, including one with features of prostatic adenocarcinoma, and cytogenetic studies. Int J Gynecol Pathol 2002;21:261–7.
93. Baker PM, Rosai J, Young RH. Ovarian teratomas with florid benign vascular proliferation: a distinctive finding associated with the neural component of teratomas that may be confused with a vascular neoplasm. Int J Gynecol Pathol 2002;21:16–21.
94. Axiotis CA, Lippes HA, Merino MJ, et al. Corticotroph cell pituitary adenoma within an ovarian teratoma. A new cause of Cushing's syndrome. Am J Surg Pathol 1987;11:218–24.
95. Kallenberg GA, Pesce CM, Norman B, et al. Ectopic hyperprolactinemia resulting from an ovarian teratoma. JAMA 1990;263:2472–4.
96. Palmer PE, Bogojavlensky S, Bhan AK, Scully RE. Prolactinoma in wall of ovarian dermoid cyst with hyperprolactinemia. Obstet Gynecol 1990;75:540–3.
97. Silver SA, Tavassoli FA. Glomus tumor arising in a mature teratoma of the ovary: report of a case simulating a metastasis from cervical squamous carcinoma. Arch Pathol Lab Med 2000;124:1373–5.
98. Lee K, Scully RE. Mucinous tumors of the ovary. A clinicopathologic study of 196 borderline tumors (of intestinal type) and carcinomas. Including an evaluation of 11 cases with 'pseudomyxoma peritonei.' Am J Surg Pathol 2000;24:1447–64.
99. Ronnett BM, Seidman JD. Mucinous tumors arising in ovarian mature cystic teratomas. Am J Surg Pathol 2003;27:650–7.
100. Davis GL. Malignant melanoma arising in mature ovarian cystic teratoma (dermoid cyst): report of two cases and literature analysis. Int J Gynecol Pathol 1996;15:356–62.
101. Smith HO, Berwick M, Verschraegen CF, et al. Incidence and survival rates for female malignant germ cell tumors. Obstet Gynecol 2006;107:1075–85.
102. Norris HJ, Zirkin HJ, Benson WL. Immature (malignant) teratoma of the ovary: a clinical and pathologic study of 58 cases. Cancer 1976;37:2359–72.
103. Gershenson DM, Del Junco G, Silva EG, et al. Immature teratoma of the ovary. Obstet Gynecol 1986;68:624–9.
104. Kawai M, Kano T, Furuhashi Y, et al. Immature teratoma of the ovary. Gynecol Oncol 1991;40:133–7.
105. Bonazzi C, Peccatori F, Colombo N, et al. Pure ovarian immature teratoma, a unique and curable disease: 10 years' experience of 32 prospectively treated patients. Obstet Gynecol 1994;84:598–604.
106. Heifetz SA, Cushing B, Giller R, et al. Immature teratomas in children: pathologic considerations: a report from the combined Pediatric Oncology Group/Children's Cancer Group. Am J Surg Pathol 1998;22:1115–24.
107. Nogales FF, Avila IR, Concha A, et al. Immature endodermal teratoma of the ovary: embryologic correlations and immunohistochemistry. Hum Pathol 1993;24:364–70.
108. Nogales Jr FF, Favara BE, Major FJ, et al. Immature teratoma of the ovary with a neural component ("solid" teratoma). A clinicopathologic study of 20 cases. Hum Pathol 1976;7:625–42.
109. O'Connor DM, Norris HJ. The influence of grade on the outcome of stage I ovarian immature (malignant) teratoma and the reproducibility of grading. Int J Gynecol Pathol 1994;13:283–9.
110. Ferguson AW, Katabuchi H, Ronnett BM, Cho KR. Glial implants in gliomatosis peritonei arise from normal tissue, not from the associated teratoma. Am J Pathol 2001;159(1):51–5.
111. Calder CJ, Light AM, Rollason TP. Immature ovarian teratoma with mature peritoneal metastatic deposits showing glial, epithelial, and endometrioid differentiation: a case report and review of the literature. Int J Gynecol Pathol 1994;13:279–82.
112. Perrone T, Steiner M, Dehner LP. Nodal gliomatosis and alpha-fetoprotein production: two unusual facets of grade I ovarian teratoma. Arch Pathol Lab Med 1986;110:975–7.
113. Zhuang Z, Devouassoux-Shisheboran M, Lubensky IA, et al. Premeiotic origin of teratomas: is meiosis required for differentiation into mature tissues? Cell Cycle 2005;4:1683–7.
114. Kraggerud SM, Szymanska J, Abeler VM, et al. DNA copy number changes in malignant ovarian germ cell tumors. Cancer Res 2000;60:3025–30.
115. Baker BA, Frickey L, Yu IT, et al. DNA content of ovarian immature teratomas and malignant germ cell tumors. Gynecol Oncol 1998;71:14–18.
116. Williams SD, Blessing JA, Liao S, et al. Adjuvant therapy of ovarian germ cell tumors with cisplatin, etoposide, and bleomycin: a trial of the Gynecologic Oncology Group. J Clin Oncol 1994;12:701–6.
117. Nogales FF, Aguilar D. Florid vascular proliferation in grade 0 glial implants from ovarian immature teratoma. Int J Gynecol Pathol 2002;21(3):305–7.
118. Dadmanesh F, Miller DM, Swenerton KD, Clement PB. Gliomatosis peritonei with malignant transformation. Mod Pathol 1997;10:597–601.
119. Riopel MA, Spellerberg A, Griffin CA, Perlman EJ. Genetic analysis of ovarian germ cell tumors by comparative genomic hybridization. Cancer Res 1998;58:3105–10.
120. Woodruff JD, Rauh JT, Markley RL. Ovarian struma. Obstet Gynecol 1966;27:194–201.
121. Simkin PH, Ramirez LA, Zweizig SL, et al. Monomorphic teratoma of the ovary: a rare cause of triiodothyronine toxicosis. Thyroid 1999;9:949–54.
122. Burg J, Kommoss F, Bittinger F, et al. Mature cystic teratoma of the ovary with struma and benign Brenner tumor: A case report with immunohistochemical characterization. Int J Gynecol Pathol 2002;21:74–7.
123. Szyfelbein WM, Young RH, Scully RE. Cystic struma ovarii: a frequently unrecognized tumor. A report of 20 cases. Am J Surg Pathol 1994;18:1102–16.
124. Szyfelbein WM, Young RH, Scully RE. Struma ovarii simulating ovarian tumors of other types: a report of 30 cases. Am J Surg Pathol 1995;19:21–9.
125. Robboy SJ, Shaco-Levy R, Peng RY, et al. Malignant struma ovarii: an analysis of 88 cases, including 27 with extraovarian spread. Int J Gynecol Pathol 2009;28:405–22.
126. Devaney K, Synder R, Norris HJ, Tavassoli FA. Proliferative and histologically malignant struma ovarii: a clinicopathologic study of 54 cases. Int J Gynecol Pathol 1993;12:333–43.
127. Willemse PH, Oosterhuis JW, Aalders JG, et al. Malignant struma ovarii treated by ovariectomy, thyroidectomy, and ^{131}I administration. Cancer 1987;60:178–82.
128. Robboy SJ, Scully RE. Strumal carcinoid of the ovary: an analysis of 50 cases of a distinctive tumor composed of thyroid tissue and carcinoid. Cancer 1980;46:2019–34.
129. Garg K, Soslow RA, Rivera M, et al. Histologically bland 'extremely well differentiated' thyroid carcinomas arising in struma ovarii recur and metastasize. Int J Gynecol Pathol 2009;28:222–30.
130. Shaco-Levy R, Bean SM, Bentley RC, et al. Natural history of biologically malignant struma ovarii: analysis of 27 cases with extraovarian spread. Int J Gynecol Pathol 2010;29:212–27.

131. Karseladze AI, Kulinitch SI. Peritoneal strumosis. Pathol Res Pract 1994;190:1086–8.
132. Roth LM, Karseladze AI. Highly differentiated follicular carcinoma arising from struma ovarii: a report of three cases, a review of the literature, and reassessment of so-called peritoneal strumosis. Int J Gynecol Pathol 2008;27:213–22.
133. Robboy SJ, Norris HJ, Scully RE. Insular carcinoid primary in the ovary: a clinicopathologic analysis of 48 cases. Cancer 1975;36:404–18.
134. Robboy SJ, Scully RE, Norris HJ. Primary trabecular carcinoid of the ovary. Obstet Gynecol 1977;49:202–7.
135. Baker PM, Oliva E, Young RH, et al. Ovarian mucinous carcinoids including some with a carcinomatous component. A report of 17 cases. Am J Surg Pathol 2001;25:557–68.
136. Davis KP, Hartmann LK, Keeney GL, Shapiro H. Primary ovarian carcinoid tumors. Gynecol Oncol 1996;61:259–65.
137. Soga J, Osaka M, Yakuwa Y. Carcinoids of the ovary: an analysis of 329 reported cases. J Exp Clin Cancer Res 2000;19:271–80.
138. Robboy SJ. Insular carcinoid of ovary associated with malignant mucinous tumors. Cancer 1984;54:2273–6.
139. Snyder RR, Tavassoli FA. Ovarian strumal carcinoid: immunohistochemical, ultrastructural, and clinicopathologic observations. Int J Gynecol Pathol 1986;5:187–201.
140. Matias-Guiu X, Forteza J, Prat J. Mixed strumal and mucinous carcinoid tumor of the ovary. Int J Gynecol Pathol 1995;14:179–83.
141. Zhao C, Bratthauer GL, Barner R, et al. Comparative analysis of alternative and traditional immunohistochemical markers for the distinction of ovarian Sertoli cell tumor from endometrioid tumors and carcinoid tumor: A study of 160 cases. Am J Surg Pathol 2007;31:255–66.
142. Sorrong B, Falkmer S, Robboy SJ, et al. Neurohormonal peptides in ovarian carcinoids: an immunohistochemical study of 81 primary carcinoids and of intraovarian metastases from six mid-gut carcinoids. Cancer 1982;49:68–74.
143. Vang R, Gown AM, Zhao C, et al. Ovarian mucinous tumors associated with mature cystic teratomas: morphologic and immunohistochemical analysis identifies a subset of potential teratomatous origin that shares features of lower gastrointestinal tract mucinous tumors more commonly encountered as secondary tumors of the ovary. Am J Surg Pathol 2007;31:854–69.
144. Rabban JT, Lerwill MF, McCluggage WG, et al. Primary ovarian carcinoid tumors may express CDX-2: a potential pitfall in distinction from metastatic intestinal carcinoid tumors involving the ovary. Int J Gynecol Pathol 2009;28:41–8.
145. Robboy SJ, Scully RE, Norris HJ. Carcinoid metastatic to the ovary. A clinocopathologic analysis of 35 cases. Cancer 1974;33:798–811.
146. Hristov AC, Young RH, Vang R, et al. Ovarian metastases of appendiceal tumors with goblet cell carcinoid-like and signet ring cell patterns: a report of 30 cases. Am J Surg Pathol 2007;31:1502–11.
147. Kleinman GM, Young RH, Scully RE. Primary ovarian neuroectodermal tumors: a report of 25 cases. Am J Surg Pathol 1993;17:764–78.
148. Kleinman GM, Young RH, Scully RE. Ependymoma of the ovary: report of three cases. Hum Pathol 1984;15:632–8.
149. Hirschowitz L, Ansari A, Cahill DJ, et al. Central neurocytoma arising within a mature cystic teratoma of the ovary. Int J Gynecol Pathol 1997;16:176–9.
150. Mikami M, Komura Y, Sakaiya N, et al. Primary ependymoma of the ovary, in which long-term oral etoposide (VP-16) was effective in prolonging disease-free survival. Gynecol Oncol 2001;83:149–52.
151. Morovic A, Damjanov I. Neuroectodermal ovarian tumors: a brief overview. Histol Histopathol 2008;23:765–71.
152. Stolnicu S, Furtado A, Sanches A, et al. Ovarian ependymomas of extra-axial type or central immunophenotypes. Hum Pathol 2011;42:403–8.
153. Ud Din N, Memon A, Aftab K, et al. Oligodendroglioma arising in the glial component of ovarian teratomas: a series of six cases and review of literature. J Clin Pathol 2012;65:631–4.
154. Carr KA, Roberts JA, Frank TS. Progesterone receptors in bilateral ovarian ependymoma presenting in pregnancy. Hum Pathol 1992;23:962–5.
155. Guerrieri C, Jarlsfelt I. Ependymoma of the ovary. A case report with immunohistochemical, ultrastructural, and DNA cytometric findings, as well as histogenetic considerations. Am J Surg Pathol 1993;17:623–32.
156. Idowu MO, Rosenblum MK, Wei XJ, et al. Ependymomas of the central nervous system and adult extra-axial ependymomas are morphologically and immunohistochemically distinct—a comparative study with assessment of ovarian carcinomas for expression of glial fibrillary acidic protein. Am J Surg Pathol 2008;32:710–18.
157. Kawauchi S, Fukuda T, Miyamoto S, et al. Peripheral primitive neuroectodermal tumor of the ovary confirmed by CD99 immunostaining, karyotypic analysis, and RT-PCR for EWS/FLI-1 chimeric mRNA. Am J Surg Pathol 1998;22:1417–22.
158. Peterson WF. Malignant degeneration of benign cystic teratomas of the ovary; a collective review of the literature. Obstet Gynecol Surv 1957;12:793–830.
159. Dos Santos L, Mok E, Iasonos A. Squamous cell carcinoma arising in mature cystic teratoma of the ovary: A case series and review of the literature. Gynecol Oncol 2007;105:321–4.
160. Hackethal A, Brueggmann D, Bohlmann MK, et al. Squamous-cell carcinoma in mature cystic teratoma of the ovary: Systematic review and analysis of published data. Lancet Oncol 2008;9:1171–80 (erratum in: Lancet Oncol 2009;10:446).
161. Hirakawa T, Tsuneyoshi M, Enjoji M. Squamous cell carcinoma arising in mature cystic teratoma of the ovary. Clinicopathologic and topographic analysis. Am J Surg Pathol 1989;13:397–405.
162. Sumi T, Ishiko O, Maeda K, et al. Adenocarcinoma arising from respiratory ciliated epithelium in mature ovarian cystic teratoma. Arch Gynecol Obstet 2002;267:107–9.
163. Song YJ, Ryu SY, Choi SC, et al. Adenocarcinoma arising from the respiratory ciliated epithelium in a benign cystic teratoma of the ovary. Arch Gynecol Obstet. 2009;280:659–62.
164. Ribeiro-Silva A, Chang D, Bisson FW, Ré LO. Clinicopathological and immunohistochemical features of a sebaceous carcinoma arising within a benign dermoid cyst of the ovary. Virchows Arch 2003;443:574–8.
165. Boyd C, Patel K, O'Sullivan B, et al. Pulmonary-type adenocarcinoma and signet ring mucinous adenocarcinoma arising in an ovarian dermoid cyst: report of a unique case. Hum Pathol 2012;43:2088–92.
166. Arora DS, Haldane S. Carcinosarcoma arising in a dermoid cyst of the ovary. J Clin Pathol 1996;49:519–21.
167. Yahata T, Kawasaki T, Serikawa T, et al. Adenocarcinoma arising from respiratory ciliated epithelium in benign cystic teratoma of the ovary: a case report with analyzes of the CT, MRI and pathological findings. J Obstet Gynaecol Res 2008;34:408–12.
168. McKenney JK, Soslow RA, Longacre TA. Ovarian mature teratomas with mucinous epithelial neoplasms: morphologic heterogeneity and association with pseudomyxoma peritonei. Am J Surg Pathol 2008;32:645–55.
169. Levine DA, Villella JA, Poynor EA, Soslow RA. Gastrointestinal adenocarcinoma arising in a mature cystic teratoma of the ovary. Gynecol Oncol 2004;94:597–9.
170. Gershenson DM, Del Junco G, Copeland LJ, et al. Mixed germ cell tumors of the ovary. Obstet Gynecol 1984;64:200–6.
171. Scully RE. Gonadoblastoma: a review of 74 cases. Cancer 1970;25:1340–56.
172. Salo P, Kaariainen H, Petrovic V, et al. Molecular mapping of the putative gonadoblastoma locus on the Y chromosome. Genes Chromosomes Cancer 1995;14:210–14.
173. Cheng L, Thomas A, Roth LM, et al. OCT4: a novel biomarker for dysgerminoma of the ovary. Am J Surg Pathol 2004;28:1341–6.
174. Li Y, Tabatabai ZL, Lee TL, et al. The Y-encoded TSPY protein: a significant marker potentially plays a role in the pathogenesis of testicular germ cell tumors. Hum Pathol 2007;38:1470–81.
175. Hersmus R, Kalfa N, de Leeuw B, et al. FOXL2 and SOX9 as parameters of female and male gonadal differentiation in patients with various forms of disorders of sex development (DSD). J Pathol 2008;215:31–8.
176. Talerman A. A distinctive gonadal neoplasm related to gonadoblastoma. Cancer 1972;30:1219–24.

30 Metastatic Tumors of the Ovary

Emanuela D'Angelo, Jaime Prat

CHAPTER OUTLINE

General Features	694	Renal Tumors	705
Mode of Spread	694	Tumors of the Urinary Tract	706
Site of Origin	696	Adrenal Gland Tumors	707
Intestinal Carcinomas	696	Malignant Melanoma	707
Krukenberg Tumor	699	Pulmonary and Mediastinal Tumors	707
Carcinoid Tumors	701	Uterine Tumors	707
Breast Carcinoma	702	Lymphoma and Leukemia	709
Tumors of the Pancreas, Biliary Tract, and Liver	703	Peritoneal Tumors	710
Tumors of the Appendix	704	Extragenital Sarcomas	711
		Summary	712

GENERAL FEATURES

The ovaries are involved by metastatic tumors more often than any other organ in the female genital tract, regardless of the location of the primary neoplasm.[1] Tumors that extend to the ovary directly from adjacent organs or tissues are also included in the category of secondary tumors; however, most ovarian carcinomas associated with uterine cancers of similar histologic type are independent primary neoplasms (see Chapter 27).

Metastatic tumors to the ovary are common and occur in approximately 30% of women dying of cancer. About 6–7% of all adnexal masses found during physical examination are actually metastatic ovarian tumors, frequently unsuspected by gynecologists.[2-4] The metastasis often masquerades as a primary ovarian tumor and may even be the initial manifestation of the patient's cancer. Pathologists also tend to mistake metastatic tumors for primary ovarian neoplasms, even after microscopic examination, because the existence of a concurrent or prior tumor in another organ is either not known or disregarded. Also, all metastatic tumors may have a functioning ovarian stroma with clinical or pathologic evidence of hyperestrogenism simulating a primary ovarian tumor.

The frequencies of various sites of origin of secondary ovarian tumors differ among different countries according to the incidence of various cancers therein. Carcinomas of the colon, stomach, breast, and endometrium, as well as lymphomas and leukemias, account for the vast majority of cases.[5] Rectal or sigmoid colon cancer accounts for 75% of the metastatic intestinal tumors to the ovary, and probably constitutes the most common cause of misdiagnosis.[2-5] The Krukenberg tumor is almost always secondary to a gastric adenocarcinoma, but may occasionally originate in the intestine, appendix, breast, or other sites.[3,5,6] Rarely, breast cancer metastatic to the ovary presents clinically as an ovarian mass. In fact, in patients with a history of breast cancer, especially *BRCA*-positive cases, clinically detected ovarian tumors are usually independent primaries and not metastases. In recent years, attention has been drawn to mucinous tumors of the appendix, pancreas, and biliary tract that often spread to the ovary and closely simulate ovarian mucinous borderline tumors or carcinomas.[7-11] Resemblance to borderline tumors or even benign cystadenofibromas is due to the so-called maturation phenomenon by which the epithelium of the metastatic carcinoma differentiates and appears flattened and benign. A wide variety of other tumors may metastasize to the ovary.

General features of ovarian metastasis include: bilaterality, multinodularity, involvement of the ovarian surface, extensive extraovarian spread, unusual patterns of dissemination, unusual histologic features, blood vessel and lymphatic invasion, and desmoplastic stromal reaction (Table 30.1).

MODE OF SPREAD

The routes of tumor spread to the ovary are variable. Lymphatic and hematogenous metastasis to the ovaries is the most common form of dissemination.[2-4] The importance of hematogenous spread is supported by the higher frequency of ovarian metastases in the well-vascularized ovaries of young patients. Embolic spread often produces multiple nodules

> **Table 30.1 Metastatic Tumors to the Ovary (Clues to the Diagnosis)**
>
> 1. Bilaterality (mucinous and endometrioid-like)
> 2. Small, superficial, multinodular tumors
> 3. Vascular invasion
> 4. Desmoplastic reaction
> 5. Unusual histology
> 6. Extensive extraovarian spread
> 7. Unusual clinical history

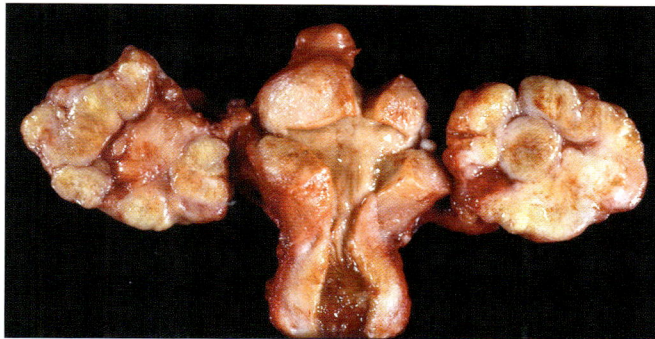

Figure 30.1 Metastatic carcinoma from the colon. The ovaries are replaced by solid multinodular tumors.

within the substance of the ovary and commonly is accompanied by prominent intravascular nests of tumor cells in the ovarian hilum, meso-ovarium, and mesosalpinx.

Direct extension is also a common form of spread from adjacent tumors of the fallopian tube, uterus, and colorectum, for mesotheliomas, and for occasional retroperitoneal sarcomas.[5] Transtubal spread provides an explanation for some surface ovarian implants from carcinomas of the uterine corpus,[12] but may also account for some cases of spread from the uterine cervix.[13,14] Neoplasms may also reach the ovary by the transperitoneal route from abdominal organs, such as the appendix.[8] The metastatic tumor is found on the surface of the ovary or in the superficial cortex. Ovulation orifices may possibly represent a portal of entry for tumor cells.

Clinical Features

Ovarian metastases can be discovered in patients during follow-up after treatment of a primary tumor, or unexpectedly diagnosed during a surgical procedure for treatment of an abdominal tumor, or fortuitously found at autopsy. The age distribution of patients with ovarian metastases depends to a great extent on that of the corresponding primary tumors, but patients with metastases to the ovaries tend to be younger than those with primary ovarian neoplasms. This partly reflects the propensity of tumors to seed to the richly vascularized ovaries of young women and partly that tumors commonly metastasizing to the ovaries, especially intestinal, gastric, and mammary carcinomas, occur in younger women.

The circumstances leading to the discovery of the ovarian metastases depend on the site of the primary tumor.[1,15] Ovarian metastases are detected before the breast cancer in only 1.5% of cases.[15] In patients with a rectal or sigmoid colon cancer, the ovarian metastases and the primary tumor are discovered simultaneously, or more often, the intestinal tumor has been resected months or, years previously (50–75% of cases). Less frequently, the colorectal adenocarcinoma is discovered several months to years after resection of the ovarian metastases (3–20% of cases).[3,16] In contrast, in about two-thirds of patients with Krukenberg tumor the diagnosis of the ovarian metastases precedes the discovery of the primary carcinoma.[17,18] When a patient presents with abdominopelvic symptoms leading to suspicion of an ovarian tumor, the symptoms are nonspecific and similar to those of ovarian cancer, i.e., pelvic masses, ascites, or vaginal bleeding.[17,19] Some patients with ovarian metastases have menstrual abnormalities, postmenopausal bleeding, and virilization, or they deliver a masculinized female fetus.

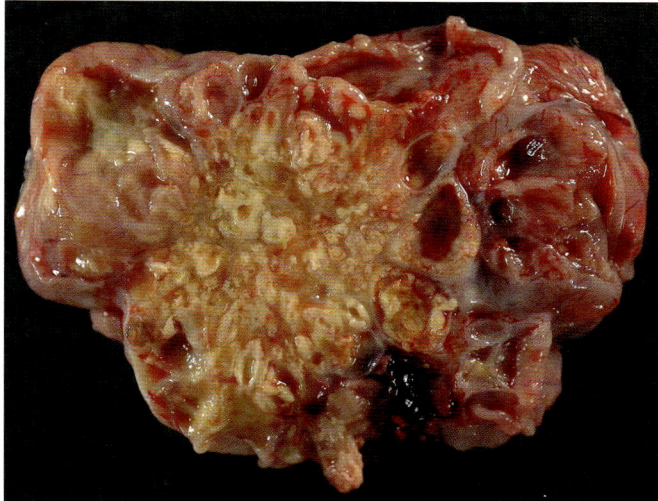

Figure 30.2 Metastatic carcinoma from the colon. Solid and cystic tumor with extensive necrosis and focal hemorrhage.

These endocrine manifestations result from hormonally active luteinized stromal cells found in approximately one-third of metastatic tumors. Stromal luteinization occurs most frequently in association with metastatic mucinous carcinomas, particularly of colorectal or gastric origin.

Approximately 80% of patients with a Krukenberg tumor have bilateral ovarian metastases, and 73% of patients with ovarian metastases from breast carcinomas have extraovarian metastases.[15,17] Radiologically, patients with a Krukenberg tumor more often have a solid mass with an intratumoral cyst, whereas primary ovarian cancers are predominantly cystic.[20,21]

Macroscopic Features

Ovarian metastases are bilateral in over 70% of cases (Figure 30.1).[3] In contrast, the ovarian carcinomas most commonly mimicked by metastases (i.e., mucinous, endometrioid, and clear cell carcinomas) are bilateral in less than 15% of cases.[22] Metastatic tumors grow as superficial or parenchymatous solid nodules or, frequently, as cysts. The size of ovarian metastases varies even from one side to the other. The ovaries may be only slightly enlarged or measure 10 cm or more. Intraoperative assessment of size and laterality may serve as a helpful guideline in distinguishing primary from metastatic mucinous tumors: bilateral tumors of any size or unilateral tumors under 10 cm have a high probability of being metastatic, whereas unilateral tumors over 10 cm are usually primary.[23] However, there are many exceptions,[24,25] especially in cases of colorectal and endocervical primaries.[26] It is also noteworthy that metastases involving the ovary are often larger than their corresponding primary tumors.

Microscopic Features

The microscopic appearance of the metastases varies depending on the nature of the primary tumor.[2–4] The identification of surface implants is extremely helpful in the recognition of secondary ovarian tumors that spread through the abdominal cavity and tubal lumen. Other features more commonly observed in metastatic tumors include multinodular infiltrative growth, single cell infiltration, follicle-like spaces (due to inadequate lymphatic drainage), and intravascular tumor emboli. Presence of a desmoplastic stroma and prominent stromal luteinization around tumor glands are also suspicious for metastasis.

SITE OF ORIGIN

INTESTINAL CARCINOMAS

Most intestinal metastases originate in the large intestine and, much less frequently, in the small bowel. Whereas at autopsy metastases from intestinal carcinomas are less common than those from gastric carcinomas (14% vs 38%, respectively), at the time of operation metastases from intestinal carcinomas are almost five times as frequent as those from gastric carcinomas.[27] Up to 45% of colorectal metastases to the ovary are clinically thought to be primary ovarian tumors, and many are misinterpreted as such on microscopic examination.[2] Metastasis from the large bowel to the ovary is seen relatively more frequently when this cancer develops in women under 40 years of age. In one large series, one-fourth of patients were less than 40 years old[28] and in another about 43% were under 50 years.[29] In the latter study, it was found that patients initially presenting

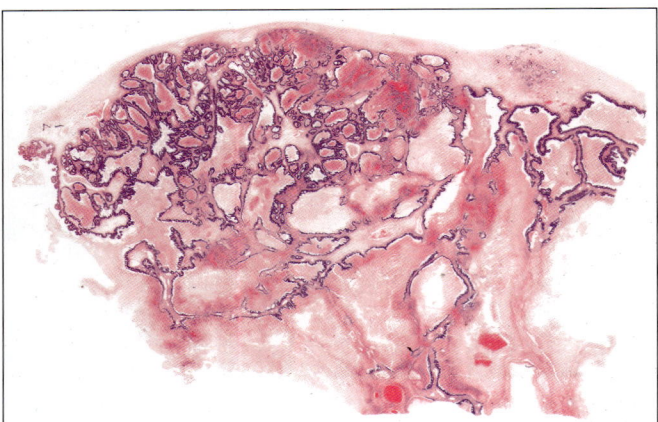

Figure 30.3 Metastatic adenocarcinoma from the colon. Garland-like glandular pattern with focal segmental necrosis of glands and abundant necrotic debris.

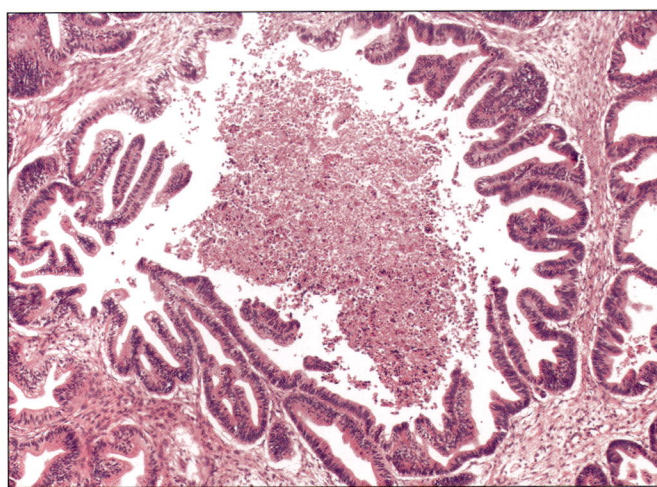

Figure 30.5 Metastatic adenocarcinoma from the colon. The glandular epithelium shows papillary growth and striking nuclear atypia (grade 3).

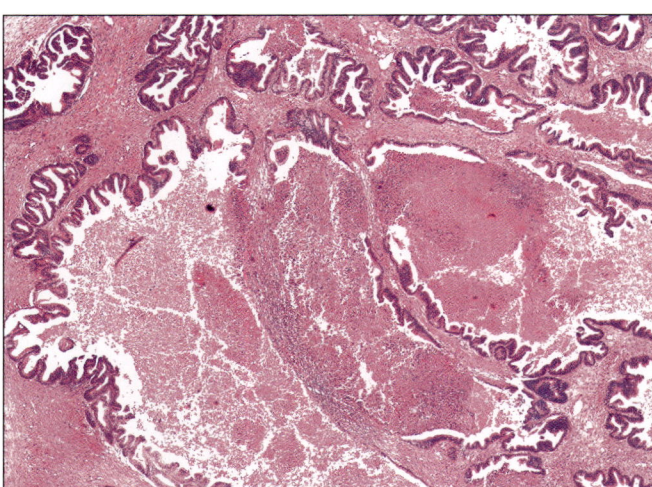

Figure 30.4 Metastatic adenocarcinoma from the colon. Focal segmental necrosis of glands and luminal necrotic debris ('dirty necrosis').

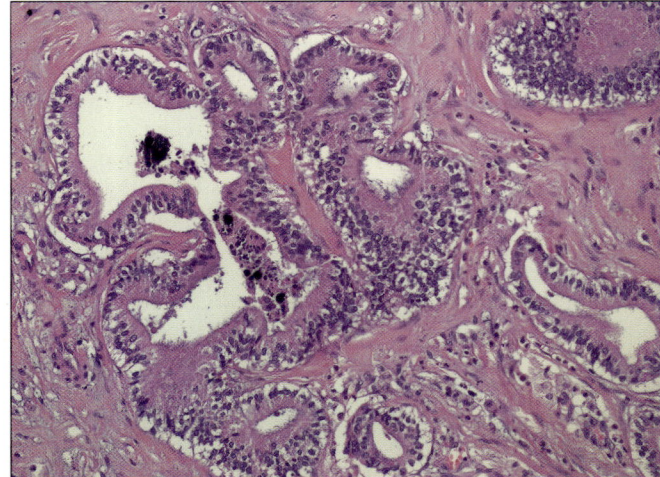

Figure 30.6 Metastatic adenocarcinoma from the colon. Neoplastic glands lying in a desmoplastic stroma.

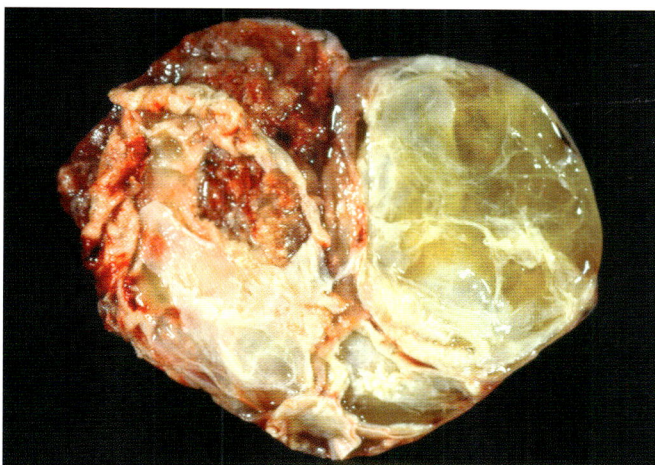

Figure 30.7 Metastatic carcinoma from the cecum. Multilocular mucinous cystic tumor with focal necrosis simulating an ovarian mucinous cystadenocarcinoma.

with an ovarian mass were significantly younger than those having ovarian spread in the setting of a known colorectal primary (average 48 vs 61 years). Not infrequently, patients have luteinized stromal cells in the ovarian tumor with resultant hormone production and endocrine symptoms.

The ovarian tumors are bilateral in approximately two-thirds of cases (Figure 30.1). Smaller tumors are usually solid, whereas larger tumors are composed of friable gray, yellow, or red tissue with cysts that contain necrotic tumor, mucinous fluid, or blood (Figure 30.2).[2,3]

Microscopically, the metastatic tumors may be confused with primary endometrioid or mucinous carcinoma depending on whether the colonic carcinoma is predominantly non-mucinous or mucinous. Features that help distinguish colon cancer from endometrioid carcinoma include luminal necrotic debris ('dirty necrosis'), focal segmental necrosis of the glands (Figures 30.3–30.5), occasional presence of goblet cells, and absence of müllerian features (squamous differentiation, an adenofibromatous component, or association with endometriosis). Also the nuclei lining the glands of metastatic colon carcinoma exhibit a higher degree of atypia than those of endometrioid carcinoma (Figure 30.5).[2,3] The stroma may be desmoplastic (Figure 30.6), edematous, or myxoid, but frequently resembles ovarian stroma. Stromal luteinization is most frequently found in metastatic colorectal carcinomas.[30]

Metastatic tumors may also resemble closely primary mucinous ovarian tumors both grossly (Figure 30.7) and microscopically. The metastases may be moderately differentiated (Figure 30.8) or so well differentiated that they can be mistaken for mucinous borderline or less often benign ovarian tumors. Generous sampling (at least one block per 1–2 cm of tumor diameter) is recommended. Metastatic mucinous tumors to the ovary can originate in the large intestine, stomach, pancreas, gallbladder, biliary tract, appendix, and even, exceptionally, urachus and lung. Features supportive of the diagnosis of a metastasis already discussed include bilaterality, histologic surface involvement by epithelial cells (surface implants) (Figure 30.9), irregular infiltrative growth with desmoplasia (Figure 30.6), single cell invasion, signet-ring cells, vascular invasion (Figure 30.10), coexistence of

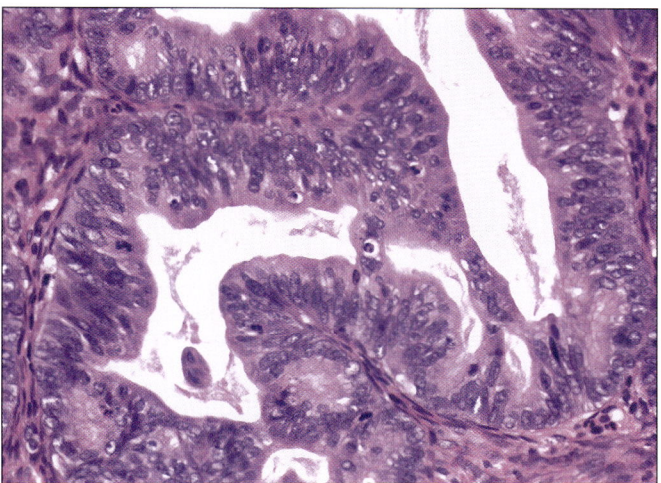

Figure 30.8 Metastatic adenocarcinoma from the colon. The mucinous glands are indistinguishable from those of a primary ovarian mucinous carcinoma. Mitotic figures are seen.

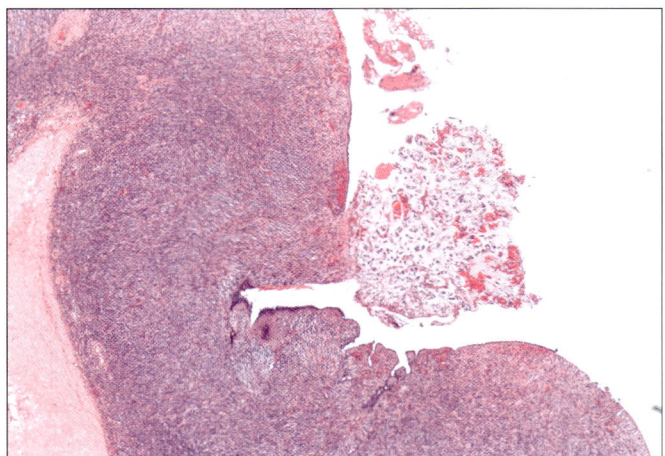

Figure 30.9 Metastatic adenocarcinoma from the colon. Ovarian surface involvement by mucinous epithelial cells (surface implant).

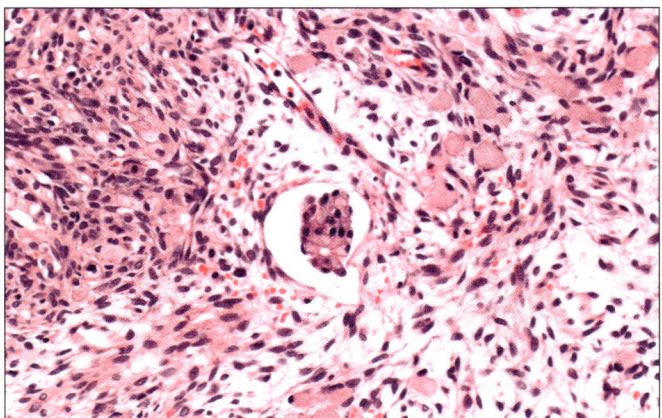

Figure 30.10 Krukenberg tumor. Vascular space invasion. Numerous signet-ring cells lie in the ovarian stroma.

benign-appearing mucinous areas with foci showing a high mitotic rate and nuclear hyperchromasia, and histologic surface mucin.[31] In some cases, the intestinal metastases contain cells with abundant clear cytoplasm and may simulate either primary clear cell carcinoma or the secretory variant of endometrioid carcinoma (Figure 30.11).[32]

Immunohistochemistry

Immunohistochemical stains can be helpful in distinguishing primary adenocarcinoma of the ovary from metastatic colorectal adenocarcinoma (Table 30.2). Cytokeratin (CK) immunostains are the most commonly used. Primary ovarian carcinomas are almost always immunoreactive for CK7 whereas colorectal adenocarcinomas are usually CK7 negative.[33,34] Mucinous adenocarcinomas of the ovary may be immunoreactive for CK20, but the reaction is typically weak and focal.[33,35] Endometrioid adenocarcinomas are almost invariably CK20 negative.[34] In contrast, colorectal adenocarcinomas are diffusely and strongly reactive for CK20. Therefore, a CK7-positive/CK20-negative immunoprofile favors a primary ovarian carcinoma, whereas a CK7-negative/CK20-positive immunoprofile suggests metastatic adenocarcinoma (Table 30.2).[35–37] Although the vast majority of colorectal adenocarcinomas express CK20, poorly differentiated and right-sided tumors can be CK20 negative.[38] Furthermore, adenocarcinomas of the appendix, small intestine, and stomach can be CK7 positive. Thus, immunostains for CK7 and CK20 should be interpreted with caution, always in the light of all clinical information, and with the understanding that no tumor shows absolute consistency in its staining with these markers.

Other immunohistochemical stains have greater overlap in their expressions and should not be used individually in this differential diagnosis. Nevertheless, after taking into account the clinicopathologic findings and the results of the CK immunostains, negative stainings for vimentin[39] CA125 and gastric mucin gene *MUC5AC*,[35] and strongly positive staining for carcinoembryonic antigen (CEA) (Figure 30.12)[33,34] favor metastatic colorectal cancer over primary ovarian adenocarcinoma (Table 30.2). Likewise, strong immunoreactivity for P53 (Figure 30.13) supports the

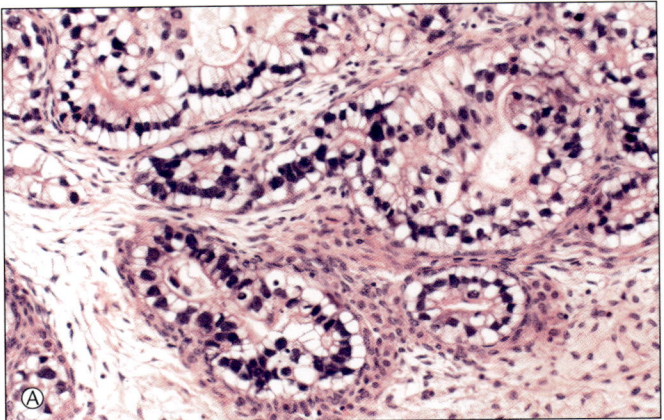
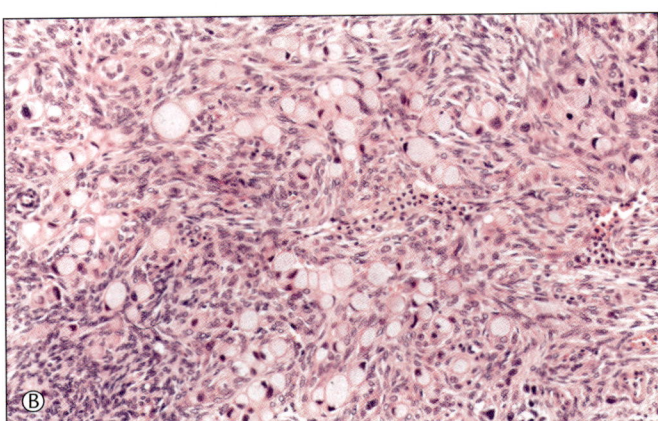

Figure 30.11 Metastatic adenocarcinoma from the small intestine. **(A)** Tubular glands lined by vacuolated cells resembling those of a secretory endometrioid carcinoma. Note the presence of stromal luteinization. **(B)** Typical Krukenberg tumor component encountered after additional sampling. Numerous signet-ring cells with eccentric nuclei and pale vacuolated cytoplasm are seen.

Table 30.2 Primary Ovarian Carcinomas versus Metastatic Gastrointestinal Carcinomas (Immunophenotypes)							
Tumor	CK7	CK20	CA125	MUC5AC	CEA	CDX2	ER
Ovarian Carcinoma							
Serous	+	−	+				
Mucinous	+	+	±	±	+	±	
Endometrioid	+	−	+		−	±	+
Metastatic Carcinoma							
Colon–rectum	−	+	−	−	+	+	−
Stomach	+	±	−	+	+	+	
Appendix	±	+	−	±	+	+	
Pancreas	+	+	−	+	+	+	

CK7, cytokeratin 7; CK20, cytokeratin 20; + usually positive; − usually negative; ± can be positive or negative, but often positive; ± can be positive or negative, but often negative.

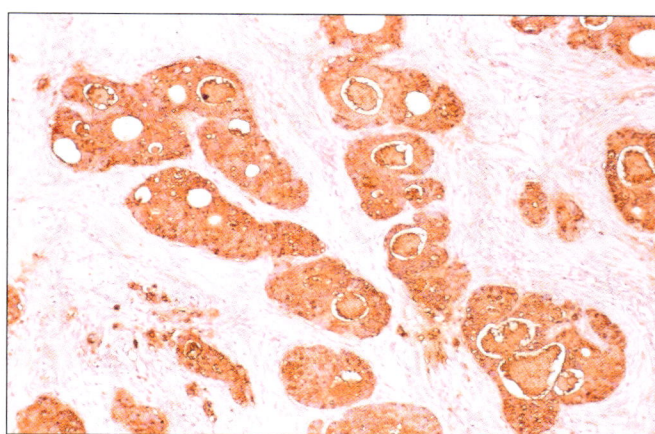

Figure 30.12 Metastatic adenocarcinoma from the colon. Strong immunoreaction for CEA.

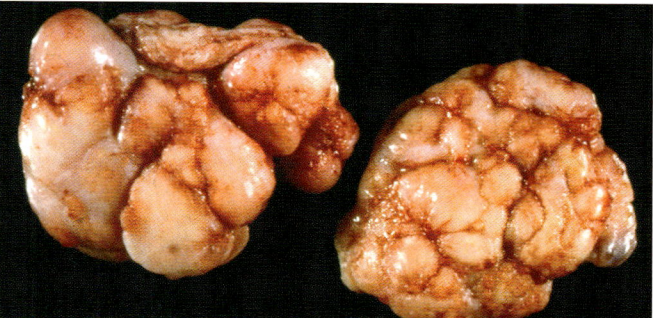

Figure 30.14 Krukenberg tumor. Bilateral multinodular tumors.

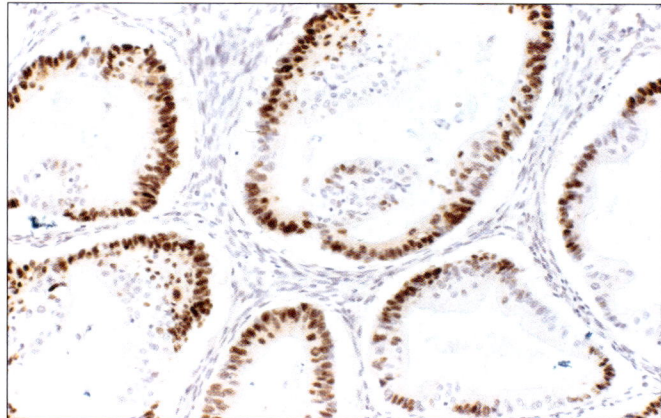

Figure 30.13 Metastatic adenocarcinoma from the colon. Positive immunoreaction for P53.

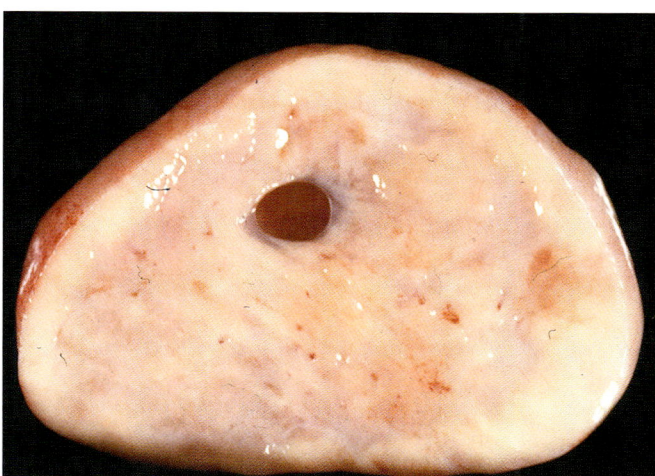

Figure 30.15 Krukenberg tumor. The cut surface shows solid beige-yellow tissue with small foci of hemorrhage.

colonic origin of the neoplasm. CDX2 is often strongly and diffusely positive in colorectal carcinomas, but it can also be positive in ovarian mucinous and endometrioid tumors.[40,41] Estrogen receptors (ERs) may be helpful for distinguishing endometrioid adenocarcinomas from metastatic intestinal carcinomas, as the former are usually positive and the latter are negative.[42]

KRUKENBERG TUMOR

Krukenberg tumors are adenocarcinomas with a distinctive histologic appearance. They consist of mucin-filled signet-ring cells and a striking proliferation of the ovarian stroma. Signet-ring cell carcinomas are associated more often with ovarian metastasis than carcinomas of other histologic types. These tumors originate in the stomach, usually in the pylorus, in the vast majority of cases. It has been demonstrated that gastric signet-ring cell carcinomas metastasize to the ovary much more often than intestinal-type carcinomas of the stomach do.[43] Sometimes, the gastric cancer may be small and remains undetected for several years after oophorectomy. Much less frequently, the primary tumor is in the large intestine, breast, gallbladder, uterine cervix, appendix, or urinary bladder. In rare cases, the site of origin of the primary tumor is unknown and a diagnosis of 'primary' Krukenberg tumor has been proposed for those cases in which either the patient survives in good health for 10 years or longer or a thorough autopsy fails to reveal an extraovarian primary tumor.[44] Possibly, some of the cases reported in the older literature as primary Krukenberg tumors represent mucinous (goblet cell) carcinoids. Patients with Krukenberg tumors tend to be younger than most patients with metastatic carcinoma; most of them are between 40 and 50 years of age. Although the symptoms are usually nonspecific, most frequently abdominal pain and swelling, endocrine manifestations, such as virilization during pregnancy, may result from stromal luteinization.[3]

Krukenberg tumors are bilateral in 60–80% of the cases.[3] They are typically solid masses with smooth nodular or bosselated outer surfaces (Figure 30.14). The cut surfaces are predominantly white or tan with areas of red or brown discoloration (Figure 30.15); the consistency may be firm, fleshy, or gelatinous. Because of the marked proliferation of the ovarian stroma, the tumors may resemble fibrothecomas on gross examination.

Microscopically, the plump, rounded carcinoma cells have a signet-ring appearance and are surrounded by a dense cellular stroma (Figure 30.16). The epithelial cells

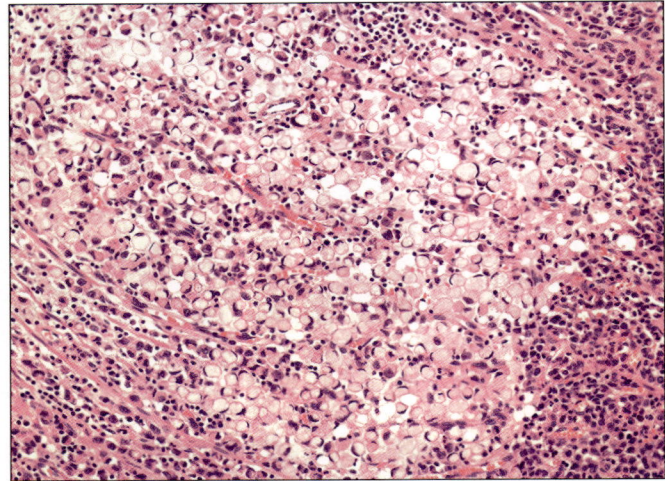

Figure 30.16 Krukenberg tumor. Numerous signet-ring cells with pale cytoplasm are arranged irregularly within a cellular stroma.

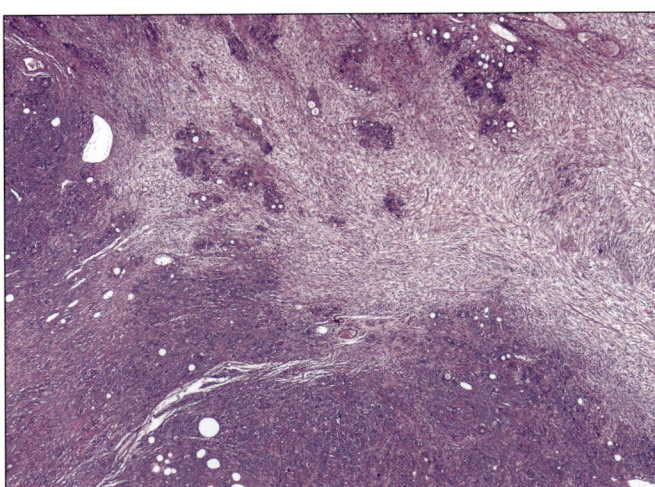

Figure 30.18 Krukenberg tumor. The ovarian stroma shows extensive edema.

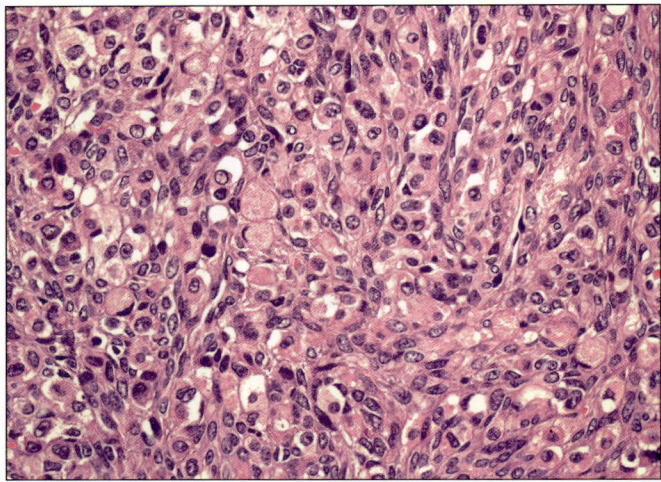

Figure 30.17 Krukenberg tumor. The signet-ring cells have eosinophilic cytoplasm and are distributed singly or in nests.

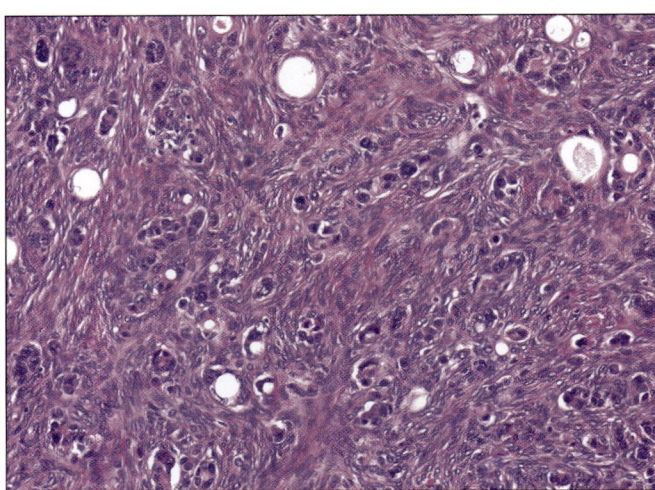

Figure 30.19 Krukenberg tumor. Small glands lined by moderately atypical epithelial cells are admixed with signet-ring cells.

may appear singly or in nests (Figure 30.17) and tend to concentrate in the dense fibroblastic areas. In some cases, the stroma is less cellular, edematous (Figure 30.18), or fibrous. Isolated small glands are usually found[45] (Figure 30.19) and, occasionally, there is a predominant tubular architecture (tubular Krukenberg tumor) (Figure 30.20).[6] The stromal cells are plump, spindle shaped, and are sometimes extensively luteinized.[3,6]

Krukenberg tumors must be distinguished from primary and other metastatic ovarian tumors including clear cell adenocarcinoma, mucinous (goblet cell) carcinoid, and a variety of ovarian tumors that contain signet-ring-like cells filled with non-mucinous material. The presence of clear cells may raise the issue of clear cell carcinoma, but the clear cells in the latter contain glycogen; mucin, when present, is typically luminal and extracellular. Rarely, clear cell carcinoma may have a signet-ring cell component that simulates a Krukenberg tumor; however, the signet-ring cells of the

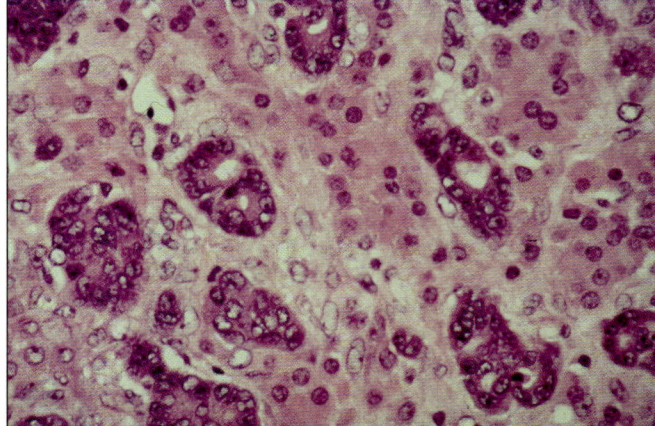

Figure 30.20 Tubular Krukenberg tumor. The tubular glands are lined by markedly atypical cells. The intervening clusters of luteinized stromal cells contribute to the resemblance to a Sertoli–Leydig cell tumor.

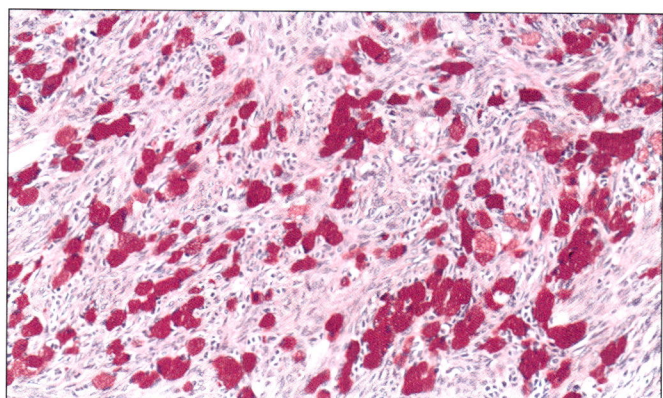

Figure 30.21 Krukenberg tumor. A PAS–diastase stain demonstrates the mucin in the vacuolated tumor cells.

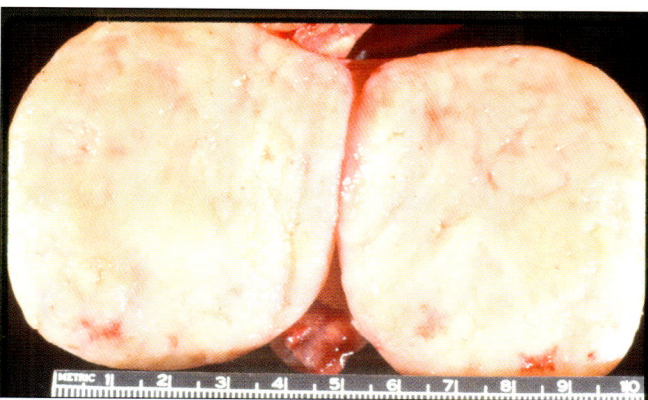

Figure 30.22 Metastatic carcinoid tumor from the pancreas. The sectioned surfaces are solid and white-yellow simulating those of a fibroma or thecoma.

former have a characteristic 'targetoid' cytoplasm (bull's eye appearance), containing a large vacuole with a central eosinophilic body. In addition, the identification of a tubulocystic pattern, as well as the presence of hobnail cells, stromal hyalinization, and eosinophilic secretion, is helpful in establishing the diagnosis. In contrast, CK immunostains are not useful, as nearly half of gastric carcinomas metastatic to the ovary are CK7 positive/CK20 negative.[38] Mucinous carcinoid, either primary or metastatic, may contain large areas of signet-ring cells; the former neoplasms, however, frequently contain other teratomatous elements, and Grimelius stains as well as immunostains for chromogranin, synaptophysin are usually positive in both.

The tubular variant of Krukenberg tumor, sometimes associated with stromal luteinization, can be confused with a Sertoli–Leydig cell tumor (Figure 30.20); however, signet-ring cells are not a feature of the latter tumor except for the heterologous form that contains mucinous intestinal glands.[6] Positive mucicarmine and periodic acid–Schiff (PAS) stains with diastase digestion (Figure 30.21) are of great value in establishing the diagnosis of a Krukenberg tumor.[6] Occasional Krukenberg tumors may closely resemble fibromas on macroscopic examination and may have relatively few signet-ring cells. Bilaterality and positive mucin stains facilitate the differential diagnosis.

Almost all patients die within a year of the diagnosis of Krukenberg tumor, but rare patients have survived for 5 or more years after gastrectomy and bilateral oophorectomy.[46] Although exceptional, this outcome justifies removal of both the stomach and the ovarian metastases in cases in which the tumor appears limited to those organs. Also, in menopausal and postmenopausal women undergoing gastrectomy for carcinoma, the ovaries should be removed routinely to prevent the later development of ovarian metastasis and avoid another operation.

CARCINOID TUMORS

Carcinoid tumors of the gastrointestinal tract, pancreas, or bronchus may metastasize to the ovary, and approximately half of the patients have the carcinoid syndrome.[47] The

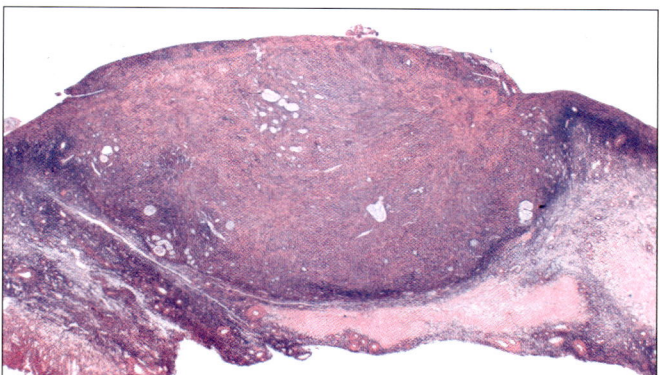

Figure 30.23 Metastatic mucinous carcinoid tumor from the appendix. The ovary is partly replaced by a nodule of dense fibrous tissue containing scattered small glands.

primary tumor is usually in the ileum. Whereas mucinous carcinoid tumors of the appendix spread to the ovary in approximately one-third of cases, typical carcinoid tumors of the appendix almost never metastasize to the ovary.[3] In the largest series reported, the age of the 35 patients ranged from 21 to 82 years, with a median of 57 years.[47] Forty percent of the women had preoperative manifestations of the carcinoid syndrome. Some of them also had clinical evidence of intestinal or ovarian involvement. Extraovarian metastases were found in at least 90% of the cases, in contrast to the rarity of similar spread in cases of primary ovarian carcinoids.

Metastatic carcinoids are typically bilateral solid tumors with smooth or bosselated surfaces. The cut section often shows firm white or yellow confluent nodules, which may simulate fibromas or thecomas (Figure 30.22). Rare carcinoid tumors are predominantly cystic.[3] Microscopically, the insular pattern is the most common, but trabecular and mucinous patterns may also be found. The carcinoid glands usually appear scattered in a dense fibrous stroma, which may be hyalinized (Figures 30.23 and 30.24). Focally, metastatic mucinous (goblet cell) carcinoids may resemble

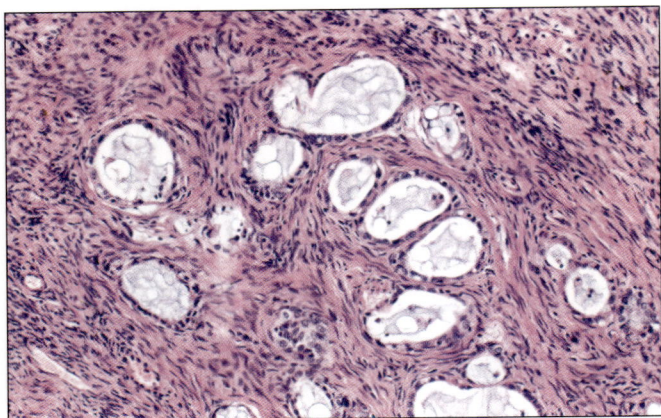

Figure 30.24 Metastatic mucinous carcinoid tumor from the appendix. Small glands lined by flat to cuboidal mucinous epithelium and occasional goblet cells. The intervening stroma appears fibromatous.

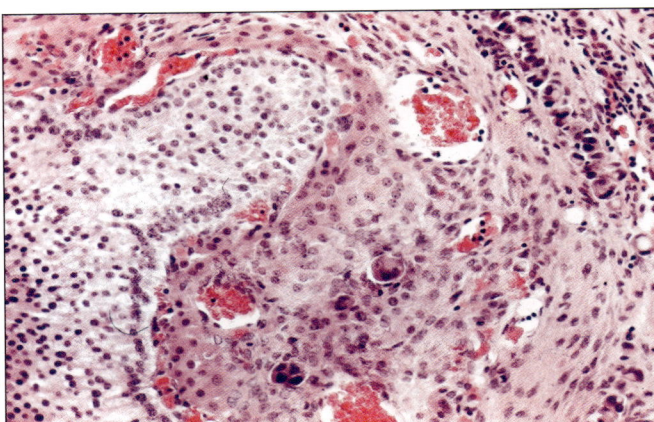

Figure 30.26 Metastatic carcinoma from the breast. Several nests of carcinoma cells are seen in the highly vascular theca layer of a Graafian follicle.

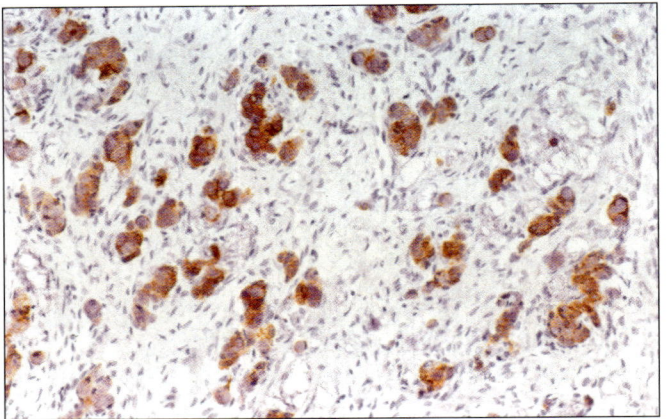

Figure 30.25 Metastatic mucinous carcinoid tumor from the appendix. Positive chromogranin immunoreaction.

Krukenberg tumors. Immunostains for chromogranin and synaptophysin are often positive (Figure 30.25).

Metastatic carcinoids can be confused with primary carcinoids (Table 30.3), granulosa cell tumors, Sertoli–Leydig cell tumors, Brenner tumors, adenofibromas, or endometrioid carcinomas.[3,5] If the diagnosis of a carcinoid tumor is difficult in any of the previous situations, more thorough sampling, and immunohistochemical staining for neuroendocrine markers can be performed. Bilaterality, extraovarian extension, and absence of teratomatous elements are important features of metastatic carcinoids. CDX-2 does not distinguish between tumors of intestinal origin and primary ovarian carcinoids.[48]

BREAST CARCINOMA

Ovarian involvement by breast cancer is usually an incidental microscopic finding without clinical significance (Figure 30.26). Historically, such tumors have been found in approximately 30% of patients who have had therapeutic oophorectomy for disseminated breast carcinoma and, at autopsy, in about 10% of cases of breast cancer. Bilateral involvement occurs in 60–80% of cases.[3]

Patients with breast cancer are at increased risk of developing primary ovarian, tubal, or pelvic peritoneal carcinoma, especially if they have a hereditary predisposition to breast and ovarian cancer due to *BRCA1* or *BRCA2* mutations. It is not surprising then that patients with a history of breast cancer who present with an adnexal or pelvic mass are more likely to have independent ovarian or tubal malignancy than metastases from the breast cancer by a 3:1 ratio.[49] The very rare cases of metastases that present clinically as primary ovarian tumors before the detection of the breast carcinoma often pose diagnostic difficulty.[50] The tumors are characteristically solid, multinodular, and firm (Figure 30.27). A larger percentage of cases of lobular carcinoma of the breast, including those of signet-ring cell type, metastasize to the ovary than do cases of ductal carcinoma; in an autopsy study 36% of the former metastasized to the ovaries in contrast to only 2.6% of the latter.[51]

Table 30.3 Primary versus Secondary Carcinoid Tumor: Differential Diagnosis

Metastatic Carcinoid	Primary Carcinoid
Clinical Profile	
Primary site apparent in 80%	No intestinal tumor
Peritoneal seeding and abdominal metastases frequent	Extraovarian spread uncommon
Early recurrence and progression	Low rate of recurrence
Macroscopic Features	
Bilateral almost always	Unilateral always
Cut surface nodular and variegated	Cut surface homogeneous
Microscopic Features	
Teratomatous elements absent	Teratomatous elements usually present

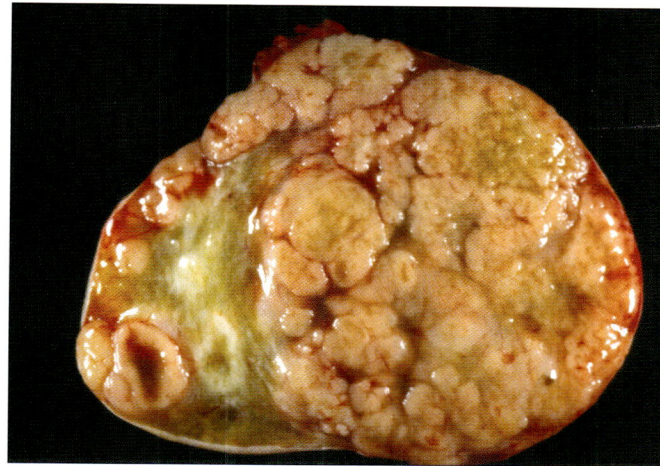

Figure 30.27 Metastatic carcinoma from the breast. The sectioned surface appears solid and multinodular.

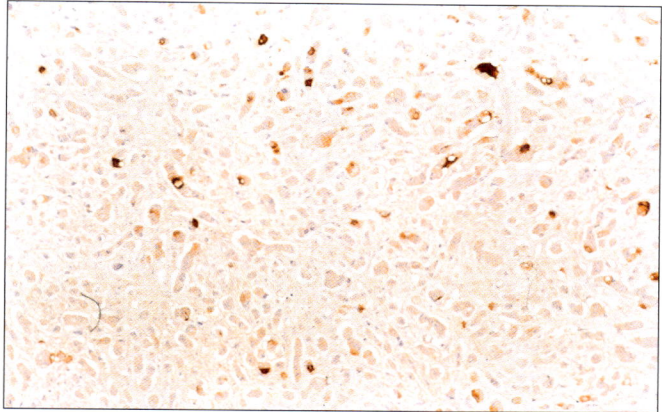

Figure 30.29 Metastatic carcinoma from the breast, lobular type. Scattered tumor cells are immunoreactive for gross cystic disease fluid protein (GCDFP-15).

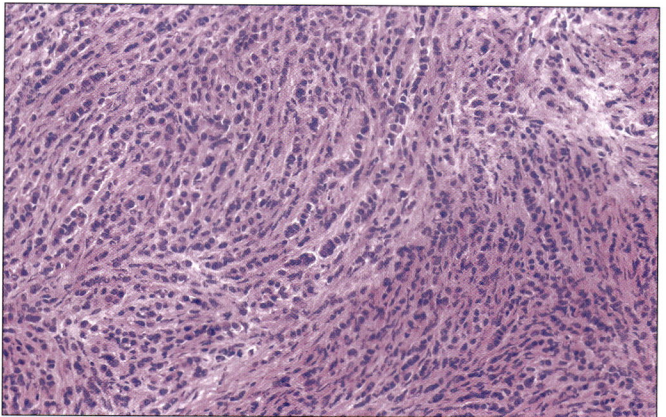

Figure 30.28 Metastatic carcinoma from the breast, lobular type. The tumor cells show a single-file arrangement.

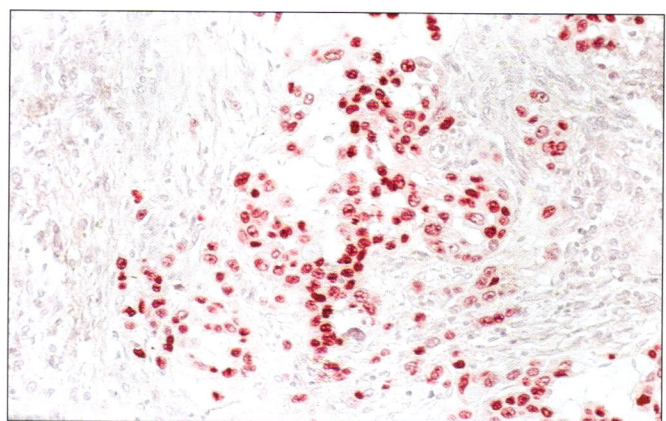

Figure 30.30 Metastatic carcinoma from the breast. Positive immunoreaction for estrogen receptor protein (ERPr).

Metastatic lobular carcinomas (Figure 30.28) usually show a diffuse pattern mimicking granulosa cell tumors, granulocytic sarcomas, or lymphomas, or even an insular pattern simulating carcinoid tumors. Rarely, metastatic ductal carcinomas may have an endometrioid-like appearance. Positive immunoreaction for gross cystic disease fluid protein (GCDFP-15) (Figure 30.29),[52] estrogen (ERPr) (Figure 30.30), and progesterone receptor proteins (ER, PR), epithelial membrane antigen (EMA), and S-100 protein, and negativity for CA12.5, CA19.9,[53] α-inhibin, myeloperoxidase, and lymphoid markers favor metastatic breast carcinoma. Mammaglobin is expressed in about 50% of breast carcinomas.[54,55] However, its expression has been demonstrated in rare ovarian serous carcinomas and in endometrioid carcinomas of the uterine corpus.[54,56] WT1 is positive in >80% of serous carcinomas of the ovary, but it is rarely positive in breast carcinomas. PAX-8 immunoreaction is seen in greater than 88% of ovarian carcinomas but not in breast carcinomas.[57] Both breast and ovarian carcinomas may be positive for CK7.[36] A panel of markers is recommended as no currently available individual marker is entirely specific for breast or ovarian carcinomas.

TUMORS OF THE PANCREAS, BILIARY TRACT, AND LIVER

Although ovarian metastases are rarely found in patients with these carcinomas, they may strikingly mimic primary ovarian tumors both grossly and microscopically.[58–60] Metastatic tumors from the pancreas are usually bilateral, large, cystic, and multiloculated (Figure 30.31), an appearance that may be indistinguishable from primary mucinous neoplasia, although in some cases surface nodules may be noted and raise suspicion for metastasis. The microscopic pattern varies considerably within individual tumors that may show areas resembling ovarian mucinous cystadenomas, borderline tumors (Figure 30.32), and well-differentiated cystadenocarcinomas as well as foci of irregular stromal infiltration.[58] In some cases, foci of high-grade adenocarcinoma appear admixed with more indolent low-grade cystic tumor and are a clue to the diagnosis. Four cases of ovarian involvement by acinar cell carcinoma of the pancreas have been recently reported[61] (Figure 30.33). Metastatic adenocarcinomas of the gallbladder and extrahepatic bile ducts are very rare.[59] Recently, however, a series of cases has been

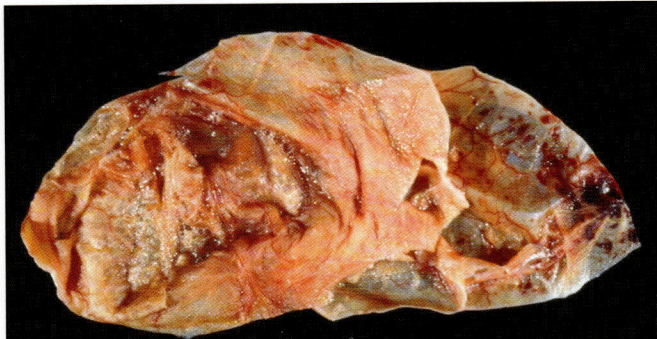

Figure 30.31 Metastatic carcinoma from the pancreas. Multiloculated cystic tumor simulating a primary mucinous tumor.

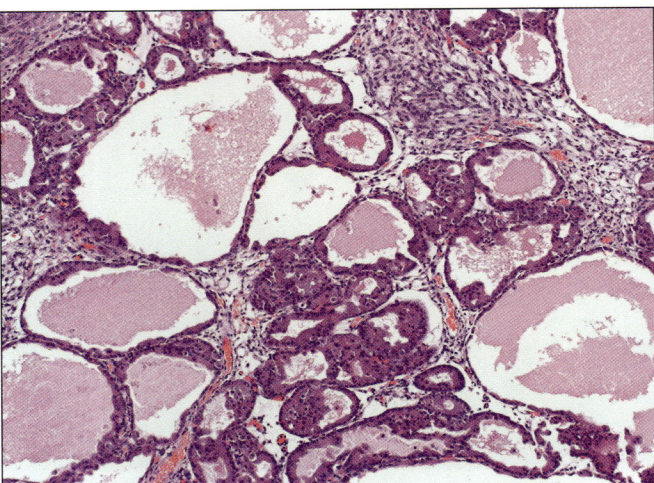

Figure 30.33 Metastatic acinar cell carcinoma from the pancreas. High-power view of typical small acini and cystic glands.

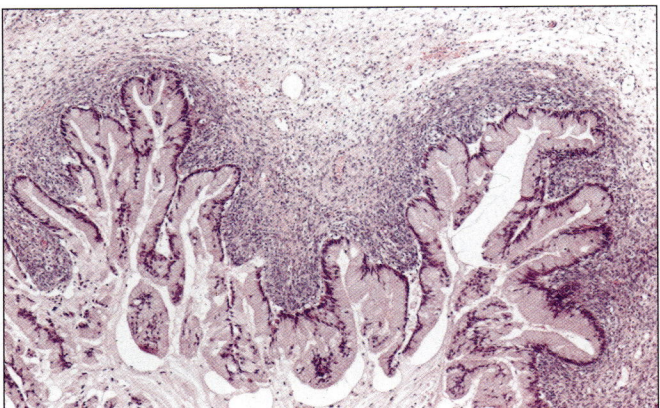

Figure 30.32 Metastatic carcinoma from the pancreas. The lining epithelium resembles that of a mucinous intestinal borderline tumor. Note the condensation of the ovarian stroma adjacent to the tumor.

reported.[62] They are usually solid tumors that microscopically may simulate ovarian mucinous (Figure 30.34) or endometrioid carcinomas, or even cystadenofibromas.[59] Rarely, Krukenberg tumors originate in the pancreas or biliary tract.[3] Features suggesting metastasis include bilaterality, extraovarian extension, ovarian surface implants, and vascular invasion. Like primary ovarian mucinous tumors, pancreatic carcinomas are diffusely immunoreactive for CK7 and MUC5AC and show focal to diffuse positivity for CK20 (Table 30.2); however, 46% of pancreatic carcinomas are negative for Dpc4.[35]

Ovarian metastases from hepatocellular carcinomas are exceedingly rare and should be distinguished microscopically from primary hepatoid carcinomas (Chapter 27), and hepatoid yolk sac tumors (Chapter 29). HepPAR1 is not useful in distinguishing among metastatic hepatocellular carcinoma, hepatoid yolk sac tumor, and hepatoid ovarian carcinoma as it is expressed in all.[63] The presence of bile in the ovarian tumor favors metastatic hepatocellular carcinoma.[60]

TUMORS OF THE APPENDIX

Metastatic tumors from the appendix are rare and represent only 1–2% of ovarian metastases.[1] Most of these cases are mucinous tumors of borderline malignancy (low-grade

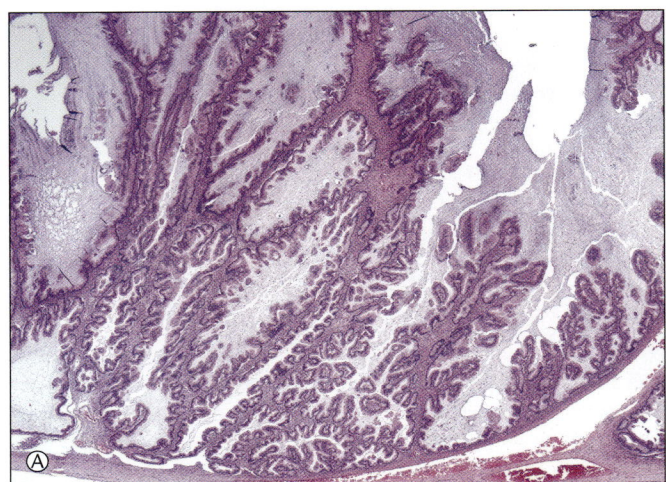

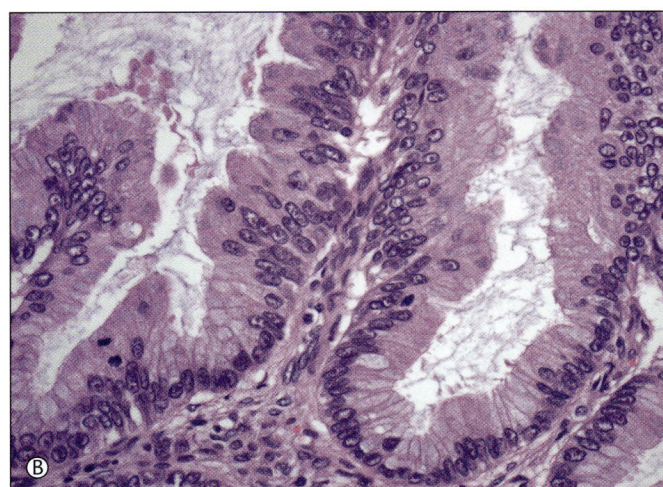

Figure 30.34 Metastatic intrahepatic cholangiocarcinoma. **(A)** Proliferation of mucinous epithelium with filiform branching papillae simulating an ovarian mucinous borderline tumor. **(B)** The mucinous intestinal epithelium shows stratified cells with moderate nuclear atypia.

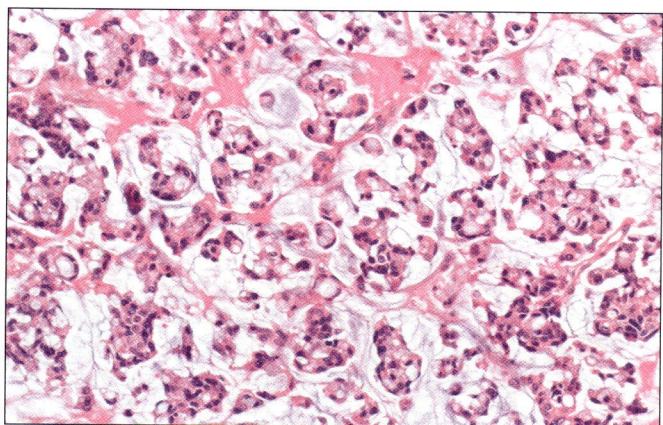

Figure 30.35 Metastatic adenocarcinoma from the appendix, signet-ring cell type.

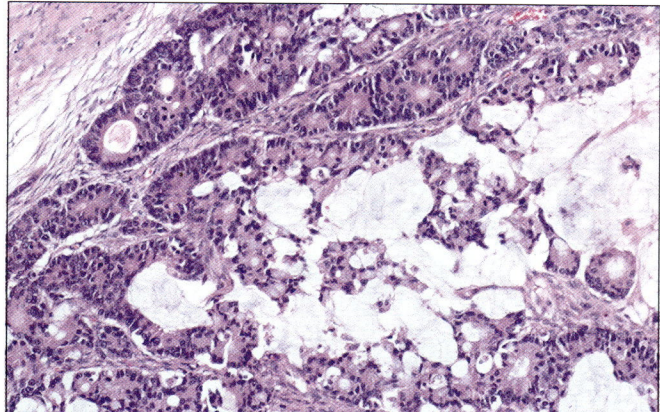

Figure 30.36 Metastatic adenocarcinoma from the appendix, colorectal type.

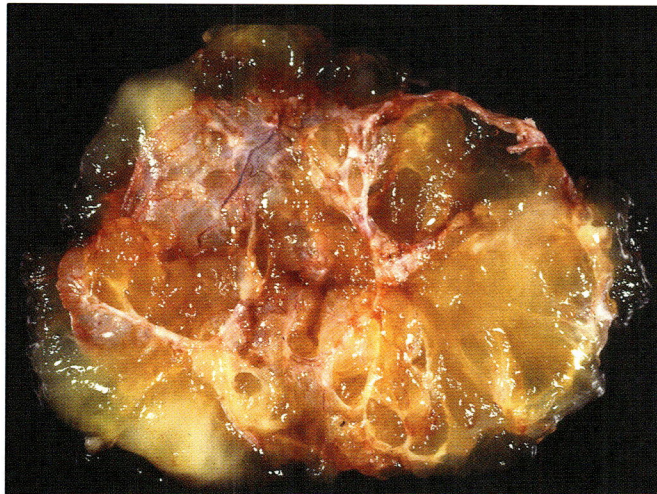

Figure 30.37 Metastatic low-grade mucinous tumor from the appendix. Multiloculated cystic tumor with abundant mucoid material.

mucinous tumors) associated with pseudomyxoma peritonei[8,64,65] (see Chapters 26 and 31). Other appendiceal tumors that may spread to the ovary include mucinous (goblet cell) carcinoids[3,66] and, less frequently, adenocarcinomas of signet-ring cell (Figure 30.35), mucinous intestinal, and colorectal types (Figure 30.36).[10] The ovarian metastases of mucinous carcinoids and signet-ring cell adenocarcinomas are generally of the Krukenberg type. The former tumors are clinically aggressive and often fail to show the characteristic immunoreactions of carcinoid tumors. A recent report on ovarian metastases of appendiceal carcinomas with neuroendocrine differentiation emphasized that the clinical features and pathologic findings support classifying the appendiceal tumors as carcinomas rather than goblet cell carcinoids. According to the authors, the presence of infiltrative and destructive growth justifies their designation as carcinomas.[67]

In patients with pseudomyxoma peritonei, low-grade mucinous tumors of the appendix often coexist with histologically similar tumors in one or both ovaries. Although these tumors were traditionally considered as independent primary neoplasms, there is now convincing clinicopathologic, immunohistochemical, and molecular genetic evidence that in most cases the ovarian tumors represent metastases from the appendiceal lesions.[8,9,64,65,68] In such cases, the ovarian tumors are frequently bilateral or, when unilateral, predominantly right-sided, and often exhibit pools of mucin dissecting through the ovarian stroma ('pseudomyxoma ovarii'). In contrast, primary ovarian mucinous borderline tumors are usually unilateral and only occasionally associated with pseudomyxoma peritonei or ovarii, even when preoperative or surgical rupture has occurred. Additional features that support the secondary nature of the ovarian tumors associated with pseudomyxoma peritonei are their jelly-like consistency on gross examination (Figure 30.37), the finding of mucin and atypical mucinous cells on the ovarian surfaces, and the presence of very tall mucinous lining cells (Figure 30.38).[3] Although appendiceal tumors are almost always diffusely positive for CK20, they may also be positive for CK7 in approximately one-third of cases.[35]

At surgery, the primary appendiceal tumor is often overlooked because the ovarian tumors are usually much larger.[10] Besides, the site of appendiceal rupture may be very small and require extensive sectioning to demonstrate it. Additionally, in some cases a rupture site heals over, and is represented only by fibrosis in the appendiceal wall.

RENAL TUMORS

Renal cell carcinoma rarely metastasizes to the ovaries; however, when it does, it must be distinguished from a primary clear cell carcinoma. Only 15 cases have been reported in detail.[69–72] Most were unilateral tumors, often large (average 12.5 cm in greatest dimension), solid and cystic, and yellow to orange. Microscopically, they showed a prominent sinusoidal vascular pattern, a homogeneous clear cell pattern without hobnail cells, absence of hyalinized papillae, and the absence of intraluminal mucin (Figure 30.39).[3,72]

A panel of antibodies may be helpful in the differential diagnosis: ovarian clear cell carcinomas are usually immunoreactive for CK7 and mesothelin and negative for CD10 and

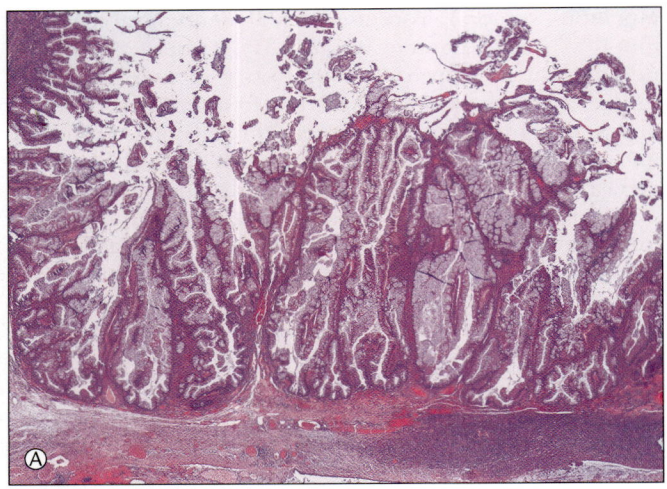

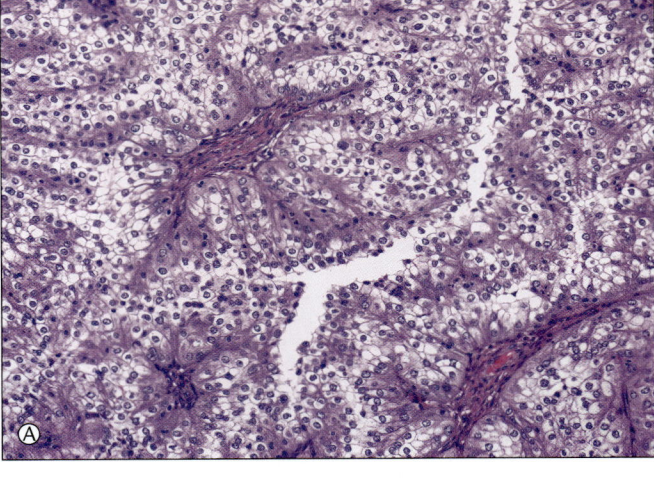

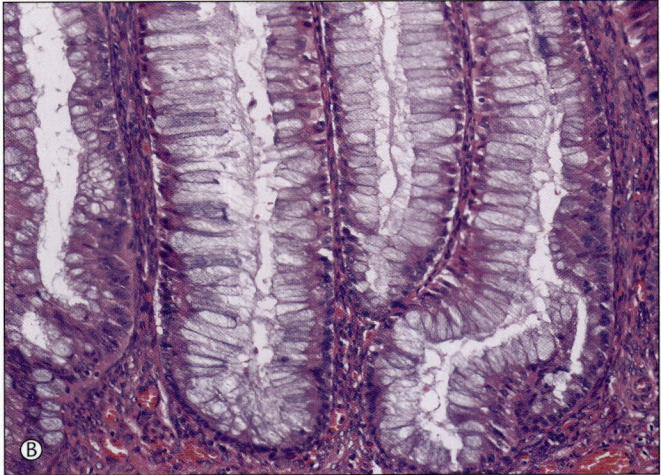

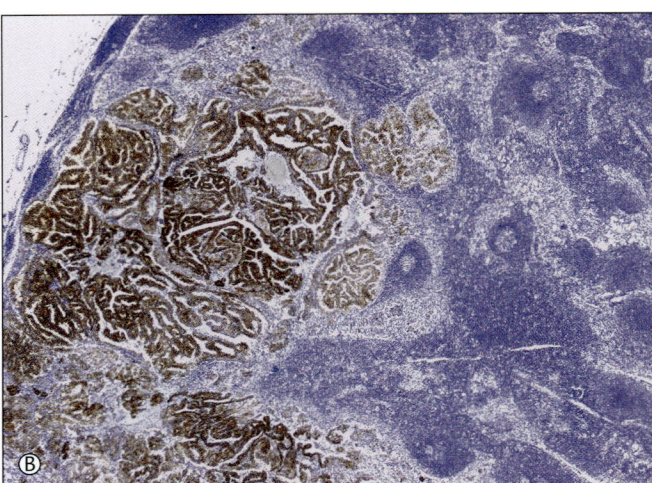

Figure 30.38 Metastatic low-grade mucinous tumor from the appendix. **(A)** The mucinous cells are tall and lack nuclear atypia. **(B)** Mucin appears to be discharged from the apical pole of the columnar cells.

Figure 30.39 Metastatic papillary renal cell carcinoma. **(A)** The renal clear cell carcinoma lacks hobnail cells, hyalinized papillae, and intraluminal mucin. **(B)** Lymph node metastasis showing a strong racemase immunoreaction.

RCCma (renal cell carcinoma marker), whereas renal cell carcinomas often show the opposite immunoprofile (CK7–/mesothelin–/CD10+/RCCma+).[73–75] Although PAX2 may be a more sensitive marker than RCCma for metastatic renal cell carcinoma, it should be noted that about 40% of ovarian clear cell carcinomas also express PAX2.[76]

TUMORS OF THE URINARY TRACT

Distinction between a transitional cell carcinoma of the urinary tract metastatic to the ovary (Figure 30.40) and a borderline or malignant Brenner tumor, or a primary ovarian transitional cell carcinoma, may be difficult.[77,78] Clinical information may be necessary to resolve the issue. In most borderline or malignant Brenner tumors, however, a benign Brenner tumor component can be found. Also, the presence of benign mucinous elements favors the diagnosis of a Brenner tumor. In contrast to primary transitional cell carcinomas of the ovary, urinary tract carcinomas are immunoreactive for CK13, CK20, uroplakin, and thrombomodulin[79] and they are typically negative for WT1.[80]

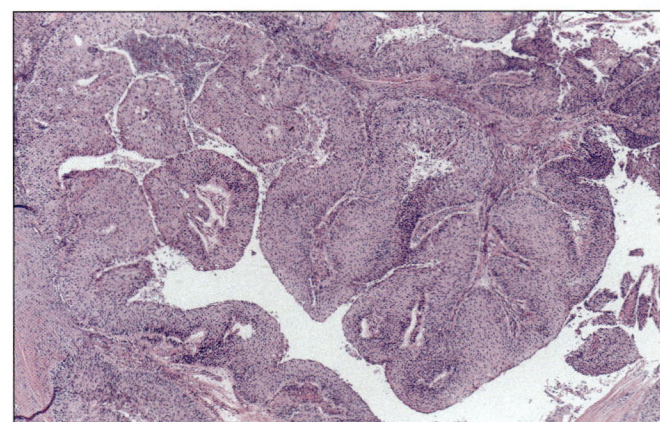

Figure 30.40 Metastatic transitional cell carcinoma from the renal pelvis. This tumor is indistinguishable from a primary transitional cell carcinoma.

ADRENAL GLAND TUMORS

Neuroblastoma is the adrenal tumor that most frequently metastasizes to the ovary.[81–83] The metastases must be distinguished from rare cases of primary ovarian neuroblastomas. In contrast to the metastatic tumors, the primary tumors are usually unilateral and are often associated with a teratoma. The prominent fibrillary background of neuroblastoma and the presence of pseudorosettes help in the distinction of metastatic neuroblastoma from other metastatic small cell tumors. Immunohistochemistry is also helpful. Metastases of adrenal cortical carcinomas to the ovary are exceedingly rare.[84] Pheochromocytomas spread to the ovary even less commonly.

MALIGNANT MELANOMA

Three series of melanomas metastatic to the ovary including 52 cases have been reported.[85–87] In the ovary metastatic malignant melanoma may be confused with primary malignant melanoma; the latter is unilateral, usually associated with a dermoid cyst, and often nonpigmented. When a melanoma is composed predominantly of large cells, it may resemble a lipid-poor steroid cell tumor or a pregnancy luteoma; sometimes, it exhibits a follicle-like arrangement resembling juvenile granulosa cell tumor; when it is composed mainly of small cells it may be confused with a small cell carcinoma of the hypercalcemic type.[87] Positive stains for melanin, S-100 protein (Figure 30.41), Melan A, and/or HMB-45 should establish the diagnosis of melanoma.

PULMONARY AND MEDIASTINAL TUMORS

Ovarian metastases from lung carcinomas account for less than 1% of ovarian metastases but are increasing in frequency as the disease becomes more common in women[88] (Figure 30.42). Most women present with symptoms of the pulmonary tumor and are subsequently found to have a pelvic tumor. All major histologic types of lung cancer can spread to the ovaries and potentially mimic a primary carcinoma. Squamous cell carcinomas, the most common form of lung cancer, rarely metastasize to ovaries.[88] Metastases from lung adenocarcinomas are slightly more frequent. Thyroid transcription factor-1 (TTF-1) immunoreactivity helps identify lungs as a potential primary site in cases of metastatic adenocarcinoma of unknown origin; it is reactive in 60–75% of primary lung adenocarcinomas, but not reactive in primary ovarian adenocarcinomas.[89] Undifferentiated small cell (oat cell) carcinomas of the lung, the most common type of pulmonary metastasis, should be distinguished from ovarian small cell carcinomas of either 'hypercalcemic type' or 'pulmonary type' (see Chapter 27), although all of the tumors have a poor prognosis. Ovarian small cell carcinomas of hypercalcemic type occur in young women and, like other ovarian tumors, are negative for TTF-1, while more than half of small cell lung carcinomas are reactive.[88,90] Primary ovarian small cell carcinoma of pulmonary type typically differs from metastatic small cell lung carcinoma in its tendency for peritoneal spread and its association with epithelial–stromal tumors, in particular endometrioid carcinoma. Interestingly, however, small cell carcinoma of the lung has been reported to metastasize to pre-existing ovarian tumors.[88,91]

Metastatic large cell carcinomas must be distinguished from morphologically similar oxyphilic tumors, both primary and secondary, including melanoma. Bronchioloalveolar carcinomas rarely are metastatic to the ovaries.[92]

Small cell carcinomas arising in sites other than lung, such as mediastinum, uterine cervix, and gastrointestinal tract, may also metastasize to the ovaries.[93,94] Isolated cases with metastases include posterior mediastinal neuroblastoma[82] and mediastinal thymoma.[95]

UTERINE TUMORS

Ovarian involvement by endometrial carcinoma has been reported in 5–15% of hysterectomy specimens. The distinction between metastatic endometrial and primary endometrioid carcinoma of the ovary has been discussed in Chapter 27. Uterine sarcomas may metastasize to the ovary and may

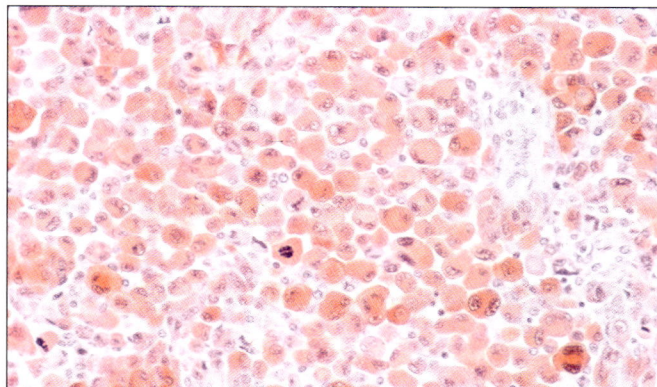

Figure 30.41 Metastatic malignant melanoma. The tumor cells are immunoreactive for S-100 protein.

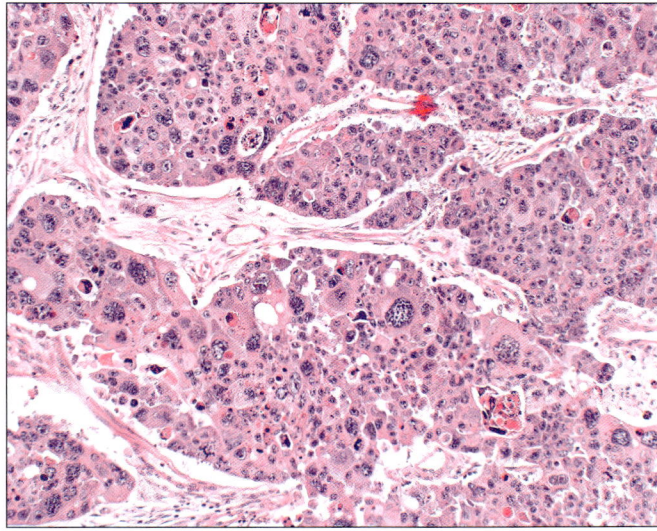

Figure 30.42 Metastatic keratinizing squamous carcinoma of lung.

occasionally be discovered before the primary tumor.[96] Metastatic epithelioid leiomyosarcoma may have an appearance that simulates a carcinoma, a malignant lymphoma, or even a Sertoli cell tumor. A positive immunoreaction for desmin may facilitate the diagnosis. Distinction between metastatic low-grade endometrial–stromal sarcoma, primary ovarian low-grade endometrioid stromal sarcoma, and sex cord–stromal tumors has been discussed in Chapter 27.

Mucinous adenocarcinomas of the cervix coexist with ovarian tumors of similar type more frequently than other adenocarcinomas.[97–99] Sometimes, it may be difficult to determine whether the tumors are metastatic from one organ to the other or independent primary neoplasms. The distinction is made by applying criteria similar to those used in diagnosing simultaneous ovarian and corpus carcinomas and in identifying metastatic tumors in general. However, the microscopic clue to the metastatic nature of the ovarian tumors is the 'hybrid' appearance of the epithelium with features of both endometrioid and mucinous differentiation, i.e., with low-power endometrioid-like features but with apical mucin seen on higher power. Additionally, the nuclei are hyperchromatic and more atypical than seen in true endometrioid or mucinous carcinomas with a similar glandular grade, and mitotic figures and apoptotic bodies are numerous (Figure 30.43).[100,101] Although nonspecific, a strong p16 immunoreaction (Figure 30.44) supports the metastatic nature of the ovarian tumor, which can be confirmed by detecting human papillomavirus (HPV) using *in situ* hybridization or polymerase chain reaction. In some cases, an occult primary cervical adenocarcinoma was discovered after resection of the ovarian metastases.[100] Subsequently, the question of whether ovarian conservation is justified in patients with cervical adenocarcinoma has been raised.

Cervical adenoma malignum may be associated with synchronous ovarian mucinous tumors, sometimes in the setting of Peutz–Jeghers syndrome. In this instance, assessing neither their HPV DNA status nor their CK immunoreactivity is of any help as adenoma malignum is not HPV related, and both primary cervical and ovarian tumors should be reactive for CK7 and unreactive for CK20.

Cervical squamous cell carcinomas metastasize to the ovary in less than 1% of cases.[102,103] Most ovarian squamous cell carcinomas arise in dermoid cysts or endometriotic cysts. Adenosquamous, neuroendocrine, undifferentiated, and transitional cell carcinomas metastatic to the ovary have also been reported.[102]

Uterine choriocarcinomas spread to the ovary in 22% of cases.[5] It may be extremely difficult to distinguish a primary ovarian choriocarcinoma of either gestational or germ cell origin from a metastatic uterine choriocarcinoma in which regression of the primary tumor has occurred. The specimen should be thoroughly sampled in an attempt to discover teratomatous elements, thus establishing a germ cell origin of the neoplasm.

Carcinomas of the fallopian tube involve the ovary in approximately 13% of cases, usually by direct extension.[1] In such cases, it may be difficult to determine whether the tumor is primary in the tube or ovary. Although the problem is usually resolved on the basis of the gross pathologic findings, in questionable cases the tumor is classified as tuboovarian carcinoma.[51] Most tubal carcinomas resemble

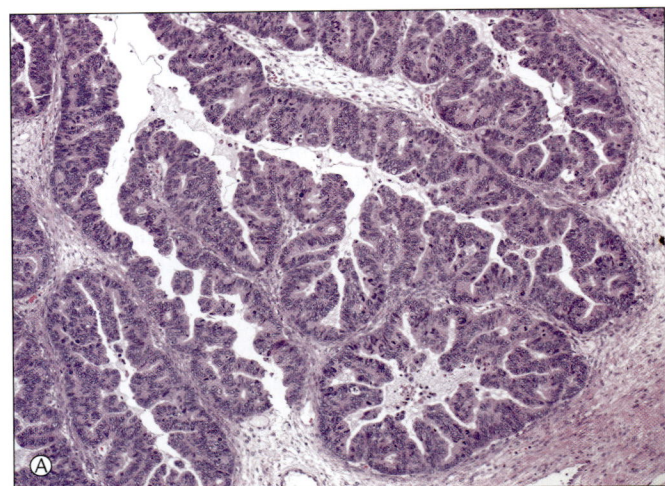
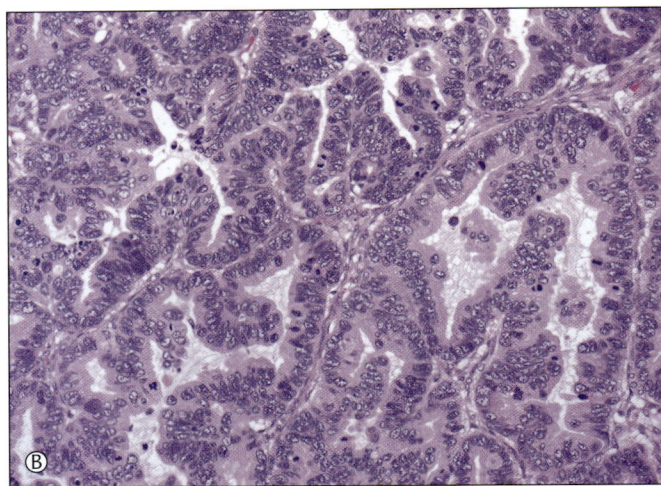

Figure 30.43 Metastatic endocervical adenocarcinoma of the usual type. **(A)** Papillary tumor resembling endometrioid carcinoma at low magnification. **(B)** Apical mucin is seen on higher power. Mitotic figures and apoptotic cells are numerous.

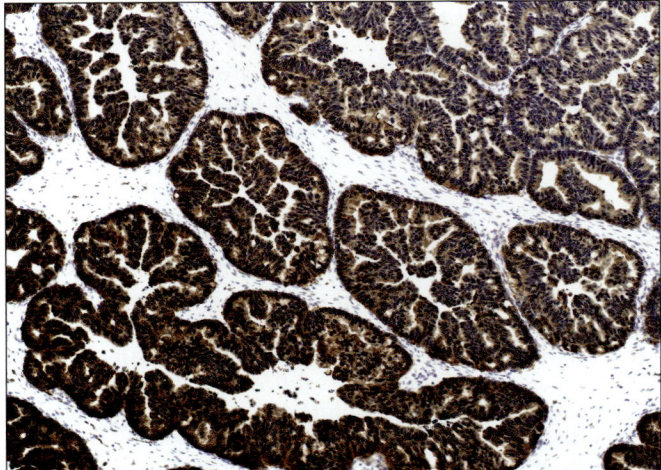

Figure 30.44 Metastatic endocervical adenocarcinoma. Strong p16 immunoreaction.

high-grade serous carcinomas of the ovary, thus microscopic examination rarely helps in deciding a primary site.[104,105] Recent studies have raised the possibility that a great number of high-grade serous carcinomas of the ovary, predominantly from *BRCA*-positive patients but also sporadic cases, may actually represent spread of fallopian tube cancers, especially those of the fimbria[106–109] (see Chapter 25).

LYMPHOMA AND LEUKEMIA

Although lymphoma and leukemia can involve the ovaries simulating various primary tumors, they rarely present clinically as an ovarian mass. In countries where Burkitt lymphoma is endemic, however, it accounts for approximately half the cases of malignant ovarian tumors in childhood.[3] On pelvic examination, unilateral or bilateral adnexal masses are palpable. Approximately two-thirds of the patients have extraovarian disease frequently involving the fallopian tubes, and the pelvic or para-aortic lymph nodes. The Ann Arbor lymphoma stage provides more prognostic information than the International Federation of Gynecologists and Obstetricians stage. With modern combination chemotherapy, patient survival is greater than 50% and is comparable to that achieved overall in nodal lymphomas.[110]

Ovarian lymphomas have an average diameter of 10–15 cm.[3] The external surface of the tumor is smooth, nodular, or bosselated. The cut surface is fleshy and tan, or gray (Figure 30.45). Microscopically, the tumor cells of Burkitt and Burkitt-like lymphomas grow in sheets punctuated by spaces that contain phagocytic histiocytes, creating a characteristic 'starry sky' appearance (Figure 30.46). The cells have scanty cytoplasm and uniform, round, medium size nuclei with coarse chromatin and 1–3 nucleoli. Mitotic figures are numerous. The tumor cells can infiltrate ovarian follicles without destroying them. In adults, large cell lymphoma is the most common type. The tumor cells show scanty to moderate amphophilic cytoplasm and round, oval, or cleaved nuclei (Figure 30.47). The nuclei are hyperchromatic with coarse chromatin or vesicular with a prominent central nucleolus. Mitotic figures are frequent. Other types of non-Hodgkin lymphoma, both follicular and diffuse, rarely involve the ovary.

Dysgerminoma is one of the most common and difficult differential diagnoses. The appearance of the cell nuclei is very important. Immunostains for lymphoid markers, such as CD45 (leukocyte common antigen), CD20 for B-cells (Figure 30.48), and CD3 for T-cells, and placental alkaline phosphatase, c-kit, and D2-40 for dysgerminoma are helpful. Dysgerminomas also react for pluripotency markers (transcription factors) SALL4 and OCT3/4. Most ovarian lymphomas have a B-cell phenotype.[111] The 'single-file' arrangement of lymphoma and leukemic cells may simulate metastatic lobular carcinoma of the breast; however, the cells of the latter tumors often contain small mucin-filled intracytoplasmic vacuoles and are immunoreactive for CKs. Carcinoid, granulosa cell tumor, or small cell carcinoma can also resemble lymphoma.

Myeloid neoplasms, including acute myeloid leukemia and myeloid (granulocytic) sarcoma, may involve the ovary and rarely constitute the initial clinical presentation of the disease. At the time of diagnosis of myeloid sarcoma,

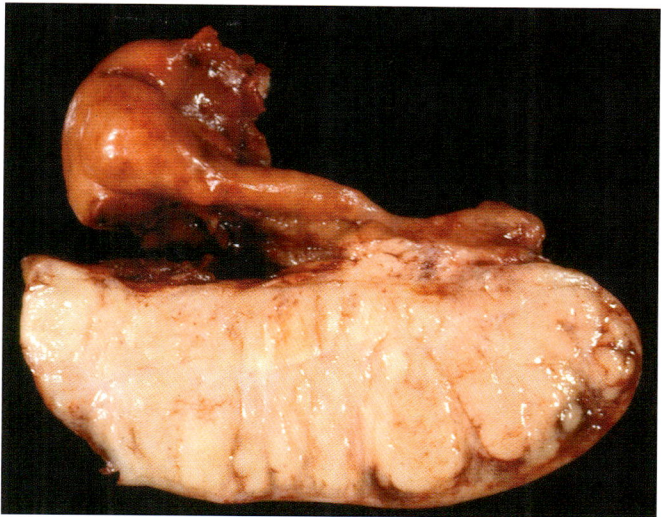

Figure 30.45 Burkitt-like lymphoma. The sectioned surface is lobulated and fleshy resembling that of a dysgerminoma. Notice the marked enlargement of the fallopian tube which is infiltrated by lymphoma.

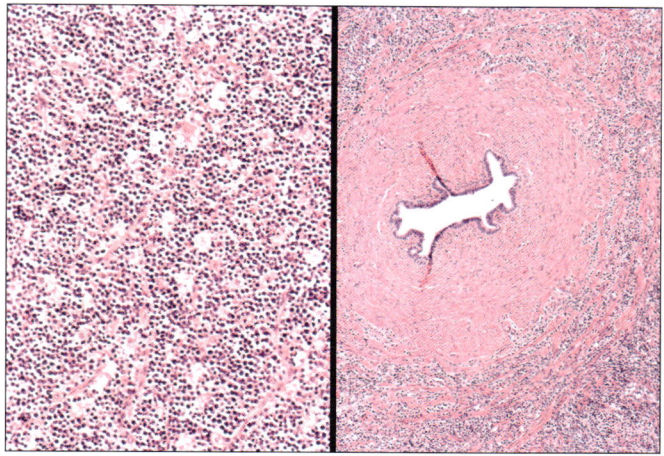

Figure 30.46 Burkitt-like lymphoma. Left: A 'starry-sky' pattern is apparent. Right: The tumor cells infiltrate the wall of the fallopian tube.

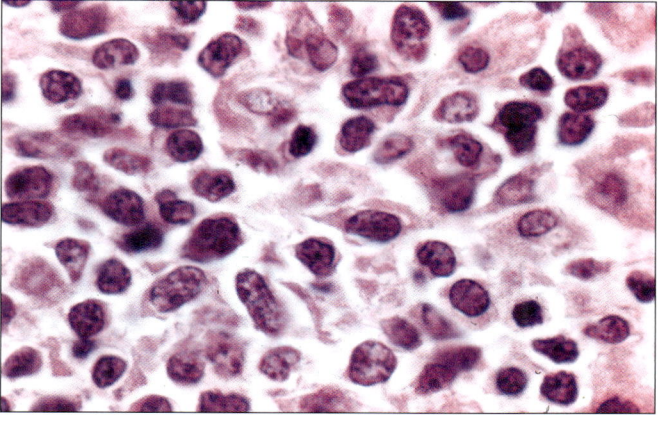

Figure 30.47 Diffuse large cell lymphoma. Large lymphoid cells exhibiting irregular nuclei.

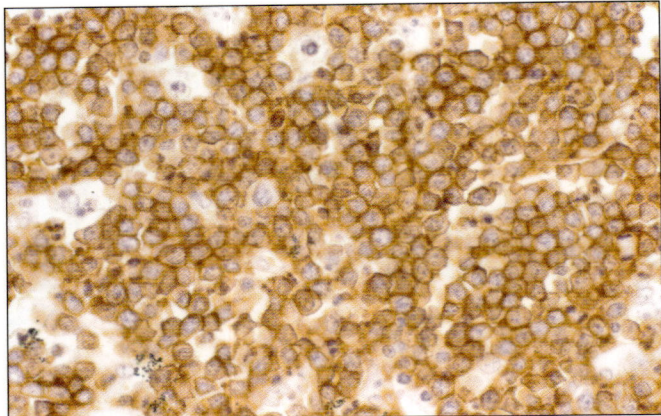

Figure 30.48 Burkitt-like lymphoma. Positive CD20 immunoreaction.

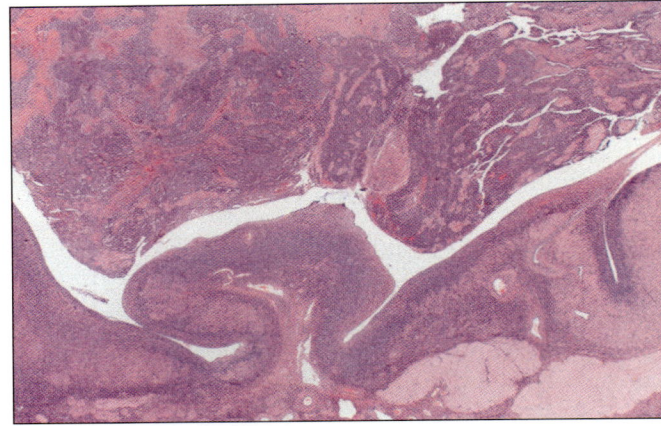

Figure 30.50 Malignant mesothelioma involving the ovary. The tumor covers the surface of the ovary.

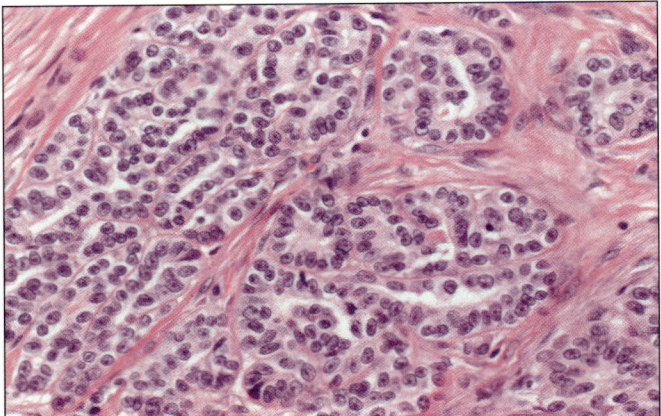

Figure 30.49 Malignant epithelial mesothelioma involving the ovary. The tumor cells have a uniform appearance and are separated by slit-like spaces.

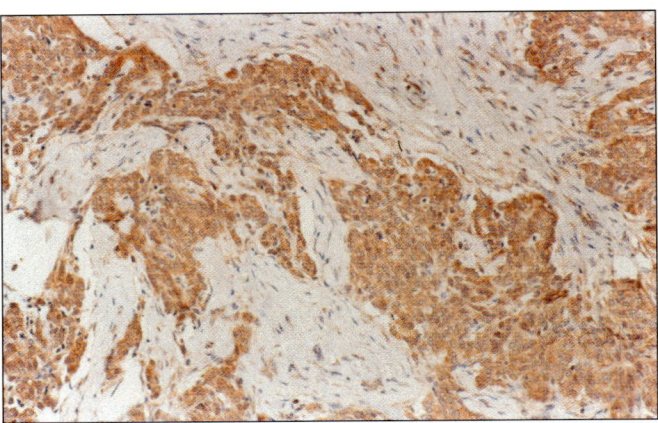

Figure 30.51 Malignant epithelial mesothelioma involving the ovary. The tumor cells are immunoreactive for calretinin.

leukemia may or may not involve the peripheral blood and bone marrow; if not present, it usually develops subsequently. Some of these tumors exhibit a characteristic green color ('chloroma'). Microscopic examination reveals a diffuse growth pattern with a prominent 'single file' arrangement of the tumor cells (Figure 30.49). In contrast to lymphoma cells, the cells of myeloid (granulocytic) sarcoma have more finely dispersed nuclear chromatin and more abundant cytoplasm. Myeloid differentiation can be demonstrated by the chloroacetate esterase stain. Immunostains for myeloperoxidase, lysozyme, and CD68 are positive.[112] B- and T-cell markers, such as CD20 and CD3, are negative.

PERITONEAL TUMORS

Secondary ovarian involvement by *malignant mesothelioma* is common and is usually limited to the surface of the ovary or the superficial stroma (Figure 30.50). Occasionally, however, the ovary is extensively involved and the clinical picture simulates that of ovarian cancer.[113] Microscopically, malignant mesotheliomas are characterized by tubular, papillary, and solid patterns and relatively uniform cells with abundant eosinophilic cytoplasm (Figure 30.49). Rare tumors with an exclusive sheet-like pattern containing polygonal cells may be confused with ectopic decidual reaction. In routinely stained sections, mesotheliomas are usually readily distinguishable from serous carcinoma by their pattern of growth and cytologic features, although histochemical or immunohistochemical stains are sometimes necessary to confirm the diagnosis. In contrast to adenocarcinomas, mesotheliomas lack neutral mucins (digested PAS negative) and contain hyaluronic acid within vacuoles (Alcian blue positive, hyaluronidase sensitive). Hyaluronic acid, however, may leach from formalin-fixed tumors, resulting in false-negative staining. The most useful immunohistochemical markers are the BerEp4-defined surface glycoprotein, which is positive in serous carcinomas but negative in mesothelioma, and calretinin (Figure 30.51), CK5/6, and thrombomodulin, all three of which are positive in mesothelioma but negative in serous carcinomas.[114,115] Additionally, no reactivity for CEA, B72.3, Leu-M1, ER, PR, and CA125 favor a diagnosis of mesothelioma over carcinoma.

Extraovarian primary *peritoneal serous carcinomas* are tumors histologically identical to serous carcinomas of the ovary that present with peritoneal carcinomatosis and minimal or no ovarian involvement. Most peritoneal serous carcinomas are high grade and fundamentally different from low-grade peritoneal serous carcinomas. The latter tumors are distinguished from serous borderline tumors by the presence of invasion. Compared with ovarian high-grade serous carcinomas, the peritoneal tumors contain less ER and PR, and exhibit a stronger expression of Ki-67, and a higher overexpression of HER-2/neu.[116]

Although desmoplastic small round-cell tumors (DSRCTs) with divergent differentiation occur mainly in young males, a few of these tumors have developed in females and have presented clinically as primary ovarian tumors.[117,118] At operation, there was extensive extraovarian disease in all the reported cases, and, despite combination chemotherapy, most patients died of tumor within 2 years of diagnosis. The tumor cells have the translocation t(11;22)(p13;q12), which results in fusion of the Ewing sarcoma and Wilms' tumor genes (EWS–WT1).[119] Microscopically, the metastatic tumor shows discrete aggregates of small cells surrounded by a desmoplastic stroma (Figures 30.52 and 30.53). The tumor cells are small with hyperchromatic nuclei, inconspicuous nucleoli, and scanty cytoplasm. Mitotic figures are numerous. Since many ovarian tumors are characterized by small cells, there is a wide range of differential diagnoses. A prominent nesting pattern of small cells in a desmoplastic stroma, as well as a young age of the patient, should lead to consideration of this tumor. The immunophenotype of the DSRCT is quite characteristic: the tumor cells stain for CKs (Figure 30.54) and epithelial membrane antigen, for neuron-specific enolase, and for desmin (Figure 30.55). Immunostain for actin is negative.

Unusual metastases to the ovary have included small cell carcinoma of the lung, adenoid cystic carcinoma of salivary gland origin, neuroblastoma, alveolar and embryonal rhabdomyosarcomas, leiomyosarcoma, angiosarcoma, Ewing sarcoma, chondrosarcoma, osteogenic sarcoma, chordoma, and ependymoma (Figures 30.56 and 30.57).[3]

EXTRAGENITAL SARCOMAS

Sarcomas rarely metastasize to the ovaries and are more likely to be primary tumors at that site. An exception to this is the gastrointestinal stromal tumor.[120] The differential

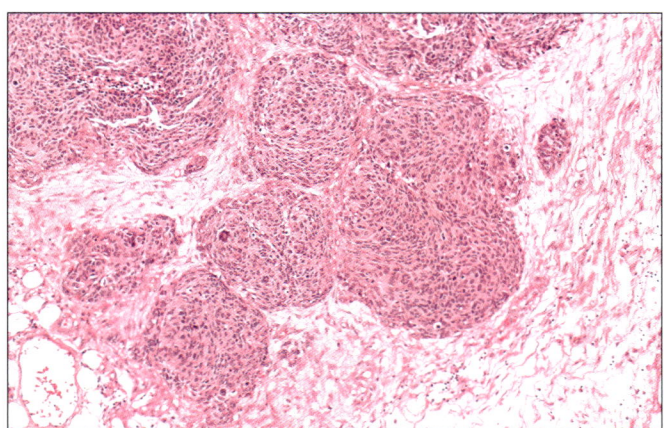

Figure 30.52 Desmoplastic small round-cell tumor involving the ovary. Round aggregates of small cells are surrounded by a fibromatous stroma.

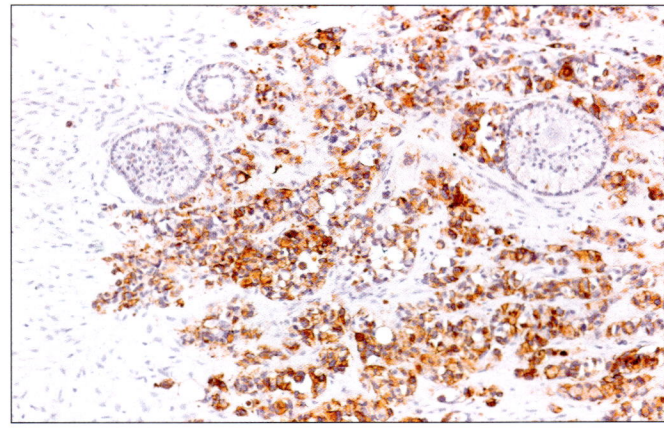

Figure 30.54 Desmoplastic small round-cell tumor involving the ovary. The tumor cells are immunoreactive for cytokeratin. Some primary follicles are seen.

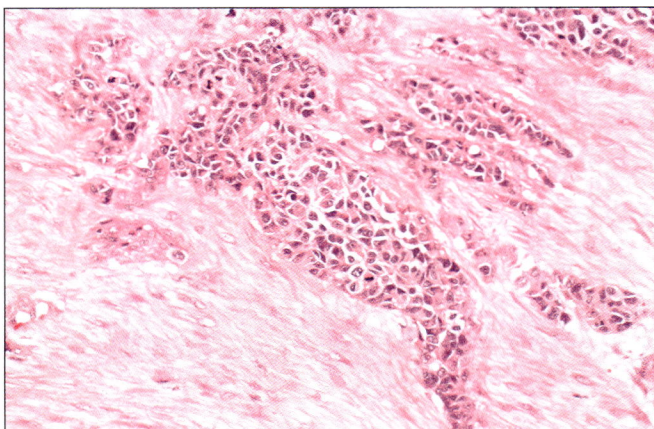

Figure 30.53 Desmoplastic small round-cell tumor involving the ovary. Elongated aggregates of small round and spindle cells are embedded in a desmoplastic stroma.

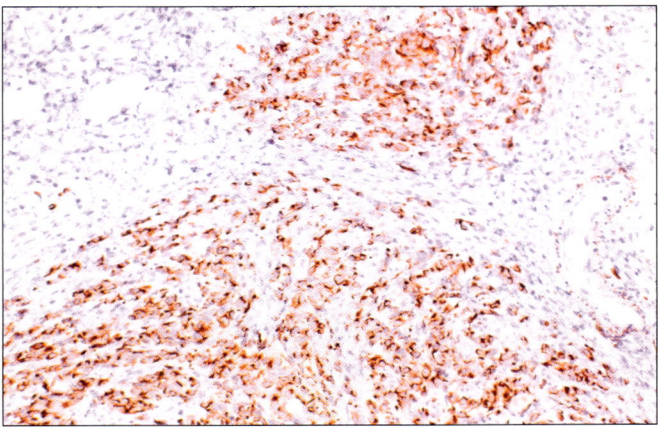

Figure 30.55 Desmoplastic small round-cell tumor involving the ovary. Positive immunoreaction for desmin.

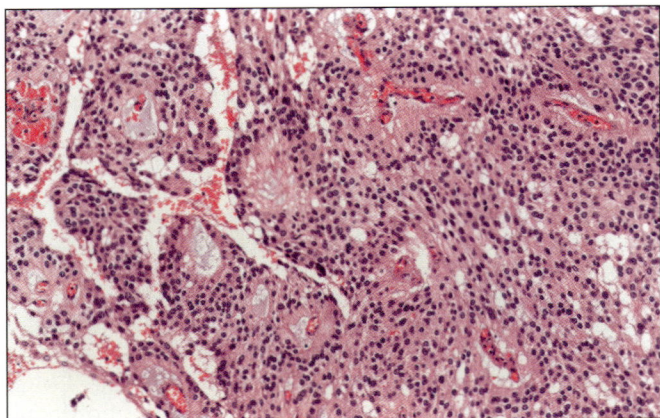

Figure 30.56 Ependymoma involving the ovary. Numerous perivascular pseudorosettes are seen. The patient had a myxopapillary ependymoma of the filum terminale removed 30 years earlier and had developed metastasis to the inguinal lymph nodes 2 years postoperatively.

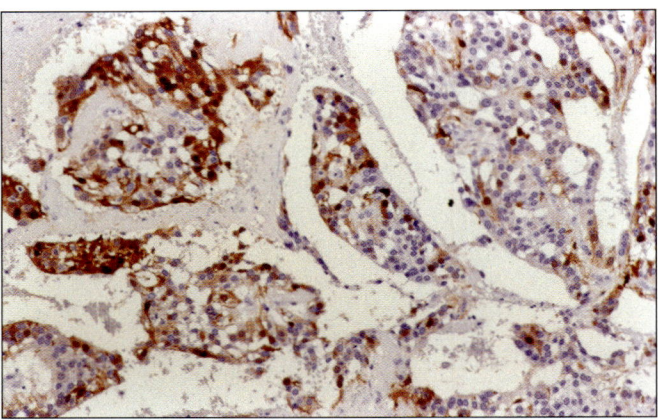

Figure 30.57 Ependymoma involving the ovary. The tumor cells are immunoreactive for glial fibrillary acidic protein (GFAP).

diagnoses include cellular and typical fibromas, smooth muscle tumors, and other primary soft-tissue-type tumors. In cases of bilateral tumors or extraovarian disease, immunohistochemistry for c-kit helps to rule out the possibility of a gastrointestinal stromal neoplasm. Leiomyosarcomas from stomach, small bowel, and retroperitoneum may occasionally metastasize to the ovary.[96] Also isolated examples of fibrosarcoma of the anterior abdominal wall, sarcoma of the mesentery, angiosarcoma of the heart, osteosarcoma of the maxilla, chondrosarcoma of the rib, Ewing sarcoma of a pubic bone, angiosarcoma,[121] alveolar rhabdomyosarcoma,[82,122] Ewing sarcoma of the fibula,[82] chordoma,[123] and malignant hemangiopericytoma.[124] In children, rhabdomyosarcoma is said to be the most common sarcoma to spread to ovary.[82] Metastatic retinoblastoma is also known.[122,125]

SUMMARY

Recognition of the secondary nature of an ovarian tumor depends on a complete clinical history, a careful operative search for a primary extraovarian tumor, and accurate evaluation of the macroscopic and histologic features of the ovarian tumor. In rare cases the primary tumor is not found until several years after resection of the ovarian metastases.

REFERENCES

1. Mazur MT, Hsueh S, Gersell DJ. Metastases to the female genital tract. Analysis of 325 cases. Cancer 1984;53:1978–84.
2. Lash RH, Hart WR. Intestinal adenocarcinomas metastatic to the ovaries: a clinicopathologic evaluation of 22 cases. Am J Surg Pathol 1987;11:114–21.
3. Scully RE, Young RH, Clement PB. Tumors of the ovary, maldeveloped gonads, fallopian tube, and broad ligament. In Atlas of tumor pathology, third series. Fascicle 23. Washington, DC: Armed Forces Institute of Pathology; 1998. p. 335–72.
4. Ulbright TM, Roth LM, Stehman FB. Secondary ovarian neoplasia. A clinicopathologic study of 35 cases. Cancer 1984;53:1164–74.
5. Young RH, Scully RE. Metastic tumours of the ovary. In: Kurman RJ, editor. Blaustein's pathology of the female genital tract. 4th ed. New York: Springer-Verlag; 1994. p. 939–74.
6. Bullón A, Arseneau J, Prat J, et al. Tubular Krukenberg tumor. A problem in histopathologic diagnosis. Am J Surg Pathol 1981;5:225–32.
7. Merino MJ, Edmonds P, LiVolsi V. Appendiceal carcinoma metastatic to the ovaries and mimicking primary ovarian tumors. Int J Gynecol Pathol 1985;4:110–20.
8. Young RH, Gilks CB, Scully RE. Mucinous tumors of the appendix associated with mucinous tumors of the ovary and pseudomyxoma peritonei. Am J Surg Pathol 1991;15:415–29.
9. Cuatrecasas M, Matias-Guiu X, Prat J. Synchronous mucinous tumors of the appendix and the ovary associated with pseudomyxoma peritonei: a clinicopathologic study of six cases with comparative analysis of c-Ki-ras mutations. Am J Surg Pathol 1996;20:739–46.
10. Ronnett BM, Kurman RJ, Shmookler BM, et al. The morphologic spectrum of ovarian metastases of appendiceal adenocarcinomas. A clinicopathologic and immunohistochemical analysis of tumors often misinterpreted as primary ovarian tumors or metastatic tumors from other gastrointestinal sites. Am J Surg Pathol 1997;21:1144–55.
11. Young RH, Hart WR. Metastases from carcinoma of the pancreas simulating primary mucinous tumors of the ovary: A report of seven cases. Am J Surg Pathol 1989;13:748–56.
12. Creasman WT, Lukeman J. Role of the fallopian tube in dissemination of malignant cells in corpus cancer. Cancer 1972;20:456–7.
13. Pins MR, Young RH, Crum CP, et al. Cervical squamous carcinoma in situ with superficial extension to corpus and tubes and invasion of tubes and ovaries. Int J Gynecol Pathol 1997;16:272–8.
14. Ronnett BM, Yemelyanova AV, Vang R, et al. Endocervical adenocarcinomas with ovarian metastases. Analysis of 29 cases with emphasis on minimally invasive cervical tumors and the ability of the metastases to simulate primary ovarian neoplasms. Am J Surg Pathol 2008;32:1835–53.
15. Gagnon Y, Tetu B. Ovarian metastases of breast carcinoma. A clinicopathologic study of 59 cases. Cancer 1989;64:892–8.
16. Petru E, Pickel H, Heydarfadai M, et al. Nongenital cancers metastatic to the ovary. Gynecol Oncol 1992;44:83–6.
17. Savey L, Lasser P, Castaigne D, et al. Krukenberg tumors. Analysis of a series of 28 cases. J Chir (Paris) 1996;133:427–31.
18. Mrad K, Morice P, Fabre A, et al. Krukenberg tumor: a clinicopathological study of 15 cases. Ann Pathol 2000;20:202–6.
19. Le Bouedec G, de Latour M, Levrel O, Dauplat J. Krukenberg tumors of breast origin. 10 cases. Presse Med 1997;26:454–7.
20. Kim SH, Kim WH, Park KJ, et al. CT and MR findings of Krukenberg tumors: comparison with primary ovarian tumors. J Comput Assist Tomogr 1996;20:393–8.
21. Ha HK, Baek SY, Kim SH, et al. Krukenberg's tumor of the ovary: MR imaging features. AJR Am J Roentgenol 1995;164:1435–9.

22. Young RH, Scully RE. Metastatic tumors in the ovary: a problem-oriented approach and review of the recent literature. Semin Diagn Pathol 1991;8:250–76.
23. Seidman JD, Kurman RJ, Ronnett BM. Incidence in routine practice with a new approach to improve intraoperative diagnosis. Primary and metastatic mucinous adenocarcinomas in the ovaries. Am J Surg Pathol 2003;27:985–93.
24. Khunamornpong S, Suprasert PS, Pojchamarnwiputh S, et al. Primary and metastatic mucinous adenocarcinomas of the ovary: evaluation of the diagnostic approach using tumor size and laterality. Gynecol Oncol 2006;101:152–7.
25. Stewart CJR, Brennan BA, Hammond IG, et al. Accuracy of frozen section in distinguishing primary ovarian neoplasia from tumors metastatic to the ovary. Int J Gynecol Pathol 2005;24:356–62.
26. Yemelyanova AV, Vang R, Judson K, et al. Distinction of primary and metastatic mucinous tumors involving the ovary: analysis of size and laterality data by primary site with reevaluation of an algorithm for tumor classification. Am J Surg Pathol 2008;32:128–38.
27. Abu-Rustum NR, Barakat RR, Curtin JP. Ovarian and uterine disease in women with colorectal cancer. Gynecol Oncol 1997;89:85–7.
28. Lewis MR, Deavers MT, Silva EG, Malpica A. Ovarian involvement by metastatic colorectal adenocarcinoma. Still a diagnostic challenge. Am J Surg Pathol 2006;30:177–84.
29. Judson K, McCormick C, Vang R, et al. Women with undiagnosed colorectal adenocarcinomas presenting with ovarian metastases: clinicopathologic features and comparison with women having known colorectal adenocarcinomas and ovarian involvement. Int J Gynecol Pathol 2008;27:182–90.
30. Scully RE, Richardson GS. Luteinization of the stroma of metastatic cancer involving the ovary and its endocrine significance. Cancer 1961;14:827–40.
31. Lee KR, Young RH. The distinction between primary and metastatic mucinous carcinomas of the ovary: gross and histologic findings in 50 cases. Am J Surg Pathol 2003;27:281–92.
32. Young RH, Hart WR. Metastatic intestinal carcinomas simulating primary ovarian clear cell carcinoma and secretory endometrioid carcinoma: a clinicopathologic and immunohistochemical study of five cases. Am J Surg Pathol 1998;22:805–15.
33. Berezowski K, Stastny JK, Kornstein MJ. Cytokeratins 7 and 20 and carcinoembryonic antigen in colonic and ovarian carcinomas. Mod Pathol 1996;9:426–9.
34. DeCostanzo DC, Elias JM, Chumas JC. Necrosis in 84 ovarian carcinomas: a morphologic study of primary versus metastatic colonic carcinoma with a selective immunohistochemical analysis of cytokeratin subtypes and carcinoembryonic antigen. Int J Gynecol Pathol 1997;16:245–9.
35. Ji H, Isacson C, Seidman J, et al. Cytokeratins 7 and 20, Dpc4, and MUC5AC in the distinction of metastatic mucinous carcinomas in the ovary from primary ovarian mucinous tumors: Dpc4 assists in identifying metastatic pancreatic carcinomas. Int J Gynecol Pathol 2002;21:391–400.
36. Wang NP, Zee S, Zarbo RJ, et al. Coordinate expression of cytokeratins 7 and 20 defines unique subsets of carcinomas. Appl Immunohistochem 1995;3:99–107.
37. Wauters CCAP, Smedts F, Gerrits LGM, et al. Keratins 7 and 20 as diagnostic markers of carcinomas metastatic to the ovary. Hum Pathol 1995;26:852–5.
38. Park SY, Kim HS, Hong EK, Kim WH. Expression of cytokeratins 7 and 20 in primary carcinomas of the stomach and colorectum and their value in the differential diagnosis of metastatic carcinomas to the ovary. Hum Pathol 2002;33:1078–85.
39. Dabbs DJ, Sturtz K, Zaino RJ. The immunohistochemical discrimination of endometrioid carcinomas. Hum Pathol 1996;27:172–7.
40. Logani S, Oliva E, Arnell PM, et al. Use of novel immunohistochemical markers expressed in colonic adenocarcinoma to distinguish primary ovarian tumors from metastatic colorectal carcinoma. Mod Pathol 2005;18:19–25.
41. Vang R, Gown AM, Wu LSF, et al. Immunohistochemical expression of CDX2 in primary ovarian mucinous tumors and metastatic mucinous carcinomas involving the ovary: comparison with CK20 and correlation with coordinate expression of CK7. Mod Pathol 2006;19:1421–8.
42. McCluggage WG. Immunohistochemical markers as a diagnostic aid in ovarian pathology. Diagn Histopathol 2008;14:335–51.
43. Lerwill MF, Young RH. Ovarian metastases of intestinal-type gastric carcinoma. A clinicopathologic study of 4 cases with contrasting features to those of the Krukenberg tumor. Am J Surg Pathol 2006;31:1382–8.
44. Scully RE, Sobin LH. World Health Organization: histological typing of ovarian tumours. 2nd ed. Berlin: Springer-Verlag; 1999. p. 39.
45. Kiyokawa T, Young RH, Scully RE. Krukenberg tumors of the ovary. A clinicopathologic analysis of 120 cases with emphasis on their variable pathologic manifestations. Am J Surg Pathol 2006;31:277–99.
46. Holtz F, Hart WR. Krukenberg tumors of the ovary. A clinicopathologic analysis of 27 cases. Cancer 1982;50:2438–47.
47. Robboy SJ, Scully RE, Norris HJ. Carcinoid metastatic to the ovary. A clinocopathologic analysis of 35 cases. Cancer 1974;33:798–811.
48. Rabban JT, Lerwill MF, McCluggage WG, et al. Primary ovarian carcinoid tumors may express CDX-2: a potential pitfall in distinction from metastatic intestinal carcinoid tumors involving the ovary. Int J Gynecol Pathol 2009;28:41–8.
49. Curtin JP, Barakat RR, Hoskins WJ. Ovarian disease in women with breast cancer. Obstet Gynecol 1994;84:449–52.
50. Young RH, Carey RW, Robboy SJ. Breast carcinoma masquerading as a primary ovarian neoplasm. Cancer 1981;48:210–12.
51. Harris M, Howell A, Chrissohou M, et al. A comparison of the metastatic pattern of infiltrating lobular carcinoma and infiltrating duct carcinoma of the breast. Br J Cancer 1984;50:23–30.
52. Monteagudo C, Merino MJ, LaPorte N, Neumann RD. Value of gross cystic disease fluid protein-15 in distinguishing metastatic breast carcinoma among poorly differentiated neoplasms involving the ovary. Hum Pathol 1991;22:368–72.
53. Brown RJ, Campagna LB, Dunn JK, Cagle PT. Immunohistochemical identification of tumor markers in metastatic adenocarcinoma: a diagnostic adjunct in the determination of primary site. Am J Clin Pathol 1997;107:12–19.
54. Bhargava R, Beriwal S, Dabbs DJ. Mammaglobin vs GCDFP-15. An immunohistologic validation survey for sensitivity and specificity. Am J Clin Pathol 2007;127:103–13.
55. Sasaki E, Tsunoda N, Hatanaka Y, et al. Breast-specific expression of MGB1/mammaglobin: an examination of 480 tumors from various organs and clinicopathological analysis of MGB1-positive breast cancers. Mod Pathol 2007;20:208–14.
56. Onuma K, Dabbs DJ, Bhargava R. Mammaglobin expression in the female genital tract: immunohistochemical analysis in benign and neoplastic endocervix and endometrium. Int J Gynecol Pathol 2008;27:418–25.
57. Nonaka D, Chiriboga L, Soslow RA. Expression of PAX8 as a useful marker in distinguishing ovarian carcinomas from mammary carcinomas. Am J Surg Pathol 2008;32:1566–71.
58. Young RH, Hart WR. Metastases from carcinomas of the pancreas simulating primary mucinous tumors of the ovary: a report of seven cases. Am J Surg Pathol 1989;13:748–56.
59. Young RH, Scully RE. Ovarian metastases from carcinoma of the gallbladder and extrahepatic bile ducts simulating primary tumors of the ovary: a report of six cases. Int J Gynecol Pathol 1990;9:60–72.
60. Young RH, Gersell DJ, Clement PB, Scully RE. Hepatocellular carcinoma metastatic to the ovary. A report of three cases discovered during life with discussion of the differential diagnosis of hepatoid tumors of the ovary. Hum Pathol 1992;23:574–80.
61. Vakiani E, Young RH, Carcangiu ML, Klimstra DS. Acinar cell carcinoma of the pancreas metastatic to the ovary. A report of 4 cases. Am J Surg Pathol 2008;32:1540–5.
62. Khunamornpong S, Lerwill MF, Siriaunkgul S, et al. Carcinoma of extrahepatic bile ducts and gallbladder metastatic to the ovary: a report of 16 cases. Int J Gynecol Pathol 2008;27:366–79.
63. Pitman MB, Triratanachat S, Young RH, Oliva E. Hepatocyte paraffin 1 antibody does not distinguish primary ovarian tumors with hepatoid differentiation from metastatic hepatocellular carcinoma. Int J Gynecol Pathol 2003;23:58–64.
64. Prayson RA, Hart WR, Petras RE. Pseudomyxoma peritonei: a clinicopathologic study of 19 cases with emphasis on site of origin and nature of associated ovarian tumors. Am J Surg Pathol 1994;18:591–603.
65. Ronnett BM, Kurman RJ, Zahn CM, et al. Pseudomyxoma peritonei in women: a clinicopathologic analysis of 30 cases with

emphasis on site of origin, prognosis, and relationship to ovarian mucinous tumors of low malignant potential. Hum Pathol 1995;26:509–24.
66. Merino MJ, Edmonds P, LiVolsi V. Appendiceal carcinoma metastatic to the ovaries and mimicking primary ovarian tumors. Int J Gynecol Pathol 1985;4:110–20.
67. Hristov AC, Young RH, Vang R, et al. Ovarian metastases of appendiceal tumors with goblet cell carcinoid-like and signet ring cell patterns: A report of 30 cases. Am J Surg Pathol 2007;31:1502–11.
68. Szych C, Staebler A, Connolly DC, et al. Molecular genetic evidence supporting the clonality and appendiceal origin of Pseudomyxoma peritonei in women. Am J Pathol 1999;154:1849–55.
69. Insabato L, DeRosa G, Franco R, et al. Ovarian metastasis from renal cell carcinoma: a report of three cases. Int J Surg Pathol 2003;11:309–12.
70. Spencer JR, Eriksen B, Garnett JE. Metastatic renal tumor presenting as ovarian clear cell carcinoma. Urology 1993;41:582–4.
71. Vara A, Madrigal B, Veiga M, et al. Bilateral ovarian metastases from renal clear cell carcinoma. Acta Oncol (Stockh) 1998;37:379–80.
72. Young RH, Hart WR. Renal cell carcinoma metastatic to the ovary: a report of three cases emphasizing possible confusion with ovarian clear cell adenocarcinoma. Int J Gynecol Pathol 1992;11:96–104.
73. Cameron RI, Ashe P, O'Rourke DM, et al. A panel of immunohistochemical stains assists in the distinction between ovarian and renal clear cell carcinoma. Int J Gynecol Pathol 2003;22:272–6.
74. Leroy X, Farine MO, Buob D, et al. Diagnostic value of cytokeratin 7, CD10 and mesothelin in distinguishing ovarian clear cell carcinoma from metastasis of renal clear cell carcinoma. Histopathology 2007;51:846–76.
75. Ohta Y, Suzuki T, Shiokawa A, et al. Expression of CD10 and cytokeratins in ovarian and renal clear cell carcinoma. Int J Gynecol Pathol 2005;24:239–45.
76. Gokden N, Gokden M, Phan DC, McKenney JK. The utility of PAX-2 in distinguishing metastatic clear cell renal cell carcinoma from its morphologic mimics. An immunohistochemical study with comparison to renal cell carcinoma marker. Am J Surg Pathol 2008;32:1462–7.
77. Young RH, Scully RE. Urothelial and ovarian carcinomas of identical cell types: Problems in interpretation. A report of three cases and review of the literature. Int J Gynecol Pathol 1988;7:197–211.
78. Oliva E, Musulén E, Prat J, Young RH. Transitional cell carcinoma of the renal pelvis with symptomatic ovarian metastases. Int J Surg Pathol 1995;2:231–6.
79. Riedel I, Czernobilsky B, Lifschitz-Mercer B, et al. Brenner tumors but not transitional cell carcinomas of the ovary show urothelial differentiation: immunohistochemical staining of urothelial markers, including cytokeratins and uroplakins. Virchows Arch 2001;438:181–91.
80. Logani S, Oliva E, Amin MB, et al. Immunoprofile of ovarian tumors with putative transitional cell (urothelial) differentiation using novel urothelial markers. Histogenic and diagnostic implications. Am J Surg Pathol 2003;27:1434–41.
81. Meyer WH, Yu GW, Milvenan ES, et al. Ovarian involvement in neuroblastoma. Med Pediatr Oncol 1979;7:49–54.
82. Sty JR, Kun LE, Casper JT. Bone scintigraphy in neuroblastoma with ovarian metastasis. Wis Med J 1980;79:28–9.
83. Young RH, Kozakewich HPW, Scully RE. Metastatic ovarian tumors in children: a report of 14 cases and review of the literature. Int J Gynecol Pathol 1993;12:8–19.
84. Kurek R, Von Knobloch R, Feek U, et al. Local recurrence of an oncocytic adrenocortical carcinoma with ovary metastasis. J Urol 2001;166:985.
85. Fitzgibbons PL, Martin SE, Simmons TJ. Malignant melanoma metastatic to the ovary. Am J Surg Pathol 1987;11:959–64.
86. Gupta D, Deavers MT, Silva EG, et al. Malignant melanoma involving the ovary. A clinicopathologic and immunohistochemical study of 23 cases. Am J Surg Pathol 2004;28:771–80.
87. Young RH, Scully RE. Malignant melanoma metastatic to the ovary: a clinicopathologic analysis of 20 cases. Am J Surg Pathol 1991;15:849–60.
88. Irving JA, Young RH. Lung carcinoma metastatic to the ovary: a clinicopathologic study of 32 cases emphasizing their morphologic spectrum and problems in differential diagnosis. Am J Surg Pathol 2005;29:997–1006.
89. Reis-Filho JS, Carrilho C, Valenti C, et al. Is TTF1 a good immunohistochemical marker to distinguish primary from metastatic lung adenocarcinomas? Pathol Res Pract 2000;196:835–40.
90. Baker PM, Oliva E. Immunohistochemistry as a tool in the differential diagnosis of ovarian tumors: an update. Int J Gynecol Pathol 2005;24:39–55.
91. Bing Z, Adegboyega PA. Metastasis of small cell carcinoma of lung into an ovarian mucinous neoplasm: immunohistochemistry as a useful ancillary technique for diagnosis and classification of rare tumors. Appl Immunohistochem Mol Morphol 2005;13:104–7.
92. Yeh KY, Chang JW, Hsueh S, et al. Ovarian metastasis originating from bronchioloalveolar carcinoma: a rare presentation of lung cancer. Jpn J Clin Oncol 2003;33:404–7.
93. Young RH, Gersell DJ, Roth LM, Scully RE. Ovarian metastases from cervical carcinomas other than pure adenocarcinomas. A report of 12 cases. Cancer 1993;71:407–18.
94. Eichhorn JH, Young RH, Scully RE. Nonpulmonary small cell carcinomas of extragenital origin metastatic to the ovary. Cancer 1993;71:177–86.
95. Bott-Kothari T, Aron BS, Bejarano P. Malignant thymoma with metastases to the gastrointestinal tract and ovary: a case report and literature review. Am J Clin Oncol 2000;23:140–2.
96. Young RH, Scully RE. Sarcomas metastatic to the ovary: a report of 21 cases. Int J Gynecol Pathol 1990;9:231–52.
97. Young RH, Scully RE. Mucinous ovarian tumors associated with mucinous adenocarcinomas of the cervix. A clinicopathological analysis of 16 cases. Int J Gynecol Pathol 1988;7:99–111.
98. Kaminski PF, Norris HJ. Coexistence of ovarian neoplasms and endocervical adenocarcinoma. Obstet Gynecol 1984;64:553–6.
99. LiVolsi VA, Merino MJ, Schwartz PE. Coexistent endocervical adenocarcinoma and mucinous adenocarcinoma of ovary: a clinicopathological study of four cases. Int J Gynecol Pathol 1983;1:391–402.
100. Elishaev E, Gilks CB, Miller D, et al. Synchronous and metachronous endocervical and ovarian neoplasms. Evidence supporting interpretation of the ovarian neoplasms as metastatic endocervical adenocarcinomas simulating primary ovarian surface epithelial neoplasms. Am J Surg Pathol 2005;29:281–94.
101. Ronnett BM, Yemelyanova AV, Vang R, et al. Endocervical adenocarcinomas with ovarian metastases. Analysis of 29 cases with emphasis on minimally invasive cervical tumors and the ability of the metastases to simulate primary ovarian neoplasms. Am J Surg Pathol 2008;32:1835–53.
102. Young RH, Gersell DJ, Roth LM, Scully RE. Ovarian metastases from cervical carcinomas other than pure adenocarcinomas. A report of 12 cases. Cancer 1993;71:407–18.
103. Nguyen L, Brewer CA, DiSaia PJ. Ovarian metastasis of stage IB1 squamous cell cancer of the cervix after radical parametrectomy and oophoropexy. Gynecol Oncol 1998;68:198–200.
104. Alvarado-Cabrero I, Young RH, Vamvakas EC, Scully RE. Carcinoma of the fallopian tube: a clinicopathological study of 105 cases with observations on staging and prognostic factors. Gynecol Oncol 1999;72:367–79.
105. Baekelandt M, Jorunn NA, Kristensen GB, et al. Carcinoma of the fallopian tube. Cancer 2000;89:2076–84.
106. Piek JM, van Diest PJ, Zweemer RP, et al. Dysplastic changes in prophylactically removed fallopian tubes of women predisposed to developing ovarian cancer. J Pathol 2001;195:451–6.
107. Piek JM, van Diest PJ, Zweemer RP, et al. Tubal ligation and risk of ovarian cancer. Lancet 2001;358:844.
108. Kindelberger DW, Lee Y, Miron A, et al. Intraepithelial carcinoma of the fimbria and pelvic serous carcinoma: evidence for a causal relationship. Am J Surg Pathol 2007;31:161–9.
109. Lee Y, Miron A, Drapkin R, et al. A candidate precursor to serous carcinoma that originates in the distal fallopian tube. J Pathol 2007;211:26–35.
110. Dimopoulos MA, Daliani D, Pugh W, et al. Primary ovarian non-Hodgkin's lymphoma: outcome after treatment with combination chemotherapy. Gynecol Oncol 1997;64:446–50.
111. Monterroso V, Jaffe ES, Merino MJ, Medeiros LJ. Malignant lymphomas involving the ovary. A clinicopathologic analysis of 39 cases. Am J Surg Pathol 1993;17:154–70.

112. Oliva E, Ferry JA, Young RH, et al. Granulocytic sarcoma of the female genital tract. A clinicopathologic study of 11 cases. Am J Surg Pathol 1997;21:1156–65.
113. Clement PB, Young RH, Scully RE. Malignant mesotheliomas presenting as ovarian masses. A report of nine cases, including two primary ovarian mesotheliomas. Am J Surg Pathol 1996;20:1067–80.
114. Ordonez NG. Role of immunohistochemistry in distinguishing epithelial peritoneal mesotheliomas from peritoneal and ovarian serous carcinomas. Am J Surg Pathol 1998;22:1203–14.
115. Yaziji H, Gown AM. Immunohistochemical analysis of gynecologic tumors. Int J Gynecol Pathol 2001;20:64–78.
116. Halperin R, Zehavi S, Hadas E, et al. Immunohistochemical comparison of primary peritoneal and primary ovarian serous papillary carcinoma. Int J Gynecol Pathol 2001;20:341–5.
117. Young RH, Eichhorn JH, Dickersin GR, Scully RE. Ovarian involvement by the intra-abdominal desmoplastic small round cell tumor with divergent differentiation: a report of three cases. Hum Pathol 1992;23:454–64.
118. Zaloudek C, Miller TR, Stern JR. Desmoplastic small cell tumor of the ovary: a unique polyphenotypic tumor with an unfavorable prognosis. Int J Gynecol Pathol 1995;14:260–5.
119. Ladanyi M, Gerald W. Fusion of the EWS and WT1 genes in the desmoplastic small round cell tumor. Cancer Res 1994;54:2837–40.
120. Irving JA, Lerwill MF, Young RH. Gastrointestinal stromal tumors metastatic to the ovary. A report of five cases. Am J Surg Pathol 2005;29:920–6.
121. Patel T, Ohri SK, Sundaresan M, et al. Metastatic angiosarcoma of the ovary. Eur J Surg Oncol 1991;17:295–9.
122. McCarville MB, Hill DA, Miller BE, Pratt CB. Secondary ovarian neoplasms in children: imaging features with histopathologic correlation. Pediatr Radiol 2001;31:358–64.
123. Zukerberg LR, Young RH. Chordoma metastatic to the ovary. Arch Pathol Lab Med 1990;114:208–10.
124. Begum M, Katabuchi H, Tashiro H, et al. A case of metastatic malignant hemangiopericytoma of the ovary: recurrence after a period of 17 years from intracranial tumor. Int J Gynecol Cancer 2002;12:510–14.
125. Moshfeghi DM, Wilson MW, Haik BG, et al. Retinoblastoma metastatic to the ovary in a patient with Waardenburg syndrome. Am J Ophthalmol 2002;133:716–18.

31 The Peritoneum

Emanuela D'Angelo, Jaime Prat

CHAPTER OUTLINE

Normal Peritoneum	716	Solitary Fibrous Tumor of Peritoneum ('Fibrous Mesothelioma')	728
Inflammatory and Reactive Lesions	716	Other Tumors	729
Granulomatous Peritonitis	717	Metastatic Tumors	729
Non-Granulomatous Histiocytic Lesions	718	Pseudomyxoma Peritonei	729
Fibrosing Lesions	718	Gliomatosis Peritonei	732
Tumor-Like Lesions	719	Strumosis Peritonei	732
Ovarian Remnant Syndrome	721	Lesions of the Secondary Müllerian System	733
Supernumerary or Accessory Ovaries	721	Endometriosis	733
Splenosis	721	Peritoneal Serous Lesions	733
Trophoblastic Implants	723	Endosalpingiosis	733
Infarcted Appendix Epiploica	723	Serous Tumors (Primary and Metastatic)	735
Mesothelial Neoplasms	723	Endocervicosis	735
Adenomatoid Tumor	723	Peritoneal Endometrioid, Clear Cell, and Transitional Cell Lesions	735
Well-Differentiated Papillary Mesothelioma	723	Deciduosis	735
Diffuse Malignant Mesothelioma	724	Disseminated Peritoneal Leiomyomatosis	735
Miscellaneous Primary Tumors	727		
Intra-Abdominal Desmoplastic, Small Round Cell Tumor	727		

NORMAL PERITONEUM

Knowledge of the peritoneum is important in understanding the pathology of the female genital tract. The uterine corpus, along with the fallopian tubes, the cervix, and the upper part of the vagina, develop from the müllerian ducts, which in turn derive from the mesenchyme of the urogenital ridge and the celomic lining epithelium (mesothelium) or primitive peritoneum. The mesothelium lining the peritoneal cavity is a single layer of flat or cuboidal cells with small round central nuclei and a single nucleolus. Cytoplasm is minimal with well-defined cell borders. On an ultrastructural basis, mesothelial cells show prominent and numerous long microvilli. This is in contrast to many müllerian epithelia, especially serous epithelia, where cilia are obvious by light microscopy and greatly overshadow the slender microvilli. The microvilli in typical müllerian adenocarcinomas tend to be shorter, stubbier, and are fewer in number than those of mesothelial cells.

Submesothelial mesenchyme anchors the mesothelium to the underlying tissue. Submesothelial stromal cells are important in the development of deciduosis, endosalpingiosis, endometriosis, and disseminated peritoneal leiomyomatosis. Microscopically, these peritoneal lesions are characterized by müllerian differentiation and are thought to derive from the so-called 'secondary müllerian system,' i.e., the pelvic and lower abdominal mesothelium and the underlying mesenchyme of females.[1] In fact, the concept of the secondary müllerian system refers to a mechanism by which benign lesions and tumors of müllerian histology might arise from the peritoneum.[1]

In females, the peritoneum is a nearly continuous membrane only interrupted in the pelvis by the fallopian tubes. The fallopian tubes are a potential passage for the transmission of pathogens, chemical and biologic, that have ascended through the genital tract from the external environment.

INFLAMMATORY AND REACTIVE LESIONS

In adult females, most infections are ascending, as in pelvic inflammatory disease, which results in localized acute peritonitis. Acute diffuse peritonitis, characterized by a serosal fibrinopurulent exudate, is most commonly associated with perforated viscera as in appendicitis or diverticulitis and is usually bacterial or chemical in origin. In addition to the acute inflammatory reaction itself, chronic changes may occur, such as are seen in granulomatous and histiocytic reactions. In some cases, the inflammatory process leads to reactive changes.

GRANULOMATOUS PERITONITIS

Both, infectious and noninfectious agents can cause granulomatous peritonitis. Among the former, *Mycobacterium tuberculosis* is the most common, and, less frequently, fungi and parasites. Granulomas are also induced by foreign material including keratin, by vernix caseosa or by meconium, in the form of necrotic pseudoxanthomatous nodules or as a post-cautery reaction.[2]

TUBERCULOSIS

Tuberculous peritonitis is still encountered in the peritoneum, usually in immunosuppressed patients.[3] It may also occur as a complication of chronic peritoneal dialysis.[4] It may be secondary to tuberculous salpingitis or result from miliary tuberculosis. Clinically, it may manifest nonspecifically as widespread carcinomatosis.[5] The presence of ascites, a pelvic mass, and marked elevation of serum levels of CA125 may lead to a false clinical suspicion of ovarian cancer.[3,6] The granulomas are characterized by caseous necrosis and Langhans type giant cells; mycobacteria may be demonstrated by acid-fast stains or immunofluorescence techniques.

SUTURE MATERIALS

Foreign-body granulomas are most commonly associated with suture material retained from prior surgical procedures. The sutures may consist of dense hyaline material in varying degrees of disintegration, or translucent threads. The foreign-body component of the granulomas can be highlighted with polarizing filters. Cellular reaction consists of macrophages, some multinucleated, and lymphocytes. There is both local fibrosis and serosal adhesions.

SURGICAL GLOVE POWDER

Surgical glove powder, either talc or starch granules, is a common cause of granulomas. At laparotomy, the peritoneal granulomas may simulate carcinomatosis or tuberculosis. Usually the starch granulomas resolve within a few months, leaving no residua or only adhesions; however, some patients develop fibrosing peritonitis. Commonly, starch granulomas exhibit a typical foreign-body reaction and, less frequently, they appear as sarcoid granulomas,[7,8] which lack necrosis, or tuberculoid granulomas, with necrosis, that simulate tuberculosis. The polyhedral and translucent starch granules are periodic acid–Schiff (PAS) positive and exhibit the typical Maltese cross under polarized light. Rarely, fat necrosis and rheumatoid-type necrotizing foci are identified as reactions to starch. Talc was once an important cause of granulomatous and fibrosing peritonitis because of its application as a lubricant on surgical gloves; however, its use has been discontinued. Talc is a greater irritant than starch and is poorly absorbed by some patients. Talc granulomas are of the typical foreign-body type. Multinucleated giant cells are numerous and contain pleomorphic crystal spicules readily seen with polarized light.

CONTRAST MEDIA

Peritoneal granulomas may result from exposure to hysterosalpingographic contrast medium, which can be associated with a lipogranulomatous reaction. These appear as foreign-body giant cell reactions around spherical vacuoles from which lipid has been removed during processing. Lipogranulomas may become confluent and focal necrosis may occur.

INTESTINAL CONTENTS

Foreign-body granulomas to intestinal contents may be seen following perforation such as in Crohn disease, diverticulitis, or malignant fistulas. These granulomas are generally confined to the serosa, but plant material and barium from a perforated colon may be identified in the wall or subserosal fat.

CYSTIC TERATOMA (DERMOID CYST) RUPTURE

Rupture of a mature cystic teratoma (dermoid cyst) is typically associated with widespread peritoneal granulomas and adhesions. The squamous cells, hairs, and sebum trigger a foreign-body reaction. This phenomenon occurs especially when the teratoma is removed by cystectomy during laparoscopic surgery.[9] On occasion the reaction may also appear as sclerosing peritonitis and mimics a neoplasm at operation.[10]

KERATIN

Peritoneal foreign-body granulomas to keratin may be found in association with uterine or ovarian endometrioid carcinomas with squamous differentiation, or, less frequently, with squamous cell carcinomas of the cervix or atypical polypoid adenomyomas.[11] Uterine examples are thought to result from retrograde transmission of acellular keratinous debris through the fallopian tubes (Figure 31.1). Granulomas have been seen on the serosa of the adnexa, uterus, colon, and appendix. These granulomas are easily misinterpreted as metastatic carcinoma. Follow-up on these patients indicates that cell-free granulomas lack prognostic significance.[11]

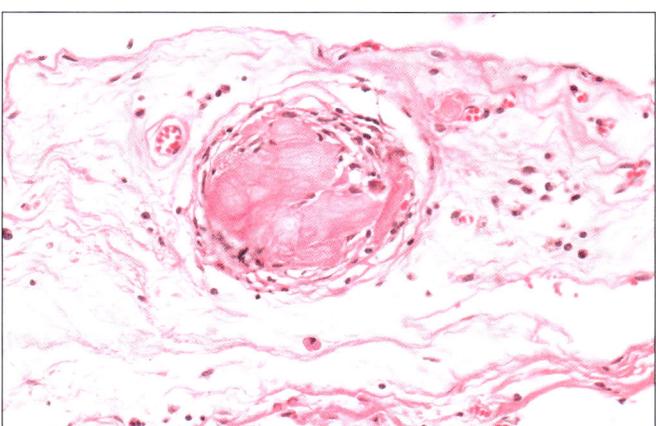

Figure 31.1 Keratin nodule in omentum. The patient had an endometrial adenocarcinoma with squamous differentiation and had received radiotherapy.

CAUTERIZED TISSUE

Foreign-body granulomatous reactions to cauterized tissue in pelvic peritoneal and ovarian biopsies are occasionally encountered in patients who have had endometriotic or other lesions treated in the weeks prior to biopsy. The lesions show central eosinophilic, focally refractile, amorphous material (representing the coagulated tissue and carbonaceous debris) palisaded by large numbers of multinucleated foreign-body giant cells and a peripheral lymphocytic infiltrate (Figure 31.2). Lesions tend to hyalinize with age and may persist for many years.

CESAREAN DELIVERY

Complicating cesarean delivery, the amniotic fluid contents may spill into the peritoneal cavity causing a syndrome clinically similar to bowel perforation.[12,13] Amniotic fluid contains squamous cells, keratin, and sometimes lanugo hair (vernix caseosa). It may also contain meconium, which itself is composed of bile, pancreatic, and intestinal secretions.[14] Grossly, the amniotic fluid contents appear as cheese-like yellow patches limited to the serosal layer of visceral organs.[15] Meconium peritonitis caused by bowel perforation *in utero* can also be a problem in newborn infants. The hallmark of meconium peritonitis is calcification, which presumably results from the action of pancreatic enzymes.

NON-GRANULOMATOUS HISTIOCYTIC LESIONS

Histiocytic infiltrates rather than discrete granulomas are occasionally found in the peritoneum.[9] Melanin-rich histiocytes are sometimes found in cases where an ovarian dermoid cyst has ruptured. The spillage contains melanin, which the peritoneal histiocytes phagocytose. Grossly, the peritoneum may appear to be stained black or display small tumor-like nodules on its surface. Distinction of benign peritoneal melanosis from metastatic malignant melanoma is usually straightforward because of the bland nuclear features of the pigmented histiocytes and the absence of mitoses. Appropriate immunohistochemical stains can further indicate that the cells are histiocytes and not atypical melanocytes.[16]

Occasionally, foci of endometriosis may disclose an abundance of histiocytes filled with ceroid, a wax-like, finely granular, and golden to yellow-brown pigment that is a form of lipofuscin, a lipid-containing residue of lysosomal digestion that is considered an aging or 'wear and tear' pigment. Ceroid is believed to be the end result of the breakdown of blood products after removal of iron. These histiocytic foci are sometimes called 'necrotic pseudoxanthomatous nodules.'[2,17,18]

FIBROSING LESIONS

Sclerosing peritonitis is a reactive process in which a thickened fibrous or myofibromatous stroma develops on the peritoneal serosa. It is often idiopathic,[19,20] although in some cases the cause is identified, such as prior peritoneal inflammation or a ruptured ovarian dermoid with spillage of the contents (see previous granulomatous reactions),[10,21] chronic dialysis,[22–26] or after surgical procedures.

In some cases, the sclerosing peritonitis has been described as part of a syndrome, often in association with a 'luteinized thecoma of the ovary.'[27–32] Clinically, most of the women are young, usually under 30 years of age. Common presenting signs include abdominal enlargement and sometimes small bowel obstruction. Ascites may be present. Even when the patients have a luteinized thecoma, none has endocrine symptoms. A significant number of patients have been exposed to propranolol-type beta-blocking agents or antiepileptics.

Grossly, opaque to light-brown 1–3 mm granules or nodules appear matted together on the peritoneum or on the serosa of the involved organs. The omentum is usually indurated. Microscopic examination discloses a fibrotic process, with various chronic inflammatory cells (Figure 31.3). There is usually some degree of mesothelial hyperplasia. Deeper tissues are relatively spared. Nodules are composed of moderately cellular fascicles of benign-appearing spindle cells resembling fibroblasts and myofibroblasts that contain occasional mitotic figures. In addition to cytokeratin reactivity, the cells also disclose immunoreactivity for vimentin and smooth muscle actin.[27,30]

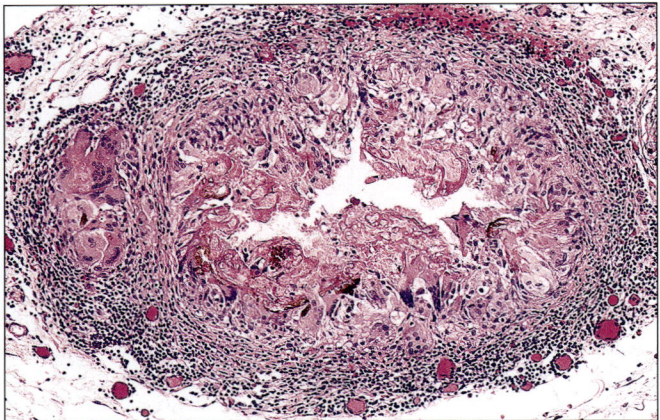

Figure 31.2 Florid foreign-body granulomatous reactions to cauterized tissue.

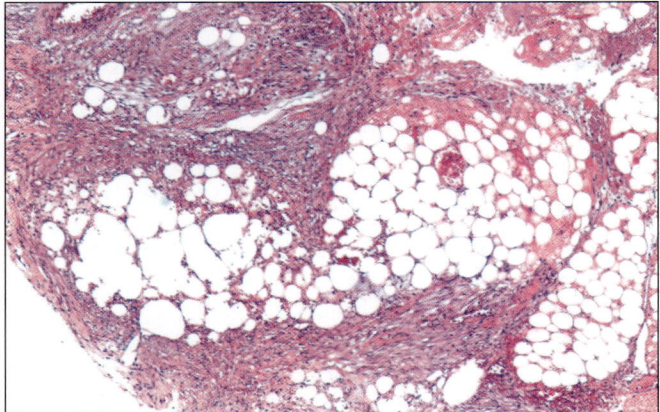

Figure 31.3 Sclerosing peritonitis. The fat lobules are surrounded by cellular fibromatous tissue.

Rarely, single or multiple fibrous nodules ranging up to 6 cm may occur in the gastrointestinal tract or mesentery in adults.[32] Microscopically, the lesions are composed of fibroblasts, collagen, and scattered mononuclear inflammatory cells. The fibroblastic cells show variable immunoreactivity for vimentin, CD117, muscle-specific actin, smooth muscle actin, and desmin, with negative staining for CD34 and ALK-1. These nodules have been designated as 'fibrous pseudotumors.'[32]

Occasionally, sclerosing lesions may be difficult to distinguish from desmoplastic mesothelioma, especially when the biopsy specimen is small. These tumors, however, are very rare in the peritoneal cavity, especially in women. Features that favor a diagnosis of mesothelioma include nuclear atypia, necrosis, organized patterns of collagen deposition (fascicular or storiform), and destructive infiltration into adjacent tissues.

Some patients with sclerosing peritonitis have been successfully treated utilizing antiestrogens and/or GnRH agonists.

TUMOR-LIKE LESIONS

MESOTHELIAL HYPERPLASIA

Mesothelial hyperplasia is a common response to inflammation that occurs in any process that leads to irritation of a serosal surface, such as ascites, hernia sacs, endometriosis, pelvic inflammatory disease, or ovarian tumors.[33-35] Grossly, the hyperplastic lesions may be seen at operation as multiple small nodules, but more commonly are incidental findings on microscopic examination. Microscopically, the changes range from a mild (Figure 31.4) to a substantial increase in the number of mesothelial cells (Figure 31.5), most of which have transformed from flat and relatively inconspicuous to cuboidal or even columnar. With marked hyperplasia, the mesothelial proliferation appears as sheets, clusters, ribbons, tubules, and sometimes as papillary formations that can be misinterpreted as metastatic adenocarcinoma (Figure 31.6). Psammoma bodies are encountered occasionally and eosinophilic elongated cells resembling rhabdomyoblasts have been described.

Reactive mesothelial cells tend to be uniform in appearance. With minor degrees of reactivity, the nuclei are small, regular, round, or oval, and exhibit central nucleoli. The cytoplasm is eosinophilic or sometimes vacuolated and contains acid mucin (predominantly hyaluronic acid). With increasing degrees of reactivity, the nuclei enlarge and the chromatin increases. Nucleoli become more apparent and, in the extreme case, may become quite large and prominent (Figure 31.7). Cells may become binucleated or multinucleated. In cytologic preparations the large macronucleoli may be mistaken as evidence for malignancy.

The immunoprofile of normal mesothelium differs from that expected of epithelial tissue. As anticipated, it expresses cytokeratin intermediate filaments typical of epithelial cells. But it also expresses vimentin and desmin, which are indicative, respectively, of mesenchymal differentiation and specialization into muscle. In contrast, ovarian surface epithelium is immunoreactive for vimentin and desmin in fewer than half of cases. Ovarian inclusion cysts are nonreactive for vimentin and desmin, as are benign and borderline ovarian tumors. Mesothelial hyperplasia can occur within the superficial ovarian stroma overlying a borderline tumor and in such cases can be misinterpreted as invasive tumor. The differential reactivity of mesothelium (and mesothelioma) and müllerian tissue (and ovarian tumors) is discussed more fully in the following sections.

With greater degrees of injury, a layer of spindle-shaped mesenchymal cells may sometimes appear below the mesothelial cells. In the resting state, this layer is inconspicuous, but, when stimulated, the cells may proliferate and produce a highly cellular desmoplastic tissue. Cells also express cytokeratin, vimentin, and desmin. These cells simulate myofibroblasts, and are thought to give rise occasionally to the muscular cells in the condition 'disseminated peritoneal leiomyomatosis' (see later).

The exuberant and sometimes pseudoinfiltrative growth that mesothelium can show, together with the increased mitotic activity that is frequently observed, may lead to a false impression of primary or metastatic carcinoma, despite the benign cytologic appearance of the cells[33] (Figure 31.6). Carcinoma cells generally demonstrate greater nuclear pleomorphism and more conspicuous mitotic activity.

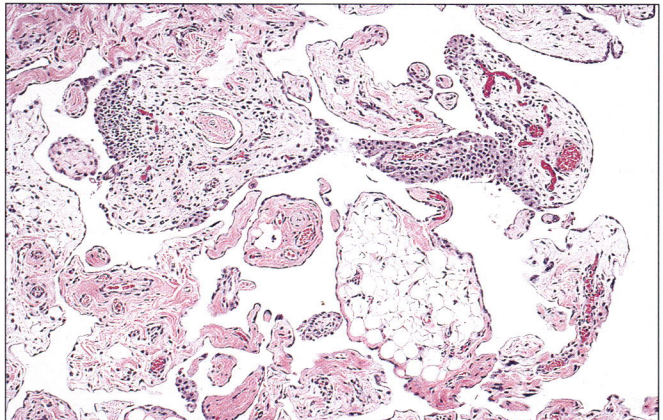

Figure 31.4 Slight mesothelial hyperplasia of peritoneum.

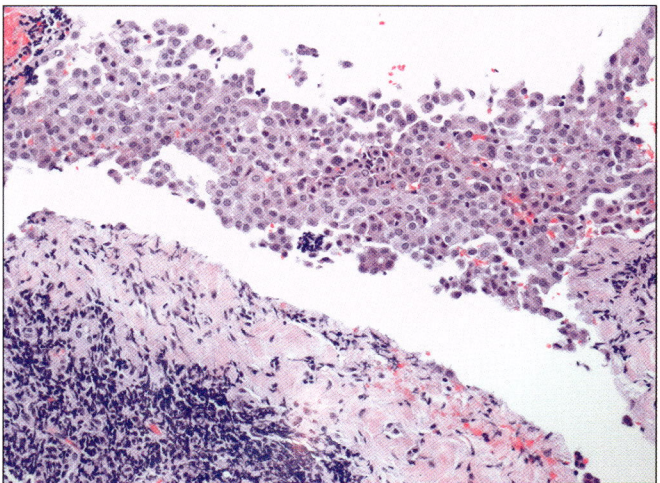

Figure 31.5 Thin layer of moderately reactive mesothelium.

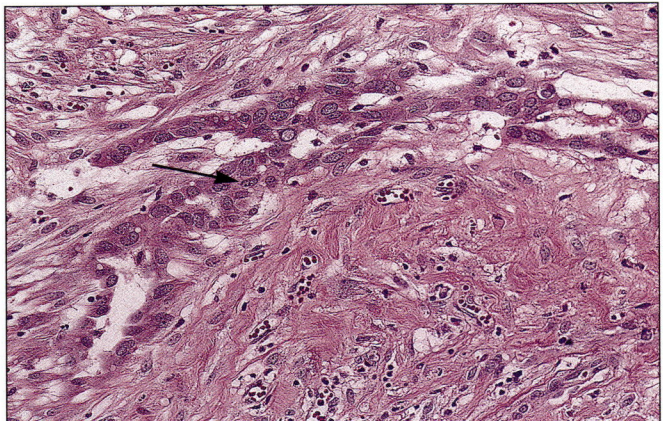

Figure 31.6 Reactive mesothelium. The enlarged mesothelial cells (arrow) that cover a focus of fibrous reaction superficially resemble metastatic adenocarcinoma.

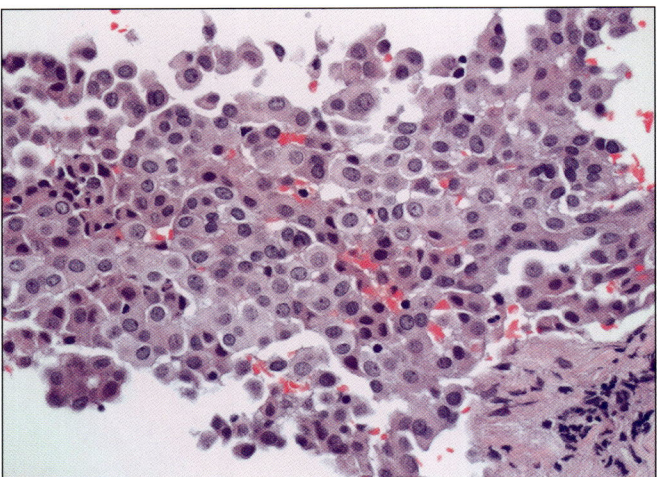

Figure 31.7 Markedly reactive mesothelial cells with prominent nucleoli.

However, clusters of mesothelial cells are easily mistaken for metastatic carcinoma. This is true especially when mesothelial cells extensively involve sinusoids in pelvic lymph nodes either as small papillary clusters or as sheets of somewhat discohesive cells.[36] Exuberant surface proliferations, sometimes forming sessile or polypoid nodules, can also simulate mesothelioma, a problem also encountered in the walls of hernia sacs. A useful morphologic feature that can help distinguish reactive mesothelial cell aggregates from metastatic carcinoma is their orientation at low-power magnification to one another (often in a line that can be traced for some considerable distance) (Figure 31.6) and their relation to the position of the original peritoneal surface (as demonstrated by the presence of the peritoneal elastic lamina).[37]

Organization of surface proliferative lesions and inflammatory exudates may leave adhesions of variable density, ranging from delicate strands of loose connective tissue to broad bands of dense, well-vascularized collagenous fibrous tissue. Entrapped inflammatory exudate within granulation tissue and proliferating sheets of mesothelial cells may lead to mesothelial (peritoneal) cyst formation. These may not become clinically apparent until months or years after the precipitating event.

Mesothelial hyperplasia must be distinguished from malignant peritoneal mesothelioma. The presence of necrosis, marked nuclear pleomorphism, and deep infiltration favors malignant mesothelioma.[38] Immunostains may help in the differential diagnosis. Strong immunoreactivities for p53[39] and epithelial membrane antigen (EMA; nuclear and cytoplasmic, respectively) are characteristic of the cells of malignant mesothelioma but not reactive mesothelial cells; in contrast, hyperplasic mesothelial cells are usually desmin positive.[40] Proliferative markers such as Ki-67 may also be helpful (approximately 25% vs 5% labeling index for malignant mesothelioma vs mesothelial hyperplasia, respectively).[41] In some cases, however, the distinction between a reactive and malignant mesothelial lesion may be difficult or impossible, particularly in a biopsy samples. An apparently benign mesothelial proliferation occasionally precedes the appearance of a malignant peritoneal mesothelioma.[38,42]

Mesothelial hyperplasia should also be distinguished from a borderline serous tumor of primary peritoneal origin. Grossly visible tumor, columnar cells with or without cilia, the presence of neutral mucin, and numerous psammoma bodies all favor a serous tumor. Immunohistochemical markers for epithelial differentiation may also be useful in the distinction (see Chapter 25).

PERITONEAL INCLUSION CYSTS

Peritoneal inclusion cysts are unilocular or multilocular mesothelial-lined lesions that occur almost exclusively in women in the reproductive age group. They usually involve the pelvis, although may occur in other abdominal locations, including the omentum and mesentery, and are frequently associated with prior abdominal surgery.[43] The origin of peritoneal inclusion cysts remains controversial; some authors consider them reactive lesions that develop in response to injury, whereas others favor their neoplastic nature.

Unilocular peritoneal inclusion cysts are usually incidental findings at laparotomy. Multilocular peritoneal inclusion cysts, also referred to as 'benign cystic mesotheliomas,' frequently form large bulky masses (Figures 31.8–31.11) simulating a cystic ovarian tumor. Cysts are thin walled, contain clear proteinaceous fluid, and are lined by a single layer of flat to cuboidal, hobnail-shaped, mesothelial cells (Figure 31.12) with bland nuclear features, although a degree of reactive atypia is occasionally seen. Tubal and squamous metaplasia of the mesothelial lining sometimes occurs. Inflammatory infiltrates, if present at all, are limited to sparse lymphocytic collections. The mesothelial cells are typically immunoreactive for calretinin, and less frequently positive for estrogen (ERs) or progesterone receptors (PRs), or both.[44]

In patients who have had peritonitis, fibrinous adhesions that are superficial to the deeper lining of normal mesothelium may develop and the underlying serosa can be mistaken for invasive serous carcinoma until attention is paid to its regularity and benign histology (Figure 31.13).

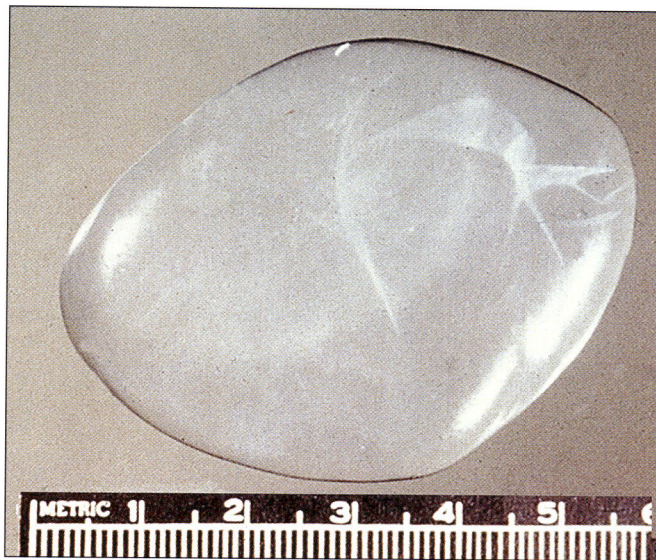

Figure 31.8 Mesothelial cyst.

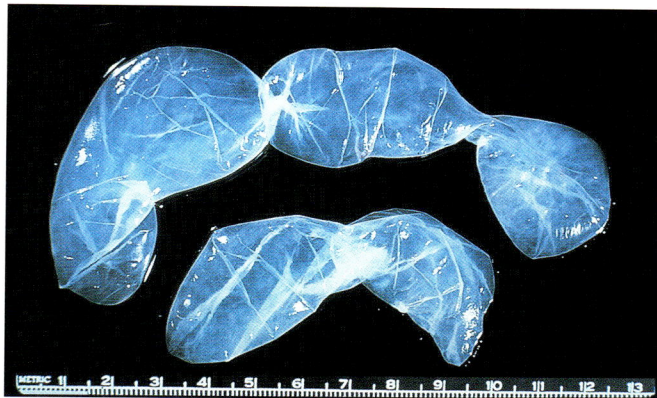

Figure 31.10 Multiple large mesothelial cysts.

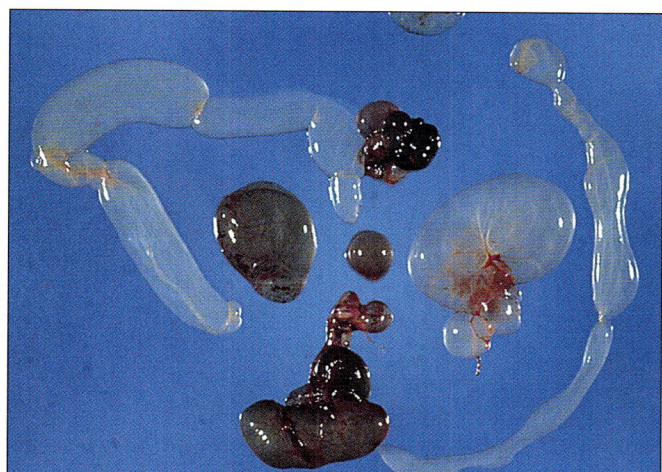

Figure 31.9 Multiple small mesothelial cysts.

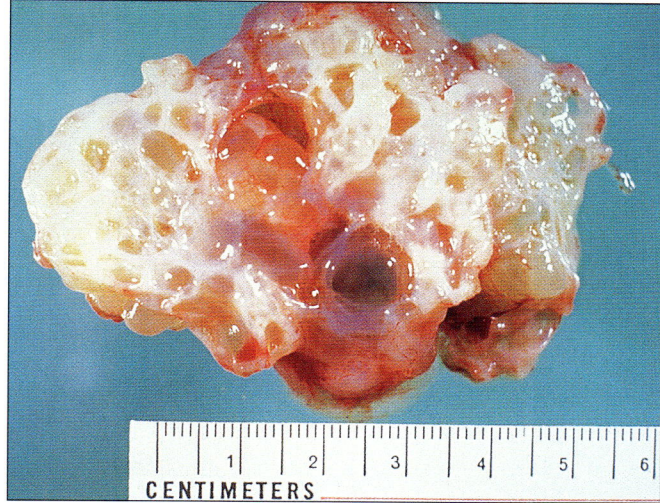

Figure 31.11 Multicystic mesothelioma.

Peritoneal inclusion cysts are confused with multilocular cystic lymphangiomas, which typically occur in children, more often in boys. Lymphangiomas are almost always localized in the mesentery of the small intestine, mesocolon, omentum, or retroperitoneum. They contain chylous material and, microscopically, show intramural lymphoid aggregates and smooth muscle, which are absent in peritoneal inclusion cysts.

Although no malignant behavior has been reported in peritoneal inclusion cysts, recurrence occurs in approximately one-half of cases from months to several years postoperatively.[45] GnRH agonists or tamoxifen have successfully been applied to some patients.[44]

OVARIAN REMNANT SYNDROME

This condition exists if a patient who has had a 'total bilateral oophorectomy' later develops a palpable mass or experiences pelvic pain or other symptoms referable to ovarian tissue that has been left behind (Figures 31.14 and 31.15). This condition is described more fully in Chapter 24.

SUPERNUMERARY OR ACCESSORY OVARIES

Supernumerary ovaries are ectopic ovaries located at some distance from the eutopic ovary. It is rare but occasional cases have been reported in the peritoneal cavity.[46] This condition is described more fully in Chapter 23.

SPLENOSIS

Nodules of splenic tissue, usually less than 1 cm in diameter, are randomly distributed in the peritoneal cavity. The etiology is trauma, most commonly a motor vehicle accident, which has resulted in splenic rupture.[47] Splenosis is generally asymptomatic but may cause abdominal or pelvic pain simulating endometriosis, or produce intestinal obstruction due to the development of adhesions. Splenosis may be encountered as an incidental finding or mistakenly interpreted as endometriosis, benign or malignant vascular tumors, or metastatic cancer.[48–50]

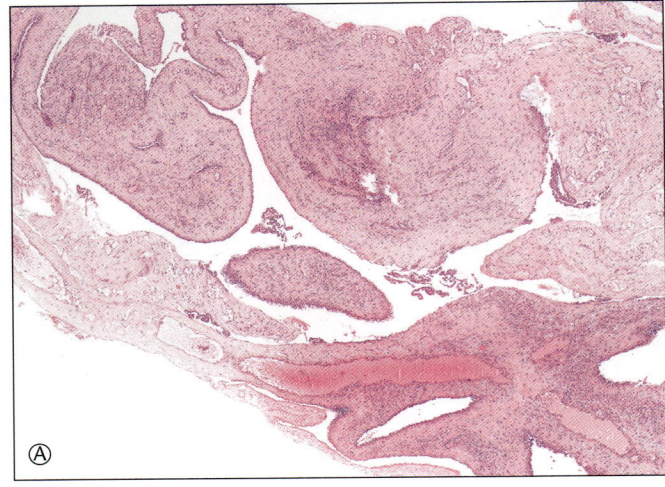

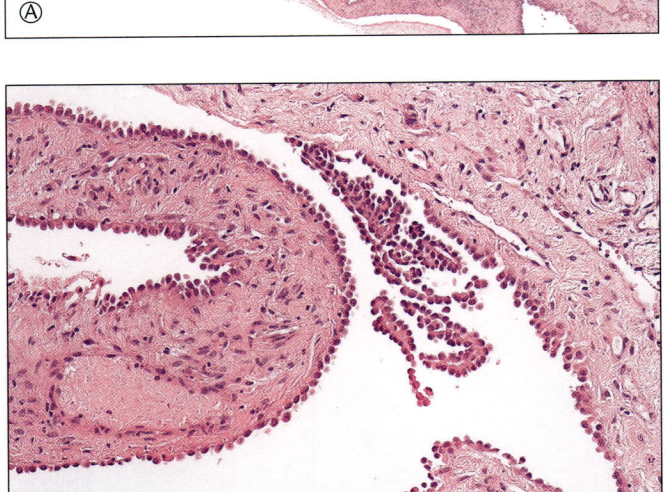

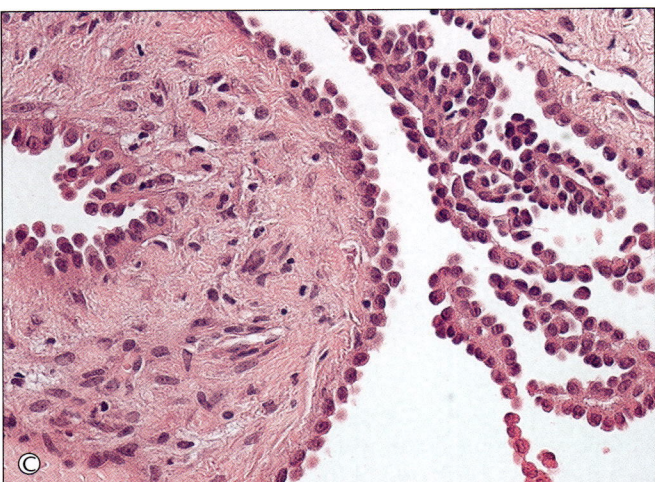

Figure 31.12 **(A)** Thin-walled mesothelial cysts in peritoneum. **(B)** The cyst is lined by numerous mesothelial cells. **(C)** Detail of the mesothelial cells.

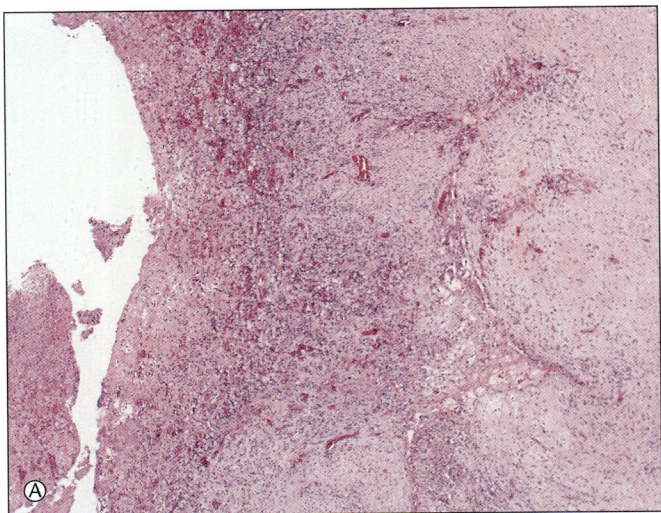

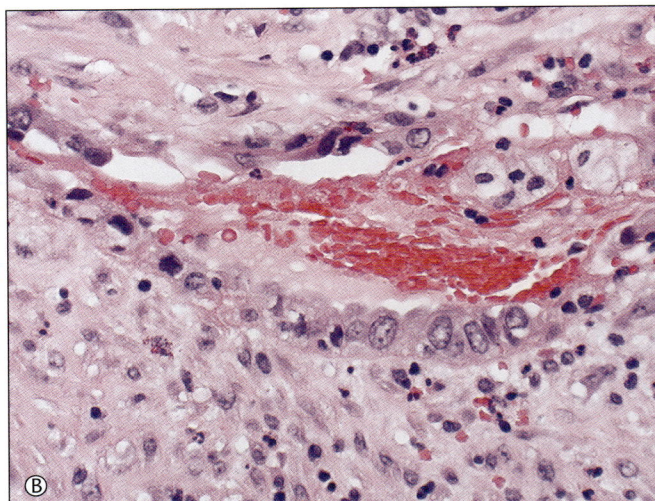

Figure 31.13 **(A)** Serosa covered by adhesions. It is easy to mistake the normal mesothelium for serous adenocarcinoma due to its location within the peritoneal wall. **(B)** Detail of mesothelial inclusion.

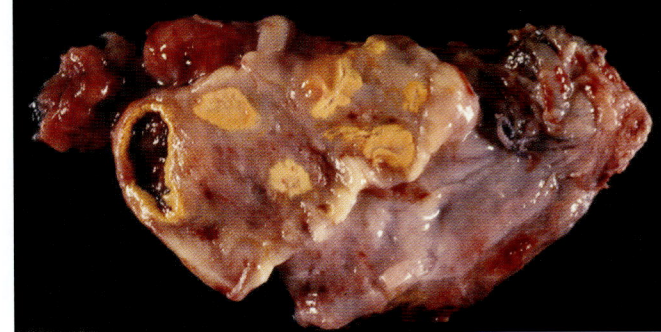

Figure 31.14 Ovarian remnant syndrome. Numerous corpora lutea appear surrounded by fibrous tissue.

CHAPTER 31 — THE PERITONEUM   723

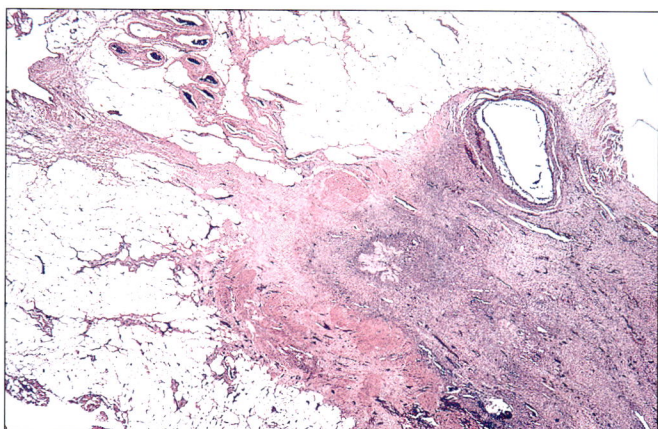

Figure 31.15 Ovarian remnant syndrome. Ovarian tissue that was left behind at the time of oophorectomy has regrown and is functional.

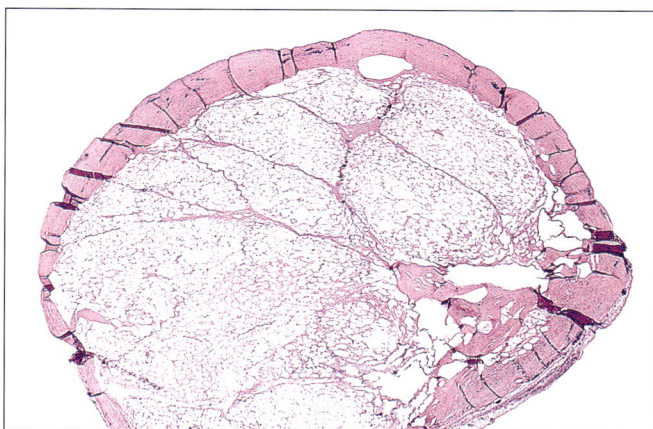

Figure 31.17 Infarcted appendix epiploica.

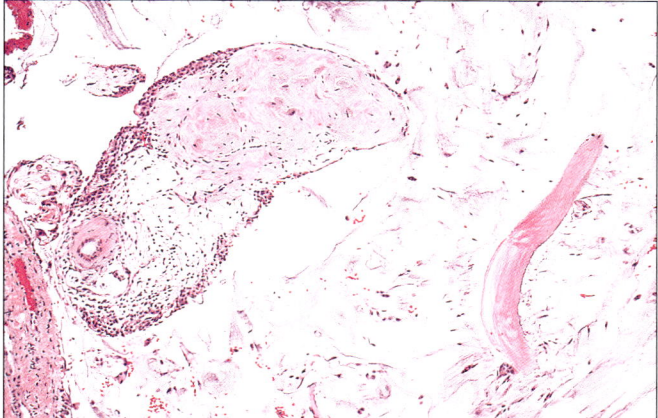

Figure 31.16 Trophoblastic implant in peritoneum. The patient had a ruptured ectopic pregnancy.

TROPHOBLASTIC IMPLANTS

Finding disseminated trophoblastic implants in the peritoneum is uncommon (Figure 31.16). They may occur on occasion with peritoneal pregnancy, or following laparoscopic treatment of tubal pregnancy, where the frequency has been estimated at 3.6%.[51,52] Viability is suggested by rising human chorionic gonadotropin concentrations following surgery. The condition is best avoided by meticulous inspection of the abdomen after resection of the tubal pregnancy. Microscopically, the implants may show trophoblastic tissue including chorionic villi. Some implants, however, may resemble a placental site nodule.

INFARCTED APPENDIX EPIPLOICA

Appendices epiploicae are small polypoid processes of adipose tissue that project from the serosa of the large intestine, especially the transverse and sigmoid colon. Occasionally, they undergo torsion, infarction, and later detachment and can be found lying free within the peritoneal cavity.[53,54] Typically in these cases, the center contains hyalinized fibrous tissue and often some residual adipose tissue that is mummified. The outer rim and variable portions of the core may calcify, resulting in a hard tumor-like mass (Figure 31.17).

MESOTHELIAL NEOPLASMS

ADENOMATOID TUMOR

Adenomatoid tumors are benign neoplasms of mesothelial origin, encountered most often in the fallopian tubes where frequently they are sieve like or multicystic. In contrast, they are also found subserosally in the uterine corpus near the fallopian tube, where they more usually simulate leiomyomas. They are seldom encountered elsewhere in the peritoneal cavity (see Chapter 21). Clinically, they are asymptomatic, and rarely recur after adequate excision. Grossly, adenomatoid tumors are usually solitary, less than 2 cm in diameter and have a white-gray appearance. Microscopically, multiple small slit-like or ovoid spaces are lined by a single layer of cells. Nuclear atypia is absent or minimal, and mitotic figures are rarely seen.

WELL-DIFFERENTIATED PAPILLARY MESOTHELIOMA

A rare form of peritoneal mesothelioma is the well-differentiated papillary mesothelioma. Most patients are of reproductive age, although an occasional patient has been postmenopausal. Also encountered in males, less common sites include the tunica vaginalis testis, pericardium, and pleura. These tumors are typically asymptomatic and often found incidentally at operation. Grossly, they are usually multiple, broad-based, wart-like excrescences that are polypoid or slightly nodular. Color and texture are similar to ovarian cortical tissue but sometimes firmer. They are generally small, usually measuring less than 2 cm in diameter.[55] An occasional tumor is solitary.[55]

On microscopic examination, the neoplasm consists of relatively thick papillae composed of dense fibrous or hyalinized tissue covered by a single layer of cytologically benign, small flattened to cuboidal cells (Figure 31.18).

Nuclei are bland, with a low nuclear grade (Figure 31.19). Mitoses are rare, usually under 1, but may be as high as 3, mitotic figures per 10 HPFs. The diagnosis should be made with caution, as malignant mesotheliomas may have foci that, viewed in isolation, resemble this tumor.[56] These lesions can usually be reliably distinguished from serous epithelial tumors, since the architecture of the latter discloses feathery irregular clusters of cells in which the nuclei are far more atypical and higher grade. Psammoma bodies may be encountered in rare cases. These tumors are nearly always benign, but rare tumors have acted aggressively.[57,58]

DIFFUSE MALIGNANT MESOTHELIOMA

Peritoneal diffuse malignant mesotheliomas are much less common than their pleural counterparts, accounting for about 10% of all malignant mesotheliomas.[59] Only one-third of these tumors occur in middle-aged or postmenopausal women and they must be distinguished from the more prevalent serous adenocarcinomas, including those arising from the peritoneum itself and those metastatic from an ovarian or fallopian tube primary. The survival rate for women with malignant mesothelioma is worse than that for women with serous adenocarcinoma, and the treatment of the two diseases currently differs.

Clinical manifestations usually are nonspecific and include ascites, abdominal discomfort, digestive disturbances, and weight loss. Ascites is present in most cases, and cytologic examination of the ascitic fluid may be diagnostic in some cases. The diagnosis, however, usually requires laparotomy or laparoscopy and biopsy. While most malignant mesotheliomas are highly aggressive, some peritoneal malignant mesotheliomas pursue a more indolent course.[60] It is generally stated in the literature that asbestos exposure is uncommon in women with peritoneal mesothelioma. In one (2003) population-based study of peritoneal malignant mesotheliomas, 29% of 96 men had asbestos-related jobs whereas none of 113 women had occupational or environmental risk factors.[61] In fact, men with peritoneal mesotheliomas typically have had a heavier burden and more prolonged exposure to asbestos than men with pleural mesotheliomas. Most males with peritoneal malignant mesotheliomas reported in the literature survived less than 2 years after diagnosis, although there have been occasional long-term survivors. A study of peritoneal malignant mesotheliomas in women,[60] however, found that 40% of the patients survived longer than 4 years. The histopathologic subtype (see later) is of prognostic significance, as biphasic peritoneal malignant mesotheliomas are associated with a much shorter survival than pure epithelial tumors[62] and deciduoid mesotheliomas are usually rapidly fatal.[63,64] Increasing nuclear and nucleolar size has been shown to correlate with shorter survival in epithelial tumors.[62] Also, p16 loss independently correlates with increased risk of death according to one study,[65] while another failed to identify any morphologic features that differentiated those cases with a highly aggressive course from indolent ones.[66] Two studies have identified a number of favorable prognostic factors including an age less than 60 years, low nuclear grade, low mitotic index, minimal residual disease after cytoreduction, and lack of deep invasion.[67,68]

Pathology

Tumors may extensively involve and diffusely thicken the peritoneum and the serosa of the various abdominal and pelvic organs and typically consist of multiple nodules measuring less than 1.5 cm in greatest dimension. Some tumors incite a striking desmoplastic reaction. On microscopic examination, most tumors have only an epithelial component, which usually has a tubulopapillary to focally solid pattern. The epithelial variant of malignant mesothelioma has polygonal or cuboidal cells with moderately abundant eosinophilic cytoplasm (Figures 31.20 and 31.21). The tumor cells usually resemble mesothelial cells, with a more or less constant nuclear:cytoplasmic ratio and only mild to moderate nuclear atypia (Figures 31.22–31.24); in some cases, however, the nuclei become larger and more bizarre as the cytoplasmic volume increases.[69] Mitotic figures usually

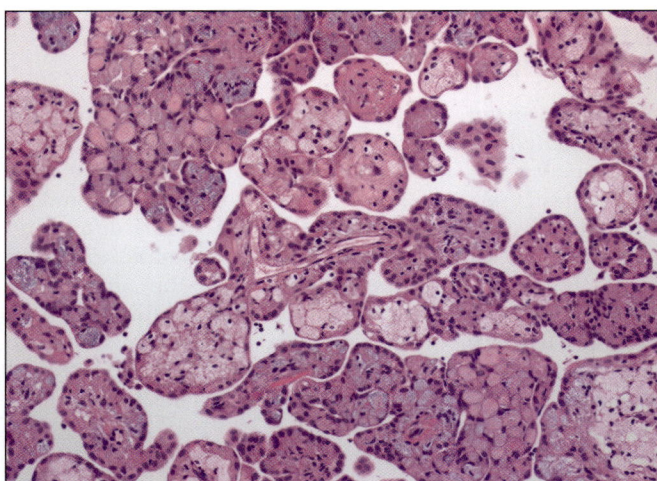

Figure 31.18 Well-differentiated peritoneal mesothelioma.

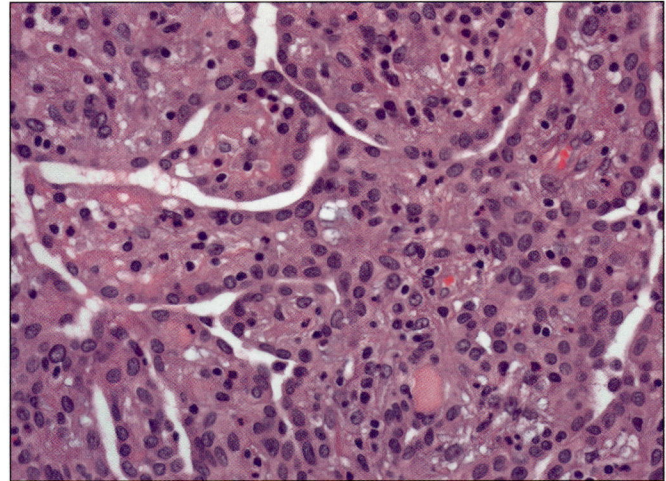

Figure 31.19 Detail of well-differentiated peritoneal mesothelioma.

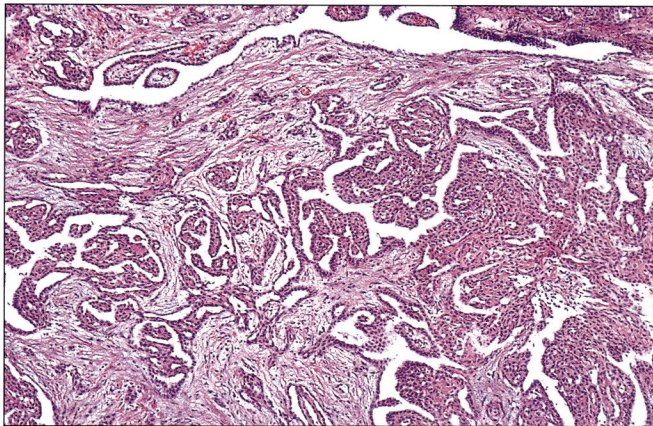

Figure 31.20 Diffuse malignant mesothelioma.

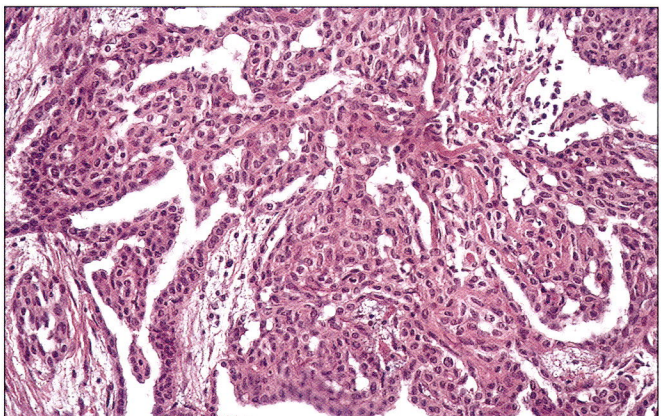

Figure 31.21 Diffuse malignant mesothelioma, detail.

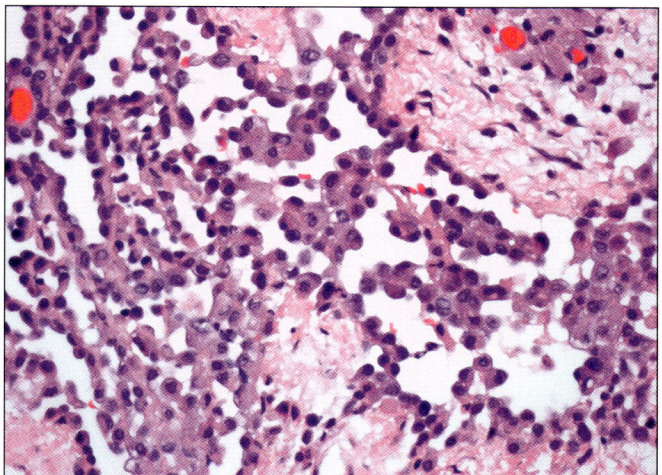

Figure 31.22 Diffuse malignant mesothelioma. Individual cells have central oval–round uniform nuclei and abundant eosinophilic cytoplasm.

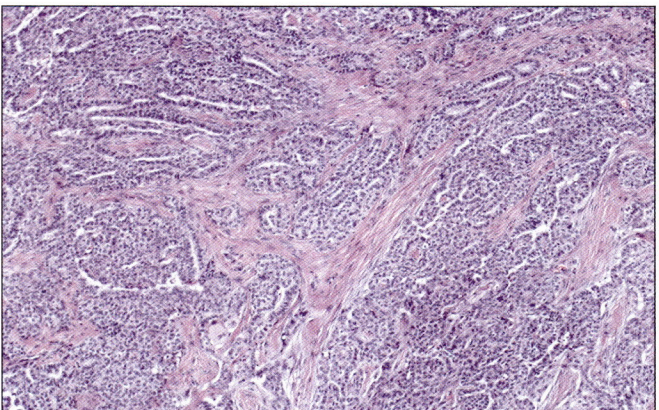

Figure 31.23 Diffuse malignant mesothelioma in which the regular-sized cells are arranged in glandular and tubular structures.

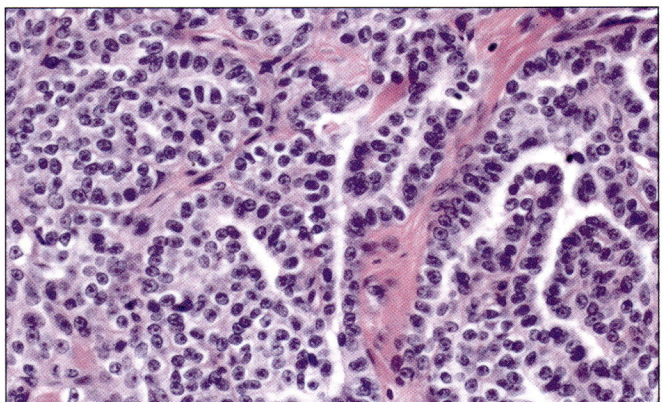

Figure 31.24 Diffuse malignant mesothelioma in which the cells display a more or less constant nuclear:cytoplasmic ratio and only mild to moderate nuclear atypia.

are present but are not numerous. In rare cases, the cytoplasm is abundant, amphophilic, and glassy, mimicking an exuberant ectopic decidual reaction (so-called 'deciduoid mesothelioma') (Figure 31.25).[56,70] Psammoma bodies are found in approximately one-third of cases (Figure 31.26), but are usually less common than in serous tumors. Unlike pleural mesotheliomas, sarcomatoid or fibrous variants are extremely rare.[56,60,68,71] Intra-abdominal lymph nodes may be involved.

Differential Diagnosis

The two types of lesions that are most difficult to distinguish from diffuse malignant mesothelioma are florid mesothelial hyperplasia and serous adenocarcinoma, whether the latter is primary in the peritoneum or metastatic from the ovary or another site. In contrast to hyperplasia, malignant mesothelioma often has grossly visible nodules, necrosis, and conspicuous large cytoplasmic vacuoles, and may have severe nuclear pleomorphism. Destructive tissue invasion should be sought as an important indicator of malignancy. Reactive mesothelial cells generally have smaller nuclei than those of malignant mesothelioma.

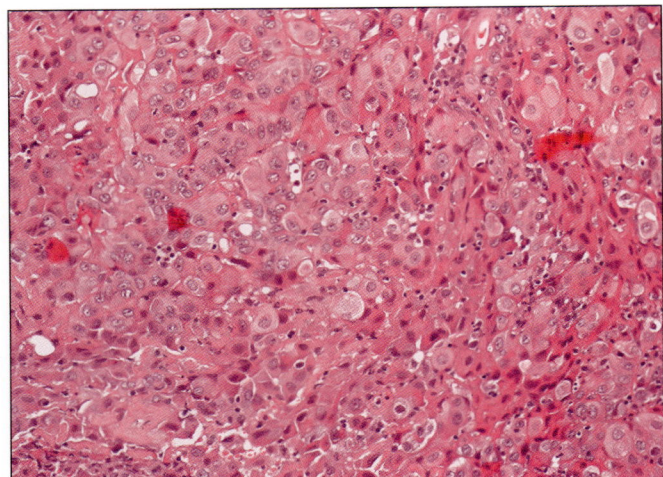

Figure 31.25 Diffuse malignant mesothelioma in which the tumor cells exhibit abundant, amphophilic cytoplasm mimicking an ectopic decidual reaction (so-called 'deciduoid mesothelioma').

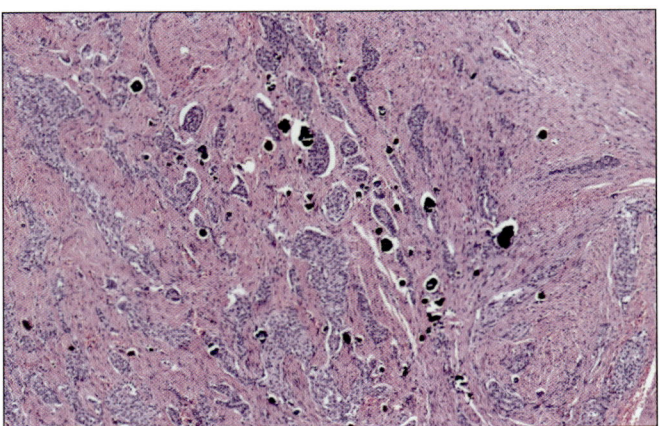

Figure 31.26 Diffuse malignant mesothelioma with numerous psammoma bodies.

Table 31.1 Malignant Mesothelioma versus Serous Carcinoma: Differential Diagnosis

Feature	Malignant Mesothelioma	Serous Carcinoma
Clinical		
History of asbestos exposure	Often positive	None
Diffuse peritoneal tumor mass	Yes	Usually dominant ovarian
Responsive to therapy	Rapidly fatal and unresponsive	Some respond
Histologic		
Sarcomatoid and adenomatoid foci	Present	Absent
Columnar cells	Rare	Numerous
Psammoma bodies	Rare	Often present
Nuclei	Round	Oval or elongate
Mucins (scanty)	Cytoplasmic acid mucin	Apical neutral mucin
Ultrastructural		
Microvilli	Abundant	Usually sparse
Cilia	Never numerous	Often numerous
Intracytoplasmic lumina	Common	Uncommon
Apical 'snouts'	Rare	Common

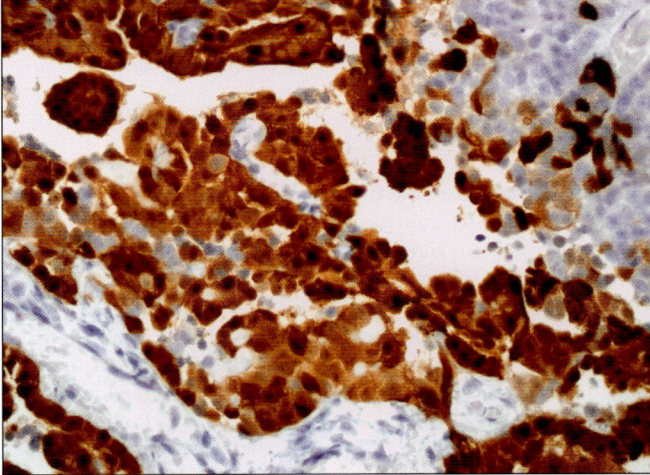

Figure 31.27 Diffuse malignant mesothelioma, calretinin immunoreaction.

The diagnosis that results in substantially differing treatment plans is the high-grade serous adenocarcinoma. Psammocarcinoma and low-grade serous carcinoma with abundant psammoma bodies are readily distinguished from mesothelioma, in which psammoma bodies are few when they are present. Mesothelial cells tend to be uniform, polygonal, and have moderate to extensive amounts of eosinophilic cytoplasm. Adenocarcinomas, in contrast, tend to have columnar cells, occasional cells with bizarre nuclear features, and variable numbers of psammoma bodies. Complicating the distinction, it is now recognized that malignant mesotheliomas can on rare occasion arise within the ovary[72] (Table 31.1).

Immunohistochemistry is important in establishing the proper diagnosis.[73-76] Differential immunoreactivities for mesothelioma and serous carcinoma are shown in Table 31.2. Calretinin, a 29 kDa calcium-binding protein, is present in nearly all epithelial mesotheliomas (Figure 31.27), but rarely in adenocarcinomas.[77] Both mesothelioma and adenocarcinoma are immunoreactive for low molecular weight cytokeratins. Cytokeratin (CK) 5/6 is usually expressed by mesotheliomas, but seldom by adenocarcinomas. Vimentin and desmin are commonly detected in mesotheliomas. Once, it was believed that vimentin expression favored a diagnosis of mesothelioma, but it is

Table 31.2 Immunohistochemical Panel to Differentiate Mesothelioma from Serous Carcinoma[a]

	Percentage Positive	
	Mesothelioma	Serous Carcinoma
h-Caldesmon	>90%	5%
Calretinin	>90%	10%[b]
CK panel (AE1/AE3 and CAM 5.2)	>90%	100%
CK5/6	>90%	25%[b]
D2-40	>90%	20%
EMA	>80%	100%
Thrombomodulin	50–75%	5%[b]
Desmin	40%	Negative
Vimentin	25%	35%
CA125	15–30%	95%
MOC-31	5%[b]	95%
S-100	0–10%	33–85%
Ber-EP4	0–10%[b]	100%
Leu-M1 (CD15)	0–10%	65%
Carcinoembryonic antigen (CEA)	>5%	15%
Placental-like alkaline phosphatase (PLAP)	>5%	65%
B72.3	>5%	85%
CA19.9	>5%	67%
ER	>5%	95%
PR	>5%	65%

Note: Mesothelial cells showing reactive atypia show an identical immunophenotype to malignant mesothelioma (with the exception of EMA immunoreactivity).
[a]The percentages for serous carcinoma of ovary and serous carcinoma primary in the peritoneum are essentially identical.
[b]Trace to focally positive.

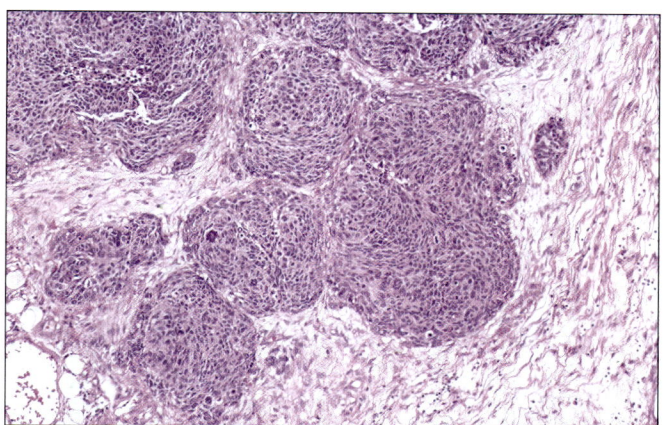

Figure 31.28 Desmoplastic small, round cell tumor. Nests of 'small, blue cells' embedded in a desmoplastic fibrous stroma.

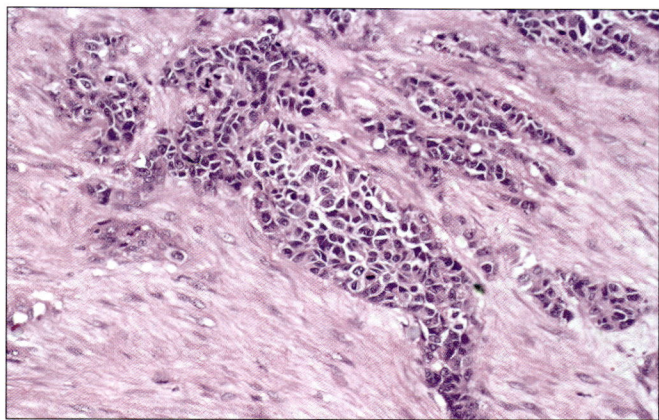

Figure 31.29 Desmoplastic small, round cell tumor. The tumor cells are uniform with scanty cytoplasm and indistinct cell borders.

now known that this intermediate filament is seen in normal and neoplastic cells of both epithelial and mesenchymal origin. Moreover, keratins and vimentin are commonly coexpressed by adenocarcinomas of müllerian type. CA125, an antigen initially identified in cell lines of ovarian serous adenocarcinomas, can be expressed by mesotheliomas. Thus, no single immunohistochemical stain is diagnostic in the separation of peritoneal malignant mesothelioma from adenocarcinoma, and a panel of antibodies should be interpreted in conjunction with the H&E and mucin stains.

MISCELLANEOUS PRIMARY TUMORS

INTRA-ABDOMINAL DESMOPLASTIC, SMALL ROUND CELL TUMOR

Desmoplastic small, round cell tumor is the descriptive designation for a rare, undifferentiated, and highly aggressive tumor that, with few exceptions, involves the peritoneal serosa[78] and contiguous organs such as the kidney and ovary.[79] It usually appears during adolescence and early adulthood, with a mean age of 25 years, but occasionally may be found in older women.[80,81] It is far more common in men than in women. The prognosis is poor.

Grossly, most tumors are bulky abdominal masses that have spread diffusely over the peritoneal surface with prominent involvement of the tunica vaginalis or the ovaries, mimicking a primary testicular or ovarian tumor.[82] The characteristic microscopic pattern is nests of 'small, blue cells' embedded in a desmoplastic fibrous stroma (Figure 31.28). The tumor cells are uniform with scanty cytoplasm and indistinct cell borders (Figure 31.29). About one-third of tumors exhibit a wider range of morphologic features, principally as spindle-shaped cells with epithelioid to focally sarcomatoid arrangements. Mitotic figures are numerous and foci of necrosis are usually present. Invasion of vascular spaces is common but lymph node involvement is rare.

Virtually all tumors are CK positive (CK monoclonal antibodies CAM 5.2, AE1/AE3), but lack CK20 expression, indicative that they are not of large intestinal origin.[66,83,84] Roughly four-fifths are also reactive with antibodies to EMA, neuron-specific enolase, desmin (with paranuclear dot-like

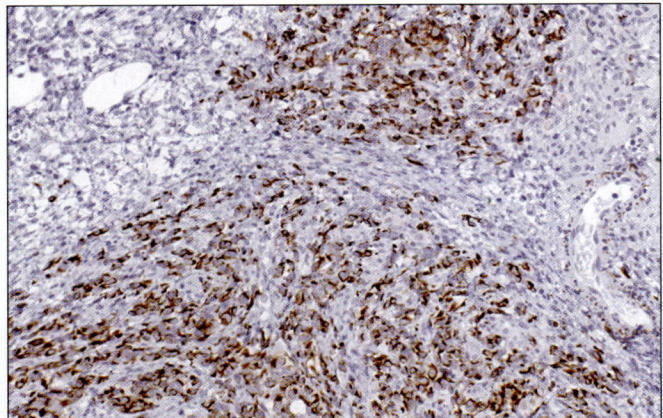

Figure 31.30 Desmoplastic small, round cell tumor. Desmin immunoreaction.

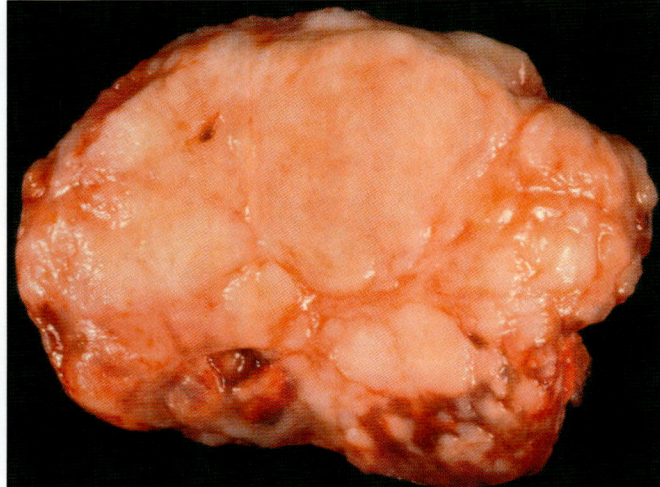

Figure 31.31 Solitary benign fibrous mesothelioma ('solitary fibrous tumor'). The cut surface appears multinodular and fleshy.

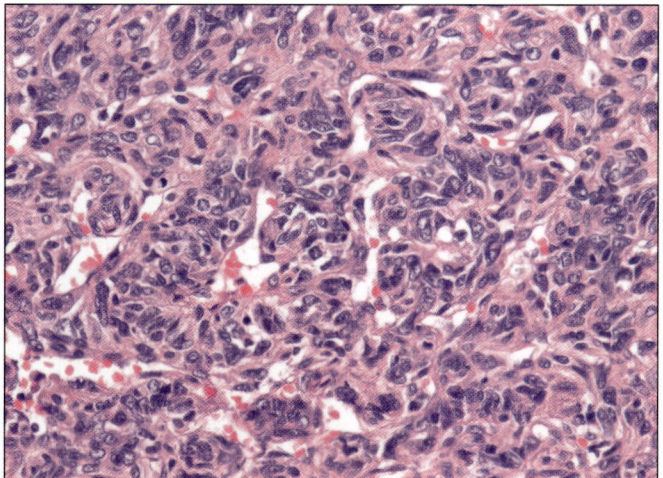

Figure 31.32 Solitary benign fibrous mesothelioma ('solitary fibrous tumor'). The tumor is composed of spindle cells arranged in a hemangiopericytoma-like pattern.

reactivity) (Figure 31.30), and vimentin, suggestive that there is both epithelial and mesenchymal (divergent) differentiation. Between two-fifths and two-thirds of tumors express Ber-EP4, CD57 (Leu-7), CD15 (Leu-M1), and CA125, suggestive that the tumor is not mesothelial in origin. Wilms' tumor (WT1) protein is detected immunohistochemically in 90% of cases.[85] Most other common immunohistochemical stains lack reactivity in most cases. Electron microscopic examination shows the tumor cells have mesenchymal–fibroblastic features.

Coexpression of epithelial and mesenchymal antigens distinguishes the desmoplastic small, round cell tumor from other small round and blue cell tumors occurring in this age group. These antigenic properties have challenged the popular notion that the intra-abdominal desmoplastic small round cell tumor is a 'blastomatous' tumor derived exclusively from the primitive mesothelium.

Desmoplastic small round cell tumor exhibits a reciprocal translocation t(11;22)(p13;q12), resulting in fusion of the *EWS1* gene on chromosome 22 and the Wilms' tumor suppressor gene (*WT1*) on chromosome 11, which appears to be unique for this tumor.[86] The translocation results in a loss of three specific amino acids[87] and appears to have an oncogenic effect. Other translocation patterns have also been described.[86,88] The fusion protein that is produced seems to function as a potent activator of transcription, suggesting that the Wilms' tumor gene gains function as a result of the fusion. Thus, the fusion gene seems to function as a dominant oncogene in this disease.[89]

After initial treatment (aggressive surgical debulking and postoperative chemotherapy, external beam radiotherapy, or both), there may be an initial response, but more than 99% of patients die of tumor progression.

SOLITARY FIBROUS TUMOR OF PERITONEUM ('FIBROUS MESOTHELIOMA')

Solitary fibrous tumors, previously called 'fibrous mesotheliomas,' are primitive tumors composed of fibroblasts and primitive mesenchymal cells that can manifest multidirectional differentiation. They are rare tumors found most often in the pleura,[90] but do occur occasionally in the peritoneum.[91,92] Most patients remain well after tumor excision, although occasional neoplasms have acted aggressively.

Grossly, the tumors vary in size from 1 cm to over 20 cm in diameter (Figure 31.31). They are usually solitary and appear encapsulated by fibrous tissue. Microscopically, tumors are composed of spindle cells in a markedly collagenized stroma, often with abundant blood vessels, in a hemangiopericytoma-like pattern (Figure 31.32). Tumor cells may have fascicular, cord-like, and irregular arrangements and are found interspersed in strands in between thick collagen bundles. Nuclei are often vesicular and the nucleoli inconspicuous. Mitoses are rare.

Tumor cells are reactive for vimentin but not for CK. CD34, a sialylated transmembrane glycoprotein found initially in endothelial cells and myeloid progenitor cells, is usually demonstrable.[90] CD31, a platelet endothelial cell adhesion molecule, is not. In contrast, desmoplastic mesotheliomas, tumors in the differential diagnosis, are reactive for CK but not for CD34.[93]

INFLAMMATORY MYOFIBROBLASTIC TUMOR

This lesion has also been referred to as inflammatory pseudotumor[94] or plasma cell granuloma.[95] Most tumors arise in the lung, mesentery, omentum, or retroperitoneum. The abdominal lesions are usually found in the mesentery of patients younger than 20 years of age who present with a mass, fever, weight loss, anemia, thrombocytosis, and polyclonal hypergammaglobulinemia. Microscopic examination reveals myofibroblastic spindle cells, mature plasma cells, and small lymphocytes. The spindle cells often show positive cytoplasmic immunoreactivity for ALK-1, with associated chromosomal translocations detected in approximately 50% of cases. Inflammatory myofibroblastic tumors are regarded as neoplasms of low-grade or intermediate biologic behavior, which can be associated with favorable outcome, but have a tendency for local recurrence and a low risk of distant metastasis. ALK-negative tumors are more likely to be associated with metastases.[96]

OTHER TUMORS

A variety of tumors arise rarely in the peritoneum. Their histogenesis is not always certain. Of the less rare tumors, adenosarcomas are often associated with endometriosis.[97] Carcinosarcomas have also been described,[98] as have the stromal sarcomas[99] and rhabdomyosarcomas.[100] Pure epithelial tumors, such as clear cell adenocarcinoma, have been described, also in association with endometriosis.[97] Any tumor usually associated with an endometrial origin could well have arisen in extrauterine endometriosis. This subject is discussed more fully in Chapter 22.

METASTATIC TUMORS

PSEUDOMYXOMA PERITONEI

Pseudomyxoma peritonei is a clinical term that refers to the accumulation of jelly-like mucus in the pelvis or abdominal cavity ('gelatinous ascites') resulting from peritoneal spread of a low-grade mucinous tumor, usually of the appendix and less commonly of other intestinal locations.[101] Unilateral or bilateral ovarian involvement is common in these cases (Figure 31.33). The ovarian and appendiceal tumors may present simultaneously or metachronously.

Pathology

Pseudomyxoma peritonei is a disease of MUC2-expressing goblet cells, which secrete voluminous quantities of mucin in a ratio of mucin:cells exceeding 10:1.[102] During the operation, it is critical for the surgeon to inspect and remove the appendix. Usually, the appendix will be enlarged (Figure 31.34) or adherent to the omentum, but in some cases it appears grossly normal and the primary tumor is found only after a thorough histologic evaluation (Figure 31.35).

The mucinous deposits may have several histologic appearances.[103–106] The mucus may be acellular ('mucinous ascites') or may contain mucinous epithelial cells (Figure 31.36). The mucinous material often contains inflammatory cells, mesothelial cells, and, if present for some time, may display capillaries and fibroblasts indicating that organization has occurred. If epithelial cells are present, the degree of nuclear atypia (variously described as low grade or high grade, or alternatively as benign, borderline, or malignant) should be indicated in the report, as well as whether the mucin dissects into tissues with a fibrous response or is merely on the surface. The finding of occasional mitoses or lack of cytoplasmic mucin suggests that the tumor is of at least borderline malignancy. Alternatively, the presence of cribriform pattern or signet-ring cells warrant a diagnosis of adenocarcinoma.[103]

Patients in whom the tumor appears benign (Figures 31.37–31.39) or borderline (peritoneal 'adenomucinosis')[103] usually have a more favorable clinical course than those in whom the tumor appears histologically malignant (peritoneal carcinomatosis).[107,108] Nevertheless, the former tumors may lead to significant morbidity and mortality (10 year survival rate of 45%)[105] and their designation as low-grade mucinous carcinomas has recently been proposed.[103]

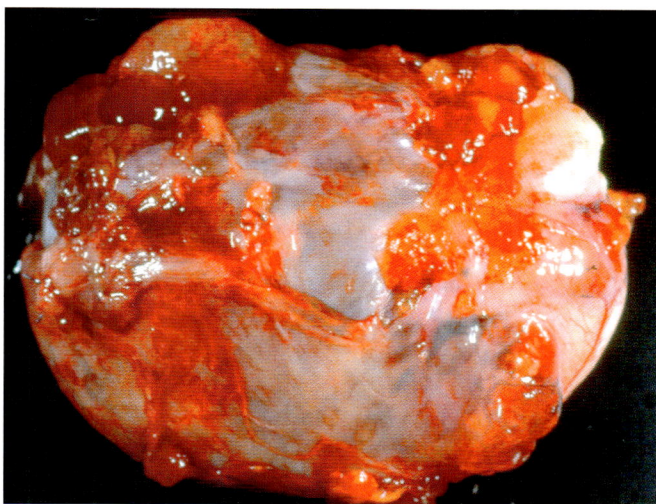

Figure 31.33 Mucinous cystic ovarian tumor associated with pseudomyxoma peritonei and a similar appendiceal tumor. Note the presence of mucin deposits on the surface of the cyst. (Reproduced with permission from Prat J. Pathology of the ovary. Philadelphia: Saunders; 2004. p. 83–109.)

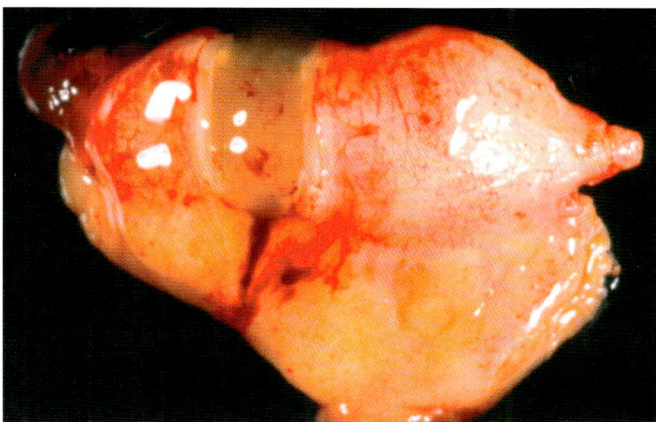

Figure 31.34 Mucinous appendiceal tumor (mucocele) associated with pseudomyxoma peritonei and bilateral ovarian mucinous tumors. (Reproduced with permission from Prat J. Pathology of the ovary. Philadelphia: Saunders; 2004. p. 83–109.)

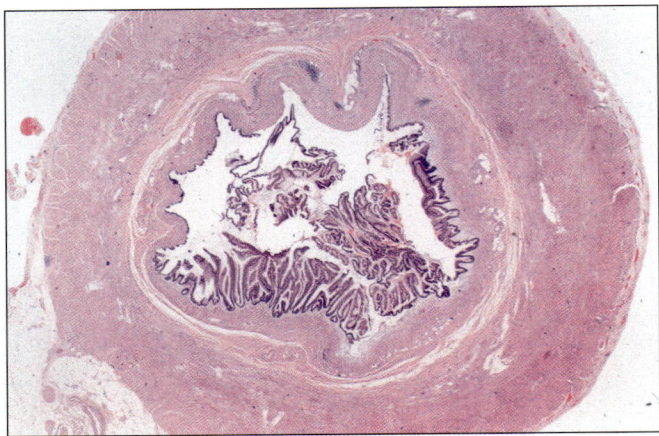

Figure 31.35 Mucinous appendiceal tumor associated with pseudomyxoma peritonei and bilateral ovarian mucinous tumors. (Reproduced with permission from Prat J. Ovarian tumors of borderline malignancy (tumors of low malignant potential): a critical appraisal. Adv Anat Pathol 1999;6:247–74.)

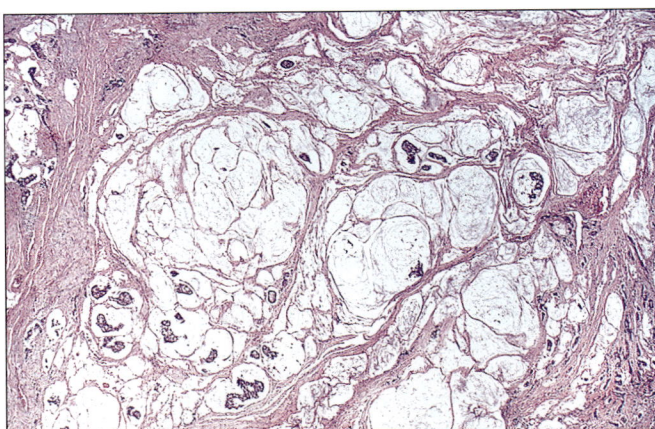

Figure 31.37 Pseudomyxoma peritonei. Multiple clusters and tumor cells are present in the mucinous material.

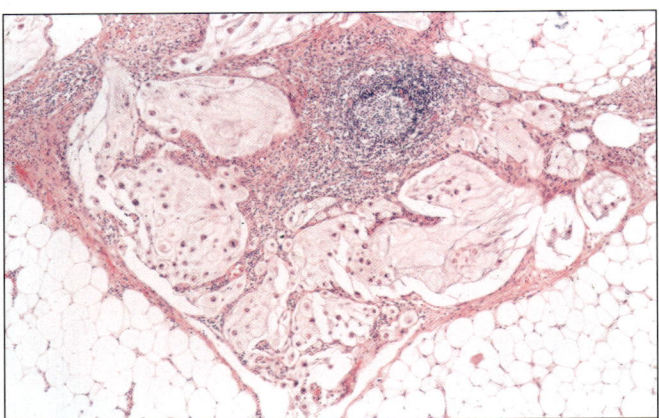

Figure 31.36 Pseudomyxoma peritonei associated with mucinous tumors of the appendix and ovaries. Note the presence of tumor cells floating in pools of mucin dissecting through the fat. (Reproduced with permission from Prat J. Pathology of the ovary. Philadelphia: Saunders; 2004. p. 83–109.)

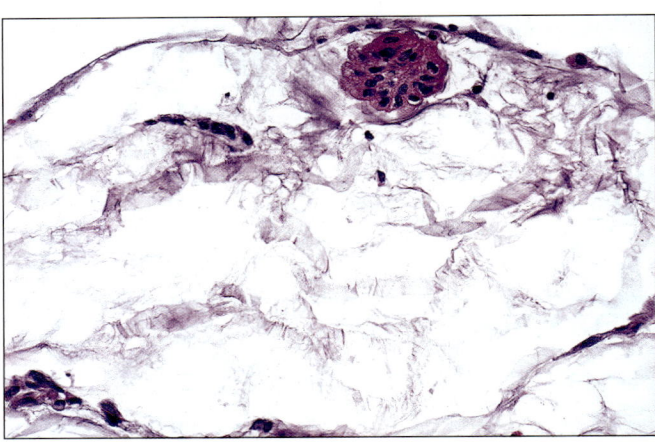

Figure 31.38 Pseudomyxoma peritonei, high magnification. Clusters of tumor cells are present in the mucin.

The secondary ovarian tumors are commonly bilateral and typically show surface involvement (Figure 31.40) and/or the presence of pools of mucin dissecting through the ovarian stroma (pseudomyxoma ovarii) (Figure 31.41). These features are in contrast to those of ovarian borderline tumors of intestinal type, which are usually unilateral and only occasionally associated with pseudomyxoma peritonei.[109–112]

Pathogenesis

The origin of pseudomyxoma peritonei has been a matter of debate.[106] Historically, most of these tumors were thought to be ovarian in origin, especially when the associated ovarian tumor was of large size or had the appearance of a mucinous borderline tumor. Over two decades ago[112] opinions began to shift toward the appendix as the site of origin in most cases. Based on genetic analyses, most cases are now believed to be of appendiceal origin,[113] and more

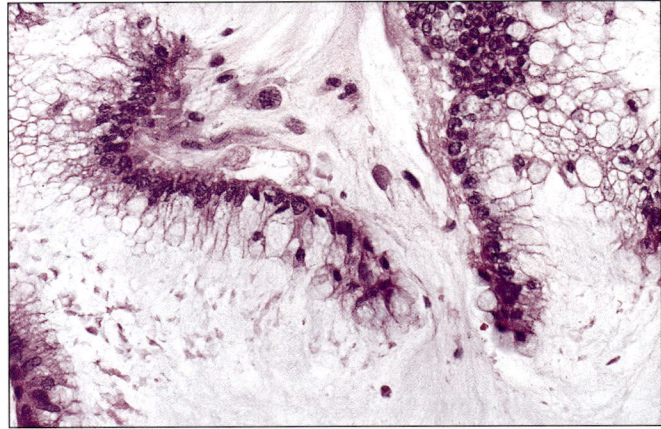

Figure 31.39 Clusters of intestinal-type epithelium in pseudomyxoma peritonei.

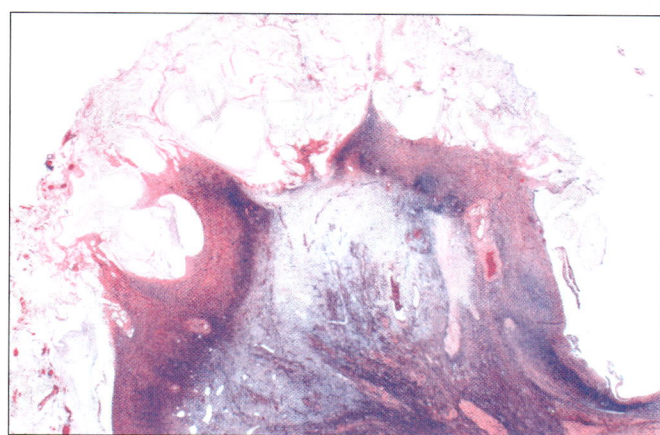

Figure 31.40 Mucinous ovarian tumor associated with a similar mucinous tumor of the appendix pseudomyxoma peritonei. Ovarian surface involvement. (Reproduced with permission from Prat J. Pathology of the ovary. Philadelphia: Saunders; 2004. p. 83–109.)

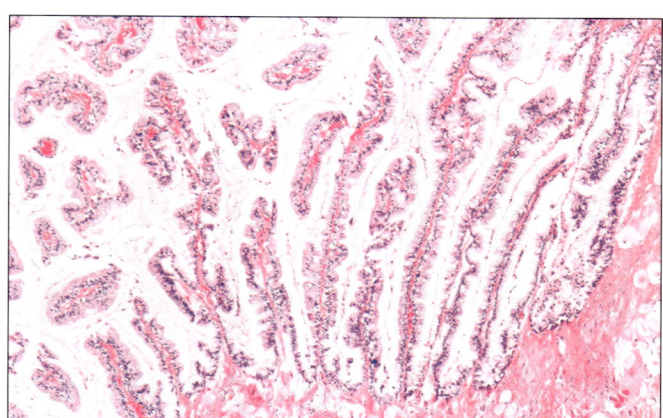

Figure 31.42 Mucinous ovarian tumor associated with pseudomyxoma peritonei and a similar appendiceal tumor. The tumor resembles a mucinous borderline tumor of the ovary. (Reproduced with permission from Cuatrecasas et al.)

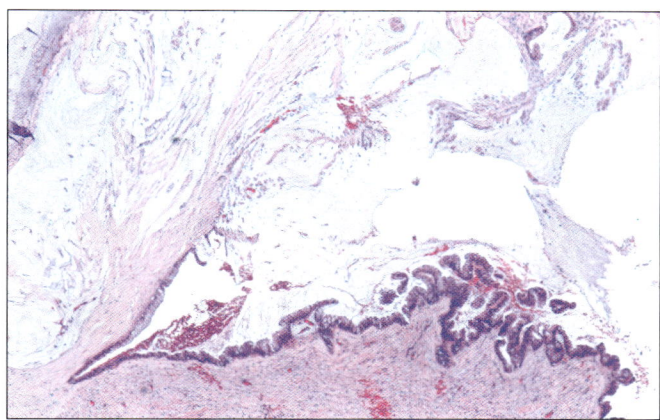

Figure 31.41 Mucinous ovarian tumor associated with mucinous tumor of the appendix and pseudomyxoma peritonei. Pools of mucin dissecting through the ovarian stroma (pseudomyxoma ovarii). (Reproduced with permission from Prat J. Pathology of the ovary. Philadelphia: Saunders; 2004. p. 83–109.)

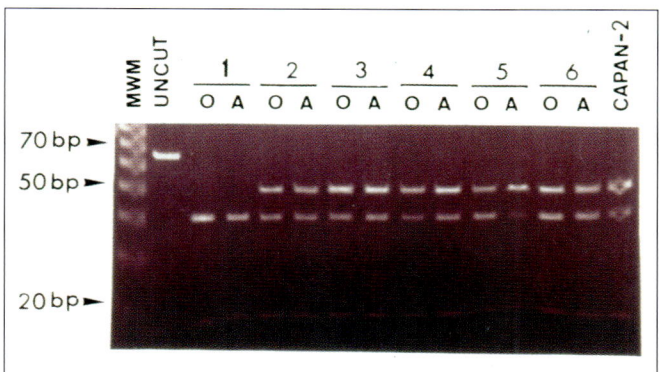

Figure 31.43 Mucinous ovarian tumors associated with mucinous tumors of the appendix and pseudomyxoma peritonei. Mutational pattern studied by RFLP-PCR. MWM, molecular weight marker, 10 bp DNA Ladder (Life Technologies Inc., Gaithersburg, MD); UNCUT, undigested 65 bp DNA amplified PCT product. Lane 15, CAPAN 2: positive control (CAPAN 2 cell line). Cases 1–6 are underlined. The mutational band (52 bp) for codon samples in five of the six cases (cases 2–6). The 40 bp fragment represents the normal allele. (Reproduced with permission from Cuatrecasas et al.)

specifically from goblet cells expressing MUC2.[114] A recent review has gone so far as to state, 'pseudomyxoma peritonei almost never results from a ruptured primary ovarian neoplasm, but often produces secondary borderline-like ovarian tumors'[109] (Figure 31.42). In an exceptional case, however, pseudomyxoma peritonei can arise from the rupture of a mucinous tumor of intestinal type that has arisen in ovarian teratomas.

Specific CK panels have been employed to distinguish ovarian mucinous tumors from gastrointestinal mucinous tumors. Tumors of müllerian origin are usually reactive for CK7 but not CK20, whereas tumors of lower intestinal origin have findings that generally are reversed, i.e., CK20 reactivity but generally not for CK7.[102,115–118] Most cases of pseudomyxoma peritonei show reaction patterns consistent with an appendiceal origin.[111,119]

Molecular genetic studies in synchronous ovarian and appendiceal tumors associated with pseudomyxoma peritonei have revealed a concordance of K-ras mutational pattern in both tumors in each patient (Figure 31.43).[113] These findings suggest their clonal nature and supports that, in the light of the clinicopathologic data, the appendix is the most likely origin.[113]

Prognosis and Treatment

Patients with pseudomyxoma peritonei containing epithelial cells that are benign or borderline appearing usually have a protracted clinical course. The 5 and 10 year survival rates are 75% and 68%, respectively. In contrast, when the epithelial cells of the pseudomyxoma peritonei appear malignant (peritoneal carcinomatosis), the clinical course is more aggressive and approximately 90% of patients die within 3 years. Cytoreductive surgery at initial presentation and repeated palliative debulking, mucolytic agents, chemotherapy and/or radiotherapy have done relatively little to modify the natural history of this disease.

GLIOMATOSIS PERITONEI

Gliomatosis peritonei is a rare condition in which peritoneal implants composed largely or exclusively of fully mature glial tissue are found in the abdominal cavity, usually in association with a solid ovarian teratoma,[120–122] which can be mature or immature.[123] Tears in the capsule of the ovarian tumor have been identified, suggesting a mechanism by which the gliomatous tissue leaks into the abdominal cavity (Figure 31.44). Nevertheless, a molecular genetic study has suggested that glial implants may also arise by metaplasia of pluripotent peritoneal stem cells.[124]

At the time of laparotomy, either when the ovarian tumor is discovered or subsequently, implants in the peritoneum are found to be composed of glial tissue only (Figures 31.44 and 31.45). Occasionally, other teratomatous elements are identified. Microscopic implants should be graded separately from the ovarian tumor, and this will determine whether subsequent therapy is needed. Usually, the implants are grade 0 or 1 (Figure 31.45). In some cases, they are grade 2 or 3. Although most patients with this condition do well, recurrences have been recorded[125] as well as subsequent malignant transformation.[126] This condition is described more fully in the section on ovarian teratomas in Chapter 29. Gliomatosis peritonei has also been reported in a patient with a ventriculoperitoneal shunt.[127]

STRUMOSIS PERITONEI

Strumosis peritonei is a rare condition in which nodules found singly or throughout the omentum are composed largely of well-differentiated thyroid tissue. The lesion most likely represents a metastatic or implanted form of malignant struma ovarii. Most cases occur in association with a solid ovarian teratoma or a struma ovarii. Nodules may be several millimeters to centimeters in size and grossly, on cut section, resemble colloid (Figure 31.46). Microscopically, the thyroid tissue may resemble a macrofollicular adenoma (Figure 31.47). Like gliomatosis peritonei, a defective

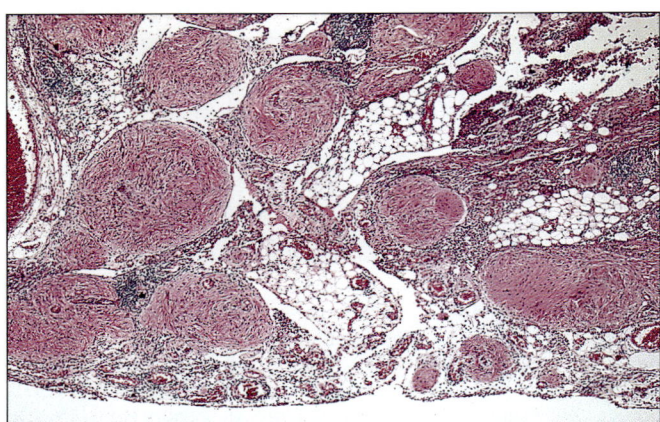

Figure 31.44 Gliomatosis peritonei. Multiple nodules of mature glial tissue are implanted within omental adipose tissue.

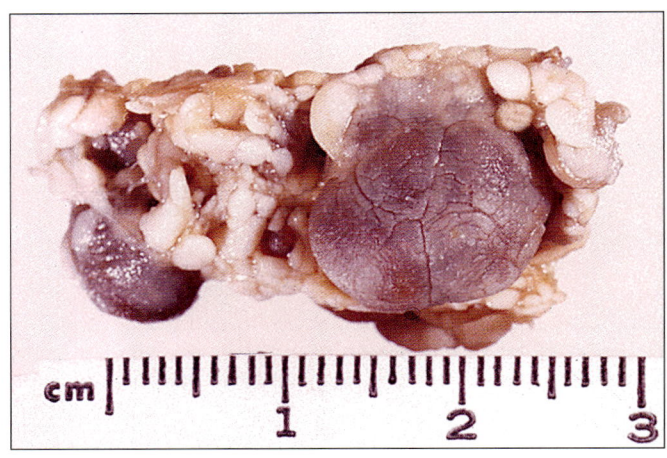

Figure 31.46 Strumosis peritonei.

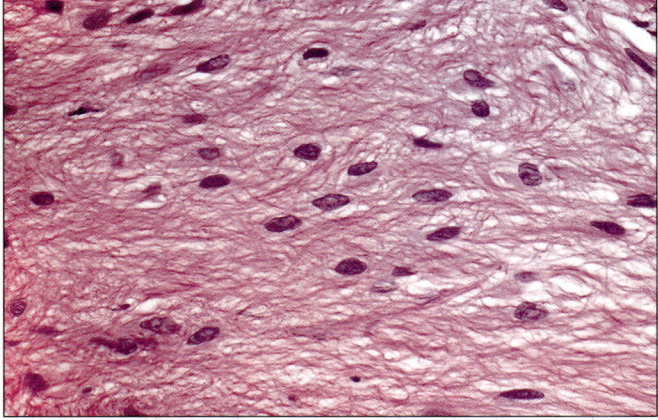

Figure 31.45 Gliomatosis peritonei. Uniform glial cells, all highly differentiated (grade 0), show an extensive neurofibrillary background.

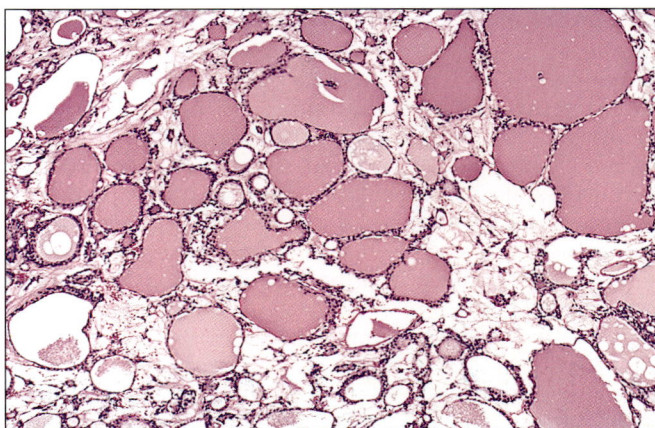

Figure 31.47 Strumosis peritonei with macrofollicular appearance.

capsule has been found in most cases with 'implants' from the ovary, suggesting a mechanism of spread into the abdominal cavity. While some patients with the condition do well, recurrence is unpredictable and some patients have had a clinically more aggressive course. This condition is described more fully on ovarian teratomas in Chapter 29.

LESIONS OF THE SECONDARY MÜLLERIAN SYSTEM

Lesions of the secondary müllerian system include those containing endometrioid, serous, and mucinous epithelium, simulating normal or neoplastic endometrial, tubal, and endocervical epithelium. Proliferation of the subjacent mesenchyme may accompany epithelial differentiation of the mesothelium or may give rise to a variety of pure mesenchymal lesions composed of endometrial stromal-type cells, decidua, or smooth muscle. Microscopically, these peritoneal lesions exhibit müllerian differentiation and share an origin from the so-called secondary müllerian system (Figure 31.48).[1] The müllerian potential of this layer is consistent with its close embryonic relation to the müllerian ducts, which arise by invagination of the celomic epithelium. The origin of many of these lesions, however, is not known with certainty, and other proposed histogenetic mechanisms are discussed in Chapter 22.

ENDOMETRIOSIS

Endometriosis is a disease principally involving the peritoneal cavity (see Chapter 22).

PERITONEAL SEROUS LESIONS

Serous lesions of the peritoneum include those that are non-neoplastic (endosalpingiosis) and neoplastic, which are morphologically analogous to their ovarian counterparts.

ENDOSALPINGIOSIS

Endosalpingiosis is the presence of benign glands lined by tubal-type epithelium involving the peritoneum, subperitoneal tissues, ovarian surface, and retroperitoneal lymph nodes. This disorder occurs almost exclusively in females, typically during their reproductive years, although occasional cases have been described in postmenopausal women. Endosalpingiosis is almost always an incidental finding at laparotomy and some cases accompany endometriosis in laparoscopic biopsies of women being investigated for infertility.[128]

An origin from the secondary müllerian system is favored by most investigators, but the association of endosalpingiosis with chronic salpingitis implicates implantation of sloughed tubal epithelium as a possible histogenetic mechanism in some cases.[129] Similarly, its association with serous borderline tumors suggests that some foci of endosalpingiosis may represent tumor implants that have undergone maturation.[130,131]

At the time of second-look laparotomy, endosalpingiosis in the absence of residual tumor does not justify additional treatment.[132]

Endosalpingiosis, if seen macroscopically, may appear as a focal granularity, with a single to few tiny bumps or cysts. Microscopically, it appears as multiple, simple glands, lined by a single layer of tubal-like epithelium (Figure 31.49) exhibiting pale ciliated cells, secretory cells, and intercalated or 'peg' cells; i.e., the three cell types of the normal epithelium of the fallopian tube. Nuclei are basally situated, mitotic activity is absent, and there is no nuclear atypia. Psammoma bodies are often present within the glandular lumens or in the surrounding stroma. If the epithelium is destroyed, the psammoma bodies may be found free in the stroma. The glands are surrounded by PAS-positive basement membranes and show PAS-positive, diastase-resistant material in their lumens. Immunoreactions for estrogen and progesterone receptors are usually positive.

The glands of endosalpingiosis may show irregular contours, crowding, and intraluminal stromal papillae.

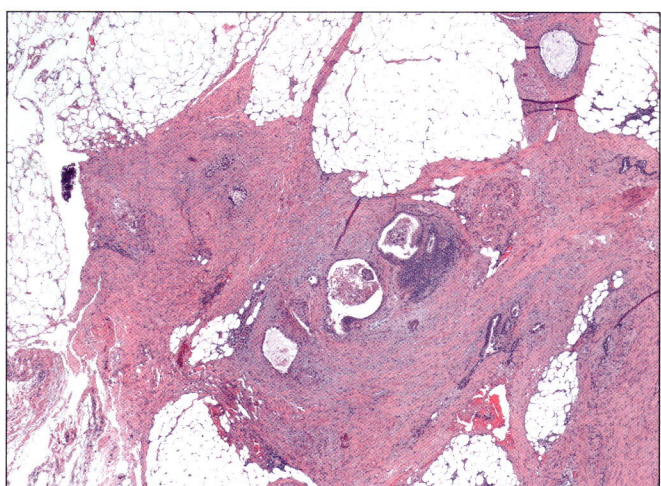

Figure 31.48 Müllerianosis. Numerous irregular müllerian glands surrounded by a prominent myofibroblastic reaction are seen in the omentum. The lesion resembles metastatic adenocarcinoma. The patient had bilateral mucinous müllerian (endocervical-type) borderline tumors of the ovary.

Table 31.3 Features Distinguishing Endosalpingiosis from Serous Borderline Tumor of the Peritoneum

	Endosalpingiosis	Serous Borderline Tumor (Primary and Implanted)
Location	Surface and subperitoneal	Surface and subperitoneal
Architecture	Simple round or oval gland	Simple glands, often with focal or complex papillary epithelial tufts, detached cell clusters, and psammoma bodies
Cytology	No atypia	Mild-to-severe atypia and often cellular stratification
Stromal reaction	None to focal hyalinization	None to exuberant desmoplasia

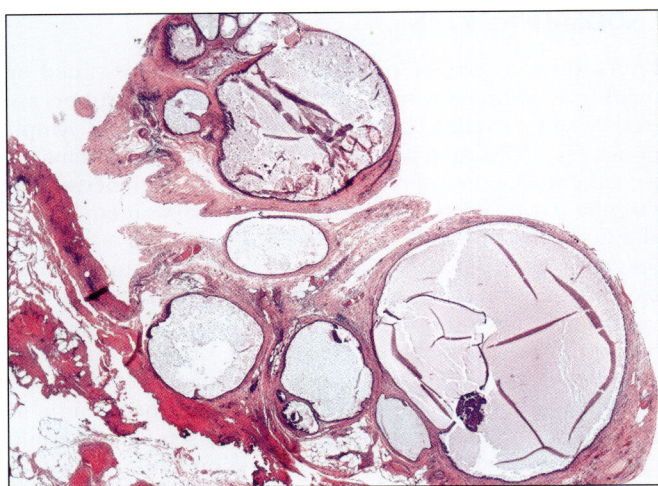

Figure 31.49 Endosalpingiosis. Numerous cystic glands lined by tubal epithelium appear in the serosa of the bladder.

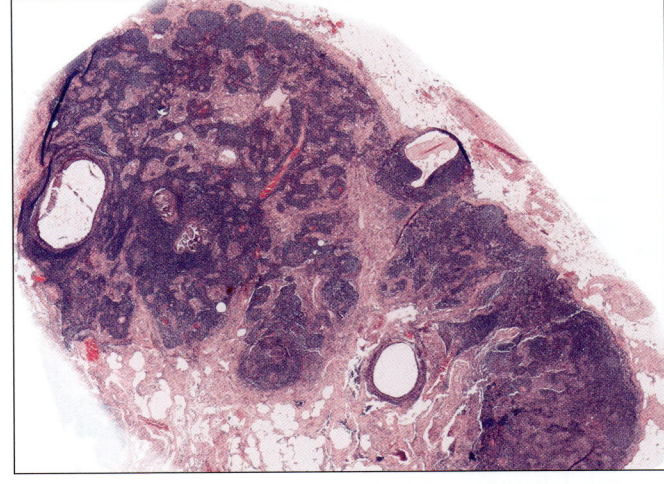

Figure 31.51 Intranodal müllerian inclusion cysts. The cyst are located in the periphery of the node.

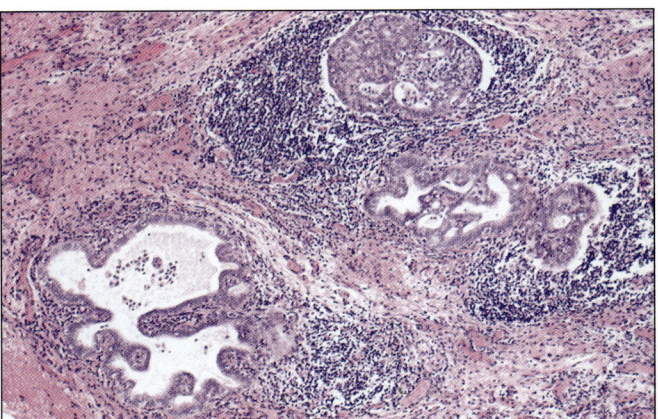

Figure 31.50 Florid endosalpingiosis mimicking adenocarcinoma. The serous glands show architectural complexity but the cells lack significant nuclear atypia.

Occasionally, the process may be so extensive as to mimic a neoplasia and the glands may be larger, exhibiting architectural complexity; however, the cells lack significant nuclear atypia (Figure 31.50).

The term atypical endosalpingiosis refers to lesions in which there is cellular stratification, including cellular buds, cribriform patterns, and varying degrees of cellular atypia, occurring in the absence of a serous borderline tumor. Histologically, such lesions merge with peritoneal serous borderline tumors (see Chapter 25).[133] Not uncommonly, the serous foci exhibit more epithelial proliferation than would be expected in benign lesions. The criteria used for assessing whether the excessive growth reflects neoplasms of borderline malignancy are identical to those for serous tumors in general and are summarized in Table 31.3. Rare extraovarian borderline and malignant serous tumors have been shown to arise from endosalpingiosis.[65,134]

Endosalpingiotic glands should be distinguished from mesonephric remnants, which are commonly found in the region of the fallopian tube. Mesonephric tubules are typically lined by a single layer of nonciliated, low columnar to cuboidal cells.

INTRANODAL GLANDS OF MÜLLERIAN TYPE (MÜLLERIAN INCLUSION CYSTS)

Benign-appearing glands of müllerian type or 'müllerian inclusion cysts' may be found in pelvic and para-aortic lymph nodes of females,[135,136] and less frequently in inguinal and femoral lymph nodes.[131] These glands are almost always incidental microscopic findings in lymph nodes removed in cases of pelvic carcinoma; therefore, their reported frequency varies from 2% to 41%, depending upon the number of lymph nodes removed and the extent of the microscopic sampling.[131] These patients often have endosalpingiosis of the peritoneum, acute and chronic salpingitis,[136] or coexistent ovarian serous tumors, which may be benign, borderline tumors, or carcinomas.[137]

Müllerian inclusion cysts are not grossly identifiable as such. The glands are usually located in the periphery of the node, most commonly within the capsule or between cortical lymphoid follicles. Histologically, the glands are identical to those of endosalpingiosis and exhibit a single layer of müllerian-type epithelium, generally with prominent cilia. Cells are cytologically bland and cuboidal to columnar. Nuclear contours are regular, the chromatin is even, and nucleoli are rarely seen. Mitoses are not identified. Intraglandular or periglandular psammoma bodies are commonly found. In rare cases, the cells can show nuclear atypia and stratification; the latter can produce an intraglandular cribriform pattern. These cases of atypical intranodal endosalpingiosis may occasionally be the site of origin of serous tumors.[138–140] In fact, müllerian inclusion cysts are more common in women with serous borderline tumors and low-grade serous carcinomas than in patients with high-grade serous carcinomas.[131]

Intranodal inclusion cysts lined by benign endometrioid epithelium, mucinous epithelium of endocervical or goblet cell type, or metaplastic squamous epithelium have also been reported[1,141,142] (Figures 31.51 and 31.52).

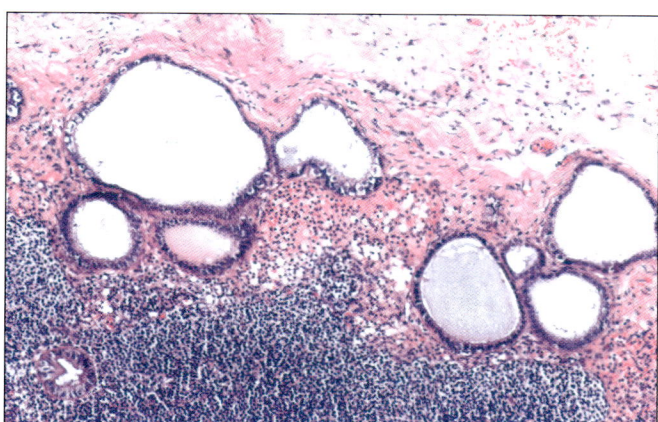

Figure 31.52 Intranodal müllerian inclusion cysts. Cysts appear within the capsule.

Differential Diagnosis

In most cases, the distinction between glandular inclusions and metastatic adenocarcinoma is not difficult. However, if an ovarian serous borderline tumor is present differential diagnosis may be difficult or even impossible. The capsular location of the glands, the presence of ciliated cells, the lack of severe nuclear atypia and mitotic activity, and the absence of a fibroblastic stromal reaction favor a benign diagnosis, i.e., endosalpingiosis. However, as indicated above, serous borderline tumors or low-grade serous carcinomas may occasionally originate within pelvic or para-aortic lymph nodes.[138–140] This diagnosis is suggested in cases in which the intranodal tumor merges with foci of atypical endosalpingiosis.

SEROUS TUMORS (PRIMARY AND METASTATIC)

SEROUS BORDERLINE TUMOR

See Chapter 25.

SEROUS CARCINOMA (OF PERITONEAL ORIGIN)

See Chapter 25.

PSAMMOCARCINOMA

See Chapter 25.

ENDOCERVICOSIS

Benign glands of endocervical type involving the peritoneum have been described as 'endocervicosis.' Nearly all reported cases involve the peritoneum overlying the posterior uterine serosa, cul-de-sac, vaginal apex, outer wall of the uterine cervix, and the urinary bladder.[143,144] Microscopically, the glands are located predominantly within the smooth muscle of the muscularis propria and mimic invasive well-differentiated adenocarcinoma. The presence of mild epithelial atypia and reactive periglandular stroma contributes to this misdiagnosis. However, the absence of a mucosal-based tumor and severe nuclear atypia facilitate the diagnosis of endocervicosis.[143,145]

PERITONEAL ENDOMETRIOID, CLEAR CELL, AND TRANSITIONAL CELL LESIONS

Occasional peritoneal cysts lined exclusively by endometrioid epithelium may occur, but it is often unclear whether these may represent endometriosis in which the stroma is absent or atrophic. Rare cases with clear cells, usually in the form of clear cell adenocarcinoma, have also been described and most likely represent clear cell adenocarcinomas arising from peritoneal endometriosis. Walthard rests, which are rests of transitional (urothelial-like) epithelium, are common occurrences on the tubal serosa, particularly the superior and posterior surfaces, and throughout the broad ligament.

DECIDUOSIS

Deciduosis, a form of 'stromal müllerianosis' disclosing foci of ectopic decidualized stromal cells, is commonly observed in association with pregnancy. Groups of decidual cells, indistinguishable from those found in gestational endometrium, occasionally appear in the pelvic and lower abdominal peritoneum, beneath the ovarian surface epithelium, and in the plicae of the fallopian tubes. It is also rarely seen in lymph nodes. Patients with trophoblastic disease also regularly exhibit deciduosis, mediated, as in a normal pregnancy, by high plasma levels of chorionic gonadotropins. Ectopic pseudodecidual reactions also occur with exogenous progesterone administration. These changes occur rarely in the absence of such histories and have mostly been identified in premenopausal women. Most lesions are incidental findings.

If seen grossly, the nodules are tan to pale brown, slightly gelatinous, and rarely more than several millimeters. Occasionally, the lesions may reach several centimeters in size and consist of multiple, tiny, soft nodules separated by thin, white, rubbery septa.[146]

In many locations, such as in fallopian tube plicae or adjacent to a corpus luteum, the decidua-like cells are pure. In the peritoneum, the decidualized cells are often admixed with smooth muscle cells, giving rise to the condition 'disseminated peritoneal leiomyomatosis,' also known as 'leiomyomatosis peritonealis disseminata.' Although the presence of the decidua in such cases has been used to argue that this condition develops by differentiation of the subcelomic mesenchyme with the formation of multiple tumor-like nodules (see later), there is no consensus that this is the true mechanism.

The decidual reaction most often appears as solid clusters of cohesive, decidualized cells with sharp cell borders (Figure 31.53). Cytoplasm may be abundant and glass like or may show some degrees of degeneration (Figure 31.54). Some cells have a clear vacuolated cytoplasm that superficially resembles the soap bubble-like physaliferous cell of chordoma (Figure 31.54). Some nodules may also show transitions between a more solid and a more myxoid pattern of decidual reaction (Figure 31.55).

DISSEMINATED PERITONEAL LEIOMYOMATOSIS

Disseminated peritoneal leiomyomatosis is a rare condition characterized by widespread nodules of benign smooth

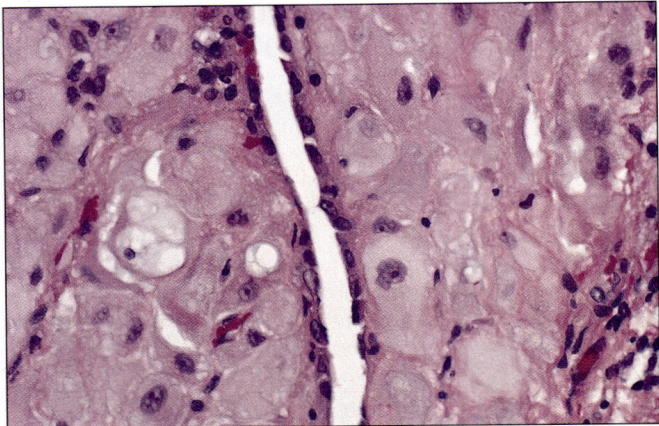

Figure 31.53 Decidual reaction of pregnancy. Several cells show sign of degeneration.

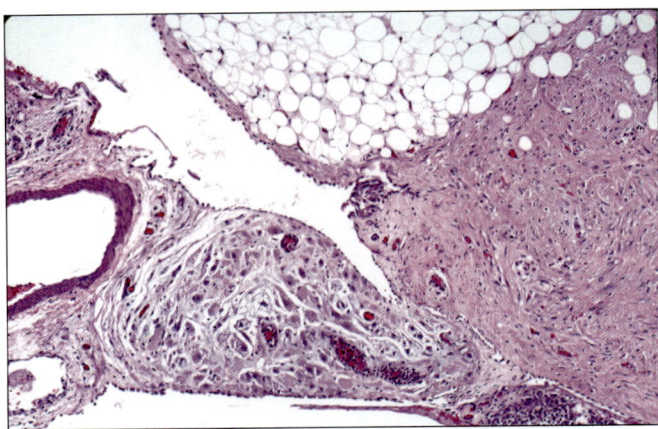

Figure 31.56 Disseminated peritoneal leiomyomatosis.

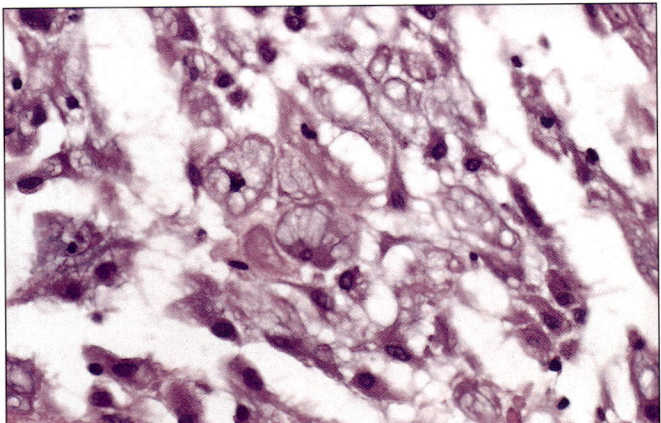

Figure 31.54 Decidual reaction of pregnancy. Numerous decidual cells are degenerative.

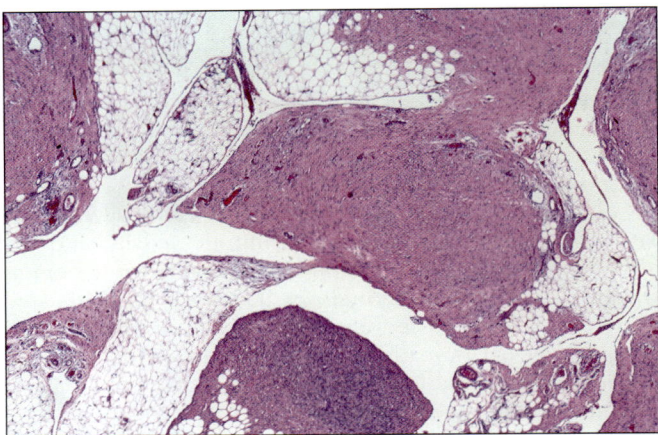

Figure 31.57 Disseminated peritoneal leiomyomatosis.

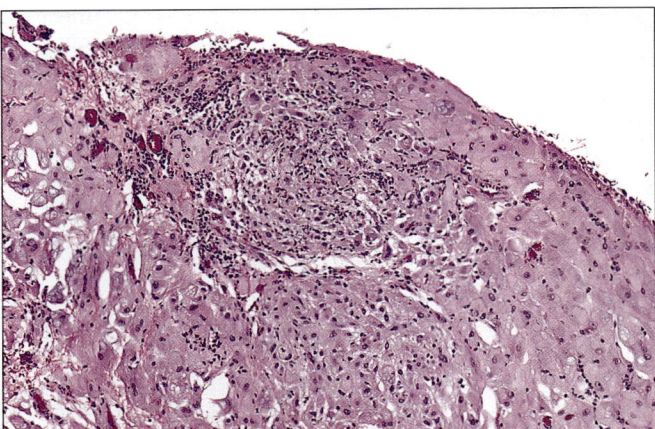

Figure 31.55 Nodules intermediate between decidua and smooth muscle proliferation. Shows features of both deciduosis and disseminated peritoneal leiomyomatosis.

muscle on the peritoneal surface of the pelvis and abdomen in women of reproductive age (see Chapter 19). Most patients have uterine leiomyomas at the time of diagnosis.[147–149] The most common presentation is as an incidental finding at the time of caesarean section. The intraoperative appearance is so alarming that frozen section examination is often requested to rule out peritoneal carcinomatosis. The peritoneal myomatous nodules develop on a background of an altered hormonal milieu, such as with pregnancy, oral contraceptive use,[150] hormonal therapy, or steroid-producing ovarian tumors.[151] While this lesion is often classified as a tumor-like condition, since it commonly regresses, the tumors in some cases persist, suggesting a neoplastic process. On rare occasions, some have shown malignant transformation.[152–154]

Pathology

Grossly, multiple gray-white nodules that may be granular to several millimeters in diameter are found covering the peritoneal surfaces of the pelvis, pelvic organs, intestines, and omentum. Microscopically, the nodules consist of smooth muscle arranged like leiomyomas (Figure 31.56). Cells usually lack atypia and mitotic activity, and only rarely have features of malignancy. In many cases, the tumor is admixed with stromal cells resembling decidua (Figure 31.57). Smooth muscle cells are markedly reactive for desmin and muscle-specific antigens, CD10, ER, and PR, but without reactivity for keratin. Although the etiology of disseminated peritoneal leiomyomatosis is unknown, this immunohistochemical profile has been used to argue in support of the hypothesis that the condition arises from multicentric differentiation of submesothelial stem cells. Ultrastructural examination discloses myofilamentous bundles with focal electron-dense bodies typical of smooth muscle cell differentiation.

Pathogenesis

Progesterone stimulation appears to be critical in the development of these tumors in nearly all cases. They are almost always strongly reactive for PRs and usually reactive for ERs although with less intensity.[155] In postpartum women, ER reactivity in decidualized nodules is either weak or absent.[156] Such an immunohistochemical profile might be expected, since ovarian and placentally derived progesterone is critical in transforming endometrial stromal cells into decidua during pregnancy and since foci of decidual cells are found with the smooth muscle cells.

Regression has been documented in cases where excess hormonal stimulation has been removed, e.g., with the cessation of oral contraceptives, oophorectomy, or following childbirth.[151] Based on the earlier observations, the general view has been that disseminated peritoneal leiomyomas are metaplastic in origin and hormonally responsive. Yet, rather than this lesion being polyclonal, one study in which 42 leiomyomatous lesions from four patients were studied found that the leiomyomas were monoclonal, which strongly suggests that the lesions are neoplastic and from the same precursor lesion.[157]

Other conditions also give rise to one or more peritoneal leiomyomas. Uterine subserosal leiomyomas may become detached and implant elsewhere on the peritoneum (parasitic leiomyomas). Leiomyomas arising in the deep retroperitoneal–abdominal soft tissue can involve the peritoneum.[158,159] Like uterine leiomyomas, they can be hormonally reactive, which is unlike leiomyomas of deep somatic soft tissue, e.g., extremities, which are hormonally unreactive.[160]

Disseminated peritoneal leiomyomatosis may regress spontaneously or after therapy with GnRH agonist. Five cases of malignant form have been reported.[152]

REFERENCES

1. Lauchlan SC. The secondary mullerian system revisited. Int J Gynecol Pathol 1994;13:73–9.
2. Clement PB. Reactive tumor-like lesions of the peritoneum. Am J Clin Pathol 1995;103:673–6.
3. Koc S, Beydilli G, Tulunay G, et al. Peritoneal tuberculosis mimicking advanced ovarian cancer: a retrospective review of 22 cases. Gynecol Oncol 2006;103:565–9.
4. Abraham G, Mathews M, Sekar L, et al. Tuberculous peritonitis in a cohort of continuous ambulatory peritoneal dialysis patients. Perit Dial Int 2001;21(Suppl):S202–4.
5. Groutz A, Carmon E, Gat A. Peritoneal tuberculosis versus advanced ovarian cancer: a diagnostic dilemma. Obstet Gynecol 1998;91(5 Pt 2):868.
6. Piura B, Rabinovich A, Leron E, et al. Peritoneal tuberculosis—an uncommon disease that may deceive the gynecologist. Eur J Obstet Gynecol Reprod Biol 2003;110:230–4.
7. Bernaciak J, Spina JC, Curros ML, et al. Case report: peritoneal sarcoidosis in an unusual location. Semin Respir Crit Care Med 2002;23:597–600.
8. Bourdillon L, Lanier-Gachon E, Stankovic K, et al. Lofgren syndrome and peritoneal involvement by sarcoidosis—case report. Chest 2007;132:310–2.
9. Rosen DMB, Lam AM, Carlton MA, Cario GM. The safety of laparoscopic treatment for ovarian dermoid tumours. Aust N Z J Obstet Gynaecol 1998;38:77–9.
10. Reich O, Kometter R, Pickel H. Chronic sclerosing peritonitis after spontaneous rupture of a cystic teratoma: a pitfall in surgical staging of ovarian tumours. Geburt Frauenheil 1999;59:94–5.
11. Wu TI, Chang TC, Hsueh S, Lai CH. Ovarian endometrioid carcinoma with diffuse pigmented peritoneal keratin granulomas: a case report and review of the literature. Int J Gynecol Cancer 2006;16:426–9.
12. Davis JR, Miller HS, Feng JD. Vernix caseosa peritonitis: report of two cases with antenatal onset. Am J Clin Pathol 1998;109:320–3.
13. Tawfik O, Prather J, Bhatia P, et al. Vernix caseosa peritonitis as a rare complication of cesarean section. A case report. J Reprod Med 1998;43:547–50.
14. George E, Leyser S, Zimmer HL, et al. Vernix caseosa peritonitis. An infrequent complication of cesarean section with distinctive histopathologic features. Am J Clin Pathol 1995;103:681–4.
15. Mahmoud A, Silapaswan S, Lin K, Penney D. Vernix caseosa: an unusual cause of post-cesarean section peritonitis. Am Surg 1997;63:382–5.
16. Jaworski RC, Boadle R, Greg J, Cocks P. Peritoneal 'melanosis' associated with a ruptured ovarian dermoid cyst: report of a case with electron-probe energy dispersive x-ray analysis. Int J Gynecol Pathol 2001;20:386–9.
17. Carey M, Kirk ME. Necrotic pseudoxanthomatous nodules of the omentum and peritoneum—a peculiar reaction to endometriotic cyst contents. Obstet Gynecol 1993;82(4 Part 2):650–2.
18. Seidman JD, Oberer S, Bitterman P, Aisner SC. Pathogenesis of pseudoxanthomatous salpingiosis. Mod Pathol 1993;6:53–5.
19. Dehner LP, Coffin CM. Idiopathic fibrosclerotic disorders and other inflammatory pseudotumors. Semin Diagn Pathol 1998;15:161–73.
20. Frigerio L, Taccagni GL, Mariani A, et al. Idiopathic sclerosing peritonitis associated with florid mesothelial hyperplasia, ovarian fibromatosis, and endometriosis: a new disorder of abdominal mass. Am J Obstet Gynecol 1997;176:721–2.
21. Stenram U. Sclerosing peritonitis in a case of benign cystic ovarian teratoma. A case report. APMIS 1997;105:414–6.
22. Afthentopoulos IE, Passadakis P, Oreopoulos DG. Sclerosing peritonitis in continuous ambulatory peritoneal dialysis patients: one center's experience and review of the literature. Adv Ren Replace Ther 1998;5:157–67.
23. Cancarini GC, Sandrini M, Vizzardi V, et al. Clinical aspects of peritoneal sclerosis. J Nephrol 2001;14(Suppl):S39–47.
24. Di Paolo N, Garosi G. Peritoneal sclerosis. J Nephrol 1999;12:347–61.
25. Garosi G, Di Paolo N, Sacchi G, Gaggiotti E. Sclerosing peritonitis: a nosological entity. Perit Dial Int 2005;25(Suppl):S110.
26. Krediet RT, Zweers MM, van Westrhenen R, et al. What can we do to preserve the peritoneum? Perit Dial Int 2003;23(Suppl):S14–9.
27. Clement PB, Young RH, Hanna W, Scully RE. Sclerosing peritonitis associated with luteinized thecomas of the ovary. A clinicopathological analysis of six cases. Am J Surg Pathol 1994;18:1–13.
28. Iwasa Y, Minamiguchi S, Konishi I, et al. Sclerosing peritonitis associated with luteinized thecoma of the ovary. Pathol Int 1996;46:510–14.
29. Nishida T, Ushijima K, Watanabe J, et al. Sclerosing peritonitis associated with luteinized thecoma of the ovary. Gynecol Oncol 1999;73:167–9.
30. Spiegel GW, Swiger FK. Luteinized thecoma with sclerosing peritonitis presenting as an acute abdomen. Gynecol Oncol 1996;61:275–81.
31. Werness BA. Luteinized thecoma with sclerosing peritonitis. Arch Pathol Lab Med 1996;120:303–6.
32. Yantiss RK, Nielsen GP, Lauwers GY, et al. Reactive nodular fibrous pseudotumor of the gastrointestinal tract and mesentery. Am J Surg Pathol 2003;27:532–40.
33. Clement PB, Young RH. Florid mesothelial hyperplasia associated with ovarian tumors—a potential source of error in tumor diagnosis and staging. Int J Gynecol Pathol 1993;12:51–8.
34. Kerner H, Gaton E, Czernobilsky B. Unusual ovarian, tubal and pelvic mesothelial inclusions in patients with endometriosis. Histopathology 1981;5:277–82.
35. Rosai J, Dehner LP. Nodular mesothelial hyperplasia in hernia sacs. A benign reactive condition stimulating a neoplastic process. Cancer 1975;35:165–75.

36. Clement PB, Young RH, Oliva E, et al. Hyperplastic mesothelial cells within abdominal lymph nodes: mimic of metastatic ovarian carcinoma and serous borderline tumor—a report of two cases associated with ovarian neoplasms. Mod Pathol 1996;9:879–86.
37. Knudsen PJ. The peritoneal elastic lamina. J Anat 1991;177:41–6.
38. Churg A, Cagle PT, Roggli VL. Tumors of the serosal membranes. Atlas of tumor pathology, ser IV. Washington, DC: Armed Forces Institute of Pathology; 2006.
39. Kafiri G, Thomas DM, Shepherd NA, et al. p53 expression is common in malignant mesotheliomas. Histopathology 1992;21:331–4.
40. Henderson DW, Shilkin KB, Whitaker D. Reactive mesothelial hyperplasia vs. mesothelioma, including mesothelioma in situ. Am J Clin Pathol 1998;110:397–404.
41. Taheri ZM, Mehrafza M, Mohammadi F, et al. The diagnostic value of Ki-67 and repp 86 in distinguishing between benign and malignant mesothelial proliferations. Arch Pathol Lab Med 2008;132:694–7.
42. Padmanabhan V, Mount SL, Eltabbakh GH. Peritoneal atypical mesothelial proliferation with progression to invasive mesothelioma: a case report and review of the literature. Pathology 2003;35:260–3.
43. Lamovec J, Sinkovec J. Multilocular peritoneal inclusion cyst (multicystic mesothelioma) with hyaline globules. Histopathology 1996;28:466–9.
44. Sawh RN, Malpica A, Deavers MT, et al. Benign cystic mesothelioma of the peritoneum: a clinicopathologic study of 17 cases and immunohistochemical analysis of estrogen and progesterone receptor status. Hum Pathol 2003;34:369–74.
45. Ross MJ, Welch WR, Scully RE. Multilocular peritoneal inclusion cysts (so-called cystic mesotheliomas). Cancer 1989;64:1336–46.
46. Kuga T, Esato K, Takeda K, et al. A supernumerary ovary of the omentum with cystic change: report of two cases and review of the literature. Pathol Int 1999;49:566–70.
47. Sarraf KM, Abdalla M, Al-Omari O, Sarraf MG. Diagnostic difficulties of pelvic splenosis: case report. Ultrasound Obstet Gynecol 2006;27:220–1.
48. Lim C, McIlroy K, Briggs G, Tan L. Splenosis mimicking lymphoma. Pathology 2007;39:183–5.
49. Peitsidis P, Akrivos T, Vecchini G, et al. Splenosis of the peritoneal cavity resembling an adnexal tumor: case report. Clin Exp Obstet Gynecol 2007;34:120–2.
50. Vydianath B, Gurumurthy M, Crocker J. Solitary ovarian splenosis. J Clin Pathol 2005;58:1224–5.
51. Rehbock J, Dimpfl T, Assemi C. Disseminated peritoneal trophoblastic implants after surgery of tubal pregnancies—a typical complication of the laparoscopic technique? Geburt Frauenheil 1997;57:155–7.
52. Tsutsumi O, Ando K, Momoeda M. Ruptured isthmal pregnancy following laparoscopic salpingostomy in the ipsilateral tube. Int J Gynecol Obstet 1997;57:187–9.
53. Ghosh P, Strong C, Naugler W, et al. Peritoneal mice implicated in intestinal obstruction—report of a case and review of the literature. J Clin Gastroenterol 2006;40:427–30.
54. Vuong PN, Guyot H, Moulin G, et al. Pseudotumoral organization of a twisted epiploic fringe or 'hard-boiled egg' in the peritoneal cavity. Arch Pathol Lab Med 1990;114:531–3.
55. Goldblum J, Hart WR. Localized and diffuse mesotheliomas of the genital tract and peritoneum in women—a clinicopathologic study of nineteen true mesothelial neoplasms, other than adenomatoid tumors, multicystic mesotheliomas, and localized fibrous tumors. Am J Surg Pathol 1995;19:1124–37.
56. Baker PM, Clement PB, Young RH. Malignant peritoneal mesothelioma in women – a study of 75 cases with emphasis on their morphologic spectrum and differential diagnosis. Am J Clin Pathol 2005;123:724–37.
57. Butnor KJ, Sporn TA, Hammar SP, Roggli VL. Well-differentiated papillary mesothelioma. Am J Surg Pathol 2001;25:1304–9.
58. Hoekstra AV, Riben MW, Frumovitz M, et al. Well-differentiated papillary mesothelioma of the peritoneum: a pathological analysis and review of the literature. Gynecol Oncol 2005;98:161–7.
59. Davidson B, Risberg B, Berner A, et al. The biological differences between ovarian serous carcinoma and diffuse peritoneal malignant mesothelioma. Semin Diagn Pathol 2006;23:35–43.
60. Kerrigan SAJ, Turnnir RT, Clement PB, et al. Diffuse malignant epithelial mesotheliomas of the peritoneum in women – a clinicopathologic study of 25 patients. Cancer 2002;94:378–85.
61. Hemminki K, Li XJ. Time, trends and occupational risk factors for peritoneal mesothelioma in Sweden. J Occup Environ Med 2003;45:451–5.
62. Cerruto CA, Brun EA, Chang D, Sugarbaker PH. Prognostic significance of histomorphologic parameters in diffuse malignant peritoneal mesothelioma. Arch Pathol Lab Med 2006;130:1654–61.
63. Shia J, Erlandson RA, Klimstra DS. Deciduoid mesothelioma: a report of 5 cases and literature review. Ultrastruct Pathol 2002;26:355–63.
64. Ordóñez NG. Deciduoid mesothelioma: report of 21 cases with review of the literature. Mod Pathol 2012;25:1481–95.
65. Carrick KS, Milvenan JS, Albores-Saavedra J. Serous tumor of low malignant potential arising in inguinal endosalpingiosis. Int J Gynecol Pathol 2003;22:412–5.
66. Ordonez NG. Desmoplastic small round cell tumor: II: an ultrastructural and immunohistochemical study with emphasis on new immunohistochemical markers. Am J Surg Pathol 1998;22:1314–27.
67. Feldman AL, Libutti SK, Pingpank JF, et al. Analysis of factors associated with outcome in patients with malignant peritoneal mesothelioma undergoing surgical debulking and intraperitoneal chemotherapy. J Clin Oncol 2003;15;21:4560–7.
68. Nonaka D, Kusamura S, Baratti D, et al. Diffuse malignant mesothelioma of the peritoneum—a clinicopathologic study of 35 patients treated locoregionally at a single institution. Cancer 2005;104:2181–8.
69. McCaughey WT, Colby TV, Battifora H, et al. Diagnosis of diffuse malignant mesothelioma: experience of a US/Canadian Mesothelioma Panel. Mod Pathol 1991;4:342–53.
70. Shanks JH, Harris M, Banerjee SS, et al. Mesotheliomas with deciduoid morphology—a morphologic spectrum and a variant not confined to young females. Am J Surg Pathol 2000;24:285–94.
71. Borczuk AC, Taub RN, Hesdorffer M, et al. P16 loss and mitotic activity predict poor survival in patients with peritoneal malignant mesothelioma. Clin Cancer Res 2005;11:3303–8.
72. Clement PB, Young RH, Scully RE. Malignant mesotheliomas presenting as ovarian masses—a report of nine cases, including two primary ovarian mesotheliomas. Am J Surg Pathol 1996;20:1067–80.
73. Attanoos RL, Webb R, Dojcinov SD, Gibbs AR. Value of mesothelial and epithelial antibodies in distinguishing diffuse peritoneal mesothelioma in females from serous papillary carcinoma of the ovary and peritoneum. Histopathology 2002;40:237–44.
74. Comin CE, Saieva C, Messerini L. h-Caldesmon, calretinin, estrogen receptor, and Ber-EP4: a useful combination of immunohistochemical markers for differentiating epithelioid peritoneal mesothelioma from serous papillary carcinoma of the ovary. Am J Surg Pathol 2007;31:1139–48.
75. Gown AM. Uses of antibody panels in the analysis of metastatic carcinomas of unknown primary. Acta Histochem Cytochem 1999;32:153–9.
76. Miller RT. Immunocytochemistry of epithelial tumors. In: ASCP National Meeting; 1999. New Orleans, LA: American Society of Clinical Pathology; 1999. p. 1–47.
77. Ordonez NG. Value of calretinin immunostaining in differentiating epithelial mesothelioma from lung adenocarcinoma. Mod Pathol 1998;11:929–33.
78. Lae ME, Roche PC, Jin L, et al. Desmoplastic small round cell tumor—a clinicopathologic, immunohistochemical, and molecular study of 32 tumors. Am J Surg Pathol 2002;26:823–35.
79. Young RH, Eichhorn JH, Dickersin GR, Scully RE. Ovarian involvement by the intra-abdominal desmoplastic small round cell tumor with divergent differentiation: a report of three cases. Hum Pathol 1992;23:454–64.
80. Fukunaga M, Endo Y, Takaki K, et al. Postmenopausal intra-abdominal desmoplastic small cell tumor. Pathol Int 1996;46:281–5.
81. Wolf AN, Ladanyi M, Paull G, et al. The expanding clinical spectrum of desmoplastic small round-cell tumor: a report of two cases with molecular confirmation. Hum Pathol 1999;30:430–5.

82. Prat J, Matias-Guiu X, Algaba F. Desmoplastic small round-cell tumor. Am J Surg Pathol 1992;16:306–7.
83. Gerald WL, Ladanyi M, de Alava E, et al. Clinical, pathologic, and molecular spectrum of tumors associated with t(11;22)(p13;q12): desmoplastic small round-cell tumor and its variants. J Clin Oncol 1998;16:3028–36.
84. Ordonez NG. Desmoplastic small round cell tumor: I: a histopathologic study of 39 cases with emphasis on unusual histological patterns. Am J Surg Pathol 1998;22:1303–13.
85. Barnoud R, Delattre O, Peoc'h M, et al. Desmoplastic small round cell tumor: RT-PCR analysis and immunohistochemical detection of the Wilm's tumor gene WT1. Pathol Res Pract 1998;194: 693–700.
86. Ordi J, de Alava E, Torne A, et al. Intraabdominal desmoplastic small round cell tumor with EWS/ERG fusion transcript. Am J Surg Pathol 1998;22:1026–32.
87. Kim J, Lee K, Pelletier J. The desmoplastic small round cell tumor t(11;22) translocation produces EWS/WT1 isoforms with differing oncogenic properties. Oncogene 1998;16:1973–9.
88. Shimizu Y, Mitsui T, Kawakami T, et al. Novel breakpoints of the EWS gene and the WT1 gene in a desmoplastic small round cell tumor. Cancer Genet Cytogenet 1998;106:156–8.
89. Benjamin LE, Fredericks WJ, Barr FG, Rauscher 3rd FJ. Fusion of the EWS1 and WT1 genes as a result of the t(11;22)(p13;q12) translocation in desmoplastic small round cell tumors. Med Pediatr Oncol 1996;27:434–9.
90. Hanau CA, Miettinen M. Solitary fibrous tumor: histological and immunohistochemical spectrum of benign and malignant variants presenting at different sites. Hum Pathol 1995;26:440–9.
91. Fukunaga M, Naganuma H, Ushigome S, et al. Malignant solitary fibrous tumour of the peritoneum. Histopathology 1996;28: 463–6.
92. Fukunaga M, Naganuma H, Nikaido T, et al. Extrapleural solitary fibrous tumor: a report of seven cases. Mod Pathol 1997;10: 443–50.
93. Flint A, Weiss SW. CD-34 and keratin expression distinguishes solitary fibrous tumor (fibrous mesothelioma) of pleura from desmoplastic mesothelioma. Hum Pathol 1995;26:428–31.
94. Day DL, Sane S, Dehner LP. Inflammatory pseudotumor of the mesentery and small intestine. Pediatr Radiol 1986;16:210–5.
95. Pettinato G, Manivel JC, De Rosa N, et al. Inflammatory myofibroblastic tumor (plasma cell granuloma). Clinicopathologic study of 20 cases with immunohistochemical and ultrastructural observations. Am J Clin Pathol 1990;94:538–46.
96. Coffin CM, Hornick JL, Fletcher CD. Inflammatory myofibroblastic tumor: comparison of clinicopathologic, histologic, and immunohistochemical features including ALK expression in atypical and aggressive cases. Am J Surg Pathol 2007;31:509–20.
97. Stern RC, Dash R, Bentley RC, et al. Malignancy in endometriosis: frequency and comparison of ovarian and extraovarian types. Int J Gynecol Pathol 2001;20:133–9.
98. Shen DH, Khoo US, Xue WC, et al. Primary peritoneal malignant mixed mullerian tumors—a clinicopathologic, immunohistochemical, and genetic study. Cancer 2001;91:1052–60.
99. Chang KL, Crabtree GS, Limtan SK, et al. Primary extrauterine endometrial stromal neoplasms—a clinicopathologic study of 20 cases and a review of the literature. Int J Gynecol Pathol 1993;12:282–96.
100. Kaplan AM, Creager AJ, Livasy CA, et al. Intra-abdominal embryonal rhabdomyosarcoma in an adult. Gynecol Oncol 1999;74:282–5.
101. Fox H. Pseudomyxoma peritonei. Br J Obstet Gynaecol 1996;103:197–8.
102. Guerrieri C, Franlund B, Fristedt S, et al. Mucinous tumors of the vermiform appendix and ovary, and pseudomyxoma peritonei: histogenetic implications of cytokeratin 7 expression. Hum Pathol 1997;28:1039–45.
103. Bradley RF, Stewart JH, Russell GB, et al. Pseudomyxoma peritonei of appendiceal origin: a clinicopathologic analysis of 101 patients uniformly treated at a single institution, with literature review. Am J Surg Pathol 2006;30:551–9.
104. Jackson SL, Fleming RA, Loggie BW, Geisinger KR. Gelatinous ascites: a cytohistologic study of pseudomyxoma peritonei in 67 patients. Mod Pathol 2001;14:664–71.
105. Misdraji J, Yantiss RK, Graeme-Cook FM, et al. Appendiceal mucinous neoplasms—a clinicopathologic analysis of 107 cases. Am J Surg Pathol 2003;27:1089–103.
106. Young RH. Pseudomyxoma peritonei and selected other aspects of the spread of appendiceal neoplasms. Semin Diagn Pathol 2004;21:134–50.
107. Lee KR, Scully RE. Mucinous tumors of the ovary. A clinicopathologic study of 196 borderline tumors (of intestinal type) and carcinomas, including an evaluation of 11 cases with 'pseudomyxoma peritonei.' Am J Surg Pathol 2000;24:1447–64.
108. Ronnett BM, Yan H, Kurman RJ, et al. Patients with pseudomyxoma peritonei associated with disseminated peritoneal adenomucinosis have a significantly more favorable prognosis than patients with peritoneal mucinous carcinomatosis. Cancer 2001;92:85–91.
109. Hart WR. Mucinous tumors of the ovary: a review. Int J Gynecol Pathol 2005;24:4–25.
110. Prayson RA, Hart WR, Petras RE. Pseudomyxoma peritonei. A clinicopathologic study of 19 cases with emphasis on site of origin and nature of associated ovarian tumors. Am J Surg Pathol 1994;18:591–603.
111. Ronnett BM, Kurman RJ, Zahn CM, et al. Pseudomyxoma peritonei in women: a clinicopathologic analysis of 30 cases with emphasis on site of origin, prognosis, and relationship to ovarian mucinous tumors of low malignant potential. Hum Pathol 1995;26:509–24.
112. Young RH, Gilks CB, Scully RE. Mucinous tumors of the appendix associated with mucinous tumors of the ovary and pseudomyxoma peritonei. A clinicopathological analysis of 22 cases supporting an origin in the appendix. Am J Surg Pathol 1991;15:415–29.
113. Cuatrecasas M, Matias-Guiu X, Prat J. Synchronous mucinous tumors of the appendix and the ovary associated with pseudomyxoma peritonei: a clinicopathologic study of six cases with comparative analysis of c-Ki-ras mutations. Am J Surg Pathol 1996;20:739–46.
114. O'Connell JT, Tomlinson JS, Roberts AA, et al. Pseudomyxoma peritonei is a disease of MUC2-expressing goblet cells. Am J Pathol 2002;161:551–64.
115. Loy TS, Calaluce RD, Keeney GL. Cytokeratin immunostaining in differentiating primary ovarian carcinoma from metastatic colonic adenocarcinoma. Mod Pathol 1996;9:1040–4.
116. Ronnett BM, Kurman RJ, Shmookler BM, et al. The morphologic spectrum of ovarian metastases of appendiceal adenocarcinomas: a clinicopathologic and immunohistochemical analysis of tumors often misinterpreted as primary ovarian tumors or metastatic tumors from other gastrointestinal sites. Am J Surg Pathol 1997;21:1144–55.
117. Ronnett BM, Shmookler B, Diener-West M, et al. Immunohistochemical evidence supporting the appendiceal origin of pseudomyxoma peritonei in women. Int J Gynecol Pathol 1997;16:1–9.
118. Vang R, Gown AM, Barry TS, et al. Cytokeratins 7 and 20 in primary and secondary mucinous tumors of the ovary: analysis of coordinate immunohistochemical expression profiles and staining distribution in 179 cases. Am J Surg Pathol 2006;30: 1130–9.
119. Ronnett BM, Zahn CM, Kurman RJ, et al. Disseminated peritoneal adenomucinosis and peritoneal mucinous carcinomatosis: a clinicopathologic analysis of 109 cases with emphasis on distinguishing pathologic features, site of origin, prognosis, and relationship to 'pseudomyxoma peritonei'. Am J Surg Pathol 1995;19:1390–408.
120. Gocht A, Lohler J, Scheidel P, Stegner H-E. Gliomatosis peritonei combined with mature ovarian teratoma. Pathol Res Pract 1995;191:1029–35.
121. Hamada Y, Tanano A, Sato M, et al. Ovarian teratoma with gliomatosis peritonei: report of two cases. Surg Today 1998;28: 223–6.
122. Nanda S, Kalra B, Arora B, Singh S. Massive mature solid teratoma of the ovary with gliomatosis peritonei. Aust N Z J Obstet Gynaecol 1998;38:329–31.
123. Schmidt D, Kommoss F. Teratoma of the ovary. Clinical and pathological differences between mature and immature teratomas. Pathologe 2007;28:203–8.
124. Ferguson AW, Katabuchi H, Ronnett BM, Cho KR. Glial implants in gliomatosis peritonei arise from normal tissue, not from the associated teratoma. Am J Pathol 2001;159:51–5.
125. Calder CJ, Light AM, Rollason TP. Immature ovarian teratoma with mature peritoneal metastatic deposits showing glial, epithelial, and endometrioid differentiation—a case report and review of the literature. Int J Gynecol Pathol 1994;13:279–82.

126. Dadmanesh F, Miller DM, Swenerton KD, Clement PB. Gliomatosis peritonei with malignant transformation. Mod Pathol 1997;10:597–601.
127. Hill DA, Dehner LP, White FV, Langer JC. Gliomatosis peritonei as a complication of a ventriculoperitoneal shunt: case report and review of the literature. J Pediatr Surg 2000;35:497–9.
128. Jansen RP, Russell P. Nonpigmented endometriosis: clinical, laparoscopic, and pathologic definition. Am J Obstet Gynecol 1986;155:1154–9.
129. Zinsser KR, Wheeler JE. Endosalpingiosis in the omentum. A study of autopsy and surgical material. Am J Surg Pathol 1982;6:109–17.
130. McCaughey WTE, Kirk ME, Lester W, et al. Peritoneal epithelial lesions associated with proliferative serous tumours of the ovary. Histopathology 1984;8:195–208.
131. Moore WF, Bentley RC, Berchuck A, Robboy SJ. Some mullerian inclusion cysts in lymph nodes may sometimes be metastases from serous borderline tumors of the ovary. Am J Surg Pathol 2000;24:710–18.
132. Copeland LJ, Silva EG, Gershenson DM, et al. The significance of müllerian inclusions found at second-look laparotomy in patients with epithelial ovarian neoplasms. Obstet Gynecol 1988;71:763–70.
133. Bell DA, Scully RE. Serous borderline tumors of the peritoneum. Am J Surg Pathol 1990;14:230–9.
134. McCoubrey A, Houghton O, McCallion K, et al. Serous adenocarcinoma of the sigmoid mesentery arising in cystic endosalpingiosis. J Clin Pathol 2005;58:1221–3.
135. Horn LC, Bilek K. Frequency and histogenesis of pelvic retroperitoneal lymph node inclusions of the female genital tract. An immunohistochemical study of 34 cases. Pathol Res Pract 1995;191:991–6.
136. Kheir SM, Mann WJ, Wilkerson JA. Glandular inclusions in lymph nodes. The problem of extensive involvement and relationship to salpingitis. Am J Surg Pathol 1981;5:353–9.
137. Prade M, Spatz A, Bentley R, et al. Borderline and malignant serous tumor arising in pelvic lymph nodes: evidence of origin in benign glandular inclusions. Int J Gynecol Pathol 1995;14:87–91.
138. Djordjevic B, Malpica A. Lymph node involvement in ovarian serous tumors of low malignant potential: with lymph node involvement: a clinicopathologic study of thirty-six cases. Am J Surg Pathol 2010;34:1–9.
139. Djordjevic B, Clement-Kruzel S, Atkinson NE, Malpica A. Nodal endosalpingiosis in ovarian serous tumors of low malignant potential with lymph node involvement: a case for a precursor lesion. Am J Surg Pathol 2010;34:1442–8.
140. Djordjevic B, Malpica A. Ovarian serous tumors of low malignant potential with nodal low-grade serous carcinoma. Am J Surg Pathol 2012;36:955–63.
141. Lauchlan SC. The secondary mullerian system. Obstet Gynecol Surv 1972;27:133–46.
142. Mills SE. Decidua and squamous metaplasia in abdominopelvic lymph nodes. Int J Gynecol Pathol 1983;2:209–15.
143. Clement PB, Young RH. Endocervicosis of the urinary bladder. A report of six cases of a benign mullerian lesion that may mimic adenocarcinoma. Am J Surg Pathol 1992;16:533–42.
144. Nazeer T, Ro JY, Tornos C, et al. Endocervical type glands in urinary bladder: a clinicopathologic study of six cases. Hum Pathol 1996;27:816–20.
145. Young RH, Clement PB. Mullerianosis of the urinary bladder. Mod Pathol 1996;9:731–7.
146. Begin LR. Florid soft-tissue decidual reaction—a potential mimic of neoplasia. Am J Surg Pathol 1997;21:348–53.
147. Altinok G, Usubutun A, Kucukali T, et al. Disseminated peritoneal leiomyomatosis—a benign entity mimicking carcinomatosis. Arch Gynecol Obstet 2000;264:54–5.
148. Heinig J, Neff A, Cirkel U, Klockenbusch W. Recurrent leiomyomatosis peritonealis disseminata after hysterectomy and bilateral salpingo-oophorectomy during combined hormone replacement therapy. Eur J Obstet Gynecol Reprod Biol 2003;111:216–8.
149. Langenberg R, Wojdat R, Volz-Koster S, Volz J. Disseminated intraperitoneal leiomyomatosis—case report of a rare differential diagnosis of metastasizing ovarian carcinoma. Geburt Frauenheil 2005;65:1074–6.
150. Scharlau LL, Scharlau J, Mathuis C, Schremmer CN. Diffuse peritoneal leiomyomatosis: a case report. Geburt Frauenheil 2000;60:225–8.
151. Hardman IWJ, Majmudar B. Leiomyomatosis peritonealis disseminata: clinicopathologic analysis of five cases. South Med J 1996;89:291–4.
152. Bekkers RLM, Willemsen WNP, Schijf CPT, et al. Leiomyomatosis peritonealis disseminata: does malignant transformation occur? A literature review. Gynecol Oncol 1999;75:158–63.
153. Fulcher AS, Szucs RA. Leiomyomatosis peritonealis disseminata complicated by sarcomatous transformation and ovarian torsion: presentation of two cases and review of the literature. Abdom Imaging 1998;23:640–4.
154. Herrero J, Kamali P, Kirschbaum M. Leiomyomatosis peritonealis disseminata associated with endometriosis: a case report and literature review. Eur J Obstet Gynecol Reprod Biol 1998;76:189–91.
155. Butnor KJ, Burchette JL, Robboy SJ. Progesterone receptor activity in leiomyomatosis peritonealis disseminata. Int J Gynecol Pathol 1999;18:259–64.
156. Buttner A, Bassler R, Theele C. Pregnancy-associated ectopic decidua (deciduosis) of the greater omentum. An analysis of 60 biopsies with cases of fibrosing deciduosis and leiomyomatosis peritonealis disseminata. Pathol Res Pract 1993;189:352–9.
157. Quade BJ, McLachlin CM, Soto-Wright V, et al. Disseminated peritoneal leiomyomatosis: clonality analysis by X chromosome inactivation and cytogenetics of a clinically benign smooth muscle proliferation. Am J Pathol 1997;150:2153–66.
158. Billings SD, Folpe AL, Weiss SW. Do leiomyomas of deep soft tissue exist? An analysis of highly differentiated smooth muscle tumors of deep soft tissue supporting two distinct subtypes. Am J Surg Pathol 2001;25:1134–42.
159. Paal E, Miettinen M. Retroperitoneal leiomyomas: a clinicopathologic and immunohistochemical study of 56 cases with a comparison to retroperitoneal leiomyosarcomas. Am J Surg Pathol 2001;25:1355–63.
160. Billings SD, Folpe AL, Weiss SW. Do leiomyomas of deep soft tissue exist? An analysis of highly differentiated smooth muscle tumors of deep soft tissue supporting two distinct subtypes. Am J Surg Pathol 2001;25:1134–42.

Implantation and Placenta

32

Eoghan E. Mooney

CHAPTER OUTLINE

Introduction	741	Architectural and Developmental Abnormalities	750
Anatomy and Embryology	741	Microscopic Lesions of the Placenta	757
Implantation and Early Pregnancy	741	Placental Inflammation and Infection	757
Functional Unit of the Placenta	745	Vascular Lesions	759
Examination of the Placenta	745	Non-Trophoblastic Tumors of the Placenta	764
Umbilical Cord	745		
Membranes	748		
Meconium on Cord and Membranes	749		

INTRODUCTION

Interest in placental examination has increased in the last two decades, with more appreciation by obstetricians and neonatologists of the contribution the report can make to understanding adverse perinatal outcomes. Not every placenta need be examined, and a triage system is essential. Indications for examination are essentially any disease of the mother, and abnormality of pregnancy, labor, delivery, or the immediate postnatal period. Placental abnormalities should prompt at least macroscopic evaluation. In most institutions, this constitutes 10–15% of deliveries. Placental examination is an integral part of the fetal or perinatal autopsy and adds conclusive or important information in between one-third and two-thirds of such cases.[1,2] While the delivery suite may be the ideal place to initiate microbiology and cytogenetic testing, full pathologic evaluation requires a laboratory-based grossing station with adequate photographic and other facilities. For those cases judged by the pathologist to only require gross examination, retention of formalin-fixed tissue can permit subsequent histologic examination in cases where an abnormality becomes apparent in neonatal life, rather than at birth. In addition to providing information to clinicians and parents, the placenta has been described as 'an amazingly good defensive witness in "bad baby" lawsuits.'[3]

In examining the placenta, the pathologist has the advantage of having the entire organ. Even so, many other variables must be taken into account to interpret the morphologic findings correctly. The gestational age may not be entirely accurate. Important data such as the infant's weight, changes in growth patterns, and other biophysical parameters are not always provided. Even with these, the variable villous patterns can make clinical correlation difficult. Proper sampling of sections for histology is also important in order to avoid false conclusions.

This chapter aims to provide the pathologist with a structured approach to the placental features most commonly encountered in routine practice. Background information on morphogenesis is provided to assist in interpretation.

ANATOMY AND EMBRYOLOGY

IMPLANTATION AND EARLY PREGNANCY

Fertilization, cell division, formation of the morula, and later formation of a blastocyst are independent of maternal contact. The blastocyst reaches the uterus on day 3 after fertilization and implants by the end of day 7.

The process of implantation has three phases: muscular, adhesive, and invasive. The muscular phase concerns transport of the conceptus to the optimal site for implantation, which in humans is the mid to high posterior wall of the uterus in the mid-sagittal plane (Figure 32.1). Implantation in different locations may be associated with different pathologies, e.g., fundal placentation shows an association with intrauterine growth retardation (IUGR).[4] During the adhesive phase, the normally repulsive interactions between two epithelial surfaces (endometrium and trophoblast) are reversed. In the invasive phase, irregular projections of syncytiotrophoblast invade into the endometrium (Figure 32.2). This phase lasts until approximately day 8 post conception and is called the prelacunar phase, based on the appearance of the blastocyst. At day 8 vacuoles appear in the syncytiotrophoblast, which become confluent to form lacunae. This change commences at the implantation pole and becomes confluent over the blastocyst by day 13. At this

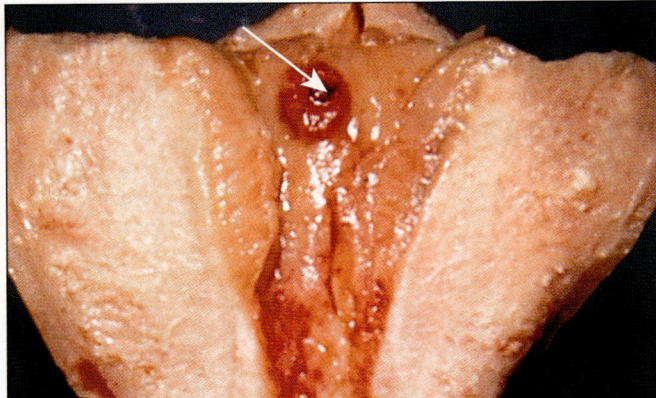

Figure 32.1 Implantation (arrow) in early pregnancy.

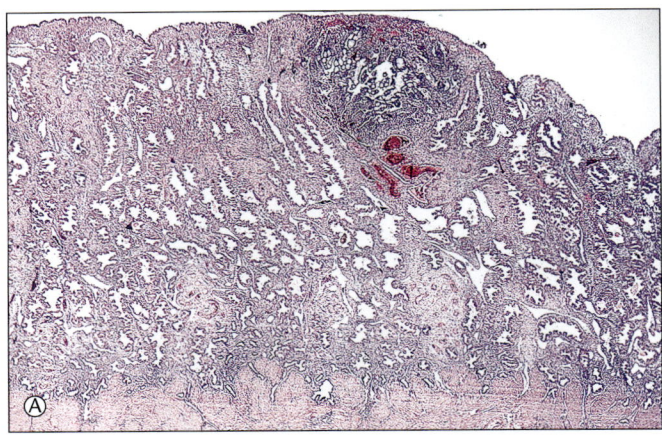

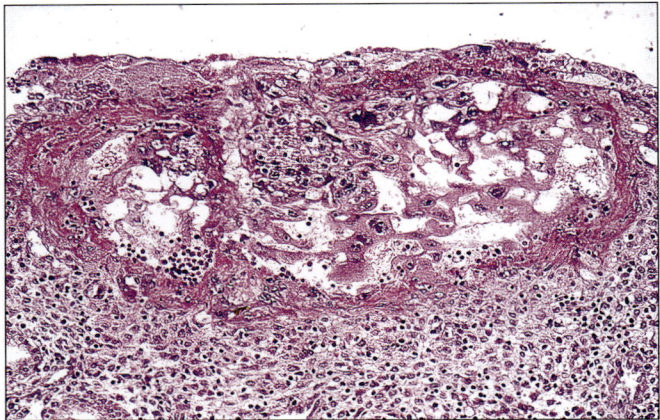

Figure 32.2 Primitive trophoblast. Chorionic villi have not yet formed in the pregnancy of about 1 week's duration.

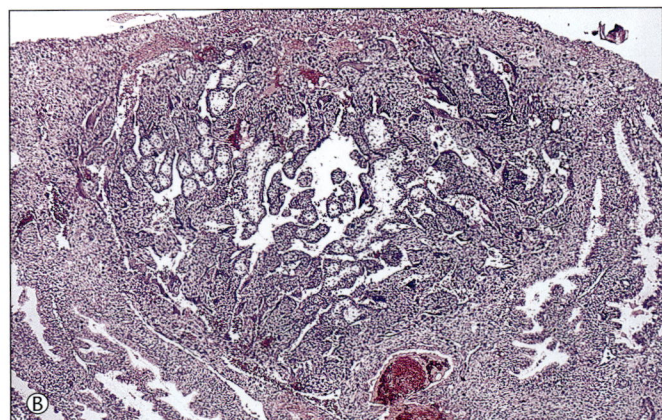

Figure 32.3 **(A)** Day 14 conceptus as a tiny implant in superficial endometrium. **(B)** Detail of the earliest stage of chorionic villous formation.

stage, the earliest forms of chorionic villi begin to form (Figure 32.3) and the primary chorionic plate consists of a continuous layer of cytotrophoblast on the embryoblast side of the lacunae. Infiltration of the pillars of syncytiotrophoblast surrounding the lacunae by cytotrophoblast from the chorionic plate is followed by expansion of these pillars as extraembryonic mesenchyme follows cytotrophoblast. The outermost layer of trophoblast (the trophoblast shell) is formed by syncytiotrophoblast, and later by cytotrophoblast as well. Cytotrophoblast continues to invade endometrium and is seen as clusters of extratrophoblast ('X' cells) and trophoblastic giant cells in what will become the basal plate. The lacunar space becomes the intervillous space, and the embryologic development of villi proceeds during gestation. These developments are maximal at the deep aspect of the blastocyst and normally only this persists to form the true placenta (chorion frondosum). The remainder atrophies (chorion laeve) (Figure 32.4).

The cytotrophoblastic shell thins and is replaced by Nitabuch's fibrin layer, which is composed of matrix-type fibrinoid and lies between the shell and the decidual boundaries. The fibrinoid between the shell and the intervillous space is called Rohr's fibrinoid and is fibrin-type fibrinoid. The two are indistinguishable on routine H&E sections, but may be differentiated immunohistochemically using antibodies directed against oncofetal fibronectin for matrix-type fibrinoid and fibrin for fibrin-type fibrinoid.

The decidua is not merely the passive recipient of the conceptus, but plays an active role in successful placentation.[5] Cytotrophoblastic cells stream out from the tips of the anchoring villi, penetrate the trophoblastic shell, and colonize the decidua and adjacent myometrium of the placental bed. These cells, which are reactive for human placental lactogen and cytokeratins, are called interstitial extravillous trophoblast. A subset of these called 'intravascular extravillous cytotrophoblast' invades and plugs the lumens of the decidual spiral arteries. The cells destroy the endothelium and the elastic and muscular tissues of the media, which are then replaced by fibrinoid material derived from fibrin and trophoblastic secretions. This produces large diameter vessels lacking intrinsic tone that allow a high-flow, low-pressure system to develop. Low oxygen tension may help control entry of cytotrophoblast into the S-phase of the cell cycle, while proliferation and high ambient oxygen tension may lead to an invasive phenotype. The higher oxygen tensions in the nontransformed spiral arteries may induce the expression of invasive integrins, a vascular adhesion molecule phenotype, and cessation of mitotic activity. This may

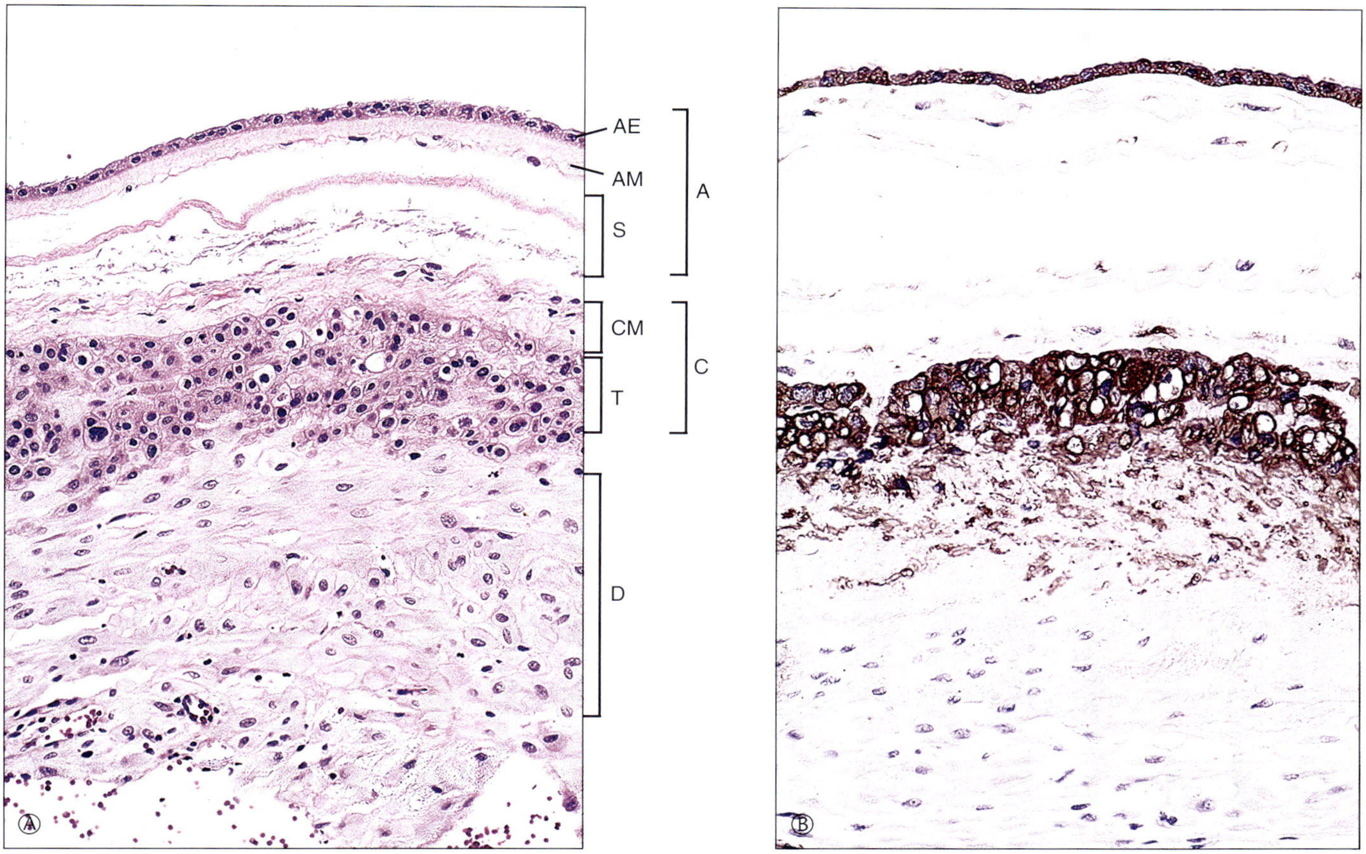

Figure 32.4 Normal membrane in a third trimester placenta. **(A)** Amnion (A), parts of which include amnionic epithelium (AE), amnionic mesoderm (AM), and spongy level (S); the chorionic plate (C) is composed of chorionic mesoderm (CM) and trophoblast (T); beneath that is the maternal decidua (D). **(B)** Both the trophoblast and amnionic epithelium are markedly reactive for cytokeratin (CAM 5.2).

explain why trophoblast only superficially invades the uterine veins. Trophoblast may switch to a noninvasive phenotype by becoming multinucleate.

Development in the first trimester takes place in a relatively hypoxic environment, and this is protective to the embryo. A trophoblast plug prevents maternal blood entering the intervillous space and early embryonic nutrition is provided by endometrial glands, perhaps facilitated by endoglandular trophoblast.[6] The trophoblast plug is seen to be deficient in many early losses (Figure 32.5). This results in the precocious onset of the maternal circulation, exposing the developing placenta to a higher oxygen concentration and to a higher arterial pressure. As spiral artery transformation is less effective peripherally, oxidative stress may be the mechanism by which villous regression occurs in the chorion laeve.[7] Patterns of regression influence placental shape and cord insertion, and localized abnormalities of flow may result in a cord that was initially paracentral becoming marginal or velamentous. Noncentral cords are associated with lower birth weights, suggesting that their vasculature is less metabolically effective.[8] Suboptimal or shallow implantation results in inadequate conversion of maternal spiral arterioles in the inner third of the myometrium. The resultant retention of vascular smooth muscle permits intermittent pulsatile contraction, resulting in

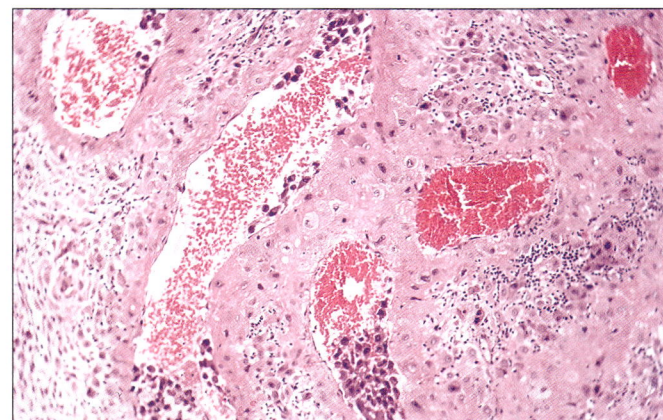

Figure 32.5 A transforming spiral artery. Intravascular trophoblast and extravillous interstitial trophoblast are present.

mechanical and oxidative stress to the developing placenta.

Placental growth trajectories are established by the end of the first trimester, with cases of IUGR having smaller placentas than normal at 12 weeks, but similar growth after that. Villous development shows a major change from

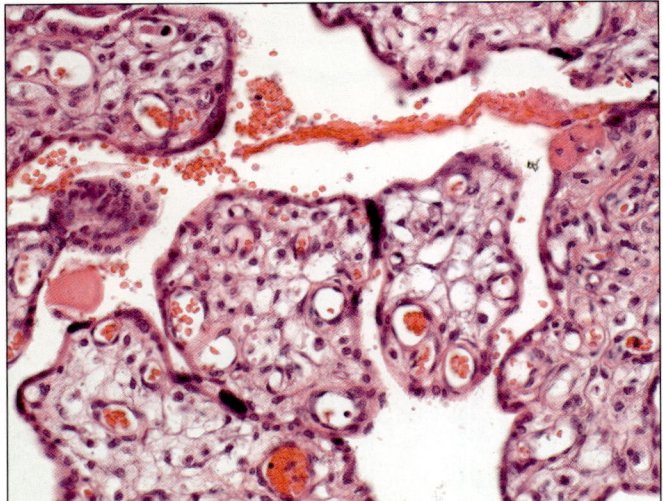

Figure 32.6 Immature intermediate villi with a reticular stroma.

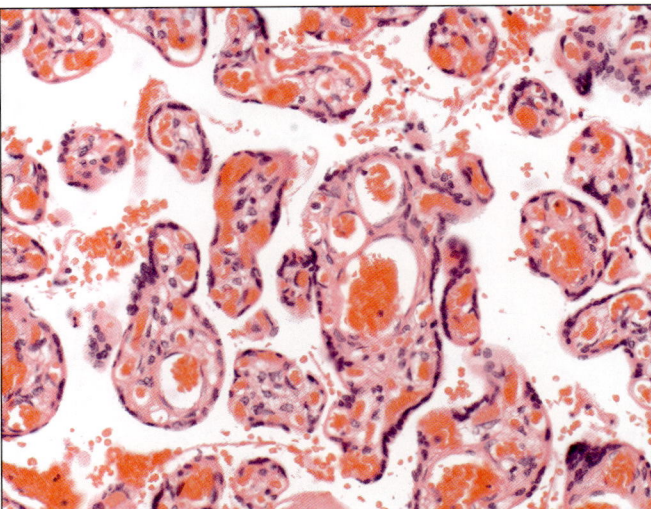

Figure 32.7 Mature intermediate villi.

growth to differentiation at the end of the second trimester. Protrusions of trophoblast (trophoblast sprouts) into the lacunae are the forerunners of villi. Initially, the sprouts consist of syncytiotrophoblast, which are followed by cytotrophoblast and by connective tissue containing fetal capillaries. The villi thus formed are termed mesenchymal villi and are the precursors of all other villous types. While they are the dominant type in the first trimester, some trophoblast sprouting and mesenchymal villous development probably occurs up to term.

Immature intermediate villi (100–200 µm in size) are formed from mesenchymal villi and are primarily responsible for placental growth (Figure 32.6). They have a complete trophoblastic mantle with many cytotrophoblastic cells present, but lack vasculosyncytial membranes. The syncytial nuclei are evenly dispersed without knots. They have a loose (reticular) stroma with abundant stromal channels containing Hofbauer cells. They are the dominant villous type seen in the second trimester and are transformed into stem villi when their production from mesenchymal villi decreases.

Stem villi are defined by 50% or more of their stroma being compact and containing vessels with media or adventitia identifiable on light microscopy. They range in size from 80 to 1500 µm and connect the chorionic plate to the remaining distal villous tree. Some stem villi connect to the basal plate (anchoring villi). They have both an arterial and a venous circulation, which (depending on size) consist of either arteries and veins or arterioles and venules. The trophoblastic cover is predominantly syncytiotrophoblast and may be replaced with fibrinoid in the mature placenta. A perivascular capillary network is more prominent in less mature stem villi and reflects their origin from immature intermediate villi. The localization of myofibroblasts and smooth muscle cells in stem villi has been defined immunohistochemically and these cells may play a role in villous vascular regulation.

Mature intermediate villi (Figure 32.7) are formed from the mesenchymal villi in the third trimester and give rise to the majority of terminal villi. They are 60–150 µm in

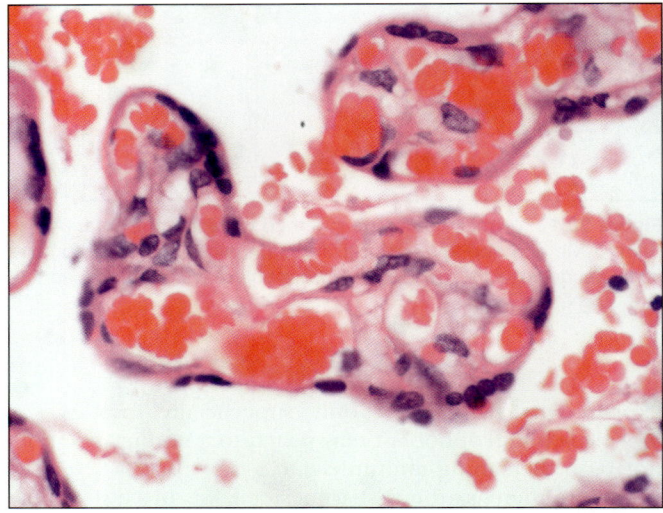

Figure 32.8 Normal terminal villi: over 50% of their area is capillary.

diameter and contain capillaries, arterioles, and venules. The stroma is loose and the vessels constitute less than half the villous cross-sectional area. The syncytiotrophoblast has a uniform structure without vasculosyncytial membranes or knots. At term, mature intermediate villi make up one-fourth of the parenchyma.

Terminal villi (40–60 µm) (Figure 32.8) are the site of gaseous exchange and derive from the mature intermediate villi. They arise as capillary growths which, in exceeding that of parent mature intermediate villi, result in trophoblastic protrusions. The capillaries are dilated and constitute over 50% of the villus cross-sectional area. Optimal gas exchange requires the formation of vasculosyncytial membranes. The syncytiotrophoblast nuclei become pushed to one side so that only an attenuated layer of syncytiotrophoblastic cytoplasm remains applied to its basement membrane, which is itself applied to the capillary's basement membrane. The capillaries are 3–5 mm long and each maintains its own nonbranching structure. They do not form a capillary network, but remain as long capillaries. In addition, the capillaries have varicosities where their diameters enlarge considerably. The exact functional significance of these varicosities is unknown, although a regulatory function where vascular deformation alters flow has been proposed. These villi appear at 27 weeks of gestation and increase in number until term, when they make up 40% of villi.

The placenta's maternal surface is partitioned by septum formation. As collections of cytotrophoblast, the so-called 'cell columns,' anchor the decidua to the villi; their growth rates differ so that slow-growing ones tend to pull up the decidual basal plate, buckling it into the placental septa. These septa are incomplete and rarely reach the chorionic plate. They have no precise anatomic relationship to the functional units of the placenta.

FUNCTIONAL UNIT OF THE PLACENTA

The placenta's functional unit is variously known as the fetal lobule, fetal cotyledon, or fetal villous tree. At term, the normal placenta contains 40–60 lobules, each 2–4 cm in diameter. The central area receives the oxygenated blood from the maternal spiral arteries and shows an increased number of immature intermediate villi. The surrounding, more densely packed villi show a predominance of mature intermediate and terminal villi. This is the area where gas exchange is maximal, as the blood slowly percolates around small villi that have vasculosyncytial membranes. At the lobule's periphery is the venous outflow area through which blood drains to the 50–200 maternal venous outlets. Despite the apparent continuity of the intervillous space, each lobule relies upon its own spiral artery. Thrombosis of that artery results in infarction in that lobule.

EXAMINATION OF THE PLACENTA

UMBILICAL CORD

Abnormalities of the cord are associated with adverse outcomes and with stasis-induced abnormalities in the fetal vasculature.[9] Cord length should be measured, but the possibility that sections of the cord may have been removed shortly after delivery should be excluded before a short cord is reported. The average cord length at term is 60 cm. Longer cords are associated with hypermotility and shorter ones with hypomotility. Neural tube defects and chromosomal abnormalities are sometimes the underlying cause of the latter. The lower limit for a normal cord varies, but seems to be around 35 cm and a short cord is associated with an increased risk of death in term infants. In an 18 year retrospective review, excessively long cords (≥70 cm) were associated with a range of gross and microscopic features, and with abnormal neurologic status in infants.[10] Clinical or pathologic abnormalities of the cord were found in 70% of infants with fetal thrombotic vasculopathy.[11] False knots (vascular loops) may be present (Figure 32.9), but usually are of no clinical significance. The maximum diameter should be measured both, sonographically[12] and pathologically; a thin cord (<8 mm) is associated with poor flow and growth restriction.

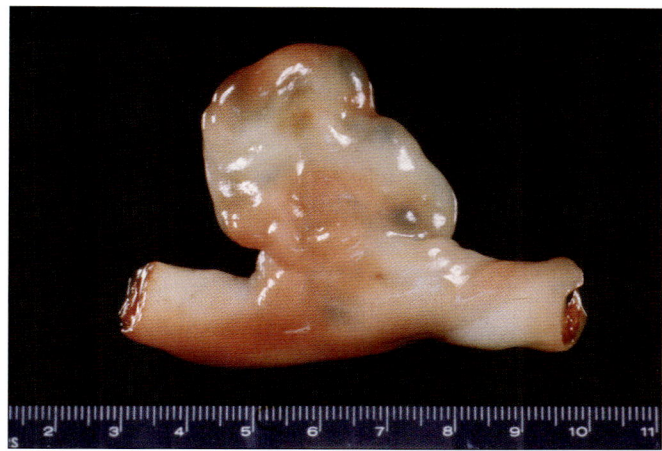
Figure 32.9 Umbilical cord with false knots (vascular loops).

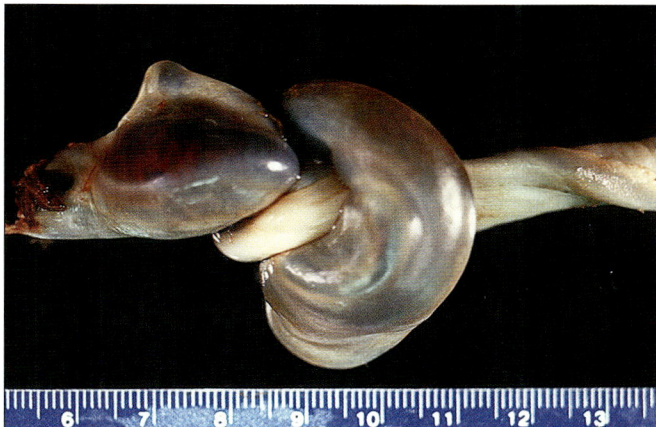
Figure 32.10 Umbilical cord with a single true knot.

True knots (Figure 32.10) occur in approximately 1% of pregnancies. They are more likely to occur with a long cord, with polyhydramnios, and with male fetuses.[13] The knots may be single or multiple. Chronic changes (grooving of the cord, edema, vascular congestion, or thrombosis) or their absence should be specifically commented on. The fetus with a long cord is less able to exert traction on the knot *in utero*. The effects of a knot are mediated by its tightening with traction, causing vascular compromise. This may happen at delivery, but then the chronic changes will be absent. Documentation of a true knot *in utero* is difficult, and a loose knot may be formed after intrauterine death. The lack of a difference in blood gas values between neonates with true knots and those without supports the interpretation that most knots are clinically insignificant.[14] However, a true knot is more commonly associated with other cord problems including nuchal cord and cord prolapse, either of which may contribute to the observed increase in antepartum (but not intrapartum) stillbirths. Cord pathology is associated with fetal thrombotic vasculopathy. A feature to be sought in such cases is an increase in nucleated red blood cells, a finding that supports a conclusion of subacute hypoxic stress.[15]

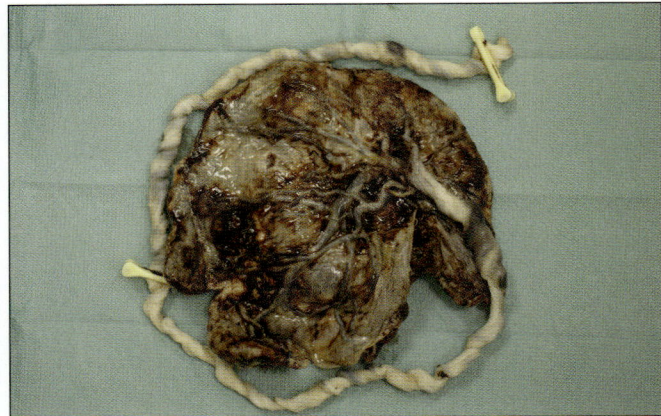

Figure 32.11 Long hypercoiled cord.

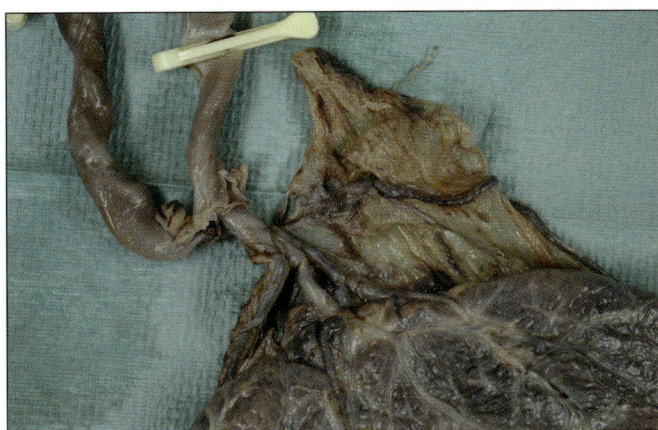

Figure 32.13 Velamentous insertion, with vessels branching to run in the membranes.

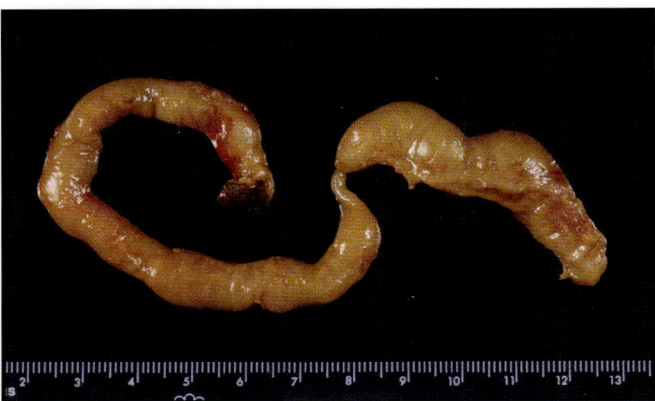

Figure 32.12 Stricture in umbilical cord.

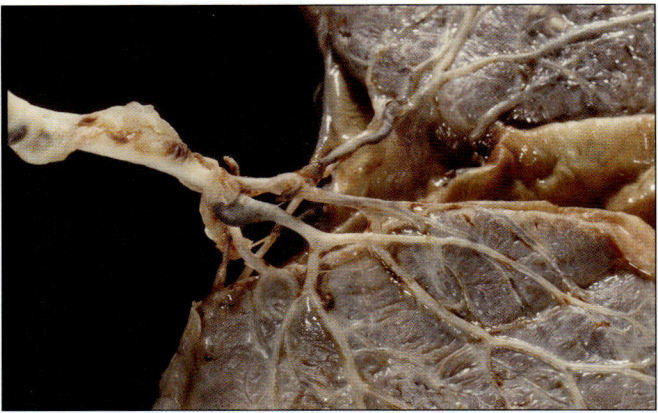

Figure 32.14 Furcate (branched) insertion of umbilical cord.

Coiling of the cord is normal. It is greater at the fetal end and is variable throughout the length of the cord. A literature review has indicated 0.17 ± 0.009 spirals completed per centimeter.[16] The 10th–90th percentile range is one per 3 cm to one per 14 cm on this basis. The mean coiling index (number of coils/length in cm) has varied from 0.13 to 0.28:[17] the 'mean of the means' of the studies listed was 0.20. A long and/or hypercoiled cord (Figure 32.11) will require a greater pressure gradient because of increased shear stresses. Both hypo- and hypercoiling of the cord are associated with a range of adverse pregnancy outcomes, including pregnancy loss and IUGR. The cord may show a stricture (Figure 32.12). Stricture and/or hypercoiling was reported in 19% of fetal deaths[18] and thrombosis of chorionic plate vessels was seen in 54% of these cases. Given the importance of the diagnosis, a thoughtful review of coiling has called for 'a return to basic but critical mensuration.'[17]

The cord may insert centrally, eccentrically, and marginally or have a velamentous insertion. The last two are the most significant. In marginal insertion, the cord joins the disc at its edge. Cord insertion directly onto the membranes (velamentous insertion) (Figure 32.13) occurs in approximately 1% of singleton deliveries. The vessels are at risk of compression and thrombosis, and rupture may lead to significant fetal blood loss and hypoxia. In addition to intrapartum events, velamentous insertion is associated with an increased risk of preterm delivery, low birth weight, and abnormalities of fetal heart rate.[19] Vessels may be present in the membranes in up to 7% of placentas, but vasa previa (vessels in the membranes in advance of the presenting part) are less common (1:2500 deliveries). In addition to velamentous insertion, other risk factors for vasa previa include a bilobed or succenturiate placenta, a low-lying placenta, and multiple IVF pregnancies. Prenatal diagnosis reduces the mortality rate, and screening of all twin pregnancies has been reported to be cost-effective.[20] When examining a placenta where this has been queried clinically, a measurement of the length of the vessels in the membranes and a comment on whether they are intact or not is appropriate. We have found that marking a torn area with ink helps in microscopic evaluation.

In the third stage of labor, avulsion of the cord may occur due to traction and this may cause subamniotic hemorrhage. However, this form of hemorrhage may also occur where a central or eccentric insertion is furcate (Figure 32.14), i.e., where cord vessels have lost their cover of Wharton's jelly and have splayed out prior to inserting into the disc. In most cases fresh subamniotic hemorrhage is of no clinical significance. In some cases there may be hematomas of the cord without apparent explanation (Figure 32.15).

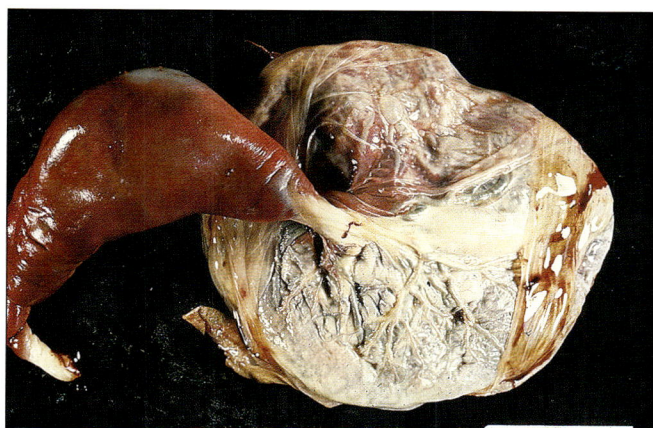

Figure 32.15 Hematoma of umbilical cord.

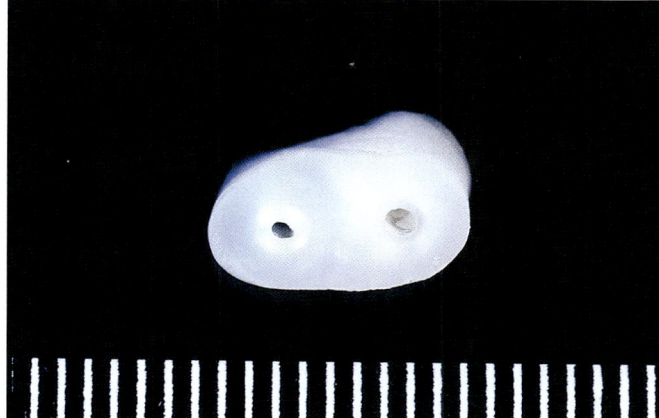

Figure 32.16 Two-vessel umbilical cord.

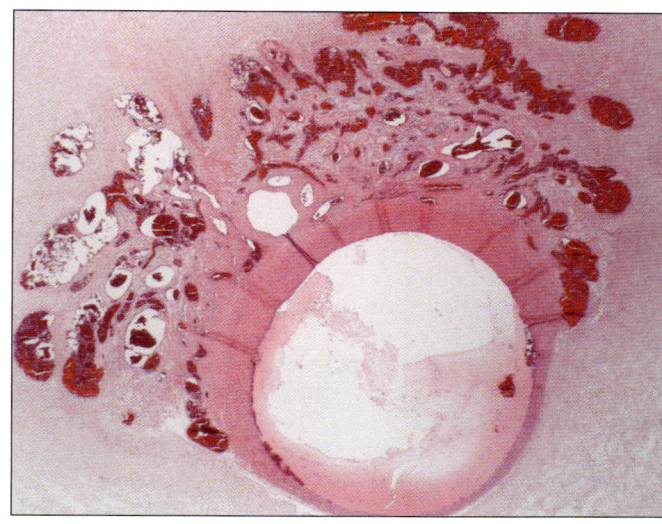

Figure 32.17 Hemangioma of the cord.

The normal cord has three vessels—two umbilical arteries and one umbilical vein. A single umbilical artery, i.e., a two-vessel cord, occurs in 0.5–1% of deliveries (Figure 32.16). As the arteries may fuse in the 5 cm before insertion into the placenta, further sections nearer the fetal end of the cord should be examined before a single artery is reported. One-third of cases of single umbilical artery are associated with other congenital abnormalities, including trisomy 18, and abnormalities of the heart, gastrointestinal and urinary tracts, and central nervous system. Isolated single umbilical artery is associated in some studies with increased preterm deliveries, growth restriction, and adverse outcomes.[21] Other studies did not show a difference in perinatal outcome or long-term development.[22]

Supernumerary vessels are rare and may be either arterial or venous. Tumors of the cord are also rare. Most are hemangiomas (Figure 32.17) but occasional angiomyxomas and teratomas have been reported. The muscularis of cord vessels may be focally thin. Confirmation of a possible association with congenital malformations is needed, given the small numbers of cases reported.[23] Grossly or sonographically visible cysts may develop from the vestigial remnants that are usually found as incidental microscopic findings. These remnants may be of the allantoic duct (possessing a flattened or transition cell-type epithelium; Figure 32.18A)

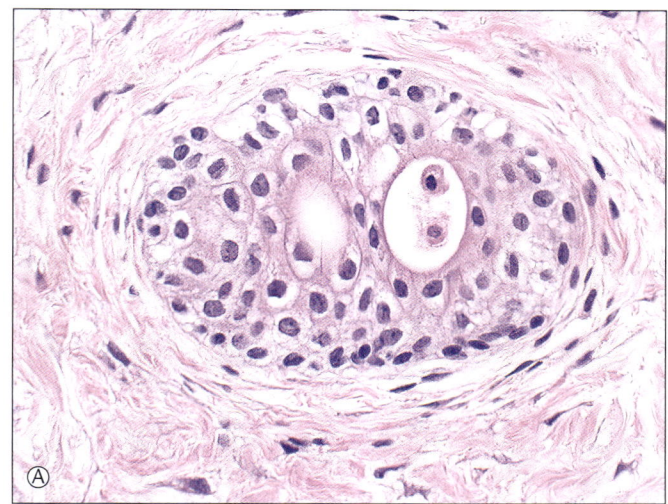

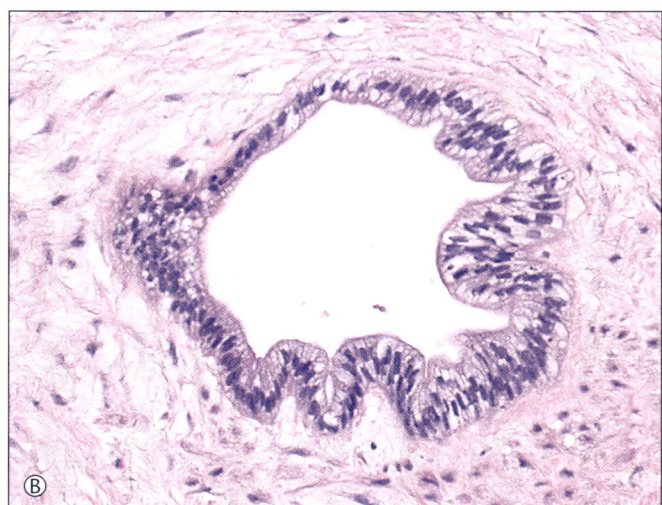

Figure 32.18 **(A, B)** Normal findings in umbilical cord. **(A)** Allantoic duct (possessing a flattened or transition cell-type epithelium), residual urinary tract system. **(B)** Omphalomesenteric duct (cuboidal epithelium with mucinous component), residual digestive system.

or omphalomesenteric duct (cuboidal epithelium with mucinous component; Figure 32.18B).

The surface of the cord may appear edematous in some cases with acute inflammation. Traction and/or clamping should be excluded. An edematous cord with a reddish discoloration typically occurs with maceration.

MEMBRANES

Acute chorioamnionitis is mainly caused by bacteria. It is the major cause of preterm birth, but it is still not clear if it is a cause or effect of either preterm rupture of membranes or preterm labor.[24] While there are clinical guidelines for recognition of infected membranes histologic chorioamnionitis is a better surrogate of intra-amniotic infection. The severity of chorioamnionitis shows a direct correlation with proteomic signatures of inflammation.[25] Organisms may or may not be cultured: group B *Streptococcus* and *Escherichia coli* are important causes of chorioamnionitis, with organisms such as *Ureaplasma urealyticum* frequently seen in mixed culture.

With early, mild acute inflammation, regardless of the organism, the membranes may be grossly normal or edematous. More advanced inflammation produces a milky opacity, altering the normal gray-purple color of the disc. There may be frank pus with an offensive odor. Meconium may obscure the alterations of the acute inflammatory infiltrate.

A section of membranes should be taken, extending from the rupture site to the margin of the disc and prepared for histologic examination as a roll. The yield is influenced by the extent of sampling, with increased yield up to four sections.[26] Criteria for categorization of the maternal and fetal inflammatory responses as early, intermediate, or advanced, and grading of both as mild/moderate or severe have been published[27] (Figures 32.19 and 32.20). These are summarized in Table 32.1. Severity of the maternal response is defined by the presence of subchorionic microabscesses, or three or more confluent polymorph bands, and in the fetal response as near-confluent bands. Amnionic inflammation is a better predictor of neonatal sepsis than funisitis in preterm gestations.[28] The inflammatory pattern and the time taken to mount an inflammatory response may primarily reflect the virulence of the infecting organism. Organisms of low virulence (e.g., *Ureaplasma*, *Mycoplasma*, and anaerobes) may cause preterm labor, but not bacteremia in the neonate. They probably take days rather than hours to reach the placenta. Virulent organisms, e.g., group B *Streptococcus*, *E. coli*, and *Listeria*, can cause bacteremia and may reach the placenta in hours rather than days. However, membrane integrity, maternal immune status, and cytokine gene polymorphisms play a role. Gestational age is also of importance; chorionic vasculitis is less prevalent with increased gestational age. Data correlating chorioamnionitis with bacterial *in situ* hybridization suggest that organisms invade through a focal area of the membranes, proliferate in the amniotic fluid, and invade the membranes from there.[29] The presence of acutely inflamed membranes should prompt a search for associated lesions, such as thrombi, and exclusion of coexistent pathology, such as

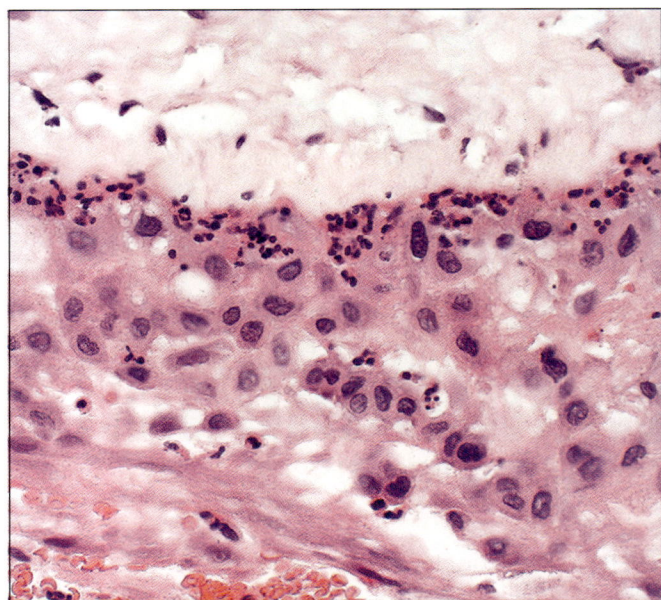

Figure 32.19 Acute chorioamnionitis, stage 1 (Table 32.1). The inflammation involves the trophoblast, but not the spongy layer of the amnion.

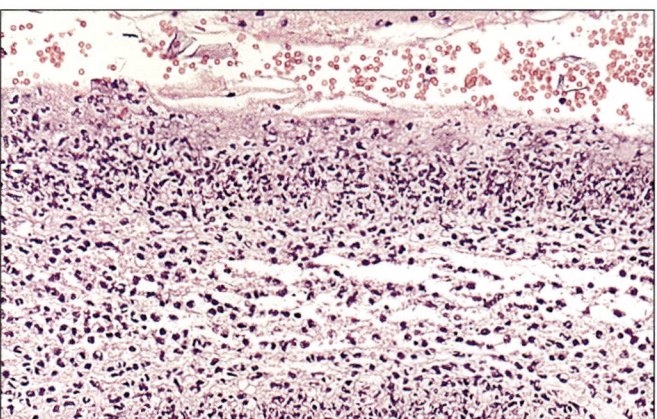

Figure 32.20 Acute chorioamnionitis, stage 3 (Table 32.1). The inflammation pervades all structures and destroys the amnionic epithelium.

Table 32.1		Categorization of Inflammatory Responses in Acute Chorioamnionitis
Response	**Stage**	**Features**
Maternal	1	PMN in subchorionic fibrin or membrane trophoblast
	2	PMN in fibrous chorion and/or amnion
	3	PMN karyorrhexis, necrosis of amnion
Fetal	1	PMN in umbilical vein or chorionic plate vessels
	2	PMN in one or more umbilical arteries
	3	PMN ± debris with perivasculitis

PMN, polymorphonuclear leukocytes.
Adapted from Redline et al.[27]

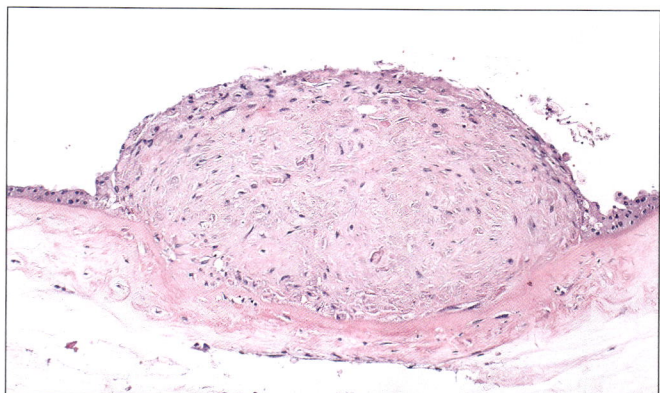

Figure 32.22 Amnion nodosum.

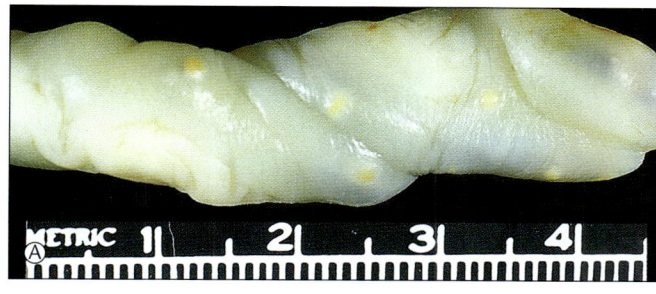

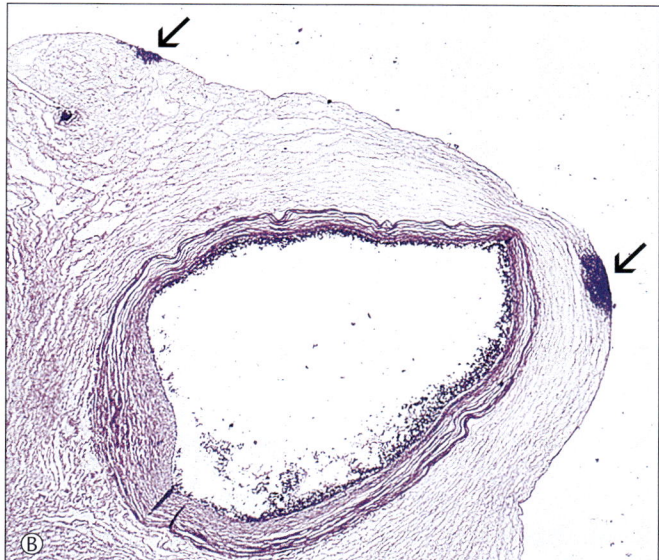

Figure 32.21 **(A, B)** *Candida* funisitis. **(A)** Small white flecks are on the surface, which **(B)** microscopically are *Candida* organisms (arrows).

retroplacental hemorrhage, where chorioamnionitis is more common.

In addition to bacteria, fungi and viruses may also cause infection via the ascending pathway. In *Candida* chorioamnionitis, numerous yellow-white spongy flecks stud the membranes and umbilical cord (Figure 32.21).

The clinical significance of chorioamnionitis and funisitis depends on gestational age and severity. Ascending infection is a major cause of preterm premature rupture of the membranes, which accounts for 30–40% of preterm births. Increasing stages of chorioamnionitis show a significant association with funisitis, preterm birth, and perinatal death. Funisitis has been directly linked with development of fetal germinal matrix hemorrhages, choroiditis with intraventricular hemorrhage, and periventricular leukomalacia.[30,31] For term infants, there is an increased risk of sepsis following chorioamnionitis, but neurologic morbidity may be related to other complications of labor.[32] In one study of very low birth weight infants, vascular thrombi associated with chorioamnionitis were felt to account for neurologic impairment.[33] An association between chorioamnionitis and adverse developmental outcome has not been demonstrated in other studies on similar groups.[34] Defining initiators of preterm birth (i.e., uteroplacental insufficiency vs inflammation) may be important in documenting their long-term

effects[35] and placental inflammation shows an association with poor neonatal growth.[36]

Decidual necrosis manifests as a shaggy, cream-yellow area, usually present near the margin of the placental disc. Nodularity of the amnion may be due to either amnion nodosum or squamous metaplasia. Amnion nodosum is a consequence of oligohydramnios and presents as 1–3 mm nodules that may be relatively easily detached. Microscopy shows aggregates of amorphous and cellular debris (Figure 32.22), and may include detached hair. With squamous metaplasia, which has no known clinical associations, the nodules are only detached with difficulty.

Abnormalities of the membranes may cause fetal malformation. Some may be fatal such as body stalk anomaly. Amniotic bands should be sought in the context of more restricted fetal abnormalities, including amputation, acral deformities, or even craniofacial abnormalities that may resemble neural tube defects. These bands are delicate strands of amnion and mesoderm whose effects may be predominantly or exclusively mechanical. They may be focal or extensive, and have been reported in Ehlers–Danlos syndrome and osteogenesis imperfecta.

MECONIUM ON CORD AND MEMBRANES

Meconium-stained amniotic fluid is seen in 14% of deliveries, and is present in approximately 1% of deliveries at 32 weeks, compared with 100% at 42 weeks. Its passage at term may be physiologic, but is generally felt to reflect hypoxic stress in the fetus.[37] We regard the presence of scanty macrophages with non-hemosiderin pigments as normal and physiologic: indeed, fetal defecation has been documented sonographically.[38] More extensive meconium passage produces a green discoloration grossly. Meconium may reach superficial amnionic macrophages (Figure 32.23) in 1 hour and chorionic macrophages in 3 hours. They may remain in the amnion or chorion for a week after the meconium is no longer visible in the amniotic fluid. Meconium acts as a vasoconstrictor on the fetoplacental vasculature, and may result in necrosis of smooth muscle cells of umbilical cord vessels (Figure 32.24) or cause ulceration of the cord.[39] The changes in muscle cells may mimic a vasculitis. The inflammation that meconium induces is maximal in the cord, but is less intense and more focal than that due to the vasculitis

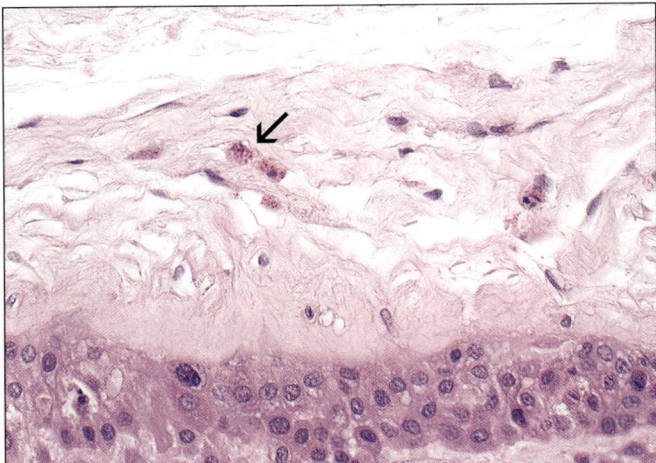

Figure 32.23 Meconium in a macrophage (arrow) is a light brown pigment usually less refractile than hemosiderin.

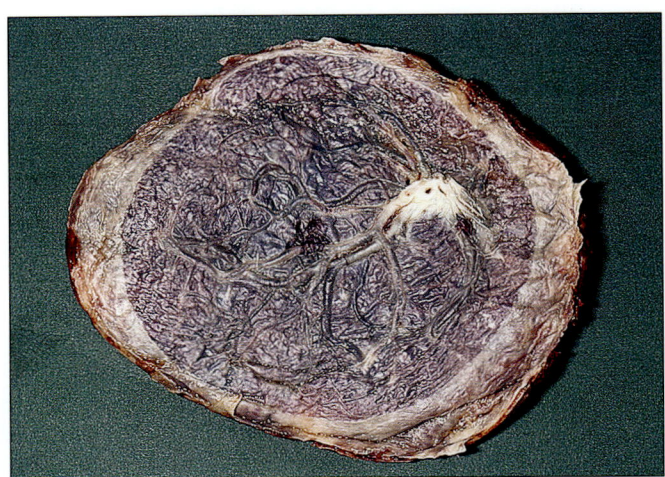

Figure 32.25 Circummarginate placenta.

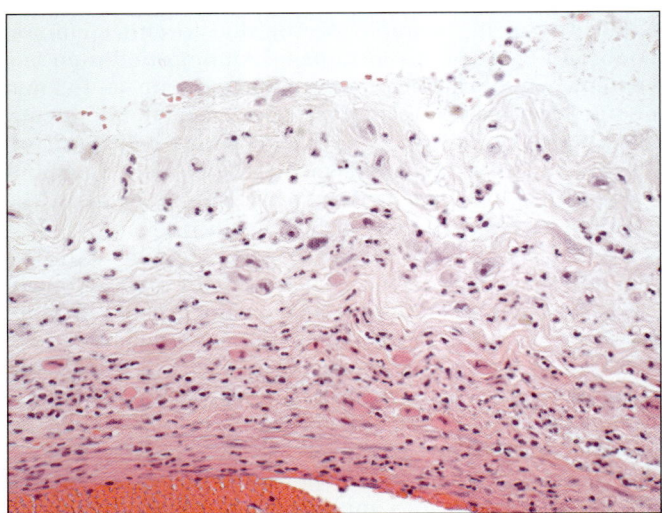

Figure 32.24 Meconium-induced vascular necrosis. Note the injured myocytes with a rounded hypereosinophilic appearance.

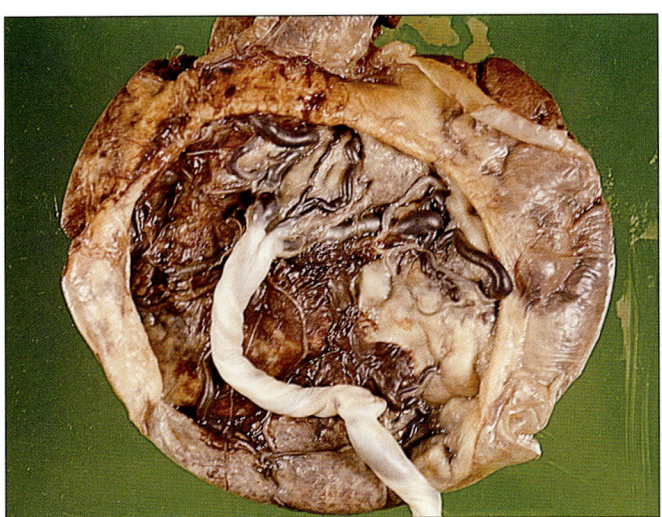

Figure 32.26 Circumvallate placenta. The membranes fold back upon themselves on the surface of the placenta.

of chorioamnionitis. Documentation of its presence is important, as thick meconium is associated with adverse pregnancy outcome. If aspirated, meconium produces significant pneumonitis.

ARCHITECTURAL AND DEVELOPMENTAL ABNORMALITIES

Extrachorial placentation is where the chorion laeve inserts at some distance inside, rather than at the rim of the placenta. The term 'extrachorial' implies that the edge of the placenta is uncovered except for fibrin and, sometimes, old clotted blood. If the transition is flat, the placenta is called 'circummarginate'; if the edge is rolled up and folded over itself ('plicated'), the placenta is then called 'circumvallate.'

The circummarginate form (Figure 32.25) has no known clinical associations. The circumvallate form (Figure 32.26), however, is associated with threatened abortion, membrane rupture, and antepartum hemorrhage leading to prematurity, but not to an increase in perinatal mortality. Circumvallation is significantly associated with iron-laden macrophages in the membranes, termed 'diffuse chorioamnionic hemosiderosis,'[40] suggesting that circumvallation may be caused by chronic peripheral separation of the placenta. Both types of extrachorial placentation are frequently partial and mixtures between the two and normal placentation are more frequently encountered.

A bilobed placenta has two nearly equal sized discs with the umbilical cord inserting between the two, either in a velamentous fashion or marginally on the larger disc. As discussed previously, inadequate blood flow leads to trophotropism and placentation on both the anterior and posterior endometrial surfaces. These placentas are associated with multiparity, older maternal age, previous history of infertility, assisted

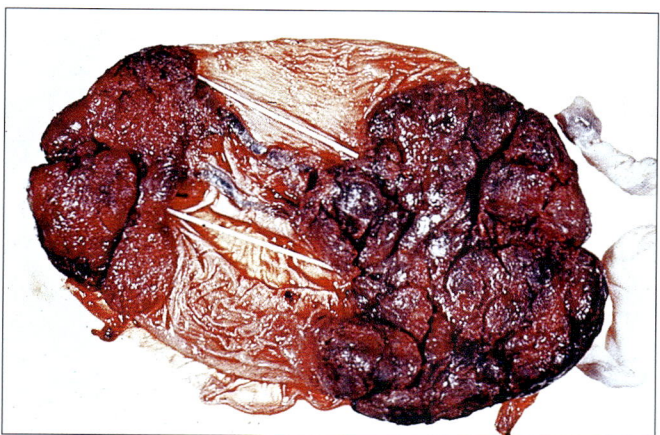

Figure 32.27 Succenturiate, or accessory, lobe of placenta.

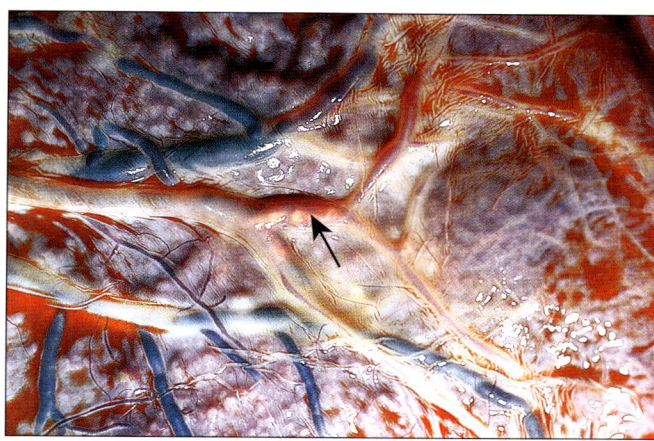

Figure 32.28 Arterial thrombus (arrow), visible on the fetal surface.

reproduction, retention, and abnormal adherence. The vessels between the two may thrombose or present as vasa previa. Higher orders of lobation are extremely rare.

Accessory (succenturiate) lobes are found in 6% of placentas and are areas of placental tissue joined by either an isthmus or velamentous vessels to the main disc (Figure 32.27). If symptomatic, they may present as placenta previa with or without fetal hemorrhage or be retained *in utero* postpartum. Placenta membranacea arises when there is failure of villous regression to form a chorion laeve. Thus, an abnormally thin placenta comes to cover an unusually large area of the uterine lining. The entire conceptual sac is covered with villi and the placenta becomes, in addition, a placenta previa. The placenta on cut section is thinned from the normal 2.5 cm or 3 cm to perhaps 1 cm or less in the fixed state. This condition is sometimes associated with mid-trimester antepartum hemorrhage. It may also sometimes show undue adherence, but normal third-stage delivery usually occurs.

A fenestrate placenta is one where a placental lobule appears to be missing. Careful inspection of the maternal aspect shows that the lobules surrounding the expected location of the missing lobule are smooth, and the featureless overlying chorion is smooth. A girdle or ring placenta is one with the membranes above and below the placental ring. They are rare in humans.

PLACENTAL WEIGHT

Placental weight combined with length, breadth, and thickness has provided valuable epidemiologic information, and is part of the evidence for the fetal origins of adult disease.[41] The placenta should be weighed trimmed of cord and membranes, with any adherent clot removed and weighed separately. Reference values for freshly delivered untrimmed placentas are also available.[42]

Placental weight depends on the *in utero* environment, timing of cord clamping, storage interval, and fixation. The timing of umbilical cord clamping at delivery will either trap a considerable quantity of blood within the placenta if early, or lead to a relatively bloodless organ if delayed. The practice of placental examination in the unfixed state will be associated with fluid loss of variable extent, but it tends to increase with storage time. Formalin fixation of the placenta will result in a gain in weight of often 8–10%, and occasionally up to 15%. There is a trend for increasing placental weight during the past century, which is most likely due to improved nutritional status and environmental factors. Twin placental weights have a ratio of 1.69 above that of the same gestational age singletons.[43] Racial and population differences exist. Recent figures for a North American population of both singletons and twins show a 50th percentile of approximately 675 g for singletons at term[44] and are almost certainly not applicable to all patient cohorts. In this study, the placental to birth weight ratio at term for the 50th percentile was 0.19 for males and 0.20 for girls.

Placentas from infants with IUGR are often small, especially if multiple pathologies are present.[45] Pre-eclamptic placentas tend to be small, as do those with fetal congenital anomalies, infection, and chromosomal abnormalities. Large placentas are found in women living at high altitude, those with diabetes mellitus, rhesus incompatibility, fetal hydrops, maternal and fetal anemia, and some chronic intrauterine infections, e.g., syphilis.

FETAL SURFACE OF PLACENTA

The normal color of the fetal surface is a gray-purple color. Stripping the amnion allows more detailed inspection of the chorionic plate vessels. Normally, fetal arteries run over (i.e., uppermost on) veins. This is valuable to note grossly, as vessels may be difficult to distinguish histologically. Thrombi, which may appear grossly as thickened white areas of the vessel wall, may be subtle and only appreciated on close examination. Thrombi may be seen in arteries (Figure 32.28) and veins (Figure 32.29). Barium gelatin injection of the umbilical arteries is one definitive method to identify arteries (Figure 32.30).

Placental mesenchymal dysplasia shows aneurysmally dilated chorionic plate vessels (Figure 32.31) and focally cystic stem villi with myxomatous stroma and cistern formation, but lacks the trophoblastic features of partial mole. Approximately one-third of cases are associated with Beckwith–Wiedemann syndrome.[46] Most fetuses are female

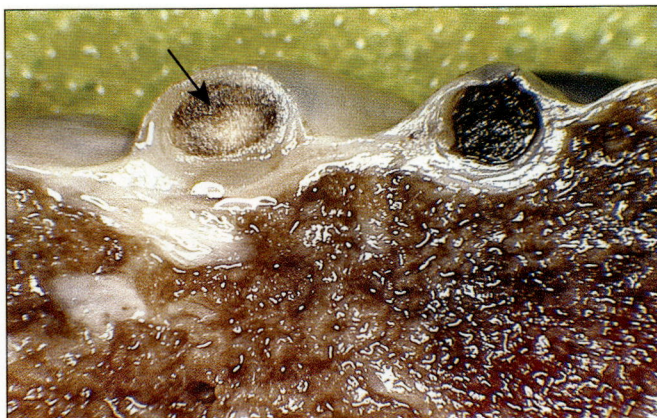

Figure 32.29 Thrombus in a chorionic plate vessel (arrow). The vessel is probably a vein.

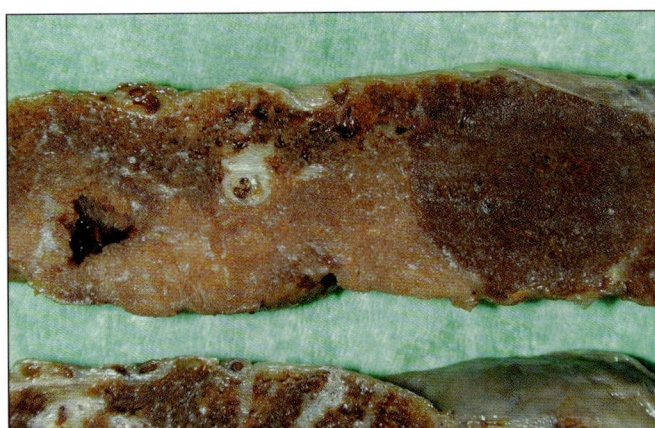

Figure 32.32 Full thickness region of avascular fetal villi appears pale upon fixation. A thrombosed vessel is also visible.

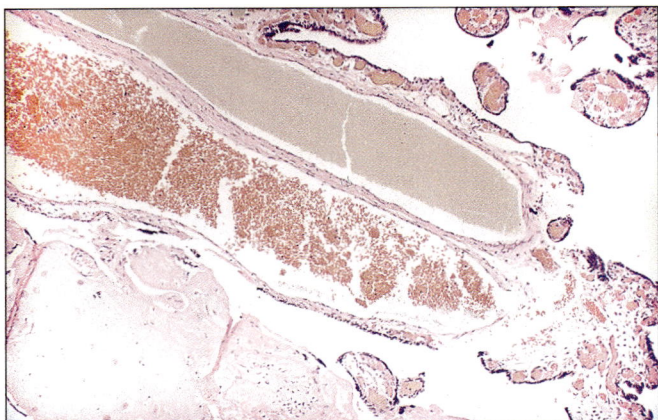

Figure 32.30 Intra-arterial injection of barium gelatin distinguishes artery from vein. (Courtesy of Dr. Peter Kelehan, National Maternity Hospital, Dublin, Ireland.)

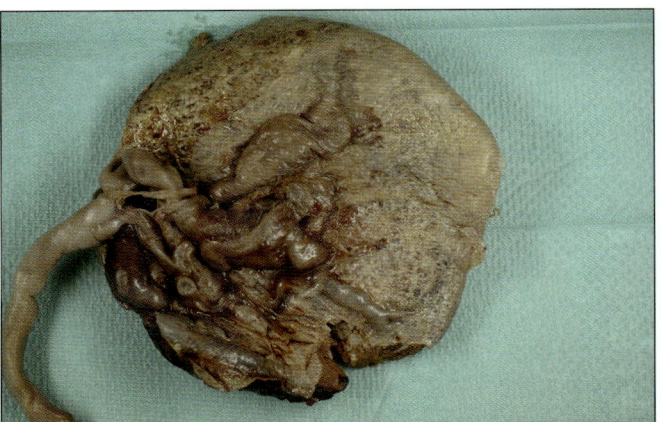

Figure 32.31 Mesenchymal dysplasia from a case of intrauterine death: aneurysmally dilated chorionic vessels are present.

and there is a strong association with IUGR and fetal and neonatal death.[47,48]

MATERNAL SURFACE OF THE PLACENTA

The cotyledons of the placenta should be examined to ensure that the placenta is intact and complete. Evidence of old hemorrhage, manifest as foci of tan-colored granularity, should be sought, especially where there is a clinical history of pre-eclampsia or extensive or central infarction. The presence of hemorrhage and the percentage of the surface affected, its location (central or peripheral), and the presence or absence of cavitation should be noted. A wrinkled gyriform pattern is characteristic of maternal floor infarction. Thrombosed spiral arteries may be detected on examination of the basal plate.[49]

CUT SURFACE

The placenta should be serially sectioned and examined at intervals of 1–2 cm. The parenchyma varies in color depending on the amount of maternal and fetal blood present. A degree of pallor is normal where the disc has been drained, e.g., following manual removal. A dramatic color change in an intact placenta, i.e., a 'two-tone' effect, may be seen in cases of retroplacental hemorrhage.[50] Any lesions should be described as central (inner two-thirds of the disc) or peripheral and the percentage of the parenchyma affected estimated and recorded. Avascular villi may be more easily detected following formalin fixation (Figure 32.32).

INFARCTION

The placenta requires both maternal and fetal blood flow for normal function. The spectrum of uteroplacental ischemia ranges from changes such as increased syncytial knots (discussed under microscopic findings) to infarction. Acute cessation of maternal blood flow results in a placental infarct. The placenta can withstand loss of a variable percentage, often given as one-third, of its tissue before this becomes clinically manifest. The clinical outcome will be influenced by how rapidly infarcts develop, and by the functional quality of the remaining parenchyma.

On cut section, an acute infarct is red and as it ages the color changes through brown, to tan, to off-white (Figure 32.33). The consistency changes from firm to hard. Central infarcts and those occurring earlier in gestation are more likely to be significant, whereas peripheral infarction of 5–10% at term may be considered physiologic. The age of

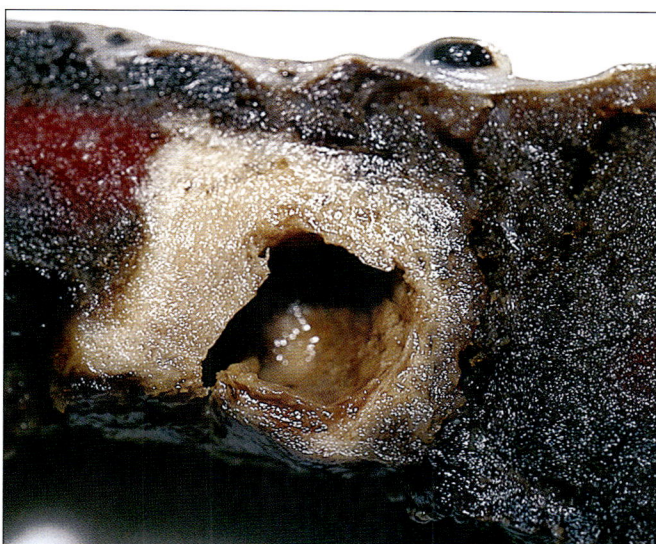

Figure 32.33 Old infarction. The cavity was due to a hematoma that caused compression. The retroplacental nature of the hematoma cannot be appreciated from this section.

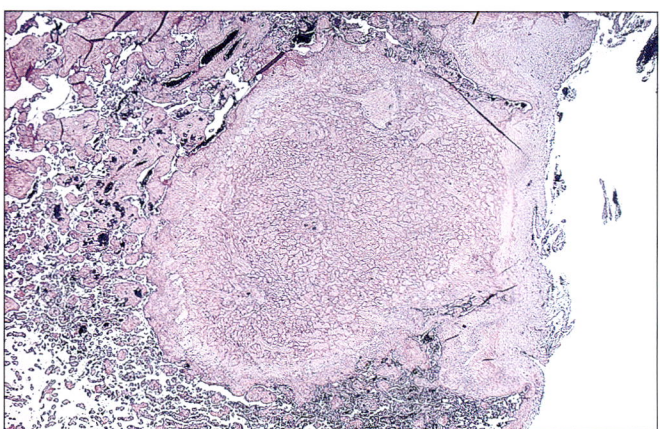

Figure 32.34 Infarct. The chorionic villi are ghost-like. No viable cells are present either in them or in the surrounding fibrin.

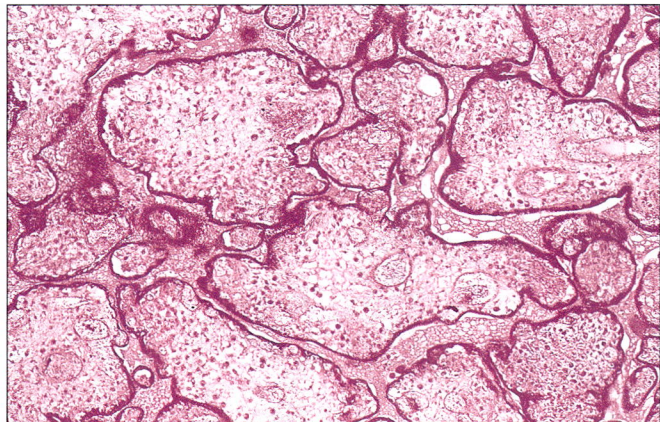

Figure 32.35 Infarct with ghost outlines of villi. As time passes, the outlines become less pronounced.

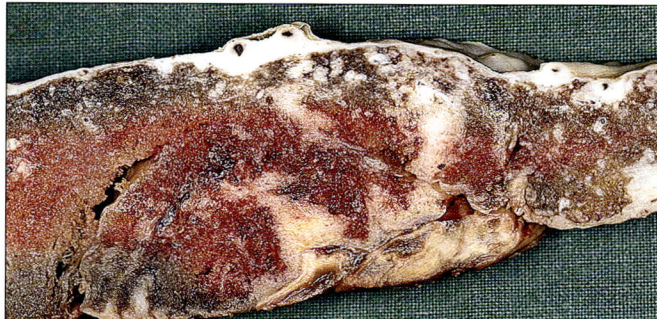

Figure 32.36 Perivillous fibrin deposition showing large waxy plaques.

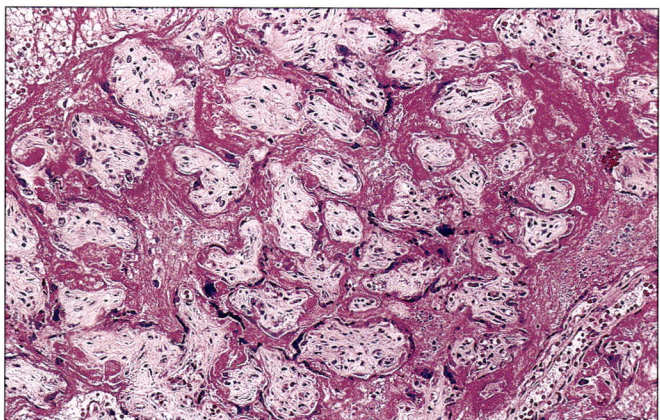

Figure 32.37 Extensive perivillous fibrin around villi.

the infarct(s), location, percentage of parenchymal involvement, and presence of associated retroplacental hemorrhage should be noted.

Histologically, the acute infarct is composed of nonviable villi with obliteration of the intervillous space. Aging lesions have ghost-like villi surrounded by fibrin (Figures 32.34 and 32.35). Infarction is associated with IUGR, fetal hypoxia, and intrauterine fetal death. A reduction in fetal blood flow may sometimes precede infarction.[51]

PERIVILLOUS FIBRIN DEPOSITION AND MATERNAL FLOOR 'INFARCTION'

Perivillous fibrin deposition is seen macroscopically as areas of firm gray-white waxy material. It may be focal or diffuse (Figure 32.36). Histologically there is eosinophilic fibrin that separates villi (Figure 32.37). There may be secondary infarction in larger lesions. Perivillous fibrin deposition is seen increasingly from 30 weeks' gestational age, but is not unduly increased in post-term deliveries. It is less prominent where maternal blood flow is reduced, i.e., with preeclampsia, essential hypertension, and diabetes. With so-called maternal floor infarction there is an increase in basal plate fibrin that exceeds 3 mm thickness on at least one histologic slide (Figures 32.38 and 32.39). Another pattern, massive perivillous fibrin deposition (≥25% of villi encased by fibrin on at least one slide), is more strongly associated

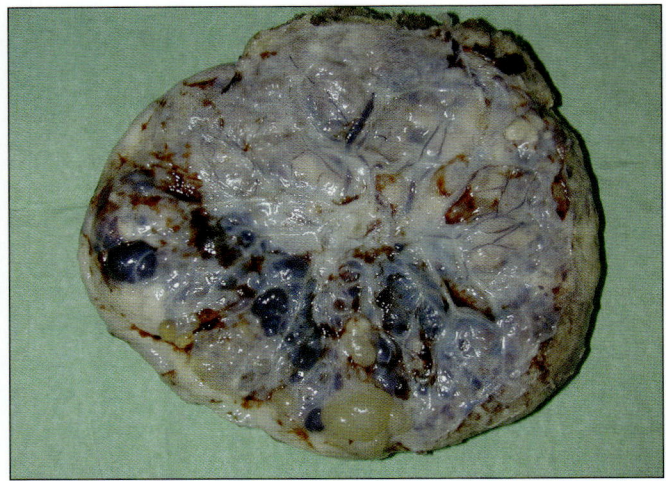

Figure 32.38 Maternal floor infarction: characteristic firm pale disc.

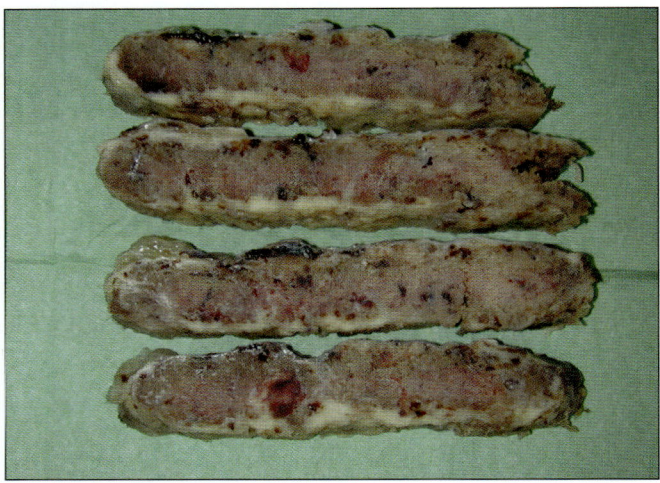

Figure 32.39 Maternal floor infarction: the basal plate is thickened by fibrin.

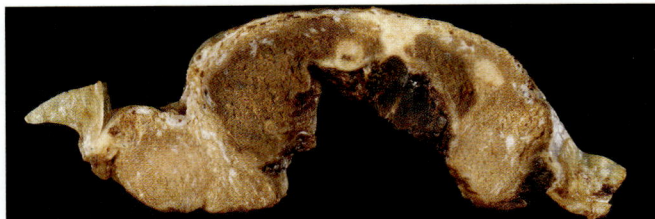

Figure 32.40 Abruptio placentae with dramatic indentation of the parenchyma. The parenchyma is infarcted between the hemorrhage and the chorionic plate.

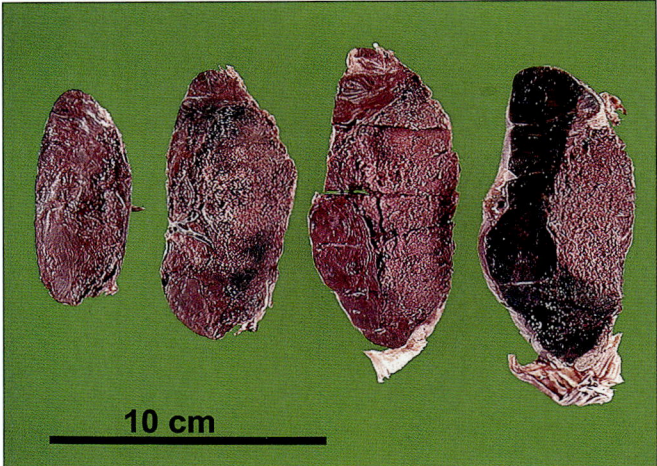

Figure 32.41 A 2 cm subchorionic hemorrhage. There was also abruption at the time of delivery of the premature infant.

with growth retardation than with maternal floor infarct.[52] Recent studies have included the additional requirement of involvement of 25% or more of the disc macroscopically.[53] It is associated with an increase in perinatal mortality and fetal growth restriction, and may recur in subsequent pregnancies.[54] Maternal serum α-fetoprotein may be raised and PAPP-A reduced, and cases may be recognized clinically by the combination of IUGR, oligohydramnios, and increased placental echogenicity. Where a diffuse increase in perivillous fibrin is seen, chronic intervillositis should be actively excluded by searching for histiocytes: an immunostain for CD68 is helpful in this.

Subchorionic fibrin deposition results from changes in blood flow and eddy currents. It is usually laminated and roughly pyramidal in shape with its base at the chorionic plate. As it lacks (or has very few) enmeshed villi, placental function is not lost.

HEMATOMA

Retroplacental hematomas separate the placenta's basal plate from the uterine wall, causing fetal anoxia and maternal hemorrhage. Retroplacental hemorrhage is found in 5% of placentas, and many small hemorrhages are clinically silent. Conversely, a dramatic abruption followed by rapid cesarean section may have no placental manifestations, and the diagnosis of abruption should be based on clinical criteria.[55] A concealed retroplacental hematoma will indent the disc and cause compression infarction of the overlying parenchyma (Figure 32.40). Small yellow flecks of decidua may be seen on the outer and inner surface of the hematoma. Acute lesions consist almost entirely of red blood cells, but with aging these degenerate and are replaced by fibrin. Neutrophils in the basal plate are found early (<4 hours) with the start of coagulative necrosis of villi following in the next 20 hours.[56] Long-standing lesions may contain hemosiderin-laden macrophages.

The following have been associated with retroplacental hematoma and abruption: pre-eclampsia, essential hypertension, obstruction of the inferior vena cava, folic acid deficiency, cigarette smoking, anticardiolipin antibodies, blunt abdominal trauma, and chorioamnionitis. An association with cocaine use may be overstated.[57] A pregnancy with abruption carries a much higher risk for adverse perinatal outcome such as stillbirth and preterm delivery and increases the risk for recurrence in a subsequent pregnancy.[58] The cause is likely to be multifactorial.[59] The extent of the hematoma, the speed of onset, and the status of the uteroplacental vasculature all interact to determine outcome: the percentage of the maternal surface involved ranges from <20% to 100%.

A marginal hematoma is a collection of blood adjacent to the margin of the placenta with stripping of the chorion laeve, usually seen as a crescent around the placental periphery. It may be associated with antepartum hemorrhage.

SUBCHORIAL THROMBOSIS (BREUS MOLE)

Subchorial thromboses are found with both abortions and live term pregnancies (Figure 32.41). The fetal surface shows numerous bosselations while the cut surface shows a laminated thrombus between the chorionic plate and the underlying villous tissue. Strands of stem villi may be found within the thrombus. Massive thrombosis defined as 1 cm or greater, measured following fixation, is associated with a poor outcome.[60] These thrombi have been described in association with coagulation abnormalities including thrombophilia and anticoagulation, but the pathogenesis is not fully understood.

INTERVILLOUS THROMBOSIS

Intervillous thrombi mark the site of fetal–maternal hemorrhage and consist of laminated blood clot comprising both fetal and maternal red cells. A rim of compressed and infarcted villi, which may be numerous, is found in about one-third of cases. Occasionally, these thrombi are found in cases of maternal–fetal rhesus incompatibility. A fresh thrombus, sometimes called a Kline's hemorrhage, may appear on section as a hole in the villous parenchyma in which the blood is easily washed out. The pathogenesis probably lies in small disruptions in the villous capillaries.

OTHER CONDITIONS

Calcification—occurring in areas of fibrin, rather than representing mineralization of villi—is common in the placentas of primigravidas, especially in those who deliver in the summer and autumn months. It is not more common in post-term placentas. Calcification occurring early preterm (i.e., less than 32 weeks) and detected sonographically is associated with an adverse outcome.[61]

Septal cysts are collections of gelatinous gray fluid seen in placental septa. They occur more frequently with similar cysts in the membranes and may be a marker of chronic placental hypoxia.[62]

MULTIPLE GESTATION

Multiple births occur normally in slightly under 1% of spontaneously conceived pregnancies and may be dizygotic or monozygotic (Figure 32.42). Dizygotic twinning has a strong hereditary component on the maternal side. The frequency of dizygotic twinning and multiple gestations is substantially increased in women who have undergone artificial induction of ovulation with hormones.

Separate placentas develop when two fertilized ova implant apart from one another. If the ova implant near one another, the two placentas show varying degrees of fusion and may appear as one. When the ova implant apart, there are discrete conceptuses, each placenta having its own amniotic sac. In the case of placental fusion, microscopic examination of the intervening membranes between the two fetuses shows two chorions and two amnions, i.e., a dichorionic diamniotic gestation (Figure 32.43).

The early division of a single fertilized ovum results in twins that are genetically identical and therefore of the same sex. If a single fertilized ovum divides within two days of fertilization, before the trophoblast has differentiated, two separate embryos develop, each with its own placenta and amniotic sac (dichorionic diamniotic twinning). Hence, scrutiny of the placenta cannot always distinguish between monozygotic and dizygotic twinning. If division occurs between days 3 and 8 after conception the trophoblast, but not the amniotic cavity, has already differentiated, and a single placenta with two amniotic sacs develops (monochorionic diamniotic twinning) (Figure 32.44). A monochorionic monoamniotic placenta forms if division occurs between days 8 and 30 after conception, because the amniotic cavity has already developed (Figure 32.45). Division at later periods results in conjoint twins.

Each placenta should be clearly designated in the delivery ward (e.g., by one clamp on the cord of twin 1, two on that of twin 2, etc.). Chorionicity should be established prior to the removal of the cords and membranes. If both amnions can be separated and pulled toward their respective cords, leaving a clear chorionic surface below, the placenta is monochorionic (Figure 32.44A). In dichorionic placentation, a low ridge formed by the junction of the two chorions is present at this point (Figure 32.43B), and attempts to remove it will expose the underlying villous parenchyma. The contents of the membranes forming this ridge can be confirmed histologically, but this is usually unnecessary.

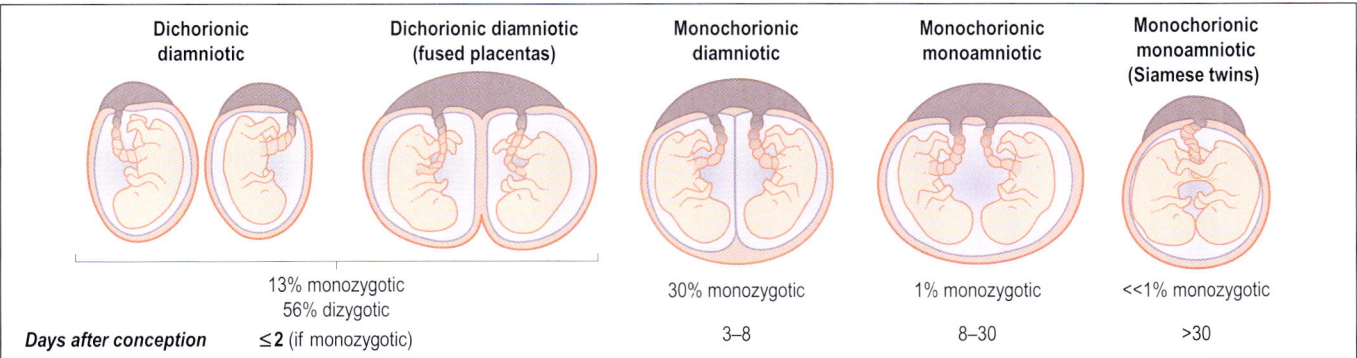

Figure 32.42 Placental structure in twin pregnancy. The listed percentages are for each variant and total 100%. (After Robboy SJ, Duggan M, Kurman R. The female reproductive system. In: Rubin E, Farber J, editors. Pathology. 3rd ed. Philadelphia: Lippincott; 1999. p. 962-1028.)

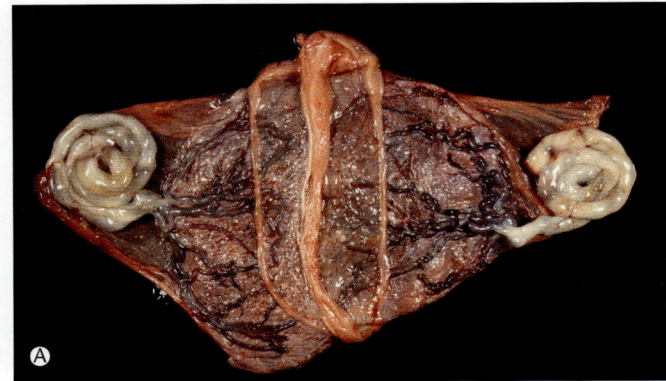

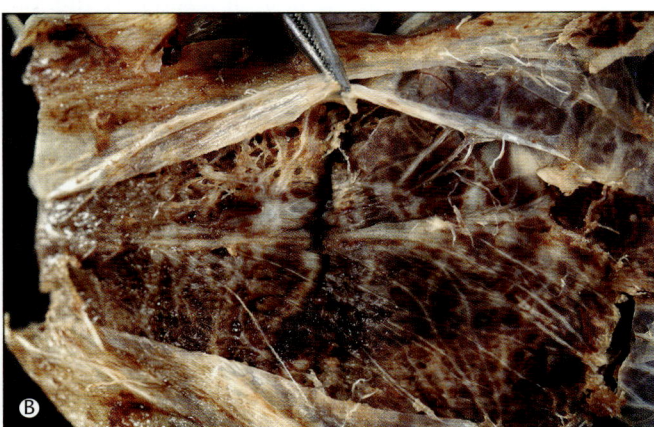

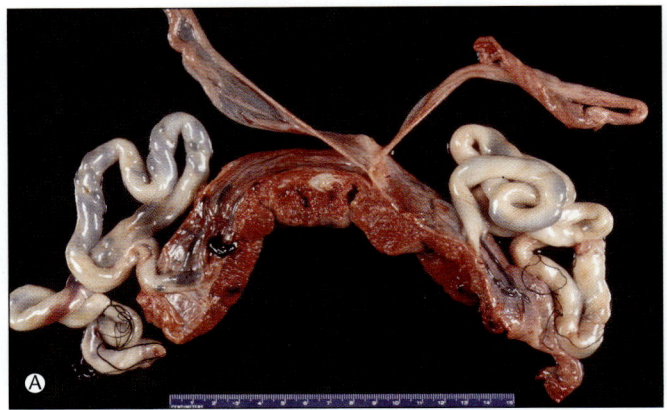

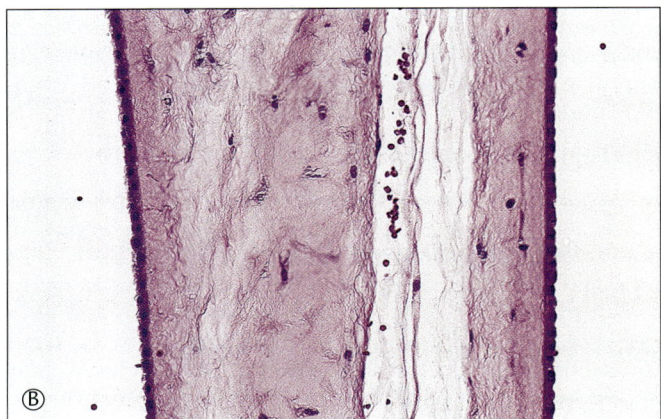

Figure 32.44 **(A, B)** Monochorionic diamniotic placenta. **(A)** Grossly, both amnions can be separated and pulled toward their respective cords, leaving a clear chorionic surface below. **(B)** Microscopically, no trophoblastic layer is present between the two amnions.

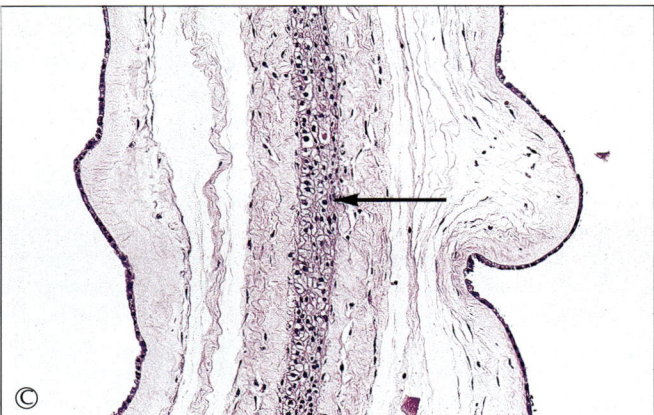

Figure 32.43 **(A–C)** Dichorionic diamniotic placenta. **(A)** Grossly, a low ridge is present at the junction of the two chorions; attempts to remove it expose the underlying villous parenchyma **(B)**. **(C)** Microscopically, a chorionic membrane separates two diamniotic fetuses, shown by the presence of trophoblast (arrow) between the two amnions.

For practical purposes, a monochorionic placenta means the twins are monozygotic, or, in common parlance, 'identical.' In view of postzygotic events, the former term is preferable, especially as discordance for sex[63] and karyotype can occur on occasion in monochorionic twins. However, it is still important to recognize that almost all monochorionic placentas are from monozygotic twins. Dichorionic placentas mean that there is a chance (approximately 10–15%) that the twins are monozygotic. Chorionicity, rather than zygosity, is the main determinant of fetal outcome.[64] Monochorionic twins are at an increased risk of complications and adverse perinatal outcome compared with dichorionic twins.[65,66] Growth discordance in twins is severe if ≥25% (calculated as a percentage of the larger twin's weight). This occurs in less than 10% of twins. Peripheral cord insertion and avascular villi are associated with abnormal growth.[67]

An important consequence of monochorionic placentation is that vascular anastomoses may be present and twin–twin transfusion syndrome may occur. Surface vessels may cross from one placenta to the other and form anastomoses (Figure 32.46). These may be demonstrated by injection of air or gelatin, but their absence does not mean that significant vascular shunting did not occur in the parenchyma during intrauterine life. The rarity of twin–twin transfusion syndrome in monochorionic monoamniotic twins has been related to arterial–arterial anastomoses in almost 100% of these cases, in contrast to the greater frequency of venoarterial anastomoses in monochorionic diamniotic twins.[68] Diagnosis may be difficult and the entity may be underrecognized in monoamniotic twins if oligohydramnios in

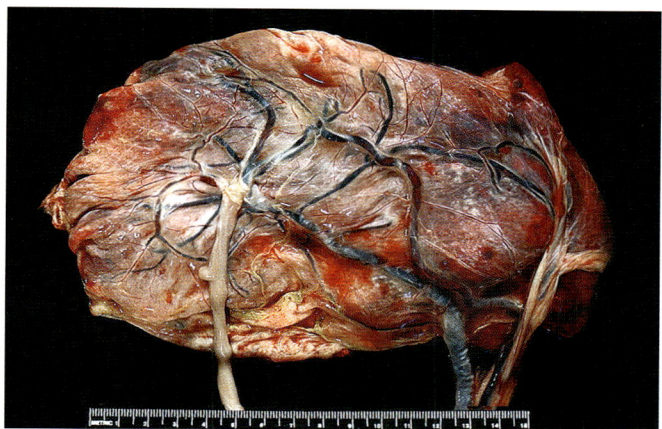
Figure 32.45 Monochorionic monoamniotic placenta.

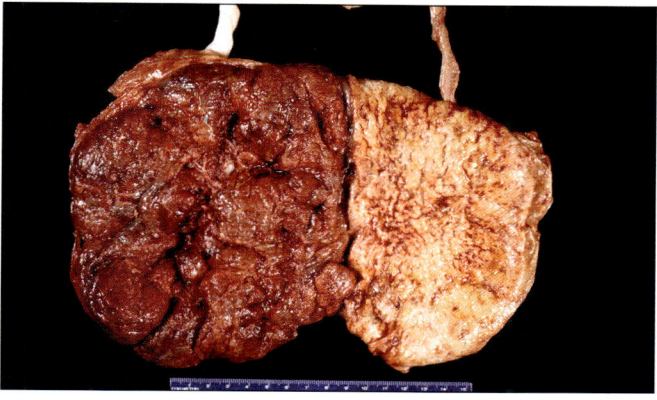
Figure 32.47 Twin–twin transfusion syndrome with pale donor placenta and congested recipient placenta.

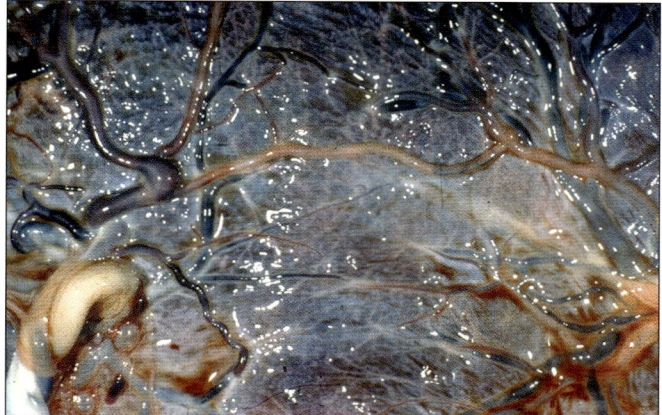
Figure 32.46 Twin–twin superficial anastomosis.

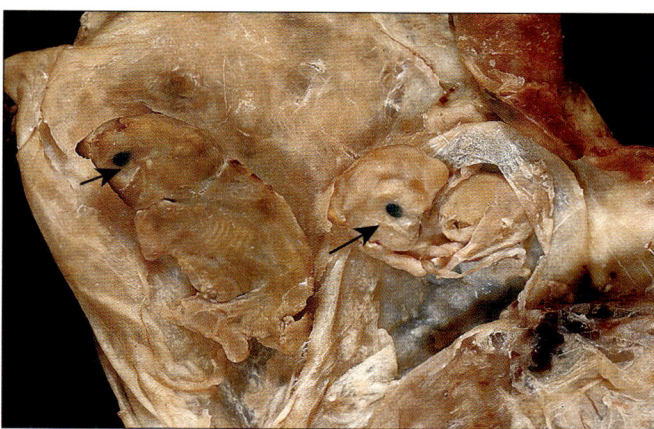
Figure 32.48 Fetus papyraceus. Two macerated fetuses (arrows) are each about 2 cm in length. This mother delivered three normal triplets.

the donor and polyhydramnios in the recipient is a criterion. The placenta of the donor twin may be pale and bulky, with edematous villi and inconspicuous vessels, whereas that of the recipient may be congested (Figure 32.47). Transfusion may be acute, but is usually chronic and the donor and the recipient may change with time. Even where both fetuses are available for autopsy, it may be difficult to be certain of the pattern of the condition.[69] Twin–twin transfusion syndrome very rarely occurs in dichorionic twins. Endoscopic laser coagulation of anastomoses results in vascular thrombosis and necrosis of the underlying parenchyma. Other complications of twin pregnancy are acardia and fetus papyraceus. Acardia occurs where one twin lacks or has only rudimentary cardiac structures, but receives its blood supply from the other twin via vascular anastomoses. The term 'twin-reversed arterial perfusion' is sometimes used for this condition. The acardiac twin usually shows a variable degree of somatic organization, sometimes with only rudimentary structures, and the donor or 'pump twin' may develop cardiac failure and hydrops. The cord of the acardiac twin usually has a single umbilical artery. The placenta is most commonly monochorionic diamniotic.

Fetus papyraceus occurs when one twin dies and becomes compressed, with some early losses appearing as thickened membranes. This occurs most commonly with triplets or more (Figure 32.48). There are various etiologies, including twin–twin transfusion, cord accidents, and, less commonly, maternal trauma.

MICROSCOPIC LESIONS OF THE PLACENTA

PLACENTAL INFLAMMATION AND INFECTION

The placenta, its membranes, and umbilical cord may become infected by numerous routes, but the two most common and clinically important are ascending infection and hematogenous spread. Maternal infection may be subclinical. Other routes include the fallopian tube itself, foci of abdominal infection using the fallopian tube as a conduit, chronic endometritis, and invasive procedures such as amniocentesis and cordocentesis (*in utero* cord blood sampling). Intrauterine transfusion of infected blood can lead to placental infection via the fetus. Ascending infection is discussed above as acute chorioamnionitis.

CHRONIC CHORIOAMNIONITIS AND DECIDUITIS

This is defined as amniotropic infiltration by maternal T-cells (Figure 32.49). It is frequent in cases with premature membrane rupture and villitis. Chronic deciduitis with plasma cells is a common finding. Together, these findings suggest that it is noninfectious, with an immunologic basis, and may play a role in some cases of preterm birth.[70-72]

MEMBRANE AND DECIDUAL HYPOXIC LESIONS

Laminar necrosis (involving at least 10% of the membrane roll) (Figure 32.50) reflects an acute hypoxic phenomenon. Chronic hypoxia may be manifest as chorionic microcysts (at least three microscopic chorionic lakes).[73] Diagnosis of diffuse decidual leukocytoclastic necrosis of the basal plate (involving 30% or more of the maternal surface on one slide) is common in preterm births and may be a marker of placental underperfusion.[74] Increased trophoblast giant cells in the deep aspect of the basal plate and increased immature intermediate trophoblast in the superficial portions of the basal plate reflect maternal underperfusion.[75]

EOSINOPHILIC/T-CELL VASCULITIS

This is an unusual lesion seen in third trimester placentas (Figure 32.51A and B). It is associated with villitis of unknown etiology and with fetal vascular occlusion. It may affect multiple vessels or be isolated.[76]

VILLITIS

Villitis is seen in approximately 10–15% of placentas. In most (95–98%) cases, no etiologic agent is found and the term 'villitis of unknown etiology' is used. The inflammatory reaction that develops in the villous stroma has been variously described as 'proliferative,' 'necrotizing,' 'granulomatous,' or 'reparative.' The end result is a sclerotic functionless villus. The demonstration that a substantial fraction of the inflammatory cells is maternal in origin[77] supports the hypothesis that villitis is frequently a maternal immunologic response to fetal tissue. Correlation between growth discordance and villitis in dizygotic twins supports this.[78]

Macroscopically, placentas with villitis may be small and pale, or normal. Villitis may be divided into four grades: grade 1 (minimal), one or two foci with few villi involved; grade 2 (mild), up to six foci of villous inflammation, each focus containing maximally 20 villi; grade 3 (moderate), multiple inflammatory foci present, each occupying up to half a low-power field; and grade 4 (severe), large areas of most sections inflamed. With use of a two-grade system, grades 3 and 4 will be high grade, and will account for approximately 20% of cases of villitis.

Villi show an infiltrate of lymphocytes, histiocytes, or both (Figure 32.52), in contrast with normal stromal cells that resemble fibroblasts. Additional signs of villitis include some disruption of the villi, destruction of the normal vasculature, and spillover of inflammatory cells into the perivillous space (Figure 32.53). There may an increase in perivillous fibrin, which should be noted. The lymphocytes are predominantly maternal, but some are of fetal origin.[77]

Villitis of grades 2–4 is associated with growth retardation, but even minimal villitis may be important in cases of premature delivery before 34 weeks.[79] Villitis with obliterative fetal vessel vasculopathy is one of the placental findings associated with neurologic impairment in term infants.[80] This is usually, but not exclusively, seen in grades 3 and 4 villitis, although we comment on its presence or absence in addition to allocating a grade. As with other entities in placental pathology, recognition of cofactors, e.g., maternal hypertension, is important.[81]

Proving recurrence of villitis is problematic, as not all subsequent placentas following an index diagnosis of villitis will be analyzed. We identified recurrence in 37% of patients whose second or subsequent placenta was examined.[82] Villitis may be more useful in explaining the outcome in the index case than in predicting recurrence.

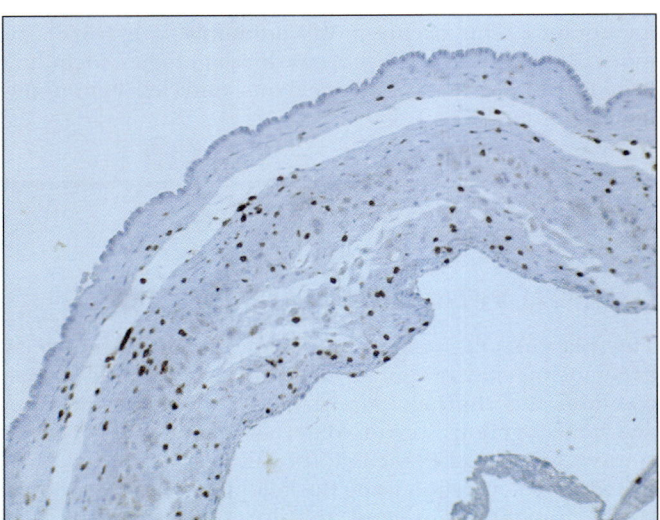

Figure 32.49 Chronic chorioamnionitis: CD3-positive T-cells in chorion and amnion.

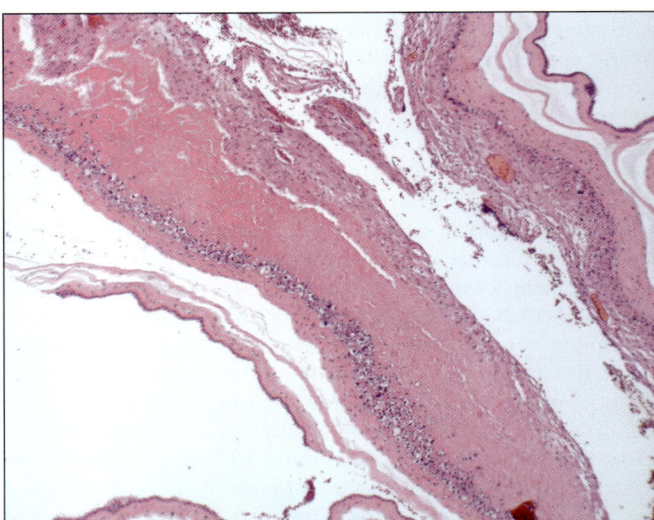

Figure 32.50 Laminar necrosis: a band of eosinophilic necrosis in over 10% of the membrane roll.

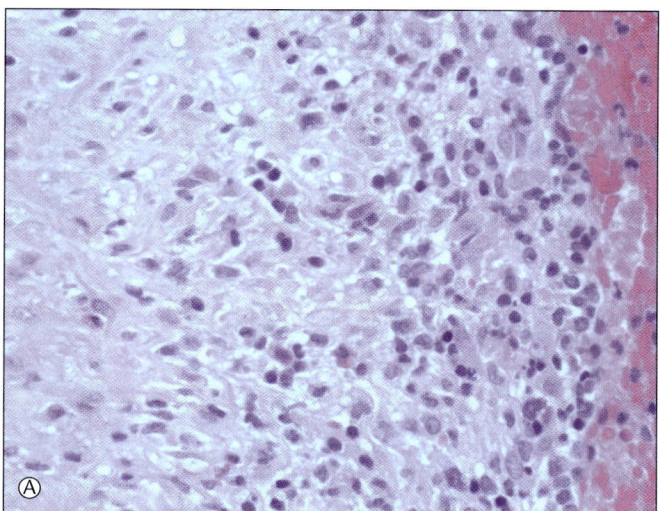 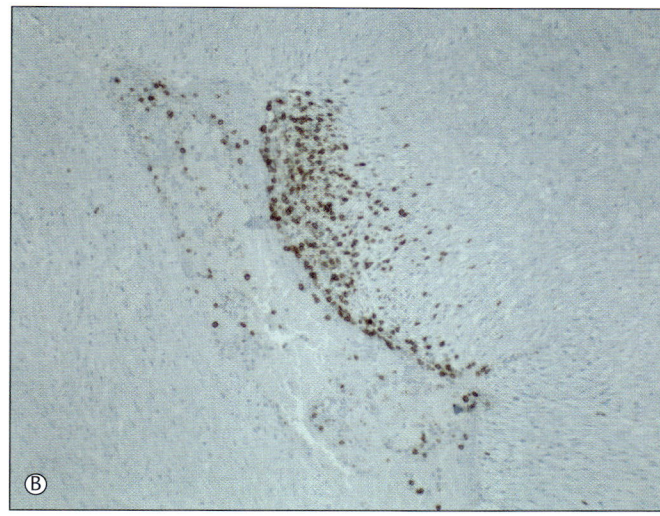

Figure 32.51 Eosinophilic/T-cell vasculitis. **(A)** High-power view of the wall of a chorionic plate vessel. **(B)** CD3-positive T-cells.

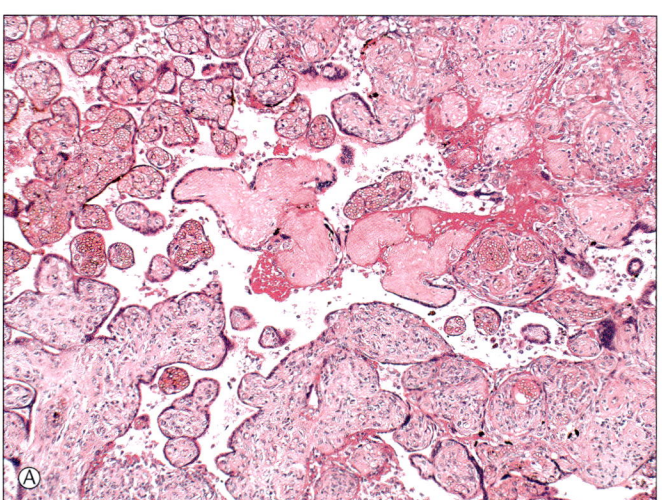 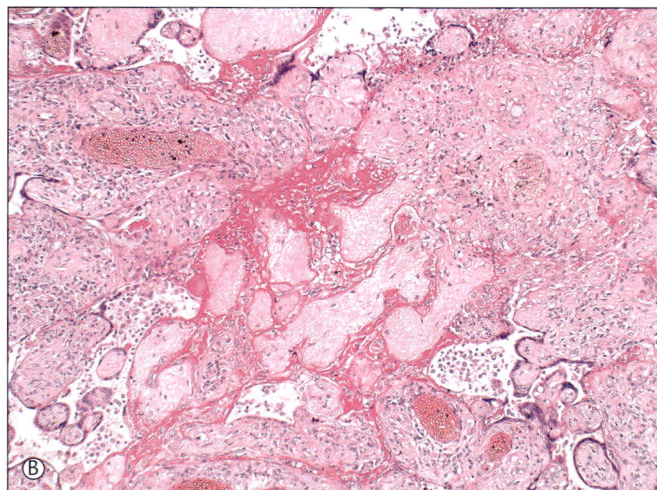

Figure 32.52 (A, B) Villitis. **(A)** Low magnification and **(B)** with swollen villi, some sclerotic, and an increase in perivillous fibrin, with adhesions among villi.

Infectious villitis is uncommon: the presence of plasma cells in villi means that organisms, especially cytomegalovirus (CMV), should be excluded. The presence of polymorphs or microabscesses means that *Listeria* should be considered. Some cases may be due to varicella or *Toxoplasma*, overlooked in the absence of clinically relevant information.[83] Many cases yield etiologic agents if modern diagnostic techniques such as immunohistochemistry, *in situ* hybridization, and polymerase chain reaction are used. The specific viruses and bacterial infections that give rise to villitis are described more fully in Chapter 33.

CHRONIC HISTIOCYTIC INTERVILLOSITIS

Chronic histiocytic intervillositis is an uncommon but important finding, with an infiltrate of mononuclear cells in the intervillous space (Figure 32.54). The infiltrate may be mild, moderate, or severe in extent, and most cells are reactive for the macrophage marker CD68. There is increased perivillous fibrin deposition. Some series exclude cases with coexistent villitis, but we have noted an overlap in about one-third of cases. It is associated with pregnancy-induced hypertension, lupus erythematosus, maternal drug use, and diabetes. Two of four cases were associated with assisted reproduction.[84] Elevated alkaline phosphatase levels have been reported.[85] Fetal outcome is poor, with early and late pregnancy loss and growth restriction. Chronic histiocytic intervillositis may recur, and should be actively excluded in cases of recurrent miscarriage before commencing assisted reproduction. Chronic intervillositis is also found in nearly 20% of cases of malaria (see later).

VASCULAR LESIONS

FETAL VESSEL THROMBI

Vascular occlusions may occur in vessels at various levels in the fetal circulation, from the umbilical cord to the villous

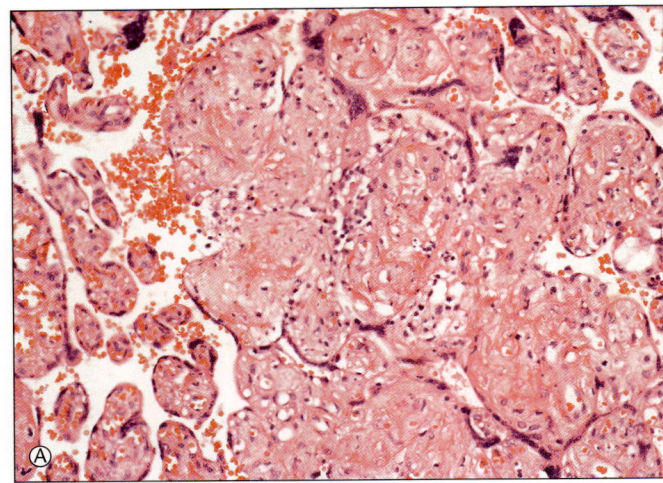
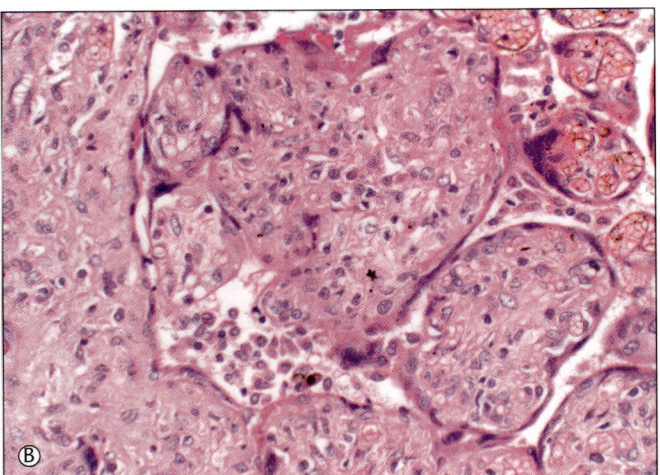
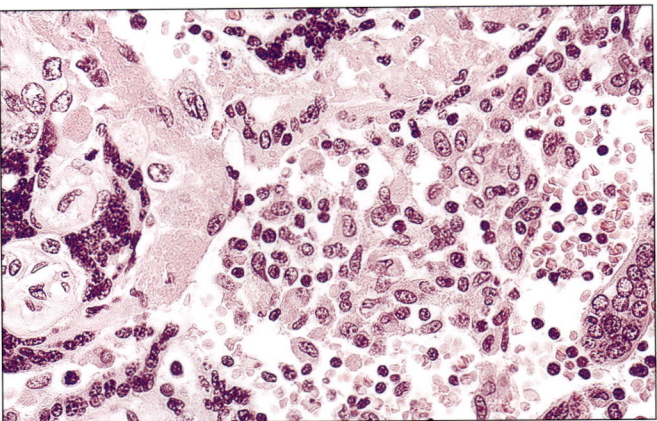

Figure 32.54 Intervillositis from an infant with growth retardation. The cells in the maternal space show a histiocytic morphology.

capillaries. Such changes, including fetal surface or stem vessel thrombi, hemorrhagic endovasculitis, stem vessel obliteration, or clusters of avascular villi, are found in approximately 3% of placentas from term deliveries.[86]

Thrombi may be seen grossly or may only be apparent microscopically (Figure 32.55). Following cessation of blood flow there is hemorrhagic endovasculitis, with vascular fibrosis with entrapment, fragmentation, and exocytosis of red blood cells into the vessel walls. Following this, the vessels fibrose (Figure 32.56). There is no associated inflammation. Many of these changes are also seen in placentas of macerated stillbirths, and only when a discrete area shows hyalinization distinct from the diffuse changes of intrauterine death can the diagnosis of antemortem thrombosis be made.

Fetal thrombotic vasculopathy is equated with severe disease and defined as more than 15 villi that are avascular or show stromal karyorrhexis in two or more slides.[87] Avascular villi are sharply demarcated from the surrounding normal villi (Figure 32.57). In some cases, often with hemorrhagic endovasculitis in the stem vessels, distal villi are bulbous and normocellular with karyorrhectic debris in vessels, rather than being small, sclerotic, and avascular. This may represent an earlier stage in the evolution of avascular villi, or, in some cases where the picture persists, a 'sublethal hit' on these villi.

Cord pathology shows an increasing association with parenchymal lesions of fetal underperfusion. Thrombi in the cord or in chorionic plate vessels may also be secondary to compression, acute inflammation, nuchal cord, and true knots. Lesions of the cord, both clinical and pathologic, were seen in two-thirds of cases with fetal thrombotic vasculopathy[11] and are more frequent with oligohydramnios and fetal cardiac anomalies.[88] Fetal thrombotic vasculopathy is found four times more commonly in placentas of infants with neonatal encephalopathy.[86] Over half of the placentas of infants with neurologic impairment showed one or more of findings of fetal thrombotic vasculopathy, villitis with vascular obliteration, chorioamnionitis with severe fetal vessel vasculitis, and meconium-induced vascular necrosis.[80]

Fibrin deposition may be seen in about 10% of placentas focally in an exophytic area of the vessel wall (Figure 32.58).

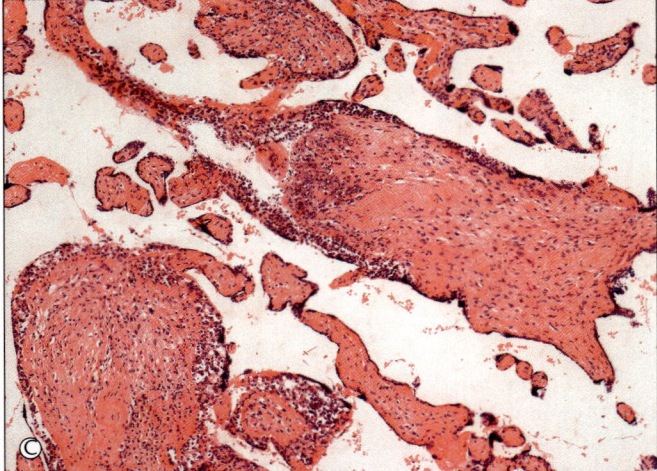

Figure 32.53 (A–C) Villitis. **(A)** Medium to high magnification, with an inflammatory infiltrate. Additionally some villi are disrupted, show **(B)** spillover of inflammatory cells into the adjacent perivillous space, and **(C)** in a stem villus, show destruction of the normal vasculature.

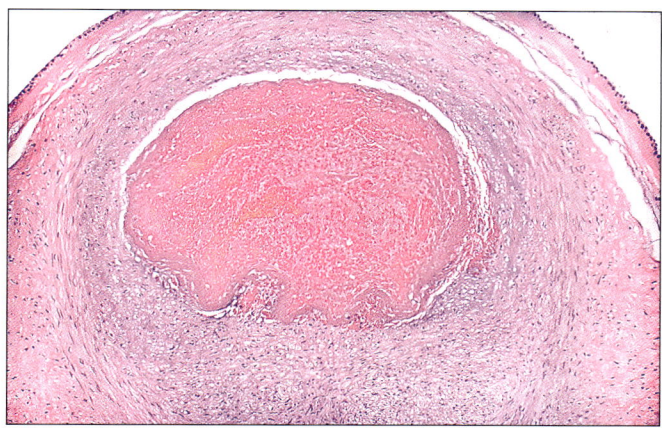

Figure 32.55 Thrombus in large surface vessels. The lumen is completely occluded, and because of its age shows peripheral organization.

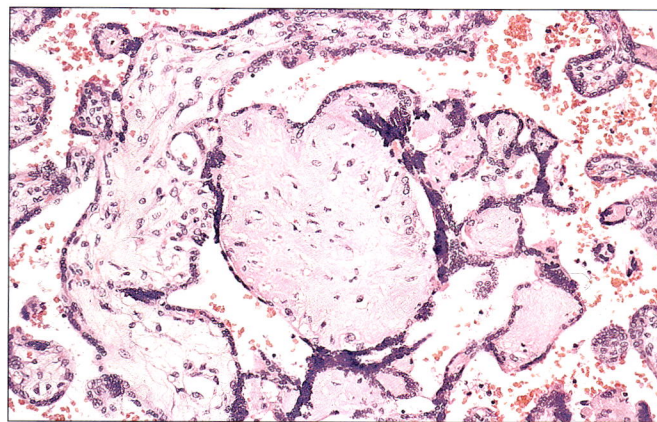

Figure 32.57 Avascular villi. The presence of hemosiderin deposits in villi such as these should alert the pathologist to the possibility of previous CMV infection.

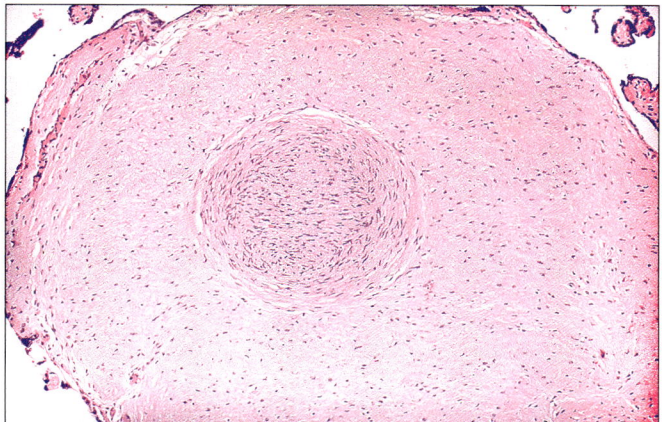

Figure 32.56 Total fibrous obliteration of a stem vessel.

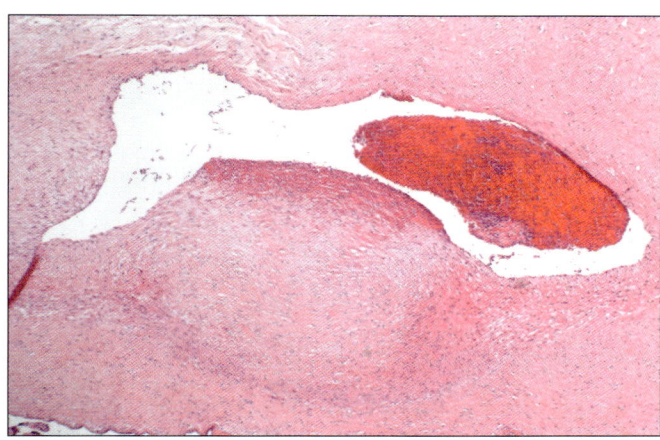

Figure 32.58 Nonocclusive mural fibrin thrombus on an endothelial cushion.

This protrusion consists of loose connective tissue and has been referred to as endothelial 'cushions' and held by some to be normal features of vascular bifurcations. Some have associated mural fibrin thrombi, seen in 8–10% of placentas.[86] These overlap with the entity termed 'fibrinous vasculosis' and may be seen in placentas with fetal thrombotic vasculopathy. However, the clinical significance of isolated lesions is unclear: it is likely that those on the chorionic plate are of more significance than those in stem vessels.

MATERNAL VESSEL PATHOLOGY

The findings of completely muscularized vessels in the basal decidua or in the decidua capsularis after 14 weeks should be considered abnormal (Figure 32.59). As implantation is deepest and most extensive in the center of the disc[7] its identification here is most significant. These arteries may subsequently undergo acute atherosis (Figure 32.60), which appears as fibrinoid necrosis of the vessel wall with subintimal accumulations of lipophages. There may be a transmural chronic inflammatory infiltrate, usually mild. Acute atherosis is pathognomonic of a uteromaternal perfusion defect. It is not specific for pre-eclampsia as it occurs in systemic lupus erythematosus with the lupus anticoagulant, diabetes, hypertension, and idiopathic IUGR. Only half of cases of pre-eclampsia will show atherosis of basal plate vessels. Acute fibrinoid necrosis of the maternal uteroplacental vessels, either marked (Figure 32.61) or slight, may also be the only histologic manifestation of maternal vascular disease.

FETAL AND MATERNAL VASCULAR DISEASE AND THROMBOPHILIA

The suggestion that maternal thrombophilias are associated with specific placental lesions, namely, fetal thrombotic vasculopathy, massive perivillous fibrin deposition, and maternal floor infarction,[89] has been disputed, with others finding no pathognomonic features of a thrombophilic mutation.[90] One study reported a 3.3-fold increase in fibrin deposition in cases with activated protein C resistance, a finding associated with thrombophilic mutations,[91] but of 108 placentas with infarction, only 13% had a positive maternal thrombophilia result.[92] Chorangiosis (villous hypervascularity), increased syncytial knots, and focal avascular villi were

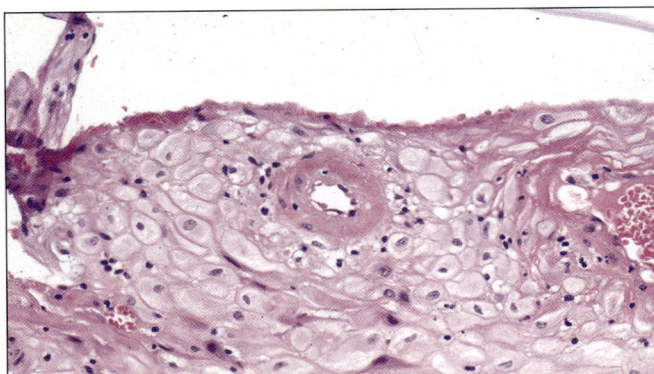

Figure 32.59 Muscularized vessel in decidua capsularis.

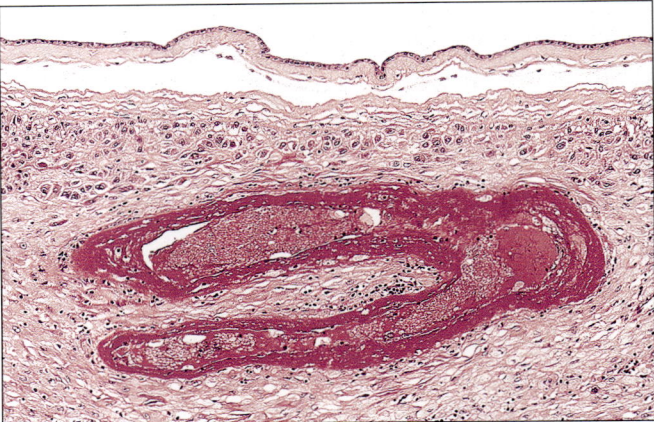

Figure 32.61 Maternal vascular disease. This is an extreme example of fibrinoid necrosis in a maternal vessel found in the decidua beneath the chorion in a woman with severe pre-eclampsia.

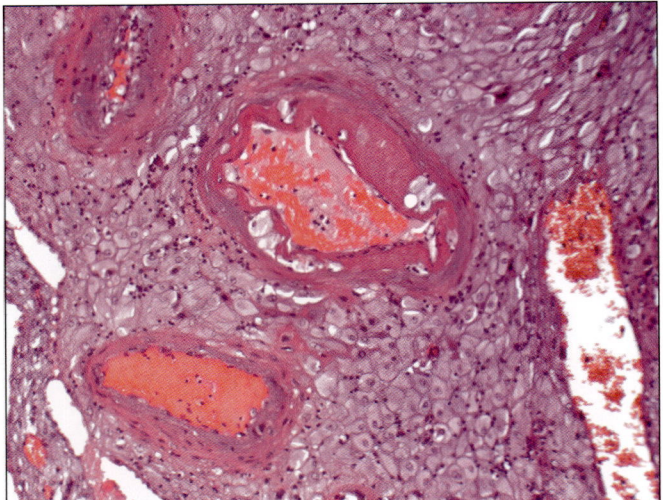

Figure 32.60 Atherosis (center) with nontransformed vascular profiles on the left.

associated with factor V Leiden gene (FVL) mutation.[93] In a systematic review, women with mutations in this gene appeared to be at a small absolute increased risk of late pregnancy loss. Neither this cohort nor those with prothrombin gene mutation appeared to be at increased risk of pre-eclampsia or birth of small for gestational age infants.[94] Many studies have been confined to the maternal genotype. The fetal genotype has been shown to modify the risk of the maternal prothrombotic state in a mouse model, and the mechanism of loss may not invariably involve thrombosis.[95]

CHORANGIOSIS

Chorangiosis is diagnosed by an increase in villous vascular profiles (Figure 32.62). It involves terminal villi, generally is not seen before 32 weeks, and is most common after 37 weeks. It is defined using a ×10 objective, with at least 10 villi with 10 or more vessels on cross section in 10 different areas on one slide in at least three different locations within the placenta. One villus should have more than 15 vascular profiles. Each capillary is surrounded by a basement membrane. It may be overdiagnosed in cases where the placenta is congested, and underdiagnosed (due to collapse of villous vessels) when umbilical cord clamping has been delayed. This condition of excessive fetal capillary growth occurs over a few weeks and signifies placental dysfunction. It may be seen with maternal smoking or anemia, and may be a marker of chronic low-grade hypoxia. It may be seen as a focal and reactive phenomenon where there has been destruction of adjacent villi due to villitis.

CHORANGIOMATOSIS

Chorangiomatosis is a rare microscopic finding. In contrast to chorangiosis, it shows a morphologic pattern typical of mature intermediate villi, with smooth-muscle actin pericytes around vessels, and a core of vimentin-positive cells (Figure 32.63). It may be found in placentas that also contain chorangiomas. Where diffuse and multifocal, it is associated with IUGR, placentomegaly, and severe congenital anomalies.[96]

VILLOUS MATURITY

Villous maturation may be disturbed chronologically by being either delayed or accelerated. Its recognition demands adequate and appropriate placental sampling, and awareness of the normal variation of the villi within the functional unit. Even experienced placental pathologists are unable to date pregnancies more accurately than within 6 weeks.[97]

We avoid the term 'dysmaturity,' preferring to characterize an abnormal pattern as either more advanced or delayed than expected. While recognizing the teleologic nature of this argument, it does provide a relatively simple and descriptive starting point in composing a report that is intelligible to the clinician. Villi should be assessed distant from the marginal areas of the disc on a number of sections, avoiding subchorionic areas, areas near infarcts, and the center of placental lobules.

Accelerated maturation is characteristic of maternal underperfusion (Figure 32.64). Syncytial knots are increased. Knots on more than 30% of villi at term represent an increase: reference values for 20–40 weeks' gestation have been published.[98] Distal villous hypoplasia is found with increasing underperfusion, and ischemic villous crowding and increased perivillous fibrin (>10% of villi encased by

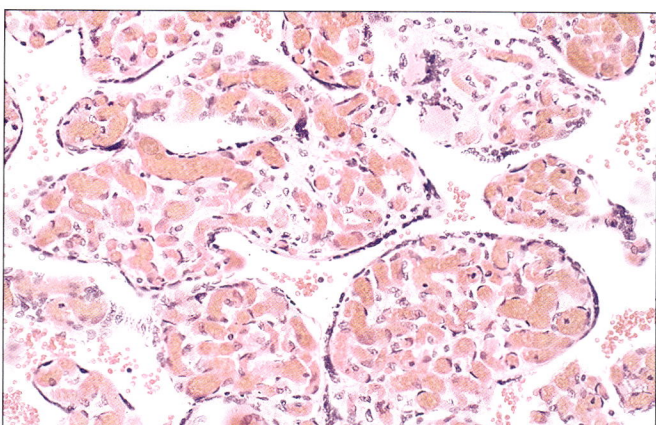

Figure 32.62 Chorangiosis. Multiple (more than 10) vascular profiles are present in a single villus.

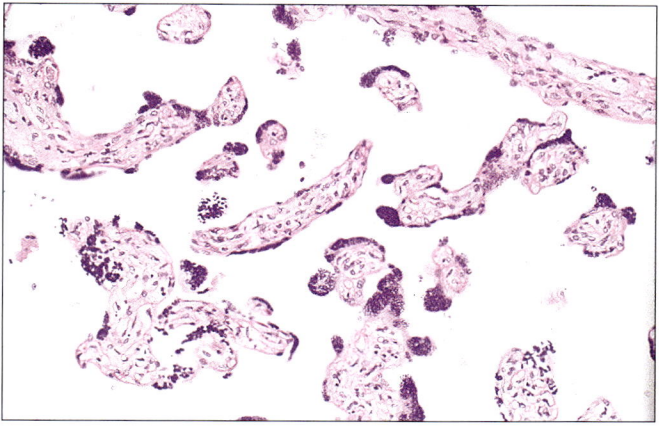

Figure 32.64 Syncytial knots (Tenney–Parker effect). Three-dimensional reconstructions have shown that the abundant syncytiotrophoblast knots are an artifact of tangential cuts through terminal villi.

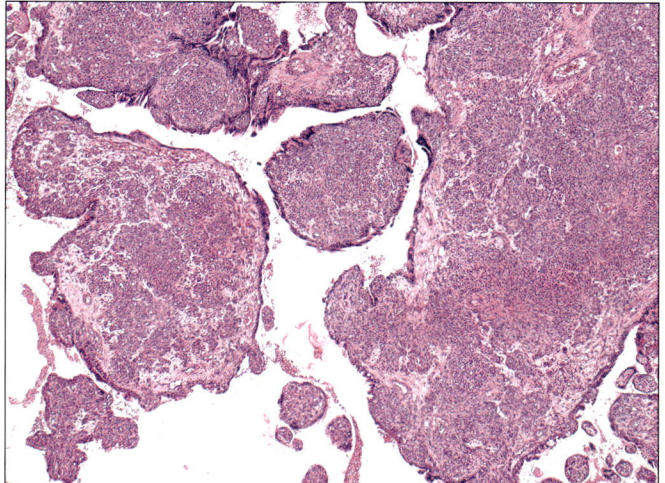

Figure 32.63 Chorangiomatosis involving multiple villi.

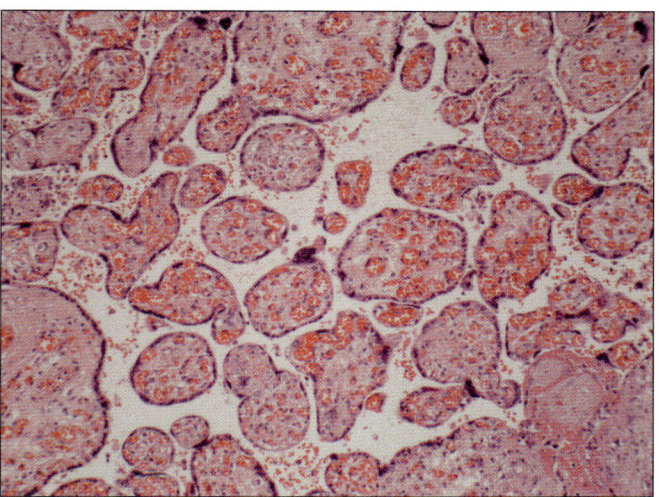

Figure 32.65 Delayed villous maturation. At low power there is a resemblance to chorangiosis.

fibrin) may be seen. When marked, these are usually accompanied by infarction.

Delayed villous maturation is classically associated with maternal diabetes mellitus, rhesus isoimmunization, syphilis, and Down's syndrome. In practice, many placentas where the diagnosis is made will have none of these associations. At low power, the villi appear less developed than expected for the gestational age (Figure 32.65). The cross-sectional profile is bulbous, and terminal villi may be reduced in number. There may be persistence of stromal channels, which are a characteristic feature of immature intermediate villi. Vasculosyncytial membrane formation is decreased (Figure 32.66). With this approach, ~5% of placentas in our practice receive a histologic diagnosis of delayed maturation. Enumeration of vasculosyncytial membranes enables classification of the lowest 10th percentile as delayed villous maturation. It is seen with congenital abnormalities, including trisomies and gastroschisis. In some cases there may be IUGR. It is the only abnormality seen in some patients with neonatal encephalopathy. One review of over 17,000 placentas found delayed maturation in 5.7%: only a minority of fetuses whose placenta showed this pattern died, but a 70-fold risk of death was claimed compared with those with a normal placenta.[99] Delayed maturation is significantly associated with antenatal or intrapartum death[100] and hypercoiling of the cord.[101]

Sometimes a mixed maturation pattern is seen, with areas of delayed maturation alternating with areas of accelerated maturation. Such a pattern may also occur in diabetes, where changes of uteroplacental ischemia are superimposed on a delayed maturation pattern. Occasional cases of pre-eclampsia show delayed maturation, instead of the advanced pattern more usually seen.

VILLOUS EDEMA

Severe villous edema is easily recognized. The placenta is pale and hydropic and the villi show stromal edema and persistent stromal channels. It may be associated with fetal

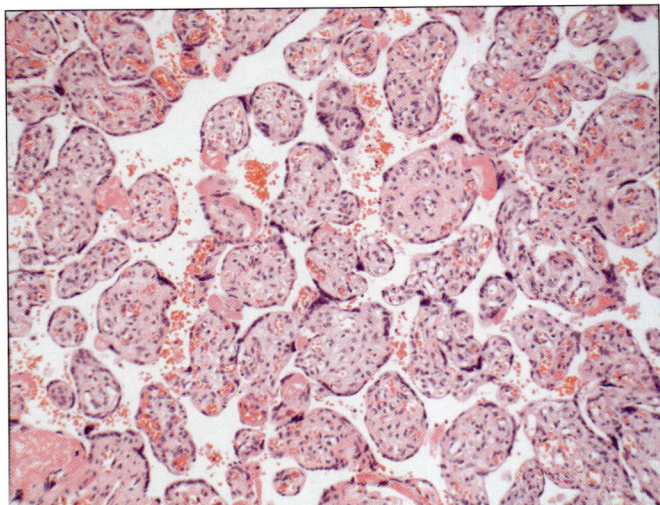

Figure 32.66 Delayed villous maturation: decreased vasculosyncytial membrane formation.

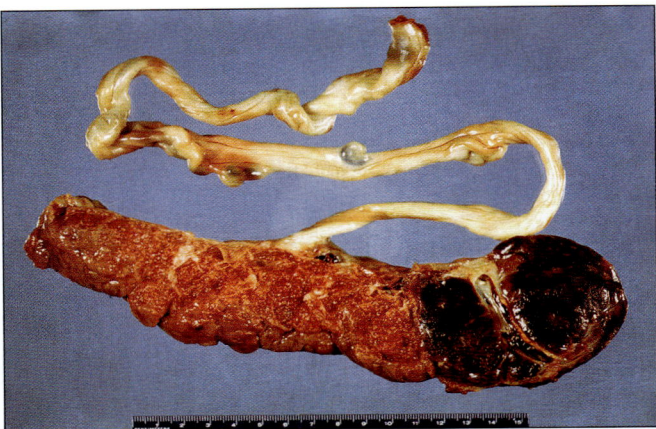

Figure 32.67 Choriangioma, cross section, large, panmural.

hydrops. Less mature villi in the center of the fetal lobule should not be used to diagnose edema. Edema may be graded. In extremely low birth weight infants (<1 kg), it correlates with abnormal neurocognitive results at 8 years of age.[102]

PERSISTANT FETAL NORMOBLASTEMIA

Nucleated red blood cells are physiologic in early pregnancy, peaking at 16 weeks. They are usually enumerated in term pregnancies, as an increase occurs 6–12 hours after onset of hypoxia, and an elevation (10/10 HPFs) correlated with subacute and chronic placental lesions.[103] They should be evaluated at high power, to distinguish them from fetal lymphocytes and other lymphoid cells.

MISCELLANEOUS VILLOUS CHANGES

Vacuolated cells in multiple tissues, including syncytiotrophoblast, intermediate trophoblast, and Hofbauer cells, should raise the suspicion of storage disease. Useful ancillary techniques include electron microscopy, fibroblast culture, and enzyme analysis. Family history and/or congenital abnormalities may accompany some cases, but, in others, placental examination may provide the first clue to the diagnosis.

NON-TROPHOBLASTIC TUMORS OF THE PLACENTA

There are relatively few non-trophoblastic tumors of the placenta.

CHORANGIOMA

The chorangioma or placental hemangioma is the most common placental tumor with a frequency of 0.6%. They are more common with increased maternal age (>30 years) and in pregnancies with hypertension and diabetes.[104] Chorangiomas may protrude from the fetal surface or less frequently the maternal surface, replacing a lobule. They may be single or multiple, varying from incidental microscopic findings to over 5 cm in size (Figure 32.67). The color of chorangiomas varies from purple-red through tan to off-white. They appear encapsulated, may appear pedunculated from the undersurface of the chorion, and are firmer than the surrounding placental parenchyma.

Histologically, chorangiomas consist of multiple vessels, usually of capillary size, although they can be cavernous, arising from a stem villus (Figure 32.68). There is a variable amount of stroma and an attenuated trophoblastic covering. Degenerative changes are common and include myxoid, hyalinized, necrotic, and calcified areas. Mitoses are occasionally seen, but, even allowing for endothelial and stromal atypia, there is no evidence that these tumors are malignant.

Complications of larger tumors include polyhydramnios with subsequent premature rupture of membranes, antepartum hemorrhage, and dystocia. The fetus may suffer growth retardation, transient cardiomegaly, bleeding disorders, hypoalbuminemia, anemia, and hydrops fetalis, the last posing the highest risk of intrauterine death.[105] The hematologic disorders may be due to entrapped red blood cells and/or platelets in the tumorous capillaries resulting in disseminated intravascular coagulation. In addition, chorangiomas have been found with fetal angiomas and hemangiomatosis,[106] Beckwith–Wiedemann syndrome, mesenchymal dysplasia, and high altitude.

CHORANGIOCARCINOMA (CHORANGIOMAS WITH TROPHOBLASTIC PROLIFERATION)

So-called chorangiocarcinoma exhibits a mantle of atypical trophoblast around a chorangioma. Among the few reported cases, all mothers and infants were well during the short periods of follow-up available. When routinely diagnosed chorangiomas were reviewed and assessed with proliferation markers, 65% could be called chorangiocarcinoma, suggesting that a better term for this group is 'chorangiomas with trophoblastic proliferation.'[107] While given a name of malignancy, there is no indication that any of these lesions are biologically malignant.

INTRAPLACENTAL CHORIOCARCINOMA

This is also known as choriocarcinoma *in situ*, and grossly resembles an infarct in a term placenta. As such, it may be

CHAPTER 32 — IMPLANTATION AND PLACENTA 765

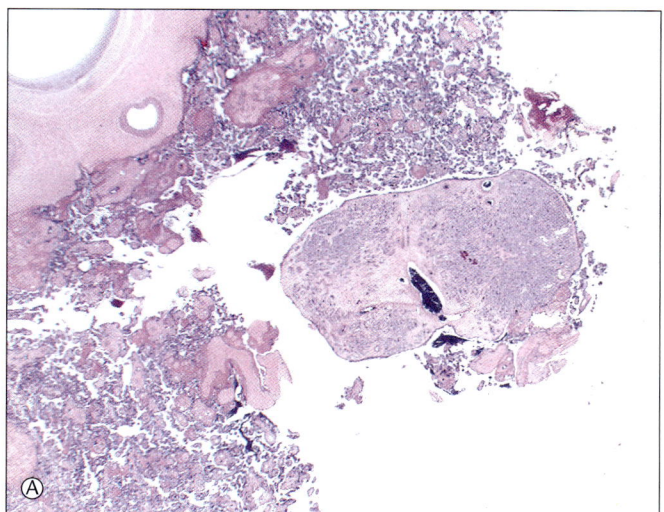

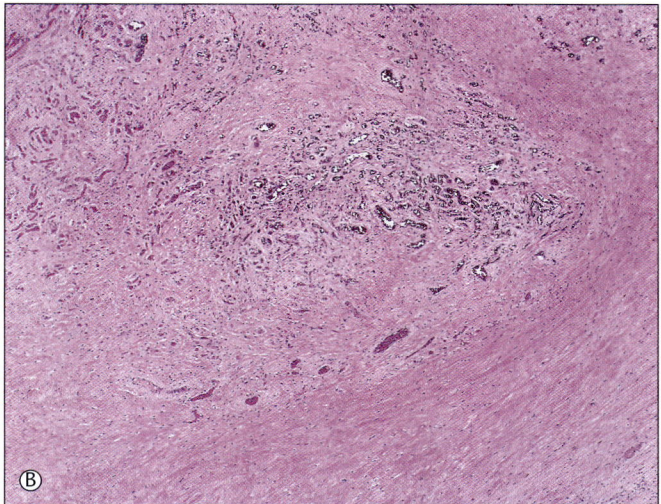

Figure 32.68 **(A, B)** Chorangioma, H&E. **(A)** Low magnification of usual nodule. **(B)** Obliterative nodule.

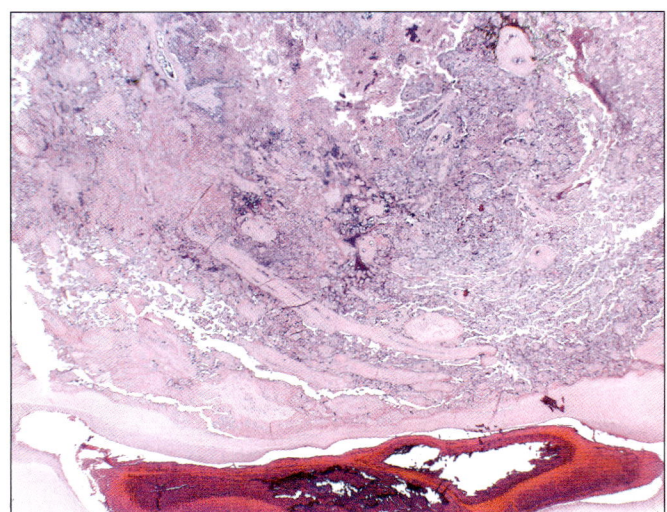

Figure 32.69 Choriocarcinoma *in situ*. Grossly, the small nodule appeared yellow as in infarct.

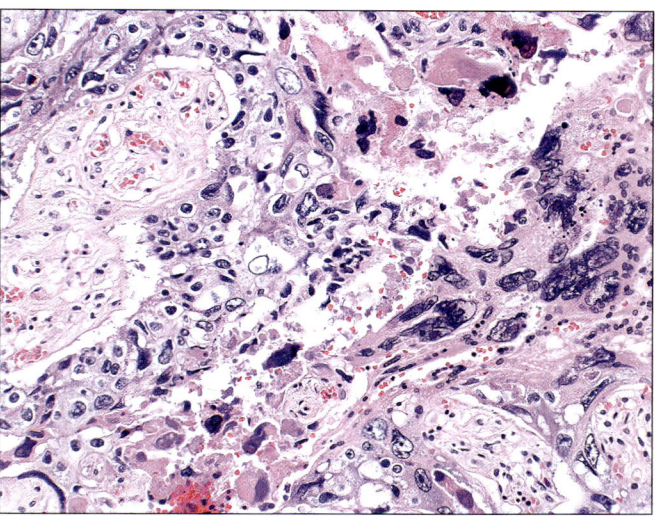

Figure 32.70 Choriocarcinoma *in situ*. The trophoblasts growing about the residual villi are in the typical pattern of choriocarcinoma.

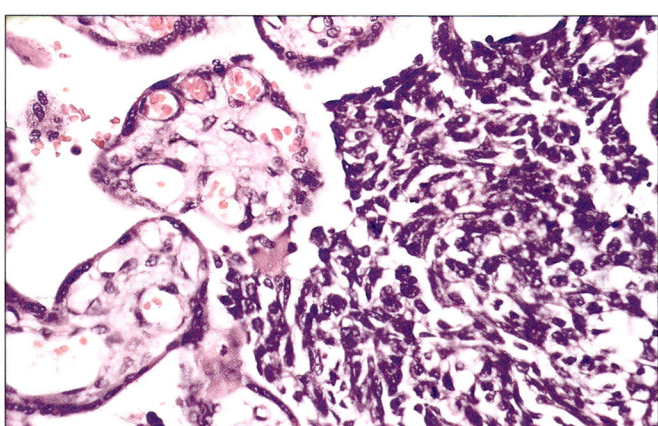

Figure 32.71 Metastatic breast carcinoma. Aggregates of poorly differentiated malignant cells lie in the intervillous space.

under-reported. Microscopically, there is central necrosis and a rim of abnormal trophoblast with choriocarcinomatous features (Figures 32.69 and 32.70). Systemic metastases are seen in some mothers or infants, but other patients appear free of disease on follow-up.[108]

TERATOMAS

Teratomas may arise in the placenta, or more accurately between the amnion and chorion, either on the placental disc or within the membranes. They contain mature elements such as skin, brain, gut, or cartilage. They probably arise from faulty migration of germ cells from the mesentery of the bowel when it is within the umbilical cord and hence may give rise to teratomas of the cord. This is the same site as the calcified yolk sac vestige that may be found, implying another possible mechanism for germ cell sequestration. Hepatocellular adenoma and an adrenal heterotopia have also been described.

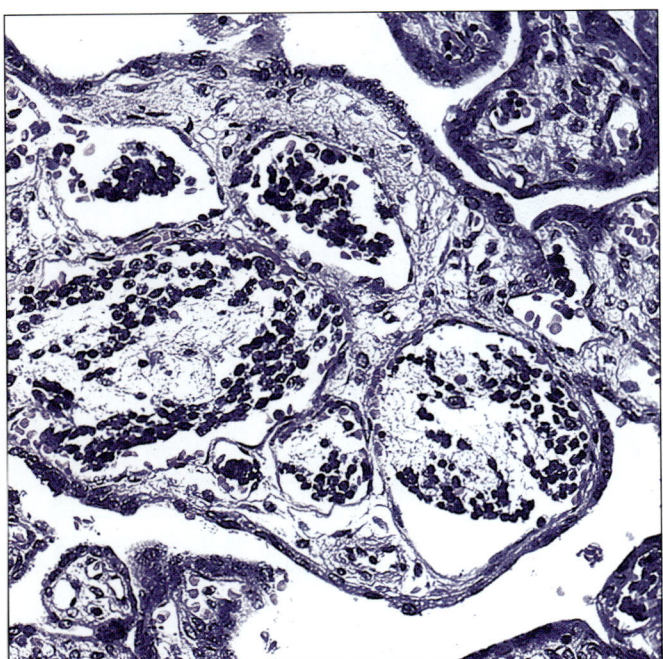

Figure 32.72 Metastatic neuroblastoma within villous blood vessels.

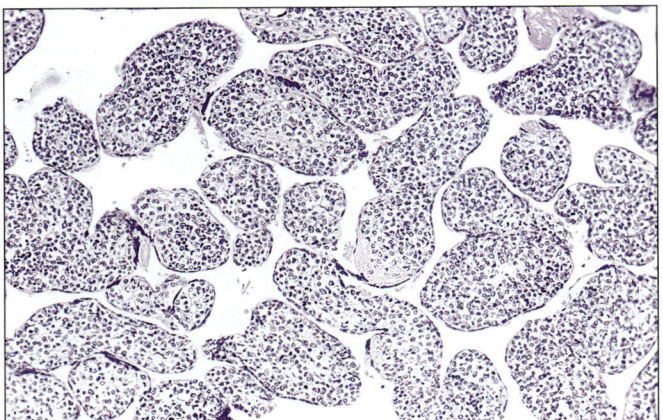

Figure 32.73 Congenital leukemia.

METASTATIC TUMOR

The placenta may rarely harbor maternal and even more exceptionally congenital fetal tumor metastases. Metastatic tumors may be seen macroscopically in 60% of involved placentas, especially in cases of pigmented melanomas. A review of metastases of maternal malignancies to placenta or baby documented 81 cases in the English-language literature from 1930.[109] Melanoma, lung carcinoma, leukemia/lymphoma, and breast carcinoma (Figure 32.71) were most common, together accounting for 74% of cases.

Neuroblastoma may present with intraplacental metastases with tumor cells being seen in villous vessels (Figure 32.72). The fetus is usually hydropic due to the large abdominal tumor load that restricts the venous return. Most fetuses are stillborn. Other malignancies that may be diagnosed primarily on placental examination include hepatoblastoma and primitive epithelial tumor of the liver. Congenital leukemia/transient myeloproliferative disease may also occasionally be seen in villous vessels (Figure 32.73). It is associated with trisomy 21, and this possibility should be suggested to the clinician or considered at autopsy.

REFERENCES

1. Larsen LG, Graem N. Morphological findings and value of placental examination at fetal and perinatal autopsy. APMIS 1999;107:337–45.
2. Korteweg FJ, Erwich JJ, Holm JP, et al. Diverse placental pathologies as the main causes of fetal death. Obstet Gynecol 2009;114:809–17.
3. Roberts DJ, Oliva E. Clinical significance of placental examination in perinatal medicine. J Matern Fetal Neonatal Med 2006;19:255–64.
4. Cooley SM, Donnelly JC, Walsh T, et al. The impact of ultrasonographic placental architecture on antenatal course, labor and delivery in a low-risk primigravid population. J Matern Fetal Neonatal Med 2011;24:493–7.
5. Pijnenborg R, Vercruysse L, Brosens I. Deep placentation. Best Pract Res Clin Obstet Gynaecol 2011;25:273–85.
6. Moser G, Gauster M, Orendi K, et al. Endoglandular trophoblast, an alternative route of trophoblast invasion? Analysis with novel confrontation co-culture models. Hum Reprod 2919;25:1127–36.
7. Burton GJ, Jauniaux E, Charnock-Jones DS. The influence of the intrauterine environment on human placental development. Int J Dev Biol 2010;54:303–12.
8. Yampolsky M, Salafia CM, Shlakhter O, et al. Centrality of the umbilical cord insertion in a human placenta influences the placental efficiency. Placenta 2009;30:1058–64.
9. Tantbirojn P, Saleemuddin A, Sirois K, et al. Gross abnormalities of the umbilical cord: related placental histology and clinical significance. Placenta 2009;30:1083–8.
10. Baergen RN, Malicki D, Behling C, Benirschke K. Morbidity, mortality, and placental pathology in excessively long umbilical cords: retrospective study. Pediatr Dev Pathol 2001;4:144–53.
11. Redline RW. Clinical and pathological umbilical cord abnormalities in fetal thrombotic vasculopathy. Hum Pathol 2004;35:1494–8.
12. Ghezzi F, Raio L, Gunter Duwe D, et al. Sonographic umbilical vessel morphometry and perinatal outcome of fetuses with a lean umbilical cord. J Clin Ultrasound 2005;33:18–23.
13. Hershkovitz R, Silberstein T, Sheiner E, et al. Risk factors associated with true knots of the umbilical cord. Eur J Obstet Gynecol Reprod Biol 2001;98:36–9.
14. Maher JT, Conti JA. A comparison of umbilical cord blood gas values between newborns with and without true knots. Obstet Gynecol 1996;88:863–6.
15. Parast MM, Crum CP, Boyd TK. Placental histologic criteria for umbilical blood flow restriction in unexplained stillbirth. Hum Pathol 2008;39:948–53.
16. de Laat MWM, Franx A, van Alderen ED, et al. The umbilical coiling index, a review of the literature. J Matern Fetal Neonatal Med 2005;17;93–100.
17. Khong TY. Evidence-based pathology: umbilical cord coiling. Pathology 2010;42;618–22.
18. Peng HQ, Levitin-Smith M, Rochelson B, Kahn E. Umbilical cord stricture and overcoiling are common causes of fetal demise. Pediatr Dev Pathol 2006;9:14–9.
19. Heinonen S, Ryynänen M, Kirkinen P, Saarikoski S. Perinatal diagnostic evaluation of velamentous umbilical cord insertion: clinical, Doppler, and ultrasonic findings. Obstet Gynecol 1996;87:112–7.
20. Cipriano LE, Barth Jr WH, Zaric GS. The cost-effectiveness of targeted or universal screening for vasa praevia at 18–20 weeks of gestation in Ontario. BJOG 2010;117:1108–18.
21. Murphy-Kaulbeck L, Dodds L, Joseph KS, Van den Hof M. Single umbilical artery risk factors and pregnancy outcomes. Obstet Gynecol 2010;116:843–50.
22. Chetty-John S, Zhang J, Chen Z, et al. Long-term physical and neurologic development in newborn infants with isolated single umbilical artery. Am J Obstet Gynecol 2010;203:368.e1–7.
23. Qureshi F, Jacques SM. Marked segmental thinning of the umbilical cord vessels. Arch Pathol Lab Med 1994;118:826–30.

24. Menon R, Taylor RN, Fortunato SJ. Chorioamnionitis—a complex pathophysiologic syndrome. Placenta 2010;31:113–20.
25. Buhimschi IA, Zambrano E, Pettker CM, et al. Using proteomic analysis of the human amniotic fluid to identify histologic chorioamnionitis. Obstet Gynecol 2008;111:403–12.
26. Winters R, Waters BL. What is adequate sampling of extraplacental membranes?: a randomized, prospective analysis. Arch Pathol Lab Med 2008;132:1920–3.
27. Redline RW, Faye-Peterson O, Heller D, et al. Amniotic infection syndrome: nosology and reproducibility of placental reaction patterns. Pediatr Dev Pathol 2003;6:435–48.
28. Park CW, Moon KC, Park JS, et al. The involvement of human amnion in histologic chorioamnionitis is an indicator that a fetal and an intra-amniotic inflammatory response is more likely and severe: clinical implications. Placenta 2009;30:56–61.
29. Kim MJ, Romero R, Gervasi MT, et al. Widespread microbial invasion of the chorioamniotic membranes is a consequence and not a cause of intra-amniotic infection. Lab Invest 2009;89:924–36.
30. Nelson KB, Dambrosia JM, Grether JK, Phillips TM. Neonatal cytokines and coagulation factors in children with cerebral palsy. Ann Neurol 1998;44;665–75.
31. Wharton KN, Pinar H, Stonestreet BS, et al. Severe umbilical cord inflammation—a predictor of periventricular leukomalacia in very low birth weight infants. Early Hum Dev 2004;77:77–87.
32. Alexander JM, McIntire DM, Leveno KJ. Chorioamnionitis and the prognosis for term infants. Obstet Gynecol 1999;94:274–8.
33. Redline RW, Wilson-Costello D, Borawski E, et al. Placental lesions associated with neurologic impairment and cerebral palsy in very low-birth-weight infants. Arch Pathol Lab Med 1998;122:1091–8.
34. Dexter SC, Malee MP, Pinar H, et al. Influence of chorioamnionitis on developmental outcome in very low birth weight infants. Obstet Gynecol 1999;94:267–73.
35. Malaeb S, Dammann O. Fetal inflammatory response and brain injury in the preterm newborn. J Child Neurol 2009;24:1119–26.
36. Mestan K, Yu Y, Matoba N, et al. Placental inflammatory response is associated with poor neonatal growth: preterm birth cohort study. Pediatrics 2010;125:e891–8.
37. Lakshmanan J, Ross MG. Mechanism(s) of in utero meconium passage. J Perinatol 2008;28(Suppl 3):S8–13.
38. Ramón y Cajal CL, Martínez RO. Defecation in utero: a physiologic fetal function. Am J Obstet Gynecol 2003;188:153–6.
39. Burgess AM, Hutchins GM. Inflammation of the lungs, umbilical cord and placenta associated with meconium passage in utero. Review of 123 autopsied cases. Pathol Res Pract 1996;192:1121–8.
40. Redline RW, Wilson-Costello D. Chronic peripheral separation of placenta. The significance of diffuse chorioamnionic hemosiderosis. Am J Clin Pathol 1999;111:804–10.
41. Barker DJP, Thornburg KL, Osmond C, et al. The prenatal origins of lung cancer. II. The placenta. Am J Hum Biol 2010;22:512–6.
42. Burkhardt T, Schäffer L, Schneider C, et al. Reference values for the weight of freshly delivered term placentas and for placental weight-birth weight ratios. Eur J Obstet Gynecol Reprod Biol 2006;128:248–52.
43. Pinar H, Sung CJ, Oyer CE, Singer DB. Reference values for singleton and twin placental weights. Pediatr Pathol Lab Med 1996;16:901–7.
44. Almog B, Shehata F, Aljabri S, et al. Placenta weight percentile curves for singleton and twins deliveries. Placenta 2011;32:58–62.
45. Redline RW, Patterson P. Patterns of placental injury. Correlations with gestational age, placental weight, and clinical diagnoses. Arch Pathol Lab Med 1994;118:698–701.
46. Sebire NJ, Sepulveda W. Correlation of placental pathology with prenatal ultrasound findings. J Clin Pathol 2008;61;1276–84.
47. Pham T, Steele J, Stayboldt C, et al. Placental mesenchymal dysplasia is associated with high rates of intrauterine growth restriction and fetal demise: a report of 11 new cases and a review of the literature. Am J Clin Pathol 2006;126:67–78.
48. Parveen Z, Tongson-Ignacio JE, Fraser CR, et al. Placental mesenchymal dysplasia. Arch Pathol Lab Med 2007;131:131–7.
49. Kraus FT. Cerebral palsy and thrombi in placental vessels of the fetus: insights from litigation. Hum Pathol 1997;28:246–8.
50. Mooney EE, al Shunnar A, O'Regan M, Gillan JE. Chorionic villous haemorrhage is associated with retroplacental haemorrhage. Br J Obstet Gynaecol 1994;101:965–9.
51. McDermott M, Gillan JE. Chronic reduction in fetal blood flow is associated with placental infarction. Placenta 1995;16:165–70.
52. Katzman PJ, Genest DR. Maternal floor infarction and massive perivillous fibrin deposition: histological definitions, association with intrauterine fetal growth restriction, and risk of recurrence. Pediatr Dev Pathol 2002;5:159–64.
53. Uxa R, Baczyk D, Kingdom JC, et al. Genetic polymorphisms in the fibrinolytic system of placentas with massive perivillous fibrin deposition. Placenta 2010;31:499–505.
54. Bane AL, Gillan JE. Massive perivillous fibrinoid causing recurrent placental failure. BJOG 2003;110:292–5.
55. Elsasser DA, Ananth CV, Prasad V, Vintzileos AM. Diagnosis of placental abruption: relationship between clinical and histopathological findings. Eur J Obstet Gynecol Reprod Biol 2010;148:125–30.
56. Bendon RW. Review of autopsies of stillborn infants with retroplacental hematoma or hemorrhage. Pediatr Dev Pathol 2011;14:10–5.
57. Mooney EE, Boggess KA, Herbert WN, Layfield LJ. Placental pathology in patients using cocaine: an observational study. Obstet Gynecol 1998;91:925–9.
58. Ananth CV, Savitz DA, Williams MA. Placental abruption and its association with hypertension and prolonged rupture of membranes: a methodologic review and meta-analysis. Obstet Gynecol 1996;88:309–18.
59. Misra DP, Ananth CV. Risk factor profiles of placental abruption in first and second pregnancies: heterogeneous etiologies. J Clin Epidemiol 1999;52:453–61.
60. Fung TY, To KF, Sahota DS, et al. Massive subchorionic thrombohematoma: a series of 10 cases. Acta Obstet Gynecol Scand 2010;89:1357–61.
61. Chen KH, Chen LR, Lee YH. Exploring the relationship between preterm placental calcification and adverse maternal and fetal outcome. Ultrasound Obstet Gynecol 2011;37:328–34.
62. Stanek, J. Placental membrane and placental disc microscopic chorionic cysts share similar clinicopathologic associations. Pediatr Dev Pathol 2011;14;1–9.
63. Souter VL, Kapur RP, Nynholt DR, et al. A report of dizygous monochorionic twins. N Engl J Med 2003;349:154–8.
64. Carroll SG, Tyfield L, Reeve L, et al. Is zygosity or chorionicity the main determinant of fetal outcome in twin pregnancies? Am J Obstet Gynecol 2005;193:757–61.
65. Hack KE, Derks JB, Elias SG, et al. Increased perinatal mortality and morbidity in monochorionic versus dichorionic twin pregnancies: clinical implications of a large Dutch cohort study. BJOG 2008;115:58–67.
66. Nikkels PGJ, Hack KEA, van Gemert MJC. Pathology of twin placentas with special attention to monochorionic twin placentas. J Clin Pathol 2008;61:1247–53.
67. Redline RW, Shah D, Sakar H, et al. Placental lesions associated with abnormal growth in twins. Pediatr Dev Pathol 2001;4:473–81.
68. Hack KEA, van Gemert MJ, Lopriore E, et al. Placental characteristics of monoamniotic twin pregnancies in relation to perinatal outcome. Placenta 2009;30:62–5.
69. Bendon RW. Twin transfusion: pathological studies of the monochorionic placenta in liveborn twins and of the perinatal autopsy in monochorionic twin pairs. Pediatr Pathol Lab Med 1995;15:363–76.
70. Edmondson N, Bocking A, Machin G, et al. The prevalence of chronic deciduitis in cases of preterm labor without clinical chorioamnionitis. Pediatr Dev Pathol 2009;12:16–21.
71. Oggé G, Romero R, Lee DC, et al. Chronic chorioamnionitis displays distinct alterations of the amniotic fluid proteome. J Pathol 2011;223:553–65.
72. Kim CJ, Romero R, Kusanov JP, et al. The frequency, clinical significance, and pathological features of chronic chorioamnionitis: a lesion associated with spontaneous preterm birth. Mod Pathol 2010;23:1000–11.
73. Stanek J. Diagnosing placental membrane hypoxic lesions increases the sensitivity of placental examination. Arch Pathol Lab Med 2010;134:989–95.
74. Goldenberg RL, Faye-Petesen O, Andrews WW, et al. The Alabama Preterm Birth Study: diffuse decidual leukocytoclastic necrosis of the decidua basalis, a placental lesion associated with preeclampsia, indicated preterm birth and decreased fetal growth. J Matern Fetal Neonatal Med 2007;20:391–5.
75. Redline RW, Boyd T, Campbell V, et al. Maternal vascular underperfusion: nosology and reproducibility of placental reaction patterns. Pediatr Dev Pathol 2004;7:237–49.

76. Jaiman S, Johansen T. Eosinophilic/T-cell chorionic vasculitis and intrauterine fetal demise at 34 weeks: case report and review of the literature. Pediatr Dev Pathol 2010;13:393–6.
77. Myerson D, Parkin RK, Benirschke K, et al. The pathogenesis of villitis of unknown etiology: analysis with a new conjoint immunohistochemistry-in situ hybridization procedure to identify specific maternal and fetal cells. Pediatr Dev Pathol 2006;9:257–65.
78. Yusuf K, Kliman HJ. The fetus, not the mother, elicits maternal immunologic rejection: lessons from discordant dizygotic twin placentas. J Perinat Med 2008;36:291–6.
79. Torrance HL, Bloemen MC, Mulder EJ, et al. Predictors of outcome at 2 years of age after early intrauterine growth restriction. Ultrasound Obstet Gynecol 2010;36:171–7.
80. Redline RW. Severe fetal placental vascular lesions in term infants with neurologic impairment. Am J Obstet Gynecol 2005;192:452–7.
81. Becroft DM, Thompson JM, Mitchell EA. Placental villitis of unknown origin: epidemiologic associations. Am J Obstet Gynecol 2005;192:264–71.
82. Feeley L, Mooney EE. Villitis of unknown aetiology: correlation of recurrence with clinical outcome. J Obstet Gynaecol 2010;30:476–9.
83. Benirschke K, Coen R, Patterson B, Key T. Villitis of known origin: varicella and toxoplasma. Placenta 1999;20:395–9.
84. Traeder J, Jonigk D, Feist H, et al. Pathological characteristics of a series of rare chronic histiocytic intervillositis of the placenta. Placenta 2010;31:1116–9.
85. Marchaudon V, Devisme L, Petit S, et al. Chronic histiocytic intervillositis of unknown etiology: clinical features in a consecutive series of 69 cases. Placenta 2011;32:140–5.
86. McDonald DG, Kelehan P, McMenamin JB, et al. Placental fetal thrombotic vasculopathy is associated with neonatal encephalopathy. Hum Pathol 2004;35:875–80.
87. Redline RW, Heller D, Keating S, Kingdom J. Placental diagnostic criteria and clinical correlation–a workshop report. Placenta 2005;26(Suppl A):S114–7.
88. Saleemuddin A, Tantbirojn P, Sirosis, K, et al. Obstetric and perinatal complications in placentas with fetal thrombotic vasculopathy. Pediatr Dev Pathol 2010;13:459–64.
89. Gogia N, Machin GA. Maternal thrombophilias are associated with specific placental lesions. Pediatr Dev Pathol 2008;11:424–9.
90. Raspollini MR, Oliva E, Roberts DJ. Placental histopathologic features in patients with thrombophilic mutations. J Matern Fetal Neonatal Med 2007;20:113–23.
91. Sedano S, Gaffney G, Mortimer G, et al. Activated protein C resistance (APCR) and placental fibrin deposition. Placenta 2008;29:833–7.
92. Franco C, Walker M, Robertson J, et al. Placental infarction and thrombophilia. Obstet Gynecol 2011;117:929–34.
93. Rogers BB, Momirova V, Dizon-Townson D, et al. Avascular villi, increased syncytial knots, and hypervascular villi are associated with pregnancies complicated by factor V Leiden mutation. Pediatr Dev Pathol 2010;13:341–7.
94. Rodger MA, Betancourt MT, Clark P, et al. The association of factor V leiden and prothrombin gene mutation and placenta-mediated pregnancy complications: a systematic review and meta-analysis of prospective cohort studies. PLoS Med 2010;7:e1000292.
95. Sood R, Zogg M, Westrick RJ, et al. Fetal gene defects precipitate platelet-mediated pregnancy failure in factor V Leiden mothers. J Exp Med 2007;204:1049–56.
96. Amer HZM, Heller DS. Chorangioma and related vascular lesions of the placenta–a review. Fetal Pediatr Pathol 2010;29:199–206.
97. Khong TY, Staples A, Bendon RW, et al. Observer reliability in assessing placental maturity by histology. J Clin Pathol 1995;48:420–3.
98. Loukeris K, Sela R, Baergen RN. Syncytial knots as a reflection of placental maturity: reference values for 20 to 40 weeks' gestational age. Pediatr Dev Pathol 2010;13:305–9.
99. Stallmach T, Hebisch G, Meier K, et al. Rescue by birth: defective placental maturation and late fetal mortality. Obstet Gynecol 2001;97:505–9.
100. Higgins MF, McAuliffe FM, Mooney E. Clinical Associations with a Placental Diagnosis of Delayed Villous Maturation: A Retrospective Study. Pediatr Dev Pathol 2011;14:273–9.
101. de Laat MWM, van der Meij JJC, Visser GHA, et al. Hypercoiling of the umbilical cord and placental maturation defect: associated pathology? Pediatr Dev Pathol 2007;10:293–9.
102. Redline RW, Minich N, Taylor HG, Hack M. Placental lesions as predictors of cerebral palsy and abnormal neurocognitive function at school age in extremely low birth weight infants (<1 kg). Pediatr Dev Pathol 2007;10:282–92.
103. Redline RW. Elevated circulating fetal nucleated red blood cells and placental pathology in term infants who develop cerebral palsy. Hum Pathol 2008;39:1378–84.
104. Guschmann M, Henrich W, Entezami M, Dudenhausen JW. Chorioangioma—new insights into a well-known problem. I. Results of a clinical and morphological study of 136 cases. J Perinat Med 2003;31:163–9.
105. Sepulveda W, Alcalde JL, Schnapp C, Bravo M. Perinatal outcome after prenatal diagnosis of placental chorioangioma. Obstet Gynecol 2003;102:1028–33.
106. Hoeger PH, Maerker JM, Kienast AK, et al. Neonatal haemangiomatosis associated with placental chorioangiomas: report of three cases and review of the literature. Clin Exp Dermatol 2009;34:e78–80.
107. Khong TY. Chorangioma with trophoblastic proliferation. Virchows Arch 2000;436:167–71.
108. Sebire NJ, Lindsay I, Fisher RA, Seckl MJ. Intraplacental choriocarcinoma: experience from a tertiary referral center and relationship with infantile choriocarcinoma. Fetal Pediatr Pathol 2005;24:21–9.
109. Al-Adnani M, Kiho L, Scheimberg I. Maternal pancreatic carcinoma metastatic to the placenta: a case report and literature review. Pediatr Dev Pathol 2007;10:61–5.

Non-Neoplastic Maternal Gestational Diseases

33

Eoghan E. Mooney, Emma M. Doyle

CHAPTER OUTLINE

Early Pregnancy Loss (Spontaneous Miscarriage)	769
Mid to Late Pregnancy Loss	771
Abruption	771
Hypertensive Disorders	772
Pre-eclampsia	772
Intrauterine Growth Restriction	773
Confined Placental Mosaicism	774
Adverse Neurologic Outcome: Neonatal Encephalopathy and Cerebral Palsy	774
Diabetes Mellitus	775
Hydrops Fetalis (Maternal Rhesus Isoimmunization)	775
Placenta Creta	775
Postpartum Hemorrhage and Subinvolution	776
Maternal Sickle Cell Trait and Disease	776
Twin Pregnancy	777
Prolonged Pregnancy	777
Maternal Infections and the Placenta	777
Cytomegalovirus	777
Parvovirus B19	778
Rubella	779
Varicella Zoster	779
Herpes Simplex	779
HIV	780
Human Papillomavirus	780
Toxoplasmosis	780
Malaria	781
Syphilis	781
Listeriosis	781
Other Organisms	781

Gross examination of the placenta by the obstetrician or midwife is a routine practice at the time of delivery. Inspection of the membranes, umbilical cord, and cotyledons can help determine whether there is any retained tissue that may result in postpartum hemorrhage, or any gross abnormalities that might prompt a closer evaluation of the newborn baby. In most institutions the decision to request a pathologic evaluation of the placenta is made by the delivering clinician.

Chapter 32 emphasizes the pathologic findings. This chapter focuses on the placental findings in common clinical scenarios. Points of particular relevance in the gross examination of the placenta are highlighted. While substantial overlap exists for some entities, e.g., intrauterine growth restriction (IUGR) and uteroplacental insufficiency, the scenarios are presented separately for ease of discussion.

Presentation of the findings in a fashion intelligible to clinicians is of major importance. The terminology proposed by the Society of Pediatric Pathology has been referred to.[1-3] A synopsis of the findings may be given as a 'one-liner' in the pathology report, and may help clinicians to categorize the histologic findings (Table 33.1).

EARLY PREGNANCY LOSS (SPONTANEOUS MISCARRIAGE)

The term 'abortion' is often replaced by the term 'miscarriage' in clinical practice. There is considerable variation in the definition of miscarriage, but 500 g birthweight or 24 weeks of gestation are frequently used as the upper limits in the definition of miscarriage (vs stillbirth). The incidence of miscarriage is difficult to ascertain as many women miscarry before they are aware of the pregnancy: as many as 78% of human conceptions do not result in term delivery. Approximately 15–25% of recognized pregnancies will end in a miscarriage.

The report on the products of conception from a miscarriage should (1) state that a pregnancy can be proven (by the presence of tissues of fetal origin, i.e., embryonic parts, chorionic villi, or trophoblast); (2) state if it is intrauterine (by the presence of decidua with implantation site); and (3) exclude a serious disease process, especially gestational trophoblastic disease.

Selected tissue from all miscarriages should be examined microscopically. Tissues felt to be present macroscopically are

Table 33.1	Classification System for Placental Reporting
1	Normal placenta
2	Placenta with chorioamnionitis
3	Placenta with villitis
4	Placenta with materno-placental circulatory disorder
5	Placenta with fetal–placental circulatory disorder
6	Placenta with maturation disturbances
7	Placenta with findings suggestive of gene aberration
8	Placenta with placentation defects
9	Placenta with other pathology

Courtesy of Professor Borghild Roald, Oslo, Norway.[4]

sometimes absent histologically, and the converse is also true. Fetal parts, when present, may be examined in accordance with parental wishes. Suction termination disrupts the fetus, but measurements of a hand or foot permit comparison against tables of growth rates. Whole fetuses and large embryos may be examined according to published protocols.

Chromosomal abnormalities in the conceptus are more frequently identified in earlier than in later fetal losses, with 65–75% of first trimester miscarriages having an abnormal karyotype.[5,6] Most will be sporadic events, but a small minority result from balanced translocations in one of the parents and hence may recur. Some of the more commonly encountered karyotypic abnormalities are trisomies, especially 16 and 13, and monosomy X (45,X). Even when the karyotype is normal, there is a clear association between congenital abnormality and miscarriage. The incidence of neural tube defects and other minor abnormalities, such as cleft lip and palate or polydactyly, is higher in abortuses than in live births. Abnormalities of chromosomes 16 and 22 are prominent in early pregnancy loss (Figure 33.1A and B), and these chromosomes are preferentially involved by confined placental mosaicism.[7]

There have been several attempts to determine the etiology of early fetal loss by morphologic examination. Villous features thought to represent karyotypic abnormalities include vesicular change, irregular villous contour, presence of trophoblastic pseudoinclusions, trophoblastic hyperplasia, abnormal stromal cells, and, in the case of monosomy X, villous fibrosis and hypoplasia. Recognition of abnormalities at the maternal–embryonic interface (i.e., absence of interstitial trophoblast columns, absence of intravascular trophoblast plugs, and absence of physiologic changes in spiral arteries) increases the sensitivity of histology for detection of chromosomal abnormalities. Recurrent and sporadic miscarriages have similar findings, and in the majority of cases it is difficult to ascertain the cause.[8] Elegant light and electron microscopic studies support the concept that many early pregnancy losses result from premature onset of the maternal–placental circulation secondary to inadequate trophoblast invasion.

Uterine abnormalities such as leiomyomas, cervical incompetence, and congenital abnormalities of müllerian duct fusion may all contribute to early pregnancy loss. Infection becomes increasingly important later in gestation as the influence of abnormal karyotype wanes. Early on, *Campylobacter* sp., *Listeria monocytogenes*, *Toxoplasma gondii*, rubella,

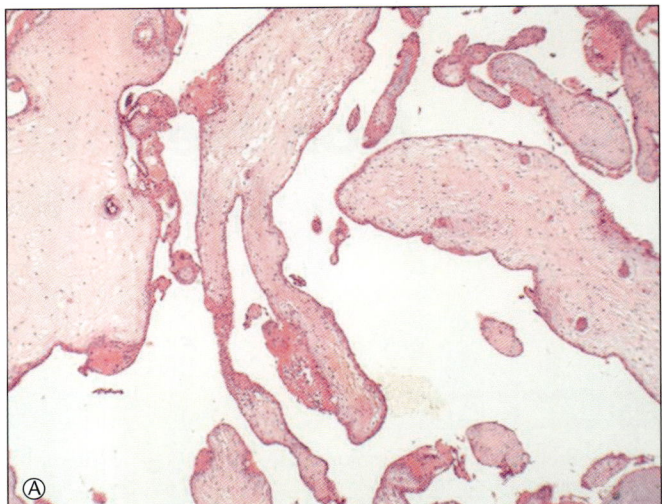

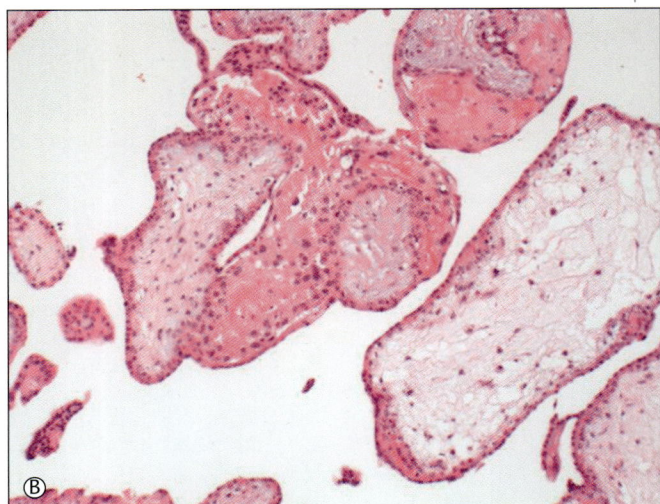

Figure 33.1 Villous changes seen in miscarriages with **(A)** trisomy 16 and **(B)** trisomy 22.

cytomegalovirus (CMV), and syphilis are important. Molecular analysis suggests that coxsackie virus is one of the most common infectious agents, but placental findings are nonspecific.[9] Similarly, human papillomavirus (HPV) is more commonly demonstrated in spontaneous pre-term delivery.[10]

The finding of a placental site trophoblastic reaction is important as it generally excludes that the pregnancy was ectopic in the fallopian tube and merely became displaced into the uterus following miscarriage. The presence of chorionic villi and decidua by themselves theoretically do not achieve this according to some reports in the literature,[11] but neither of the authors has encountered an example of chorionic villi in the uterus where the origin proved to be an ectopic pregnancy. In summary, examination of the early pregnancy loss will:

- Confirm intrauterine gestation in most cases
- Exclude hydatidiform mole in the vast majority of cases
- Identify an occasional case of chronic histiocytic intervillositis
- Not identify the etiology in most cases.

MID TO LATE PREGNANCY LOSS

The 9–12 week period sees the highest rate of miscarriage. Miscarriages may be retained for some time before detection, when advanced maceration can make precise dating and definitive diagnosis difficult.

If a miscarriage at 18–22 weeks is fresh, infection is a likely cause and examination should focus on the membranes. A small placenta is frequently found in trisomies and should prompt cytogenetic analysis, as karyotypic abnormalities can be expected from over 85% of placental cultures even when maceration is present.[12] Second trimester miscarriages may occur following abnormal implantation, with ischemic changes up to and including infarction. Any infarction in the second trimester is likely to be clinically significant, and should be confirmed histologically. Placental infarction is associated with cerebral ischemia in the fetus, particularly in growth-restricted infants.[13] The mean gestational age of pregnancy loss due to intervillositis in our practice is 25 weeks, and any increase in fibrin should prompt careful evaluation for this entity. Villitis of unknown etiology is uncommon before the third trimester.

Caution must be exercised in making the diagnosis of fetal thrombotic vasculopathy in macerated fetuses, unless there is unequivocal evidence of antemortem vascular pathology, such as clearly defined avascular villi (Figure 33.2). This is usually not possible, but, where present, enables antemortem pathology to be distinguished from the secondary effects of intrauterine death.

Abnormal cord coiling, assessed as both under- and over-coiled cords, is associated with fetal death.[14,15] Cord coiling is frequently presented as an explanation for fetal death. Features of vascular compromise such as avascular villi, vascular ectasia, and mural fibrin thrombi should be sought in this context.

The role of an individual placental finding in stillbirth may be problematic. A National Institute of Child Health and Human Development workshop in 2007 evaluated maternal, fetal, and placental conditions as a cause of stillbirth.[16] The proceedings also include useful overviews of the role of infectious organisms in stillbirth.

ABRUPTION

Abruption, a condition in which the placenta detaches if not tears away from the uterine wall, can be a dramatic obstetric event. Although abruption and retroplacental hemorrhage are sometimes used interchangeably, abruption signifies a clinical event with signs and symptoms, whereas retroplacental hemorrhage is a pathologic finding, often with no clinical correlation (see Chapter 32). Occurring in 1% of pregnancies, abruption is a leading cause of vaginal bleeding in the latter half of pregnancy, and an important cause of perinatal morbidity. It accounts for 12% of perinatal deaths.[17] The effect on the mother depends primarily on the severity of the abruption, whereas the effect on the fetus depends both on the severity of the abruption as well as on the fetus's gestational age. Risk factors include prior abruption, smoking, trauma, multifetal gestation, hypertension, pre-eclampsia, thrombophilias, advanced maternal age, preterm premature rupture of the membranes, intrauterine infections, and polyhydramnios.[18] Cocaine abuse may also be a cause. From the pathologist's viewpoint, chorionic villus hemorrhage and villus edema are more frequent in cocaine users.

Questions frequently posed to the pathologist include: does an abruption exist, how extensive is it, and is it recent or old? More often than not, none of these questions can be answered solely on the pathologic examination, leading the pathologist to come away disappointed at not being able to add much of clinical use. Most are peripheral (Figure 33.3) and, if recent, will not be detected by pathologic examination, since the hemorrhage will have escaped peripherally and presented as vaginal bleeding. Retroplacental hemorrhage toward the center is far more significant (Figure 33.4), since the displaced placenta can no longer support fetal functions. In a study of over 53,000 pregnancies[19] the extent of placental separation determined

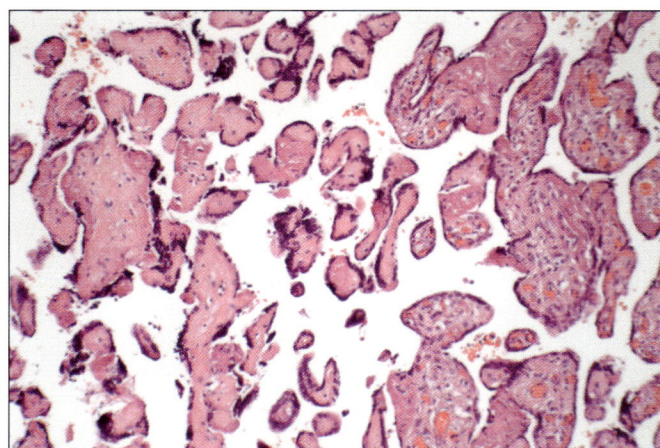

Figure 33.2 Despite changes of intrauterine death, avascular villi can be discerned (left of picture).

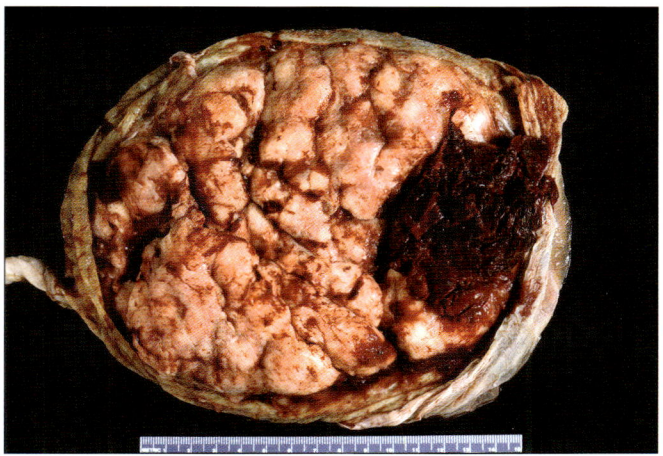

Figure 33.3 Peripheral and probably clinically insignificant abruption/retroplacental hemorrhage.

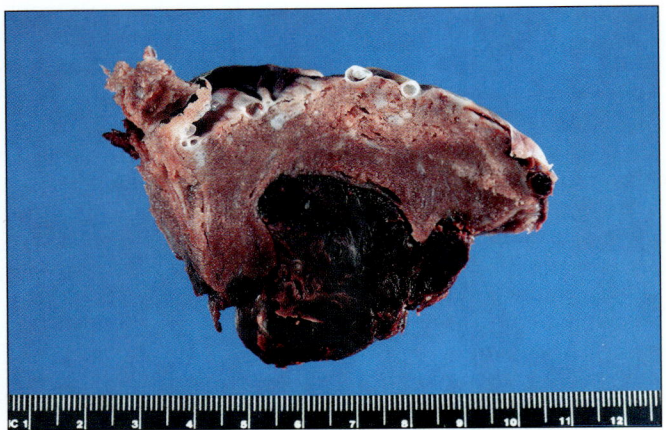

Figure 33.4 Abruption with parenchymal compression nearly half the placental thickness.

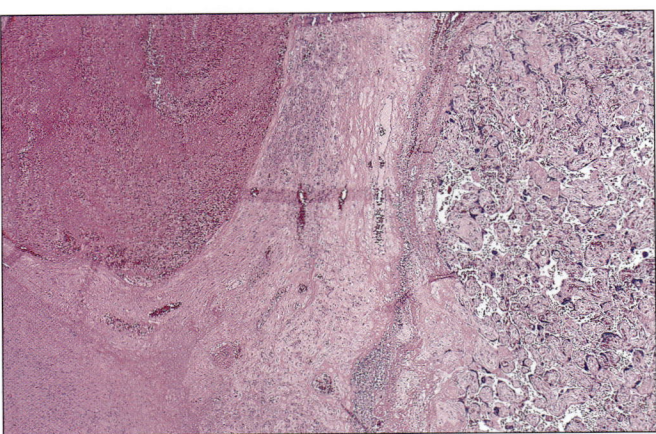

Figure 33.5 Abruption, clinically of 1 day's duration. An acute inflammatory infiltrate has developed at the interphase of the bleeding and parenchyma.

the chance of stillbirth. With a 75% separation, the risk of fetal death was increased 31-fold. Even a 50% separation showed profound effects. The risk for preterm delivery was also substantially increased when the separation was mild (with a separation of 25%, the relative risk was 5). The amount of bleeding is best gauged by the volume of retroplacental clot found at cesarean section, or secondarily by the amount of blood clot that accompanies the placenta to the pathology laboratory. The duration of the bleeding is best gauged by whether the parenchyma has been displaced by the blood, whether the junction of the blood and parenchyma shows discoloration from pigment breakdown, and whether the parenchyma near the abruption is infarcted.

Macroscopically, the location, diameter of the involved area, depth of the crater, and thickness of the normal placenta above should be recorded, as these measurements will help determine the significance of the abruption. Microscopic sections should be taken at several areas of the junction between the blood and placental parenchyma, as the tissue reaction can help date the abruption. Neutrophils in the basal plate above the hemorrhage are the earliest finding, occurring in <4 hours.[20] Nearly a day will have passed before the villi degenerate and an inflammatory response appears at the edge of the hemorrhage (Figure 33.5). Within several days there will be evidence of hemoglobin breakdown. Some placentas will show different changes at different areas. Placental abruption is generally regarded as an acute event, but it is often the end result of chronic processes that have begun earlier in pregnancy, even near the time of conception.[21] In a cohort of extremely low birth weight infants (<1000 g), placental abruption was found more commonly with histologic chorioamnionitis and funisitis.[22]

HYPERTENSIVE DISORDERS

PRE-ECLAMPSIA

Pre-eclampsia, a disorder unique to pregnancy, occurs in about 5–8% of pregnant women. Risk factors include nulliparity, women who are at the extremes of reproductive age, multiple gestation, and chronic diseases such as diabetes mellitus, kidney disease, and chronic hypertension. It usually begins insidiously after week 20 of pregnancy with excessive weight gain, marked fluid retention, increase in maternal systemic blood pressure, and the appearance of proteinuria. Pre-eclampsia is diagnosed when the blood pressure is sustained at or above 140 mmHg systolic or 90 mmHg diastolic and the urinary protein excretion exceeds 300 mg/day, but classification systems differ somewhat.[23]

Progression of mild pre-eclampsia can be slow or rapid and can manifest in many different ways. With increasing blood pressure and declining renal function the resulting fluid retention may result in pulmonary edema. The systemic vasospasm that occurs is particularly noticeable in organs with microvasculature. Hence the classic signs and symptoms of pre-eclampsia, including: visual disturbances from retinopathy, headache from cerebral vasculature changes, chest pain and shortness of breath from cardiopulmonary changes, right upper quadrant discomfort from hepatic dysfunction, proteinuria and glomerulopathy from decreased renal blood flow, systemic edema from peripheral vasospasm, and oligohydramnios and non-reassuring fetal testing from decreased placental perfusion.

Pre-eclampsia can be fatal for both the mother and the fetus. Maternal complications include eclamptic seizure, the syndrome of hemolysis, elevated liver enzymes, and low platelets (HELLP syndrome), subcapsular liver hematoma, pulmonary edema, acute renal failure, intracerebral hemorrhage, and death. The disseminated intravascular coagulation that sometimes develops is not part of the pre-eclampsia itself as much as a consequence of the developing HELLP syndrome, abruption, or hematoma. Fetal complications include non-reassuring fetal testing, placental abruption, oligohydramnios, IUGR, and death. Pre-eclampsia is treated with magnesium sulfate and antihypertensive agents, but the definitive therapy is the removal of the placenta, usually by induction of labor or by cesarean delivery.

Pre-eclampsia is classified as early onset (<34 weeks) or late onset. While late onset is by far the more common, it is not associated with placental disease and usually does not result in fetal growth restriction. The points below relate to early onset pre-eclampsia, which has been described as 'a disease of failed interaction between two genetically different organisms."[24] Along with understanding of the role of implantation has been its description as a two-stage disease.[24] Stage 1 is inadequate implantation and stage 2 is the clinical manifestations of endothelial activation in the third trimester. The sequence of events is outlined in Figure 33.6. Decidual natural killer cells, which constitute the majority of decidual white cells in the first trimester, play a key role in trophoblast invasion and successful implantation.[25] Persistence of smooth muscle in uterine spiral arteries results in irregular pulsatile flow, with consequent mechanical and oxidative stress to the placenta. This results in increased shedding of trophoblast by necrosis and aponecrosis, which facilitates an inflammatory response in the mother.[26] The complex interaction of abnormal placental flow and pre-eclampsia suggests that impaired invasion of deep spiral arteries might result from, rather than cause, maternal flow defects.[23]

Examination of the placenta from early onset pre-eclampsia should include evaluation of acute and chronic hypoxic changes, with a comment as to the degree of severity. Expected findings include a small placenta with accelerated maturation, ischemic villous crowding, and infarction. Atherosis (Figure 33.7) will be seen in only 50% of cases, but nontransformed vessels (i.e., those whose muscularis has not been replaced by trophoblast and fibrin) (Figures 33.8 and 33.9), and hypertrophic decidual arteriopathy may be present. Laminar decidual necrosis is common. Thrombotic disease in the fetal circulation is three to four times more common when there is uteroplacental ischemic disease, and may be focal or extensive.

INTRAUTERINE GROWTH RESTRICTION

Intrauterine Growth Restriction (IUGR), also known as fetal growth restriction, is where the infant fails to achieve its biologic growth potential. This category overlaps with those who are small for gestational age. Both entities are commonly defined as fetal weight below the 10th percentile for gestational age, but approximately 70% of infants in this

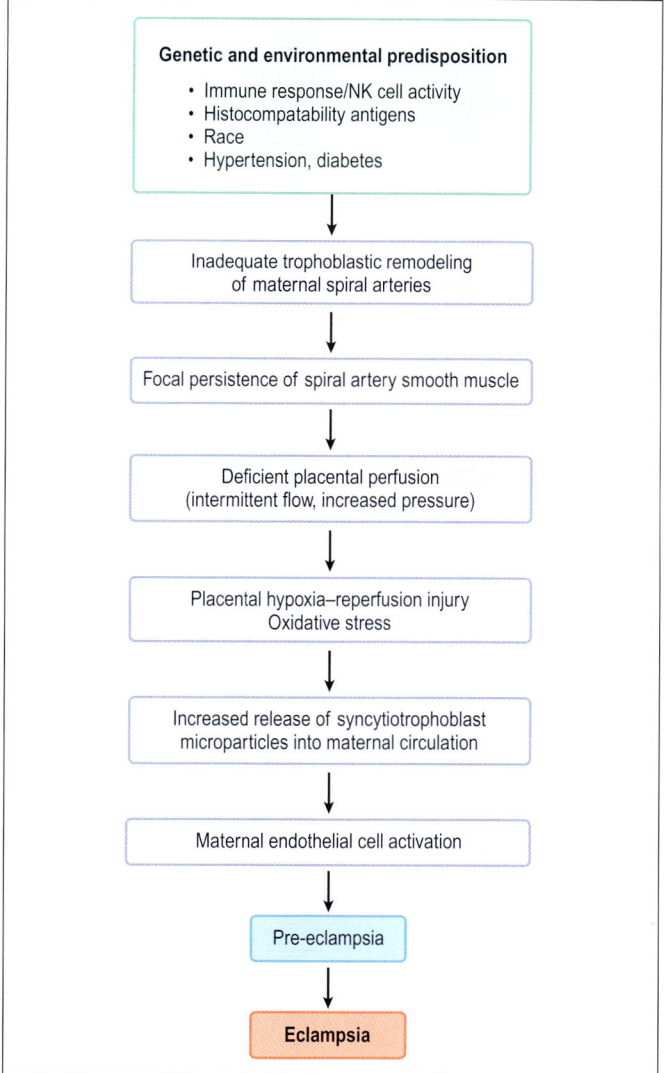

Figure 33.6 Pathogenesis of pre-eclampsia and eclampsia. (Data from Robboy SJ, Duggan M, Kurman RT. The female reproductive system. In: Rubin E, Farber J, editors. Pathology. 3rd ed. Philadelphia: Lippincott; 1999. p. 962–1028.)

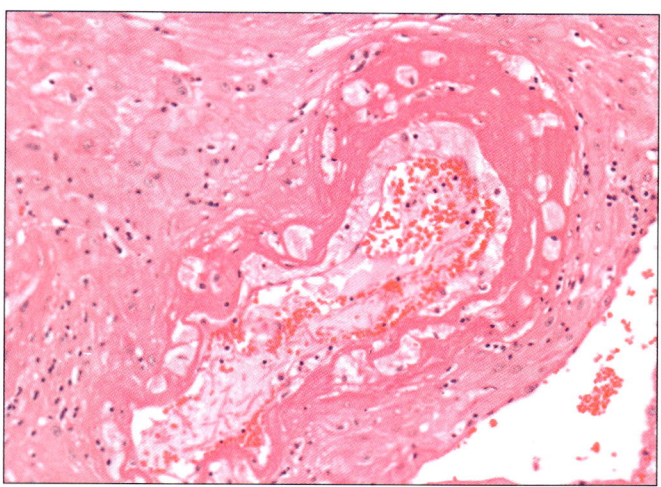

Figure 33.7 Maternal hypertension. Untransformed vessel wall, but with atherosis.

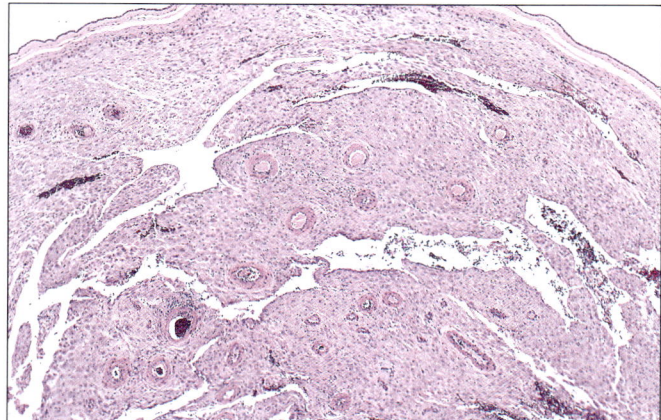

Figure 33.8 Maternal hypertension with a vessel showing atherosis (left) contrasted with untransformed vessels (right).

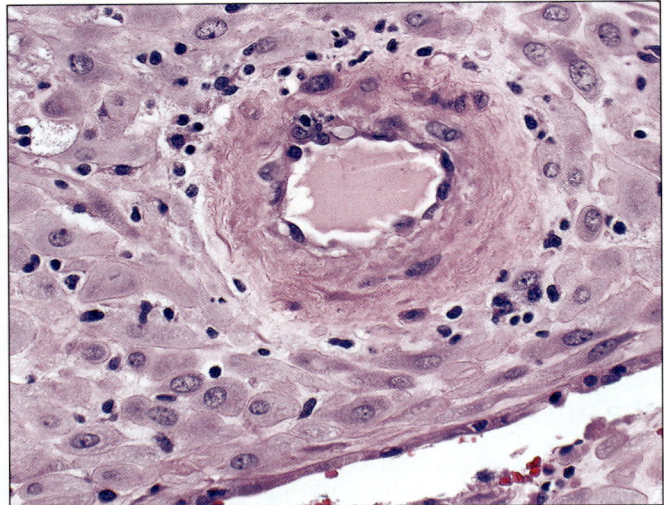

Figure 33.9 Maternal hypertension with untransformed vessel wall.

group are constitutionally small and have no pathology. Data on race, birth order, and parental body characteristics can help improve identification of true growth restriction.[27] Agreement between customized standards and a population standard on growth restriction can be expected in approximately two-thirds of births. Birth weight below the 3rd percentile shows the strongest correlation with perinatal mortality.

IUGR is a late stage manifestation of several disease states. The etiologies can be divided into maternal causes and fetal factors. Chronic maternal hypoxia is an important cause, seen in high altitude, pulmonary hypertension, anemia, hemoglobinopathies, and cardiac failure.[28] Fetal factors include fetal genetic disorders, chromosomal abnormalities, and congenital malformations. Mothers who have a history of a prior pregnancy with IUGR are also at risk for recurrence in subsequent pregnancies, including an increased risk of stillbirth.[29]

Pre-eclampsia is accompanied by IUGR in up to one-third of cases, but IUGR may occur in normotensive pregnancies. Differences in the pathways of spiral artery remodeling may result in the development of IUGR alone, or PET with IUGR.[25]

Placental pathology may cause or contribute to IUGR. The fetal surface should be examined for vascular thrombosis and the maternal surface for infarcts. The cut surface may show infarcts or increased perivillous fibrin. However, many diseases responsible for causing IUGR can only be diagnosed microscopically, such as villitis. In our practice over a recent 3 year period, placental findings in 126 cases of IUGR below the 3rd percentile were uteroplacental ischemia 44%, fetal thrombotic vasculopathy 8%, villitis 14% (with two-thirds of these being moderate to severe), and intervillositis or increased perivillous fibrin 4%. Ten percent of placentas were small, but histologically normal.

Morphologic findings in IUGR in some cases reflect the effects of stress on the placenta. Placental function is compromised by oxidative stress and complement activation, causing a decrease in the functioning trophoblast mass. This is manifest by syncytiotrophoblast apoptosis, syncytial knots, and increased perivillous fibrin.[30]

Early onset IUGR is less common than late onset. It is characterized by absence or reversal of end-diastolic flow in umbilical artery Doppler studies. Histologic examination shows poor peripheral villous development with nonbranching angiogenesis and increased syncytial knots.[31] This cohort with persistent absence or reversal of end-diastolic flow represents a severely affected group in whom early intervention is warranted. Other abnormalities of Doppler flow include abnormalities of the systolic/diastolic ratio and of the pulsatility index. These correlate strongly with placental abnormalities, not just those reflecting maternal underperfusion, but also villous abnormalities and fetal vascular obstruction.[32] Epigenetic regulation of the placenta occurs, with imprinted and nonimprinted genes influencing development.[33] Overexpression of *PHLDA2*, a paternally imprinted gene that regulates placental growth, correlates with histologic features of maternal vascular underperfusion.[34]

CONFINED PLACENTAL MOSAICISM

Confined placental mosaicism occurs when the placenta's karyotype differs from that of the fetus. This may cause both IUGR and fetal loss. In one study of IUGR with matched controls, confined placental mosaicism was significantly higher (15.7% vs 1.4% in controls).[35] While these placentas often showed decidual vasculopathy and infarction, there are no criteria for diagnosis by light microscopy. The diagnosis depends on awareness of the condition and ancillary tests such as fluorescent *in situ* hybridization or comparative genomic hybridization. Involvement of the cytotrophoblast as well as the mesenchymal core is required for adverse outcomes and low birth weight.[7]

ADVERSE NEUROLOGIC OUTCOME: NEONATAL ENCEPHALOPATHY AND CEREBRAL PALSY

The area of neonatal neurologic disability is a contentious one, and the erroneous attribution of such damage to 'birth asphyxia' has led to obstetricians becoming uninsurable in many Western jurisdictions. The incidence of cerebral palsy has remained between 2 and 3 per 1000 live births over the last three decades, with similar figures from many centers.[36] Only 4% (2 of 46) of cases of cerebral palsy in one center were related to birth asphyxia when the objective American College of Obstetricians and Gynecologists/American Academy of Pediatrics criteria were used.[37]

Placental examination, when combined with relevant clinical information, can add much to the understanding of a bad outcome. Any center wishing to examine such placentas must first have a mechanism in place for identifying, retrieving, and processing them, without producing an impossibly large workload. A diagnosis of cerebral palsy may often not be made until the nonprogressive nature of the impairment is clear, and, as such, placental analysis may have to proceed with a less definitive label. For term infants, neonatal encephalopathy is the best predictor of long-term neurologic disability. Over 90% of placentas from term infants who later develop cerebral palsy have a finding that may have contributed to the abnormality.[38] IUGR may offer protection against the development of brain injury.[39]

Macroscopic description should include any findings (and relevant negatives) of the cord, membranes, fetal surface vessels, parenchyma, and basal plate. At a minimum, a section of parenchyma, cord, and membranes should be available for microscopy. Gross examination of the fixed tissue by the trained observer may identify foci of avascular villi that can be missed at a busy grossing station and may require additional sections. The key lesions to be sought, graded, and reported are those of inflammation and thrombosis.[40–42] The presence of both, with lesions of different age and duration, appears to increase the risk of cerebral palsy. The coexistence of subacute and chronic pathology was significantly more likely to be identified in a cohort of medicolegal cases than in controls (24% vs 2%, respectively).[42] In a series of 12 cases of neonatal stroke from a national registry, placental pathology was found in 10 (83%), with five (42%) showing mixed lesions.[43] Infection plays an important role in the genesis of cerebral palsy. Clinical and histologic chorioamnionitis both increase the risk of development of cerebral palsy.[44] Bacteria and other microorganisms may not be cultured, due either to antibiotic treatment or to their fastidious nature. Not uncommonly, infectious agents may exist in the placenta without histologic findings—nearly three-fourths of neonates with poor outcomes in one study had viral or bacterial disease (coxsackievirus 46%, bacteria 38%, herpes 8%, parvovirus 4%, and picornavirus 4%) when tested with *in situ* hybridization or reverse transcriptase polymerase chain reaction (RT-PCR), compared with none of the controls.[45] In a population-based study, perinatal exposure to neurotropic viruses, in particular herpes B viruses, showed an association with cerebral palsy.[45] Given the prevalence of viral nucleic acids in the control population (almost 40%), the need for a cofactor or trigger might be necessary to result in damage. Histologic findings may suggest chronic infection, with capsular deciduitis associated with periventricular leukomalacia in infants born between 23 and 34 weeks of gestation.[46]

DIABETES MELLITUS

Both placental weight and macrosomia increase with poor control. Delayed villous maturation (villous immaturity) is significantly associated with pregestational and gestational diabetes.[47] Other changes include chorangiosis. Maternal hypertensive disorders also impact on the placental morphology.[48] With good control and without macrosomia, placental weight may be normal and there may be no discernible changes by routine light microscopy. With stereologic assessment, more subtle changes may be detected, even in type 1 diabetics with good glycemic control, with enhanced angiogenesis, and increased capillary length and volume.[49,50]

HYDROPS FETALIS (MATERNAL RHESUS ISOIMMUNIZATION)

Maternal rhesus (Rh) isoimmunization and to a lesser extent anti-Kell, Duffy, and other minor antibodies and ABO incompatibility produce similar placental changes. However, with modern obstetric practice, full-blown cases of immune hydrops fetalis are uncommon. The Rh-negative mother may be sensitized in her first pregnancy, either before birth from fetal–maternal hemorrhage or during birth. The risk of sensitization increases in cases of operative removal of the placenta.

Macroscopically, the placenta ranges from normal to enlarged and bulky. The villi may show appropriate or delayed maturity, with an increase in immature intermediate villi. Generally, the placental changes are inconstant in any given placenta, appearing as a mosaic of normal areas admixed with others that are edematous. Cytotrophoblasts are mildly increased and there is focal basement membrane thickening. Up to 30% of cases show increased numbers of intervillous thromboses and fibrinoid necrosis of villi. The villous capillaries (which tend to be sparser than normal) contain nucleated fetal red blood cells. The villous stroma is edematous and macrophages (Hofbauer cells) are easily identified. The cause of the edema is believed to be a consequence of fetal anemia leading to high-output cardiac failure. These changes are not pathognomonic for Rh isoimmunization.

PLACENTA CRETA

Placenta accreta, which occurs in about 0.9% of deliveries,[51] substantially increases the risk of preterm delivery and small for gestational age babies. Previous cesarean section is the most common cause of a morbidly adherent placenta (Figure 33.10). The disorder is also associated with prior manual removal of the placenta, cornual implantation, leiomyomas, and prior endometrial scarring. It is frequently diagnosed clinically when there is a difficult delivery of the placenta and relates to undue adherence of the placenta to the uterine myometrium. Ultrasound with Doppler imaging of the placental vasculature and MRI of the placenta can confirm these suspicions, thus helping to guide management of the delivery. The term 'accreta' is used to mean an attached placenta without myometrial invasion. Increta implies a moderate degree of myometrial penetration and percreta means penetration by chorionic villi through the entire wall to the level of the serosa (Figure 33.11),

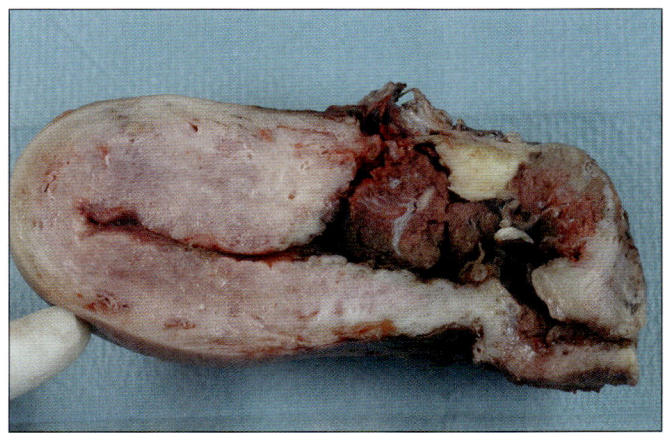

Figure 33.10 Placenta accreta: note the old cesarean section scar. (Reproduced with permission from Kelehan P, Mooney EE. Pathology of the uterus. In: Sir S. Arulkumaran et al., editors. A comprehensive textbook of postpartum hemorrhage. 2nd ed. Kirkmahoe, UK: Sapiens Publishing; 2012.)

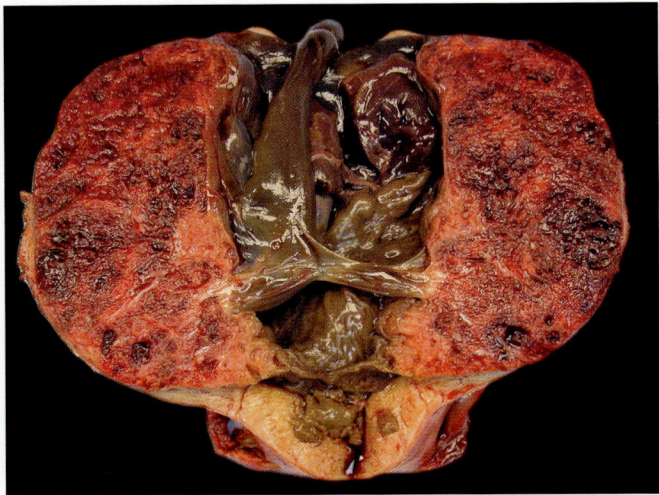

Figure 33.11 Placenta percreta. The placenta penetrates the myometrium to the level of the serosal covering.

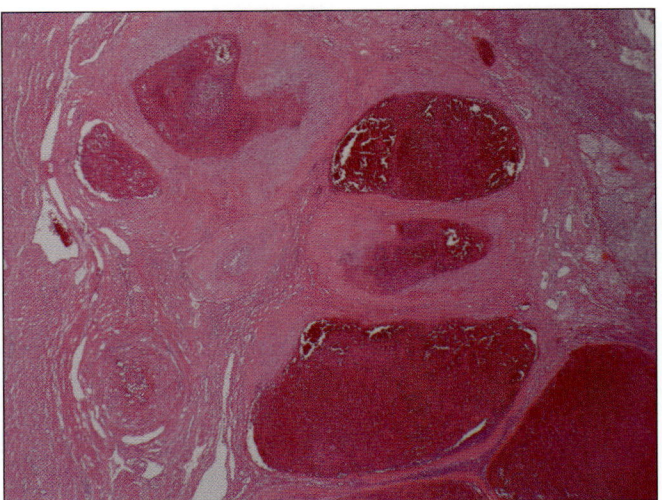

Figure 33.12 Subinvolution: affected vessels are dilated and filled with blood, in contrast with the normally involuted vessel (center left).

sometimes with invasion of adjacent pelvic organs. In practice, all types are sometimes referred to as 'placenta creta.'

The primary defect is deficiency of the decidua basalis with consequent apposition of chorionic villi and myometrium. The significance of myometrial cells in the basal plate in the absence of clinical evidence of placenta accreta is controversial, and the frequency of this finding will be influenced by sampling. The term 'placenta adhesiva' has been used for an abnormally adherent placenta that has a clear plane of separation on manual removal.[52] Myometrial fibers in the basal plate were found in 78% of these placentas and multinucleate trophoblast is reduced. The term 'occult placenta accreta'[53] has been used for cases where there are myometrial fibers in the basal plate without intervening decidua. An increase in intermediate trophoblast was seen and there was an association with features of placental hypoxia.

Morbid adherence of the placenta is one of the most common indications for postpartum hysterectomy and this scenario is most likely when there is a prior cesarean section and current placenta previa. The placenta will have a markedly disrupted maternal surface and careful dissection is needed to identify chorionic villi adjacent to or admixed with myometrial fibers. The finding of only trophoblast admixed with superficial myometrial fibers is insufficient for the diagnosis, as this occurs normally in the uncomplicated state. In a hysterectomy specimen with placenta accreta the chorionic villi are found lying directly on the surface of the myometrium or in the uterine wall.

Alterations in the myometrial wall seen following cesarean section include distortion and widening, inflammation, and adenomyosis. A grossly visible defect may be present in the anterior wall. Implantation on either a normally healed or a diseased scar will not have the protective effect provided by the presence of fundal decidua, and normal postpartum separation cannot occur. Implantation in the lower segment (adjacent to the defect) can cause expansion of the defect, dehiscence of the wall, and the formation of a sac that will further enlarge and progress with growth of the placenta.

POSTPARTUM HEMORRHAGE AND SUBINVOLUTION

Postpartum hemorrhage may be immediate or delayed. Immediate causes include atony, where there are few or no pathologic findings. Implantation on a cesarean section scar leading to placenta accreta will show morbid adherence. Delayed hemorrhage may be due to retained products of conception. Subinvolution of the blood vessels of the placental bed is an important and probably under-recognized cause of secondary postpartum hemorrhage.

Normal arterial involution involves a decrease in the lumen size, disappearance of trophoblast, thickening of the intima, regrowth of endothelium, and regeneration of internal elastic lamina. These changes occur within 3 weeks of delivery. With subinvolution, arteries remain distended and contain red cells or fresh thrombus (Figure 33.12), and trophoblast persists in a perivascular location. In some cases, endovascular trophoblast may be present. Hemorrhage from subinvolution is maximal in the second week postpartum, although it may occur up to several months later. It is more common in older, multiparous women and may recur in subsequent deliveries. Subinvolution is not related to the method of delivery and may be regarded as a specific entity, possibly due to an abnormal immunologic relationship between trophoblast and the uterus.[54] The changes may be recognized on curettage specimens, and retained products may or may not be present. The hysterectomy specimen will show a uterus that is soft and larger than expected. As normally involuted vessels may be present adjacent to subinvoluted ones, multiple blocks of placental bed should be taken to exclude this process.

MATERNAL SICKLE CELL TRAIT AND DISEASE

The heterozygous trait (sickle cell trait) appears not to be associated with placental pathology. In the homozygous form, maternal anemia and veno-occlusive disease result in

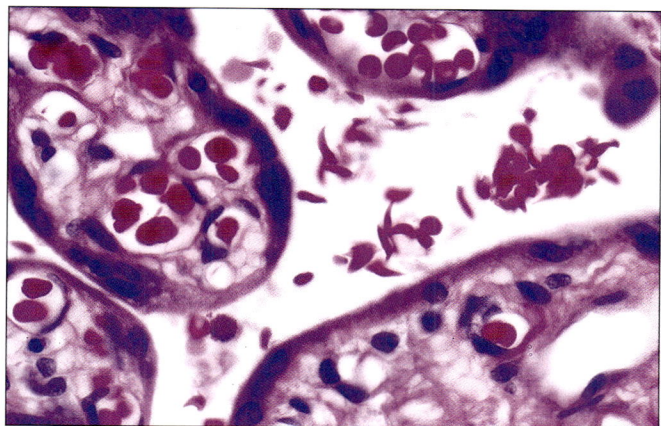

Figure 33.13 Sickled red cells. Compare the sickled red cells in the perivillous space with the perfectly round and smooth fetal red cells in chorionic villi.

a preplacental type of fetal hypoxia. Alterations in the endothelium of the umbilical vein, demonstrable by scanning and transmission electron microscopy, may also be due to hypoxia.[55] The initial clue that the disease exists may be from the finding of sickled cells in the intervillous space of the placenta (Figure 33.13).

TWIN PREGNANCY

As discussed in Chapter 32, establishing chorionicity (e.g., monochorionic or dichorionic) is critical in assessing the pathology that may be present in a twin pregnancy. Twins have a higher incidence of perinatal morbidity and mortality than singleton pregnancies, and monochorionic twins are at higher risk than dichorionic. Ten percent of twins with dichorionic placentas are monozygotic, and fetal outcome is related to chorionicity rather than to zygosity. Monoamniotic monochorionic twins (MoMo) have a 20% fetal mortality rate.[56] This is usually attributed to prematurity, congenital abnormalities, and rarely twin–twin transfusion syndrome. Cord entanglement is seen in 40% of MoMo twins. Monochorionic twins weigh less than twins from dichorionic gestations. Severe growth discordance between the twins (>25%) has an overall prevalence of approximately 9% in twin pregnancies[57] but is more common in MoMo twins where it is associated with an increased perinatal mortality. MoMo placentas have significantly greater numbers of both superficial and deep anastomoses than do uncomplicated monochorionic diamniotic pregnancies, which may provide a vascular basis for the twin–twin transfusion syndrome that occurs on rare occasions in monoamniotic pregnancies. Monochorionic twins have an increased risk of fetal death and neurologic injury.[58]

Assessing growth restriction in twins may be problematic, and use of a twin nomogram with allowance for chorionicity is advised. Peripheral cord insertion reflective of a spatially limited intrauterine compartment and avascular villi indicative of occluded fetal vessels in the placenta are associated with moderate growth discordance (>15% of birth weight) or low birth weight (<10th percentile).[59] Decreased placental weight, velamentous insertions, and a single umbilical artery have also been associated with severe growth discordance.[60] Other findings such as thrombotic lesions differ according to chorionicity; nonocclusive mural thrombi in fetal vessels are more common in monochorionic than in dichorionic twins or in singletons, and are associated with avascular villi in the last two groups.[61]

A systematic review of observational studies over a 15 year period has shown that, following death of one twin, monochorionic and dichorionic twins have a death risk of 12% and 4%, respectively, with a risk of neurologic disability of 18% and 1%.[62] The likelihood of survival of the co-twin decreases with increasing gestational age of the first fetal death, with mortality higher for same-sex twins.

PROLONGED PREGNANCY

Prolonged pregnancy is generally defined as a gestation, based on menstrual age, exceeding 42 weeks. With the estimated date of confinement, or due date, for normal pregnancies calculated as 38 weeks after conception, or 40 weeks from the first day of the last normal menstrual period, about 18% of pregnancies in the United States extend 1 week beyond the normal due date and 7% beyond 2 weeks. (Some differences between statistics in the United States and Canada seem to relate to whether menstrual or clinical dates are used.[63,64]) In general, the risks of post-term pregnancy include increased meconium aspiration, macrosomia, and perinatal death, with small for gestational age infants at increased risk.[65] Postmature placentas may be normal. Delayed villous maturation is important to recognize in this cohort. It typically permits normal growth, but by unknown mechanisms may culminate in a normally formed macerated term stillbirth.

MATERNAL INFECTIONS AND THE PLACENTA

The possible effects of exposure to infections during pregnancy are a cause of great anxiety. In addition to serologic evaluation during pregnancy, examination of the placenta may help to confirm or refute intrauterine infection.

CYTOMEGALOVIRUS

Cytomegalovirus (CMV) is considered one of the most common and important congenital infections in developed nations with approximately 1% of pregnant women acquiring a primary infection.[66] It is also the most common agent of the **t**oxoplasmosis, **o**ther infections, **r**ubella, CMV infection, and **h**erpes simplex (TORCH) group to infect the placenta and fetus.

With 40% of the women transmitting the infection to their fetuses, the risk of serious fetal injury is great. While the risk of transmission is greatest if the infection is acquired during the third trimester, the risk of serious fetal injury is greatest if acquired during the first or early part of the second trimester. The virus is transmitted in blood and body fluids, including saliva. Infection in a pregnant woman is usually asymptomatic. The virus can be transmitted following a primary infection in the mother during pregnancy or a recrudescence of a latent infection acquired at a time before pregnancy. Most (75–85%) infants suffer no adverse effects. Those that do may suffer from IUGR and serious neurologic impairment, including deafness and ocular damage. Co-infection with HIV may enhance CMV transmission and lead to more severe tissue damage.

The fetus and placenta may be hydropic. The combination of a lymphoplasmacytic villitis (Figure 33.14), villous sclerosis, and hemosiderin deposition (Figure 33.15) is commonly found. The characteristic deposition of hemosiderin pigment in sclerotic villi reflects the virus's endotheliotropic nature, although syncytiotrophoblasts are also infected.[67] Intranuclear inclusions (Figure 33.16) may be seen adjacent to necrotic debris in the villous stroma, although these may be few or absent, even with immunohistochemistry (Figure 33.17).

The diagnosis can be otherwise confirmed by serologic testing, viral culture, and PCR assay to detect CMV DNA in fetal and placental tissues.[68] Demonstration of CMV and parvovirus B19 DNA was more common in placentas from stillbirths than controls, but does not prove causality.[69]

PARVOVIRUS B19

Parvovirus B19 causes erythema infectiosum, also called 'slapped cheek syndrome.' Approximately 50–75% of adult women are immune. Primary infection in adults is usually subclinical or causes nonspecific flu-like symptoms and arthralgia. Maternal infection with parvovirus B19 occurs in 1–6% of susceptible pregnancies. Transplacental transmission occurs in 25–50% of cases and appears to increase in later gestations. The virus is a recognized cause of first trimester miscarriage and hydrops fetalis. It is frequently diagnosed by detection of maternal IgM as part of a work-up for an ultrasound diagnosis of hydrops.

The primary site of parvovirus B19 infections is within erythroid precursor cells and it has an affinity for the late normoblast stage (Figure 33.18). Cardiac myocytes are also infected. Hydrops is due to fetal anemia, myocarditis, and resulting cardiac failure.

The placenta is usually bulky, pale, and edematous. Histologically, there is villous edema with villous tissue dysmaturity, villitis, and intervillitis. A fetal nucleated red cell

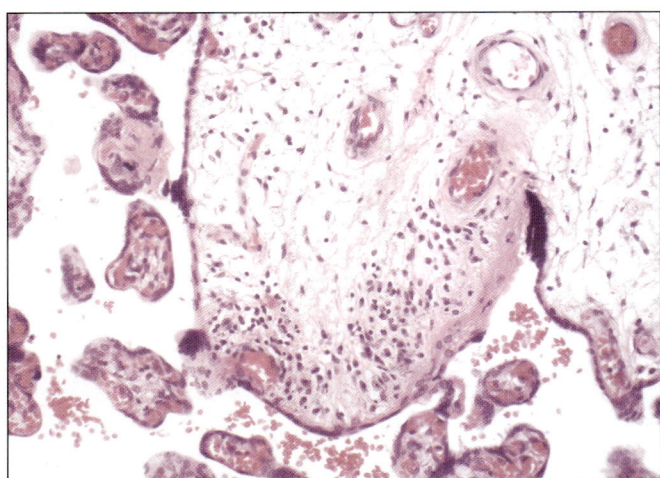

Figure 33.14 CMV villous edema and chronic inflammatory cells.

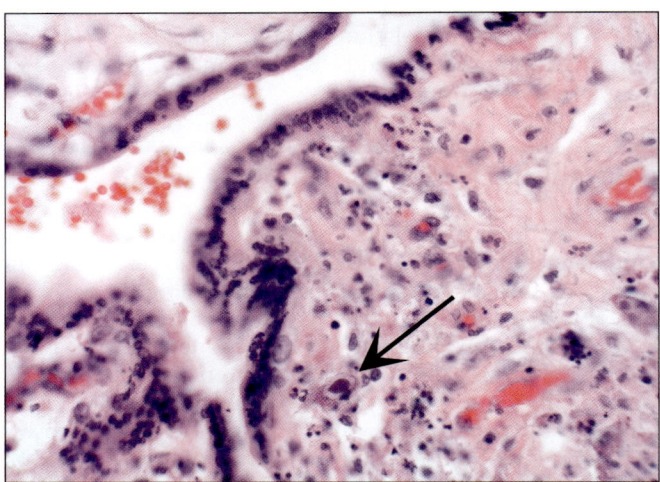

Figure 33.16 CMV inclusion.

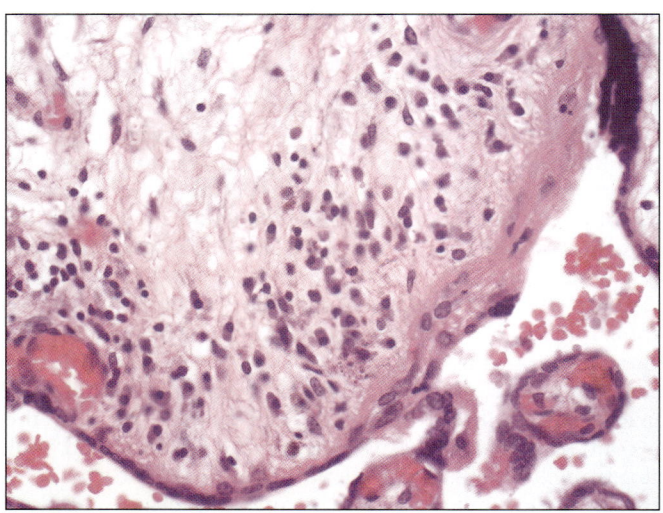

Figure 33.15 CMV plasma cells and hemosiderin prominent in villus.

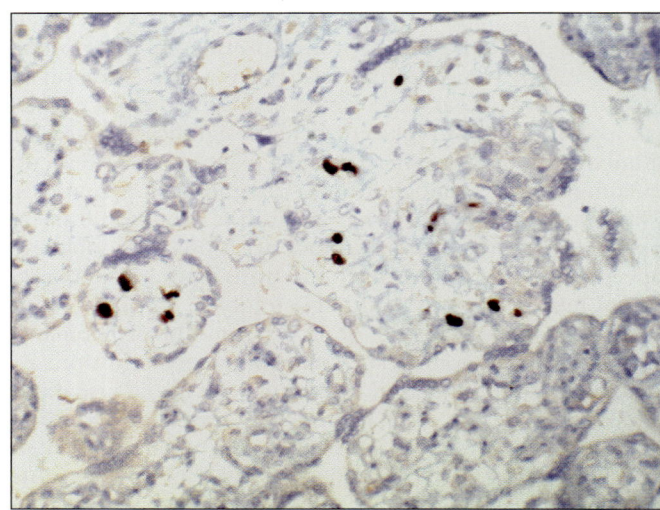

Figure 33.17 CMV (immunoperoxidase stain).

response (erythroblastosis) is seen in capillaries. Some nucleated red blood cells show a characteristic appearance of marginated chromatin with central nuclear clearing.[70] Diagnosis can also be made by immunohistochemistry (Figure 33.19).

RUBELLA

Rubella is transmitted via droplet spread from respiratory tract secretions of infected individuals. Clinical disease exhibits a generalized maculopapular rash, lymphadenopathy, and fever, although nearly one-half of those infected are asymptomatic. The virus can be transmitted to the fetus through the placenta and is capable of causing serious congenital defects, miscarriages, and stillbirths. With immunization, rubella infection and congenital rubella syndrome are rarely seen today. The risk of fetal infection varies according to the time of onset of maternal infection. It is about 80% if the fetal infection occurs in the first trimester, 67% in the second, and 35% in the third. Serologic tests and viral cultures are useful in confirming the diagnosis. Serious complications, such as deafness and ocular, cardiovascular, and neurologic damage, result almost exclusively from infection in the first 16 weeks of gestation.

Placental changes reflect the time of the infection. Early on, there is a focal necrotizing villitis with endarteritis, focal trophoblastic necrosis with or without neutrophilic infiltration, and perivillous fibrin deposition. Rarely, eosinophil inclusions may be seen in trophoblast or endothelial cells. Hofbauer cells are increased and there may be a perivasculitis. Infection during later pregnancy causes chronic inflammatory infiltrates in the placental membranes, cord, and deciduas. These features are nonspecific and may be seen in cases of infection by herpes viruses or CMV. The end stage is stromal fibrosis, although both acute and chronic features may be present simultaneously.

VARICELLA ZOSTER

Primary infection with varicella zoster virus causes chickenpox. The virus remains dormant in the dorsal root ganglion and may reactivate as shingles at a later time. Chickenpox is highly contagious and is spread by droplet transmission or by direct personal contact with vesicular fluid. Primary infection in pregnancy is associated with an increased risk of complications, including maternal death and the fetal varicella syndrome. Women from tropical and subtropical areas are more likely to be seronegative for varicella zoster virus IgG and therefore are more susceptible to developing chickenpox. The risks to the fetus are greatest when the primary infection occurs prior to the 20th week of gestation or after 36 weeks. Fetal varicella syndrome does not occur at the time of the initial fetal infection, but is believed to result from subsequent herpes zoster reactivation *in utero* and only occurs in a minority of infected fetuses. It occurs in 1–2% of maternal varicella infections that take place prior to 20 weeks' gestation. Placental histologic findings include chronic villitis with multinucleated giant cells, granulomatous inflammation, and fetal vessel occlusion.[71] The diagnosis can be confirmed by immunohistochemistry.

HERPES SIMPLEX

Herpes simplex virus (HSV) type 1 and 2 cause genital herpes. Direct contact with infected maternal secretions can lead to neonatal herpetic infection. The risks are greatest when a woman acquires a new infection (primary genital herpes) during late pregnancy, before the development of protective maternal antibodies. Most maternal infections are asymptomatic or go unrecognized and it may be difficult to distinguish clinically between primary and recurrent HSV infection. If primary genital herpes is present at the time of delivery and the baby is delivered vaginally, the risk of neonatal herpes is about 40%.[72] Recurrent genital herpes does not pose a significant risk for the development of neonatal herpes infection. Occasionally, *in utero* infection of the fetus and placenta does occur, and morphologic placental features include giant cell change, usually in the decidua and extravillous trophoblast. There is often marked immaturity of the placenta with inflammatory changes in all

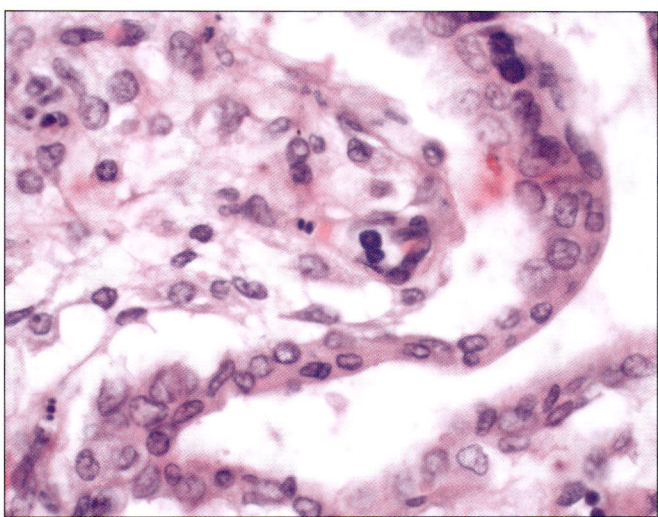

Figure 33.18 Nucleated red blood cells with parvovirus inclusions.

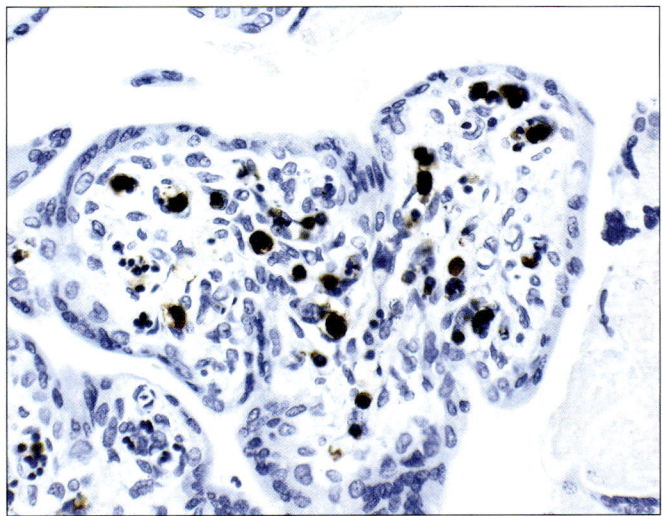

Figure 33.19 Parvovirus in nucleated red blood cells (immunohistochemical stain).

placental areas. A heavy plasma cell infiltrate in the chorion should raise the suspicion of herpes, and there may be a chronic villitis with necrosis. Diagnosis is confirmed by any of immunohistochemistry, viral culture, or PCR.

HIV

Before the era of highly active antiretroviral therapy, the risk of mother to child transmission of HIV neared 20% in non-breastfeeding women in Europe and up to 40% in breastfeeding African populations. The principal obstetric risk factors for mother–child transmission are maternal plasma viral load, vaginal delivery, duration of membrane rupture, chorioamnionitis, preterm delivery, and breastfeeding. Mother–child transmission is largely preventable with universal antenatal screening, antiretroviral therapy, delivery by cesarean section in certain circumstances, and artificial formula feeding. In women who do not breastfeed, over 80% of HIV transmissions from mother to child occur late in the third trimester (from 36 weeks) and during labor and at delivery. Fewer than 2% of transmissions occur during the first and second trimesters.

Placentas from cases with fetal transmission of HIV-1 subtype E (the type most frequently seen in Southeast Asia) show chorioamnionitis, chronic deciduitis, and decidual necrosis.[73] No specific features are seen.[74] Histologic chorioamnionitis is the most common pathologic finding in placentas of HIV-1 infected women, and this may increase the risk of viral transmission to the fetus.[75]

HUMAN PAPILLOMAVIRUS

Human Papillomavirus (HPV) is a DNA virus trophic for squamous epithelium, but may be found in the placenta. *In vitro* studies show that HPV can infect extravillous trophoblast and decrease extracellular matrix invasion.[10] Infection with HPV was demonstrated in 6% of cases between 11 and 13 weeks' gestation,[76] and a higher rate of spontaneous abortion (60% vs 20% of controls) has been reported in HPV-positive women. HPV has been demonstrated in cord blood:[77] the placentas were macroscopically normal, and no microscopic features of HPV infection have been described.

TOXOPLASMOSIS

Toxoplasmosis, an infection caused by the protozoan parasite *T. gondii,* may be acquired by eating contaminated meat or from exposure to contaminated soil or cat litter. Immunocompetent individuals are usually asymptomatic. Acute infections in pregnant women can be transmitted to the fetus, although approximately 75% of congenitally infected newborns are asymptomatic.[78] Consequences include mental retardation, blindness, and epilepsy, but, today, the classic triad of chorioretinitis, hydrocephalus, and cerebral calcifications is relatively rare. The risk of maternal–fetal transmission increases with gestational age at the time of exposure, whereas the incidence of severe disease decreases. If infection occurs just before or during the first trimester, it may cause miscarriage, intrauterine death, or severe neurologic lesions, whereas fetal infection occurring late in pregnancy may result in either congenital disease or a subclinical state. The classic finding in the placenta is villitis (Figure 33.20),

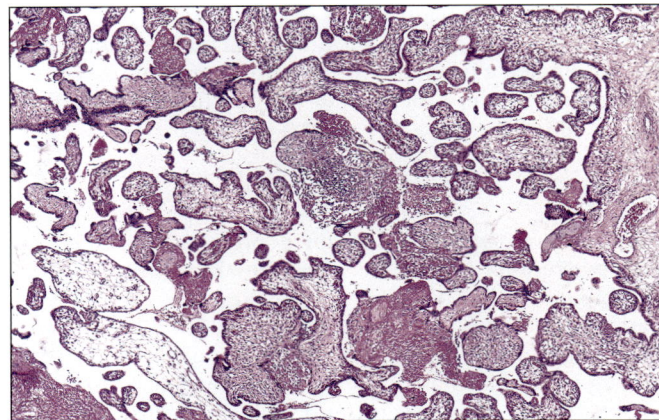

Figure 33.20 Toxoplasmosis manifest on low power as villitis.

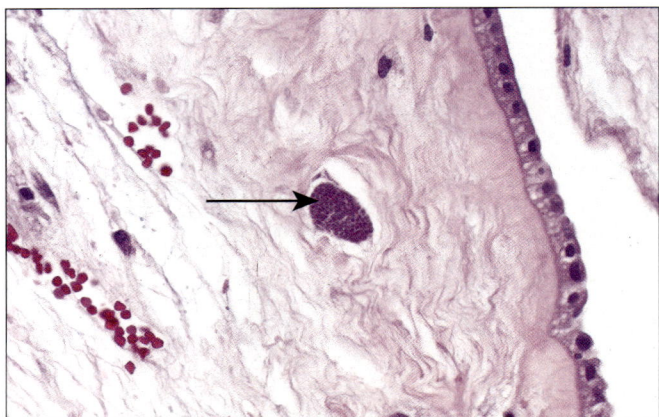

Figure 33.21 Toxoplasma cysts in amniotic membrane (arrow).

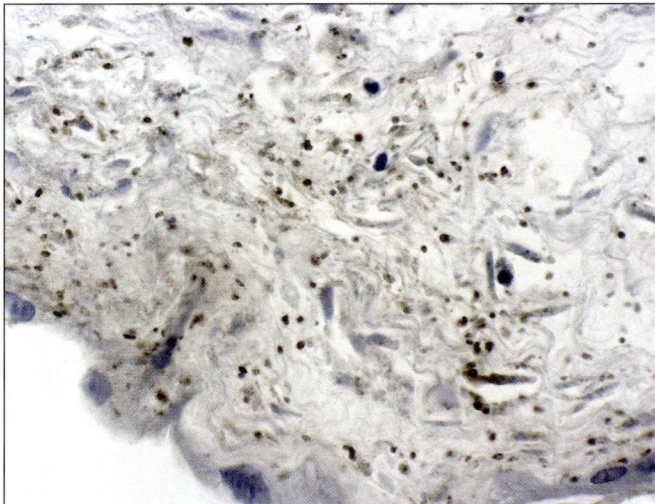

Figure 33.22 Toxoplasma (immunoperoxidase stain).

but manifestations range from no sign of inflammation to necrotizing inflammation. Toxoplasma cysts may be seen in the cord and membranes (Figures 33.21 and 33.22), and fetal vessel calcification may be found.[71] Toxoplasmosis is a rare cause of granulomatous villitis.[79]

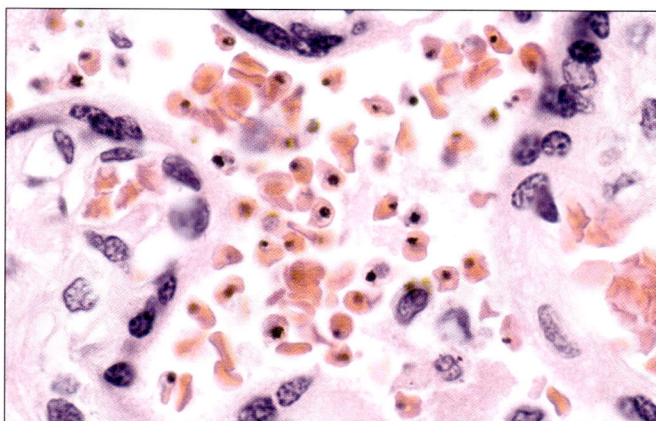

Figure 33.23 Malaria parasites in red blood cells.

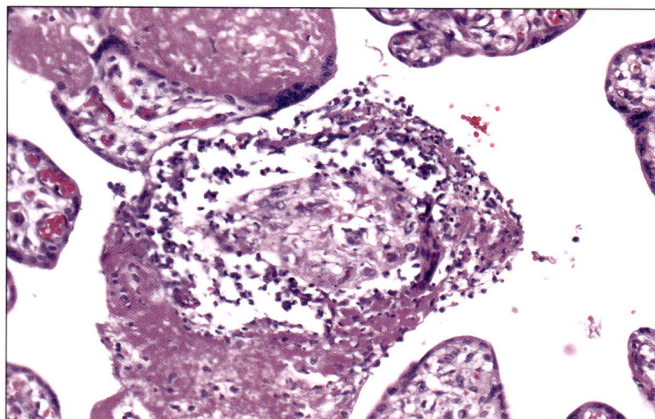

Figure 33.24 Syphilis with necrotizing villitis.

MALARIA

Pregnant women from endemic areas (especially primiparous women, who have more severe disease and significantly higher prevalence rates of malarial infection) are more prone to develop malaria than non-pregnant women. Infection in pregnancy is associated with extensive parasitic infection of the placenta, maternal anemia, a reduction in birth weight, miscarriage, preterm birth, and neonatal and maternal death.[80]

A mononuclear inflammatory infiltrate (intervillositis), malarial pigment, and an increase in perivillous fibrin is characteristic (Figure 33.23). In active infection, the parasitized cells attach to villi in areas of syncytiotrophoblast damage. Fibrinoid necrosis, basal membrane thickening, and increased numbers of syncytial knots are features also associated with malarial infection. Chronic infections show the most severe changes whereas placentas with acute infections exhibit a mild increase in inflammatory cells only and those with past infections show only minimal differences compared with noninfected placentas. A histologic grading system assessing the presence of pigment and inflammation in *Plasmodium falciparum* infection shows a correlation with birth weight.[81] HIV co-infection will increase both viral and parasitic loads and decrease birth weight.

SYPHILIS

Congenital syphilis is caused by transplacental transmission of the spirochete *Treponema pallidum*. Congenital syphilis remains a major cause of stillbirth and long-term morbidity globally. If untreated, the sequelae of congenital syphilis can be lifelong, including neurologic abnormalities, bone and joint malformations, and deafness secondary to nerve VIII involvement. The transmission rate from mother to fetus approaches 100% if the primary or secondary syphilis in the mother remains untreated during pregnancy. Perinatal death may result from congenital infection in more than 40% of untreated pregnancies. A pregnant woman with syphilis who has not received therapy or who has received inadequate therapy may transmit the infection to the fetus at any clinical stage of the disease, although this more frequently occurs following early syphilis.

Grossly, the placenta may be pale, bulky, and hydropic, and necrotizing funisitis lends a 'barber's pole' appearance to the cord. Classic gummas are rare today. The syphilitic 'triad' includes enlarged hypercellular (immature) villi, proliferative vascular changes (obliterative endarteritis), and acute or chronic villitis with plasma cells. Other features may be present, such as granulomatous, proliferative, and necrotizing villitis (Figure 33.24) with multinucleated giant cells. The decidua may have a plasma cell infiltrate. These findings are present to varying degrees in an affected placenta and are not specific for syphilis. In one cohort, necrotizing funisitis, villous enlargement, and acute villitis were significantly more common in both stillborn and liveborn infants with congenital syphilis. Placental examination improved the detection rate in both liveborn and stillborn infants.[82]

Diagnosis may be confirmed by PCR for treponemal DNA. In untreated cases, Warthin–Starry silver stain, or more recently introduced immunohistochemical methods for tissue in paraffin, may demonstrate spirochetes in placental and umbilical cord tissue. As with villitis of unknown etiology, the predominant inflammatory cells are maternal in origin and are CD8-positive T-lymphocytes.[83]

LISTERIOSIS

This is due to infection with the bacterium *L. monocytogenes*. The placentas are frequently studded with microabscesses on their maternal and cut surfaces and usually have an associated chorioamnionitis. Histologically, there are multiple microabscesses with associated necrosis within the intervillous space and villi (Figures 33.25 and 33.26). *Listeria* may infect the placenta via the hematogenous and ascending routes. Although maternal infection produces little systemic upset, it causes devastating fetal sepsis with congenital pneumonia, gastritis, and esophagitis. Immunohistochemical[84] or PCR detection of *Listeria* antigens may be useful in cases where culture has not been possible.

OTHER ORGANISMS

Mycobacterium tuberculosis may infect the placenta, and produces granulomatous inflammation in the placenta and decidua.

Other parasitic infections include trypanosomiasis, schistosomiasis and cryptococcosis.

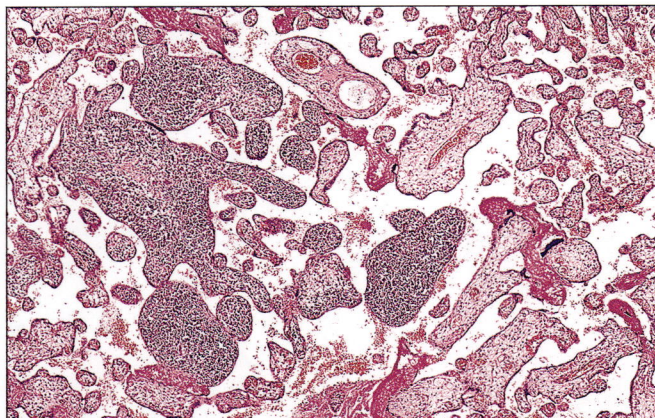

Figure 33.25 *Listeria* villitis. A low-power view shows hypercellular villi.

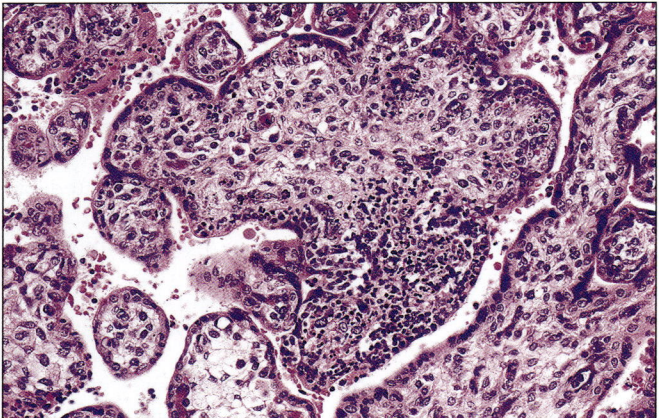

Figure 33.26 *Listeria* villitis. Inflamed villi show disrupted trophoblast lining, fibrin accumulation, and adhesion to adjacent villi.

REFERENCES

1. Redline RW, Fay-Petersen O, Heller D, et al. Amniotic infection syndrome: nosology and reproducibility of placental reaction patterns. Pediatr Dev Pathol 2003;6:435–48.
2. Redline RW, Boyd T, Campbell V, et al. Maternal vascular underperfusion: nosology and reproducibility of placental reaction patterns. Pediatr Dev Pathol 2004;7:237–49.
3. Redline RW, Ariel I, Baergen RN, et al. Fetal vascular obstructive lesions: nosology and reproducibility of placental reaction patterns. Pediatr Dev Pathol 2004;7:443–52.
4. Turowski G, Berge LN, Helgadottir LB, et al. A new, clinically oriented, unifying and simple placental classification system. Placenta 2012;33:1026–35.
5. Philipp T, Philipp K, Reiner A, et al. Embryoscopic and cytogenetic analysis of 233 missed abortions: factors involved in the pathogenesis of developmental defects of early failed pregnancies. Hum Reprod 2003;18:1724–32.
6. Lathi RB, Mark SD, Westphal LM, Milki AA. Cytogenetic testing of anembryonic pregnancies compared to embryonic missed abortions. J Assist Reprod Genet 2007;24:521–4.
7. Toutain J, Labeau-Gaüzere C, Barnetche T, et al. Confined placental mosaicism and pregnancy outcome: a distinction needs to be made between types 2 and 3. Prenat Diagn 2010;30:1155–64.
8. Jindal P, Regan L, Fourkata EO, et al. Placental pathology of recurrent spontaneous abortion: the role of histopathological examination of products of conception in routine clinical practice: a mini review. Hum Reprod 2007;22:313–6.
9. Nuovo GJ, Cooper LD, Bartholomew D. Histologic, infectious, and molecular correlates of idiopathic spontaneous abortion and perinatal mortality. Diagn Mol Pathol 2005;14:152–8.
10. Gomez LM, Ma Y, Ho C, et al. Placental infection with human papillomavirus is associated with spontaneous preterm delivery. Hum Reprod 2008;23:709–15.
11. Gruber K, Gelven PL, Austin RM. Chorionic villi or trophoblastic tissue in uterine samples of four women with ectopic pregnancies. Int J Gynecol Pathol 1997;16:28–32.
12. Doyle EM, McParland P, Carroll S, et al. The role of placental cytogenetic cultures in intrauterine and neonatal deaths. J Obstet Gynaecol 2004;24:878–80.
13. Burke C, Sinclair K, Cowin G, et al. Intrauterine growth restriction due to uteroplacental vascular insufficiency leads to increased hypoxia-induced cerebral apoptosis in newborn piglets. Brain Res 2006;1098:19–25.
14. de Laat MWM, van Alderen ED, Franx A, et al. The umbilical coiling index in complicated pregnancy. Eur J Obstet Gynecol Reprod Biol 2007;130:66–72.
15. Peng HQ, Levitin-Smith M, Rochelson B, Kahn E. Umbilical cord stricture and overcoiling are common causes of fetal demise. Pediatr Dev Pathol 2006;9:14–9.
16. Reddy UM, Goldenberg R, Silver R, et al. Stillbirth classification—developing an international consensus for research: executive summary of a National Institute of Child Health and Human Development workshop. Obstet Gynecol 2009;114:901–14.
17. Ananth CV, Wilcox AJ. Placental abruption and perinatal mortality in the United States. Am J Epidemiol 2001;153:332–7.
18. Oyelese Y, Ananth CV. Placental abruption. Obstet Gynecol 2006;108:1005–16.
19. Ananth CV, Berkowitz GS, Savitz DA, Lapinski RH. Placental abruption and adverse perinatal outcomes. JAMA 1999;282:1646–51.
20. Bendon RW. Review of autopsies of stillborn infants with retroplacental hematoma or hemorrhage. Pediatr Devel Pathol 2011;14:10–5.
21. Ananth CV, Oyelese Y, Prasad V, et al. Evidence of placental abruption as a chronic process: associations with vaginal bleeding early in pregnancy and placental lesions. Eur J Obstet Gynecol Reprod Biol 2006;128:15–21.
22. Verma RP, Kaplan C, Southerton K, et al. Placental histopathology in the extremely low birth weight infants. Fetal Pediatr Pathol 2008;27:53–61.
23. Steegers EAP, von Dadelszen P, Duvekot JJ, Pijnenborg R. Preeclampsia. Lancet 2010;376:631–44.
24. Roberts JM, Hubel CA. The two stage model of preeclampsia: variations on the theme. Placenta 2009;30(Suppl. A):S32–7.
25. James JL, Whitley GS, Cartwright JE. Pre-eclampsia: fitting together the placental, immune and cardiovascular pieces. J Pathol 2010;221:363–78.
26. Huppertz B. IFPA Award in Placentology Lecture: biology of the placental syncytiotrophoblast—myths and facts. Placenta 2010;31(Suppl.):S75–81.
27. Clausson B, Gardosi J, Francis A, Cnattingius, S. Perinatal outcome in SGA births defined by customised versus population-based birth-weight standards. BJOG 2001;108:830–4.
28. Hutter D, Kingdom J, Jaeggi E. Causes and mechanisms of intrauterine hypoxia and its impact on the fetal cardiovascular system: a review. Int J Pediatr 2010;401323.
29. Surkan PJ, Stephansson O, Dickman PW, Cnattingius S. Previous preterm and small-for-gestational-age births and the subsequent risk of stillbirth. N Engl J Med 2004;350;777–85.
30. Scifres CM, Nelson DM. Intrauterine growth restriction, human placental development and trophoblast cell death. J Physiol (Lond) 2009;587:3453–8.
31. Kingdom J, Huppertz B, Seaward G, Kaufmann P. Development of the placental villous tree and its consequences for fetal growth. Eur J Obstet Gynecol Reprod Biol 2000;92:35–43.
32. Dicke JM, Huettner P, Yan S, et al. Umbilical artery Doppler indices in small for gestational age fetuses: correlation with adverse outcomes and placental abnormalities. J Ultrasound Med 2009;28:1603–10.
33. Nelissen ECM, van Montfoort APA, Dumoulin JCM, Evers JLH. Epigenetics and the placenta. Hum Reprod Update 2010;17:397–417.
34. McMinn J, Wei M, Schupf N, et al. Unbalanced placental expression of imprinted genes in human intrauterine growth restriction. Placenta 2006;27:540–9.

35. Wilkins-Haug L, Quade B, Morton CC. Confined placental mosaicism as a risk factor among newborns with fetal growth restriction. Prenat Diagn 2006;26:428–32.
36. Clark SL, Hankins GDV. Temporal and demographic trends in cerebral palsy–fact and fiction. Am J Obstet Gynecol 2003;188:628–33.
37. Strijbis EMM, Oudman I, van Essen P, MacLennan AH. Cerebral palsy and the application of the international criteria for acute intrapartum hypoxia. Obstet Gynecol 2006;107:1357–65.
38. Redline RW. Disorders of placental circulation and the fetal brain. Clin Perinatol 2009;36:549–59.
39. Wintermark P, Boyd T, Gregas MC, et al. Placental pathology in asphyxiated newborns meeting the criteria for therapeutic hypothermia. Am J Obstet Gynecol 2010;203:579.e1–9.
40. Keogh JM, Badawi N. The origins of cerebral palsy. Curr Opin Neurol 2006;19:129–34.
41. McDonald DG, Kelehan P, McMenamin JB, et al. Placental fetal thrombotic vasculopathy is associated with neonatal encephalopathy. Hum Pathol 2004;35:875–80.
42. Redline RW. Cerebral palsy in term infants: a clinicopathologic analysis of 158 medicolegal case reviews. Pediatr Dev Pathol 2008;11:456–64.
43. Elbers J, Viero S, MacGregor D, et al. Placental pathology in neonatal stroke. Pediatrics 2011;127:e722–9.
44. Shatrov JG, Birch SC, Lam LT, et al. Chorioamnionitis and cerebral palsy: a meta-analysis. Obstet Gynecol 2010;116:387–92.
45. Genen L, Nuovo GJ, Krilov L. Davis JM. Correlation of in situ detection of infectious agents in the placenta with neonatal outcome. J Pediatr 2004;144:316–20.
46. Maleki Z, Bailis AJ, Argani CH, et al. Periventricular leukomalacia and placental histopathologic abnormalities. Obstet Gynecol 2009;114;1115–20.
47. Higgins M, McAuliffe FM, Mooney E. Clinical Associations with a Placental Diagnosis of Delayed Villous Maturation: a retrospective study. Pediatr Dev Pathol 2011;14:273–9.
48. Jauniaux E, Burton GJ. Villous histomorphometry and placental bed biopsy investigation in Type I diabetic pregnancies. Placenta 2006;27:468–74.
49. Mayhew TM. Enhanced fetoplacental angiogenesis in pregestational diabetes mellitus: the extra growth is exclusively longitudinal and not accompanied by microvascular remodelling. Diabetologia 2002;45:1434–9.
50. Higgins M, Felle P, Mooney EE, et al. Stereology of the placenta in type 1 and type 2 diabetes. Placenta 2011;32:564–9.
51. Gielchinsky Y, Rojansky N, Fasouliotis SJ, Ezra Y. Placenta accreta—summary of 10 years: a survey of 310 cases. Placenta 2002;23:210–4.
52. van Beekhuizen HJ, Joosten I, de Groot AN, et al. The number of multinucleated trophoblastic giant cells in the basal decidua is decreased in retained placenta. J Clin Pathol 2009;62:794–7.
53. Stanek J, Drummond Z. Occult placenta accreta: the missing link in the diagnosis of abnormal placentation. Pediatr Dev Pathol 2007;10:266–73.
54. Andrew AC, Bulmer JN, Wells M, et al. Subinvolution of the uteroplacental arteries in the human placental bed. Histopathology 1989;15:395–405.
55. Decastel M, Leborgne-Samuel Y, Alexandre L, et al. Morphological features of the human umbilical vein in normal, sickle cell trait, and sickle cell disease pregnancies. Hum Pathol 1999;30:13–20.
56. Heyborne KD, Porreco RP, Garite TJ, et al. Improved perinatal survival of monoamniotic twins with intensive inpatient monitoring. Am J Obstet Gynecol 2005;192:96–101.
57. Tan H, Wen SW, Fung Kee Fung K, et al. The distribution of intra-twin birth weight discordance and its association with total twin birth weight, gestational age, and neonatal mortality. Eur J Obstet Gynecol Reprod Biol 2005;121:27–33.
58. Hack KE, Derks JB, Elias SG, et al. Increased perinatal mortality and morbidity in monochorionic versus dichorionic twin pregnancies: clinical implications of a large Dutch cohort study. BJOG 2008;115:58–67.
59. Redline RW, Shah D, Sakar H, et al. Placental lesions associated with abnormal growth in twins. Pediatr Dev Pathol 2001;4:473–81.
60. Victoria A, Mora G, Arias F. Perinatal outcome, placental pathology, and severity of discordance in monochorionic and dichorionic twins. Obstet Gynecol 2001;97:310–5.
61. Sato Y, Benirschke K. Increased prevalence of fetal thrombi in monochorionic-twin placentas. Pediatrics 2006;117:e113–7.
62. Ong SSC, Zamora J, Khan KS, Kilby MD. Prognosis for the co-twin following single-twin death: a systematic review. BJOG 2006;113:992–8.
63. Joseph KS, Huang L, Liu S, et al. Reconciling the high rates of preterm and postterm birth in the United States. Obstet Gynecol 2007;109:813–22.
64. Klebanoff MA. Gestational age: not always what it seems. Obstet Gynecol 2007;109:798–9.
65. Nakling J, Backe B. Pregnancy risk increases from 41 weeks of gestation. Acta Obstet Gynecol Scand 2006;85:663–8.
66. Duff P. A thoughtful algorithm for the accurate diagnosis of primary CMV infection in pregnancy. Am J Obstet Gynecol 2007;196:196–7.
67. Chow SS, Craig ME, Jacques CF, et al. Correlates of placental infection with cytomegalovirus, parvovirus B19 or human herpes virus 7. J Med Virol 2006;78:747–56.
68. Satosar A, Ramirez NC, Bartholomew D, et al. Histologic correlates of viral and bacterial infection of the placenta associated with severe morbidity and mortality in the newborn. Hum Pathol 2004;35:536–45.
69. Syridou G, Spanakis N, Konstantinidu A, et al. Detection of cytomegalovirus, parvovirus B19 and herpes simplex viruses in cases of intrauterine fetal death: association with pathological findings. J Med Virol 2008;80:1776–82.
70. Rogers BB, Over CE. Parvovirus B19 in fetal hydrops. Hum Pathol 1999;30:247.
71. Benirschke K, Coen R, Patterson B, Key T. Villitis of known origin: varicella and toxoplasma. Placenta 1999;20:395–9.
72. Brown ZA, Selke S, Zeh J. The acquisition of herpes simplex virus during pregnancy. N Engl J Med 1997;337:509–15.
73. Bhoopat L, Khunamornpong S, Sirivatanapa P, et al. Chorioamnionitis is associated with placental transmission of human immunodeficiency virus-1 subtype E in the early gestational period. Mod Pathol 2005;18:1357–64.
74. Goldenberg RL, Mudenda V, Read JS, et al. HPTN 024 study: histologic chorioamnionitis, antibiotics and adverse infant outcomes in a predominantly HIV-1-infected African population. Am J Obstet Gynecol 2006;195:1065–74.
75. Al-Husaini AM. Role of placenta in the vertical transmission of human immunodeficiency virus. J Perinatol 2009;29:331–6.
76. Weyn C, Thomas D, Jani J, et al. Evidence of human papillomavirus in the placenta. J Infect Dis 2011;203:341–3.
77. Sarkola ME, Grénman SE, Rintala MAM, et al. Human papillomavirus in the placenta and umbilical cord blood. Acta Obstet Gynecol Scand 2008;87:1181–8.
78. Rorman E, Zamir CS, Rilkis I, Ben-David H. Congenital toxoplasmosis—prenatal aspects of Toxoplasma gondii infection. Reprod Toxicol 2006;21:458–72.
79. Yavuz E, Aydin F, Seyhan A, et al. Granulomatous villitis formed by inflammatory cells with maternal origin: a rare manifestation type of placental toxoplasmosis. Placenta 2006;27:780–2.
80. Mens PF, Bojtor EC, Schallig HDFH. Molecular interactions in the placenta during malaria infection. Eur J Obstet Gynecol Reprod Biol 2010;152:126–32.
81. Muehlenbachs A, Fried M, McGready R, et al. A novel histological grading scheme for placental malaria applied in areas of high and low malaria transmission. J Infect Dis 2010;202:1608–16.
82. Sheffield JS, Sánchez PJ, Wendel Jr GD, et al. Placental histopathology of congenital syphilis. Obstet Gynecol 2002;100:126–33.
83. Kapur P, Rakheja D, Gomez AM, et al. Characterization of inflammation in syphilitic villitis and in villitis of unknown etiology. Pediatr Dev Pathol 2004;7:453–8; discussion 421.
84. Parkash V, Morotti RA, Joshi V, et al. Immunohistochemical detection of Listeria antigens in the placenta in perinatal listeriosis. Int J Gynecol Pathol 1998;17:343–50.

34 Gestational Trophoblastic Disease

Kyu-Rae Kim

CHAPTER OUTLINE

Introduction	784	Partial Hydatidiform Mole	795
Overview of Early Placental Development	784	Adverse Clinical Outcomes in Molar Disease	798
Villous Trophoblast	784	Trophoblastic Neoplasia	800
Extravillous (Intermediate) Trophoblast	785	Choriocarcinoma	800
Trophoblast Immunohistochemical Markers	787	Choriocarcinoma Associated with Full-term Pregnancy and Intraplacental Choriocarcinoma	802
Molar Gestational Trophoblastic Disease	788	Placental Site Trophoblastic Tumor	803
Complete Hydatidiform Mole	788	Epithelioid Trophoblastic Tumor	805
Early (First Trimester) Complete Hydatidiform Moles	791	Non-Neoplastic Trophoblastic Lesions	807
		Placental Site Nodule or Plaque	807
Advanced (Second Trimester) Complete Hydatidiform Moles	791	Exaggerated Placental Site (Reaction)	809

INTRODUCTION

Gestational trophoblastic disease is a spectrum of disorders ranging from unusual presentations of normal implantation, through premalignant hydatidiform moles (complete, partial, and invasive mole) to malignant disorders including choriocarcinoma, placental site trophoblastic tumor, and epithelioid trophoblastic tumor (Table 34.1). Often, trophoblast remnants of normal gestations, including placental site nodules, and exaggerated placental site reaction may cause clinical symptoms, which can be clinically and histologically confused with trophoblastic tumors. Although each of these entities has its own clinical and pathologic characteristics, they may be grouped under the single umbrella of gestational trophoblastic disease because they are all related to pregnancy, and may progress from one to another.

OVERVIEW OF EARLY PLACENTAL DEVELOPMENT

Histologic findings in trophoblastic disease often recapitulate those of the early placenta, causing difficulty in distinction between a disease state and normal gestational or postgestational trophoblast remnants. For this reason, it will be helpful to review early phases of normal placental development to understand the cells of origin, and those cytomorphologic features that are useful to distinguish normal from abnormal trophoblast.

VILLOUS TROPHOBLAST

At the end of the first week following conception, trophectoderm of the blastocyst implants in the endometrial surface and invades the endometrial stroma. The mononuclear trophoblastic shell, composed of previllous trophoblast, has not yet formed villous structures. This is responsible for erosion of maternal tissue by production of various hormones, cytokines, a number of extracellular matrix receptors, and matrix-degrading proteases and their inhibitors.[1] The previllous trophoblast of the implanting embryonic pole differentiates into two components, the outer syncytiotrophoblast located at the maternal–fetal interface and the inner cytotrophoblast (Figure 34.1). The cytotrophoblast is an inner layer of ovoid, mononuclear cells with high proliferative activity that functions as the trophoblastic stem cell. Syncytiotrophoblast, the first differentiated trophoblast lineage, produces human chorionic gonadotropin (hCG) and proteolytic enzymes, and secretes factors that cause

Table 34.1	World Health Organization Classification of Gestational Trophoblastic Disease

Non-Neoplastic, Non-Molar Trophoblastic Lesions

Placental site nodule
Exaggerated placental site

Hydatidiform Moles (Abnormally Formed Placentas)

Complete mole
Partial mole
Invasive mole

Trophoblastic Tumors (Neoplastic Diseases)

Choriocarcinoma
Placental site trophoblastic tumor
Epithelioid trophoblastic tumor

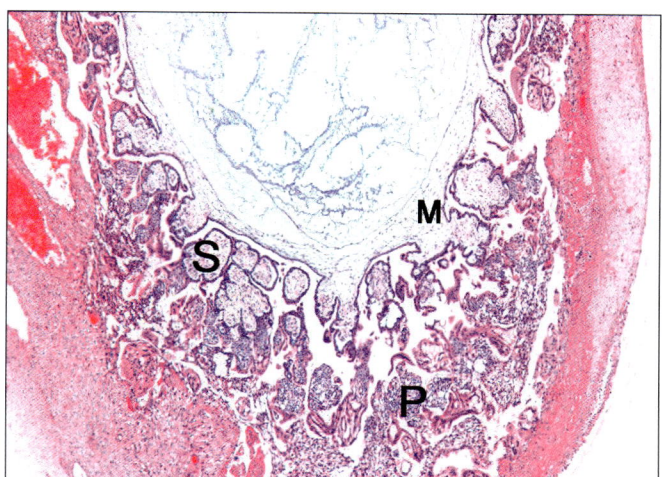

Figure 34.2 Villous stage in placental development. Mesenchymal cells derived from extraembryonic mesoderm (M) invade the villi, transforming the primary villi (P) into secondary villi (S).

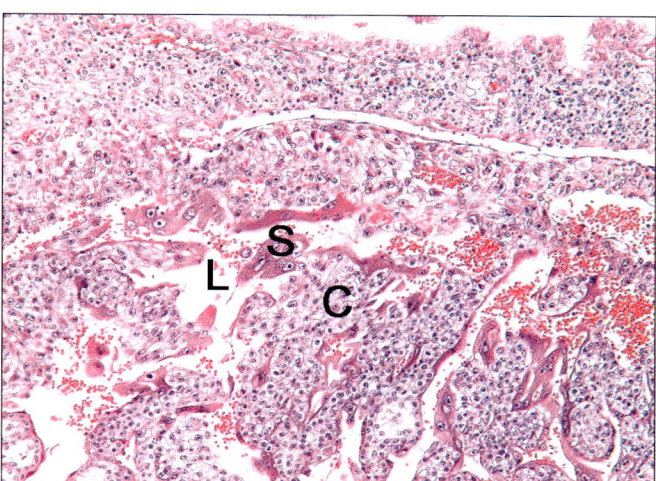

Figure 34.1 Lacunar stage in early placental development. As the trophoblastic cells invade the endometrium, they differentiate to form a double layer of cytotrophoblast (C) and syncytiotrophoblast (S) and intervening lacunar space (L).

apoptosis of the endometrial epithelial cells and decidua. Penetration and erosion of the adjacent maternal capillaries results in the formation of lacunae within the syncytiotrophoblast,[2] and these structures enlarge to form the intervillous space.

Early in the third week, extraembryonic mesoderm grows into the solid primary villous trabeculae of cytotrophoblast and syncytiotrophoblast (Figure 34.2), forming secondary villi. These consist of an outer layer of syncytiotrophoblast, a middle layer of cytotrophoblast, and an inner connective tissue core. At this stage secondary chorionic villi cover the entire surface of the chorionic sac.[2]

Active vasculogenesis begins within the secondary villous stroma, transforming them into tertiary villi (Figure 34.3A–D). Early primitive capillaries in the villous core are formed by *in situ* differentiation of pluripotent mesodermal tissue into hemangioblastic stem cells that give rise to committed endothelial progenitors (angioblast) and hematopoietic stem cells. Angioblasts form angiogenic cell cords (Figure 34.3A), which develop slit-like vascular lumens during the third to fourth week (Figure 34.3B). Subsequently, distinct vascular lumens with variable numbers of immature hematopoietic cells begin to appear (Figure 34.3C). Frequent mitotic figures and occasional karyorrhexis are identified among the angiogenic cell cords and the stromal cells at this stage. After that, new blood vessels in the villous stroma are derived by sprouting, elongation, and remodeling of already existing blood vessels. Villous stroma is basophilic and myxomatous until the end of the fourth week when the ground substance gradually assumes an edematous and reticular appearance (Figure 34.3D).

As active vasculogenesis is occurring, the villi branch, trophoblast proliferates at the implanting embryonic pole, and forms a confluent shell along the external circumference of the chorionic villi (Figure 34.4). This cytotrophoblastic shell of early pregnancy mimics the trophoblastic hyperplasia of hydatidiform moles, with which it should not be confused.

EXTRAVILLOUS (INTERMEDIATE) TROPHOBLAST

Extravillous trophoblast is a general term for the entire population of trophoblast residing outside the villi, including implantation site (basal plate), chorion laeve, chorionic plate (subchorionic area), and placental septum. It is commonly designated as 'intermediate trophoblast' by pathologists. The terms extravillous and intermediate trophoblast will be used interchangeably in this chapter.

While one group of cytotrophoblast fuses to form multinucleated syncytiotrophoblast, which encases the free villi of the placenta, another differentiates into extravillous trophoblast and develops invasive properties.[3] At the basal end of anchoring villi, cytotrophoblast proliferates to form columns of 'villous intermediate trophoblast,' a cohesive mass of cells with high proliferative activity (Figure 34.5A). As the cells in the trophoblastic column come into contact with decidua, these cells exit the cell cycle, thereby losing

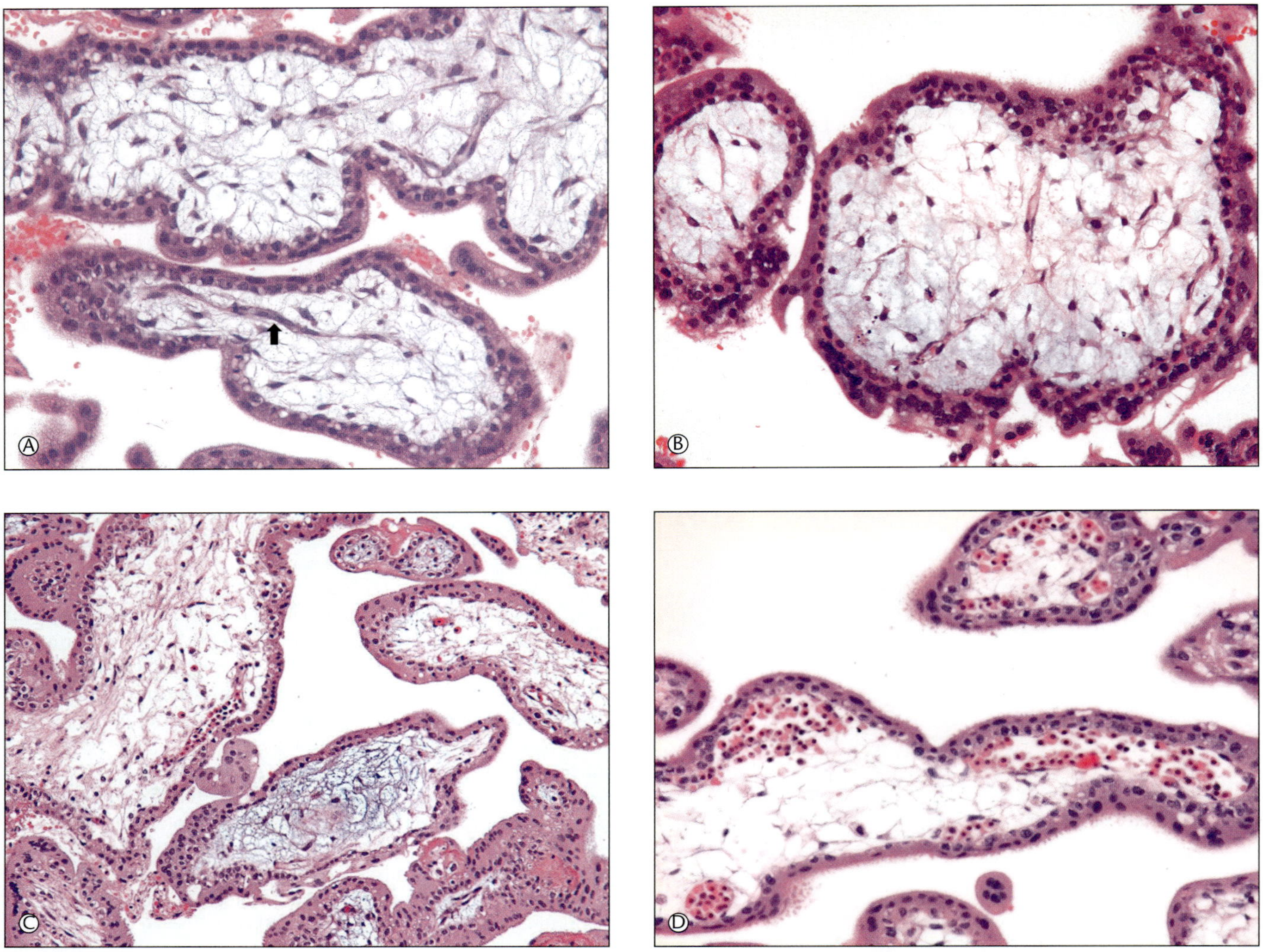

Figure 34.3 Vasculogenetic steps in chorionic villi during early pregnancy **(A–D)**. Stromal vessels are differentiated from **(A)** immature angiogenic cell cords (arrow) within basophilic stroma to **(B)** immature blood vessels containing primitive slit-like vascular lumens and immature hematopoietic components to **(C, D)** mature blood vessels containing distinct vascular lumens and hematopoietic components. Note stromal changes from basophilic to edematous stroma.

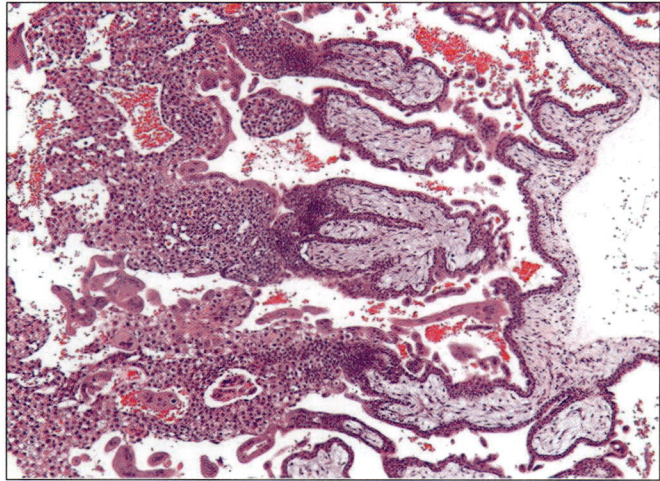

Figure 34.4 Normal placenta during the early gestation showing exuberant polarized and circumferential trophoblastic proliferation merging into a peripheral cytotrophoblastic shell (left).

their proliferative activity, detach from the cell column, and acquire migratory and invasive properties. Subsequently, the cells move into the decidua and superficial myometrium (interstitial trophoblast) (Figure 34.5B) and penetrate the decidual spiral arteries (endovascular trophoblast) (Figure 34.5C). These are collectively referred to as 'implantation site intermediate trophoblast.'[4]

In a normal implantation site, endovascular trophoblast displaces the endothelial lining and musculoelastic tissue of spiral arteries, increasing the luminal diameter and allowing greater transport of maternal blood to the intervillous space. Proliferative and invasive ability do not coexist in one and the same cell of normal trophoblast, but rather are seen in mutually exclusive populations. This contrasts with 'malignant' trophoblast, where the invasive cells also proliferate.

Interstitial (intermediate) trophoblast cytology is similar to that of surrounding decidualized stromal cells (Figure 34.5A–D), but the trophoblast nuclei are slightly larger, irregular, and hyperchromatic. Trophoblastic spindle cells

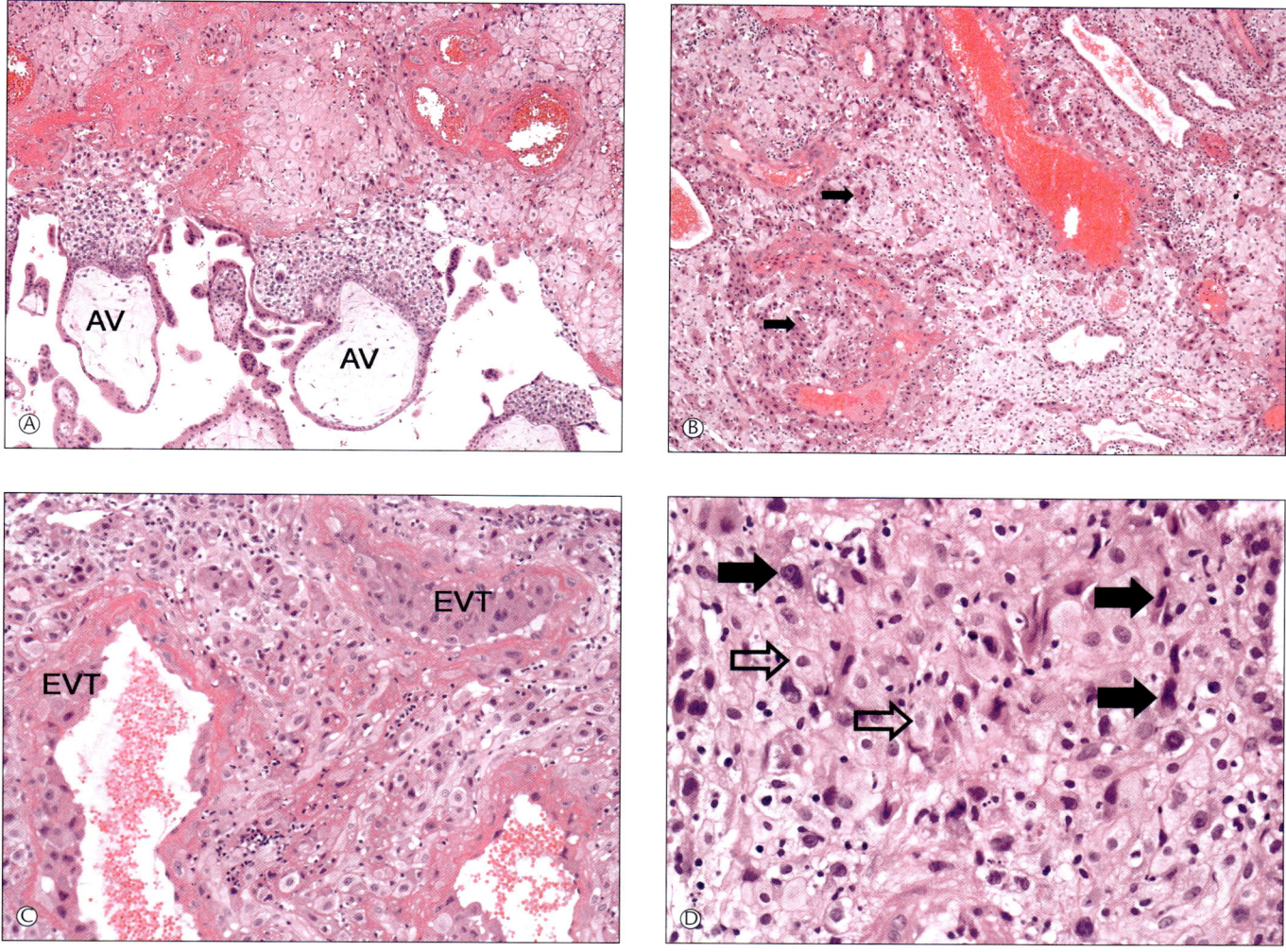

Figure 34.5 Villous and extravillous trophoblast at the implantation site. **(A)** Anchoring villi (AV) are attached to the decidua of the implantation site. **(B)** Extravillous (interstitial) trophoblast (closed arrows) infiltrating into the decidua have densely eosinophilic or amphophilic cytoplasm. **(C)** Extravillous (endovascular) trophoblast (EVT) infiltrating into the blood vessels. **(D)** Close-up view of extravillous trophoblast (closed arrows) shows slightly larger, irregular, and hyperchromatic nuclei with more eosinophilic or amphophilic cytoplasm than the admixed decidual cells with paler cytoplasm (open arrows).

often have angular dark nuclei as they dissect individually or in small clusters between decidual cells (Figure 34.5D).

Chorionic villi cover the entire chorionic sac until the beginning of the eighth week but become asymmetrical as those associated with the decidua capsularis begin to degenerate. A variable thickness of trophoblastic cells persists in the chorion laeve until term, but this extravillous trophoblast is not invasive. Therefore, the fetal membrane is composed of amniotic epithelium sitting on thin connective tissue layers of amnion and chorion, maternal decidua parietalis with interposed extravillous trophoblast, and occasional ghost villi (Figure 34.6A). Microscopically, intermediate trophoblast in the chorion laeve of term placentas are composed of two populations with differing cytology and immunophenotypes (Figure 34.6A–F).[4,5] These two types of intermediate trophoblast are not strictly separated into different compartments, but rather are admixed to some extent.

TROPHOBLAST IMMUNOHISTOCHEMICAL MARKERS

Non-neoplastic trophoblastic lesions can be confused with a variety of trophoblastic and nontrophoblastic tumors because of their inherent cytologic atypia and pleomorphism. Immunohistochemical markers can be helpful in resolving the differential diagnosis.

All trophoblastic cells, including cytotrophoblast, syncytiotrophoblast, and intermediate trophoblast, possess epithelial antigens detected by antibodies for cytokeratin (AE1 and AE3), epithelial membrane antigen, and low molecular weight cytokeratins (CAM 5.2 and Ber-P4). Although not specific to the trophoblast, these common antibodies are useful to distinguish trophoblastic from nonepithelial tumors, such as epithelioid smooth muscle neoplasia. Some antibodies, including HSD3β1, HLA-G, and β-hCG, are used in the differential diagnosis between trophoblastic and

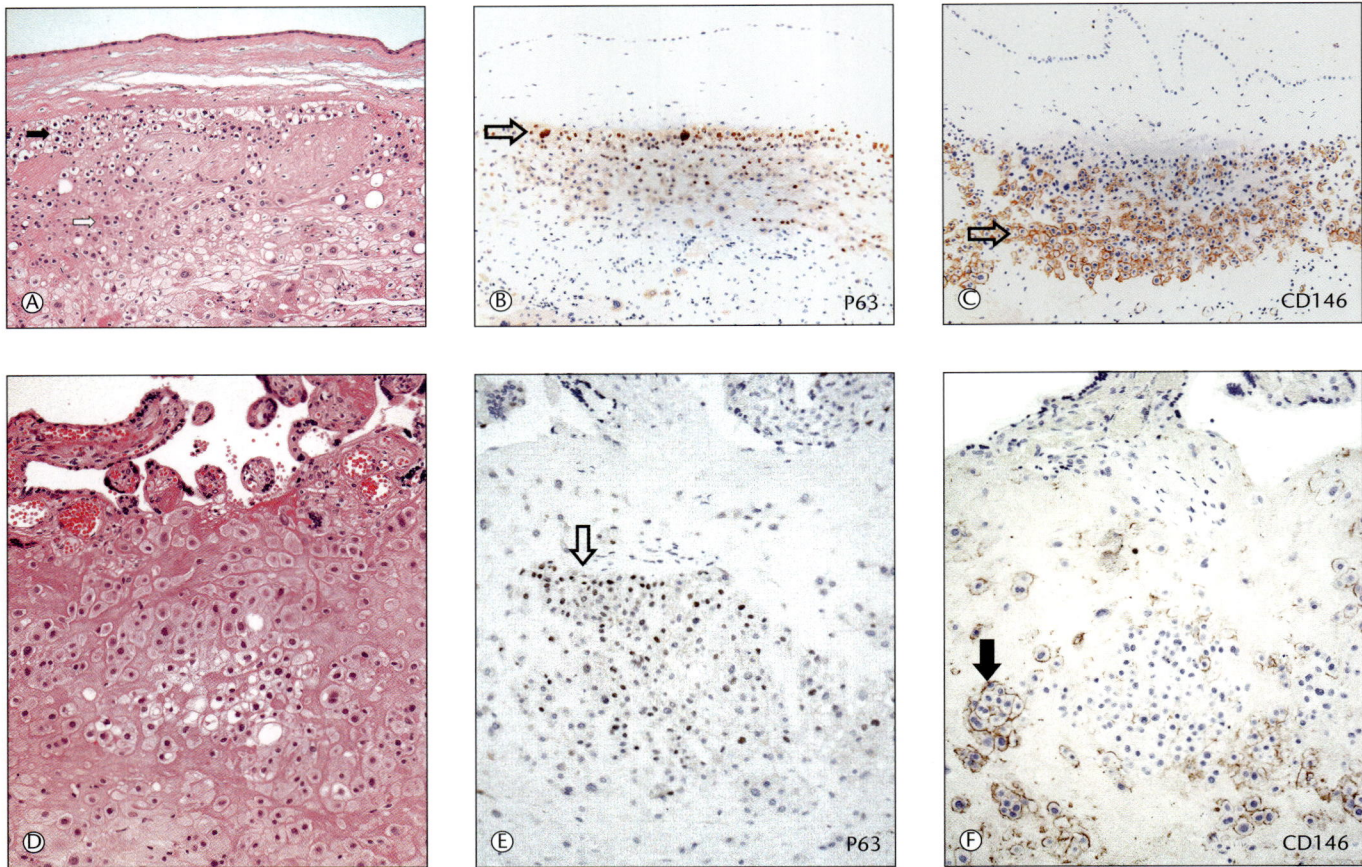

Figure 34.6 Cytomorphologic features and immunophenotypes of extravillous trophoblast. Trophoblast contacting chorionic stroma are relatively smaller and uniform with clear cytoplasm (**A**, closed arrow), while those directly contacting decidua have slightly larger nuclei and amphophilic cytoplasm (**A**, open arrow). P63 is only expressed in the former (**B**, open arrow), whereas CD146 (Mel-CAM) is mostly expressed in the latter (**C**, open arrow). Extravillous trophoblast in the implantation site (basal plate) is also composed of two populations (**D**). P63 is expressed in the smaller trophoblasts with clear cytoplasm (**E**, open arrow) and CD146 (Mel-CAM) is expressed in the larger trophoblasts with amphophilic cytoplasm (**F**, closed arrow).

nontrophoblastic lesions. Others, including P63, placental alkaline phosphatase, human placental lactogen, and CD146 (Mel-CAM), are useful to infer 'chorionic-type' or 'implantation site' differentiation among intermediate trophoblast. Expressions of various trophoblastic markers in subpopulations of trophoblast are summarized in Panel A of Table 34.2, and their use in resolving various differential diagnoses is shown in Panel B.

MOLAR GESTATIONAL TROPHOBLASTIC DISEASE

Hydatidiform moles are abnormal gestations created by an imbalance of parental genomes secondary to abnormal fertilization events, most commonly androgenetic diploid (complete moles) or biparental triploid (partial moles). They are significant as examples of failed pregnancy that may recur at heightened risk, and as premalignant lesions that justify observational or therapeutic intervention. Depending on the nature of the genomic imbalance, which is reflected in the histologic appearance, some may display invasive or metastatic behavior, or progress to overtly malignant choriocarcinoma. All hydatidiform moles have an edematous villous stroma, with a tendency to form drop-like fluid cisternae, or 'hydatids,' that have conferred the designation of this class of diseases. Discrimination between degenerative and molar pregnancies can be difficult, and accurate subclassification as complete or partial mole directly impacts clinical prognosis and management.

COMPLETE HYDATIDIFORM MOLE

Incidence

Epidemiologic studies have reported wide regional variation in the incidence of hydatidiform mole, of 0.57–1.6 per 1000 pregnancies[6,7] in North America and Europe, rising to 2.0–8.5 in Asia, Africa, and Latin America.[8,9] Although trophoblastic diseases occur more frequently in Asia than in North America or Europe, considerable difficulty exists in determining true incidence rates. Since these diseases are directly related to pregnancy, incidence ratios have been expressed per total number of pregnancies, number of deliveries, or live births in population-based or hospital-based studies. However, it is hard to obtain data regarding clinically unrecognized pregnancies, spontaneous and

Table 34.2 Trophoblast Immunomarkers (Panel A) and a Diagnostic Algorithm for Their Use in Differential Diagnosis (Panel B)

Panel A

Differential Diagnosis	Trophoblastic Versus Nontrophoblastic			Chorionic-Type Versus Implantation Site IT			
Marker	HSD3β1	HLA-G	β-hCG	P63	PLAP	hPL	CD146
Cytotrophoblast	−	−	−	+	+	−	−
Syncytiotrophoblast	+	−	+	−	+	+	−
Implantation site IT	+	+	±	−	−	+	+
Chorionic-type IT	+	+	−	+	+	−	−
Nontrophoblastic epithelial cells	−	±	−	Variable	−	−	Variable

IT, intermediate trophoblast; PLAP, placental alkaline phosphatase; hPL, human placental lactogen.

Panel B

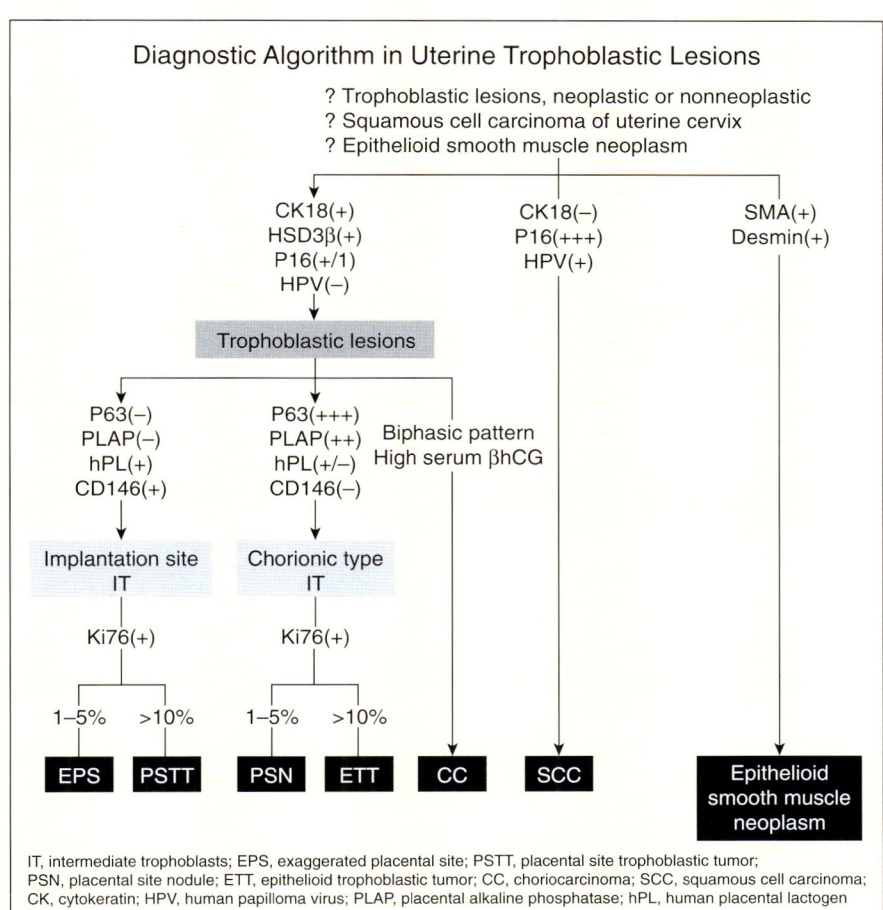

IT, intermediate trophoblasts; EPS, exaggerated placental site; PSTT, placental site trophoblastic tumor; PSN, placental site nodule; ETT, epithelioid trophoblastic tumor; CC, choriocarcinoma; SCC, squamous cell carcinoma; CK, cytokeratin; HPV, human papilloma virus; PLAP, placental alkaline phosphatase; hPL, human placental lactogen

---

induced abortions, ectopic pregnancies, and uncomplicated live births and pregnancies that did not receive hospital-based care. Moreover, histopathologic examination of evacuated tissue is infrequent in some parts of the world and the diagnosis of hydatidiform mole can be missed, especially early in gestation.

Even in the high-incidence areas, overall incidence rates have significantly decreased over the last few decades with improved socioeconomic status of women, suggesting that environmental factors including dietary or nutritional factors are as important as ethnic or genetic factors.[10-12] In the Netherlands, the incidence of trophoblastic disease increased significantly in recent years, partially explained by increased maternal age, increased proportion of live births of Asian descent, and improved diagnostic techniques.[7]

Risk Factors

Extremes of maternal age and prior molar pregnancy are established risk factors.[7,13] Conceptions occurring at extreme reproductive age, women over 45 and girls under 15, have higher risks of molar pregnancy than those for women aged 16–40.[6,14]

Pathogenetic Mechanism

The genetic origin of hydatidiform moles was first suggested by the observation that about 90% have sex chromatin.[15] Cytogenetic studies confirmed that about 90% of hydatidiform moles had a 46,XX karyotype[16] and others triploid karyotypes.[17] Based on the correlation of the histologic findings of hydatidiform moles and their karyotypes, existence of the two genetically distinct entities of complete and partial mole were suggested.[18,19]

Most complete hydatidiform moles are a diploid androgenetic pregnancy in which all 46 chromosomes are paternally derived. Usually these arise following endoreduplication of a haploid sperm (Figure 34.7), but a minor proportion result from fertilization of an anucleate egg by two sperms (dispermy)[20] (Figure 34.7). The fate of the missing maternal chromosomes is unclear, but may be caused by extrusion of both maternal sets of chromosomes into one of the polar bodies during meiosis, giving rise to an anucleate egg. Alternatively, retained maternal chromosomes may degenerate and thus fail to participate in postfertilization cell division. Triploid and tetraploid complete moles have been reported; however, these are still generally androgenetic in origin, having three or four paternal sets of chromosomes.

Rarely, complete moles are biparental diploid with both a maternal and paternal chromosome complement.[21,22] This corroborates the suggestion that fertilization of an empty egg is not mandatory for the creation of a hydatidiform mole. Studies have shown that these biparental moles are frequently associated with patients with recurrent or familial molar disease.[22] Biparental complete hydatidiform moles are now recognized as a clinically important subgroup, caused by maternal autosomal recessive mutation of *NLRP7*, located in a 1.1 Mb region on chromosome 19q13.4. Mutation in this gene may result in dysregulation of imprinting in the female germ line with abnormal development of both embryonic and extraembryonic tissue.

Clinical Features

Molar pregnancies are now diagnosed at an earlier gestational age due to routine use of first trimester ultrasonography. Formerly, the majority of patients presented by 20 weeks of gestation with vaginal bleeding, symptomatic anemia, passage of molar tissue, excessive uterine size, hyperemesis, and markedly elevated hCG levels. Preeclampsia was observed in approximately 27%, and clinically evident hyperthyroidism in about 7% of the cases. Abdominal pain and pelvic pain resulting from enlarged theca lutein cysts of the ovary were commonly associated, and pelvic ultrasound examination revealed a characteristic 'snowstorm appearance.' Recently, however, the gestational age at the time of ultrasound diagnosis ranges from 5.0 to 12.5 weeks (median 8–9 weeks). Accordingly, the clinical presentation has changed considerably; excessive uterine size, anemia, hyperemesis, and metastatic disease are less common, and earlier stage molar tissues are submitted for examination. Today 40% of women are asymptomatic, and most symptomatic patients present with vaginal bleeding or suspected miscarriage in early pregnancy. In the first trimester, a significant proportion of complete moles demonstrate minimal ultrasound findings and are missed by this modality.[23] Overall sensitivity for the ultrasound diagnosis of molar gestations is 40–60%.[23]

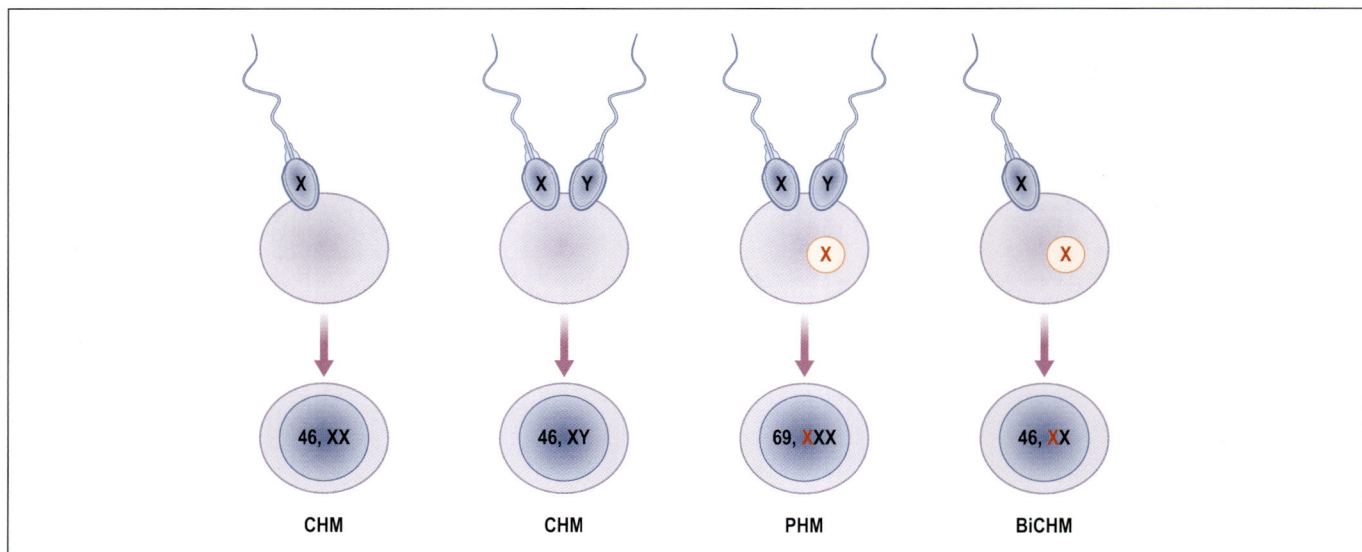

Figure 34.7 Genetic origins of hydatidiform moles. Endoreduplication of a haploid sperm or fertilization of two sperm in a functionally 'empty' ovum results in androgenetic complete hydatidiform mole (CHM). Fertilization of a normal ovum by two sperm results in triploid partial hydatidiform mole (PHM). Presence of biparental genome, but with mutation, results in biparental complete hydatidiform mole (BiCHM).

Gross and Microscopic Findings

Pathologic findings of first trimester moles are more commonly encountered over the past decade due to the current practice of very early uterine evacuation. Thus, it is important for pathologists to recognize the subtle, but distinctive, histopathologic features unique to both early and late complete hydatidiform moles.

Grossly, the amount of tissue from early moles is less than that of advanced moles. The chorionic villi of early moles have smaller mean maximal villous diameter, and may not be grossly hydropic, unlike the more characteristically grape-like hydrops seen in late moles.

Microscopically, variable degrees of trophoblastic proliferation and hydropic change are identified in all complete moles, but the histopathologic presentation differs by gestational age.

EARLY (FIRST TRIMESTER) COMPLETE HYDATIDIFORM MOLES

Early moles in which trophoblastic proliferation and hydropic change is minimal (Figure 34.8) are easily confused with non-molar hydropic abortions. At this early phase, molar chorionic villi have bulbous outlines resembling blunt finger-like projections, and the villous stroma may not have appreciable hydropic change. Villous trophoblastic proliferation is minimal or is frequently proliferated in a polar fashion (Figure 34.9), resembling polar proliferation of normal anchoring villi in early developing placentas. Trophoblastic pseudoinclusions, although often present, are not diagnostic, as they also may be seen in partial moles and aneuploid gestations. It is a combination of hypercellular basophilic stroma, immature blood vessels, and abnormal villous profiles that characterizes early complete moles, as these individual features may be seen separately and to a lesser extent in normal early developing placentas.

Poorly formed immature blood vessels in the villous stroma are characteristic of early moles. Vascular structures, when present (Figure 34.10), are linear cords in basophilic stroma, similar to the angiogenic cell cords of normal placentas (Figure 34.3A). Rarely, there are cleft-like spaces within the vascular structures, but unlike normal placentas they almost never contain hematopoietic components or red blood cells. There is characteristic karyorrhexis and apoptosis of stromal cells and immature vascular structures, scattering karyorrhectic nuclear debris throughout the villous stroma (Figure 34.11). Karyorrhexis and apoptosis within the villous stroma of non-molar hydropic abortuses and normal placentas are limited to a few cells within small terminal villi.

ADVANCED (SECOND TRIMESTER) COMPLETE HYDATIDIFORM MOLES

The cellular and mildly edematous basophilic stroma of early moles progressively changes to form hydropic villi with

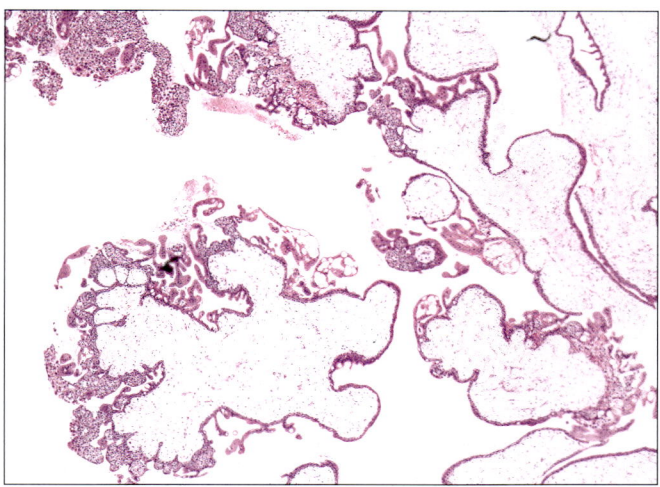

Figure 34.9 Early complete hydatidiform mole during the first trimester. Note the bulbous outlines of the chorionic villi and polar proliferation of villous trophoblast, resembling those of normal anchoring villi.

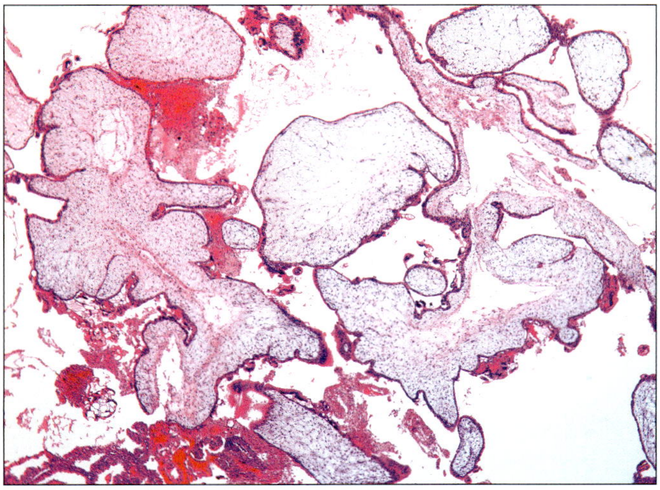

Figure 34.8 Early (first trimester) complete hydatidiform mole during the first trimester. Trophoblastic proliferation or hydropic change is nearly absent, which may cause underdiagnosis as non-molar hydropic abortion.

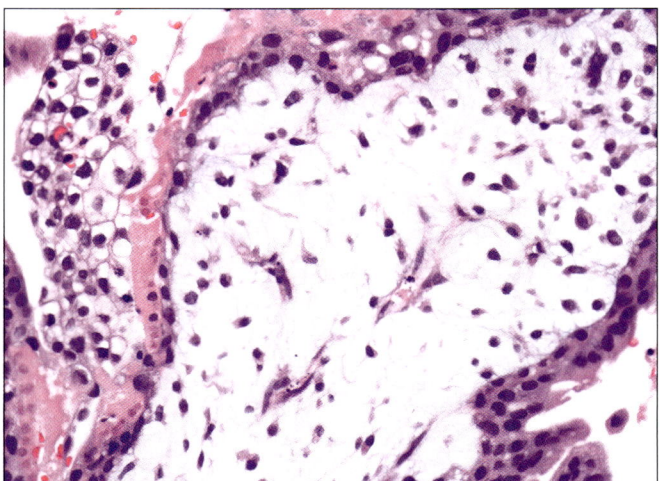

Figure 34.10 Early complete hydatidiform mole during the first trimester. Immature vascular structure with apoptotic nuclear debris in basophilic stroma is a characteristic feature of early moles.

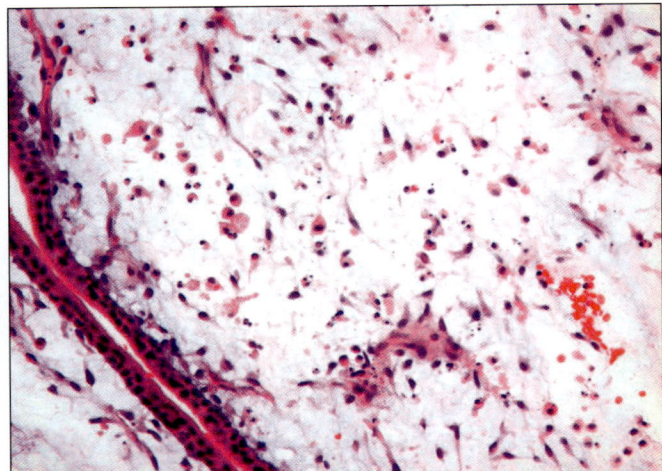

Figure 34.11 Early complete hydatidiform mole, first trimester. Markedly increased apoptosis in the stromal cells as well as in the immature blood vessels is a frequent feature of early moles.

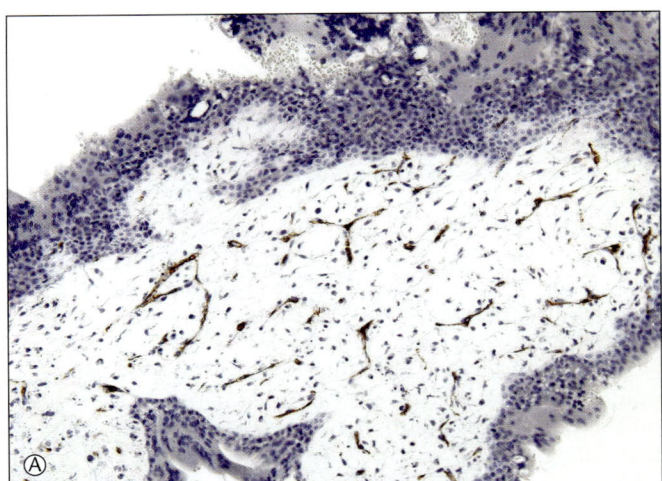
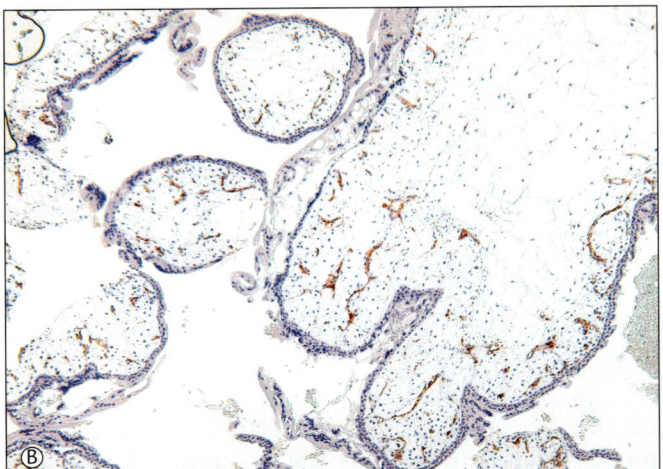
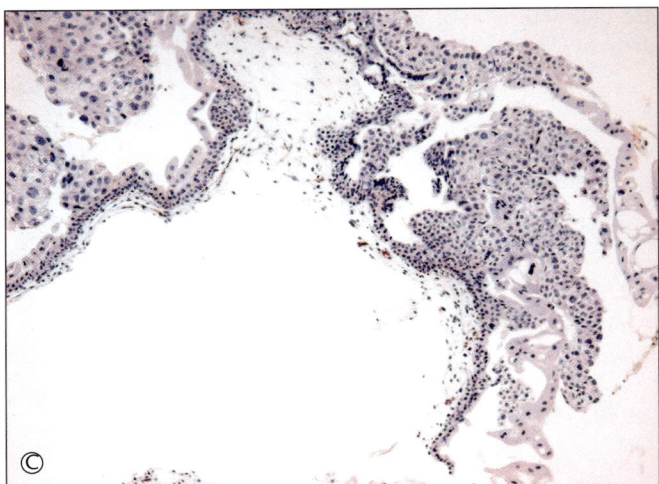

Figure 34.12 Progressive hydropic changes in the villous stroma of complete hydatidiform mole shown by blood vessel (CD31) immunostain. Numerous brown staining immature blood vessels are present in the cellular nonhydropic stroma during the first trimester **(A)**, soon to be displaced. A cisterna is formed by accumulation of fluid in the center of the cellular nonhydropic stroma **(B)**. In the second trimester, avascular hydropic villi are formed by extensive accumulation of vesicular fluid in vesicular cisternae **(C)**.

central acellular cisternae, and eventually, diffusely hydropic hypocellular villi (Figure 34.12A–C). Stroma is progressively displaced from the central part of the villi by accumulated fluid. These hydropic vesicles have grossly visible 'bunch of grapes' appearance filling the entire uterine cavity (Figure 34.13). Circumferential proliferation of cytotrophoblast, intermediate trophoblast, and syncytiotrophoblast is prominent (Figures 34.14 and 34.15), sometimes forming large sheets of trophoblast around the edematous villi. The trophoblast of complete moles has variable degrees of cytologic atypia, which may include nuclear pleomorphism and heterochromasia, often accompanied by cytoplasmic vacuoles (Figure 34.16). The vacuoles are relatively more prominent than seen in normal trophoblast at the same gestational age. The degree of trophoblastic proliferation and hydropic change appears to be a time-dependent phenomenon that varies by gestational age, and is not related to the risk of subsequent persistent trophoblastic neoplasia.

Molar implantation sites are almost always exaggerated, in that intermediate trophoblastic cells are more atypical and the Ki-67 labeling index is higher than for a normal pregnancy.[24] Biparental, triploid, or tetraploid complete moles and 46,XX and 46,XY complete moles are histologically and immunohistochemically indistinguishable from the more common androgenetic diploid mole.[25]

Differential Diagnosis and Special Studies

Complete hydatidiform moles can be, and usually are, diagnosed based on the histopathologic findings alone using the above-described criteria. However, significant interobserver and intraobserver variability is observed, especially during early pregnancy. Distinction of molar from non-molar pregnancy and subclassification of moles into complete and partial types is important because subsequent management and the risk of persistent disease are different. Formerly, diagnostic difficulty was most frequently observed between complete and partial moles, but distinguishing complete moles from non-molar hydropic abortion is more problematic these days because most of the placental tissues are evacuated in the first trimester.

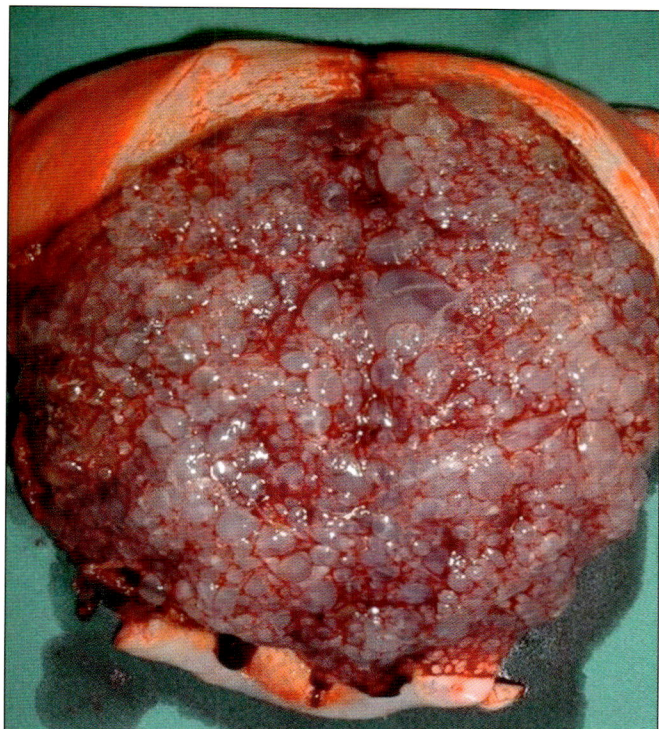

Figure 34.13 Complete hydatidiform mole in the second trimester of pregnancy. Molar tissue has a grossly visible 'bunch of grapes' appearance filling the entire uterine cavity

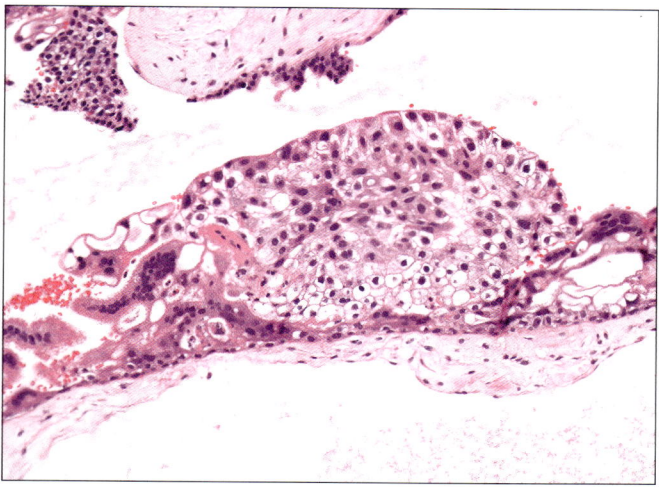

Figure 34.15 Complete hydatidiform mole in the second trimester of pregnancy. Proliferating trophoblast are composed of cytotrophoblast, intermediate trophoblast, and syncytiotrophoblast.

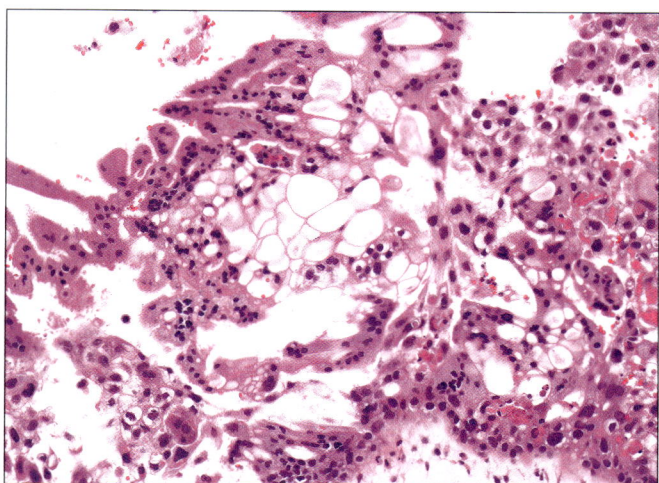

Figure 34.16 Complete hydatidiform mole in the second trimester of pregnancy. The trophoblast has variable degrees of cytologic atypia and frequent cytoplasmic vacuoles, although vacuoles themselves are not a diagnostic feature.

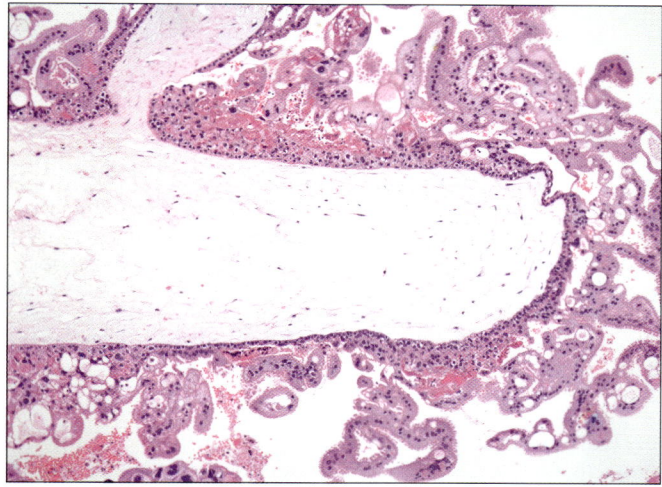

Figure 34.14 Complete hydatidiform mole in the second trimester of pregnancy. Circumferential trophoblastic proliferation and hydropic change of villous stroma are evident.

Introduction of immunostaining for $p57^{kip2}$ (CDKN1C), a paternally imprinted biomarker expressed only from the maternal genome of villous trophoblast, permits distinction between androgenetic (complete mole) and biparental (normal placenta, hydropic abortion, partial mole) tissues. Lack of $p57^{kip2}$ immunohistochemical staining is thus a clinically useful feature of complete moles, contrasting with positive expression in all biparental gestations. Interpretation should be based solely on scoring of the villous cytotrophoblast as extravillous trophoblast relax the imprint and thus may demonstrate variable expression even in androgenetic cells (Figure 34.17A–C).

If both histologic features and the $p57^{kip2}$ result are equivocal, DNA ploidy analysis by flow cytometry or image analysis and chromosomal enumeration by fluorescent or chromogenic *in situ* hybridization (Figure 34.18A and B) are of great value in making the distinction between a diploid complete (Figure 34.18A) and triploid partial hydatidiform mole (Figure 34.18B). Even with those ancillary studies, diagnosis of hydatidiform mole can sometimes be difficult. Recently, DNA genotyping has been used to confirm their unique parental chromosomal compositions of complete and partial hydatidiform moles except for rare biparental complete moles and complete moles arising from a twin gestation.[26] However, decidual tissue should be carefully removed during the preparation.

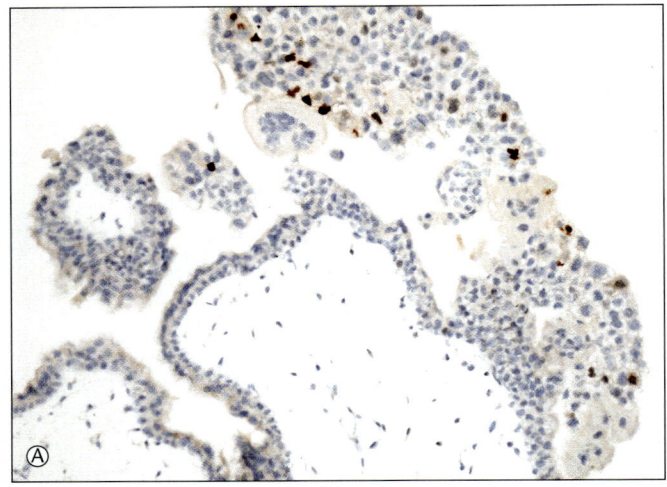
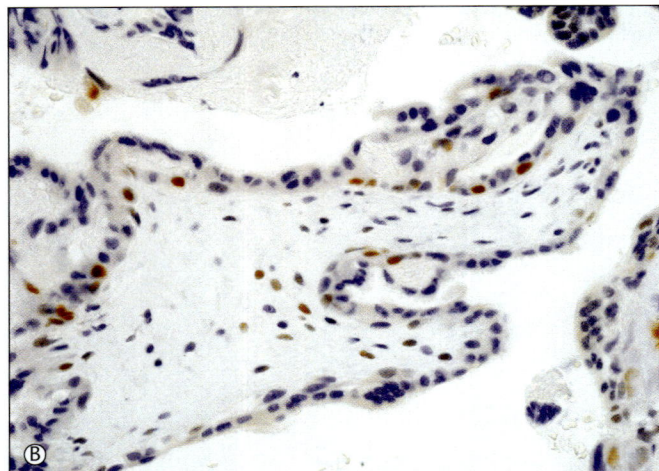
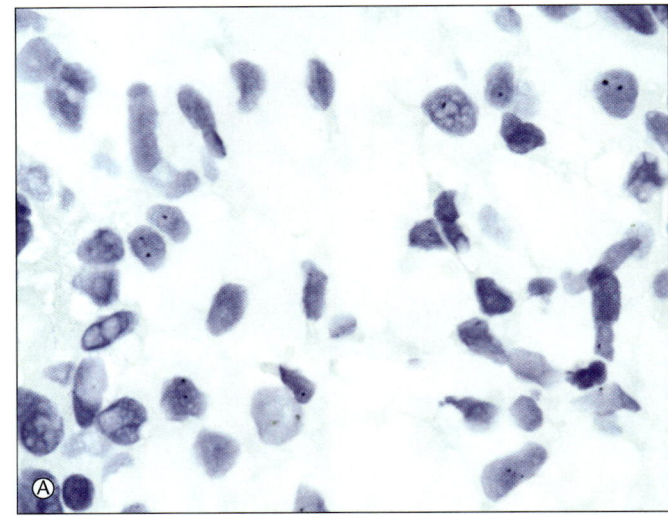
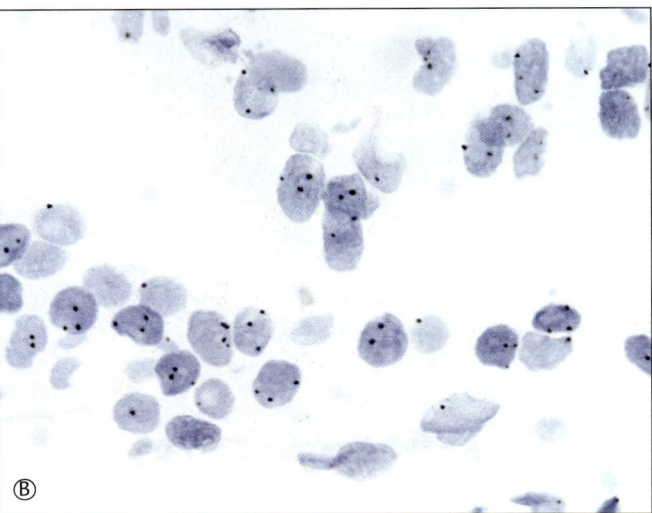
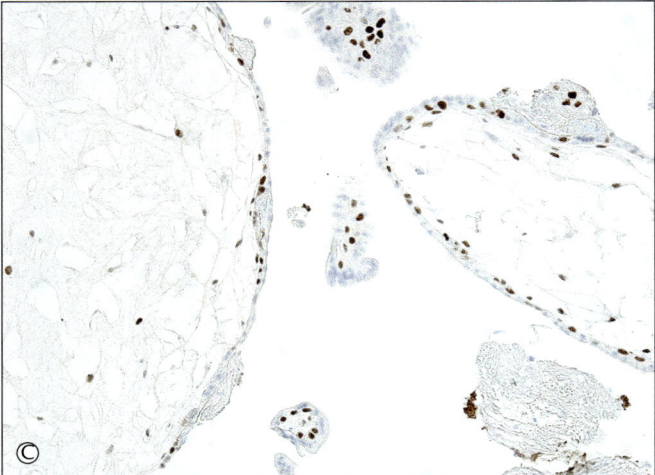

Figure 34.17 p57^{kip2} immunostaining patterns in complete and partial hydatidiform moles, and hydropic abortion **(A–C)**. Immunonegativity for p57^{kip2} in the villous stromal cells and villous cytotrophoblastic cells of complete hydatidiform mole **(A)** is contrasted with the immunopositivities in those cell components in partial hydatidiform mole **(B)** and non-molar abortion **(C)**. Diagnostic intrepetation should be based on villous surface trophoblast only, as solid columns of extravillous trophoblast emerging from the villous tips maintain p57 staining even in complete moles (A).

Figure 34.18 Chromogenic *in situ* hybridization using a centromere probe. Complete hydatidiform mole shows less than two signals in most of the cells **(A)**, whereas a significant number of cytotrophoblast and villous stromal cells demonstrate three signals in partial hydatidiform mole **(B)**. Although trisomy and triploid status cannot be distinguished, it is a simple and useful method to confirm the diagnosis of partial mole in conjunction with histologic features.

Hydropic non-molar abortion is often histologically difficult to differentiate from early complete mole because of hydropic stroma. Mature blood vessels containing hematopoietic components, if present, are a helpful feature for the exclusion of mole. However, hydropic abortuses in early pregnancy may lack mature vascular structures. In hydropic abortuses, trophoblastic cells lining the chorionic villi are frequently stretched and thin, and the villous outline is usually smooth and rounded (Figure 34.19). Although significant hydropic change is observed in hydropic abortion, central cisterna formation is less frequent, and extensive stromal karyorrhexis is rare. If the tissue is well preserved the diagnosis can easily be resolved with p57^{kip2} immunostaining.

Nonhydropic normal early gestations may also be confused with complete moles because of prominent and confluent trophoblast along the external circumference of the

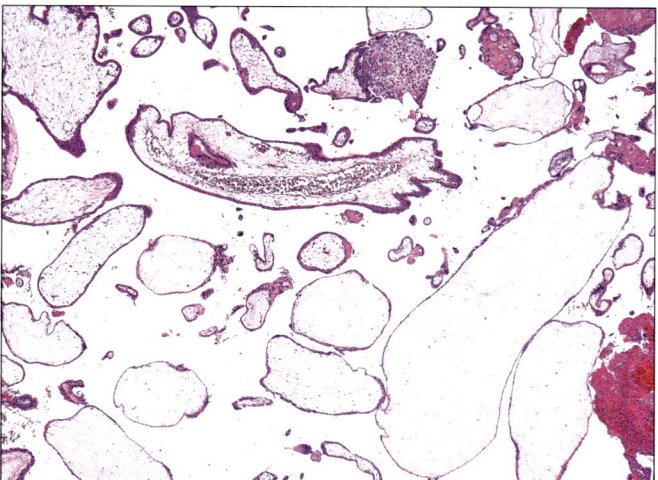

Figure 34.19 Non-molar hydropic abortion. The villous stroma has an edematous and myxoid appearance, but stromal blood vessels are well formed. The trophoblastic layer is thin, and the villous outline is usually smooth and rounded.

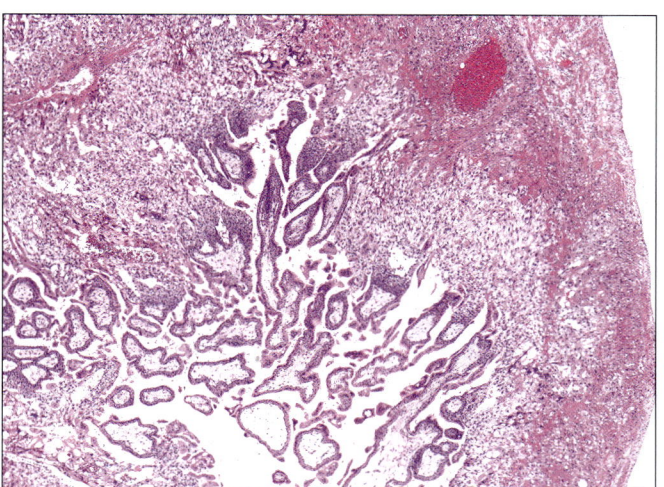

Figure 34.20 Ectopic tubal pregnancy. Exuberant trophoblastic proliferation in the early gestational period may cause misdiagnosis of tubal pregnancy as a hydatidiform mole in an ectopic site.

chorionic villi (Figure 34.4). Mature stromal blood vessels containing distinct lumens and hematopoietic components, if present, and immunopositivity for p57^{kip2} antibody are helpful features for the exclusion of complete moles.

Although hydatidiform moles, either complete or partial, do occur in ectopic sites, molar pregnancies in ectopic locations should be diagnosed using strict histologic criteria. Non-molar ectopic gestations typically present early, when sheets of particularly prominent extravillous trophoblast and degenerative hydropic changes can easily be mistaken for molar disease (Figure 34.20).[27,28] When the diagnosis is equivocal, positive immunohistochemical staining for p57^{kip2} will exclude complete mole.

Treatment and Prognostic Factors

Once molar pregnancy is suspected by clinical history, physical examination, serum β-hCG level, or ultrasonographic findings, diagnostic tissue is obtained by dilatation and curettage and clinical course monitored by biochemical (hCG) follow-up. Since molar pregnancies are very vascular and commonly invade the myometrium, suction curettage is recommended to minimize the risk of uterine perforation. Non-metastatic complete hydatidiform mole can be successfully treated with preservation of fertility in approximately 80% of patients.

PARTIAL HYDATIDIFORM MOLE

Partial hydatidiform mole is defined as a conceptus with a fetus (alive or dead) and a single placenta with focal hydatidiform change of the villi in the presence of trophoblastic hyperplasia. Although an embryo or fetus often can be demonstrated, sometimes this is not represented in the available specimen, either because of sampling error or prior passage or degeneration of fetal parts.

There is continuing uncertainty regarding the frequency and natural history of partial moles because of difficulty of histopathologic diagnosis, and variable access to ploidy and molecular genetic analysis.

Pathogenetic Mechanism

Partial moles differ from complete moles in that they are almost always triploid, having a 69,XXX, 69,XXY, or 69,XYY karyotype.[31] In almost all cases, the additional chromosome set is paternally derived, or diandric.[32] The most common mechanism is fertilization of an ovum by a diploid sperm or by two haploid sperm (Figure 34.7). However, only a portion of paternally derived triploid (diandric triploidy) placentas develop partial molar phenotype, indicating that the mere presence of two paternal haploid genomes is insufficient for molar development.[33,34] Additionally, non-molar maternally derived triploidy (digynic triploids) may be accompanied by degenerative hydropic change but lack other histologic features of partial moles.[32,35] Sometimes, a triploid placenta is associated with a grossly visible fetus,[36] but most are digynic and thus not a partial mole[32] or confined placental mosaicism with a diploid fetus. Thus, in the absence of pathognomonic histologic features, triploidy alone is not diagnostic of partial mole. This is especially the case with first trimester spontaneous abortions having degenerative hydropic change, as non-molar digynic triploidy is the most common form of triploidy in this subset of conceptuses.[32] Occasionally, trisomies 2, 7, 15, 16, and 22 may share some features with partial mole, such as villous hydrops and trophoblastic proliferation.[37] Tetraploid partial moles have also been reported and they usually have an excess of paternal genomes.[38]

Clinical Features

Symptoms and signs of patients with partial moles are not different from those of complete moles. Vaginal bleeding is the main presenting symptom. The main clinical diagnosis is threatened or incomplete abortion. They tend to have much less uterine enlargement and relatively lower concentration of hCG than those of complete moles. Patients with partial mole also have a risk of pre-eclampsia and hyperthyroidism. Hydropic change in partial moles is minimal in the first trimester of pregnancy, becoming prominent only in the second or third trimester. Therefore, most first trimester partial moles escape detection by ultrasound or macroscopic examination, and when encountered are difficult to distinguish from more common digynic triploid spontaneous abortions.[39] Intraplacental choriocarcinoma directly arising from triploid partial molar gestations has been described.[40]

Gross and Microscopic Findings

Partial moles may or may not have grossly recognizable hydropic villi. The size of hydropic villi is usually smaller than that of complete moles, ranging from 1.2 to 6.5 mm.[41]

Microscopically, partial mole is characterized by variably sized hydropic or fibrotic villi, mild to moderate trophoblastic hyperplasia, and irregular villous contour with or without trophoblastic inclusions (Figure 34.21). They tend to have considerably less trophoblastic proliferation than complete moles. Angulated irregular villous outline frequently produces trophoblastic nests or islands within the stroma, which is called 'trophoblastic inclusion,' but it is by no means a diagnostic feature. In contrast to complete moles, the stromal blood vessels may contain fetal hematopoietic elements or nucleated red blood cells. Central cisternae are consistently identified, and frequently have a characteristic maze-like angiomatoid pattern in the stroma[42] (Figure 34.22). The villous stroma often has extensive stromal fibrosis, which is prominent especially in the later gestational period.[42] Accurate diagnosis of partial moles in the first trimester remains a challenge, as characteristic features are not yet sufficiently developed to reliably distinguish them from hydropic abortion.

Immunostaining for $p57^{kip2}$ shows diffuse expression in all cellular components including cytotrophoblast and villous stromal cells, but is noncontributory in the differential diagnosis of partial mole from degenerated spontaneous abortion.

Differential Diagnosis

There is significant interobserver and intraobserver variability in the histologic diagnosis of partial moles, even among placental pathologists.[41] There can be confusion in the application of diagnostic criteria, which has led to both overdiagnosis of hydropic abortuses and underdiagnosis of complete moles. Frequently, differential diagnosis between partial mole and non-molar hydropic abortion is difficult. Immunostaining for $p57^{kip2}$ is not helpful in those cases, and trophoblastic hyperplasia is an essential feature for the diagnosis of partial mole. Confirmatory evidence can be obtained by DNA ploidy analysis, chromosomal enumeration by fluorescent or chromogenic *in situ* hybridization, and DNA genotyping.[26] In general, diploid gestations are not partial moles, but triploid conceptuses can be either diandric partial moles or digynic spontaneous abortions. Therefore, triploidy is an expected, but nonspecific, feature of the partial mole.

Twin pregnancy with a complete mole and normal conceptus should also be differentiated from partial mole because both conditions have an embryo, amniotic membrane, and admixed populations of hydropic and non-hydropic chorionic villi. Microscopic findings will be discussed in more detail in the following sections.

Placental mesenchymal dysplasia is a rare condition of placental vascular malformation that should be differentiated from partial mole. Antenatal ultrasonographic examination shows multiple cysts with anechoic regions. Clinically, it can be associated with slightly elevated levels of serum β-hCG.[43] Grossly, there are grape-like vesicles in the parenchyma, which mimics molar pregnancy (Figure 34.23). Microscopic findings are characterized by placentomegaly, multicystic placenta, and large edematous stem villi interspersed with normal villi (Figure 34.24). Many have loose hydropic stem villi with myxoid stroma, rich in hyaluronic acid, cisterna formation, and chorangiomatoid change, but others have a fibromatous core (Figure 34.25). Extravillous (intermediate) trophoblast can be prominent in the intervillous spaces. However, irregular villous outline with trophoblastic pseudoinclusions, which is a diagnostic feature of partial mole, is not observed. Stem villi are mainly involved by the hydropic change in mesenchymal dysplasia, while terminal villi are mostly affected in partial moles.[44]

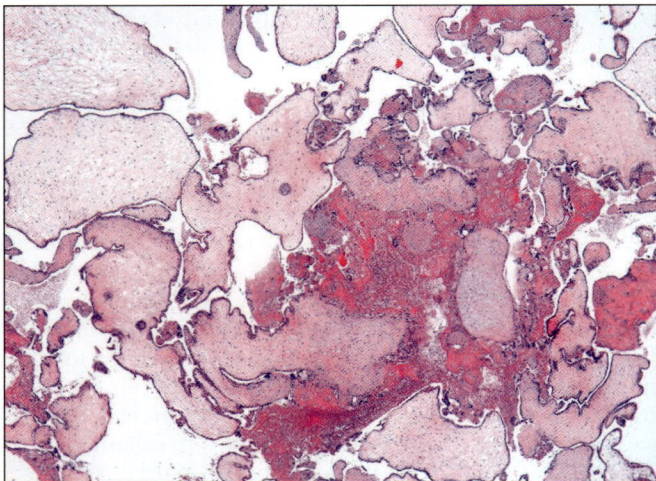

Figure 34.21 Triploid partial hydatidiform mole. It is characterized by variably sized hydropic or fibrotic villi, irregular villous contour with trophoblastic inclusions, and minimal trophoblastic proliferation.

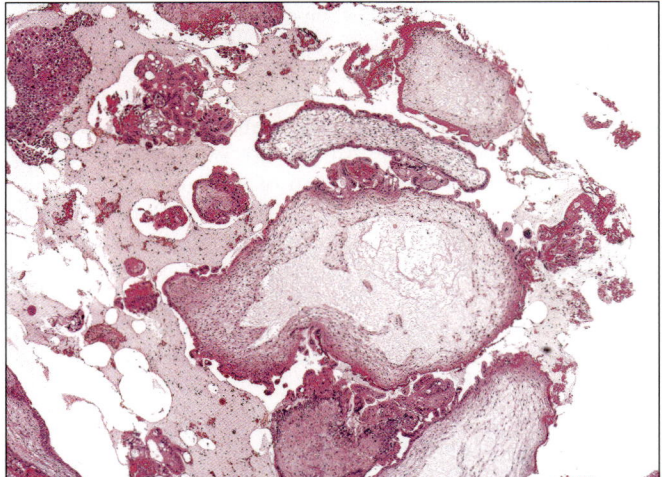

Figure 34.22 Triploid partial hydatidiform mole. This triploid, first trimester mole has a well-formed maze-like angiomatoid cisterna.

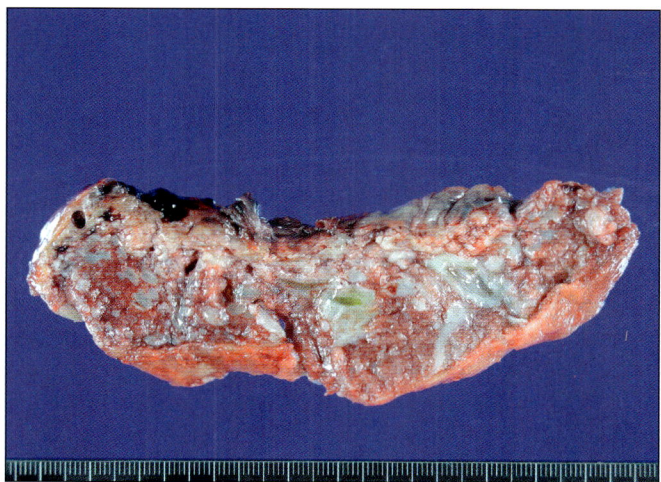

Figure 34.23 Placental mesenchymal dysplasia. Cut surface of the placenta shows multiple grossly visible cysts in otherwise normal placental parenchyma.

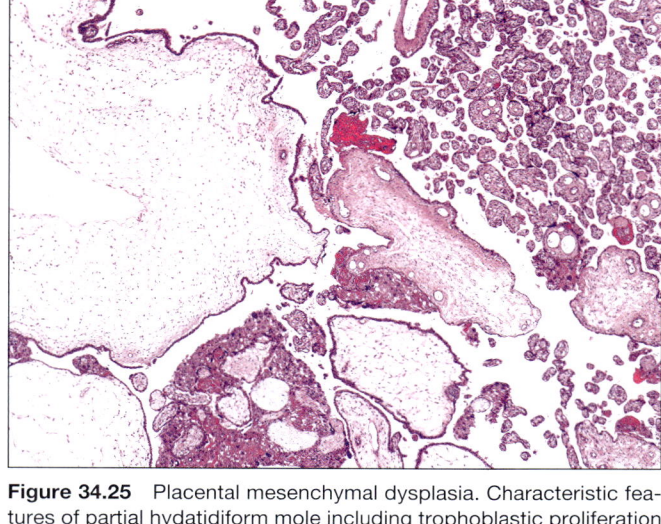

Figure 34.25 Placental mesenchymal dysplasia. Characteristic features of partial hydatidiform mole including trophoblastic proliferation or inclusion are not seen.

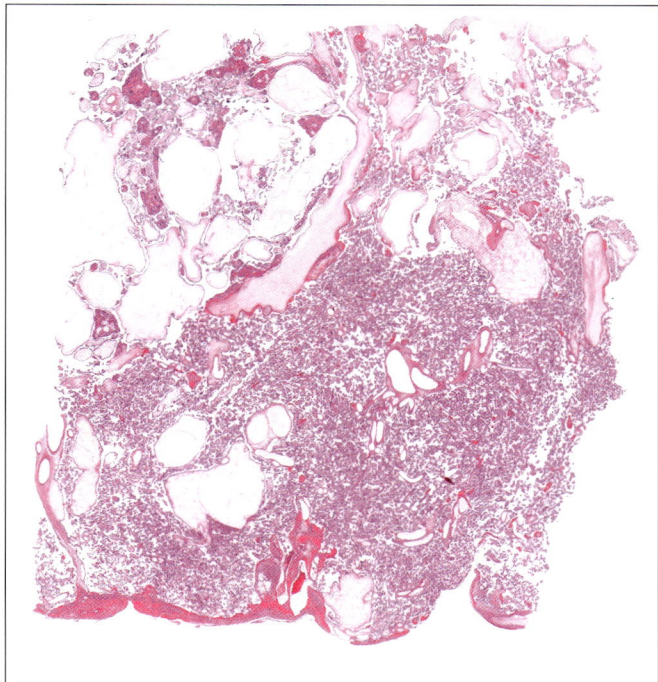

Figure 34.24 Placental mesenchymal dysplasia. Dilated hydropic stem villi are interspersed within normal villi, mimicking partial hydatidiform mole.

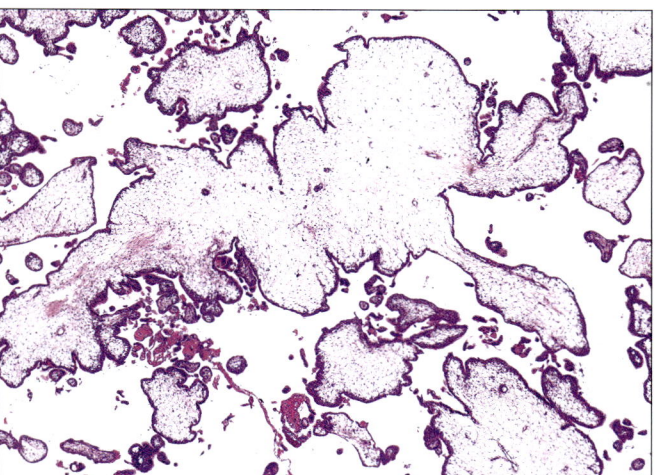

Figure 34.26 Aneuploid placenta from trisomy. Prominent scalloping of villous outlines with frequent intravillous trophoblastic pseudoinclusions mimic those of partial hydatidiform mole, but trophoblastic proliferation is not identified.

Aneuploid placenta or placenta with structural chromosomal abnormalities including trisomy may show prominent scalloping of villous outlines, which may produce many intravillous trophoblastic pseudoinclusions. Microscopic findings are similar to those of partial mole, but trophoblastic proliferation is not identified[45] (Figure 34.26).

Twin pregnancies with one complete mole and one normal gestation are rare, but when they occur, they can be confused with partial mole.[50,51] The existence of such cases was proven by DNA polymorphism studies demonstrating sole paternal origin of the molar tissues and biparental origin of the normal gestation. The mortality rate for the coexistent twin fetus is high, usually attributed to spontaneous abortion or early pregnancy termination due to severe pre-eclampsia or vaginal bleeding,[52] but the chances of a live birth have also been estimated as 21–40%.[50,51] There is a 20–55% risk of persistent trophoblastic disease after twin pregnancy with complete mole, which is similar to or higher than that after a complete mole alone.[51] Microscopically, two different populations of chorionic villi are identified in a well-sampled single specimen (Figure 34.27A–E). In cases of twin pregnancy composed of complete mole and normal gestation, the histologically different populations of villi are usually not intimately admixed, but separated (Figure 34.27A). Histologic findings vary with gestational age. Immunostaining for $p57^{kip2}$ will show different staining patterns between molar and non-molar villi.

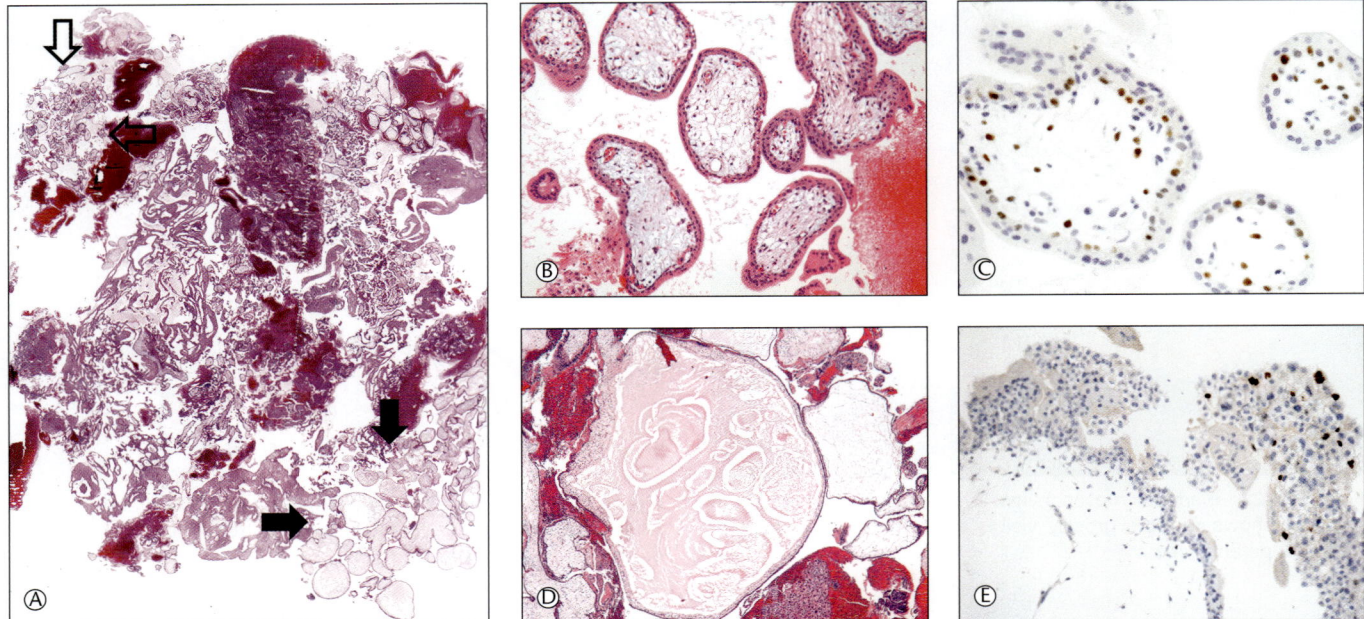

Figure 34.27 Twin pregnancy with complete hydatidiform mole and coexisting normal pregnancy. **(A)** There are two separate and distinct populations of chorionic villi from normal placenta (open arrows) and complete hydatidiform mole (closed arrows). **(B, C)** Chorionic villi in normal placenta show well-formed blood vessels in the stroma **(B)** and expression of p57^{kip2} in the cytotrophoblast and stromal cells **(C)**. **(D, E)** Complete hydatidiform mole shows central cisternae, immature blood vessels within cellular stroma at the periphery **(D)**, and immunonegativity for p57^{kip2} **(E)**.

Treatment and Prognosis

Because of ambiguities in diagnosis, and lack of standardized outcome measures, there is disagreement regarding treatment of partial moles. Some have questioned whether women with partial moles need any β-hCG follow-up. However, approximately 0.2% to 4% of partial moles are followed by recurrent molar pregnancies, which is a significantly higher incidence than in women having a normal pregnancy.[46] Rarely, histologically verified invasive mole, choriocarcinoma, or metastatic disease requiring chemotherapy have been described.[47,48] All patients with molar gestations should be followed irrespective of type, although the absolute risk of persistent trophoblastic neoplasia is much lower for partial than for complete mole. There is no universally accepted protocol for β-hCG surveillance following evacuation of partial mole, as these have varied in both sampling frequency and recommended follow-up interval.

Recurrent partial mole is a very rare clinical disorder, but a second molar pregnancy occurs in 1.7%, of which two-thirds are partial and one-third complete.[49]

ADVERSE CLINICAL OUTCOMES IN MOLAR DISEASE

PERSISTENT TROPHOBLASTIC DISEASE

The terms persistent trophoblastic disease and posthydatidiform gestational trophoblast neoplasia have been used interchangeably to indicate persistent mole, invasive mole, and choriocarcinoma. The reported frequency of persistent trophoblastic disease is 15–20% in complete and 0.2–4% in partial hydatidiform mole.[29] When a patient has persistent

Table 34.3	Criteria for the Diagnosis of Post-Hydatidiform Mole Trophoblastic Neoplasia
1.	Plateau of β-hCG lasts for four measurements over a period of 3 weeks or longer (days 1, 7, 14, and 21)
2.	A rise of β-hCG of 10% or greater on 3 consecutive weekly measurements over at least 2 weeks (days 1, 7, and 14)
3.	The presence of histologic choriocarcinoma
4.	Persistence of β-hCG 6 months after molar evacuation

trophoblastic disease by defined criteria (Table 34.3) immediate work-up and treatment are indicated. Treatment should be individualized according to the prognostic factors and clinical stage.

Over the years various anatomic, clinical, and prognostic scoring systems have been used. The response to treatment with chemotherapy, surgery, and radiotherapy is influenced by several clinical factors that form the basis of the World Health Organization (WHO) scoring system.[13] On the other hand, pure anatomic staging systems have not been universally adopted because the prognosis of patients in the same anatomic stage varies greatly and is affected by a number of clinical features.

In 2002, the International Federation of Obstetrics and Gynecology (FIGO) ratified a revised classification system for trophoblastic disease, which combines anatomic staging (pre-2002 FIGO) with clinical risk factors (WHO clinical score). A patient's anatomic stage is first summarized by Roman numeral as I, II, III, or IV (Table 34.4). This is then separated by a colon from the sum of all the clinical risk factor scores, expressed in Arabic numerals (Table 34.5), e.g., stage II:4, stage IV:9.[30] For purposes of reporting, patients with persistent trophoblastic disease are divided into high-risk and low-risk groups. Those with non-metastatic (stage I) and low-risk metastatic disease (stage II or III, metastases to lung and/or vagina) with total clinical score <7 can be treated with single agent chemotherapy: methotrexate with or without folinic acid or actinomycin. Patients with high-risk metastatic gestational trophoblastic neoplasia (stage IV, clinical score ≥7) need intensive chemotherapy with multiple combination chemotherapy. Relapse after first-line chemotherapy for high-risk disease can often be treated by platinum-containing chemotherapy regimens. Almost 100% cure rate can be achieved in the majority of patients with optimal treatment.

RECURRENT HYDATIDIFORM MOLE

Molar recurrence should be distinguished from persistence, and the risk in sporadic cases ranges from 1% to 4.3%.[49,53] Women who have experienced one molar pregnancy have a 20-fold increased risk of a further molar pregnancy in comparison with other women in the general population.[49] Second molar pregnancies are of the same type (complete vs partial) as the first in approximately three-quarters of cases.[49] Multiple occurrences may be sporadic or familial. After two molar pregnancies, the risk of developing molar disease in a subsequent conception rises to 15–20%.[14] The frequency of familial recurrent hydatidiform mole is not known, but more than 40 different familial cases, in which two or more individuals have molar pregnancies, have been reported in the English literature.

INVASIVE MOLE

Invasive mole is defined as molar villi invading into the myometrium, cervical stroma, and blood vessels or metastasizing to an extrauterine site. The most common sites of metastasis are lung, liver, brain, vagina, and vulva. Rarely spinal cord and urinary bladder have been described. The diagnosis is usually made on a hysterectomy specimen. Since both invasive mole and choriocarcinoma have an elevated β-hCG titer and may produce metastatic lesions, these are often indistinguishable clinically when biopsied tissue only contains a scanty amount of atypical trophoblast without intact villi. According to FIGO 2000 criteria, patients with plateaued or rising consecutive β-hCG titers following molar evacuation are clinically classified as having persistent gestational trophoblastic disease and treated with chemotherapy irrespective of anatomic documentation of invasion or metastasis.

Initial presentation as an invasive mole is rare; rather, it is preceded by complete or partial mole in 75% and 18.5% of cases, respectively.[54] Bleeding is the main cause of morbidity and mortality in patients with invasive or metastatic moles. Grossly, molar vesicles are usually identified in myometrium of hysterectomy specimens (Figure 34.28). Microscopically, invasive and metastatic villi are similar in appearance to those of noninvasive moles, except they can be identified within myometrium, blood vessels, or distant tissues (Figure 34.29). Adjacent myometrium around the invasive villi usually contains florid proliferation of extravillous trophoblasts, which are reminiscent of placental site trophoblastic tumor.

Treatment of Invasive Mole

Patients with invasive mole have a good prognosis. Even if disease has spread, single agent chemotherapy might be sufficient as long as the diagnosis is histologically confirmed. Approximately 80% of young patients treated with chemotherapy alone conceive after recovery. If untreated, invasive mole can result in uterine rupture or heavy bleeding. Metastatic lesions can successfully be treated by minimally invasive angiographic embolization.

Differential Diagnosis of Invasive Mole

Metastatic invasive mole needs to be differentiated from displacement of normal placental elements into the lung, known as trophoblastic pulmonary embolization, or villotrophoblastic nodule.[55] Most cases have been identified during postmortem examination performed in patients with sudden death in mid-gestation due to unrelated causes, but rare cases have been detected in asymptomatic patients.[55] Careful examination of villous structure is useful in these cases, and immunopositivity for p57^{kip2} in the cytotrophoblast lining chorionic villi is helpful to exclude invasive complete moles.

Table 34.4 FIGO (2002) Anatomical Staging System

Stage	Description
Stage I	Disease confined to the uterus
Stage II	GTN extends outside of the uterus, but is limited to the genital structures (adnexa, vagina, broad ligament)
Stage III	GTN extends to the lungs, with or without known genital tract involvement
Stage IV	All other metastatic sites

Table 34.5 FIGO (2002) Clinical Risk Factor Score

Scores	0	1	2	4
Age	<40	≥40	—	—
Antecedent pregnancy	Mole	Abortion	Term	—
Interval months from index pregnancy	<4	4 to <7	7 to <13	≥13
Pretreatment serum hCG (IU/ml)	$<10^3$	10^3 to $<10^4$	10^4 to $<10^5$	$≥10^5$
Largest tumor size (including uterus)	—	3 to <5 cm	≥5 cm	—
Site of metastases	Lung	Spleen, kidney	Gastrointestinal	Liver, brain
Number of metastases	—	1–4	5–8	>8
Previous failed chemotherapy	—	—	Single drug	Two or more drugs

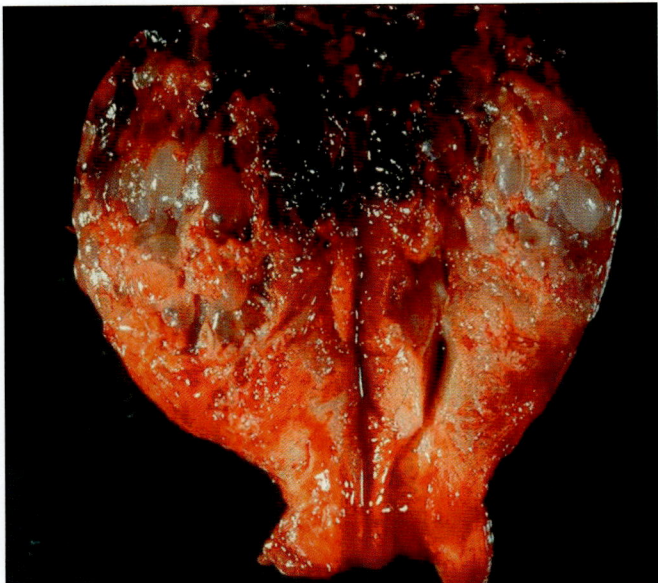

Figure 34.28 Invasive mole. Hydropic villi invade the entire myometrium.

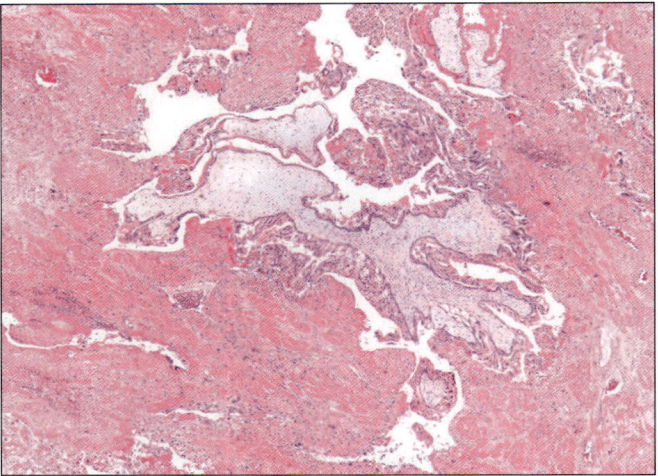

Figure 34.29 Invasive mole. Molar villi within the myometrium show circumferential trophoblastic proliferation.

TROPHOBLASTIC NEOPLASIA

CHORIOCARCINOMA

Choriocarcinoma is a highly malignant tumor of gestational trophoblastic origin. The incidence in Europe and North America is 1 in 20,000 to 50,000 pregnancies,[6,56–58] whereas in Asia, Africa, and Latin America, the rates are variable and generally higher.[59,60] Incidence rates, however, are imprecise both because of uncertainty of the total number of pregnancies and because of difficulty in clinical distinction between postmolar choriocarcinoma and invasive mole. Nongestational choriocarcinoma, a rare primary germ cell tumor of the ovary, is discussed in Chapter 29.

Choriocarcinoma is a disease of the reproductive years, especially at the upper and lower extremes. Very rarely, however, it can develop in postmenopausal women long after pregnancy.[61] The incidence increases with maternal age, with women aged 40–44 years at an 8.6-fold increased risk compared with those aged 20–24 years, and parous teenagers have an elevated risk.[62] It presents usually within 1 year of the antecedent pregnancy (molar or non-molar).[6,9] Choriocarcinoma may occur in association with any pregnancy event; approximately 25% of cases follow abortion or tubal pregnancy, and 25% are associated with intrauterine gestation. The remaining half arise from hydatidiform moles, although only 0.4–3% of hydatidiform moles progress to choriocarcinoma.[6,63]

Clinical Presentation

Clinical symptoms and signs of choriocarcinoma are variable depending on the presence or absence, and the site of, metastases. It can metastasize to any organ in the body, but the most common sites are lung, vagina, central nervous system, liver, kidney, and gastrointestinal tract.[64] The symptoms of metastases frequently result from spontaneous bleeding at metastatic foci.

The most frequent presentation is vaginal bleeding from the uterus or from vaginal metastases. Vaginal metastases usually appear as highly vascular, red to violaceous patches. In rare cases following full-term pregnancy, patients complain of persistent heavy vaginal bleeding and have persistently elevated postpartum β-hCG levels. Cough, dyspnea, hemoptysis, and pleuritic chest pain can be manifested in cases of pulmonary metastases, which occur in over 80% of patients with choriocarcinoma. Brain can be involved in 10% of patients, usually with concurrent pulmonary and/or vaginal metastases. In reproductive age women with neurologic symptoms including headaches, seizures, loss of consciousness and hemiplegia, or postpartum cerebrovascular accidents, choriocarcinoma should be included in the differential diagnosis. Liver metastasis occurs in 10% of patients and it may cause epigastric or right upper quadrant pain due to stretching of Glisson's capsule, or hemoperitoneum due to spontaneous rupture of hepatic metastasis.[65] Rarely, metastatic spread to the fetus or infant from maternal gestational choriocarcinoma has been reported.

Primary extrauterine choriocarcinoma is extremely rare, but has been described in various organs including lung, ovary, fallopian tube, stomach, small intestine, omentum, and peritoneum. Extrauterine choriocarcinoma may develop in several different ways: (1) as a metastatic gestational choriocarcinoma from a regressed or occult primary gestational tumor, (2) as a nongestational germ cell tumor, (3) as a primary gestational choriocarcinoma associated with ectopic pregnancy, or (4) as a dedifferentiated tumor from a somatic carcinoma.[66]

Genetics

The genetic make-up of choriocarcinoma is dependent on the antecedent pregnancy.[67] Those that result from term pregnancies, non-molar abortions, or partial moles have both maternal and paternal chromosomes, while those from complete moles are androgenetic in origin.[67] Sole maternal contribution indicates nongestational origin. Karyotype shows a range of abnormalities; however, frequent losses in

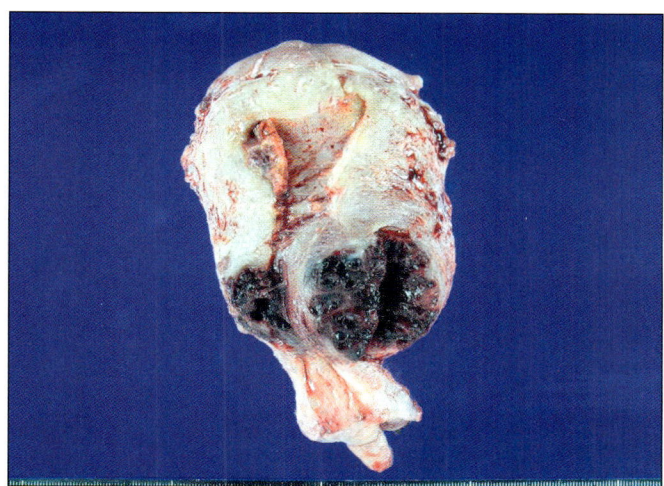

Figure 34.30 Choriocarcinoma of the uterus. The tumor consists of a hemorrhagic mass in the uterine wall.

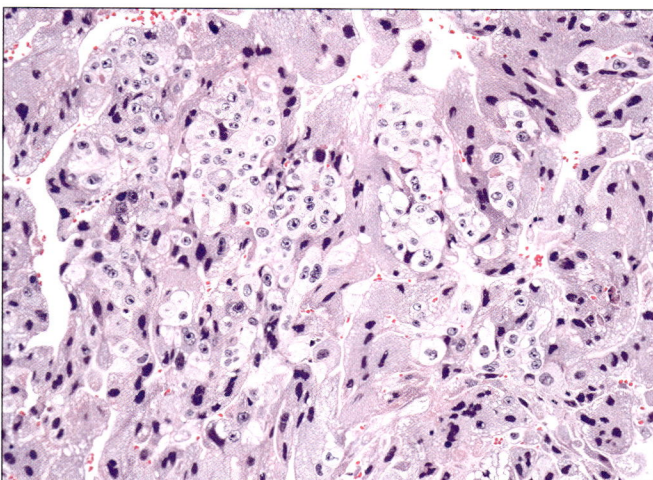

Figure 34.31 Choriocarcinoma of the uterus showing the characteristic biphasic pattern of cytotrophoblast and syncytiotrophoblast.

chromosome 7 and 8q suggest that 7p12–7q11.23 and 8p12–p21 may contain putative tumor suppressor genes.[68,69]

Gross and Microscopic Findings

Grossly, choriocarcinoma forms variable sized, friable, dark red and hemorrhagic masses in the uterus with an infiltrating border (Figure 34.30). There are variable proportions of necrosis.

Microscopically, choriocarcinoma is composed of variable amounts of atypical cytotrophoblast, syncytiotrophoblast, and extravillous (intermediate) trophoblast. Cytotrophoblast are large polygonal cells with round nuclei and one or several prominent nucleoli and abundant clear or faintly eosinophilic cytoplasm. Both cytotrophoblast and syncytiotrophoblast in choriocarcinoma usually have severe nuclear pleomorphism and large nucleoli compared to normal villi or intermediate trophoblast on anchoring villi. Chorionic villi are not observed except in cases of intraplacental choriocarcinoma. Cytotrophoblast nests surrounded by syncytiotrophoblast often recapitulate the normal 'biphasic' relationship of previllous trophoblast (Figure 34.31). Although cytotrophoblast and syncytiotrophoblast within choriocarcinoma have an alternating arrangement, syncytiotrophoblastic differentiation is often identified in the middle of cytotrophoblast or intermediate trophoblast instead of encasing cytotrophoblast (Figure 34.32). Occasionally, the syncytiotrophoblastic component is indistinct, and the lesions are difficult to differentiate from placental site trophoblastic tumor or even squamous cell carcinoma, especially when it occurs in the lower uterine segment or cervix[70] (Figure 34.33A). Immunostaining for β-hCG can be helpful in demonstrating indistinct syncytiotrophoblast (Figure 34.33B).

Differential Diagnosis

Choriocarcinoma can easily be overlooked when small amounts are present in a curettage specimen. When cytotrophoblast and syncytiotrophoblast are present without any obvious villous structure, a possibility of choriocarcinoma

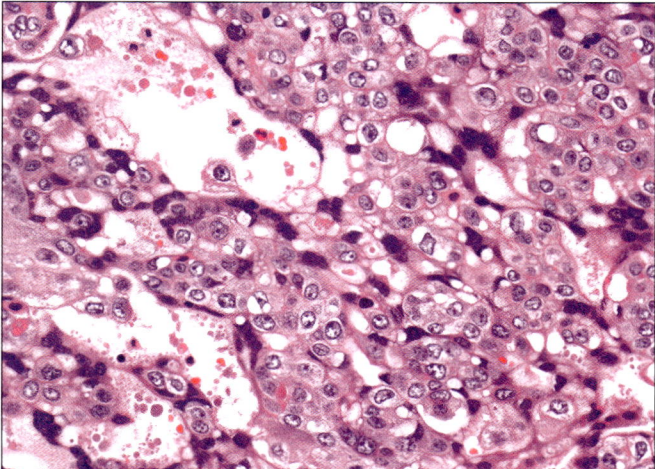

Figure 34.32 Choriocarcinoma. Syncytiotrophoblastic component is often identified in the middle of cytotrophoblast or intermediate trophoblast instead of encasing the cytotrophoblastic component.

should always be considered. Since chorionic villi at hemorrhagic ectopic pregnancy sites are often displaced or obscured, it is easy to overdiagnose the remaining degenerating and proliferative trophoblastic cells as choriocarcinoma (Figure 34.34A). Complete sampling, and occasionally deeper sections, may reveal chorionic villi in the vicinity (Figure 34.34B). A regular biphasic arrangement of rather uniform cytotrophoblastic cells without significant pleomorphism or tumor necrosis are key features to differentiate it from choriocarcinoma.

Choriocarcinoma has a similar histologic appearance whether nongestational (germ cell) or gestational. This distinction is especially important in extrauterine sites because nongestational choriocarcinoma more frequently metastasizes through lymphatics and spreads intra-abdominally, and is often chemoresistant. Recently, DNA polymorphism analysis has been used to confirm nongestational origin.[71]

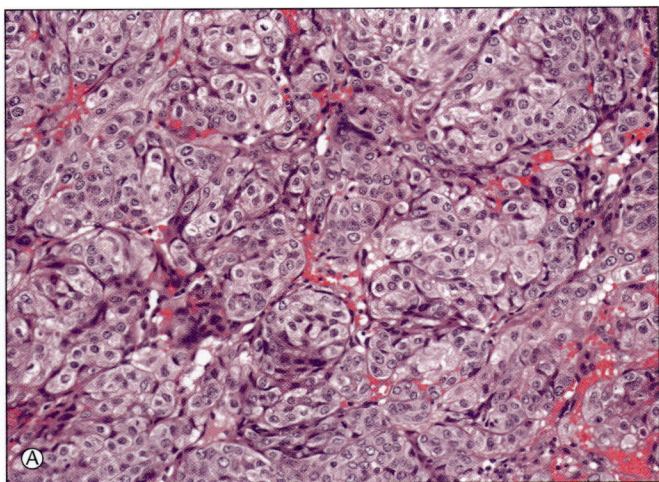 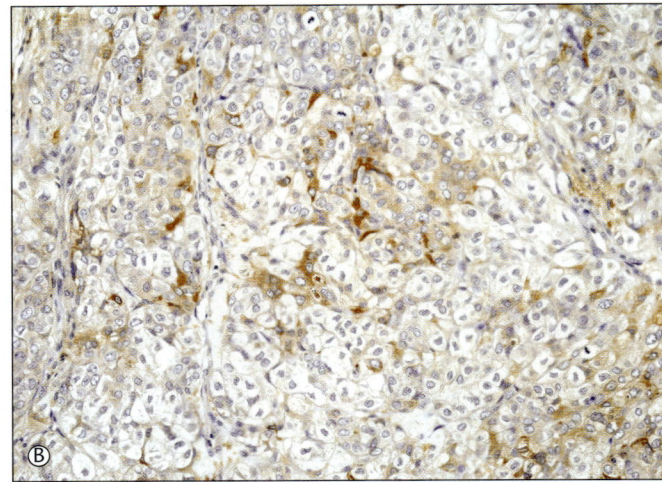

Figure 34.33 Choriocarcinoma predominantly composed of a monotonous sheet of cytotrophoblast with an indistinct syncytiotrophoblastic component **(A)**, mimicking poorly differentiated carcinoma. Immunostaining for β-hCG **(B)** can be helpful in demonstrating attenuated syncytiotrophoblast.

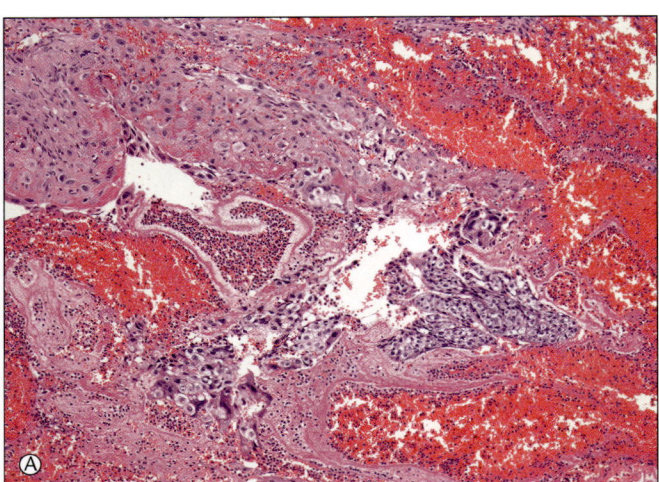 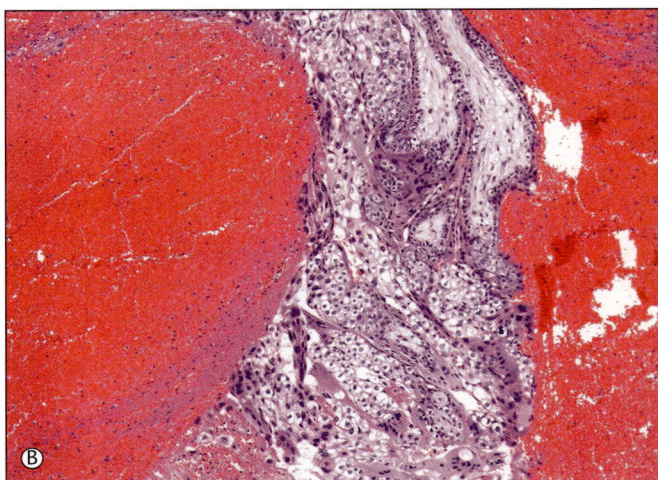

Figure 34.34 Ectopic ovarian pregnancy. **(A)** A portion of proliferating trophoblastic cells at ectopic sites can be easily overdiagnosed as choriocarcinoma because of the biphasic arrangement of the trophoblast. **(B)** Villous structure is often identified in an adjacent area or deeper sections.

Ordinary somatic carcinoma with syncytiotrophoblastic differentiation in various organs which secretes hCG into the blood should be differentiated from a choriocarcinoma, but microscopically they do not form biphasic arrangement of cytotrophoblast and syncytiotrophoblast. Choriocarcinomas elaborating low hCG levels should be differentiated from placental site trophoblastic tumor by histology because of the low chemotherapy sensitivity and need for surgical treatment of the latter.

CHORIOCARCINOMA ASSOCIATED WITH FULL-TERM PREGNANCY AND INTRAPLACENTAL CHORIOCARCINOMA

Choriocarcinoma following term pregnancy is a rare form of gestational trophoblastic disease with an estimated occurrence of 1 per 160,000 pregnancies.[72] It probably arises from asymptomatic intraplacental choriocarcinoma, which is often missed because placental examination is not routine in all deliveries. The usual presentation is persistent postpartum hemorrhage, and a significantly elevated postpartum hCG level. Choriocarcinoma should be suspected when hCG levels fail to decrease to undetectable levels within 3 weeks after a normal delivery. Rarely spontaneous uterine perforation may occur. Lung, liver, and brain metastases are common at the time of initial diagnosis.

Although term pregnancy is an adverse prognostic factor, multiagent systemic chemotherapy has a comparable survival rate for choriocarcinoma irrespective of associated term pregnancy.[73] Rarely, metastases to the fetus or infant from maternal gestational choriocarcinoma have been reported.

Intraplacental choriocarcinoma can be an incidental finding at the placental examination. When visible, it appears as well-circumscribed, single or multiple, whitish nodules resembling infarcts in the placental parenchyma.

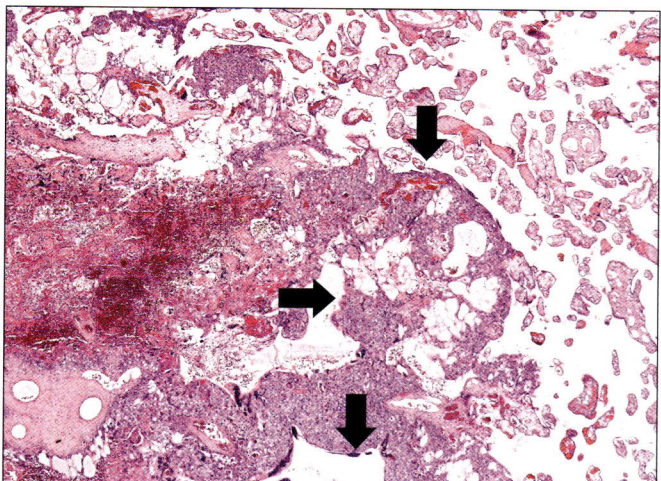

Figure 34.35 Intraplacental choriocarcinoma. There is a distinct transition from normal placenta to malignant trophoblast (arrows).

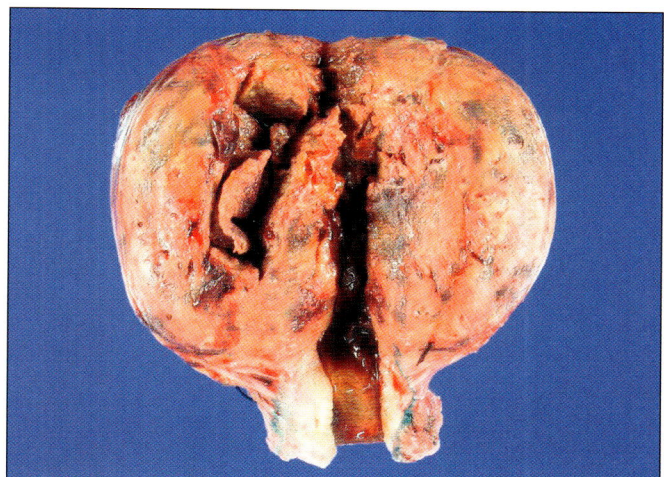

Figure 34.37 Placental site trophoblastic tumor. The tumor diffusely infiltrates the uterine wall forming an ill-defined mass in the myometrium.

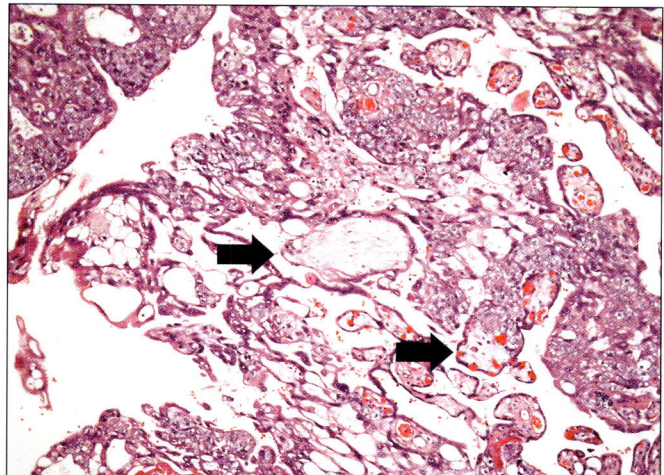

Figure 34.36 Intraplacental choriocarcinoma. Highly atypical cytotrophoblast and syncytiotrophoblast are in direct contact with chorionic villi (arrows), suggesting that the tumor arises from villous trophoblast.

Hemorrhage and necrosis may or may not be present. Microscopic examination demonstrates morphologically normal, non-molar third trimester chorionic villi mixed with a distinct area of florid atypical pleomorphic trophoblastic proliferation occupying the intervillous space (Figure 34.35). Biphasic proliferation of tumor cells composed of highly atypical cytotrophoblast and syncytiotrophoblast imperceptibly merge with normal trophoblast, suggesting that the tumor arises from villous trophoblast (Figure 34.36). Entrapped normal villi are common among the malignant trophoblast. Tumor cells frequently invade blood vessels, where they spread hematogenously and result in metastases.

PLACENTAL SITE TROPHOBLASTIC TUMOR

General

Placental site trophoblastic tumor is an uncommon form of gestational trophoblast neoplasia composed of neoplastic proliferation of extravillous (intermediate) trophoblast. It was first described as a 'trophoblastic pseudotumor,' thought to be an exaggerated reaction at the implantation site because of its uneventful clinical course after curettage and a close structural resemblance to the trophoblastic components in normal human placenta. Subsequently, malignant behavior including recurrences and distant metastasis have been reported.

Clinical Presentation

It can occur in any reproductive age group, but has been reported in postmenopausal women. The majority follow a normal full-term or terminated pregnancy, suggesting that it may arise from a malignant transformation of previously healthy trophoblastic cells. Ectopic or molar antecedent pregnancy is also seen. The interval from antecedent pregnancy ranges from 5 to 131 months (mean, 34).[74] Patients with placental site trophoblast tumor present with only mildly elevated levels of serum β-hCG, which rarely exceeds 1000 mIU/ml. The most common presenting symptom is vaginal bleeding and/or amenorrhea, occasionally with symptoms related to the site of tumor metastasis, including hemoptysis, pneumothorax, and cutaneous masses. Proteinuria,[75] galactorrhea, virilization,[76] and polycythemia[77] have been described.

Gross and Macroscopic Findings

The tumor usually forms an ill-defined intramural or protruding mass in the uterine corpus, sometimes extending to the cervix. More rarely, it involves the cervix, ovary, and fallopian tube as a primary site. Usually it is deeply invasive into the myometrium. The cut surface is yellow or tan, and solid with frequent hemorrhage and necrosis (Figure 34.37).

Microscopically, tumors are highly infiltrative, separating myometrial fibers with confluent sheets of epithelioid cells (Figure 34.38) that may become spindle shaped as they infiltrate between myometrium. Tumor cells are predominantly mononucleated large polygonal cells with abundant amphophilic, eosinophilic, or clear cytoplasm (Figure 34.39). Syncytiotrophoblast-like multinucleated

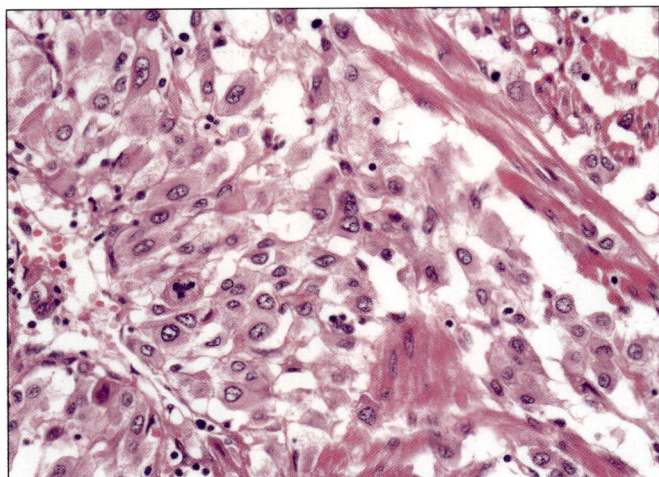

Figure 34.38 Placental site trophoblastic tumor. Sheets of monomorphic intermediate trophoblast characteristically separate smooth muscle bundles of the uterus as they infiltrate the myometrium. Note the abundant eosinophilic or amphophilic cytoplasm and well-defined cell border.

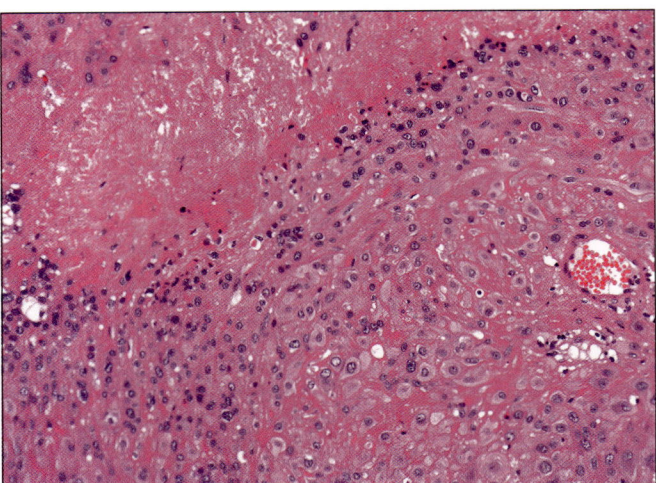

Figure 34.40 Placental site trophoblastic tumor. Extensive necrosis or abundant extracellular eosinophilic fibrinoid material around the tumor cells is a frequent feature.

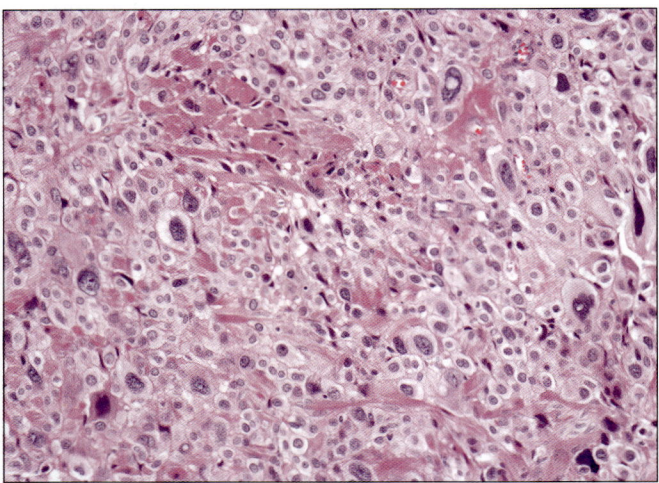

Figure 34.39 Placental site trophoblastic tumor. The tumor cells have variable degrees of cytologic atypia, frequent nuclear grooves, and intranuclear cytoplasmic pseudoinclusions. Scattered multinucleated intermediate trophoblast can be misinterpreted as syncytiotrophoblast of choriocarcinoma. However, the trophoblast do not form a biphasic arrangement.

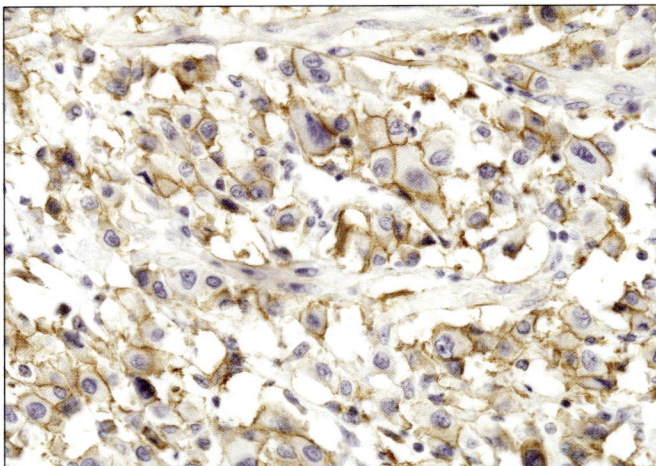

Figure 34.41 Placental site trophoblastic tumor showing strong expression of CD146 (Mel-CAM).

cells can be identified, but are individually scattered among the mononucleated cells without forming a typical biphasic pattern of choriocarcinoma. Nuclei have variable degrees of atypia, inconspicuous nucleoli, frequent nuclear grooves, and intranuclear cytoplasmic pseudoinclusions. The mitotic count is variable between cases, and from field to field even in the same case, ranging from 0 to 20 (average 5.0) per 10 HPF.[74] Atypical mitotic figures are frequent. Coagulative necrosis and deposition of extracellular eosinophilic fibrinoid material around the tumor cells is a frequent feature (Figure 34.40), often leaving islands of tumor cells only around blood vessels. Chorionic villi are absent in almost all cases, except in a rare case associated with molar pregnancy.

Rarely, this tumor is admixed with other components such as epithelioid trophoblastic tumor or choriocarcinoma.[78,79] The immunophenotype resembles that of extravillous (intermediate) trophoblast at the implantation site, so-called 'implantation site' intermediate trophoblast, including positive human placental lactogen, CD146 (Mel-CAM) (Figure 34.41). Differential diagnosis with normal extravillous (intermediate) trophoblast is possible by demonstration of a high Ki-67 labeling index (range 10–25%) of the intermediate trophoblastic cells[24] (Figure 34.42). Ultrastructurally, the placental site trophoblast tumor is composed primarily of intermediate trophoblast with prominent paranuclear filaments not seen in choriocarcinoma.

Pathogenetic Mechanism

Occurrence following normal gestation, combined with the presence of a Y chromosomal locus and/or paternal alleles

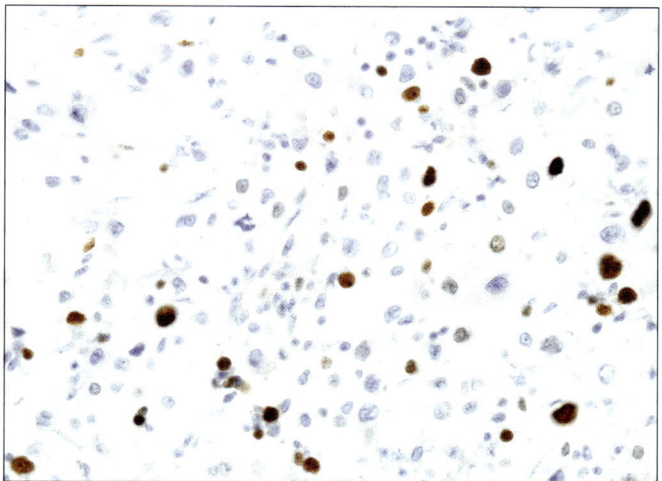

Figure 34.42 Placental site trophoblastic tumor showing an increased Ki-67 labeling index. The number of proliferating cells is higher than in an exaggerated placental site, but it is significantly lower than in choriocarcinoma.

in the tumor, suggests a biparental fetal trophoblastic origin.[80] However, they may also arise from germ cells, presenting in the testis[81,82] or mediastinum of male patients with or without a teratomatous component,[83] or in the ovary.[84]

Clinical Behavior and Treatment

Most placental site trophoblastic tumors show benign behavior with 5 year overall survival of 80%,[85] whereas 10–15% are clinically malignant with recurrence, metastasis, and a fatal outcome.[86,87] The most common metastatic sites are the lung, liver, and vagina; lymph nodes; and rarely ovary.[74,88,89] There are no consistent and reliable means of predicting clinical outcome, but advanced FIGO stage (III or IV) is the single most important adverse prognostic indicator.[90]

Surgery is the mainstay of treatment. It is important to differentiate placental site trophoblast tumor from other trophoblast diseases because they tend to be less sensitive to chemotherapy. However, young patients who wish to preserve fertility may be treated by conservative surgery or dilatation and curettage with postoperative chemotherapy.[91] Metastatic tumors have a poor prognosis because of a poor response to chemotherapy compared to other types of trophoblastic disease, but there have been many cases of recurrent or metastatic disease controlled by chemotherapy.[87]

Long-term follow-up is essential as placental site trophoblast tumor may progress after years of remission. Serum β-hCG levels are the best available marker of disease, but the disease may still progress even if hCG levels are not raised. Despite high serum human placental lactogen production within lesional tissues, the serum human placental lactogen level is not a useful tumor marker due to a short half-life in the circulation.

Differential Diagnosis

Placental site trophoblastic tumor should be differentiated from non-neoplastic trophoblastic lesions and a variety of tumors, including exaggerated placental site, placental site nodule, choriocarcinoma, cervical squamous cell carcinoma, epithelioid smooth muscle neoplasm, and malignant melanoma. Appreciation of the morphologic features and immunophenotype can lead to a correct diagnosis in most cases.

Since both exaggerated placental sites and placental site trophoblastic tumor lesions show exuberant infiltration of intermediate trophoblast into the endometrium and myometrium and cellular differentiation toward 'implantation site' intermediate trophoblast, immunostain panels with trophoblastic markers are not helpful. The Ki-67 labeling index of intermediate trophoblast in normal implantation sites and exaggerated placental sites is close to zero, while those in the placental site trophoblastic tumor and choriocarcinoma averages 14% and 69%, respectively.[24] However, careful interpretation is required not to include the Ki-67-positive lymphocytes within the lesion.

A placental site nodule can be confused with placental site trophoblastic tumor especially in the curettage specimen, because the former often has atypical cytomorphologic features in the nodule. The differential diagnosis is described in the section on placental site nodules.

Choriocarcinoma contains alternating zones of cytotrophoblast and syncytiotrophoblast and can generally be distinguished from placental site trophoblastic tumor by a high serum β-hCG level.

When considering the differential diagnosis of cervical squamous cell carcinoma and placental site trophoblast tumor, cautious interpretation of p16 is needed, because weak and focal p16 expression can also be identified in the latter.[92] Only strong diffuse p16 staining should be considered helpful for the diagnosis of cervical squamous cell carcinoma.[92]

Epithelioid smooth muscle tumor lacks the angioinvasive growth and the deposition of eosinophilic fibrinoid material seen in placental site trophoblastic tumors. Immunonegativity for smooth muscle markers and positivity for cytokeratin 18, human placental lactogen, and CD146 (Mel-CAM) are helpful in the differential diagnosis.

EPITHELIOID TROPHOBLASTIC TUMOR

Epithelioid trophoblastic tumor is a distinctive but rare gestational trophoblastic tumor of extravillous (intermediate) trophoblastic origin. Initially, the tumor was described as a solitary metastatic lesion in the lung following multiple courses of chemotherapy for gestational choriocarcinoma and was originally termed 'atypical choriocarcinoma.' More recently, it has been considered an independent disease entity because similar tumors have been described in the uterus without history of antecedent trophoblastic disease or without prior chemotherapy.

Clinical Presentation

The tumor mostly occurs in women of reproductive age, but very rarely it can occur in postmenopausal women. The interval between the preceding gestational event and the diagnosis of epithelioid trophoblastic tumor is variable, ranging from 1 month to 18 years.[93,94] The preceding gestational event may be full-term delivery, spontaneous abortion, hydatidiform mole, or invasive mole.

Most patients present with abnormal vaginal bleeding and in some cases with a mildly elevated serum β-hCG level during the follow-ups of antecedent hydatidiform mole.[93] Lung masses can be incidentally identified in asymptomatic patients years after chemotherapy for uterine trophoblastic disease,[95] or may present as primary lung carcinomas without an identified primary site.[96] In the latter cases, P63 immunopositivity and similar histologic features may lead to misdiagnosis as a squamous cell carcinoma of the lung.

Gross and Microscopic Findings

The tumor involves the uterine fundus, lower uterine segment, or endocervix. Rarely, occurrences in unusual locations including ovary, fallopian tube, gallbladder, and broad ligament have been reported.

Grossly, the tumor usually has a well-circumscribed and expansile border, and the cut surface shows a partly solid and partly cystic, tan to dark-brown mass that deeply invades the myometrium or cervical wall (Figure 34.43). The presence of varying amounts of hemorrhage and necrosis is quite characteristic.

Microscopically, it has generally well-circumscribed borders, frequently surrounded by an abundant lymphocytic infiltration (Figure 34.44). However, it is not uncommon to find some focal infiltrative peripheral areas. The neoplastic cells are composed of a relatively uniform population of mononucleated cells with abundant clear or eosinophilic cytoplasm lying in sheets, nests, cords, and islands which resemble extravillous trophoblast in the chorion laeve (Figure 34.45). Binucleated cells and multinucleate syncytiotrophoblast-like cells can also be intermingled with mononucleate tumor cells, but they do not form a biphasic arrangement as in choriocarcinoma. Frequently, hyaline material is present between the tumor cells, and islands of trophoblastic cells surrounded by hyaline-like matrix and extensive necrosis create a 'geographic' pattern. In some cases, dense eosinophilic, fibrinoid material within and around the tumor cells closely simulates the keratin of squamous cell carcinoma of the cervix. The mitotic count is relatively low, averaging 2 per 10 HPF.[5]

Immunohistochemically, tumor cells are diffusely positive for P63, placental alkaline phosphatase, cytokeratin 18 (Figure 34.46A–C), and inhibin-α, and but only focally positive for β-hCG, human placental lactogen, and CD146 (Mel-CAM). The Ki-67 proliferative index ranges from 10% to 25%.

Pathogenetic Mechanism

Although trophoblastic in nature, the cell of origin and the histogenetic relationship with other types of gestational trophoblastic neoplasia have not been clarified.

Clinical Behavior and Treatment

Although resection can be curative, distant metastasis occurs in 25% of cases. The most frequent metastatic sites are lung,

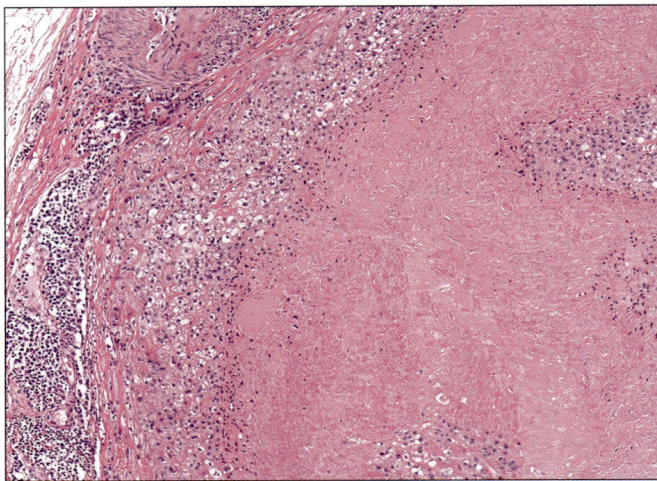

Figure 34.44 Epithelioid trophoblastic tumor. The tumor has generally well-circumscribed margins, frequently surrounded by an abundant lymphocytic infiltration.

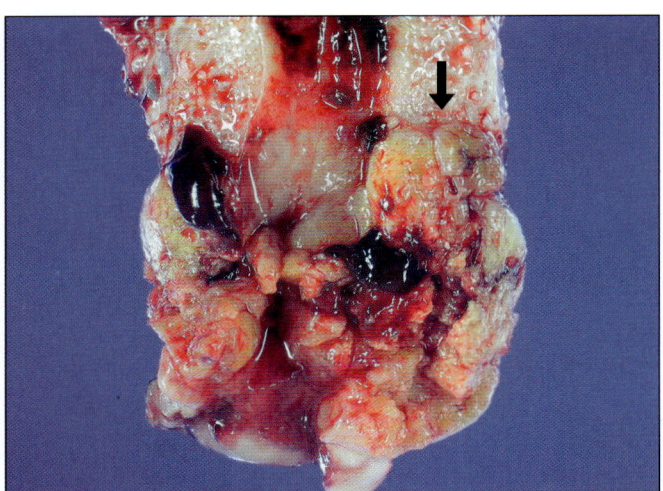

Figure 34.43 Epithelioid trophoblastic tumor in uterine cervix showing a well-circumscribed margin (arrow).

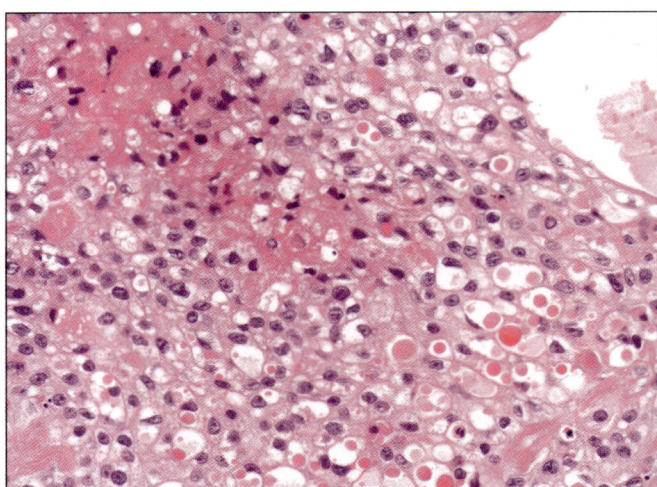

Figure 34.45 Epithelioid trophoblastic tumor. The tumor cells have relatively smaller, uniform, and less pleomorphic nuclei than placental site trophoblastic tumor and abundant clear or eosinophilic cytoplasm growing in sheets. Frequently, eosinophilic hyaline material is present within the tumor.

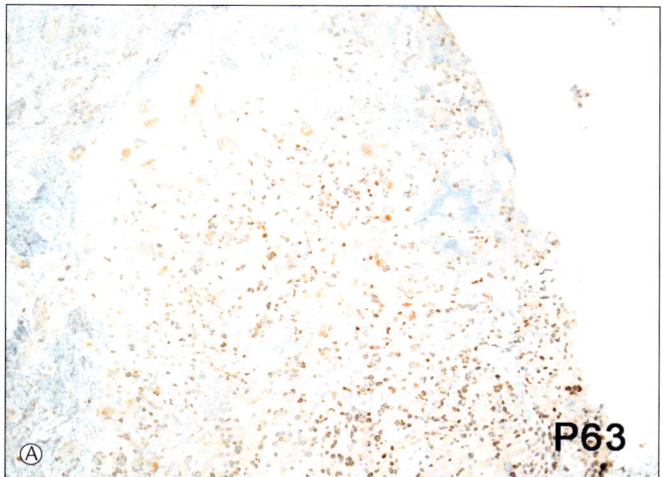
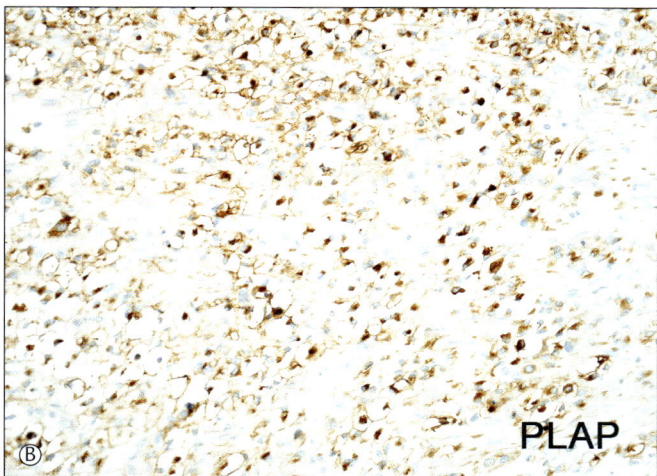
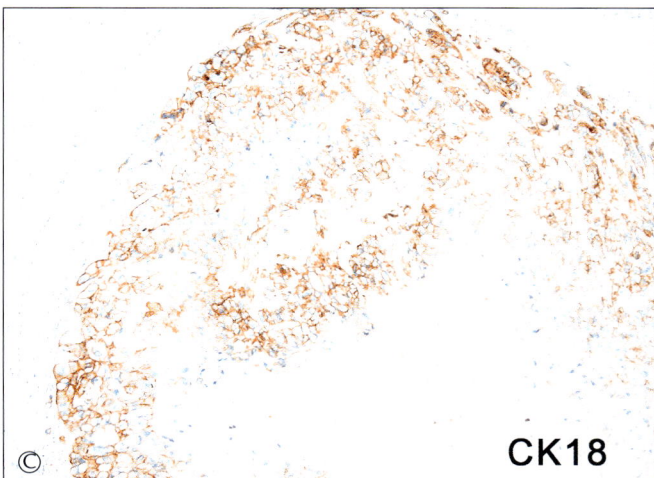

Figure 34.46 Immunohistochemical features of epithelioid trophoblastic tumor. The tumor cells show diffuse immunopositivities for P63 **(A)**, PLAP **(B)**, and cytokeratin 18 **(C)**.

brain, vagina, and bone.[97] It appears to be less aggressive than choriocarcinoma, but the behavior is closer to that of placental site trophoblastic tumor.

Since epithelioid trophoblastic tumors are chemoresistant and they have a propensity for lymphatic spread, surgical intervention including hysterectomy and lymph node dissection is the recommended primary treatment.[98] Combination chemotherapy has been used in patients with metastatic disease.

Differential Diagnosis

Diagnosis of epithelioid trophoblastic tumor at extrauterine sites can be challenging. In the uterine cervix or lung, it can resemble squamous cell carcinoma because of its epithelioid cytomorphology and misinterpretation of hyaline-like material as keratin. When the neoplastic cells focally replace the endocervical surface and glandular epithelium, it may mimic a cervical squamous intraepithelial lesion. These can be recognized by cytokeratin 18 and inhibin-α stainings, which are not seen in squamous lesions. When the tumor occurs primarily or metastasized to the ovary, it can be misdiagnosed as clear cell carcinoma of the ovary.[99] A diffuse and intense immunostaining pattern of cytokeratin 18 and HSD3β1 in the majority of trophoblastic lesions distinguishes them from other nontrophoblastic carcinomas, specifically uterus, lung, and breast, which are rarely positive for these markers.

A placental site nodule must be differentiated from epithelioid trophoblastic tumor as both are well-circumscribed nodular lesions and show cellular differentiation toward 'chorionic type' intermediate trophoblast. The differential diagnosis can be difficult, especially in the curettage specimen. A low Ki-67 proliferating index (less than 5%) in the placental site nodule can be helpful in the differential diagnosis.

Epithelioid trophoblastic tumor can resemble monomorphic variants of choriocarcinoma (Figure 34.33A) and placental site trophoblastic tumor. The cells of epithelioid trophoblastic tumor are smaller and less pleomorphic than either of these. Absence of characteristic biphasic growth pattern and significantly lower mitotic counts (2/10 HPF vs >10/10 HPF) assist in exclusion of choriocarcinoma. Placental site trophoblastic tumor is essentially negative for P63 expression, whereas 45–80% of cells in epithelioid trophoblastic tumor express P63.

Epithelioid smooth muscle tumors, especially epithelioid leiomyosarcomas, can cytologically resemble epithelioid trophoblastic tumor but these can usually be distinguished with smooth muscle markers.

NON-NEOPLASTIC TROPHOBLASTIC LESIONS

PLACENTAL SITE NODULE OR PLAQUE

Placental site nodule or plaque is a non-neoplastic lesion of intermediate trophoblast from a previous gestation that failed to involute. It is almost always found in the endometrium or endocervix; however, rarely, it occurs at sites of ectopic gestation. In most cases, long-term follow-up results are uneventful after dilatation and curettage.[100,101]

Clinical Presentation

The lesions usually occur in reproductive age women. The majority of patients present with menorrhagia, irregular uterine bleeding, or abnormal Pap smear, but it can be an incidental finding in curettage or hysterectomy specimens.[100,101] It is often detected several months to years after the pregnancy.

Gross and Microscopic Findings

Placental site nodule is usually detected microscopically but does not form a grossly apparent mass. Oval, variably cellular nodules or plaques are mostly well circumscribed from the surrounding endometrium (Figure 34.47). The nodule is composed of mononucleated or binucleated epithelioid trophoblastic cells forming small clusters in an abundant acellular, hyaline background (Figure 34.48). Cystic changes are common. The trophoblastic cells in the nodules closely resemble those in the chorion laeve, suggesting that they are remnant of extravillous trophoblast of fetal membrane. They are composed of two populations of cells; one with eosinophilic and the other with clear (glycogen-rich) cytoplasm. The eosinophilic cells tended to be larger with more pleomorphic nuclei, but often have pyknotic and degenerative-appearing nuclei, whereas the clear cells were smaller with more uniform nuclei. Mitotic figures can be observed, but are rare. At the periphery of the nodules and the surrounding endometrium, there are frequent inflammatory infiltrates composed of plasma cells and lymphocytes that may cause intermittent bleeding in patients.

Immunohistochemically, the cellular components in the nodule are diffusely and strongly positive for placental alkaline phosphatase, P63, inhibin-α, and cytokeratin 18, but are negative or weakly and focally positive for human placental lactogen and CD146 (Mel-CAM). The immunophenotype of the cellular components in a placental site nodule are equivalent to those of 'chorionic-type' intermediate trophoblast. A minority of cases are positive for hCG. Ki-67 proliferating activity is usually low, ranging from 1% to 5%.

Differential Diagnosis

Placental site nodules should be distinguished from other aggressive lesions such as placental site trophoblastic tumor, epithelioid trophoblastic tumor, and squamous cell carcinoma. The differential diagnosis from placental site trophoblastic tumor is often difficult especially in the curettage specimens because the periphery is not well preserved, and the overall size is hard to estimate. However, extensive hyalinization, degenerative appearance of nuclei, low cellularity, and rare or absent mitotic inactivity favor placental site nodule. Absence of CD146 (Mel-CAM) staining and a low Ki-67 labeling index in the placental site nodule may be helpful to differentiate from placental site trophoblastic tumor. At times, placental site nodules can be confused with squamous cell carcinoma of the cervix (Figure 34.49), but these can be distinguished using trophoblast markers.

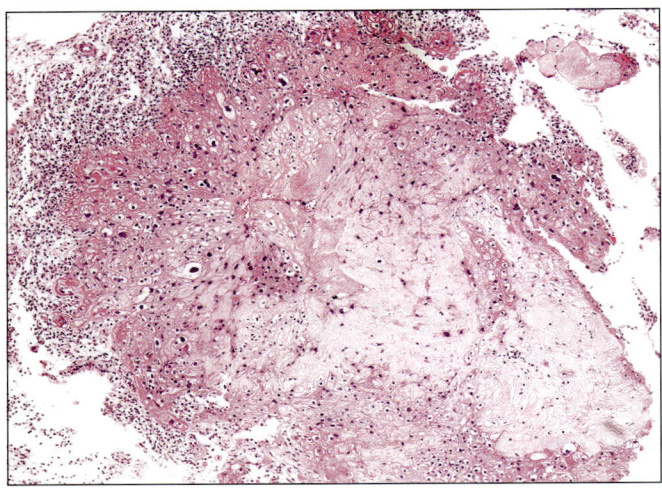

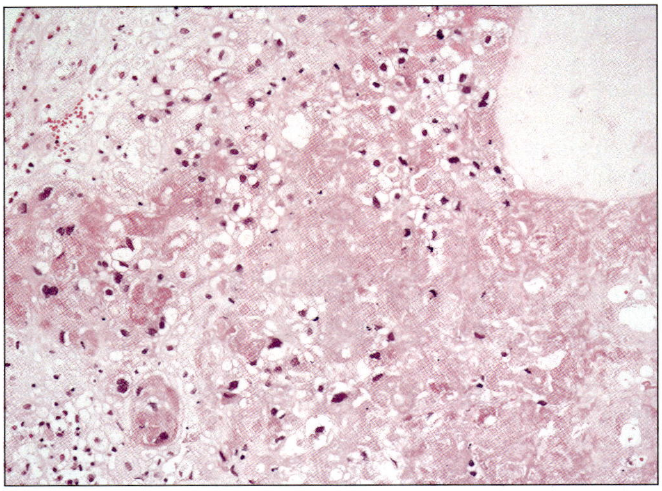

Figure 34.47 Placental site nodule in endometrial curettings. A small, discrete hyalinized nodule in the endometrium contains intermediate trophoblast that are histologically similar to those in chorion laeve.

Figure 34.48 Placental site nodule. Intermediate trophoblast in hyalinized background have variable degrees of nuclear atypia, but they are mostly of smudged or degenerated nature. Mitotic figures are rare or absent.

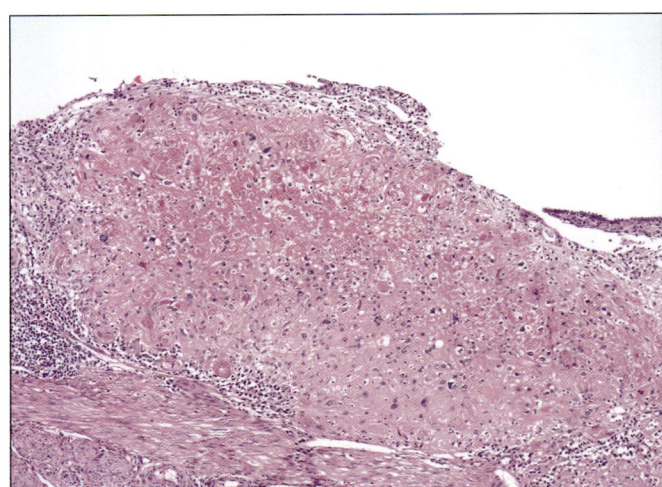

Figure 34.49 Placental site nodule in a lower uterine segment. It is often misdiagnosed as a squamous cell carcinoma of uterine cervix because of irregular nuclei and eosinophilic fibrinoid material misinterpreted as keratin.

EXAGGERATED PLACENTAL SITE (REACTION)

Exaggerated placental site, previously known as syncytial endometritis, is a non-neoplastic trophoblastic lesion showing exuberant infiltration of extravillous (intermediate) trophoblast and syncytiotrophoblast into the endometrium and myometrium. Normally, intermediate trophoblast invades the inner third of the myometrium in the first trimester of pregnancy and then undergoes progressive regression. Thus, the distinction between a normal and exaggerated placental site is somewhat arbitrary and reliable data quantifying the amount and extent of trophoblastic infiltration at different stages of normal gestation has not been determined.[4]

An exaggerated placental site can occur following normal or ectopic pregnancy, abortion, or hydatidiform mole.

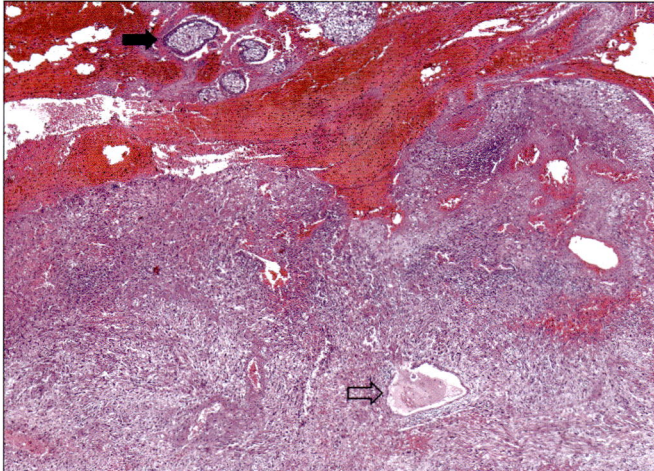

Figure 34.50 Exaggerated placental site. The infiltrative growth of the intermediate trophoblast is reminiscent of placental site trophoblastic tumor, but the presence of chorionic villi (closed arrow), preservation of the normal architecture of the endometrium (open arrow), and the absence of mitotic figures in the trophoblast are distinguishable histologic features.

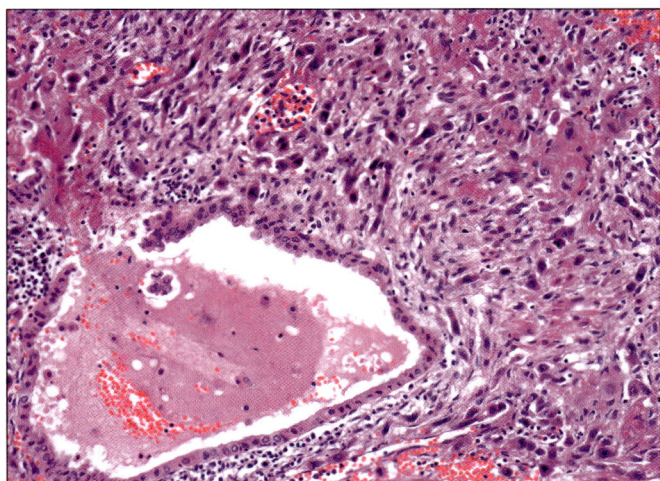

Figure 34.51 Exaggerated placental site. Infiltrating extravillous trophoblast are epithelioid or spindle-shaped cells with frequently smudged or degenerated nuclei. Mitotic figures are rare.

Microscopically, the lesion is characterized by abundant noninvoluted intermediate trophoblastic cells, which are of an identical type to those of a normal implantation site, but the glandular architecture is usually not disrupted (Figures 34.50 and 34.51). Chorionic villi are frequently seen, which helps the differential diagnosis from placental site trophoblastic tumor.

Differential Diagnosis

Placental site trophoblastic tumor is the most important differential diagnosis of exaggerated placental site, because the latter can be cured by simple curettage or endometrial ablation. The pleomorphism of extravillous (intermediate) trophoblastic cells along with the invasion into the blood vessels and myometrium may lead to diagnostic confusion with neoplastic conditions, especially when they are found in locations outside the endometrium, such as the ovary, fallopian tube, or cervix. Exaggerated placental site is usually associated with the presence of chorionic villi, mitosis is usually absent, and the Ki-67 labeling index is less than 5% (usually 0–1%), whereas placental site trophoblastic tumor is a massively infiltrating lesion with solid sheets and cords of cells that replace the normal architecture of the endometrium, with occasional mitotic figures and an increased Ki-67 labeling index. In the evaluation of the Ki-67 labeling index, it is important not to count activated lymphocytes in the placental site, which are positive for Ki-67. Therefore, a double-staining technique using MIB1 and CD146 (Mel-CAM) can be useful to identify proliferating intermediate trophoblastic cells.

There are cases in which a differential diagnosis between an exaggerated placental site and placental site trophoblastic tumor is extremely difficult in the curettage specimen since the infiltrated cells have quite a high Ki-67 labeling index, exceeding 5%. In those cases, monitoring of β-hCG is required.

REFERENCES

1. Carson DD, Bagchi I, Dey SK, et al. Embryo implantation. Dev Biol 2000;223:217–37.
2. Moore KL, Persaud TVN. Formation of germ layers and early tissue and organ differentiation: third week. In: Moore KL, Persaud TVN, editors. The developing human. New York: Saunders; 2003. p. 60–76.
3. Cartwright JE, Fraser R, Leslie K, et al. Remodelling at the maternal-fetal interface: relevance to human pregnancy disorders. Reproduction 2010;140:803–13.
4. Shih IM, Kurman RJ. The pathology of intermediate trophoblastic tumors and tumor-like lesions. Int J Gynecol Pathol 2001;20:31–47.
5. Shih IM, Kurman RJ. Epithelioid trophoblastic tumor: a neoplasm distinct from choriocarcinoma and placental site trophoblastic tumor simulating carcinoma. Am J Surg Pathol 1998;22:1393–403.
6. Salehi S, Eloranta S, Johansson AL, et al. Reporting and incidence trends of hydatidiform mole in Sweden 1973–2004. Acta Oncol 2011;50:367–72.
7. Lybol C, Thomas CM, Bulten J, et al. Increase in the incidence of gestational trophoblastic disease in The Netherlands. Gynecol Oncol 2011;121:334–8.
8. Kim SJ, Bae SN, Kim JH, et al. Epidemiology and time trends of gestational trophoblastic disease in Korea. Int J Gynaecol Obstet 1998;60(Suppl. 1):S33–8.
9. Soares PD, Maesta I, Costa OL, et al. Geographical distribution and demographic characteristics of gestational trophoblastic disease. J Reprod Med 2010;55:305–10.

10. Matsui H, Kihara M, Yamazawa K, et al. Recent changes of the incidence of complete and partial mole in Chiba prefecture. Gynecol Obstet Invest 2007;63:7–10.
11. Kim SJ, Lee C, Kwon SY, et al. Studying changes in the incidence, diagnosis and management of GTD: the South Korean model. J Reprod Med 2004;49:643–54.
12. Khashoggi TY. Prevalence of gestational trophoblastic disease. A single institution experience. Saudi Med J 2003;24:1329–33.
13. Bagshawe KD. Risk and prognostic factors in trophoblastic neoplasia. Cancer 1976;38:1373–85.
14. Bagshawe KD, Dent J, Webb J. Hydatidiform mole in England and Wales 1973–83. Lancet 1986;2:673–7.
15. Altaras MM, Rosen DJ, Ben-Nun I, et al. Hydatidiform mole coexisting with a fetus in twin gestation following gonadotrophin induction of ovulation. Hum Reprod 1992;7:429–31.
16. Dautenhahn L, Babyn PS, Smith CR. Metastatic choriocarcinoma in an infant: imaging appearance. Pediatr Radiol 1993;23:597–600.
17. Makino S, Sasaki MS, Fukuschima T. Triploid chromosome constitution in human chorionic lesions. Lancet 1964;2:1273–5.
18. Vassilakos P, Kajii T. Letter: Hydatidiform mole: two entities. Lancet 1976;1:259.
19. Szulman AE, Surti U. The syndromes of hydatidiform mole. II. Morphologic evolution of the complete and partial mole. Am J Obstet Gynecol 1978;132:20–7.
20. Ohama K, Kajii T, Okamoto E, et al. Dispermic origin of XY hydatidiform moles. Nature 1981;292:551–2.
21. El-Maarri O, Seoud M, Riviere JB, et al. Patients with familial biparental hydatidiform moles have normal methylation at imprinted genes. Eur J Hum Genet 2005;13:486–90.
22. Fisher RA, Hodges MD, Newlands ES. Familial recurrent hydatidiform mole: a review. J Reprod Med 2004;49:595–601.
23. Fowler DJ, Lindsay I, Seckl MJ, et al. Routine pre-evacuation ultrasound diagnosis of hydatidiform mole: experience of more than 1000 cases from a regional referral center. Ultrasound Obstet Gynecol 2006;27:56–60.
24. Shih IM, Kurman RJ. Ki-67 labeling index in the differential diagnosis of exaggerated placental site, placental site trophoblastic tumor, and choriocarcinoma: a double immunohistochemical staining technique using Ki-67 and Mel-CAM antibodies. Hum Pathol 1998;29:27–33.
25. Bewtra C, Frankforter S, Marcus JN. Clinicopathologic differences between diploid and tetraploid complete hydatidiform moles. Int J Gynecol Pathol 1997;16:239–44.
26. Hui P. Molecular diagnosis of gestational trophoblastic disease. Expert Rev Mol Diagn 2010;10:1023–34.
27. Burton JL, Lidbury EA, Gillespie AM, et al. Over-diagnosis of hydatidiform mole in early tubal ectopic pregnancy. Histopathology 2001;38:409–17.
28. Sebire NJ, Lindsay I, Fisher RA, et al. Overdiagnosis of complete and partial hydatidiform mole in tubal ectopic pregnancies. Int J Gynecol Pathol 2005;24:260–4.
29. Berkowitz RS, Goldstein DP, Bernstein MR. Natural history of partial molar pregnancy. Obstet Gynecol 1985;66:677–81.
30. FIGO staging for gestational trophoblastic neoplasia 2000. FIGO Oncology Committee. Int J Gynaecol Obstet 2002;77:285–7.
31. Procter SE, Gray ES, Watt JL. Triploidy, partial mole and dispermy. An investigation of 12 cases. Clin Genet 1984;26:46–51.
32. McFadden DE, Langlois S. Parental and meiotic origin of triploidy in the embryonic and fetal periods. Clin Genet 2000;58:192–200.
33. Zaragoza MV, Surti U, Redline RW, et al. Parental origin and phenotype of triploidy in spontaneous abortions: predominance of diandry and association with the partial hydatidiform mole. Am J Hum Genet 2000;66:1807–20.
34. Sergi C, Schiesser M, Adam S, et al. Analysis of the spectrum of malformations in human fetuses of the second and third trimester of pregnancy with human triploidy. Pathologica 2000;92:257–63.
35. Redline RW, Hassold T, Zaragoza MV. Prevalence of the partial molar phenotype in triploidy of maternal and paternal origin. Hum Pathol 1998;29:505–11.
36. Sanchez-Ferrer ML, Ferri B, Almansa MT, et al. Partial mole with a diploid fetus: case study and literature review. Fetal Diagn Ther 2009;25:354–8.
37. Zaragoza MV, Millie E, Redline RW, et al. Studies of non-disjunction in trisomies 2, 7, 15, and 22: does the parental origin of trisomy influence placental morphology? J Med Genet 1998;35:924–31.
38. Surti U, Szulman AE, Wagner K, et al. Tetraploid partial hydatidiform moles: two cases with a triple paternal contribution and a 92,XXXY karyotype. Hum Genet 1986;72:15–21.
39. Jauniaux E, Kadri R, Hustin J. Partial mole and triploidy: screening patients with first-trimester spontaneous abortion. Obstet Gynecol 1996;88:616–9.
40. Medeiros F, Callahan MJ, Elvin JA, et al. Intraplacental choriocarcinoma arising in a second trimester placenta with partial hydatidiform mole. Int J Gynecol Pathol 2008;27:247–51.
41. Fukunaga M, Katabuchi H, Nagasaka T, et al. Interobserver and intraobserver variability in the diagnosis of hydatidiform mole. Am J Surg Pathol 2005;29:942–7.
42. Fukunaga M. Early partial hydatidiform mole: prevalence, histopathology, DNA ploidy, and persistence rate. Virchows Arch 2000;437:180–4.
43. Matsui H. Re: 'Twin pregnancy consisting of a complete hydatidiform mole and co-existent fetus: report of two cases and review of literature.' Gynecol Oncol 2006;100:218; author reply 218–219.
44. Chan YF, Sampson A. Placental mesenchymal dysplasia: a report of four cases with differentiation from partial hydatidiform mole. Aust N Z J Obstet Gynaecol 2003;43:475–9.
45. Rakheja D, Wilson KS, Rogers BB. Dysmorphic villi mimicking partial mole in a case with del(18)(q21). Pediatr Dev Pathol 2004;7:546–8.
46. Sebire NJ. Histopathological diagnosis of hydatidiform mole: contemporary features and clinical implications. Fetal Pediatr Pathol 2010;29:1–16.
47. Zou L, Zhao X, Li Z, et al. Four repetitive partial hydatidiform moles followed by malignant transformation to an invasive mole. Acta Obstet Gynecol Scand 2010;89:1364–5.
48. Cheung AN, Khoo US, Lai CY, et al. Metastatic trophoblastic disease after an initial diagnosis of partial hydatidiform mole: genotyping and chromosome in situ hybridization analysis. Cancer 2004;100:1411–7.
49. Sebire NJ, Fisher RA, Foskett M, et al. Risk of recurrent hydatidiform mole and subsequent pregnancy outcome following complete or partial hydatidiform molar pregnancy. BJOG 2003;110:22–6.
50. Dolapcioglu K, Gungoren A, Hakverdi S, et al. Twin pregnancy with a complete hydatidiform mole and co-existent live fetus: two case reports and review of the literature. Arch Gynecol Obstet 2009;279:431–6.
51. Massardier J, Golfier F, Journet D, et al. Twin pregnancy with complete hydatidiform mole and coexistent fetus: obstetrical and oncological outcomes in a series of 14 cases. Eur J Obstet Gynecol Reprod Biol 2009;143:84–7.
52. Xue WC, Guan XY, Ngan HY, et al. Malignant placental site trophoblastic tumor: a cytogenetic study using comparative genomic hybridization and chromosome in situ hybridization. Cancer 2002;94:2288–94.
53. Kim JH, Park DC, Bae SN, et al. Subsequent reproductive experience after treatment for gestational trophoblastic disease. Gynecol Oncol 1998;71:108–12.
54. Martaadisoebrata D. Invasive mole: Indonesian perspective. J Reprod Med 2007;52:839–42.
55. Song DE, Jang SJ, Kim KR. Villotrophoblastic pulmonary nodule with implantation site intermediate trophoblasts after induced abortion. Int J Gynecol Pathol 2007;26:305–9.
56. Smith HO, Wiggins C, Verschraegen CF, et al. Changing trends in gestational trophoblastic disease. J Reprod Med 2006;51:777–84.
57. Loukovaara M, Pukkala E, Lehtovirta P, et al. Epidemiology of choriocarcinoma in Finland, 1953 to 1999. Gynecol Oncol 2004;92:252–5.
58. Smith HO, Qualls CR, Hilgers RD, et al. Gestational trophoblastic neoplasia in American Indians. J Reprod Med 2004;49:535–44.
59. Cagayan MS. Changing trends in the management of gestational trophoblastic diseases in the Philippines. J Reprod Med 2010;55:267–72.
60. Harma M, Yurtseven S, Gungen N. Gestational trophoblastic disease in Sanliurfa, southeast Anatolia, Turkey. Eur J Gynaecol Oncol 2005;26:306–8.

61. O'Neill CJ, Houghton F, Clarke J, et al. Uterine gestational choriocarcinoma developing after a long latent period in a postmenopausal woman: the value of DNA polymorphism studies. Int J Surg Pathol 2008;16:226–9.
62. Brinton LA, Bracken MB, Connelly RR. Choriocarcinoma incidence in the United States. Am J Epidemiol 1986;123:1094–100.
63. Thapa K, Shrestha M, Sharma S, et al. Trend of complete hydatidiform mole. JNMA J Nepal Med Assoc 2010;49:10–3.
64. Lok CA, Ansink AC, Grootfaam D, et al. Treatment and prognosis of post term choriocarcinoma in The Netherlands. Gynecol Oncol 2006;103:698–702.
65. Gulati A, Vyas S, Lal A, et al. Spontaneous rupture of hepatic metastasis from choriocarcinoma: a review of imaging and management. Ann Hepatol 2009;8:384–7.
66. Olson MT, Gocke CD, Giuntoli RL, et al. Evolution of a trophoblastic tumor from an endometrioid carcinoma—a morphological and molecular analysis. Int J Gynecol Pathol. 2011;30(2):117–20, 1170–20.
67. Zhao J, Xiang Y, Wan XR, et al. Molecular genetic analyses of choriocarcinoma. Placenta 2009;30:816–20.
68. Matsuda T, Sasaki M, Kato H, et al. Human chromosome 7 carries a putative tumor suppressor gene(s) involved in choriocarcinoma. Oncogene 1997;15:2773–81.
69. Burke B, Sebire NJ, Moss J, et al. Evaluation of deletions in 7q11.2 and 8p12-p21 as prognostic indicators of tumour development following molar pregnancy. Gynecol Oncol 2006;103:642–8.
70. Horn LC, Bilek K, Nenning H. Postpartal gestational choriocarcinoma fatally misdiagnosed as squamous cell cancer of the uterine cervix. Gen Diagn Pathol 1997;143:191–6.
71. Nakayama M, Namba A, Yasuda M, et al. Gestational choriocarcinoma of Fallopian tube diagnosed with a combination of p57(KIP2) immunostaining and short tandem repeat analysis: Case report. J Obstet Gynaecol Res 2011;37:1493–6.
72. Ganapathi KA, Paczos T, George MD, et al. Incidental finding of placental choriocarcinoma after an uncomplicated term pregnancy: a case report with review of the literature. Int J Gynecol Pathol 2010;29:476–8.
73. Park JS, Cho MH, Nam JS, et al. Adiponectin is independently associated with apolipoprotein B to A-1 ratio in Koreans. Metabolism 2010;59:677–82.
74. Baergen RN, Rutgers JL, Young RH, et al. Placental site trophoblastic tumor: a study of 55 cases and review of the literature emphasizing factors of prognostic significance. Gynecol Oncol 2006;100:511–20.
75. Bonazzi C, Urso M, Dell'Anna T, et al. Placental site trophoblastic tumor: an overview. J Reprod Med 2004;49:585–8.
76. Nagamani M, Kaspar HG, Van Dinh T, et al. Hyperthecosis of the ovaries in a woman with a placental site trophoblastic tumor. Obstet Gynecol 1990;76:931–5.
77. Brewer CA, Adelson MD, Elder RC. Erythrocytosis associated with a placental-site trophoblastic tumor. Obstet Gynecol 1992;79:846–9.
78. Shen DH, Khoo US, Ngan HY, et al. Coexisting epithelioid trophoblastic tumor and choriocarcinoma of the uterus following a chemoresistant hydatidiform mole. Arch Pathol Lab Med 2003;127:e291–3.
79. Knox S, Brooks SE, Wong-You-Cheong J, et al. Choriocarcinoma and epithelial trophoblastic tumor: successful treatment of relapse with hysterectomy and high-dose chemotherapy with peripheral stem cell support: a case report. Gynecol Oncol 2002;85:204–8.
80. Hui P, Wang HL, Chu P, et al. Absence of Y chromosome in human placental site trophoblastic tumor. Mod Pathol 2007;20:1055–60.
81. Petersson F, Grossmann P, Vanecek T, et al. Testicular germ cell tumor composed of placental site trophoblastic tumor and teratoma. Hum Pathol 2010;41:1046–50.
82. Suurmeijer AJ, Gietema JA, Hoekstra HJ. Placental site trophoblastic tumor in a late recurrence of a nonseminomatous germ cell tumor of the testis. Am J Surg Pathol 2004;28:830–3.
83. Went PT, Dirnhofer S, Stallmach T, et al. Placental site trophoblastic tumor of the mediastinum. Hum Pathol 2005;36:581–4.
84. Arroyo MR, Podda A, Cao D, et al. Placental site trophoblastic tumor in the ovary of a young child with isosexual precocious puberty. Pediatr Dev Pathol 2009;12:73–6.
85. Bower M, Paradinas FJ, Fisher RA, et al. Placental site trophoblastic tumor: molecular analysis and clinical experience. Clin Cancer Res 1996;2:897–902.
86. Ohmaru T, Yamakawa H, Netsu S, et al. Placental site trophoblastic tumor (PSTT) with multiple metastases and extremely poor prognosis. Int J Clin Oncol 2009;14:452–6.
87. Ayas S, Gurbuz A, Karateke A, et al. Placental site trophoblastic tumor with multiple metastases and complete response to salvage BEP regimen: a case report and review of the literature. Med Oncol 2009;26:96–100.
88. Lan C, Li Y, He J, et al. Placental site trophoblastic tumor: lymphatic spread and possible target markers. Gynecol Oncol 2010;116:430–7.
89. Milingos D, Doumplis D, Savage P, et al. Placental site trophoblastic tumor with an ovarian metastasis. Int J Gynecol Cancer 2007;17:925–7.
90. Piura B, Rabinovich A, Meirovitz M, et al. Placental site trophoblastic tumor: report of four cases and review of literature. Int J Gynecol Cancer 2007;17:258–62.
91. Numnum TM, Kilgore LC, Conner MG, et al. Fertility sparing therapy in a patient with placental site trophoblastic tumor: a case report. Gynecol Oncol 2006;103:1141–3.
92. Chew I, Post MD, Carinelli SG, et al. p16 expression in squamous and trophoblastic lesions of the upper female genital tract. Int J Gynecol Pathol 2010;29:513–22.
93. Li J, Shi Y, Wan X, et al. Epithelioid trophoblastic tumor: a clinicopathological and immunohistochemical study of seven cases. Med Oncol 2011;28:294–9.
94. Fadare O, Parkash V, Carcangiu ML, et al. Epithelioid trophoblastic tumor: clinicopathological features with an emphasis on uterine cervical involvement. Mod Pathol 2006;19:75–82.
95. Hamazaki S, Nakamoto S, Okino T, et al. Epithelioid trophoblastic tumor: morphological and immunohistochemical study of three lung lesions. Hum Pathol 1999;30:1321–7.
96. Lewin SN, Aghajanian C, Moreira AL, et al. Extrauterine epithelioid trophoblastic tumors presenting as primary lung carcinomas: morphologic and immunohistochemical features to resolve a diagnostic dilemma. Am J Surg Pathol 2009;33:1809–14.
97. Chohan MO, Rehman T, Cerilli LA, et al. Metastatic epithelioid trophoblastic tumor involving the spine. Spine (Phila Pa 1976) 2010;35:E1072–5.
98. Lurain JR. Gestational trophoblastic disease II: classification and management of gestational trophoblastic neoplasia. Am J Obstet Gynecol 2011;204:11–8.
99. Khunamornpong S, Settakorn J, Sukpan K, et al. Ovarian involvement of epithelioid trophoblastic tumor: a case report. Int J Gynecol Pathol 2011;30:167–72.
100. Huettner PC, Gersell DJ. Placental site nodule: a clinicopathologic study of 38 cases. Int J Gynecol Pathol 1994;13:191–8.
101. Young RH, Kurman RJ, Scully RE. Placental site nodules and plaques. A clinicopathologic analysis of 20 cases. Am J Surg Pathol 1990;14:1001–9.

35 Gross Description and Processing of Specimens

Brooke Howitt, George L. Mutter

CHAPTER OUTLINE

Introduction	812	Uterine Corpus	818
Section Codes and the Report	813	Endometrial Biopsies and Curettings	818
Section Codes	813	Uterus Removed for Benign or Functional Disease	818
Location of Section Codes in the Report	813	Supracervical Hysterectomy	820
Specimen and Site Identification	814	Malignant Uterine Disease	820
General Aspects of Gross Decription and Cutting in of Specimens	814	Endometrial Sampling for Products of Conception	821
Gross Description	814	Uterus Removed during Obstetric Procedures	821
Inking	815	Fallopian Tube	821
Drawings and Photographs	815	Sterilization	822
Fixatives	815	Tubal Ectopic Pregnancy	822
Number of Sections Required	815	Prophylactic Salpingectomy (with or without Oophorectomy)	822
Synoptic Checklists	815	Tubal Neoplasm	822
Vulva	815	Ovary	822
Excisional Biopsies	815	General Rules	822
Wide Local Excision	815	Large Cystic or Neoplastic Ovaries	823
Skinning Vulvectomy	816	Microscopic Sections	823
Simple (or Total) Vulvectomy	816	Staging Operations	824
Radical Vulvectomy	816	Fetus and Placenta	824
Cervix	817	Second Trimester Fetus	824
Punch Biopsies	817	Placenta	825
Endocervical Curettage	817		
Cervical Cone Biopsy/Excision and Trachelectomy	817		
Hysterectomy for Malignant Cervical Disease	818		

INTRODUCTION

The surgical pathologist reports the histopathologic diagnosis and specific information relating to prognosis and treatment. Therefore, one must have sufficient familiarity with the management of gynecologic and obstetric disorders to assure that the pathology report communicates the clinically relevant information. This chapter provides an approach to the processing of gynecologic and obstetric tissue specimens. The techniques of gross examination and the method of reporting the pathologic findings are guided by the clinical principles on which patient management is based. Several textbooks are now devoted entirely to this topic.[1-3]

In general, most tissue specimens submitted to the surgical pathology laboratory fall into one of three categories:

- Diagnostic biopsy
- Therapeutic resections
- Obstetrical specimens.

The main purpose of a biopsy is to provide a histologic diagnosis that will guide management. Since biopsy specimens tend to be small and without specific gross features, the major pathology resides in the histology. The gross description is important mainly to ensure that what is received in the pathology laboratory and submitted for microscopic examination matches the slides returned from the histology laboratory for the pathologist to examine. Disparity between the findings on a slide and those expected based on the gross description is often the only clue that a slide or block may have been mislabeled. A good gross description therefore should be precise and brief. Examples of good descriptions are '3 ovoid fragments 2 to 4 mm in diameter,' 'multiple shreds of tissue 5 cm in aggregate,' or the exact size given in three dimensions. For some specimens, it is also useful to note whether it is largely blood, mucin, or tissue.

In contrast, the gross description that the pathologist provides in therapeutic resections may be the most important aspect of the entire report. These are usually larger operative specimens and, after the specimen is examined in the gross state and dissected, it is normally discarded after several weeks. There is no way to return to the specimen and determine the position and size of any lesion, its margins, its relation to neighboring organs, or any other facets about its growth pattern after this time.

For operative specimens, particularly those containing a malignancy, information in the surgical pathology report should describe the extent of the tumor and specific features that relate to prognosis and staging. The adequacy of the surgical treatment as well as the need for additional therapy depends on these findings. Since the gynecologic surgeon has seen the pathology *in vivo*, it is important that the surgeon communicate the operative findings, since these will bear directly on how the pathologist processes the specimen. For example, adequacy of resection margins requires an appreciation of the orientation of the specimen to certain anatomic landmarks that are obvious to the surgeon, but which the pathologist cannot always reconstruct in the laboratory.

A good gross description enables the reader to reconstruct an image that corresponds to the specimen and its lesion. Since the histologic diagnosis for many tumors has been made by biopsy before the operative procedure, the gross description of the specimen should focus on the site and extent of the lesion and its relationship to adjacent structures. Key findings should be suggested from the gross examination of the specimen. Microscopic findings should be complementary to those identified grossly, and it should be uncommon for them to be in conflict. A careful gross examination is mandatory to ensure that the appropriate microscopic sections are obtained. Conversely, an inattentive gross examination often leads to preparation of needless 'representative' slides (read: 'haphazard' or 'taken without thinking'), or, worse yet, an incorrect diagnosis. An accurate pathology report and microscopic evaluation is dependent on an accurate evaluation of the specimen in the gross state.

The final diagnosis of a tumor includes its histologic type, grade, dimensions, location, and extent, as well as the adequacy of the resection margins, presence of lymphatic or vascular invasion, and status of the regional lymph nodes. Since 2004, all hospitals wishing to achieve certification/designation as a cancer institute by the American College of Surgeons must issue pathology reports listing all of the data points deemed mandatory by the College of American Pathologists (CAP). An appropriate gross description and selection of blocks for microscopy requires a full understanding of what should be in the final report for each specimen type, and why.

SECTION CODES AND THE REPORT

Many operations result in two or more separate specimens being submitted to the pathology department. Cervical examinations often produce two or three colposcopically directed biopsies plus endocervical curettage. Twenty or more specimens from a staging laparotomy are not uncommon. As a first step, each container received should be numbered and checked to ensure that all specimens removed have in fact reached the pathologist. This information is usually listed on the requisition sheet ('specimens submitted'). Each specimen should be uniquely labeled (see later). Payment issues also require that each container be given an identifiable diagnosis.

SECTION CODES

It is important that every department settle on a numbering system that is clear and used consistently throughout the specimen. The most common systems in use today are computer generated, providing the accession number for the overall case, the container sub-number for each portion of the specimen when it is received in multiple parts, an identifier for each paraffin block, the level within each paraffin block, and the type of stain used with any given slide.

Most systems use a one- or two-letter prefix to identify the general type of case received (S = surgical, C = cytology, A = autopsy), followed by a two-digit number designating the year (00 = 2000), followed by a sequential digit number. One system, in common use worldwide, then assigns a unique letter to each container received, starting at the beginning of the alphabet, i.e., 'A.' Each block sampled from that specimen/container then receives a sequential number, e.g., A1, A2,...An. Each subsequent specimen/container receives the next available letter, e.g., B, with multiple blocks from the container having sequential numbers, B1...Bn. If multiple levels of a single paraffin block are made, a practice for cervical biopsies in many institutions, the letter 'L' is appended with the designation of the slide level, e.g., -L2 for the second level of the block. Thus a typical specimen number might be SG-00-02167 B4-L2, which translates to 'Surgical specimen of a gynecologic nature, received in year 2000, accession number 2167, container B, fourth block taken from specimen B, and second slide prepared from that paraffin block.' Variants of the above system typically utilize letters in upper and lower case, Roman numerals, and Arabic numbers, usually in some combination and defined sequence. Of course, multiple numbering systems exist, and it is not the purpose of this chapter to pick which is best; the purpose is rather to help ensure clarity in whatever system is used.

LOCATION OF SECTION CODES IN THE REPORT

Most pathologists prefer a section code summary at the end of the gross text while some prefer entering block codes within the gross text. In either case, the report must be clear, both to the pathologist and to any person who at a later time will need to utilize the report. Block summaries, if used, may duplicate substantial parts of the gross, but cannot be used in its place. Including the block submission within the body of the gross description may be easier and more efficient for the person cutting in the specimen: 'The borders in one region are sharp and distinct from the surrounding myometrium (Block B10) while elsewhere it blends into the adjacent myometrium (Block B11).' However, having a section key at the end of the dictation may make histologic examination easier and more efficient. If the block codes are listed sequentially at the end of the report, the specific site and feature identified require presentation in sufficient detail so that the reader can easily link the gross description with the slide. Using the example above, it would be inappropriate for the coding block at the end to state that B10 and B11 are myometrium as it is unclear which section has the sharp borders and which has blurred borders. A section code at the end might better read, 'B10 Myometrium, sharply circumscribed medial border, B11 Myometrium, blurred indistinct borders.'

SPECIMEN AND SITE IDENTIFICATION

Regardless of the section code method used, it is critical that the reader can link the tissues received to the sections processed and both to the final diagnoses. For example, four cervical biopsies from the same patient are received in separate containers, but from the same operation. Information on the requisition slip indicates that the colposcopically directed specimens are from 3, 6, 9, and 12 o'clock, respectively. In this example, the accession number might be SG-00-02167, and the containers labeled A, B, C, and D, respectively. Since the paraffin block usually is identified solely by the code, then this same code should appear throughout. Thus, the gross might read 'A. 3:00 bx' (the wording exactly replicating what the clinician wrote on the container itself) while the final diagnosis would include 'A. Cervix, Biopsy at 3 o'clock: Diagnostic finding.' Obviously, the label on the slide must provide all of the necessary identifiers.

A most perplexing problem we encounter in referred specimens is where the label assigned to the container in the gross description differs from that given in the microscopic description to that given in the final diagnosis. For example, the container might be 'A' in the gross description, which refers to a specimen consisting of uterus, ovaries, and fallopian tubes, whereas the final diagnosis is '1. Endometriosis of the ovary.' Such cases require substantial effort on the part of the consultant pathologist to determine (and sometimes guess) which gross description truly belongs to which slide and both to the listed final diagnosis.

GENERAL ASPECTS OF GROSS DECRIPTION AND CUTTING IN OF SPECIMENS

GROSS DESCRIPTION

If possible, describe specimens received in the fresh state before fixation. Formalin alters natural color and consistency of tissue. The opening sentence of the gross description should indicate how the tissue is received (fresh or fixed) and labeled. Does the specimen received correspond with its label? For example, the container received states 'Uterus, tubes, and ovaries,' yet the left adnexa is absent. Such a gross description might read, 'Received fresh is a uterus and right ovary and fallopian tube. The left ovary and fallopian tube are absent.' Give measurements and weights of the individual diseased organs (e.g., 'the 710 g, $18 \times 15 \times 8$ cm uterus'). Conglomerate measurements and weights are meaningless (uterus, tubes, and ovaries which together weigh 710 g and measure $18 \times 15 \times 8$ cm) since they are ambiguous as to the role played by each organ and where the pathology resides.

The gross description should proceed in an orderly fashion, focusing on the primary lesion. Several common methods are in use. In one, the pathology in any given container/specimen is emphasized first. This highlights the pathology and de-emphasizes the normal. In practice, descriptions are full but economical in words and space. The second method is to follow a routine pattern whereby the same order is followed in every case, e.g., ovary, fallopian tube, uterine corpus, cervix, etc. This method, while usually easier for the novice, lends itself to loquacious reports filled with tedious description. All too often the true pathology is treated least well or even inadequately, as it is buried deep in the description. Not uncommonly, such travelogues lead to reports several pages long, but with a description of the tumor under several lines *in toto*. With the novice, detailed descriptions force careful examination, but, with experience, can be refined to a more concise and readable form.

Avoid elaborate descriptions of normal incidental anatomy. In a radical hysterectomy for cervical cancer, there is no need for an overly elaborate description of a normal fallopian tube. The following is excessive, '7 cm long, elongate structure with a 1 mm internal diameter and 4 mm external diameter with a tan, smooth, glistening serosa, a 2 mm thick wall, and a lumen without identifiable abnormality.' Simply 'the fallopian tube is 7 cm long, 4 mm in diameter and unremarkable' will do.

Similarly, we believe experience should allow the pathologist to describe grossly obvious lesions in diagnostic terms rather than nonspecific and frequently long-winded descriptions, a practice with which many also disagree. Leiomyoma, or, where useful, the diagnostic term with one or two adjectives ('well-circumscribed, whorled leiomyoma lacking hemorrhage or necrosis'), is far more useful than the excessive description ('numerous, discrete, circumscribed, rounded lesions with a bulging whorled cut surface, white in color, and compressing the adjacent myometrium'), which is tedious to read. At worst the description is vague ('rounded lesions'). Purposeful uncertainty, where it exists, can also be introduced with adjectives ('5 cm soft, focally necrotic leiomyomatous nodule with irregular borders suspicious for sarcomatous change').

The gross description, especially of small specimens, should conclude by stating how much of the tissue has been processed for microscopic examination. This is especially important in the case of endometrial curettings removed for a suspected intrauterine pregnancy where neither chorionic villi nor other tissues of fetal origin are found and all of the tissue has been submitted. Specify the number of each type of block sampled and from where each was obtained. An example of a useful gross description is 'The endometrium, which is 2 mm thick, discloses no obvious tumor. The entire endometrium including the superficial myometrium is blocked and submitted *in toto*.'

INKING

Application of ink, often in multiple colors, can be useful to identify various surgical margins, which on histologic sections is helpful to determine if the lesion is truly present at the margin or is present only where the tissue has been cut on a bias, thus simulating a margin (ink absent). If used, apply ink sparingly and blot dry to prevent spillover or running. Acetone or distilled white vinegar can be used to set the ink. As inking is a procedure all too often done indiscriminately, determine first whether it is even useful. There is no need to ink a uterine serosa in cases of cervical squamous intraepithelial lesions (SIL) or in cases where the endometrial cancer is small and noninvasive and the serosa is obviously normal and uninvolved. Ink sometimes is helpful (and sometimes the only clue) in identifying the surface of the ovary when replaced by tumor. Ensure also that the ink does not inadvertently conceal disease, e.g., endometriosis or a metastasis on the serosa.

DRAWINGS AND PHOTOGRAPHS

The inclusion of drawings and/or photographs may simplify portrayal of complicated relationships and permits better orientation, especially of surgical resection margins. Today, most photographs use digital technology. Document scanners can also be used for this purpose and can create surprisingly high-quality images. Block diagrams made from digital photographs or Xerox copies are particularly useful in complex cases. In the absence of actual photographs, diagrammatic drawings of the specimen and sections taken can also be helpful.

FIXATIVES

Formalin-based fixatives are generally the most practical and commonly used today. Tissue submitted in blocks for processing should be less than 3 mm thick. Thicker fragments are difficult to dehydrate and inhibit paraffin infiltration, thus leading to suboptimal slides. Sometimes, it is much easier to cut sections from tissue that has been fixed for several hours instead of attempting to cut 3 mm thick slices directly from a fresh specimen. Large specimens should be cross sectioned and cut at intervals 1 cm thick or less. This permits adequate penetration by formalin, after which the tissue can be trimmed into 3 mm thick sections. For large specimens, e.g., uteri removed for leiomyomata, placing the tissue blocks into cassettes (with all labeling complete) and retaining them in the fluid fixative for an extra day facilitates better sections. If fresh or frozen tissue is required for special studies, this should be collected prior to fixation.

NUMBER OF SECTIONS REQUIRED

Judging what must be sampled to optimally examine a specimen is one of the more controversial subjects not only in gynecologic pathology, but in all branches of surgical pathology. In general, the authors believe that far too many blocks are usually taken, adding expense without furthering diagnostic information gained. A useful exercise is to determine what single slide would be taken if the entire prosection permitted were limited to the single slide. This forces thinking about which single slide would demonstrate the lesion as well as pertinent margins or neighboring relations. Such forethought often has a major influence on how a specimen is opened and/or sampled. For example, an excisional biopsy of vulvar tumor might be best sampled by six equidistant perpendicular blocks sampling the central tumor, deep margin, and lateral margins rather than eight parallel lateral margins, shave margins of the base, and only several of the tumor. Leiomyomas/equivocal leiomyosarcomas should include not only the tumor but also the border with neighboring tissue and margins if possible. Endometrial tumors can easily be sampled to include the adjacent 'normal' endometrium.

SYNOPTIC CHECKLISTS

As the complexity of information contained in reports increases and tumor cases are accessioned into trials with specific entry criteria, checklists are being used with increasing frequency to record and evaluate the details of operative and pathologic findings consistently. A full listing of College of American Pathologists specimen processing protocols, including synoptic checklists, is available online at www.cap.org.

VULVA

EXCISIONAL BIOPSIES

Biopsies of the vulva should be handled like skin biopsies. Assess the deep and lateral resection margins. If the surgeon has placed a suture for orientation, inking (often in several colors) facilitates recognition on microscopic examination.[4]

WIDE LOCAL EXCISION

In general, wide local excisions are performed for noninvasive neoplasms such as vulvar intraepithelial neoplasm (VIN) 3 or Paget disease of the vulva, as well as superficially invasive (less than 1 mm) stage 1 carcinomas. Lymph node dissections are added for stage 1B carcinomas (greater than 1 mm invasive). Orientation is critical in these specimens and, if not clearly indicated, consultation with the surgeon may be required. Operative specimens often include labia minora and majora, clitoris, perineal body, and perianal tissue (Figure 35.1). Describe and measure the lesions, distances to resection margins, and the anatomic structures involved. Examine the coloration and surface texture carefully as intraepithelial lesions are subtle, typically red-brown to white and roughened.

As intraepithelial lesions are often multifocal and difficult to discern macroscopically, all surgical peripheral and deep resection margins should be evaluated microscopically. Sections parallel to margins ('tangential') may be taken to

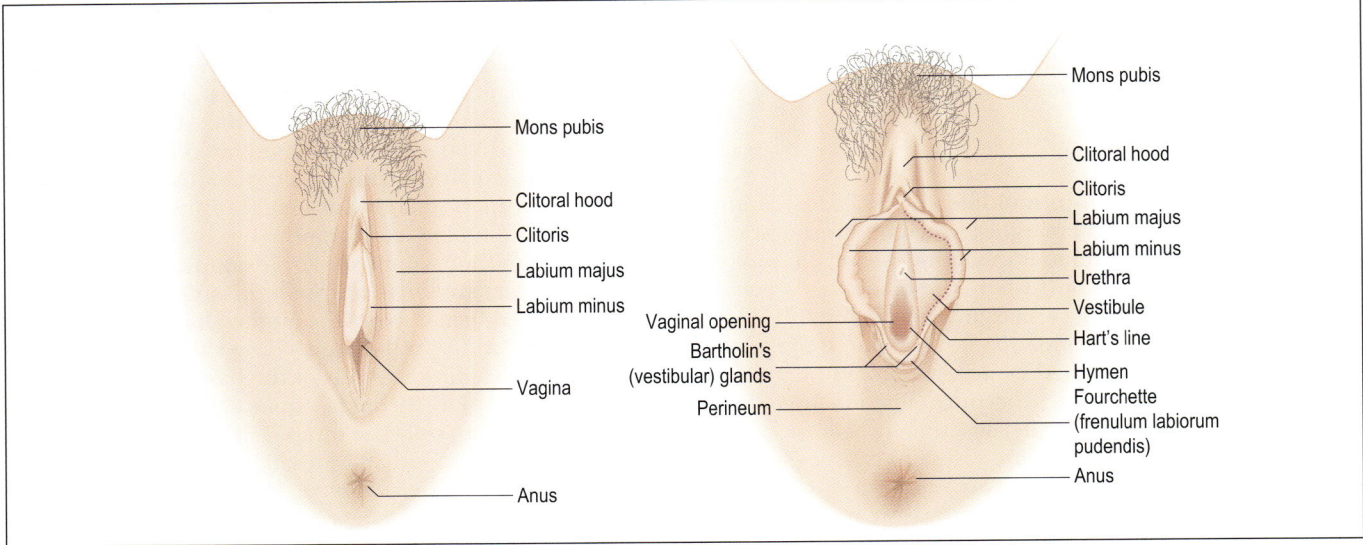

Figure 35.1 External genitalia.

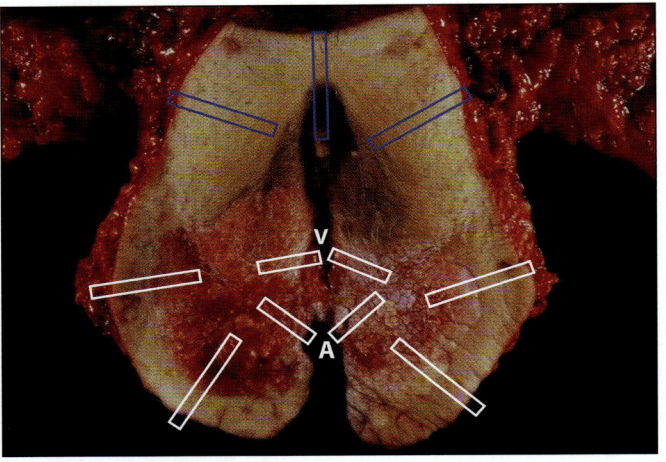

Figure 35.2 Perpendicular sections for examination of vulvar cancer. Sections, which are full thickness, include tumor and all margins (white), in addition to random samples of uninvolved areas (blue). Vaginal (V) and perianal (A) margins are closest to the gross lesion.

SKINNING VULVECTOMY

This is by definition a superficial excision of the vulvar skin at the level of the dermis, meaning it is performed almost entirely for noninvasive neoplasms (VIN 3 and Paget disease). The gross description and sections taken will be similar to those of wide local excision.

SIMPLE (OR TOTAL) VULVECTOMY

This includes the entire vulva and subcutaneous fat (dissection to deep fascia). It is typically performed for noninvasive neoplasms that widely involve the vulva. Pin, fix, and section the specimen at 0.5 cm intervals to evaluate for invasive carcinoma. Typically, the extent of Paget disease exceeds that visible macroscopically as occult foci are often present within normal-appearing skin. The resection margins must be thoroughly evaluated.[2,5]

RADICAL VULVECTOMY

Radical vulvectomy consists of vulva excised to the deep fascia of the thigh, the periosteum of the pubis, and the inferior fascia of the urogenital diaphragm. It is most commonly performed together with at least an inguinal lymph node dissection, which may be included en bloc with the vulvectomy. Total radical vulvectomies have largely been replaced in favor of more limited excisions, but sufficient to completely excise the primary tumor with a minimum 2 cm margin. Radical total vulvectomies are now performed primarily for large and/or aggressive tumors. The gross description should include the size, location, depth of invasion, and all resection margins, including perianal and vaginal margins. Sections should include the tumor, showing the maximum depth of invasion, labia majora and minora, clitoris, distal urethra, resection margins including the vaginal margin, and all lymph nodes. Separate lymph nodes into superficial and deep groups, and submit all lymph nodes entirely for histologic examination (unless grossly positive;

evaluate the excision lines; however, one difficulty commonly encountered in parallel sections for evaluation of margins is to determine if tumor found in the slide truly involves the margin or was from the inner face, and therefore not a true representation of the margin.

For discrete tumors, such as squamous cell carcinoma, multiple full thickness sections perpendicular to the skin surface and radiating outward from the lesion are advantageous as the central lesion, margins, and intervening areas can be included in one slide and tumor close to the margin is easy to evaluate (Figure 35.2). Facilitate sectioning by pinning the specimen on a corkboard or a block of paraffin and fix for several hours or overnight. Diagrams or photographs are often useful.

in that case a representative section is sufficient). Invasive vulvar neoplasms are typically solitary in contrast to intraepithelial lesions, which are often multifocal. Consequently, evaluation of resection margins can be largely limited to the margins closest to the tumor. The report should include microscopic diagnosis, tumor grade, dimensions, location and maximum depth of invasion, presence of lymphatic invasion, number and location of involved lymph nodes, and distance to resection margins. Diagrams and/or photographs may be useful aids.

CERVIX

The cervix may be sampled as punch biopsies, endocervical curettages, or cone biopsies (various methods), or removed entirely in total hysterectomy specimens or radical hysterectomy specimens.[6]

PUNCH BIOPSIES

Biopsies are usually colposcopically directed. The best specimens are at least several millimeters long with underlying stroma to a depth of 2–4 mm. If the fragments are tiny, they can be placed in a mesh bag for processing. Record the number of pieces received. The fixed, curled biopsy may be bisected transversely to produce two pieces that are approximately pyramidal in shape. These are then embedded with the flat, cut surface downward so that this surface is cut by the microtome. Step-serial sectioning is not necessary routinely.

ENDOCERVICAL CURETTAGE

Endocervical curettage is performed to evaluate the presence of glandular neoplasms, cervical squamous neoplasia involving the endocervical canal, or to determine whether endometrial carcinoma has spread into the cervix. Endocervical scrapings should be submitted as a separate specimen in a mesh bag before being placed into the cassette to avoid loss of small fragments of tissue during processing.

CERVICAL CONE BIOPSY/EXCISION AND TRACHELECTOMY

Cone biopsy is the standard procedure performed for women with high-grade SIL and glandular lesions. The cone biopsy can be a diagnostic or a therapeutic procedure. Commonly, it is both simultaneously. The conventional cone biopsy is obtained using a scalpel ('cold knife') but, today, is often done with laser or low-voltage, large-loop diathermy methods (LEEP). Excision with loop diathermy has the advantage that there is usually less bleeding and the cervix heals with better preservation of anatomy. It can also be performed as an outpatient procedure without the need for general anesthetic. One disadvantage, especially if the instrument is used at suboptimal power levels, is thermal damage that may make diagnosis and, in particular, the examination of margins difficult. Trachelectomy may also be performed as a therapeutic procedure for early stage invasive carcinomas of the cervix. A trachelectomy is a more extensive version of a cone excision, as the entire cervix is removed, with or without a vaginal cuff.

The cone biopsy is a roughly cone-shaped excision of the uterine cervix to include a portion of exocervix, external os with the entire transformation zone (T-zone), and endocervical canal with varying amounts of deep tissue. We ask the surgeon to note the 12 o'clock position with a black suture. If the specimen is not oriented, the 12 o'clock position may be arbitrarily assigned.

The surgical pathologist can limit the gross description to the measurements of the specimen and any obvious lesion. The measurements should include the cranial–caudal distance (the height or length of the cone specimen), the diameter if the specimen is not opened (Figure 35.3), or circumference and thickness if received opened. For a trachelectomy specimen, the presence of vaginal cuff should be documented and measured.

Blot dry the tissue and apply ink sparingly. Open the specimen at 12 o'clock, and pin the tissue on a corkboard with the mucosa facing up. Fixation for 3 hours before cutting is usually adequate. Serially cut sections should be sequentially submitted in cassettes numbered consecutively. Submit the entire specimen in a clockwise direction beginning at 12 o'clock (Figure 35.3). Convenience and economy dictate placing two or three sections per cassette.

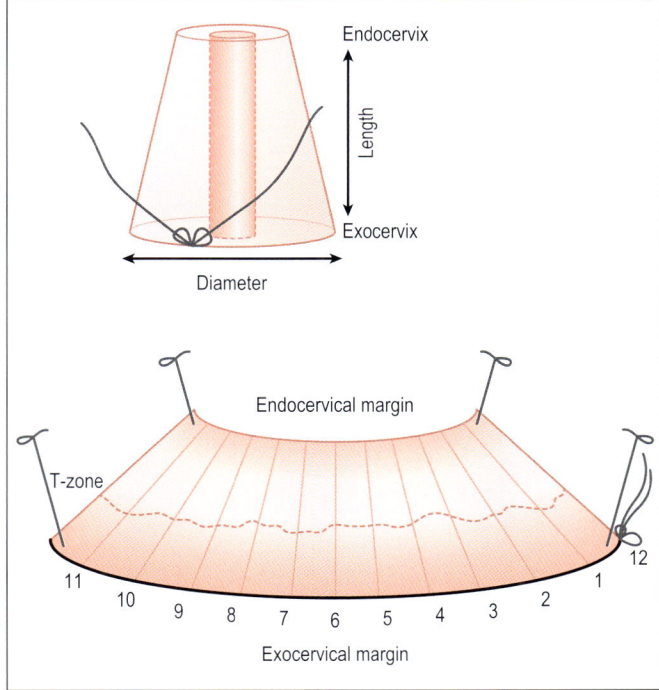

Figure 35.3 Cervical cone biopsy. The craniocaudal length and exocervix (portio) diameter should be measured. The exocervical and endocervical margins need to be separately assessed (with differential inking). Open the cone along its length through the canal, at the 12 o'clock position marked by the surgeon with a suture, or a random starting point if not oriented. Block in the entire specimen sequentially cut so each piece represents the canal lining, and surgical margins. The specimen is shown here endocervical mucosa up, with a dashed line marking the T-zone.

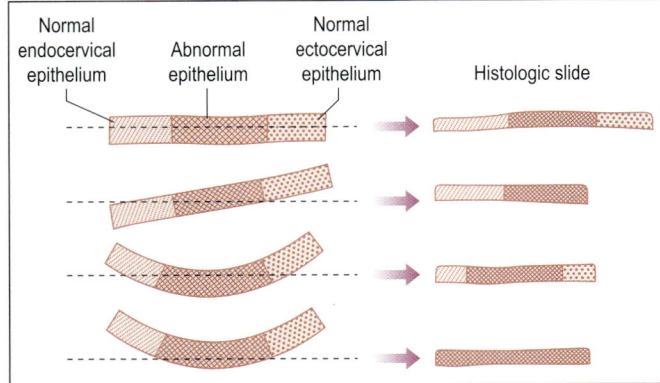

Figure 35.4 Examples of potential errors introduced if paraffin blocks are embedded and cut tangentially or on a bias.

Both the ectocervical and endocervical edges of the cone specimen need to be assessed. This can prove to be problematic if a specimen is bowed and cut tangentially (Figure 35.4).

HYSTERECTOMY FOR MALIGNANT CERVICAL DISEASE

Simple hysterectomy is commonly performed for high-grade intraepithelial neoplasms and many microinvasive cancers. Radical hysterectomy, which refers to the removal of paracervical soft tissue, is common for stage 1 squamous carcinomas, depending on size and configuration of the tumor in the endocervical canal, and for some stage 2A tumors.

For uteri removed for the treatment of squamous intraepithelial lesion, amputate the cervix at least 1 cm above the level of the external os and process in the way that has been described above for a cone biopsy. Often, one section from each quadrant may be sufficient. Each section should be full thickness to include the endocervical mucosa, squamo-columnar junction, exocervix, and outer adventitia. If a vaginal cuff has been submitted, measure the distance from the exocervix to the line of resection. We prefer sections perpendicular to the line of resection.

The gross description from a radical hysterectomy needs to include tumor dimensions and location—especially with respect to the vaginal fornix and the vaginal margin—depth of invasion, and an impression of whether the lymph nodes contain metastases. Sections of the cervix need to demonstrate both the maximum depth of invasion and the relationship of the tumor to the surgical margins. One or more blocks should contain a complete section from the mucosal surface of the uterus through to the serosa. Additional sections of the tumor to the non-neoplastic mucosa interface will often demonstrate SIL. The region of the internal os–lower uterine segment (LUS) should also be sampled. These sections may be taken longitudinally (upper endocervix to LUS). Submit all of the parametrial tissue since this represents the lateral and most significant resection margin. Inking the parametrium is useful. The surgeon will usually group lymph nodes by areas. If received intact and oriented, separate and group as right and left, further by location (internal iliac, external iliac, obturator, etc.).

UTERINE CORPUS

ENDOMETRIAL BIOPSIES AND CURETTINGS

Tissue from an endometrial biopsy (curettage or outpatient sample) should be submitted in its entirety. The gross description should estimate the aggregate volume. The cassettes should be packed loosely to permit proper fixation and dehydration. Wrap specimens in fine Shandon mesh/tea bags or equivalent and document in the dictation that the whole specimen is included.[7]

Sampling of hysteroscopically evident lesions must always be accompanied by a broader and representative sampling of the remaining otherwise unremarkable endometrial lining.

UTERUS REMOVED FOR BENIGN OR FUNCTIONAL DISEASE

This includes hysterectomy for leiomyomas, endometrial hyperplasia, persistent abnormal bleeding, uterine prolapse, or intractable pelvic pain, the last sometimes due to unrecognized organic causes, e.g., adenomyosis or endometriosis on the serosa.

List specimens received, including whether the adnexae are attached or separate. Several methods are available for orientation. One easy method to determine laterality is to lift the specimen by the two ovaries, which will be posterior to the fallopian tubes (Figure 35.5). Another method that is useful in the absence of adnexae is to observe the peritoneal reflections. The posterior uterine peritoneal surface covers a larger area and extends farther down toward the cervix in a V-shaped configuration, whereas, anteriorly, it ends higher over the bladder and in a more flat or smooth U shaped reflection edge.

Weigh the specimen without adnexae (i.e., subtract the estimated adnexal weight). Nomenclature is given in Figure 35.6.

Normal weights
 Nulliparous: 30–40 g
 Parous: 75–100 g
 After eight pregnancies: 240 g
 Postmenopausal: 20–40 g
Normal measurements
 Top of fundus to exocervix: 5–8 cm
 Cornu to cornu: 3–5 cm
 Anterior to posterior surface: 2–4 cm
 Cervical length and diameter: 3 cm each

Examine the uterine serosa, particularly the posterior surface, for adhesions or brown hemosiderin deposits, so-called 'powder burns,' which may indicate endometriosis, and small vesicles or gritty implanted foci suggestive of borderline serous tumor, endosalpingiosis, ovarian cancer, or psammoma body implants. Examine the exocervix for lacerations, scarring, ulcerations, and nabothian cysts.

Before opening the uterus, probe the cervical canal and endometrial cavity to establish the canal's patency; this also facilitates opening the uterus. With scissors cut from the cervical os to the cornu along one lateral margin to the fundal top and then repeat on the opposite side. Another option is to pass a pair of long fine forceps through the

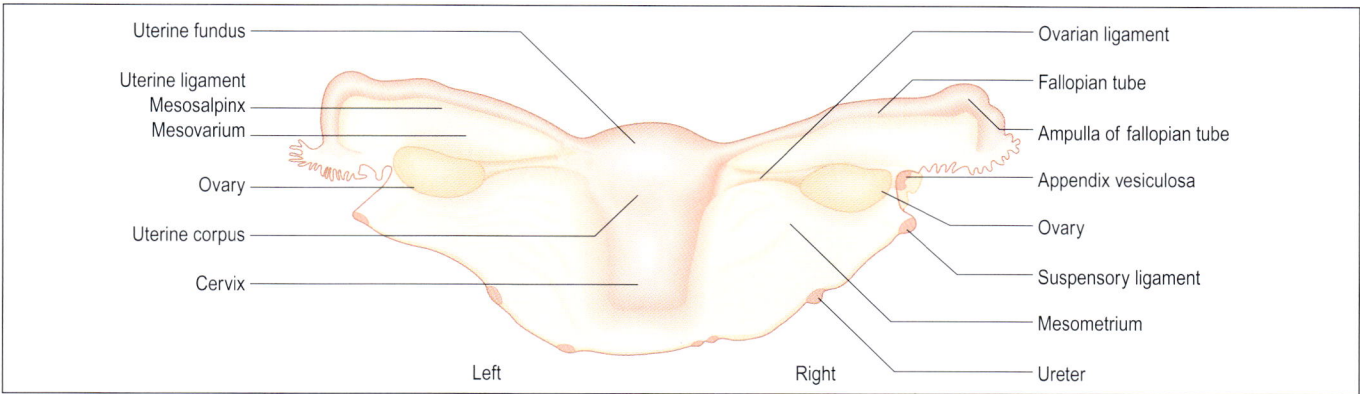

Figure 35.5 The uterus and adnexa, posterior aspect. One easy method for determining laterality is to suspend the two ovarian ligaments, which are posterior to the fallopian tube and therefore define right from left.

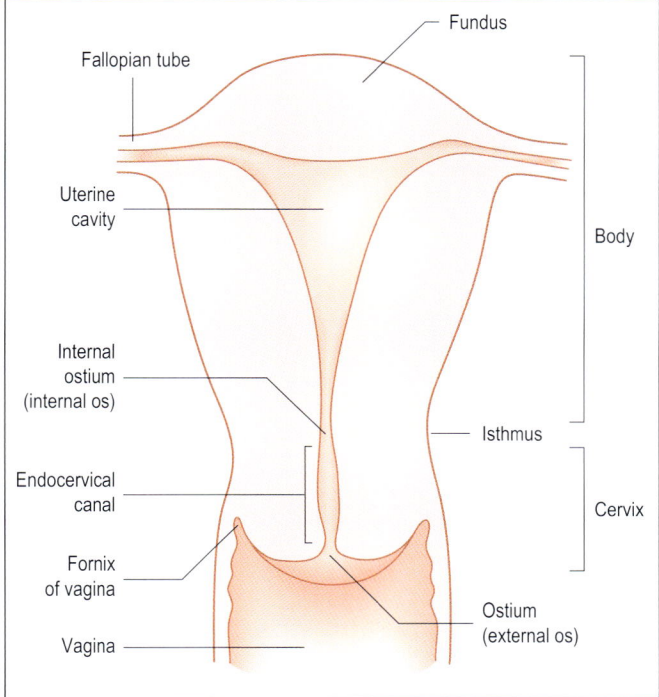

Figure 35.6 Components of the human uterus.

cervical os all the way to the fundus and cut the uterus open by using a long knife between the forceps blades. These methods ensure that the endometrial cavity will be exposed, with the anterior and posterior endomyometrium intact.

Measure the average thickness of the endometrium and assess whether it is atrophic, polypoid, lush, or hemorrhagic, and smooth or rough surfaced. Record polyp measurements and location (fundic, anterior/posterior, near LUS, etc.). Evaluate the myometrium and state its average and maximum thickness. Focally or asymmetrically thickened myometrium, small cysts, or hemorrhage suggests adenomyosis. For a normal cervix, usually one section is adequate if it includes the entire wall to involve the endocervix, squamocolumnar junction, exocervix, and paracervical soft tissue. Some pathologists prefer one section each of the anterior and posterior lips. The section through the endometrium, if the lesion is benign, should be 2 cm long and include the full endometrial thickness and a wedge of myometrium with serosa if not too thick. Generally, two sections, one each from the anterior and posterior (or right and left) corpus, suffice if the woman is in reproductive years and one if the uterus is atrophic and the woman is in the postmenopausal years (Figure 35.7). If there is no apparent pathology and the preoperative diagnosis is pain or dysfunctional uterine bleeding, then increase the number of sections to at least four that are full thickness, and include a posterior LUS section with peritoneal reflection. It is surprising how frequently adenomyosis is confined to only a single area in a single slide.

Uteri removed for endometrial hyperplasia or precancerous lesions require multiple sections of the endomyometrium to exclude carcinoma. For example, six sections, each 2 cm long and cut as wedges, can usually fit into two or three cassettes (Figure 35.8). If the uterus is not enlarged, this number of sections often samples 75% of the endometrium. Some pathologists prefer to block in the entire endometrium with sections through to the serosa so as not to miss the possibility of invasive cancer and be able to measure the depth of invasion.

Uteri removed for leiomyomas should have documented the number of leiomyomas present, their location (submucosal, intramural, subserosal) and size (e.g., 'ten measuring ≤ 1 cm and two measuring 13 and 18 cm in diameter'). If submucosal, state whether the tumor distorts the endometrial cavity or protrudes into the lower uterine canal or cervix. Each leiomyoma should be sectioned and examined grossly, but not necessarily microscopically. If all are small, white, firm, whorled, with well-circumscribed margins, and lack areas that are soft, necrotic, or hemorrhagic, even one block can be sufficient. Routine microscopic examination of every typical leiomyoma is unnecessary. Conversely, as leiomyosarcomas generally grow as a single nodule or mass and exhibit soft and degenerative areas, any suspicious areas should be thoroughly sampled. As a rule, of the suspicious regions take one microscopic section per 1 cm of the nodule's greatest dimension, for these areas usually yield more useful information. The transition between smooth muscle tumors and surrounding myometrium is the preferred site for histologic sampling. 'Random' sections of grossly typical

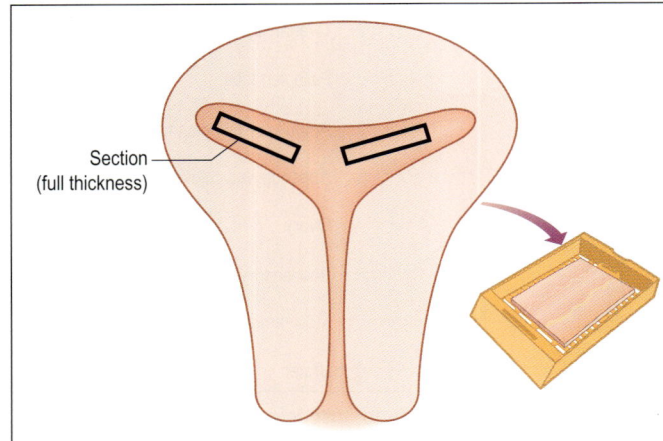

Figure 35.7 Sampling of the uterine body for complaint of bleeding where no obvious gross disease is present (e.g., occult adenomyosis). Two full thickness sections anteriorly and two posteriorly (shown here) extensively and efficiently sample the endometrium and myometrial wall.

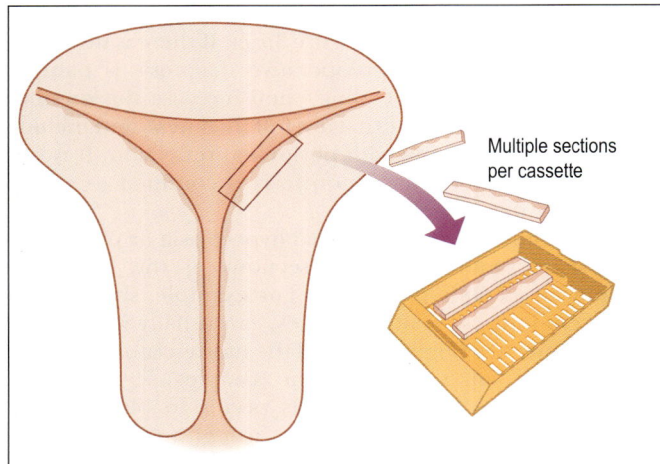

Figure 35.8 Efficient but extensive sampling of the uterine body for endometrial hyperplasia or endometrial intraepithelial neoplasia.

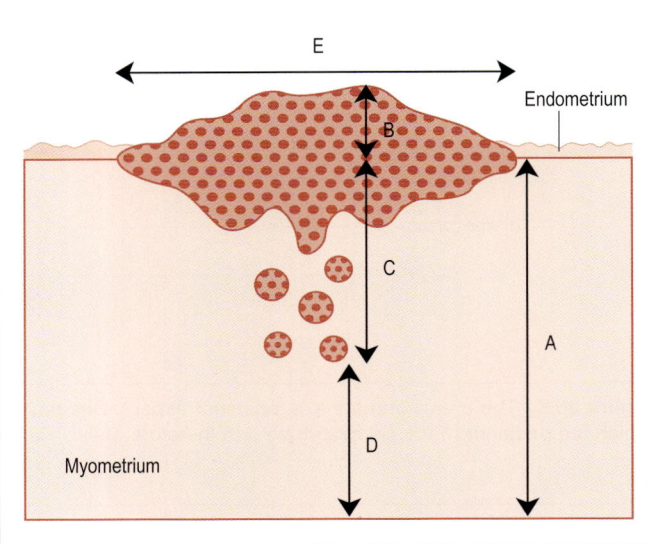

Figure 35.9 Measurements of depth to which tumor invades. **A**, full thickness of myometrial wall, measured from the native endometrial–myometrial junction. This landmark may require examination of the endometrium–myometrium interface adjacent to the tumor. **B**, component of tumor exophytic and rising above an imaginary line drawn between adjacent normal endometrium. **C**, depth of invasion. **D**, tumor-free zone. **E**, width of tumor. We generally report a tumor as measuring $n \times n \times n$ and 'invading through X percentage of the myometrial thickness' (percentage of myoinvasion = $100 \times C/A$).

leiomyomas generally are of little use. For myomectomy specimens, transect each leiomyoma and take one section of each if the number is not excessive, or more if any areas are suspicious. More commonly, hysterectomies for benign conditions are being performed laparoscopically with morcellation. In this situation, the morcellated uterus should be weighed and examined to identify fragments with endometrium, serosa, cervix if present, and lesional tissue (leiomyomas, adenomyosis, etc.), and a conservative number of blocks submitted.

SUPRACERVICAL HYSTERECTOMY

Supracervical hysterectomy is sometimes performed for benign uterine disease such as leiomyomas. These may be processed as discussed earlier; however the 'endocervical' margin of excision must be inked to document the level of transection, and representative sections of this margin submitted for histologic examination.

MALIGNANT UTERINE DISEASE

Evaluate all specimens with a preoperative diagnosis of malignancy for residual tumor. If present, determine the maximum depth of myometrial invasion and cervical involvement (mucosal or stromal) and take sections to document these findings.

The gross description must include the size, location, distribution (focal or diffuse), and shape (sessile or polypoid) of the lesion. For example, 'a 6 × 5 cm sessile anterior endometrial tumor involves the anterior LUS but not the endocervix. The tumor grossly invades 5 mm and maximally 10 mm into a 23 mm thick wall (approximately 45% of the myometrial thickness).' If the tumor is polypoid and protrudes into the endometrial cavity, identify the borders of the adjacent normal endometrium, draw an imaginary line between, and then report measurements above and below the line. Thus the 1 cm thick tumor, which protrudes 7 mm into the endometrial cavity, penetrates 3 mm into the superficial myometrium (Figure 35.9). Describe and sample the uninvolved endometrium, including its relationship with the tumor and adjacent myometrium. At least one microscopic section should permit measurement of the greatest depth of tumor invasion, and may be submitted as two blocks if the full myometrial thickness does not fit in one cassette (Figure 35.10). For intramural tumors, describe and sample the interface between the tumor and myometrium

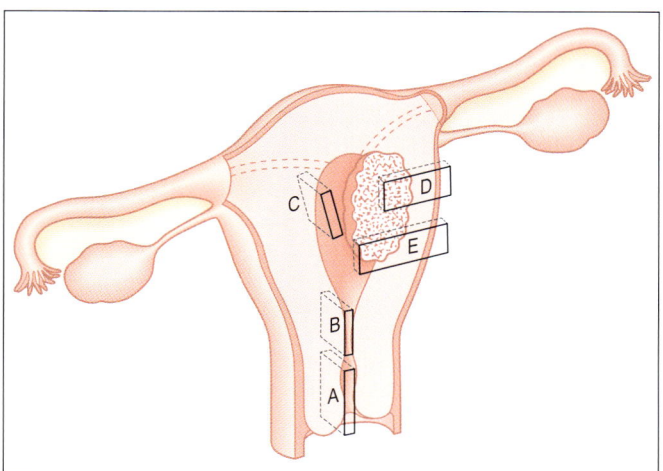

Figure 35.10 Technique for sectioning the uterus. The sampling shown is for the posterior half, and would be mirrored in the anterior half, producing double the number of sections. It includes cervix (**A**); margins adjacent and deep to a cancer (**D, E**); LUS and uppermost endocervix (**B**), for example, to determine whether an endometrial cancer involves the cervix, thus upstaging it; the wall for adenomyosis (**C**); and endometrium with areas partially or totally seemingly free of tumor. In sampling the LUS, a posterior midline section extending to include the peritoneum (**B**) will enable evaluation of potential 'drop metastases' within the cul-de-sac peritoneal reflection.

(circumscribed, irregular, or infiltrative) and note any worm-like extrusions of tumor in surrounding tissues that could represent grossly involved lymphatic/vascular channels (seen most commonly in endometrial stromal sarcomas and intravenous leiomyomatosis). An endometrium previously ablated for precancerous disease need not be entirely submitted; representative sections in addition to any grossly identifiable lesion should be submitted for microscopic examination.

Lymphadenectomy may be included in the staging of endometrial carcinoma. Studies have shown that higher numbers of removed pelvic and para-aortic lymph nodes (12 or greater) are more prognostically powerful, particularly when negative.[8] Thus, careful dissection of lymphadenectomy specimens, with submission of all possible lymph nodes, is necessary.

ENDOMETRIAL SAMPLING FOR PRODUCTS OF CONCEPTION

For specimens with obvious aborted products of conception, evaluate completeness of fetal and placental removal when possible. Therapeutic abortions, if performed after week 8, will more often show fetal fragments than spontaneous abortions. Single small samples of fetal parts and placenta suffice for sectioning. When fetal parts are absent, pay particular attention to finding chorionic villi. Chorionic villi are soft gray-white tissue fragments that arborize when submerged in fluid. Soft, tan, solid, and often shiny gray tissue is decidua and, in itself, does not diagnose the presence of an intrauterine pregnancy.

At times, the specimen may consist of a uterine cast. Look for an intact or ruptured gestational sac in spontaneous abortions especially. Embedding a portion of the sac with the embryo in agar may improve the chances of observing it microscopically. When a fetus or fetal parts are identified grossly, usually one section is sufficient for documentation, unless there is a gross abnormality. Note crown–rump length and head circumference of the fetus, if possible, and obtain the weight. Since the fetus is often disrupted in therapeutic abortions, another measurement useful to assess fetal age is the toe–heel (foot) length. Only if microscopic examination fails to reveal tissues of fetal origin should additional tissue be processed. Avoid submitting blood clots; in contrast to ectopic pregnancy in the fallopian tube where blood clots typically contain chorionic villi, uterine blood clots almost always lack chorionic villi, even when villi are abundant elsewhere.

Curettings from hydatidiform moles often come in two parts: suction curettage and sharp curettage. Examine carefully for fetal parts. Submitting three blocks is usually sufficient. Tissue from the sharp curettage should be processed entirely, since it must be evaluated for myometrial invasion. It should also be remembered that, with suction curettage, most vesicles will have been forcibly disrupted and the classic gross appearance will not be present.

UTERUS REMOVED DURING OBSTETRIC PROCEDURES

Hysterectomy during delivery is performed for intractable hemorrhage, placenta accreta, uterine rupture, or cervical neoplasia. For the last, process the specimen as described previously. For the other conditions, focus the gross description and sectioning on the relation of the placenta and membranes to the uterus. Describe lacerations, usually lateral, carefully as to location, extent, and depth of penetration. Uterine rupture may have occurred at the site of a previous lower segment cesarean section scar and sections across the site of rupture should be oriented to optimize its identification as a predisposing factor. Also, placenta previa, placenta accreta, and previous cesarean section in the lower segment not infrequently go together. Obtain sections from these sites. A prosector should be aware that occasionally a fetus/baby might have been delivered through the site of uterine rupture, which subsequently was sutured. If no obvious site of rupture is identified, the sutured wound should be sampled for microscopic examination after inking of the serosal surface. For placenta previa, sample carefully the zone of the internal os to identify associated placenta accreta. Suspected placental retention sites identified by strongly adherent placenta are useful in defining placenta accreta, increta, and percreta. Full thickness sections of these areas should be submitted.

FALLOPIAN TUBE

Many fallopian tube specimens (salpingectomy) are performed in conjunction with oophorectomy and hysterectomy, especially in older women in whom it is no longer necessary to preserve fertility. Typically in these cases, there is no grossly identifiable lesion in the fallopian tubes. The overall length and diameter of the tube should be measured. Peritubal cysts and adhesions should be documented. The fimbriae should be examined for thickening or irregularities. Small, grossly undetectable carcinomas have been

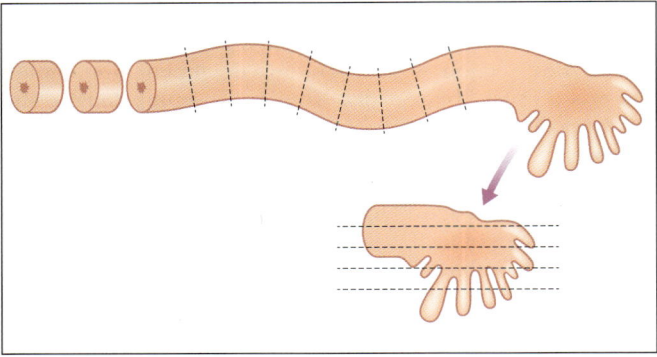

Figure 35.11 SEE-FIM protocol for cutting in a fallopian tube where comprehensive sampling is desired to assess possible occult epithelial lesions, such as those seen in *BRCA* patients. Cross sections cut at ~3 mm intervals of the length of the tube, and the fimbriated end amputated and cut in the longitudinal axis at 1–2 mm intervals. The entire fimbria is submitted.

shown to occur in the fimbriated end of the fallopian tube not infrequently. For this reason, regardless of the indication for salpingectomy, portions of the fimbria should be included in microscopic sampling. If there is significant concern for an occult tubal carcinoma, the entire fimbriated end can be submitted for histologic examination according to the SEE-FIM (sectioning and extensively examining the fimbriated end) protocol (Figure 35.11).[6]

STERILIZATION

When removed for ligation, the single most important finding is that indeed the tube has been ligated. This requires that a complete cross section of the tube, which includes the lumen, be identified grossly and confirmed microscopically. Measure the length and the diameter of each tube. One method for sampling is to slice the tube into sections 1–3 mm long and to submit all for microscopic examination, each piece being cut on end. Even if per chance some sections are cut tangentially, usually at least some will be intact to document that the lumen is present. This saves substantial time and effort by not having to request additional recuts.

TUBAL ECTOPIC PREGNANCY

Record the site and location of the pregnancy, which is often seen as a bulging area of hematosalpinx. A rupture site, if present, should be described and sampled. If the ectopic pregnancy is not obvious, a focal enlargement or swelling should be sought, and the entire tube sectioned extensively. Blood distending the lumen should be documented, as it is unlikely to result from any other cause. A tubal abortion leaves foci of trophoblast at the implantation site. Blood clot in the tube, sometimes submitted as a separate specimen, should be examined carefully for gray-white tissue and sampled microscopically for trophoblast or chorionic villi. Multiple cross sections of the fallopian tube at the site of swelling or bleeding demonstrate chorionic villi efficiently. Sections of fallopian tube, even slightly away from the swelling, may be normal, but should be sampled to confirm or exclude pre-existing pathology such as agglutinated plicae in healed salpingitis.

PROPHYLACTIC SALPINGECTOMY (WITH OR WITHOUT OOPHORECTOMY)

Another increasingly common indication for salpingectomy is prophylaxis for patients who have *BRCA1/2* mutations, a personal history of breast cancer, or strong family history of breast and/or tubo-ovarian cancer. Typically the specimen is grossly unremarkable; however, these fallopian tubes, along with the corresponding ovaries, should be submitted entirely for histologic examination according to the SEE-FIM protocol.[9] The proximal fallopian tube is serially sectioned at ~3 mm intervals, stopping approximately 1 cm before the distal-most portion of the fallopian tube. The fimbria should be sectioned longitudinally to maximize fimbrial plicae histologic examination (Figure 35.11).

TUBAL NEOPLASM

Recent studies have shown that tubal cancer is more common than was initially appreciated, partly due to the fact that fallopian tubes historically were not thoroughly sampled for histologic examination.[9] Tubal carcinomas behave similarly to ovarian carcinoma and frequently appear as a solid mass in the wall of a grossly dilated tube, but may sometimes only be identified upon microscopic examination. When grossly identifiable, its size, location, and extent, with reference to other pelvic structures, should be documented. Transverse sections through the full tubal wall permit determination of the depth of penetration/invasion, which is an essential component to the pathology report.

OVARY

The pathologist may receive ovarian tissue from patients in a variety of clinical circumstances, each of which determines the manner in which the specimen is handled. If oophorectomy is performed in association with a hysterectomy with no expectation or realization of ovarian pathology, a simple 'routine' pathologic examination will usually suffice. In contrast, ovaries excised for prophylaxis or suspected or proven neoplasms may require several different specialized analyses in addition to histologic assessment. In some circumstances, e.g., ovarian failure, it may be appropriate to have a preoperative consultation to discuss the appropriate site and size of the biopsy and its immediate handling in the operating room in order to optimize analysis of the clinical problem.[10]

GENERAL RULES

Several general rules can be applied when the specimen is small, incidental, or where no substantial pathology is anticipated:

- The specimen should be examined fresh or at most fixed for a short period.
- It should be weighed and measured.
- The external surface should be inspected for adhesions, excrescences, hemorrhage, or hemosiderin.

- Sections should be taken perpendicularly through the adhesions to include the capsule and parenchyma to determine whether or not the adhesions are due to inflammation or neoplasm. Note the presence of a corpus luteum, cystic follicles (if excessive in number), or cysts. Their combined absence may indicate an otherwise unexpected diffuse metastasis.
- Residual uninvolved ovary should be incised by parallel transverse cuts (Figure 35.12).
- One block is sufficient from a macroscopically normal ovary, but this should include cortex, medulla, and hilus, conveniently sampled by a single section through the middle of the ovary. An exception to this rule is in prophylactic bilateral salpingo-oophorectomy specimens, in which case the entire specimen should be submitted for histologic examination.

LARGE CYSTIC OR NEOPLASTIC OVARIES

Weighing large ovarian tumors may provide a more readily appreciable assessment of the size of the lesion. Document whether the ovarian tumor is received intact or ruptured and learn whether the rupture occurred intraoperatively (preoperative rupture can upstage the patient). If a tubo-ovarian mass is submitted, careful dissection may be necessary to identify its components. In pelvic inflammatory disease the ovary is relatively spared and should be readily recognized once the surrounding adhesions have been teased away. The course of the fallopian tubes should be identified and the condition of the fimbriae noted. A hydrosalpinx or para-ovarian cyst, especially if associated with adhesions, may cause confusion if diligent efforts are not made to establish the anatomic relationships.

Pay attention to the capsule, inking the outer surface before slicing the ovary at 1 cm or less intervals. Document if adhesions, inflammation, or tumor involve the surface. This is important in staging. Include the capsule and tumor, and include tumor with adjacent normal parenchyma. Many ovarian tumors are cystic and all locules should be opened with scissors or sliced through with a sharp long-bladed knife. Note the character of the cyst contents (serous, mucoid, bloodstained, oily, gelatinous, pultaceous) and the smoothness of its lining. A smooth shiny lining usually indicates a benign lesion, whereas solid areas or papillary excrescences may suggest a more worrisome lesion and thus should be extensively sampled. Ragged hemorrhagic cyst linings suggest endometriosis. Mature cystic teratomas (dermoid cysts) should be emptied as completely as possible of the trapped hair and sebaceous material. Remove sebum by washing with hot water (liquefies the sebum).

Look for the fallopian tube, which may be incorporated in or stretched over the tumor mass/cyst. It may contain coexistent neoplasia.

For small tumors, identify the location as cortical, medullary, or hilar. If mucinous, find the most solid regions and sample extensively. The cystic areas will be benign or microscopically disclose little more than borderline tumor. Only the solid areas generally show areas definable as adenocarcinoma.

If the ovary has undergone torsion, the tissues may be extremely edematous, hemorrhagic, or even necrotic. Slice the ovary finely, looking for any viable tissue or residua of a cyst or solid tumor that may have undergone torsion. Reticulin stains on suspicious areas may help to highlight the underlying pathology. The accompanying fallopian tube, if also involved, should be closely examined because it may be, albeit rarely, the site of the inciting lesion. In children, torsion of normal adnexa is not uncommon.

MICROSCOPIC SECTIONS

Ink can be useful to document the tumor's serosal surface. The best blocks of tumor are where the tissue is viable. Generally, about one block per 2 cm of greatest tumor dimension will suffice to document the tumor process. It is common in cystic mucinous neoplasms for any single tumor to have large areas that are benign or borderline, with only few areas that are unequivocally malignant. Commonly, areas with multilocular thin-walled cysts are benign, or at most of borderline malignancy. Areas that are more solid are usually borderline and sometimes frankly malignant. Quite commonly, only 10% of solid areas may show unequivocal malignancy, which in a 10 cm tumor translates to only two slides with malignancy out of 20 sampled. Search diligently for solid areas and sample them thoroughly. Unilocular cysts with a smooth inner-wall lining may be large, but require few sections. Membrane rolls composed of extensive quantities of cyst wall tissue can be examined if the wall is made into a membrane roll and a cross-section slide prepared (Figure 35.13).

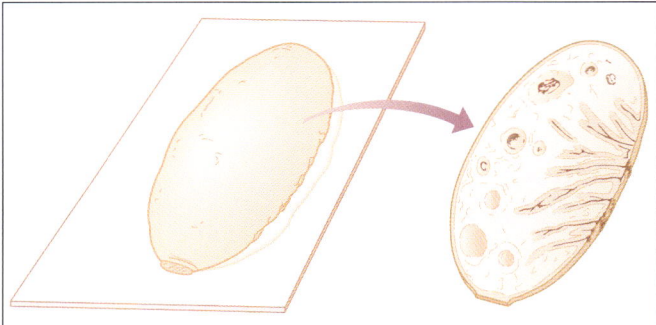

Figure 35.12 Technique for sectioning ovary in the absence of abnormalities. The cross section shows cortex, medulla, and hilum.[1]

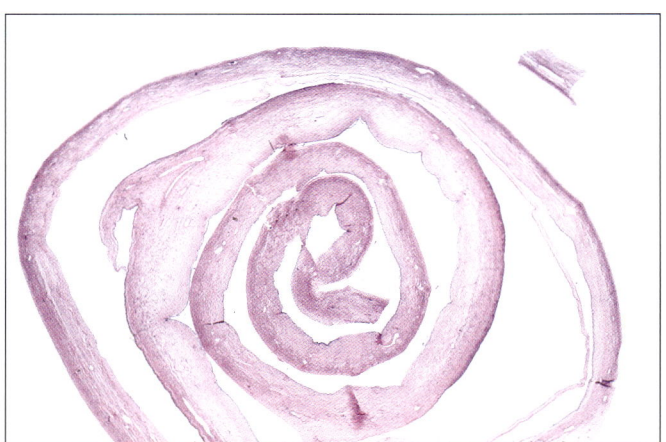

Figure 35.13 'Membrane-roll' made from thin-walled ovarian cyst.

Germ cell tumors should be sampled extensively, especially if they appear grossly heterogeneous. If there is a history or clinical suspicion of intersex an X-ray for calcifications may indicate an area of gonadoblastoma. These regions should be sampled thoroughly. All variations in the gross appearance such as foci of hemorrhage or necrosis should be specifically sampled as they may represent different tumor types, e.g., foci of embryonal carcinoma or yolk sac tumor (YST) arising in association with a dysgerminoma.

Dermoid cysts should have microscopic sections taken from the solid tissue. These are the business components, and the ones that will disclose the carcinoid, strumas, etc.

STAGING OPERATIONS

There is need for close cooperation between surgeon and pathologist in the staging operations for assessment of both primary ovarian carcinoma and for previously treated cancer. These may involve intraoperative assessment of excised tissues, including frozen section, as well as the histologic examination of multiple specimens and cytologic assessment of peritoneal washings and ascitic fluid. General guidelines for the surgeon include the following:

1. Evaluate the ovarian mass to exclude metastasis from colon, stomach, or elsewhere. Note penetration through capsule and biopsy areas of adherence.
2. Obtain ascitic fluid or saline washings for cytology.
3. Inspect all peritoneal surfaces. Prove that apparent implants are malignant by frozen section, or submit multiple samples for permanent section, or both. Inspect the diaphragm, with biopsy of visible lesions or scrapings for cytology.
4. Confirm accuracy of apparent stage 1 or 2 disease by generous omental biopsy and biopsy of palpable pelvic and para-aortic nodes.
5. After excision, mark the specimen, indicating for the pathologist the site of rupture and/or area(s) of adherence. Record residual disease location and estimate extent.

Specimens submitted for pathologic examination are likely to include the following:

- Uterus with attached or separately submitted adnexa, preferably delivered fresh to the pathologist immediately. Carefully examine the whole specimen noting the excisional margins if necessary. Complete the assessment of the ovaries as recommended previously. Before fixation, open the uterine cavity, keeping in mind the possibility of a coexisting endometrial carcinoma or hyperplasia. Scrutinize the uterine serosal surface for tumor deposits and section any adhesions to exclude microscopic metastases (since these will raise the International Federation of Gynecologists and Obstetricians stage from at least stage 1 to at least stage 2A).
- Omentum. Slice finely, looking for tumor deposits and block these. If none is found, sample any unusually firm areas (usually fibrous adhesions which may or may not be associated with microscopic tumor deposits). One or two blocks should be sufficient. In over 20% of cases, the grossly normal omentum will disclose microscopic foci of tumor.
- Pelvic and/or para-aortic lymph nodes. Submit all lymphoid tissue.
- Peritoneal biopsies. These are often very small and should be handled accordingly, using a mesh bag if necessary.
- Peritoneal washings. The surgeon collects these by saline irrigation from the left and right paracolic gutters, subdiaphragmatic region, and pouch of Douglas. These fluids should be processed by cytology; evaluation of cytospins, smears, liquid-based cytology techniques (e.g. ThinPrep), and cell block as deemed appropriate by the laboratory. Ascitic fluid is treated similarly.

FETUS AND PLACENTA

SECOND TRIMESTER FETUS

In many institutions, special permission is required to examine a fetus nearing viability. Statutes variously define the cut-off as a fetus older than 20 weeks' gestation, greater than 15 cm crown–rump length, or greater than 300 g weight. Regardless of gestational age, the placenta can be submitted as a surgical pathology specimen.[11]

Pathologic examination of fetuses varies by clinical context and local resources. Generally, a voluntarily aborted 'normal' fetus will be handled differently than intrauterine demise for unknown reasons or a fetus that carries a specific antenatal diagnosis. In particular, formal fetopsy may be indicated when the intent is to discover cause of death or evaluate a suspected congenital syndrome. If indicated, sterile samples for cytogenetics or culture should be taken prior to fixation. Whenever possible in these cases the placenta should be evaluated in conjunction with the fetus. This section reviews generally applicable grossing and sampling procedures, which will be modified by clinical circumstance.

Physical integrity (intact, fragmented) and autolytic state (well preserved, macerated) of the fetus should be recorded. Extent of fetal maceration may be helpful in documentation of the time frame of fetal demise. Measure and record the fetal weight, crown–heel length, crown–rump length, and head circumference. Other common measurements include foot length, thorax, and abdominal circumferences. Sex can usually be determined by external examination. If the genitalia are ambiguous, then describe them as such. Never give a 'best guess' for sex assignments. Look for obvious external anomalies, and if present consider whether they may be part of a multi-feature syndrome that requires targeted examination of visceral abnormalities. More subtle ones are difficult to observe in early gestation. Measure the attached cord length and state the number of blood vessels. Describe the skin surface and, after the body is opened, observe the organs *in situ*. Determine situs and note any obvious abnormalities. Retrieve the gonads and place them in a mesh bag at this point. Take sections of various organs. Weighing organs that are part of a fragmented surgical specimen is often a futile exercise. Microscopic sampling should include each lobe of lung, both gonads, and small sections of every other organ including stomach and other various parts of gastrointestinal tract and skin. Macerated fetuses are difficult to sample adequately because of the severe softening of the tissues; submit sections of more solid tissue (lungs, heart, kidneys). Often the entire examination consists of no more than three cassettes filled with tissue.

PLACENTA

Abnormalities of the placenta are frequently associated with adverse outcomes in either the fetus or the mother.[11,12] Examination of the placenta is not routinely performed in most institutions unless specific indications are present. The CAP practice guidelines include recommendations of indications for placental examination (Table 35.1). To determine which placentas should be examined, remember the three funnies: funny mother, funny infant, funny disease. This should lead to the examination of about one in three placentas, although in practice fewer are examined (about one in five).[11]

If indicated, sterile samples for cytogenetics or culture should be taken prior to fixation. Fresh samples should also be taken for metabolic/biochemical studies and/or electron microscopy.

Identify the site of membrane rupture. If far from the placenta proper, consider it to be unremarkable and make no comment. If there is a membranous cord insertion or large fetal vessels traverse the membranes, note their relation to rupture site. Record the presence or absence of hemorrhage in the membranes, and the approximate distance of it to the margin of the placenta.

Remove the free membranes and cord, leaving the fetal side of the disc undisturbed, and weigh the placenta (Table 35.2). Measure the disc diameter. Systematically describe all parts (Figure 35.14).

- *Fetal surface.* Describe the color, surface characteristics (smooth, roughened, opaque, etc.), vascularity. Note the margins. Are the membranes inserted in the usual manner? Is there thickening, circummarginate or circumvallate insertion, etc.? If present, estimate the percentage of circumference affected.
- *Umbilical cord.* Describe insertion (central, eccentric, marginal, velamentous); measure length and cross-sectional diameter (state as average or range); state number of blood vessels. Look for varicosities, excessive coiling, false knots, true knots, edema, discoloration, thrombosis, hemorrhage, etc.
- *Membranes.* The amnion is the layer adjacent to the fetus. Usually the chorion and amnion are loosely fused (easily separated), but may be completely separate. Look for thickening, opacity, and adherent blood clot. Describe color, clarity, edema, etc. Make a membrane roll to include the area of rupture. There are several methods of membrane rolling, of which one is to:
  1. Cut a 10 cm long strip to include both chorion and amnion extending from the edge that was attached to the placenta to the edge where the rupture occurred.
  2. Grasp the placental edge with non-toothed forceps and roll the membranes around the forceps with the amnion (which is smoother) on the outside of the roll.
  3. Relax the grip on the forceps slightly and use the blunt side of a knife blade to remove the roll from the forceps.
  4. Pin the membrane roll onto cork and cut sections with a sharp blade, or fix the membrane roll overnight and cut sections the next day.

Table 35.1 Examination of the Placenta

Recommended Maternal Indications (General Agreement)

Systemic disorders with clinical concerns for mother or infant (e.g., severe diabetes, impaired glucose metabolism, hypertensive disorders, collagen disease, seizures, severe anemia; <9 g)
Premature delivery ≤34 weeks' gestation
Peripartum fever and/or infection
Unexplained third trimester bleeding or excessive bleeding >500 cm^3
Clinical concern for infection during this pregnancy (e.g., human immunodeficiency virus, syphilis, cytomegalovirus, primary herpes, toxoplasma, rubella)
Severe oligohydramnios
Unexplained or recurrent pregnancy complication (e.g., intrauterine growth retardation, stillbirth, spontaneous abortion, premature birth)
Invasive procedures with suspected placental injury
Abruption
Non-elective pregnancy termination
Thick and/or viscous meconium

Other Maternal Indications (Less General Agreement)

Premature delivery >34–37 weeks' gestation
Severe unexplained polyhydramnios
History of substance abuse
Gestational age ≥42 weeks
Severe maternal trauma
Prolonged (>24 hours) rupture of membranes

Recommended Fetal/Neonatal Indications

Admission or transfer to other than a level 1 nursery
Stillbirth or perinatal death
Compromised clinical condition defined as any of the following: cord blood pH, <7.0; Apgar score, ≤6 at 5 minutes; ventilatory assistance, >10 minutes; or severe anemia, hematocrit <35%
Hydrops fetalis
Birthweight <10th percentile
Seizures
Infection or sepsis
Major congenital anomalies, dysmorphic phenotype, or abnormal karyotype
Discordant twin growth >20% weight difference
Multiple gestation with same-sex infants and fused placentas

Other Fetal/Neonatal Indications (Less General Agreement)

Birthweight >95th percentile
Asymmetric growth
Multiple gestation without other indication
Vanishing twin beyond the first trimester

Recommended Placental Indications

Physical abnormality (e.g., infarct, mass, vascular thrombosis, retroplacental hematoma, amnion nodosum, abnormal coloration, or opacification, malodor)
Small or large placental size or weight for gestational age
Umbilical cord lesions (e.g., thrombosis, torsion, true knot, single artery, absence of Wharton's jelly)
Total umbilical cord length <32 cm at term

Other Placental Indications (Less General Agreement)

Abnormalities of placental shape
Long cord (>100 cm)
Marginal or velamentous cord insertion

Table 35.2 Placenta Weight Standards, Percentile by Gestational Age

Gestational Age (weeks)	Singletons (g)			Twins (Combined Weight, g)		
	10%	50%	90%	10%	50%	90%
12		56				
14		83				
16		110				
18		137.8				
20		145		166	218	270
22	122	157	191	191	251	310
24	145	189	233	232	307	382
26	175	227	280	284	380	475
28	210	270	331	345	464	584
30	249	316	384	409	554	700
32	290	364	438	472	644	815
34	331	411	491	531	727	923
36	372	457	542	582	798	1011
38	409	499	589	619	850	1082
40	442	537	632	638	879	1118

Placentas weighing less than the 10th percentile or greater than the 90th percentile are abnormal (cut-off weights in bold), and this should be included in the report, even in the absence of other gross or microscopic findings.

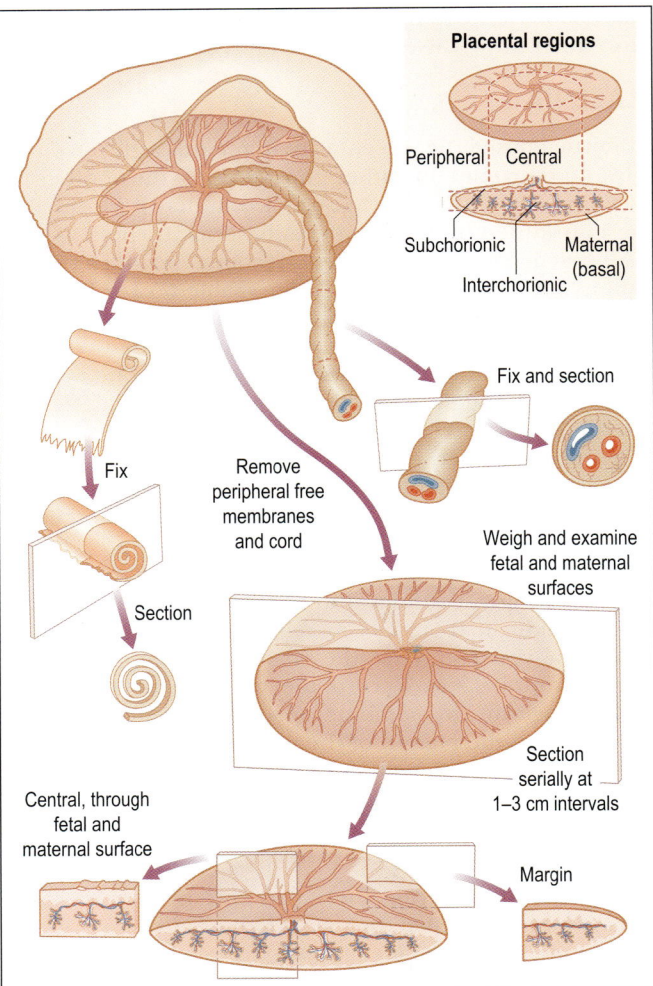

Figure 35.14 Placental examination. Adequate sampling for histologic study includes membrane roll, cross section of cord, and full thickness placental parenchyma, specifically cut to display fetal and maternal surfaces.[1]

- *Maternal surface.* Is the surface intact or disrupted? If disrupted, estimate whether all tissue is present. Record and describe any subchorionic fibrin, calcification, or blood clot. Describe well-defined depressions. Give the average thickness of the placental disc. Describe any succenturiate (accessory) lobes. Cross section the specimen and look for and describe lesions, infarcts, blood clots, masses, etc. For any abnormality identified, estimate the percentage of the area involved.
- *Tissue sections.* It is our preference to submit at least three sections for microscopic examination: (1) cross section of the umbilical cord; (2) membrane roll; and (3) cross section of full thickness normal parenchyma somewhere centrally. Other sections should be taken as appropriate.

TWIN PLACENTA

Determine the type of twin placenta, i.e., dichorionic diamniotic, monochorionic diamniotic, and monochorionic monoamniotic. Unless it is a monochorionic monoamniotic placenta, take a strip of the dividing membranes, roll it, fix, and then section (Figure 35.15). Sections of membrane away from the dividing membranes should also be rolled, fixed, and submitted. Examine, weigh, and cut the placenta (or placentas if not fused) as for a singleton placenta. If the placentas are fused, estimate the percentage each placenta constitutes of the total area, and note any differences in color between each placenta.

Monoamniotic twin placentas are uncommon and result in a high rate of fetal morbidity and mortality. These twins are always identical (monozygotic).

Monochorionic diamniotic placentas have two layers of amnion separating the two fetal sacs. These membranes are thin and can be easily stripped from the fetal surface leaving no trace. Careful examination of the fetal surface often reveals vascular anastomoses between the two fetal circulations. Injection of colored dye is a useful way to demonstrate vascular anastomoses before fixation. These twins are always identical.

Fused dichorionic diamniotic or separate twin placentas have amnion–chorion–amnion layers, which can be divided into three or sometimes four layers and are more opaque/white, often with visible blood vessels in the membranous position. The amnion layers can be easily stripped away, but the chorion is firmly attached and cannot easily be pulled away from the placental surface. Removal leaves a thin low ridge of firm tan tissue. Vascular anastomoses are absent. These twins may be identical or fraternal (dizygotic). If of the same sex, approximately 75% will be fraternal and 25% monozygotic or identical.

Similar principles apply to the examination of placentas from gestations greater than two (triplets, etc.).

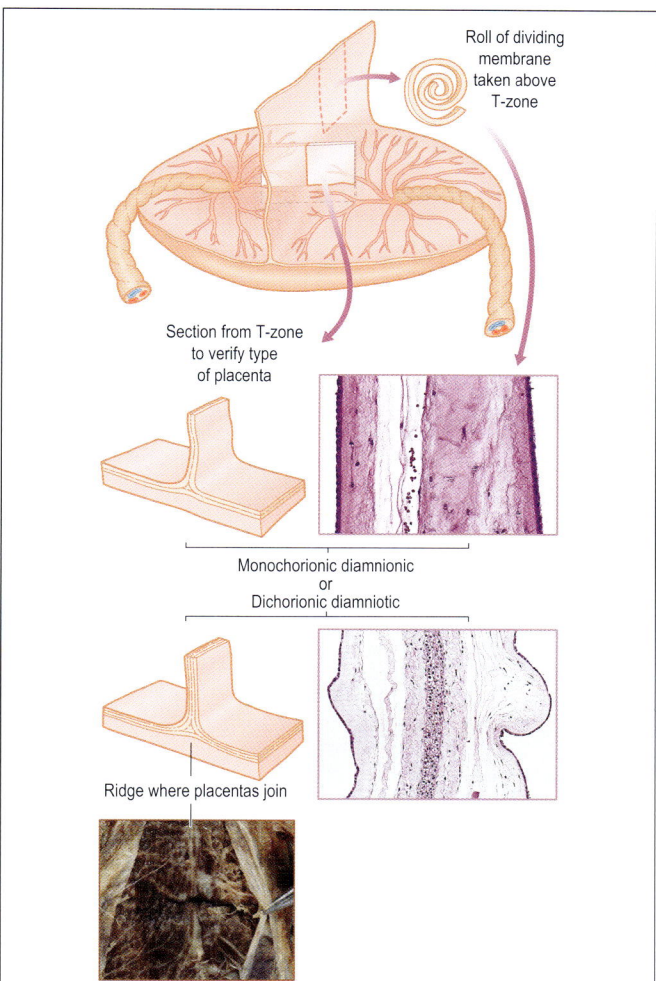

Figure 35.15 Examination of placenta of twins. Sampling of a twin placenta includes a section of septal membrane dividing the amniotic cavities, cut to display the T-zone, where the septal membrane attaches to the placental surface.[1]

REFERENCES

1. Lester SC. Manual of surgical pathology. 3rd ed. Philadelphia: Saunders; 2010.
2. Schmidt WA. Principles and techniques of surgical pathology. Menlo Park: Addison-Wesley; 1983.
3. Westra WH, Hruban RH, Phelps TH, Isacson C. Surgical pathology dissection: an illustrated guide. New York: Springer; 2003.
4. Greene LA, Branton P, Montag A, et al. Protocol for the examination of specimens from patients with carcinoma of the vulva. <http://www.cap.org/apps/docs/committees/cancer/cancer_protocols/2012/Vulva_12protocol_3101.pdf>/; 2012.
5. Black D, Tornos C, Soslow RA, et al. The outcomes of patients with positive margins after excision for intraepithelial Paget's disease of the vulva. Gynecol Oncol 2007;104:547–50.
6. Kalof AN, Dadmanesh F, Longacre TA, et al. Protocol for the examination of specimens from patients with carcinoma of the uterine cervix. <http://www.cap.org/apps/docs/committees/cancer/cancer_protocols/2012/Cervix_12protocol.pdf>; 2012.
7. Movahedi-Lankarani S, Gilks CB, Soslow R, et al. Protocol for the examination of specimens from patients with carcinoma of the endometrium. <http://www.cap.org/apps/docs/committees/cancer/cancer_protocols/2012/Endometrium_12protocol.pdf>; 2012.
8. Lutman CV, Havrilesky LJ, Cragun JM, et al. Pelvic lymph node count is an important prognostic variable for FIGO stage I and II endometrial carcinoma with high-risk histology. Gynecol Oncol 2006;102:92–7.
9. Crum CP, Drapkin R, Miron A, et al. The distal fallopian tube: a new model for pelvic serous carcinogenesis. Curr Opin Obstet Gynecol 2007;19:5.
10. Oliva E, Branton PA, Scully RE. Protocol for the examination of specimens from patients with carcinoma of the ovary. <http://www.cap.org/apps/docs/committees/cancer/cancer_protocols/2012/Ovary_12protocol.pdf>; 2012.
11. Kraus FT. Introduction: the importance of timely and complete placental and autopsy reports. Semin Diagn Pathol 2007;24:1–4.
12. Curtin WM, Krauss S, Metlay LA, Katzman PJ. Pathologic examination of the placenta and observed practice. Obstet Gynecol 2007;109:35–41.

36 Practical Biomarkers for Female Genital Tract Lesions

W. Glenn McCluggage

CHAPTER OUTLINE

Introduction	828	Neuroendocrine Markers	833
Broad Spectrum Differentiation Markers	828	Lymphoid Markers	834
Epithelial Markers	828	Markers Of Altered Function In Disease States	834
Mesenchymal Cell Markers	831	Tumor Markers	834
Smooth Muscle Markers	831	Tumor Suppressor Genes	836
Skeletal Muscle Markers	832	Proto-oncogenes	838
Endometrial Stromal Markers	832	Cell Cycle And Nuclear Proliferation	838
Mesothelial Markers	832	Hormone Receptors	839
Blood Vessel Markers	832	Cell Adhesion Markers	840
Narrow Spectrum Differentiation Markers	832	Other Markers	840
Trophoblastic Markers	833		
Melanocytic Markers	833		

INTRODUCTION

Recent years have witnessed a marked expansion in the use of immunohistochemical markers in gynecologic pathology.[1,2] Most relate to the use of antibodies in the diagnosis of gynecologic neoplasms but some markers have prognostic or predictive value. In general when immunohistochemistry is used diagnostically, panels of markers provide better information than reliance on a single antibody. As anticipated historically, most antibodies, although initially thought specific for a given tumor, later have proven to have a broader range of reactivity than is initially suspected, with reactivity in a more diverse set of tumor types. This chapter provides an overview of the antibodies commonly used in the diagnosis of gynecologic lesions grouped as to function or type. The value of markers as prognostic or predictive factors is discussed where appropriate, understanding only a handful are sufficiently informative to be used in routine practice. Different markers result in different staining patterns, for example nuclear, membranous, cytoplasmic, or a combination (Figure 36.1), and knowledge of the expected staining patterns is essential when interpreting immunohistochemical slides.

BROAD SPECTRUM DIFFERENTIATION MARKERS

The following biomarkers are commonly expressed in many cell types and are useful in a wide variety of settings and in differential diagnoses. In some cases, their combinations may be unique to a particular entity.

EPITHELIAL MARKERS

CYTOKERATINS

Cytokeratins (CKs) belong to the group of intermediate filament proteins that are intermediate between microfilaments and microtubules. They constitute the cytoskeletal structure of virtually all epithelial cells, both benign and malignant. Some nonepithelial cell types and tumors derived from these may also express CKs. The cytokeratin family of proteins, which are coded by different genes, has been numbered (numbers 1–20).[3] The expression of the various CKs in cells and tumors depends on their embryonic origin and also the degree of cellular differentiation.[3] One broad group of CKs, type I (CK9–20), has an acidic isoelectric point. The other group, type II (CK1–8), has a basic neutral

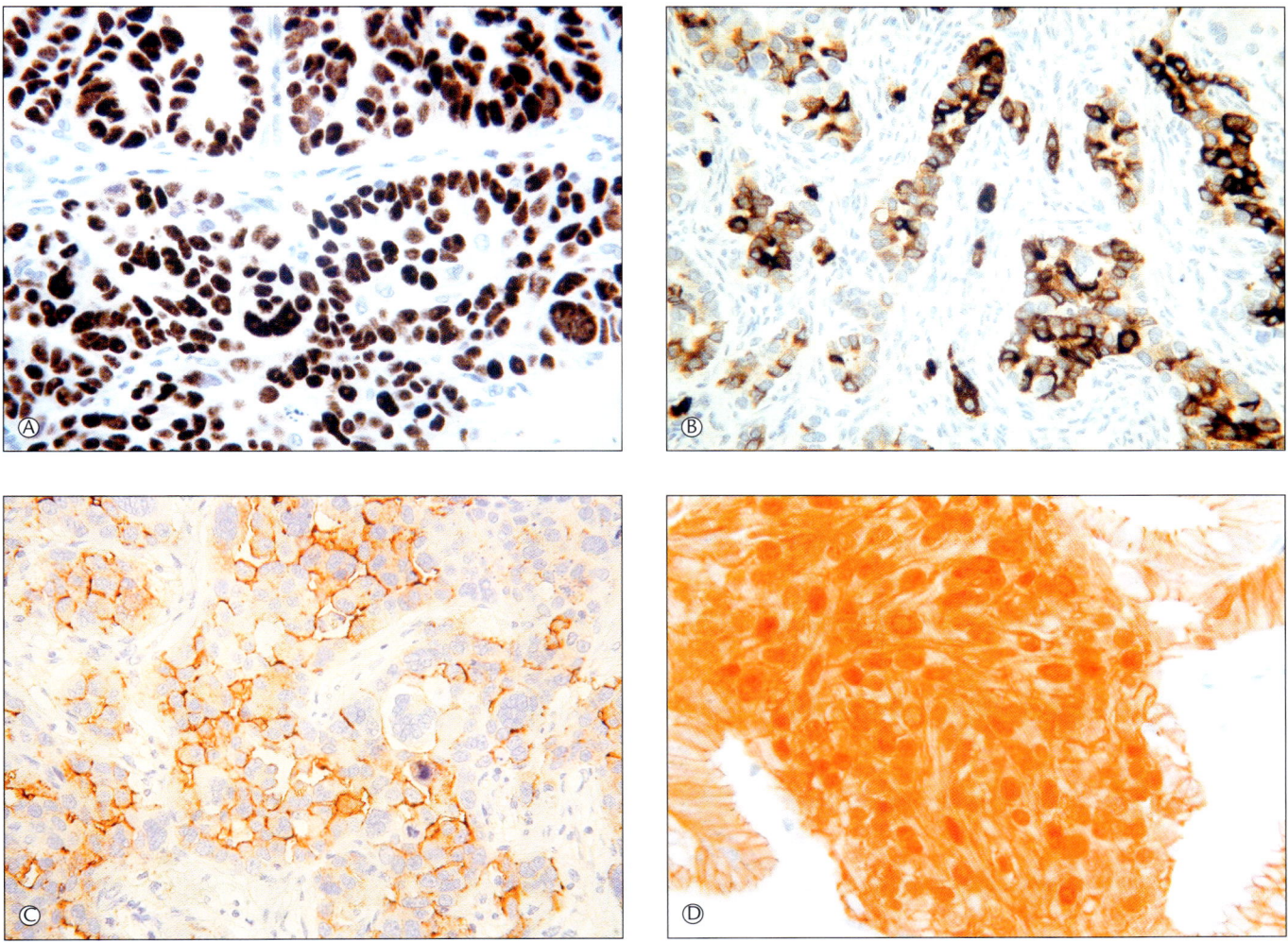

Figure 36.1 Different antibodies characteristically result in different patterns of immunoreactivity such as nuclear **(A)**, cytoplasmic **(B)**, membranous **(C)**, and a combination of nuclear, cytoplasmic, and membranous **(D)**.

isoelectric point. Antibodies against CKs help confirm the epithelial lineage of a neoplasm. In this regard, monoclonal antibodies, such as AE1/3 and CAM 5.2, are available that recognize multiple members of the CK family. AE1/3 reacts against almost all of the CK family of proteins (AE1 recognizes most of the type 1 CKs whereas AE3 reacts against most of the type II CKs) while CAM 5.2 reacts against CK8 and CK18. Additionally, antibodies are available that react against specific CKs, for example, CK7, CK20, or CK5/6. The following sections detail the use of various anti-CK antibodies in the diagnosis of female genital tract lesions.

BROAD SPECTRUM CYTOKERATINS

Broad spectrum anti-CK antibodies, such as AE1/3, often prove of value in confirming the epithelial lineage of a neoplasm. For example, in distinguishing a poorly differentiated carcinoma from sarcoma, melanoma, or lymphoma, reactivity with AE1/3, especially if widespread, favors a diagnosis of carcinoma. However, anti-CK antibodies, such as AE1/3, occasionally react with tumors of melanocytic, mesenchymal, and lymphoid origin.[4] Smooth muscle tumors may also react with anti-CK antibodies.[5] This may result in diagnostic difficulties, especially if dealing with an epithelioid smooth muscle neoplasm, and underscores the necessity of using panels of antibodies.

Endometrial stromal neoplasms may also be CK positive.[6] Broad spectrum anti-CK antibodies are reactive with trophoblastic cells and may be useful in distinguishing intermediate trophoblast from decidua, thus confirming the presence of a placental site.

CAM 5.2

CAM 5.2 does not react against normal squamous epithelium but is reactive against most glandular epithelia. It may help in the diagnosis of vulvar Paget disease, as the Paget cells usually react (the residual squamous cells do not), and this may help to exclude mimics such as melanocytic tumors, pagetoid Bowen's disease, and mycosis fungoides.

CK7 AND 20

A combination of antibodies against CK7 and 20 (differential CK staining) has been widely used in ovarian and peritoneal pathology to distinguish between a primary ovarian or peritoneal adenocarcinoma and a metastatic adenocarcinoma, especially of colorectal origin.[1,2,7–9] In general, primary ovarian carcinomas of serous, endometrioid, and

Table 36.1 Typical Reaction Patterns in Primary Ovarian and Metastatic Colorectal Adenocarcinoma

Antibody	Endometrioid Ovarian Adenocarcinoma	Mucinous Ovarian Adenocarcinoma	Colorectal Adenocarcinoma
CK7	Diffuse +	Diffuse or focal +	−
CK20	−	Neg, focal or diffuse +	Diffuse +
CA125	Diffuse +	−	−
CEA	−	Neg, focal or diffuse +	Diffuse +
β-Catenin	Neg, focal or diffuse +	−	Focal or diffuse +
CDX2	−	Neg, focal or diffuse +	Diffuse +
Villin	−	Neg, focal or diffuse +	Diffuse +
MUC5AC	Diffuse +	Diffuse +	−

clear cell type exhibit diffuse CK7 reactivity and are negative with CK20. Primary ovarian mucinous neoplasms exhibit a more variable immunophenotype. In general, they are diffusely reactive with CK7 and nonreactive or focally reactive with CK20. However, there are exceptions with occasional primary ovarian mucinous neoplasms, especially those of intestinal type, being diffusely CK20 positive. In the distinction between a primary ovarian endometrioid adenocarcinoma and a metastatic colorectal adenocarcinoma with an endometrioid appearance, differential CK staining is very useful alone or as part of a larger panel (Table 36.1). Endometrioid adenocarcinoma is usually diffusely CK7 reactive and CK20 negative while colonic carcinoma generally exhibits the opposite immunophenotype. In the case of an ovarian mucinous neoplasm, differential CK staining is not uncommonly difficult to interpret since many primary ovarian mucinous neoplasms may be CK20 reactive and mucinous colorectal adenocarcinoma may be focally CK7 positive. Rectal adenocarcinomas may also be CK7 positive. Additionally mucinous tumors arising in a teratoma often exhibit a large intestinal immunophenotype with diffuse CK20 immunoreactivity. In this regard, other antibodies (discussed in the following sections) are sometimes of value.

Differential CK staining is of limited value in distinguishing between a primary ovarian carcinoma and a metastatic adenocarcinoma from other organs, since many of these tumors exhibit a CK7-positive/CK20-negative or focally positive immunophenotype (Table 36.2). However, dual CK7 and CK20 reactivity raises the possibility of a primary neoplasm in the stomach, pancreas, biliary tree, or urinary bladder.[1,2,7–9] Breast, pulmonary, endometrial, and endocervical adenocarcinomas are most commonly CK7 positive and CK20 negative.

CK7 and CK20 staining also helps to confirm that most cases of pseudomyxoma peritonei in women are of appendiceal (or more rarely colorectal) origin rather than originating from a ruptured ovarian mucinous neoplasm.[10] In cases of pseudomyxoma peritonei with coexistent appendiceal and ovarian mucinous neoplasms, the epithelial elements in all locations, i.e., the appendix, ovary, and peritoneum, are usually diffusely CK20 positive and negative or focally positive with CK7, in keeping with an intestinal origin.

CK7 may be of value in the vulva in confirming a diagnosis of Paget disease and excluding mimics such as malignant

Table 36.2 Typical Differential Cytokeratin Reaction Patterns in Tumors

	CK7	CK20
Mucinous ovarian adenocarcinoma	+	− or +
Non-mucinous ovarian adenocarcinoma	+	−
Colorectal adenocarcinoma	−	+
Cervical adenocarcinoma	+	−
Endometrial adenocarcinoma	+	−
Pancreatic/biliary adenocarcinoma	+	+ or −
Gastric adenocarcinoma	+	+ or −
Renal cell carcinoma	−	−
Bladder adenocarcinoma	+	+ or −
Breast adenocarcinoma	+	−
Pulmonary adenocarcinoma	+	−
Mesothelioma	+	−

melanoma and mycosis fungoides. The cells of primary vulvar Paget disease are usually intensely CK7 positive,[11,12] a feature that may assist in assessment of margins. Strong CK20 reactivity should result in consideration of secondary Paget disease, from either the colorectum or urinary tract.[11,12]

CK5/6

CK5/6 is often reactive in mesothelial cells (benign or malignant) and is helpful to distinguish a mesothelial from a serous epithelial proliferation (benign, borderline, or malignant); the latter is usually negative.[13] In this regard, CK5/6 should be used as part of a panel that may include Ber-EP4 (an epithelial marker reactive in most epithelial lesions and generally negative in mesothelial lesions). Other antibodies generally reactive in mesothelial lesions are calretinin, HBME1, thrombomodulin, D2-40, and CD44H (generally negative in epithelial lesions).[13,14] CK5/6 is more likely to be positive in squamous than glandular neoplasms and this may be useful in diagnosis.

OTHER CYTOKERATINS

Although the remaining specific CKs have found little place in diagnostic gynecologic pathology, there are a few exceptions. Staining with the high molecular weight CK34β E12 may assist in highlighting the basal cell layer in ectopic prostatic tissue within the cervix.[15] CK18 is especially likely to be positive in undifferentiated endometrial carcinoma and this marker may be useful in distinguishing undifferentiated endometrial carcinoma from undifferentiated sarcoma.[16]

EPITHELIAL MEMBRANE ANTIGEN AND BER-EP4

Epithelial membrane antigen (EMA), a glycoprotein found in human milk fat globule membranes, and Ber-EP4, an epithelial-specific antigen to a membrane-bound glycoprotein, help to confirm that a neoplasm has an epithelial lineage. Trophoblast and trophoblastic neoplasms are also reactive. Both markers are commonly used in panels to distinguish an ovarian adenocarcinoma (reactive) from a sex cord–stromal tumor (negative).[1,2,17] Ber-EP4 is useful in distinguishing a serous proliferation of the ovary or peritoneum (reactive) from mesothelial derived lesions (negative). Although EMA reactivity is rare in ovarian sex cord–stromal tumors, focal immunoreactivity has been found in 50% of a small series of juvenile granulosa cell tumors.[18] EMA is generally negative in female adnexal tumor of wolffian origin (FATWO). This is diagnostically useful since FATWO may be confused with an epithelial neoplasm, which is usually EMA reactive. EMA is often positive in undifferentiated endometrial carcinoma and may be useful in distinguishing this from undifferentiated sarcoma.[16]

MESENCHYMAL CELL MARKERS

VIMENTIN

Vimentin is the most widely distributed of the intermediate filament proteins and is expressed in virtually all mesenchymal cells, and most mesenchymal neoplasms in the female genital tract. In most cases the distinction of whether a tumor is mesenchymal or epithelial is apparent from the H&E-stained slide, but, when this is not obvious, vimentin staining may be useful, although vimentin positivity is not uncommon in epithelial neoplasms.

In the cervix, vimentin may be used as an aid to distinguish between tuboendometrial metaplasia and endometriosis (usually vimentin reactive) and adenocarcinoma *in situ* (AIS) (usually vimentin negative).[19] Vimentin may also be useful in differentiating between an endometrial adenocarcinoma of endometrioid type and an endocervical adenocarcinoma of usual type.[20] The former usually exhibits diffuse vimentin reactivity whereas endocervical adenocarcinomas are generally negative.

Vimentin may help distinguish between a microglandular variant of endometrioid or mucinous adenocarcinoma of the endometrium (usually vimentin reactive) and cervical microglandular hyperplasia (vimentin negative).[21]

SMOOTH MUSCLE MARKERS

The three most common smooth muscle markers are alpha smooth muscle actin (α-SMA), desmin, and h-caldesmon. These are helpful in several diagnostic scenarios, especially in confirming smooth muscle differentiation within a neoplasm within the female genital tract. Some smooth muscle neoplasms, especially malignant and epithelioid variants, are negative or only focally reactive.[22] h-Caldesmon is the most specific, but is less sensitive than desmin. However, it

Table 36.3 Typical Reaction Patterns in Endometrial Stromal and Smooth Muscle Neoplasm

Antibody	Smooth Muscle Neoplasm	Endometrial Stromal Neoplasm
Desmin	Diffuse +	– or focal +
α-SMA	Diffuse +	Neg, focal or diffuse +
h-Caldesmon	Diffuse +	–
CD10	Neg, focal or diffuse +	Diffuse +
Oxytocin receptor	Diffuse +	–

should be kept in mind that some tumors that may mimic smooth muscle neoplasms, such as gastrointestinal stromal tumor (GIST), may be h-caldesmon positive.[23] Desmin is not a specific smooth muscle marker, as it also stains skeletal muscle.

In the uterus, the main value of smooth muscle markers is in establishing a diagnosis of a smooth muscle neoplasm, either benign or malignant. An antibody panel composed of desmin, h-caldesmon, and CD10 (discussed later) helps distinguish cellular and other morphologically problematic leiomyomatous neoplasms from endometrial stromal neoplasms[24,25] (Table 36.3). In general, leiomyomatous neoplasms are diffusely reactive with desmin and h-caldesmon. CD10 is usually negative or focally reactive, although some cellular leiomyomatous neoplasms and leiomyosarcomas may be diffusely reactive. Endometrial stromal neoplasms are usually diffusely CD10 reactive and desmin and h-caldesmon usually negative. Sometimes, desmin and h-caldesmon, are focally positive, although occasional examples are diffusely positive, especially with desmin. α-SMA is of limited value since many endometrial stromal neoplasms are diffusely reactive. Uterine tumor resembling ovarian sex cord tumor, sex cord-like areas within endometrial stromal neoplasms, and uterine perivascular epithelioid cell tumor (PEComa) are also variably reactive with smooth muscle markers.[26]

In the cervix, α-SMA may be useful in distinguishing normal endocervical glands or non-neoplastic endocervical glandular lesions from the well-differentiated glands of adenoma malignum. The presence of many α-SMA reactive stromal cells suggests a desmoplastic response to tumor.[27]

In the vulvovaginal region, many of the wide range of relatively site-specific mesenchymal neoplasms such as angiomyofibroblastoma, aggressive angiomyxoma, and superficial myofibroblastoma of the lower female genital tract react with smooth muscle markers, especially desmin.[28] Thus, none of these markers are of value in confirming that a mesenchymal lesion represents a leiomyomatous neoplasm. However, negative staining with smooth muscle markers is of value in diagnosing cellular angiofibroma which, in contrast to most other neoplasms in the differential diagnosis, does not usually react.[28]

Another tumor that commonly shows reactivity with desmin is intra-abdominal desmoplastic small round cell tumor (IADSRCT; in females this may clinically mimic a primary ovarian neoplasm), usually with paranuclear dot-like immunoreactivity.[29] This is useful in diagnosis, especially in differentiating this neoplasm from the wide range of 'small blue cell tumors' that may involve the ovary and peritoneum. Desmin sometimes assists in the distinction between benign and malignant mesothelial proliferations. Benign mesothelial cells are usually desmin reactive while the cells of malignant mesothelioma are generally negative, although there is significant overlap.

SKELETAL MUSCLE MARKERS

A variety of skeletal muscle markers are available, including myoglobin, myogenin, myoD1, and sarcomeric actin. These assist in confirming rhabdomyosarcomatous differentiation within a neoplasm such as carcinosarcoma. Embryonal rhabdomyosarcomas are rare in general in the female genital tract and are most common in the vagina where the differential diagnosis usually includes the 'small blue cell tumors of childhood.' Rhabdomyosarcomas of embryonal, alveolar, and pleomorphic types rarely arise in the cervix, uterine corpus, or ovary. Myogenin and myoD1 are markers which have been generated against intranuclear transcription factors.[30] They are relatively specific nuclear markers of skeletal muscle and are the antibodies of choice in demonstrating skeletal muscle differentiation within a neoplasm, having superseded myoglobin and sarcomeric actin.

ENDOMETRIAL STROMAL MARKERS

CD10

CD10, or the common acute lymphoblastic leukemia antigen, is a cell-surface neutral endopeptidase expressed by lymphoid precursor cells and B-lymphoid cells of germinal center origin. Antibodies against CD10 are widely used in lymphoma panels.

CD10 is useful in diagnosing an endometrial stromal neoplasm, since most endometrial stromal nodules and endometrial stromal sarcomas (low-grade endometrial stromal sarcomas) exhibit diffuse intense reactivity, although fibrous variants may be negative.[24,25] In the distinction between an endometrial stromal and a smooth muscle neoplasm, CD10 should be used as part of a panel (Table 36.3), since conventional uterine smooth muscle tumors may be focally reactive and it is not uncommon for cellular and highly cellular leiomyomas (which are not infrequently mistaken for endometrial stromal neoplasms) and leiomyosarcomas to be diffusely reactive.

CD10 is also characteristically reactive in mesonephric glandular lesions within the female genital tract. Mesonephric remnants throughout the female genital tract usually exhibit luminal CD10 reactivity.[31,32] CD10 reactivity in a benign cervical glandular lesion is good evidence of a mesonephric origin,[31] although so-called ectopic prostatic tissue may also be reactive.[15] However, CD10 is of limited value in confirming a mesonephric origin for an adenocarcinoma since many cervical and endometrial adenocarcinomas are also reactive.[31] FATWO may be CD10 reactive.[33]

Other uses of CD10 staining in gynecologic pathology include the distinction between a metastatic renal clear cell carcinoma involving the ovary (CD10 reactive)[34] and a primary ovarian clear cell carcinoma (usually CD10 negative). In addition, most trophoblastic cell populations and trophoblastic neoplasms are reactive.[32] A wide range of other gynecologic neoplasms may be CD10 reactive, including leiomyosarcoma, carcinosarcoma, undifferentiated uterine sarcoma, ovarian sex cord–stromal tumors, uterine tumors resembling ovarian sex cord tumor, and mixed tumor of the vagina.[35] However, CD10 immunoreactivity in these neoplasms is inconsistent and unlikely to be of diagnostic value. In summary, CD10 is expressed in a much wider range of gynecologic neoplasms than was originally appreciated and, when used as an aid to diagnosis, should always be part of a panel, which will depend on the differential diagnoses under consideration.

MESOTHELIAL MARKERS

CALRETININ

Calretinin is a 29 kDa calcium-binding protein, best known for its role in the diagnosis of mesothelioma. In the distinction between a mesothelioma and an adenocarcinoma, calretinin should be used as part of a panel. Calretinin and Ber-EP4 are the two most useful antibodies to distinguish between a serous epithelial and a mesothelial proliferation.[14] Most serous proliferations are Ber-EP4 reactive and calretinin negative; the converse is the rule for mesothelial lesions. Nuclear reactivity with calretinin is more specific than cytoplasmic staining for mesothelial cells.[14]

Calretinin is also expressed in most ovarian sex cord–stromal tumors, being more sensitive but less specific than inhibin.[36,37] Calretinin is more likely to be reactive in an ovarian fibroma than inhibin.

In general, neoplasms reactive for inhibin also show reactivity with calretinin. Other gynecologic neoplasms that may show calretinin reactivity include FATWO, uterine tumor resembling ovarian sex cord tumor, sex cord-like areas within endometrial stromal neoplasms, and adenomatoid tumor. Mesonephric lesions, both benign and malignant, within the cervix and elsewhere in the female genital tract may show reactivity.[31]

BLOOD VESSEL MARKERS

CD34

CD34, a single chain transmembrane glycoprotein, leukocyte differentiation antigen, is expressed by hematopoietic progenitor cells, endothelial cells, and connective tissue cells, such as skin fibroblasts. CD34 is variably expressed in several vulvovaginal mesenchymal lesions, including aggressive angiomyxoma, cellular angiofibroma, and superficial myofibroblastoma of the lower female genital tract.[28] Solitary fibrous tumors rarely occur at various sites within the female genital tract and are CD34 reactive. Endometrial stromal neoplasms are usually CD34 negative, which may be of use in differential diagnosis in that many mimics are reactive.[38] Metastatic GIST in the ovary is usually CD34 positive,[23] as are rare primary GISTs arising in the rectovaginal septum or elsewhere in the female genital tract.[39]

NARROW SPECTRUM DIFFERENTIATION MARKERS

These are cell-type specific (pathognomonic) markers that are often useful to confirm or exclude specific lineage.

TROPHOBLASTIC MARKERS

A major application of broad spectrum CKs, as discussed previously, is simple confirmation of the presence or absence of an implantation site. Because trophoblastic cells are reactive for keratin and decidual stroma is not, keratin reactivity is an easy method to identify trophoblast in uterine or extra-uterine products of conception. CK is more robust than beta human chorionic gonadotropin (β-hCG) or human placental lactogen (hPL), and the intensity is uniform throughout gestation. The value of inhibin and CD10 as trophoblastic markers is discussed elsewhere.

β-hCG

hCG is a glycoprotein comprising a protein core and a carbohydrate side chain, and composed of two dissimilar subunits, α and β. The α-subunits are indistinguishable from the α-subunits of luteinizing hormone, follicle-stimulating hormone, and thyroid-stimulating hormone. The β-subunits differ and confer specificity.

β-hCG reacts against syncytiotrophoblast but not cytotrophoblast. Choriocarcinoma shows the strongest and most diffuse reactivity. Placental site trophoblastic tumor (PSTT) and epithelioid trophoblastic tumor are less reactive. Trophoblastic elements in mixed germ cell tumors show reactivity, as do isolated syncytiotrophoblast cells in neoplasms such as dysgerminoma and endometrial carcinoma. β-hCG may be reactive on occasions in a variety of nontrophoblastic neoplasms, such as cervical squamous carcinoma.[40]

PLACENTAL ALKALINE PHOSPHATASE

Placental alkaline phosphatase (PLAP) is a dimer of 65 kDa subunits and is synthesized during the G_1 phase of the cell cycle. PLAP is expressed in syncytiotrophoblast and in some intermediate trophoblastic populations. Reactivity is stronger in lesions derived from chorion-type intermediate trophoblast, such as placental site nodule, than in lesions of implantation site intermediate trophoblast which are usually only focally positive. Ovarian dysgerminoma is also reactive.

HUMAN PLACENTAL LACTOGEN

Human placental lactogen (hPL), a member of the gene family that includes human growth hormone and human prolactin, is expressed in intermediate trophoblast, and is useful in panels to diagnose trophoblastic neoplasms. In general, expression is stronger and more diffuse in placental site trophoblastic tumor than in choriocarcinoma.

Mel-CAM (CD146)

Mel-CAM is expressed in implantation site intermediate trophoblastic cells.[41] Chorion-type intermediate trophoblastic cells are usually negative or focally reactive. Placental site trophoblastic tumor and exaggerated placental site, lesions of implantation site intermediate trophoblast, express Mel-CAM, whereas placental site nodule and epithelioid trophoblastic tumor, lesions of chorion-type intermediate trophoblast, are usually negative. In distinguishing placental site trophoblastic tumor from exaggerated placental site, double immunohistochemical staining with Mel-CAM and MIB1 is of value.[41] In exaggerated placental site, the MIB1 index in intermediate trophoblastic cells is close to zero whereas it is significantly elevated (14 ± 6.9%) in placental site trophoblastic tumor.[41]

HLA-G

HLA-G is expressed in all known trophoblastic tumors, including choriocarcinoma, placental site trophoblastic tumor, and epithelioid trophoblastic tumor, as well as in benign trophoblastic lesions, such as placental site nodule and exaggerated placental site.[42] HLA-G is generally negative in nontrophoblastic uterine neoplasms.[64] HLA-G reactivity has been demonstrated in some ovarian carcinomas.[43]

MELANOCYTIC MARKERS

HMB45

HMB45 is probably the most specific marker of malignant melanoma, and it is melanosome associated. HMB45 reactivity is useful to confirm the diagnosis of malignant melanoma at any site within the female genital tract, most commonly in the vulva or vagina. Metastatic melanoma in the ovary can assume an unusual array of morphologic appearances and easily fool the pathologist if there is no history of melanoma. HMB45 may assist in this regard. However, occasional ovarian steroid cell tumors, which may mimic melanoma, are HMB45 reactive.[44] Another neoplasm characteristically reactive with HMB45 is PEComa.[26] This is an uncommon neoplasm, which in the female genital tract most often involves the myometrium.[41] Uterine epithelioid leiomyosarcomas with a clear cell appearance may also express HMB45.[45]

MELAN-A (MART-1)

Melan-A, also known as MART-1, is another melanocytic marker of value in the diagnosis of malignant melanoma. Ovarian sex cord–stromal tumors are also commonly reactive.[46]

S-100

S-100 is useful in the diagnosis of malignant melanoma, either primary or metastatic, at various sites within the female genital tract. Other neoplasms in the female genital tract that may be S-100 positive include ovarian sex cord–stromal tumors and cartilaginous areas within carcinosarcomas.

NEUROENDOCRINE MARKERS

There are various neuroendocrine markers in widespread use, including chromogranin, CD56, synaptophysin, and PGP9.5. These vary in their specificity and sensitivity. For example, chromogranin is a highly specific but poorly sensitive marker while CD56 is sensitive but lacks specificity. Reactivity with neuroendocrine markers is not necessary to establish a diagnosis of a small cell neuroendocrine carcinoma since many of these are sparsely granulated and negative with neuroendocrine markers. In contrast, reactivity with neuroendocrine markers is a prerequisite for a diagnosis of large cell neuroendocrine carcinoma. Rarely paraganglioma and typical and atypical carcinoid occur within the female genital tract and are reactive. A high percentage of ovarian sex cord–stromal tumors are CD56 positive.[47]

Undifferentiated uterine carcinomas may be focally positive with neuroendocrine markers.[16]

LYMPHOID MARKERS

Markers against lymphoid cells are of value in diagnosing rare hematopoietic malignancies, either lymphoma or leukemia, within the female genital tract.

Several markers may assist in the diagnosis of a low-grade endometritis, which usually depends on the morphologic identification of plasma cells that may be difficult to visualize with H&E when few in number. In the normal endometrium, most lymphoid cells are of T-cell or natural killer (NK) cell lineage. B-lymphocytes account for less than 1% of endometrial leukocytes, and are mainly located in lymphoid aggregates. In endometritis, the number of T-lymphocytes and NK cells does not differ from controls. However, the use of B-lymphoid markers, such as CD20 and CD79a, reveals substantially increased numbers of B-cells in unusual locations such as beneath the surface epithelium and intraepithelially.[48] Markers against plasma cells, such as syndecan and VS38, may also assist in diagnosing endometritis.[49]

MARKERS OF ALTERED FUNCTION IN DISEASE STATES

The expression of the following markers usually indicates a disease state and therefore helps in distinguishing normal from disease states. The pattern of aberrant expression may be pathognomonic for a particular disease state, and thus useful in resolving a differential diagnosis.

TUMOR MARKERS

CA19.9

CA19.9, an antigen of sialyl Lewis(a) containing glycoprotein, is usually reactive in pancreatic, biliary, and colorectal adenocarcinoma metastatic to the ovary whereas most primary ovarian adenocarcinomas of serous, endometrioid, or clear cell type are negative, although some serous carcinomas are focally positive. Primary ovarian mucinous neoplasms are commonly focally or diffusely reactive.

CARCINOEMBRYONIC ANTIGEN

Carcinoembryonic antigen (CEA) consists of a heterogeneous family of related oncofetal glycoproteins secreted into the glycocalyceal surface of gastrointestinal cells.

Monoclonal CEA helps distinguish non-mucinous ovarian adenocarcinomas (usually negative) from colorectal adenocarcinoma (usually reactive), when used as part of a panel.[1,2] Primary ovarian mucinous neoplasms are often reactive. Adenocarcinomas from other organs, such as pancreas and stomach, are variably reactive.

CEA is useful as part of a panel to help distinguish endometrioid-type endometrial adenocarcinoma from endocervical adenocarcinoma of usual type.[20] Endocervical adenocarcinomas are usually, but not always, diffusely reactive with CEA. Primary endometrioid adenocarcinomas of the corpus are negative or focally reactive, although the associated squamous elements may be diffusely reactive. CEA staining patterns of primary mucinous adenocarcinoma of the endometrium are not well studied, but at least a proportion are reactive. CEA is usually reactive in cervical AIS and negative in benign endocervical glandular lesions.[50]

CEA is usually reactive in primary vulvar Paget disease and, like CK7 and CAM 5.2, helps exclude mimics and assess margins.

CA125 (OC125)

CA125 is a mucin-like glycoprotein, commonly elevated in patients with ovarian cancer, especially of serous type. Although elevated levels are not specific for an ovarian cancer, serum CA125 measurements may be useful in diagnosis and especially in the follow-up of patients with ovarian cancer.

Immunohistochemical staining with CA125 helps to distinguish between a primary and a metastatic ovarian adenocarcinoma and in the evaluation of a disseminated peritoneal tumor in a female.[1,2] In general, primary ovarian (or peritoneal) adenocarcinomas of serous, endometrioid, and clear cell types exhibit diffuse CA125 reactivity. Primary ovarian mucinous carcinomas are usually negative, as are colorectal adenocarcinomas. In distinguishing primary ovarian adenocarcinoma from a metastatic colorectal adenocarcinoma, CA125 should be used in a panel (Table 36.2) that could include CK7, CK20, estrogen receptor (ER), CDX2, and CEA. CA125 reactivity is not specific for an ovarian adenocarcinoma, as primary adenocarcinomas of many other organs, including pancreas, breast, lung, cervix, and uterine corpus exhibit reactivity in a proportion of cases. Mesotheliomas are commonly reactive, as are benign mesothelial cells.[51]

INHIBIN

Inhibin is a dimeric 32 kDa peptide hormone composed of an α- and a β-subunit and produced by ovarian granulosa and theca cells. Individual antibodies are available against each subunit. Most ovarian sex cord–stromal tumors show focal to diffuse cytoplasmic reactivity with inhibin (antibody against α-subunit), although fibroma, poorly differentiated Sertoli–Leydig, and sarcomatoid granulosa cell tumors are sometimes negative.[52,53] Since ovarian sex cord–stromal neoplasms may be morphologically confused with a wide range of neoplasms, especially endometrioid carcinomas, immunohistochemical evaluation with inhibin (and other sex cord–stromal markers such as calretinin) may be extremely useful in primary diagnosis and also when confirming a metastatic neoplasm, which may occur years or decades later. In distinguishing between a sex cord–stromal tumor and an endometrioid carcinoma, the former is almost always negative with EMA[17] (Table 36.4). Ovarian sex cord–stromal tumors are usually negative with CK7 but may be focally positive with broad spectrum anti-CK antibodies. Most carcinomas are negative with inhibin, although occasional tumors are focally reactive. Activated ovarian stromal cells that occur in association with and at the periphery of any ovarian neoplasm may be reactive with sex cord–stromal markers, so close attention must be paid to the cellular morphology of the particular clusters that are immunohistochemically reactive.

Inhibin staining may also be of use in the evaluation of aspirates of ovarian cysts.[54] Reactivity of the cells in an aspirate with inhibin and negative staining with EMA helps

Table 36.4 Antibodies of Value in Distinguishing between Ovarian Endometrioid Adenocarcinoma and Sex Cord–Stromal Tumor

Antibody	Endometrioid Adenocarcinoma	Sex Cord–Stromal Tumor
CK7	+	−
EMA	+	−
α-Inhibin	−	+
Calretinin	− or +	+
Steroidogenic factor 1	−	+
Broad spectrum CKs	Diffuse +	− or focal +

confirm the presence of granulosa cells, indicating a follicular rather than an epithelial lined cyst. Inhibin may also help to demonstrate luteinized stromal cells in cases of ovarian stromal hyperthecosis, or in association with ovarian neoplasms of non-sex cord–stromal type that have resulted in androgenic or estrogenic manifestations.[55]

Other gynecologic neoplasms that are variably reactive with inhibin include FATWO, cervical mesonephric adenocarcinoma, uterine tumor resembling ovarian sex cord tumor, and sex cord-like areas within endometrial stromal neoplasms.[31,56] Inhibin also stains some trophoblastic cell populations, syncytiotrophoblast, and some intermediate trophoblastic cells showing reactivity while cytotrophoblast is negative.[57] Choriocarcinoma and other trophoblastic neoplasms, such as placental site trophoblastic tumor and epithelioid trophoblastic tumor, may be inhibin reactive. β-Inhibin is less useful diagnostically than α-inhibin since many ovarian and extraovarian carcinomas are reactive.[58]

OCT3/4

OCT3/4 is an octamer binding transcription factor expressed in both mouse and human embryonic stem and germ cells. Nuclear reactivity is present in ovarian dysgerminoma and embryonal carcinoma and in the germ cell component of gonadoblastoma.[59] Most ovarian epithelial and sex cord–stromal tumors are unreactive, although occasional clear cell carcinomas are positive.[59] As clear cell carcinoma and dysgerminoma often superficially resemble each other, OCT3/4 reactivity must be assessed with caution.

HIK1083

HIK1083, a monoclonal antibody against gastric/pyloric gland mucins, is reactive in cervical minimal deviation adenocarcinoma of mucinous type (adenoma malignum) and primary cervical adenocarcinoma of gastric type.[60,61] Focal reactivity may be present in ordinary endocervical adenocarcinomas and less well-differentiated areas in adenoma malignum may be negative.

The benign endocervical glandular lesion lobular endocervical glandular hyperplasia, which can mimic adenoma malignum and which is also considered to exhibit gastric differentiation, may also be reactive with HIK1083.[60]

CDX-2

CDX-2 is a gene that encodes for a transcription factor involved in the development and differentiation of the small and large intestines. Colorectal adenocarcinomas usually exhibit diffuse nuclear reactivity with antibodies against *CDX-2*[62] and this may be useful, as part of a panel, in distinguishing between a primary ovarian adenocarcinoma and a metastatic colorectal adenocarcinoma. However, occasional primary ovarian endometrioid adenocarcinomas exhibit *CDX-2* reactivity, as do some primary ovarian mucinous tumors, chiefly those of intestinal type.[62] *CDX-2* is also commonly expressed in intestinal type AIS in the cervix and in some cervical adenocarcinomas, including those of intestinal type.[63] *CDX-2* has been shown to be almost invariably expressed in squamous morules in endometrioid proliferative lesions of the uterus or ovary.[64] *CDX-2* positivity in the cells of vulvar Paget disease suggests secondary Paget disease from a primary colorectal adenocarcinoma.

ALPHA-FETOPROTEIN

Alpha-fetoprotein (α-FP) is a glycoprotein composed of 590 amino acid residues present in yolk sac tumors and some cases of hepatocellular carcinoma. In the female genital tract, α-FP helps to establish a diagnosis of yolk sac tumor. Primary hepatoid carcinomas of the ovary, metastatic hepatocellular carcinoma, and metastatic hepatoid carcinomas from other organs may also be reactive. Some Sertoli–Leydig cell tumors in the ovary express α-FP and are associated with an elevated α-FP serum level.[65]

Hep-PAR1

Hep-PAR1 is expressed in most ovarian hepatoid yolk sac tumors, primary ovarian hepatoid carcinomas, and hepatoid carcinomas metastatic to the ovary.[66] Hep-PAR1 is of no value in distinguishing any of these tumors from each other. Occasional cervical carcinomas, of either glandular or squamous type, also express Hep-PAR1.[67]

MUC ANTIBODIES

Mucins are high molecular weight glycoproteins. Several mucin genes have been identified or cloned (*MUC1–MUC12*) and monoclonal antibodies to these are available. Expression of the mucin gene *MUC5AC* helps distinguish colonic adenocarcinoma metastatic to the ovary (nonreactive) from a primary ovarian adenocarcinoma (reactive).[7,68] Appendiceal and pancreatic adenocarcinomas typically express *MUC5AC*.[7,68] Colorectal adenocarcinomas express *MUC2*. *MUC2* expression in vulvar Paget's disease favors an underlying colorectal adenocarcinoma.[69] *MUC2* reactivity is also useful to confirm that pseudomyxoma peritonei is of appendiceal origin.[71] *MUC6* (along with HIK1083) is often positive in so-called primary cervical adenocarcinomas of gastric type.[60,61]

CD99

The CD99 antigen, or MIC2 gene product, is a cell-surface glycoprotein that is involved in cell adhesion. CD99 is important in antibody panels used to diagnose small round blue cell tumors.

In the female genital tract, CD99 helps establish the diagnosis of a tumor in the Ewing family or peripheral primitive neuroectodermal tumor, which has rarely been described in the ovary, uterus, cervix, and vulva.[72] The reactivity should be membranous. Cytoplasmic reactivity is less specific. Ovarian sex cord–stromal tumors also commonly exhibit membranous CD99 reactivity, as may uterine tumor resembling ovarian sex cord tumor and sex cord-like areas within endometrial stromal neoplasms.[73]

THYROID TRANSCRIPTION FACTOR 1

Thyroid transcription factor 1 (TTF1) is a 38 kDa nuclear protein member of the NKx2 family of homeodomain transcription factors, which is positive in thyroid neoplasms and in primary pulmonary adenocarcinomas and neuroendocrine neoplasms. It may be useful in the ovary (in combination with thyroglobulin) in diagnosing unusual morphologic variants of struma ovarii. It may also be useful in helping to confirm a diagnosis of a metastatic pulmonary adenocarcinoma. In the female genital tract, TTF1 is often positive in cervical small cell and large cell neuroendocrine carcinomas, sometimes with diffuse immunoreactivity,[74] and is of no value in distinguishing these from a lung metastasis. Studies have shown that a not insignificant proportion of primary gynecologic adenocarcinomas of uterine, cervical, and ovarian origin may be TTF1 positive, including some with diffuse immunoreactivity.[75] Cervical mesonephric adenocarcinomas may also be positive.[76] This illustrates that TTF1 nuclear immunoreactivity in an adenocarcinoma is not always indicative of a pulmonary primary. Some normal epithelia in the female genital tract may be TTF1 positive.[77]

PROSTATIC-SPECIFIC ANTIGEN AND PROSTATIC ACID PHOSPHATASE

Prostatic-specific antigen and prostatic acid phosphatase are positive in cases of so-called ectopic prostatic tissue in the cervix and in vaginal tubulosquamous polyp.[15,78] It is probable that these are part of the same spectrum of lesions and derived from misplaced periurethral Skene glands.[79] The latter are the female equivalent of prostatic glands in the male and may exhibit immunoreactivity with prostatic markers.

GLYPICAN 3

Glypican 3 has emerged as a useful marker of yolk sac tumor or yolk sac areas in a mixed gonadal or extragonadal germ cell tumor.[80] Positive staining is cytoplasmic and membranous. Glypican 3 appears a more sensitive and specific marker of yolk sac tumor than α-FP. Positive staining is restricted to areas of yolk sac tumor, all patterns of yolk sac tumor are positive, staining is more widespread than with α-FP, and there is less background staining. Some ovarian clear cell carcinomas (44% in one study) are also glypican 3 positive.[81]

SALL 4

SALL 4 is a marker of primitive gonadal and extragonadal germ cell tumors.[82] There is nuclear immunoreactivity in yolk sac tumor, embryonal carcinoma, dysgerminoma, and some immature teratomas. SALL 4 is a more sensitive marker of yolk sac tumor than α-FP; all patterns of yolk sac tumor are positive, staining is more widespread, and there is less background staining.

STEROIDOGENIC FACTOR 1

Steroidogenic factor 1 (SF-1) is a sensitive and useful nuclear marker of ovarian sex cord–stromal tumors with all morphologic subtypes positive while most mimics, such as endometrioid adenocarcinoma and carcinoid tumor, are negative.[83]

ALK1

Occasional inflammatory myofibroblastic tumors of the uterus have been described and these are ALK1 positive with cytoplasmic staining.[84]

HER-2/NEU

Human epidermal growth factor receptor 2 (HER-2/NEU) is a 185 kDa transmembrane tyrosine kinase receptor with close homology to the epidermal growth factor receptor. Many cases of primary vulvar Paget disease overexpress HER-2/NEU, and anti- HER-2/NEU antibodies such as trastuzumab may be a treatment option.[85] Similarly some uterine serous carcinomas overexpress HER-2/NEU,[86] as well as some ovarian carcinomas, especially of mucinous type.[87]

TUMOR SUPPRESSOR GENES

WT1

The *WT1* gene is a tumor suppresser gene located on the short arm of chromosome 11 at p13. It was first reported as a candidate for the main gene implicated in Wilms' tumor development and *WT1* immunohistochemical expression is found in normal tissues of ovary, kidney, testis, spleen, and mesothelium. *WT1* is expressed in a number of malignancies, including malignant mesothelioma and IADSRCT.

Antibodies are available against both the C terminal and the N terminal of *WT1* and nuclear staining is regarded as positive. Nonspecific cytoplasmic staining may be seen in many diverse neoplasms as well as in endothelial cells and mesenchymal tissues. IADSRCT, in most cases, is reactive with antibodies against the C terminal rather than the N terminal. This may be useful in diagnosis and in the distinction of IADSRCT from the other small blue cell tumors that rarely may involve the ovary and peritoneum.[88]

Primary ovarian, peritoneal, and tubal serous carcinomas are usually *WT1* positive (antibody against N terminal).[89,90] In a poorly differentiated ovarian carcinoma, nuclear *WT1* reactivity, especially when diffuse, favors a serous neoplasm since most endometrioid, clear cell, and mucinous carcinomas are negative. Transitional and undifferentiated carcinomas of the ovary are also commonly *WT1* reactive, providing evidence that many are variants of high-grade serous carcinoma.[91] With a disseminated serous carcinoma involving more than one site, diffuse reactivity with *WT1* favors an ovarian, peritoneal, or tubal primary. Most uterine serous carcinomas are unreactive or only focally reactive, although the literature is somewhat contradictory and some cases are positive.[89,90,92]

When disseminated adenocarcinoma involves the abdomen and peritoneal cavity in a female, diffuse nuclear *WT1* reactivity strongly favors a serous carcinoma arising from the ovary, peritoneum, or fallopian tube. Most pancreatic, biliary, gastric, breast, and colorectal carcinomas are *WT1* negative. In this regard *WT1* should be employed as one element of a panel of markers.

Table 36.5 Antibodies of Value in Distinguishing between Ovarian Small Cell Carcinoma of Hypercalcemic Type and Juvenile Granulosa Cell Tumor

Antibody	Ovarian Small Cell Carcinoma of Hypercalcemic Type	Juvenile Granulosa Cell Tumor
WT1 (N terminal)	Diffuse + (intense)	– or focal + (weak)
α-Inhibin	–	Diffuse or focal +
EMA	Focal +	– or focal +

Ovarian small cell carcinoma of hypercalcemic type is usually reactive with an antibody against the N terminal of *WT1* (Table 36.5).[88] As this small cell tumor can morphologically resemble adult or juvenile granulosa cell tumor, a panel of antibodies to *WT1*, inhibin, and EMA may be of value. However, it is cautioned that some ovarian granulosa cell tumors of adult and juvenile type are *WT1* positive.

Other neoplasms involving the female genital tract that may be *WT1* reactive include malignant mesothelioma, adenomatoid tumor, endometrial stromal neoplasms, leiomyomatous tumors, and a variety of ovarian sex cord–stromal tumors.[93]

WT1 is commonly positive with nuclear immunoreactivity in müllerian smooth muscle neoplasms and may be useful in distinguishing between a müllerian and non-müllerian smooth muscle tumor.[94]

DPC4

Deleted in Pancreatic Cancer, locus 4 (*DPC4*; also known as *SMAD4*), is a tumor suppressor gene that is inactivated by allelic loss in approximately 50% of pancreatic cancers. Such cases lack immunohistochemical staining.[7] In contrast, primary ovarian, colorectal, and appendiceal carcinomas are usually *DPC4* reactive since there is no allelic loss.[7] Since pancreatic adenocarcinoma metastatic to the ovary may closely mimic a primary ovarian mucinous neoplasm, evaluation of *DPC4* reactivity is helpful diagnostically.

p53

p53 is a tumor suppressor gene, located on the short arm of chromosome 17, which encodes a 35 kDa nuclear protein involved in regulating cell growth. Mutated *p53* gene (*TP53* mutation) is among the most commonly detected genetic abnormalities in human neoplasia. Mutations result in a conformational change of the protein, which becomes stabilized, thus allowing for immunohistochemical detection. The most widely used anti-*p53* antibody is D07. Usually, but not always, diffuse intense nuclear reactivity is found whenever *TP53* mutation occurs. It has also been shown that totally absent *p53* staining may be associated with underlying *TP53* mutation (usually nonsense mutation, in contrast to missense mutation, which results in diffuse staining) and that it is this 'all or nothing' staining that is aberrant and of diagnostic importance and associated with *TP53* mutation.[95,96] In contrast, 'wild-type' staining with a focal, weak, and heterogeneous pattern occurs in many tumors and in normal tissues and is not associated with *TP53* mutation.

Diffuse intense nuclear *p53* reactivity or total absence of staining is characteristic of uterine serous carcinoma.[1,2,97] *p53* may also help identify the presumed precursor lesion of serous carcinoma, namely serous endometrial intraepithelial carcinoma (serous EIC), which exhibits diffuse or totally absent staining. This is often a subtle lesion that not uncommonly involves an endometrial polyp. *p53* helps distinguish serous carcinoma and serous EIC from benign papillary endometrial proliferations and metaplasias, a problem most likely to be encountered in small endometrial biopsies. Diffuse *p53* reactivity is much more common in uterine leiomyosarcomas than benign leiomyomatous neoplasms, including symplastic or atypical leiomyoma.[98]

In ovarian carcinomas, aberrant *p53* function (diffuse *p53* reactivity or total absence of staining) is more common in high-grade serous and undifferentiated carcinomas than in other morphologic subtypes.[99–101] *TP53* mutation occurs early in the evolution of high-grade ovarian serous carcinoma, having been identified in microscopic ovarian or tubal high-grade serous carcinomas, and in its putative precursor lesion, serous tubal intraepithelial carcinoma (serous TIC).[102]

In the vulva, *p53* helps distinguish classic (undifferentiated, usual) vulvar intraepithelial neoplasia (VIN; 'wild-type' staining) from differentiated (simplex) VIN. Strong *p53* reactivity extending above the basal cell layer favors differentiated VIN,[103] although *p53* reactivity may also be seen in the basal cell layers in lichen sclerosus in the absence of differentiated VIN.[104]

p63

The *p63* gene is a transcription factor that belongs to the *p53* family. The *p63* protein has six isoforms, three each classified into two groups, designated TA and Δ N *p63*.[105] Cytotrophoblast expresses the Δ N *p63* isoform whereas chorion-type intermediate trophoblast in the fetal membranes, placental site nodule, and epithelioid trophoblastic tumor express the TA *p63* isoform.[105] Intermediate trophoblast in the implantation site and placental site trophoblastic tumor do not express *p63*. Most commercially available antibodies react against all *p63* isoforms. In the cervix, *p63* is preferentially expressed in immature cells of squamous lineage and in basal and reserve cells.[106]

p63 helps distinguish cervical small cell neuroendocrine carcinoma (negative or focally reactive) from poorly differentiated and small cell nonkeratinizing squamous carcinoma (positive).[106] However, in one study a small number of cervical neuroendocrine carcinomas were *p63* positive.[74]

In ovarian neoplasms, *p63* reactivity is largely confined to transitional neoplasms, including benign, borderline, and some malignant Brenner tumors.[107]

PTEN

PTEN (phosphatase and tensin homolog deleted on chromosome 10) is a tumor suppresser gene mutated in a high percentage of endometrioid adenocarcinomas of the endometrium.[108] *PTEN* mutation is generally associated with loss of *PTEN* immunohistochemical staining.[109] *PTEN* is also mutated in some endometrioid adenocarcinomas of the ovary.[110] *PTEN* mutation occurs early in the development of endometrioid-type endometrial adenocarcinoma since mutation with associated absence of staining has been found in 66% of the cases of the precursor lesion, termed endometrial intraepithelial neoplasia (EIN) in one classification scheme and atypical endometrial hyperplasia in another. *PTEN*-null glands also occur not uncommonly in normal cyclical endometrium[109] and therefore a lack of reactivity cannot be used to diagnose EIN or atypical endometrial hyperplasia. Furthermore, not all cases of EIN exhibit an absence of *PTEN* reactivity and in other cases loss of expression precedes the development of morphologic features of EIN. The most widely used anti-*PTEN* antibody is 6H2.1. The *PTEN*-null rate in endometrial adenocarcinoma varies by tumor subtype, ranging from a low of 13% of serous cancers to 83% of those endometrioid tumors preceded by an EIN lesion.[109]

PROTO-ONCOGENES

Bcl-2

Bcl-2, a proto-oncogene located on chromosome 18, encodes a 25 kDa protein mainly localized to the inner mitochondrial membrane. This extends cell survival by blocking apoptosis.

In proliferative endometrium, bcl-2 is diffusely expressed in the glandular cytoplasm. The activity is reduced in the glands of both atypical hyperplasia and endometrioid-type adenocarcinomas.[111] In the cervix, bcl-2 is normally expressed in the basal cell layer of the squamous epithelium. Normal fallopian tube epithelium is bcl-2 reactive,[112] as are foci of ciliated metaplasia involving the ovarian surface epithelium and the epithelium of cortical inclusion cysts.[112]

Tuboendometrial metaplasia and endometriosis in the cervix generally exhibit diffuse cytoplasmic reactivity, which helps distinguish them from AIS, which is generally negative.[113] Endometrial stromal neoplasms are commonly bcl-2 reactive, but this is of limited value since many other tumors included in the differential diagnosis are also reactive.[38] A subset of uterine leiomyosarcomas overexpressed bcl-2 may be associated with a good prognosis.[114]

CD117 (C-Kit)

CD117, a transmembrane tyrosine kinase receptor, is expressed in metastatic GIST within the ovary[23] and in rare primary GISTs arising in the rectovaginal septum, uterine corpus, or elsewhere in the female genital tract.[39] Some gynecologic sarcomas, including leiomyosarcoma,[115,116] may focally express CD117, as occasionally do other tumors, including uterine carcinosarcoma and ovarian serous carcinoma. Dysgerminoma commonly exhibits diffuse membranous immunoreactivity.

CELL CYCLE AND NUCLEAR PROLIFERATION

KI-67 (MIB1) AND PROLIFERATING CELL NUCLEAR ANTIGEN

The best known markers of cell proliferation are MIB1 (reactive against the Ki-67 antigen) and proliferating cell nuclear antigen (PCNA). MIB1 identifies all cells in non-G_0 phases of the cell cycle, in other words in all proliferating cells. PCNA expression is highest during the S-phase of the cell cycle but due to a relatively long half-life persists in cells that are no longer cycling and are in G_0.

Cervical squamous intraepithelial lesions exhibit an increased MIB1 proliferation index.[117] In normal squamous epithelium, MIB1 reactivity is largely confined to the basal and parabasal layers, with substantial to nearly full thickness reactivity in high-grade squamous intraepithelial lesion (HSIL). Its major use is to distinguish between HSIL and benign mimics such as atrophic squamous epithelium, transitional metaplasia, and immature squamous metaplasia.

Similarly in endocervical AIS the proliferation index is in excess of 30%, in comparison with its benign mimics such as tuboendometrial metaplasia, endometriosis, and microglandular hyperplasia, which usually exhibit a proliferation index <10%.[113] Because there may be quantitative overlap at the lower end of the AIS and upper end of the benign spectrum, MIB1 should form part of a panel including p16.

In the vulva, MIB1 has some utility in evaluating squamous lesions.[118] Human papillomavirus (HPV) infection of the vulva is associated with clusters of MIB1 reactive cells in the middle and upper thirds of the epithelium,[118] which helps to definitively categorize a lesion in which an equivocal diagnosis of condyloma might be made. The cells of high-grade VIN of classic type express MIB1 throughout much of the full epithelial thickness, which helps distinguish high-grade VIN from atrophic squamous epithelium.

Proliferation markers have been used in the assessment of trophoblastic lesions. In chorionic villi, reactivity with proliferation markers is largely confined to villous cytotrophoblast. MIB1 aids in distinguishing PSTT from an exaggerated placental site.[41] In the former, the MIB1 index is significantly elevated (14 ± 7%) whereas it is nearly zero in the latter.[41] Care should be taken to exclude reactivity in small lymphocytes. MIB1 also helps distinguish PSTT from choriocarcinoma, since the latter exhibits a much higher proliferation index.[41]

p16

p16, also known as cyclin-dependent kinase-4 inhibitor (CDK4-I), is the product of the *INK4-A* gene and specifically binds to cyclin D-CDK4/6 complexes to control the cell cycle at the G_1–S interphase. In the cervix, diffuse p16 staining usually, but not always, correlates with the presence of high-risk HPV; in other words, diffuse p16 staining is a surrogate for the presence of high-risk HPV.[119,120] Thus, there is diffuse p16 expression (usually a combination of nuclear and cytoplasmic staining) in most HSILs.[119,120] In cervical squamous lesions, p16 may help identify small focal areas of HSIL and distinguish immature squamous metaplasia from HSIL involving immature metaplastic squamous epithelium.[120]

p16 may be useful in diagnosing endocervical AIS, which is usually diffusely reactive, and distinguishing this from mimics such as tuboendometrial metaplasia and endometriosis, which are either negative or focally reactive.[113,121] In this regard, p16, MIB1, and bcl-2 can be used as part of a panel (Table 36.6).

p16 helps distinguish endocervical adenocarcinoma of usual type, which exhibits diffuse reactivity, from endometrial adenocarcinoma of endometrioid type, which is generally negative or focally reactive.[122] The squamous elements

Table 36.6 Antibodies of Value in Distinction between Cervical Tuboendometrial Metaplasia and Endometriosis and AIS

Antibody	Tuboendometrial Metaplasia/ Endometriosis	Cervical AIS
MIB1	<30%	>50%
Bcl-2	Diffuse +	–
p16	– or focal +	Diffuse +

in endometrial adenocarcinomas may be strongly reactive. Some cases of uterine corpus endometrioid adenocarcinoma will exhibit diffuse reactivity with p16 but even in these cases there are usually admixed positive and negative areas, a so-called mosaic staining pattern. Many endometrial and ovarian high-grade serous carcinomas also react diffusely with p16.[123]

p16 is useful to distinguish metastatic cervical adenocarcinoma in the ovary (p16 reactive) from primary ovarian endometrioid or mucinous adenocarcinoma (usually, but not always, p16 negative).[124] In the vulva, p16 reactivity is characteristic of classic VIN, since this disease is associated with HPV infection. Differentiated VIN is usually p16 negative since there is no association with HPV. Similarly, HPV-associated vulvar squamous carcinomas are p16 reactive while those not associated with HPV are negative.[125] p16 is much more strongly expressed in uterine leiomyosarcomas than leiomyomas, including morphologically problematic variants, and this may be useful in diagnosis.[97]

p57

p57, also known as Kip2, is a cell cycle inhibitor of cell proliferation and tumor suppressor encoded by a strongly paternally imprinted, maternally expressed gene. p57 is only expressed when maternal DNA is present. A particular use is in the distinction of complete hydatidiform mole from partial hydatidiform mole and hydropic abortion. p57 is expressed in the nuclei of the cytotrophoblast and villous mesenchyme in the normal placenta, hydropic abortion, and partial mole since all have a maternal component.[126,127] In contrast, p57 is absent in the complete mole, since these villi are paternally derived and lack maternal DNA. Positive reactivity in decidua and extravillous trophoblast (it is not known why extravillous trophoblast reacts) acts as an internal positive control.

CYCLIN D1

Cyclin D1 is positive in normal endocervical glands while staining is typically lost in premalignant and malignant endocervical glandular lesions.[128] However, there may be focal nuclear immunoreactivity in adenocarcinomas, especially at the invasive front.[129] A similar staining pattern is seen in some endometrial adenocarcinomas and it has been suggested that cyclin D1 is upregulated in areas of epithelial–mesenchymal transition at the advancing edge of endometrial and cervical adenocarcinomas. In the former, these often correspond to glands exhibiting a microcystic, elongated, and fragmented (MELF) pattern of myometrial invasion.[130]

CYCLIN E

Cyclin E is useful in the distinction between an epithelioid trophoblastic tumor and a placental site nodule, two lesions derived from the intermediate trophoblast of the chorion laeve (chorionic-type intermediate trophoblast).[131] There is much higher cyclin E immunostaining in epithelioid trophoblastic tumor than in placental site nodule.[131]

ProExC

ProExC is a cocktail of antibodies against minichromosome maintenance protein 2 (MCM2) and topoisomerase II-α, which are key proteins overexpressed in the nucleus during aberrant S-phase induction of the cell cycle. ProExC is useful in the evaluation of premalignant cervical squamous lesions (reliable marker of HSIL) and glandular lesions (useful in distinction between AIS and benign glandular mimics).[132,133] It may also be useful in the diagnosis of high-grade VIN of classic type. Positive staining is limited to the basal and parabasal layers of normal cervical and vulvar squamous epithelium but extends higher in the squamous epithelium in accordance with the degree of cervical intraepithelial neoplasia or VIN.[134]

HORMONE RECEPTORS

ESTROGEN RECEPTOR AND PROGESTERONE RECEPTOR

Many native normal tissues and tumors arising within the female genital tract exhibit reactivity with antibodies against estrogen receptor (ER) and progesterone receptor (PR). There are several situations in which these markers have diagnostic value.

Most of the vulvovaginal mesenchymal lesions react with ER and PR, including aggressive angiomyxoma, angiomyofibroblastoma, cellular angiofibroma, superficial myofibroblastoma of the lower female genital tract, and smooth muscle neoplasms.[28,135] Therefore, ER and PR do not assist in distinguishing between these neoplasms, most of which are thought to arise from the zone of hormone receptor-positive subepithelial cells that extend from the cervix to the vulva. The fact that aggressive angiomyxoma is often hormone receptor positive is the rationale for treating these neoplasms with gonadotropin-releasing hormone agonists, especially recurrent neoplasms and those tumors not amenable to surgical resection.[136]

Endometrial cancers of endometrioid type are commonly ER and PR reactive, whereas serous and clear cell carcinomas are often negative. However, there is considerable immunophenotypic overlap and a significant percentage of serous carcinomas are ER and/or PR positive, especially ER.[92] In spite of this, diffuse strong nuclear reactivity with ER and PR favors an endometrioid adenocarcinoma whereas negative staining or focal reactivity suggests a serous carcinoma. In practice it is useful to combine ER and PR with *p53*, the latter usually being diffusely reactive or totally negative in serous carcinomas and exhibiting 'wild-type' staining in endometrioid cancers. Similarly, a combination of ER, PR, and *p53* may help distinguish problematic benign papillary proliferations from a small uterine serous carcinoma or

Table 36.7 Typical Reaction Patterns of Endometrial Adenocarcinoma of Endometrioid Type and Endocervical Adenocarcinoma

Antibody	Endometrioid Type Endometrial Adenocarcinoma	Endocervical Adenocarcinoma
ER	Diffuse +	− or focal +
Vimentin	Diffuse +	−
Monoclonal CEA	− or focal +	Diffuse or focal +
p16	− or focal +	Diffuse +

serous EIC. Endometrial metaplasias usually exhibit a weak heterogeneous pattern of *p53* staining whereas serous EIC generally exhibits diffuse intense reactivity. Many other uterine neoplasms may be ER and PR positive, including endometrial stromal and smooth muscle neoplasms, both benign and malignant.

ER, as part of a panel (Table 36.7), helps differentiate endometrioid adenocarcinoma of the endometrium from endocervical adenocarcinoma.[20] This may be a difficult distinction to make when tumor is present in both endometrial and cervical biopsies or in a hysterectomy specimen where tumor involves both the corpus and cervix. Endometrial adenocarcinomas of endometrioid type are generally diffusely ER reactive while endocervical adenocarcinomas are negative or at most focally reactive, although occasional well-differentiated cervical adenocarcinomas are diffusely positive. In a panel with vimentin, monoclonal CEA, and p16,[20] endometrioid-type endometrial adenocarcinomas are usually vimentin reactive, CEA negative, or focally reactive and p16 negative, or focally reactive. In contrast, endocervical adenocarcinomas are usually vimentin negative and diffusely reactive with CEA and p16. Squamous elements in endometrioid adenocarcinomas of the uterus may be both CEA and p16 reactive. Molecular techniques, such as *in situ* hybridization or polymerase chain reaction, to demonstrate HPV may also be of value. Endometrioid adenocarcinoma of the corpus is HPV negative, whereas endocervical adenocarcinoma of usual type is usually positive.[137]

Another situation in which ER and PR may be of diagnostic value is the distinction between a primary ovarian adenocarcinoma and a secondary adenocarcinoma from outside the female genital tract. In general, ER and/or PR reactivity suggests an ovarian primary, although some primary ovarian adenocarcinomas are negative. Approximately 70–80% of ovarian serous carcinomas are positive with ER and/or PR (more commonly ER), as are most endometrioid adenocarcinomas. Most clear cell and mucinous carcinomas are negative. However, ER and PR are of no value in the distinction between a primary ovarian adenocarcinoma and a metastasis from the breast or from elsewhere within the female genital tract. Many mucinous carcinomas of ovarian or non-ovarian origin exhibit nonspecific cytoplasmic staining with PR.

ANDROGEN RECEPTOR

In both the cervix and vagina, androgen receptor is reactive in mesonephric remnants and ectopic prostatic tissue.[15] Normal endocervical glands are usually negative, although the expression of androgen receptor in the wide range of benign endocervical glandular lesions has not been extensively studied. Normal cervical and vaginal stromal fibroblasts are androgen receptor positive.[15] Other neoplasms in the female genital tract found to express androgen receptor in a variable percentage of cases include endometrial adenocarcinoma, endometrial stromal sarcoma, cervical mesonephric adenocarcinoma, and FATWO.[138]

OXYTOCIN RECEPTOR

Oxytocin receptor is present in the nonpregnant uterus, in both the endometrium and myometrium. An antibody against oxytocin receptor helps to distinguish a uterine smooth muscle tumor (oxytocin receptor reactive) from an endometrial stromal neoplasm (oxytocin receptor negative).[139]

CELL ADHESION MARKERS

β-CATENIN

β-Catenin may be a useful addition to the panel of antibodies employed to distinguish between a primary ovarian adenocarcinoma and a metastatic colorectal adenocarcinoma.[140] Most, but not all, colorectal adenocarcinomas exhibit nuclear reactivity while the majority of primary ovarian mucinous neoplasms are negative. Primary ovarian endometrioid adenocarcinomas may exhibit nuclear reactivity since they can be associated with β-catenin gene mutation and the squamous morules are almost invariably positive, as are squamous morules in endometrioid proliferations within the uterus.[64] Membranous β-catenin staining is the norm in epithelial cells and only nuclear reactivity is of diagnostic value. β-Catenin nuclear staining occurs in a significant percentage of uterine low-grade endometrial stromal sarcomas.[141]

E-CADHERIN

There is loss of E-cadherin membranous staining at the invasive front of some uterine endometrioid adenocarcinomas exhibiting a MELF pattern of myometrial invasion and this may be a form of epithelial–mesenchymal transition. E-cadherin (but not β-catenin) nuclear staining has been demonstrated in a high percentage of ovarian adult granulosa cell tumors and in the granulosa cells of developing ovarian follicles.[142]

OTHER MARKERS

PAX8

PAX8 is a paired-box gene important in embryogenesis of the thyroid, müllerian, and renal/upper urinary tracts. In the female genital tract, PAX8 is typically positive with nuclear immunoreactivity in non-mucinous ovarian carcinomas, including those of serous, endometrioid, and clear cell types, and endometrial and cervical adenocarcinomas.[143] It may be useful as part of a panel in the distinction between an ovarian carcinoma of serous or endometrioid type (PAX8 positive) and a breast carcinoma (PAX8 negative).[143,144] It may also be useful in the distinction between a serous neoplasm (PAX8 positive) and a mesothelial proliferation (PAX8 negative).[145] Cervical mesonephric adenocarcinomas are commonly positive.[76]

PAX2

PAX2 encodes a transcription factor necessary in the development of the wolffian and müllerian duct systems. In the cervix, *PAX2* is strongly and diffusely expressed with nuclear immunoreactivity in mesonephric remnants, normal endocervical glands, and in benign glandular lesions.[146] In contrast, most cervical adenocarcinomas and AIS are negative. Inactivation of the *PAX2* gene with loss of expression has been demonstrated in endometrial precancers and cancers.[147]

HMGA2

The architectural transcription factor *HMGA2* (formerly known as HMGIC), a high-mobility group AT-hook (HMGA) protein, is a nonhistone DNA-binding factor and binds to AT-rich sequences in the minor groove of the DNA helix. *HMGA2* is expressed in embryonic tissues, but not in most adult tissues. It is an important regulator of cell growth, differentiation, apoptosis, and malignant transformation. *HMGA2* is overexpressed in a variety of epithelial and mesenchymal neoplasms.

The best known application of *HMGA2* staining in surgical pathology is in the diagnosis of vulvovaginal aggressive angiomyxoma. In this lesion, rearrangements involving the *HMGA2* gene at chromosome 12q15 can cause overexpression. In one study, 11 of 13 aggressive angiomyxomas exhibited nuclear positivity, usually diffuse, with this marker.[148] It has also been shown that there is *HMGA2* nuclear reactivity in most cases of ovarian and uterine serous carcinoma and in serous tubal intraepithelial carcinoma.[149,150] Since serous EIC is also positive, *HMGA2* abnormalities may be involved early in the pathogenesis of uterine serous carcinoma. Cervical mesonephric adenocarcinomas may be positive with this marker.[75]

HEPATOCYTE NUCLEAR FACTOR 1-β

Hepatocyte nuclear factor 1-beta (HNF1-β) was identified from large-scale gene expression studies as being a useful marker of ovarian and uterine clear cell carcinomas.[151] Both tumor types exhibit nuclear immunoreactivity with this marker while most, but not all, of the other morphologic subtypes are negative.

FOXL2

Mutation of the *FOXL2* gene is present in a high percentage of ovarian adult granulosa cell tumors and only rarely in other variants of ovarian sex cord–stromal tumors.[152] Mutations have not been demonstrated in ovarian epithelial neoplasms. There is nuclear staining with *FOXL2* in a high percentage (80%) of ovarian sex cord–stromal tumors, including many without the mutation.[153] In one large study, all epithelial neoplasms were negative and *FOXL2* staining was found to be 99% specific for a sex cord–stromal tumor.[153] Occasional FATWO origin and uterine tumors resembling ovarian sex cord tumor were positive.[153]

IMP-3 AND IMP-2

Insulin-like growth factor II mRNA-binding protein 3 (IMP-3) is an oncofetal protein highly expressed in fetal tissue and malignant tumors but rarely found in adult benign tissues. It is highly expressed in uterine serous carcinomas and, when used as part of a panel, is useful in the distinction from an endometrioid adenocarcinoma.[154] It has also been shown that IMP-2 may be of value in this scenario since uterine serous carcinomas are diffusely positive while there is variable loss of staining in endometrioid adenocarcinomas.[155]

DOG1

Discovered on gastrointestinal stromal tumor 1 (DOG1) is a sensitive and specific marker of gastrointestinal stromal tumors and may be useful, combined with CD117, in the diagnosis of primary and metastatic gastrointestinal stromal tumor within the female genital tract, although a variety of other neoplasms are occasionally positive.[70]

REFERENCES

1. McCluggage WG. Recent advances in immunohistochemistry in the diagnosis of ovarian neoplasms. J Clin Pathol 2000;53:327–34.
2. McCluggage WG. Recent advances in immunohistochemistry in gynaecological pathology. Histopathology 2002;40:309–26.
3. Heatley MK. Cytokeratins and cytokeratin staining in diagnostic histopathology. Histopathology 1996;28:479–83.
4. Ben-Izhak O, Stark P, Levy R, et al. Epithelial markers in malignant melanoma. A study of primary lesions and their metastases. Am J Dermatopathol 1994;16:241–6.
5. Norton AJ, Thomas JA, Isaacson PG. Cytokeratin-specific monoclonal antibodies are reactive with tumours of smooth muscle derivation. An immunocytochemical and biochemical study using antibodies to intermediate filament cytoskeletal proteins. Histopathology 1987;11:487–99.
6. Adegboyega PA, Qiu S. Immunohistochemical profiling of cytokeratin expression by endometrial stromal sarcoma. Hum Pathol 2008;39:1459–64.
7. Ji H, Isacson C, Seidman JD, et al. Cytokeratins 7 and 20, DPC4, and MUC5AC in the distinction of metastatic mucinous carcinomas in the ovary from primary ovarian mucinous tumors: Dpc 4 assists in identifying metastatic pancreatic carcinomas. Int J Gynecol Pathol 2002;21:391–400.
8. Ladendijk JA, Mullink EH, van Diest PJ, et al. Tracing the origin of adenocarcinomas with unknown primary using immunohistochemistry. Differential diagnosis between colonic and ovarian carcinomas as primary sites. Hum Pathol 1998;29:491–7.
9. Chu P, Wu E, Weiss LM. Cytokeratin 7 and cytokeratin 20 expression in epithelial neoplasms: a survey of 435 cases. Mod Pathol 2000;13:962–72.
10. Ronnett BM, Shmookler BM, Diener-West M, et al. Immunohistochemical evidence supporting the appendiceal origin of pseudomyxoma peritonei in women. Int J Gynecol Pathol 1997;16:1–9.
11. Goldblum JR, Hart WR. Vulvar Paget's disease: a clinicopathologic and immunohistochemical study of 19 cases. Am J Surg Pathol 1997;21:1178–87.
12. Goldblum JR, Hart WR. Perianal Paget's disease—a histologic and immunohistochemical study of 11 cases with and without associated rectal adenocarcinoma. Am J Surg Pathol 1998;2:170–1.
13. Cury PM, Butcher DN, Fisher C, et al. Value of the mesothelium-associated antibodies thrombomodulin, cytokeratin 5/6, calretinin, and CD44H in distinguishing epithelioid pleural mesothelioma from adenocarcinoma metastatic to the pleura. Mod Pathol 2000;13:107–12.
14. Attanoos RL, Webb R, Dojcinov SD, Gibbs AR. Value of mesothelial and epithelial antibodies in distinguishing diffuse peritoneal

mesothelioma in females from serous papillary carcinoma of the ovary and peritoneum. Histopathology 2002;40:237–44.
15. McCluggage WG, Ganesan R, Hirschowitz L, et al. Ectopic prostatic tissue in the uterine cervix and vagina: report of a series with a detailed immunohistochemical analysis. Am J Surg Pathol 2006;30:209–15.
16. Silva EG, Deavers MT, Malpica A. Undifferentiated carcinoma of the endometrium: a review. Pathology 2007;39:134–8.
17. Costa MJ, De Rose PB, Roth LM, et al. Immunohistochemical phenotype of ovarian granulosa cell tumors: absence of epithelial membrane antigen has diagnostic value. Hum Pathol 1994;25:60–6.
18. McCluggage WG. Immunoreactivity of ovarian juvenile granulosa cell tumours with epithelial membrane antigen. Histopathology 2005;46:235–6.
19. Marques T, Andrade LA, Vassallo J. Endocervical tubal metaplasia and adenocarcinoma in situ: role of immunohistochemistry for carcinoembryonic antigen and vimentin in differential diagnosis. Histopathology 1996;28:549–50.
20. McCluggage WG, Sumathi VP, McBride HA, et al. A panel of immunohistochemical stains, including carcinoembryonic antigen, vimentin and estrogen receptor aids the distinction between primary endometrial and endocervical adenocarcinomas. Int J Gynecol Pathol 2002;21:11–5.
21. Qiu W, Mittal K. Comparison of morphologic and immunohistochemical features of cervical microglandular hyperplasia with low-grade mucinous adenocarcinoma of the endometrium. Int J Gynecol Pathol 2003;22:261–5.
22. Oliva E, Young RH, Amin MB, Clement PB. An immunohistochemical analysis of endometrial stromal and smooth muscle tumors of the uterus: a study of 54 cases emphasizing the importance of using a panel because of overlap in immunoreactivity for individual antibodies. Am J Surg Pathol 2002;26:403–12.
23. Irving JA, Lerwill MF, Young RH. Gastrointestinal stromal tumors metastatic to the ovary: a report of five cases. Am J Surg Pathol 2005;29:920–6.
24. Nucci MR, O'Connell JT, Huettner PC, et al. h-Caldesmon expression effectively distinguishes endometrial stromal tumors from uterine smooth muscle tumors. Am J Surg Pathol 2001;25:253–8.
25. McCluggage WG, Sumathi VP, Maxwell P. CD10 is a sensitive and diagnostically useful immunohistochemical marker of normal endometrial stroma and of endometrial stromal neoplasms. Histopathology 2001;39:273–8.
26. Vang R, Kempson RL. Perivascular epithelioid cell tumour (PEComa) of the uterus : a subset of HMB-45 positive epithelioid mesenchymal neoplasms with an uncertain relationship to pure smooth muscle tumors. Am J Surg Pathol 2002;26:1–13.
27. Mikami Y, Kiyokawa T, Moriya T, Sasano H. Immunophenotypic alteration of the stromal component in minimal deviation adenocarcinoma ('adenoma malignum') and endocervical glandular hyperplasia: a study using oestrogen receptor and alpha-smooth muscle actin double immunostaining. Histopathology 2005;46:130–6.
28. McCluggage WG. A review and update of morphologically bland vulvovaginal mesenchymal lesions. Int J Gynecol Pathol 2004;24:26–38.
29. Ordonez NG. Desmoplastic small round cell tumour. II: An ultrastructural and immunohistochemical study with emphasis on new immunohistochemical markers. Am J Surg Pathol 1998;22:1314–27.
30. Morotti RA, Nicol KK, Parham DM, et al. An immunohistochemical algorithm to facilitate diagnosis and subtyping of rhabdomyosarcoma: the Childrens Oncology Group experience. Am J Surg Pathol 2006;30:962–8.
31. McCluggage WG, Oliva E, Herrington CS, et al. CD10 and calretinin staining of endocervical glandular lesions, endocervical stroma and endometrioid adenocarcinoma of the uterine corpus: CD10 positivity is characteristic of, but not specific for, mesonephric lesions and is not specific for endometrioid stroma. Histopathology 2003;43:144–50.
32. Ordi J, Romagosa C, Tavassoli FA, et al. CD10 expression in epithelial tissues and tumors of the gynecologic tract; a useful marker in the diagnosis of mesonephric, trophoblastic and clear cell tumors. Am J Surg Pathol 2003;27:78–186.
33. Devouassoux-Shisheboran M, Silver SA, Tavassoli FA. Wolffian adnexal tumor, so-called female adnexal tumor of probable Wolffian origin (FATWO): immunohistochemical evidence in support of a Wolffian origin. Hum Pathol 1999;30:856–63.
34. Cameron RI, Ashe P, O'Rourke DM, et al. A panel of immunohistochemical stains assists in the distinction between ovarian and renal clear cell carcinoma. Int J Gynecol Pathol 2003;22:272–6.
35. Oliva E. CD10 expression in the female genital tract: does it have useful diagnostic applications? Adv Anat Pathol 2004;11:310–5.
36. McCluggage WG, Maxwell P. Immunohistochemical staining for calretinin is useful in the diagnosis of ovarian sex cord-stromal tumours. Histopathology 2001;38:403–8.
37. Shah VI, Freites ON, Maxwell P, McCluggage WG. Inhibin is more specific than calretinin as an immunohistochemical marker for differentiating sarcomatoid granulosa cell tumor of the ovary from other spindle cell neoplasms. J Clin Pathol 2003;56:221–4.
38. Bhargava R, Shia J, Hummer AJ, et al. Distinction of endometrial stromal sarcomas from 'hemangiopericytomatous' tumors using a panel of immunohistochemical stains. Mod Pathol 2005;18:40–7.
39. Lam MM, Corless CL, Goldblum JR, et al. Extragastrointestinal stromal tumors presenting as vulvovaginal/rectovaginal septal masses: a diagnostic pitfall. Int J Gynecol Pathol 2006;25:288–92.
40. Hameed A, Miller DS, Muller CY, et al. Frequent expression of beta-human chorionic gonadotropin (beta-hCG) in squamous cell carcinoma of the cervix. Int J Gynecol Pathol 1999;18:381–6.
41. Shih IM, Kurman RJ. The pathology of intermediate trophoblastic tumors and tumor-like lesions. Int J Gynecol Pathol 2001;20:31–47.
42. Singer G, Kurman RJ, McMaster MT, Shih IM. HLA-G immunoreactivity is specific for intermediate trophoblast in gestational trophoblastic disease and can serve as a useful marker in differential diagnosis. Am J Surg Pathol 2002;26:914–20.
43. Davidson B, Elstrand MB, McMaster MT, et al. HLA-G expression in effusions is a possible marker of tumor susceptibility to chemotherapy in ovarian carcinoma. Gynecol Oncol 2005;96:42–7.
44. Deavers MT, Malpica A, Ordonez NG, Silva EG. Ovarian steroid cell tumors: an immunohistochemical study including a comparison of calretinin with inhibin. Int J Gynecol Pathol 2003;22:162–7.
45. Silva EG, Deavers MT, Bodurka DC, Malpica A. Uterine epithelioid leiomyosarcomas with clear cells: reactivity with HMB-45 and the concept of PEComa. Am J Surg Pathol 2004;28:244–9.
46. Stewart CJR, Nandini CL, Richmond JA. Value of A103 (melan-A) immunostaining in the differential diagnosis of ovarian sex cord tumours. J Clin Pathol 2000;53:206–11.
47. McCluggage WG, McKenna M, McBride HA. CD56 is a sensitive and diagnostically useful immunohistochemical marker of ovarian sex cord-stromal tumors. Int J Gynecol Pathol 2007;26:322–7.
48. Disep B, Innes BA, Cochrane HR, et al. Immunohistochemical characterization of endometrial leucocytes in endometritis. Histopathology 2004;45:625–32.
49. Bayer-Garner IB, Korourian S. Plasma cells in chronic endometritis are easily identified when stained with syndecan-1. Mod Pathol 2001;14:877–9.
50. Cina SJ, Richardson MS, Austin RM, Kurman RJ. Immunohistochemical staining for Ki-67 antigen, carcinoembryonic antigen, and p53 in the differential diagnosis of glandular lesions of the cervix. Mod Pathol 1997;10:176–80.
51. Bateman AC, al-Talib RK, Newman T, et al. Immunohistochemical phenotype of malignant mesothelioma: predictive value of CA125 and HBME-1 expression. Histopathology 1997;30:49–56.
52. Deavers MT, Malpica A, Liu J, et al. Ovarian sex cord-stromal tumors : an immunohistochemical study including a comparison of calretinin and inhibin. Mod Pathol 2003;16:584–90.
53. McCluggage WG, Maxwell P, Sloan JM. Immunohistochemical staining of ovarian granulosa cell tumors with monoclonal antibody against inhibin. Hum Pathol 1997;28:1034–8.
54. McCluggage WG, Patterson A, White J, Anderson NH. Immunocytochemical staining of ovarian cyst aspirates with monoclonal antibody against inhibin. Cytopathology 1998;9:336–42.
55. McCluggage WG. The value of inhibin staining in gynecological pathology. Int J Gynecol Pathol 2001;20:79–85.
56. McCluggage WG. Uterine tumours resembling ovarian sex cord tumours: immunohistochemical evidence for true sex cord differentiation. Histopathology 1999;34:373–80.
57. McCluggage WG, Ashe P, McBride H, et al. Localisation of the cellular expression of inhibin in trophoblastic tissue. Histopathology 1998;32:252–6.

58. McCluggage WG, Maxwell P. Adenocarcinomas of various sites may exhibit immunoreactivity with anti-inhibin antibodies. Histopathology 1999;35:216–20.
59. Cheng L, Thomas A, Roth CM, et al. OCT4. A novel biomarker for dysgerminoma of the ovary. Am J Surg Pathol 2004;18:1341–6.
60. Mikami Y, Kiyokawa T, Hata S, et al. Gastrointestinal immunophenotype in adenocarcinomas of the uterine cervix and related glandular lesions: a possible link between lobular endocervical glandular hyperplasia/pyloric gland metaplasia and adenoma malignum. Mod Pathol 2004;17:962–72.
61. Kojima A, Mikami Y, Sudo T, et al. Gastric morphology and immunophenotype predict poor outcome in mucinous adenocarcinoma of the uterine cervix. Am J Surg Pathol 2007;31664–72.
62. Werling RW, Yaziji H, Bacchi CE, Gown AM. CDX2, a highly sensitive and specific marker of adenocarcinomas of intestinal origin: an immunohistochemical survey of 476 primary and metastatic carcinomas. Am J Surg Pathol 2003;27:303–10.
63. McCluggage WG, Shah R, Connolly LE, McBride HA. Intestinal-type cervical adenocarcinoma in situ and adenocarcinoma exhibit a partial enteric immunophenotype with consistent expression of CDX2. Int J Gynecol Pathol 2006;27:92–100.
64. Houghton O, Connolly LE, McCluggage WG. Morules in endometrioid proliferations of the uterus and ovary consistently express the intestinal transcription factor CDX2. Histopathology 2008;53:156–65.
65. Gagnon S, Tetu B, Silva EG, McCaughey WT. Frequency of alpha-fetoprotein production by Sertoli-Leydig cell tumors of the ovary: an immunohistochemical study of eight cases. Mod Pathol 1989;2:63–7.
66. Pitman MB, Triratanachat S, Young RH, Oliva E. Hepatocyte paraffin 1 antibody does not distinguish primary ovarian tumors with hepatoid differentiation from metastatic hepatocellular carcinoma. Int J Gynecol Pathol 2004;23:58–64.
67. Thamboo TP, Wee A. Hep Par 1 expression in carcinoma of the cervix: implications for diagnosis and prognosis. J Clin Pathol 2004;57:48–53.
68. Albarracin CT, Jafri J, Montag AG, et al. Differential expression of MUC2 and MUC5AC mucin genes in primary ovarian and metastatic colonic carcinoma. Hum Pathol 2000;31:672–7.
69. Kuan SF, Montag AG, Hart J, et al. Differential expression of mucin genes in mammary and extramammary Paget's disease. Am J Surg Pathol 2001;25:1469–77.
70. Miettinen M, Wang ZF, Lasota J. DOG1 antibody in the differential diagnosis of gastrointestinal stromal tumors: a study of 1840 cases. Am J Surg Pathol 2009;33:1401–8.
71. O'Connell JT, Hacker CM, Barsky SH. MUC2 is a molecular marker for pseudomyxoma peritonei. Mod Pathol 2002;15:958–72.
72. McCluggage WG, Sumathi V, Nucci M, et al. Ewing family of tumours involving the vulva and vagina: report of a series of four cases. J Clin Pathol 2007;60:674–80.
73. Loo KT, Leung AKF, Chan JKC. Immunohistochemical staining of ovarian granulosa cell tumours with MIC2 antibody. Histopathology 1995;27:388–90.
74. McCluggage WG, Kennedy K, Busam KJ. An immunohistochemical study of cervical neuroendocrine carcinomas: Neoplasms that are commonly TTF1 positive and which may express CK20 and P63. Am J Surg Pathol 2010;34:525–32.
75. Siami K, McCluggage WG, Ordonez NG, et al. Thyroid transcription factor 1 expression in endometrial and endocervical adenocarcinomas. Am J Surg Pathol 2007;31:1759–63.
76. Kenny SL, McBride HA, Jamison J, McCluggage WG. Mesonephric adenocarcinomas of the uterine cervix and corpus: HPV-negative neoplasms that are commonly PAX8, CA125, and HMGA2 positive and that may be immunoreactive with TTF1 and Hepatocyte Nuclear Factor 1-β. Am J Surg Pathol 2012;36:799–807.
77. Niu HL, Pasha TL, Pawel BR, et al. Thyroid transcription factor-1 expression in normal gynecologic tissues and its potential significance. Int J Gynecol Pathol 2009;28:301–7.
78. McCluggage WG, Young RH. Tubulo-squamous polyp: a report of 10 cases of a distinctive hitherto uncharacterized vaginal polyp. Am J Surg Pathol 2007;31:1013–9.
79. Kelly P, McBride HA, Kennedy K, et al. Misplaced Skene's glands: glandular elements in the cervix, vagina and vulva which are variably prostate marker positive and which encompass vaginal tubulosquamous polyp and cervical ectopic prostatic tissue. Int J Gynecol Pathol 2011;30:605–12.
80. Zynger DL, McCallum JC, Luan C, et al. Glypican 3 has a higher sensitivity than alpha-fetoprotein for testicular and ovarian yolk sac tumour: immunohistochemical investigation with analysis of histological growth patterns. Histopathology 2010;56:750–7.
81. Maeda D, Ota S, Takazawa Y, et al. Glypican-3 expression in clear cell adenocarcinoma of the ovary. Mod Pathol 2009;22:824–32.
82. Cao D, Guo S, Allan RW, et al. SALL4 is a novel sensitive and specific marker of ovarian primitive germ cell tumors and is particularly useful in distinguishing yolk sac tumor from clear cell carcinoma. Am J Surg Pathol 2009;33:894–904.
83. Cao D, Guo S, Allan RW, et al. Identification of the most sensitive and robust immunohistochemical markers in different categories of ovarian sex cord-stromal tumors. Am J Surg Pathol. 2009;33:894–904.
84. Rabban JT, Zaloudek CJ, Shekitka KM, Tavassoli FA. Inflammatory myofibroblastic tumor of the uterus: a clinicopathologic study of 6 cases emphasizing distinction from aggressive mesenchymal tumors. Am J Surg Pathol 2005;29:1348–55.
85. Richter CE, Hui P, Buza N, et al. HER-2/NEU overexpression in vulvar Paget disease: the Yale experience. J Clin Pathol 2010;63:544–7.
86. Singh P, Smith CL, Cheetham G, et al. Serous carcinoma of the uterus-determination of HER-2/neu status using immunohistochemistry, chromogenic in situ hybridization, and quantitative polymerase chain reaction techniques: its significance and clinical correlation. Int J Gynecol Cancer 2008;18:1344–51.
87. Gilks CB, McAlpine J. Human epidermal growth factor 2 overexpression and amplification in mucinous tumours of ovary. Histopathology 2011;58:1173–4.
88. McCluggage WG. Ovarian neoplasms composed of small round cells. A review. Adv Anat Pathol 2004;11:288–96.
89. Al-Hussaini M, Stockman A, Foster H, McCluggage WG. WT-1 assists in distinguishing ovarian from uterine serous carcinoma and in distinguishing serous and ovarian endometrioid carcinoma. Histopathology 2004;44:109–15.
90. McCluggage WG. WT1 is of value in ascertaining the site of origin of serous carcinomas within the female genital tract. Int J Gynecol Pathol 2004;23:97–9.
91. Logani S, Oliva E, Amin MB, et al. Immunoprofile of ovarian tumors with putative transitional cell (urothelial) differentiation using novel urothelial markers: histogenetic and diagnostic implications. Am J Surg Pathol 2003;27:1434–41.
92. Hirschowitz L, Ganesan R, McCluggage WG. WT1, p53 and hormone receptor expression in uterine serous carcinoma. Histopathology 2009;55:478–82.
93. Sumathi VP, Al-Hussaini M, Connolly LE, et al. Endometrial stromal neoplasms are immunoreactive with WT-1 antibody. Int J Gynecol Pathol 2004;23:241–7.
94. Patil DT, Laskin WB, Fetsch JF, Miettinen M. Inguinal smooth muscle tumors in women- a dichotomous group consisting of Mullerian-type leiomyomas and soft tissue leiomyosarcomas: an analysis of 55 cases. Am J Surg Pathol 2011;35:315–24.
95. Kobel M, Reuss A, Du Bois A, et al. The biological and clinical value of p53 expression in pelvic high-grade serous carcinomas. J Pathol 2010;222:191–8.
96. Yemelyanova A, Vang R, Kshirsagar M, et al. Immunohistochemical staining patterns of p53 can serve as a surrogate marker for TP53 mutations in ovarian carcinoma: an immunohistochemical and nucleotide sequencing analysis. Mod Pathol 2011;24:1248–53.
97. Alkushi A, Lim P, Coldman A, et al. Interpretation of p53 immunoreactivity in endometrial carcinoma: establishing a clinically relevant cut-off level. Int J Gynecol Pathol 2004;23:129–37.
98. O'Neill CJ, McBride HA, Connolly LE, McCluggage WG. Uterine leiomyosarcomas are characterized by high p16, p53 and MIB1 expression in comparison with usual leiomyomas, leiomyoma variants and smooth muscle tumours of uncertain malignant potential. Histopathology 2007;50:851–8.
99. Russell SE, McCluggage WG. A multistep model for ovarian tumorigenesis: the value of mutation analysis in the KRAS and BRAF genes. J Pathol 2004;203:617–9.
100. O'Neill CJ, Deavers MT, Malpica A, et al. An immunohistochemical comparison between low grade and high grade ovarian

serous carcinomas: significantly higher expression of p53, MIB1, bcl2, HER-2/neu and C-KIT in high grade neoplasms. Am J Surg Pathol 2005;29:1034–41.
101. Herrington CS, McCluggage WG. The emerging role of the distal fallopian tube and p53 in pelvic serous carcinogenesis. J Pathol 2010;220:5–6.
102. Lee Y, Medeiros F, Kindelberger D, et al. Advances in the recognition of tubal intraepithelial carcinoma: applications to cancer screening and the pathogenesis of ovarian cancer. Adv Anat Pathol 2006;13:1–7.
103. Yang B, Hart WR. Vulvar intraepithelial neoplasia of the simplex (differentiated) type: a clinicopathologic study including analysis of HPV and p53 expression. Am J Surg Pathol 2000;24:429–41.
104. Liegl B, Regauer S. p53 immunostaining in lichen sclerosus is related to ischaemic stress and is not a marker of differentiated vulvar intraepithelial neoplasia (d-VIN). Histopathology 2006;48:268–74.
105. Shih IM, Kurman RJ. p63 expression is useful in the distinction of epithelioid trophoblastic and placental site trophoblastic tumors by profiling trophoblastic subpopulations. Am J Surg Pathol 2004;28:1177–83.
106. Wang TY, Chen BF, Yang YC, et al. Histologic and immunophenotypic classification of cervical carcinomas by expression of the p53 homologue p63: a study of 250 cases. Hum Pathol 2001;32:479–86.
107. Liao XY, Xue WC, Shen DH, et al. p63 expression in ovarian tumours: a marker for Brenner tumours but not transitional cell carcinomas. Histopathology 2007;51:477–83.
108. Bussaglia E, del Rio E, Matias-Guiu X, Prat J. PTEN mutations in endometrial carcinomas: a molecular and clinicopathologic analysis of 38 cases. Hum Pathol 2000;31:312–7.
109. Mutter GL, Ince TA, Baak JP, et al. Molecular identification of latent precancers in histologically normal endometrium. Cancer Res 2001;61:4311–4.
110. Catasus L, Bussaglia E, Rodrguez I, et al. Molecular genetic alterations in endometrioid carcinomas of the ovary: similar frequency of beta-catenin abnormalities but lower rate of microsatellite instability and PTEN alterations than in uterine endometrioid carcinomas. Hum Pathol 2004;35:1360–8.
111. Henderson GS, Brown KA, Perkins SL, et al. bcl-2 is down-regulated in atypical endometrial hyperplasia and adenocarcinoma. Mod Pathol 1996;9:430–8.
112. Piek JM, Verheijen RH, Menko FH, et al. Expression of differentiation and proliferation related proteins in epithelium of prophylactically removed ovaries from women with a hereditary female adnexal cancer predisposition. Histopathology 2003;43:26–32.
113. Cameron RI, Maxwell P, Jenkins, D, McCluggage WG. Immunohistochemical staining with MIB-1, bcl2 and p16 assists in the distinction of cervical glandular intraepithelial neoplasia from tubo-endometrial metaplasia, endometriosis and microglandular hyperplasia. Histopathology 2002;41:313–21.
114. D'Angelo E, Spagnoli LG, Prat J. Comparative clinicopathologic and immunohistochemical analysis of uterine sarcomas diagnosed using the World Health Organization classification system. Hum Pathol 2009;40:1571–85.
115. Raspollini MR, Amunni G, Villanucci A, et al. c-Kit expression in patients with uterine leiomyosarcomas: a potential alternative therapeutic treatment. Clin Cancer Res 2004;10:3500–3.
116. Winter 3rd WE, Seidman JD, Krivak TC, et al. Clinicopathological analysis of c-kit expression in carcinosarcomas and leiomyosarcomas of the uterine corpus. Gynecol Oncol 2003;91:3–8.
117. Pirog EC, Baergen RN, Soslow RA, et al. Diagnostic accuracy of cervical low-grade squamous intraepithelial lesions is improved with MIB1 immunostaining. Am J Surg Pathol 2002;26:70–5.
118. Logani S, Cu D, Quint WGV, et al. Low-grade vulvar and vaginal intraepithelial neoplasia: correlation of histologic features with human papillomavirus DNA detection and MIB1 immunostaining. Mod Pathol 2003;16:735–41.
119. Kalof AN, Evans MF, Simmons-Arnold L, et al. p16INK4A immunoexpression and HPV in situ hybridization signal patterns: potential markers of high-grade cervical intraepithelial neoplasia. Am J Surg Pathol 2005;29:674–9.
120. Klaes R, Benner A, Friedrich T, et al. p16INK4a immunohistochemistry improves interobserver agreement in the diagnosis of cervical intraepithelial neoplasia. Am J Surg Pathol 2002;26:1389–99.
121. Negri G, Egarter-Vigi E, Kasal A, et al. p16 (INK4a) is a useful marker for the diagnosis of adenocarcinoma of the cervix uteri and its precursors. Am J Surg Pathol 2003;27:187–93.
122. McCluggage WG, Jenkins D. Immunohistochemical staining with p16 may assist in the distinction between endometrial and endocervical adenocarcinoma. Int J Gynecol Pathol 2003;22:231–5.
123. Chiesa-Vottero AG, Malpica A, Deavers MT, et al. Immunohistochemical overexpression of p16 and p53 in uterine serous carcinoma and ovarian high-grade serous carcinoma. Int J Gynecol Pathol. 2007;26:328–33.
124. Elishaev E, Gilks CB, Miller D, et al. Synchronous and metachronous endocervical and ovarian neoplasms: evidence supporting interpretation of the ovarian neoplasms as metastatic endocervical adenocarcinomas simulating primary ovarian surface epithelial neoplasms. Am J Surg Pathol 2005;29:281–94.
125. Quddus MR, Xu C, Steinhoff MM, et al. Simplex (differentiated) type VIN: absence of p16INK4 supports its weak association with HPV and its probable precursor role in non-HPV related vulvar squamous cancers. Histopathology 2005;46:718–20.
126. Castrillon DH, Sun DQ, Weremowicz S, et al. Discrimination of complete hydatidiform mole from its mimics by immunohistochemistry of the paternally imprinted gene product p57 (KIP2). Am J Surg Pathol 2001;25:1225–30.
127. Genest DR, Dorfman DM, Castrillon DH. Ploidy and imprinting in hydatidiform moles. Complementary use of flow cytometry and immunohistochemistry of the imprinted gene product p57 KIP2 to assist molar classification. J Reprod Med 2002;47:342–6.
128. Little L, Stewart CJ. Cyclin D1 immunoreactivity in normal endocervix and diagnostic value in reactive and neoplastic endocervical lesions. Mod Pathol 2010;23:611–8.
129. Stewart CJ, Crook ML, Little L, Louwen K. Correlation between invasive pattern and immunophenotypic alterations in endocervical adenocarcinoma. Histopathology 2011;58:720–8.
130. Stewart CJ, Crook ML, Leung YC, Platten M. Expression of cell cycle regulatory proteins in endometrial adenocarcinoma: variations in conventional tumor areas and in microcystic, elongated and fragmented glands. Mod Pathol 2009;22:725–33.
131. Mao TL, Seidman JD, Kurman RJ, Shih IEM. Cyclin E and p16 immunoreactivity in epithelioid trophoblastic tumor- an aid in differential diagnosis. Am J Surg Pathol 2006;30:1105–10.
132. Pinto AP, Schlecht NF, Woo TYC, et al. Biomarker (ProExC, p16, and MIB1) distinction of high-grade squamous intraepithelial lesion from its mimics. Mod Pathol 2008;21:1067–74.
133. Aximu D, Azad A, Ni R, et al. A pilot evaluation of a novel immunohistochemical assay for Topoisomerase II-α and minichromosome maintenance protein 2 expression (ProExC) in cervical adenocarcinoma in situ, adenocarcinoma, and benign glandular mimics. Int J Gynecol Pathol 2009;28:114–9.
134. Chen H, Gonzalez JL, Brennick JB, et al. Immunohistochemical patterns of ProExC in vulvar squamous lesions. Am J Surg Pathol 2010;34:1250–7.
135. McCluggage WG, Patterson A, Maxwell P. Aggressive angiomyxoma of pelvic parts exhibits oestrogen and progesterone receptor positivity. J Clin Pathol 2000;53:603–5.
136. Fine BA, Muñoz AK, Litz CE, Gershenson DM. Primary medical management of recurrent aggressive angiomyxoma of the vulva with a gonadotropin-releasing hormone agonist. Gynecol Oncol 2001;81:120–2.
137. Staebler A, Sherman ME, Zaino RJ, et al. Hormone receptor immunohistochemistry and human papillomavirus in situ hybridisation are useful for distinguishing endocervical and endometrial adenocarcinomas. Am J Surg Pathol 2002;26:998–1006.
138. Moinfar F, Regitnig P, Tabrizi AD, et al. Expression of androgen receptors in benign and malignant endometrial stromal neoplasms. Virchows Arch 2004;444:410–4.
139. Loddenkemper C, Mechsner S, Foss H-D, et al. Use of oxytocin receptor expression in distinguishing between uterine smooth muscle tumors and endometrial stromal sarcoma. Am J Surg Pathol 2003;27:1458–62.
140. Logani S, Oliva E, Arnell PM, et al. Use of novel immunohistochemical markers expressed in colonic adenocarcinoma to distinguish primary ovarian tumors from metastatic colorectal carcinoma. Mod Pathol 2005;18:19–25.
141. Jung C-K, Jung J-H, Lee A, et al. Diagnostic use of β-catenin expression for the assessment of endometrial stromal tumors. Mod Pathol 2008;21:756–63.
142. Ohishi Y, Oda Y, Kurihara S, et al. Nuclear localization of E-cadherin but not beta-catenin in human ovarian granulosa cell

tumours and normal ovarian follicles and ovarian stroma. Histopathology 2011;58:423–32.
143. Laury AR, Perets R, Piao H, et al. A Comprehensive Analysis of PAX8 Expression in Human Epithelial Tumors. Am J Surg Pathol 2011;35:816–26.
144. Nonaka D, Chirboga L, Soslow RA. Expression of pax8 as a useful marker in distinguishing ovarian carcinomas from mammary carcinomas. Am J Surg Pathol 2008;32:1566–71.
145. Laury AR, Hornick JL, Perets R. PAX8 reliably distinguishes ovarian serous tumors from malignant mesothelioma. Am J Surg Pathol 2010;34:627–35.
146. Rabban JT, McAlhany S, Lerwill MF, et al. PAX2 distinguishes benign mesonephric and mullerian glandular lesions of the cervix from endocervical adenocarcinoma, including minimal deviation adenocarcinoma. Am J Surg Pathol 2010;34:137–46.
147. Monte NM, Webster KA, Neuberg D, et al. Joint loss of PAX2 and PTEN expression in endometrial precancers and cancer. Cancer Res 2010;70:6225–32.
148. McCluggage WG, Connolly L, McBride HA. HMGA2 is a sensitive but not specific immunohistochemical marker of vulvovaginal aggressive angiomyxoma. Am J Surg Pathol 2010;34:1037–42.
149. McCluggage WG, Connolly LE, McBride HA, et al. HMGA2 is commonly positive in uterine serous carcinomas and is a useful adjunct to diagnosis. Histopathology 2012;60:547–53.
150. Wei JJ, Wu J, Luan C, et al. HMGA2: a potential biomarker complement to p53 for detection of early-stage high-grade papillary serous carcinoma in fallopian tubes. Am J Surg Pathol 2010;34:18–26.
151. Yamamoto S, Tsuda H, Aida S, et al. Immunohistochemical detection of hepatocyte nuclear factor 1beta in ovarian and endometrial clear-cell adenocarcinomas and nonneoplastic endometrium. Hum Pathol 2007;38:1074–80.
152. Shah SP, Kobel M, Senz J, et al. Mutation of FOXL2 in granulosa-cell tumors of the ovary. N Engl J Med 2009;360:2719–29.
153. Al-Agha OM, Huwait HF, Chow C, et al. FOXL2 is a sensitive and specific marker for sex cord-stromal tumors of the ovary. Am J Surg Pathol 2011;35:484–94.
154. Zheng W, Yi X, Fadare O, et al. The oncofetal protein IMP3: a novel biomarker for endometrial serous carcinoma. Am J Surg Pathol 2008;32:304–15.
155. Zhang L, Liu Y, Hao S, et al. IMP2 expression distinguishes endometrioid from serous endometrial adenocarcinomas. Am J Surg Pathol 2011;35:868–72.

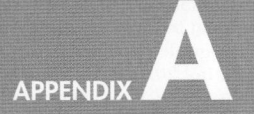

APPENDIX A

FIGO Staging of Cancers of the Female Genital Tract

George L. Mutter, Jaime Prat

The purpose of tumor staging is two-fold: to provide standardized terminology that allows comparison of patients between centers; and to distribute patients and their tumors into prognostic groups requiring specific treatments. Thus, as new data become available diagnostic methods improve and therapeutic options change, staging systems evolve over time. This appendix lists anatomic staging criteria by primary site effective at the time of publication.

The most widely used staging system for gynecologic malignancies, as presented here, is that of the International Federation of Gynecology and Obstetrics (FIGO). FIGO staging recommendations are endorsed by the American Joint Committee on Cancer (AJCC), the International Union against Cancer (UICC), and the World Health Organization (WHO), who promote concordance with FIGO by incorporating parallel staging elements into their own published systems.

Staging is based upon a variety of information sources including clinical, imaging, surgical-pathological, and biomarker parameters. Individual pathologic specimens are often inadequate for comprehensive staging, either because they lack the full repertoire of required samples or because the pathologist does not have access to relevant ancillary information. In all cases of primary tumor excision, the pathologist should clearly indicate in the pathology report involvement of included anatomic structures that define different disease stages.

Tables are organized, in anatomic sequence, from upper to lower genital tract, with gestational disease at the end.

Cancer of the Ovary, Fallopian Tube, and Peritoneum: Chapters 21 and 25–31

Stage	Anatomic Distribution
Stage I	Tumor confined to ovaries or fallopian tube(s).
IA	Tumor limited to 1 ovary (capsule intact) or fallopian tube. Surface free of tumor and washings negative.
IB	Tumor limited to both ovaries (capsules intact) or fallopian tubes. Surface free of tumor and washings negative.
IC	Tumor limited to 1 or both ovaries or fallopian tubes, with any of the following:
IC1	Surgical spill.
IC2	Capsule ruptured before surgery or tumor on ovarian or fallopian tube surface.
IC3	Malignant cells in the ascites or peritoneal washings.
Stage II	Tumor involves 1 or both ovaries or fallopian tubes with pelvic extension (below pelvic brim) or primary peritoneal cancer.
IIA	Extension and/or implants on the uterus and/or fallopian tubes and/or ovaries.
IIB	Extension to other pelvic intraperitoneal tissues.
Stage III	Cytologically or histologically confirmed spread to the peritoneum outside the pelvis and/or metastasis to the retroperitoneal lymph nodes.
IIIA	Positive retroperitoneal lymph nodes (cytologically or histologically proven).
IIIA1	
IIIA1 (i)	Nodal metastasis ≤10 mm in greatest dimension.
IIIA1 (ii)	Nodal metastasis >10 mm in greatest dimension.
IIIA2	Microscopic extrapelvic (above the pelvic brim) peritoneal involvement with or without positive retroperitoneal lymph nodes.
IIIB	Macroscopic peritoneal metastases beyond the pelvic brim ≤2 cm in greatest dimension with or without positive retroperitoneal lymph nodes.
IIIC	Macroscopic peritoneal metastases beyond the pelvic brim >2 cm in greatest dimension with or without positive retroperitoneal lymph nodes (includes extension of tumor to capsule of liver and spleen without parenchymal involvement of either organ).
Stage IV	Distant metastasis excluding peritoneal metastases.
IVA	Pleural effusion with positive cytology.
IVB	Metastases to extra-abdominal organs (including inguinal lymph nodes and lymph nodes outside of abdominal cavity).

Notes:
- The primary site should be designated as ovary (OV), fallopian tube (FT), peritoneum (P), or cannot be assessed ("undesignated").
- Involvement of abdominal organs such as spleen and liver must be distinguished as surface peritoneal spread (Stage III) compared with isolated parenchymal metastases (Stage IVB).

FIGO, 2014.[1]

Cancer of the Endometrium, including Carcinosarcoma: Chapter 18

Stage	Anatomic Distribution
Stage I	Tumor confined to the corpus uteri.
IA	No myometrial invasion or invasion ≤50% of myometrium thickness.
IB	Tumor invades >50% of myometrium thickness.
Stage II	Tumor invades cervical stroma, but does not extend beyond the uterus.
Stage III	Local and/or regional spread of the tumor.*
IIIA	Tumor invades the serosa of the corpus uteri and/or adnexa.*
IIIB	Vaginal and/or parametrial involvement.*
IIIC	Metastases to pelvic and/or para-aortic lymph nodes.*
IIIC1	Positive pelvic nodes.
IIIC2	Positive para-aortic lymph nodes with or without positive pelvic lymph nodes.
Stage IV	Tumor invades bladder and/or bowel mucosa, and/or distant metastases.
IVA	Tumor invasion of bladder and/or bowel mucosa.
IVB	Distant metastases, including intra-abdominal metastases and/or inguinal lymph nodes.

*In Stage III disease, positive peritoneal cytology should to be reported separately without changing the stage.
FIGO, 2009.[2]

Uterine Leiomyosarcomas and Endometrial Stromal Sarcomas: Chapters 19 and 20

Stage	Anatomic Distribution
Stage I	Tumor limited to uterus.
IA	Tumor ≤5 cm.
IB	Tumor >5 cm.
Stage II	Tumor extends to the pelvis.
IIA	Adnexal involvement.
IIB	Tumor extends to extrauterine pelvic tissue.
Stage III	Tumor invades abdominal tissues.
IIIA	One site.
IIIB	More than one site.
IIIC	Metastasis to pelvic and/or para-aortic lymph nodes.
Stage IV	Tumor invades bladder and/or rectum and/or distant metastasis.
IVA	Tumor invades bladder and/or rectum.
IVB	Distant metastasis.

Notes:
- Stratification of stage 1 tumors at a size cut-off of 5 cm is based on data from non-uterine sites, and will be reassessed as more uterine data becomes available.
- Simultaneous endometrial stromal sarcomas of the uterine corpus and ovary/pelvis in association with ovarian/pelvic endometriosis should be classified as independent primary tumors.

FIGO, 2009.[3]

Uterine Adenosarcomas: Chapter 20

Stage	Anatomic Distribution
Stage I	Tumor limited to uterus.
IA	Tumor limited to endometrium/endocervix (without myometrial invasion).
IB	Tumor invades <50% of myometrium thickness.
IC	Tumor invades ≥50% of myometrium thickness.
Stage II	Tumor extends to the pelvis.
IIA	Adnexal involvement.
IIB	Tumor extends to extrauterine pelvic tissue.
Stage III	Tumor invades abdominal tissues.
IIIA	One site.
IIIB	More than one site.
IIIC	Metastasis to pelvic and/or para-aortic lymph nodes.
Stage IV	Tumor invades bladder and/or rectum and/or distant metastasis.
IVA	Tumor invades bladder and/or rectum.
IVB	Distant metastasis.

Notes:
- As these tumors usually arise primarily from the uterine lining, stratification of stage I tumors is based on depth of myoinvasion.
- Carcinosarcomas should be staged as carcinomas of the endometrium.

FIGO, 2009.[3]

Cancer of the Cervix Uteri: Chapters 11 and 12

Stage	Anatomic Distribution
Stage I	Carcinoma confined to the cervix.
IA	Invasive carcinoma that can be diagnosed only by microscopy, with deepest invasion ≤5 mm and largest extension ≤7 mm.
IA1	Measured stromal invasion of ≤3.0 mm in depth and extension of ≤7.0 mm.
IA2	Measured stromal invasion of >3.0 mm and <5.0 mm with an extension of not more than 7.0 mm.
IB	Clinically visible lesions limited to the cervix uteri or preclinical cancers greater than stage IA.
IB (i)	Clinically visible lesion ≤4.0 cm in greatest dimension.
IB (ii)	Clinically visible lesion >4.0 cm in greatest dimension.
Stage II	Tumor invades beyond the uterus, but not to the pelvic wall or to the lower third of the vagina.
IIA	Without parametrial invasion.
IIA (i)	Clinically visible lesion ≤4.0 cm in greatest dimension.
IIA (ii)	Clinically visible lesion >4 cm in greatest dimension.
IIB	With obvious parametrial invasion.
Stage III	Tumor extends to the pelvic wall and/or involves lower third of the vagina and/or causes hydronephrosis or nonfunctioning kidney.
IIIA	Tumor involves lower third of the vagina, with no extension to the pelvic wall.
IIIB	Tumor extension to the pelvic wall and/or hydronephrosis or nonfunctioning kidney.
Stage IV	Tumor has extended beyond the true pelvis or has involved (biopsy proven) the mucosa of the bladder or rectum.
IVA	Spread to adjacent organs.
IVB	Spread to distant organs.

Notes:
- Extension from the cervix to uterine corpus is disregarded in stage I tumors.
- All grossly visible lesions (even with superficial invasion) are stage IB.
- The depth of invasion should always be reported in millimeters.
- Lymphovascular involvement is not a staging parameter.
- The LAST working group[4] has recommended the term 'superficially invasive squamous cell carcinoma' for stage IA1 squamous cell carcinoma that has been completely excised and is thus potentially amenable to conservative surgical therapy.

FIGO, 2009.[3]

Cancer of the Vagina: Chapter 7

Stage	Anatomic Distribution
Stage I	Carcinoma limited to the vaginal wall.
Stage II	Tumor extends to subvaginal tissue but has not extended to the pelvic wall.
Stage III	Tumor extends to the pelvic wall.
Stage IV	Tumor has extended beyond the true pelvis or has clinically involved the mucosa of the bladder or rectum.
IVA	Tumor invades bladder and/or rectal mucosa and/or direct extension beyond the true pelvis.
IVB	Spread to distant organs.

FIGO, 2009.[5]

Cancer of the Vulva: Chapters 4 and 5

Stage	Anatomic Distribution
Stage I	Tumor confined to the vulva.
IA	Lesions ≤2 cm in size, confined to the vulva or perineum and with stromal invasion ≤1.0 mm.
IB	Lesions >2 cm in size, or with stromal invasion >1.0 mm, confined to the vulva or perineum.
Stage II	Tumor with extension to adjacent perineal structures (⅓ lower urethra, ⅓ lower vagina, anus).
Stage III	Tumor with positive inguinofemoral lymph nodes.
IIIA	
IIIA (i)	With one lymph node metastasis ≥5 mm.
IIIA (ii)	With one or two lymph node metastases <5 mm.
IIIB	
IIIB (i)	With two or more lymph node metastases ≥5 mm.
IIIB (ii)	With three or more lymph node metastases <5 mm.
IIIC	Any positive node(s) with extracapsular spread.
Stage IV	Tumor invades other regional (⅔ upper urethra, ⅔ upper vagina), or distant structures.
IVA	Tumor invades regional structures.
IVA (i)	Tumor invades upper urethral and/or vaginal mucosa, bladder mucosa, rectal mucosa, or fixed to pelvic bone.
IVA (ii)	Fixed or ulcerated inguinofemoral lymph nodes involved by tumor.
IVB	Any distant metastasis including pelvic lymph nodes.

Notes:
- The depth of invasion is defined as the measurement of the tumor from the epithelial stroma junction of the adjacent most superficial dermal papilla to the deepest point of invasion.

FIGO, 2009.[3]

Gestational Trophoblastic Neoplasia: Chapter 34

Stage	Anatomic Distribution
Stage I	Disease confined to the uterus.
Stage II	Disease extends outside of the uterus, but is limited to genital structures (adnexa, vagina, broad ligament).
Stage III	Lung involvement, with or without known genital tract tumor.
Stage IV	All other metastatic sites.

Note:
- The anatomic staging system above has been modified by WHO in a prognostic scoring system (Table 34.5),[6] which incorporates additional tumor distribution and clinical information for improved outcome prediction. This prognostic scoring system has also been endorsed by FIGO.

FIGO, 2000.[5,6]

REFERENCES

1. Prat J. Staging classification for cancer of the ovary, fallopian tube, and peritoneum. Int J Gynecol Obstet 2014;124:1–5.
2. Creasman W. Revised FIGO staging for carcinoma of the endometrium. Int J Gynecol Obstet 2009;105:109.
3. Mutch DG. The new FIGO staging system for cancers of the vulva, cervix, endometrium and sarcomas. Gynecol Oncol 2009;115:325–8.
4. Darragh TM, Colgan TJ, Cox JT, et al. The Lower Anogenital Squamous Terminology Standardization Project for HPV-Associated Lesions: Background and consensus recommendations from the College of American Pathologists and the American Society for Colposcopy and Cervical Pathology. Arch Pathol Lab Med 2012;136:1266–97.
5. Current FIGO staging for cancer of the vagina, fallopian tube, ovary, and gestational trophoblastic neoplasia. Int J Gynecol Obstet 2009;105:3–4.
6. FIGO staging for gestational trophoblastic neoplasia 2000. FIGO Oncology Committee. Int J Gynaecol Obstet 2002;77:285–7.

APPENDIX B: Online Resources

George L. Mutter

Online resources have exploded in the last decade, providing a sometimes bewildering array of information, which varies greatly in quality and annotation. Although this provides free access to an unparalleled depth and breadth of content, search engines yield indiscriminate lists unfiltered for accuracy, and some of the best sites cannot be appreciated without exploration. Many online resources have added value beyond what was ever possible in static printed format, such as real-time updates and customized assembly of mixed content in response to a custom query. When developed or curated by a recognized authority or specialized nonprofit organization, these achieve a level of accuracy, timeliness, and stability well suited to the demanding standards of clinical practice.

This appendix lists specific Web-based resources that the author has found to be useful and meet the following criteria:

- The content is unique or unusually comprehensive.
- Authorship by a recognized authority in the field or curation by an established nonprofit organization or group.
- Available as open access. Commercial and paid access sites are excluded.
- The site must be stable over time (no temporary postings).

PATHOLOGY PRACTICE AND GENERAL EDUCATIONAL RESOURCES

Atlas of Human Embryology
http://www.embryo.chronolab.com/

Nice graphics of human embryology with tables of developmental benchmarks. Interactive timeline slider shows date-specific events. Placenta included.

College of American Pathologists
http://www.cap.org/

Look in their Reference Resources Tab for protocols for processing and reporting of cancer specimens. They also have a Lower Anogenital Squamous Terminology Project page that is excellent but buried deep. Do a search for 'LAST Project' in the site search box.

Endometrium.org
http://www.endometrium.org/

Endometrial precancer educational Web site for pathologists by G. Mutter.

Global Library of Women's Medicine
http://www.glowm.com/

An excellent online-only textbook with expert contributors and a good search engine that retrieves well-organized articles.

The Virtual Human Embryo
http://www.ehd.org/virtual-human-embryo/

Electronic version of a Carnegie-staged atlas with many enhancements. Photographic and artwork representations of actual embryos. Excellent tables and lookup of various stages by organ search.

U.S. and Canadian Academy of Pathology
http://www.uscap.org/home.htm

Online educational materials, including a virtual slide box of digital slides with histories and discussion.

MEDICAL LITERATURE

Coremine
http://www.coremine.com/medical/#search

Self-organized graphic display of Pubmed literature retrieved in response to your search term(s). Each search term is first associated with most frequent nearby terms, and results displayed as a web with strands between original search and associated terms. Clicking on a strand or node retrieves literature, organized by topic and discipline.

Pubmed
http://www.ncbi.nlm.nih.gov/pubmed/

The standard for retrieval of medical literature. National Library of Medicine (U.S.).

Pubmed Central
http://www.ncbi.nlm.nih.gov/pmc/

Free public access to full text versions of all papers resulting from work supported by the U.S. government.

DISEASE AND CODING DATABASES

Diagnostic Billing Codes (ICD9)
http://www.cms.gov/Medicare/Coding/ICD9Provider DiagnosticCodes/codes.html

These billing codes are issued by the Centers for Medicare and Medicaid Services. Requires data download in one of several formats such as .txt or spreadsheet, after which you can search locally on your computer. ICD10 version is coming in 2014.

National Center for Biotechnology Information
http://www.ncbi.nlm.nih.gov/

U.S. government clearinghouse and master portal for access to many curated and constantly updated resources. Published literature, specialty databases, genetics, proteomics, and more.

Online Mendelian Inheritance in Man (OMIM)
http://www.ncbi.nlm.nih.gov/omim

OMIM is a searchable electronic database of syndromic developmental and cancer syndromes. Customized queries of co-occurring features retrieves comprehensive clinical and genetic information of candidate syndromes. You can also search by genetic lesion and retrieve details of all clinical phenotypes. Classic example of a print resource that had to go online to accommodate voluminous data.

Snoflake Browser
http://www.snoflake.co.uk/

Online lookup of Snomed terms and ICD10 codes by diagnosis. Requires registration but is free. Lean interface takes some getting used to.

CLINICAL PRACTICE STANDARDS IN OBSTETRICS AND GYNECOLOGY

American College of Obstetricians and Gynecologists
http://www.acog.org/Resources_And_Publications/Committee_Opinions_List

ACOG practice guidelines, which provide peer group reviews of changing practice for gynecologic disorders.

American Society for Reproductive Medicine (ASRM)
http://www.asrm.org/Guidelines/

ASRM practice committee guidelines include peer consensus opinions on diagnosis and management of fertility-related disorders.

Royal College of Obstetricians and Gynaecologists (UK)
http://www.rcog.org.uk/guidelines

Consensus guidelines for obstetrics and gynecology practice in the UK.

Society of Gynecologic Oncologists
https://www.sgo.org/

Need to refer a patient to a board-certified gynecologic oncologist in the United States? The Society of Gynecologic Oncologists has a nice referral search engine by geographic location. They also publish clinical practice guidelines for gynecologic cancers.

CANCER-RELATED CLINICAL INFORMATION

American Association of Cancer Research
http://www.aacr.org/

Sponsors several cancer-related meetings and has a searchable online 'clinical trials finder.'

Division of Cancer Prevention, NIH (U.S.)
http://prevention.cancer.gov/prevention-detection/cancers

Excellent precancer summaries by organ site. Includes review of susceptibility testing and core documents for common topics such as tamoxifen risk in endometrial cancer, and data from the cervix ALTS trial.

National Cancer Institute (U.S.)
http://www.cancer.gov/cancertopics/types/womenscancers

U.S. government mega-portal for comprehensive updated summaries of women's cancers. Includes statistical, pathobiologic, and clinical information.

PDQ Cancer Summaries
http://www.cancer.gov/cancertopics/pdq

'PDQ' cancer summaries by the U.S. government organize critical data by cancer type. Reviewed by a panel of listed experts, with formal assessments of level of evidence for stated conclusions. Includes prevention, treatment, screening, and genetics components by site. FIGO staging tables are included.

CANCER EPIDEMIOLOGY AND STATISTICS

American Cancer Society
http://www.cancer.org/

Organization that publishes annual summary of cancer statistics by disease site. See 'Cancer Facts and Figures' in the Explore Research section on the Web site.

International Agency for Research on Cancer
http://www.iarc.fr/

This is the cancer arm of the World Health Organization, which maintains online incidence databases and cancer staging (FIGO and non-FIGO). Interesting international incidence comparisons, but for a limited repertoire of disease. Use their search box, as menus are confusing.

Surveillance Epidemiology and End Results
http://seer.cancer.gov/

The SEER queryable database is a pan-U.S. cancer registry that allows user-friendly customization of disease-specific queries. You can, for example, easily create a plot of changing cancer rates by year and age.

MOLECULAR MARKERS AND GENOMICS

Cancer Genome Anatomy Project
http://cgap.nci.nih.gov/

Many tools for exploration and display of structural and expression changes in human cancers. Instant meta-analysis across multiple studies with a few clicks.

Catalog of Somatic Mutations in Cancer
http://cancer.sanger.ac.uk/cancergenome/projects/cosmic/

Pull lists of mutated genes by specified tissue or tissues by specified genes. Results can be downloaded for further analysis or compilation of figures.

Gene Expression Omnibus Profiles
http://www.ncbi.nlm.nih.gov/geoprofiles

Integrated database of gene expression data annotated by tissue type. Allows comparison of normal-disease state expression profiles across multiple independently published studies.

Genetic Testing Registry
http://www.ncbi.nlm.nih.gov/gtr/

Searchable disease database that returns syndromic and non-syndromic occurrences. These can be individually selected for a live report of which laboratories are doing which molecular tests for the disorder, complete with a report of interpretation and evidence level.

Kyto Encyclopedia of Genes and Genomics
http://www.genome.jp/kegg/

This site has gene molecular pathway maps organized by different diseases ('pathways in cancer'). Allows creation of customized diagrams from curated hierarchy of relationships.

National Center for Biotechnology Information
http://www.ncbi.nlm.nih.gov/

Pan-genomic databases for protein, RNA, DNA, and related literature across multiple species. Curated by the U.S. government.

Unigene
http://www.ncbi.nlm.nih.gov/unigene/

Enter your favorite gene and get genomic and protein/RNA expression structural details.

Index

Page numbers followed by 'f' indicate figures, 't' indicate tables, and 'b' indicate boxes.

A

Abdominal wall endometriosis, 500
Abortion
   endometritis following, 331
   tubal, 470
Abortus, hydropic, 794
Abruptio placenta, 754f, 771, 771f–772f
Acantholysis, 75–76
Acantholytic dermatitis, 50f–52f
Acanthosis, 75
   nigricans, 66
   psoriasiform, 76
Acardia, 756–757
Accessory
   ovaries, 721
   placental lobe, 751, 751f
Accreta, placenta, 346, 775–776, 775f
Acetowhite epithelium, 227–228, 227f–228f
Acrochordon, 109, 109f
Actinomyces spp., 140, 140f, 524
Actinomyces israelii, 330
   endometritis, 329f–330f
Actinomycosis, 525–526, 526f
Activin, 515–516
Adenocarcinoma in situ (AIS), 251–257
   biologic behavior and treatment of, 256–257
   cytologic findings of, 254, 254f
   definition of, 251
   differential diagnosis of, 254–256, 255f–256f
   etiology of, 252
   general features of, 252
   immunohistochemistry of, 253–254, 254f
   pathology of, 252–253, 252f–254f
Adenocarcinoma of cervix, 257–270, 499–500
   adenoma malignum of, 263
   endocervical-type, 259, 708f
   gastric-type, minimal deviation adenocarcinoma, adenoma malignum, 263–265
      biologic behavior and treatment of, 265
      clinical features of, 263
      cytologic diagnosis of, 264
      definition of, 263
      differential diagnosis of, 265
      immunohistochemistry of, 264
      pathology of, 263–264, 264f–265f
   intestinal-type, 262, 263f
   invasive, 259, 259t
   mesonephric, 269–270, 269f–270f
   microinvasive (early invasive), 257–259
   villoglandular, 265–267
Adenosquamous carcinoma, 270
   Glassy cell carcinoma, 271
Adenocarcinoma of endometrium, 370–401
   carcinosarcoma, 393–394, 393f–394f
   ciliated, 385, 385f
   clear cell, 391–393, 392f–393f, 616, 626–629
   endometrioid, 370, 371f–372f, 371t, 374–387
   glassy cell, 394
   histopathologic classification of, 372, 373t
   metastatic tumors, 395–396, 396f
   mixed, 393
   mucinous, 383, 383f–384f
      intestinal type, 394
   non-endometrioid, 370, 371f–372f, 371t
   prognostic factors in, 396–398
   risk factors for, 373
   secretory, 384, 384f, 616
   serous, 387–391, 388f–391f
   sertoliform, 385, 386f
   signet-ring, 394
   spread of, 398
   squamous cell, 394–395, 394f–395f
   synchronous with ovarian carcinoma, 395
   transitional cell, 394
   with trophoblastic differentiation, 395
   types of, 370–372, 371f
   undifferentiated, 394
   villoglandular, 385, 385f
Adenocarcinoma of ovary in dermoid cyst, 688
Adenocarcinoma of vagina, clear cell, 150–153, 151f–152f
Adenofibroma, 281, 281f, 478
   mixed Müllerian, 438–439
Adenoid basal carcinoma, 275–277, 276f
Adenoid cystic carcinoma, 277, 277f
Adenoma
   rete ovarii, 636
   Sertoli cell, 27–28, 27f–29f
Adenoma malignum, 380f
Adenomatoid tumor
   fallopian tube, 477–478, 478f
   ovary, 636–637
   peritoneum, 723
Adenomyoma, 281, 411, 447–452
   atypical polypoid, 345, 345f, 386, 386f, 449–450, 449f–450f
   endocervical- and endometrial type, 447–448, 448f
Adenomyosis, 378, 446–447, 446f–447f
   clinical features of, 446
   definition of, 446
   gross features of, 446, 446f
   microscopic features of, 446f–447f, 447
   pathogenesis of, 446
Adenosarcoma
   cervix, 281–282, 281f
   in endometriosis, 504
   Müllerian, 502, 620–621, 620f
   staging, 501
Adenosis of vagina, 136–139, 137f–138f
   fetal (embryonic), 138f
   mucinous, 138f
   tuboendometrial, 138f, 152f
Adenosquamous carcinoma of cervix, 270–271, 271f
Adjuvanted peptide and proteins, 195
Adnexal tumors, female, of Wolffian origin, 637
Adrenal gland tumors metastatic to the ovary, 707
Adrenal hyperplasia, forms of, affecting the external genitalia, 21t
Adrenal rest, 475, 475f
Adrenogenital syndrome, 18–22, 20t, 21f
Adult granulosa cell tumors (AGCTs), 643–647
Adult linear IgA bullous dermatosis, 59t, 61, 61f
AE1, granulosa cell tumors, 645
Age, and endometrial carcinoma prognosis, 397
Agenesis
   ovary, 523
   vagina, 139
ALK1, 836
Allergic contact dermatitis, 53–54, 53f
   common causes of, 54t
Alveolar soft part sarcoma, 453–454, 453f
Amenorrhea, 643–644
American Society for Clinical Pathology (ASCP), 200
AMH, 6t, 12
AMHR2, 6t
Amnion nodosum, 749, 749f
Anastrozole, 319
Anchoring villi, 742–743
Androgen insensitivity syndrome, 25–30, 27f–28f
Androgen receptor, 840
Androgen receptor insensitivity, 15
Androgen receptor insufficiency
   complete, 26–29, 26f
   incomplete, 29–30
Androgens, maternal ingestion of, 22
Aneuploid placenta, 797
   from trisomy, 797f
Angiofibroma, cellular, 119–120, 119f–120f, 120t
Angiogenesis, 491
Angiokeratoma, 124, 124f
Angiolipoma, 110
Angiomyofibroblastoma
   vagina, 145–146, 146f
   vulva, 118–119, 118f–119f, 120t
Angiomyxoma
   deep (aggressive), 120t, 125–126, 125f–126f
   superficial (cutaneous), 120t, 126–127, 126f–127f
Angiosarcoma, 454, 454f
'Anovulatory bleeding/shedding', 310–312

855

Antibodies
    for distinction between cervical tuboendometrial metaplasia and endometriosis and AIS, 839t
    patterns of immunoreactivity of, 829f
Anti-Müllerian hormone (AMH), 11, 13f
Apoplectic leiomyoma. *See* Hemorrhagic cellular leiomyoma
Appendix
    metastatic adenocarcinoma from, 705f
    metastatic low-grade mucinous tumor, 705f–706f
    tumors of, 704–705
Appendix epiploica infarction, 723, 723f
ARID1A mutation, 595
Arias-Stella reaction, 152–153, 181, 181f, 268, 333t, 339, 339f, 628–629
Aromatase inhibitors, endometrial effects of, 319
Artifact, in cervix, 217, 218f
ASCUS, 215
Asherman's syndrome, 305, 345–346
Atherosis, 762f
Atopic dermatitis, 53
Atopy, 74–75
Atretic follicular cysts, 538
Atrophic squamous epithelium, 162f–163f
Atrophic vaginitis, 140
Atrophy, 135f
'Atypical hyperplasia', 312
Atypical polypoid adenomyoma, 345, 345f
Atypical squamous metaplasia, 215, 216f
Atypical vessels, 226f, 228, 228f
Autoimmune oophoritis, 520–522, 521f–522f, 530
Autoimplants, 569, 569f
Avascular villi, 760, 761f, 771, 771f
    fixation of, 752f

B

Bacterial infections of vulva, 67–69
    chancroid, 69
    chlamydial infection, 69
    gonorrhea, 68
    granuloma inguinale, 69
    staphylococcal infections, 67
    streptococcal infections, 67
    syphilis, 67–68
Bacterial oophoritis, 524–526, 524f–525f
    actinomycosis, 525–526, 526f
    malacoplakia, 525
    pelvic inflammatory disease, 524
    tuberculosis, 526, 526f
    xanthogranulomatous oophoritis, 524–525
Bacterial vaginosis, 139
Bacteroides spp., 524
Band-like plasmacytic infiltrate, 50f–52f
Barium gelatin, intra-arterial injection of, 752f
Barr bodies, 31f
Bartholin cyst, 96–97, 96f–97f, 142
Bartholin gland, tumors of, 112–113, 112f
Basal cell carcinoma of vulva, 92–93, 92f
Basal cell hyperplasia of cervix, 163–164, 163f, 215, 215f
Basal cell nevus syndrome, 653
Basal layer hydropic degeneration, 75
Basaloid squamous cell carcinoma
    cervix, 241, 241f
    vulva, 90f
Basket-weave pattern, cervical squamous epithelium, 169
Bcl-2 proto-oncogene, 838
Beckwith-Wiedemann syndrome, 751–752, 764

Behçet disease, 63–64, 63f
Benign familial pemphigus, 50f–52f
'Benign mesothelioma', 477
Benign mixed tumor of vagina, 144, 144f
Benign squamous neoplasms of vulva, 79–81
    condyloma acuminatum, 79, 80f
    keratoacanthoma, 80–81, 81f
    seborrheic keratosis, 79–80, 80f
BER-EP4 antigen, 831
Bilobed placenta, 750–751
Biomarkers, 828–845, 829f
    broad spectrum differentiation markers, 828–832
        epithelial markers, 828–831
        mesenchymal cell markers, 831
    cell adhesion markers, 840
    cell cycle and nuclear proliferation, 838–839
    CIN, 218–219, 219f
    EIN, 367
    hormone receptors, 839–840
        androgen receptor, 840
        estrogen receptor, 839–840
        oxytocin receptor, 831t
        progesterone receptor, 839–840
    narrow spectrum differentiation markers, 832–834
        lymphoid markers, 834
        melanocytic markers, 833
        neuroendocrine markers, 833–834
        trophoblastic markers, 833
    proto-oncogenes, 838
    tumor markers, 834–836
Biopsy, 812–813
    cervix
        cone, 817–818, 817f–818f
        punch, 817
    endometrial, 818
    LEEP, 237–238
        thermal artifacts, 217, 218f, 237–238
    Pipelle, 305, 307f
    vulva, 815
Bizarre nuclei, in endometrial stromal tumors, 431
Black cohosh, 319
Blastocyst, 741
Blood vessel markers, 832
'Blue balls', 297f
Blue nevus, 284, 284f
    cervix, 284
    vulva, 102, 103f
Borderline tumors of the ovary, 565
BRCA1, 584
BRCA2, 584
BRCA abnormalities, 628
Breast, heterotopic, 109
Breast cancer, 20t
Breast carcinoma, metastatic, 702–703, 702f–703f, 765f
Brenner nests, 629
Brenner tumors, 684
    benign, 629–630
        clinical features of, 629
        immunohistochemistry and somatic genetics of, 630
        macroscopic features of, 629, 630f
        microscopic features of, 629–630, 630f
    borderline and malignant, 630–633
        clinical features of, 630
        differential diagnosis of, 632–633
        genetic profile of, 632
        immunohistochemistry of, 632, 632f
        macroscopic features of, 630–631, 631f

        microscopic features of, 631–632, 631f–632f
        treatment and prognosis of, 633, 633f
    differential diagnosis of, 616
Breslow thickness, 105
Breus mole, 754f, 755
Broad ligament, 492f
    adrenal rests, 475
    cysts, 473
    endometriosis, 488t, 492f
Broad spectrum differentiation markers, 828–832
    epithelial markers, 828–831, 829f
        BER-EP4, 831
        CAM 5.2, 829
        cytokeratins, 828–829
        epithelial membrane antigen, 831
    mesenchymal cell markers, 831
        blood vessel markers, 832
        endometrial stromal markers, 832
        mesothelial markers, 832
        skeletal muscle markers, 832
        smooth muscle markers, 831–832
        vimentin, 831
Brooke-Spiegler syndrome, 107
Bulky specimen, 352t
Bullae, 75
Bullous disorders, 58–61
    adult linear IgA bullous dermatosis, 59t, 61, 61f
    bullous pemphigoid, 59t, 61
    chronic bullous dermatosis, 59t, 61, 61f
    cicatricial pemphigoid, 59t, 61
    pemphigus vegetans, 59t, 60–61, 60f
    pemphigus vulgaris, 58–60, 59t
Bullous pemphigoid, 50f–52f, 59t, 61
Burkitt lymphoma, starry-sky pattern, 709f

C

CA19.9, 834
CA125, 834
E-Cadherin, 840
Calcific degeneration, 407
h-Caldesmon, 831t
    cellular leiomyoma, 406
    endometrial stromal tumors, 433t
Call-Exner bodies, 612–613, 643f, 644–645
    differential diagnosis of, 646–647
Calretinin, 437, 645, 832
    mesothelioma, 710f
Calymmatobacterium granulomatis, 69
CAM 5.2, 276, 829
Canal of Nuck, cysts of, 98
Candida, 140f
Candida albicans, 69, 170
Candida chorioamnionitis, 749
Candida funisitis, 749f
Candidiasis, 69, 69f
Capsid/virion production, 209–210
Carcinoembryonic antigen (CEA), 176, 834
Carcinoid syndrome, 666
Carcinoid tumor
    cervix
        atypical, 277–278, 278f
        typical (classic), 277, 278f
    differential diagnosis of, 702t
    metastatic, 697f, 701–702
    ovary, 646, 686f
Carcinoids, 684–686, 685f–686f
Carcinoma
    embryonal, 671f, 678, 678f
    undifferentiated, *versus* diffuse AGCT, 646–647
Carcinoma of cervix
    adenoid basal, 275–277, 276f

adenoid cystic, 277, 277f
glassy cell, 271, 271f
large cell neuroendocrine, 280, 280f
small cell neuroendocrine, 278–279, 278f–279f
Carcinoma of colon, 616
Carcinoma of ovary arising in dermoid cyst, 565
Carcinoma of vagina
small cell, 150, 150f
verrucous, 149, 149f
warty, 150
Carcinomatosis, peritoneal, 598
Carcinosarcoma
cervix, 282–283
endometrium, 393–394, 393f–394f, 443–446, 443f–445f
fallopian tube, 483, 484f
β-Catenin, 840
gene mutations, 610–611
Cauterized tissue, granuloma, 718
Cavernous hemangioma, 108
CD4+, 521
CD10, 282, 831t, 832
endometrial stromal tumors, 431–432, 433t
CD30, 673t
CD34, 832
CD56, 833–834
CD99, 835–836
granulosa cell tumors, 645
CD117, 3, 838
dysgerminoma, 673
CDX-2, 835
Cell adhesion markers, 840
Cellular angiofibroma, 119–120, 119f–120f, 120t
Cellular endometrial polyp, 442
Cellular fibroma, 646, 653–654, 654f
Cellular intravenous leiomyomatosis, 434
Cellular leiomyoma, 405–406, 405f
Centers for Disease Control, 195
Cerebral palsy, placenta in, 774–775
Ceroid, 718
Cervarix, 195
Cervical adenocarcinoma, 257
adenoma malignum gastric-type or minimal deviation, 263
biologic behavior and treatment of, 265
clinical features of, 263
cytologic diagnosis of, 264
definition of, 263
differential diagnosis of, 265
immunohistochemistry of, 264
pathology of, 263–264, 264f–265f
clear cell, 245, 267–268
biologic behavior and treatment of, 268
definition of, 267
differential diagnosis of, 268
pathology of, 267–268, 267f–268f
gastric type, minimal deviation of, 263–265
intestinal-type, 262, 263f
invasive, 259, 259t
mesonephric, 269–270
biologic behavior and treatment of, 269
definition of, 269
differential diagnosis of, 269–270
pathology of, 269, 269f–270f
microinvasive (early invasive)
biologic behavior and treatment of, 258–259
cytologic correlation of, 258
definition of, 257
pathology of, 257–258, 257f–258f
serous, 268–269

usual-type, 259–262
biologic behavior and treatment of, 262
cytologic correlation of, 261, 262f
definition of, 259
differential diagnosis of, 261–262
immunohistochemistry of, 261, 261f
pathology of, 259–260, 259f–260f, 260t
in situ hybridization of, 261
Cervical carcinoma
adenosquamous, 270–271
biologic behavior and treatment of, 270–271
clinical features of, 270
definition of, 270
differential diagnosis of, 270
pathology of, 270, 270f–271f
Cervical glandular intraepithelial neoplasia (CGIN), 251
Cervical glandular neoplasia (CGN), 251–274
Cervical intraepithelial neoplasia (CIN), 251, *see also* Squamous intraepithelial lesions, cervical
cytologic findings on, 254
definition of, 251
Cervical neoplasia, 275–289
adenoid basal carcinoma, 275–277, 276f
epithelioid trophoblastic tumor, 245
leukemia, 285–286
lymphoma, 285–286
metastatic, 286–287, 287f
squamous type, 188–199
early detection of, 194–195
epidemiology of, 188
immune-based therapies for, 195
public health significance of, 188
vaccines for, 194–196
Cervical neuroendocrine tumors, 277–280
carcinoid tumor, 277
atypical, 277–278, 278f
typical (classic), 277, 278f
large cell, 280
small cell, 278–279, 278f–279f
Cervical sarcoma
adenosarcoma, 281–282
carcinosarcoma, 282–283
embryonal rhabdomyosarcoma, 283, 283f
Cervical squamocolumnar junction, 224
Cervical squamous cell carcinoma, 232–250
cervical stump, 245
invasive, 232–233
biomarkers of, 244
clinical behavior of, 243, 243f
clinicopathologic correlation of, 242–243
cytology of, 242, 242f
definition of, 239t
differential diagnosis of, 244–245
epidemiology of, 232–233
gross features of, 238–239, 239f–240f
microscopic features of, 239–242, 242f
basaloid type, 241, 241f
keratinizing type, 239–240, 240f
nonkeratinizing type, 240, 240f–241f
microscopic grading of, 241
prognostic features of, 243–245, 243t
histopathologic, 243–244, 243t, 244f
peritumoral lymphatic vessel density, 244
tumor size, 244
staging of, 233, 233t
lymphoepithelioma, 247–248, 247f
microinvasive, 233–238
definition of, 233–234
depth of invasion of, 234–237, 234t
histopathologic features of, 236t
history of, 233–234

morphologic features of, 235–238
clinical management of, 238
confluent growth pattern, 235–236, 236f
cytologic findings, 238
diagnosis of, 238
extent of spread, 236–237
lymphovascular space involvement, 237, 237f
spray-bud growth pattern, 235–236, 235f
stromal invasion, 235–236, 235f–237f
surgical margins, 237–238
micrometastasis, 246
mucin-secreting, 246, 246f
papillary squamotransitional cell carcinoma, 248
radiotherapy effects on, 245–246, 246f
verrucous, 246–247, 247f
warty, 247
Cervical squamous intraepithelial lesions (CIN, HSIL, LSIL), 200–231, 201f
Cervical stump carcinoma, 245
Cervicitis, 171f–172f
cytologic correlation, 171
infective, 170–174, 171f–172f
inflammatory, 170–176
Cervix, 499–500
anatomy of, 160, 161f
Arias-Stella reaction, 181
blue nevus, 284
decidual change, 182, 182f
deep Nabothian cysts, 179, 179f
diffuse laminar endocervical glandular hyperplasia, 180, 180f
ectopic tissue, 186, 186f
endocervical glandular epithelium, 177–180
endocervical tunnel clusters, 177–178, 261
endocervical villi, 164f
endometriosis, 183, 183f, 499–500
exogenous stimuli, lesions related to, 180–183
external os, 160
glandular epithelium, 179f–180f
healing/regenerating epithelium, 175–176, 175f–176f
inflammatory changes, 170–176
Chlamydia trachomatis, 170–172
cytomegalovirus, 173–174, 174f
epithelial, 175–176, 175f
herpes simplex virus, 170
infective cervicitis, 170–174
mesonephric duct hyperplasia, 184–185
mesonephric duct remnants, 183–184
microglandular hyperplasia, 180–181
schistosomiasis, 174, 175f
syphilis, 172–173, 173f
tuberculosis, 172, 173f
metaplasias, 176–177
native (original) glandular epithelium, 164–165, 164f
native (original) squamous epithelium, 160–164
non-neoplastic changes, 160–187
intestinal metaplasia, 177, 177f
tubal, endometrioid, and tuboendometrioid metaplasia, 176–177
normal structure of, 160–165
physiologic changes, 165–170
eversion, 166f
inversion, 166
polyp, 185–186, 185f
postmenopausal atrophy, 163, 167f
radiation changes, 182–183, 182f

specimen processing, 817–818
   cone biopsy, 817–818, 817f–818f
   endocervical curettage, 817
   malignant disease, 818
   punch biopsies, 817
squamous epithelium, 161f
   basal cell hyperplasia, 163–164, 163f
   basket-weave pattern, 161
   differentiation of, 161
   endometrial cells, 163, 163f
   hormonal influences on, 162–163, 162f
   intermediate squamous cells, 162, 162f
   keratinization of, 162
   maturation of, 161
   parabasal squamous cells, 162, 162f
   picket-fence appearance, 161
   postmenopausal atrophy, 163
   squamous cell hyperplasia, 164
   stratification of, 161–162
   superficial squamous cells, 162, 162f
squamous metaplasia, 166–169, 168f–169f
structural changes of, 136, 137f
transformation zone, 165–170, 170f
   histogenesis, 169–170
Cesarean delivery causing granulomatous peritonitis, 718
Chancroid, 69
Chaste tree berry, 319
Chemotherapy, ovarian effects, 558
Chlamydia trachomatis, 69, 170–172
   cytologic correlation, 172
   endometritis, 328
Chlamydial cervicitis, 172f
Chlamydial infection, 69
Chloroma, 709–710
Chocolate cyst, 493, 494f
Cholesterol synthesis defects, 24
Chondrosarcoma, 454
Chorangiocarcinoma, 764
Chorangioma, 764, 764f–765f
Chorangiomatosis, 762, 763f
Chorangiosis, 762, 763f
Chorioamnionitis
   acute, 748, 748f
      inflammatory responses in, 748t
   chronic, 758, 758f
Choriocarcinoma, 800–802, 801f–802f
   clinical presentation of, 800
   differential diagnosis of, 801–802
   extrauterine, 800
   full-term pregnancy, 802–803
   genetics of, 800–801
   gross and microscopic findings of, 801
   intraplacental, 764–765, 802–803, 803f
   of uterus, 801f
Choriocarcinoma *in situ*, 765f
Chorion frondosum, 741–742
Chorion laeve, 741–742, 743f
Chorionic gonadotropin, 13
Chorionic plate vessel, thrombus in, 752f
Chorionic vasculitis, 748–749
Chorionic villi, 741–742, 770, 787
Chorionic villous, 742f
Chromogranin, 278–279, 279f
Chronic bullous dermatosis, 59f, 61, 61f
Cicatricial pemphigoid, 50f–52f, 59t, 61
Ciliated cyst, 97, 97f
CIN, Cervical Intraepithelial Neoplasia. *See* squamous intraepithelial lesions
Circummarginate placenta, 750, 750f
Circumvallate placenta, 750, 750f
Civatte bodies, 58, 58f
   see also Basal layer hydropic degeneration
CK7, 829–830
CK20, 829–830

C-kit, 3, 7f, 674
   endometrial stromal tumors, 432
Clark nevus, 102–103
Clear cell adenocarcinoma, 150–153, 151f–152f
   of cervix, 245, 267–268
   endometriosis, 504–505, 504f
   endometrium, 267, 391–393
      behavior and treatment of, 393
      biologic behavior and treatment, 268
      clinical features of, 391
      definition of, 267
      differential diagnosis of, 268, 392, 393f
      gross features of, 391
      immunochemistry of, 391–392
      microscopic features of, 391, 392f
      pathology, 267–268, 267f–268f
   of ovary, 504, 504f–505f, 626–629, 626f–627f
      differential diagnosis of, 628–629
      genetic susceptibility of, 628
      immunohistochemistry of, 627–628, 627f
      somatic genetics of, 628
      treatment and prognosis of, 629
      tumor spread and staging of, 629
Clear cell carcinoma, fallopian tube, 482
Clear cell leiomyoma, 409–410, 410f
Clear cell lesions, 735
Clear cell ovarian tumors, 624–629
   adenocarcinomas, 626–629
   benign, 625
   borderline, 625, 625f
   general features of, 624
   macroscopic features of, 624–625, 625f
   SNOMED classification of, 624
Clinical Practice Committee of the Society of Gynecologic Oncologists, 349
Clomiphene citrate, 559
   endometrial effects of, 320, 320f
Clue cells, 139, 140f, 171, 171f
C-myc, 419
Coagulative necrosis, 417–418
Colloid bodies. *See* Civatte bodies
Colonic adenocarcinoma, metastatic, 616
Colonic tumors, metastatic, 695f–697f, 699f
Colorectal adenocarcinoma, metastatic, reaction patterns in, 830t
Colposcopy, 224–229
   abnormal findings of, 226–229, 226f–229f, 226t
      acetowhite epithelium, 227–228, 227f–228f
      acuminate warts, 228–229, 229f
      atypical vessels, 226f, 228, 228f
      congenital transformation zone, 228
      glandular lesions, 229, 229f
      leukoplakia, 228, 228f
      mosaic and punctation, 226–227, 226f–227f
      subclinical HPV infection, 229
      suspect frank invasive carcinoma, 228, 229f
   normal findings of, 225–226, 225f–226f
      columnar epithelium, 225, 225f
      original squamous epithelium, 225, 225f
      squamous metaplasia, 225–226
   vagina and, 229
Common acute lymphoblastic leukemia antigen. *See* CD10
Condyloma acuminatum, 72–73, 73f–74f, 79, 80f, 208–210, 208f–211f
   flat lesions (CIN1), 211–212, 212f
   histologic features of, 219–221

Confluent growth pattern superficially invasive squamous cell carcinoma of cervix, 235–236, 236f
Congenital disorders, miscellaneous, 139
Congenital leukemia, 766f
Congenital lipoid adrenal hyperplasia, 20t, 24
Congenital transformation zone (CTZ), 169, 170f, 218, 228
   histogenesis of, 169–170
Contact dermatitis
   allergic, 53–54
   irritant, 53
Contrast media granuloma, 717
Cord
   hemangioma of, 747f
   hypercoiled, 746f
Corpus albicans cysts, 539
Corpus luteum, 512–513
   cysts, 536, 536f, 538–539, 539f
   formation of, 512–513, 513f
   involution of, 513–514, 514f
   persistent, 538
Corticosteroids, endometrial effects of, 321
Corynebacterium minutissimum, 69–70
Crohn disease, 64
   cutaneous, 64f
   ovary, 529–530
   vulvar, 64f
Crystalloids of Reinke, 11f
CTNNB1, 615, 655–656
   mutations, 610–611
Cushing syndrome, 667
Cutaneous myxoma. *See* Superficial angiomyxoma
Cutaneous neuroendocrine carcinoma, 110–112
Cyclin D1, 615, 839
Cyclin E, 839
CYP21A2, 19–21
Cystadenofibroma, mucinous, 592f–593f
Cystadenoma
   mucinous, 592f
   rete, 567
   serous, 478, 566f
Cystic degeneration, 406–407
Cystic granulosa cell tumors, 538
Cystic teratoma, rupture, 717
Cysts, 95–98
   atretic follicular, 538
   Bartholin, 96–97
   of canal of Nuck, 98
   chocolate, 493, 494f
   ciliated, 97, 97f
   corpus albicans, 539
   corpus luteum, 536, 536f, 538–539, 539f
   epidermoid (squamous cell), 633
   fallopian tube, 472–474
      mesonephric, 473, 473f
      paramesonephric, 473, 473f
   follicular (epidermoid), 95–96, 96f
   granulosa lutein, 536–537, 536f, 538f
   of introitus, 142
   luteinized follicular, 537, 542–543, 543f–544f
   mesonephric-like, 97–98
   mesothelial, 499, 721f–722f
   mucinous, 97
   ovarian serosal inclusion, 498–499
   paraurethral (Skene) gland, 97
   peritoneal inclusion, 720–721, 722f
   rete ovarii, 636
   simple (unclassified), 540, 540f
   steatocystoma multiplex, 96
   theca-lutein, 536–537, 536f, 538f, 542, 543f

unluteinized follicular, 536–537, 536f–537f
urothelial, 142
vaginal, 141–142
Cytogenetics, 419
Cytokeratin reaction patterns, in tumors, 830t
Cytokeratins (CKs), 245–246, 276–277, 828–829, 830t
  BER-EP4, 831
  broad spectrum, 829
  CAM 5.2, 829
  CK5/6, 830
  CK7, 829–830
  CK20, 829–830
  epithelial membrane antigen, 831
Cytologic atypia, 205
Cytomegalovirus
  cervix, 173–174, 174f
  endometritis, 327t, 328–329, 329f
  placenta in, 777–778, 778f
Cytotrophoblast, 741–742, 784–785
  cell columns, 745
  intravascular extravillous, 742–743

D

D2-40, 673t
Daidzein, 319–320
Danazol
  endometrial effects of, 321
  ovarian effects of, 559
Darier disease, 59t, 62, 62f
DAX1, 2–3, 6t
DAZ, 9–10
Decidua capsularis, vessel in, 762f
Deciduitis, 758
Deciduosis, 543–544, 544f, 735, 736f
Deep angiomyxoma, 120t, 125–126, 125f–126f
Deep lymphatic malformation, 108–109, 109f
Degenerated leiomyoma, 406–407, 406f
Denys-Drash syndrome, 20t, 36
Dermal infiltrate, 54
Dermal-epidermal junctional split, 50f–52f
Dermatitis medicamentosa, 66–67
Dermatofibroma, 121–122, 121f–122f
Dermatofibrosarcoma protuberans, 127–128, 127f
Dermatolipoma, 109, 109f
Dermatosis, 75
Dermoid cyst, 717
Desmin, 831t
  cellular leiomyoma, 406
  endometrial stromal tumors, 433t
  granulosa cell tumors, 645
17,20-desmolase enzyme, deficiency of, 24–25
Desmoplastic small round cell tumor, 711f, 727–728, 727f–728f
Desogestrel, 312t–313t
Diabetes mellitus
  endometrial adenocarcinoma risk, 373
  placenta in, 775
DICER1 gene, 659
Diethylstilbestrol, 311t
  vaginal effects of, 136–139, 137f
Diffuse chorioamnionic hemosiderosis, 750
Dihydrotestosterone, 15
Dilatation and curettage, 304
Dimpling sign, 121
Diploid androgenetic pregnancy, 790
Dissociation artifact, 307–308, 307f–308f
DMRT1, 6t
DMRT2, 6t
DOG1, 841
Dong quai, 319

DPC4, 837
Drawings, 815
Drospirenone, 312t–313t
D-score, 367–368
Dysesthetic vulvodynia, 65
Dysgerminoma, 628, 671–674
  clinical features of, 671–672
  differential diagnosis of, 628, 674
  genetic susceptibility of, 674
  immunohistochemistry of, 673–674, 673f–674f, 673t
  macroscopic features of, 672, 672f
  metastatic, 709
  microscopic features of, 672–673, 672f–673f
  in mixed gonadal dysgenesis, 40f
  somatic genetics of, 674
  treatment and prognosis of, 674
Dyskaryotic cells, 206–207
Dyskeratosis, 210
Dysplasia, 202
  placental mesenchymal, 796
Dysplasia-free koilocytes, 209

E

E6 oncoprotein, 192
E7 oncoprotein, 193
Early pregnancy loss, 769–770, 770f
Eclampsia, pathogenesis of, 773f
Ectocervix, 161f
Ectopic decidua. See Pseudodecidual change
Ectopic hydatidiform mole, 795
Ectopic pregnancy
  ovarian, 545, 545f–546f, 802f
  tubal, 471f–472f, 795f, 822
Eczematous, 75
Edema, ovarian, 552–556, 655
EIN. See Endometrial intraepithelial neoplasia (EIN)
Embryology, 1–17, 4t–5t
  external genitalia, 15–16, 16f
  external influence on, 12–14
  gonadal development, 1–11
  Müllerian duct development, 11–15
  role of germ cells in, 11
  Wolffian duct development, 11–15
Embryonal carcinoma, 678f
Embryonal rhabdomyosarcoma, 117, 154–155, 155f, 283, 283f
Embryonic ovary, 34f
Emphysematous vaginitis, 140, 141f
Endocervical adenocarcinoma, reaction patterns of, 840t
Endocervical cells, 165, 165f
Endocervical crypts, 165f
Endocervical curettage, 817
Endocervical like mucinous borderline tumors, 593–595
  immunohistochemistry and somatic genetics of, 595
  macroscopic features of, 594, 594f
  microscopic features of, 594–595, 594f–595f
  treatment and prognosis of, 595
Endocervical tunnel clusters, 177–178, 178f, 256, 261, 265
Endocervicosis, 735
Endometrial ablation, 347, 347f
Endometrial adenocarcinoma, 370–401
  carcinosarcoma, 393–394, 393f–394f
  ciliated, 385, 385f
  clear cell, 391–393, 392f–393f
  endometrioid, 370, 371f–372f, 371t, 374–387

  precursor lesions EIN, 381–382, 381f
  secretory, 616
  histopathologic classification of, 372, 373t
  invasion, reaction patterns of, 840t
  metastatic tumors, 395–396, 396f
  mixed, 393
  mucinous, 383, 383f–384f
  non-endometrioid, 370, 371f–372f, 371t
  prognostic factors in, 396–398
    age, 397
    histological grade, 396
    lymphovascular invasion, 397
    stage and depth of myometrial invasion, 396–397, 396t, 397f
    steroid hormone receptors, 397–398
    tumor type, 396
  risk factors for, 373
    diabetes, 373
    estrogens, 373
    ovarian granulosa tumor, 643–644
    obesity, 373
    polycystic ovary syndrome (PCOS), 373
    reproductive factors, 374
    sex cord-stromal tumors, 373
    smoking, 374
    tamoxifen, 374
  secretory, 384, 384f, 616
  serous, 387–391, 388f–391f
  sertoliform, 385, 386f
  signet-ring, 394
  spread of, 398
  squamous cell, 394–395, 394f–395f
  synchronous with ovarian carcinoma, 395
  transitional cell, 394
  with trophoblastic differentiation, 395
  types of, 370–372, 371f
  undifferentiated, 394
  villoglandular, 385, 385f
Endometrial cells in PAP, 163, 163f
Endometrial extramedullary hemopoiesis, 342
Endometrial granular cells, 294–295
Endometrial hyperplasia, 350, 609
  atypical, see Endometrial intraepithelial neoplasia (EIN)
  non-atypical, 350–357, 353f–355f
    clinical features of, 351
    cytology of, 353–354
    differential diagnosis of, 356
      disordered proliferative endometrium, 352–353
      endometrial intraepithelial neoplasia, 357
      normal endometrium, 356, 356f
      postmenopausal cystic atrophy, 356–357
    etiology of, 351
    general features of, 350f
    gross features of, 351, 352f
    histologic features of, 352t
    microscopic features of, 351–352
      cysts and tubal metaplasia, 352t
      remodeling, fibrin thrombi and microinfarcts, 352t
      superimposed progestin effect, 355, 355f–356f
      withdrawal shedding, 355–356, 356f
    treatment of, 357
Endometrial intraepithelial neoplasia (EIN), 312, 350t, 357–367
  biomarkers, 367
  cancer outcomes in women with, 358, 358f
  with ciliated tubal differentiation, 333f–334f
  clinical features of, 357
  diagnostic criteria for, 360–364, 360t

architecture, 361, 361f
cytology, 361–362, 361f–362f
exclusion of benign mimics, 362–363, 363f
exclusion of carcinoma, 363–364, 364f
size, 362, 362f
diagnostic problems with, 364–365
EIN within endometrial polyp, 365, 365f
excessively fragmented tissue, 365
hormonally treated EIN, 366–367, 367f
localizing lesions subdiagnostic for EIN, 365, 365f
non-endometrioid EIN, 366, 366f
non-localizing EIN, 364–365, 364f
differential diagnosis of, 356
with eosinophilic differentiation, 340
gross features of, 359
management of, 368
hormonal therapy, 368
hysterectomy, 368
with micropapillary differentiation, 340–341, 341f
microscopic features of, 359–360, 360f
molecular etiology of, 358–360
clonal growth, 358–359, 359f
latent precancers, 359–360
mutation, 358–359, 359f
with mucinous differentiation, 336–339
natural history of, 358–360
neoplastic character of, 350
quantitative histomorphometry, 367–368
with secretory differentiation, 339–340, 340f
special studies for, 367–368
with squamous morules, 333–336
Endometrial metaplasias, 331–342
eosinophilic, 340
epithelial, 332, 332t–333t
mesenchymal, 342
endometrial extramedullary hemopoiesis, 342
osseous metaplasia, 342, 342f
micropapillary "hobnail", 341–342, 342f
to mucinous epithelium, 336–339
benign mucinous changes, 337–338, 337f–338f
EIN and adenocarcinoma with mucinous differentiation, 338–339, 338f–339f
papillary, 340–341, 341f
papillary syncytial, 332t, 341, 341f–342f
to secretory epithelium, 339–340
to squamous epithelium, 333–336
EIN with squamous morules, 334–335, 335f–336f
ichthyosis uteri, 334, 334f
isolated squamous morules, 335–336, 337f
to tubal epithelium, 332–333, 333f–334f
Endometrial polyps, 342–344
clinical features of, 343
etiology and natural history of, 342–343, 343f
gross features of, 343, 343f
microscopic features of, 343–344, 344f–345f
Endometrial replacement, 474f
Endometrial stromal markers, 832
Endometrial stromal neoplasm (ESN), 433t
reaction patterns in, 831t
Endometrial stromal sarcoma, 429, 429f–430f
Endometrial stromal tumors, 425–435
high-grade and undifferentiated sarcoma, 432f, 434f, 435, 436f

low-grade sarcoma, 427–435, 427f–429f, 431f, 434f
clinical features of, 427
cytogenetics of, 434
definition of, 427
differential diagnosis of, 432–434
gross features of, 427
immunohistochemical features of, 431–432
microscopic features of, 427–428, 427f–428f
treatment and prognosis of, 434–435
resembling ovarian sex cord tumor, 411, 436–438, 437f–438f
with sex cord-like elements, 429, 430f
with smooth muscle tumor elements, 428–429
stromal nodules, 425–426
clinical features of, 425
definition of, 425
differential diagnosis of, 426
gross features of, 425, 426f
microscopic features of, 426, 426f–427f
treatment and prognosis of, 426
variants features of, 428–435, 428t
Endometrialization, 290
Endometrioid adenocarcinoma of cervix, 267, 350t, 609f
Endometrioid adenocarcinoma of endometrium, 370, 371f–372f, 371t, 374–387
behavior and treatment of, 387
with ciliated differentiation, 385, 385f
clinical features of, 374
cytological correlation of, 381–382, 381f–382f
definition of, 374
differential diagnosis of, 385–387
gross features of, 374–375, 375f
histologic grading of, 377–378, 377f–378f, 377t–378t
microscopic features of, 375–377, 375f–377f
with mucinous differentiation, 383, 383f–384f
myoinvasion of, 378–381, 379f–380f
post-radiation appearance, 387, 387f
with secretory differentiation, 384, 384f
with sertoliform differentiation, 385, 386f
with squamous differentiation, 382, 382f–383f, 383t
villoglandular, 385, 385f
Endometrioid adenofibroma of ovary
borderline, 610f
differential diagnosis of, 616
with well-differentiated (grade 1) intraepithelial carcinoma, 610f
Endometrioid carcinoma of fallopian tube, 481
Endometrioid carcinoma of ovary, 611–618, 614f
differential diagnosis of, 616
genetic susceptibility of, 614
grading of, 614, 614f
immunohistochemistry of, 614, 614f
macroscopic features of, 611, 611f
microscopic features of, 611–614, 611f–612f
mucin-rich, 612, 612f
somatic genetics of, 615–616, 615f–616f
spread and metastasis of, 614
treatment and prognosis of, 616–618
Endometrioid carcinoma of ovary and endometrium, 617f, 618, 619f
Endometrioid metaplasia, 176–177, 177f

Endometrioid stromal sarcomas, 620–623
clinical features of, 621
definition of, 621
differential diagnosis of, 622
versus diffuse AGCT, 646
immunohistochemistry and somatic genetics of, 621–622
macroscopic features of, 621, 621f
microscopic features of, 621, 621f–622f
prognosis of, 622, 622f
treatment of, 623
Endometriosis, 487–508
abdominal wall, 500
as benign solid tumor, 501–502
cervix, 183, 183f, 499–500
classification of, 501
clinical features of, 487–488
distribution of, 488, 488t
epidemiology of, 488–489
etiologic factors in, 490–491
angiogenesis, 491
congenital anatomic abnormalities, 491
genetics factors, 490–491
peritoneal environment, 491
systemic hormonal factors, 491
fallopian tube, 474, 474f, 499, 499f
gastrointestinal tract, 500, 500f
gross features of, 492–493, 492f
infertility in, 501
intrinsic abnormalities of, 490, 490f
lymph nodes, 500–501, 501f
malignancy in, 502–505, 503f, 505f–506f
microscopic features of, 493–498, 494f–498f
morphologic features of, 491–498, 498f
mulberry lesions, 492–493, 493f
ovary, 498–499
pathogenesis of, 489–490
metaplastic theory, 490
transplantation, 489, 489f
peritoneal surfaces, 499
peritoneum, 733
powder burn lesion, 492–493, 493f
specific anatomic locations of, 498–501
urinary tract, 500
vagina, 144, 502
vulva, 109, 503
Endometritis, 326–331
Actinomyces israelii, 329f–330f, 330
acute, 327, 327f
Chlamydia trachomatis, 328
chronic, 326, 328f
classification of, 327t
cytomegalovirus, 327t, 328–329, 329f
granulomatous, 327t, 330
herpes simplex virus, 327t, 329
histiocytic, 330, 330f
histologic features of, 328t
Mycoplasma, 328
Neisseria gonorrhoeae, 328, 331
nonspecific, 327–328
postabortal, 327t, 330–331, 331f
postpartum, 327t, 330–331
pyometra, 327t, 331, 331f
tuberculous, 329, 329f
Endometrium, 290–309
blood vessels in, 295
components of, 290–295, 291f–292f
disordered proliferative, 352–353, 353f
glandular cells of, 292–293, 292f–293f
hormonal effects in, 310–325
aromatase inhibitors, 319
clomiphene, 320, 320f
corticosteroids, 321
danazol, 321
estrogens, 310–312, 311f, 311t

gonadotropin-releasing hormone agonists, 321
gonadotropins, 321
hormone replacement therapy, 315–317, 316f–317f
mifepristone, 320–321
oral contraceptives, 313–315, 313t
ovulation induction therapy, 320, 320f
phytoestrogens, 319–320
progestins, 312–313, 312f–313f, 312t, 321–322
tamoxifen, 318–319, 318f–319f
treatment of hyperplasia, EIN and carcinoma, 322, 322f–323f
intrauterine contraceptive device, 346–347, 346f
isthmic, 291f
lymphocytes, 294–295, 294f–295f
menopause, 303–304, 303f–304f
menstrual cycle, 295–303, 296f
  interval phase, 299, 299f
  menstrual phase, 297–298, 297f–298f
  proliferative phase, 298, 298f–299f
  secretory exhaustion, 301–303, 301f–303f
  secretory phase, 299–301, 300f–301f
normal, 356, 356f
'pill', 312–313, 314f
polyps, 342–344, 356
radiation effect on, 346, 346f
sampling, 304–307
  cytologic evaluation, 305, 305f
  dilatation and curettage, 304
  hysteroscopy, 305
  Pipelle biopsy, 305, 307f
  resection (ablation), 305–307, 306f
  Vabra aspirator, 304–305
specimen interpretation, 307–309
  adequacy, 307, 307f
  dissociation artifact, 307–308, 307f–308f
  fixation artifact, 308, 308f
  telescoping artifact, 308, 308f
  tissue contaminants, 308–309
stratum basalis, 291f
stratum compactum, 291–292, 292f
stratum functionalis, 291–292, 292f
stratum spongiosum, 291–292, 292f
stromal cells of, 293–294, 293f–294f
surface epithelium, 292, 292f
  ciliated, 292f
"Swiss cheese", 303–304, 356–357
see also Endometrial
Endosalpingiosis, 474, 494, 499, 499f, 573f, 733–735, 733t, 734f
Endovascular trophoblast
  infiltrating into blood vessels, 787f
  in normal implantation site, 786
Eosinophilic metaplasia, 340
Eosinophilic/T-cell vasculitis, 758, 759f
Epidermoid (squamous cell) cysts, 633
Epidermolysis bullosa, 59t, 62
  acquisita, 50f–52f
Epithelial inflammatory changes, 175–176, 175f
Epithelial markers, 828–831
  BER-EP4, 831
  CAM 5.2, 276, 829
  cytokeratins, 828–829
  epithelial membrane antigen, 831
Epithelial membrane antigen, 831
  dysgerminoma, 673–674
  granulosa cell tumors, 645
Epithelioid appearance, in endometrial stromal tumors, 430, 431f
Epithelioid leiomyoma, 409–410, 409f–410f

Epithelioid leiomyosarcoma, 415, 415f
Epithelioid smooth muscle tumor, 805
Epithelioid trophoblastic tumor, 245, 805–807, 806f–807f
Epstein-Barr virus, cervical changes, 204–205
Erythema, 75
Erythema infectiosum, 778
Erythema multiforme, 50f–52f, 63
Escherichia coli, 524
  endometritis, 331
Estradiol, 311t
Estradiol valerate, 311t
Estrogen receptors, 839–840
  endometrial stromal tumors, 432
Estrogens
  and benign endometrial hyperplasia, 350
  conjugated equine, 311t
  endometrial adenocarcinoma risk, 373
  endometrial effects of, 310–312, 311f
  synthetic conjugated, 311t
Estropipate, 311t
Ethinyl estradiol, 311t, 313t
Evening primrose oil, 319
Ex vivo manipulation, 196
Exemestane, 319
Exocytosis, 75
Extensive warty VIN 3, 82f
Extragenital sarcomas, 711–712
Extrauterine choriocarcinoma, 800
Extravillous trophoblast, 785–787
  cytomorphologic features and immunophenotypes of, 788f
  at implantation site, 787f

F

Fabry disease, 124
Factor V Leiden gene, 761–762
Fallopian tube, 459–486, 499
  adrenal rests, 475, 475f
  anatomy of, 459–462
  benign tumors in, 477–479, 478f–479f
  borderline tumors in, 479, 499
  carcinosarcoma, 483, 484f
  cysts, 472–474
    mesonephric, 473, 473f
    paramesonephric, 473
  endometriosis, 474, 474f, 499, 499f
  examining tubal specimens, 462–463
  female adnexal tumor of probable Wolffian origin, 484–485, 484f–485f
  function of, 462
    ovum transport, 462
    sperm transport, 462
  histology of, 459–462, 460f
  inflammation of, 463–464
    infectious salpingitis, 464, 464f–469f
    pelvic inflammatory disease, 467
    salpingitis isthmica nodosa, 469–470, 469f–470f
  malignant tumors of, 479–484
    clear cell, 482
    clinical features of, 479–480
    definition of, 479
    endometrioid, 481
    general features of, 479
    gross features of, 480, 480f
    metastatic, 483–484
    microscopic features of, 480–482, 481f
    serous, 480–481, 482f
    spread, treatment and prognosis of, 482–483
    squamous cell carcinoma, 482, 483f
    transitional cell, 481–482
  mucinous metaplasia, 474
  non-neoplastic lesions, 463–476

epithelial proliferation associated with salpingitis, 476, 476f–477f
  metaplasias, 474–475, 474f
  mucosal epithelial proliferation, 461–462
prolapse, 476
specimen processing, 821–822
  neoplasm, 822
  SEE-FIM protocol, 822f
  sterilization, 822
  tubal ectopic pregnancy, 822
squamous cell carcinoma, 482, 483f
torsion, 475–476
tubal pregnancy, 470–472, 471f–472f
tubal sterilization, 462, 463f
tumors of, 477–485
see also Tubal
Fatty degeneration, 407
Federation International of Gynecologists and Obstetricians (FIGO), 598
Female adnexal tumor of probable Wolffian origin (FATWO), 484–485, 484f–485f
Female pelvis, 133f
Female pseudohermaphroditism, 18–22
  fetal defects, 18–22, 20t
  maternal influence, 22
Fenestrate placenta, 751
Fetal growth restriction, 773–774
Fetal normoblastemia, persistant, 764
Fetal vessel thrombi, 759–761, 761f
α-Fetoprotein, 613, 835
  dysgerminoma, 671f
Fetus, specimen processing, 824–826
Fetus papyraceus, 757, 757f
Fibrin thrombi, 352f
Fibroepithelial polyps
  vagina, 142–143, 142f
  vulva, 109, 109f
Fibroepithelial-stromal polyps, vulva, 116–117, 117f
Fibroma, ovarian, 652–654
  cellular, 653–654, 654f
  differential diagnosis of, 653
  fibrosarcoma, 654, 654f
  general features of, 652–653
  macroscopic features of, 653, 653f
  microscopic features of, 653, 653f
  treatment and prognosis of, 653
Fibroma, prepubertal vulvar, 120–121, 121f
Fibromatosis, ovarian, 554–556
  definition of, 554
  differential diagnosis of, 556
  etiology of, 554–555, 554f
  gross features of, 555
  microscopic features of, 555–556, 555f–556f
Fibronectin, 293–294
Fibrosarcoma of ovary, 654, 654f
Fibrosing lesions, 718–719
Fibrous histiocytoma, 121–122
Fibrous mesothelioma, 728–729
FIGO staging, 587
  anatomical staging system, 799t
  clinical risk factor score, 799t
  see also International Federation of Gynecology and Obstetrics (FIGO)
Fixation artifact, 308, 308f
Fixatives, 815
Fixed drug eruptions, 66–67, 67f
Flat warts, 73
Florid endometriosis, 501–502, 502f
Flow cytometry, 419
Foamy histiocytes, endometrial stromal tumors, 433t

Follicles
  Graafian, 511f, 512
  preovulatory, 511–512, 511f
  primary, 11f
  primordial, 7–9
Follicle-stimulating hormone (FSH), 510
Follicular atresia, 514–515, 515f
Follicular cysts, unluteinized, 536–537, 536f–537f
Follicular (epidermoid) cyst, 95–96, 96f
Follicular failure, 517–523
  follicular dysgenesis, 517, 517f
  hypogonadotrophic hypogonadism, 522–523, 523f
  ovarian failure, 517–522, 518t
Follicular salpingitis, 465–467, 466f
Folliculogenesis, 510
Foreign body granulomas, 616–618, 717
  florid, reactions, 718f
FOXL2, 6t, 10, 643, 645, 646f, 841
Frasier syndrome, 20t, 36
Fungal infections of vulva, 69–70
  candidiasis, 69
  pityriasis versicolor, 69–70
  tinea cruris, 70
Fungal oophoritis, 529
  blastomycosis, 529
  coccidioidomycosis, 529

G

Gardasil, 195
Gardner syndrome, 95
Gardnerella vaginalis, 139, 170
  endometritis, 330–331
Gartner ducts, 135–136
Gastrointestinal tract, endometriosis, 500, 500f
Genistein, 319–320
Genital differentiation disorders, 18–30, 19t
  female pseudohermaphroditism, 18–22
  genes involved in, 20t
  gonadal tumors involved in, 20t
  male pseudohermaphroditism, 22–30
Genital rhabdomyoma, 124, 124f–125f
Genital tract development, pathophysiology of, 2f
Germ cells
  intratubular, 9f
  primordial, 11
  role of, in embryology, 11
Germinoma, 20t
Gestational trophoblastic disease, 784–811
  choriocarcinoma. *See* Choriocarcinoma
  classification of, 785t
  definition of, 784
  epithelioid trophoblastic tumor, 784
  exaggerated placental site, 809
  invasive mole, 799
  molar. *See* Molar gestational trophoblastic disease
  placental site trophoblastic tumor, 784
  trophoblast immunohistochemical markers, 787–788
  see also Hydatidiform moles
Giant cell arteritis, 531
Ginseng, 319
Gland-poor adenomyosis, 433f
Glandular elements, in endometrial stromal sarcoma, 429, 430f
Glandular lesions, 229, 229f
  preinvasive, 251
Glassy cell carcinoma of cervix, 271, 271f
Glassy cell carcinoma of endometrium, 394
Glial tissue, 186

Gliomatosis peritonei, 732, 732f
Global breakdown, 352t
Glucocorticoids, biosynthesis of, 21f
Glypican 3, 613, 673t, 836
GnRHa. *See* Gonadotrophin-releasing hormone agonists (GnRHa)
Goblet cells, 252–253, 262, 263f, 337
Gonad, undifferentiated, 8f
Gonadal development, 1–11
Gonadal dysgenesis
  mixed, 36–39, 37f–40f
  pure, 35–36
Gonadal ridge, 7f
Gonadoblastoma, 20t, 40–42, 42f, 688–689, 689f–690f, 689t
  calcified, 41f
  clinical features of, 40–41
  differential diagnosis of, 646
  genetic changes in, 41
  with immature granulosa/Sertoli cells, 43f
  with multifocal 'mulberry-like' calcifications, 40f–41f
  pathology of, 41–42
  with superimposed dysgerminoma, 41f
Gonadotrophin insensitivity syndrome, 520
Gonadotrophin-releasing hormone agonists (GnRHa)
  endometrial effects of, 321
  leiomyoma treated with, 406, 406f
  ovarian effects of, 559
Gonadotrophin-releasing hormone (GnRH), 510
Gonadotropins, endometrial effects of, 321
Gonorrhea, vulva, 68
Gorlin syndrome, 652
Graafian follicles, 511f, 512
Granular cell tumor, 122, 122f
Granulation tissue nodule, 143
Granulocytes, endometrial, 294–295
Granulocytic sarcoma, 709–710
Granuloma inguinale, 69
Granulomatous endometritis, 327t, 330
Granulomatous peritonitis, 717–718
  cauterized tissue, 718
  cesarean delivery, 718
  contrast media, 717
  cystic teratoma rupture, 717
  intestinal contents, 717
  keratin, 717
  surgical glove powder, 717
  suture materials, 717
  tuberculosis, 717
Granulomatous salpingitis, 467–469, 468f–469f
  gross features of, 467, 468f
  microscopic features of, 467–469, 469f
Granulosa cell tumors, 542, 616, 643–650
  adult type, 643–647
    clinical features of, 643–644
    differential diagnosis of, 616, 646–647, 646f
    genetic profile of, 645–646
    immunohistochemistry of, 645, 646f
    macroscopic features of, 643f, 644
    microscopic features of, 643f–645f, 644–645
    spread and metastasis of, 647
    treatment and prognosis of, 647
  differential diagnosis of, 622
  juvenile type, 628, 647–650
    clinical features of, 647
    differential diagnosis of, 649, 649t
    immunohistochemistry and genetic profile of, 648, 649f
    macroscopic features of, 647f, 648
    microscopic features of, 647f–649f, 648
    prognosis of, 649t

Granulosa cells
  primitive, 10, 10f
  proliferations of pregnancy, 544, 545f
Granulosa lutein cysts, 536–537, 536f, 538f
Granulosa-theca cell tumor, 645, 645f
Gynandroblastoma, 661
Gynecologic Oncology Group, 586
Gynecomastia, 32f

H

Haemophilus ducreyi, 69
Hailey-Hailey disease, 50f–52f, 59t, 61–62, 62f
Hamartomas, Sertoli cell, 20t
Hand-Schüller-Christian disease, 110
Hart's line, 75
β-HCG, 833
Hemorrhage
  ovarian, 560, 560f
  tubal, 470
Hemorrhagic cellular leiomyoma, 406
Hemosiderin-laden macrophages, 497f
Hepatocyte nuclear factor 1-β, 841
Hepatoid carcinoma
  differential diagnosis of, 628–629
  of ovary, 637, 637f
Hepatoid yolk sac tumor, 628–629, 675–676
Hep-PAR1, 835
Hereditary non-polyposis colorectal carcinoma syndrome (HNPCC), 373–374
Hermaphroditism, true, 20t, 43–44, 43f
HER-2/NEU, 836
Hernia uteri inguinale, 25, 37
Herpes simplex virus
  cervix, 170, 173, 173f–174f
  endometritis, 327t, 329
  placenta in, 779–780
Herpes virus infection, 70–71, 70f–71f
Heterologous elements, 411, 411f
Heterotopic breast, 109
Hidradenitis suppurativa, 64, 64f
Hidradenoma papilliferum, 106, 107f
High-grade serous carcinoma of ovary, 582
  differential diagnosis with endometrioid carcinoma, 616
  differential diagnosis with clear cell carcinoma, 628
  Transitional cell variant, 629
High-grade squamous intraepithelial lesions (HSILs), 200, 212–214
  vaginal, 147, 148f
  differentiated or simplex type, 86–87, 87f
  of vulva (VIN 2-3), 82–83, 83f, 86f
    basaloid type, 84f
    differentiated type, 86f
    elongated rete ridges of, 86f
    mixed basaloid and warty, 84f
    with skin appendage involvement, 84f
HIK1083, 835
Hilus cell hyperplasia, 20t
Hilus cells, 11, 11f
Histiocytic endometritis, 330, 330f
Histiocytic non-granulomatous lesions, 718
Histiocytosis X, 110
HIV, placenta in, 780
HLA-G, 833
HMB45, 833
HMGA2, 841
HNF-1β, 628
HNPCC. *See* Hereditary non-polyposis colorectal carcinoma syndrome (HNPCC)
Hobnail cells, 624

Hofbauer cells, 744
Hormone receptors, 839–840
Hormone replacement therapy
　endometrial effects of, 315–317
　　combined estrogen-progesterone, 317, 317f–318f
　　cyclic estrogen-progesterone, 316f–317f
　types of, 315
HOX genes, 332
hPL, 833
HPV-related low- and high-grade squamous intraepithelial lesions of vulva (VIN1-3), 81–85
HSIL. *See* High grade squamous intraepithelial lesion, and Squamous intraepithelial lesion
Human chorionic gonadotrophin, dysgerminoma, 673t
Human chorionic gonadotrophin (hCG), 647
Human papillomavirus (HPV), 188, 189f–190f, 200
　cervical pathogenesis of, 189f
　classification of, 189t, 201t
　cofactors of, 190t
　DNA assessment of, 602
　gene expression of, 191f
　genome of, 192, 192f
　immune response to, 193–194
　infection, 72–73
　integration of, 191–192
　life cycle of, 191, 191f
　oncoproteins of, 192–193
　placenta in, 780
　prevalence of, 190f
　tissue-resident immune cells, 194
　type frequency of, 202t
　vaccines for, 194–196
　vagina, 146
Hyaline bodies, 512–513, 513f, 637
Hyaline degeneration, 406–407, 406f
Hydatidiform moles, 785t, 788
　complete, 788–791
　　advanced/second trimester, 791–795, 792f–793f
　　chromogenic in situ hybridization, 794f
　　clinical features of, 790
　　differential diagnosis of, 792–795
　　early/first trimester, 791, 791f–792f
　　genetic origin of, 790, 790f
　　gross and microscopic findings of, 791
　　incidence of, 788–790
　　p57 immunostaining pattern of, 794f
　　risk factors of, 790
　　treatment and prognostic factors of, 795
　ectopic, 795
　invasive, 799, 800f
　ovarian, 545–546
　partial, 795–798
　　clinical features of, 795–796
　　differential diagnosis of, 796–797
　　gross and microscopic findings of, 796
　　p57 immunostaining pattern of, 794f
　　pathogenetic mechanism of, 795
　　treatment and prognosis of, 798
　　triploid, 796f
　recurrent, 799
Hydropic degeneration, 406–407
Hydropic non-molar abortion, 794, 795f
　p57 immunostaining pattern of, 794f
Hydrops fetalis, placenta in, 775
Hydrosalpinx, 467
　follicularis, 465–467, 467f
21-Hydroxylase deficiency, 19–21
Hydroxyprogesterone, 312t
3β-Hydroxysteroid dehydrogenase, 19

17-Hydroxysteroid dehydrogenase, 24–25
Hylutin. *See* Hydroxyprogesterone
Hymen, imperforate, 139
Hyperaldosteronism, 667
Hypercalcemia, 666
Hyperinsulinemia, 547
Hyperpigmentation
　postinflammatory, 65
　vulvar skin, 65
Hyperplasia without atypia, 350t
Hyperprolactinemia, 667
Hyperreactio luteinalis, 542
Hypertensive disorders, 772–776
Hyperthecosis, 548–551
　behavior and treatment of, 551
　definitions and clinical features of, 548–549
　differential diagnosis of, 549–551, 551f
　gross features of, 549, 549f
　microscopic features of, 549, 549f–551f
Hyperthyroidism, 666
Hypoglycemia, 667
Hypopigmentation, 66
　postinflammatory, 66
Hysterectomy, 220
　EIN, 368
　for malignant cervical disease, 818
　supracervical, 820
Hysteroscopy, 305

I

Ichthyosis uteri, 334, 334f, 394, 395f
Idiopathic acquired pigmentation of Laugier, 65, 65f
Imiquimod, 196
Immature squamous metaplasia, 168f, 215, 216f, 216t
IMP-2, 841
IMP-3, 841
Imperforate hymen, 139
Implantation, and placenta, 741–768
Implantation site intermediate trophoblast, 785–786
In vitro stimulation, 193–194
Increta, placenta, 775–776
Infantile hemangioma, 108, 108f
Infarct, 753f
Infectious salpingitis, 464
　granulomatous, 467–469, 468f–469f
　non-granulomatous, 464–467, 464f–466f
Infertile male syndrome, 30
Infertility in endometriosis, 501
Inflammatory and infectious processes, 326
Inhibin, 437, 834–835
　granulosa cell tumors, 645, 646f
　ovarian mucinous tumors, 591
α-Inhibin, 645, 646f
Inking, 815
Insulin, and PCOS, 547
Interface dermatitis, 50f–52f
Interferon regulatory factor 3 (IRF-3), 193
International Federation of Gynecology and Obstetrics (FIGO), 233, 233t, 798–799
International Society for the Study of Vulvovaginal Disease (ISVVD), 48–49
Intersexual disorders, classification of, 19t
Interstitial cells, 11
Interstitial extravillous trophoblast, 742–743
Interstitial trophoblast, 786–787, 787f
Interval phase of menstrual cycle, 299, 299f
Intervillositis, 760f
　chronic, 759
Intestinal carcinoma, 696–699, 696f, 698t
Intestinal contents, granuloma, 717

Intraplacental choriocarcinoma, 764–765
Intratubular germ cell neoplasia, 20t
Intrauterine contraceptive device
　endometrial changes, 346–347, 346f
　endometritis, 327t, 329f–330f, 330
Intravascular extravillous cytotrophoblast, 742–743
Invasive squamous cell carcinoma, 148–149, 148t, 217
Irritant contact dermatitis, 53, 53t
Isosexual pseudoprecocity, 643–644
Itch/scratch cycle, 53–54
IUGR, placenta in, 773–774

J

JAZF1
　JJAZ1 gene fusion, 436
　SUZ12 gene fusion, 434
Juvenile colonic polyp, 110
Juvenile granulosa cell tumors (JGCTs), 628, 647–650, 647f–649f, 649t
　antibodies of, 837t

K

Karyopyknotic index, 134–135
Karyorrhexis, 791
Karyotype, 1
K-cells, 294–295
Keratin, 279–280, 286
　granuloma, 717, 717f
　hyperpigmentation, 65–66
Keratin changes, 54
Keratin pearls, 334
Keratinocytes, 54
Keratoacanthoma, 80–81, 81f
Keratohyalin granules, 134
Keratosis follicularis, 59t, 62, 62f
Keratotic warts, 73
Ki-67, 134, 134f, 419, 838
　CIN, 218, 219f
　staining, 215
Kip2. *See* P57
Klebsiella granulomatis, 69
Klinefelter syndrome, 20t, 31–32, 32f
　gynecomastia in, 32f
　Leydig cells in, 33f
　neoplasm, 33f
　testis in, 32f
　　postpubertal end-stage, 33f
Kline's hemorrhage, 755
Koilocytes, 203, 204f–205f, 204t
　atypia, 203, 210
K-ras, 419
　mutations, 576, 580, 591–592
Krukenberg tumors, 628, 653, 697f, 699–701, 699f–701f
　tubular, 700f

L

Labioscrotal folds, 16
Lactate dehydrogenase, 671–672
Lactobacillus acidophilus, 133–134
Lamina propria, 135
Laminar necrosis, 758, 758f
Laminin, 293–294
Langerhans cell histiocytosis, 110, 110f–111f
Langerhans cells, dendritic cells, 135, 135f
Laparoscopic salpingostomy, 472
LEEP. *See* Loop electrosurgical excision procedure (LEEP)
Leiomyoblastoma, 409–410, 410f
Leiomyoma, 283
　fallopian tube, 479, 499

highly cellular, 433f, 433t
ovary, 499, 623, 623f
uterus, 402–405
atypical, 408–409, 408f–409f, 420–421, 420f, 420t
benign metastasizing, 412–413, 412f
cellular, 405–406, 405f
definition of, 402
degenerated, 406–407, 406f
epithelioid, 409–410, 409f–410f
etiology of, 403–404
gross features of, 404, 404f
hemorrhagic cellular, 406
with heterologous elements, 411, 411f
incidence of, 402–403
microscopic features of, 404–405, 404f–405f
mitotically active, 405, 405f
myxoid, 410
treated by interventional radiology, 407
treated with GnRHa, 406, 406f
unusual growth patterns of, 411–414
vagina, 145, 145f
vulva, 122–123, 123f
Leiomyomatosis
diffuse, 411
disseminated peritoneal, 413–414, 413f, 546, 719, 722f, 736f
intravenous, 411–412, 412f
vulvar, 124
Leiomyosarcoma, 283
ovary, 623–624, 623f
mixed, 624, 624f
uterus, 414–420
clinical features of, 414
definition of, 414
diagnostic criteria for, 417–418
atypia, 417
factors that favor malignancy, 418
immunochemistry of, 418, 418f–419f
mitotic activity, 417, 417f
necrosis, 417–418, 417f–418f
epithelioid, 415, 415f
gross features of, 414, 414f
histologic diagnosis of, 416, 416f
incidence of, 414
microscopic features of, 414–416, 414f–415f
molecular genetics of, 418–419
myxoid, 416, 416f
prognosis and treatment of, 419–420
vagina, 154, 154f
vulva, 128, 128f
Lentigo, 101, 101f
Lesional stroma, 196
Letrozole, 319
Letterer-Siwe disease, 110, 110f
Leukemia
cervix, 285–286
ovary, 709–710
Leukoderma, 66
Leukoplakia, 228, 228f
Levonorgestrel, 312t–313t
Leydig cell deficiency, 24
Leydig cell nodules, 20t, 27–28, 29f
Leydig cell tumors, 20t, 29f, 542, 663, 663f–664f
Leydig cells, 9, 11, 13
hyperplasia, 20t, 543, 551–552, 552f
in Klinefelter syndrome, 33f
neoplasm, 33f
Lichen planus, 57–58, 57f–58f
cutaneous, 57–58
erosive, 57f
mucosal, 57–58
reticulate, 57–58

Lichen sclerosus, 55–57, 56f
Lichen simplex chronicus, 54, 54f–55f
Lichenification, 49–54, 75
Lichenoid, 75
Lichenoid dermatitis, 50f–52f
Lichenoid infiltrate, 76
Ligneous vaginitis, 141
LIN28, 673t
Lipoblastoma-like tumor of vulva, 124, 125f
Lipoleiomyoma, 411, 411f
Lipoma, 110
Liposarcoma, 129, 129f, 454
Listeria monocytogenes, placenta in, 781, 782f
Listeriosis, placenta in, 781
Lobular endocervical glandular hyperplasia, 179–180, 179f
Loop electrosurgical excision procedure (LEEP), 177, 237–238
thermal artifacts, 217, 218f, 237–238
Loop excision of the transformation zone (LETZ), thermal artifacts, 217, 218f
Loss of heterozygosity (LOH), 615
Low estrogen states, 216
Low or absent mitoses, 352t
Low-grade serous carcinoma of the ovary, 580
Low-grade squamous intraepithelial lesions (LSILs), 200, 208–212
vaginal (VaIN 1), 147
of vulva (VIN 1), 82, 82f
LSIL. See low-grade squamous intraepithelial lesions, and squamous intraepithelial lesions
Lumens, 135–136
Lutein, 651–652
Luteinized follicular cysts, 537, 542–543, 543f–544f
Luteinized thecoma of ovary, 556, 651–652, 651f–652f, 718
Luteinized unruptured follicle syndrome, 536, 536f
Luteinizing hormone (LH), 510
theca-lutein cysts, 536
Luteoma of pregnancy, 20t, 540–542
clinical features of, 540
definition of, 540
differential diagnosis of, 541–542, 541f, 542t, 665
etiology of, 540
microscopic features of, 541, 541f
Lymph nodes
endometriosis, 500–501, 501f
serous borderline tumors in, 576, 577f–579f, 578–579
Lymphangioma circumscriptum, 123–124, 124f
Lymphocytes, endometrial, 294–295, 294f–295f
Lymphoepithelioma-like squamous cell carcinoma, 247–248, 247f
Lymphoid markers, 834
Lymphoma
Burkitt-like, 709f–710f
cervix, 285–286, 285f–286f
diffuse large cell, 709f
metastatic, 709–710
vagina, 156, 156t
Lynch syndrome, 373–374

M

Macrophages, 294
Maffuci syndrome, 647
Magma reticulare, 677
Malakoplakia, 140–141, 141f, 330
Malaria, placenta in, 781, 781f

Malassezia furfur, 67
Malassezia globosa, 69–70
Male pseudohermaphroditism, 22–30
end-organ defects, 25–30
androgen insensitivity syndrome, 25–30, 27f–28f
primary gonadal defects, 22–25
Leydig cell deficiency, 24
persistent Müllerian duct syndrome, 25, 25f
testicular regression syndrome, 22–23, 23f
testosterone synthesis defects, 24–25
Malignant melanoma, 153–154, 154f
cervix, 284–285, 284f–285f
metastatic, 707, 707f
vulva, 103–106, 104f, 105t, 106f
Breslow thickness, 105
Malignant mesodermal mixed tumors, 618–620
definition of, 618
differential diagnosis of, 620
general features of, 618
histogenesis of, 620
immunohistochemistry of, 620
macroscopic features of, 618, 619f
microscopic features of, 618–620, 619f
somatic genetics of, 620
tumor spread and diagnosis of, 620
Malignant mesothelioma, 710f
Malignant mixed Müllerian tumor, 282–283, 282f
see also Carcinosarcoma
Malignant peripheral nerve sheath tumor, 283–284
Malignant rhabdoid tumor, 454
Marchand rests, 475, 475f
Massive edema of ovary, 552–556, 653
Maternal gestational diseases, non-neoplastic, 769–783
Maternal hypertension, 773f–774f
see also Pre-eclampsia
Maternal infections, 777–781
Maternal rhesus isoimmunization, placenta in, 775
Maternal sickle cell trait, and disease, 776–777, 777f
Maternal vascular disease, 762f
Maternal vessel, 761
Maternal virilizing lesions, 22
Maternal virilizing tumor, 20t
Matrix metalloproteinase-7 *(MPP-7)*, 615
Mature adipose tissue, in endometrial stromal tumors, 431
Mature metaplasia, 168f, 169
Mayer-Rokitansky-Hauser-like syndrome, 10
Mayer-Rokitansky-Kuster-Hauser syndrome, 139
McCune-Albright syndrome, 536–537
Meconium, 750f
on cord/membranes, 749–750
Meconium-induced vascular necrosis, 750f
Mediastinal germ cell tumors, 20t
Mediastinal tumors, metastatic, 707
Medroxyprogesterone, 312t
Medusa head-like appearance, 570f
Megestrol acetate, 312t
Meigs syndrome, 652
Melan-A, 833
Melanin-rich histiocytes, 718
Melanocytic lesions, 101–106
blue nevus, 102
lentigo, 101
malignant melanoma, 103–106
Melanocytic markers, 833
HMB45, 833

melan-A, 833
S-100, 833
Melanocytic nevus
    atypical, 102–103, 103f
    atypical of genital type, 102, 102f
    common acquired, 101, 102f
Mel-CAM, 833
Menopause, endometrial changes, 303–304, 303f–304f
    cystic atrophy, 356–357
    polyps, 345
Menstrual cycle
    endometrium, 295–303, 296f
        interval phase, 299, 299f
        menstrual phase, 297–298, 297f–298f
        proliferative phase, 298, 298f–299f
        secretory exhaustion, 301–303, 301f–303f
        secretory phase, 299–301, 300f–301f
    histologic features, 296f
    secretory exhaustion, 312–313
Merkel cell carcinoma, 105t, 110–112, 111f
Merkel cell polyomavirus (MCV), 110
Mesenchymal cell markers, 831
    blood vessel markers, 832
    endometrial stromal markers, 832
    mesothelial markers, 832
    skeletal muscle markers, 832
    smooth muscle markers, 831–832
    vimentin, 831
Mesenchymal dysplasia, placenta, 751–752, 752f, 796
Mesenchymal villi, 743–744
Mesonephric duct hyperplasia, 184–185, 184f–185f
Mesonephric ducts, 11, 12f, 135–136, 135f–136f
    remnants, 183–184, 184f
Mesonephric glomeruli, 8f, 12f
Mesonephric-like cyst, 97–98
Mesonephros, 7f
Mesothelial hyperplasia, 569, 569f, 719–720, 719f
Mesothelial inclusion cysts, 473–474
Mesothelial lesions, 561
Mesothelial markers, 832
Mesothelioma
    diffuse malignant, 724–727, 725f–726f
        differential diagnosis of, 725–727
        pathology of, 724–725
    fibrous, 728–729
    malignant, 726t–727t
    ovary, 636–637, 710f
    peritoneum
        deciduoid, 724–725
        well-differentiated papillary, 723–724, 724f
Mestranol, 311t
Metaplastic papillary tumor, 479, 479f
Metastatic carcinoids, 701–702
    tumors, 701f–702f
Metastatic renal cell carcinoma, 628
Metropathia hemorrhagica, 643–644
Michaelis-Gutmann bodies, 140–141, 141f, 330
Microcystic stromal tumors, 655–656, 656f
Microglandular hyperplasia, 143–144, 143f–144f, 180–181, 180f–181f
Microinfarcts with epithelial change, 352t
Microinvasive squamous cell cancer, of vulva, 85f
Micropapillary "hobnail" metaplasia, 341–342, 342f
Mifepristone, endometrial effects of, 320–321
Mineralocorticoids, biosynthesis of, 21f
Minichromosome maintenance 7 (MCM7), 192–193
Minimal deviation adenocarcinoma of cervix, 263–265

'Mini-pill', 315
MIS, 6t
'Miscarriage', 769
    spontaneous, 769–770, 770f
MISR II, 6t
Mitotic activity, 352t
Mitotically active leiomyoma, 405, 405f
Mixed gonadal dysgenesis, 36–39, 37f–40f
Mixed Müllerian tumors, 438–446
    adenofibroma, 438–439
    adenosarcoma, 439–443, 439f–442f
    carcinosarcoma, 443–446, 443f–445f
    contrasting features of, 442t
Mobiluncus species, 139
Molar disease, adverse clinical outcomes in, 798–799
Molar gestational trophoblastic disease, 788–799
Molluscum contagiosum virus infection, 71–72, 72f
Monoamniotic monochorionic twins (MoMo), 777
Monochorionic twins, 777
Monoclonal carcinoembryonic antigen, 276
Monodermal teratomas, 591
Mononuclear trophoblastic shell, 784–785
Motherwort, 319
MSH-1, 614
MSH-2, 614
MUC antibodies, 835
Mucin droplets, 138f, 337
Mucinous adenocarcinoma
    of cervix metastatic to the ovary, 708
    of endometrium, 383, 383f–384f
    intestinal type, 262
    metastatic to the ovary, 600
    primary ovarian, 600–604
Mucinous borderline tumors (MBTs), 593–598, 593f, 594t
    endocervical like, 593–595, 594f–595f
    gastrointestinal type, 595–598, 596f
    with intraepithelial carcinoma (IEC), 591
Mucinous carcinoids, 685
Mucinous cyst, 97
Mucinous cystadenofibroma, 592f–593f
Mucinous cystadenoma, 592f
Mucinous metaplasia, 474, 474f
Mucinous ovarian adenocarcinoma, reaction patterns in, 830t
Mucinous tumors of ovary, 591–607
    benign, 592–593, 592f–593f
    borderline, 593–598
        endocervical like, 593–595, 594f–595f
        gastrointestinal type, 595–598, 596f
    carcinomas, 600–604, 600f
        differential diagnosis of, 602
        expansile type, 600–601, 601f
        immunohistochemistry of, 601–602
        infiltrative type, 600–601, 601f
        macroscopic features of, 600, 600f
        microscopic features of, 600–601
        somatic changes of, 602–603, 602f–603f
        treatment and prognosis of, 603–604, 603t, 604f
    general features of, 591–592
    mural nodules, 604–606, 604f–605f, 620
    pseudomyxoma peritonei associated, 598–600, 598f–599f
Mucin-secreting cervical carcinoma, 246, 246f
Mucoid degeneration, 406–407
Muir-Torre syndrome, 614
Müllerian adenofibroma, 438–439
Müllerian adenosarcoma, 439–443, 439f–442f, 620–621, 620f

Müllerian agenesis, 139
Müllerian duct, 8f, 12f–13f
    after week 8, 14, 14f–15f
    development of, 11–15
    during the second trimester, 14–15
    to week 8, 11, 15f
Müllerian inclusion cysts, 734–735, 734f
    benign, 499
    differential diagnosis of, 735
Müllerian inhibiting substance (MIS), 11
Müllerian papilloma, 144–145, 145f
Müllerianosis, 561, 733–737, 733f
    endocervicosis, 735
    endometrioid, clear cell and transitional cell lesions, 735
    endosalpingiosis, 733–735, 733t, 734f
    peritoneal serous lesions, 733
Multipolar mitosis, 206f
Munro abscesses, 55
Mural fibrin thrombus, nonocclusive, 761f
Mural nodules, 604–606, 604f–605f, 620
Mycoplasma endometritis, 328
Mycoplasma hominis, 139
Myofibroblastic tumor, inflammatory, 729
Myometrial hypertrophy, 411
Myometrium, 290–291
Myxoid degeneration, 406–407
Myxoid leiomyoma of uterus, 410
Myxoid leiomyosarcoma
    ovary, 624, 624f
    uterus, 416, 416f

N

Nabothian cysts, 179, 179f
Narrow spectrum differentiation markers, 832–834
    lymphoid markers, 834
    melanocytic markers, 833
    neuroendocrine markers, 833–834
    trophoblastic markers, 833
Natural killer cells, decidual, 772–773
Necrobiosis, 407, 407f
Necrotic pseudoxanthomatous nodules, 718
Necrotizing arteritis, 530–531, 530f
Necrotizing fasciitis, 67
Neisseria gonorrhoeae, 68, 170
    endometritis, 328, 331
Neonatal encephalopathy, adverse neurologic outcome, 774–775
Neoplastic atypia, 205
Neurilemmomas (schwannomas), 287
Neuroblastoma, metastatic, 707, 766f
Neuroectodermal-type tumors, 686–688, 687f
Neuroendocrine adenocarcinoma of endometrium, 394
Neuroendocrine markers, 833–834
Neuroendocrine tumors of cervix, 277–280
    carcinoid tumor, 277
        atypical, 277–278, 278f
        typical (classic), 277, 278f
    large cell, 280
    small cell, 278–279, 278f–279f
Neurofibroma, 110
Neuron-specific enolase, 277
    dysgerminoma, 671–672
Nevus
    blue
        cervix, 284
        vulva, 102

melanocytic
  atypical, 102–103
    of genital type, 102
  common acquired, 101
Nidation, 290, 293–294
Nitabuch's fibrin layer, 742
Nodular fasciitis, 117–118, 118f
Nodular hyperthecosis, 662–663
Nodular stromal hyperthecosis, 541
Nodular theca-lutein hyperplasia of pregnancy, 540–542
Non-clear cell adenocarcinoma of the vagina, 153, 153f
Nongestational choriocarcinoma, 679, 679f
Non-granulomatous salpingitis, 464–467, 464f–466f
  gross features of, 465
  microscopic features of, 465–467, 465f–466f
Non-molar trophoblastic lesions, 785t
Non-neoplastic maternal gestational diseases, 769–783
Non-neoplastic trophoblastic lesions, 785t, 807–809
Norethindrone, 312t–313t
Norethynodrel, 312t
Norgestimate, 312t–313t
Norgestrel, 312t–313t
Nuclear atypia, 204f, 205
Nuclear β-catenin, endometrial stromal sarcomas, 432

O

Obesity
  endometrial adenocarcinoma risk, 373
  and PCOS, 547
'Occult placenta accreta', 776
OCT3/4, 835
  dysgerminoma, 673, 673t
Ollier disease, 647
Oncogenesis, mechanisms of, 192
Oogonia, 9f
Oophorectomy/hysterectomy, for salpingectomy, 463
Oophoritis, 527t
  autoimmune, 520–522, 521f–522f
  bacterial, 524–526, 524f–525f
    actinomycosis, 525–526, 526f
    malacoplakia, 525
    pelvic inflammatory disease, 524
    tuberculosis, 526, 526f
    xanthogranulomatous oophoritis, 524–525
  viral, 526–527
    cytomegalovirus, 527, 527f
    mumps, 526–527
Oral contraceptives
  endometrial effects, 313–315, 313t
    combined oral contraceptives, 314–315, 314f–315f
    long-term progestin-only contraception, 315, 315f
    pure progestin oral contraceptives, 315
  ovarian effects of, 558–559
Original squamous epithelium, 225, 225f
Orthohyperkeratosis, 65
Osseous metaplasia, 342, 342f
Osteoclast-type cells, in endometrial stromal tumors, 431
Osteosarcoma, 454
Ovarian cycle, 515–516, 515f
Ovarian cysts
  classification of, 536t
  corpus albicans, 539
  corpus luteum, 536, 536f, 538–539, 539f
  definitions of, 535–536
  dysfunctional, 535–540
    classification of, 536t
  follicular, 536–538
    clinical features of, 536–537
    differential diagnosis of, 538
    etiology of, 536
    gross features of, 537
    microscopic features of, 537–538, 537f
    of pregnancy, 542–543, 543f–544f
  granulosa lutein, 536–537, 536f, 538f
  simple (unclassified), 540, 540f
  theca-lutein, 536–537, 536f, 538f
Ovarian development, 10f, 510
Ovarian "drilling", 557, 557f
Ovarian edema, 552–554
  behavior and treatment of, 553–554
  clinical features of, 552
  definition of, 552
  differential diagnosis of, 553
  etiology of, 552
  gross and microscopic features of, 552–553, 553f–554f
Ovarian endometrioid adenocarcinoma
  antibodies of, 835t
  reaction patterns in, 830t
Ovarian endometrioid tumors, 608–618
Ovarian adenomatoid tumors, 636
  benign, 609–610
  borderline, 610–611, 610f–611f
    immunohistochemistry and somatic changes of, 610–611
    pathologic features of, 610
  definition of, 608
  epithelial, 609–618
    clinical features of, 609
    pathogenesis of, 609
Ovarian female adnexal tumors of Wolffian origin, 637
  with sarcomatous component, 618–623
    endometrioid stromal sarcomas, 621–623, 621f–622f
    malignant mesodermal mixed tumors, 618–620, 619f
    Müllerian adenosarcomas, 620–621, 620f
Ovarian Smooth muscle tumors, 623–624
  leiomyomas, 623
  leiomyosarcomas, 623–624, 623f
  myxoid leiomyosarcoma, 624, 624f
  SNOMED classification of, 608–609
  synchronous with endometrial adenocarcinoma, 395
Ovarian failure, follicular, 520
Ovarian germ cell tumors
  carcinoids, 684–686
  carcinoma, 688
  dysgerminoma, 628, 671–674
  embryonal carcinoma, 678, 678f
  general features of, 670–671, 671f, 672t
  mixed germ cell sex cord-stromal tumor, 688–689
  mixed MGCTs, 688
  neuroectodermal-type tumors, 686–688, 687f
  nongestational choriocarcinoma, 679, 679f
  polyembryoma, 678–679, 678f
  teratomas, 679–688
    immature, 620, 681–683
    mature, 679–680
  yolk sac tumors, 616, 674–678
Ovarian hemorrhage, 560, 560f
Ovarian hyperstimulation syndrome, 559
Ovarian ligament, 510f
Ovarian neoplasia, 564–590
  borderline tumors, 565
  carcinoid tumors, 646
  carcinomas, 565
  carcinosarcomas, 618–620
  clear cell ovarian tumors, 624–629
    adenocarcinomas, 626–629
    benign, 625
    borderline, 625
    general features of, 624
    macroscopic features of, 624–625
    SNOMED classification of, 624
  endocrine syndromes associated with, 665–667
  epithelial/stromal tumors, 564–565
  hepatoid carcinoma, 637, 637f
  leukemia, 709–710
  malignant mesothelioma, 710f
  mesotheliomas, 636–637
  metastatic, 600
    from extragenital sarcomas, 711–712
    from gastrointestinal tract
      appendix, 704–705
      carcinoid tumors, 701–702
      pancreas, 703–704
    from gastrointestinal tract, Krukenberg tumor, 628
  mixed epithelial tumors, 633
  mucinous tumors, 591–607
    associated with pseudomyxoma peritonei, 598–600, 598f–599f
    benign, 592–593, 592f–593f
    borderline, 593–598, 594t
      endocervical like, 593–595, 594f–595f
      gastrointestinal type, 595–598, 596f–597f
    carcinomas, 600–604, 600f
    general features of, 591–592
    mural nodules, 604–606, 604f–605f, 620
    sarcoma-like mural nodules, 604, 604f–605f
  peritoneal implants, 572–578
  in pregnancy, 546, 546t
  rete ovarii cysts and adenomas, 636
  serous tumors, 565–580
    benign, 565–567, 566f
    borderline, 567–578, 567f–568f
      immunohistochemistry, 572
      in lymph nodes, 576, 577f–579f, 578–579
      microinvasion, 571–572, 571f–572f, 572t
      micropapillary pattern, 569–570, 569f–570f, 571t
      peritoneal implants, 572–578, 573f–575f, 575t
      of peritoneum, 579–580, 579f
      pseudoinvasion, autoimplants, and mesothelial cell hyperplasia, 569, 569f
    carcinomas, 580–587, 580f
    Low-grade serous carcinomas, 580
    High-grade serous carcinomas, 582
    definition of, 565
    SNOMED classification, 565
  sex cord-stromal tumors
    fibrosarcoma, 654
    granulosa cell tumors, 622
    sex cord-stromal tumors, 642–669
  small cell
    pulmonary type, 636
    undifferentiated hypercalcemic type, 635–636, 635f–636f, 646
  squamous cell, 633
    epidermoid (squamous cell) cysts, 633
    squamous cell carcinomas, 633

transitional cell tumors, 629–633
  benign Brenner tumor, 629–630, 630f
  borderline and malignant Brenner tumors, 630–633, 631f–632f
  SNOMED classification of, 629
undifferentiated carcinomas, 634, 634f
  definition of, 634
  differential diagnosis of, 634
  immunohistochemistry of, 634
  of non-small cell (neuroendocrine) type, 636
  pathologic features of, 634, 634f
  prognosis of, 634
Ovarian pregnancy, 544–545
  ectopic, 802f
Ovarian remnant syndrome, 556–557, 557f, 721, 722f–723f
Ovarian sex cord-stromal tumors. *See* Sex cord-stromal tumors
Ovarian small cell carcinoma of hypercalcemic type, antibodies of, 837t
Ovarian transitional cell carcinoma (TCC), 584
Ovarian tumors with functioning stroma (OTFS), 665–666, 665f–666f
Ovary, 498–499, 509–534
  agenesis, 523
  anatomy of, 509
  chemotherapy, 558
  clinical features of, 695
  corpus luteum, 498, 510
    formation, 512–513, 513f
    involution, 513–514, 514f
  danazol, 559
  development of, 510
  dystopic, 523
  ectopic ovarian tissue, 523, 523f
  ectopic pregnancy, 527–528
  endometrioma, 493, 493f–497f, 498
  endometriosis in, 498–499
  ependymoma, 712f
  fibromatosis, 517, 554–556
  follicular atresia in, 514–515, 515f
  follicular failure of, 517–523
    follicular dysgenesis, 517, 517f
    hypogonadotrophic hypogonadism, 522–523, 523f
    ovarian failure, 517–522, 518t
  follicular maturation of, 511–512, 512f
  folliculogenesis of, 510, 511f
  formation of corpus luteum in, 512–513, 513f
  GnRH analogs, 559
  Graafian follicle of, 498f
  hilum in, 516–517, 516f–517f
  histology of, 509–510, 510f
  hydatidiform mole, 545–546
  immunosuppressive drugs affecting, 521–522, 558
  infectious inflammatory diseases of, 524–529
    bacterial oophoritis, 524–526, 524f–525f
      actinomycosis, 525–526, 526f
      malacoplakia, 525
      pelvic inflammatory disease, 524
      tuberculosis, 526, 526f
      xanthogranulomatous oophoritis, 524–525
    fungal oophoritis, 529
      blastomycosis, 529
      coccidioidomycosis, 529
    parasitic oophoritis, 527–529, 528f
      echinococcosis, 529
      enterobiasis, 528–529
      schistosomiasis, 527–528
    viral oophoritis, 524–529

luteinized thecoma, 651–652, 718
macroscopic features of, 695–696
metastatic tumors of, 694–715, 695t
  general features, 694
  origin, 696–712
  spread, 694–696
microscopic features of, 696
non-infectious inflammatory diseases of, 529–531
  cortical granulomas, 530
  Crohn disease, 529–530
  giant cell arteritis, 531
  isolated noninfectious granulomas, 530
  necrotizing arteritis, 530–531, 530f
  polyarteritis nodosa, 531, 531f
  postpartum ovarian vein thrombophlebitis, 531
  sarcoidosis, 529, 530f
non-neoplastic and tumor-like conditions of, 535–563
  adnexal torsion, 560–561, 561f
  dysfunctional cysts, 535–540
  hemorrhage, 560–561
  iatrogenic disorders, 558–560
  reactive mesothelial lesions, 561
  sequelae of surgery or trauma, 556–558
  tumor-like lesions
    associated with pregnancy, 540–546
    reactive stromal, 546–556
non-neoplastic and tumor-like conditions of Müllerianosis, 561
oral contraceptives, 558–559
physiologic function of, 510–517
polycystic, 510
  see also Polycystic ovary syndrome
progesterone effects on, 516, 559, 559f
radiotherapy damage on, 558
  etiology of, 524, 558
  microscopic features of, 524–525, 558, 558f
replacement by uterus-like mass, 523–524
sequelae of surgery/trauma, 522
serous carcinoma of, 20t
sex cord-stromal tumor, 515
specimen processing, 822–824, 823f
  large cystic or neoplastic ovaries, 823
  microscopic sections, 823–824, 823f
  staging operations, 824
splenogonadal fusion, 523
streak, 519, 519f
tamoxifen, 560
torsion, 523, 546, 560–561, 561f
trophoblastic disease, 545–546
white lesion, 526f
  see also Ovarian
Ovotestis, 43, 43f
Ovulation induction therapy, 559–560
  clomiphene citrate, 559
  endometrial effects, 320, 320f
Ovum transport, 462
Oxytocin receptor, 831t, 840

P

P16, 218, 219f, 419, 838–839
P53, 576, 837
P57, 839
P63, 245, 837
Paget disease, extramammary, 98–100, 98f–100f, 101t
Pancreatic tumors, metastatic, 704f
Paneth cells, 252–253, 262
Papanicolaou smear, 194–195, 201f
  Bethesda classification system, 202–203, 207
  staining, 207

Papillae and pseudopapillae, in endometrial stromal tumors, 430–431, 431f
Papillary squamotransitional cell carcinoma, 150, 248
Papillary syncytial metaplasia, 332t, 341, 341f–342f
Papillomatosis, 75–76
Papular warts, 73
Paradoxical maturation, 85f
Paraendocrine hypercalcemia, 666
Paramesonephric duct, 11, 12f
Parasitic oophoritis, 527–529, 528f
  echinococcosis, 529
  enterobiasis, 528–529
  schistosomiasis, 527–528
Paratubal cyst, 472f–473f
Paraurethral (Skene) gland, cyst, 97
Parvilocular cystoma, 624–625, 624f
Parvovirus B19, placenta in, 778–779, 779f
PAX2, 841
PAX8, 840–841
PCNA. *See* Proliferating cell nuclear antigen (PCNA)
PCOS. *See* Polycystic ovary syndrome; Polycystic ovary syndrome (PCOS)
PEComa, endometrial, 450–452, 450f–452f
Pelvic inflammatory disease (PID), 326
Pemphigoid gestationis, 59t
Pemphigus vegetans, 59t, 60–61, 60f
Pemphigus vulgaris, 58–60, 59t
Percreta, placenta, 775–776, 776f
Periglandular cuffing, 439, 620
Peritoneal carcinomatosis, 598
Peritoneal inclusion cysts, 720–721, 722f
Peritoneal tumors, 710–711
Peritoneum, 716–740
  desmoplastic small round cell tumor, 727–728, 727f–728f
  disseminated peritoneal leiomyomatosis, 546, 735–737
  implants, 572–578, 573f–575f, 575t
  inflammatory/reactive lesions, 716–723
    fibrosing lesions, 718–719
    granulomatous peritonitis, 717–718
    histiocytic non-granulomatous lesions, 718
    reactive mesothelial, 719, 720f
  mesothelial neoplasms, 723–727
    diffuse malignant mesothelioma, 724–727, 725f–726f
    well-differentiated papillary mesothelioma, 723–724, 724f
  metastatic tumors, 729–733
    gliomatosis peritonei, 732, 732f
    pseudomyxoma peritonei, 729–732, 729f–731f
    strumosis peritonei, 732–733, 732f
  miscellaneous primary tumors, 727–729
  Müllerian inclusion cysts, 734–735
  Müllerianosis, 733–737, 733f
    endocervicosis, 735
    endometrioid, clear cell and transitional cell lesions, 735
    endosalpingiosis, 733–735, 733t, 734f
  normal, 716
  serous tumors, 735
    serous carcinoma, 726t–727t
  solitary benign fibrous mesothelioma, 728f
  solitary fibrous tumor of, 728–729
  tumor-like lesions of, 719–721
    appendix epiploica infarction, 723
    deciduosis, 735, 736f
    disseminated peritoneal leiomyomatosis, 719, 722f, 735–737, 736f

ovarian remnant syndrome, 721, 722f–723f
splenosis, 721
supernumerary/accessory ovaries, 721
trophoblastic implants, 723, 723f
Perivillous fibrin
deposition, 753–754, 753f
of villi, 753f
Persistent Müllerian duct syndrome, 25, 25f
Persistent trophoblastic disease, 798–799, 798t
Peutz-Jeghers syndrome, 263, 591, 656
PHLDA2 gene, 774
Photographs, 815
Phytoestrogens, endometrial effects of, 319–320, 320f
Picket-fence appearance, 161
PIK3CA mutations, 615, 632
'Pill' endometrium, 312–313, 314f
Pipelle biopsy, 305, 307f
Pityriasis versicolor, 69–70
Placenta, 741–768
abruption, 754f, 771–772, 771f–772f
absence or reversal of end diastolic flow, 774
accreta, 346
bilobed, 750–751
calcification, 755
cerebral palsy, 774–775
circummarginate, 750, 750f
circumvallate, 750, 750f
classification system for, 770t
confined mosaicism, 774
creta, 775–776
cut surface of, 752
development of, 784–788, 785f
diabetes mellitus, 775
early pregnancy, 741–745, 742f
early pregnancy loss, 769–770, 770f
fenestrate, 751
fetal normoblastemia, persistant, 764
fetal surface of, 751–752, 751f
functional unit of, 745
fused, 755f
during gestational period, 786f
hematoma, 754–755
hydrops fetalis, 775
hypertensive disorders, 772–776
IUGR, 773–774
pre-eclampsia, 772–773, 773f–774f
infarction of, 752–753, 753f
maternal floor, 753–754, 754f
inflammation/infection, 757–759
chronic chorioamnionitis, 758, 758f
chronic intervillositis, 759
deciduitis, 758
eosinophilic/T-cell vasculitis, 758, 759f
hypoxic lesions, 758
villitis, 758–759, 759f–760f
intervillous thrombosis, 755
maternal infections, 777–781
CMV, 777–778, 778f
herpes simplex, 779–780
HIV, 780
HPV, 780
listeriosis, 781
malaria, 781, 781f
Mycobacterium tuberculosis, 781
parvovirus B19, 778–779, 779f
rubella, 779
syphilis, 781, 781f
toxoplasmosis, 780, 780f
varicella zoster, 779
maternal rhesus isoimmunization, 775
maternal surface of, 752
maternal vessel, 761, 762f

membranes of, 743f, 748–749
meconium on, 749–750, 750f
mesenchymal dysplasia, 752f, 796, 797f
mid to late pregnancy loss, 771, 771f
multiple gestation, 755–757
neonatal encephalopathy, 774–775
non-trophoblastic tumors, 764–766
chorangiocarcinoma, 764
chorangioma, 764, 764f–765f
intraplacental choriocarcinoma, 764–765
metastatic, 765f–766f, 766
teratoma, 765
perivillous fibrin deposition, 753–754, 753f
postpartum hemorrhage, 776
prolonged pregnancy, 777
retroplacental hemorrhage, 754
septal cysts, 755
sickle cell trait/disease, 776–777, 777f
specimen processing, 825–826
examination of, 825t, 826f
twin, 826, 827f
weight standards, 826t
subchorial thrombosis, 755
subinvolution, 776, 776f
succenturiate lobe, 751, 751f
twin pregnancy, 777
umbilical cord, 745–748, 745f–747f
vascular lesions, 759–764
chorangiosis, 762, 763f
fetal vessel thrombi, 759–761
maternal vascular disease and thrombophilia, 761–762
villous edema, 763–764
villous maturity, 762–763, 763f–764f
weight, 751
'placenta adhesiva', 776
'placenta creta', 775–776
Placental alkaline phosphatase, 833
Placental aromatase defect, 22
Placental site
exaggerated, 809, 809f
nodule/plaque, 807–808, 808f
Placental site trophoblastic tumor, 803–805, 803f–805f
clinical behavior and treatment of, 805
clinical presentation of, 803
differential diagnosis of, 805
gross and macroscopic findings of, 803–804
pathogenetic mechanism of, 804–805
Placental-like alkaline phosphatase, 3
dysgerminoma, 671–672
Plan B. *See* Levonorgestrel
PLAP, 3, 673t
Plaque of warty VIN 3, 82f
Plasma cell vulvitis, 63, 63f
Pleomorphic rhabdomyosarcoma, 453f
Plexiform leiomyoma, 409–410
Podoplanin, dysgerminoma, 673
Polyarteritis nodosa, 531, 531f
Polycystic ovary syndrome (PCOS), 515, 546–548
definition of, 546–547
differential diagnosis of, 548
endometrial adenocarcinoma risk, 373
etiology of, 547
gross features of, 548, 548f
investigation profile of, 547–548
microscopic features of, 548, 548f
string of pearls, 548
Polyembryoma, 678–679, 678f
Polymerase chain reaction (PCR) analysis, 216
Polypoid adenomyoma, atypical, 345, 345f

Polypoid endometriosis, 442, 502, 502f–503f
Polyps
cervix, 185–186, 185f
endometrium, 342–344, 356
Polyvesicular vitelline tumors, 675–676
Portal vein tumor thrombosis (PVTT), 678
Postabortal endometritis, 327t, 330–331, 331f
Postadolescent cervix, 166f
Postinflammatory hyperpigmentation, 65
Postinflammatory hypopigmentation, 66
Postmenopausal bleeding, 643–644
Postoperative spindle cell nodule, 143
Postpartum endometritis, 327t, 330–331
Postpartum hemorrhage, placenta in, 776
Postpartum ovarian vein thrombophlebitis, 531
PRb, 218
Pre-eclampsia, placenta in, 772–773, 773f–774f
Pregnancy
early, 741–745, 742f
persistant fetal normoblastemia, 764
ectopic, tubal, 471f–472f
follicular cysts of, 537, 542–543, 543f–544f
luteoma of, 20t, 540–542
ovarian, 544–545
ovarian granulosa cell proliferations of, 544, 545f
ovarian neoplasms, 546, 546t
prolonged, 777
twin, placenta in, 755, 755f, 777
vasculogenetic steps in chorionic villi during, 786f
Premature follicular depletion, 518–520, 519f
Premature ovarian failure, 517
Prepubertal cervix, 166f
Prepubertal vulvar fibroma, 120–121, 121f
Previllous trophoblast, of implanting embryonic pole, 784–785
Primary carcinoma, of fallopian tube, 479–483
Primary follicles, 11f
Primitive neuroectodermal tumors, 284, 453, 453f
Primordial follicles, 7–9
Primordial germ cells, 11
Products of conception, 769
ProExC, 839
Progesterone, 312t
ovarian effects of, 559, 559f
Progesterone receptor modulators, 320–321, 321f
Progesterone receptors, 839–840
endometrial stromal tumors, 432
Progestins
in EIN, 368
endometrial effects of, 312–313, 312f–313f, 312t, 321–322
maternal ingestion of, 22
Prolapse of fallopian tube, 143, 143f, 476
Proliferating cell nuclear antigen (PCNA), 419, 838
Proliferation markers, 419
Proliferative index, 806
Proliferative phase of menstrual cycle, 298, 298f–299f
Prophylactic salpingectomy, 822, 822f
Prostaglandins, in endometriosis, 488
Prostatic acid phosphatase, 836
Prostatic specific antigen, 836
Prostatic tissue, 186, 186f
Proto-oncogenes, 838
Protozoal infections of vulva, 73
trichomoniasis, 73

Pruritus, 50f–52f
Psammocarcinoma, 581
Psammoma bodies, 499, 565, 724–725
Pseudoautosomal pairing region, 1–2
Pseudodecidual change, 475, 476f
Pseudohermaphroditism
　female, 18–22
　male, 22–30
Pseudoinvasion, 569
Pseudomonas, 67
Pseudomyxoma ovarii, 596–597, 705
Pseudomyxoma peritonei, 729–732, 729f–731f
　mucinous tumors associated with, 598–600, 598f–599f
Pseudopolyp, 136, 137f
Pseudosarcoma botryoides, 116–117
Psoriasiform, 75
Psoriasiform acanthosis, 76
Psoriasiform dermatitis, 50f–52f
Psoriasis, 54–55, 55f
PTCH gene, 652
PTEN, 359, 614–615, 837–838
Pubic (crab) lice, 74
Punch biopsies, 817
Pure gonadal dysgenesis, 35–36
Pustule, 76
Pyometra, 327t, 331, 331f
Pyosalpinx, 466f

R

Radiation effects
　cervix, 182–183, 182f
　endometrium, 346, 346f
Radiotherapy, cervical carcinoma, 245–246
Raloxifene, endometrial effects of, 319
Red clover, 319
Red degeneration (necrobiosis), 407, 407f
5α–Reductase, 15
5α-Reductase type 2 deficiency, 30
Reed syndrome, 403
Reifenstein syndrome, 30
Reinke crystalloids, 11f, 542, 552, 657
Renal cell carcinoma, metastatic, 156f, 628, 705, 706f
Renal tumors, 705–706
Repair (reactive epithelial changes of cervix), 216, 216f
Reserve cells, 167f
Resistant ovary syndrome, 520, 520f
Rete ovarii, 499
　cysts and adenomas, 636
Reticulin, 542
Retinoblastoma gene, 218
Retroplacental hemorrhage, 754
Rhabdoid morphology, in endometrial stromal tumors, 430
Rhabdomyoma of vagina, 145, 145f
Rhabdomyosarcoma, 129, 283, 452–453
　embryonal, 117, 283, 283f
Rohr's fibrinoid, 742
Rokitansky's protuberance, 680
Rubella, placenta in, 779

S

S-100 protein, 277, 833
SALL4, 673t, 682, 836
Salpingectomy, prophylactic, 822, 822f
Salpingitis
　mucosal epithelial proliferation of, 461–462, 461f–462f
　non-granulomatous, 464–467, 464f–466f

Salpingitis isthmica nodosa, 469–470, 469f–470f, 499
　definition of, 469
　differential diagnosis of, 470
　histogenesis of, 469–470
　pathology of, 469, 469f–470f
Sarcoidosis, 529, 530f
Sarcoma
　cervix
　　adenosarcoma, 281–282
　　alveolar soft part, 284, 284f
　　carcinosarcoma, 282–283
　　embryonal rhabdomyosarcoma, 283, 283f
　　endometrioid stromal, 621–623, 621f–622f
　　ovary, stromal, 504, 654–655, 655f
　　stromal, 504, 504f
　　uterine, 503
　　vulva, 503
　　　leiomyosarcoma, 128, 128f
　　　liposarcoma, 129, 129f
　　　proximal-type epithelioid, 128–129, 128f–129f
Sarcomeric actin, 832
Savage syndrome, 520
'Saw-tooth pattern', 302–303
Scabies, 73–74, 74f
Scant endocervical curettage, 214–215
Schiller-Duval bodies, 268, 675–676, 675f
Schistosoma haematobium, 170
Schistosomiasis, cervix, 174, 175f
Schwannoma, 110
Sclerosing peritonitis, 718, 718f
Sclerosing stromal tumors, 654–655, 655f
Sebaceous carcinoma, 93, 93f
Sebaceous glands, 186, 186f
Seborrheic dermatitis, 53
Seborrheic keratosis, 79–80, 80f
Secondary Müllerian system, 490
Secretory carcinoma of endometrium, 384, 384f, 616
Secretory change, in non-atypical hyperplasia, 352t
Secretory phase of menstrual cycle
　changing vacuolar patterns, 299–300, 300f
　increasing stromal edema, 300–301, 300f–301f
　predecidual change, 301–303, 301f–303f, 463, 464f
SEE-FIM (sectioning and extensively examining the fimbriated end) protocol, for fallopian tube, 822f
Seminiferous tubules, 9f
　in mixed gonadal dysgenesis, 40f
Seminoma, 20t, 29f–30f
Senile polyps, 344, 345f
Senile vaginitis, 140
Septal cysts, of placenta, 755
Serous carcinoma of endometrium, 268–269, 387–391
　behavior and treatment of, 390–391
　biologic behavior and treatment, 268–269
　clinical features of, 388
　definition of, 268
　differential diagnosis of, 390, 390f–391f
　gross features of, 388
　immunohistochemistry of, 389, 389f
　microscopic features of, 388–389, 388f–389f
　pathology of, 268
Serous carcinoma of fallopian tube, 480–481, 482f
Serous carcinomas of ovary, 20t, 580–587, 580f
　clinical features of, 582–583
　differential diagnosis of, 581–582, 586–587

　genetic susceptibility of, 584
　histogenesis and genetic profile of, 584–585
　immunohistochemistry and somatic genetics of, 581, 584
　macroscopic features of, 582f, 583
　microscopic features of, 580–581, 581f–584f, 583–584
　pathogenic model of, 585, 586f
　treatment and prognosis of, 582, 587
Serous endometrial intraepithelial carcinoma (serous EIC), 389–391, 389f–390f
Serous tubal intraepithelial carcinomas, 480, 481f
Serous tumors of ovary, 565–580
　benign, 565–567, 566f
　borderline, 567–578, 567f–568f
　　immunohistochemistry of, 572
　　in lymph nodes, 576, 577f–579f, 578–579
　　microinvasion of, 571–572, 571f–572f, 572t
　　micropapillary pattern of, 569–570, 569f–570f, 571t
　　peritoneal implants, 572–578, 573f–575f, 575t
　　of peritoneum, 579–580, 579f
　　pseudoinvasion, autoimplants, and mesothelial cell hyperplasia, 569, 569f
　carcinoma
　　low-grade serous carcinoma, 580
　　high-grade serous carcinoma, 582
　carcinoma definition of, 565
　SNOMED classification of, 565
Serous tumors of peritoneum, 735
Sertoli cell adenoma, 27–28, 27f–29f
Sertoli cell hamartomas, 20t
Sertoli cell tumors, 656, 656f–657f
Sertoli cells, 2–3
Sertoli-Leydig cell tumors, 576, 591, 602, 612–613, 613f, 620, 656–661, 657f, 659f, 660t
　moderately/poorly differentiated, 658, 658f
　retiform variants, 657f, 658, 659f–660f
　well-differentiated, 657, 658f–660f
Sertoli-stromal cell tumors, 616, 656–661
Sex cord tumor with annular tubules (SCTAT), 661, 661f
Sex cords, 642
　primary, 7, 8f
Sex cord-stromal tumors, 642–669
　androblastoma, Sertoli-Leydig cell tumors, poorly differentiated, 620
　with annular tubules (SCTAT), 661, 661f
　antibodies of, 835t
　endometrial adenocarcinoma risk, 373
　fibroma, 652–654
　fibrosarcoma, 654
　granulosa cell tumors, 643–650
　　adult type, 643–647
　　juvenile type, 628, 647–650
　gynandroblastoma, 661
　microcystic stromal tumors, 655–656, 656f
　sclerosing stromal tumors, 654–655, 655f
　Sertoli-stromal cell tumors, 656–661
　　Sertoli cell tumors, 656, 656f–657f
　　Sertoli-Leydig cell tumors, 656–661
　　　moderately/poorly differentiated, 658
　　　retiform variants, 658
　　　well-differentiated, 657
　signet-ring cell tumors, 655, 655f
　steroid cell tumors, 662–665, 662f, 662t
　thecoma, 650–652
Sex determination, genes involved in, 6t

Sex determination disorders, 30–44
  Denys-Drash syndrome, 20t, 36
  Frasier syndrome, 20t, 36
  Klinefelter syndrome, 20t, 31–32, 32f
  mixed gonadal dysgenesis, 36–39, 37f–41f
  pure gonadal dysgenesis, 35–36
  Turner syndrome, 20t, 32–35, 33f
  XX male, 35
  XY female, 42–43
Sex reversal
  XX male, 35
  XY female, 42–43
Sex steroids, biosynthesis of, 21f
Sexual ambiguity, frequent, 36–44
Sexual development, normal, 1, 3f
Sexual development disorders, 18–47
  genital differentiation disorders, 18–30, 19t
    female pseudohermaphroditism, 18–22
    genes involved in, 20t
    gonadal tumors involved in, 20t
    male pseudohermaphroditism, 22–30
  sex determination disorders, 30–44
    Denys-Drash syndrome, 20t, 36
    Frasier syndrome, 20t, 36
    Klinefelter syndrome, 20t, 31–32, 32f
    mixed gonadal dysgenesis, 36–39, 37f–41f
    pure gonadal dysgenesis, 35–36
    Turner syndrome, 20t, 32–35, 33f
    XX male, 35
    XY female, 42–43
SF1, 2–7, 6t
Siamese twins, 755f
Signet-ring carcinoma of endometrium, 394
Signet-ring cell tumors, 655, 655f
Signet-ring cells, 262–263, 263f, 624, 626f–627f
Simple (or total) vulvectomy, 816
Simple (unclassified) cysts, 540, 540f
Skeletal muscle differentiation, in endometrial stromal tumors, 430
Skeletal muscle markers, 832
Skin appendages, 106–107
  hidradenoma papilliferum, 106
  syringoma, 106–107
  trichoepithelioma, 107
Skin tags, 109
'slapped cheek syndrome', 778
Small cell adenocarcinoma of endometrium, 394, 394f
Small cell carcinoma
  cervix, 245
  ovary
    hypercalcemic type, 635–636, 635f–636f, 646
    pulmonary type, 636
  skin, 110–112
  vagina, 150, 150f
Small intestine, metastatic adenocarcinoma of, 698f
Smith-Lemli-Opitz syndrome, 24
Smoking, endometrial adenocarcinoma risk, 374
Smooth muscle actin (α–SMA), 645, 831
Smooth muscle markers, 831–832
Smooth muscle neoplasm, reaction patterns in, 831t
Smooth muscle tumors of uncertain malignant potential (STUMP), 402, 420–421, 420f, 420t
Solitary fibrous tumor of peritoneum, 728–729, 728f
SOX2, 673t, 682
SOX9, 2–3, 6t

Specimen processing, 812–827
  cervix, 817–818
    cone biopsy, 817–818, 817f–818f
    endocervical curettage, 817
    malignant disease, 818
    punch biopsies, 817
  drawings and photographs, 815
  fallopian tube, 821–822
    neoplasm, 822
    sterilization, 822
    tubal ectopic pregnancy, 822
  fetus and placenta, 824–826
    placenta, 825–826, 825t–826t, 826f
    second trimester fetus, 824–825
    twin, 826, 826t, 827f
  fixatives, 815
  gross description and, 814–815
  inking, 815
  number of sections required, 815
  ovary, 822–824, 823f
    large cystic or neoplastic ovaries, 823
    microscopic sections, 823–824, 823f
    staging operations, 824
  section codes and the report, 813–814
    location of section codes in the report, 813–814
    specimen and site identification, 814
    types of section codes, 813
  synoptic checklists, 815
  uterine corpus, 818–821, 819f
    benign or functional disease, 818–820, 819f
    endometrial biopsies and curettings, 818
    malignant disease, 820–821, 820f
    sampling, 820f–821f, 821
    supracervical hysterectomy, 820
  vulva, 815–817
    excisional biopsies, 815
    radical vulvectomy, 816–817
    simple (or total) vulvectomy, 816
    skinning vulvectomy, 816
    wide local excision, 815–816, 816f
Sperm transport, 462
Spiral arterioles, 295f
Spiral artery of placenta, 743f
Splenogonadal fusion, 523
Splenosis, 557–558, 557f, 721
Spongiform pustule of Kogoj, 55
Spongiosis, 54, 76
Spongiotic dermatitis, 49–54, 50f–52f
  acute, 49
  chronic, 49
  clinical patterns of, 49–54
  endogenous, 49–53
  exogenous, 53–54
  general clinical and pathologic features of, 49
  subacute, 52f
Spontaneous miscarriage, 769–770, 770f
Spray-bud growth pattern, 235–236, 235f
Squamocolumnar junction, 165f
Squamous cell adenocarcinoma of endometrium, 394–395, 394f–395f
Squamous cell carcinoma of cervix, 232–250
  cervical stump, 245
  invasive, 232–233
  lymphoepithelioma, 247–248, 247f
  microinvasive, 233–238
  micrometastasis, 246
  mucin-secreting, 246f
  papillary, 247
  papillary squamotransitional cell carcinoma, 248
  radiotherapy effects on, 245–246, 246f
  verrucous, 246–247, 247f
  warty, 247

Squamous cell carcinoma of fallopian tube, 482, 483f
Squamous cell carcinoma of ovary, 633, 688, 688f, 707
Squamous cell carcinoma of vulva, 85f, 87–91, 88f–89f
  survival rates for, by stage, 91t
  uncommon subtypes of, 91–93
    basal cell carcinoma, 92–93, 92f
    sebaceous carcinoma, 93, 93f
    verrucous carcinoma, 91–92, 91f–92f
Squamous epithelium, hormonal influences on, 162–163
Squamous intraepithelial lesions (SILs), 202–223
  Cervical, 202–223
    biomarkers of, 218–219, 219f
      HPV typing, 219
      Ki-67 cell clusters, 218, 219f
      p16, 218, 219f
      ProExC, 218–219
    CIN1 (flat lesions), 211–212, 212f
    CIN2, 212–214, 212f–214f
    CIN3, 212–214, 214f, 219f–220f
    colposcopy and, 224–229
      abnormal findings, 226–229, 226f–229f, 226t
      normal findings, 225–226, 225f–226f
    correlation between cytology and histology, 223–224
    diagnostic difficulty of, 214–218
      artifact, 217, 218f
      basal cell hyperplasia, 215, 215f
      congenital transformation zone, 218
      immature/atypical squamous metaplasia, 215, 216f, 216t
      invasive squamous cell carcinoma, 217
      low estrogen states and atrophy, 216
      miscellaneous conditions, 218
      repair, 216, 216f
      scant endocervical curettage, 214–215
      stratified mucin-producing intraepithelial lesion, 217–218
      thin epithelium, 216–217, 217f
    disease states of, 207–212, 207f–208f
      condyloma acuminatum, 208–210, 208f–211f
    distribution and site of origin of, 224
    features of, 203–207, 203f
      differentiation, maturation and stratification, 203t, 206–207
      mitotic activity, 203t, 205–206, 206f
      nuclear abnormalities, 203t, 205
    histological features of, 219–221
      endocervical gland crypts, 219–220, 219f–220f
      invasive disease, 221, 221t
      resection margins, 220–221, 220f–221f
    management and prognosis of, 219–221
    natural history of, 222t
    nomenclature of, 201f, 202–203
    regression and progression of, 221–223, 222t–223t, 223f
Squamous Intraepithelial Lesions, of vagina (VaIN), 146–148
Squamous intraepithelial lesions, of vulva (VIN), 81–87
  classification schemes for, 81t
  definition of, 81
  high-grade VIN, differentiated or simplex type, 86–87
  HPV-related low- and high grade, 81–85
Squamous metaplasia of cervix, 225–226, 226f

Squamous neoplasia
  cervix, 188–199
    early detection of, 194–195
    epidemiology of, 188
    immune-based therapies for, 195
    public health significance of, 188
    vaccines for, 194–196
  vagina, 146–153
    HPV infection, 146
    invasive, 148–149
    papillary squamotransitional cell carcinoma, 150
    small cell carcinoma, 150, 150f
    squamous intraepithelial lesion (VaIN), 146–148
    verrucous carcinoma, 149, 149f
    warty carcinoma, 150
Squamous papilloma, vulva, 109
SRY, 1–2, 6t
Staging
  of cervical squamous cell carcinoma, 233, 233t, 848
  of carcinomas of ovary, 846
Staphylococcal infections, 67
Staphylococcus aureus, 67, 141
  endometritis, 331
STAR, 24
Starch granuloma, 717
Steatocystoma multiplex, 96, 96f
Stein-Leventhal syndrome, 546, 547t
Stem vessel, fibrous obliteration of, 761f
Stem villi, 744
Sterilization, 822
Steroid cell tumors, 542, 628–629, 642–669, 662f, 662t
  adrenal cortical type, 664
  differential diagnosis of, 664–665
  Leydig cell tumor, 663, 663f–664f
  NOS, 664–665, 664f
  stromal luteoma, 662–663, 663f
  treatment and prognosis of, 665
Steroid hormone receptors, and endometrial adenocarcinoma prognosis, 397–398
Steroidogenic factor-1, 3–7, 836
Stevens-Johnson syndrome, 63
STK11 gene, 652
Stratified mucin-producing intraepithelial lesion, 217–218
Strawberry hemangioma, 108
Streak ovaries, 34f, 519, 519f
Streptococcal infections, 67
Streptococcus viridans endometritis, 331
String of pearls, 548
Stromal hyperplasia, 548–551
  behavior and treatment of, 551
  definitions and clinical features of, 548–549
  differential diagnosis of, 549–551, 551f
  gross features of, 549, 549f
  microscopic features of, 549, 549f–551f
Stromal luteoma, 20t, 662–663, 663f
Stromal nodule of endometrium, 425–426
Stromal pre-decidualization, 352t
Struma ovarii, 683–684
  clinical features of, 683
  cystic, 567
  differential diagnosis of, 567, 684
  macroscopic features of, 683, 683f
  microscopic features of, 683–684, 683f
  treatment and prognosis of, 684
Strumal carcinoids, 685
Strumosis peritonei, 732–733, 732f

STUMP. *See* Smooth muscle tumors of uncertain malignant potential (STUMP)
Subchorial thrombosis, 755
Subchorionic hemorrhage, 754f
Subinvolution, in placenta, 776, 776f
Superficial angiomyxoma, 120t, 126–127, 126f–127f
Superficially invasive squamous cell carcinoma (SISCCA), 233–238
Supernumerary/accessory ovaries, 721
Suprabasal split, 50f–52f
Surgical glove powder granuloma, 717
Suspect frank invasive carcinoma, 228, 229f
Suture materials, granuloma, 717
'Swiss cheese endometrium', 303–304, 356–357
Swyer syndrome, 22
Synaptophysin, 278–279, 279f
Syncytial knots, 762–763, 763f
Syncytiotrophoblast, 741–742, 744, 784–785
Synoptic checklists, 815
Syphilis, 67–68
  cervix, 172–173, 173f
  placenta in, 781, 781f
  secondary, 68f
Syringoma, 106–107, 107f

T

Talc granulomas, 717
Tamoxifen
  endometrial adenocarcinoma risk, 374
  endometrial effects of, 318–319, 318f–319f
  ovarian effects of, 560
Tampon-related lesions, 141
Tao Brush, 305, 305f
Telescoping artifact, 308, 308f
Telomerase, 193
Teratoma, 679–688
  immature, 681–683
    clinical features of, 681
    differential diagnosis of, 682
    immunohistochemistry of, 682
    macroscopic features of, 681, 681f
    microscopic features of, 681–682, 681f–682f, 682t
    somatic genetics of, 682
    treatment and prognosis of, 683
  mature, 679–680
    clinical features of, 679–680
    macroscopic features of, 680, 680f
    microscopic features of, 680
    treatment and prognosis of, 680
  monodermal, 683–688
  placental, 765
Terminal villi, 744–745, 744f
Testicular development, 8f
Testicular feminization
  complete, 26–29, 26f
  incomplete, 29–30
Testicular regression syndrome, 22–23, 23f
Testis, in Klinefelter syndrome, 32f
Testis capsule, 9, 9f
Testis determining factor, 1
Testosterone, 13
  synthesis defects in, 24–25
Theca-lutein cysts, 536–537, 538f
  microscopic appearance of, 536f
  multiple (hyperreactio luteinalis), 538f, 542, 543f
Theca-lutein (paralutein) cells, 536
Thecoma, 542, 650–652
  versus diffuse AGCT, 646
  luteinized, 554–556, 651–652, 651f–652f

  malignant, 650
  typical form, 650–651, 650f–651f
Three-group metaphase mitosis, 206f
Thyroid transcription factor 1 (TTF1), 707, 836
Tinea cruris, 70
Tissue contaminants, 308–309
Tissue-resident immune cells, 194
T-lymphocytes, antigen-experienced, 194
Toker cells, 100, 101f
Torsion
  fallopian tube, 475–476, 476f
  ovary, 523, 546, 560–561, 561f
Toxic shock syndrome, 141
Toxoplasmosis, placenta in, 780, 780f
Trabecular carcinoma, 110–112
Transformation zone, 224
Transitional cell adenocarcinoma of endometrium, 394
Transitional cell carcinoma
  fallopian tube, 481–482
  metastatic, 706f
  ovary, 629
Transitional cell lesions, 735
Transitional cell tumors of ovary, 629–633
  benign Brenner tumor, 629–630, 630f
  borderline and malignant Brenner tumors, 630–633, 631f–632f
  SNOMED classification of, 629
Transitional metaplasia, 474–475, 475f
Transverse vaginal septum, 139
Trastuzumab, 98
Treponema pallidum, 67–68, 68f
  see also Syphilis
Triaster (tripolar) mitosis, 206f
Trichoepithelioma, 107, 108f
Trichomonas vaginalis, 73, 139, 140f, 170
Trichomoniasis, 73
Trichophyton rubrum, 70
Trisomy, aneuploid placenta from, 797f
Trisomy 12, 654
Trisomy 16, villous changes seen in miscarriages with, 770f
Trisomy 22, villous changes seen in miscarriages with, 770f
Trophoblast, 741–742
  interstitial extravillous, 742–743
  primitive, 742f
  sprouts, 743–744
Trophoblast immunohistochemical markers, 787–788, 789t
Trophoblastic disease
  gestational. *See* Gestational trophoblastic disease
  ovaries, 545–546
  persistent, 798–799, 798t
Trophoblastic implants, 723, 723f
Trophoblastic inclusion, 796
Trophoblastic lesions
  non-neoplastic, 807–809
  uterine, diagnostic algorithm in, 789f
Trophoblastic markers, 833
Trophoblastic neoplasia, 800–807
  criteria for diagnosis of, 798t
Trophoblastic pseudoinclusions, 791
Trophoblastic tumors, 785t
  choriocarcinoma. *See* Choriocarcinoma
  epithelioid, 805–807
  placental site, 803–805
TSPY1, 688–689
Tubal abortion, 470
Tubal ectopic gestation, salpingectomy for, 463
Tubal hemorrhage, 470
Tubal metaplasia, 176–177, 176f, 352t

Tubal pregnancy, 470–472, 471f–472f
  etiology and pathogenesis, 470
  natural history, 470–471
  pathology, 471–472, 471f–472f
Tubal rupture, 470–471
Tubal sterilization, 462, 463f
Tuberculosis
  cervix, 172, 173f
  granulomatous peritonitis, 717
Tuberculous endometritis, 329, 329f
Tuberculous salpingitis, 468f–469f
Tuboendometrioid metaplasia, 176–177
Tubo-ovarian abscess, 466f
Tumor markers, 834–836
Tumor suppressor genes, 836–838
Tumors metastatic to the ovary
  of adrenal gland, 707
  of appendix, 704–705
  of biliary tract, 703–704
  carcinoid, 701–702
  cytokeratin reaction patterns in, 830t
  diagnosis of, 813
  of liver, 703–704
  metastatic to fallopian tube, 483–484
  of pancreas, 703–704
  peritoneal, 710–711
  pulmonary, 707
  uterine, 707–709
Tunica albuginea, 9, 9f, 40f
  in PCOS, 548
Turner syndrome, 20t, 32–35, 33f, 518–519
  embryonic ovary, 34f
  streak ovary, 34f
Twin placenta, 826, 827f
Twin pregnancy, 796, 798f
  dizygotic twinning, 755
  placenta in, 755, 755f, 777
    dichorionic diamniotic placenta, 756f
    fused placenta, 755f
    monochorionic diamniotic placenta, 756f
    monochorionic monoamniotic placenta, 757f
  Siamese twins, 755f
  twin-twin superficial anastomosis, 757f
Twin-reversed arterial perfusion, 756–757
Twin-twin transfusion syndrome, 756–757, 757f, 777

U

Umbilical cord, 745–748, 745f–747f
  avulsion, 746
  coiling of, 746
  furcate (branched) insertion of, 746f
  hematoma of, 747f
  knots, 745, 745f
  meconium on, 749–750, 750f
  stricture in, 746, 746f
  velamentous insertion of, 746f
  vessels of, 747, 747f
Undervirilized male syndrome, 30
Ureaplasma urealyticum, 748
  endometritis, 328, 330–331
Urethral carcinoma, 113
Urethral caruncle, 113
Urinary tract, endometriosis, 500
Urogenital sinus, 15–16
Urticaria, 76
Uterine corpus, specimen processing, 818–821, 819f–820f
  benign or functional disease, 818–820, 819f
  endometrial biopsies and curettings, 818
  malignant disease, 820–821, 820f
  sampling, 820f–821f, 821
  supracervical hysterectomy, 820
Uterine tumor resembling ovarian sex cord tumor (UTROSCT), 411, 436–438, 437f–438f
Uterine tumors
  atypical smooth muscle tumor, 408–409, 408f–409f, 420–421, 420f, 420t
  leiomyoma, 402–405, 404f–405f
    benign metastasizing, 412–413, 412f
    cellular, 405–406, 405f
    degenerated, 406–407, 406f
    epithelioid, 409–410, 409f–410f
    hemorrhagic cellular, 406
    with heterologous elements, 411, 411f
    mitotically active, 405, 405f
    myxoid, 410
    treated by interventional radiology, 407
    treated with GnRHa, 406, 406f
    unusual growth patterns of, 411–414
  leiomyosarcoma, 414–420
    clinical features of, 414
    diagnostic criteria for, 417–418, 417f–419f
    epithelioid, 415, 415f
    gross features of, 414, 414f
    histologic diagnosis of, 416, 416f
    incidence of, 414
    microscopic features of, 414–416, 414f–415f
    molecular genetics of, 418–419
    myxoid, 416, 416f
  smooth muscle, 402–424, 402f, 403t
Uterus, 14f
  components of, 819f
  myometrium, 290–291
  normal structure of, 290–295, 291f
  removed during obstetric procedures, 821
  removed for benign or functional disease, 818–820
  see also Endometrium
UTROSCT. *See* Uterine tumor resembling ovarian sex cord tumor (UTROSCT)

V

Vabra aspirator, 304–305
Vaccines
  for cervical cancer, 194–196
  immunogenicity of, 195–196
Vagina, 132–159
  adenosis, 136–139, 137f
  anatomy of, 133
  benign tumors, 144–146
    angiomyofibroblastoma, 145–146, 146f
    benign mixed tumor, 144, 144f
    leiomyoma, 145, 145f
    Müllerian papilloma, 144–145, 145f
    rhabdomyoma, 145, 145f
  cysts, 142
    of introitus, 142
  development of, 132–133
  developmental disorders of, 136–139
    imperforate hymen, 139
    miscellaneous congenital, 139
    transverse septum, 139
    vaginal agenesis, 139
  diethylstilbestrol effects, 136–139
  histology of, 133–136
  inflammatory disorders of, 139–141
    malakoplakia, 140–141, 141f
    tampon-related lesions, 141
    toxic shock syndrome, 141
    vaginitis, 139–140, 140f
  mesonephric ducts, 135–136, 135f–136f
  noninfectious inflammatory diseases of, 141–142
    ligneous vaginitis, 141
    vaginal cysts, 141–142
  normal, 134f
  physiology of, 133–136
  primary malignant tumors of, 153–154
  secondary tumors of, 156f, 157
  squamous neoplasia of, 146–153
  structural changes of, 136, 137f
  tumor-like conditions of, 142–144
    endometriosis, 144
    fibroepithelial polyps, 142–143, 142f
    granulation tissue nodule, 143
    microglandular hyperplasia, 143–144, 143f–144f
    postoperative spindle cell nodule, 143
    prolapsed fallopian tube, 143, 143f
Vagina SIL (VaIN), 229
  and *see* Squamous intraepithelial lesions, vaginal.
Vaginal agenesis, 139
Vaginal epithelium, normal, 134f
Vaginal muscularis, 133f
Vaginal neoplasia
  childhood malignant tumors, 154–156
    embryonal rhabdomyosarcoma, 154–155, 155f
    yolk sac tumor, 156
  leiomyosarcoma, 154, 154f
  lymphoma, 156, 156t
  malignant melanoma, 153–154, 154f
  secondary tumors, 156f, 157
  squamous, 146–153
    HPV infection, 146
    invasive, 148–149
    papillary squamotransitional cell carcinoma, 150
    small cell carcinoma, 150, 150f
    verrucous carcinoma, 149, 149f
    warty, 150
Vaginal plate, 14f
Vaginal wall, 133f
Vaginitis, 139–140, 140f
Valergen. *See* Estradiol valerate
Variable gland density, 352t
Varicella zoster virus
  placenta in, 779
  vulva, 71, 71f–72f
Vascular endothelial growth factor (VEGF), 244
Vascular lesions, 108–109
  cavernous hemangioma, 108
  deep lymphatic malformation, 108–109
  infantile hemangioma, 108
Vasculogenesis, active, 785
Verrucous carcinoma
  cervix, 246–247, 247f
  vagina, 149, 149f
  vulva, 91–92, 91f–92f
Vesicles, 76
Villi
  anchoring, 742–744
  chorionic, 741–742
  endocervical, 164f
  immature intermediate, 744, 744f
  mature intermediate, 744, 744f
  mesenchymal, 743–744
  terminal, 744–745, 744f
Villin, 677
Villitis, 758–759, 759f–760f
Villoglandular adenocarcinoma of endometrium, 385, 385f
Villoglandular carcinoma of cervix, 265–267

biologic behavior and treatment of, 266–267
definition of, 265
immunohistochemistry of, 266
pathology of, 265–266, 266f–267f
Villoglandular lesions, 248
Villous changes, miscellaneous, 764
Villous trophoblast, 784–785
  at implantation site, 787f
  intermediate, 785–786, 787f
Vimentin, 831
  dysgerminoma, 673
  granulosa cell tumors, 645
VIN, Vulvar intraepithelial neoplasia. *See* squamous intraepithelial leions, vulva.
Viral infections of vulva, 70–71
  herpes virus, 70–71, 70f–71f
  human papillomavirus, 72–73
  molluscum contagiosum, 71–72, 72f
  varicella zoster, 71, 71f–72f
Viral oophoritis, 524–529
  cytomegalovirus, 527, 527f
  mumps, 526–527
Virilizing lesions, maternal, 22
Virilizing tumor, maternal, 20t
Vitiligo, 66
Vulva
  specimen processing, 815–817
    excisional biopsies, 815
    radical vulvectomy, 816–817
    simple (or total) vulvectomy, 816
    skinning vulvectomy, 816
    wide local excision, 815–816, 816f
  tumor-like conditions of, 110–112, 116–118
    fibroepithelial-stromal polyp, 116–117, 117f
    nodular fasciitis, 117–118, 118f
Vulvar dermatoses, 48–78
  bacterial infections, 67–69
    chancroid, 69
    chlamydial infection, 69
    gonorrhea, 68
    granuloma inguinale, 69
    staphylococcal infections, 67
    streptococcal infections, 67
    syphilis, 67–68
  Behçet disease, 63–64, 63f
  bullous disorders, 58–61
    adult linear IgA bullous dermatosis, 59t, 61, 61f
    bullous pemphigoid, 59t, 61
    chronic bullous dermatosis, 59t, 61, 61f
    cicatricial pemphigoid, 59t, 61
    pemphigus vegetans, 59t, 60–61, 60f
    pemphigus vulgaris, 58–60, 59t
  chronic dermatitides, 54
    lichen simplex chronicus, 54
  classification of, 49t
  Crohn disease, 64
  differential diagnoses of, 50f–52f
  drugs, 66–67
  dysesthetic vulvodynia, 65
  erythema multiforme, 63
  fungal infections, 69–70
    candidiasis, 69
    pityriasis versicolor, 69–70
    tinea cruris, 70
  hidradenitis suppurativa, 64, 64f
  infestations, 73–74
    pubic (crab) lice, 74
    scabies, 73–74
  inherited, 61–62
    Darier disease, 62, 62f
    epidermolysis bullosa, 62
    Hailey-Hailey disease, 61–62, 62f
    warty dyskeratoma, 62
  lichenoid dermatoses, 55–58
    lichen planus, 57–58
    lichen sclerosus, 55–57
  pigmentary alterations, 65–66
    hyperpigmentation, 65–66
    hypopigmentation, 66
  plasma cell vulvitis, 63, 63f
  protozoal infections, 73
    trichomoniasis, 73
  psoriasis, 54–55, 55f
  spongiotic dermatitis, 49–54
    acute, 49, 52f
    chronic, 49
    endogenous, 49–53
    exogenous, 53–54
    subacute, 52f
  viral infections, 70–71
    herpes virus, 70–71, 70f–71f
    human papillomavirus, 72–73
    molluscum contagiosum, 71–72, 72f
    varicella zoster, 71, 71f–72f
  vulvar vestibulitis, 65
  Zoon vulvitis, 63, 63f
Vulvar leiomyomatosis, 124
Vulvar lesions
  malignant keratinocytic, extramammary Paget disease, 98–100
  melanocytic, 101–106
    blue nevus, 102
    lentigo, 101
    malignant melanoma, 103–106
    melanocytic nevus
      atypical, 102–103
      atypical of genital type, 102
      common acquired, 101
  metastatic, 112
  skin appendages, 106–107
    hidradenoma papilliferum, 106
    syringoma, 106–107
    trichoepithelioma, 107
  vascular lesions, 108–109
    cavernous hemangioma, 108
    deep lymphatic malformation, 108–109
    infantile hemangioma, 108
Vulvar melanosis, 65, 65f
Vulvar neoplasia
  benign, 118–124
    angiokeratoma, 124, 124f
    angiomyofibroblastoma, 118–119, 118f–119f
    cellular angiofibroma, 119–120, 119f–120f, 120t
    dermatofibroma, 121–122, 121f–122f
    genital rhabdomyoma, 124, 124f–125f
    granular cell tumor, 122, 122f
    leiomyoma, 122–123, 123f
    lipoblastoma-like tumor of vulva, 124, 125f
    lymphangioma circumscriptum, 123–124, 124f
    prepubertal vulvar fibroma, 120–121, 121f
    vulvar leiomyomatosis, 124
  locally recurrent, 125–128
    deep angiomyxoma, 120t, 125–126, 125f–126f
    dermatofibrosarcoma protuberans, 127–128, 127f
    superficial angiomyxoma, 120t, 126–127, 126f–127f
  malignant, 128–129
    leiomyosarcoma, 128, 128f
    liposarcoma, 129, 129f
    epithelioid sarcoma, 128–129, 128f–129f
Vulvar squamous lesions, 79–94
  benign squamous neoplasms, 79–81
    condyloma acuminatum, 79, 80f
    keratoacanthoma, 80–81, 81f
    seborrheic keratosis, 79–80, 80f
  squamous cell carcinoma, 87–91
    subtypes of, 91–93
  squamous intraepithelial lesions, 81–87
    high-grade VIN, differentiated or simplex type, 86–87
    HPV-related low- and high-grade, 81–85
Vulvar tumor pathologic staging, 90t
Vulvar vestibule, 75
Vulvar vestibulitis, 65
Vulvectomy
  radical, 816–817
  simple (or total), 816
  skinning, 816

W

Walthard rests, 475f, 629
Warthin-Starry silver stain, 781
Warty carcinoma, vagina, 150
Warty dyskeratoma, 62
Warty squamous cell carcinoma, 247
'Watered-silk' appearance, 644f
Wilms' tumor, 20t
Wilms' tumor suppressor gene defect, 36
WNT4, 6t, 10
Wolffian duct, 8f, 11, 12f–13f, 135–136
  development of, 11–15
Wolffian tumors, 616
World Health Organization (WHO), 349, 565
  classification of tumors of fallopian tube, 477t
  diagnostic entities and terminology, 350t
WT1
  endometrial stromal tumors, 432
  granulosa cell tumors, 645
WT1, 3–7, 6t, 7f, 10–11, 836–837

X

XX male, 35
XY female, 42–43

Y

Yolk sac, 3, 5f
Yolk sac tumors
  differential diagnosis of, 616, 628
  glandular, 675–676
  hepatoid, 628–629, 675–676
  ovary, 674–678
    clinical features of, 674–675
    differential diagnosis of, 677
    immunohistochemistry of, 677, 677f
    macroscopic features of, 675, 675f
    microscopic features of, 675–677, 675f–677f
    treatment and prognosis of, 678

Z

Zollinger-Ellison syndrome, 591, 666–667
Zoon vulvitis, 63, 63f